Holland–Frei Cancer Medicine

Tenth Edition

Dedication

The 10th edition of *Cancer Medicine* has grown from the vision and dedication of James F. Holland and his fellow pioneer Emil "Tom" Frei. Jim and Tom were among the founding fathers of medical oncology and life-saving combination chemotherapy for which they shared the Albert Lasker Award for Clinical Medical Research. Jim had originally planned a career in cardiology after graduating from Princeton and Columbia University College of Physicians and Surgeons. When he returned from the United States Army Medical Corps in 1951, he took what was to be a temporary position at Frances Delafield Hospital where he cared for children with leukemia, drawing him to the mission of making pre-curable cancers curable for more than six decades. After conducting research at the National Cancer Institute, he became the chief of medicine at Roswell Park Memorial Institute at the age of 28. With Tom Frei, then at NCI, Jim created the first cancer chemotherapy cooperative trials group, the Acute Leukemia Group B, that became the Cancer and Leukemia Group B (CALGB) and now Alliance for Clinical Trials in Oncology. In 1972, he had represented the United States in a Mission to Russia studying Soviet oncology and training of Soviet oncologists. The next year he established a department of neoplastic diseases at the Tisch Cancer Institute at Mt. Sinai in New York where he was later named a distinguished professor. Having served as the president of the American Association for Cancer Research and the American Society of Clinical Oncology, he inspired the creation of the T.J. Martell Foundation for Cancer Research. With his wife Jimmie Holland, founder of the field of onco-psychiatry, Jim helped to found and nurture AORTIC, the African Organization for Research and Training in Cancer, promoting cancer control and palliation in Africa for more than 25 years. Jim's contributions to oncologic research extended beyond treatment of leukemia to therapy of breast cancer and to the possible role of viruses in the development of that disease. A master clinician and extraordinary human being, Jim Holland inspired generations of oncologists and the editors of this text with his wisdom and insatiable drive to continue to help people with cancer. He was indeed a giant who we miss, but who will be remembered by everyone who had the privilege of knowing him.

Waun Ki Hong was born in 1942, the sixth of seven children, in a small suburb of Seoul, North Korea. After attending medical school at Yon Sei University, Ki served as a flight surgeon in the Vietnam War prior to training in internal medicine residency at the Boston VA medical center. After completing a medical oncology fellowship at Memorial Sloan Kettering Cancer Center, Ki headed back to Boston in 1976 as chief of oncology and hematology at the Boston VAMC where he led the first clinical chemoprevention studies in solid tumors while launching the VA Larynx preservation study with Greg Wolf. In 1984, he moved to the University of Texas MD Anderson Cancer Center as chief of the head and neck cancer division, soon combined with the lung cancer section to become the first department of lung and head and neck (aerodigestive cancers) in the country. Over a 30-year career at MD Anderson, Ki led as senior author dozens of seminal papers in premiere journals such as the *New England Journal of Medicine*, establishing himself with Bernard Fischer as fathers of clinical cancer chemoprevention. Ki led major collaborative program projects and SPORE grants, establishing a series of biomarker-based clinical trials that helped unlock our understanding of the impact of molecular agents on premalignancies, while providing substantial contributions to targeted therapy. Over the course of his career, Ki Hong mentored a veritable who's who of lung and aerodigestive track clinical and translational investigators and received numerous major honors. He served as the president of AACR and was one of very few individuals to deliver AACR's Joseph Burchenal Award and ASCO's David Karnofsky Lecture in the same academic year. Ki joined the editorial leadership of *Cancer Medicine* for the seventh edition and was remarkably persistent and effective at recruiting many of the world-class authors who have led its chapters. Perhaps even more notable than his stellar scientific contributions was his unstinting devotion to his proteges, trainees and friends, and especially his wife Mihwa, children Burt and Ed, and their families.

We editors who treasure these oncology giants miss them sorely and dedicate this 10th Edition of *Cancer Medicine* to these preeminent leaders in cancer practice, research, education, and training and diversity, equity, and inclusion.

Robert C. Bast Jr.
John C. Byrd
Carlo M. Croce
Ernest Hawk
Fadlo R. Khuri
Raphael E. Pollock
Apostolia M. Tsimberidou
Christopher G. Willett
Cheryl L. Willman

Holland–Frei Cancer Medicine

Tenth Edition

EDITORS

Robert C. Bast Jr., MD
Vice President for Translational Research
Professor of Medicine
Harry Carothers Wiess Distinguished University Chair for Cancer Research
Division of Cancer Medicine
Department of Experimental Therapeutics
The University of Texas MD Anderson Cancer Center
Houston, Texas

John C. Byrd, MD
The Gordon and Helen Hughes Taylor Professor and Chair
Department of Internal Medicine
University of Cincinnati College of Medicine
Cincinnati, Ohio

Carlo M. Croce, MD
Distinguished University Professor
John W. Wolfe Chair in Human Cancer
Department of Cancer Biology and Genetics
The Ohio State University
Comprehensive Cancer Center
Columbus, Ohio

Ernest Hawk, MD, MPH
Vice President and Head
Division of Cancer Prevention & Population Sciences
The University of Texas MD Anderson Cancer Center
Houston, Texas

Fadlo R. Khuri, MD
President
Professor of Internal Medicine
American University of Beirut
Beirut, Lebanon

Raphael E. Pollock, MD, PhD
Klotz Family Chair in Cancer Research
Professor and Director
Ohio State University Comprehensive Cancer Center
The Ohio State University Medical Center
Columbus, Ohio

Apostolia M. Tsimberidou, MD, PhD
Professor
Department of Investigational Cancer Therapeutics
The University of Texas MD Anderson Cancer Center
Houston, Texas

Christopher G. Willett, MD
Professor and The Mark W. Dewhirst Distinguished Professor of Radiation Oncology
Department of Radiation Oncology
Duke University School of Medicine
Durham, North Carolina

Cheryl L. Willman, MD
Executive Director
Mayo Clinic Cancer Programs: Rochester, Minnesota/Midwest, Arizona, Florida, London, Abu Dhabi
Director
Mayo Clinic Comprehensive Cancer Center
Professor of Laboratory Medicine and Pathology
College of Medicine
Mayo Clinic Cancer Center
Rochester, Minnesota

ASSOCIATE EDITORS

Jene' Reinartz
Administrator
Department of Translational Research
The University of Texas MD Anderson Cancer Center
Houston, Texas

Michael S. Ewer, MD, JD, PhD
Professor of Medicine
Department of Cardiology
The University of Texas MD Anderson Cancer Center
Houston, Texas

Anthea Hammond, PhD
Science Writer/Editor
Department of Hematology and Medical Oncology
Emory University
Atlanta, Georgia

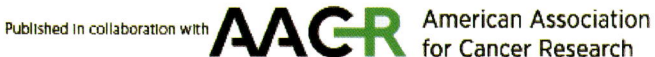
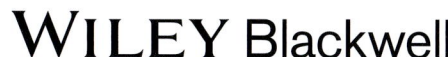

This edition first published 2023
© 2023 John Wiley & Sons, Inc.

© 2016 John Wiley & Sons, Inc (9e); © 2010 John Wiley & Sons, Inc (8e)

Published by John Wiley & Sons, Inc., Hoboken, New Jersey.
Published simultaneously in Canada.

No part of this publication may be reproduced, stored in a retrieval system, or transmitted in any form or by any means, electronic, mechanical, photocopying, recording, scanning, or otherwise, except as permitted under Section 107 or 108 of the 1976 United States Copyright Act, without either the prior written permission of the Publisher, or authorization through payment of the appropriate per-copy fee to the Copyright Clearance Center, Inc., 222 Rosewood Drive, Danvers, MA 01923, (978) 750-8400, fax (978) 750-4470, or on the web at www.copyright.com. Requests to the Publisher for permission should be addressed to the Permissions Department, John Wiley & Sons, Inc., 111 River Street, Hoboken, NJ 07030, (201) 748-6011, fax (201) 748-6008, or online at http://www.wiley.com/go/permission

Limit of Liability/Disclaimer of Warranty
While the publisher and author have used their best efforts in preparing this book, they make no representations or warranties with respect to the accuracy or completeness of the contents of this book and specifically disclaim any implied warranties of merchantability or fitness for a particular purpose. No warranty may be created or extended by sales representatives or written sales materials. The advice and strategies contained herein may not be suitable for your situation. You should consult with a professional where appropriate. Further, readers should be aware that websites listed in this work may have changed or disappeared between when this work was written and when it is read. Neither the publisher nor authors shall be liable for any loss of profit or any other commercial damages, including but not limited to special, incidental, consequential, or other damages.

For general information on our other products and services or for technical support, please contact our Customer Care Department within the United States at (800) 762-2974, outside the United States at (317) 572-3993 or fax (317) 572-4002.

Wiley also publishes its books in a variety of electronic formats. Some content that appears in print may not be available in electronic formats. For more information about Wiley products, visit our web site at www.wiley.com

Library of Congress Cataloging-in-Publication Data has been applied for:

Print ISBN: 9781119750680

Cover Design: Wiley
Cover Image(s): Hiep T. Vo and Apostolia Maria Tsimberidou

Set in 9/11pt MinionPro by Straive, Chennai, India

Printed in Singapore
M112757_300123

Contents

List of contributors xi

Preface xxvii

Acknowledgments xxix

Part 1: INTRODUCTION

1. Cardinal manifestations of cancer 3
   James F. Holland, Robert C. Bast, Jr., John C. Byrd, Carlo M. Croce, Ernest Hawk, Fadlo R. Khuri, Raphael E. Pollock, Apostolia M. Tsimberadou, Christopher G. Willett, and Cheryl L. Willman

2. Biological hallmarks of cancer 7
   Douglas Hanahan and Robert A. Weinberg

Part 2: TUMOR BIOLOGY

3. Molecular biology, genetics, and translational models of human cancer 19
   Benno Traub, Florian Scheufele, Srinivas R. Viswanathan, Matthew Meyerson, and David A. Tuveson

4. Oncogenes 49
   Marco A. Pierotti, Milo Frattini, Samantha Epistolio, Gabriella Sozzi, and Carlo M. Croce

5. Tumor suppressor genes 73
   Fred Bunz and Bert Vogelstein

6. Epigenetic contributions to human cancer 89
   Stephen B. Baylin

7. Cancer genomics and evolution 101
   William P. D. Hendricks, Aleksandar Sekulic, Alan H. Bryce, Muhammed Murtaza, Pilar Ramos, Jessica D. Lang, Timothy G. Whitsett, Timothy K. McDaniel, Russell C. Rockne, Nicholas Banovich, and Jeffrey M. Trent

8. Chromosomal aberrations in cancer 125
   Megan E. McNerney, Ari J. Rosenberg, and Michelle M. Le Beau

9. MicroRNA expression in cancer 143
   Serge P. Nana-Sinkam, Mario Acunzo, and Carlo M. Croce

10. Aberrant signaling pathways in cancer 151
    Luca Grumolato and Stuart A. Aaronson

11. Differentiation therapy 161
    Sai-Juan Chen, Xiao-Jing Yan, Guang-Biao Zhou, and Zhu Chen

12. Cancer stem cells 177
    Grace G. Bushnell, Michael D. Brooks, and Max S. Wicha

13. Cancer and cell death 187
    John C. Reed

14. Cancer cell immortality: targeting telomerase and telomeres 201
    Ilgen Mender, Zeliha G. Dikmen, and Jerry W. Shay

15. Cancer metabolism 211
    Natalya N. Pavlova, Aparna D. Rao, Ralph J. DeBerardinis, and Craig B. Thompson

16. Tumor angiogenesis 223
    John V. Heymach, Amado Zurita-Saavedra, Scott Kopetz, Tina Cascone, Monique Nilsson, and Irene Guijarro

Part 3: QUANTITATIVE ONCOLOGY

17. Cancer bioinformatics 247
    John N. Weinstein

18. Systems biology and genomics 261
    Saima Hassan, Joe W. Gray, and Laura M. Heiser

19. Statistical innovations in cancer research 269
    J. Jack Lee and Donald A. Berry

20. Biomarker based clinical trial design in the era of genomic medicine 285
    R. Donald Harvey, Yuan Liu, Taofeek K. Owonikoko, and Suresh S. Ramalingam

21. Clinical and research informatics data strategy for precision oncology 293
    Douglas Hartman, Uma Chandran, Michael Davis, Rajiv Dhir, William E. Shirey, Jonathan C. Silverstein, and Michael J. Becich

Part 4: CARCINOGENESIS

22. Chemical carcinogenesis 305
    Lorne J. Hofseth, Ainsley Weston, and Curtis C. Harris

23. Ionizing radiation 325
    David J. Grdina

24. Ultraviolet radiation carcinogenesis 333
    James E. Cleaver, Susana Ortiz-Urda, and Sarah Arron

25. Inflammation and cancer 339
    Jelena Todoric, Atsushi Umemura, Koji Taniguchi, and Michael Karin

26. RNA tumor viruses 347
    Robert C. Gallo and Marvin S. Reitz

27. Herpesviruses 359
    Jeffrey I. Cohen

28 Papillomaviruses and cervical neoplasia 367
Michael F. Herfs, Christopher P. Crum, and Karl Munger

29 Hepatitis viruses and hepatoma 373
Hongyang Wang

30 Parasites 379
Mervat El Azzouni, Charbel F. Matar, Radwa Galal, Elio Jabra, and Ali Shamseddine

Part 5: EPIDEMIOLOGY, PREVENTION, AND DETECTION

31 Cancer epidemiology 391
Veronika Fedirko, Kevin T. Nead, Carrie Daniel, and Paul Scheet

32 Hereditary cancer syndromes: risk assessment and genetic counseling 403
Rachel Bluebond, Sarah A. Bannon, Samuel M. Hyde, Ashley H. Woodson, Nancy Y.-Q. You, Karen H. Lu, and Banu Arun

33 Behavioral approaches to cancer prevention 425
Roberto Gonzalez and Maher Karam-Hage

34 Diet and nutrition in the etiology and prevention of cancer 433
Steven K. Clinton, Edward L. Giovannucci, Fred K. Tabung, and Elizabeth M. Grainger

35 Chemoprevention of cancer 453
Ernest Hawk, Karen C. Maresso, Powel Brown, Michelle I. Savage, and Scott M. Lippman

36 Cancer screening and early detection 473
Otis W. Brawley

Part 6: CLINICAL DISCIPLINES

37 Clinical cancer genomic diagnostics and modern diagnostic pathology 493
Katherine Roth, Stephen B. Gruber, and Kevin McDonnell

38 Molecular diagnostics in cancer 505
Zachary L. Coyne, Roshni D. Kalachand, Robert C. Bast Jr., Gordon B. Mills, and Bryan T. Hennessy

39 Principles of imaging 519
Lawrence H. Schwartz

40 Interventional radiology for the cancer patient 521
Zeyad A. Metwalli, Judy U. Ahrar, and Michael J. Wallace

41 Principles of surgical oncology 531
Todd W. Bauer, Kenneth K. Tanabe, and Raphael E. Pollock

42 Principles of radiation oncology 543
Scott R. Floyd, Justus Adamson, Philip P. Connell, Ralph R. Weichselbaum, and Christopher G. Willett

43 Principles of medical oncology 553
Apostolia M. Tsimberidou, Robert C. Bast, Jr., Fadlo R. Khuri, and John C. Byrd

44 Pain and palliative care 567
Laura Van Metre Baum and Cardinale B. Smith

45 Psycho-oncology 577
Diya Banerjee and Andrew J. Roth

46 Principles of cancer rehabilitation medicine 585
Michael D. Stubblefield, Miguel Escalon, Sofia A. Barchuk, Krina Vyas, and David C. Thomas

47 Integrative oncology in cancer care 593
Gabriel Lopez, Wenli Liu, Santhosshi Narayanan, and Lorenzo Cohen

48 Health services research 599
Michaela A. Dinan and Devon K. Check

Part 7: INDIVIDUALIZED TREATMENT

49 Precision medicine in oncology drug development 613
Apostolia M. Tsimberidou, Elena Fountzilas, and Razelle Kurzrock

Part 8: CHEMOTHERAPY

50 Drug development of small molecule cancer therapeutics in an Academic Cancer Center 631
Christopher C. Coss, Jeffrey T. Patrick, Damien Gerald, Gerard Hilinski, Reena Shakya, and John C. Byrd

51 Principles of dose, schedule, and combination therapy 641
Joseph P. Eder and Navid Hafez

52 Pharmacology of small-molecule anticancer agents 655
Zahra Talebi, Sharyn D. Baker, and Alex Sparreboom

53 Folate antagonists 667
Lisa Gennarini, Peter D. Cole, and Joseph R. Bertino

54 Pyrimidine and purine antimetabolites 679
Robert B. Diasio and Steven M. Offer

55 Alkylating agents and platinum antitumor compounds 693
Zahid H. Siddik

56 DNA topoisomerase targeting drugs 701
Anish Thomas, Susan Bates, William D. Figg, Sr., and Yves Pommier

57 Microtubule inhibitors 717
Giuseppe Galletti and Paraskevi Giannakakou

58 Drug resistance and its clinical circumvention 731
Jeffrey A. Moscow, Shannon K. Hughes, Kenneth H. Cowan, and Branimir I. Sikic

Part 9: BIOLOGICAL AND GENE THERAPY

59 Cytokines, interferons, and hematopoietic growth factors 739
Narendranath Epperla, Walter Hanel, and Moshe Talpaz

60 Monoclonal antibody and targeted toxin therapy 755
Robert C. Bast, Jr. and Michael R. Zalutsky

61 Vaccines and immunomodulators 781
Jeffrey Schlom, Sofia R. Gameiro, Claudia Palena, and James L. Gulley

62 T cell immunotherapy of cancer   789
    M. Lia Palomba, Jae H. Park, and Renier Brentjens

63 Cancer immunotherapy   799
    Padmanee Sharma, Swetha Anandhan, Bilal A. Siddiqui, Sangeeta Goswami, Sumit K. Subudhi, Jianjun Gao, Karl Peggs, Sergio Quezada, and James P. Allison

64 Cancer gene therapy   817
    Haruko Tashiro, Lauren Scherer, and Malcolm Brenner

65 Cancer nanotechnology   825
    Xingya Jiang, Yanlan Liu, Danny Liu, Jinjun Shi, and Robert Langer

66 Hematopoietic cell transplantation   833
    Qaiser Bashir, Elizabeth J. Shpall, and Richard E. Champlin

Part 10: SPECIAL POPULATIONS

67 Principles of pediatric oncology   847
    Theodore P. Nicolaides, Elizabeth Raetz, and William L. Carroll

68 Cancer and pregnancy   867
    Jennifer K. Litton

69 Cancer and aging   877
    Ashley E. Rosko, Carolyn J. Presley, Grant R. Williams, and Rebecca L. Olin

70 Disparities in cancer care   885
    Otis W. Brawley

71 Neoplasms in people living with human immunodeficiency virus   895
    Chia-Ching J. Wang and Elizabeth Y. Chiao

72 Cancer survivorship   911
    Lewis Foxhall

Part 11: DISEASE SITES

73 Primary neoplasms of the brain in adults   921
    Matthew A. Smith-Cohn and Mark R. Gilbert

74 Neoplasms of the eye and orbit   933
    Erica R. Alvarez, Claudia M. Prospero Ponce, Patricia Chevez-Barrios, and Dan S. Gombos

75 Neoplasms of the endocrine glands and pituitary neoplasms   943
    Rui Feng, Chirag D. Gandhi, Margaret Pain, and Kalmon D. Post

76 Neoplasms of the thyroid   949
    Matthew D. Ringel

77 Malignant tumors of the adrenal gland   961
    Jeffrey E. Lee, Mouhammed A. Habra, and Matthew T. Campbell

78 Tumors of the diffuse neuroendocrine and gastroenteropancreatic system   971
    Evan Vosburgh

79 Neoplasms of the head and neck   981
    Robert L. Ferris, Adam S. Garden, and Nabil F. Saba

80 Cancer of the lung   1005
    Daniel Morgensztern, Daniel Boffa, Alexander Chen, Andrew Dhanasopon, Sarah B. Goldberg, Roy H. Decker, Siddhartha Devarakonda, Jane P. Ko, Luisa M. Solis Soto, Saiama N. Waqar, Ignacio I. Wistuba, and Roy S. Herbst

81 Malignant pleural mesothelioma   1029
    Michele Carbone, Daniel R. Gomez, Anne S. Tsao, Haining Yang, and Harvey I. Pass

82 Thymomas and thymic tumors   1043
    Mayur D. Mody, Gabriel L. Sica, Suresh S. Ramalingam, and Dong M. Shin

83 Tumors of the heart and great vessels   1055
    Moritz C. Wyler von Ballmoos and Michael J. Reardon

84 Primary germ cell tumors of the thorax   1061
    John D. Hainsworth and Frank A. Greco

85 Neoplasms of the esophagus   1065
    Max W. Sung and Virginia R. Litle

86 Carcinoma of the stomach   1083
    Carl Schmidt, Nour Daboul, Carly Likar, and Joshua Weir

87 Primary neoplasms of the liver   1095
    Hop S. Tran Cao, Junichi Shindoh, and Jean-Nicolas Vauthey

88 Gallbladder and bile duct cancer   1109
    Mariam F. Eskander, Christopher T. Aquina, and Timothy M. Pawlik

89 Neoplasms of the exocrine pancreas   1123
    Robert A. Wolff, Donghui Li, Anirban Maitra, Susan Tsai, Eugene Koay, and Douglas B. Evans

90 Neoplasms of the appendix and peritoneum   1139
    Annie Liu, Diana Cardona, and Dan Blazer

91 Carcinoma of the colon and rectum   1147
    Yota Suzuki, Douglas S. Tyler, and Uma R. Phatak

92 Neoplasms of the anus   1169
    Alexandre A. A. Jácome and Cathy Eng

93 Renal cell carcinoma   1181
    Claude M. Grigg, Earle F. Burgess, Stephen B. Riggs, Jason Zhu, and Derek Raghavan

94 Urothelial cancer   1191
    Derek Raghavan, Richard Cote, Earle F. Burgess, Derek McHaffie, and Peter E. Clark

95 Neoplasms of the prostate   1201
    Ana Aparicio, Patrick Pilie, Devaki S. Surasi, Seungtaek Choi, Brian F. Chapin, Christopher J. Logothetis, and Paul G. Corn

96 Tumors of the penis and the urethra   1239
    Jad Chahoud, Andrea Necchi, and Philippe E. Spiess

97 Testis cancer   1245
    Michael Hawking, Gladell Paner, Scott Eggener, and Walter M. Stadler

98 Neoplasms of the vulva and vagina   1261
    Michael Frumovitz and Summer B. Dewdney

99 Neoplasms of the cervix 1275
Anuja Jhingran

100 Endometrial cancer 1299
Shannon N. Westin, Karen Lu, and Jamal Rahaman

101 Epithelial ovarian, fallopian tube, and peritoneal cancer 1311
Jonathan S. Berek, Malte Renz, Michael L. Friedlander, and Robert C. Bast, Jr.

102 Nonepithelial ovarian malignancies 1329
Jonathan S. Berek, Malte Renz, Michael L. Friedlander, and Robert C. Bast, Jr.

103 Molar pregnancy and gestational trophoblastic neoplasia 1343
Neil S. Horowitz, Donald P. Goldstein, and Ross S. Berkowitz

104 Gynecologic sarcomas 1351
Jamal Rahaman and Carmel J. Cohen

105 Neoplasms of the breast 1361
Debu Tripathy, Sukh Makhnoon, Banu Arun, Aysegul Sahin, Nicole M. Kettner, Senthil Damodaran, Khandan Keyomarsi, Wei Yang, Kelly K. Hunt, Mark Clemens, Wendy A. Woodward, Melissa P. Mitchell, Rachel Layman, Evthokia A. Hobbs, Bora Lim, Megan Dupuis, Rashmi Murthy, Omar Alhalabi, Nuhad Ibrahim, Ishwaria M. Subbiah, and Carlos Barcenas

106 Malignant melanoma 1413
Michael J. Carr, Justin M. Ko, Susan M. Swetter, Scott E. Woodman, Vernon K. Sondak, Kim A. Margolin, and Jonathan S. Zager

107 Other skin cancers 1437
Stacy L. McMurray, William G. Stebbins, Eric A. Millican, and Victor A. Neel

108 Bone tumors 1451
Timothy A. Damron

109 Soft tissue sarcomas 1477
Katherine A. Thornton, Elizabeth H. Baldini, Robert G. Maki, Brian O'Sullivan, Yan Leyfman, and Chandrajit P. Raut

110 Myelodysplastic syndromes 1501
Uma M. Borate

111 Acute myeloid leukemia in adults: mast cell leukemia and other mast cell neoplasms 1517
Richard M. Stone, Charles A. Schiffer, and Daniel J. DeAngelo

112 Chronic myeloid leukemia 1537
Jorge Cortes, Richard T. Silver, and Hagop Kantarjian

113 Acute lymphoblastic leukemia 1547
Elias Jabbour, Nitin Jain, Hagop Kantarjian, and Susan O'Brien

114 Chronic lymphocytic leukemia 1559
Jacqueline C. Barrientos, Kanti R. Rai, and Joanna M. Rhodes

115 Hodgkin lymphoma 1569
David J. Straus and Anita Kumar

116 Clonal hematopoiesis in cancer 1579
Philipp J. Rauch and David P. Steensma

117 Non-Hodgkin's lymphoma 1587
Arnold S. Freedman and Ann S. LaCasce

118 Mycosis fungoides and Sézary syndrome 1603
Walter Hanel, Catherine Chung, and John C. Reneau

119 Plasma cell disorders 1611
Andrew J. Yee, Teru Hideshima, Noopur Raje, and Kenneth C. Anderson

120 Myeloproliferative disorders 1633
Jeanne Palmer and Ruben Mesa

Part 12: MANAGEMENT OF CANCER COMPLICATIONS

121 Neoplasms of unknown primary site 1647
John D. Hainsworth and Frank A. Greco

122 Cancer cachexia 1659
Assaad A. Eid, Rachel Njeim, Fadlo R. Khuri, and David K. Thomas

123 Antiemetic therapy 1673
Michael J. Berger and David S. Ettinger

124 Neurologic complications of cancer 1683
Luis Nicolas Gonzalez Castro, Tracy T. Batchelor, and Lisa M. DeAngelis

125 Dermatologic complications of cancer chemotherapy 1701
Anisha B. Patel, Padmavathi V. Karri, and Madeleine Duvic

126 Skeletal complications 1715
Michael A. Via, Ilya Iofin, Jerry Liu, and Jeffrey I. Mechanick

127 Hematologic complications and blood bank support 1729
Roger Belizaire and Kenneth C. Anderson

128 Coagulation complications of cancer patients 1739
Tzu-Fei Wang and Kristin Sanfilippo

129 Urologic complications related to cancer and its treatment 1747
Omar Alhalabi, Ala Abudayyeh, and Nizar M. Tannir

130 Cardiac complications 1757
Michael S. Ewer, Steven M. Ewer, and Thomas M. Suter

131 Respiratory complications 1779
Vickie R. Shannon, George A. Eapen, Carlos A. Jimenez, Horiana B. Grosu, Rodolfo C. Morice, Lara Bashoura, Ajay Sheshadre, Scott E. Evans, Roberto Adachi, Michael Kroll, Saadia A. Faiz, Diwakar D. Balachandran, Selvaraj E. Pravinkumar, and Burton F. Dickey

132 Gastrointestinal and hepatic complications in cancer patients 1811
Robert S. Bresalier, Emmanuel S. Coronel, and Hao Chi Zhang

133 Oral complications of cancer and their treatment 1827
Stephen T. Sonis, Anna Yuan, and Alessandro Villa

134 Gonadal complications 1839
Robert W. Lentz and Catherine E. Klein

135 Sexual dysfunction   1849
Leslie R. Schover

136 Endocrine complications and paraneoplastic syndromes   1855
Sai-Ching J. Yeung and Robert F. Gagel

137 Infections in patients with cancer   1869
Harrys A. Torres, Dimitrios P. Kontoyiannis, and Kenneth V.I. Rolston

138 Oncologic emergencies   1883
Sai-Ching J. Yeung and Carmen P. Escalante

Part 13: THE FUTURE OF ONCOLOGY

139 A vision for twenty-first century healthcare   1907
Leroy Hood, Nathan D. Price, and James T. Yurkovich

Index   1915

PART 11

Disease Sites

73 Primary neoplasms of the brain in adults

Matthew A. Smith-Cohn, DO ■ Mark R. Gilbert, MD

Overview

In 2021, it is expected that at least 700,000 people in the United States will be living with a primary brain tumor.

Primary brain tumors are a heterogeneous group of neoplasms arising from nervous system tissue and the surrounding meninges. Unique to these cancers is a presentation of neurologic symptoms such as seizures, worsened headaches, weakness, personality changes, impaired cognition, and speech difficulty. It is estimated that 70% of brain tumors are benign (most commonly meningiomas), while 30% are malignant (most commonly gliomas). Malignant brain tumors are among the most challenging cancers to treat, due to limited effective therapies and difficulty of drug delivery across the blood–brain barrier. Despite the challenges, there has been a tremendous amount of knowledge gained about these neoplasms over the past decade. The 2016 World Health Organization (WHO) classification of central nervous system tumors (CNS) introduced the integration of histologic evaluation and molecular alterations to make a more informed diagnosis of these alterations, which have prognostic implications. This article will review the most encountered primary brain neoplasms and their management approaches.

Introduction

Primary tumors of the central nervous system (CNS) are a heterogeneous group of both benign and malignant neoplasms of the brain and spinal cord. CNS tumors are classified into two groups: those that grow within the parenchyma of the brain or spinal cord (intracerebral or intramedullary) and those that grow outside the brain (extracerebral or extramedullary). Historically, the malignant primary CNS tumors have been incurable despite surgical resection, radiotherapy (RT), and chemotherapy. However, over the past several decades, advances in diagnostic imaging, surgical techniques, radiation oncology, and chemotherapy have improved survival and quality of life. One of the most promising developments has been gaining a better understanding of the molecular events associated with the malignant phenotype of a brain tumor, which has led to several novel chemotherapeutic approaches to treatment.

Epidemiology

Primary CNS tumors are uncommon. The overall annual incidence of brain tumors, both benign and malignant, in the United States is estimated at 23.41 cases per 100,000 person-years leading to an estimated 86,010 new cases diagnosed each year [Central Brain Tumor Registry of the United States Statistical Report (CBTRUS), 2012–2016].[1] Gliomas represented 25.5% of all CNS tumors and 80.8% of malignant tumors. Of malignant brain tumors, Grade 4 astrocytoma or glioblastoma (GBM) accounts for 48.3%.[1] The incidence and histologic type of intracranial tumors differ by race, gender, and age.[1] Incidence rates for astrocytoma are over two times greater in individuals who are Caucasians than in individuals who are African-American. In contrast, meningioma and pituitary adenoma are more frequent in individuals who are African-American than Caucasians. Pituitary, lymphoma, and other hematopoietic neoplasms are the only CNS histologies that have a higher incidence in individuals who are Hispanic. Primary brain tumors that are more common in men include oligodendroglioma, astrocytoma including GBM, primary CNS lymphoma, and germ cell tumors. There are over twice as many women with meningioma.

Risk factors

There have been many studies that examine the relationship between the environment and the occurrence of brain tumors. Still, only two definite risk factors have been identified: ionizing radiation and immune suppression.[1-3] Irradiation for intracranial tumors, for example, medulloblastoma or extracranial head and neck cancers, including prophylactic irradiation for leukemia, increase the incidence of both gliomas and sarcomas sevenfold in those who survive more than 3 years. The cumulative relative risk of secondary brain tumors in patients treated with cranial irradiation ranges from 5.65 to 10.9; approximately two-thirds of the tumors are gliomas, and one-third are meningiomas.[4] Congenital or acquired immune suppression, such as human immunodeficiency virus (HIV) infection, or the use of immunosuppressive drugs after organ transplantation, increases the incidence of primary central nervous system lymphoma (PCNSL).[2,5] No other environmental risk factors have been found to have an association with brain tumors. Familial brain tumor syndromes are a heterogeneous group of uncommon disorders characterized by an association of brain tumors with systemic features, primarily dermatologic including neurofibromatosis 1, neurofibromatosis 2, tuberous sclerosis, von Hippel–Lindau disease, Li–Fraumeni, and Turcot syndrome (Table 1).

Classification of CNS tumors

Previously, the criterion used by pathologists for the diagnosis and grading of brain tumors were defined by histopathologic evaluation, organized by their patterns of differentiation and presumed cell of origin. Limitations of this approach include reliance on adequate tissue sampling and interobserver variability.[6] Investigations into the molecular biology of CNS tumors identified distinct subclassifications with therapeutic and prognostic implications. Subsequently, in 2016, the WHO published a new classification of

Table 1 CNS tumor syndromes.

Disorders	CNS tumors	Tumors of other organs and tissues	Skin lesions	Genes	Chromosomes
Neurofibromatosis-1	Glioma, neurofibroma	Iris hamartoma, osseous lesions, pheochromocytoma, leukemia, MPNST, breast cancer	Café au-lait spots, cutaneous axillary freckling, neurofibromas	NF1	17q11.2
Neurofibromatosis-2	Vestibular, Schwannoma, Meningioma, ependymoma	Posterior lens opacities, retinal hamartoma	None	NF2	22q12.2
von Hippel–Lindau disease	Hemangioblastoma	Retinal hemangioblastoma, renal cell carcinoma, pheochromocytoma, visceral cysts, endolymphatic sac tumor	None	VHL	3p25–p26
Tuberous sclerosis	Subependymal giant cell astrocytoma (SEGA)	Cardiac rhabdomyoma, adenomatous polyps of the duodenum and small intestine, cysts of the lung and kidney, lymphangioleiomyomatosis, renal angiomyolipoma	Cutaneous Angiofibroma ("adenoma sebaceum"), peau de chagrin, subungual fibromas	TSC1, TSC2	9q34.14, 16p13.3
Li–Fraumeni syndrome	Gliomas (10%)	Breast carcinoma; bone and soft tissue sarcoma; adrenocortical, lung, and GI carcinoma; leukemia	None	P53	17p13.1
Cowden disease	Dysplastic gangliocytoma of cerebellum	Hamartomatous polyps of the eye, colon, and thyroid; breast carcinoma, thyroid cancer	Multiple trichilemmomas, fibromas	PTEN	10q22.3
Brain tumor-polyposis syndrome type 1	Malignant glioma	Colorectal adenomas, colon carcinoma, no polyps		MLH1 MSH2 MSH6 PMS2	3p21.3 2p21–22 2p16 7p22.1
Brain tumor-polyposis syndrome type 2	Medulloblastoma	Colon cancer, colonic polyps		APC	5q21
Nevoid basal cell carcinoma syndrome (Gorlin syndrome)	Medulloblastoma (anaplastic)	Jaw cysts, ovarian fibromas, skeletal abnormalities	Multiple basal cell carcinomas, palmar and plantar pits	PTCH	9q22.3–31
Retinoblastoma	Pineal tumor	Retinal tumor, osteosarcomas, and other tumors	None	RB1	13q14
Bloom syndrome	Medulloblastoma meningioma	Characteristic face and voice, gonadal failure, diabetes, immunodeficiency	Sun sensitivity, patches of hyper- and hypopigmentation	BLM	15q26.1
Fanconi anemia	Astrocytoma, medulloblastoma	Anemia, skeletal malformations, enlarged cerebral ventricles, gastrointestinal malformations	Café au-lait spots, hyper- and hypopigmentation	FANCA	16q24.3
Familial melanoma	Astrocytoma	Melanoma, pancreas, breast	Patches of hyperpigmentation Nevi	MLM CDKN2A p16(1NK4)	1p36 9p21.3
Rhabdoid, predisposition, syndrome	Atypical teratoid/rhabdoid tumor, choroid plexus carcinoma	Renal tumors, extrarenal malignant rhabdoid tumors	None	HSNFA/INH1	22q11
Multiple endocrine neoplasia (MEN-1 Carney complex)	Pituitary adenomas	Hyperparathyroidism, gastrinoma, insulinoma, thyroid/bronchial carcinoid	Facial angiofibroma, lipoma, collagenoma	MEN1	11q13
Ataxia-telangiectasia	Astrocytoma, medulloblastoma cerebellar ataxia	Lymphomas, hypogonadism, radiation sensitivity, insulin resistance, premature aging, small stature	Telangiectasias	ATM	11q22–q23

Abbreviation: MPNST, malignant peripheral nerve sheath tumor.

CNS tumors which was subsequently updated by cIMPACT-NOW (the Consortium to Inform Molecular and Practical Approaches to CNS Tumor Taxonomy) which restructured and integrated histology and molecular features (Table 2).[7–9] Next-generation sequencing of brain tumors is recommended to improve diagnostic accuracy, since immunohistochemistry staining can have false-negative rates leading to an incorrect diagnosis.[6,10] The classification of brain tumors is an ongoing effort that will likely have many revisions as new technologies emerge, such as those associated with methylation profiling and proteomic evaluation.[11,12] Clinical trials conducted before the new molecular classification should be approached with caution, as many of these studies now include subgroups with different biologic features that were previously evaluated together. As the biology of brain tumors becomes more clearly understood, clinical trials will include a more homogenous patient population to delineate subgroups that can respond to particular therapies. The next section describes in more detail the classifications of astrocytic, oligodendroglial, ependymal, and embryonal neoplasms.

Classification of astrocytic and oligodendroglial tumors

The 2016 classification of CNS tumors integrates the identification of molecular alterations to identify subtypes of astrocytomas, including isocitrate dehydrogenase (IDH) and histone mutations of H3K27M as well as defining oligodendrogliomas harboring both an IDH mutation and 1p/19q codeletion.

GBM, IDH (isocitrate dehydrogenase)-wild-type and astrocytoma, IDH-mutant, Grade 4 are characterized by hypercellularity with nuclear pleomorphism, mitotic figures, endothelial proliferation, and necrosis. The term GBM is now reserved for Grade 4 IDH-wildtype astrocytomas.[8] Gliosarcomas display the typical

Table 2 Partial list of tumors of neuroepithelial tissue from the 2016 WHO with cIMPACT-NOW updates.

I. Diffuse astrocytic tumors
1. Diffuse astrocytoma, IDH-mutant, Grade 2
2. Diffuse astrocytoma, IDH-wildtype, Grade 2
3. Diffuse astrocytoma, NOS, Grade 2
4. Anaplastic astrocytoma, IDH-mutant, Grade 3
5. Anaplastic astrocytoma, IDH-wildtype, Grade 3
6. Anaplastic astrocytoma, NOS, Grade 3
7. Glioblastoma, IDH-wildtype (giant cell, gliosarcoma variants), Grade 4
8. Astrocytoma, IDH-mutant, Grade 4
9. Glioblastoma, NOS, Grade 4
10. Diffuse glioma, H3.3 G34-mutant, Grade 4

II. Other astrocytic tumors
1. Subependymal giant cell astrocytoma, Grade 1
2. Pilocytic astrocytoma (pilomyxoid variant), Grade 1
3. Pleomorphic xanthoastrocytoma, Grade 2
4. Pleomorphic xanthoastrocytoma, Grade 3
5. Astroblastoma, *MN1*-altered (NOS and NEC variants)

III. Oligodendroglial tumors
1. Oligodendroglioma, IDH-mutant and 1p/19q-codeleted, Grade 2
2. Oligodendroglioma, NOS, Grade 2
3. Anaplastic Oligodendroglioma, IDH-mutant and 1p/19q-codeleted, Grade 3
4. Anaplastic Oligodendroglioma, NOS, Grade 3
5. Oligoastrocytoma, NOS, Grade 2
6. Anaplastic oligoastrocytoma, NOS, Grade 3

IV. Ependymal tumors
1. Myxopapillary ependymoma, Grade 2
2. Subependymoma, Grade 1
3. Ependymoma, Grade 2
4. Anaplastic ependymoma, Grade 3
5. Supratentorial ependymoma, RELA fusion-positive, Grade 2 or 3
6. Supratentorial ependymoma, *YAP1-MAMLD1* fusion-positive
7. Posterior fossa ependymoma, pediatric-type/PFA
8. Posterior fossa ependymoma, adult-type/PFB
9. Spinal ependymoma, MYCN-amplified

V. Choroid plexus tumors
1. Choroid plexus papilloma, Grade 1
2. Atypical Choroid plexus papilloma, Grade 2
3. Choroid plexus carcinoma, Grade 3

VI. Neuronal and mixed neuronal-glial tumors
1. Dysembryoplastic neuroepithelial tumor (DNET), Grade 1
2. Gangliocytoma, Grade 1
3. Dysplastic gangliocytoma of the cerebellum (Lhermitte-Duclos)
4. Ganglioglioma, Grade 1
5. Multinodular and vacuolating neuronal tumor (MVNT), Grade 1
6. Central neurocytoma, Grade 2
7. Anaplastic ganglioglioma, Grade 3
8. Diffuse leptomeningeal glioneuronal tumor (DLGNT)

VII. Pineal tumors
1. Pineocytoma, Grade 1
2. Pineal parenchymal tumor of intermediate differentiation, Grade 2
3. Pineoblastoma, Grade 3

VIII. Embryonal tumors
1. Medulloblastoma, genetically defined, Grade 4
   a. WNT-activated
   b. SHH-activated and TP53-mutant
   c. SHH-activated and TP53-wild-type
   d. Group 3
   e. Group 4
2. Medulloblastoma, histologically defined, Grade 4
   a. Classic
   b. Desmoplastic/nodular
   c. with extensive nodularity
   d. Large cell/anaplastic
   e. NOS
3. Embryonal tumor with multilayered rosettes, C19MC altered, Grade 4
4. Embryonal tumor with multilayered rosettes, NOS
5. Atypical teratoid/rhabdoid tumor
6. CNS embryonal tumor, NOS

Abbreviation: NOS, not otherwise specified; NEC, not elsewhere classified.

pathologic features of Grade 4 astrocytomas in combination with densely packed spindle-shaped cells in herringbone patterns. Anaplastic astrocytomas (AA), Grade 3 also have increased cellularity, nuclear atypia, and mitoses, but necrosis and microvascular proliferation are absent. WHO Grade 2 astrocytomas typically comprise a fairly uniform group of astrocytes in a background of a fibrillary matrix. There is less cellular pleomorphism, and mitoses are rare.[13]

IDH mutations are found in 80% of Grade 2 and 3 gliomas.[14] IDH mutations have also been identified in myeloid leukemia, myelodysplastic syndrome, chondrosarcoma, angioimmunoblastic T cell lymphoma, cholangiocarcinoma, thyroid carcinoma, and rare subsets of breast cancer.[15] The most common IDH mutation is at position 132 in IDH1 from arginine to histidine (R132H) followed by substitution at position 172 in IDH2 from arginine to lysine (R172K). This mutation results in the conversion of α-ketoglutarate to the putative oncometabolite 2-hydroxyglutarate (2HG) and leads to epigenetic changes that contribute to oncogenesis.[6] Diffuse astrocytic tumors in the current WHO classification are defined by the presence or absence of an IDH mutation and are more likely to be found in younger adults compared to IDH wild-type gliomas as exemplified by the median age for a diagnosis in Grade 4 astrocytomas being 44 years and 62 years, respectively.[7] Gliomas with an IDH mutation typically have a significantly better prognosis than IDH-wildtype; and mutant Grade 4 astrocytomas, for example, have a median survival of 31 months versus 15 months, respectively.[7] Further molecular insights introduced in the cIMPACT updates are expected to be incorporated in the next updated WHO classification for astrocytic tumors.[8] In IDH-wild type diffuse astrocytoma, emerging data demonstrate that Grade 2 and 3 tumors with telomerase reverse transcriptase (TERT) promoter mutation, epidermal growth factor receptor (*EGFR*) gene amplification, or with +7/−10 chromosome copy number changes have similar behavior and prognosis of a histologic IDH-wild type GBM and should be designated as the histologic grade, IDH-wildtype "with molecular features of GBM, Grade 4". Due to aggressive behavior, a histologic Grade 2 IDH-mutant diffuse astrocytomas and the presence of CDKN2A/B homozygous deletion is now defined as a Grade 4 neoplasm.

Oligodendrogliomas are now defined by the simultaneous presence of an IDH mutation, and concurrent deletion of chromosome 1p/19q.[7] Oligodendrogliomas are characterized by a relatively uniform array of small round cells with artifactual perinuclear halos in a background of fine capillary ("chicken-wire") vasculature. They are typically described as having a "fried-egg" appearance. Occasionally, oligodendrogliomas have features of anaplasia, pleomorphism, and necrosis and are classified as Grade 3 anaplastic oligodendrogliomas (AO). As discussed later, patients with oligodendrogliomas have a better prognosis than most patients with diffuse astrocytic brain tumors. The previous histologic diagnosis of oligoastrocytoma is now only made in the absence of molecular testing and should prompt next-generation sequencing of any remaining tissue.[7]

Diffuse midline glioma, H3 K27M mutant [previously diffuse intrinsic pontine glioma (DIPG)] is an astrocytic tumor that is Grade 4 by definition and is a new entity in the 2016 WHO classification. It is thought to most often occur in children, although with routine molecular analysis, the discovery of these mutations in adults with glioma is increasing. These cancers commonly have a midline location and are associated with a poor prognosis with proven treatment options limited to radiation therapy.[16] Currently, the use of imipridone (ONC201), a dopamine receptor (DRD2) antagonist that has shown clinical activity, is being evaluated in a clinical trial in patients older than 16 years of age (NCT02525692).[17] Recently, an alternative histone mutated GBM, with a histone G35 mutation has been described primarily in adolescents and young adults and most commonly present in the cerebral hemisphere.[18]

Grade 1 tumors, juvenile pilocytic astrocytomas (JPA), occur most commonly in children. They are characterized by low cellularity, Rosenthal fibers, cysts, and they do not infiltrate surrounding tissue extensively. In young children, they occur more frequently in the cerebellar hemispheres, and the 5-year progression-free survival (PFS) rate is 95% after complete resection. The other low-grade glial tumors also tend to be discreet and less infiltrative. These include pleomorphic xanthoastrocytoma (PXA), ganglioglioma, neurocytoma, and dysembryoplastic neuroepithelial tumor (DNET). Up to 66%, 50%, and 10% of PXA, ganglioglioma, and JPA respectively have *BRAFV600E* mutations or other alterations in *BRAF*, such as gene fusions. Detection of this mutation can assist in the clarification of the diagnosis, and there are ongoing investigations in targeting this mutation with BRAF and MEK inhibitors in disease refractory to surgery and radiation with case reports and a small basket trial showing clinical benefit.[6,19]

Classification of ependymal and embryonal tumors

Ependymomas arise from ependymal cells that line the ventricles and spinal canal. They occur wherever ependymal cells are present and have a predilection for the fourth ventricle. They are the most frequent neuroepithelial tumor of the spinal cord, accounting for more than 50% of spinal gliomas in both children and adults. They are histologically characterized by perivascular pseudorosettes (tumor cells arranged radially around blood vessels), and Homer-Wright (true) rosettes. These tumors are either low grade (WHO Grade 2) or anaplastic (WHO Grade 3) and are aggressive and spread along cerebrospinal fluid (CSF) pathways. They are classified by the anatomic site and by molecular group/genetic alteration.[9] This includes supratentorial ependymomas including REL-associated protein (RELA) fusion-positive and Yes1 associated transcriptional regulator (YAP1) fusion-positive (both of which are less common in adults) and posterior fossa ependymoma including pediatric-type (PFA) and adult-type (PFB) which have unique epigenetic signatures.[7,8] Spinal cord ependymomas are more common in adults, frequently have an *NF2* mutation, and are associated with a better prognosis except for those with *MYCN* amplification, which have poor outcomes.[9] Myxopapillary and subependymomas are Grade 2 and Grade 1, respectively. They have different biology than ependymomas and are best treated with gross total resection when possible.[9,20]

Embryonal tumors, previously designated primitive neuroectodermal tumors (PNET), are a group of neoplasms characterized by undifferentiated small blue cells with Homer–Wright rosettes (cells arranged around a true lumen). They are usually fast-growing and often disseminate along CSF pathways. They occur more frequently in children and are often found in the cerebellum (medulloblastoma) and the pineal gland (pineoblastoma). Although these lesions are histologically similar, medulloblastoma is generally more amenable to treatment and has a better outcome.[21]

Clinical presentation

Patients with brain tumors may present with generalized, nonfocal symptoms and signs or with focal manifestations related to the specific location of the tumor in the brain.[22] Factors that contribute to the presenting symptoms and signs include tumor location, size, and growth rate. Supratentorial tumors are more likely to present with seizures, whereas infratentorial tumors more often present with headache, nausea, and vomiting. Superficial cortical tumors are more likely to cause seizures, whereas more deep-seated tumors are more likely associated with personality and cognitive changes. A seizure is the presenting symptom in approximately 40% of patients with GBM, 60–75% in low-grade gliomas (LGGs), and 20–50% in meningioma.[23] Tumors in eloquent areas of the brain will cause focal symptoms such as aphasia, hemiparesis, or sensory loss; and tumors in the brainstem typically present with cranial nerve deficits such as diplopia or facial weakness. Tumors of the cerebellum may cause ipsilateral ataxia, unsteady gait, and nystagmus. Symptoms usually evolve over several weeks; sometimes, the symptoms begin acutely, corresponding to hemorrhage, or a seizure with a prolonged postictal state.

Diagnostic neuroimaging

Patients with symptoms and signs suggestive of an intracranial lesion should have a magnetic resonance imaging (MRI) study with intravenous contrast. This is the modality of choice for CNS tumors and CT should be used only in those patients who are intolerant of MRI scanning.

High-grade tumors such as GBM disrupt the blood–brain barrier and have the characteristic appearance of a hypointense center surrounded by a hyperintense irregular rim of contrast enhancement (Figure 1). Approximately 95% of GBMs will enhance heterogeneously with gadolinium. Anaplastic gliomas enhance less frequently, particularly in younger adults, and they may be confused with LGGs radiographically (Figure 2). GBMs also have a greater tendency to spread along white matter tracts, particularly the corpus callosum, and to cross to the contralateral cerebral hemisphere. In contrast, low-grade tumors have an intact blood–brain barrier and usually do not contrast enhance. An exception is the JPA, a Grade 1 tumor that has areas of dense enhancement. Fluid-attenuated inversion recovery (FLAIR)

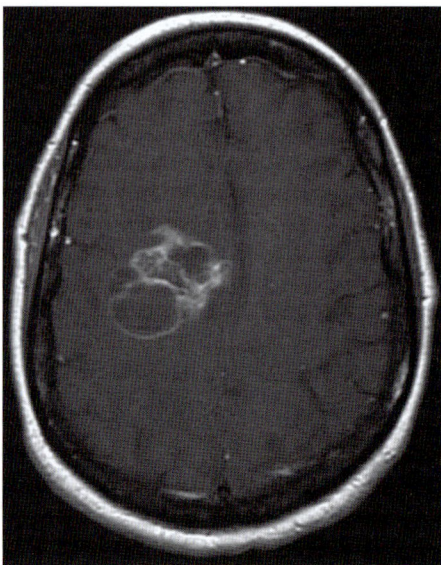

Figure 1 Glioblastoma. This is a postgadolinium *T*1-weighted MRI of a right posterior frontal glioblastoma. There is irregular contrast enhancement with focal areas of necrosis.

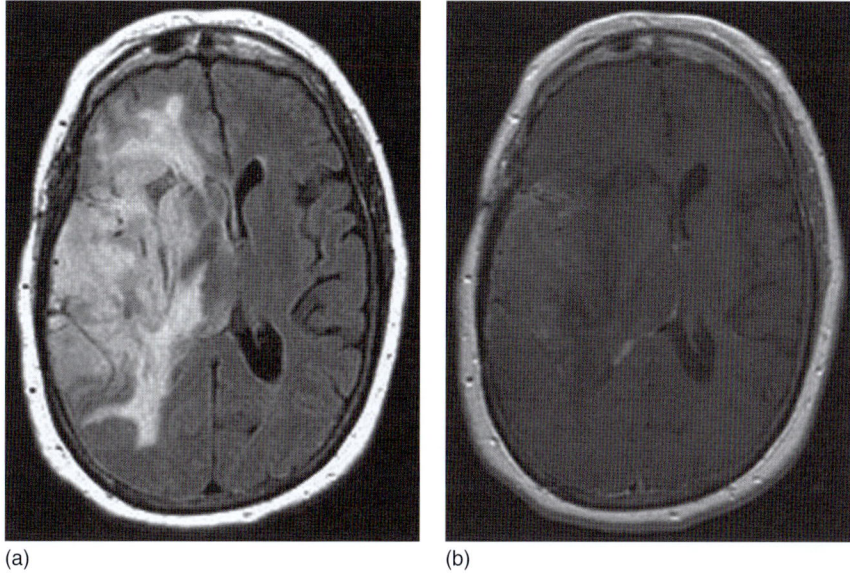

Figure 2 Anaplastic oligodendroglioma. (a) FLAIR image showing extensive tumor-infiltrating the right hemisphere. (b) Patchy enhancement is seen throughout the tumor.

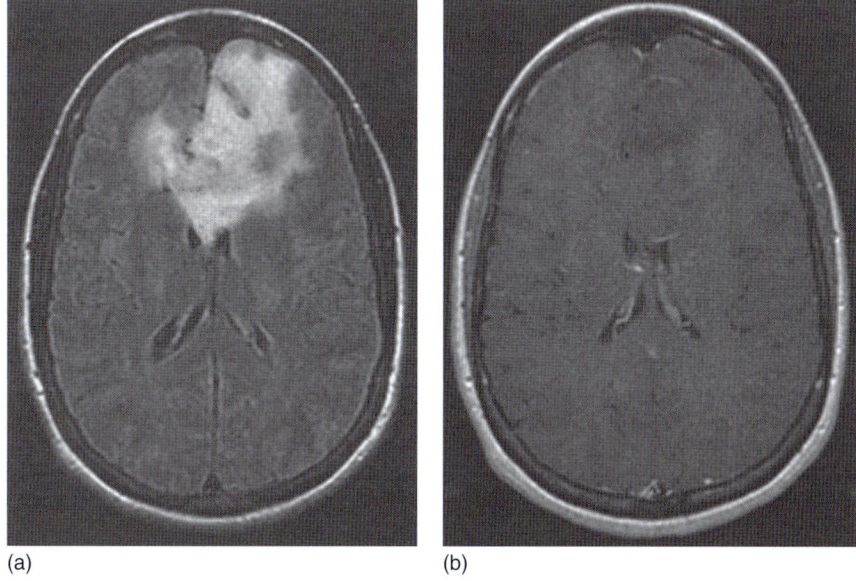

Figure 3 Low-grade glioma. (a) FLAIR image demonstrating extensive infiltrative disease predominantly of the left frontal lobe extending across the anterior corpus callosum and involving the deep right frontal white matter. (b) Postcontrast images show no evidence of enhancement of this large lesion.

sequences provide a rapid distinction between normal brain tissue and brain tumor or edema and provide the best images to delineate the radiographic extent of the lesion (Figure 3). On FLAIR imaging, however, an infiltrative tumor cannot be differentiated from edema. Diffusion-weighted imaging (DWI) assesses the mobility of water molecules and may distinguish between ischemia and tumor. Perfusion images measure blood volume and vascularity and correlate with tumor grade and with fluorodeoxyglucose (FDG) positron emission tomography (PET) studies. There are some limitations to MRI, and the differential diagnosis of a primary brain tumor includes radiation necrosis, ischemic stroke, infection, inflammatory process, and demyelination. Re-resection or biopsy is frequently required to determine tumor reoccurrence or treatment effect.

CT and MRI readily diagnose meningiomas. On CT imaging, meningiomas are hyperdense extra-axial masses and demonstrate dense, uniform contrast enhancement. Calcification is present in 25% of these cases. Atypical, malignant, and large meningiomas more commonly cause surrounding brain edema. On T1- and T2-weighted MRI images, most meningiomas have a signal intensity similar to surrounding grey matter. They enhance diffusely, and a "dural tail" seen on contrast-enhanced images is characteristic (Figure 4). Some tumors may have flow voids indicating marked vascularity.

Functional magnetic resonance imaging (fMRI) maps the functional organization of the brain, particularly the primary motor, sensory, and language cortices, and is useful in presurgical planning. It allows a surgeon to map eloquent cortex and then plan

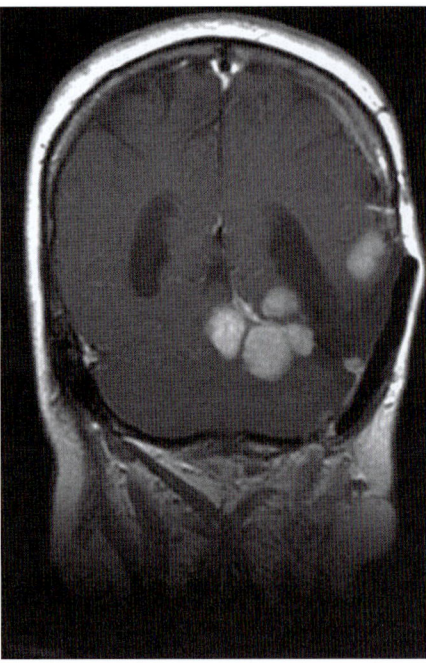

Figure 4 Meningioma. A coronal postgadolinium MRI of a multilobulated meningioma extending below and above the tentorium. There is a second lesion in the left occipito-parietal cortex.

resection while preserving neurologic function thereby facilitating maximal resection without neurologic deficit.

Principles of therapy

Treatment of a brain tumor includes both definitive and supportive therapy. Definitive therapy encompasses surgery, RT, and chemotherapy. Supportive therapy considers the management of tumor symptoms such as treatment of focal and general symptoms with corticosteroids, seizure control with antiepileptic medication, treatment of deep venous thrombosis (DVT) with anticoagulants, and the provision of psychosocial support when needed.

Supportive therapy

In addition to surgery, RT, and chemotherapy, where the goal of treatment is to extend survival, various types of supportive therapy are required to treat a patient's neurologic symptoms and improve their quality of life.

All seizures from a brain tumor begin as a focal seizure even if the focality is not observed clinically. Patients with brain tumors who have had a seizure either at presentation or during their treatment should be treated with an antiepileptic drug (AED). The optimal AED does not affect the hepatic microsomal system, which can alter the metabolism of chemotherapeutic agents; common choices include levetiracetam, lacosamide, topiramate, or zonisamide.[24,25] It is controversial if AEDs should be used to prevent seizures in patients with brain tumors who have never had a seizure. Current guidelines discourage prophylactic anticonvulsant use. This decision should be made with consideration of medication side effects, higher seizure risk clinical profiles including tumors that are located superficially in the temporal or insular lobes, and presence of IDH mutation as well as concern about losing the ability to drive after a seizure.[22,23,26]

Corticosteroids dramatically relieve the symptoms from edema caused by brain tumors, thus reducing intracranial pressure. Symptomatic improvement usually takes hours, and patients may be symptom-free within 24–48 h. Corticosteroids are indicated in all symptomatic patients with brain tumors, except those with presumed PCNSL where corticosteroids may cause tumor necrosis owing to their lympholytic effect, compromising a histologic diagnosis if the steroids are administered before biopsy.

The optimal dose of corticosteroids has not been established, but the dose should be titrated to the lowest dose commensurate with good neurologic function. For patients on steroids greater than 6 weeks, prophylactic treatment for *Pneumocystis jirovecii* infection is indicated. There are also some concerns when corticosteroids are administered before the initiation of immunotherapies because of their impact on select aspects of an immune response.[27]

DVT is a common complication of brain tumors with approximately 30% of patients with high-grade gliomas develop venous thromboembolic events.[28] Factors that contribute to its development include immobility, neurosurgery, the release of thromboplastins from the brain, and hypercoagulability related to cancer and chemotherapy. The use of prophylactic and therapeutic anticoagulation generally has an acceptable safety profile. It is useful in patients with primary brain tumor, although there are studies showing a greater than threefold increased risk of intracerebral hemorrhage.[28,29] Anticoagulants, including low molecular weight heparin and the newer inhibitors of thrombin or factor Xa, are the agents of choice.[30] Vena cava filters should be reserved for those with contraindications to anticoagulation.

Surgery

There are multiple goals of surgery, including establishment of a tissue-based diagnosis, decompression of the tumor mass, alleviate symptoms, and reduction of corticosteroid requirements. The ultimate goal of surgery is to achieve a gross total resection. Biopsy, in particular stereotactic needle biopsy, is indicated for: (1) surgically inaccessible tumors such as those in the brainstem, basal ganglia, or thalamus; (2) multifocal tumors; (3) patients with medical comorbidities resulting in a high surgical/anesthetic risk. Needle biopsies have several limitations, including obtaining a small tissue sample that may compromise diagnostic accuracy as well as not providing sufficient tumor for molecular analyses. Benign tumors or Grade 1 gliomas may be cured by complete removal. For incurable tumors, such as all infiltrative gliomas, the extent of resection is often a significant prognostic factor, and biopsy alone confers inferior survival compared with more extensive resection. A retrospective analysis of three prospective Radiation Therapy Oncology Group (RTOG) randomized trials of 645 patients with GBM revealed a statistically significant improvement in overall survival between patients who had gross total resection versus those who had biopsy alone (median 11.3 vs 6.6 months; $p < 0.001$).[31] Even more compelling data are available for LGGs supporting the prognostic benefit of extensive resection. In 2017, the FDA-approved 5-aminolevulinic acid (5-ALA) to aid in the visualization of malignant tissue during surgery for malignant glioma to allow complete resection. 5-ALA is a nonfluorescent prodrug that leads to intracellular accumulation of fluorescent porphyrins in malignant gliomas that are visualized with blue light.[32] Furthermore, resection, when done with concern for eloquent areas of the brain, often improves neurologic function. In a prospective multi-institutional series, among 408 patients undergoing craniotomy for newly diagnosed malignant glioma the rates of morbidity and mortality were 24% and 1.5%, respectively. After craniotomy, 53% of patients had improvement, and only 8% had worsening of neurologic symptoms.[33] Preoperative fMRI (see earlier text) and awake intraoperative cortical mapping are techniques that facilitate tumor removal without neurologic injury.

Radiation therapy

RT is an effective adjuvant treatment for malignant glioma.[34] For selected tumors, such as germinomatous germinomas, RT is curative.[35] In prospective trials of high-grade gliomas, RT is associated with higher rates of overall survival than surgery alone, or surgery plus chemotherapy. In the original 1978 Brain Tumor Study Group report of high-grade glioma, the median overall survival duration of patients treated by surgery alone was 14 weeks. In contrast, the overall survival duration of those receiving postoperative whole-brain RT (WBRT) of 50–60 Gy was 36 weeks.[36] Improved RT techniques now allow for higher doses to the tumor while sparing normal brain. Focal RT is delivered to the area of abnormal FLAIR signal on an MRI scan with a margin of 2–3 cm, followed by a cone down to the enhancing area. Standard fractionated external beam RT involves delivering the optimum dose of 60 Gy in daily fractions of 1.8–2.0 Gy/day over 6 weeks.[37] Modern techniques include intensity-modulated radiation therapy (IMRT), which conforms the dose to the shape of the target volume, sparing adjacent critical structures.[38]

Stereotactic radiosurgery (SRS) is another technique indicated for the treatment of selected brain tumors. SRS delivers highly focal RT to a clearly defined small target, typically in a single dose. SRS can be delivered by a gamma knife (cobalt 60 sources), linear accelerator, or Cyberknife with similar results.[39] A steep dose gradient is maintained with a small target volume of less than 4 cm. Radiosurgery is primarily used to treat small lesions such as metastatic tumors, meningiomas, vestibular schwannomas, and pituitary adenomas. It is rarely used in the treatment of malignant glioma because this infiltrative disease does not lend itself to focused RT.

Protons, neutrons, and heavy charged particles have also been used to treat CNS tumors. Proton beams interact with nuclei of atoms rather than their electrons. Large doses of radiation are deposited in a targeted area sparing adjacent tissue. Charged particles can have an abrupt fall off, sparing sensitive structures that could not withstand therapeutic irradiation. This technique is ideal for skull base tumors such as chordomas, meningiomas, and chondrosarcomas, lesions adjacent to the optic nerves, chiasm, and brainstem. Proton therapy is also used to a greater extent in pediatrics to limit RT exposure to developing organs, but its superiority to standard RT has not yet been established.[40]

Chemotherapy

Chemotherapeutic drugs have traditionally been unsuccessful in the treatment of most brain tumors. Some exceptions include PCNSL, germinomas, and some oligodendrogliomas. The role of chemotherapy in the treatment of astrocytomas is limited for extending survival compared with surgery and radiation alone.

There are several limitations associated with chemotherapy for the treatment of brain tumors, including the role of the blood–brain barrier, the paucity of lymphatics in the brain, the heterogeneity of gliomas, the intrinsic resistance of gliomas, and a low therapeutic/toxic ratio.[41] Most chemotherapeutic agents cannot penetrate a tumor in the brain owing to an intact blood–brain barrier, particularly in the margins beyond contrast enhancement.[42] Many attempts have been made to disrupt the blood–brain barrier in the treatment of brain tumors, such as opening the blood–brain barrier with a hyperosmolar agent such as intraarterial mannitol. Other attempts include intra-arterial infusions, intratumoral injections via catheters, implanting drug-impregnated wafers, and drugs altered to cross the blood–brain barrier. None has yet proved to be more effective, and many are more toxic than conventional routes.[43]

In addition to the blood–brain barrier, primary brain tumors have intrinsic resistance to conventional chemotherapeutic agents. Therefore, most are ineffective, even if they achieve adequate concentrations in tumor tissue. When RT or chemotherapy does succeed in killing tumor cells, the deficiency of a lymphatic system in the brain prevents the efficient removal of detritus caused by treatment. Thus, necrotic tissue may serve as a nidus for edema and worsening neurologic function. Specific drugs will be discussed by tumor type.

Diffuse astrocytic tumors, IDH-*wildtype*

Glioblastoma, IDH-*wildtype*, and gliosarcoma (Grade 4)

GBM, IDH wild-type, is a disease of advancing age where the mean age is 54 years. The median survival of patients with GBM is approximately 14–18 months. Favorable prognostic factors include younger age, a high Karnofsky Performance Score (KPS), methylation of the promoter region of the *O*-6-methylguanine-DNA methyltransferase (MGMT) gene, and surgical resection versus biopsy alone.[22,44]

For newly diagnosed GBM, the standard treatment following surgical resection is RT (60 Gy in 1.8–2.0 fractions) with concurrent daily temozolomide followed by six cycles of adjuvant temozolomide. Published in 2005, a prospective randomized trial of 573 patients aged ≤70 years with newly diagnosed GBM demonstrated that patients treated with RT plus continuous daily temozolomide (75 mg/m^2/day) followed by six months of adjuvant temozolomide ($150–200$ mg/m^2/day for 5 days of a 28-day cycle) had a median overall survival of 14.6 months compared with 12.1 months in patients treated with RT alone ($p < 0.001$). More importantly, the 2-year survival rate was 26.5% compared with 10.4%.[37] There was minimal toxicity in the combined RT/chemotherapy group, aside from 11% of patients who experienced Grade 4 thrombocytopenia. The significance of the DNA repair enzyme, MGMT, was also demonstrated in approximately one-half of patients from the Phase III study.[45] There was a distinct overall survival advantage for any patient whose promoter was methylated. The overall survival durations of patients treated with RT plus temozolomide with and without a methylated *MGMT* promoter were 21.7 months and 15.3 months, respectively ($p = 0.007$). Although patients whose tumors have a methylated promoter benefitted the most from the addition of temozolomide, there was a modest benefit from the addition of temozolomide even in patients whose tumor had an unmethylated *MGMT* promoter. The use of adjuvant temozolomide beyond six cycles has not shown to prolong overall survival and is associated with more toxicity, although this has not been formally evaluated in a randomized clinical trial.[46,47] Recent recommendations suggest that given the limited efficacy of alkylating chemotherapy, patients harboring GBM with unmethylated *MGMT* promoter should be considered for clinical trials omitting temozolomide.[48]

Elderly patients (>70 years of age) treated with surgery and RT survive longer than those treated with surgery alone, but the prognosis remains poor.[49] Reducing the dose and duration of RT for patients over 70 years (40 Gy/15 fractions) has comparable efficacy to the more protracted regimens and can be considered with patients with a low-performance status.[50] Alternatively, temozolomide alone can be offered to elderly patients with MGMT methylated GBM based on two randomized trials comparing single-agent temozolomide chemotherapy versus RT. These studies suggest that treating MGMT unmethylated tumors with temozolomide is associated with worse outcomes.[49,51]

Tumor treating fields (TTFields) act as an antimitotic treatment modality that interferes with cell division and organelle assembly by delivering low-intensity alternating electric fields to the tumor. This treatment is administered using a device that requires patients to wear it at least 16 h a day. A trial in 237 heavily pretreated patients with GBM showed no benefit with this modality. A follow-up randomized controlled trial of 695 patients with newly diagnosed GBM who had completed radiochemotherapy, demonstrated that the median PFS from randomization was 6.7 months in the TTFields plus temozolomide group compared with 4.0 months in the temozolomide-alone group (hazard ratio, 0.63). This subsequently led to its FDA approval, although the treatment is controversial within the neuro-oncology community regarding the trial study design.[52,53]

Despite standard therapy, almost all patients will have disease recurrence, typically at the original location. Treatment options at relapse include re-resection, re-irradiation with or without bevacizumab, and a change in systemic chemotherapy. Bevacizumab is FDA approved for recurrent GBM as a single agent. However, two large randomized phase III trials of standard chemoradiation with or without bevacizumab for patients with newly diagnosed GBM demonstrated a statistically significant prolongation of PFS (median, 6–7 months to 10.7 months), but no difference in overall survival (median, 15–16 months).[54,55] However, the two studies differed in their patient outcomes data with one study showing an increase in symptom burden, a decline in formal neurocognitive testing, and a worse quality of life with bevacizumab and the second which only measured health-related quality of life (not symptom burden or neurocognitive function) showed equal maintenance of quality of life with bevacizumab. Based on these data, the incorporation of bevacizumab into initial therapy is not recommended. Nitrosoureas (i.e., carmustine, lomustine) are a potential treatment option in recurrent GBM, particularly in the presence of MGMT promoter methylation.[56] Bevacizumab can be used as a steroid-sparing agent in recurrent GBM but does not confer a survival advantage based on a Phase II trial evaluating concurrent treatment with bevacizumab and lomustine over lomustine alone.[57,58]

Gliosarcomas have similar age of onset and prognosis as GBM but have a greater propensity to metastasize systemically via a hematogenous route, most often to the lung and liver and occasionally bone and other organs.[59] Some patients with gliosarcoma have tumor MGMT promoter methylation and are currently treated the same as GBM aside from a going trial evaluating the use of sunitinib (NCT03641326).[60]

Anaplastic (Grade 3) and diffuse (Grade 2) astrocytoma, IDH-*wildtype*

AA are less frequent than GBM, and consequently, there have been few trials studying Grade III tumors exclusively.[1] IDH-wildtype AA and GBM have similar outcomes suggesting that the established histopathological grading criteria lose their prognostic significance.[61,62] Emerging data show that diffuse astrocytomas that are IDH wild-type have clinical and molecular features of their Grade 4 counterparts and likely represent an early stage of GBM.[63] Retrospective data supporting the use of RT plus temozolomide of AA at diagnosis and treatment approaches at recurrence are identical to GBM.[64] If not treated with chemoradiation upon diagnosis, diffuse astrocytomas, IDH-wild type should be monitored with close interval imaging and treated when tumor growth or contrast enhancement is seen on imaging.

Diffuse astrocytic tumors, IDH-mutant

Grade 4 astrocytoma and anaplastic astrocytoma (Grade 3), IDH-mutant

IDH-mutant Grade 4 astrocytomas comprise 10% of all Grade 4 gliomas, patients have a median age at diagnosis of 44 years (compared with 62 years for those with wild type IDH), and treatment with chemoradiation after surgery is associated with better prognosis (median overall survival, 31 months vs 15 in their IDH wild type counterparts). Treatment is identical to IDH-wildtype GBMs.[45,62] For AA, IDH mutant, the RTOG 9402 study showed an overall survival benefit of 2.2 months (5.5 years vs 3.3 years; $p < 0.05$) with radiation followed by adjuvant chemotherapy procarbazine, lomustine, and vincristine (PCV) compared with RT alone.[65] Alternatively, the preliminary results of the CATNON intergroup trial of concurrent and adjuvant temozolomide chemotherapy in newly diagnosed non-1p/19q deleted anaplastic glioma demonstrated that the application of chemoradiation and up to 12 cycles adjuvant temozolomide in the same manner as GBM is an effective treatment.[66] Due to better tolerability, a temozolomide-based approach is most commonly used.

Diffuse astrocytoma, IDH-mutant (Grade 2)

Diffuse astrocytomas with IDH mutation are associated with a median overall survival of 11 years and comprise less than 10% of all gliomas.[1,67] The timing of postoperative chemoradiation is unclear and typically has an individualized approach and must be weighed against the long-term side effects of RT given the long-term survival of this patient population. Factors to consider earlier treatment include the following higher risk factors: age ≥ 40 years, preoperative tumor size of greater than 5 cm, subtotal resection, neurologic deficit related to the tumor, and uncontrolled seizures. Those with a favorable risk profile could be monitored clinically and radiographically, although increasingly early therapeutic interventions are being used.[68–71] Although similar to Grade 3 and 4 IDH-mutant astrocytomas, chemoradiation with temozolomide is often utilized, there are concerns that this regimen may increase risk of treatment-related brain injury; and therefore some specialists do not recommend concurrent temozolomide and radiation.[72] Currently, there are ongoing investigations with IDH inhibitors and vaccines (NCT02193347) in these patients.[73]

Oligodendrogliomas

Oligodendrogliomas tend to arise in the white matter of the frontal (40%), parietal (30%), and temporal (20%) lobes of young adults. They represent 10% of all LGGs in adults and 5% of LGGs in children. AO are typically treated after pathologic diagnosis following surgery with radiation and chemotherapy. Grade 2 oligodendrogliomas, on the other hand, are frequently monitored clinically and radiographically to mitigate the cognitive side effects of radiation therapy unless patients are symptomatic with focal neurologic deficits, seizures, or there is radiographic evidence of significant progression. However, in light of increasing evidence that early treatment may prolong overall survival, particularly in patients whose gross total tumor resection was not possible, more patients are receiving radiation therapy followed by chemotherapy [temozolomide or procarbazine/CCNU/vincristine (PCV)]. There have been two large randomized trials of patients with newly diagnoses AO, RTOG 9402 and European Organization for Research and Treatment of Cancer (EORTC) 26961.[74,75] Both studies investigated the administration of RT +/− PCV chemotherapy; the RTOG trial used PCV in the neoadjuvant setting, and the EORTC used it following RT. Both studies demonstrated dramatic prolongation in overall survival with RT and PCV compared with RT (e.g., median 14.7 and 7.3 years in the RTOG trial; $p = 0.03$) in the 1p19q co-deleted group. This disease is now classified as oligodendroglioma (WHO 2016). Therefore, the standard of care is to treat such patients with RT and chemotherapy. Similarly, radiation followed by adjuvant PCV has demonstrated success in Grade 2 oligodendrogliomas with a median PFS of 10.4 years and a median overall survival of 13.3 years.[71] Typically, six adjuvant cycles of PCV are used, but in practice due to tolerability and myelosuppression, most patients receive three to four cycles after dose reductions.

Whether PCV must be the regimen of choice is unknown, as temozolomide is clearly effective and better tolerated. The EORTC is currently leading a Phase III trial randomizing patients with LGG to radiation or temozolomide. Many investigators suggest that temozolomide can replace PCV when administered in combination with RT in a schedule similar to the treatment of GBM because of its markedly lower toxicity profile.[76]

Ependymoma

Ependymomas account for approximately 2% of all intracranial tumors in adults and 5% in children; they are the most common intracranial tumor in children under the age of 5 years.[20] Ependymomas have a bimodal incidence with a significant peak in the 0 to 4-year age group and a smaller peak at the third to the fifth decade of life.[77] Ependymomas are tumors comprising ependymal cells that tend to occur along the surfaces of the ventricles. They may also occur in the brain parenchyma adjacent to the ventricles or anywhere along the spinal canal.[20] More than 60% of ependymomas arise in the posterior fossa and arise from the caudal floor of the fourth ventricle.[78] Supratentorial ependymomas are typically located in the parenchyma rather than intraventricularly and most commonly in the frontal and parietal lobes. They can extend along the subarachnoid space and seed the CSF.[20]

The initial treatment of ependymomas is surgical. A gross total resection prolongs overall survival, but it may not always be possible depending upon the location of the tumor. Whether a completely resected Grade II tumor requires additional treatment remains controversial. A retrospective analysis of adult patients with ependymoma in the posterior fossa showed that regional radiation after complete resection prevented any recurrence within 10 years.[79] However, subtotal resection of a Grade II lesion or identification of an anaplastic ependymoma (Grade III), regardless of the extent of resection, should be followed by focal RT.

RT is delivered to the tumor bed and not to the entire neuroaxis unless CSF spread is documented at diagnosis on spine MRI or CSF cytology, which should be done in all patients for staging. Ependymomas are primarily chemoresistant tumors, and there is currently no role for routine adjuvant chemotherapy. Chemotherapy may be considered at recurrence. Some investigators have reported response rates of up to 65% with platinum drugs; others have reported responses with nitrosoureas, etoposide, or even bevacizumab, but temozolomide is now the agent of choice.[80] Recently, a Phase II trial of temozolomide 125 mg–150 mg/m^2 7 days on and 7 days off combined with lapatinib 1250 mg daily in recurrent ependymoma demonstrated beneficial activity and improvement in the quality of life measures with minimal toxicity leading to incorporation of this regimen into the National Comprehensive Cancer Network® guidelines.[81]

Primary central nervous system lymphoma

PCNSL is a non-Hodgkin lymphoma restricted to the brain, CSF, spinal cord, or eyes. It has an estimated incidence of 0.43/100,000/year and accounts for 4% of all brain tumors.[1,82] It has a higher incidence in the immunosuppressed patients, and in this subpopulation, PCNSL is usually associated with the Epstein–Barr virus.[82]

The median age at PCNSL diagnosis is 65 years, although immunocompromised patients are younger.[82,83] Older age and poor performance status are associated with shorter overall survival.[82] The majority of PCNSLs are diffuse large cell, or large cell immunoblastic lymphomas and exhibit a B-cell immunophenotype with less than 3% of T-cell origin.[84] The tumor cells have a characteristic perivascular growth pattern, forming concentric rings around vessel walls without invading the vascular lumen.[82] Multiple lesions occur in 30–40% of sporadic cases. PCNSL is a rapidly growing tumor, so symptoms are usually present for only a few weeks before diagnosis. The most common presenting symptoms are cognitive deficits or personality changes that can be attributed to tumor's predilection for the frontal lobe and its tendency for multifocality (Figure 5).[83] The ocular involvement of PCNSL is common. It may be the initial manifestation of the disease or it may occur at relapse. Patients who develop ocular lymphoma first have a 50–80% chance of developing cerebral lymphoma.[85] The diagnosis of isolated ocular lymphoma can be difficult because symptoms often mimic benign inflammatory conditions such as uveitis. The most frequent symptoms are floaters and visual blurring. Diagnosis is made by slit-lamp examination, ocular ultrasound, and often vitreous biopsy.[83,85] Staging evaluation should include an ocular examination and lumbar puncture for cytologic evaluation in every patient with cerebral PCNSL as well as a systemic examination that includes whole-body PET scan and bone marrow biopsy.[82,83]

PCNSL is a highly treatable disease and is very sensitive to chemotherapy and radiation. Despite this high initial response to treatment, PCNSL has a high recurrence rate with a 5-year survival of 30–50%.[82] There are conflicting reports on the therapeutic value of surgical resection, but most patients are diagnosed by biopsy alone as resection is usually not feasible. Steroids should be held before surgical biopsy in order to avoid interference with the pathologic diagnosis due to their oncolytic effect on malignant lymphocytes, often resulting in a nondiagnostic biopsy.[82,83]

The treatment of PCNSL is based upon high-dose methotrexate (HD-MTX) regimens (doses of 3–8 g/m^2), which produces response rates of 60–90% when used as a single agent or in combination with other drugs. A wide range of HD-MTX regimens are reported in the literature, and they are associated with a median overall survival of 30–60 months.[82,83,86] Other drugs commonly administered with methotrexate include cytarabine, procarbazine, and temozolomide.[82,87] Methotrexate-based regimens have been consolidated using various approaches, including autologous stem cell transplantation (highly selected patients), low-dose

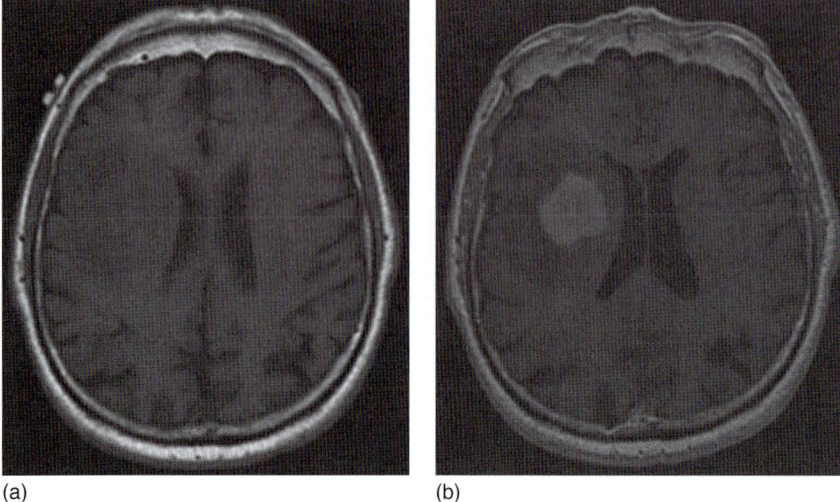

Figure 5 PCNSL. Pregadolinium (a) and postgadolinium (b) images of a right frontal diffusely enhancing PCNSL. Note the edema that surrounds the enhancing mass.

WBRT of 2340 cGy (theoretic potential for neurotoxicity), and continuous infusion of etoposide and high-dose cytarabine (severe systemic toxicity).[87–89] Rituximab has been added to most regimens despite its poor penetration into the CNS; and efficacy has been observed.[82,90] The optimal therapeutic approach will be determined after the completion of multiple ongoing randomized studies. A large Phase III trial failed to demonstrate a survival benefit when full dose WBRT RT of 4500 cGy was added to methotrexate, and this approach has largely been abandoned due to the enhanced neurotoxicity noted in long-term survivors, especially among older patients.[91] Standard chemotherapy regimens for systemic lymphoma such as CHOP (cyclophosphamide, doxorubicin, vincristine, and prednisone) are not beneficial and should be avoided.[82,83] Refractory and recurrent PCNSL have no uniform standard of care, and the relatively large number of treatment options based small trials and include re-challenge with HD-MTX-based therapy or single agent and combinational approaches with ibrutinib, lenalidomide, pomalidomide, pemetrexed, and temozolomide.[86]

Meningioma

Meningiomas account for approximately 25% of intracranial tumors. They are extra-axial and arise from arachnoid cap cells rather than the dura itself. Their incidence is higher in women than in men, but the gender distribution is equal in malignant meningiomas.[1] Approximately 85% of meningiomas are supratentorial, and multiple meningiomas occur in 10% of sporadic cases. Ionizing radiation is the only established environmental risk factor, and these meningiomas are more often atypical or malignant and are often multifocal.[92]

A recent molecular profiling analysis study demonstrated that the tumor suppressor NF2 was inactivated in about one-half of patients. Approximately 25% had *TRAF7* mutations with co-occurrence of the K409Q mutation in KLF4, a transcription factor. Approximately 20% had an E17K mutation in *AKT1*, which often co-occurred with *TRAF7* mutations. Additionally, about 5% had mutations in smoothened (SMO), which activates the Hedgehog signaling pathway. Each of the mutations conferred geographic localization of the tumor at the skull base, usually anterior and distinct from the NF2 mutations, which had no genetic overlap and occurred in the posterior skull base.[93,94] These interesting biologic insights have led to an innovative, pathway-driven clinical trial (NCT02523014).

The prognosis after treatment of meningiomas depends upon the histology of the tumor and the extent of resection. Age at diagnosis and tumor size may also play a role. Younger patients have a better prognosis than the elderly. The recurrence rate for a completely resected typical meningioma is 20% at 5 years and 25% at 10 years. Tumors that are incompletely resected have about a 60% chance of recurrence without RT. McCarthy et al. published a survey of more than 9000 patients with meningiomas treated in the United States and were included in the National Cancer Data Base.[95] The 5-year overall survival rate was 60%; 81% for patients <65 years and 56% for patients >65 years. The estimated 5-year survival rates for benign and malignant tumors were 75% and 55%, respectively. Population-based studies reported a 5-year survival rate of approximately 90%.

Typically, meningiomas produce symptoms and signs by compressing brain structures and causing edema or hydrocephalus, rather than invading the adjacent brain. However, they may invade venous structures such as the superior sagittal sinus. The histologic appearance of meningiomas may vary, but only those with rhabdoid or clear cell features are more aggressive and are associated with poor prognosis. Atypical meningiomas have a higher mitotic index as well as increased cellularity, a high nucleus/cytoplasm ratio, prominent nucleoli, necrosis, patternless growth, and brain invasion.[7] A malignant meningioma must have at least 20 mitoses per 10 high power fields or histology resembling carcinoma or sarcoma. Whereas only 1% of meningiomas metastasize, about one-half of malignant meningiomas metastasize, usually to liver, bone, and lung.[96]

Most meningiomas are very slow-growing and may be asymptomatic; many are found incidentally on imaging studies performed for other reasons.[97] Although most meningiomas do not cause significant brain edema, secretory meningiomas may cause edema resulting in substantial neurologic symptoms.[98] Convexity meningiomas may cause seizures. Meningiomas in particular locations may have typical clinical syndromes, such as cavernous sinus meningiomas that cause diplopia, proptosis, and other oculomotor abnormalities.[99]

The first step in managing a patient with a meningioma is to decide whether treatment is necessary. Many meningiomas are incidental findings and may be followed for years if they do not exhibit growth or cause neurologic symptoms. If seizures are the only symptom and are well controlled with medication, surgical resection may not be necessary. Some meningiomas are not resected because tumor removal may be associated with significant risk, especially in the case of those located at the skull base and cavernous sinus due to proximity of the intracavernous carotid artery and multiple cranial nerves.[99]

Surgery can be definitive, and if the tumor can be removed completely, a cure may be achieved. Meningiomas with the best potential for complete removal are those located along the convexity. Preoperative embolization may be done to reduce the size and vascularity of the tumor, making resection easier. Even in those patients in whom a complete resection has been accomplished, the 5-year recurrence rates after gross total resection in Grade I meningiomas range between 7% and 23%, in Grade II they are 50–55%, and in Grade III 72–78%, and with all grades, recurrence may require additional surgery or RT.[100]

RT is used in the treatment of inoperable meningiomas in partially resected tumors in some patients at recurrence, and in all malignant (Grade 3) tumors regardless of the extent of resection.[101] The role of RT in atypical (Grade 2) meningiomas is unclear. Recent data suggest that RT can be effective, particularly in prolonging PFS for patients with atypical tumors, but this is true for a minority of patients, and the effect on overall survival is less clear.[100,101] In addition, 3D planning techniques and stereotactically guided conformational RT allow for reductions in the volume of normal tissue irradiated and decreased neurotoxicity. The use of protons in the treatment of some meningiomas has also been of benefit in reducing toxicity and delaying recurrence.[102]

Stereotactic RT is an important treatment option for atypical, malignant, and recurrent meningioma. Radiosurgery has also become an option for small typical meningiomas measuring less than 3 cm. In a retrospective comparison of outcomes of 198 adult patients who underwent either surgical resection or radiosurgery as initial treatment of their meningioma, both modalities had equivalent tumor control.[103] Tumor control rates with SRS are higher than 90% in most series, with complication rates less than 5%.[100,104]

There is a small group of patients in whom, despite multiple surgical resections and RT, the meningioma recurs. In these patients, medical therapy may be considered but is generally ineffective.[105] Sunitinib and bevacizumab are reportedly effective, but these data are derived from small reports.[106,107] Pasireotide may be helpful in those patients whose tumors express somatostatin receptors.[108]

Conclusion

Continued research into primary brain tumors is anticipated to reveal new insights from genomic, epigenomic, proteomic, and immunologic perspectives. Future editions of CNS tumor classification will provide even more diagnostic precision. Patients should be encouraged to participate in clinical trials. Current trials utilizing targeted molecular therapies, immunotherapies, and gene therapies provide hope and are underway. Increasingly these studies have correlative components to develop robust molecular markers which will enable better patient selection while preclinical and early clinical trials will increasingly explore tumor pharmacokinetics and pharmacodynamics to ensure that there is both adequate drug delivery and impact on the drug target. These concerted efforts are essential to achieve significant therapeutic advances.

Key references

The complete reference list can be found on Vital Source version of this title, see inside front cover.

1. Ostrom QT, Cioffi G, Gittleman H, et al. CBTRUS statistical report: primary brain and other central nervous system tumors diagnosed in the United States in 2012–2016. *Neuro-Oncology*. 2019;**21**(Supplement_5):v1–v100.
4. Marta GN, Murphy E, Chao S, et al. The incidence of second brain tumors related to cranial irradiation. *Exp Rev Anticancer Ther*. 2015;**15**(3):295–304.
7. Louis DN, Perry A, Reifenberger G, et al. The 2016 World Health Organization classification of tumors of the central nervous system: a summary. *Acta Neuropathol*. 2016;**131**(6):803–820.
8. Louis DN, Wesseling P, Aldape K, et al. cIMPACT-NOW update 6: new entity and diagnostic principle recommendations of the cIMPACT-Utrecht meeting on future CNS tumor classification and grading. *Brain Pathol*. 2020;**30**: 844–856.
9. Ellison DW, Aldape KD, Capper D, et al. cIMPACT-NOW Update 7: advancing the molecular classification of ependymal tumors. *Brain Pathol*. 2020. doi: 10.1111/bpa.12866.
16. Bailey S, Howman A, Wheatley K, et al. Diffuse intrinsic pontine glioma treated with prolonged temozolomide and radiotherapy--results of a United Kingdom phase II trial (CNS 2007 04). *Eur J Cancer*. 2013;**49**(18):3856–3862.
19. Maraka S, Janku F. BRAF alterations in primary brain tumors. *Discov Med*. 2018;**26**(141):51–60.
20. Wu J, Armstrong TS, Gilbert MR. Biology and management of ependymomas. *Neuro-Oncology*. 2016;**18**(7):902–913.
23. Englot DJ, Chang EF, Vecht CJ. Epilepsy and brain tumors. In: *Handbook of Clinical Neurology [Internet]*. Elsevier; 2016:267–285. https://linkinghub.elsevier.com/retrieve/pii/B9780128029978000165.
25. Smith-Cohn M, Chen Z, Peereboom D, et al. Maximizing function and quality of life of patients with glioblastoma after surgical resection: a review of current literature. *J Cancer Ther*. 2016;**07**(12):857–888.
26. Armstrong TS, Grant R, Gilbert MR, et al. Epilepsy in glioma patients: mechanisms, management, and impact of anticonvulsant therapy: table 1. *Neuro-Oncology*. 2016;**18**(6):779–789.
27. Giles AJ, Hutchinson M-KND, Sonnemann HM, et al. Dexamethasone-induced immunosuppression: mechanisms and implications for immunotherapy. *J Immunother Cancer*. 2018;**6**(1):51.
28. Lin RJ, Green DL, Shah GL. Therapeutic anticoagulation in patients with primary brain tumors or secondary brain metastasis. *The Oncol*. 2018;**23**(4):468–473.
31. Simpson JR, Horton J, Scott C, et al. Influence of location and extent of surgical resection on survival of patients with glioblastoma multiforme: results of three consecutive radiation therapy oncology group (RTOG) clinical trials. *Int J Radiat Oncol Biol Phys*. 1993;**26**(2):239–244.
32. Stummer W, Pichlmeier U, Meinel T, et al. Fluorescence-guided surgery with 5-aminolevulinic acid for resection of malignant glioma: a randomised controlled multicentre phase III trial. *Lancet Oncol*. 2006;**7**(5):392–401.
34. Ziu M, Kim BYS, Jiang W, et al. The role of radiation therapy in treatment of adults with newly diagnosed glioblastoma multiforme: a systematic review and evidence-based clinical practice guideline update. *J Neuro-Oncol*. 2020;**150**(2):215–267.
36. Walker MD, Alexander E, Hunt WE, et al. Evaluation of BCNU and/or radiotherapy in the treatment of anaplastic gliomas. A cooperative clinical trial. *J Neurosurg*. 1978;**49**(3):333–343.
37. Stupp R, Hegi ME, Mason WP, et al. Effects of radiotherapy with concomitant and adjuvant temozolomide versus radiotherapy alone on survival in glioblastoma in a randomised phase III study: 5-year analysis of the EORTC-NCIC trial. *Lancet Oncol*. 2009;**10**(5):459–466.
40. Merchant TE, Farr JB. Proton beam therapy: a fad or a new standard of care. *Curr Opin Pediatr*. 2014;**26**(1):3–8.
41. Smith-Cohn MA, Celiku O, Gilbert MR. Molecularly targeted clinical trials. *Neurosurg Clin N Am*. 2021. doi: 10.1016/j.nec.2020.12.002.
42. Grossman SA, Romo CG, Rudek MA, et al. Baseline requirements for novel agents being considered for Phase II/III brain cancer efficacy trials: conclusions from the adult brain tumor consortium's first workshop on CNS drug delivery. *Neuro-Oncology*. 2020. doi: 10.1093/neuonc/noaa142.
44. Hegi ME, Genbrugge E, Gorlia T, et al. *MGMT* promoter methylation cutoff with safety margin for selecting glioblastoma patients into trials omitting temozolomide: a pooled analysis of four clinical trials. *Clin Cancer Res*. 2019;**25**(6):1809–1816.
46. Balana C, Vaz MA, Sepúlveda JM, et al. A phase II randomized, multicenter, open-label trial of continuing adjuvant temozolomide beyond six cycles in patients with glioblastoma (GEINO 14-01). *Neuro-Oncology*. 2020. doi: 10.1093/neuonc/noaa107.
49. Malmström A, Grønberg BH, Marosi C, et al. Temozolomide versus standard 6-week radiotherapy versus hypofractionated radiotherapy in patients older than

49. 60 years with glioblastoma: the Nordic randomised, phase 3 trial. *Lancet Oncol.* 2012;**13**(9):916–926.

50. Perry JR, Laperriere N, O'Callaghan CJ, et al. Short-course radiation plus temozolomide in elderly patients with glioblastoma. *N Engl J Med.* 2017;**376**(11):1027–1037.

51. Wick W, Platten M, Meisner C, et al. Temozolomide chemotherapy alone versus radiotherapy alone for malignant astrocytoma in the elderly: the NOA-08 randomised, phase 3 trial. *Lancet Oncol.* 2012;**13**(7):707–715.

52. Stupp R, Taillibert S, Kanner A, et al. Effect of tumor-treating fields plus maintenance temozolomide vs maintenance temozolomide alone on survival in patients with glioblastoma: a randomized clinical trial. *JAMA.* 2017;**318**(23):2306.

54. Chinot OL, Wick W, Mason W, et al. Bevacizumab plus radiotherapy–temozolomide for newly diagnosed glioblastoma. *N Engl J Med.* 2014;**370**(8):709–722.

55. Gilbert MR, Dignam JJ, Armstrong TS, et al. A randomized trial of bevacizumab for newly diagnosed glioblastoma. *N Engl J Med.* 2014;**370**(8):699–708.

57. Wick W, Gorlia T, Bendszus M, et al. Lomustine and bevacizumab in progressive glioblastoma. *N Engl J Med.* 2017;**377**(20):1954–1963.

59. Han SJ, Yang I, Tihan T, et al. Primary gliosarcoma: key clinical and pathologic distinctions from glioblastoma with implications as a unique oncologic entity. *J Neuro-Oncol.* 2010;**96**(3):313–320.

68. Dhawan S, Patil CG, Chen C, et al. Early versus delayed postoperative radiotherapy for treatment of low-grade gliomas. *Cochrane Database Syst Rev.* 2020;**20**(1):CD009229.

72. Fisher BJ, Hu C, Macdonald DR, et al. Phase 2 study of temozolomide-based chemoradiation therapy for high-risk low-grade gliomas: preliminary results of radiation therapy oncology group 0424. *Int J Radiat Oncol Biol Phys.* 2015;**91**(3):497–504.

74. Cairncross G, Wang M, Shaw E, et al. Phase III trial of chemoradiotherapy for anaplastic oligodendroglioma: long-term results of RTOG 9402. *J Clin Oncol.* 2013;**31**(3):337–343.

75. van den Bent MJ, Brandes AA, Taphoorn MJB, et al. Adjuvant procarbazine, lomustine, and vincristine chemotherapy in newly diagnosed anaplastic oligodendroglioma: long-term follow-up of EORTC brain tumor group study 26951. *J Clin Oncol.* 2013;**31**(3):344–350.

80. Green RM, Cloughesy TF, Stupp R, et al. Bevacizumab for recurrent ependymoma. *Neurology.* 2009;**73**(20):1677–1680.

81. Gilbert ME, Yuan Y, Wani K, et al. A phase II study of dose-dense temozolomide and lapatinib for recurrent low-grade and anaplastic supratentorial, infratentorial, and spinal cord ependymoma. *Neuro-Oncology.* 2021;**23**(3):468–477.

82. Grommes C, DeAngelis LM. Primary CNS lymphoma. *J Clin Oncol.* 2017;**35**(21):2410–2418.

83. Batchelor TT. Primary central nervous system lymphoma. *Hematology.* 2016;**2016**(1):379–385.

84. Camilleri-Broët S, Martin A, Moreau A, et al. Primary central nervous system lymphomas in 72 immunocompetent patients: pathologic findings and clinical correlations. *Am J Clin Pathol.* 1998;**110**(5):607–612.

85. Chan C-C, Wallace DJ. Intraocular lymphoma: update on diagnosis and management. *Cancer Control.* 2004;**11**(5):285–295.

86. Holdhoff M, Wagner-Johnston N, Roschewski M. Systemic approach to recurrent primary CNS lymphoma: perspective on current and emerging treatment strategies. *OncoTargets Ther.* 2020;**13**:8323–8335.

87. Rubenstein JL, Hsi ED, Johnson JL, et al. Intensive chemotherapy and immunotherapy in patients with newly diagnosed primary CNS lymphoma: CALGB 50202 (Alliance 50202). *J Clin Oncol.* 2013;**31**(25):3061–3068.

88. Morris PG, Correa DD, Yahalom J, et al. Rituximab, methotrexate, procarbazine, and vincristine followed by consolidation reduced-dose whole-brain radiotherapy and cytarabine in newly diagnosed primary CNS lymphoma: final results and long-term outcome. *J Clin Oncol.* 2013;**31**(31):3971–3979.

89. Omuro A, Correa DD, DeAngelis LM, et al. R-MPV followed by high-dose chemotherapy with TBC and autologous stem-cell transplant for newly diagnosed primary CNS lymphoma. *Blood.* 2015;**125**(9):1403–1410.

90. Holdhoff M, Ambady P, Abdelaziz A, et al. High-dose methotrexate with or without rituximab in newly diagnosed primary CNS lymphoma. *Neurology.* 2014;**83**(3):235–239.

91. Thiel E, Korfel A, Martus P, et al. High-dose methotrexate with or without whole brain radiotherapy for primary CNS lymphoma (G-PCNSL-SG-1): a phase 3, randomised, non-inferiority trial. *Lancet Oncol.* 2010;**11**(11):1036–1047.

92. Saraf S, McCarthy BJ, Villano JL. Update on meningiomas. *Oncologist.* 2011;**16**(11):1604–1613.

93. Clark VE, Erson-Omay EZ, Serin A, et al. Genomic analysis of non-NF2 meningiomas reveals mutations in TRAF7, KLF4, AKT1, and SMO. *Science.* 2013;**339**(6123):1077–1080.

94. Brastianos PK, Horowitz PM, Santagata S, et al. Genomic sequencing of meningiomas identifies oncogenic SMO and AKT1 mutations. *Nat Genet.* 2013;**45**(3):285–289.

95. McCarthy BJ, Davis FG, Freels S, et al. Factors associated with survival in patients with meningioma. *J Neurosurg.* 1998;**88**(5):831–839.

96. Adlakha A, Rao K, Adlakha H, et al. Meningioma metastatic to the lung. *Mayo Clin Proc.* 1999;**74**(11):1129–1133.

97. Näslund O, Skoglund T, Farahmand D, et al. Indications and outcome in surgically treated asymptomatic meningiomas: a single-center case-control study. *Acta Neurochir.* 2020;**162**(9):2155–2163.

98. Regelsberger J, Hagel C, Emami P, et al. Secretory meningiomas: a benign subgroup causing life-threatening complications. *Neuro-Oncology.* 2009;**11**(6):819–824.

99. Huntoon K, Toland AMS, Dahiya S. Meningioma: a review of clinicopathological and molecular aspects. *Front Oncol.* 2020;**10**:579599.

100. Buerki RA, Horbinski CM, Kruser T, et al. An overview of meningiomas. *Future Oncol.* 2018;**14**(21):2161–2177.

105. Kaley T, Barani I, Chamberlain M, et al. Historical benchmarks for medical therapy trials in surgery- and radiation-refractory meningioma: a RANO review. *Neuro-Oncology.* 2014;**16**(6):829–840.

74 Neoplasms of the eye and orbit

Erica R. Alvarez, MD ■ Claudia M. Prospero Ponce, MD ■ Patricia Chevez-Barrios, MD, FCAP ■ Dan S. Gombos, MD, FACS

Overview

Cancers of the eye and orbit are associated with diverse pathological conditions, disease prognosis, and significant mortality. The survival rates vary among patients from different countries and have been reported to be significantly lower in those from developing countries compared to those noted in the United States owing mainly to delay in diagnosis associated with advanced-stage disease and unavailability of treatments. In this article, we provide an overview of the most common and rare ophthalmic malignancies that include ocular surface, external and adnexal diseases, and orbital and intraocular malignancies. We summarize the incidence, histopathology, risk factors, molecular alterations, clinical presentation, diagnostic evaluation, and therapeutic approaches for these diseases. We also describe the first-line and salvage treatments and their complications. These treatments depend on disease stage at presentation and include pathology-guided excision, Mohs microsurgery, chemo-reduction, chemoprophylaxis, adjuvant chemotherapy after enucleation, and/or neoadjuvant chemotherapy. Complications include symblepharon, scarring, and limbal stem cell deficiency while incomplete excision of eyelid tumors may result in recurrence of larger and more aggressive tumors. Currently, identification of genetic abnormalities identified in genomic profiling of patient tumors improves treatment selection. Early diagnosis and involvement of an ocular oncologist at the time of diagnosis will optimize the therapeutic management of patients with these diseases.

Introduction

Cancers of the eye cause significant disease morbidity and mortality. Starting with the ocular adnexa-eyelid, the most challenging tumor is sebaceous cell carcinoma (SBC) which can be easily misdiagnosed as eyelid inflammation and can rapidly spread to the entire orbit. The most common eyelid cancer is basal cell carcinoma which is associated with a favorable prognosis when complete surgical excision is feasible. For orbital and optic nerve tumors, imaging studies and tumor biopsies remain the cornerstone for accurate diagnosis and appropriate therapeutic management.

The prognosis of ocular malignancies is highly dependent on timely clinical suspicion, diagnosis, and complete surgical excision with possible chemotherapy and radiation. Referral to ocular oncologists to determine the appropriate management that may include multidisciplinary collaboration is essential. Scientific advancements in molecular alterations of patients with primary intraocular tumors, such as lymphoma, melanoma, and retinoblastoma (RB) tumors have led to patient-tailored treatment strategies. In this article, we review the most common neoplasms of the eye from an anatomical perspective: external, ocular surface, intraocular, and orbital and their therapeutic management.

External/adnexal disease

Basal cell carcinoma (BCC) is the most common eyelid malignancy. It affects men more frequently than women and typically presents at the age of 60 years.[1-3] Risk factors include ultraviolet (UV) sun exposure, lighter complexion, and immunosuppression.[4,5] BCC is related to Gorlin–Goltz syndrome and xeroderma pigmentosum.[6] BCC presents as an opalescent nodule with overlying telangiectatic vessels and central ulceration,[6,7] either pigmented or nonpigmented.[1] The disease is seen on the lower lid (>50%), medial canthus (30%), upper lid (15%), and lateral canthus (5%).[2,4,7]

The most common type is nodular disease, followed by nodulo-ulcerative, pigmented, cystic, and morpheaform (or infiltrative) disease.[1] Subtypes of BCC that demonstrate aggressive cellular behavior (such as infiltrative) portend higher recurrence and poorer prognosis.[2,7] Histology is characterized by medium-sized cells, that are basophilic and have scant cytoplasm forming prominent peripheral palisading, with mitosis and apoptosis. Morpheaform BCC, an uncommon variant in which tumor cells induce a proliferation of fibroblasts within the dermis, is characterized by small finger-like projections that extend into deep dermis allowing easy spread of the disease. The histological diagnosis of BCC is challenging as it can resemble trichoepithelioma, sebaceous, or squamous cell carcinoma (SCC).[8]

Mohs surgery or excision utilizing frozen or permanent pathology confirmation are associated with high curative rates.[9] Incomplete excision is associated with tumor recurrence that is often larger and more aggressive.[10] Treatment with carbon dioxide laser or cryotherapy[1] can lead to scarring and is reserved for small/superficial tumors only.[7] External beam radiotherapy (EBRT) combined with surgical excision or exenteration is considered for patients with highly aggressive BCC lesions with orbital invasion,[9] or for patients who cannot tolerate other treatments.[5] In addition, surface brachytherapy is useful in patients at risk for functional disability after surgical excision.[11-13] In recent years, vismodegib, a hedgehog inhibitor has demonstrated favorable results in both locally advanced and metastatic BCC.[5,6,14,15] Metastases from lesions in the lower lid or inner canthus may rarely occur.[2] Invasion of the orbit or sinuses should be considered on initial evaluation.[2,10] Physical examination to assess lymphadenopathy and fat-suppressed magnetic resonance imaging (MRI) or bone window computed tomography (CT) scan are used to determine orbital extension.[1,2] Due to the risk of recurrence, surveillance is recommended for a minimum of 5 years.[4,6]

SCC is the second most common eyelid cancer,[16] and it occurs mostly in men over 60 years; risk factors are UV sun exposure, radiation, and immunosuppression.[17-19] It affects the lower lid, medial canthus, upper lid, and lateral canthus.[9,18] The clinical presentation is characterized by a painless pearlescent plaque or elevated lesion with rolled edges but can also have overlying telangiectasia, ulceration, and scaling.[9,19] Metastatic disease develops via lymphatic dissemination along with hematogenous spread, leading to regional and distant disease.[18,20] Perineural involvement reported in 7–14% of cases, via cranial nerves II, III, IV, V, and VII may lead to orbital, retroorbital, and intracranial invasion.[9,17,19] Orbital invasion is treated with exenteration.[20]

Pathology-guided excision or Mohs microsurgery remains the standard of care.[19,21] Histopathology is characterized by keratinocytes with atypia, dyskeratosis, sometimes intercellular bridges, or anaplasia, high rate mitosis, pleomorphism, and loss of keratin/cellular bridges. Notably, keratoacanthoma is now identified as a SCC variant, presenting as a crater-shaped tumor with central keratinization and peripheral inflammation.[10] Immunohistochemical (IHC) staining with high-molecular-weight cytokeratins (HMWC), p63, p40 help confirm the diagnosis, especially in the metastatic setting.[8] Sentinel lymph node biopsy (SLNB) is vital to determine the stage of the disease and the need for adjuvant treatment.[16] The tumor/lymph node/metastasis (TNM) staging system includes biopsy of preauricular and submandibular lymph nodes and of distant organs. Patients with SCC should be staged according to the American Joint Committee on Cancer staging (AJCC) system.[22]

Complimentary radiation therapy (RT) is used after wide excision or exenteration to prevent recurrence. It is also used when perineural invasion and lymph node metastasis are present or palliatively for inoperable tumors.[13,17,19] RT is applied to the tumor bed along the nerve tracks back to the cavernous sinus and Meckel's cave.[18] In inoperable SCC tumors epidermal growth factor receptor (EGFR) inhibitor, such as erlotinib and the EGFR monoclonal antibody panitumumab, have been used as single agents and in combination therapy with RT.[6,23] The adverse events of EGFR-targeted therapies include skin rash, conjunctivitis, corneal erosion, and very unique eyebrow and eyelash overgrowth that spontaneously resolve upon medication discontinuation.[23] Patients with SCC require lifelong monitoring for local recurrence or perineural invasion.[18,21]

SBC is the third most common eyelid malignancy worldwide, with higher prevalence in Asia.[6] It typically presents in patients older than 70 years of age, and it affects men and women equally. SBC is often misdiagnosed as blepharoconjunctivitis or chalazion,[5,24] and it may appear as a diffuse or nodular eyelid thickening,[9,25] often in the upper eyelid where meibomian/Zeiss glands are denser compared to the lower lid.[25] Differentiating features of SBC include madarosis (loss of lashes) and treatment resistance, that are not present in blepharoconjunctivitis or chalazion.[10] SBC is associated with prior RT,[10] hereditary nonpolyposis colorectal cancer subtype—Muir Torre syndrome, and multiple sebaceous neoplasms with visceral malignancies that include colorectal and genitourinary cancers and breast cancer.[6,24,26,27] Delay in diagnosis may lead to local extension of SBC into the bulbar conjunctiva, orbit, or sinus and may allow the disease to metastasize to distant organs.[24,28]

High-risk histopathologic features include poorly differentiated tumor (anaplasia, pleomorphism, and high mitotic rate), perineural invasion, and pagetoid spread (independent spread of malignant cells to the epithelium)[10] which is pathognomonic.[5,6,9] SBC requires wide surgical margins of primary tumor, map biopsies of conjunctiva and pathologic examination to rule out additional cancer foci.[9,24,27] Oil Red O staining (only in fresh tissue), and IHC staining for adipophilin are used to confirm the diagnosis.[29] Surgical treatment guided by Mohs ensures adequate margins.[11,13] Conjunctival lesions require excision via no touch technique and cryotherapy.[6,9] Extensive orbital invasion is treated by orbital exenteration.[9,11,28,30] SLNB is recommended in SBC due to higher risk of regional and distant metastasis.[5,16] Adjuvant RT (EBRT or brachytherapy) has been shown to lower the rate of disease recurrence in stage T3 or higher SBC tumors.[6,11,27] RT is beneficial for tumors with aggressive histologic features such as perineural invasion or nodal metastasis at presentation, for tumors that are incompletely resected or for patients who are unfit for surgery.[5,9,13] Systemic chemotherapy is used for extensive nodal disease and distant metastases.[16,24,26] Pembrolizumab, a programmed cell death protein 1 (PD-1) inhibitor, may have antitumor activity in patients with SBC whose tumors have mismatch repair gene mutations. The use of pembrolizumab is investigational and additional studies are needed.[27] The disease usually recurs after 2 years. Lymph node metastasis (8–18%) and more distant metastases (3–8%) necessitate vigilant long-term follow-up.[6]

Eyelid melanoma (EM): Risk factors include UV exposure, both from sun and artificial tanning. EM is rare compared with other tumors such as BCC and SCC and accounts for <1% of all eyelid tumors.[6] EM staging is similar to that of cutaneous melanoma. Lymph node involvement is present in 11% of the cases and early resection is shown to be associated with longer survival.[6] Surgical excision is the primary treatment. Topical therapy, such as imiquimod (non-FDA approved), is reserved for small confined lesions or for the treatment of patients who are refusing surgery. Imiquimod has shown benefit in EM.[31] The Collaborative Skin Melanoma Group evaluated surgical intervention, most with excision margins of ≤5 mm, yielding 25% local recurrence. Most tumors had <1 mm Breslow thickness, whereas those with 2 mm thickness showed a higher rate of recurrence and progression to metastasis.[32]

Ocular surface neoplasms

Ocular surface squamous neoplasia (OSSN) represents a spectrum of diseases from cellular dysplasia to carcinoma in situ to SCC. It can be noninvasive or invasive. OSSN typically presents in Caucasians at the sixth to seventh decade and affects men more than women. In younger patients, it is associated with xeroderma pigmentosum and human immunodeficiency virus (HIV).[33–35] Risk factors include exposure to UV light, smoking, chronic surface irritation, vitamin A deficiency, mutations or deletions of p53, and immunosuppression. OSSN is associated with human papillomavirus (HPV) 16 & 18,[33,36,37] and latitude of 16° South.[8,17,20,21]

OSSN is the most common nonpigmented tumor of the ocular surface[38,39] and arises from limbal stem cells mainly at intrapalpebral cornea and bulbar conjunctiva.[34] Fleshy conjunctival lesions can be gelatinous, leukoplakic, or papillary and they present as flat, raised, localized, or diffuse with large feeder vessels.[29,34] Findings suggestive of invasion are neovascularization of the iris/cornea, tumor cells in the anterior chamber (iridocyclitis), or secondary glaucoma from involvement of the trabecular meshwork.[36,40] Clinical diagnosis can be supported by staining devitalized epithelial cells with rose bengal, lissamine green, methylene blue, and fluorescein.[29,41]

Confocal microscopy is a noninvasive method to identify pleomorphic epithelial cells, prominent bright nucleoli, and a demarcation line between normal and neoplastic changes, while monitoring treatment response.[34,38,42] Drawbacks include limited field of view, artifacts, difficulty with reproducibility, and require equipment and training.[42] Cytology does not require a biopsy, therefore, protecting limbal stem cell integrity, but it requires adequate sampling/processing and cytopathology expertise.[34,43]

A biopsy is required to evaluate local invasion of corneal/conjunctival SCC; however, distant metastasis may also occur. OSSN is categorized by the degree of epithelial dysplasia. Carcinoma *in situ* displays mitotically active, pleomorphic, keratinizing, epithelial cells with intercellular bridges confined to the epithelium only (a precursor of SCC). Once the basement membrane has lost its integrity, "stromal invasion" of the tumor is reported as SCC. IHC staining for HMWC and p63 is helpful in diagnosing poorly differentiated carcinomas.[8]

Anterior segment optical coherence tomography (OCT) is a noninvasive method that is used to evaluate epithelial compromise, to delineate equivocal lesions and to monitor treatment response, coined an "optical biopsy."[41,44,45] High frequency ultrasound is used to assess tumor thickness, internal reflectivity, and scleral or deeper orbital invasion.[37,40]

Topical chemotherapy is now recommended by some ophthalmologists as a primary treatment modality for OSSN,[38,46] because it can reduce tumor bulk prior to surgical excision, prevent tumor recurrence postoperatively, and help manage large multifocal disease, recurrent lesions, and microscopic disease.[34] Therapeutic agents used for topical chemotherapy include interferon alpha-2b, 5-fluorouracil, and mitomycin C. They are delivered as intralesional injections or ophthalmic drops.[41] Various concentrations and regimens have been reported and they are determined according to patient characteristics, tolerance, and disease status (first-line or at recurrence).[6,34,35,37–39,46–48] Excision is performed via a "no-touch technique" alcohol epitheliectomy, and surgical edge cryotherapy (double freeze thaw) obtaining 2–4 mm clear margins.[1,34,36,48] Complications associated with surgery include symblepharon, scarring, and limbal stem cell deficiency.[46] If corneoscleral invasion is present, a globe-sparing deep lamellar keratoplasty/sclerokeratoplasty is advised or plaque brachytherapy can be used, as it has shown efficacy. If intraocular invasion is present, a modified enucleation is recommended and if orbital extension is found, exenteration with or without adjuvant EBRT is warranted.[33,36,48]

Conjunctival melanoma (CM) typically arises from a precursor lesion such as primary acquired melanosis (PAM) [World Health Organization (WHO) classification—intraepithelial melanocytic lesion—high grade (IML-HG)] (75%), novel melanoma (5%), and nevi (20%).[48–51] CM presents as an elevated pigmented mass often found on the interpalpebral bulbar conjunctiva and less commonly in the fornices and palpebral conjunctiva.[51] The forniceal location of CM is associated with a higher suspicion for malignancy. Non-pigmented tumors are seen in 20% of the cases.[8] CM commonly presents with metastatic disease (distant and regionally) at the time of initial diagnosis.[52] CM activation by the MAPK pathway via proto-oncogene B-Raf (*BRAF*) (27–50%), NRAS proto-oncogene (*NRAS*) (18–20%), and proto-oncogene c-KIT (*KIT*) (<7%) mutations[53]; or by neurofibromatosis 1 (*NF1*) mutation are seen in CM.[49,54,55] *BRAF* 10q26.3 deletion has been correlated with increased metastatic risk.[55] Melanoma cells are spindle cells with polyhedral or epithelioid shape and have prominent nucleoli. IHC staining for S100, Melan-A, SOX10, HMB-45 (melanocytic markers) is used. Ki-67 staining demonstrates a high proliferation index (>5%).[8]

Excision is performed *via* no touch technique.[52] Large extensive disease may require enucleation or even exenteration, but this radical surgery is not associated with improved overall survival.[48,53] Local recurrence occurs in approximately 50% of patients at 5 years and metastatic disease is noted in 30% of patients at 10 years.[52,53,55,56] SLNB sensitivity in CM remains lower and is less predictive than other pathologies. Clinically confounding distant metastatic disease is noted in the presence of negative regional lymph nodes.[51,53] SLNB is paramount, given that micro-metastatic disease is identified in nearly one-fifth of cases. Micro-metastatic disease is associated with large and histologically aggressive tumors.[57] Proper excision with cryotherapy, no touch technique, and tumor-free margins can prevent tumor recurrence, metastasis, and death.[48]

Adjuvant treatment (topical chemotherapy, or RT) is advantageous in incomplete excisions or extensive tumor.[38] Mitomycin C has the longest and most favorable track record as ophthalmic chemotherapy for CM, while interferon alpha-2b has shown early promise.[51,54] Brachytherapy shows favorable local tumor control and decreased radiation sequalae compared with EBRT. However, EBRT remains useful for more widespread tumors.[38,52] BRAF inhibitors have shown promise in cutaneous metastatic melanoma and are associated with improved overall survival rates; however, they are not FDA-approved for CM.[38,55] In a literature review, the use of off-label BRAF or BRAF/mitogen-activated protein kinase (MEK) inhibitors was used in patients with CM induced favorable responses that ranged from local tumor control (that allowed additional surgical excision) to complete tumor control.[58] Prospective clinical trials are required to confirm this data. Checkpoint inhibitors (pembrolizumab, or nivolumab) have demonstrated favorable responses in advanced metastatic CM not amenable to surgery.[50]

Intraocular neoplasms

Uveal melanoma (UM) is the most common primary ocular cancer in adults, and typically presents after 60 years of age, without gender predilection.[59,60] Patients with nevus of ota and dysplastic nevus syndrome have a higher incidence of UM. Fair complexion and lighter colored irises are risk factors for UM, but UV exposure is not a risk factor.[60] UM is common in Caucasians, closely followed by Hispanics, with a lower incidence reported in Asians, Native Americans, Pacific Islanders, and African Americans.[52]

UM can arise from choroid, iris, and ciliary body. UM of the ciliary body is associated with poor prognosis. Pathologic staging and classification can be clinical or pathologic. Staging by size and location is directly proportional to the risk of metastasis (Table 1). Compared with UM classified as AJCC stage 1, the rate of metastasis and/or death was three times higher for stage 2, and 9 to 10 times higher for stage 3 UM. This rate could not be assessed for stage 4 due to lack of follow-up[22,61] (Table 2). Tumors are classified from lower to higher risk as Class 1A, Class 1B, and Class 2.

The therapeutic management of UM includes surgical excision, laser, radiation, adjuvant therapy, and immunotherapy. Enucleation is the treatment of choice for very large UM, not amenable to other eye-sparing therapies. Transpupillary thermotherapy (TTT) is not used any longer as a primary treatment alone due to high recurrence rate (up to 30%). TTT is still used as a complimentary treatment with plaque brachytherapy. Radiotherapy is the preferred treatment modality and includes brachytherapy, proton beam therapy, and stereotactic radiotherapy. Proton beam therapy employs charged particles that yield ionizing radiation, bypassing external tissues, and delivers high-dose targeted radiation to the tumor, minimizing collateral damage.[60] Stereotactic RT uses gamma knife or cyberknife to deliver multidirectional radiation while protecting surrounding structures.[62] In a prospective randomized trial (Collaborative Ocular Melanoma Study, COMS) in patients with medium-size UM, no difference in overall survival was found between plaque brachytherapy and enucleation.[63] These results generated a shift in the treatment paradigm for UM, favoring brachytherapy for small and medium tumors that allow

Table 1 AJCC uveal melanoma tumor classification per size.

AJCC classification of posterior Uveal Melanoma (choroid, ciliary body) Thickness in mm							
>15.0	4	4	4	4	4	4	4
12.1–15.0	3	3	3	3	3	4	4
9.1–12.0	3	3	3	3	3	3	4
6.1–9.0	2	2	2	2	3	3	4
3.1–6.0	1	1	1	2	2	3	4
<3.0	1	1	1	1	2	2	4
Either pathological (enucleation) or clinical (US) measurements	<3.0	3.1–6.0	6.1–9.0	9.1–12.0	12.1–15.0	15.1–18.0	>18.0
	Largest basal diameter in mm						

Table 2 Uveal melanoma 10-year survival percentage per tumor AJCC 8th edition staging.

Uveal Melanoma AJCC 8th edition staging[a]				
1a	N0	M0	I	94%
T1b-d	N0	M0	IIA	84%
T2a	N0	M0	IIA	
T2b	N0	M0	IIB	70%
T3a	N0	M0	IIB	
T2c-d	N0	M0	IIIA	60%
T3b-c	N0	M0	IIIA	
T4a	N0	M0	IIIA	
T3d	N0	M0	IIIB	50%
T4b-c	N0	M0	IIIB	
T4d-e	N0	M0	IIIC	NA
Any T	N1	M0	IV	
Any T	Any N	M1a	IV	

10-year survival

Abbreviations: N, lymph node; M, metastasis; I–IV staging.
[a]T = Size (see Table 1).

for eye sparing and in some cases, vision sparing treatment.[59,60] However, patients treated with RT should be monitored for radiation-induced complications such as cataract, retinopathy, optic neuropathy, and neovascular glaucoma.[60]

Fine needle aspiration to obtain tissue for genomic analysis has become the standard diagnostic test. GNAQ and GNA11 gene mutations and amplifications (potential drivers of MAPK activation) are often identified in tumor molecular analysis.[59] Other abnormalities include monosomy 3 and 6p gain. Monosomy 3 is associated with poor prognosis, whereas 6p gain alterations are associated with favorable outcomes. The genomic profile of UM is different from cutaneous melanoma that is often linked to BRCA1-associated protein-1 (BAP1) inactivating mutations, and it may confer predisposition for the development of UM later in life. In addition, RNA-based gene expression profiling is used to categorize tumors based on risk of metastasis to other tissues over time. However, neither RNA nor DNA-based genetic testing can determine whether the tissue sample is derived from the tumor or from the adjacent tissue and therefore a rapid on-site cytologic evaluation is recommended by some investigators to determine that adequate tumor cells are present. The interval of screening for metastases is determined by the individual patient's unique genetic profile. UM metastasizes to the liver, lung, and bone. Surveillance of UM includes ultrasound and/or MRI of the liver. High-risk patients should be screened for metastases every 3–6 months for the first 5 years, and every 6–12 months afterward.[59]

UM metastasizes to other organs in approximately 50% of patients.[60] Tumor characteristics that favor metastatic spread include large tumors, epithelioid cell predominance, ciliary body involvement, extraocular spread, monosomy 3, 8q gain, RNA class 2, and BAP-1 mutation.[60] Treatment of liver metastases includes liver resection, radiofrequency ablation, hepatic artery chemoembolization, and hepatic arterial infusion of chemotherapy. However, none of these treatments were shown to be associated with survival benefit.

Metastatic UM is highly resistant to systemic single-agent and combination chemotherapy; yielding response rates of <1%.[59] Checkpoint inhibitors and PDL-1 inhibitors have demonstrated limited clinical benefit in the metastatic setting. MEK inhibitors have shown early promising results, but additional studies are needed. The MET-inhibitor crizotinib is undergoing clinical testing as an adjuvant prophylactic treatment in patients whose genetic profile is associated with high risk for developing metastatic disease.

Retinoblastoma (RB) is the most common primary intraocular malignant tumor in children.[8] Approximately 8000 new cases are diagnosed annually worldwide. The disease is often diagnosed before the age of 5 years and the highest incidence is reported in Africa, India, and in areas of low socioeconomic status.

RB presents as leukocoria (white pupil), ocular deviation (esotropia, exotropia), glaucoma, heterochromia, iritis, pseudohypopyon, or spontaneous hyphema. The differential diagnosis includes retinocytoma, medulloepithelioma, Coats disease, and ocular toxocariasis. Children may present with vitreous hemorrhage, intraocular mass, hyphema/hypopyon, or retinal detachment without an apparent tumor. Vitrectomy/vitreous tap should be avoided to prevent iatrogenic extraocular extension. Clinically, RB presents as a nonpigmented, tan-white mass that extends into subretinal space often with retinal detachment (exophytic), or as a fungating tumor that extends toward the vitreous cavity (endophytic). Three types of vitreous seeds are noted and include spheres (compact viable tumor cells), dust (scattered individual tumor cells), and clouds (necrotic material). Tumor seed identification is critical because spheres, namely "translucent centers" confer high risk for recurrence and clouds show relative resistance to treatment.[64] If orbit involvement is suspected, MRI of the orbits is required.

RB is histologically characterized by small blue tumor cells, scant cytoplasm, and a pleomorphic nucleus with neuroendocrine type chromatin forming rosettes (Homer Wright and Flexner–Winterseiner) or fleurettes (photoreceptor differentiation). Rosettes are more common in younger children. RB has central tumor vessels, surrounded by viable cells, adjacent to geographic necrosis. The rapid turnover of tumor cells results in tumor necrosis and calcification; and basophilic DNA deposits are occasionally noted in vessel walls. Exophytic tumors are associated with retinal detachment and increased choroidal invasion, while endophytic growth yields vitreous seeds and optic nerve invasion.[8,22] Intracranial recurrence extends from the nerve. IHC

Table 3 Comparison table for Retinoblastoma: Resse–Ellsworth versus International Classification for Retinoblastoma.

Reese–Ellsworth scheme for intraocular retinoblastoma		Prognosis		International classification for retinoblastoma
a. Solitary tumor <4DD at or behind the equator b. Multiple tumors, none >4DD, all at or behind the equator	I	Very favorable	A	Rb ≤ 3 mm (basal dimension or thickness)
a. Solitary tumor, 4-10DD, at or behind the equator b. Multiple tumors, 4-10DD, behind the equator	II	Favorable	B	Rb > 3 mm or: – Macular Rb (≤3 mm to foveola) – Juxtapapillary Rb(≤1.5 mm to optic nerve) – Subretinal fluid (≤3 mm from margin)
a. Any lesion anterior to the equator b. Solitary tumors > 10DD behind the equator	III	Doubtful	C	Rb with seeds: – Subretinal ≤3 mm – Vitreous ≤3 mm – Both subretinal and vitreous seeds ≤3 mm
a. Multiple tumors, some >10DD b. Any lesion extending anteriorly to the ora serrata	IV	Unfavorable	D	Rb with seeds: – Subretinal >3 mm – Vitreous >3 mm – Both subretinal and vitreous seeds >3 mm
a. Massive tumors involving over half the retina b. Vitreous seeding	V	Very unfavorable	E	Extensive Rb > 50% of globe or: – Neovascular glaucoma – Opaque media from vitreous hemorrhage (anterior chamber, vitreous, or subretinal space) – Invasion of postlaminar optic nerve, choroid (>2 mm), sclera, orbit, or anterior chamber – Tumor touching lens – Diffuse infiltrating tumor – Phthisis or prephthisis

is negative for RB1 protein in approximately 85% of tumors and positive for synaptophysin.

Prior classification schemes, such as the Reese–Ellsworth or International Classification of Retinoblastoma (ICRB), stratified tumors according to their size and location (Table 3).[65] The new TNM classification system is a universally accepted validation that correlates with prognosis (Table 4). It utilizes clinical and pathological staging that incorporates tumor size and extraocular extension, lymph node involvement, metastatic disease, and hereditary traits.[22] The treatment of RB is selected based on tumor classification, genetic predisposition, and access to drugs (Table 5).[66]

Germline or somatic mutations in the *RB1* gene or less frequently amplification of the N-myc proto-oncogene protein (*MYCN*) are identified in RB.[8,51] The *RB1* tumor suppression gene (13q14.2) is a result of the "two-hit" oncogenic process, where the "first-hit" is either sporadic/somatic or germline. Germline *RB1* tumors present at an earlier age (~12 mo), are frequently bilateral and multifocal, and are associated with extraocular tumors (i.e., neuroblastic or pineal, etc.).[8,67,68] In somatic mutations, the first and second hit occur after the germ cell division and they appear at the age of 2 years as unilateral tumors.

Genetic testing of all patients is necessary for accurate genetic counseling. Germline mutations occur in 40% of patients. *RB1* autosomal dominant mutations have a 50% chance of passing the mutation to the offspring. If parents carry the mutation, the next sibling has a risk of 45% of developing RB tumor because the tumor has a 95% penetrance. Approximately 60% of tumors are sporadic or unilateral cases. Retinocytomas that carry an *RB1* gene mutation require an additional mutation to manifest the tumor.[8] The AJCC 8th edition included genetic/hereditary status to TNM classification for prognostication with "H1-hereditary retinoblastoma" conferring a risk for secondary tumors.[22] Molecular analysis for *RB1* mutations can be performed using tumor tissue or peripheral blood (cell-free DNA analysis).

Extraocular extension generally occurs when diagnosis is delayed, or surgical intervention is inappropriate (i.e., intravitreal surgery). Late-stage tumors (extraocular extension, choroidal, lamina cribrosa/optic nerve involvement) are associated with a high risk for metastases and their enucleation should be followed by adjuvant chemotherapy. Cerebrospinal fluid studies are helpful in metastatic evaluation. The Children's Oncology Group (COG) reported that massive uveal invasion (>3 mm in maximum dimension) and post lamina cribrosa optic nerve invasion are associated with poor prognosis. Tumor anaplasia has been described as a risk factor for metastasis.[8] Attempts to salvage tumor-eyes with high-risk features (older age, delay in enucleation, bilateral advanced intraocular RB group D/E and advanced TNM group) are associated with high risk for extraocular disease and early metastases.

Early diagnosis and treatment are associated with favorable prognosis. For instance, small tumors confined to the eye have a cure rate of >97%.[51,67] Although the 5-year survival rate in the United States is >95%, the survival rates in developing countries range from 30% to 50% due to delay in diagnosis leading to advanced metastatic disease, and limited access to treatment. Currently, the overall survival rates in patients with RB are improving as new resources for diagnosis and treatment are becoming available to patients. The One RB World initiative (www.1rbw.org) guides patients to treatment centers. ECancerCareRB (eCCRB) is a shared database among RB centers. The Disease-specific, electronic Patient Illustrated Clinical Timeline (DePICT) provides patient education and care resources.[68]

Primary vitreoretinal lymphoma (PVRL) is a high-grade lymphoma arising from the retina and vitreous, and it is considered a *masquerader* since it can present as many entities that include uveitis, vasculitis, retinal infiltrate, and glaucoma. Clinical symptoms include blurry vision, floaters, and contrast loss; as well as altered mental status, headache, and seizures,

Table 4 Retinoblastoma Clinical tumor node metastasis clinical and pathological classification and staging by AJCC 8th edition.

Retinoblastoma clinical tumor node metastasis (c, clinical; p, pathological)					
cTX		Unknown evidence of intraocular tumor	pTX		Unknown evidence of intraocular tumor
cT0		No evidence of intraocular tumour	pT0		No evidence of intraocular tumor
cT1		Intraocular tumor(s) with sub-retinal fluid ≤ 5mm from the base of any tumor	pT1		Intraocular tumor(s) without any local invasion, focal choroidal invasion, or pre- or intralaminar involvement of the optic nerve head
	cT1a	Tumors ≤ 3mm and further than 1.5 mm from the disc and fovea	pT2		Intraocular tumor(s) with local invasion
	cT1b	Tumors > 3 mm or closer than 1.5 mm to the disc and fovea		pT2a	Concomitant focal choroidal invasion and pre- or intralaminar involvement of the optic nerve head
cT2		Intraocular tumour(s) with retinal detachment, vitreous seeding, or subretinal seeding		pT2b	Tumor invasion of stroma of iris or trabecular meshwork or Schlemm's canal
	cT2a	Subretinal fluid > 5 mm from the base of any tumor	pT3		Intraocular tumor(s) with significant local invasion
	cT2b	Tumors with vitreous seeding and/or subretinal seeding		pT3a	Massive choroidal invasion (>3 mm in largest diameter, or multiple foci of focal choroidal involvement totaling >3 mm, or any full-thickness choroidal involvement)
cT3		Advanced intraocular tumor(s)		pT3b	Retrolaminar invasion of the optic nerve head, not involving the transected end of the optic nerve
	cT3a	Phthisis or prephthisis bulbi		pT3c	Any partial-thickness involvement of the sclera within the inner two-thirds
	cT3b	Tumor invasion of the pars plana, ciliary body, lens, zonules, iris, or anterior chamber		pT3d	Full-thickness invasion into the outer third of the sclera or invasion into or around emissary channels
	cT3c	Raised intraocular pressure with neovascularization and/or buphthalmos	pT4		Evidence of extraocular tumor: tumor at the transected end of the optic nerve, tumor in the meningeal spaces around the optic nerve, full-thickness invasion of the sclera with invasion of the episclera, adjacent adipose tissue, extraocular muscle, bone, conjunctiva, or eyelids
	cT3d	Hyphema and/or massive vitreous hemorrhage			
	cT3e	Aseptic orbital cellulitis			
cT4		Extraocular tumor(s) involving the orbit, including the optic nerve			
	cT4a	Radiological evidence of retrobulbar optic nerve involvement or thickening of the optic nerve or involvement of the orbital tissues			
	cT4b	Extraocular tumor clinically evident with proptosis and orbital mass			

Staging

Clinical TNM			H	S
cT1,cT2,cT3	cN0	cM0	Any H	I
cT4a	cN0	cM0	Any H	II
cT4b	cN0	cM0	Any H	III
Any T	cN1	cM0	Any H	III
Any T	Any N	cM1 or pM1	Any H	IV

N1= Preauricular, submandibular, cervical.

M1= Distant metastasis without microscopic confirmation involving distant site (bone marrow, liver, on clinical or radiologic test) or CNS (other than pineoblastoma; on radiologic image)

H= Hereditary. Bilateral Rb, trilateral Rb, family h/o Rb, molecular test of RB1 gene mutation

S= Stage

Pathological TNM			H	S
pT1,pT2, pT3	pN0	cM0	Any H	I
pT4	pN0	cM0	Any H	II
Any T	pN1	cM0	Any H	III
Any T	Any N	cM1 or pM1	Any H	IV

N1 = Regional lymph node.

M1 = Distant metastasis with histopathologic confirmation involving any organ (bone marrow, liver, other) or CSF/brain parenchyma

H = Hereditary. Bilateral Rb, trilateral Rb, family h/o Rb, molecular test of RB1 gene mutation

S = Stage

Table 5 Retinoblastoma treatment paradigm.

Disease stage or presentation	Treatment options
Naïve tumor ("primary treatment")	1. Chemoreduction (Group B–D) 2. Chemoprophylaxis (anterior chamber- scleral- choroidal- optic nerve involvement) 3. Adjuvant chemo after enucleation (extrascleral- optic nerve involvement) 4. Neoadjuvant chemo (orbital- extraorbital involvement)
Eye saving treatment ("salvage therapy")	1. Chemoreduction (Group B–D) 2. Chemoprophylaxis (anterior chamber- scleral-choroidal- optic nerve involvement) 3. Adjuvant chemo after enucleation (extrascleral- optic nerve involvement) 4. Neoadjuvant chemo (orbital- extraorbital involvement)

Intraocular disease only	1. Enucleation: tumors group D, E (cT3-4 TNMH). Most commonly used worldwide. A long optic nerve sample is required to identify tumor extension. If high risk histopathological features are found adjuvant therapy – Intravenous chemotherapy (IVC) is recommended to avoid metastasis. Prosthetic eye placement contributes to quality of life and psychological well-being.
	2. Intravenous chemotherapy (IVC) with focal therapy (which includes laser therapy, or cryotherapy)
	3. Intra-arterial chemotherapy (IAC) with focal therapy
	4. Intravitreal chemotherapy
	5. Focal therapy, usually as adjuvant therapy:
	  a. Laser photocoagulation: <2 mm RB, isolated to posterior equator.
	  b. Thermotherapy: <3 mm RB 42°–60°, coagulation threshold.
	  c. Cryotherapy: <3 mm RB, 42°–60°, freezes the tumor.
	  d. Chemothermotherapy: >15 mm diameter. "transpupillary thermotherapy and chemotherapy"
	6. Radiation
	- Types of radiation treatment that release energy both before and after they hit the intended target.
	  a. External Beam Radiation Therapy (EBRT)[a]: given 5 days a week for several weeks.
	  b. Intensity modulated radiation therapy (IMRT): limit the dose while reducing side effects
	  c. Brachytherapy (BT)
	- Type of radiation that releases its energy after traveling a certain distance.
	  a. Proton Beam (PB)

[a]EBRT previously first line therapy until an increase in secondary cancers were noted.

if the central nervous system (CNS) is involved (most common, frontal lobe).[8,69,70] The disease is frequently associated with CNS lymphoma, either concurrent (~15% at initial PVRL diagnosis)[8] or consecutive (42–92%) 8–29 months later.[70] Risk factors associated with PVRL include HIV and Epstein–Barr virus (EBV) infection. Its incidence 0.46/100,000 people and it often presents in patients >60 years of age with no gender predilection.

Vitreoretinal biopsy is challenging due to fragility of lymphoma cells upon removal. In some cases, lymphoma cells can be confined exclusively to the subretinal space and a deep retinal biopsy is required to make the diagnosis. The diagnosis of PVRL is made by cytologic, morphologic, IHC, flow cytometric studies and with the use of elevated cytokine levels (high IL-10/IL-6 ratio) and molecular testing.[71] Alterations identified by polymerase chain reaction (PCR) include rearrangements in *IGH/BCL2* – t (14;18) translocation, gains on chromosomes 1q, 18q, and 19q and frequent losses on 6q. These alterations are also frequently identified in PCNSL. *MYD88* mutation is seen in ~70% of PRVL without CNS involvement. PVRL microRNA (miRNA) and epigenetic alterations are also found and include downregulation of miR-155 and upregulation of miR-92, miR-19b, and miR-21.[69] Next-generation sequencing (NGS) has shown gain of function mutations in *MYD88*, chromosome 19q loss in *CDKN2A* and *AKT1*. PVRL aggressiveness is attributed to extranodal non-Hodgkin mainly B-cells that arise from postgerminal center cells. MRI brain and lumbar puncture are needed to assess the CNS involvement.

Treatment includes local radiation if confined to eye, whole-brain radiation (WBRT) with or without systemic chemotherapy if CNS disease is present,[72] intravitreal methotrexate and/or rituximab,[69,70] intravitreal melphalan,[73] systemic methotrexate, myeloablative chemotherapy, and immunotherapy. The role of preventive WBRT is controversial.[69,70] The prognosis of PVRL is poor and the overall survival is approximately 5 years.[69]

Orbital neoplasms

Rhabdomyosarcoma (RMS) is the most common mesenchymal malignancy in children, manifesting in the orbit (10%)[74,75] or conjunctiva/caruncle (12%)[8] and represents approximately 4.5% of cranial sarcomas in children.[75] Clinically, RMS is seen as a pink-orange vascular mass that is fast growing within 2 months.

The prognosis of RMS depends on histology and molecular profiling. Botryoid RMS is associated with the most favorable prognosis, followed by the embryonal RMS that represents >90% of cases and has less favorable prognosis.[75] Pleomorphic RMS has intermediate prognosis and it typically spares the periorbital area.[8] Alveolar RMS with translocations of *PAX* and *FOX01* genes is associated with poor prognosis. Embryonal RMS is characterized by tumor cells that are spindle-shaped with hyperchromatic nuclei and with cytoplasmic processes that resemble a *tadpole*. Alveolar RMS is characterized by small blue cell tumors with nests separated by fibrovascular septa. IHC studies demonstrate positivity for MYOD1 (myoblast determination protein 1) that is specific and MYF4 (myogenin).

The initial treatment of RMS includes chemotherapy typically followed by EBRT.[76] The most commonly used chemotherapeutic agents are vincristine and cyclophosphamide, but dactinomycin, ifosfamide, and etoposide have also been used. Treatment with tyrosine kinase inhibitors has also been reported. Combination surgery and systemic therapy with and without RT has been associated with improved overall survival in patients with intermediate-risk (at 5 years, 70%) and low-risk (at 5 years, 90%) RMS, specifically in combination with IGF1R and mTOR inhibitors. However, the 5-year overall survival for the high-risk RMS was <40%.[77,78] Salvage therapy is recommended for recurrent disease and includes RT and surgery, often exenteration.[79] Salvage therapy after EBRT in patients with orbital RMS includes ablative surgery, mold technique brachytherapy, and reconstruction.[78]

Ocular adnexal lymphoma (OAL) is a type of lymphoma that includes the orbit, conjunctiva, lacrimal gland, drainage system, and other surrounding tissues such as lymph nodes (submandibular, preauricular, cervical). The classification of OAL is addressed in AJCC 8th edition[22] that excludes secondary lymphomatous involvement. The Ann Arbor system is preferred for addressing nodal lymphomas but not OAL. Children rarely develop OAL, but this disease is common in adults and elderly and has a slight female predominance.[1,8] Risk factors include autoimmune disease and HIV.[8] The presentation of OAL varies by location and includes skin redness and elevation, a painless, pink, slow-growing salmon patch of conjunctiva or fornix, and exophthalmos or epiphora. Clinically, it can present unilaterally (>70%) or bilaterally (10–20%). Bilateral disease is associated with extraocular disease.[80] Primary non-Hodgkin extranodal marginal zone mucosa-associated lymphoid tissue lymphoma (MALT) is the most common OAL (60%) followed by follicular (10%), diffuse large B-cell lymphomas (DLBCL) (~9%),[8] mantle cell lymphoma (MCL), and lymphoplasmacytic lymphoma (LPL).[22] The most common disease site if the eyelid (tarsal conjunctiva), followed by orbit and bulbar conjunctiva. The primary conjunctival lymphoma accounts for 2% of extranodal lymphomas and approximately 30% of OAL.[8] Laboratory tests include complete blood count, lactate dehydrogenase levels, liver enzymes, bone marrow (BM) aspiration, and biopsy. MRI or CT imaging and PET scans are required to assess tissue and bone involvement and radiographic bowing of bone is pathognomonic.[22] Definitive diagnosis is via histological assessment, IHC, and genomic analysis.

Treatment is determined by the TNM staging and type of lymphoma. For localized OAL, surgery, RT, and cryotherapy are preferred. As lymphoma is highly radiosensitive, RT is associated with favorable results. The use of 30 Gy hyperfractionated RT for patients with MALT OAL induces total tumor control in >80% of patients for >5 years.[1] Systemic chemotherapy with B-cell targeted therapy[8] or CHOP (Cytoxan, Hydroxyrubicin [Adriamycin], Oncovin [Vincristine], and Prednisone) are preferred for aggressive OAL. MALT OAL is associated with the most favorable prognosis (5-year survival rate, 97%) followed by follicular, DLBCL and mantle cell OAL.[1,80] Evaluation of prognostic indexes per tumor type (i.e., DLBCL, follicular, or mantle cell) is recommended.[22]

Adenoid cystic carcinoma (ACC) is the most common lacrimal gland malignancy, with bimodal distribution in teenagers and adults (≥40 years of age). It has no gender, race, or geographic predisposition. ACC comprises 20% of lacrimal gland epithelial tumors and 2–16% of malignancies of the orbit. The time from occurrence to presentation of symptoms is approximately 7 months.[8,81] Clinically, ACC is seen as a progressive painful proptosis with displacement medially and inferiorly. CT imaging shows bone destruction/sclerosis while MRI shows hyperintense, well-demarcated tumors with calcification and moderate enhancement with contrast. If necrosis is present, increased tumor signal intensity is noted. A-wave ultrasonography demonstrates medium-to-high internal reflectivity.[81]

Histology demonstrates several patterns, including the "swiss cheese" pattern that shows different sizes of neoplastic glands, myoepithelial and ductal luminal cells with high nuclear-cytoplasmic ratio, the tubular, sclerosing, comedocarcinomatous, and solid type patterns. The later pattern is associated with a high rate of mitosis and poor prognosis.[8,82] Intraoperative sections are evaluated with caution as pleomorphic adenoma can resemble ACC in frozen sections.[83] Perineural invasion is typical in ACC. Cells are zinc finger protein PLAG1 (pLAG1)-negative. Tumor analysis may show MYB-NFIB fusion gene via chromosome 6q loss and genetic mutations in the survivin (*BIRC5*), *KRAS*, *NRAS*, or *MET* genes. Tumor staging is used to determine prognosis and T3 tumors or above are associated with poor prognosis.[8,81,82,84]

Treatment is generally exenteration.[8,84] Eye salvage is *via* tumor-only resection followed by adjuvant therapy that includes RT (EBRT, brachytherapy, and proton therapy), or chemotherapy (systemic or intra-arterial chemotherapy). Cisplatin and doxorubicin used as adjuvant intra-arterial chemotherapy in one study demonstrated improved survival. However, the role of adjuvant therapy is still unclear.[82,84] *In vitro* studies demonstrated that the use of Gingko Biloba[85,86] and arsenic trioxide[86] resulted in suppression of growth of human ACC cells. Other investigators suggested that EGFR and ErbB1/ErbB2 inhibition may be promising in patients with ACC of the salivary gland.[87] The presence of basaloid predominance, perineural invasion, bone invasion, and recurrence after extensive resection and local treatment are associated with poor prognosis.[84] The rates of overall survival at 5 years in patients with ACC with and without basaloid patterns were 21% and 71%, respectively.[81] Patients should be monitored with serial MRI and CT scans.[8]

Optic nerve glioma [pilocytic astrocytoma (PA)] accounts for approximately 66% of all nerve tumors.[8] It occurs within the first two decades and the female to male ratio is 3:2 ratio. However, if chiasmal location is present, there is no gender predominance.[88] Clinically, PA presents as optic neuropathy (color vision loss, visual acuity loss) and proptosis with or without pain. Visual field (VF) defects are common, but it is difficult to quantify them in children. Malignant gliomas or glioblastomas are rare in adults. PA (WHO grade 1) is seen in NF1 (~70%), and therefore, a detailed familial history is recommended. PA is bilateral in 20% of cases. Findings of NF1 include skin neurofibromas, torso café-au-lait spots, axila/groin freckling, iris hamartomas (lisch nodules), and bone dysplasia. High-grade glioblastomas extend intracranially and spread posteriorly along the optic radiations and have a high mortality risk. MRI brain/orbits with and without contrast (fat suppression) is recommended.[88]

Histologic examination shows bipolar astrocytic cells, biphasic growth (dense and loose arrangements), and many eosinophilic beads with corkscrew shape (Rosenthal fibers). Glioblastomas show extensive mitosis and microvascular proliferation with "palisading necrosis." All glioblastomas are positive for glial fibrillary acidic protein (GFAP).[8]

Treatment depends on clinically significant visual loss (≥0.2 logMAR) or VF progression. Observation is recommended for slowly growing tumor. Surgical resection is considered in the presence of rapid extension or high-risk location (mass effect). Standard treatment consists of chemotherapy with vincristine and carboplatin. MEK inhibitors with or without antivascular endothelial growth factor (VEGF) may represent an alternative therapy.[88] RT combined with chemotherapy is preferred in unresectable cases (i.e., optic nerve radiations and chiasm). RT may be associated with adverse events such as hypothalamic dysfunction, and visual and cognitive impairments. Fractionated stereotactic RT, proton beam therapy, and gamma knife treatment are more targeted approaches.[88] The treatment of glioblastoma includes RT and chemotherapy, but the prognosis is poor, and the median overall survival is less than a year.

The prognosis of PA remains fair. Malignant transformation is rare and spontaneous regression may occur. In cases associated with NF1, the prognosis depends on involvement of other organs.[8]

Orbital metastases are very rare. The most common primary tumors associated with orbital metastases are breast carcinoma in women followed by "cancer of unknown primary."[89,90] Other primary tumors in both genders include cutaneous melanoma,[91] carcinoid tumor and kidney, lung, liver (hepatocellular carcinoma),[92] prostate, and rarely penial cancers.[90,93] Diagnostic procedures include PET/CT scans and orbital biopsy if possible. The prognosis depends on the prognosis of the primary cancer.

Conclusion

This article provides an overview of Ophthalmic Oncology based on anatomical location focusing on clinical presentation, diagnostic procedures, and treatment. Common risk factors associated with eyelid cancers include exposure to UV light, irradiation, and immunosuppression. Factors associated with ocular surface diseases also include smoking, chronic surface irritation, vitamin A deficiency, molecular alterations in tumor suppressor p53, and viral infection. Tumor molecular profiling can identify genomic mutations that can be used to select treatment. Neoplasms of the eye are classified using a clinical and pathological staging system that integrates tumor size and extraocular extension, lymph node involvement, metastatic disease, and hereditary trait. Targeted and immunomodulating therapies have demonstrated encouraging results in selected patients with advanced, metastatic tumor-including BCC and CM. Further investigations are warranted.

Early diagnosis and complete surgical excision or early initiation of treatment are associated with favorable outcomes. The therapeutic management of ocular neoplasms should be multidisciplinary and it should include ocular oncologists, ophthalmic pathologists, medical and radiation oncologists.

Key references

The complete reference list can be found on Vital Source version of this title, see inside front cover.

1. Maheshwari A, Finger PT. Cancers of the eye. *Cancer Metastasis Rev*. 2018;**37**(4):677–690.
2. Shi Y, Jia R, Fan X. Ocular basal cell carcinoma: a brief literature review of clinical diagnosis and treatment. *Onco Targets Ther*. 2017;**10**:2483–2489.
4. Leibovitch I, McNab A, Sullivan T, et al. Orbital invasion by periocular basal cell carcinoma. *Ophthalmology*. 2005;**112**(4):717–723.
5. Rene C. Oculoplastic aspects of ocular oncology. *Eye (Lond)*. 2013;**27**(2):199–207.
6. Yin VT, Merritt HA, Sniegowski M, et al. Eyelid and ocular surface carcinoma: diagnosis and management. *Clin Dermatol*. 2015;**33**(2):159–169.
7. Margo CE, Waltz K. Basal cell carcinoma of the eyelid and periocular skin. *Surv Ophthalmol*. 1993;**38**(2):169–192.
8. Grossniklaus HE, Eberhart CG, Kivela TT. In: Grossniklaus HE, Eberhart CG, Kivela TT, eds. *WHO Classification of Tumours of the Eye*, 4th ed. World Health Organization Book and Report Series International Agency for Research on Cancer (IARC) Publications; 2018.
9. Cook BE Jr, Bartley GB. Treatment options and future prospects for the management of eyelid malignancies: an evidence-based update. *Ophthalmology*. 2001;**108**(11):2088–2098; quiz 99-100, 121.
10. Pe'er J. Pathology of eyelid tumors. *Indian J Ophthalmol*. 2016;**64**(3):177–190.
13. Laskar SG, Basu T, Chaudhary S, et al. Postoperative interstitial brachytherapy in eyelid cancer: long term results and assessment of Cosmesis After Interstitial Brachytherapy scale. *J Contemp Brachytherapy*. 2015;**6**(4):350–355.
15. Sagiv O, Nagarajan P, Ferrarotto R, et al. Ocular preservation with neoadjuvant vismodegib in patients with locally advanced periocular basal cell carcinoma. *Br J Ophthalmol*. 2019;**103**(6):775–780.
16. Mendoza PR, Grossniklaus HE. Sentinel lymph node biopsy for eyelid and conjunctival tumors: what is the evidence? *Int Ophthalmol Clin*. 2015;**55**(1):123–136.
20. Reifler DM, Hornblass A. Squamous cell carcinoma of the eyelid. *Surv Ophthalmol*. 1986;**30**(6):349–365.
21. Gayre GS, Hybarger CP, Mannor G, et al. Outcomes of excision of 1750 eyelid and periocular skin basal cell and squamous cell carcinomas by modified en face frozen section margin-controlled technique. *Int Ophthalmol Clin*. 2009;**49**(4):97–110.
22. Amin MB, Edge S, Greene F, et al. (eds). *AJCC Cancer Staging Manual*, 8th ed. Springer International Publishing; 2017:1032.
23. Rafailov L, Leyngold IM. EGF-R inhibitors for squamous cell carcinoma. *Int Ophthalmol Clin*. 2020;**60**(2):31–38.
24. Shields JA, Shields CL. Sebaceous adenocarcinoma of the eyelid. *Int Ophthalmol Clin*. 2009;**49**(4):45–61.
27. Lin AC, Shriver EM. The role of pembrolizumab in the treatment of sebaceous carcinoma. *Int Ophthalmol Clin*. 2020;**60**(2):39–46.
32. Esmaeli B, Youssef A, Naderi A, et al. Margins of excision for cutaneous melanoma of the eyelid skin: the Collaborative Eyelid Skin Melanoma Group Report. *Ophthal Plast Reconstr Surg*. 2003;**19**(2):96–101.
33. Kamal S, Kaliki S, Mishra DK, et al. Ocular surface squamous neoplasia in 200 patients: a case-control study of immunosuppression resulting from human immunodeficiency virus versus immunocompetency. *Ophthalmology*. 2015;**122**(8):1688–1694.
34. Sayed-Ahmed IO, Palioura S, Galor A, et al. Diagnosis and medical management of ocular surface squamous neoplasia. *Expert Rev Ophthalmol*. 2017;**12**(1):11–19.
36. Mendoza PR, Craven CM, Ip MH, et al. Conjunctival squamous cell carcinoma with corneal stromal invasion in presumed pterygia: a case series. *Ocul Oncol Pathol*. 2018;**4**(4):240–249.
37. Theotoka D, Morkin MI, Galor A, et al. Update on diagnosis and management of conjunctival papilloma. *Eye Vision (Lond, Engl)*. 2019;**6**:18.
38. Cicinelli MV, Marchese A, Bandello F, et al. Clinical management of ocular surface squamous neoplasia: a review of the current evidence. *Ophthalmol Therapy*. 2018;**7**(2):247–262.
39. Venkateswaran N, Mercado C, Galor A, et al. Comparison of topical 5-fluorouracil and interferon alfa-2b as primary treatment modalities for ocular surface squamous neoplasia. *Am J Ophthalmol*. 2019;**199**:216–222.
40. Finger PT, Tran HV, Turbin RE, et al. High-frequency ultrasonographic evaluation of conjunctival intraepithelial neoplasia and squamous cell carcinoma. *Arch Ophthalmol (Chicago, IL: 1960)*. 2003;**121**(2):168–172.
43. Barros Jde N, Almeida SR, Lowen MS, et al. Impression cytology in the evaluation of ocular surface tumors: review article. *Arq Bras Oftalmol*. 2015;**78**(2):126–132.
45. Davila JR, Mruthyunjaya P. Updates in imaging in ocular oncology. *F1000Research*. 2019;**8**:1706.
46. Polski A, Sibug Saber M, Kim JW, et al. Extending far and wide: the role of biopsy and staging in the management of ocular surface squamous neoplasia. *Clin Exp Ophthalmol*. 2019;**47**(2):193–200.
47. Chaugule SS, Park J, Finger PT. Topical chemotherapy for giant ocular surface squamous neoplasia of the conjunctiva and cornea: is surgery necessary? *Indian J Ophthalmol*. 2018;**66**(1):55–60.
48. Shields CL, Shields JA. Tumors of the conjunctiva and cornea. *Surv Ophthalmol*. 2004;**49**(1):3–24.
50. Cohen VML, O'Day RF. Management issues in conjunctival tumours: conjunctival melanoma and primary acquired melanosis. *Ophthalmol Ther*. 2019;**8**(4):501–510.
51. Vasalaki M, Fabian ID, Reddy MA, et al. Ocular oncology: advances in retinoblastoma, uveal melanoma and conjunctival melanoma. *Br Med Bull*. 2017;**121**(1):107–119.

52 Mahendraraj K, Shrestha S, Lau CS, et al. Ocular melanoma-when you have seen one, you have not seen them all: a clinical outcome study from the Surveillance, Epidemiology and End Results (SEER) database (1973-2012). *Clin Ophthalmol (Auckland, NZ)*. 2017;**11**:153–160.

53 Blum ES, Yang J, Komatsubara KM. et al., Clinical management of uveal and conjunctival melanoma. *Oncology (Williston Park)*. 2016;**30**(1):29–32, 4-43, 8.

55 Kenawy N, Kalirai H, Sacco JJ, et al. Conjunctival melanoma copy number alterations and correlation with mutation status, tumor features, and clinical outcome. *Pigment Cell Melanoma Res*. 2019;**32**(4):564–575.

56 Finger PT, Pavlick AC. Checkpoint inhibition immunotherapy for advanced local and systemic conjunctival melanoma: a clinical case series. *J Immunother Cancer*. 2019;**7**(1):83.

57 Pfeiffer ML, Ozgur OK, Myers JN, et al. Sentinel lymph node biopsy for ocular adnexal melanoma. *Acta Ophthalmol*. 2017;**95**(4):e323–e328.

59 Chattopadhyay C, Kim DW, Gombos DS, et al. Uveal melanoma: from diagnosis to treatment and the science in between. *Cancer*. 2016;**122**(15):2299–2312.

60 Dogrusoz M, Jager MJ, Damato B. Uveal melanoma treatment and prognostication. *Asia Pac J Ophthalmol (Philadelphia, PA)*. 2017;**6**(2):186–196.

61 Baron ED, Nicola MD, Shields CL. Updated AJCC Classification for Posterior Uveal Melanoma A case example of a patient with choroidal melanoma is discussed in light of the latest edition of this cancer staging manual. *Retin Today*. 2018:30–34.

62 Krema H, Heydarian M, Beiki-Ardakani A, et al. A comparison between ^{125}Iodine brachytherapy and stereotactic radiotherapy in the management of juxtapapillary choroidal melanoma. *Br J Ophthalmol*. 2013;**97**(3):327–332.

63 Diener-West M, Earle JD, Fine SL, et al. The COMS randomized trial of iodine 125 brachytherapy for choroidal melanoma, III: initial mortality findings. COMS Report No. 18. *Arch Ophthalmol (Chicago, IL: 1960)*. 2001;**119**(7):969–982.

64 Amram AL, Rico G, Kim JW, et al. Vitreous seeds in retinoblastoma: clinicopathologic classification and correlation. *Ophthalmology*. 2017;**124**(10):1540–1547.

65 Reese AB. *Tumors of the Eye*, 3rd ed. New York: Harper and Row; 1976.

66 cancer.org (2021) *Radiation Therapy for Retinoblastoma*, https://www.cancer.org/cancer/retinoblastoma/detailedguide/retinoblastoma-treating-radiation-therapy (accessed 19 April 2021).

68 Dimaras H, Corson TW, Cobrinik D, et al. Retinoblastoma. *Nat Rev Dis Primers*. 2015;**1**:15021.

69 Araujo I, Coupland SE. Primary vitreoretinal lymphoma – a review. *Asia Pac J Ophthalmol (Philadelphia, PA)*. 2017;**6**(3):283–289.

70 Sagoo MS, Mehta H, Swampillai AJ, et al. Primary intraocular lymphoma. *Surv Ophthalmol*. 2014;**59**(5):503–516.

71 Cani AK, Hovelson DH, Demirci H, et al. Next generation sequencing of vitreoretinal lymphomas from small-volume intraocular liquid biopsies: new routes to targeted therapies. *Oncotarget*. 2017;**8**(5):7989–7998.

72 de la Fuente MI, Alderuccio JP, Reis IM, et al. Bilateral radiation therapy followed by methotrexate-based chemotherapy for primary vitreoretinal lymphoma. *Am J Hematol*. 2019;**94**(4):455–460.

73 Shields CL, Sioufi K, Mashayekhi A, et al. Intravitreal melphalan for treatment of primary vitreoretinal lymphoma: a new indication for an old drug. *JAMA Ophthalmol*. 2017;**135**(7):815–818.

76 Oberlin O, Rey A, Anderson J, et al. Treatment of orbital rhabdomyosarcoma: survival and late effects of treatment–results of an international workshop. *J Clin Oncol*. 2001;**19**(1):197–204.

77 van Erp AEM, Versleijen-Jonkers YMH, van der Graaf WTA, et al. Targeted therapy-based combination treatment in rhabdomyosarcoma. *Mol Cancer Ther*. 2018;**17**(7):1365–1380.

79 Shields CL, Shields JA. Tumors of the conjunctiva and cornea. *Indian J Ophthalmol*. 2019;**67**(12):1930–1948.

80 Shields CL, Chien JL, Surakiatchanukul T, et al. Conjunctival tumors: review of clinical features, risks, biomarkers, and outcomes–The 2017 J. Donald M. Gass Lecture. *Asia Pac J Ophthalmol (Philadelphia, PA)*. 2017;**6**(2):109–120.

81 Proia AD, Ranjit-Reeves R, Woodward JA. Lacrimal gland tumors. *Int Ophthalmol Clin*. 2018;**58**(2):197–235.

87 Bell D, Sniegowski MC, Wani K, et al. Mutational landscape of lacrimal gland carcinomas and implications for treatment. *Head Neck*. 2016;**38**(Suppl 1):E724–e9.

88 Farazdaghi MK, Katowitz WR, Avery RA. Current treatment of optic nerve gliomas. *Curr Opin Ophthalmol*. 2019;**30**(5):356–363.

90 Bonavolontà G, Strianese D, Grassi P, et al. An analysis of 2,480 space-occupying lesions of the orbit from 1976 to 2011. *Ophthal Plast Reconstr Surg*. 2013;**29**(2):79–86.

75 Neoplasms of the endocrine glands and pituitary neoplasms

Rui Feng, MD ■ Chirag D. Gandhi, MD, FACS, FAANS ■ Margaret Pain, MD ■ Kalmon D. Post, MD, FACS, FAANS

> **Overview**
>
> Pituitary neoplasms represent a phenotypically and pathologically diverse family of tumors. Symptoms may derive from abnormal hormone production, compression of adjacent nervous system structures, and in rare cases, metastases. New cell lineage classification based on transcription factors brings new insights into pathogenesis and treatment. Transsphenoidal surgery represents a command well-tolerated treatment for most pituitary adenomas; however, advances in radiation and chemotherapy have increased treatment options enhancing treatment efficacy and eligibility.

Pituitary adenomas are epithelial tumors arising from the adenohypophysis that can manifest with neurological symptoms from local mass effect such as headaches, visual disturbances, increased intracranial pressure, and cranial nerve palsies, or as a variety of clinical entities depending on the hormones they secrete. In rare cases (<1%), patients can also present with diabetes insipidus. Pituitary adenomas constitute 10–20% of intracranial tumors,[1] although the incidence is as high as 24% in autopsy series. They are most common in the third and fourth decades of life and overall affect both sexes equally. However, there are differences in frequency of certain subtypes between the sexes. Cushing's disease, for example, is more common in women. Prolactin (PRL)-secreting adenomas are more common in young women. Gonadotropin-secreting adenomas are more common in men.

Classification of pituitary adenomas

Recently, there was significant progress in refining the classification systems to better distinguish between pituitary neoplasm subtypes.[2] Prior to 2017, tumors are most commonly categorized based on the predominant hormone that they secrete.[3,4] Tumors are further categorized as hormonally active or inactive based on if the amount of hormone they secrete exceeds normal levels in the blood and is clinically evident. In 2017, the World Health Organization (WHO) after incorporating recent advances in molecular and immunohistochemical advances in pituitary research, proposed a new classification system.[5] The fourth edition of the WHO classification system no longer uses the concept of "a hormone-producing pituitary adenoma" and adopted a pituitary adenohypophyseal cell lineage designation. The different histological variants are categorized according to hormone content and specific histological and immunohistochemical features including but not limited to pituitary transcription factors. The steroidogenic factor 1 (SF1) staining identifies the gonadotroph lineage, and its utilization has shown that many hormone-negative adenomas are, in fact, silent gonadotroph adenomas.[6] DAX1 (dosage-sensitive sex reversal, adrenal hypoplasia critical region, on chromosome X, gene 1) is a member of the nuclear receptor superfamily involved with pituitary gonadotroph differentiation, which was also shown to be expressed in clinically defined nonfunctional pituitary adenomas even with absent immunostaining for SF1.[7] The pituitary-specific positive transcription factor 1 (PIT1) identifies the growth hormone, PRL, and TSH lineage.[8] Some studies suggest that PIT1-positive plurihormonal adenomas are a distinct entity with aggressive behavior.[9] The TPIT (coded by the T-box transcription factor 19 gene) staining is used for identifying the corticotroph lineage (Figure 1).[10]

Previously null cell adenomas were defined as hormone-negative adenoma, which was thought to account for approximately 10% of all pituitary adenomas.[11,12] Studies have, however, demonstrated that the majority of the null cell tumors, in fact, demonstrate positive immunohistochemical results for transcription factors and true transcription factor-negative adenomas only account for less than 1% of all pituitary adenomas.[8] Recognizing these findings, the new WHO 2017 classifications system definition of the null cell adenoma requires the demonstration of immuno-negativity for pituitary transcription factors and adenohypophyseal hormones and is a diagnosis of exclusion. The distinction of null cell adenoma has also become clinically relevant. Studies suggest these tumors to have an unfavorable outcome compared with hormone-negative but transcription factor-positive adenomas,[8] with higher rates of early recurrence, cavernous sinus invasion, and a higher Ki-67 labeling index.[13,14] As immunohistochemical staining for transcription factors regulating pituitary development becomes better studied and more widely available, future efforts will hopefully be able to address whether and how the management of silent pituitary adenomas would change with an accurate pathological diagnosis.

Furthermore, the new classification system eliminated "atypical adenoma," which in previous editions was defined as tumor cells with "extensive" nuclear staining for p53, "elevated" mitotic index, and Ki-67 labeling index greater than 3%.[5,15] It does recognize some subtypes of pituitary neuroendocrine tumors as "high-risk" pituitary adenomas with clinical aggressive behavior. The new system recommends full assessment of the tumor proliferative potential to include mitotic count and Ki-67 index, and other clinical parameters such as tumor invasion, in addition to accurate tumor subtyping. Since its introduction, many clinicopathological studies have been published based on the new WHO classification system.[16–20] Several studies have shown that the new

---

Holland-Frei Cancer Medicine, Tenth Edition. Edited by Robert C. Bast, John C. Byrd, Carlo M. Croce, Ernest Hawk, Fadlo R. Khuri, Raphael E. Pollock, Apostolia M. Tsimberidou, Christopher G. Willett, and Cheryl L. Willman.
© 2023 John Wiley & Sons, Inc. Published 2023 by John Wiley & Sons, Inc.

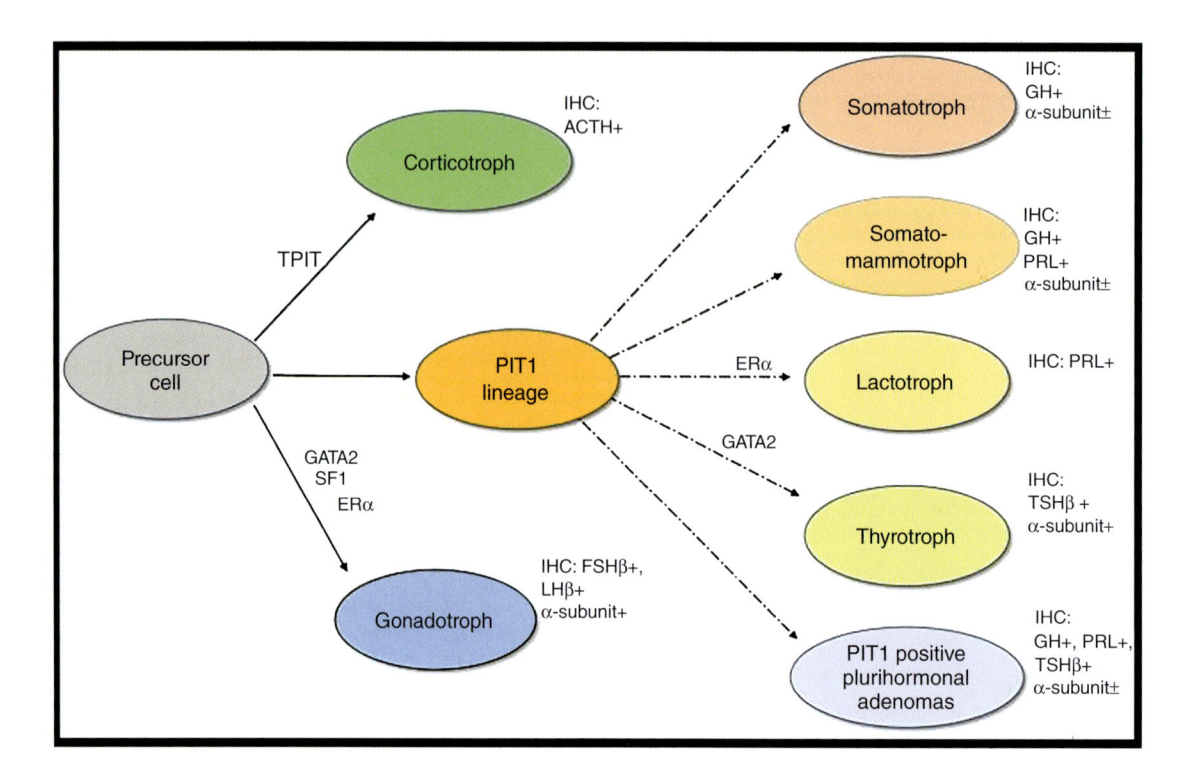

Figure 1 During pituitary development, specific transcription factors are fundamental to the complex process of adenohypophyseal cell differentiation. The three main pathways of cell differentiation and the immunoprofile of each cell lineage are illustrated. GATA2, GATA-binding protein-2; PROP1, PROP paired-like homeobox 1 (also called prophet of PIT1); PIT1, POU class 1 homeobox 1 (PUO1F1) or pituitary-specific positive transcription factor 1; TPIT, T-box transcription factor 19 (TBX19). Source: Adapted from Drummond et al.[2]

WHO 2017 classification categorizes less null cell adenoma compared with previous classifications.[8,16,17] Most studies found the new classification system to be practical and reasonable. Further investigations with large sample sizes and long-term data on tumor outcomes and patient prognosis are still needed to provide more accurate understanding and application of this latest classification system for clinical diagnosis and treatment.

Tumors can also be classified anatomically and radiologically based on their relationship to and involvement within the cavernous sinus. Magnetic resonance imaging (MRI) is the modality of choice, with T2-weighted thin slices through the pituitary in the coronal plane. Gadolinium contrast enhancement is also essential, as in general, pituitary adenomas appear as a hypointense lesion on a T1 precontrast image and will enhance less than normal pituitary tissue on T1 postcontrast series. Radiographic appearance has been used to further categorize parasellar invasive tumors. The Knosp classification scheme, in brief, stratifies the likelihood of invasion based on the tumor's preoperative MRI appearance and influence on the medial wall of the sinus relative to the position of the intracavernous internal carotid artery. Increasing mass effect of the tumor on the medial wall correlates with increased likelihood of invasiveness. When compared with noninvasive tumors, invasive tumors are more likely to demonstrate aggressive behavior (Figure 2).[21] A recent study of 106 consecutive Knosp high-grade pituitary adenomas with parasellar extension who underwent endoscopic transsphenoidal surgery further demonstrated that adenomas with extension into the superior cavernous sinus compartment have a lower rate of invasive growth than adenomas extending into the inferior cavernous sinus compartment or encasing the carotid artery.[22]

Prolactin-secreting pituitary adenomas

Prolactinomas are the most commonly diagnosed pituitary adenoma, representing approximately 30% of cases,[23,24] and 50% of cases requiring medical attention.[25,26] Overall prevalence is between 25 and 63 per 100,000.[27-29] In women of reproductive age, hyperprolactinemia may cause oligomenorrhea, secondary amenorrhea, galactorrhea, and sterility. In men and postmenopausal women, symptomatic hyperprolactinemia can be much more subtle. The tumor may grow to much larger sizes and are detected only when they begin to produce symptoms related to mass effect. Macroadenoma-related mass effects may include headaches, visual disturbances (typically bitemporal hemianopsia from chiasmatic compression), hypopituitarism, ophthalmoplegia. Men may also experience diminished libido, impotence, gynecomastia, and infertility from decreased androgen production. Although autopsy studies have demonstrated that prolactinomas have similar prevalence between the genders, women are four times more likely than men to become symptomatic.

Prolactinomas can be difficult to diagnose, and in most cases require radiographic evidence in addition to elevated PRL levels. In men, a basal PRL value greater than 100 ng/mL is almost always indicative of a prolactinoma but could be from stalk effect. In women, PRL levels of 100–200 ng/mL should raise suspicion, while a level of over 200 ng/mL is highly suggestive.[30,31] For patients with PRL level between 50 and 100 ng/mL, there can be diagnostic uncertainty due to "stalk effect" where mass of a tumor interferes with the flow of prolactin-inhibitory factor from the hypothalamus.[32] Serum PRL levels are an index of secretory activity and have been shown to be associated with the size of the prolactinoma. For very large tumors, however, the laboratory value may be falsely low due to the Hook effect, which results from

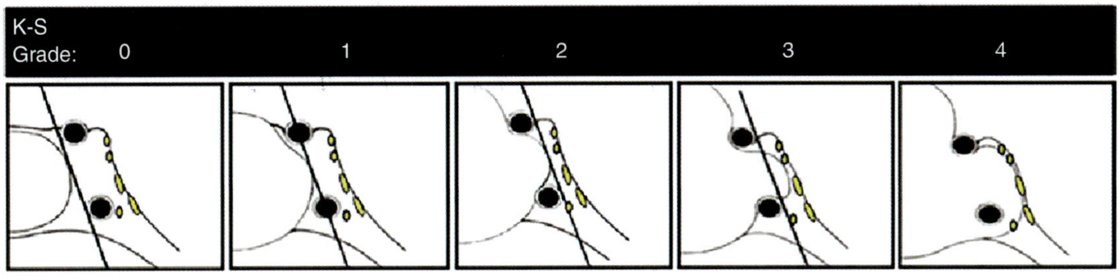

Figure 2 Knosp-Steiner classification scheme: Grade 0, no invasion, the lesion does not reach the medial aspect of the CCA; Grade 1, invasion extending to, but not past, the intercarotid line; Grade 2, invasion extending to, but not past, the lateral aspect of the CCA; Grade 3, invasion past the lateral aspect of the CCA but not completely filling the CS; and Grade 4, completely filling the CS both medial and lateral to the CCA. Source: Knosp et al.[21]

saturation of the antibody binding sites during radioimmunoassay and therefore distorting the binding curve. This effect should be considered in all giant pituitary adenomas and serial dilutions should be performed.

Treatment options for prolactinoma include observation, medical therapy, surgery, and radiotherapy. Majority of microprolactinoma (<10 mm) does not increase in size and can be observed in the absence of clinical hyperprolactinemia, normal pituitary function, and no desire for pregnancy. Dopamine is an endogenous inhibitor of PRL production, and dopamine agonists have been shown to be highly effective in suppressing tumor growth and PRL production. Bromocriptine was the first to be used, and newer agents include cabergoline, quinagolide, lisuride, and terguride. Dopamine agonists (DA) have been shown to have a high response rate with normalization of PRL levels in 70–80% of patients, tumor shrinkage in 80–90%, and restoration of ovulation in 80–90%.[33] It remained the first-line treatment for most prolactinomas. Surgery, due to recent advances in imaging and surgical techniques and better surgical outcomes, has been gaining traction. Indications can include resistance or intolerance to DA, women planning a pregnancy, young patients with a high likelihood of complete resection and who do not wish to undergo prolonged medical treatment, or predominantly cystic tumors.[34] Even with incomplete resections, surgical debulking may improve hormonal control with lower postoperative dose of DA.[35,36] For tumors larger than 2 cm or with PRL levels between 200 and 500 ng/mL, neoadjuvant treatment with dopamine agonists appears to reduce tumor volume, followed by surgery. Any residual tumor can then be treated medically. For very large, invasive, or tumors associated with PRL levels of greater than 500 ng/mL, medical therapy should be the primary treatment modality.[37]

Growth hormone-secreting pituitary adenomas

GH-secreting pituitary adenomas account for approximately 30% of all endocrine-active pituitary tumors, with overall prevalence between 3 and 14 per 100,000.[38] Patients typically present in their third to fifth decade, with classic symptoms of acromegaly or gigantism, marked by insidious coarsening of features with frontal bossing and prognathism, macroglossia, exaggerated acral growth.[39] More severe medical consequences can include organomegaly, hypertension, cardiomyopathy, congestive heart failure, restrictive lung disease, sleep apnea, impaired glucose metabolism, and diabetes mellitus.[39–41] Untreated patients have a high rate of early mortality, 50% at 50 years old and two to three times of the general population.[40,42] The goals of treatment are to normalize GH and insulin-like growth factor-1 (IGF-1) levels and prevent tumor growth.[43–45]

Elevated basal fasting GH levels greater than 2.5 ng/mL suggest acromegaly. However, GH has a short half-life and is secreted in a pulsatile manner. Thus, the assessment of IGF-1 often generates a more accurate diagnosis of GH excess.[46,47] Clinical symptoms of GH-secreting tumors also have been found to correlate better with IGF-1 levels than with GH levels. Dynamic testing is typically reserved for monitoring therapeutic efficacy. The oral glucose tolerance test (OGTT) tracks GH response to a large oral glucose load (75–100 g). Normal patients respond to the glucose load with GH suppression and levels fall below 1 ng/ml. Loss of glucose-induced suppression is diagnostic for a GH-secreting tumor.[46,47]

Transsphenoidal surgery remains the first-line therapy for GH-secreting tumors.[48,49] The advantages of surgery include a prompt decrease in GH levels and a tissue diagnosis. In a 14-year review of 115 patients demonstrated that surgery alone produced biochemical remission in 61% of cases.[50] The rate was 88% for microadenomas and 53% for macroadenomas. There was a negative correlation of surgical outcome with tumor size and preoperative GH levels. Immediate postoperative GH levels were found to correlate with long-term outcome. In cases where the postoperative GH level was less than 3 ng/mL, the chance of a favorable long-term outcome was 89%. Postoperative radiotherapy was given to 32 patients and led to remission in 31% of these patients. Three additional patients achieved remission with a combination of surgery, radiotherapy, and medical treatment. The overall complication rate was 6.9% with no CSF leaks, meningitis, permanent diabetes insipidus, or new hypopituitarism. The recurrence rate was 5.4%. Other published studies reflect similar results.[51,52]

Radiosurgery has largely replaced radiation therapy and is currently used as adjective therapy after transsphenoidal surgery.[53] A recent meta-analysis demonstrated an overall disease control rate of 73%.[54] Common complications can include pituitary hormone deficiency, visual disturbance.[53] Medical management can include somatostatin analogs,[55,56] dopamine agonists,[57–59] and GH-receptor blockers.[60] Somatostatin analogs currently are often used as first-line treatment for patients after unsuccessful surgery. Recent data suggest that response to treatment may be associated with certain gene expression, particularly somatostatin receptors 2.[55] Medical treatments, although they are well-tolerated and efficacious, require lifelong compliance to avoid recurrence. Additionally, in the context of the significant long-term morbidity associated with acromegaly, surgery remains the first-line treatment with adjuvant medical or radiotherapy if needed. Future investigation incorporating biochemical and molecular genetic characteristics will likely elucidate new potential therapies and appropriate target patient populations.

Adrenocorticotropic hormone-secreting adenomas

The majority of ACTH-secreting tumors present with clinical hypercortisolism, or "Cushing's syndrome". Cushing's disease is nine times more common in women with a peak incidence in the third and fourth decades of life. Common presenting features include central obesity, moon facies, buffalo hump, hirsutism, purple abdominal striae, and acne. Other medical findings include hypertension, osteopenia, proximal myopathy, diabetes mellitus, and very frequently psychiatric disorders. Affected patients experience significant morbidity from the condition with a 5-year mortality rate of 50% in those left untreated.[61] Only 10–20% of ACTH-secreting adenomas are large enough to produce mass effect with resultant visual field deficits, cranial neuropathies, or hypopituitarism.[62]

Accurate diagnosis of Cushing's disease depends on identifying evidence of hypercortisolism and localizing the pathology to the pituitary gland. Hypercortisolism can be demonstrated through elevation in 24-hour urinary free cortisol and 17-OH corticosteroids, as well as midnight salivary cortisol levels. The etiology of hypercortisolism should be assessed first with a low-dose dexamethasone suppression test. Patients with Cushing's disease will have hypercortisolism that persists in spite of a low-dose bolus of dexamethasone. However, 95% of Cushing's disease patients demonstrate a 50% decrease in plasma cortisol when a high dose of dexamethasone is used. Plasma ACTH levels should be assessed to differentiate a diagnosis of Cushing's disease from adrenal causes of hypercortisolism. Diagnostic sensitivity for Cushing's disease can be further increased if a corticotrophin-releasing hormone (CRH) stimulation test is added to the workup.[62,63] Finally, inferior petrosal sinus sampling (IPSS) can be performed to improve tumor localization and diagnostic specificity if the previous workup is not definitive.[64,65] Recent advances in imaging technology and high definition sequences also allow more small size tumors to be visualized on MRI scans, although as many as 50% of ACTH secreting adenomas will be large enough to be evident on MRI scans.[66,67]

Transsphenoidal surgery is the first-line treatment for Cushing's disease. The overall remission rate following surgery ranges from 76% to 91%.[68,69] Microadenomas tend to be associated with slightly better outcomes and their remission rates range between 84% and 94%.[70] The major determining factor for success is the ability to localize the tumor on MRI.[71,72] In contrast, remission rates for macroadenomas appear to depend chiefly on the degree of invasiveness. Surgery alone can induce remission in 64% of patients and when combined with adjuvant radiotherapy or radiosurgery this figure improves to 83% or 70%, respectively.[73–75] Postoperatively most patients require replacement cortisol therapy for up to 1 year. Favorable prognostic factors for full postoperative remission include lower than normal serum levels of cortisol and ACTH. However, even with immediate improvement in serum cortisol, 15–25% of patients experience a recurrence.[63,76,77] Long-term follow-up is essential in these patients, as delayed recurrences and hypopituitarism are not infrequent. Radiotherapy and radiosurgery are frequently used as adjuvant treatment when surgical results are inadequate.[76]

Conventional radiotherapy cure rates are as high as 90% at 5 years posttreatment. However, the effect takes years to develop, and a large proportion of these patients began to experience hypopituitarism in later years and 5% developed Nelson's syndrome. Radiosurgery for Cushing's disease produces results much sooner. Remission is achieved in 35–90% of patients with much lower rates of hypopituitarism.[70,73,74,78]

While medical therapy is not recommended as a primary treatment of Cushing's disease it may be suitable for patients who do not experience improvement after surgery or who are otherwise not good candidates for surgery. Pasireotide, a somatostatin analog with high specificity for the somatostatin receptor 5, has been shown to be clinically efficacious in decreasing cortisol levels, and it should be considered the preferred medication to treat Cushing's disease.[79] Ketoconazole is often used to temporize patients with severe hypercortisolism as they await surgery. It inhibits adrenal steroid synthesis. Up to 90% of patients experience normalization of serum cortisol and ACTH while taking ketoconazole.[80,81] Other medical treatments for Cushing's disease include aminoglutethimide, metyrapone, mitotane, and cyproheptadine. Dopamine agonists such as cabergoline have also been shown to be successful in the treatment of ACTH-secreting tumors.[82] Total adrenalectomy, as a more radical surgical option for patients who do not respond to the above measures, offers absolute control of cortisol secretion but requires lifelong dependence on exogenous glucocorticoid and mineralocorticoid replacement.

TSH-secreting pituitary adenomas

TSH-secreting adenomas are the least common variant of pituitary tumors, representing only 1–2% of cases.[83,84] Patients typically present with signs and symptoms of hyperthyroidism, which often triggers a workup and presumptive diagnosis of Graves' disease. As a result, patients are often diagnosed later in their disease course and can develop symptoms related to mass effect from large and invasive tumors. Nowadays ultrasensitive immunometric assays for TSH and the measurement of circulating free thyroid hormones (FT4 and FT3) are routinely used and TSH-secreting adenomas are detected much earlier.[84,85] The majority of TSH-secreting adenomas are associated with elevated levels of TSH, in spite of elevated levels of T3 and free T4.[86]

Transsphenoidal surgery is the primary treatment for this type of tumor but is associated with low rates of remission (35–70%).[83,87] Prior to surgery, beta-blockade or antithyroid drugs are commonly used to decrease anesthesia and surgical risk. When adjuvant medical therapy or radiotherapy is added, the rate of remission increases to 55–86%.[87–89] External radiation is used if clinical remission is not attained with surgery alone but is not used as first-line treatment. Octreotide has demonstrated clinical efficacy in 92% of cases and is associated with a normalization of TSH and tumor shrinkage for the vast majority. Lanreotide, a long-acting octreotide analogue, may have similar efficacy while avoiding the downsides of octreotide in terms of long-term costs and compliance.[84,85] In a recent meta-analysis of 536 patients, Cossu et al. report biochemical remission rate of 66% after adjuvant radiation therapy and 76% after adjuvant medical treatment. The combination of both allowed remission in 67% of cases. Overall biochemical remission rate at final follow-up was significantly better (85.8%) when compared to the postoperative biochemical remission.[83]

Key references

The complete reference list can be found on Vital Source version of this title, see inside front cover.

2. Drummond J, Roncaroli F, Grossman AB, et al. Clinical and pathological aspects of silent pituitary adenomas. *J Clin Endocrinol Metab*. 2019;**104**(7):2473–2489.
5. Lloyd RV, Osamura RY, Klöppel G, et al. *WHO Classification of Tumours of Endocrine Organs*, 4th ed. IARC; 2017.
6. Gomez-Hernandez K, Ezzat S, Asa SL, et al. Clinical implications of accurate subtyping of pituitary adenomas: perspectives from the treating physician. *Turk Patoloji Derg*. 2015;**31**(Suppl 1):4–17.
10. Asa SL, Mete O. Immunohistochemical biomarkers in pituitary pathology. *Endocr Pathol*. 2018;**29**(2):130–136.
11. Inoshita N, Nishioka H. The 2017 WHO classification of pituitary adenoma: overview and comments. *Brain Tumor Pathol*. 2018;**35**(2):51–56.
13. Balogun JA, Monsalves E, Juraschka K, et al. Null cell adenomas of the pituitary gland: an institutional review of their clinical imaging and behavioral characteristics. *Endocr Pathol*. 2015;**26**(1):63–70.
16. Liu J, He Y, Zhang X, et al. Clinicopathological analysis of 250 cases of pituitary adenoma under the new WHO classification. *Oncol Lett*. 2020;**19**(3):1890–1898.
17. Batista RL, Trarbach EB, Marques MD, et al. Nonfunctioning pituitary adenoma recurrence and its relationship with sex, size, and hormonal immunohistochemical profile. *World Neurosurg*. 2018;**120**:e241–e246.
18. Lee JYK, Cho SS, Zeh R, et al. Folate receptor overexpression can be visualized in real time during pituitary adenoma endoscopic transsphenoidal surgery with near-infrared imaging. *J Neurosurg*. 2018;**129**(2):390–403.
21. Knosp E, Steiner E, Kitz K, et al. Pituitary adenomas with invasion of the cavernous sinus space: a magnetic resonance imaging classification compared with surgical findings. *Neurosurgery*. 1993;**33**(4):610–617; discussion 7–8.
37. Melmed S, Casanueva FF, Cavagnini F, et al. Guidelines for acromegaly management. *J Clin Endocrinol Metab*. 2002;**87**(9):4054–4058.
38. Lavrentaki A, Paluzzi A, Wass JA, et al. Epidemiology of acromegaly: review of population studies. *Pituitary*. 2017;**20**(1):4–9.
39. Vilar L, Vilar CF, Lyra R, et al. Acromegaly: clinical features at diagnosis. *Pituitary*. 2017;**20**(1):22–32.
40. Dekkers OM, Biermasz NR, Pereira AM, et al. Mortality in acromegaly: a metaanalysis. *J Clin Endocrinol Metab*. 2008;**93**(1):61–67.
43. Giustina A, Chanson P, Kleinberg D, et al. Expert consensus document: a consensus on the medical treatment of acromegaly. *Nat Rev Endocrinol*. 2014;**10**(4):243–248.
46. Bernabeu I, Aller J, Alvarez-Escola C, et al. Criteria for diagnosis and postoperative control of acromegaly, and screening and management of its comorbidities: expert consensus. *Endocrinol Diabetes Nutr*. 2018;**65**(5):297–305.
48. Melmed S, Bronstein MD, Chanson P, et al. A consensus statement on acromegaly therapeutic outcomes. *Nat Rev Endocrinol*. 2018;**14**(9):552–561.
49. Donoho DA, Bose N, Zada G, et al. Management of aggressive growth hormone secreting pituitary adenomas. *Pituitary*. 2017;**20**(1):169–178.
50. Freda PU, Wardlaw SL, Post KD. Long-term endocrinological follow-up evaluation in 115 patients who underwent transsphenoidal surgery for acromegaly. *J Neurosurg*. 1998;**89**(3):353–358.
51. Phan K, Xu J, Reddy R, et al. Endoscopic endonasal versus microsurgical transsphenoidal approach for growth hormone-secreting pituitary adenomas-systematic review and meta-analysis. *World Neurosurg*. 2017;**97**:398–406.
55. Venegas-Moreno E, Vazquez-Borrego MC, Dios E, et al. Association between dopamine and somatostatin receptor expression and pharmacological response to somatostatin analogues in acromegaly. *J Cell Mol Med*. 2018;**22**(3):1640–1649.
57. Melmed S. Acromegaly pathogenesis and treatment. *J Clin Invest*. 2009;**119**(11):3189–3202.
61. Pivonello R, De Martino MC, De Leo M, et al. Cushing's disease: the burden of illness. *Endocrine*. 2017;**56**(1):10–18.
62. Lonser RR, Nieman L, Oldfield EH. Cushing's disease: pathobiology, diagnosis, and management. *J Neurosurg*. 2017;**126**(2):404–417.
63. Molitch ME. Diagnosis and treatment of pituitary adenomas: a review. *JAMA*. 2017;**317**(5):516–524.
64. Bekci T, Belet U, Soylu AI, et al. Efficiency of inferior petrosal sinus sampling in the diagnosis of Cushing's disease and comparison with magnetic resonance imaging. *North Clin Istanb*. 2019;**6**(1):53–58.
65. Bonelli FS, Huston J 3rd, Carpenter PC, et al. Adrenocorticotropic hormone-dependent Cushing's syndrome: sensitivity and specificity of inferior petrosal sinus sampling. *AJNR Am J Neuroradiol*. 2000;**21**(4):690–696.
66. Chowdhury IN, Sinaii N, Oldfield EH, et al. A change in pituitary magnetic resonance imaging protocol detects ACTH-secreting tumours in patients with previously negative results. *Clin Endocrinol (Oxf)*. 2010;**72**(4):502–506.
68. Baig MZ, Laghari AA, Darbar A, et al. Endoscopic transsphenoidal surgery for Cushing's disease: a review. *Cureus*. 2019;**11**(7):e5254.
70. Shirvani M, Motiei-Langroudi R, Sadeghian H. Outcome of microscopic transsphenoidal surgery in Cushing disease: a case series of 96 patients. *World Neurosurg*. 2016;**87**:170–175.
73. Gupta A, Xu Z, Kano H, et al. Upfront gamma knife radiosurgery for Cushing's disease and acromegaly: a multicenter, international study. *J Neurosurg*. 2018;**131**(2):532–538.
74. Mehta GU, Ding D, Patibandla MR, et al. Stereotactic radiosurgery for Cushing disease: results of an international, multicenter study. *J Clin Endocrinol Metab*. 2017;**102**(11):4284–4291.
76. Bunevicius A, Laws ER, Vance ML, et al. Surgical and radiosurgical treatment strategies for Cushing's disease. *J Neurooncol*. 2019;**145**(3):403–413.
80. Tritos NA, Biller BMK. Medical management of Cushing disease. *Neurosurg Clin N Am*. 2019;**30**(4):499–508.
82. Pivonello R, Ferone D, de Herder WW, et al. Dopamine receptor expression and function in corticotroph pituitary tumors. *J Clin Endocrinol Metab*. 2004;**89**(5):2452–2462.
83. Cossu G, Daniel RT, Pierzchala K, et al. Thyrotropin-secreting pituitary adenomas: a systematic review and meta-analysis of postoperative outcomes and management. *Pituitary*. 2019;**22**(1):79–88.
84. Beck-Peccoz P, Giavoli C, Lania A. A 2019 update on TSH-secreting pituitary adenomas. *J Endocrinol Invest*. 2019;**42**(12):1401–1406.
85. Kirkman MA, Jaunmuktane Z, Brandner S, et al. Active and silent thyroid-stimulating hormone-expressing pituitary adenomas: presenting symptoms, treatment, outcomes, and recurrence. *World Neurosurg*. 2014;**82**(6):1224–1231.
87. Herguido NG, Fuentes ED, Venegas-Moreno E, et al. Surgical outcome and treatment of thyrotropin-secreting pituitary tumors in a tertiary referral center. *World Neurosurg*. 2019;**130**:e634–e639.
88. Malchiodi E, Profka E, Ferrante E, et al. Thyrotropin-secreting pituitary adenomas: outcome of pituitary surgery and irradiation. *J Clin Endocrinol Metab*. 2014;**99**(6):2069–2076.

76 Neoplasms of the thyroid

Matthew D. Ringel, MD

Overview

Thyroid cancer is the most common malignancy of a classical endocrine organ. The most common forms of thyroid cancer derive from follicular thyroid cells, are characterized by cellular and histological patterns (e.g., papillary and follicular thyroid cancer), and are associated with outstanding overall survivorship but a high frequency of disease persistence. Less commonly, thyroid cancers can derive from thyroid neuroendocrine C-cells (medullary thyroid cancer) that can occur as part of defined genetic syndromes (e.g., multiple endocrine neoplasia type 2). Thyroid cancers can present as or develop into poorly differentiated or dedifferentiated (anaplastic thyroid cancer) that are associated with highly aggressive courses and poor outcomes. Over the past decade, a more individualized approach has been taken for patients with early-stage thyroid cancer, with reduced emphasis on aggressive surgical approaches, expansion of active surveillance approaches, and reduced use and/or dosing strategies for radioiodine therapy (RAI) using I-131. RAI, TSH suppression therapy, and for selected local recurrence, reoperation, and external beam radiation therapy remain cornerstones of therapy for patients with progressive or nonremitting forms of thyroid cancer. For those who do not respond to those treatments, or those with specific gene mutations, there has been expansion of options including the use of targeted inhibitors of mutated driver oncogenes in all forms of thyroid cancer, anti-angiogenic multikinase inhibitors in patients with progressive differentiated thyroid cancers, and immune checkpoint inhibitors.

Historical perspective

Historically when considered as a single population, patients with thyroid cancer have an outstanding prognosis. Over the past several decades, it has become clear that individual prognosis and consequent treatment recommendations must be considered in the context of tumor and patient characteristics. The frequency of the diagnosis of thyroid cancer, particularly papillary thyroid cancer (PTC), has been increasing steadily over decades with a more recent very rapid increase in diagnosis with the advent of more sensitive techniques such as thyroid ultrasound and ultrasound-guided fine-needle aspiration (FNA).[1] The development and use of these technologies allowed for identification and evaluation of small nonpalpable thyroid nodules and resulted in a marked increase in the diagnosis of small subclinical thyroid cancers across the globe. This led to large population studies demonstrating an increase in diagnosis without improved mortality, consistent with overtreatment.[2,3] This situation has resulted in new guidelines over the past 5 years that recommend limiting FNA to larger or growing nodules that are more likely clinically significant thyroid cancers based in part on studies demonstrating safety of active surveillance rather than intervention for the smallest of thyroid cancers.[3–6] Adoption of these approaches has reduced the incidence of thyroid cancer over the past several years.[7] However, for uncertain reasons, there also has been a steady rise in the incidence of larger thyroid cancers since the 1970s, and in increase in the number of patients (although a stable disease-specific death rate) who die from thyroid cancer annually.[8–10] Thus, there are two components when considering thyroid cancer incidence over time; (1) a large number of patients with subclinical thyroid cancer who have an outstanding prognosis for whom overtreatment is concerned; and (2) a smaller but rising number of individuals with more aggressive disease for whom aggressive therapy is appropriate, cure has been elusive, and new therapies are needed. These two populations create the clear need for individualized approaches to thyroid cancer diagnosis and management that have been a focus over the past decade.

Incidence and epidemiology

In the United States alone, it is estimated by the American Cancer Society that 52,890 will be diagnosed in 2020 with disease-related mortality of 2180 individuals (www.cancer.org/cancer/thyroid-cancer). The former number has stabilized or reduced but the latter has continued to rise. Similar patterns have been seen worldwide, with the highest reported incidence in South Korea when thyroid ultrasound was offered as part of the cancer screening for women. This has led to thyroid cancer being the second most common form of cancer in women in that country.[2,7,11] The rise incidence associated with screening has been dubbed as "overdiagnosis" due to the preponderance of small, intrathyroidal, mostly PTCs that have been diagnosed.[3] In addition to this increase in small tumors, a consistent increase in diagnosis of larger tumors also has occurred, perhaps related to imaging or greater attention to thyroid nodules.[8–10] These are felt to represent a true increase in diagnosis that requires active therapy.

Thyroid cancer can derive from either follicular thyroid cells that are responsible for making thyroid hormone and thereby concentrate iodine, express thyroid stimulating hormone (TSH) receptors, and secrete thyroglobulin (Tg); or from parafollicular C-cells that are neuroendocrine and secrete calcitonin but do not have the other features of follicular thyroid cells.[12] Follicular-cell-derived thyroid cancers account for ~90% of all thyroid cancers. They are further subdivided into differentiated thyroid cancers (DTCs) that maintain most of the features of normal thyroid follicular cells, poorly differentiated thyroid cancers (PDTCs) that lose some of the growth patterns and expression patterns of DTC, and anaplastic thyroid cancer (ATC) that are recognized as thyroid cancer only by the site of origin, evidence of development from a DTC or PDTC, or clinical history.[13] These tumors account for ~5% of call cases. DTCs are subdivided into PTC (~85%); follicular thyroid cancer

---

Holland-Frei Cancer Medicine, Tenth Edition. Edited by Robert C. Bast, John C. Byrd, Carlo M. Croce, Ernest Hawk, Fadlo R. Khuri, Raphael E. Pollock, Apostolia M. Tsimberidou, Christopher G. Willett, and Cheryl L. Willman.
© 2023 John Wiley & Sons, Inc. Published 2023 by John Wiley & Sons, Inc.

(FTC, ~10%); or Hurthle Cell thyroid cancer (HCC, ~5%). Finally, medullary thyroid cancer (MTC) are neuroendocrine tumors of the thyroid derived from the parafollicular C-cell population and account for ~2–3% of all thyroid cancer cases.[14]

Risk factors for thyroid cancer

Most patients with DTC have apparently sporadic disease from a genetic perspective.[15] There are rare patients with DTC that occurs as part of identifiable genetic syndromes. This includes Cowden syndrome, caused mostly by germline mutations in the gene encoding phospatase and tensin homolog (PTEN), in which a greater percentage of patients have FTC or benign follicular adenomas than other sporadic thyroid cancers (although most still have forms of PTC), Carney complex, caused by mutations in the gene encoding protein kinase CAMP-dependent type 1 regulatory subunit alpha (PRKAR1A), familial adenomatous polyposis (FAP), DICER1 syndrome, and Werner syndrome.[1] These situations are rare but should be considered in patients with either multiple cancers, or first-degree family members with related cancers, and genetic counseling is recommended. Often, patients are identified in thyroid ultrasound screening performed after a family member is diagnosed with thyroid cancer. These individuals and patients diagnosed clinically who have family history of thyroid cancer are categorized as having familial non-MTC when it occurs in three or more close family members.[15] In rare large affected families, culpable genes have been identified.[15–18] However, in all of these rare families, the mutations have been unique and whether the identified cancers have unique characteristics has been debated. Thus, to date, there are no specific screening recommendations for family members of patients diagnosed with DTC, PDTC, or ATC as the frequency is not common and there is no clear advantage of prophylactic surgery.

In contrast to these tumor types, 25% of all MTCs occur in patients with multiple endocrine neoplasia type 2A and 2B syndromes.[14] These syndromes are caused by germline mutations in ret proto-oncogene (RET) and associate MTC with pheochromocytoma, hyperparathyroidism, and in MEN2B, ganglioneuromas and marfanoid habitus.[14] Even in patients with clinically sporadic MTC diagnoses (including older patients), germline screening for RET mutations is recommended due to the variable phenotypes associated with the different mutations, and the opportunity for prophylactic thyroidectomy to prevent MTC from occurring in affected family members.[19] It is recommended that patients with MTC should be referred to a cancer genetic counselor to assist with germline testing, counsel patients, and enable cascade family screening if a patient is diagnosed with MEN2.[14]

The most well-defined environmental risk factor for thyroid cancer is exposure to radiation, particularly in childhood. Data from individuals exposed to radiation from the Chernobyl nuclear disaster in 1986 and from the nuclear bomb test sites in the Marshall Islands clearly demonstrate that exposure to radioiodine at an early age increases the risk of thyroid cancer as one ages.[20–23] In addition, children treated with external radiation for hematological or other malignancies also are at increased risk for developing thyroid nodules and cancer with a peak at about 10 Gy of exposure.[24–26] Iodine deficiency is associated with a higher incidence of FTC as well as nodular goiter.[27–29] The relationship between obesity and thyroid cancer is less certain with some, but not all studies associating obesity with increases in risk of thyroid cancer while most studies have not shown an association with poor prognosis.[30–34]

Pathology

The eighth edition of the American Joint Commission on Cancer (AJCC)/Union for International Cancer Control (UICC) update on endocrine organ tumors is recommended worldwide for tumor staging and the most updated WHO guidelines are utilized to classify histological subtypes of thyroid cancer.[1,35–38] The histological subtypes of DTC are ascribed based on a combination of specific nuclear features along with growth patterns (Figure 1). PTCs are comprised of cells that contain intranuclear cytoplasmic pseudoinclusions, nuclear grooves, and light hypodense chromatin that classically occur surrounding fibrovascular cores leading to a papillary growth pattern. PTCs also can occur in a "follicular pattern" in which the cells occur in round structures surrounding a colloid core that are termed follicular variant of PTC (FVPTC). Variants of PTC that are often approached in a similar manner to PDTC due to their more aggressive clinical courses include

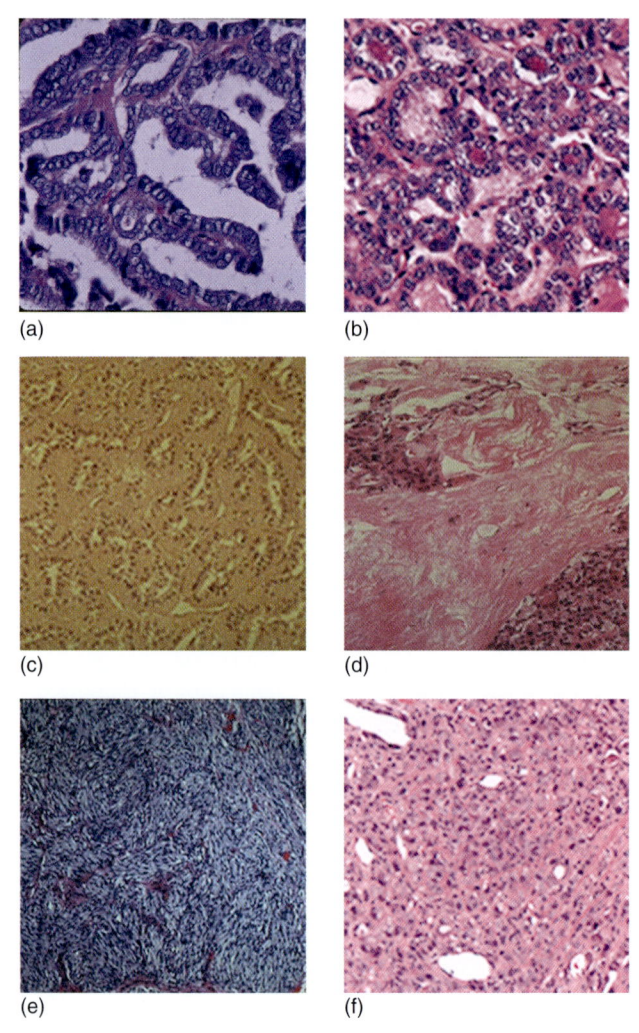

Figure 1 Pathologic features of thyroid carcinoma. (a) Papillary carcinoma, with characteristic fibrovascular papillary formation, crowded nuclei, and nuclear clearing. (b) Follicular variant of papillary carcinoma, with typical cells of papillary carcinoma in follicular formations. (c) Tall cell variant of papillary carcinoma, with cells at least twice as tall as they are wide and eosinophilic cytoplasm. (d) Follicular carcinoma, demonstrating invasion across a thick capsule into neighboring thyroid. (e) Medullary thyroid carcinoma, with nests of spindle-shaped cells. Such nests are often interspersed with clusters of round-to-oval cells. (f) Anaplastic carcinoma, showing large, discohesive, pleomorphic tumor cells. Source: Courtesy of Michelle D. Williams M.D.

tall and columnar cell variants in which the tumors have typical PTC patterns but the height of the cells at least twice the width. Importantly, most PTCs (with the exception of some FVPTCs) are not surrounded by a tumor capsule and do not appear to have a premalignant lesion. Local invasion through the thyroid and vascular invasion can occur, as well as robust peritumoral immune responses. PTCs also commonly can occur in a background of Hashimoto's thyroiditis.

FTCs have a pattern similar to that described above for FVPTCs except that the nuclear features of PTC are absent. In contrast to PTCs, FTCs are characterized by having a tumor capsule and must be distinguished from benign follicular adenomas and noninvasive follicular tumors with papillary features (NIFT-P) that are classified as benign but premalignant. FTCs are diagnosed by the presence of vascular invasion, lymphatic invasion, or capsular invasion. They are further subdivided into minimally invasive and widely invasive subtypes based on the extent of invasion. In general, those tumors with minimal capsular invasion only are clinically handled as minimally invasive FTC and are associated with an outstanding prognosis.

HCC had once been included as a variant of FTC but more recently has been recognized genomically and clinically to be an individual entity.[39–41] HCC cells are characterized by an abundant eosinophilic cytoplasm that is derived of a large number of mitochondria. HCC cells can have either papillary or follicular growth patterns. They typically do not concentrate iodine but make abundant levels of Tg.

PDTCs are felt to derive from well-differentiated FTC or PTCs but still express thyroid differentiated proteins (albeit at lower levels) and do not have anaplastic features.[13] Growth patterns of these tumors are often solid or nested and often are termed as insular forms of thyroid cancer. They are not characterized by typical papillary cellular features and often have necrosis, at least three mitoses per high-powered field, and have abnormal and variably sized nuclei.[13] They typically retain some level of expression of thyroid cells such as Tg.

ATCs are usually large and infiltrative in at diagnosis. They often are highly fibrotic and firm and have extensive evidence of an active immune environment with tumor macrophages, lymphocytes, fibroblasts, and other elements accounting for more than 50% of the cellular mass of the cancer. The thyroid cancer cells themselves have bizarre nuclei and often a spindle cell or giant cell appearance with the absence of expression of all thyroid-specific markers. ATCs are carcinomas and stain for epithelial markers in general. They can occur alone but often the tumors contain regions of DTC and/or PDTC or a variant of PTC that can be either a major or a minor component of the tumor.[42] The presence of ATC, even if a minor component, confers the diagnosis.

MTCs, when they occur in the context of MEN2, derive from regions of hyperplastic C-cells found throughout the thyroid as premalignant lesions. Sporadic MTCs typically present as a thyroid nodule similar to other forms of thyroid cancer. Histologically, MTCs are nests of neuroendocrine cells that have an eosinophilic cytoplasm in association with fibrosis and amyloid deposition, the latter assists in MTC diagnosis. These tumor stain for neuroendocrine markers and are similar in appearance to neuroendocrine tumors from other organs, with the exception of high levels of calcitonin expression.[43]

Pathology staging

The eighth edition of the AJCC/UICC (www.cancerstaging.org) is recommended by most guidelines committees to standardize the approach to thyroid cancer[1,37,38] (Table 1). This system, used for most cancer types, is based on mortality risk for tumors. For thyroid cancer, staging is broken into two groups based on age (greater or less than age 55) to account for the importance of this parameter on 5 and 10-year disease-specific survival rates. The staging system is shown in Table 1 and the system predicts mortality with good accuracy. However, because of the relatively low mortality of DTC, PDTC, and MTC during that time frame and the relatively high risk for residual or clinically recurrent disease (~15–20%), there is concern that this system underestimates clinical risk for younger patients and may overestimate risk for some older patients.[36,37,44–46] Based on these concerns, the American Thyroid Association proposed clinical definitions based on imaging and biochemical evaluations after therapy to assess risk of progressive residual disease that are now validated.[1,47–51] Thus, most clinicians utilize TNM (tumor, node, metastases) to assess risk of tumor-specific mortality but the clinical definitions to assess risk of residual/recurrent disease and to guide active therapy.

Genomics of thyroid cancer

The drivers for most DTCs can be identified (~90%) as has been demonstrated in large genomic studies. One study of PTC performed as part of the NCI Cancer Genome Atlas program serves as an example.[51] In this and many prior studies, it was shown that the majority of sporadic PTCs in adults with classical growth patterns, including Tall and Columnar cell variants, express $BRAF^{V600E}$, a constitutively activating mutation in the mitogen activated protein kinase (MAPK) pathway. By contrast, gene rearrangements involving the Ret receptor tyrosine kinase (RET/PTC) are particularly common after thyroidal exposure to radiation and in children with PTC.[52,53] Tumors with follicular growth patterns (FVPTC, NIFT-P, FTC, and benign follicular adenomas) are more commonly associated with mutations in RAS oncogenes (most commonly NRAS), PPARγ/PAX8 rearrangements or mutations in PIK3CA or PTEN that activate the phosphoinositide 3-kinase (PI3K) pathway and, for RAS, also MAPK signaling.[12] Less common rearrangements and genomic fusions also occur in genes such as neurotrophin receptor tyrosine kinase (NTRK), anaplastic lymphoma kinase (ALK), and thyroid adenoma associated (THADA) that also are bonafide thyroid oncogenes based on experimental models.[51,54,55] As one might predict from their typical slow growth and maintenance of thyroid cell features, DTCs (both PTC and FTCs), are among the most genomically stable forms of cancer. HCCs are genomically unique among thyroid cancers with a near-haploid genotype and higher frequency of mutations in mTOR signaling and mitochondrial DNA.[39,40,54,55]

Uncommon aggressive PTC and FTCs, PDTC, and ATC all are associated with greater degrees of genomic complexity versus smaller well-DTCs. The co-occurrence of a driver mutation with one of two mutations in the promoter of hTERT, the gene that encodes the active domain of telomerase, results in overexpression of telomerase and when paired with BRAF or RAS activating mutations, is associated with worse prognosis.[56] PDTCs and ATCs are more genomically complex than DTCs in general. They often maintain the original driver mutation but gain not only hTERT promoter mutations but also mutations in TP53, in genes involved in DNA damage repair (e.g., ataxia telangetasia mutated 9ATM), chromosomal stability (e.g., SWI/SNF complex members), and mutations that activate PI3K signaling if the driver was $BRAF^{V600E}$.[42,57,58] These result together in greater genomic instability, increased growth rate, and increased immune activation leading to cancer progression.

In MEN2 syndromes, the MTCs are caused by expression of oncogenic RET in the C-cells of the thyroid. Nearly all patients

Table 1 TNM (tumor, node, metastases): The AJCC (American Joint Committee on Cancer) staging scheme for thyroid carcinomas (eighth edition) (www.cancerstaging.org)[a].

T: definition of primary tumor	
TX	Primary tumor cannot be assessed
T0	No evidence of primary tumor
T1	Tumor ≤2 cm in greatest dimension limited to the thyroid
T1a	Tumor ≤1 cm in greatest dimension limited to the thyroid
T1b	Tumor >1 cm but ≤2 cm in greatest dimension, limited to the thyroid
T2	Tumor >2 cm but ≤4 cm in greatest dimension, limited to the thyroid
T3	Tumor >4 cm in greatest dimension limited to the thyroid or gross extrathyroidal extension invading only strap muscle
T3a	Tumor >4 cm limited to the thyroid
T3b	Tumor any size with gross extrathyroid extension invading only strap muscles (sternohyoid, sternothyroid, thyrohyoid, or omohyoid muscles)
T4	Includes gross extrathyroidal extension beyond the strap muscles
T4a	Tumor of any size with gross extrathyroidal extension invading subcutaneous soft tissues, larynx, trachea, esophagus, or recurrent laryngeal nerve
T4b	Tumor of any size with gross extrathyroidal extension invading prevertebral fascia or encasing carotid artery or mediastinal vessels
N: definition of regional lymph nodes	
Nx	Regional lymph nodes cannot be assessed
N0	No evidence of locoregional lymph node metastasis
N0a	One or more cytologically or histologically confirmed benign nodes
N0b	No radiographic or clinical evidence of locoregional nodal metastasis
N1	Metastasis to regional lymph nodes
N1a	Metastases to Level VI or VII (pretracheal, paratracheal, or prelaryngeal/Delphian, or upper mediastinal) lymph nodes. This can be unilateral or bilateral
N1b	Metastases to unilateral, bilateral, or contralateral cervical (Levels I, II, III, IV, or V) or retropharyngeal lymph nodes
M: Definition of Distant metastases	
cM0	No distant metastasis
cM1	Distant metastasis
pM1	Distant metastasis, microscopically confirmed

Prognostic factors required for stating				
Age at diagnosis: <55 Years or ≥ Years				
When age at diagnosis is…	And T is…	And N is…	And M is…	Then the stage group is…
DTC AJCC Prognostic Stage Groups				
<55 years	Any T	Any N	M0	I
<55 years	Any T	Any N	M1	II
≥55 years	T1	N0/NX	M0	I
≥55 years	T1	N1	M0	II
≥55 years	T2	N0/NX	M0	I
≥55 years	T2	N1	M0	II
≥55 years	T3a/T3b	Any N	M0	II
≥55 years	T4a	Any N	M0	III
≥55 years	T4b	Any N	M0	IVA
≥55 years	Any T	Any N	M1	IVB
ATC AJCC prognostic stage groups				
N/A	T1–T3a	N0/NX	M0	IVA
N/A	T1–T3a	N1	M1	IVB
N/A	T3b	Any N	M0	IVB
N/A	T4	Any N	M0	IVB
N/A	Any T	Any N	M1	IVC
MTC AJCC prognostic stage groups				
N/A	T1	N0	M0	I
N/A	T2	N0	M0	II
N/A	T3	N0	M0	II
N/A	T1-3	N1a	M0	III
N/A	T4a	Any N	M0	IVA
N/A	T1-3	N1b	M0	IVA
N/A	T4b	Any N	M0	IVB
N/A	Any T	Any N	M1	IVC

[a]Source: Tuttle et al.[37] with permission from UICC.

with MEN2 will develop MTC over the course of their lives and there are strong genotype–phenotype correlations between particular germline mutations and aggressiveness and age of onset of MTC.[14] These have led to recommendations regarding the timing for prophylactic thyroidectomy that also incorporate family wishes enabling shared decision-making.[14] In the 75% of MTC that are sporadic, approximately 50% will have a *RET* activating mutations, most commonly at codon 918, the same site in that causes MEN2B when inherited in the germline.[59] The majority of the remaining MTCs harbor activating mutations in the *RAS* oncogenes, most commonly *HRAS*.[59]

Diagnostic evaluation and initial imaging of thyroid cancer

Approximately 5% of all thyroid nodules harbor a thyroid cancer.[1] The frequency of thyroid nodules depends on the mode of evaluation and patient demographics. Most studies show that ~5% of patients have palpable thyroid nodules but the frequency of nodules on ultrasound is much higher particularly in older patients.[1,60] Initial evaluation of patients with thyroid nodules includes a patient history and exam as well as a TSH level to assess thyroid function. If a nodule is rock hard, fixed to local structures and/or rapidly growing, there is a higher likelihood of thyroid cancer. Associated neck adenopathy and family history should also be assessed and TSH should be measured. If a patient has thyrotoxicosis, the next step in evaluation is an I-131 thyroid scan and uptake to assess if the nodule is hyper- or hypo-functioning.[1] If the former, malignancy is extremely rare and FNA is not indicated.

The selection of nodules for FNA in patients with normal or elevated TSH levels (or cold nodule iodine scan if hyperthyroid) depends on the risk of cancer as defined by the size and ultrasound features of the nodule. These include the presence or absence of calcifications, the regularity of the borders, degree of echogenicity relative to the normal thyroid, and other features that can be quantified as part of a radiological staging system such as TiRADs or that developed by the American Thyroid Association.[61] In all cases, neck lymph nodes should be assessed because the presence of malignant-appearing nodes may influence the site of FNA (node rather than nodule for a more clear result). Additional studies prior to FNA, such as fluorodeoxyglucose positron emission tomography (FDG/PET) is not recommended as it does not add to the sensitivity of ultrasound and the negative predictive values are lower than FNA.[62,63] Thus, the decision to perform FNA of a particular nodule is based on the clinical and radiographic parameters noted above and most FNAs are performed under ultrasound guidance to ensure accurate sampling of the target nodule. In settings where this technology is not available, palpation-guided FNA is still occasionally performed.

In general, FNA is not recommended for nodules <1 cm even with high-risk features (in the absence of abnormal nodes) or <1.5–2 cm for those with low-risk features or low TiRADs scores. Nodules with intermediate or high TiRADs scores or those with concerning features >1 or 1.5 cm or those nonpurely cystic nodules >2 cm are generally planned for FNA.[1,61,64,65]

The so-called "Bethesda criteria" developed at a consensus panel at NIH is generally utilized for cytopathology readings of thyroid FNA.[66] The first step is to determine if a sufficient sample has been obtained (90–95% of cases) based on the number of clusters containing thyroid cells and the number of thyrocytes per cluster. If sufficient, readings are characterized as benign, atypical cells of undetermined significance or follicular lesion of undetermined significance (ACUS/FLUS), follicular neoplasm or suspicious for follicular neoplasm, suspicious for malignancy, or malignant. The risk of malignancy for these categories varies between cytologists and by the selection criteria used by clinicians to perform a FNA. In general, the false-negative rate (i.e., rate of a benign FNA being malignant) is ~2–5%; the false-positive rate of a malignant FNA being benign is ~1%. The frequency of thyroid cancer in ACUS/FLUS or follicular neoplasia readings is highly variable ranging from ~10 to 35% while those that are suspicious for malignancy are ~80–90% likely to have thyroid cancer.[66] From a practical perspective, benign FNA results lead to monitoring and suspicious or malignant FNA results lead to surgery. Insufficient results lead to repeat FNA or surgery depending on the radiographic and clinical features. ACUS/FLUS or follicular neoplasia results are considered indeterminate and can be addressed by diagnostic surgery, a decision to monitor over time and readdress if there is growth, or by performing additional commercially available molecular diagnostic tests based on mutation profiling, gene expression analysis, or pattern of microRNA expression.[67] In general, these molecular tests have a very high negative predictive value that is similar to that of a benign FNA, and depending on the genes identified as mutated have either very high prediction of cancer (e.g., BRAF^{V600E} or RET^{M918T}) or modest prediction (e.g., RAS) that may influence the decision to send patients to surgery.[67] To date, there is no compelling evidence a particular mutation profile should alter the surgical approach, although there is much ongoing research in this area. MTC also can be difficult to diagnose on cytology. In addition to molecular analysis, in some countries, a random serum calcitonin is obtained in indeterminate or benign nodules due to data suggesting that a level >100 pg/mL is suggestive of this diagnosis.[1,60,68]

Once a thyroid cancer has been diagnosed or is suspected, a CT of the neck with contrast also may be obtained for large tumors or if there are large abnormal nodes, to assist in evaluating for nodes in the superior mediastinum or posterior to the thyroid that are difficult to image by ultrasound.[69] Further staging in the preoperative setting (e.g., CT of chest or PET/CT) is performed only in selected patients with poorly differentiated, very large, or that have extensive nodal disease at diagnosis. In these settings, imaging focuses mostly in the lungs (the most common site of distant metastases in DTC and PDTC) but may include liver and bones in selected patients with MTC. Patients with ATC are typically staged with a PET/CT due to the high sensitivity and potential for metastasis in multiple locations at diagnosis.[70] Brain MRI is also performed for initial staging in ATC.

Initial management of thyroid cancer

Surgery and active surveillance

DTC and PDTC: Surgical removal of the thyroid cancer has long been the mainstay of initial therapy and often is curative for patients with intrathyroidal tumors or those with microscopic nodal metastases. In addition, published data worldwide demonstrate the importance of a higher volume thyroid surgeon, when available, to minimize complications.[69] The extent of initial surgery has been studied for decades, mostly retrospectively, with a long-standing debate in the literature on the need for total thyroidectomy or if hemithyroidectomy is adequate. More recently, for small intrathyroidal PTCs that are easily visualized on ultrasound, active surveillance without initial surgery has been reported, mostly for patients with PTCs <1.0.[5,71,72] For patients either diagnosed with PTCs <1.0 cm or with highly suspicious nodules <1.0 cm and no visible abnormal nodes, active surveillance has been shown to be a safe approach in several retrospective series with up to 10 years of follow-up. During that time ~10–15% of patients underwent surgery either due to growth of the thyroid cancer by >20% or the detection of a new node.[5,71,72] Outcomes were similar between this group and historical controls treated with upfront surgery.[5,71,72] Importantly, it should be recognized that this approach requires joint decision-making with a patient and confidence in the ultrasound follow-up that is required.[73,74] Advantages of active surveillance include the absence of surgical risks of general anesthesia, recurrent laryngeal nerve damage, or hypoparathyroidism, and no requirement for levothyroxine. Disadvantages include patient anxiety, the high frequency of required ultrasound monitoring, and concerns that therapy for rare more aggressive cases might be inadvertently delayed.

Historically, the advantages of total thyroidectomy versus total thyroidectomy included a presumed lower rate of recurrence due to the potential for recurrence in the remaining lobe, enabling radioiodine (RAI) therapy, avoiding reoperation, and creating a more clear baseline for subsequent monitoring.[75] Recent data point to similar recurrent rates for patients with T1 thyroid cancers (<2 cm) between the two surgeries with lower incidences of recurrent laryngeal nerve damage and hypoparathyroidism supporting a greater role for initial hemithyroidectomy,[69] although long-term follow up, cost analyses, and patient-reported outcomes data are less certain. In addition, the need for lifelong levothyroxine therapy following hemithyroidectomy occurs in ~50% of patients, rather than all patients following total thyroidectomy.[69]

To date, there are no large randomized prospective studies to determine optimal cut-points to help clarify the optimal extent of initial surgery. Thus, a practical and experiential approach is generally recommended at the present time: (1) total thyroidectomy for tumors >4 cm, those with local invasion, or those with PDTC; (2) for intrathyroidal solitary thyroid tumors <1 cm either active surveillance or hemithyroidectomy is recommended; (3) for patients with intrathyroidal tumors between 1 and 4 cm, either hemithyroidectomy of total thyroidectomy can be performed and an individualized decision-making approach is recommended.[1,69] Exceptions may occur for patients with multiple contralateral nodules or those with a history of radiation exposure in whom a more aggressive surgical approach might be recommended.

One additional aspect is patient concern about the neck scar that occurs following traditional thyroid surgery. To minimize or alleviate this concern, a number of surgical approaches have been developed to minimize the size of the scar using robotic approaches. In addition, axillary and transoral approaches all have been developed and their potential roles are highlighted in recent surgical guidelines.[69]

With regard to nodal dissection, it is important to recognize that microscopic (<2–3 mm) nodal metastasis occur in the majority of patients with PTC, many patients are cured with surgery that does not include nodal dissection (presumably due to loss of vascular supply after surgery) and that surgical risks are increased by performing this procedure.[69] Thus, "prophylactic" central neck dissection is not generally recommended other than in selected cases with large and/or invasive PDTCs. In contrast, it is generally recommended that clinically enlarged nodes detected preoperatively or in the operating room result in resection of the involved compartments (e.g., central or lateral).[69] In general, the goal of thyroid cancer surgery is to remove all visible tumor in a manner that maximized functional outcomes, unless the disease is unresectable or if a patient refuses the proposed surgery.

MTC: Patients who have newly diagnosed MTC should have a negative *RET* germline sequencing result or be screened for other components of MEN2 prior to surgery. If *RET* mutation-positive or if *RET* sequencing is delayed prior to neck surgery, serum calcium, and plasma-free metanephrine should be performed.[14] If pheochromocytoma is suspected, it should be imaged and addressed prior to neck surgery. If hyperparathyroidism is present, the surgical approach and intraoperative testing may be altered. For patients with MTC, there is a very high frequency of bilateral tumors, even in sporadic cases, there is no I-131 treatment for residual disease, and the prognosis is worse than for DTC. Thus, for patients with known MTC who do not have identified nodal metastases prior to surgery, total thyroidectomy, and bilateral prophylactic central neck and mediastinal dissection are indicated.[14] Previously, prophylactic ipsilateral lateral neck dissections in the absence of identifiable metastases were performed, but this does not clearly improve outcomes and can be associated with surgical complications.[14,76–78]

It has been shown that prophylactic thyroidectomy in children with RET mutation can prevent MTC in the vast majority of cases.[14,19] The age at diagnosis for RET mutation carriers depends on the specific mutation, the family history, and preference of the parents. In general, the more aggressive the mutation, and the more aggressive the family history, the younger age of surgery is recommended.[12,14,19] For MEN2B, for example, prophylactic surgery in children <1 year of is recommended, while in some families with a more benign genotype (e.g., codon 804) and a history of less aggressive disease, monitoring even into adulthood using thyroid ultrasound and calcitonin levels has been successfully employed and is included in guideline recommendations.[12,14,19,69]

ATC: In ATC, it is important to recognize that in most studies, total thyroidectomy does not improve survivorship with the exception of patients with intrathyroidal ATCs.[69,70] In cases where there is locally invasive ATC, surgery may be performed with palliative rather than curative intent. More recently, for selected patients with ATC that have a $BRAF^{V600E}$ mutation, there is potential for neoadjuvant therapy with a BRAF/MEK inhibitor combination to improve surgical outcomes, an approach that is being studied at present.[79,80] Preoperative imaging generally using PET/CT, neck CT with contrast, and brain MRI is recommended when the diagnosis is clear preoperatively.[38,70]

Postsurgical assessment of disease status

With the exception of rare patients who present with distant metastases, the goal of surgery is to remove all visible tumor. The typical approach after surgery is to place the patient on levothyroxine at a dose estimated to fully replace the thyroid (~1.6 mcg/kg) and assess the status 2–3 months after surgery.[1] The rationale is to determine if the patient had an excellent, incomplete, or indeterminate response to surgery. This assessment relies primarily on two features, measurement of serum levels of Tg, and radiographic imaging primarily consisting of neck ultrasound for patients with PTC and for other patients to assess for residual thyroid tissue.[1] More extensive imaging based on tumor histology, Tg levels, or other features are individually recommended as detailed in the subsequent sections.

Thyroglobulin measurement: Tg is a thyroid-specific protein that serves as the backbone for thyroid hormones.[81] It is stored in colloid in the normal thyroid but also is secreted and can be measured. In the early 1980s after development of an assay that could detect circulating Tg, its potential utility in monitoring patients with thyroid cancer was recognized and reported.[82,83] Over the years, there have been improvements in Tg assays; however, there remain several caveats for measuring Tg. The first is that up to 20% of patients harbor circulating anti-Tg antibodies.[84] The antibodies interfere with measurements of Tg; they falsely lower Tg levels when measured by immunochemiluminescent assay or immunoradiometric assay (ICMA and IRMA, respectively) or falsely elevate radioimmunoassay measurements (RIA).[1,84,85] Because ICMA assays are most commonly used, they can cause false-negative results in many patients. Thus, Tg measurement should always be paired with an anti-Tg antibody measurement on the same sample. Several methods have been developed to circumvent this issue including commercially available measurements using liquid chromatography/tandem mass spectroscopy (LC/MSMS), measurements of different thyroids-specific mRNA transcripts in blood, and measures of circulating free DNA for specific mutations.[86–89] Of these, the Tg LC/MSMS has been most widely employed, but it suffers from low sensitivity in many patients.[90,91] Finally, anti-Tg Ab levels themselves can serve as tumor markers but often can take years to disappear in patients in a complete remission (CR).[84,92] The second caveat is that Tg itself is not thyroid cancer specific, but rather is thyroid specific. Therefore, it must be paired with imaging such as a neck ultrasound to ascertain if there is residual thyroid tissue remaining that may account for measurable Tg levels.[1] The limited accuracy of Tg levels for thyroid cancer monitoring after hemithyroidectomy should be considered prior to opting for this surgical approach. Finally, it is important to recognize that PDTCs may express and secrete Tg but perhaps at a lower level per cell than DTCs. Thus, in such cases, lower Tg levels may reflect a larger residual tumor burden. The half-life of Tg is ~8 days, thus 6–12 weeks after surgery is usually an adequate time to assess postoperative baseline.[1]

Calcitonin and CEA measurement: Serum calcitonin is a useful highly specific and sensitive marker for identifying residual MTC after surgery.[76–78] It is not expressed to a significant degree in other tissues. Although levels can increase by proton pump inhibitors that increase gastrin or acute changes in calcium levels, it is generally undetectable following total thyroidectomy and central neck dissection. MTCs also typically express carcinoembryonic antigen (CEA) and this measure, while not specific for MTCs also is useful in monitoring patients with MTC following thyroidectomy and central neck dissection.[14] Calcitonin is a small peptide with a short half-life, thus it can be measured several weeks after surgery to assess baseline.[77]

Postoperative imaging: Postoperative imaging for patients with PTC is generally directed at the neck due to its predilection for nodal spread, most commonly using neck ultrasound if a skilled operator is available.[1] This will assess for any residual thyroid cancer, abnormal nodes, and determine the amount of any residual thyroid tissue that might be present to help interpret laboratory evaluations. Typically, it will take ~3 months for postoperative swelling and changes to resolve. Imaging for other forms of thyroid cancer, and more aggressive PTCs, typically includes the neck but may be more extensive depending on marker levels or histological subtype.[1] If Tg is very high, the thyroid cancer is poorly differentiated suggesting Tg may under-represent the amount of thyroid cancer, or calcitonin levels in MTC are elevated then systemic imaging, if not already performed, should be performed after surgery. Because patients with FTC rarely develop local nodal metastasis, if an FTC with extensive vascular invasion is removed, a chest CT is generally performed. Whether or not a chest CT should be performed in all patients with anti-Tg antibodies is an area of debate in the literature. The extent of imaging for MTC is determined by the postoperative calcitonin level with systemic imaging limited to those with calcitonin levels >150 pg/mL.[14] Systemic imaging with FDG-PET/CT and brain MRI is recommended for all patients with ATC if not performed prior to surgery.[38,70]

Assignment of postoperative response: The ATA guidelines initially adopted a risk-adaptive approach to determine the status of patients with DTC at various time points and use that status to clarify the roles of therapy.[1] This approach has been validated in a number of populations and is combined with the UJC/UICC staging to estimate the likelihood of residual or recurrent thyroid cancer and predict outcomes.[47–50] After surgery, one can achieve an excellent response (Tg < 1.0 ng/mL and a negative neck ultrasound); an incomplete response (positive imaging or a Tg > 10 ng/mL with negative imaging); or an indeterminate response (Tg 1–10 ng/mL with negative imaging or anti-Tg Ab positive with negative imaging).[1] These assignments are useful constructs, when combined with the pathology staging, to determine the best approach for additional therapy such as TSH suppression, RAI. A similar approach can be used for patients with MTC using calcitonin and CEA as the biochemical markers.[14]

TSH suppression therapy

In comparison to patients who have thyroidectomy for benign thyroid disease, classically, patients with DTC or PDTC have been treated with mildly higher doses of thyroid hormone to suppress TSH levels while maintaining normal circulating free T4 levels.[1] Studies over the past 20 years have demonstrated overall and disease-free survival benefit for TSH suppression for patients with stage III and IV disease while more modest, or no benefits have been shown for patients with stage I and II disease.[1,93–95] In all cases, there are potential side effects of TSH suppression that become more significant as patients age and with greater degrees of TSH suppression, principally an increased risk of heart palpitations and atrial fibrillation and acceleration of osteoporosis in postmenopausal women.[96] These side effects can be mitigated by use of beta-blockers and antiresorptive agents but concerns for these side effects have led to a more individualized approach to long-term TSH suppression. In general, patients with stage III, IV, or stage II patients with distant metastases or growing local residual disease are treated to achieve TSH <0.1 mU/L; those with residual Tg levels and/or at higher risk of recurrence goal TSH is 0.1–0.5 mU/L, and those who have achieved an excellent response (see above) with stage I disease, or with stage II or III disease that is durable for 5 years, TSH in the lower part of the normal range is adequate.[1,96] Most patients with ATC also do not benefit from TSH suppression as they do not express TSH receptor, although some patients may benefit from this if the tumors have a component of PDTC or DTC but the impact may still be more modest.[70,97] Similarly, TSH suppression is not appropriate for patients with MTC because the cancer cells do not express the TSH receptor.[14]

RAI therapy

RAI therapy is likely the first every targeted therapy use to treat cancer in a systemic manner. In the 1940s, it was first recognized that radioactive forms of iodine could be used to detect and treat Graves' disease.[98,99] This approach was extended subsequently to thyroid cancer therapy.[100,101] Since then, it has been a pillar of thyroid cancer medial therapy and historically, most or nearly all patients with DTC or PDTC were treated with RAI. RAI is not appropriate for MTC, which does not express the Na. I symporter (NIS) or for ATC other than in selected cases in which there is a major component of DTC or PDTC in the tumor.[70]

Over the past decade, with the improvement of Tg assays, neck ultrasound, and CT scans, there has been a greater recognition of the low sensitivity of RAI scanning to detect thyroid cancer a greater understanding of the side-effects of therapy.[1] Thus, there has been emphasis on defining the rationale for the use of RAI in an effort to avoid overtreatment of patients who have had an excellent response to surgery while focusing efforts to maximize efficacy in patients with progressive metastatic disease. Current guidelines categorize the use of RAI by clinical goal: (1) *remnant ablation* where therapy is planned to ablate residual presumed normal thyroid tissue to enable easier monitoring long term. This term is mostly for individual who have achieved an excellent response to surgery with lower risk thyroid cancers, or those with significant normal tissue remnants that may impair monitoring; (2) *adjuvant therapy*, when patients with either an indeterminate response or those with an excellent response but high-risk pathology parameters are treated for presumed residual thyroid cancer; (3) *RAI therapy* for patients with known residual thyroid cancer with distant metastases or other incomplete response parameter following surgery.[1] Dosing strategies follow the rationale used for the therapy with progressively higher doses used for patients more likely or known to have thyroid cancer.

Treatment with RAI requires meticulous patient preparation and the efficacy relies in effective delivery of I-131 to the target cells that depends on the amount of RAI uptake that can be achieved.[1] RAI uptake occurs through the function of the NIS, which is a cell membrane transporter. NIS expression and function are regulated by TSH with higher expression and function achieved with higher TSH levels, and lower levels of circulating iodide to minimize competition for the I-131 and reduce endogenous iodide stores. Thus, patients are typically prepared for RAI with a low iodine diet for ~2 weeks and either taken off of thyroid hormone to increase endogenous TSH levels, or administered recombinant human TSH (rhTSH) so they can continue thyroid hormone.[1] Several prospective randomized studies have demonstrated similar efficacy for thyroid hormone withdrawal or rhTSH preparation for first therapy after surgery.[102–104] Retrospective studies have suggested rhTSH is also effective preparation for long-term benefit and for patients with distant metastases but this is not part of its FDA approval.[1,105–107] Most centers, although not all, perform a diagnostic I-131 whole body scan with 2–5 mci of I-123 or I-131 to identify unexpected areas of uptake that might influence dosing strategies. The patient is typically then treated within 24–48 hours with the treatment dose of I-131. This is followed by resumption of a regular diet and thyroid hormone (if prepared with L-T4 withdrawal) two days later, and by a period of home, quarantine to avoid exposing others to excreted radiation. Depending on the administered dose, rate of secrtionl, local/national laws, and patient-specific social factors, hospital admission may be required. Most centers perform a posttherapy scan to complete that component of staging and document areas of uptake a 7–14 days after the treatment after which time patients are able to resume normal activities.

Side effects of I-131 are generally dose-related. This includes those related to NIS expression in nonthyroid tissues, such as episodes of sialoadenitis that can result in permanent damage with resultant dry mouth or dental issues, and lacrimal duct stenosis. In addition, there are complications related to systemic radiation exposure, such as transient oligospermia and leukopenia, particularly when higher or repeated doses are administered.[108,109] Higher doses of cumulative RAI therapies are associated with secondary malignancies. The most common in large population series is acute myelogenous leukemia (AML) and salivary cancers that occur at ~0.05% estimated rate greater in thyroid cancer patients treated with RAI versus those not treated with RAI, although there is heterogeneity in the reported numbers and study designs.[110–114] Individual centers have described higher incidences of some solid tumors such as colorectal, bladder, and breast cancers, but these have not been consistently identified in larger population-based studies.[114] Finally, patients with high levels of diffuse lung uptake can develop radiation-induced pulmonary fibrosis.

The general concept of dosing I-131 at present is to use it only to treat patients who will benefit, and use the lowest dose needed in order to minimize the risk of off-target toxicity.[1,60] Thus, many patients with early-stage thyroid cancer who have achieved an excellent response are no longer treated with I-131 therapy. Pts for whom remnant ablation is selected, typically a dose in the 30–100 mCi range is selected. A similar range is utilized for patients treated with adjuvant therapy with occasionally higher dose depending on the pathology and if there are positive surgical margins. Finally, for patients with known residual thyroid cancer, particularly those with distant metastases, higher doses up to ~200 mCi may be employed.[1] Whole-body dosimetry is performed at some centers to ensure that administered doses do not exceed safety recommendations for lung or bone marrow exposure while lesional dosimetry can be performed at some centers to maximize delivered dose.[115,116]

Reoperation

Reoperation prior to RAI therapy is sometimes performed in several scenarios. One is when a patient has a diagnostic hemithyroidectomy and surgical pathology identifies a thyroid cancer for whom RAI is likely to be recommended. In that case, a completion hemithyroidectomy is generally recommended.[1,69] A second scenario occurs if residual nodes are identified on postoperative imaging. This may include tissue in the superior mediastinum, the lateral neck, or in the posterior central neck that were difficult to identify and remove at the initial surgery. In these situations, particularly if nodes are >1 cm in size, reoperation (compartmental resection) is often recommended prior to I-131 therapy.[69]

External beam radiation therapy (EBRT)

External beam radiation therapy (EBRT) is utilized in selected patients with locally aggressive, PDTC with aerodigestive invasion. It is most commonly administered using intensity-modified strategies to minimize toxicities. There is evidence from nonrandomized studies that EBRT can reduce the frequency of progression of residual disease in older patients with incompletely resected PTC and PDTC.[117–119] In general, EBRT is considered in patients with inoperable residual locally aggressive thyroid cancer with aerodigestive invasion and/or with positive margins. Typical doses for DTC and PDTC are in the 50 Gy range.

EBRT may have a role in MTC treatment in similar circumstances to that described in DTC/PDTC in which further surgery is not possible and local invasion and progression is present. However, retrospective studies suggest benefit that is more modest for this selected group of patients.[117,118,120] For MTC, doses are typically in 50–60 Gy range to achieve local control.

In ATC, EBRT combined with chemotherapy is one of the frequently used treatment options to attain local control of disease and have some benefit on distant metastases. Despite some data suggesting local control rates are transiently improved, survival benefits have not been reported.[121–123]

Monitoring after completion of initial therapy

Patients are typically monitored using the same biochemical and radiographic tests as outlined above for assessing status after surgery. For DTC/PDTC serum Tg with anti-Tg antibodies; and for MTC, plasma calcitonin levels and serum CEA levels.[1,14] Typically, these are performed at 3 months intervals after completion of initial therapy and imaging is performed after 12 months, unless there is concern with changes in biochemical parameters. For patients with ATC, for whom Tg is insensitivity, there is greater reliance on imaging at 3 month intervals.[70]

Tg assays that now measure to a sensitivity of 0.1 ng/mL have made the prior requirement for TSH stimulation for adequate sensitivity unnecessary for most patients.[90,124,125] The pattern of Tg, calcitonin, or CEA changes over time are strong predictors of outcome from thyroid cancer.[126–133] The "doubling times" for all of these markers, in conjunction with the absolute levels, are useful parameters to predict outcomes (poor for doubling times <6 months; excellent for >2 years) and in determining timing for subsequent imaging and/or therapy. In addition, based on the frequency of identifying anatomical lesions, systemic imaging for residual/recurrent MTC is not recommended until calcitonin levels are >100–150 pg/mL.[14] When following Tg doubling times, it is important to recognize not only that it cannot be reliably used in the context of anti-Tg Ab even if detectable but also that TSH levels also influence Tg levels. Thus, it is necessary to use Tg levels with relatively consistent TSH levels on L-T4 when calculating doubling times.

The choice of diagnostic imaging depends on the type of thyroid cancer and the level of the biomarker. For PTC, where neck nodes and lung lesions predominate, lower levels of Tg leads to neck ultrasound and if negative or if levels are higher, chest CT often is employed. FTC, which is most associated with hematogenous spread, earlier performance of chest CT and potentially spine MRI is performed.[1] Brain MRI may also be used in patients with bone or large volume lung metastases, or those with high Tg levels and negative imaging.[134,135] Diagnostic whole-body I-131 scanning, a long-standing mainstay of monitoring, is much less frequently performed due to its lower sensitivity, although there is a high specificity for DTCs. ATCs and PDTCs may make little or no Tg and often are followed by FDG PET/CT and imaging may include brain MRI.[70] FDG-PET/CT scanning is often useful in HCCs that typically have high levels of FDG uptake.[136,137] Lastly, for MTC, three-phase contrast CT or MRI of the liver and axial skeleton MRI are often employed in addition to neck and chest imaging due to the higher frequency of liver and bone metastases, particularly at higher calcitonin levels.[14] Newer PET imaging modalities such as DOTATATE-PET/CT that binds to somatostatin receptors may have utility in MTC based on a number of recent reports.[138,139] Bone scanning has low utility in patients with DTC and MTC owing to the frequent lytic nature of the metastases.

Long-term remission

Continued biomarker and imaging results consistent with excellent response over time define CR from thyroid cancer. Typically, once this response level is achieved for 1–2 years, the frequency of biochemical and imaging is reduced depending on the initial pathology prediction of recurrence risk. Other than in aggressive DTC, PDTC, or ATC, patients with a persistent excellent response after 5 years are followed generally with annual Tg, or calcitonin/CEA levels for MTC, with neck ultrasound at 5 years intervals or as driven by biochemical markers. Similarly, for patients with DTC in a remission, the degree of TSH suppression is typically reduced after 3–5 years depending on the initial tumor staging for a goal TSH in the 0.1–0.5 mU/L or low/normal ranges. This less aggressive monitoring and treatment approach is based upon data demonstrating that the frequency of clinical recurrence is low after 5 years, particularly for individual with early-stage DTC.[1]

Management of clinically recurrent, progressive, or metastatic disease

Residual and recurrent thyroid cancer: general approach

With the improved sensitivity of Tg measurement and neck ultrasound over the years, there has been a greater recognition that much of what has been referred to as "recurrent" disease in the literature frequently reflects progression of nonanatomically defined residual disease.[140] This does not imply incomplete efforts to eradicate all thyroid cancer, but that subclinical residual thyroid tissue, often in very small nodes, is common. Moreover, patients with DTC who later are found to have pulmonary metastases, for example, likely had subclinical metastases at diagnosis since in distinction for many other tumor types, the entire thyroid gland is removed and residual tissue is often ablated or treated with RAI. A recent autopsy study further suggests that is the case as a surprisingly high proportion of patients with incidentally identified thyroid cancer at autopsy also harbored small lung metastases that were subclinical.[141] Thus, it is likely that most clinically recurrent thyroid cancer represents subclinical residual thyroid cancer that remains after initial therapy.

Because of its slow growth pattern, the overall excellent long-term disease-specific survivorship, and typical absence of symptoms, the decision of when or how to treat clinically recurrent or residual DTC has evolved over the years.[1] The decision to treat again with RAI, surgery, EBRT, or a systemic medical therapy depends on the rate and location of growth, the presence or absence of symptoms balance, and predicted outcomes without therapy beyond TSH suppression balanced by the anticipated outcome and side-effects from treatment to balance quality of life. Many patients with stable or slowly growing asymptomatic metastases to the neck and lungs are treated with TSH suppression, and perhaps RAI if there was prior uptake, and are monitored without further therapy unless the rate of progression changes or larger tumor volumes occur. Data for DTC and MTC using either biochemical or radiographic doubling times point to a consistent rate of progression (log/linear curves) over time for most patients.[126,128–133,142,143] Interestingly, the duration of clinical dormancy with stable low volume disease can last for decades, thus, this monitoring approach is usually acceptable to patients.

PDTCs and some MTCs have variable clinical courses that can range from slow progression to much more aggressive behaviors. Thus, a more aggressive therapeutic approach often is utilized. For MTC in particular, symptoms may develop due to hormone secretion from the cancer-causing watery diarrhea, flushing, and Cushing syndrome for which symptomatic therapy may be employed.[14]

Patients with ATC and some with PDTC, with residual disease in the neck, distant metastases, or progression have a poor prognosis. While individuals with a BRAF^{V600E} mutation-positive ATC may have remarkable initial responses to ATC, even these patients typically relapse and succumb to the disease.[144] Thus, treatment strategies for ATC include less aggressive approaches to maintain patient quality of life and comfort.[70]

Isolated or limited recurrence locations

Surgery and interventional radiology
For residual or recurrent thyroid cancer identified in the neck, typically a compartmental resection including the involved regions on imaging and/or FNA is performed if the nodes are large, symptomatic, or at risk of complications such as invasion into local structures (e.g., trachea or esophagus).[69] Risk of complications from reoperation, particularly in the central neck, is higher than primary surgeries. In selected patients, alternative local therapies such as ethanol injection, radiofrequency ablation (RFA), LASER, and others have been reported.[145–147] In some cases, re-treatment and treatment side effects occur. It is important for patients and physicians to recognize that data from a number of large centers demonstrated that the most outcome from surgery for recurrent thyroid cancer is local control and/or reductions in biochemical markers and reduced tumor volume, not complete remission (CR rates ~50% depending on the stringency of the definition).[69] The tumor outcome depends in part on the completeness of surgical resection and anatomical and pathology factors. Similar results have been published for MTC, thus reoperation is recommended only for patients with more bulky disease in the neck.

Surgery is sometimes employed for distant metastases to alleviate local symptoms, prevent catastrophic complications such as in the vertebral column or hip, or to great rapidly growing metastatic lesions. These procedures usually are performed either for palliation, or in an effort to delay systemic therapies. Isolated or dominant brain metastases are often treated surgically, or with stereotactic radiosurgery (SRS) methods.[1] Bone metastases also can be treated with interventional radiology techniques such as RFA, TACE in liver metastases, cryo-treatment, and others.[1] These are considered on an individual case bases and are highly dependent on access to skilled physicians to perform these procedures.

EBRT

Similar to some cases of primary cancer therapy, local/regional metastases also are often treated using EBRT. In the neck, this is often employed after surgery for aggressive disease in the central neck in patients with PDTC and often can achieve local control with rates as high as 55% at 10 years reported.[122] EBRT is administered in most cases for symptomatic growing bone metastases or those with impending fracture, depending on the location. SRS for isolated brain metastases and whole-brain radiation for patients with multifocal and higher volume brain metastases also is employed with some benefit.[1]

Progressive multi-location/distant disease

RAI therapy

RAI has been a mainstay of therapy for patients with residual thyroid cancer when detected after initial therapy. RAI has been shown to be effective in inducing CR in selected patients with iodine avid micrometastatic (<1 cm) lung metastases using repeated doses, particularly in younger patients.[148] Some institutions prefer to administer larger doses of I-131 based on either safety profiles defined using whole blood dosimetry and/or delivered radioactivity to selected targets (lesion dosimetry) with some suggestion of benefit from this approach in nonrandomized studies.[115,116,149] Despite years of use, a prospective study of RAI versus monitoring with TSH suppression in patients with progressive thyroid cancer has not been performed. Thus, many patients are treated who have stable RAI avid disease and it is not known if early therapy is beneficial for all both those selected patients noted above.

RAI refractory disease is generally defined in several manners: (1) the absence of uptake on diagnostic or post-RAI therapy whole-body scanning in patients with certain metastatic disease (biopsy or prior RAI uptake); (2) progression within 1–2 years of a therapeutic dose of RAI despite uptake; (3) in some clinical trials, the absence of partial response or therapeutic benefit despite a cumulative dose of >600 mCi.[1] The latter is based on data showing relatively low efficacy of doses >600 mCi; however, it is important to recognize that although potential risks do increase with higher doses, higher cumulative doses may be employed in selected cases depending on responses to prior therapies, degree of I-131 uptake, or other considerations.

Over the past several years, there has been a renewed interest in "redifferentiation" approaches where a RAI-resistant thyroid cancer can be pretreated to increase NIS expression and RAI uptake thereby improving therapeutic response. This has been driven by basic and translational studies demonstrating that activation of the MAPK pathway by RAS or BRAF activation causes dedifferentiation of thyroid cells *in vivo*, reducing expression of both the TSH receptor and NIS thereby reducing iodine uptake.[150] Disruption of this pathway using BRAF and MEK inhibitors in the context of a BRAF^{V600E} mutation, or MEK inhibition alone in the context of either a BRAF^{V600E} or RAS mutation reversed this effect in thyroid cells and mouse models.[150,151] Several clinical trials have shown benefit of this approach for patients with DTC or PDTC that harbor RAS activating mutations or BRAF^{V600E} treated with either MEK inhibitors or a combination of BRAF^{V600E} and MEK inhibitors, respectively.[152–154] Larger clinical trials are ongoing. How and if this approach should be incorporated into clinical care remains an area of active research that holds promise.

Medical therapy

Medical therapy is considered for selected patients with progressive RAI-refractory thyroid cancer, particularly those with progressive or symptomatic distant metastases.[80,155] Medical therapy also is considered for patients with progressive and/or symptomatic MTC and for patients with ATC.[14,38,70,79] Thyroid cancer is relatively resistant to cytotoxic chemotherapy, despite an FDA approval for doxorubicin for ATC in the early 1970s.[70] There is evidence that ATCs may have transient partial responses to taxane-based chemotherapies but no survival benefit has been demonstrated.[70,156] Thus, while some patients with ATC are treated with cytotoxic chemotherapy, expectations are for transient partial responses but not major or complete responses.

Over the past decade, there has been emphasis on treating patients with progressive thyroid cancer with kinase inhibitors, ranging from multikinase inhibitors (MKIs) that are relatively nonspecific, to highly specific inhibitors of thyroid cancer oncogenes[80] (Figure 2). For MTC, the FDA approved the MKIs vandetanib and cabozantinib, that inhibit RET, VEGF receptors, and other angiogenic kinase receptors, based on prolonged progression-free survivals and partial response rates in the 30% range with duration or response in the 18–30 month ranges.[157–160] Side effects with the medications were common and there was a suggestion of greatest benefit in patients with *RET*^{M918T}-mutated MTC for cabozantinib.[158] The medications have side effects such as weight loss, nausea, fatigue, and hypertension, prolongation of QT intervals on electrocardiogram, and rarely, perforations and fistula formation. Thus, use is limited for patients with progressive MTC whose life expectance is <50% at 5 years or who have a high degree of symptoms.[79,157–160] A second generation of RET inhibitors with much greater specificity (selpercatinib and pralsetinib) have been developed with impressive antitumor effects in those harboring *RET* mutations with fewer side effects; both of which were FDA approved for RET-mutated or RET-rearranged cancers including MTC and PTC.[161–163] Thus, while not appropriate for patients with *RET*-wild-type MTCs (such as those with RAS mutations), this offers a new alternative for appropriately selected patients. Resistance mechanisms including overexpression of C-MET or the development of "solvent front" mutations in RET have been identified.[164–166] Finally, nonrandomized studies of peptide receptor radionuclide therapy (PRRT) driven by somatostatin analogs have demonstrated promising results.[80,167–170]

In DTC, the MKIs sorafenib and lenvatinib are approved in the United States for patients with progressive metastatic and/or symptomatic RAI-refractory DTC and PDTC.[159,171–176] Similar to vandetanib and cabozantinib, these compounds lead to improved progression-free survivorship, PR in a minority of patients, side effects that can be limiting, and a several-year duration of action.[79,159,171–177] Occasionally, rearrangements involving Ret (e.g., RET/PTC) NTRK, or ALK are identified in DTC and PDTC. FDA-approved therapies that are disease agnostic are in place for several of these targets and have been reported to be effective for patients with thyroid cancer in the setting of clinical trials or case reports.[79,177] These data have led to recommendations for genomic analysis of growing metastatic thyroid cancer tissues or from blood

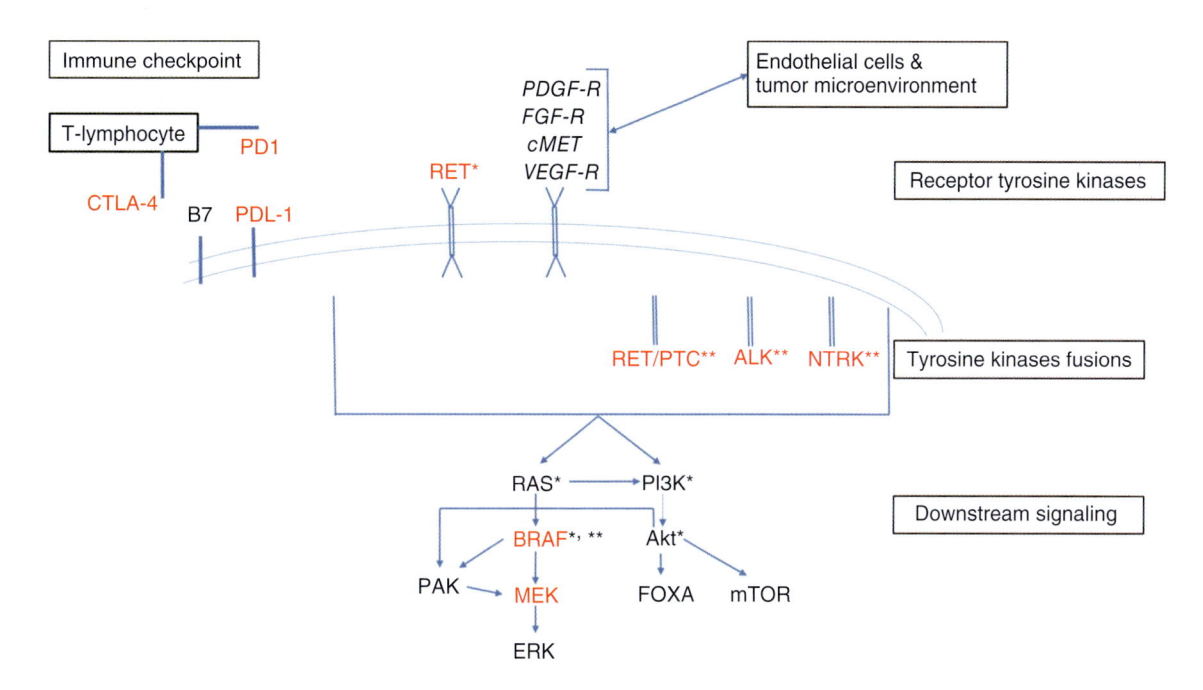

Figure 2 Therapeutic Targets in Thyroid Cancer. Genomic drivers of thyroid cancer include mutations (*) or rearrangements (**) in genes that result in enhanced activity of signaling pathways. Mutational activation occurs at the level of receptor tyrosine kinases (e.g., RET) and in signaling molecules such as BRAF, RAS, PI3K, and AKT. Chromosomal rearrangements that lead to fusion proteins linking the promoter and exons of one gene to the kinase domain of a tyrosine kinase (e.g., RET, NTRK, ALK) or serine-threonine kinase (e.g., BRAF) result in overexpression and activation of the wild type kinase. Additional therapeutic targets include proteins that regulate the immune checkpoint and those that control tumor cell interactions with the microenvironment. Red notates the proteins with FDA-approved compounds with specific targeting. Bold and italicized names indicate receptor tyrosine kinases that are inhibited by FDA-approved multikinase inhibitors. Source: Ringel[80] (reproduced with permission).

to allow for selection of therapies for patients selected for medical therapy.[38,155]

In 2019, the FDA approved combination therapy with dabrafenib (BRAF^{V600E} inhibitor) and trametinib (MEK inhibitor) for BRAF^{V600E}-mutated ATC based on case reports and a cohort nonrandomized experience that all reported occasional dramatic initial responses with possible disease-specific survival benefit vs historical controls.[144,177] Thus, it is now standard to perform BRAF^{V600E} genotyping or BRAF^{V600E}- specific immunohistochemistry on ATC samples at diagnosis.[38] Studies are ongoing to determine the potential use of this combination in a preoperative manner to facilitate surgery, and as a radiation sensitizer in this context.[79,178] Clinical trials using less specific MKIs have not shown benefit in ATC.

A robust immune response, genomic instability, and high levels of programmed death-1 (PD1) and programmed death ligand-1 (PDL1), all of which predict response to immune checkpoint inhibitors (ICIs) therapy, are common in ATC. Thus, ICI therapies have been used in ATC with reported benefits.[179] Efficacy in progressive DTC and PDTC has been reported in selected patients.[180] Clinical trials are ongoing using combinations of MKI with ICI and with multiple ICIs. Finally, there has been interested in pursuing immune therapies including ICI and cellular therapies in MTC and ATC as the search for more effective therapies continues.[80,181]

Key references

The complete reference list can be found on Vital Source version of this title, see inside front cover.

1 Haugen BR, Alexander EK, Bible KC, et al. 2015 American Thyroid Association Management Guidelines for Adult Patients with Thyroid Nodules and Differentiated Thyroid Cancer: The American Thyroid Association Guidelines Task Force on Thyroid Nodules and Differentiated Thyroid Cancer. *Thyroid*. 2016;**26**(1):1–133.

4 Davies L, Morris L, Hankey B. Increases in thyroid cancer incidence and mortality. *JAMA*. 2017;**318**(4):389–390.

5 Ito Y, Miyauchi A. Active surveillance of low-risk papillary thyroid microcarcinomas in Japan and other countries: a review. *Expert Rev Endocrinol Metab*. 2020;**15**(1):5–12.

6 Cibas ES, Alexander EK, Benson CB, et al. Indications for thyroid FNA and pre-FNA requirements: a synopsis of the National Cancer Institute Thyroid Fine-Needle Aspiration State of the Science Conference. *Diagn Cytopathol*. 2008;**36**(6):390–399.

13 Volante M, Collini P, Nikiforov YE, et al. Poorly differentiated thyroid carcinoma: the Turin proposal for the use of uniform diagnostic criteria and an algorithmic diagnostic approach. *Am J Surg Pathol*. 2007;**31**(8):1256–1264.

14 Wells SA Jr, Asa SL, Dralle H, et al. Revised American Thyroid Association guidelines for the management of medullary thyroid carcinoma. *Thyroid*. 2015;**25**(6):567–610.

19 Skinner MA, Moley JA, Dilley WG, et al. Prophylactic thyroidectomy in multiple endocrine neoplasia type 2A. *N Engl J Med*. 2005;**353**(11):1105–1113.

20 Baverstock K, Egloff B, Pinchera A, et al. Thyroid cancer after Chernobyl. *Nature*. 1992;**359**(6390):21–22.

26 Veiga LH, Lubin JH, Anderson H, et al. A pooled analysis of thyroid cancer incidence following radiotherapy for childhood cancer. *Radiat Res*. 2012;**178**(4):365–376. doi: 10.1667/rr2889.1.

30 Paes JE, Hua K, Nagy R, et al. The relationship between body mass index and thyroid cancer pathology features and outcomes: a clinicopathological cohort study. *J Clin Endocrinol Metab*. 2010;**95**(9):4244–4250.

32 Kitahara CM, Pfeiffer RM, Sosa JA, Shiels MS. Impact of overweight and obesity on US papillary thyroid cancer incidence trends (1995-2015). *J Natl Cancer Inst*. 2020;**112**(8):810–817.

37 Tuttle RM, Haugen B, Perrier ND. Updated American Joint Committee on cancer/tumor-node-metastasis staging system for differentiated and anaplastic thyroid cancer (eighth edition): what changed and why? *Thyroid*. 2017;**27**(6):751–756.

39 Ganly I, Makarov V, Deraje S, et al. Integrated genomic analysis of hurthle cell cancer reveals oncogenic drivers, recurrent mitochondrial mutations, and unique chromosomal landscapes. *Cancer Cell*. 2018;**34**(2):256–70.e5.

40. Gopal RK, Kubler K, Calvo SE, et al. Widespread chromosomal losses and mitochondrial DNA alterations as genetic drivers in hurthle cell carcinoma. *Cancer Cell*. 2018;(2):34, 242–55.e5.
47. Pitoia F, Jerkovich F, Urciuoli C, et al. Implementing the modified 2009 American Thyroid Association Risk Stratification System in thyroid cancer patients with low and intermediate risk of recurrence. *Thyroid*. 2015;**25**(11):1235–1242.
51. Cancer Genome Atlas Research Network. Integrated genomic characterization of papillary thyroid carcinoma. *Cell*. 2014;**159**(3):676–690.
56. Xing M, Liu R, Liu X, et al. BRAF V600E and TERT promoter mutations cooperatively identify the most aggressive papillary thyroid cancer with highest recurrence. *J Clin Oncol*. 2014;**32**(25):2718–2726.
57. Landa I, Ibrahimpasic T, Boucai L, et al. Genomic and transcriptomic hallmarks of poorly differentiated and anaplastic thyroid cancers. *J Clin Invest*. 2016;**126**(3):1052–1066.
61. Angell TE, Maurer R, Wang Z, et al. A cohort analysis of clinical and ultrasound variables predicting cancer risk in 20,001 consecutive thyroid nodules. *J Clin Endocrinol Metab*. 2019;**104**(11):5665–5672.
66. Cibas ES, Ali SZ. The 2017 Bethesda system for reporting thyroid cytopathology. *J Am Soc Cytopathol*. 2017;**6**(6):217–222.
69. Patel KN, Yip L, Lubitz CC, et al. The American Association of Endocrine Surgeons Guidelines for the definitive surgical management of thyroid disease in adults. *Ann Surg*. 2020;**271**(3):e21–e93.
70. Smallridge RC, Ain KB, Asa SL, et al. American Thyroid Association guidelines for management of patients with anaplastic thyroid cancer. *Thyroid*. 2012;**22**(11):1104–1139.
73. Ito Y, Miyauchi A, Kudo T, et al. Trends in the implementation of active surveillance for low-risk papillary thyroid microcarcinomas at Kuma hospital: gradual increase and heterogeneity in the acceptance of this new management option. *Thyroid*. 2018;**28**(4):488–495.
76. Machens A, Dralle H. Surgical cure rates of sporadic medullary thyroid cancer in the era of calcitonin screening. *Eur J Endocrinol*. 2016;**175**(3):219–228.
80. Ringel MD. New horizons: emerging therapies and targets in thyroid cancer. *J Clin Endocrinol Metab*. 2020;**106**(1):e382–e388.
90. Netzel BC, Grebe SK, Carranza Leon BG, et al. Thyroglobulin (Tg) testing revisited: Tg assays, TgAb assays, and correlation of results with clinical outcomes. *J Clin Endocrinol Metab*. 2015;**100**(8):E1074–E1083.
93. Cooper DS, Specker B, Ho M, et al. Thyrotropin suppression and disease progression in patients with differentiated thyroid cancer: results from the National Thyroid Cancer Treatment Cooperative Registry. *Thyroid*. 1998;**8**(9):737–744.
102. Schlumberger M, Catargi B, Borget I, et al. Strategies of radioiodine ablation in patients with low-risk thyroid cancer. *N Engl J Med*. 2012;**366**(18):1663–1673.
104. Ladenson PW, Braverman LE, Mazzaferri EL, et al. Comparison of administration of recombinant human thyrotropin with withdrawal of thyroid hormone for radioactive iodine scanning in patients with thyroid carcinoma. *N Engl J Med*. 1997;**337**(13):888–896.
108. American Thyroid Association Taskforce On Radioiodine S, Sisson JC, Freitas J, et al. Radiation safety in the treatment of patients with thyroid diseases by radioiodine 131I: practice recommendations of the American Thyroid Association. *Thyroid*. 2011;**21**(4):335–346.
114. Yu CY, Saeed O, Goldberg AS, et al. A systematic review and meta-analysis of subsequent malignant neoplasm risk after radioactive iodine treatment of thyroid cancer. *Thyroid*. 2018;**28**(12):1662–1673.
119. Jacomina LE, Jacinto JKM, Co LBA, et al. The role of postoperative external beam radiotherapy for differentiated thyroid carcinoma: a systematic review and meta-analysis. *Head Neck*. 2020;**42**(8):2181–2193.
132. Ito Y, Miyauchi A, Kihara M, et al. Calcitonin doubling time in medullary thyroid carcinoma after the detection of distant metastases keenly predicts patients' carcinoma death. *Endocr J*. 2016;**63**(7):663–667.
141. Hugen N, Sloot YJE, Netea-Maier RT, et al. Divergent metastatic patterns between subtypes of thyroid carcinoma results from the Nationwide Dutch Pathology Registry. *J Clin Endocrinol Metab*. 2020;**105**(3):e299–e306.
144. Subbiah V, Kreitman RJ, Wainberg ZA, et al. Dabrafenib and trametinib treatment in patients with locally advanced or metastatic BRAF V600-mutant anaplastic thyroid cancer. *J Clin Oncol*. 2018;**36**(1):7–13.
152. Ho AL, Grewal RK, Leboeuf R, et al. Selumetinib-enhanced radioiodine uptake in advanced thyroid cancer. *N Engl J Med*. 2013;**368**(7):623–632.
160. Wells SA Jr, Robinson BG, Gagel RF, et al. Vandetanib in patients with locally advanced or metastatic medullary thyroid cancer: a randomized, double-blind phase III trial. *J Clin Oncol*. 2012;**30**(2):134–141.
162. Wirth LJ, Sherman E, Robinson B, et al. Efficacy of selpercatinib in RET-altered thyroid cancers. *N Engl J Med*. 2020;**383**(9):825–835.
171. Brose MS, Nutting CM, Jarzab B, et al. Sorafenib in radioactive iodine-refractory, locally advanced or metastatic differentiated thyroid cancer: a randomised, double-blind, phase 3 trial. *Lancet*. 2014;**384**(9940):319–328.
176. Schlumberger M, Tahara M, Wirth LJ, et al. Lenvatinib versus placebo in radioiodine-refractory thyroid cancer. *N Engl J Med*. 2015;**372**(7):621–630.

77 Malignant tumors of the adrenal gland

Jeffrey E. Lee, MD ■ Mouhammed A. Habra, MD ■ Matthew T. Campbell, MD

Overview

Optimal evaluation and treatment of malignant or potentially malignant adrenal tumors including pheochromocytoma/paraganglioma and adrenal cortical carcinoma can be complex. It requires appropriate diagnostic imaging and endocrine hormone evaluation, and benefits from expert multidisciplinary coordination, by medical oncologists, endocrinologists, and surgeons, as well as additional specialists, for example genetic counselors. Recent advances in diagnostic imaging, including functional imaging such as PET, have facilitated early detection and diagnosis, enhanced the accuracy of staging, and improved treatment planning. Good-risk patients with resectable localized, recurrent, or limited metastatic disease are usually recommended to undergo either minimally invasive or open surgery. Advances in minimally invasive and open surgical techniques have improved surgical outcomes. There is no defined role for adjuvant therapy following resection of pheochromocytoma/paraganglioma. Adjuvant therapy for patients with adrenal cortical carcinoma, most commonly single-agent mitotane, is considered selectively. Systemic treatment options for patients with locally recurrent, unresectable, or metastatic malignant adrenal carcinoma include targeted treatments for patients with metastatic pheochromocytoma/paraganglioma, and combination chemotherapy with or without mitotane for patients with adrenal cortical carcinoma. Radiation therapy for patients with malignant adrenal tumors of either histology is also employed selectively. Emerging genetic and molecular data, as well as clinical trials, increasingly inform treatment strategies and choice of systemic therapy.

Introduction

Malignant neoplasms of the adrenal gland and related organs include metastatic pheochromocytoma/paraganglioma and adrenal cortical carcinoma. Due to the rare nature of these cancers, there have been relatively few clinical trials conducted to inform care. However, evolving data regarding the frequency and spectrum of inherited pheochromocytoma/paraganglioma syndromes increasingly informs management of patients with or at risk for developing these tumors. Furthermore, recent comprehensive molecular analyses of both pheochromocytoma/paraganglioma and adrenal cortical carcinoma identify relevant prognostic subgroups and suggest targets for therapeutic development. Finally, emerging information from more common histologically, molecularly and/or mechanistically related cancers is being increasingly leveraged to inform treatment for these rare tumors, including application of targeted and immune-based strategies.

Benign adrenal tumors

Benign tumors of the adrenal cortex and medulla are much more common than malignant tumors. Metastasis to the adrenal gland also occurs commonly, especially in renal cell carcinoma, lung cancer, and melanoma. However, presentation of unknown primary cancer as an asymptomatic, isolated adrenal metastasis is exceedingly rare.[1] Common hormonally functioning benign adrenal tumors include cortisol-producing adrenal adenomas, pheochromocytomas, and aldosteronomas. Nonfunctioning adrenal tumors include nonfunctioning adrenal adenomas or "incidentalomas," metastases to the adrenal gland, and other benign primary tumors including angiomyelolipomas. Treatment of functioning benign adrenal tumors is generally surgical (total unilateral adrenalectomy) in good-risk patients, with a minimally invasive approach preferred.[2] Patients with an inherited syndrome (e.g., MEN2, VHL) and bilateral pheochromocytoma may be considered for partial, cortical-sparing operations to preserve cortical function and to avoid an Addisonian state and associated chronic steroid hormone dependence.[3] Management of nonfunctioning adrenal tumors clinically thought to represent a benign adrenal cortical adenoma is selective, with observation recommended for those with small, stable tumors without suspicious radiographic features, and resection for those that are larger, growing progressively, or with other suspicious features. Percutaneous biopsy is generally not indicated in the management of benign adrenal tumors and should be avoided prior to documenting that the tumor does not represent a pheochromocytoma to avoid inducing malignant hypertension.[1]

Pheochromocytoma and paraganglioma

Pheochromocytomas are neuroectodermal tumors that arise from the chromaffin cells of the adrenal medulla, while paragangliomas arise from neuroectodermal chromaffin cells in an extra-adrenal site (carotid bulb, mediastinum, abdomen, pelvis, urinary bladder, renal hilum, and organ of Zuckerkandl, located between the inferior mesenteric artery and aortic bifurcation). The estimated incidence of pheochromocytoma and paraganglioma is between 0.005% and 0.1% of the general population and between 0.1% and 0.6% of the adult hypertensive population.[4] Approximately 10% of adrenal pheochromocytomas are bilateral, with some patients presenting with multiple tumors. Pheochromocytomas represent 5% of incidentally discovered adrenal masses. Invasion of adjacent organs and/or the presence of metastatic disease are the defining features of malignancy, which can be impossible to distinguish histologically[5]; the Pheochromocytoma of the Adrenal Scaled System (PASS) and the Grading System for Adrenal Pheochromocytoma and Paraganglioma (GAPP) represent attempts to do so. Malignancy has been reported to range from 2% to 13% in patients with pheochromocytoma and 2.4% to 50% in patients with paraganglioma.[6] Metastatic disease most commonly develops in the bones, liver, lungs, kidneys, and lymph nodes. Local recurrence after surgical resection occurs in 6.5–16.5% of patients. Metastatic disease has been documented to occur as late as 40 years

Holland-Frei Cancer Medicine, Tenth Edition. Edited by Robert C. Bast, John C. Byrd, Carlo M. Croce, Ernest Hawk, Fadlo R. Khuri, Raphael E. Pollock, Apostolia M. Tsimberidou, Christopher G. Willett, and Cheryl L. Willman.
© 2023 John Wiley & Sons, Inc. Published 2023 by John Wiley & Sons, Inc.

Table 1 American Joint Committee on Cancer 8th edition staging system for pheochromocytoma/paraganglioma.

Stage	TNM status
I	T1 (pH < 5 cm, no extra-adrenal invasion), N0, M0
II	T2 (pH ≥ 5 cm or PG-sympathetic of any size, no invasion into surrounding tissues), N0, M0
III	T1 or T2, N1 (regional lymph node metastasis), M0 T3, Any N, M0
IV	Any T, Any N, M1 (distant metastasis)

or more after initial diagnosis. The 8th Edition of the American Joint Committee on Cancer (AJCC) Staging Manual is the first to include staging for pheochromocytomas and paragangliomas (Adrenal—Neuroendocrine Tumors) (Table 1).[7]

Genetics and molecular characterization

Historically, familial pheochromocytomas account for approximately 10% of cases ("the 10% rule"). However, recent data suggest that 40% or more of unselected cases of apparently sporadic pheochromocytomas are, in fact, hereditary. Genetic alterations associated with pheochromocytoma are listed in Table 2. Multiple endocrine neoplasia (MEN) type 2A and 2B are some of the most common genetic conditions associated with pheochromocytoma. The likelihood of pheochromocytoma occurring in MEN2A is mutation-specific, with penetrance of pheochromocytoma in patients with an *MEN2A C634* mutation of nearly 100%. The risk, however, of malignant pheochromocytoma occurring in patients with MEN2A is very low, less than 1%.[8] Neuroectodermal dysplasias including neurofibromatosis, tuberous sclerosis, Sturge–Weber syndrome, and von Hippel–Lindau disease (VHL) are also associated with pheochromocytoma, with observed penetrance of up to 20% in VHL. Malignancy occurs, however, in less than 10% of cases.

Pheochromocytomas and paragangliomas also occur in hereditary paraganglioma syndromes (mutations in succinate dehydrogenase *SDHD*, *SDHB*, *SDHC*, and *SDH5* genes), with patients harboring mutations in subunit B (*SDHB*) at particularly high risk for malignancy (50%). Other reported pheochromocytoma susceptibility genes include *TMEM127*, *MAX*, *SDHAF2*,[9] and *SLC25A11*.[10]

Multi-platform, integrated molecular characterization of pheochromocytomas and paragangliomas by The Cancer Genome Atlas Research Network confirmed diverse etiologic genes and pathways are associated with these tumors, including eight previously identified germline susceptibility genes, along with *CSDE1* as a somatically mutated driver gene, and four additional known drivers, *HRAS*, *RET*, *EPAS1*, and *NF1*. Four molecularly defined groups were identified, suggesting important targets for precision medicine and targeted therapy.[11]

Clinical presentation

Hypertension, sustained or paroxysmal, is the most common clinical presentation of pheochromocytoma or paraganglioma, whether benign or malignant. Other common symptoms include excessive sweating, palpitations, arrhythmias, tremulousness, anxiety, headache, chest pain, nausea, and vomiting. More than half of patients with pheochromocytomas have impaired glucose tolerance and may have symptoms of diabetes mellitus, including polydipsia or polyuria.[12] Nonfunctioning adrenal pheochromocytomas are rare; extra-adrenal paragangliomas, however, may be nonfunctioning; function is mutation-specific.

Diagnosis and evaluation

Diagnosis of pheochromocytoma is usually made by documenting excess secretion of catecholamines, which is present in >90% of patients. Plasma-free metanephrine determination is a very sensitive screen for the presence of catecholamine elevation and is more convenient than timed urine collection. Computed tomography (CT) remains the initial imaging study of choice for primary evaluation of patients with known or

Table 2 Major genetic alterations associated with pheochromocytoma/paraganglioma.

Syndrome	Gene	Features	Frequency of pheo/PGL	Malignant potential
NF1	NF1	Von Recklinghausen disease: peripheral nervous system tumors, gastrointestinal stromal tumors, malignant gliomas, breast cancer, leukemia	1–14%	1–9%
VHL	VHL	von Hippel–Lindau disease: retinal and cerebellar hemangioblastoma, renal cell carcinoma, pheo/PGL (multiple, bilateral), pancreatic neuroendocrine tumors	20%	1–9%
MEN2	RET	MEN2A: medullary thyroid carcinoma, pheochromocytoma (bilateral), hyperparathyroidism MEN2B: medullary thyroid carcinoma, pheochromocytoma (bilateral), mucosal neuromas	50%	<1%
PGL1	SDHD	Multiple pheo and PGL (particularly head and neck), nonmedullary thyroid carcinoma, GIST	>50%	1–9%
PGL2	SDHAF2	Pheo and PGL	1–9%	Not reported
PGL3	SDHC	Pheo and PGL (particularly head and neck), nonmedullary thyroid carcinoma, GIST	1–9%	Not reported
PGL4	SDHB	Solitary pheo and PGL, renal cell carcinoma, nonmedullary thyroid carcinoma, GIST	25–50%	25–50%
PGL5	SDHA	Pituitary adenoma, GIST, renal cell carconima	25–50%	1–12%
No name	MAX	Renal cell carcinoma	>50%	1–9%
No name	TMEM127	Not reported	>50%	10–24%
No name	SLC25A11	Not reported	>50%	71%
No name	HIF2A	Polycythemia	Unknown	Not reported
No name	PHD	Polycythemia	Unknown	50%

Pheo, pheochromocytoma; PGL, paraganglioma; GIST, gastrointestinal stromal tumor.

suspected primary pheochromocytoma or paraganglioma. Magnetic resonance imaging (MRI) may be useful in selected cases because the T2-weighted images can identify chromaffin tissue. ^{68}Ga-DOTATATE Positron Emission Tomography (DOTATATE PET), ^{18}F-Fluorodeoxyglucose (^{18}F-FDG) Positron Emission Tomography (FDG PET), or ^{131}I-metaiodobenzylguanidine (^{131}I-MIBG) imaging can be helpful in identifying metastatic, extra-adrenal, or bilateral pheochromocytomas, and are therefore useful in patients with biochemical evidence of pheochromocytoma whose tumors cannot be localized by CT or MRI and in the evaluation of patients with suspected or documented recurrent or metastatic disease. FDG PET has been found to be equally effective in detecting nonmetastatic pheochromocytomas and paragangliomas when compared to MIBG but more sensitive in detecting metastatic disease, and FDG PET is superior in localizing bone metastases when compared to both CT and MRI.[13] Furthermore, DOTATATE PET has a greater lesion-to-background contrast than FDG PET.[14] For these reasons, DOTATATE PET or FDG PET have become the imaging procedures of choice for staging of patients with recurrent or metastatic pheochromocytoma or paraganglioma. Percutaneous biopsy is generally not indicated in patients suspected of having primary pheochromocytoma/paraganglioma. If needed to establish a tissue diagnosis and guide treatment when the initial plan does not include surgery (e.g., in the setting of distant metastatic disease), it should be performed only after hormone evaluation and appropriate biochemical blockade.

Surgical treatment of localized disease

After diagnosis and localization of the pheochromocytoma, preoperative preparation is required to prevent a cardiovascular crisis during surgery caused by excess catecholamine secretion. The focus of preoperative preparation is traditionally adequate alpha-adrenergic blockade (phenoxybenzamine or doxazosin) followed selectively by beta-adrenergic blockade (e.g., metoprolol) and restoration of fluid and electrolyte balance, although some experienced clinical teams have had success with selectively avoiding preoperative alpha blockade in good-risk patients, with excellent outcomes and the possibility of fewer associated side effects, less postoperative hypotension, and quicker postoperative recovery.[15]

If preoperative imaging suggests a modestly sized, benign-appearing unilateral pheochromocytoma with a radiographically normal contralateral gland, a minimally invasive approach (e.g., laparoscopic or posterior retroperitoneoscopic) is appropriate and preferred.[16] Cortical-sparing adrenalectomy, either open or minimally invasive, has been performed successfully in patients with MEN 2A or VHL with bilateral pheochromocytomas, avoiding chronic steroid hormone replacement and the risk of Addisonian crisis in most patients.[17,18] Paragangliomas may also be selectively approached in a minimally invasive fashion from either a retroperitoneoscopic or an anterior laparoscopic/robotic approach, depending on the size and location of the tumor, patient anatomy, and the surgeon's experience.

While follow-up after resection of pheochromocytoma or paraganglioma has not been completely standardized, a commonly accepted schedule includes measurement of plasma-free metanephrines at 1, 6, and 12 months postoperatively, then annually thereafter, in addition to periodic cross-sectional imaging.[19] Biochemical testing of functioning pheochromocytoma/paraganglioma typically includes a plasma-free metanephrine level for catecholamine determination. If recurrence is identified, evaluation should include assessment for metastatic disease, and resection of isolated recurrent or metastatic tumor is indicated when feasible (discussed below).

Treatment of advanced disease

While patients with benign pheochromocytoma have a 97% 5-year survival rate, the 5-year survival rate for patients with malignant pheochromocytoma is approximately 43%, with no significant difference in survival between malignant adrenal and extra-adrenal pheochromocytomas. The most common sites of metastases from malignant pheochromocytoma/paraganglioma are lymph nodes, bone, liver, and lung.[20] Patients with known or suspected malignant pheochromocytoma/paraganglioma should be staged, with cross-sectional imaging as described above. Therapy is individualized based upon the extent of disease and benefits from the expertise of multidisciplinary coordination. Resection of malignant pheochromocytoma, including resection of oligo-metastases, may be considered in good-risk individuals. Surgical debulking can be used to achieve interim biochemical control, potentially to improve response to systemic therapies through diminished tumor burden, and to palliate symptoms (Figure 1).[21] When extra-regional disease is present, a sustained biochemical response is unlikely after resection, stressing the importance of patient selection and determination of treatment goals preoperatively. Localized nonsurgical treatment, for example, radiation therapy or radiofrequency ablation, has an accepted role in the treatment of symptomatic and asymptomatic isolated sites of metastasis, including bone metastases.[22]

Since metastatic pheochromocytoma/paraganglioma may be indolent in up to 50% of patients and effective systemic therapies are limited, observation remains an acceptable management strategy in asymptomatic patients.[23] Palliative treatment options for adrenergic symptoms include α-methyl-*para*-tyrosine, which directly inhibits catecholamine synthesis. However, it is expensive, can be difficult to obtain, and has significant side effects including anxiety, fatigue, and diarrhea. Management with α- and β-blockade, or calcium channel antagonists, angiotensin receptor blockers, and angiotensin-converting enzyme inhibitors is usually at least initially more straightforward.

Targeted radionuclide therapy

Targeted radionuclide therapy with high specific activity, carrier-free ^{131}I-MIBG is currently recommended as first-line treatment for patients with metastatic pheochromocytoma/paraganglioma and MIBG-avid slowly growing tumors.[24] Fifty percent of patients with metastatic pheochromocytoma/paraganglioma have tumors that concentrate MIBG and can potentially benefit from this therapy. The newer formulation has a much higher reported overall response rate (92%)[25] than the older, less specific agent (30–40%), while also avoiding cardiovascular toxicity, although high-dose regimens may result in bone marrow suppression.

Chemotherapy

The most commonly used systemic chemotherapy regimen is the combination of cyclophosphamide, vincristine, and dacarbazine. The overall response rates with this regimen are approximately 37%.[26] As for all treatments of metastatic pheochromocytoma/paraganglioma, chemotherapy is palliative rather than curative, with durations of response reported in the range of 20–40 months. For this reason, combination chemotherapy is usually reserved for patients with rapidly progressive and/or symptomatic disease.

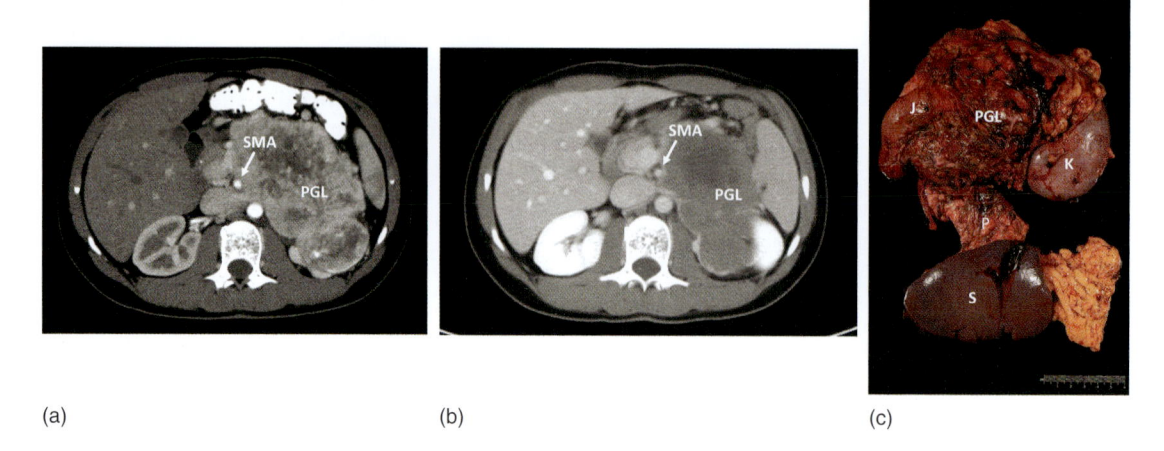

Figure 1 Patient with germline SDHB mutation and metastatic paraganglioma, including bone metastases and (a) a large borderline resectable primary tumor of the left retroperitoneum (PGL), including with long-segment abutment of the superior mesenteric artery (SMA) and involvement of multiple adjacent organs. The patient received a total of seven cycles of cisplatin/vinblastine/doxorubicin, initially with stable disease, then overlapped with cabozantinib with partial biochemical and radiographic response, then additional single-agent cabozantinib with continued response (b). Resection of the primary left retroperitoneal tumor was subsequently performed (c), en bloc with the involved adjacent organs including the left adrenal gland and kidney (K), spleen (S), tail of pancreas (P), and proximal jejunum (J); the SMA was preserved.

Targeted and immunotherapy

Since the molecular pathogenesis of malignant pheochromocytoma/paraganglioma importantly includes hypoxia-inducible factors and angiogenesis, there has been significant interest in the potential utility of tyrosine kinase inhibitors including sunitinib, cabozantinib, and lenvatinib. The results of a recent phase 2 trial of sunitinib in patients with progressive pheochromocytoma/paraganglioma found a low overall response rate (13%), with all objective responses occurring in patients with germline *RET* or *SDH* mutations,[27] suggesting that molecularly defined subgroups of patients with pheochromocytoma/paraganglioma are more likely to benefit from TKI therapy. Evaluation of axitinib and cabozantinib are ongoing (NCT03839498, NCT02302833).

Since molecularly defined cluster-1 pheochromocytomas/paragangliomas, including SDH- and VHL-associated tumors demonstrate an immunosuppressive molecular phenotype, investigators have been interested in the potential role of immune checkpoint inhibitors in these patients.[28] A trial of pembrolizumab is under way (NCT02721732).

Pheochromocytomas and paragangliomas express high levels of somatostatin receptor,[29] however, organized investigation of the potential efficacy of somatostatin analogs has not previously been carried out. A trial of lanreotide in patients with advanced or metastatic pheochromocytoma/paraganglioma has been initiated.

Adrenal cortical carcinoma

Adrenal cortical carcinoma is a rare endocrine malignancy with an incidence of 0.5–2 cases per 1 million people each year in the United States. There is a bimodal age distribution, with incidence peaking in young children less than five years old and then again between 40 and 50 years of age. Prognosis tends to be poor because diagnosis is usually delayed, with one-third of patients presenting with metastatic disease, and there have been limited effective systemic treatment options. Surgical resection remains the mainstay of curative therapy. Even after surgical resection, rates of locoregional recurrence and metastasis are as high as 85%. Five-year survival rates range from 16% to 50%.[30]

Genetics and molecular characterization

The inherited genetic syndrome best characterized as associated with adrenal cortical carcinoma is Li Fraumeni (germline TP53 mutations). Other reported associated or potentially associated syndromes with much lower penetrance of adrenal cortical carcinoma include Beckwith-Wiedemann, MEN1, Familial Adenomatous Polyposis (FAP), Hereditary Nonpolyposis Colorectal Cancer (HNPCC), and Neurofibromatosis Type 1 (NF1).[31]

Integrated molecular analyses of adrenal cortical carcinoma have identified a number of genetic alterations associated with adrenal cortical carcinoma.[32–34] Driver genes identified include *TP53, CTNNB1, ZNRF3, PRKAR1, CCNE1, TERF2, CDKN2A, RB1, MEN1, DAXX, TERT, MED12, RPL22,* and *NF1*. Two very common molecular alterations found in adrenal cortical carcinoma are overexpression of IGF-2, occurring in nearly 90% of cases, and activation of the Wnt/β-catenin pathway. The presence of β-catenin nuclear staining is associated with worse overall survival in patients with adrenal cortical carcinoma. Germline mutations in the tumor suppressor gene TP53 are seen in up to 80% of pediatric adrenal cortical carcinomas but in only 4% of adult cases. Multiple mutations, alterations in DNA methylation, and massive DNA loss/whole-genome doubling are also associated with a more aggressive phenotype.

Clinical presentation

Patients with adrenal cortical carcinoma commonly present with vague abdominal symptoms secondary to an enlarging retroperitoneal mass and/or with clinical manifestations of overproduction of one or more adrenal cortical hormones. At least one-third are hormonally functional, most commonly secreting cortisol and producing Cushing syndrome. Another 10–20% of adrenal cortical carcinomas produce androgens, estrogens, or aldosterone, often in combination with cortisol, which can cause virilization in females, feminization in males, or hypertension, respectively.[35]

Diagnosis, evaluation, and pathology

Evaluation of patients with known or suspected adrenal cortical carcinoma includes biochemical screening for hormone overproduction. Standard preoperative staging includes high-resolution

Table 3 American Joint Committee on Cancer 8th edition staging system for adrenal cortical carcinoma.

Stage	TNM status
I	T1 (≤5 cm, no extra-adrenal invasion), N0, M0
II	T2 (>5 cm, no extra-adrenal invasion), N0, M0
III	T1 or T2, N1 (regional lymph node metastasis), M0
	T3 (tumor of any size with local invasion, but not invading adjacent organs), Any N, M0
	T4 (tumor of any size that invades adjacent organs or large blood vessels), Any N, M0
IV	Any T, Any N, M1 (distant metastasis)

abdominal CT or MRI. MRI may be especially helpful in delineating tumor extension into the inferior vena cava. FDG PET, when combined with CT imaging, may be helpful in detecting metastasis. Chest CT is necessary prior to surgery or initiation of systemic therapy to evaluate for pulmonary metastasis; in addition, chest CT allows for the evaluation of occult pulmonary emboli in these patients, which is common. Primary adrenal cortical carcinomas are typically large at presentation (median 11 cm). Considering the rarity of brain metastasis in adrenal cortical carcinoma, brain imaging is only needed in case of clinical suspicion of brain metastasis.[36]

Percutaneous biopsy should not be performed in patients suspected of having primary adrenal cortical carcinoma when the initial treatment plan would be surgery. However, fine-needle aspiration biopsy can be safely performed when necessary to establish a tissue diagnosis and guide treatment when surgery is not planned or systemic therapy is preferred prior to consideration for surgery (neoadjuvant approach).[37] Pheochromocytoma should always be clinically excluded prior to biopsy. Staging of patients with adrenal cortical carcinoma is now internationally concordant, as the 8th edition update of the AJCC Staging System for adrenal cortical carcinoma brought the AJCC staging system into alignment with the European Network for the Study of Adrenal Tumors (ENSAT) staging system (Table 3).[7]

Adrenal cancer histology is heterogeneous and includes several variants (oncocytic, myxoid, and sarcomatoid). The most commonly applied and best validated histopathologic diagnostic and prognostic scoring system is that defined by Weiss, which includes nine criteria (nuclear grade; mitotic rate; atypical mitoses; clear or vacuolated cytoplasm; diffuse architecture; necrosis; and venous, sinusoid, or capsular invasion); the presence of three or more suggests malignant clinical behavior.[38–40]

Surgical treatment of localized disease

Complete surgical resection is the only potentially curative therapy for localized adrenal cortical cancer. Approximately 50% of adrenal cortical carcinomas are localized to the adrenal gland at initial presentation. The appropriateness of minimally invasive versus open resection for such patients has been a subject of controversy and has been evaluated by multiple investigators.[41–43] Donatini et al.[44] proposed that laparoscopic resection for Stage I and II tumors (≤10 cm with no extra-adrenal invasion) can be performed without compromising oncologic outcomes. However, several other groups have reported higher rates of local and peritoneal recurrence, positive margins, shorter time to recurrence, and worse overall survival in patients undergoing laparoscopic compared to open resection, particularly in patients referred to major centers following resection elsewhere.[45–49] These unfortunate outcomes are likely due at least in part to poor patient selection and technical deficiencies, including high rates of tumor fracture and peritoneal contamination of the typically soft adrenal cancers during the laparoscopic procedure. For these reasons, open adrenalectomy continues to be recommended by most experts for patients with known or suspected adrenal cortical carcinoma.[50,51] An open transabdominal approach facilitates adequate exposure to ensure complete resection, minimizes the risk of tumor spillage, and allows for vascular control of the inferior vena cava, aorta, and renal vessels when necessary. Radical en bloc resection of adrenal cortical carcinoma that includes adjacent organs involved by tumor provides the only chance for long-term survival and should be performed when possible. Routine nephrectomy or resection of other adjacent organs however without radiographic or macroscopic evidence of invasion is generally not warranted.[52] Tumor thrombectomy of the renal vein or inferior vena cava may be required.[53] Lymph node invasion is common in patients with adrenal cortical carcinoma and is associated with worse overall survival. Patients who undergo lymphadenectomy have been reported to have improved survival and recurrence rates[54,55] and therefore it has been suggested that resection of clinically and radiographically normal lymph nodes (elective lymphadenectomy) should routinely be performed, potentially to include celiac, renal hilum, and ipsilateral aortic lymph nodes. While radiographically or clinically suspicious lymph nodes should always be resected, elective lymphadenectomy is not routinely performed at most centers in the United States and remains controversial; however, based on the retrospective data at least selective consideration for including lymph nodes as part of the regional operation is reasonable.[56]

Risk factors for local recurrence include the center at which surgery is performed (tertiary referral center vs. other hospitals), age, stage at presentation, and incomplete resection.[30] Patients who undergo a complete resection have a 5-year survival rate of approximately 40% and a median survival of 43 months; those who undergo incomplete resection have a median survival of less than 12 months. Therefore, the strongest predictor of outcome in is the ability to perform a complete resection.[57,58]

Surveillance after surgery for adrenal cortical carcinoma is typically by CT or MRI of the abdomen and CT of the chest every 3–4 months, with biochemical testing for those who had hormonally active tumors. After 2 years of follow-up, the frequency of surveillance may be decreased but should continue for at least 10 years.[35]

Treatment of advanced disease

Expert multidisciplinary management of patients with recurrent or metastatic adrenal cortical carcinoma is essential. Care of these patients is typically complex, with frequent co-existence of tumor-related hormone production, the frequent presence of cancer-related co-morbidities including a hypercoagulable state and risk for pulmonary emboli, side effects of therapy including an Addisonian state induced by mitotane therapy, and challenges in selection and administration of multiple potential treatment options including combination chemotherapy but also investigational agents.

The most common sites of metastasis of adrenal cortical carcinoma include lungs, lymph nodes, liver, peritoneum, and bone. Surgery should be considered following multidisciplinary evaluation in good-risk patients with potentially resectable local recurrence, especially in the setting of a longer disease-free interval, the absence of distant metastasis, and limited disease progression following an interval of systemic therapy (Figure 2).[59–62] Complete resection of recurrent disease, including pulmonary metastases, is associated with prolonged survival in select patients and can help control symptoms related to excess hormone production.[63–66]

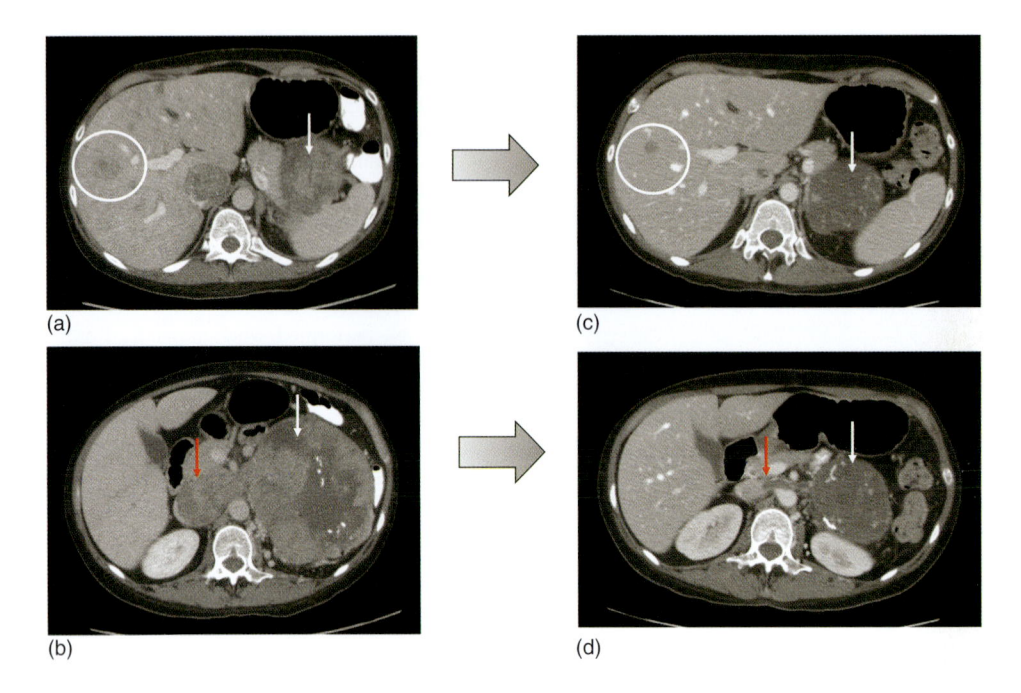

Figure 2 (a) Patient with a large hormonally active left-sided adrenal cortical carcinoma (white arrow) and liver metastasis (circle) together with (b) extension of disease into the left renal vein and vena cava (red arrow). (c) Images after nine cycles of neoadjuvant therapy with mitotane together with etoposide/doxorubicin/cisplatin illustrate shrinkage of primary tumor and liver metastasis as well as (d) improvement in the burden of tumor thrombus with delineation of renal vein allowing for en bloc resection of left kidney together with vena cava tumor thrombectomy and segment VIII liver resection.

For those with unresectable local recurrence, distant metastatic disease, or poor performance status, treatment is generally palliative, complex, and individualized, and can include combinations of hormonal therapy, the adrenolytic agent mitotane, combination chemotherapy, radiation therapy, and targeted radionuclide therapy. While results with molecularly targeted therapies have so far been largely disappointing, checkpoint immunotherapies have had some activity. Evaluation at specialized centers, along with consideration for experimental protocol-based therapy, is encouraged.

Hormonal therapy

Patients with adrenal cortical carcinoma frequently require specific treatment for symptoms related to steroid hormone excess. Endocrinology expertise is essential in managing such patients. In addition to risks associated with hormone excess, clinicians must be vigilant to the risk of an Addisonian state induced by mitotane therapy (discussed below) or by surgery (due to prior chronic suppression of cortisol production of the remaining contralateral adrenal gland by the now-resected adrenal cancer). Patients with adrenal cortical carcinoma and Cushing syndrome require prompt treatment. In addition to the adrenolytic agent mitotane, the steroidogenesis inhibitors ketoconazole and metyrapone can be helpful. The glucocorticoid antagonist mifepristone can assist with the management of hyperglycemia. Patients with hyperaldosteronism can benefit from treatment with the mineralocorticoid receptor antagonists spironolactone or eplerenone. Androgen-secreting adrenal cortical carcinomas may require treatment with spironolactone, bicalutamide, or flutamide, while in the rare case of estrogen excess, estrogen receptor antagonists or aromatase inhibitors can be used.[67]

Mitotane

Mitotane has been one of the most commonly used systemic agents in patients with advanced adrenal cortical carcinoma. This drug is an isomer of dichlorodiphenyltrichloroethane (DDT) and not only inhibits steroid production but also leads to atrophy of adrenal cortical cells. Mitotane is associated with several side effects, most notably gastrointestinal and neuromuscular symptoms. The drug has a relatively narrow therapeutic range (ideal plasma level >14–20 mg/L) and requires close monitoring of serum levels to minimize toxicity.[68–70] Furthermore, provision of exogenous steroid hormone replacement following initiation of mitotane therapy is essential to avoid symptoms associated with adrenal insufficiency due to suppression of cortisol production in the remaining normal contralateral gland.[67] Glucocorticoid replacement doses required are often higher than in patients with other causes of adrenal insufficiency. Furthermore, mitotane induces cytochrome P450-3A4 (CYP3A4), resulting in significant drug–drug interactions.[71] Mitotane is most commonly used as a single agent in the adjuvant setting, or in combination with systemic chemotherapy for treatment of unresectable local-regionally advanced or metastatic disease.

Adjuvant mitotane

The role of mitotane in the adjuvant setting after radical resection of adrenal cortical carcinoma remains controversial.[69,72] A 2007 nonrandomized retrospective study by Terzolo et al.[73] examined the role of adjuvant mitotane postoperatively with respect to overall and recurrence-free survival. The authors examined 177 patients with adrenal cortical carcinoma who had undergone resection in 55 centers in Italy and Germany over a period of 20 years. The study included a group of 47 Italian patients treated at a single center with adjuvant mitotane and compared these patients to a group of 55 Italian patients as well as another group of 75 German patients who had not received adjuvant mitotane. While there was no significant difference in overall survival, recurrence-free survival was prolonged in the mitotane group (median 42 months) compared to the Italian (10 months) and German (25 months) controls. Limitations of the study included lack of details regarding

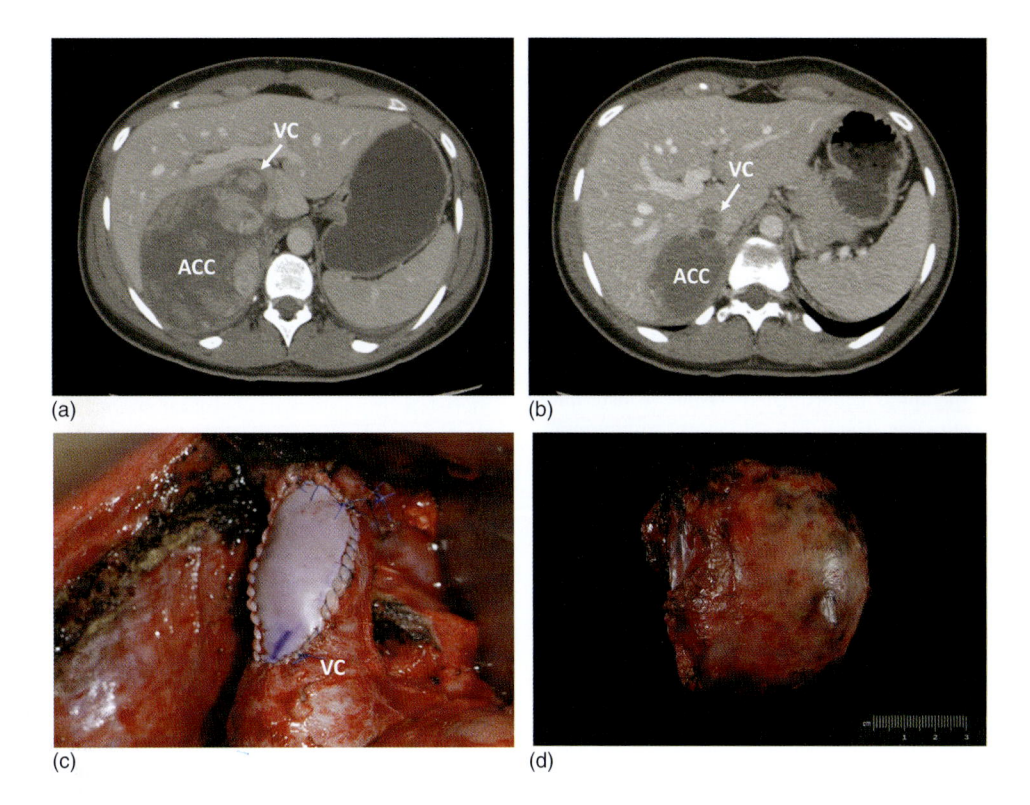

Figure 3 (a) Patient with a large hormonally active right-sided adrenal cortical carcinoma (ACC) with evidence for vena cava involvement including extensive retro-hepatic vena cava tumor thrombus (VC). (b) The patient received five cycles of neoadjuvant therapy with mitotane together with etoposide/doxorubicin/cisplatin. Posttreatment images show a significant decrease in tumor size, including major response of the vena cava tumor. (c) At surgery, the patient underwent en bloc complete resection including the lateral wall of the vena cava and tumor thrombectomy with bovine pericardium patch graft reconstruction. The resected specimen demonstrated negative margins (d).

the mitotane regimen and potential inconsistencies in surgery and follow-up evaluation among the various institutions over the span of two decades, resulting in an ascertainment or lead-time bias in the detection of recurrences. Importantly, the relatively high recurrence rate of the Italian control group suggests that some patients may not have had a complete resection.[17] Differences in outcomes between the patient groups in the Terzolo mitotane study may have been related at least in part to quality and completeness of surgery rather than adjuvant mitotane therapy.[58] For example, the US Adrenocortical Carcinoma Group examined the outcomes of 207 patients who received adjuvant mitotane after surgical resection. After adjusting for tumor factors, the receipt of mitotane was not associated with improved recurrence-free or overall survival.[74] The Efficacy of Adjuvant Mitotane Treatment (ADIUVO and ADIUVO-2) trials are currently underway and will provide additional insight into the utility of adjuvant mitotane.[75] Until then, risk estimations such as the nomogram proposed by Kim et al.[30] to predict recurrence and survival after resection of adrenal cortical carcinoma that includes variables included are tumor size, nodal status, T stage, cortisol secretion, capsular invasion, and resection margins can be used to help select high-risk patients who may be candidates for adjuvant therapy following resection of adrenal cortical carcinoma.

Chemotherapy

The FIRM-ACT (First International Randomized Trial in Locally Advanced and Metastatic Adrenocortical Carcinoma Treatment) trial established combination chemotherapy with mitotane as the standard of care for patients with unresectable adrenal cortical carcinoma.[76] This study randomized 304 patients to receive etoposide, doxorubicin, cisplatin, and mitotane (EDP-M) or streptozocin and mitotane (Sz-M). Response rates were higher with EDP-M compared to Sz-M (23.2% vs 9.2%, $P < 0.001$), and median time to progression with EDP-M was longer (5.0 months vs 2.1 months; hazard ratio 0.55; 95% confidence interval, 0.43–0.69; $P < 0.001$) The median survival of the EDP-M group was 14.8 months versus 12 months for patients in the Sz-M group, which was not statistically significant (hazard ratio 0.79; 95% confidence interval, 0.61–1.02; $p = 0.07$), emphasizing the need for improved systemic therapies for patients with adrenal cortical carcinoma. Gemcitabine-based chemotherapy (gemcitabine + capecitabine) represents an alternative, second-line treatment regimen for adrenal cortical carcinoma. It is well tolerated, modestly active, and can be administered with or without mitotane.[77]

Neoadjuvant therapy

Patients with adrenal cortical carcinoma often present with features that indicate a particularly aggressive tumor biology and argue against initial surgical treatment (Figure 3), including the presence of oligometastatic disease, local tumor extension that will be requiring multiorgan resection such as extensive vena cava tumor thrombus, and/or potentially correctable co-morbidities such as severe Cushing syndrome or pulmonary emboli. In a retrospective study of fifteen patients deemed borderline resectable,[78] 38% had a partial response to neoadjuvant therapy, and six of seven patients with a vena cava tumor thrombus experienced at least a 30% reduction in the extent of the tumor thrombus. Thirteen of fifteen patients were able to undergo surgical resection, with a 92.3% negative margin rate (R0). Median disease-free survival was 27.6 months for patients who underwent neoadjuvant chemotherapy compared to 12.6 months for a contemporary cohort of adrenal cortical carcinoma patients who underwent upfront surgery ($p = 0.48$), while actuarial 5-year overall survival was 65% and 57%, respectively. Based on this limited experience, neoadjuvant chemotherapy may be an attractive option for selected patients with borderline resectable adrenal cortical carcinoma who are considered candidates for initial chemotherapy followed by surgery.

Targeted therapy

With the emergence of information revealing molecular drivers in adrenal cortical carcinoma, there has been increased investigation of targeted therapies. Unfortunately, results to date have been generally discouraging. The IGF1R inhibitors cixutumumab, figitumumab, and linsitinib have been investigated with modest or no benefit documented. The anti-angiogenic VEGFR (vascular endothelial growth factor receptor) inhibitor bevacizumab did not show benefit. The multikinase inhibitors sorafenib, sunitinib, dovitinib, and axitinib, have all been evaluated, with very few or no objective responses. In a phase II study of sunitinib, an inverse correlation was identified between mitotane levels and the active metabolite of sunitinib.[79] Mitotane induces the CYP34A hepatic metabolism which leads to rapid clearance of most targeted agents. A trial with the multikinase inhibitor cabozantinib is ongoing (NCT03370718). The EGFR inhibitors gefitinib and erlotinib have been investigated, without demonstrated benefit. The mTOR inhibitor temseirolimus (in combination with the immunomodulatory agent lenalidomide or cixutumumab) has been evaluated without clear benefit.

Immunotherapy

Multiple clinical trials are currently evaluating the role of immune checkpoint inhibitors in adrenal cortical carcinoma. The rationale for pursuing such treatment includes the observation of adrenalitis in patients receiving immune checkpoint inhibitors, the presence of programmed death-ligand 1 (PD-L1), and tumor-infiltrating lymphocytes (TIL) in adrenal cortical cancers.[80]

In a phase 1b trial of avelumab (anti-PD-L1) in patients with previously treated adrenal cortical carcinoma, 3 of 50 patients had an objective response (6%) and an additional 21 patients (42%) had stable disease.[81] Importantly, almost half of the study participants were on concomitant mitotane therapy that could have influenced the findings of this trial. In a phase 2 trial of nivolumab (anti-PD1) in 10 patients with metastatic adrenal cortical carcinoma, 2 patients had stable disease for 11 and 48 weeks.[82] In a phase 2 trial of pembrolizumab (anti-PD1) in patients with previously treated, advanced rare cancers including a prespecified cohort of adrenal cortical carcinoma, among 14 previously evaluable patients with adrenal cortical carcinoma, there were 2 partial responses (14%) and an additional 7 patients with stable disease (50%). A second phase 2 study with pembrolizumab reported 9 of 39 evaluable patients (23%) experienced a partial or complete response.[80] Toxicities have generally been in line with that seen with these treatments in other cancers.[83,84] Ipilimumab (anti-CTLA-4) in combination with nivolumab is being evaluated in two phase 2 trials that include patients with adrenal cortical carcinoma (NCT03333616 and NCT02834013).

Since IL-13Rα2 is overexpressed on adrenal cortical carcinoma, a trial of IL-13-PE, a recombinant cytokine consisting of human interleukin-13 (IL-13) and a truncated form of pseudomonas endotoxin A (PE) was administered in a phase 1 trial of patients with adrenal cortical carcinoma and IL-13Rα2 expression; 1 of 5 patients treated had stable disease.[85]

Targeted radionuclide therapy

Since 30% of adrenal cortical carcinomas demonstrate significant iodometomidate uptake, treatment with ^{131}I-iodometomidate may offer a targeted radionuclide therapeutic option. In 11 patients with advanced adrenal cortical carcinoma who had high ^{123}I-iodometomidate uptake on diagnostic scans, administration of ^{131}I-iodometomidate resulted in partial response in 1 patient and stable disease in 5. Toxicities included adrenal insufficiency and bone marrow suppression.[86]

Radiation therapy

Radiation therapy has an established role for treatment of isolated metastasis from adrenal cortical carcinoma, including as palliative therapy for bone metastasis.[87] The potential role of radiation therapy as adjuvant treatment following primary resection for adrenal cortical carcinoma remains controversial[88]; it is more commonly used selectively (delivered via external beam or as brachytherapy) following resection for locoregional recurrence.

Conclusion

Despite the rare nature of malignant adrenal tumors which has limited scientific and clinical progress, recent advances in genetics, molecular biology, diagnostic imaging, surgery, targeted therapies including targeted radionuclide therapies, and immunotherapies have improved both care and clinical options for patients with these challenging diseases. Continued emphasis on informed multidisciplinary management, coordinated care, multiinstitutional and international collaboration on translational and clinical investigation, and commitment to clinical trial enrollment will be critical to accelerating progress.

Key references

The complete reference list can be found on Vital Source version of this title, see inside front cover.

6 Hamidi O, Young WF Jr, Iniguez-Ariza NM, et al. Malignant pheochromocytoma and paraganglioma: 272 patients over 55 years. *J Clin Endocrinol Metab*. 2017;**102**(9):3296–3305.

9 Bausch B, Schiavi F, Ni Y, et al. Clinical characterization of the pheochromocytoma and paraganglioma susceptibility genes SDHA, TMEM127, MAX, and SDHAF2 for gene-informed prevention. *JAMA Oncol*. 2017;**3**(9):1204–1212.

11 Fishbein L, Leshchiner I, Walter V, et al. Comprehensive molecular characterization of pheochromocytoma and paraganglioma. *Cancer Cell*. 2017;**31**(2):181–193.

13 Timmers HJ, Chen CC, Carrasquillo JA, et al. Staging and functional characterization of pheochromocytoma and paraganglioma by 18F-fluorodeoxyglucose (18F-FDG) positron emission tomography. *J Natl Cancer Inst*. 2012;**104**(9):700–708.

21 Roman-Gonzalez A, Zhou S, Ayala-Ramirez M, et al. Impact of surgical resection of the primary tumor on overall survival in patients with metastatic pheochromocytoma or sympathetic paraganglioma. *Ann Surg*. 2018;**268**(1):172–178.

25 Pryma DA, Chin BB, Noto RB, et al. Efficacy and safety of high-specific-activity (131)I-MIBG therapy in patients with advanced pheochromocytoma or paraganglioma. *J Nucl Med*. 2019;**60**(5):623–630.

27 O'Kane GM, Ezzat S, Joshua AM, et al. A phase 2 trial of sunitinib in patients with progressive paraganglioma or pheochromocytoma: the SNIPP trial. *Br J Cancer*. 2019;**120**(12):1113–1119.

30 Kim Y, Margonis GA, Prescott JD, et al. Nomograms to predict recurrence-free and overall survival after curative resection of adrenocortical carcinoma. *JAMA Surg*. 2016;**151**(4):365–373.

31 Else T. Association of adrenocortical carcinoma with familial cancer susceptibility syndromes. *Mol Cell Endocrinol*. 2012;**351**(1):66–70.

32 Assie G, Letouze E, Fassnacht M, et al. Integrated genomic characterization of adrenocortical carcinoma. *Nat Genet*. 2014;**46**(6):607–612.

33 Zheng S, Cherniack AD, Dewal N, et al. Comprehensive pan-genomic characterization of adrenocortical carcinoma. *Cancer Cell*. 2016;**29**(5):723–736.

34. Assie G, Jouinot A, Fassnacht M, et al. Value of molecular classification for prognostic assessment of adrenocortical carcinoma. *JAMA Oncol.* 2019;**5**(10): 1440–1447.
35. Kim Y, Margonis GA, Prescott JD, et al. Curative surgical resection of adrenocortical carcinoma: determining long-term outcome based on conditional disease-free probability. *Ann Surg.* 2017;**265**(1):197–204.
36. Fassnacht M, Dekkers OM, Else T, et al. European Society of Endocrinology Clinical Practice Guidelines on the management of adrenocortical carcinoma in adults, in collaboration with the European Network for the Study of Adrenal Tumors. *Eur J Endocrinol.* 2018;**179**(4):G1–G46.
43. Gaujoux S, Mihai R, joint working group of E, Ensat. European Society of Endocrine Surgeons (ESES) and European Network for the Study of Adrenal Tumours (ENSAT) recommendations for the surgical management of adrenocortical carcinoma. *Br J Surg.* 2017;**104**(4):358–376.
44. Donatini G, Caiazzo R, Do Cao C, et al. Long-term survival after adrenalectomy for stage i/ii adrenocortical carcinoma (ACC): a retrospective comparative cohort study of laparoscopic versus open approach. *Ann Surg Oncol.* 2013;**21**(1):284–291.
47. Miller BS, Gauger PG, Hammer GD, Doherty GM. Resection of adrenocortical carcinoma is less complete and local recurrence occurs sooner and more often after laparoscopic adrenalectomy than after open adrenalectomy. *Surgery.* 2012;**152**(6):1150–1157.
49. Mir MC, Klink JC, Guillotreau L, et al. Comparative outcomes of laparoscopic and open adrenalectomy for adrenocortical carcinoma: single, high-volume center experience. *Ann Surg Oncol.* 2012;**20**(5):1456–1461.
51. Dickson PV, Kim L, Yen TWF, et al. Evaluation, staging, and surgical management for adrenocortical carcinoma: an update from the SSO Endocrine and Head and Neck Disease Site Working Group. *Ann Surg Oncol.* 2018;**25**(12):3460–3468.
52. Smith P, Kiernan CM, Tran TB, et al. Role of additional organ resection in adrenocortical carcinoma: analysis of 167 patients from the U.S. Adrenocortical Carcinoma Database. *Ann Surg Oncol.* 2018;**25**(8):2308–2315.
54. Gerry JM, Tran TB, Postlewait LM, et al. Lymphadenectomy for adrenocortical carcinoma: is there a therapeutic benefit? *Ann Surg Oncol.* 2016;**23**(Suppl 5):708–713.
55. Reibetanz J, Jurowich C, Erdogan I, et al. Impact of lymphadenectomy on the oncologic outcome of patients with adrenocortical carcinoma. *Ann Surg.* 2012;**255**(2):363–369.
58. Grubbs EG, Callender GG, Xing Y, et al. Recurrence of adrenal cortical carcinoma following resection: surgery alone can achieve results equal to surgery plus mitotane. *Ann Surg Oncol.* 2010;**17**(1):263–270.
59. Gonzalez RJ, Tamm EP, Ng C, et al. Response to mitotane predicts outcome in patients with recurrent adrenal cortical carcinoma. *Surgery.* 2007;**142**(6):867–875; discussion -75.
63. Dy BM, Strajina V, Cayo AK, et al. Surgical resection of synchronously metastatic adrenocortical cancer. *Ann Surg Oncol.* 2015;**22**(1):146–151.
65. Howell GM, Carty SE, Armstrong MJ, et al. Outcome and prognostic factors after adrenalectomy for patients with distant adrenal metastasis. *Ann Surg Oncol.* 2013;**20**(11):3491–3496.
71. Hermsen IG, Fassnacht M, Terzolo M, et al. Plasma concentrations of o,p'DDD, o,p'DDA, and o,p'DDE as predictors of tumor response to mitotane in adrenocortical carcinoma: results of a retrospective ENS@T multicenter study. *J Clin Endocrinol Metab.* 2011;**96**(6):1844–1851.
72. Berruti A, Grisanti S, Pulzer A, et al. Long-term outcomes of adjuvant mitotane therapy in patients with radically resected adrenocortical carcinoma. *J Clin Endocrinol Metab.* 2017;**102**(4):1358–1365.
73. Terzolo M, Angeli A, Fassnacht M, et al. Adjuvant mitotane treatment for adrenocortical carcinoma. *N Engl J Med.* 2007;**356**(23):2372–2380.
76. Fassnacht M, Terzolo M, Allolio B, et al. Combination chemotherapy in advanced adrenocortical carcinoma. *N Engl J Med.* 2012;**366**(23):2189–2197.
77. Henning JEK, Deutschbein T, Altieri B, et al. Gemcitabine-based chemotherapy in adrenocortical carcinoma: a multicenter study of efficacy and predictive factors. *J Clin Endocrinol Metab.* 2017;**102**(11):4323–4332.
78. Bednarski BK, Habra MA, Phan A, et al. Borderline resectable adrenal cortical carcinoma: a potential role for preoperative chemotherapy. *World J Surg.* 2014;**38**(6):1318–1327.
79. Kroiss M, Quinkler M, Johanssen S, et al. Sunitinib in refractory adrenocortical carcinoma: a phase II, single-arm, open-label trial. *J Clin Endocrinol Metab.* 2012;**97**(10):3495–3503.
80. Raj N, Zheng Y, Kelly V, et al. PD-1 blockade in advanced adrenocortical carcinoma. *J Clin Oncol.* 2020;**38**(1):71–80.
82. Carneiro BA, Konda B, Costa RB, et al. Nivolumab in metastatic adrenocortical carcinoma: results of a phase 2 trial. *J Clin Endocrinol Metab.* 2019;**104**(12): 6193–6200.
83. Habra MA, Stephen B, Campbell M, et al. Phase II clinical trial of pembrolizumab efficacy and safety in advanced adrenocortical carcinoma. *J Immunother Cancer.* 2019;**7**(1):253.
84. Naing A, Meric-Bernstam F, Stephen B, et al. Phase 2 study of pembrolizumab in patients with advanced rare cancers. *J Immunother Cancer.* 2020;**8**(1).
86. Hahner S, Kreissl MC, Fassnacht M, et al. [131I]iodometomidate for targeted radionuclide therapy of advanced adrenocortical carcinoma. *J Clin Endocrinol Metab.* 2012;**97**(3):914–922.
87. Polat B, Fassnacht M, Pfreundner L, et al. Radiotherapy in adrenocortical carcinoma. *Cancer.* 2009;**115**(13):2816–2823.
88. Fassnacht M, Hahner S, Polat B, et al. Efficacy of adjuvant radiotherapy of the tumor bed on local recurrence of adrenocortical carcinoma. *J Clin Endocrinol Metab.* 2006;**91**(11):4501–4504.

78 Tumors of the diffuse neuroendocrine and gastroenteropancreatic system

Evan Vosburgh, MD

Overview

The diffuse neuroendocrine system (DES) is represented by a small number of cells spread through the body, and the tumors that derive from these cells present a wide spectrum of epidemiologic, pathologic, biologic, genetic, and clinical features. Clinical and scientific investigation of the inherited multiple endocrine neoplasia (MEN) syndromes, and the various unique clinical syndromes secondary to secretion of specific peptides (e.g., insulinomas, glucagonomas, VIPomas) are challenging. Clinical presentation can be dramatic, nonspecific, or incidentally noted in absence of symptoms. Tumors might be small, difficult to detect tumors (<1 cm in size), or bulky hepatic metastases in a well patient. Cancer registry data show 5-year survivals for tumors of the neuroendocrine system that have not improved in the past several decades, and that remain about 30–60%. The same registry data documents a rising and unexplained incidence of these tumors, particularly the neuroendocrine tumors of the gastroenteropancreatic system (GEP-NETs), that when coupled with the long average survival results in prevalence figures similar to cancers such as testicular, ovarian, and multiple myeloma and pancreatic adenocarcinoma.

Recent advances in understanding of the genetics, biology, clinical features, and response to therapy are better defining subtypes of neuroendocrine tumors once clustered and studied as "carcinoids." Revised histologic grouping and staging are informing ongoing clinical trials and are providing more informed clinical care of these diverse tumors. Surgery remains the best opportunity for cure at presentation and experience suggests a major role in local control of hepatic metastases. Recent trials of somatostatin analogs have better defined their utility. Results of a series of randomized trials of peptide receptor radiotherapy (PRRT) as well as chemotherapy and targeted therapies have expanded the therapeutic options for patients. Despite advances, the choice and sequencing of specific therapies remains poorly supported by clinical data.

system have not improved in the past several decades, leading many to argue stridently for the avoidance of the term "benign" for NET as a group.

Advances in characterizing the genetics, biology, clinical features, and response to therapy are better defining subtypes of NET once clustered and studied as "carcinoids." Revised histologic grouping and staging are informing ongoing clinical trials and are providing more informed clinical care of these diverse tumors. Not long ago, it was assumed the low incidence of NET and the clinical heterogeneity would preclude randomized trials. However, an impressive number of randomized clinical trials involving over 2000 patients have resulted in recent approvals of peptide receptor radiotherapy (PRRT), several targeted therapies, and demonstrated benefits of certain chemotherapy combinations. Many landmark clinic papers defined this fascinating group of tumors, yet space allows for inclusion of only a few. Rather, this article will focus on more recent epidemiology, diagnosis, and therapy of the more prevalent NETs:

- Gastroenteropancreatic neuroendocrine tumors (GEP-NET), representing the majority of all NET.
- GI-NETs—including the small intestinal NETS (Si-NETS), in years past referred to by the term "carcinoid."
- PNET (pancreatic neuroendocrine tumors)—both nonsecretory and those defined by secretion of specific peptides (i.e., insulinomas).
- MEN (multiple endocrine neoplasia syndromes) and MTC (medullary thyroid carcinoma) and other inherited syndromes with defined gene mutations and associated neuroendocrine cancers.
- Pheochromocytoma and parathyroid tumors—both as sporadic cases and in association with MEN syndromes.

Introduction

The diffuse neuroendocrine system (DES) is represented by several cell types of common embryologic origin, in small numbers spread through the body, and the collection of tumors that derive from these cells present a bewildering spectrum of epidemiologic, pathologic, biologic, genetic, and clinical features. Clinical and scientific investigation of these rare tumors, which include sporadic and inherited syndromes with associated neuroendocrine tumors (NET), unique clinical syndromes secondary to secretion of specific peptides, and a wide spectrum of morbidity and mortality, are challenging. Clinical presentation can be dramatic, nonspecific, or incidentally noted on imaging or at surgery. Tumors might be small, difficult to detect tumors (<1 cm in size), or bulky hepatic metastases in a well patient. Cancer registry data show 5-year survivals of about 30–60% for most tumors of the neuroendocrine

Epidemiology

In comprehensive epidemiologic reviews of *carcinoid* tumors, Modlin et al.[1] and Yao et al.[2] report SEER (Surveillance, Epidemiology, and End Results) cancer registry data of incidence and prevalence spanning over a half-century. One of the challenges facing the classification systems over the past century for *carcinoid* and related NET is that the histology is not particularly informative and tends to be similar for localized and metastatic tumors. One distinction that has been maintained with some consistency over time has been the separation of classic *carcinoid* tumors of the GI tract from the pancreatic islet cell tumors or PNETs. The multidecade analysis of over 13,000 and 35,000 cases respectively show an increase in overall incidence for the past 30 years. Over 65% of NET are in the two broad groups of tumors, *carcinoid* (now referred to as GI-NET), and islet cell tumors (now referred to as PNET), together referred to as GEP-NET. Within the GI-NET, the

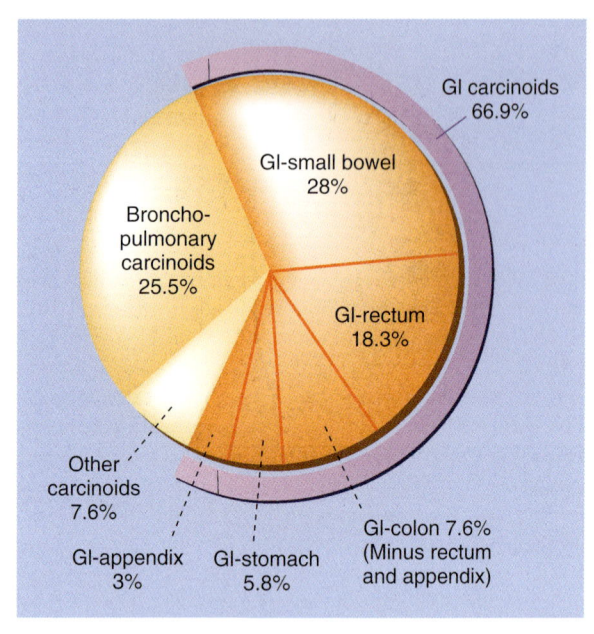

Figure 1 Estimated relative incidence of neuroendocrine tumors (NET) by anatomical site. Compiled for illustrative purpose from numerous publications and estimated by combining classification systems that have varied over time and by source. Source: Data from Modlin et al.[1]; Yao et al.[2]; Dasari et al.[3]

small bowel remains the most common site with a stable incidence over time, as opposed to the gastric and rectal carcinoids that have increased in recent decades (Figure 1). The PNET are divided into nonfunctional PNET and functional PNET. Functional PNET in order of decreasing incidence are gastrinoma, insulinoma, VIPoma, glucagonoma, and the rare neurotensinoma, somatostatinoma, and other ectopic hormone-secreting tumors. The changes in gastric and rectal incidence are thought to represent an increased detection rate with the increasing use of upper and lower endoscopies. Over the same period, the incidence of carcinoids of the appendix decreased, perhaps reflecting the decrease in open abdominal procedures and bystander appendectomies.[1] The gastric, rectal, and appendicle NET are often diagnosed incidentally and are not discussed in this article.

The over 50 years of data documents little change in overall survival, survival by site, and extent of disease, including documentation of metastatic disease at diagnosis in a relatively constant 10–12%. Overall, the general prognosis for NET is favorable compared with that of many tumors. The low incidence of GEP-NET tumors is somewhat deceptive, as Yao et al.[2] and Dasari et al.[3] demonstrated that the overall survival that exceeds many other tumors types translates to *prevalence* figures of GEP-NET that exceed other gastrointestinal tumors including esophageal, gastric, pancreatic, and hepatobiliary. NET patients are well represented in most oncology practice. Further refinements include the clear distinction of well-differentiated neuroendocrine tumors (WDNET) from poorly differentiated neuroendocrine carcinomas (NECs) along with grading based on mitotic rate and/or Ki-67 staining. Defining distinct patient groups continues to inform translational and clinical studies.

The diffuse neuroendocrine system

The DES had its descriptive origins in early histology and cell biology that defined a population of normal chromium-avid epithelial cells widely scattered through the intestinal tract (enterochromaffin cells) and organs including brain, parathyroid, pituitary, thyroid, lungs, adrenal glands (chromaffin or clear cells). In the GI tract, cells of the DES are found from the stomach to rectum and represent less than 1% of the surrounding cell population. The cells of the gut DES share phenotypic and biochemical features with neural cells. Along with the large core dense vesicles (LCDV) of endocrine cells, the DES cells also contain synaptic-like microvesicles (SLMV) characteristic of the synaptic regions of neural cells. The complex and diverse biochemistry and control of secretion of over 100 amines, peptides, and eicosanoids from the LCDV and SLMV of the DES cells are discussed in detail by Weidenmann et al.[4] All four epithelial cell types of the gut, including neuroendocrine cells, are derived from a common pluripotential stem cell found in the intestinal crypts,[5] a stem cell characterized by expression of leucine-rich repeat-containing G-protein coupled receptor 5 (LGR5).[6] The pancreatic neuroendocrine cells are most often derived from pluripotent cell of the islets of Langerhans.

The genetic, epigenetic characterization of normal NE cells, inherited syndrome [MEN, von Hippel–Lindau (VHL), tuberous sclerosis (TS), neurofibromatosis-1 (NF-1)] and germline and somatic tumors cells of NET have better defined distinct tumor subtypes that are informing screening, (early) diagnosis, and clinical trials for new therapeutics.

Neuroendocrine markers

Neuroendocrine markers are utilized in the histologic and immunohistochemical categorization of NETs, and to some degree as clinical markers for diagnosis and assessment of response and relapse. Markers include

Serotonin and metabolites—The rate-limiting step in NETs that synthesize and secrete serotonin is the conversion of tryptophan into 5-hydroxytryptophan (5-HTP). 5-HTP is rapidly converted to 5-hydroxytryptamine that is either stored in the neurosecretory granules or may be secreted directly into the vascular compartment where it is converted into the urinary metabolite 5-hydroxyindoleacetic acid (5-HIAA). The quantification of 5-HIAA in a 24-h urine collection is well characterized and most frequently used clinical assay for diagnosis and follow-up for those NETs that synthesize and secrete serotonin.[7] A more recent serum assay of 5-HIAA appears to be comparable to urinary 5-HIAA and more convenient.[8]

Chromogranin A (CgA) is a member of the chromogranin family of glycoproteins that are stored along with numerous peptide hormones in LDCV of endocrine and neuroendocrine cells. It therefore can serve as an immunohistochemical marker for tissue staining and a plasma marker. CgA was long accepted as the most useful diagnostic marker for both secretory and nonsecretory GEP-NET patients with sensitivity in some studies above 90%.[9] More recent studies have questioned its sensitivity and specificity as a prognostic, progression, relapse marker.[10]

Synaptophysin (p38) is a major neuronal protein concentrated in the membrane of small synaptic vesicles of nerve cells. Weidenmann et al.[11] demonstrated the presence of synaptophysin in a wide range of normal neuroendocrine cells and NET. Its expression is seen across well and poorly differentiated tumors.

Neuron-specific enolase (NSE) is considered a general cytosolic marker of normal neuroendocrine cells and tumors.

CD56, TTF-1, and other immunohistochemical assays provide additional data on NET cell type and tissue/organ derivation.[12]

Though well characterized as monoanylates in the diagnosis of various NET, these biomarkers have not been validated as providing prognostic information, or as accurate measures of response. Both circulating tumor cells (CTC) and multianalyte tests are in development as potential assays to provide more refined prognostic and response data.[13]

Somatostatin and somatostatin receptors

The biology of somatostatin and the somatostatin receptors (SSTRs) and their expression on GEP-NET have yielded information that remains central to the diagnosis and therapy of this group of tumors.

Somatostatin is a peptide that inhibits a wide variety of physiologic activities, the most relevant for the treatment of NET being the inhibition of hormone secretion. Somatostatin is found in the central nervous system, hypothalamic-pituitary system, GI tract, exocrine and endocrine pancreas, and immune effector cells. It exists as somatostatin-28 and somatostatin-14.[14]

The GEP-NET, particularly tumors of the small bowel and pancreatic islets, express multiple SSTR subtypes, the most common and highest density being SSTR-2 in over 80% of cases, followed by SSTR-5.[15] The expression of SSTR-2 has been central to the development of somatostatin analogs as *targeted* therapy to control secretory symptoms, for diagnostic and follow-up nuclear imaging, and for the more recent therapeutic options of tumor control and PRRT.

Histology and staging of neuroendocrine tumors

Modlin[16] detailed the rich history of NET dating from Siegfried Oberndorfer's 1907 description of a group of monotonous-appearing GI tumors labeled "karzinoide" (carcinoid = carcinoma-like), as distinct from the more aggressive adenocarcinomas. The term *carcinoid* has, for over 100 years, been applied to all tumors of the DES that share a similar histological appearance described as monotonous small cells with regular, well-rounded nuclei with insular, trabecular, glandular, undifferentiated, and mixed growth patterns. With an increased understanding of the DES, more specifically the GEP cells, and the parallels between normal cell types and specific tumor types, the description and classification of "carcinoids" has evolved, and a series of revised classifications systems have been proposed to further classify tumors into more biologically and clinically relevant groups.

Histology and staging

A series of revised classifications from the WHO, UICC/AJCC recognized the importance of site of origin, differentiation, adapted the term *(neuro) endocrine* to avoid the inconsistent historical definitions of *carcinoid*, introduced the term GEP-NET and defined three broad groups based on differentiation, leaving site of origin as the lead descriptor to accommodate the breadth of NET subtypes (Table 1). More recent modifications by the European Neuroendocrine Society (ENETS) and North American Neuroendocrine Tumor Society (NANETS)[17] recognize the common and shared importance of histologic *differentiation* and placed further emphasis on *grade* as determined by mitotic rate and/or Ki67 percentage. The most recent classification modification is the WHO 2017 classification that includes pancreatic well-differentiated grade 3-grade tumors as distinct from poorly differentiated grade 3 pancreatic NEC.[18]

Table 1 Classification of GEP-NET.[a]

WHO 2010 Nomenclature	WHO/IARC 2017
Neuroendocrine neoplasm, grade 1	Neuroendocrine tumor, grade 1
Neuroendocrine neoplasm, grade 2	Neuroendocrine tumor, grade 2
	Neuroendocrine tumor, grade 3
Neuroendocrine carcinoma, grade 3	Neuroendocrine carcinoma, grade 3
• Small-cell carcinoma	• Small-cell carcinoma
• Large-cell neuroendocrine carcinoma	• Large-cell neuroendocrine carcinoma

Both systems emphasize the importance of grade, as determined by mitoses/hpf or Ki-67 percentage.[17,18]
[a]Source: Klimstra et al.[17]; Lloyd et al.[18]

Molecular alterations

Genetic/epigenetic studies of NETs have clearly distinguished NETs into separate subtypes. High-grade carcinomas from various organs are characterized by frequent mutations in p53 and Rb.[19] Most studies have focused on well-differentiated grade 1 or 2 GI-NETs and/or PNETs given their higher incidence, and a clear separation of these two GEP-NETs has been demonstrated.

PNET molecular alterations were first suggested by the inherited syndromes associated with PNETS, that is, MEN, VHL, TS, and NF-1. The gene mutations and altered proteins/pathways in the inherited syndromes were later confirmed in large whole-exome and next-generation sequencing studies of sporadic tumors, starting with the initial report by Jiao et al.[20] MEN-1 is mutated in 44% of PNETs, VHL and its regulated gene HIF-1α is inactivated in 24% of PNETs, TSC2 is inactivated in about 35% of PNETs.[21] The study that defined the MEN-1 gene mutations also demonstrated mutations in chromatin remodeling genes ATRX (18%), DAXX (25%), and the PI3K/mTOR pathway inhibitor PTEN (7%). Combined studies to date of defined mutations only account for about 50% of PNETs, and whether these represent driver mutations is under investigation.

GI-NETs, in contrast to PNETs, were not informed by familial/inherited syndromes. First discovered were large chromosomal losses and gains, most prominent being loss of chromosome 18. The genetic consequences of the chromosome 18 loss are still undefined. One whole exome study of GI-NETS found no driver mutations and documented a low mutation rate, three times less than PNETs.[22] A second whole exome study reported mutations (8%) and locus deletions (14%) in the gene CDKN1B, perhaps defining a driver mutation of up to 20% of GI-NETS.[23] Pathway analysis of these studies suggests dysregulation of the PI3K/mTOR pathway.

In summary, molecular studies have begun to unravel the genetic/epigenetic determinants of various NETs. GI-NET, PNETS, and high-grade NEC appear as distinct molecular types. Interestingly they may converge on several signaling pathways and chromatin modifiers, as has been suggested in therapeutic trials in which various NET subtypes respond to the same agents.

Clinical features of tumors of the DES

Tumors of the DES are difficult to recognize at initial presentation. Pulmonary nodules, pancreatic masses, hepatic metastases, and gastric and rectal lesions at endoscopy often are thought to be more common malignancies prior to pathology reports being issued. The early symptoms are often nonspecific (i.e., abdominal pain and diarrhea), and even when more dramatic or classic secretory symptoms occur, the primary tumors are often small and difficult to localize. Patients often have long-standing symptoms and are diagnosed following the development of symptoms related to more advanced local or distant metastatic disease. However, once the diagnosis is considered, advancements in nonspecific (i.e., CgA) and specific tumor markers (i.e., 5-HIAA, gastrin) along with the imaging capabilities with radio-labeled somatostatin analogs, complemented by ultrasound, computed tomography (CT), magnetic resonance imaging (MRI), and positron emission tomography (PET) scanning, permit a strong presumptive or confirmed diagnosis to guide medical and surgical management. Once largely based on consensus, recent Phase II and Phase III clinical trials have informed clinical practice guidelines by NCCN,[24] ENETS,[25] and NANETS.[26]

Imaging

Somatostatin receptor scintigraphy (SRS) is central to the diagnosis and localization of most cases of GEP-NET. The OctreoScan™, ([^{111}Indium-DPTA-pentreotide]), was for decades the scan of choice, now just recently being replaced in many institutions by the increased specificity and sensitivity of ^{68}Ga-PET/CT.[27] CT and MRI generally provide further anatomical definition of SRS-documented disease and are more useful than SRS in following tumor growth or response.[28] Most reports support SRS as the initial imaging modality for locating both primary and metastatic lesions (including bone) in patients with confirmed and suspected GEP-NET, except those with insulinoma. The low detection rate (46%) noted for insulinomas is related to the lower density of SSTR2 on insulinoma cells. Fasting insulin levels coupled with endoscopic ultrasound (EUS) is the most sensitive method of preoperative localization for insulinomas.[29]

Gastrointestinal neuroendocrine tumors (GI-NETS)

In a classic publication Moertel[30] published that WDNET of the small bowel (GI-NETs) are the most common of all the NET, and in the small bowel, where tumors, in general, are rare, they account for 13–34% of all tumors and 17–46% of all malignant tumors.

GI-NETs have been reported from the first to the tenth decade. Modlin et al.[1] reported the average age at diagnosis has increased from 59.9 years to 61.4 years over several decades. Except for the small percentage of patients who present with undifferentiated NECs, GI-NETs are generally slow growing, often remain undiagnosed for many years, and sometimes are recognized only by symptoms related to metastatic spread to lymph nodes, liver, and, less often, bone.

GI-NET can present with small bowel obstruction, abdominal pain, diarrhea, iron deficiency, and GI bleeding. Because tumors located in the distal small bowel in most cases have a low intramural profile (Figure 2), it is not surprising that many of these tumors can grow to larger than 2 cm and remain undiagnosed. The ability of small tumors to cause significant local symptoms is in part related to the development of events such as ischemia, strangulation, and intussusception from the marked fibrotic reaction they produce. The likelihood of metastases relates to tumor size. The incidence of metastases associated with ileal GI-NET is less than 15% with a tumor smaller than 1 cm, but increases to 95% with tumors larger than 2 cm. When not diagnosed incidentally during a surgical or endoscopic procedure, the confirmation of GI-NET tumors might be made only after lengthy evaluation of abdominal complaints or iron-deficiency anemia, or astute recognition of the *carcinoid syndrome*.

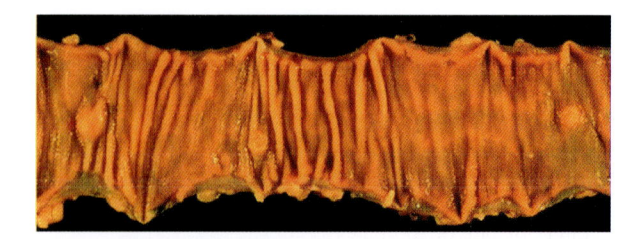

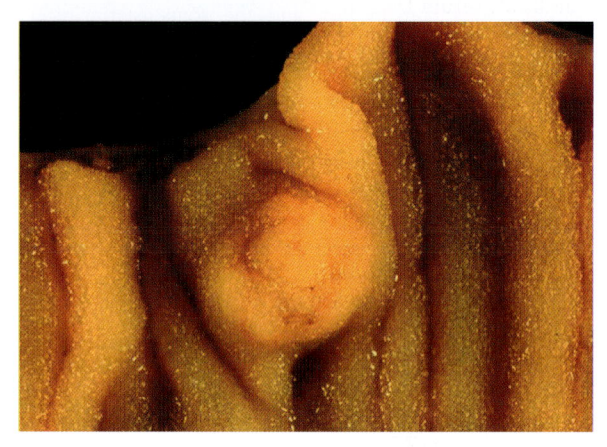

Figure 2 Multiple carcinoids of the small bowel. Three small (<1 cm) intestinal carcinoids found in a young male on inspection of the terminal ileum at colonoscopy. Source: Courtesy of Ed Uthman, MD.

Carcinoid syndrome

Carcinoid syndrome occurs at diagnosis in less than 10% of patients with small bowel GI-NET tumors, but small bowel GI-NET account for upwards of 90% of patients with the carcinoid syndrome.[31] Over 90% of cases of carcinoid syndrome occur only after metastatic spread to the liver, with principal features of diarrhea (83%), flushing (49%), wheezing (6%), abdominal pain, and very rarely, pellagra.[32] No single measurement detects all cases of carcinoid syndrome, although the urine 5-HIAA appears to be the best screening procedure, detecting about 84% of patients with NET-related carcinoid syndrome.[8] Serotonin and its metabolites are thought to account for most carcinoid syndrome symptoms, but other mediators, such as prostaglandins, substance P, kallikrein, dopamine, and neuropeptide K, may also be involved.[7]

Carcinoid heart disease

Carcinoid heart disease has been shown to develop in half to two-thirds of patients with the *carcinoid syndrome*[33] and is characterized by predominantly right-sided valvular lesions described as plaques with proliferation of myofibroblasts and dense extracellular collagen and myxoid deposits.[34] More recently, presumably due to better control of serotonin secretion, the incidence of carcinoid heart disease has decreased.[35] The cardiac disease is a structural disease with thickening and retraction of the valves causing regurgitation (followed later by fusion of fibrous changes to cause stenosis) resulting most often in right-sided congestive heart failure.

Pancreatic NET (PNET) (ISLET-cell tumors)

The second most common GEP-NET occurs in the pancreas. As a group, they have histologic features similar to other GEP-NET. The PNET represent about 15% of all GEP-NET but represent only

1–2% of all pancreatic tumors. Nonfunctioning PNET and gastrinoma are the most common PNETs, followed by insulinoma and a list of increasingly rare tumors defined by the clinical syndromes associated with their specific secretory products (Table 2).

Nonfunctioning PNET

Nonfunctioning PNET have no specific clinical syndrome, despite staining for one or more peptides and amines and often having quantifiable serum levels of certain neuroendocrine markers. As imaging use and sensitivity have increased, nonfunctioning PNETs represent about 90% of all PNETS.[37] The increased detection is raising issues on the proper clinical management of the small incidental lesions.[38] SRS, CT, and MRI are all used to stage and follow for recurrence and development of metastatic disease.

As for most GEP-NET, the treatment of choice and the only therapy that can achieve a cure is surgery. In addition, procedures such as surgical debulking and relief of biliary obstruction can provide significant palliation. The impact of earlier detection due to increased use of imaging has yet to be documented. Therapies for advanced, progressive disease are discussed in later sections.

Less common GEP-NETS

Gastrinoma: The gastrinoma syndrome, also named the Zollinger–Ellison syndrome (ZES), originated with a report of two patients with severe peptic ulcer disease and non-β islet-cell tumors of the pancreas, with later identification of gastrin as the secreted hormone.[39] Gastrinomas account for about 25% of all PNET, are found primarily in the duodenum (70%) and pancreas (25%), and demonstrate malignant behavior in approximately 50% of cases. Patients have a severe ulcer diathesis and persistently elevated basal gastric acid hypersecretion that also accounts for diarrhea.[40] About 20% of gastrinoma patients are eventually found to have germline mutations in *MEN-1*,[41] and their presentation and course differ from sporadic cases (see MEN-1 Syndrome).

The diagnosis requires the demonstration of an elevated fasting serum gastrin and elevated basal acid output, both also seen in *Helicobacter pylori* infection, antisecretory/PPI therapy, chronic gastritis, pernicious anemia, atrophic gastritis, and postvagotomy states. The most sensitive and specific test remains the secretin stimulation test.[42]

Treatment of the gastrinoma syndrome with medical therapy (i.e., omeprazole) is successful in about 95% of patients, such that the long-term survival of patients with slow-growing gastrinomas is now determined largely by the eventual malignant behavior of the tumor rather than ulcer diathesis and diarrhea.[43] Surgery has evolved from gastric resections to control ulcer disease to complex surgery using pre- and intraoperative imaging to localize and resect often small local and regional metastatic disease. The overall survival rate for gastrinomas at 5 years, excluding patients with MEN-1, is between 60% and 80%, and at 10 years is between 45% and 75%.[44]

Insulinomas: were first described by Whipple in a 1938 report of 30 patients with pancreatic adenomas and hypoglycemia.[45] Insulinomas are the most common functioning PNET, and the incidence of metastatic disease, about 5–15%, is low compared with other PNET. The tumors are often well encapsulated as a single solitary nodule, or multiple nodules evenly distributed throughout the pancreas. The finding of multiple insulinomas should prompt testing for MEN-1 given a prospective study of patients operated for insulinomas, 88% of MEN-1 patients had multifocal lesions versus only 4% of non-MEN-1 patients.[30,45]

Almost all cases of insulinoma present with symptoms of hypoglycemia, with neuroglycopenic symptoms (visual complaints, altered consciousness, weakness) more common than adrenergic symptoms alone (sweating, tremulousness). Diagnosis of suspected cases is made by a supervised fast, where over 90% of patients will develop a serum glucose of <50 mg/dL during a 48-h fast, and the corresponding serum insulin level at the time of hypoglycemia will equal or exceed 5 U/mL.[46]

With surgery, 80–90% of all insulinoma patients will be cured.[30] EUS, which has a reported sensitivity of 80%, can localize tumors less than 1 cm, and intraoperative ultrasound (IOUS) can be used to avoid blind pancreatic resections when EUS cannot localize a lesion.[29]

VIPoma: Vasoactive intestinal polypeptide (VIP)oma was first described by Verner and Morrison followed by a review of 55 patients with the WDHA syndrome (watery diarrhea, hypokalemia, and achlorhydria).[47] The VIPomas are quite rare, about 5% of PNET, and have distinct adult and pediatric subsets of patients. In adults, 90% of the tumors are found in the pancreas, often as solitary nodules, and upwards of 60% present with or develop metastatic disease. In children, most VIP-secreting tumors are extrapancreatic and are neurogenic in origin. Long et al.[48] reported that in 52 patients with pancreatic VIPomas, the average lesion was 9 cm in diameter, and thus readily visible by CT or ultrasound. The diagnosis requires the documentation of elevated plasma VIP concentrations and documentation of large volume secretory diarrhea.

Octreotide controls symptoms in over 80% of patients, corresponding with a drop in the VIP plasma level.

Complete resections have resulted in long-term control of symptoms in 30–50% of adult patients.[49]

Glucagonoma: First reported in 1966 by McGavran et al.[50] who called attention to a syndrome that included acquired diabetes and glucagon-producing tumors. This rare tumor, estimated to account for 1% of GEP-NET, was later recognized to include a characteristic skin rash labeled *necrolytic migratory erythema* (NME).[51]

The largest single-institution experience by the Mayo Clinic reported on 21 patients seen between 1975 and 1991.[52] The main presenting features of the glucagonoma syndrome included weight loss (71%), NME rash (67%), mild diabetes mellitus (38%), diarrhea (29%), and painful glossitis and angular stomatitis (29%).

If the diagnosis is made while the tumor is still localized, surgical resection can be curative. Due to the slow growth of tumors and available therapies, the 10-year survival is 51% for patients with metastases and 64% for patients without metastases at diagnosis. Both the NME rash and diarrhea, but generally not the glucose intolerance/diabetes, respond to octreotide in over 50% of the patients, with complete disappearance of symptoms in about 30% of patients.[53]

Somatostatinomas: The first cases were reported in 1977 by Ganda et al.[54] and Larsson et al.[55] To date, a total of about 50 cases have been reported.

Despite a defined clinical syndrome of diabetes, diarrhea, steatorrhea, gallbladder disease, hypochlorhydria, and weight loss, most cases are diagnosed at laparotomy or laparoscopy, or identified on imaging studies for abdominal complaints or jaundice. The tumors tend to present as large masses, reflecting the high levels of somatostatin thought necessary to create symptoms. At diagnosis, 85% of the pancreatic and 50% of the intestinal primaries have evidence of metastatic spread.[56]

Therapy for GEP-NET

In general, GEP-NET are slow growing, and symptoms are most often attributable to secretory products or pain from bulky disease.

Table 2 The clinical syndromes.[a]

Clinical syndrome	Tumor type	Site	Hormone(s)
Flushing/diarrhea/wheezing	Carcinoid	Mid foregut	Serotonin, substance P
		Pancreas/foregut Adrenal medulla	NKA, TCT, PP, CGRP, VIP
Ulcer disease	Gastrinoma	Pancreas (85%), duodenum (15%)	Gastrin
Hypoglycemia	Insulinoma sarcomas	Pancreas/uterus	Insulin/TNF
	Hepatoma	Retroperitoneal liver	IGF/BP
Dermatitis/dementia	Glucagonoma	Pancreas	Glucagon
Diabetes/DVT			
Diabetes/steatorrhea	Somatostatinoma	Pancreas	Somatostatin
Cholelithiasis/neurofibromatosis	Somatostatinoma	Duodenum	Somatostatin
Silent/liver mets	PPoma	Pancreas	PP
Acromegaly	GEP	Pancreas	GH (GHRH)
Cushing	GEP	Pancreas	ACTH/CRF
Hypercalcemia	VIPoma	Pancreas	VIP
	GEP	Pancreas	PTHrP
Pigmentation	GEP	Pancreas	MSH

Abbreviations: ACTH, adrenocorticotropic hormone (corticotrophin); BP, binding protein; CGRP, calcitonin gene, related peptide; CRF, corticotropin-releasing factor; DVT, deep venous thrombosis; GEP, gastroenteropancreatic; GH, growth hormone, somatotropin; GHRH, growth hormone-releasing hormone; IGF, insulin-like growth factor; MSH, melanocyte-stimulating hormone; NKA, neurokinin A; PP, pancreatic polypeptide; PTHrP, parathyroid hormone-related peptide; TCT, thyrocalcitonin; TNF, tumor necrosis factor; VIP, vasoactive intestinal peptide; WDHHA, watery diarrhea, hypokalemia, hypochlorhydria, and acidosis.
[a]Source: Solcia et al.[36]

Surgery remains central for localized disease. For those patients, whose tumors are not resectable at diagnosis or who later develop recurrent/metastatic disease, significant tumor responses are rare, and the focus is on control of symptoms. Proper use of the long-acting somatostatin analogs or a THP inhibitor to decrease secretion of vasoactive and other hormones, combined with bulk-reducing procedures primarily directed at hepatic lesions, the quantity and quality of life of GEP-NET patients can be maintained for extended periods of time. Given that GEP-NET are rare, and the rate of progression is slow, it was formerly thought large Phase III trials could not be completed. Through an organized community of investigators, centers of excellence, NANETS, ENETS, NCCN[24–26] there are well-developed guidelines enriched by Phase I, II, III clinical trials. Table 3 outlines the drug approvals in past years, following a several decades pause after approval of octreotide. One of the challenges that remains, with unfortunately little evidence at present, is the sequencing of these therapies.

Liver-directed therapies

Resection: Given the high frequency of metastatic spread to the liver, several liver-directed therapies have been used in the management of GEP-NETs. Current guidelines support surgical resection with curative intent as initial management of liver.[58] However, it is estimated that >90% of patients with hepatic metastases have lesions that are too large, too numerous, or too diffuse to permit resection and thus other methods have been pursued.

Radiofrequency ablation: Radiofrequency ablation (RFA) has been used in patients to reduce bulk of disease and control symptoms. The largest series to date of RFA in metastatic NET involving patients treated over a 10-year period at a single institution demonstrated perioperative morbidity of <5%, a 90% partial and 72% complete relief of symptoms, and median duration of symptom control of approximately one year.[59]

Hepatic artery vasoocclusive therapy: Overall, vascular-occlusion therapies have led to biochemical responses as high as 50%, and tumor reduction as high as 40%, all generally of short duration.[60] Hepatic arterial occlusion combined with sequential chemotherapy has resulted in biochemical responses as high as 80%, with a median duration of response of 18 months or more.[61]

Hepatic transplantation: Restrictive transplant criteria, significant morbidity and mortality of the procedure and the general lack of transplantable organs make transplant a limited therapeutic option.[62]

There are no randomized trials comparing various methods of control of liver metastases. The numerous reports of these methods have been collected in published meta-analyses[63] and these reports, though acknowledging limitations in data, support overall survival benefits of resection versus no resection, any surgery versus chemotherapy alone, any surgery versus embolization. Consideration for aggressive management of liver metastases at presentation and throughout disease progression should be considered on a case-by-case basis in multidisciplinary evaluations.

Somatostatin analogs

Somatostatin analogs have had a major impact on the flushing, diarrhea, and wheezing in patients with metastatic carcinoid and the carcinoid syndrome and can control many of the other secretory symptoms associated with various NET. Yao's analysis of SEER data[2] has shown an increase in survival in GEP-NET following the introduction of octreotide in the United States in 1998, perhaps reflecting an antiproliferative effect combined with reduced risks of surgery, allowing patients to benefit from more aggressive approach to metastatic disease. Kvols et al.[64] established early on that a positive SRS (OctreoScan™) predicts for patient symptomatic response to somatostatin analogs. Octreotide, a long-acting formulation (somatostatin-LAR) and more recently approved lanreotide are available in the United States.

Use of somatostatin analogs over many decades, both short and long-acting formulations, are associated with biochemical responses in 70–80% of patients, symptomatic control of diarrhea and flushing in over 80% of patients, and a decrease in 5-HIAA levels (if elevated at baseline) in over 70% of patients.[65] Telotristat ethyl, an inhibitor of tryptophan hydroxylase, was shown in the randomized Phase 3 TELESTAR trial in NET patients to significantly reduce the number of daily bowel movements and reduced urinary 5-HIAA in patients refractory to octreotide.[66]

Studies of somatostatin analogs in *asymptomatic* GEP-NET patients with significant tumor burden have shown clinical benefit beyond symptom control. The PROMID trial was a Phase III, randomized, placebo-controlled, double-blind study of small bowel GI-NET patients with minimally or asymptomatic metastatic

Table 3 Following the approval of octreotide several decades elapsed before a rapid series of approvals for GEP-NET therapy followed.[a]

Timeline of Advances in GEP-NET

1980 → 1985 → 1990 → 1995 → 2000 → 2005 → 2010 → 2015 → 2018

- Streptozocin (1982)
- Octroetide (1992)
- Everolimus, Sunitinib in PNET 2011
- Lanreotide in GEP-NET 2014
- Everolimus in GI/Lung NET 2014
- Telotristat in CS 2017
- ^{177}LU-DOTATATE CAPE-TEM 2018

[a]Source: Kunz.[57]

disease that compared long-acting octreotide to placebo. The median time to progression for octreotide was 14.3 months and placebo was 6.0 months. Median overall survival was not assessed due to a crossover design.[67] The CLARINET trial was a Phase III, randomized, placebo-controlled, double-blind study of both well-differentiated GI-NET and PNET patients with asymptomatic but progressive metastatic disease. The trial compared long-acting lanreotide to placebo. The primary end point of progression-free survival was significantly greater for lanreotide ("not reached") versus 18 months for placebo, with no significant difference in overall survival.[68]

Peptide receptor radiotherapy (PRRT)

SSTR targeting provided by somatostatin analogs has led to the development of PRRT reagents for GEP-NET for selective delivery of a radiopharmaceutical at the site of SSTR2, 5 expressing tumors.[69] A series of developments over several decades combining various somatostatin analogs, chelators, and radionuclides resulted in the Phase 3 randomized NETTER1 trial of ^{177}LU (lutetium)-DOTATATE versus high dose octreotide in GI-NETS with progressive disease and positive SRS.[70] At initial report, the ^{177}LU-DOTATATE group had an ORR of 18% versus 3% in the octreotide group, and there is an early signal of an overall survival benefit. Both Octreoscan™ and ^{68}Ga-DOTATATE PET/CT uptake correlate with PRRT response, allowing selection among all GEP-NET patients for the FDA approved Lutathera®.[71] The adverse effects of PRRT have been limited, and fortunately, the renal toxicities of earlier generation PRRT are not seen with ^{68}GA-DOTATATE, and the incidence of marrow toxicity including myelodysplasia and acute leukemia is <2% in follow-up to date.

Cytotoxic chemotherapy

Several authors have reviewed the history of treatment of GEP-NET, with single-agent and multi-agent chemotherapy.[72] In the absence of randomized trials that contain a no-treatment arm, there was no persuasive evidence that single-agent or combination chemotherapy provided any significant impact on disease progression or on survival in patients with metastatic NET. The long-approved agents, DTIC and Streptozocin, have significant toxicities and questionable benefit. Trials selecting for high-grade NEC patients have shown significant, though often of short duration, responses with platinum and etoposide regimens.[73] For well-differentiated GEP-NET patients, recent studies of temozolomide, in combination with thalidomide,[74] or capecitabine[75] provided data for an ECOG randomized Phase 2 trial of temozolomide versus temozolomide plus capecitabine (CAPTEM). The trial in PNET grade 1,2 patients showed a significant improvement in progression free survival (PFS) and OS for the combination arm.[76]

Targeted therapies

Early phase trials have been completed for several targeted therapies. Minimal or no response was seen in Phase II studies of the tyrosine kinases inhibitors imatinib[77] and gefitinib.[78] More encouraging responses were seen in Phase II trials of the VEGF inhibitor bevacizumab,[79] yet to be confirmed in Phase III trials.

A series of clinical trials has led to FDA approval in 2011 for both everolimus and sunitinib for PNET. GI-NET patients were included in the trials and responded, but below the level required for approval.

Everolimus, an oral inhibitor of m-TOR, was studied in a series of RADIANT Phase III, randomized, placebo-controlled studies of well-differentiated PNETs. The RADIANT-2 Phase III, randomized, placebo-controlled study of well-differentiated GI-NET patients with advanced and progressive disease and carcinoid syndrome, demonstrated a nonsignificant difference in median PFS of 16.4 months for everolimus versus 11.3 months for placebo.[80] RADIANT-3 studied PNET patients with advanced and progressive disease and demonstrated a significant difference in median PFS of 11.0 months for everolimus versus 4.6 months for placebo, without a clear OS benefit on early follow-up.[81] RADIANT-4 studied advanced, progressive, nonfunctioning lung and GI-NET and demonstrated a significant difference in median PFS of 11 months for everolimus versus 3.9 months for placebo.[82] Everolimus is FDA approved for lung and GI-NETS and based on significant toxicities is generally reserved for patients with demonstrated disease progression.

Sunitinib, and oral multi-tyrosine kinase inhibitor, was shown in a Phase III, randomized, placebo-controlled study of well-differentiated PNET that were locally advanced or metastatic and with recent progression, to have a PFS of 11.1 versus 5.5 months for placebo. Though assessments were confounded by early closure by a data safety committee, and possible bias from investigator response assessment, the FDA-approved sunitinib for this indication after an independent data review.[83] No data is available for sunitinib use in GI NETS. With the growth of therapeutic opportunities in minimal access surgery, interventional procedures, radiopharmaceuticals, chemotherapy, and targeted therapies, a multidisciplinary approach would benefit treatment decisions for most patients.

Inherited syndromes with associated neuroendocrine tumors

Most NET occur sporadically. However, several inherited syndromes are well described and have provided numerous insights into sporadic NET.

The MEN syndromes, currently named as MEN1,2,3,4, were initially referred to as Werner syndrome, based on the author's observation of groups of individuals with multiple adenomas that appeared to be inherited in an autosomal dominant pattern.[84] The MEN syndromes differ in genetics, clinical presentation, the type, and frequency of involvement of certain endocrine tissues, preventive and therapeutic surgery, and follow-up of affected individuals and family members. The NET that occur within the MEN syndromes have both similarities and differences to the same tumors when they occur sporadically.

MEN-1 syndrome

A somewhat unpredictable cluster of neuroendocrine and nonendocrine tumors from a total of about 20 different histologic types characterizes MEN-1 syndrome cases and families (Table 4). Though there is no "typical" grouping of NET, data from many families show that the most common tumors are parathyroid (including hyperplasia) (90%), enteropancreatic (70%), and anterior pituitary (25%).[86]

About 80% of familial MEN-1 individuals and about 50% of sporadic MEN-1 individuals have a heterozygous germline mutation in the *MEN-1* gene. A recent update described 1336 mutations spread across the coding region of the *MEN-1* gene.[87] MENIN, the product of the *MEN-1* gene, acts as a tumor suppressor with the various mutations resulting in loss-of-function. MEN-4 represents a group of patients originally characterized as "mutation-negative" MEN-1 families. Later sequencing has identified mutations in CDKN1B (p27 protein) in many of the families.[88] Of interest is the finding that CDKN1B is the most frequent mutation identified in GI-NETs, though in only 8% of tumors.[23]

MEN-1 and parathyroid lesions

Most patients first present with symptoms of hyperparathyroidism (HPT), asymptomatic hypercalcemia, or if in a known MEN-1 family undergoing screening, with biochemical or imaging evidence of parathyroid tumor(s). The average age of onset is 25–30 years old, and by age 50, nearly 100% of the MEN-1 patients will have evidence of HPT. In contrast, only 2–4% of cases of sporadic HPT investigated will be found to have mutations in the *MEN-1* gene and the average age of onset is 55–60 years old.

MEN-1 and gastrinoma

Gastrinomas are the next most common "tumor" to follow HPT in MEN-1 patients. Approximately 20% of gastrinomas are associated with the MEN-1 syndrome,[41] present at an earlier age, often are multiple small or undetectable primaries, and are less frequently (7–12%) malignant than sporadic gastrinomas. When there is no evidence of metastatic disease and venous sampling demonstrates an anatomically localized source of gastrin, enucleation (pancreatic head) or resection (body or tail) may offer excellent palliation, but rarely a cure. It is generally recommended to avoid surgery and manage medically with periodic evaluations for radiological progression of tumors.

MEN-1 medical and surgical management

The clinical features of patients with MEN-1 depend entirely upon the natural history of the individual tumors and endocrine hyperfunction. Treatment of the MEN-1 syndrome is dependent on the phenotypic expression in the individual patient. Most patients with MEN-1 pancreatic disease requiring surgical intervention present with a syndrome caused by hypersecretion of a specific hormone such as gastrin, insulin, VIP, or glucagon. Overall, patients with familial MEN-1 neoplasms have longer survival than patients with sporadic endocrine pancreatic tumors. Regardless of initial findings, MEN-1 patients must be followed for life for involvement of the pituitary gland, parathyroid glands, endocrine pancreas or duodenum, adrenal glands, thymus, and lungs (bronchial carcinoids). Family members who are screened with *MEN-1* gene sequencing and are found to be positive should undergo similar lifelong surveillance.[89]

MEN-2 and MEN-3 syndromes

The MEN-2 syndromes represent several distinct clusters of NET with an association between specific gene mutations of the *RET* proto-oncogene and phenotype. MEN-2 (formerly MEN-2A) patients are characterized by MTC (95%), pheochromocytoma (50%), and hyperplasia/adenoma of the parathyroid glands (15–30%) of cases.[90] MEN-3 (formerly MEN-2B) patients have medullary thyroid (MTC) (100%), pheochromocytoma (50%), and varied reported incidences of mucosal neuromas and marfanoid body habitus.[90,91] In MEN-3, approximately 95% of patients harbor the aggressive, highly specific M918T mutation, associated with a high risk of early MTC metastasis, aggressive growth, and poor prognosis. Approximately half of all MEN-3 patients have *de novo* RET germline mutations.[92]

Medullary thyroid carcinoma

MTC represents about 5–10% of new cases of thyroid cancers, or about 1000 cases per year in the United States. Of these, about 75% have no family history of MTC (sporadic MTC) and are generally diagnosed around the age of 50–60 years. In known MEN-2 families, biochemical evidence of MTC usually occurs between the ages of 5 and 25 years. The MEN-3 patients have an earlier age of onset of cancers and a more aggressive phenotype of MTC leading to a worse prognosis compared with MEN-2 patients.[93] MTC is suspected in the presence of elevated serum calcitonin levels, a sensitive and specific marker. Patients not identified by genetic testing or biochemical screening, about 30% of MTC patients, will present with a (painful) neck mass, and/or diarrhea associated with high calcitonin levels, and often have local or distant spread of their tumors.

Treatment of medullary thyroid carcinoma

Prophylactic thyroidectomy (and auto-transplant of parathyroid tissue) is accepted therapy for MEN-2 patients with documented *RET* germline mutations. The timing of the surgery, still controversial, can in fact be guided by the specific *RET* codon affected.[93] Of these patients, approximately 50% will develop recurrent disease,[94] necessitating yearly screening with a calcitonin stimulation test.

Table 4 MEN-1 tumor type distribution and estimated penetrance (%) by age 40 years.[a]

Endocrine tumors (common)	Endocrine tumors (less common)	Nonendocrine features
Parathyroid adenoma (90%)	Thymic carcinoid (2%)	Collagenomas (70%)
Gastrinoma (40%) PP (nonfunctioning) oma (20%)	Bronchial carcinoid (2%)	Facial angiofibromas (85%)
	PNET (VIPoma, glucagonoma, etc) (2%)	
Prolactinoma (20%)	ACTH, GH (2%)	Lipomas (30%)
Insulinoma (10%)	Pheochromocytoma (<1%)	
ECL tumor (10%)	TSH (rare)	

Nonfunctioning adrenal tumors are found in as high as 25% of MEN-1 patients on full evaluation.
[a]Source: Data from Giusti et al.[85]

Vandetanib is an oral inhibitor of VEGF2-3, RET, EGFR that in a Phase III randomized, placebo-controlled trial that achieved the primary endpoint of an increase in PFS of 30.5 versus 19.3 months for placebo.[95] Partial response of 45% was seen, with even higher biochemical responses in calcitonin and CEA. No overall survival benefit has been demonstrated yet, and significant toxicity including QTc prolongation requiring a *black box warning* was required at FDA approval in 2011.

Cabozantinib is an oral inhibitor VEGF2-3, RET, MET that in a Phase III randomized, placebo-controlled trial of patients (with documented recent progression) achieved the primary endpoint of an increase in PFS of 11.2 versus 4.0 months for placebo. Partial response was 28%, with no overall survival benefit yet demonstrated. Toxicities were similar to vandetanib, excluding effects on QTc.[96]

Clinical trials of vandetanib, cabozantinib, and several other multikinase inhibitors alone and in combination are ongoing.[97]

von Hippel–Lindau (VHL), tuberous sclerosis (TS), neurofibromatosis-1 (NF-1)

Though rare, VHL/TS/NF-1 syndromes and associated NET have provided genetic and clinical insight relevant to NET in general.

VHL syndrome is caused by mutations in the VHL gene, resulting in a decrease in HIF-1α and hypoxia-induced cytokine activation. Patients develop a variety of benign and malignant tumors, including PNETs in about 10% of cases.[98]

NF-1 syndrome is caused by mutations in the *neurofibromin* gene, resulting in aberrant signaling in the mTOR and RAS pathways. In addition to the classic neurofibromas and café-au-lait skin lesions, a small percentage of NF-1 patients develop pheochromocytomas and PNETs.[99]

TS syndrome is caused by mutations in either *TSC1* or *TSC2*, and respective proteins hamartin and tuberin inhibit mTOR signaling. Numerous hamartomas and benign tumors are distributed through multiple organs, including brain, causing significant clinical manifestations. A small percentage, about 1%, develop PNETs.[100]

Pheochromocytoma

Pheochromocytomas arise in the chromaffin cells of the adrenal medulla. Mayo Clinic data estimates that approximately 800 cases of pheochromocytoma are diagnosed in the United States each year.[101]

Clinical features and diagnosis

Previously, it was generally taught that 10% of pheochromocytomas were familial, but recent updates document that over 40% of pheochromocytoma patients without personal or family history of associated endocrine neoplasia have a germ-line mutation in one of the following genes: *VHL, RET, NF-1, MEN-1*, succinate dehydrogenase subunits D, B, C (*SDHD, SDHB, SDHC, SDHAF2*), *SMAD4, ENG, ALK1, TMEM127, MAX, HIF2A*.[102] Nölting et al.[103] detail the complexities of genotype-dependent diagnosis, evaluation, treatment, and surveillance of patient and families.

MEN-2 and pheochromocytoma

Pheochromocytomas in MEN-2 patients are diagnosed between the ages of 20–30 years, earlier than the sporadic pheochromocytomas diagnosed between 35 and 45 years old,[103] in part due to MEN-2 patients being actively screened. About 25% of MEN-2 patients present with pheochromocytoma as their first tumor. MEN-2 patients with pheochromocytomas develop bilateral tumors and appear to have a lower incidence of malignant transformation than patients with sporadic tumors.[104] The MEN-2 patients are often asymptomatic but can develop hypertensive crises during surgery undertaken for HPT or MTC. Therefore, all patients with MEN-2 should be carefully screened for the presence of pheochromocytoma before any surgery or invasive procedure and, if present, treated with α-adrenergic blockade to control blood pressure.

Within MEN-2 families, the specific *RET* mutation at codon 634 is highly associated with the presence or eventual development of pheochromocytoma and should be considered in following these patients. Overall, the general recommendation is to screen all MEN-2 patients for pheochromocytoma on a yearly basis.

Key references

The complete reference list can be found on Vital Source version of this title, see inside front cover.

3 Dasari A, Shen C, Halperin D, et al. Trends in the incidence, prevalence, and survival outcomes in patients with neuroendocrine tumors in the United States. *JAMA Oncol.* 2017;**3**:1335–1342.

6 Clevers H. The intestinal crypt, a prototype stem cell compartment. *Cell.* 2013;**154**:274–284.

7 Oberg K, Couvelard A, Delle Fave G, et al. Antibes consensus conference participants. ENETS consensus guidelines for standard of care in neuroendocrine tumours: biochemical markers. *Neuroendocrinology.* 2017;**105**:210–211.

13 Oberg K, Modlin IM, De Herder W, et al. Consensus on biomarkers for neuroendocrine tumour disease. *Lancet Oncol.* 2015;**16**(9):e435–e446.

17 Klimstra DS, Modlin IR, Coppola D, et al. The pathologic classification of neuroendocrine tumors. A review of nomenclature, grading, and staging systems. *Pancreas.* 2010;**39**:707–712.

20 Jiao Y et al. DAXX/ATRX, MEN1, and mTOR pathway genes are frequently altered in pancreatic neuroendocrine tumors. *Science.* 2011;**331**:1199–1203.

21 Scarpa A et al. Whole-genome landscape of pancreatic neuroendocrine tumours. *Nature.* 2017;**543**:65–71.

22 Banck MS et al. The genomic landscape of small intestinal neuroendocrine tumors. *J Clin Invest.* 2013;**123**:2502–2508.

23 Francis JM et al. Somatic mutation of CDKN1B in small intestinal neuroendocrine tumors. *Nat Genet.* 2013;**45**:1483–1486.

25 ENETS *European Neuroendocrine Tumour Society (ENETS) guidelines website.* https://www.enets.org/current_guidelines.html (accessed 1 February 2020).

26 NANETS *North American Neuroendocrine Tumors Society (NANETS) guideline website*. https://nanets.net/net-guidelines-library (accessed 2 February 2020).
27 Hope TA, Bergelsand E. Appropriate use criteria for somatostatin receptor PET imaging in neuroendocrine tumors. *J Nucl Med*. 2018;**59**:66.
31 Clement D, Ramage J, Srirajaskanthan R. Update on pathophysiology, treatment, and complications of carcinoid syndrome. *J Oncol*. 2020;**2020**:8341426.
56 Vinik A, Pacak K, Feliberti E, Perry RR. Somatostatinoma. In: Feingold KR, Anawalt B, Boyce A, et al., eds. *Endotext [Internet]*. South Dartmouth, MA: MDText.com, Inc.; 2017, 2021 (accessed 21 January 2021).
57 Kunz PL. Gastrointestinal Cancer Symposium; 2021.
58 Pavel M, O'Toole D, Costa F, et al. ENETS consensus guidelines update for the management of distant metastatic disease of intestinal, pancreatic, bronchial neuroendocrine neoplasms (NEN) and NEN of unknown primary site. *Neuroendocrinology*. 2016;**103**:172–185.
60 Eriksson BK, Larson EG, Skogseid BM, et al. Liver embolization of patients with malignant neuroendocrine gastrointestinal tumors. *Cancer*. 1998;**83**:2293–2302.
61 Del Prete M, Fiore F, Modica R, et al. Hepatic arterial embolization in patients with neuroendocrine tumors. *J Exp Clin Cancer Res*. 2014;**33**:43–51.
62 Moris D, Tsilimigras DI, Ntanasis-Stathopoulos I, et al. Liver transplantation in patients with liver metastases from neuroendocrine tumors: a systematic review. *Surgery*. 2017;**162**:525–536.
63 Kaçmaz E, Heidsma CM, Besselink MGH, et al. Treatment of liver metastases from midgut neuroendocrine tumours: a systematic review and meta-analysis. *J Clin Med*. 2019;**8**:403.
65 Delaunoit T, Rubin J, Neczyporenko F, et al. Somatostatin analogues in the treatment of gastroenteropancreatic neuroendocrine tumors. *Mayo Clin Proc*. 2005;**80**:502–506.
66 Pavel M, Gross DJ, Benavent M, et al. Telotristat ethyl in carcinoid syndrome: safety and efficacy in the TELECAST phase 3 trial. *Endocr Relat Cancer*. 2018;**25**:309–322.
67 Rinke A, Mueller H-H, Schade-Brittinger C, et al. Placebo-controlled, double-blind, prospective, randomized study on the effect of octreotide LAR in the control of tumor growth in patients with metastatic neuroendocrine midgut tumors: report from the PROMID study group. *J Clin Oncol*. 2009;**27**:4656–4663.
68 Caplin ME, Pavel M, Cwikla JB, et al. Lanreotide in metastatic enteropancreatic neuroendocrine tumors. *NEJM*. 2014;**371**:224–233.
69 Kwekkeboom DJ, Bakker WH, Kam BL, et al. Treatment with Lu-177 DOTA-Tyr3-octreotate in patients with neuroendocrine tumors: interim results. *Eur J Nucl Med Mol Imaging*. 2003;**30**:S231.
70 Strosberg J, El-Haddad G, Wolin E, et al. Phase 3 trial of 177Lu-dotatate for midgut neuroendocrine tumors. *N Engl J Med*. 2017;**376**:125–135.
74 Kulke MH, Stuart K, Enzinger PD, et al. Phase II study of temozolomide and thalidomide in patients with metastatic neuroendocrine tumors. *J Clin Oncol*. 2006;**24**:401–406.
75 Strosberg JR, Fine RL, Choi J, et al. First-line chemotherapy with capecitabine and temozolomide in patients with metastatic pancreatic endocrine carcinomas. *Cancer*. 2011;**117**:268–275.
76 Kunz PL, Catalano PJ, Nimieri HS, et al. A randomized study of temozolomide or temozolomide and capecitabine in patients with advanced pancreatic neuroendocrine tumors: a trial of the ECOG-ACRIN Cancer Research Group (E2211). *J Clin Oncol*. 2018;**33**(15S):4004.
80 Pavel ME, Hainsworth JD, Baudin E, et al. Everolimus plus octreotide long-acting repeatable for the treatment of advanced neuroendocrine tumours associated with carcinoid syndrome (RADIANT- 2): a randomized, placebo-controlled, phase 3 study. *Lancet*. 2011;**378**:2005–2012.
81 Yao JC, Shah MH, Ito T, et al. Everolimus for advanced pancreatic neuroendocrine tumors. *N Engl J Med*. 2011;**364**:514–523.
82 Yao JC, Fazio N, Singh S, et al. Everolimus for the treatment of advanced, non-functional neuroendocrine tumours of the lung or gastrointestinal tract (RADIANT-4): a randomized, placebo-controlled, phase 3 study. *Lancet*. 2016;**387**:968–977.
83 Raymond E, Dahan L, Raoul J-L, et al. Sunitinib maleate for the treatment of pancreatic neuroendocrine tumors. *N Engl J Med*. 2011;**364**:501–513.
86 Brandi ML, Gagel RF, Andeli A, et al. CONSENSUS: guidelines for diagnosis and therapy of MEN type I and type 2. *J Clin Endocrinol Metab*. 2001;**86**:5658–5671.
88 Thakker RV. Multiple endocrine neoplasia type 1 (MEN1) and type 4 (MEN4). *Mol Cell Endocrinol*. 2014;**386**(1-2):2–15.
90 Ponder BA. The phenotypes associated with ret mutations in the multiple endocrine neoplasia type 2 syndrome. *Cancer Res*. 1999;**59**:1736s–1741s.
91 Hansford JR, Mulligan LM. Multiple endocrine neoplasia type 2 and RET: from neoplasia to neurogenesis. *J Med Genet*. 2003;**37**:817–827.
97 Haraldsdottir S, Shah MH. An update on clinical trials of targeted therapies in thyroid cancer. *Curr Opin Oncol*. 2014;**26**:36–44.
103 Nölting S, Ullrich M, Pietzsch J, et al. Current management of pheochromocytoma/paraganglioma: a guide for the practicing clinician in the era of precision medicine. *Cancers (Basel)*. 2019;**11**(10):1505.

79 Neoplasms of the head and neck

Robert L. Ferris, MD, PhD ■ *Adam S. Garden, MD* ■ *Nabil F. Saba, MD, FACP*

Overview

Head and neck cancers (HNCs) comprise a diverse group of malignancies affecting the upper aerodigestive tract. The most common tumor type is squamous cell carcinoma. While the main risk factors for HNC remain tobacco and alcohol abuse, oncogenic viruses such as human papilloma virus and Epstein–Barr virus play a major carcinogenic role in tumors of the oropharynx and nasopharynx respectively. The management of head and neck malignancies is site and histology specific and requires a multi-disciplinary team approach. Immunotherapy has become the standard of care in the treatment of advanced metastatic squamous cell cancers. In this article, we will review the current knowledge of HNC, with focus on squamous and salivary cancers, and discuss ongoing and future research aiming to improve the management and outcomes of patients with these malignancies.

Introduction

Approximately 65,630 new cases of head and neck cancer (HNC) were diagnosed in the United States and over 14,500 Americans were estimated to die from these malignancies in 2020, accounting for 3% of all new cancer cases and 2% of cancer deaths annually.[1,2] Tobacco and alcohol are the primary etiologic agents for squamous cell carcinomas (SCCs).[3] However, a rising proportion of these cancers (particularly those found in the oropharynx) are attributable to oncogenic human papilloma virus (HPV)[3] and the preventive efficacy of population-wide HPV vaccination on incidence rates has yet to be determined. HNCs have a much greater impact in certain parts of the world, especially where cigarette smoking and/or chewing of carcinogenic stimulants is more prevalent.[1,4] The more widespread adoption of multidisciplinary care likely underlies improvements in survival rates for some sites (nasopharynx and oropharynx).[5]

Despite marked advances in imaging, reconstructive surgery, rehabilitation, and radiation treatment delivery, head, and neck squamous cell carcinoma (HNSCC) patients continue to have significant functional deficits which affect quality of life. Combined-modality approaches involving chemotherapy and radiation are now standards of care for "nonsurgical" locally advanced disease with objectives of disease eradication and organ preservation. This article reviews the current status of and future investigative directions for the epidemiology, biology, diagnosis, and therapy of HNC.

Descriptive epidemiology

Incidence

In the United States, estimates for 2020 are for approximately 53,260 new cases of oral cavity and oropharynx cancer, and 12,370 new cases of laryngeal cancer.[2] The United States has benefited from tobacco control efforts with declining smoking prevalence beginning in the 1960s and subsequent declines in incidence rates for most HNC beginning in the 1980s.[6] Approximately 1 in 2 oral cavity cancers occur in women, while only 1 in 4 pharyngeal and laryngeal cancers occur in women. Death rates from oral cavity and pharyngeal cancers have declined among whites and blacks over the years from 1993 to 2007, the largest changes in black men and women with 12 years of education. Although blacks and whites have similar rates of oral cavity/pharyngeal cancer, black men have double the rate of laryngeal cancer of white men; and black women have a 40% higher rate of laryngeal cancer than that of white women. Hispanics have the lowest incidence of oral cavity/pharyngeal cancer, and Asians have the lowest rates of laryngeal cancer.[7] The median age at diagnosis for HNSCC is approximately 60 years, but the incidence of these cancers in young adults (age <45 years) appears to be increasing, related to increasing numbers of oropharyngeal cancers associated with oncogenic HPV.[8] HPV-positive oropharyngeal cancers are more common in white men, presumably related to the prevalence of oral sexual practices.[6]

Worldwide, HNC incidence was over 900,000 cases in 2020.[4] Melanesia has the highest incidence of oral cavity cancer (36:100,000), followed by South-Central Asia, and Central and Eastern Europe.[7] While mortality rates attributed to oral cavity cancer have been decreasing in most countries in Europe and Asia, rates continue to increase in Eastern European countries, particularly in females, reflecting the tobacco epidemic in that region. Although 80% of HNC cases in South Central Asia are oral cavity and pharyngeal (excluding nasopharyngeal), in other regions of the world, laryngeal and nasopharyngeal cancers are more common. Laryngeal cancer accounts for approximately one-third of HNC in the developed world, and approximately 40% of cases in Southern and Eastern Europe. In South-Eastern Asia, nasopharynx carcinoma is the sixth most common malignancy overall in males, accounting for ~70% of all HNC in Malaysia, Indonesia, and Singapore.[7]

Mortality

In 2015 in the United States, 8650 deaths were attributed to oral cavity and oropharyngeal cancer, and 3640 to laryngeal cancer.[9]

Holland-Frei Cancer Medicine, Tenth Edition. Edited by Robert C. Bast, John C. Byrd, Carlo M. Croce, Ernest Hawk, Fadlo R. Khuri, Raphael E. Pollock, Apostolia M. Tsimberidou, Christopher G. Willett, and Cheryl L. Willman.
© 2023 John Wiley & Sons, Inc. Published 2023 by John Wiley & Sons, Inc.

Broader use of and improvements in multidisciplinary care, and the declining incidence attributable to tobacco control, likely underlie the significantly improved survival rates for nasopharyngeal, oropharyngeal, and hypopharyngeal cancer patients, and trends toward improved oral cavity cancer survival rates; however, laryngeal cancer survival rates appear to be worsening.[5,10] As with other cancer sites, mortality/incidence ratios for HNC are much higher in developing countries as compared with the United States.[7,11]

Risk factors

Tobacco
The strength and consistency of the association between smoking and HNSCC have been demonstrated in numerous case-control and cohort studies with significant relative risks or odds ratios in the 5–25-fold range.[3,12] Furthermore, a dose–response effect is consistently shown between the duration and dose of smoking with increasing risk of HNSCC and between the time since quitting and the decreasing risk of HNSCC. Other mucosal malignancies of the head and neck such as nasopharyngeal carcinoma (NPC) and sinonasal malignancies have a weaker association with tobacco smoking.[13]

Alcohol, too, is an important promoter of carcinogenesis in at least 30% of HNSCCs.[7] Furthermore, alcohol appears to have an effect on HNSCC risk independent of tobacco smoking, but these effects are consistently significant only at the highest level of alcohol consumption.

In contrast to nonoropharyngeal cancers, the incidence of oropharyngeal squamous cell carcinoma (OPSCC) has increased in recent decades, specifically among younger age groups,[14–18] given the rising incidence of oropharyngeal cancers associated with HPV infection.[19,20] HPV is associated with approximately 70% of OPSCC in the United States.[21] HPV may also play a role in the etiology of SCCs arising in the sinonasal tract.[22]

Over 120 different HPV types have been isolated, with low-risk types (e.g., HPV 6, 11) inducing benign hyperproliferation of the epithelium, leading to lesions such as papillomas and warts, and high-risk types (e.g., HPV 16, 18, 31, 33, 35) associated with carcinogenesis.[23] The prototypical oncogenic types 16 and 18 account for over 90% of HPV-related OPSCC, and are capable of malignant transformation of primary human keratinocytes from genital or upper respiratory tract epithelia.[24] The transforming potential of HPV is attributed to the two HPV oncoproteins, E6 and E7, that inactivate two human tumor-suppressor proteins, p53 and pRb, respectively.[25] These viral oncoproteins are not only necessary for transformation, but also stimulate cellular proliferation, delay cellular differentiation, increase the frequency of spontaneous and mutagen-induced mutations, and promote focal and broad chromosomal instability in transfected cell lines.[26] Furthermore, in order to maintain a malignant phenotype, a transcriptionally active viral genome appears to be necessary.[27–30]

Pathologic assessment and biology
Aside from stating that a particular tumor is SCC, additional information reported by the pathologist usually includes tumor grade or differentiation. Unfortunately, differentiation factors have not been consistently accurate in reflecting the biologic aggressiveness of HNSCC.[31] Prognosis is influenced by many factors other than grade.[32,33] These include tumor size, nodal status, site, surface expression of epidermal growth factor receptor (EGFR), host immune response, age, and performance status. P16 expression/HPV status is the strongest independent prognostic factor for survival among patients with OPSCC.[34]

Features reflecting aggressive disease include lymphatic invasion, perineural invasion, lymph node metastases, and penetration of the tumor through the capsule of involved lymph nodes (extracapsular spread [ECS]). A complete discussion of the molecular pathology underpinning HNSCC is beyond the scope of this article, and the reader is referred to some of the many reviews on this area.[35,36] Intense investigation is ongoing regarding the complex interplay of cellular and genetic alterations that contribute to carcinogenesis and the metastatic phenotype in HNSCC. The fundamental roles of p53, dysregulated receptor tyrosine kinase signaling, apoptotic resistance, angiogenesis, and chemotherapeutic resistance are under active study.

Anatomy
The term "cancer of the head and neck" refers to a diverse collection of neoplasms arising from the anatomic sites that make up the upper aerodigestive tract (UADT). This article, however, deals predominantly with SCC, as it accounts for approximately 90% of malignanciesin this region. The UADT consists of a complex mucosa-covered conduit for food and air that extends from the vermilion surface of the lips to the cervical esophagus. In common usage, the term HNC has been applied primarily to those cancers arising from the mucosal surfaces of the lips, oral cavity, pharynx, larynx, and cervical esophagus. Included in this designation, however, are other important sites, such as the nose and paranasal sinuses, and salivary glands (major and minor). Some cancers arising in this region are typically excluded from the generic designation of HNC. Examples are tumors of the central nervous system, ocular neoplasms, and primary tumors of lymphatic origin.

Because of the diversity of sites and tissues of origin, the biology of tumor growth, patterns of metastases, and natural boundaries for tumor extension, signs, and symptoms of disease are quite varied. Although the anatomic structures are only millimeters apart, the low metastatic potential and high curability of vocal cord cancers stand in contrast to the early dissemination and poor prognosis of stage-matched pyriform sinus cancers.[37] Clinical differences between cancers in different sites are explained by anatomic factors and major biologic differences. Regrettably, the relatively small number of HNC patients often requires grouping patients for trials. Associated morbidities of disease and treatment involve the special senses to varying degrees, notably speech, mastication and swallowing, smell, and respiratory function, all critically important for social interaction, a good quality of life, and ultimately, survival.

Diagnosis and staging
Since site and stage of disease at the time of diagnosis are the most important prognostic factors in the treatment of HNSCC, the identification and treatment of early-stage cancers generally correlate with excellent survival. Most dysplastic lesions or *in situ* carcinomas of the oral mucosa occur as red (erythroplasia) or white (leukoplakia) patches that may be readily apparent on visual examination. In areas less easily visualized directly, such as the larynx and hypopharynx, early lesions cause such symptoms as

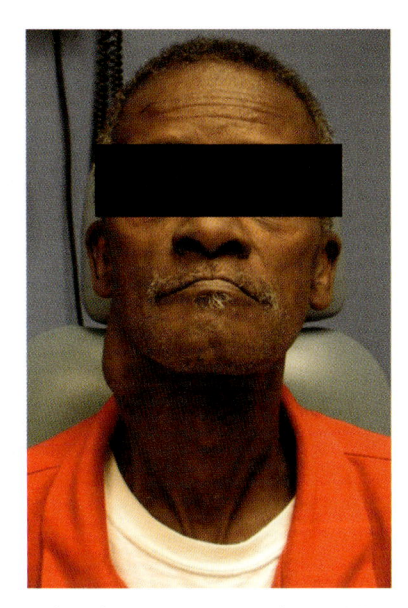

Figure 1 Untreated N3 disease in a patient with HNSCC.

chronic hoarseness and sore throat and, with progression, referred otalgia or dysphagia. Such symptoms demand visualization of the larynx and hypopharynx usually by fiber-optic approaches.

Dysphagia, odynophagia, otalgia, hoarseness, mucosal irregularities and ulceration, oral or oropharyngeal pain, weight loss, and the presence of an unexplained neck mass are the most common presenting symptoms of invasive HNSCC. The predominant symptoms vary with the site: chronic dysphagia or odynophagia demand thorough visualization of the oropharynx, hypopharynx, and esophagus; chronic hoarseness demands visualization of the larynx; chronic unilateral serous otitis media in an adult may be a result of cancer of the nasopharynx blocking the eustachian tube; and unilateral nasal polyps, nasal obstruction, or epistaxis is a common presenting sign of nasal cavity or paranasal sinus neoplasms. A firm or hard unilateral cervical mass represents malignancy until proven otherwise. In persons older than 20 years, such a mass represents neoplasm more than 80% of the time, and 60% of these neoplasms are due to metastatic spread from an UADT primary.

In patients presenting with a suspicious neck mass, a complete head and neck examination usually reveals the primary malignant tumor (Figure 1). If it does not, a thorough search for occult primary cancers both above and below the clavicles is warranted. Technologic advances in fiber optics and in flexible and rigid endoscopes now provide excellent upper airway visualization and biopsy capabilities that can be performed routinely in the clinic setting.[38] Endoscopic evaluation should include the nasopharynx, oropharynx, hypopharynx, larynx, and upper esophagus. Endoscopic evaluation should be accompanied by chest radiography and axial imaging of the head and neck. If these fail to reveal a primary, then consideration should be given for esophagoscopy as well, since it is more sensitive for mucosal lesions of the esophagus than is computerized tomography. Most commonly, occult primaries responsible for neck metastases occur in the nasopharynx, tongue base, tonsil, or hypopharynx. In the absence of an identifiable mass, directed biopsies of these sites are indicated during endoscopic evaluation, and, if present, bilateral tonsillectomies should be performed if a primary is not identified. Metastasis to a solitary left supraclavicular lymph node (Virchow's node) is occasionally seen with infraclavicular cancer, especially colon cancer. Generally, isolated metastatic supraclavicular masses (level IV)

derive from breast, lung, or infradiaphragmatic neoplasms. Thyroid malignancies may also metastasize to this area.

Imaging with computed tomography (CT) and magnetic resonance imaging (MRI) is frequently used to supplement the clinical evaluation and staging of the primary tumor and regional lymph nodes. Ultrasonography, when combined with fine-needle aspiration (FNA) technique, is an effective means for staging the neck, thyroid, and salivary glands. Open biopsies should be performed only after attempts by FNA of suspicious nodes are nondiagnostic. If an excisional biopsy is required because FNA is inconclusive or not feasible, then the surgeon and patient should discuss the advisability of neck dissection if the mass should prove to be metastatic SCC. The potential ramifications of false-negative results on FNA are inherently obvious. Accuracy of the cytological interpretation of the aspirate is directly dependent on the skill and experience of the ultrasonographer and pathologist.

Positron emission tomography (PET) imaging has a demonstrated role in management of HNC. Highly elevated primary tumor fluorodeoxyglucose standardized uptake values (FDG SUVs) may predict for more aggressive disease and inferior treatment outcomes.[39–41] FDG-PET can provide over 90% sensitivity and specificity for upfront staging of both primary and cervical neck nodal disease,[42] and can localize occult local primary disease[43,44] or distant metastases[45] not elicited by anatomic imaging or physical exam. Combined FDG-PET/CT imaging may further improve neck staging accuracy results.[46,47] Incremental superiority of FDG-PET for regional staging of the neck relative to CT or MRI alone was confirmed by a meta-analysis of retrospective and prospective studies encompassing over 1200 FDG-PET imaging cases with confirmatory neck dissection pathology.[48] Analysis of this dataset revealed FDG-PET to be sensitive (79%) and specific (86%) for this indication. Recent prospective series in early-intermediate T-stage oral cavity and oropharyngeal cancer patients suggest that FDG-PET can potentially guide more appropriate management of clinically N0 patients when directly correlated with CT and sentinel node biopsy[49] or with CT/MRI findings.[50]

Considerable interest has recently focused on FDG-PET monitoring of disease response to radiotherapy or chemoradiotherapy. A number of groups have found that FDG-PET posttreatment restaging provides high negative predictive power[51–53]; accordingly, there is now growing acceptance of withholding consolidative neck dissection following radiotherapy in the absence of residual FDG-avid adenopathy,[54] although others argue that expert clinical interpretation of serial CT imaging could achieve similar results.[55,56] FDG-PET/CT may eventually prove useful for improving delineation of disease targets for advanced radiotherapy planning.[57] However, challenges for this remain, particularly for identification of validated thresholding techniques to precisely distinguish FDG-avid disease from bystander tissues.[58,59]

Staging criteria for cancers arising in the UADT, paranasal sinuses, and salivary glands have been developed by the American Joint Committee on Cancer (AJCC) (Table 1). Except for tumors arising in the nasopharynx and those of the thyroid, there is uniformity in the nodal staging criteria and stage grouping (Table 2).

Careful documentation of tumor extent and accurate staging classification is crucial for discussions of the results of different treatment approaches. Restaging after treatment or for recurrent cancers must be clearly designated and separate from the primary staging of previously untreated cancers. Postsurgical, or pathologic, staging is important in the primary treatment of HNC because of the increasing use of postoperative radiation therapy

Table 1 Clinical tumor stage and groupings for head and neck cancer.[a]

Stage 0	Tis	N0	M0
Stage I	T1	N0	M0
Stage II	T2	N0	M0
Stage III	T3	N0	M0
	T1	N1	M0
	T2	N1	M0
	T3	N1	M0
Stage IVA	T4a	N0, N1 or N2	M0
	Any T	N2	M0
Stage IVB	Any T	N3	M0
	T4b	Any N	M0
Stage IVC	Any T	Any N	M1

[a]Source: Edge et al.[60]

Table 2 Clinical tumor staging characteristics for regional lymph nodes and distant metastases.[a]

Regional lymph nodes	
Nx	Regional lymph nodes cannot be assessed
N0	No evidence of regional lymph node metastases
N1	Metastasis in single, ipsilateral regional lymph node <3 cm in greatest dimension
N2a	Metastasis in single, ipsilateral regional lymph node between 3 and 6 cm in greatest dimension
N2b	Metastasis in multiple ipsilateral regional lymph nodes, none >6 cm in greatest dimension
N2c	Metastasis in bilateral or contralateral regional lymph nodes, none >6 cm in greatest dimension
N3	Metastasis to regional lymph node >6 cm in greatest dimension
Distant metastases	
Mx	Presence of distant metastasis cannot be assessed
M0	No evidence of distant metastasis
M1	Distant metastases are present in one or more locations

[a]Source: Edge et al.[60]

(PORT) and/or adjuvant chemotherapy for patients with locally aggressive tumors, ECS into the soft tissues of the neck, close or positive margins, and perineural invasion.

Moreover, the recent emergence of HPV-positive cancers presents an essentially distinctive group of patients for whom some of the older baseline staging data may not be fully applicable.[61] Recent revisions to the AJCC 8 staging have mostly impacted HPV-related OPSCC.

General principles of treatment

After a histological diagnosis has been established and tumor extent determined, the selection of appropriate treatment of a specific cancer depends on a complex array of variables, including tumor site and stage, HPV status, prognosis, relative morbidity of various treatment options, patient performance and nutritional status, concurrent health problems, social and logistic factors, therapeutic options for potential recurrences or second primaries, and patient preference. These variables are each considered with respect to the established effectiveness of various treatment regimens available.

The overall management goals in treating patients with HNC are to achieve the highest cure rates at the lowest cost in terms of functional and cosmetic morbidity. The achievement of these goals requires the close cooperation of an interdisciplinary team of practitioners representing surgery, radiation and medical oncology, prosthodontics, dentistry, speech-language pathology, social services, dietetics, physical and rehabilitative medicine, pathology, nursing, and often psychiatry.

Effective rehabilitation is an important part of the overall treatment of HNC. Modern advances in surgical reconstruction, microvascular free-tissue transfer, and prosthodontics have significantly improved posttreatment function.[62] Rehabilitation concerns must be addressed at initial treatment planning and carefully integrated with the various treatment modalities used. Pretreatment dental evaluations and speech and swallowing assessments should be routinely performed. Needed dental care and/or extractions should be performed prior to radiation to reduce the risks of dental-associated mucositis and osteoradionecrosis. The overall impact of treatment and rehabilitation on patient quality of life is an important issue that may require specialized social or psychiatric support systems for the patient and family. Furthermore, attention must be paid to nutritional support, and early intervention with the placement of enteral access for gastrostomy feeding should be entertained in selected patients. Co-morbidities may affect the choice of systemic therapy to be administered in the concurrent setting. For example, renal insufficiency or significant hearing are generally considered contraindications for cisplatin administration. Recent clinical trials are investigating the appropriate choice of systemic agents in platinum ineligible patients and investigating the role of immune-checkpoint inhibitors (ICI) versus targeting the EGFR receptor with cetuximab. Contemporary combined approaches of chemotherapy and radiotherapy are often associated with severe mucocutaneous treatment effects that must be addressed. Finally, the prolonged nature of treatment for advanced disease, which may extend over many months, requires consideration of the social and financial impact of treatment decisions on the patient, the family, and the patient's career.

Biopsies of primary tumors need not be excisional unless the biopsy procedure is sufficient for local control. Oncologic principles of surgical resection must not be compromised by ill-conceived reconstructive efforts or attempts at modifying the necessary resection in order to minimize functional or cosmetic morbidity. Gross residual cancer or positive surgical margins after tumor resection portend high risk for treatment failure. Appropriate management must also include the use of precise modern techniques of conservative surgical resection (e.g., partial laryngectomy and functional neck dissection) that, in selected patients, have cure rates similar to those of more radical techniques.

Oral premalignancy

Appropriate management of leukoplakia and erythroplakia lesions includes a high index of suspicion, particularly in high-risk individuals. Despite aggressive local therapy, complete surgical resection (as defined by the absence of dysplasia at the margins) does not prevent oral carcinoma development in cases of aneuploid dysplastic leukoplakia.[63] In this context, a targeted therapy prevention approach has been tested in a phase II randomized trial (Erlotinib for prevention of oral cancer (EPOC)). This study compared erlotinib, an EGFR inhibitor, versus placebo in patients with high-risk oral premalignant lesions harboring loss of heterozygosity (LOH). Despite the negative results for the overall population, there was a trend towards improved oral cancer-free survival in patients that did not have a prior oral cancer.[64] Future research in this area should evaluate the roles of optimal surgical margin width and complete resection as confirmed by molecular analyses in reducing the cancer risk associated with molecularly defined high-risk oral intraepithelial neoplasia (IEN). Additional research has focused on combining EGFR targeting with other agents including COX-2 inhibitors such as celecoxib or natural compounds such as green tea extract polyphenon E (PPE).[65–67]

Overview of natural history and treatment by site

Oral cavity

Both tumor and treatment may significantly compromise speech and deglutition, particularly for those patients in whom cancer involves the tongue, floor of the mouth, or mandible. Despite the fact that this region is readily amenable to visual examination and bimanual palpation, more than 50% of patients are diagnosed in advanced stages. The current T-staging of oral cavity primaries is presented in Table 3.

Lips

Considerations in the treatment of lip cancers include (1) oncological control of the disease, (2) a functional oral sphincter with oral competence, and (3) acceptable cosmetic outcome. These goals may be achieved with either primary radiation or surgery when the tumors are less than 2 cm in size or very superficial. Larger or deeply invasive lesions, however, are best treated with surgical resection and reconstruction, which allow for greater accuracy in evaluating the extent of tumor and nerve or lymphatic involvement.

Radiation therapy techniques for management of lip cancers include external irradiation, interstitial implants, and combinations of both. Local tumor control rates with irradiation exceed 80%,[68,69] with determinant survival at 5 years (including surgical salvage) in excess of 95%. Similar tumor control and survival rates are reported with primary surgical excision.[70] Regional metastasis decreases the survival rates to approximately 55%.[71,72] The 5-year survival rates for patients with carcinomas of the upper lip are lower than for those with similar lower-lip lesions and range from 40 to 60%.[73] Involvement of both lips and the lateral commissure is uncommon. The prognosis for commissure lesions is not as good as for cancers of other areas of the lip.

Tongue

Tongue cancers account for approximately 25% of oral cavity SCCs and most commonly arise in the anterior two-thirds of the tongue on the lateral or ventral surface. Infiltration of the underlying tongue musculature occurs early. The management of carcinomas of the tongue has been significantly influenced by an increased appreciation of the aggressiveness of seemingly small but deeply infiltrative lesions, the high rate of occult lymph node metastases, and improvements in soft tissue and bony reconstruction. Although surgical excision alone has been the mainstay of treatment, combined surgery, and adjuvant radiation therapy to include the primary site and regional nodes is commonly used for advanced cancers (stages III and IV) and is being used increasingly for small stage II cancers that exhibit pathologic indicators of lymph node metastasis or perineural invasion (Figure 2). Postoperative chemoradiotherapy is indicated for adverse pathologic findings of perineural invasion, nodal ECS, or close surgical margins.[74]

For stage I cancers, surgical excision is effective and expeditious, with excellent preservation of function. For stage II lesions that are infiltrative, hemiglossectomy or partial glossectomy achieves excellent tumor control rates and should be combined with dissection of neck nodes at risk (supraomohyoid dissection) to provide accurate information about staging and determine the need for PORT. Free-tissue transfer reconstruction can significantly offset the morbidity of hemiglossectomy.

Extension of cancer to the floor of mouth (FOM) or the mandible may necessitate partial mandibulectomy or segmental mandibular resection. Modern reconstructive techniques with vascularized

Table 3 Primary tumor staging characteristics for oral cavity and oropharynx carcinoma.

Tx	Primary tumor cannot be assessed (as occurs after excisional biopsy)
T0	No evidence of primary (as in unknown primary tumors)
Tis	Carcinoma *in situ*
T1	Tumor is 2 cm or less in greatest dimension
T2	Tumor is between 2 and 4 cm in greatest dimension
T3	Tumor is >4 cm in greatest dimension
T4	A: moderately advanced local disease (T4a and T4b were removed from HPV related OPCA in AJCC 8): Tumor invades adjacent structures (through cortical bone, maxillary sinus, skin, tongue musculature, deep tissue, nerves B: very advanced local disease: Oral cavity: tumor invades masticator space, pterygoid plates, skull base, encase carotid artery Oropharynx: tumor invades prevertebral fascia, encases carotid artery, or involve mediastinal structures

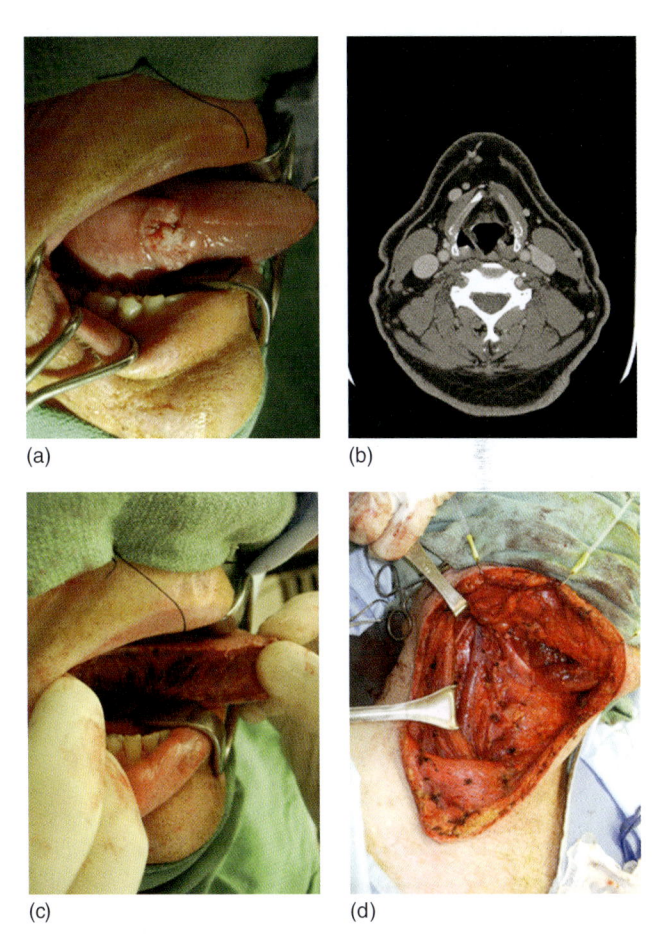

Figure 2 (a) T1 N0 SCCA of the oral cavity. (b) CT scan revealing no lymphatic metastasis. (c) Hemiglossectomy resection. (d) Staging supraomohyoid neck dissection.

composite bone and soft tissue-free flaps, titanium metal prostheses, and dental implants have improved the functional and cosmetic results of major mandibular resections. An elective neck dissection is recommended for lesions with >4 mm of invasion owing to the risk of occult nodal disease.

For more advanced primary lesions (stages III and IV), surgery and postoperative external beam radiation are generally used. No prospective controlled trials have proved the superiority of combined therapy over surgery alone for disease without nodal metastases, but retrospective studies indicate improved locoregional control rates. When tumors extend to the midline or involve the tongue base, subtotal or total glossectomy may be necessary. Continued advances in reconstructive techniques have improved the functional results of these aggressive resections. Provision for temporary tracheostomy and prolonged enteral nutrition should be made. Total glossectomy or sacrifice of both hypoglossal nerves frequently necessitates permanent feeding gastrostomy. Current experience indicates that total glossectomy can, in highly select patients, be accomplished without the need for laryngectomy although prolonged or even permanent parenteral feeding will likely be required.[75] PORT is generally administered within 4–6 weeks of surgery. High-risk surgical margins or ECS can be treated to a high dose or with concomitant chemoradiotherapy. For advanced oral cavity cancers, both ipsilateral and contralateral necks are irradiated, with the dosage determined by the extent of disease. Even with combined therapy, estimated 2-year disease-free survival (DFS) and overall survival (OS) rates for advanced disease are about 50%. The 5-year survival rates range from 50–70% for stages I and II to 15–30% for stages III and IV.[76–80]

Floor of mouth (FOM)
Small cancers (T1, T2) are generally treated effectively by wide resection. More advanced FOM cancers (T3, T4) are generally treated with resection combined with similar approaches to that described for oral tongue cancers in the prior section (Figure 3).

Treatment results are influenced by the size of the primary tumor, presence of lymph node metastases, degree of mandibular involvement, and adequacy of resection. The 5-year survival rates for stage I and II FOM carcinomas range around 80%.[81] Cancers that cross the midline or involve the tongue or the mandible are associated with 5-year survival rates of 50–60%.[82] Survival rates for more advanced lesions (stages III and IV) are less than 50%. The major advantage of combined treatment (radiation and surgery) in these patients is improved control of neck disease. Recurrence in the untreated, clinically negative neck is the most frequent site of failure in patients treated only with surgery.[83] For patients with multiple nodal metastases, induction chemotherapy is under study[84] as there is high risk for later development of distant metastases. Continuing surveillance for metachronous second primary cancers in the head and neck, esophagus, or lungs is advised.[85,86]

Gingival and buccal mucosa
Gingival cancers occur most commonly (80%) in the lower gingiva, posterior to the bicuspids. For both sites, trismus is an ominous sign indicating extension to the masseter or pterygoid muscles. Elective neck dissection should be performed for advanced lesions of the mandibular gingival, as these lesions tend to have occult metastases. Limited data are available on the behavior of maxillary ridge and hard palate cancers, but these lesions can metastasize to the lateral neck nodes, and thus elective management of the neck is strongly encouraged, whether with neck dissection or neck irradiation.[87] Clinically positive neck nodes warrant neck dissection at the time of the resection of the primary tumor.

OS rates for gingival and buccal cancers depend on tumor size, bone involvement, and node metastases. Surgical results are clearly superior to those of radiation when bone involvement is present.[88,89]

Retromolar trigone
Cancers arising in the retromolar trigone are rarely confined to that gingiva, but often involve adjacent buccal mucosa, anterior tonsillar pillar, the FOM, and/or posterior gingiva. Primary radiation therapy is reserved for superficial lesions that cover a large surface area, such as extension to the soft palate or buccal mucosa, and remain mobile. Moderately advanced or deeply invasive lesions are best treated with surgical resection (mandibulectomy and neck dissection), followed by postoperative adjuvant therapy, as indicated.

Oropharynx
The clinical staging of oropharyngeal cancers has been redefined in the latest edition of the AJCC (8th edition). The division is based on separating HPV-associated tumors. The staging of HPV-negative tumors is similar to the staging of oral cavity cancers (Table 3). Staging of HPV-positive tumors has largely been modified in nodal staging, such that it closely resembles NPC staging and includes pathologic staging. This has resulted in a dramatic group downstaging of these cancers.

Tumors arise most commonly from the palatine arch, which includes the tonsillar fossa and base of the tongue. The recent identification of HPV as the major etiological factor in the development of OPSCC has led to a recognition of a distinct disease phenotype.

(a)

(b)

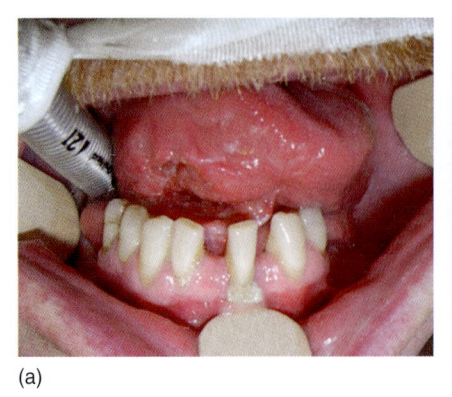

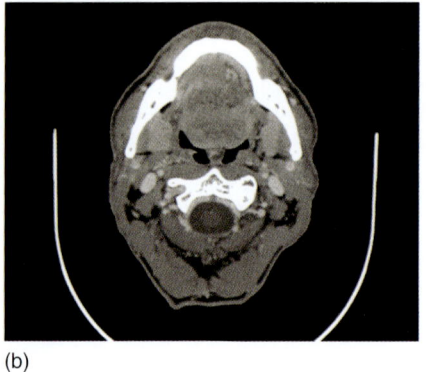

Figure 3 (a) T3 N0 floor of mouth SCCA. (b) Deep infiltration of the intrinsic tongue musculature on axial imaging.

Clinically, HPV-associated tumors are small, but the nodal burden is more robust.[90] Aside from a cervical mass of unknown etiology, the most common presenting symptom is chronic odynophagia (often unilateral) and referred otalgia. Change in voice, dysphagia, and trismus are late signs. Regional lymphatic metastases occur frequently and are related to the depth of tumor invasion and tumor size.

Management of oropharyngeal cancers is very challenging, given the essential role this anatomic site plays in breathing, speech, and swallowing. Therefore, the goal of treatment is to not only achieve oncologic cure but also to preserve the multi-modal function of the oropharynx. Traditional surgical approaches to the oropharynx are associated with significant morbidity, which prompted a shift toward nonsurgical modalities in the 1990s, specifically utilizing radiation or chemoradiation, which have been the mainstay therapeutic approaches for the past 15–20 years.[91] However, recent technological innovations have led to a resurrection of surgical options through a transoral robotic approach (Transoral robotic surgery (TORS)), which allows for adjuvant therapy to be modified based on the pathological findings of disease.

Tumor-related contraindications for TORS include unresectable cervical lymphadenopathy, mandibular invasion, pharyngeal wall or tongue base involvement requiring resection of greater than 50% of these sites, radiologic evidence of carotid involvement, and fixation to the prevertebral fascia. The other limitation of TORS is accessed, and therefore a thorough preoperative assessment of the patient and tumor characteristics is essential. This should include an evaluation of the dentition, presence of trismus or tori, tongue size, degree of neck extension, sequelae of previous treatment, and the tumor extent. The oncologic outcomes for robotic surgery have been favorable thus far with OS and DFS rates ranging 82–100% and 86–96%, respectively. Although the role of TORS is still being determined, early oncologic results from several case series are comparable to the outcomes observed with radiation or concurrent chemoradiation.[92]

Radiation therapy is a standard approach for definitive treatment for the oropharynx which combines the goal of an oncological cure with organ preservation. The current XRT regimens are the results of several large randomized trials that have demonstrated favorable OS and DFS.[93]

The classic pattern of relapse after RT in OPSCC has been locoregional recurrence. To overcome radiation resistance, chemotherapy has been added to sensitize the tumor cells to the damaging effects of ionizing radiation. For patients with locally advanced oropharyngeal cancer, a pivotal randomized phase III trial by the French GORTEC group revealed an improvement in both progression-free survival (PFS) and 5 year OS for patients receiving combined modality therapy (42% and 51%) versus radiation therapy alone (22.4% and 15.8%) and improvement in locoregional control rates in the chemoradiation arm (66%) versus radiation therapy alone (42%). Despite these benefits, more significant side effects were observed in the chemotherapy arm.[94,95] These toxicities led to a higher rate of temporary gastrostomy tube usage in the combination arm compared to the radiation therapy alone arm. Taken together, these results suggest that the addition of chemotherapy concurrently to radiation therapy improves locoregional control, which translates into both a PFS and OS benefit for these patients, at the expense of more acute toxicities. With modern radiation techniques, the incidence of dysphagia and permanent G-tube usage has decreased substantially. More recent experiences include a pooled analysis of over 2300 patients with OPC treated with intensity-modulated radiotherapy (IMRT), where the 2-year G-tube dependency rate was 4.4%[96] and several randomized trials with rates ranging from 5 to 10%.[97]

The risk of recurrence for locally advanced OPSCC following surgical resection has traditionally been high. PORT often with the addition of chemotherapy has been shown to decrease locoregional recurrences. Whether this treatment paradigm is necessary for HPV-positive patients is currently under investigation.

Tonsil

The traditional treatment of stage I and II tonsillar neoplasms is radiation therapy as a single modality. Transoral wide local excision of small, superficial lesions may be locally effective but does not address the high potential of occult lymph node metastasis. For patients with early-stage HPV-positive tumors, TORS with neck dissection offers excellent local-regional control, without the need for adjuvant radiotherapy.[92] For patients with small primary but nodal disease (N1-2), the addition of PORT to TORS is associated with excellent oncological and functional outcomes, and spares the need for concurrent chemoradiotherapy. Surgical management of advanced cancers results in poor patient function and thus combined chemotherapy and radiotherapy approaches are utilized (Figure 4). There is a growing rationale for avoiding or reducing XRT particularly among patients with p16 positive (HPV-related) small tumors (T1-2) and small volume neck disease (N1), and this approach is currently under investigation in a multi-institutional clinical trial (ECOG 3311).

Alternatively, radiation for early tonsillar cancers offers the advantage of treating upper echelon lymph nodes along with the primary tumor. Treatment is usually unilateral unless extension to the tongue base or midline soft palate is present.[98] Ipsilateral treatment portals allow sparing of the contralateral mucosa and

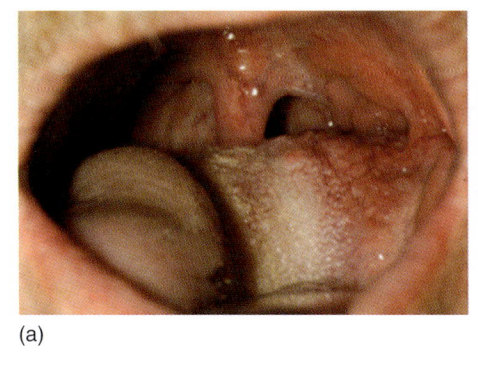

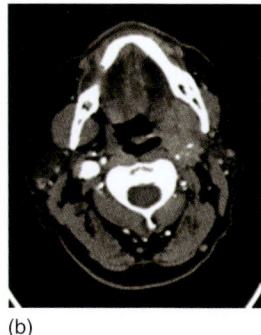

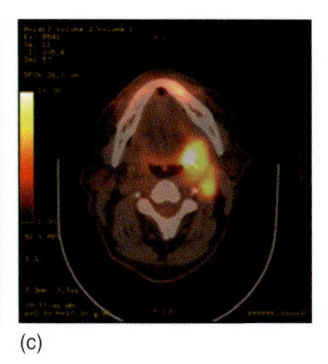

Figure 4 (a) T2 N2b SCCA of the oropharynx, clinically small lesion. (b) Deep infiltration into the parapharyngeal space is evident on CT scanning. (c) On PET-CT imaging, two distinct lesions are evident, the primary tumor and a posterior lymphatic metastasis.

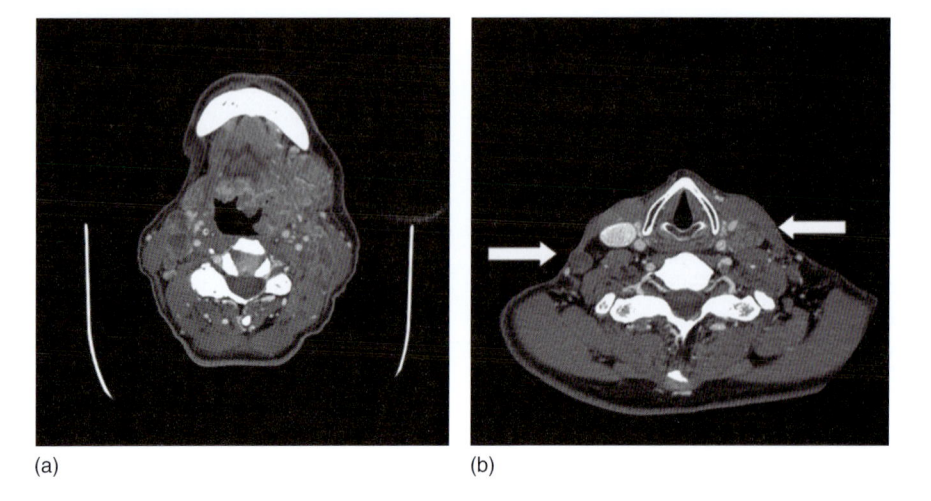

Figure 5 (a) Massive T4 N2c SCCA of the oropharynx (left base of tongue). (b) Multilevel bilateral nodal metastases present.

salivary glands. Modern treatment techniques, such as IMRT, permit conformal dose delivery which can reduce the potential morbidity of radiation treatment, particularly by reducing radiation-related xerostomia.

Survival rates for patients with advanced (stage III/IV) tumors vary according to HPV/p16 expression status and smoking history. Patients with HPV-positive tumors and less than 10 pack-year smoking history (low-risk) treated with the combination of chemotherapy and radiotherapy have a 3-year survival rate of 93%; while those with a smoking history of more than 10 pack-years and HPV/p16 negative tumor undergoing chemoradiation have a 3-year survival rate of 46.2%.[34] In general, surgery is rarely recommended for advanced tonsillar tumors unless the mandible is grossly invaded. When surgery is planned, postoperative concurrent therapy should be anticipated in the properly selected patient.

Tongue base

Due to the aggressive nature of HPV-negative tumors, most are treated with definitive radiation with or without chemotherapy, although a role for TORS is currently under clinical investigation. Owing to the rich network of lymphatics present in the base of the tongue, 75% of patients will present with stage III or IV disease (Figure 5). Under-staging of the primary tumor is common because these cancers tend to be diffusely infiltrative beyond their clinical appearance.[99]

The results of radiation therapy alone as definitive treatment of small primary tumors (T1, T2) are better for exophytic than for deeply invasive tumors.[100] Radiation alone is generally reserved for those patients without clinical nodal metastases but can be combined with planned neck dissection for patients with clinically positive nodes that persist after the completion of radiation-based approaches.

Surgical management of early primary tongue-base tumors (T1-2) achieves results similar to those from radiation alone. Advances in robotic surgery have prompted the application of this technology in the management of tongue-base cancers, and it is now a well-established approach in the HPV-positive population.[101] Elective neck dissection can serve as a staging procedure, thereby providing a rationale for adjuvant radiation therapy. To date, no prospective randomized trial data are available that compare surgery alone with combined surgery with either preoperative or postoperative radiation.

The approach for patients with locally advanced base of tongue cancer is similar to tonsillar cancer. Selected patients, particularly those with large tumors that are exophytic with limited invasion may benefit from surgical resection with PORT based on pathologic findings. Most patients though are treated with combined chemotherapy and radiation.

Soft palate and pharyngeal wall

Radiation-based approaches as curative treatment are preferred in most cases, even for T3 primary tumors. Resection of most soft-palate lesions is associated with severe functional disability. The rates of occult regional metastases are difficult to determine because elective irradiation of bilateral nodal groups is included as part of primary treatment and must include the retropharyngeal lymphatics. Clinically positive lymph nodes at presentation occur in 30% of patients.[102] Small primary tumors with positive nodes can be effectively treated with definitive radiation to the primary tumor and neck. Overall 5-year survival rates for soft-palate and faucial pillar cancers are 60–70% and range from 80–90% for T1 and T2 lesions to 30–60% for stages III and IV lesions.[103]

Hypopharynx

The hypopharynx represents one of the most lethal sites for HNSCC. Lymph node metastases are clinically evident at time of diagnosis in 70–80% of patients.[104] Primary tumor extension beyond the hypopharynx is common.[105] More than 75% of hypopharyngeal cancers arise in the pyriform sinus, while 20% occur in the posterior pharyngeal wall (Figure 6). Postcricoid cancers are rare (less than 5%). Because of the locale of hypopharyngeal cancers, their growth patterns, and proximity to the larynx, surgical management often entails total laryngopharyngectomy. Extension to the esophagus will necessitate a cervical esophagectomy.

The staging of hypopharyngeal cancer is based on the subsite involved, the size of the tumor, the presence of vocal cord fixation, and the extent of lymph node metastases.[60] Staging is critical for treatment planning and must include endoscopic evaluation.[106]

Because of the necessity to remove the larynx as part of the surgical treatment of most hypopharyngeal cancers, radiation therapy for early T1 and T2 and in combination with chemotherapy for T3 disease has been investigated.[107] Retrospective analyses have consistently demonstrated that survival rates are lower and

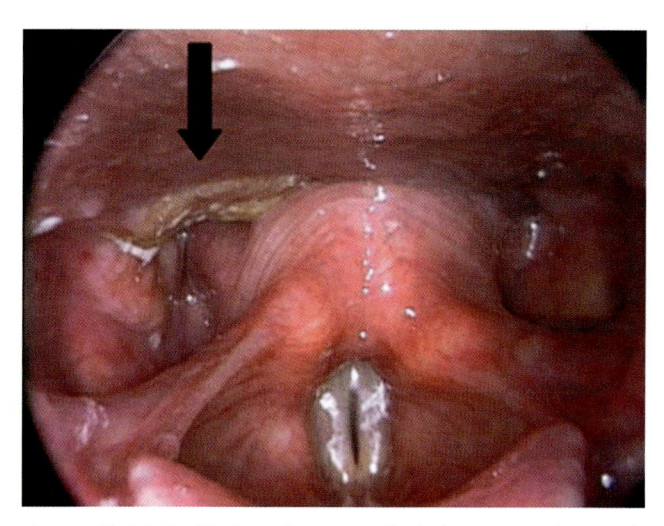

Figure 6 T1 SCCA of the hypopharynx, involving the posterior pharyngeal wall and extending into the esophageal inlet.

locoregional failure rates higher with radiation alone as compared with surgery or surgery and radiotherapy.[108,109]

Tumors arising in the lower hypopharynx or postcricoid mucosa often spread to involve the esophagus. Distal submucosal spread into the esophagus can be extensive and requires partial or total esophagectomy. Reconstruction with transposition of the stomach (gastric pull-up), jejunal free graft, or tubed fasciocutaneous free flap is currently recommended.[110-112] With improved locoregional control following the advent of total laryngopharyngectomy and PORT, disease recurrence more commonly occurs in distant sites (i.e., the lung).

Overall 5-year survival rates range from 10% to 30% for posterior pharyngeal wall cancers and from 20% to 40% for pyriform sinus cancers. The rates of distant metastases could reach up to 60%[104] and increase with the extent of lymph node disease.[104,113-115]

Larynx

Because of the prominent role, the larynx plays in communication, swallowing, respiration, and protection of the lower airway, the treatment of cancer of the larynx presents formidable dilemmas regarding functional consequences in addition to the intrinsic threat to life posed by these cancers. More so than with any other site of HNC, quality-of-life issues have been incorporated into treatment decisions and have echoed throughout the management strategy of the other head and neck sites.

Early diagnosis is critical for achieving high survival rates and larynx preservation. Most cancers that are diagnosed at an early stage arise in the glottic larynx. This is because minimal changes of the vibrating vocal cord from tumor growth result in dysphonia or hoarseness. Supraglottic cancers are usually more advanced than glottic cancers at the time of diagnosis because they do not generally produce early symptoms of hoarseness. Rather, the earliest symptoms of a supraglottic cancer are usually sore throat, dysphagia, referred otalgia, or the development of a neck mass representing regional metastasis. Airway compromise may be an early symptom with subglottic cancer.

Early tumors of the larynx are often confined to their respective subsite (though stage 2 glottic cancers will often have minimal spread superiorly or inferiorly to involve the supra- or sub-glottis), and their management is addressed for each subsite. Management of local-regional advanced laryngeal cancer, with few exceptions, tends to have a more general paradigm.

Supraglottic cancers

Supraglottic primary tumors account for approximately 35% of all laryngeal cancers.[10] The staging of supraglottic cancers is based on the subsite or region of the supraglottis involved. Subsites include the false vocal cords, arytenoids, lingual and laryngeal surfaces of the epiglottis, and aryepiglottic folds. The epiglottis itself is also subdivided into the region extending above the plane of the hyoid and that below the hyoid. Suprahyoid tumors tend to have a better prognosis than infrahyoid with the exception of those invading the aryepiglottic fold to involve the pyriform sinus. Early cancers (T1 and T2) can involve one or more subsites but have normal vocal cord motion. Those cancers that cause fixation of the arytenoid or involve the postcricoid region, medial wall of the pyriform sinus, or preepiglottic space are staged T3. Those that extend beyond the larynx or invade thyroid cartilage are staged T4.

Important factors in selecting therapy for supraglottic cancers are tumor location, cord fixation, and preepiglottic extension. Tumors limited to the suprahyoid epiglottis are amenable to radiation with fields that encompass neck regions at risk of lymphatic metastases. In addition, some proponents of limited surgical interventions recommend endoscopic laser excision separate from management of the neck. Radiation alone is less effective than surgery for tumors involving the aryepiglottic folds, pyriform sinuses, or infrahyoid epiglottis, resulting in more frequent local recurrences that require surgical salvage. The addition of systemic concurrent chemotherapy will positively impact the outcomes of patients with these tumors. Persistent postradiation edema of the supraglottic larynx is not uncommon and contributes to difficulty in detecting recurrence, which occurs in 40–50% of cases.[116,117] Most patients who recur will ultimately require a salvage total laryngectomy.

In any patient undergoing partial laryngectomy, preoperative consent should be obtained for total laryngectomy in case the surgical findings dictate that more extensive surgery is needed. Approximately 20% of patients require prolonged tracheostomy, and this is usually related to edema secondary to PORT. The rates of persistent swallowing difficulties are low, however, and the need for completion laryngectomy for persistent aspiration ranges only from 0% to 5%.[118,119]

The frequency of neck node metastases is at least 20% with T2 or greater tumors. Treatment of the clinically negative neck may be accomplished with surgery or radiation.[120] Cure rates range from 73% to 75% for radiotherapy and increase to 80–85% with the addition of surgical salvage.[121-123] Most recurrences are local, and preservation of voice is successful in 65–70% of patients when salvage surgery is included.[121]

While distant metastases are relatively uncommon for laryngeal cancer, distant spread is approximately four times more common with supraglottic than with glottic cancers.[124] Rates of distant metastases associated with glottic cancer have increased, however, with the use of combined therapy and have been reported in approximately 20% of patients with advanced disease. Rates appear to be directly related to the extent of nodal disease, with reported rates as high as 40–50% in patients with N2 or N3 disease.[125]

Glottic cancers

Functional and anatomic features determine the staging of glottic carcinomas. Cancers limited to the true vocal cords are T1, those with extension to an adjacent site or with impaired cord mobility are T2, arytenoid fixation and vocal cord immobility upstages a lesion to a T3. Those tumors with cartilage involvement or extension outside the larynx are T4.

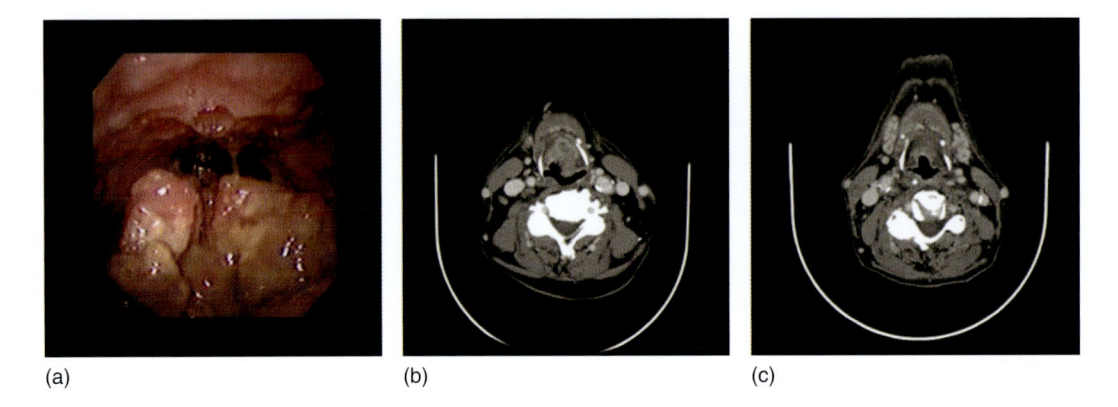

Figure 7 (a) T3 N0 SCCA of the supraglottis. Destruction of the epiglottis is evident. (b) Invasion of the preepiglottic space is seen on CT scan, prior to concurrent chemoradiotherapy. (c) Posttreatment imaging, demonstrating a complete response at the primary site.

The treatment of glottic cancer is greatly influenced by the secondary goal of voice preservation. For small cancers (T1, T2) with mobile vocal cords, radiation therapy alone achieves excellent local control rates of 80–95% and OS rates similar to those for surgical resection.[126,127] Voice quality, although often impaired by radiation, is generally better than that following surgical resection.[128] Local recurrences after definitive radiation can often be salvaged by subsequent surgery. Conservation laryngeal surgical salvage is effective in those 10–20% of cases. Tumor involvement of the anterior commissure or arytenoids has been associated with higher local recurrence rates for radiation alone, but this may have been related to understaging.

In some instances, conservation laryngeal surgery is preferred over radiation. Lesions that are mid-cord are particularly favorable for this approach. Techniques include laser excision or partial laryngeal surgery. Both require frozen-section analysis of margins if the patient and tumor factors support such an approach. Recurrence rates with these approaches are uncommon. In addition, conservation laryngeal surgical salvage is effective in those 10–20% of cases in which external beam therapy has been unsuccessful for stages I and II cancers.

The design of radiation treatment must be tailored to the individual patient, but some general comments can be made. Early-stage (T1-2, N0) glottic lesions are treated with conventional fields localized to the larynx only; for T2 tumors with significant subglottic spread, the upper trachea is also included. T1 tumors are typically treated once-daily to doses of approximately 6300–6600 cGy, while T2 tumors are treated more aggressively with twice-daily or concurrent-boost fractionation.[129] T2 tumors with bulky subglottic extension or with anterior involvement with potential extralaryngeal spread outside the thyroid cartilage are at higher risk for treatment failure and can be considered for concurrent chemoradiotherapy. There has been recent interest in using IMRT to minimize dose to the adjacent carotid vessels, and for very early lesions, there have also been reports of single vocal cord irradiation[130] to further reduce the volume of irradiated tissue.

Subglottic cancers

True subglottic cancers that are limited to the subglottic region (T1) or to the subglottis and true vocal cords (T2) are early cancers. Fixation of the vocal cord (T3) and cartilage invasion or extension outside the larynx (T4) is associated with a worse prognosis. The nodal classification for staging is the same as for other HNSCC sites.

Subglottic carcinomas are a rare variant of squamous carcinomas of the larynx possessing a high risk for paratracheal metastases, local recurrence, and death from disease. Surgery is the preferred therapy except in early superficial diseases of this site.[131,132] Tumors originating from or involving the subglottic larynx can spread to the upper paratracheal nodes as well as to the nodes in the cervical chain.

Advanced laryngeal cancer

The treatment of advanced cancers that are T3 is controversial, with laryngeal preservation remaining a focus of treatment (Figure 7). Combined chemoradiotherapy is often curative, but toxicities remain significant.

Management of advanced T3 cancers has historically consisted of total laryngectomy with or without PORT. With proper selection, radiotherapy control rates for supraglottic T3 lesions can approach 70–80%,[133,134] which is enhanced by the addition of platinum-based chemotherapy.

Induction chemotherapy has long been recognized as highly active with clinical partial and complete responses observed in 80–90% of patients.[135–137] It was postulated that a substantial response to initial treatment with chemotherapy would lead to an improvement of therapeutic efficacy for surgery or radiotherapy. This led to the Department of Veterans Affairs Laryngeal Cancer Study,[138] in which 332 patients with stage III or IV SCC of the larynx were randomized to receive either induction chemotherapy consisting of cisplatin and fluorouracil followed by radiotherapy or surgery and PORT. Patients who experienced no tumor response to chemotherapy or those who had locally persistent or recurrent cancer underwent salvage laryngectomy. Two-year survival for both treatment groups was 68%, and 41% of patients randomly assigned to the experimental arm were alive with a functional larynx at 2 years. Thus, the efficacy of chemotherapy followed by radiotherapy (with surgical salvage) was similar to that of surgery followed by radiotherapy and established organ preservation as a realistic goal of nonsurgical treatment administered with curative intent. Lefebvre and colleagues[107] later reported the potential for effective sequential induction chemotherapy followed by radiotherapy in a European trial involving patients with cancers of the hypopharynx.

In the Veterans Affairs study, there were observed trends in patterns of tumor relapse, with 20% of patients in the chemotherapy arm having locoregional recurrence versus 7% in the surgery arm. Distant disease recurrence was more commonly observed the surgical arm, affecting 17% of patients versus 11% in the chemotherapy/radiotherapy group.

The Veterans Affairs Larynx study prompted further investigations of sequential chemotherapy and radiotherapy in the treatment of intermediate-stage larynx cancer. These trials indicate that for patients with intermediate-stage SCC of the larynx, a combined treatment program with the objectives of tumor eradication and laryngeal preservation is appropriate. It is also important to recognize that patients with locally advanced destructive primary laryngeal cancers were not included in the multi-institutional trial. These patients may require total laryngectomy for optimal tumor control and to preserve swallowing function.

Prospective randomized studies have shown convincingly that chemotherapy and radiation therapy (including surgical salvage) are equally effective in the long-term survival of patients with T3 laryngeal cancers as compared with surgery with or without radiation therapy. It is important to note that approximately 60% of patients may preserve their larynx, and thus quality of life has significantly improved.[139-141] Speech communication profiles are clearly better in the group of patients randomized to the larynx preservation arm, but there was no determination of swallowing function.[142]

One area of controversy surrounds the management of patients with bulky T3 lesions and poor pretreatment function. These patients may require long-term or permanent enteral nutrition and tracheostomy for significant aspiration, and may ultimately require a laryngectomy for pulmonary toilet. One novel approach that has been advocated is to utilize induction chemotherapy to assess both tumor and functional responses. Those with improvement of their function after one cycle of chemotherapy may tolerate concurrent chemoradiotherapy and avoid laryngectomy. Alternatively, those with minimal or no response would be best managed with surgery and PORT.

The laryngeal preservation studies have suggested that a nonsurgical approach results in higher rates of local failure for patients with T4 lesions. In the Veterans Affairs Laryngeal Study, salvage laryngectomy was required in 56% of patients with T4 cancers compared with 29% of patients with smaller primary tumors ($p = 0.001$). It is therefore still recommended that these patients are best managed with laryngectomy and radiotherapy, as cartilage and bone invasion are difficult to control with radiation. However, some experienced centers have treated patients with minimal laryngeal framework invasion with combined chemoradiotherapy with high success.

Many surgical procedures for laryngeal carcinoma involve the creation of a tracheal stoma. This area is at significant risk of tumor recurrence, which is most likely associated with paratracheal nodal metastases. For this reason, bilateral paratracheal dissections should be performed in T4 glottic cancers and radiation therapy provided postoperatively if metastases to this echelon of nodes are found pathologically. Once a stomal recurrence has developed, the prognosis is grave regardless of salvage treatment, with a reported 5-year survival of 17%.[143] If risk factors for stomal recurrence are present, then the tracheal stoma should be irradiated as part of the initial management.

Although the stigma of laryngectomy remains, contemporary postoperative laryngeal rehabilitation offers quite acceptable functional outcomes. The advent of tracheoesophageal punctures (TEP), in conjunction with intense rehabilitation, has markedly improved the functional outcomes of laryngectomized patients. Alaryngeal speech can be realized within 2 weeks after surgery. In the salvage surgical setting, TEP placement should be deferred for at least 3 months while the surgical site matures. Early TEP placement resulted in fistula formation and poor wound healing.

Because rates of occult regional metastases approach 30% in patients with advanced glottic (T3, T4) cancers, elective modified or selective node dissections for staging purposes are recommended when surgery is performed for primary disease. Demonstration of histologically positive nodal metastases has been used as an indication for PORT. Surgery alone is curative in 50–80% of patients without nodal metastases,[144-148] but this decreases to less than 40% if metastases are present.[146,149,150]

Nasopharynx

Presentation and staging

In the United States, NPC accounts for 2% of all HNSCC. Its unusual epidemiologic and natural history features include a remarkable tendency toward early regional and distant dissemination. NPC is also extremely sensitive to radiotherapy and cytotoxic chemotherapy.

The nasopharynx is a chamber bounded anteriorly by the choana of the nasal cavity, superiorly by the clivus, and inferiorly by the soft palate. Its posterior wall is the mucosa that overlies the superior constrictor muscles of the pharynx and the C1 and C2 vertebral bodies. The lateral walls contain the eustachian tube orifices. The region is richly endowed with lymphatics that drain to the retropharyngeal and deep cervical nodes.

Malignant neoplasms of the nasopharynx are primarily epithelial, with the presence of keratin associated with a poorer prognosis. The World health organization (WHO) recognizes three histopathologic types of NPC: type 1, differentiated SCC (of varying degrees); type 2, nonkeratinizing carcinoma; and type 3, undifferentiated lymphoepithelial carcinoma. Mixed patterns are common.

Evaluation of the nasopharynx should consist of direct visualization with a fiber-optic scope. An MRI scan is important in evaluating base-of-skull involvement and the possible presence of occult-involved lymph nodes.

The most recent revision of the AJCC/Union Internationale Contre le Cancer (UICC) staging system recognizes the uniqueness of NPC among other head and neck tumors.[60]

Treatment

Standard treatment of NPC is radiation therapy or concurrent chemoradiotherapy for early and locally advanced disease, respectively. The role of the surgeon is limited to obtaining tissue for diagnosis, resecting residual adenopathy after definitive radiotherapy, and surgery for rare non-WHO histologies such as adenoid cystic carcinoma.[151]

For patients with stage III or IV at diagnosis, platinum-based concurrent chemoradiotherapy is the standard of care. More recently, a sequential approach consisting of gemcitabine and cisplatin induction chemotherapy significantly improved recurrence-free survival (RFS) and OS, as compared with chemoradiotherapy alone. In this phase III randomized trial, 480 patients (242 patients in the induction and 238 in the standard arms, respectively) were randomized. With a median follow-up of 42.7 months, the 3-year RFS was 85.3% in the induction arm versus 76.5% in the standard arm. The 3-year OS was 94.6% and 90.3%, respectively.[152] Preceding these findings, chemoradiotherapy followed by adjuvant chemotherapy was the standard of care. The Intergroup Cooperative Study (IG0099) tested a radiotherapy-alone arm versus an experimental arm consisting of concurrent cisplatin given on days

Table 4 Selected concurrent chemoradiotherapy trials in locally advanced NPC.

Study	N	Treatment arms	Outcomes
Al-Sarraf et al.[153]	78	cddp 100 mg/m^2 weeks 1,4,7-RT + adj cddp/fu	5-yr PFS 58% and OS 67% CM versus 29%
	69	RT	29% and 37% RT
			($p < 0.001$)
Lin et al.[156]	141	cddp 20 mg/m^2/d + fu 400 mg/m^2/d 96 h infusion weeks 1 + 5-RT	5-yr PFS 72% and OS 72% CM versus 53% and 54% RT
	143	RT	($p = 0.001 + 0.002$)
Chan et al.[154,155]	174	cddp 40 mg/m^2 weekly-RT	5-yr PFS 60% and OS 70% CM versus 52% and 59% RT
	176	RT	($p = 0.06 + 0.05$)
Hui et al.[157]	34	Doc 75 mg/m^2 + cddp 75 mg/m^2 x2 → CRT	3-yr PFS 88% and OS 94% versus 60% ($p = 0.12$) and 68% ($p = 0.01$)
	31	CRT	

Abbreviations: cddp, cisplatin; CM, combined modality; doc, docetaxel; fu, fluorouracil; OS, overall survival; PFS, progression-free survival; RT, radiotherapy.

1, 22, and 43 during radiotherapy followed by three courses of adjuvant cisplatin and 5-FU chemotherapy.[153] A total of 147 evaluable patients with stages III and IV tumors were enrolled. Notably, approximately one-third of patients were classified WHO 1, unlike most reports from the Pacific Rim in which >95% of patients are WHO 2/3. At 3 years there was improved PFS (69% vs 24%, $p = 0.001$), improved OS (76% vs 46%, $p = 0.005$), and reduced distant metastases (13% vs 35%, $p = 0.002$) for the experimental arm. These data were corroborated by another randomized phase III trial, which compared concurrent cisplatin (40 mg/m^2 weekly) and radiotherapy with radiotherapy alone in 350 patients with local and regionally advanced (N2 and N3, or N1 with nodal disease ≥4 cm) NPC.[154] This study found that treatment with combined chemotherapy plus radiotherapy prolonged PFS. The treatment effect had a notable covariate interaction with tumor stage, and subgroup analysis showed a significant difference in patients with T3 disease in favor of the concurrent therapy arm ($p = 0.0075$). The time to first distant failure also was statistically prolonged in patients with T3 tumors in the concurrent-treatment arm ($p = 0.016$). An updated report[155] concludes that OS benefit after chemoradiotherapy was most clearly obtained in patients with T3/4 staging ($p = 0.013$). Lin and colleagues[156] conducted a prospective phase III trial with randomization to radiation therapy alone or XRT with two cycles of concurrent cisplatin and fluorouracil administered during weeks 1 and 5 of XRT. OS again favored the combined treatment arm (Table 4).

Alternatively, strategies with induction chemotherapy had much appeal because of the high risk of systemic tumor dissemination in patients with NPC. Chua and colleagues[158] analyzed pooled data from two large phase III trials investigating the role of induction chemotherapy in NPC. In these trials, a total of 784 patients were randomized to receive 2–3 cycles of cisplatin-based combination therapy followed by radiotherapy alone. The 5-year relapse-free survival was 50.9% and 42.7%, respectively ($p = 0.014$), and disease-specific survival was 63.5% and 58.1% ($p = 0.029$). OS was not found to be significantly different between the arms ($p = 0.092$). Hui et al.[157] have recently reported favorable PFS and OS results in a phase II study of induction cisplatin and docetaxel followed by chemoradiotherapy. With the recent findings of the Zhang et al. NEJM trial,[152] sequential therapy has now become a standard of care.

Rather than treat all patients with upfront chemotherapy, some have suggested that a better approach may be to identify the subset of patients who would benefit most from adjuvant treatment. NRG-HN001 is an ongoing phase II/III study investigating the value of measuring plasma Epstein–Barr virus deoxyribonucleic acid (EBV DNA) as a marker of efficacy of concurrent chemoradiotherapy. With undetectable DNA, patients are randomized to observation or adjuvant chemotherapy. Patients with detectable DNA after chemoradiotherapy receive additional treatment, testing alternative regimens consisting of paclitaxel and gemcitabine versus cisplatin and fluorouracil.

Nose and paranasal sinuses

Cancer of the nose and paranasal sinuses is relatively rare. It accounts for approximately 3% of cancers of the UADT and tends to occur in the fifth decade of life.[159] These tumors tend to be asymptomatic and usually contained within either a sinus or the nasal cavity. Early symptoms usually include nasal airway obstruction, rhinorrhea, sinusitis, epistaxis, and, occasionally, dental problems such as dental pain, numbness, and loose teeth. Late symptoms include cranial nerve deficits, proptosis, facial pain and swelling, ulceration through the palate, and trismus, all of which are ominous signs (Figure 8).

Treatment

Treatment of neoplasms of the sinonasal cavity is primarily determined by the histology. Traditionally, surgery with PORT has been advocated for many of these tumors. Although very effective for smaller tumors of selected histologies, this approach provides poor control for advanced disease involving the orbit, skull base, and soft tissues of the face. An induction chemotherapy-based approach, with patients triaged to either concurrent chemoradiotherapy or surgery with PORT based upon the response to chemotherapy is currently under investigation among patients with advanced tumors (clinical trial registration number NCT00707473).[160]

Radiotherapy plays a major role in the management of sinonasal malignancies. It is used both preoperatively and postoperatively and in select cases as definitive therapy for small T1 and T2 lesions, especially those limited to the nasal vestibule and anterior nasal cavity.[161] In this situation, high locoregional control rates and good cosmetic outcome should be expected. With the increased use of radiotherapy in combination with surgery, ever-improving rates of locoregional control have been achieved. Surgery with PORT remains the standard of care for advanced sinonasal cavity tumors. As mentioned above, concurrent chemoradiotherapy can be utilized in selected patients. Patients with inoperable tumors or those who are not considered good surgical candidates may be best treated with radiation therapy alone for local control and palliation.

Although chemotherapy as a component of concurrent treatment with radiation is covered more extensively in a separate section, some aspects of chemotherapy will be mentioned briefly here. The use of induction chemotherapy in selected patients with

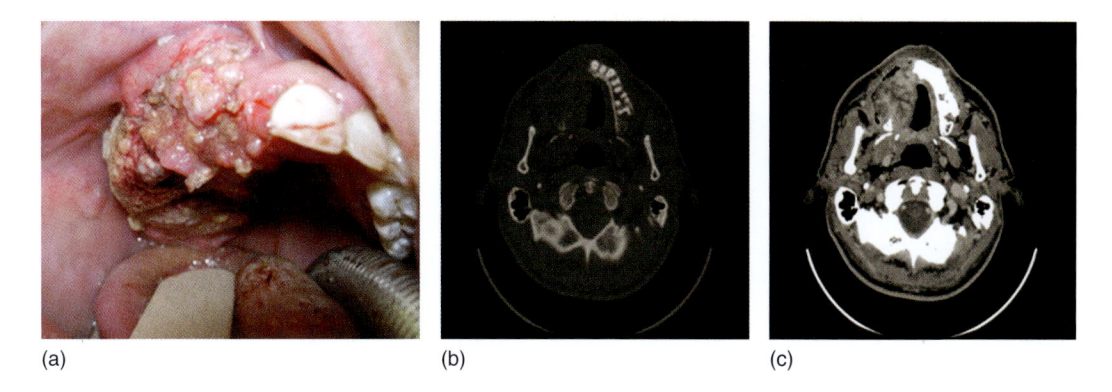

Figure 8 (a) T4 SCCA of the maxillary sinus, with extension into the oral cavity. (b) Bone windows on CT scan reveal complete replacement of the maxillary sinus with tumor and destruction of the pterygoid plates. (c) Soft tissue windows reveal extra-osseous extension into the midface.

involvement of the eye has shown promising results in preserving the orbit.[162] These results remain based on single-institution series. The recently activated EA3163 study is asking the question of whether intensification with a preoperative systemic therapy approach could impact the rate of structure preservation (in this case orbit or base of skull) or affect OS in sino-nasal SCCs. Choi and colleagues reported results of concurrent chemoradiotherapy and investigators at the University of Chicago have used induction chemotherapy with cisplatin and infusional 5-FU to achieve improved rates of locoregional control and preserve the eye.[162,163] Studies at various centers are currently ongoing to validate the use of this approach for advanced sinonasal malignancies. Some investigators have utilized intra-arterial chemotherapy followed by surgery and/or radiation therapy for advanced sinonasal malignancies.[164–166] Although these studies have shown some benefit with regard to locoregional control, the morbidity associated with intra-arterial therapy does not appear to justify this approach. For patients with unresectable skull-base neoplasms, concurrent chemoradiotherapy is a reasonable approach that may offer locoregional control in up to 50% of patients.[162] Sinonasal undifferentiated carcinoma (SNUC), neuroendocrine carcinoma, and esthesioneuroblastoma represent a spectrum of tumors with neuroendocrine differentiation that can be difficult to distinguish histologically. Immunohistochemistry is often necessary to accurately diagnose these lesions, which may also be confused with sinonasal melanoma, rhabdomyosarcoma, PNET, or lymphoma. An experienced head and neck pathologist should be consulted prior to determining a treatment plan.

SNUC is a rare but lethal cancer typically presenting as advanced disease in elderly patients. Traditional treatment has been surgery followed by PORT, but this has provided poor long-term control. These tumors may be chemosensitive and a response to induction chemotherapy may identify patients for concurrent chemoradiotherapy as definitive treatment.[167–169] Surgical salvage has a uniformly dismal prognosis, but in light of the poor locoregional control achieved with traditional surgery and PORT, most agree that study of concurrent chemoradiotherapy is warranted.

Esthesioneuroblastoma is a rare neoplasm emanating from the olfactory neurofilaments at the cribriform plate. Invasion of the anterior cranial fossa occurs early in the disease process, and eventually involves the brain parenchyma (Figure 9). Patients often present with nasal obstruction and epistaxis. Treatment centers around surgical resection and PORT, which offers effective locoregional control and favorable survival outcomes.[170] Chemotherapy is reserved for patients with extensive intracranial or orbital disease that would otherwise require an extensive resection. It may also be used in the neoadjuvant setting as a cytoreductive approach to allow complete surgical resection.[171]

Salivary glands

Anatomy

Salivary gland tissue is ubiquitous in the submucosa of the upper gastrointestinal tract and with three major salivary glands: parotid, submaxillary (or submandibular), and sublingual glands. The most common sites of tumors of minor salivary glands are the palate, the base of the tongue, and the buccal mucosa.[172]

The majority of salivary gland tumors arise in the parotid glands, and although nearly 80% of these are benign, these glands are the origin of the majority of malignant tumors. Tumors arising in the submandibular, sublingual, or minor salivary glands are more likely to be malignant.

Histopathology

Benign lesions are the most frequent tumor of the parotid gland. The histological classification of malignant salivary tumors has been reviewed and expanded over the years and the present WHO classification is the most often quoted (Table 5).[173] Mucoepidermoid carcinoma (MEC) is the most frequent cancer of the parotid gland and is classified into high-grade, intermediate, and low-grade tumors (Figure 10).[174,175] Low-grade MEC is characterized by a slow growth rate, a low recurrence rate after complete surgical excision (about 15%), and rare incidence of metastasis. High-grade tumors are more aggressive, and the local recurrence rate after surgery alone approaches 60%.[176] Local recurrences and distant metastases may occur many years after treatment. About 50% of patients with high-grade MEC present with regional metastases, and 30% develop metastases at distant sites.[174,177] Acinic cell carcinomas are usually well differentiated and account for approximately 13% of the cancers arising from the parotid glands. Lymph node metastases occur in about 15% of cases. Local recurrence and distant metastases may occur many years after treatment.[178] Adenoid cystic carcinoma accounts for approximately 10% of parotid gland malignancies but 60% of malignant neoplasms of the submandibular or minor salivary glands.[172,179] Three subtypes have been identified that correlate to biological behavior: cribriform, tubular, and solid (most aggressive). A remarkable feature of this neoplasm is its propensity to invade major nerves and spread along the endoneural and perineural sheaths. This has significant prognostic importance and must be taken into account when deciding treatment and, specifically, when considering PORT. Although

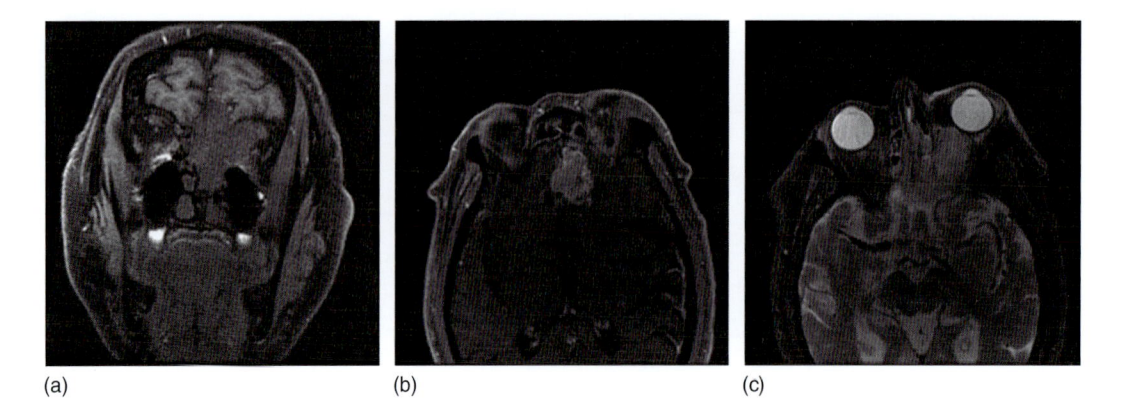

Figure 9 (a) Esthesioneuroblastoma involving the central skull base, with intracranial extension. (b) Involvement of the left frontal lobe on MRI. (c) Invasion of the left orbital apex.

Table 5 Most common malignant tumors of salivary glands.[a]

Mucoepidermoid carcinoma (low, intermediate, or high grade)
Acinic cell carcinoma
Adenoid cystic carcinoma
Adenocarcinoma
Malignant mixed tumor (carcinoma-expleomorphic adenoma)
Squamous cell carcinoma

[a]Source: Modified from Seifert and Sobin.[173]

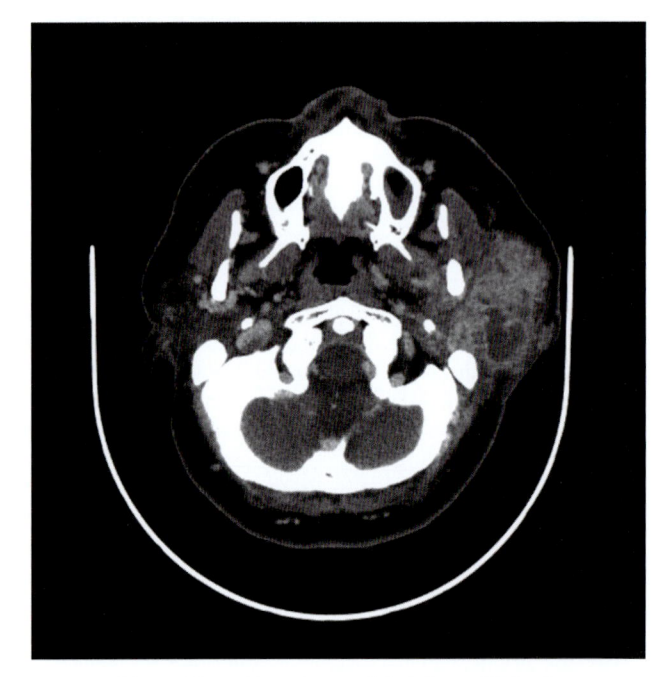

Figure 10 Mucoepidermoid carcinoma of the left parotid gland.

these tumors often follow an indolent course, as many as 40% of patients ultimately develop regional and distant metastases.[179]

Adenocarcinomas are more common in the minor salivary glands. The majority of them are high-grade tumors. About 36% of patients either present with or subsequently develop regional lymph node metastases; therefore, the regional lymph nodes need to be addressed in treatment strategies for high-grade adenocarcinomas.[180] Lung and bone are frequent sites of distant metastases.

Carcinoma ex-pleomorphic arises from preexisting benign pleomorphic adenoma. The risk of malignant transformation increases with time and age of the patient. Of adenomas of less than 5 years duration, 1.6% can dedifferentiate; when present for more than 15 years, the dedifferentiation rate increases to 9.4%.[181] True malignant mixed tumors are rare, constituting only 2–5% of all malignant salivary gland tumors. These are typically aggressive tumors. A histology that deserves mention is salivary ductal carcinoma, which appears microscopically similar to breast carcinoma. Primary SCC of the salivary gland is rare, accounting for less than 3% of parotid neoplasms. This lesion must be distinguished from metastatic SCC to the parotid lymph nodes from cutaneous malignancies or from other sites. Primary SCCs of the parotid gland may develop regional lymph node metastases in 50% of patients, a clinical feature that must be considered when patients are treated by surgery and PORT.

Treatment

The accepted staging system for salivary gland tumors can be found in the monographs of the AJCC and UICC.[60] The treatment of benign and malignant salivary gland tumors is surgery. Early-stage (T1 or T2) and especially low-grade tumors should be treated with comprehensive excision with free surgical margins. Such tumors arising in the parotid gland are generally treated by parotidectomy with preservation of the facial nerve. Early-stage high-grade tumors of any histology are treated with surgical resection of the primary site, with an attempt to achieve free surgical margins. This often is not possible, and microscopic spread, especially of adenoid cystic carcinoma, may occur along tissue planes, submucosal spaces, and perineural pathways. The dissection of regional lymph nodes should be done judiciously; elective nodal dissection is seldom indicated except in high-grade malignancies, especially salivary duct carcinoma, MEC, and SCC.[182] Salivary glands malignancies were thought to be resistant to conventional photon radiation, but over the years it has become established that postoperative irradiation is highly effective for eradicating subclinical disease.[179,183,184]

PORT is also indicated for major and minor salivary gland cancers when: (1) the tumor is high grade or is metastatic SCC, regardless of surgical margins; (2) the surgical margins are close or microscopically positive, regardless of grade; (3) a resection has been performed (in a radiation naïve patient) for a recurrent cancer, regardless of the histology or margin status; (4) the tumor has invaded beyond the capsule of the gland into skin, bone, nerve, or glandular tissue; (5) regional lymph nodes contain metastatic cancer; or (6) if there is gross residual or unresectable disease. In addition, preoperative radiotherapy prior to planned surgery may facilitate parotidectomy in advanced cases and allow preservation of the facial nerve.[183,185] If the facial nerve is involved at presentation, surgery, and PORT is favored.

For T3 and T4 parotid cancer, unless the facial nerve is circumferentially encompassed by tumor or grossly enlarged by cancer, nerve-sparing surgery may be used followed by radiotherapy. Radiation therapy doses to the primary site and involved structures are in the range of 55–65 Gy. Generally, for low-grade MEC and acinic cell carcinomas, it is not necessary to treat the clinically uninvolved neck. For all other high-grade histologies, the neck nodal drainage is generally treated to doses in the range of 50 Gy. In the case of adenoid cystic carcinomas, the radiation fields should include the anatomic course of named nerve trunks to the base of the skull.[179] Management of the facial nerve is one of the more controversial and complex issues surrounding the treatment of salivary gland cancers. Resection of the nerve results in profound cosmetic and functional deficits. Even resection of a single branch, particularly the frontal branch, can lead to significant morbidity. Thus, patients must be extensively counseled preoperatively regarding the intraoperative management of the nerve. Compromised function preoperatively portends for poor functional outcome, even with nerve grafting. When the normally functioning facial nerve is found intraoperatively to be involved by cancer and cannot be preserved, resection and primary nerve grafting should be performed. PORT can be administered to nerve grafts, although the long-term functional outcomes remain suboptimal.

The results of treatment depend on histological type and tumor site. In a series from the University of Texas MD Anderson Cancer Center, 5-year survival rates were 100% for patients with acinic cell carcinoma, 95% for patients with adenoid cystic carcinoma, 90% for patients with low-grade MEC, 80% for patients with high-grade MEC, 70% for patients with adenocarcinoma, and 59% for patients with malignant mixed tumors.[180,183] At the Princess Margaret Hospital, primary parotid disease was controlled by surgery alone in 24% of cases and by surgery and radiotherapy in 74% of cases.[186]

Minor salivary gland tumors, especially tumors in the paranasal sinuses, often present with advanced-stage disease. In the MD Anderson series, the 2-year local control rate was 47% in patients treated with surgery alone and 76% in patients treated with surgery and PORT.[183,187,188]

For patients with large inoperable salivary gland tumors or who are at high risk of local recurrence after an incomplete resection, as neutron therapy is only available in very few centers and with mixed results that are dependent on the site of disease, other alternatives for inoperable salivary gland cancers have been studied, albeit in very small retrospective series. Samant and colleagues describe encouraging results in patients with unresectable adenoid cystic carcinoma treated with concurrent chemoradiation.[189] A team from Massachusetts General Hospital[190] have described encouraging outcomes of patients with adenoid cystic carcinoma involving the skull base treated with proton therapy, and similarly, the MD Anderson Cancer Center team has reported early results of proton therapy in the treatment of adenoid cystic carcinoma of the head and neck.[191] Intrigued with the role of high energy particle therapy, German investigators have performed a small phase II trial (COSMIC) combining IMRT with a carbon ion boost. Results are very preliminary, but the response rate in 16 patients with unresected malignant salivary gland tumors was 69%.[192]

Systemic therapy
Systemic therapy for salivary cancer remains an investigational endeavor, with no standard regimen universally accepted. Previous studies have demonstrated single-agent activity for methotrexate, doxorubicin, cisplatin, 5-FU, vinca alkaloids, and taxanes. Response rates are in the range of 15–20%. Combination therapy provides some increase in response but with no clear survival advantages. A regimen with cyclophosphamide, doxorubicin, and cisplatin (CAP) has produced responses in 40–50% of patients treated, with duration 4–6 months.[193] Cisplatin and vinorelbine render responses in 44–54% of patients.[194,195] Responses are more often observed in patients with adenocarcinomas, and less likely in adenoid cystic carcinoma. Antivascular endothelial growth factor (VEGF) inhibitors as sunitinib and axitinib have demonstrated minimum activity with mostly disease stabilization in metastatic adenoid cystic carcinomas.[196,197]

Taxanes are active as single agents and are being tested in combination chemotherapy regimens.[198] A recent report suggested significant clinical activity of lenvatinib in treating advanced metastatic adenoid cystic carcinoma.[199] More recently, NOTCH1 mutations were noted to define a clinical behavior in adenoid cystic carcinomas phenotype characterized by solid histology, liver and bone metastasis, and potential responsiveness to Notch1 inhibitors.[200] Clinical trials are currently underway to define the role of NOTCH inhibitors in treating this subtype of adenoid cystic carcinomas.[201]

A high level of c-KIT expression has been identified in adenoid cystic carcinoma, but preliminary trials with imatinib mesylate, a tyrosine kinase inhibitor (TKI) against KIT, have not demonstrated clinical benefit.[202] Salivary duct carcinomas overexpress HER2 in up to 50% of cases, and approximately 20% are HER2 amplified.[203] Androgen receptor overexpression is seen in 80% of salivary duct carcinomas. Responses to trastuzumab, a monoclonal antibody that targets HER2, and to androgen blockage have been reported.[204–207]

Radiation therapy

Radiotherapy plays an integral role in the treatment of most HNCs. Used as the sole modality for the treatment of selected early-stage disease, radiation gives comparable results to a surgical resection, often with less morbidity. Radiation therapy is the treatment of choice for early staged NPC. It is also a very effective therapy for early-stage oropharynx cancers.

For advanced-sized lesions, radiation is used as a component of multimodality therapy. For patients planned for surgery, radiation is often used as an adjuvant in order to improve locoregional control. The sequencing for radiation, when combined with surgery, has been a topic of debate, as preoperative and postoperative radiation has advantages and disadvantages. The Radiation Therapy Oncology Group (RTOG) conducted a randomized trial comparing preoperative and postoperative radiation, and concluded that postoperative radiation resulted in improved local-regional control with a suggestion of an improvement in survival.[208] The results of this study combined with general practice patterns have led to performing radiation postoperatively. A principle advantage of performing surgery first is that pathology can be assessed. Based on the presence of varying pathologic findings, a trichotomous risk assessment system is used. Patients are assigned into "low", "intermediate" and "high" risk categories that estimate their likelihood of developing local and/or regional recurrence. Low-risk patients have pathology without adverse features and recurrence is uncommon; therefore, the benefits of adjuvant treatment may not be warranted. Intermediate risk patients have pathologic findings including large tumor size, perineural invasion, and lymphovascular invasion of the primary tumor. The degree of depth of invasion in oral cavity cancers is also taken into consideration. High-risk patients are those with inadequate surgical margins or extracapsular nodal disease and have a very high probability of recurrence. Studies have demonstrated concurrent cisplatin chemotherapy added to adjuvant radiation lowers the risk of recurrence,[209] and current research efforts are evaluating multi-drug regimens (including cytotoxins, targeted therapies, and immunotherapy) combined with radiation.

When used as an adjuvant, it is important that there is good communication between the surgeon and the radiation oncologist in order to avoid inadvertent delays that can compromise outcome. Several groups have highlighted the importance of minimizing the treatment "package" time, the time from surgery to the completion of PORT, to maximize local and regional control.[210,211]

For advanced tumors arising in certain sites, such as the pharynx and larynx, nonoperative therapy, consisting of combined radiation and chemotherapy may be preferred. Combination chemotherapy and radiation is the standard treatment for advanced NPC and often chosen to treat locally advanced oropharyngeal cancer. In particular, HPV-associated cancers of the oropharynx have been demonstrated to be very responsive to chemotherapy and radiation, with high survival rates seen in patients treated with concurrent chemoradiation.[34]

HNSCC are generally characterized as being "moderately radiosensitive," meaning that fairly large amounts of radiation must be delivered in order to achieve a high probability of tumor control. Fortunately, the required doses are within the tolerance range of most tissues in the head and neck.

Photon radiation, the most common type of radiation used worldwide, interacts with matter in subtle ways.[212] Tumors and normal tissues vary in their ability to repair the cellular damage caused by ionizing radiation. This differential repair capability led to the concept of fractionated radiation, whereby radiation is delivered in modest doses on a daily basis to ultimately result in tumoricide with normal tissue recovery. Traditional regimens used consist of giving 180–200 cGy once a day for 5 days a week. Curative dose in the definitive setting is generally 7000 cGy, though small tumors may be treated with a lower dose. PORT doses typically range from 6000 to 6600 cGy. Thus, most courses of radiation take 6–7 weeks to deliver.[213]

The above radiation fractionation schemas are generally referred to as "standard" or "conventional" fractionation. While generally considered to be effective, many have studied modifying fractionation to achieve greater gains in tumor control while balancing the challenge of maintaining normal tissue recovery. There are three basic strategies: hyperfractionation, accelerated fractionation, and hypofractionation. Hyperfractionation is a strategy where the total time (i.e., 6–7 weeks) is maintained, but more fractions with smaller fractionation doses (typically 110–120 cGy) are used. Keeping the overall time the same and increasing the fraction number requires multiple daily fractions. Ultimately this leads in theory to a higher tumoricidal dose, without compromising normal tissue recovery.

Accelerated fractionation is a technique used to decrease the overall time. However, compared to hypofractionation, it maintains fractional doses that are similar to or slightly lower than those of standard fractionation. Thus, similar to hyperfractionation, it also depends on delivering multiple fractions per day. Accelerated schedules have ranged from 12 days to 6 weeks; the latter is accelerated in comparison to a standard 7 week schedule. A meta-analysis of 33 randomized trials evaluating altered fractionation (8 trials of hyperfractionation, 25 trials of accelerated fractionation) revealed an approximate 3% benefit in OS with altered fractionation compared to conventional radiation.[214] Ultimately, these small gains with fractionation are less than the gains seen with concurrent chemoradiation, and further altering radiation fractionation with chemotherapy does not appear to result in synergistic gains.[97] Fractionation issues have been relegated to patients who can or should not receive chemotherapy.

Hypofractionation has been less formally studied than the other two types of altered fractionation. Hypofractionation uses larger doses per fraction while also shortening the overall time; it is differentiated from the accelerated strategy where the principal goal is related to time rather than dose. Historically, a larger fractional dose was concerning for increased toxicity, and ultimately the radiation community settled on 2 Gy as the safe standard. However, as radiation techniques improve, limiting the amount of normal tissue exposed to radiation, consideration for larger fractional doses is being reconsidered. One established example is the treatment of early glottic cancer. As the volume of tissue treated is small, fractional doses of 220–240 cGy are accepted. A schedule of 6300 cGy in 28 fractions is widely used for stage 1 glottic cancer and is supported by randomized data.[215] Using extremely conformal radiation techniques, such as stereotactic radiotherapy, studies are ongoing evaluating treatments with significantly greater dose per fraction delivered in only a few treatments.

Patients receiving radiation therapy must be monitored closely to ensure that they maintain adequate nutrition during therapy, and often a feeding tube is required. Placement of such a tube is preferable to giving the patient a break in therapy, which can lower the tumor control probability due to repopulation.[216-218] A reaction can occur in the skin in the treatment portals, giving rise to a severe sunburn-like reaction. Radiation to the head and neck area can cause significant changes in salivary gland function and taste perception.[219-221] The severity and duration of these changes are dose dependent. There is transient loss of saliva and taste after doses of 1000–1500 cGy, however, these lower doses often do not cause permanent late effects. Doses of 7000 cGy almost always cause permanent changes. Studies by the Universities of Michigan and Utrecht[222] have demonstrated the absence of a threshold dose for gland damage, and the TD(50), or dose leading to 50% complication probability in the parotid gland is 40 Gy. Radioprotectors and salivary stimulants have been extensively studied and have limited success in minimizing xerostomia. The more significant advances in xerostomia reduction have been in using conformal techniques to lower the dose to the salivary glands.[223]

Both the decrease in the amount of saliva and the changes in its chemical composition allow changes in the distribution of microorganisms inhabiting the mouth, which in turn can markedly increase the risk of dental caries. Aggressive dental prophylaxis prior to beginning radiotherapy is mandatory in the dentulous patient because the incidence of osteoradionecrosis can be considerably reduced if the necessary repairs and/or extractions are done prior to treatment rather than in heavily irradiated tissues.[224] If extractions are necessary, a delay of 2–3 weeks between the extractions and the initiation of radiotherapy is necessary in order to allow for adequate healing. If extractions or other invasive procedures are required after high-dose XRT, hyperbaric oxygen treatments are helpful in reducing the risk of osteoradionecrosis, particularly if the mandible is involved.[225,226]

Technologic advances

Modern radiotherapy centers use sophisticated linear accelerators producing photon beams of different energies and megavoltage electron beams that can easily treat posterior neck lymph nodes without risk of spinal cord damage. Computer-controlled multileaf collimators facilitate custom blocking techniques to spare uninvolved normal tissues. CT and MRI are used to localize tumors, with many radiation oncology centers having dedicated scanners used exclusively for simulation and treatment planning. CT, MRI, and PET scans are fused to give the clinician a broader perspective in locating regions at risk of tumor.

Intensity-modulated radiotherapy (IMRT)

The principle goal of radiation is to deliver the appropriate dose to areas harboring cancer, while avoiding radiation to adjacent normal tissues. This concept is referred to as conformal therapy. IMRT was developed during the last decade of the twentieth century and is currently an accepted standard for achieving conformal therapy in HNC. In this approach, many different treatment fields are used, with each field being divided into multiple segments, and each segment delivering a prescribed amount of radiation.[227] Recently, these techniques have further evolved in that the treatment can be delivered dynamically, with either treatment accelerators built with computerized tomographic units, or with arc-rotational techniques (volumetric modulated arc therapy (VMAT)). These techniques allow for a continued rotation of the therapy machine as well as a fluid change in the field collimation, ideally achieving even more conformality.

These IMRT systems are further enhanced by software innovations that allow for inverse treatment planning. This form of planning enables the clinician to specify normal tissue dose constraints in combination with specific dose goals to be delivered to the treatment target. In HNCs, there often are critical normal structures in close proximity to the tumor, and achieving a sharp dose gradient around the target while limiting the normal tissue dose offers the potential for significant therapeutic gain. The initial applications of IMRT were principally to reduce the dose to the parotid glands and to reduce the subsequent xerostomia experienced by the patient. IMRT also allows for dose reduction, which is an important advantage of this technique and has been demonstrated in several trials including the randomized phase III PARSPORT trial.[223] Likewise, additional anatomic regions important for functional swallowing, including the larynx, pharyngeal constrictor muscles, and esophagus could be spared with IMRT leading to improvement in functional recovery following treatment.[228]

Nowadays, IMRT is the standard technique for radiation treatment planning and delivery of HNC. Many series published in the last 10–15 years have reported encouraging locoregional disease-control rates for oropharyngeal disease often with favorable toxicity profiles.[229-232] Gillison et al. reported the results of radiotherapy with either cetuximab or cisplatin from the NRG Oncology RTOG 1016 phase III randomized trial.[232] Over 800 patients with HPV-associated OPC were treated, and the vast majority were treated with IMRT. The estimated 5-year survival in the control arm was 84.6%; the incidence of grade 2–3 dry mouth was 32.1% and <5% of patients had a feeding tube at 5 years after treatment. Similar excellent results are seen for NPC, a disease that often approximates critical neural structures adding to the complexity of treatment. The RTOG phase II study 0225 tested the feasibility of transporting IMRT for NPC to a multi-institutional setting. The estimated 2-year PFS was nearly 93%.[233] More recently, large series, particularly from China where NPC is endemic, reported similar high rates of disease control.[234]

Given the complexity of IMRT treatment planning and delivery, rigorous quality assurance and technical support, as well as adequate clinician experience are critical to its ultimate effectiveness.[235]

Particle therapy

Atomic particles, including electrons, neutrons, and protons, and atomic ions can be used for radiation therapy, and all have found a role in treating patients with HNC, Electrons, with their negligible mass are generally not grouped with the heavier atomic particles but have been used for decades. They have a limited range of radiation deposition dependent on their energy. While not suited for deeply seated tumors, in HNC they have a variety of roles. They are very useful for treating parotid malignancies and nasal cancers, particularly those of the anterior nasal cavity. They are also very effective for treating skin cancers of the face, particularly cancers near the nose and eyes where cosmesis can be a concern. They had been used frequently for supplementing dose to cervical nodal beds lateral to the spinal cord. However, with technological advances, and the use of IMRT as a standard, the role of electrons has diminished.

Neutron therapy was studied decades ago for multiple tumor sites. It was believed that neutrons interacted with tissues in a different manner than photons, causing more direct DNA damage and thereby having a greater radiobiologic effectiveness (RBE). Studies did not demonstrate an advantage for neutrons for most tumors, but there did appear to be an advantage for neutrons in the management of inoperable salivary gland tumors.[236]

Proton therapy has also been available for decades, but it has only been recently that the technology has advanced to allow for protons to be more than just a niche treatment. The principal goal of radiation treatment planning is to conform the shape of the radiation dose to maximize dose in the tumor while avoiding dose delivery to normal tissues. Photons continually deposit dose through tissues, and to compensate for this, IMRT essentially uses arcs to spread the dose out. Normal tissues receive lower doses to minimize side effects, but a greater amount of normal tissue receives some dose. The dose distribution of protons forms a Bragg peak, where maximal dose is deposited at a defined finite range, followed by a dramatic dose fall-off.

The recent technological advances have been to develop machines that can actively deliver protons in "pencil-beams" and akin to IMRT, these beams can also be modulated to deliver intensity-modulated proton therapy (IMPT). The theoretical ability to deliver a more conformal radiation is particularly exciting in the treatment of HNC, and numerous small studies have suggested a benefit for IMPT in the treatment of OPC, NPC, paranasal sinus cancers, salivary gland cancers, and in the re-irradiation setting.[237] Larger trials including randomized phase 3 trials are ongoing to further define the role of IMPT in HNC management.

Heavy-ion therapy is also gaining interest in the radiation community, with Carbon–ion therapy the most common form. The first heavy ion accelerator for clinical use opened in 1994 in Japan, and currently, there are over 10 centers worldwide. The theoretical benefit of Carbon–ion therapy is that it has the benefits of both protons and neutrons. The benefit of protons is the physical properties of rapid dose fall off after deposition in the target, and the benefit of neutrons is the higher linear energy transfer (LET) that results in a greater degree of direct DNA damage and less cellular capability for repair. Carbon–ion therapy has been evaluated in numerous organ sites, including HNC. Studies, however, remain small, and it will likely be years before the true benefit of this therapy will both be understood and available.

Combined surgery and radiotherapy

Radiotherapy is often given as an adjuvant to surgery for moderately advanced but resectable tumors. For most head and neck sites, giving adjuvant radiotherapy improves local control for T3 or T4 primaries or in situations where there is pathologic involvement of cervical lymph nodes.

In the postoperative setting, the surgical procedure has disrupted the regional blood supply. Generally, 5500–6000 cGy in 180–200 cGy fractions are given for microscopic residual disease. If the surgical margins are grossly positive or if there is a high likelihood of macroscopic residual disease, higher doses are used (6300–6600 cGy). Peters and colleagues[238] have shown that at least 6300 cGy should be given if extracapsular nodal extension is found in the operative specimen.

Although it is generally felt that there is little use for a debulking surgical procedure, there may be situations where a gross total resection followed by high-dose radiotherapy is preferable to treatment with radiotherapy alone. An analysis by the Head and Neck Intergroup (IG0034) showed that excluded patients with positive surgical margins had improved locoregional tumor control compared with matched cohorts from the RTOG databases of patients treated with radiotherapy alone.[239] At 4 years, respective locoregional control rates were 44% versus 24% ($p = 0.007$). Since this was not a randomized study, the authors do not argue for changing traditional resectability criteria, but, rather, testing this concept in the context of a controlled clinical trial.

Locoregional disease relapse following surgery is particularly common in patients with positive surgical margins, extracapsular nodal disease, or multiple positive nodes. Based on retrospective analyses,[240,241] adjuvant radiation reduces the relative risk of relapse by approximately 50%, however, locoregional recurrence rates remain as high as 35–60% in this population.[242] Two landmark multi-institutional phase III trials demonstrated improved outcomes with concurrent chemoradiation in patients with high risk of recurrence following surgery. In the first trial,[243] the European Organization for Research and Treatment of Cancer (EORTC) randomized 334 subjects to 6600 cGy with or without cisplatin 100 mg/m^2 × 3 cycles. Estimated 3-year local control (85% vs 70%), DFS (60% vs 40%), and OS (65% vs 50%) were improved by the addition of cisplatin. Acute toxicity was exacerbated by chemotherapy, but severity of late effects purportedly remained equivalent. The RTOG conducted a complementary trial,[74] randomizing 459 patients to nearly identical treatment arms as the EORTC trial: 6000–6600 cGy with or without cisplatin 100 mg/m^2 × 3 cycles. Chemotherapy improved estimated 2-year local control (82% vs 72%, $p = 0.01$) and DFS (70% vs 60%, $p = 0.05$). As with the EORTC trial, this was at the cost of higher acute grade 3 or greater toxicity. The trials had different inclusion criteria, study populations, and follow-up intervals. However, joint reanalysis of both trials strongly suggested significant clinical benefit to combined adjuvant therapy for patients with either positive surgical margins or extra-capsular nodal disease.[243]

Systemic therapy

Chemotherapy and radiation for locally advanced disease

Induction chemotherapy
Treatment with chemotherapy used in sequence before surgery or radiotherapy—known as induction or neoadjuvant chemotherapy—has potential advantages. It is feasible. Drug activity may be optimal because there has been no disruption of normal vascularity. Effective systemic therapy in this setting is likely to induce a favorable tumor response and there is a reduction in the risk of distant disease recurrence.[138,141,244,245] The potential for induction chemotherapy to affect local disease control following surgery or radiotherapy continues under study. Early trials demonstrated that PF is a highly active regimen;[246] a substantial response to chemotherapy predicts for tumor sensitivity to radiotherapy; and that there appeared to not be a major adverse effect on surgical or radiotherapy morbidity.[245]

To build on the more modern IC platform of incorporating a taxane, GORTEC conducted the TREMPLIN phase 2 randomized trial comparing concurrent cisplatin versus concurrent cetuximab following a partial response to induction TPF.[247] OS was equivalent in both arms, and the authors concluded they could not determine the optimal regimen to test against a control of IC followed by radiation alone.

While the addition of docetaxel to the PF backbone chemotherapy regimen improved outcomes in TAX323 and 324, it remained undetermined if the three-drug IC regimen was superior to concurrent chemoradiation. At least four clinical trials attempted to answer this question. The PARADIGM study randomized 145 unresectable stage III or IV HNSCC patients to receive TPF followed by concurrent chemoradiation with carboplatin (for patients who responded to IC) or docetaxel (for nonresponders to IC), versus concurrent radiation therapy with cisplatin (100 mg/m^2 every 3 weeks × 2 doses). The 3-year OS was not statistically different between the two groups (73% in the IC arm vs 78% in the concurrent chemoradiation arm). Higher hematological toxicity and one treatment-related death were seen in the IC arm. Given slow accrual, the study did not meet its patient target number limiting its power and interpretation.[248] The DeCIDE trial included 285 patients with N2 or N3 nodal status (therefore, with a higher risk of distant recurrence). Patients were randomized to receive two cycles of TPF followed by concurrent chemoradiation with DFHX (docetaxel, 5-fluorouracil, and hydroxyurea) versus the same concurrent definitive chemoradiation regimen. Once again, due to slow accrual, sample size was adjusted and the study was closed early. The 3-year OS rates were similar between the two groups with 75% in the IC arm and 73% in the concurrent chemoradiation arm. Significantly lower distant metastasis was seen in the group that received IC (10% vs 19%, $p = 0.025$) and there was a trend to survival benefit for the patients with N2c and N3 disease who received IC ($p = 0.19$).[249] Both PARADIGM and DeCIDE were underpowered studies. Patients' outcomes were better than historical control, most likely because the majority of the population had oropharynx carcinoma primaries, possibly HPV related. Hitt et al. evaluated in a randomized phase III trial IC with either PF or TPF followed by concurrent chemoradiation with high dose cisplatin versus the same concurrent chemoradiation schema. There was no difference in median PFS, time to treatment failure, or OS between the two arms.[250] Preliminary results of a phase II/III European trial presented at the 2014 American Society of Clinical Oncology (ASCO) meeting, evaluated induction TPF versus no induction chemotherapy followed by chemoradiation with either cetuximab or PF in 415 patients. The median survival was of 53.7 months in the induction arm versus 30.3 months in the upfront chemoradiation arm (HR 0.72, $p = 0.025$) with a reduced risk of distant metastases in patients who received induction chemotherapy. The difference in outcomes observed in this trial versus DeCIDE and PARADIGM is likely due to different patient populations and inclusion criteria.[251]

Based on the results of these trials, together with the meta-analysis of chemotherapy in head and neck cancer (MACH-NC) meta-analysis,[93] concurrent chemoradiation with cisplatin remains as standard of care treatment for locally advanced HNSCC.

Concurrent chemotherapy and radiation

A sequence of randomized trials[94,141,252–259] and meta-analysis[260] demonstrate that the concurrent administration of chemotherapy and radiation leads to improved local control and OS in patients with locally advanced SCC, particularly of the oropharynx. However, most reported trials include patients with invasive SCC from a mix of primary sites. Scrutiny of these manuscripts is advised as the percentage of patients with oral cavity, pharyngeal, and laryngeal primary sites may vary in reports from different centers, and this may markedly affect study outcomes. It should be emphasized that concurrent chemoradiotherapy is associated with marked, acute mucocutaneous toxicity requiring expert supportive medical care. Speech and swallow rehabilitation consultation is routinely needed. Gastrostomy feeding tubes are placed in a high percentage of patients. The risk of long-term complications such as osteonecrosis and oropharyngeal fibrosis is under study.

Oral cavity primary tumors are most often approached surgically if there are no medical contraindications. Depending upon tumor histology, size, pathologic margins, and the extent of nodal involvement, PORT is administered. Patients with positive surgical margins or nodal ECS are more likely to benefit from adjuvant concurrent chemoradiation rather than radiotherapy administered as a single modality, as previously discussed.[74,209,243]

With regard to toxicity, usually, a brisk mucocutaneous reaction occurs with chemoradiation, necessitating the use of oral rinses for hygiene, analgesics, attention to fluid and calorie intake, and involvement of speech and swallowing rehabilitation specialists. Moreover, there is concern that long-term xerostomia, fibrosis, and related swallowing dysfunction may be more likely after concurrent chemoradiotherapy than radiation therapy alone. Long-term functional data for most patients have not been routinely reported. In the Intergroup larynx trial[141] and the postoperative chemoradiotherapy trials,[74,209,243] there appeared not to be a high risk of chronic deleterious effects of combined therapy relative to control groups treated with radiotherapy alone. Setton and colleagues[96] reported on nearly 1500 oropharyngeal cancer patients treated with concurrent chemotherapy and radiation. The 2-year gastrostomy tube dependence rate was 4.4%.

In a landmark study, Bonner and colleagues[261] conducted a prospectively randomized trial in which previously untreated patients with locally advanced SCC of the oropharynx, hypopharynx, or larynx received definitive radiotherapy with or without cetuximab. Cetuximab is a chimeric human and murine monoclonal antibody directed against the EGFR. In this phase III trial, 424 patients were entered and median duration of follow-up was 38 months. Notably, there was no increase in severe-grade radiation-related mucocutaneous toxicity. Moreover, median survival (28 months vs 54 months) and 3-year survival (44% vs 57%) favored the combined therapy arm with a significant advantage in locoregional tumor control. This study led to the approval of cetuximab to be administered concurrently with radiation therapy for locally advanced HNSCC.

A follow-up phase III study, RTOG 0522, evaluated the addition of cetuximab to the standard concurrent cisplatin and radiotherapy treatment in 891 patients with stage III or IV HNSCC. Patients were randomized to receive radiation and cisplatin with or without cetuximab. The addition of cetuximab to cisplatin-radiation led to significantly more interruptions in treatment, an increased rate of acute grade 3 and 4 toxicity, and was not associated with improved patient outcomes.[262] Concert 1 and 2 trials have further explored bioradiotherapy with panitumumab (Table 6)[263,264] showing no OS or local disease control advantage after matching chemoradiotherapy with the addition or substitution of the antibody.

Thus, the current standard of care for patients with stage III and IV HNSCC, who are not candidates for surgery, is to be treated with definitive concurrent chemoradiotherapy. Cisplatin 100 mg/m² administered on weeks 1, 4, and 7 with once-daily radiotherapy, or cisplatin 40 mg/m² weekly, are widely accepted (Table 7).

Table 6 EGFR-based bioradiotherapy with panitumumab (P).[a]

	N	2-yr LRC (%)
Concert 1		
CT–RT	63	68
CT–RT + P	87	61
Concert 2		
CT–RT	61	61
P–RT	90	51

[a]Source: Mesia et al.[263]; Giralt et al.[264]

Table 7 Single-agent activity in recurrent head and neck cancer.

Agent	Approximate response (%)
Methotrexate	25
Bleomycin	15
Cisplatin	25
Carboplatin	20
5-Fluorouracil	15
Paclitaxel	30
Docetaxel	30
Ifosfamide	20
Cetuximab	13

Recurrent and metastatic disease

Cytotoxics

Combination chemotherapy may produce responses in 30–40% of patients but without significant survival advantages over single-agent therapy, which is usually in the range of 6–9 months (Table 8). Gibson and colleagues[270] conducted a prospective phase III trial comparing cisplatin and infusional fluorouracil with cisplatin and paclitaxel in 218 patients. There was no difference in response rate (27% and 26%, respectively) or median survival (8.7 months vs 8.1 months). Toxicity was similar.

In a randomized phase III prospective trial, Vermorken and colleagues[274] evaluated the addition of cetuximab to the platin-fluorouracil combination in 442 patients with recurrent or metastatic HNSCC. A response advantage and improved median survival from 7.4 to 10.1 months were observed. There was no unusual toxicity. This regimen has become the standard of care first-line therapy for suitable patients.

OS for patients with recurrent or metastatic HNSCC remains poor. Only approximately 30% of patients survive 1 year, highlighting the pressing need for new drug development and more efficacious systemic therapy strategies.

Novel therapeutics

Invasive SCCs emerge after the accumulation of multiple genomic events in a multistep process. A detailed and comprehensive

Table 8 Selected randomized phase 3 trials of chemotherapy in recurrent or metastatic squamous cell carcinoma of the head and neck.

Trial	No. of patients	Regimen	Response rate (%)	Survival (p value)
Jacobs et al.[265]	79	cddp/fu	32	NS
	83	cddp	17	
	83	fu	13	
Forastiere et al.[266]	87	cddp/fu	32	NS
	86	cbdca/fu	21	
	88	mtx	10	
Clavel et al.[267]	127	cddp/mtx/bleo/vcr	34	NS
	116	cddp/fu	31	
	122	cddp	15	
Schrijvers et al.[268]	122	cddp/fu/ifnα-2b	47	NS
	122	cddp/fu	38	
Forastiere et al.[269]	101	cddp/pac (high dose)	35	NS
	98	cddp/pac (low dose)	36	
Gibson et al.[270]	104	cddp/fu	22	NS
	100	cddp/pac	28	
Vermorken et al.[271]	215	platin/fu	20	7.4 mos median
	219	platin/fu—cet	36	10.1 mos med 7.5 mo
Ferris et al.[272]	361	Nivo-	13	
		Chemo	5.8	5.5 mo ($p = 0.01$)
Burtness et al.[273]	882	Pembro	20	14 (PDL1+) ($p < 0.01$)
		Pembro platin/5FU	35	13 ($p < 0.01$)
		Platin/fu-Cet	35	11

Abbreviations: bleo, bleomycin; cbdca, carboplatin; cddp, cisplatin; fu, fluorouracil; ifnα-2b, interferon alfa-2b; mtx, methotrexate; NS, not statistically significant; pac, paclitaxel; vcr, vincristine.

genomic characterization of HNC has been recently reported through The Cancer Genome Atlas (TCGA) network effort. Even though no clear alteration in the standard of care has resulted from this effort as of yet, it opened the door for research efforts focused on the most frequent of the observed alterations.[275] Preceding this effort, there appeared to be essential molecular alterations that are biologically significant, which confer a survival advantage for cancer cells and which constitute the process of carcinogenesis.[276] As we understand better the underlying cancer biology, potential therapeutic targets have been identified and are leading to innovative treatment strategies.

Epidermal growth factor receptor

EGFR is a transmembrane glycoprotein, activation of which triggers a cascade of downstream intracellular signaling events important for regulation of epithelial cell growth.[277–281] EGF and transforming growth factor-alpha (TGF-α) are ligands for the receptor. Overexpression of EGFR or TGF-α has been observed in approximately 90% of HNSCC.[280]

Gefitinib and erlotinib are small molecule inhibitors of EGFR. Both agents have been tested as single agents in recurrent or metastatic HNSCC showing minimum clinical activity.[282,283] Afatinib and dacomitinib, second-generation EGFR inhibitors, are under investigation in platinum-refractory metastatic HNSCC. Results demonstrated some activity with responses rates around 10%.[284]

Cetuximab is a monoclonal antibody directed against the extracellular portion of EGFR. Binding of the monoclonal antibody competes with ligand activation and prevents receptor dimerization, with consequent abrogation of multiple downstream signals. Vermorken and colleagues[285] have reported responses in 13% of platin-refractory patients treated with cetuximab single agent. As previously mentioned, Vermorken et al.[274] demonstrated in a phase III trial that the addition of cetuximab to cisplatin or carboplatin and fluorouracil favorably affects tumor response and improved overall median survival by 2.7 months (from 7.4 to 10.1 months in the cetuximab group). Bonner and colleagues[261] have also reported, as discussed earlier, an increase in local tumor control and OS in the radiotherapy plus cetuximab combination arm versus radiotherapy alone.

An association between skin rash and tumor response has been repeatedly observed[244,286] and needs further exploration, possibly by escalating cetuximab dose until rash or dose-limiting toxicities develop. To date, cetuximab is the only Food and Drug Administration (FDA)-approved targeted therapy for the treatment of HNSCC.

Angiogenesis

New blood vessel formation is a necessary process for tumor growth. VEGF is a multifunctional cytokine and a potent stimulator of the growth of endothelial cells. Increased VEGF protein expression is seen in many cancers, including HNSCC.[287,288]

Bevacizumab prevents VEGF binding to receptor tyrosine kinases (VEGFR1 and VEGFR2) with resultant inhibition of tumor cell growth. Argiris et al.[289] evaluated in a single-arm phase II trial the activity of cetuximab and bevacizumab in 46 patients with recurrent or metastatic HNSCC that received up to one line of systemic therapy. The overall response rate was 16% and median PFS and OS were 2.8 and 7.5 months, respectively. A large phase III trial (E1305) with platin and docetaxel or platin and 5-fluorouracil plus or minus bevacizumab for patients with recurrent or metastatic HNSCC has been conducted and even though it fell short of showing an improvement in OS with the addition of bevacizumab, it did reveal a significant improvement in PFS favoring the bevacizumab group.[290] These results are considered a step in the right direction as far as the role of VEGF inhibitors in the management of recurrent and metastatic HNSCC, especially in the era of immunotherapy (clinical trial reference number NCT00588770). Newer generation small molecule VEGFR inhibitors axitinib and pazopanib are currently being investigated clinically. Sorafenib and sunitinib are small-molecule pan-receptor TKIs, with multiple targets including VEGFR. They have been tested in metastatic HNSCC with modest activity.[291,292]

Phosphatidylinositol-3 kinase (PI3K)
Advances in next-generation sequencing have revealed recurrent genetic alterations in HNSCC. The most frequent potentially targetable alterations consist of activation of the PI3K pathway, either by PIK3CA mutations or amplification (~35%) or PTEN loss (~5%).[293,294] The PI3K/AKT/mTOR pathway is important in regulating the cell cycle and its deregulation is involved in cancer cell proliferation. Various clinical trials with PI3K inhibitors as single agent or combined with other targeted therapy (e.g., EGFR inhibitors or MEK inhibitors) are being conducted in HNSCC.

Gene therapy
Approaches utilizing adenovirus-mediated wild-type *TP53* gene transfer have generated excitement following the demonstration of tumor responses in some patients.[295] Khuri and colleagues[296] conducted a multicenter phase II trial combining ONYX-015, which is a selective replicating adenovirus, with cisplatin and 5-FU in treating patients with advanced HNSCC. A response rate of 52% was observed in 30 patients with fully evaluable tumors. In a subset analysis of patients with tumors injectable and not accessible for injection, there was a substantial difference with tumor responses observed more often after chemotherapy and ONYX-015 administration ($p = 0.006$).

Immunotherapy
Recently, a new class of drugs that enhances antitumor immunity has emerged and is transforming the medical oncology field. One of the most promising pathways for manipulation involves programmed death-ligand 1 (PD-L1). PD-L1 can be overexpressed in solid tumors, and upon binding to PD-1 expressing tumor-infiltrating T cells, it inhibits its activity and promotes immune tolerance, protecting the tumor cells from apoptosis. Blockage of PD1–PD-L1 interaction enhances immune function and has shown meaningful clinical activity.[297–299] Further dissection of the tumor microenvironment in HNC continues to elucidate the complexity of the interaction between different immune-effector components including innate immunity.[300] Pembrolizumab and nivolumab, humanized monoclonal antibodies that target PD-1, were approved initially for the treatment of metastatic refractory melanoma. More recently, nivolumab and pembrolizumab were approved for the treatment of recurrent or metastatic HNSCC.

The first trial exploring ICI in HNSCC was the KEYNOTE-012 phase I trial which showed that 78% of the 104 patients with refractory metastatic/recurrent HNSCC screened expressed PD-L1 in at least 1% of the cells in the tumor microenvironment. Out of the 51 patients evaluable for response, 51% experienced decreased tumor burden, with an overall response rate by RECIST of 20%, irrespective of HPV status.[301] Eight patients had disease stability over 6 months, and seven remained on treatment when the preliminary data of the study was presented. Treatment was overall well tolerated with main side effects being fatigue, pruritus, and rash. The ORR was 18% and 71% of responders maintained a response for greater than 1 year. The PFS was 2.1 months and the 1-year OS rate was 38%. The first phase III randomized trial establishing a superior outcome to ICI compared to cytotoxic chemotherapy or cetuximab was the checkmate 141 trial.[272] In this randomized, open-label, phase 3 trial, 361 patients with recurrent HNSCC who had disease progression within 6 months after platinum-based chemotherapy were randomized in a 2 : 1 design to receive nivolumab (at a dose of 3 mg per kilogram of body weight) every 2 weeks or single-agent systemic methotrexate, docetaxel, or cetuximab. The OS was significantly longer with nivolumab (hazard ratio for death, 0.70; 97.73% CI, 0.51–0.96; $P = 0.01$), and the 1-year survival rate was approximately 19% greater with nivolumab than with standard therapy (36.0% vs 16.6%). These trials led to the approval in 2016 of pembrolizumab and nivolumab in patients with advanced HNSCC who fail platinum-based therapy.

Multiple subsequent reports analyzing data from checkmate 141 revealed a maintained superiority of nivolumab in terms of patient-reported outcomes, a possible continued role of ICI in the treatment of some patients with initial radiographic disease progression, as well as maintained activity regardless of patient's age or HPV tumor status.[302–304] Furthermore the Keynote 055 and 040 studies established pembrolizumab as a standard of care in the same patient population. In Keynote 055, platinum- and cetuximab-pretreated patients received single-agent pembrolizumab. The overall response rate was 16% (95% CI, 11–23%), with a median duration of response of 8 months.[305] Keynote 055 built on the results of Keynote 012 and confirmed the response rate of 18% with single-agent pembrolizumab in patients whose disease had failed platinum-based therapy as well as cetuximab. Keynote 040 compared single-agent pembrolizumab to investigator choice systemic therapy in patients who had failed platinum in a phase III randomized design and showed a superior outcome with single-agent pembrolizumab over chemotherapy or cetuximab in patients who had failed platinum-based therapy, confirming the results of checkmate 141. More recently, Keynote 048 established the role of PD-1 inhibitors in the first-line management of recurrent or metastatic HNSCC. This study enrolled patients who are candidates for first-line therapy and established a superior survival to single-agent pembrolizumab over the Extreme regimen in biomarker positive disease (PD-L1 by CPS score > or = 1); for biomarker unselected patients chemo-immunotherapy resulted in improved OS compared to the Extreme regimen. This trial has set the new standard of care for recurrent or metastatic disease that is untreated with immunotherapy.[273]

Given these encouraging early results, numerous immunotherapy clinical trials with checkpoint inhibitors, co-stimulatory agonists, vaccines, and adoptive T cell transfer are being conducted in HNSCC and hold great promise for the near future (Figure 11). In addition, immunotherapy applications are now moving to the

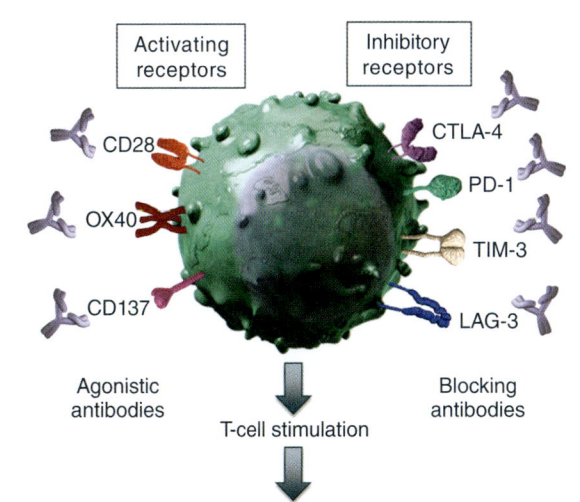

Figure 11 Activating and inhibitory receptor in T-cells. Source: Mellman et al.[306] and Pardoll.[307]

definitive management setting and are being combined with radiation therapy or radiation and chemotherapy. Furthermore, a possible role of immunotherapy was noted in preoperative window of opportunity trials revealing a significant response to single-agent PD-1 inhibitors in this setting. These findings have opened the door to larger more definitive studies looking testing these approaches against the current standard of care.

Current directions

Systemic therapy is an integral part of HNC treatment. Many patients with locally advanced disease are treated with chemotherapy and radiation. The increasing appreciation of HPV as an etiologic and favorable prognostic factor can be expected to affect patient management and de-escalation clinical studies are currently ongoing. Options for the treatment of recurrent disease now include re-irradiation, cytotoxic chemotherapy, and molecularly targeted therapy. In the era of immunotherapy, a re-examination of these different modalities is required and is being pursued namely in the salvage setting, combining ICI with re-irradiation and revisiting the role of various targeted agents with otherwise modest clinical activities in combination with ICI. Of note here are several trials looking at the combination of ICI with TKIs (NCT 02501096) (NCT 03468218). Insights into the genomics of HNC are leading to multiple targeted therapy trials in specific subgroups. It is clear that ICI have revolutionized the treatment of recurrent and metastatic HNSCC and are poised to change the standard of care in the definitive therapy setting. Along those lines, several clinical trials are investigating the role of these agents in the definitive therapy setting. Of note here is the phase III Javelin trial, which tested the addition of avelumab (a PD-L1 inhibitor) to the backbone of platinum and radiation in the definitive concurrent therapy setting. The results of the Javelin trial, unfortunately, revealed no evidence of improved PFS in the avelumab arm, as reported at the ESMO 2020 meeting. RTOG 3504 tested the feasibility of adding nivolumab to the backbone of radiation and chemotherapy and suggested this to be a fairly well-tolerated approach. Furthermore, the question of the role of maintenance therapy with ICI following completion of definitive therapy is being examined in the atezolizumab phase III Invoke 10 trial (NCT 03452137). Given that the outcome in these studies is driven mostly by HPV unrelated disease, an approach to test maintenance with ICI in HPV related disease is being investigated in the EA3161 study randomizing patients who have intermediate-risk HPV-related OPSCC to maintenance nivolumab following definitive radiation and platinum therapy versus observation following definitive therapy (NCT 03811015).

Key references

The complete reference list can be found on Vital Source version of this title, see inside front cover.

16 D'Souza G, Kreimer AR, Viscidi R, et al. Case-control study of human papillomavirus and oropharyngeal cancer. *N Engl J Med*. 2007;**356**(19):1944–1956.

17 Gillison ML, Koch WM, Capone RB, et al. Evidence for a causal association between human papillomavirus and a subset of head and neck cancers. *J Natl Cancer Inst*. 2000;**92**(9):709–720.

27 Lin JC, Chen KY, Wang WY, et al. Detection of Epstein-Barr virus DNA the peripheral-blood cells of patients with nasopharyngeal carcinoma: relationship to distant metastasis and survival. *J Clin Oncol*. 2001;**19**(10):2607–2615.

28 Lin JC, Wang WY, Chen KY, et al. Quantification of plasma Epstein-Barr virus DNA in patients with advanced nasopharyngeal carcinoma. *N Engl J Med*. 2004;**350**(24):2461–2470.

29 Lo YM, Chan AT, Chan LY, et al. Molecular prognostication of nasopharyngeal carcinoma by quantitative analysis of circulating Epstein-Barr virus DNA. *Cancer Res*. 2000;**60**(24):6878–6881.

34 Ang KK, Harris J, Wheeler R, et al. Human papillomavirus and survival of patients with oropharyngeal cancer. *N Engl J Med*. 2010;**363**(1):24–35.

55 Liauw SL, Mancuso AA, Amdur RJ, et al. Postradiotherapy neck dissection for lymph node-positive head and neck cancer: the use of computed tomography to manage the neck. *J Clin Oncol*. 2006;**24**(9):1421–1427.

65 Saba NF, Hurwitz SJ, Kono SA, et al. Chemoprevention of head and neck cancer with celecoxib and erlotinib: results of a phase ib and pharmacokinetic study. *Cancer Prev Res (Phila)*. 2014;**7**(3):283–291.

66 Shin DM, Zhang H, Saba NF, et al. Chemoprevention of head and neck cancer by simultaneous blocking of epidermal growth factor receptor and cyclooxygenase-2 signaling pathways: preclinical and clinical studies. *Clin Cancer Res*. 2013;**9**(5):1244–1256.

67 Shin DM, Nannapaneni S, Patel MR, et al. Phase Ib study of chemoprevention with green tea polyphenon E and erlotinib in patients with advanced premalignant lesions (APL) of the head and neck. *Clin Cancer Res*. 2020;**26**(22):5860–5868.

74 Cooper JS, Pajak TF, Forastiere AA, et al. Postoperative concurrent radiotherapy and chemotherapy for high-risk squamous-cell carcinoma of the head and neck. *N Engl J Med*. 2004;**350**(19):1937–1944.

93 Pignon JP, le Maitre A, Maillard E, et al. Meta-analysis of chemotherapy in head and neck cancer (MACH-NC): an update on 93 randomised trials and 17,346 patients. *Radiother Oncol*. 2009;**92**(1):4–14.

94 Calais G, Alfonsi M, Bardet E, et al. Randomized trial of radiation therapy versus concomitant chemotherapy and radiation therapy for advanced-stage oropharynx carcinoma. *J Natl Cancer Inst*. 1999;**91**(24):2081–2086.

97 Nguyen-Tan PF, Zhang Q, Ang KK, et al. Randomized phase III trial to test accelerated versus standard fractionation in combination with concurrent cisplatin for head and neck carcinomas in the Radiation Therapy Oncology Group 0129 trial: long-term report of efficacy and toxicity. *J Clin Oncol*. 2014;**32**(34):3858–3866.

101 O'Malley BW Jr, Weinstein GS, Snyder W, Hockstein NG. Transoral robotic surgery (TORS) for base of tongue neoplasms. *Laryngoscope*. 2006;**116**(8):1465–1472.

138 Department of Veterans Affairs Laryngeal Cancer Study Group, Wolf GT, Fisher SG, et al. Induction chemotherapy plus radiation compared with surgery plus radiation in patients with advanced laryngeal cancer. The Department of Veterans Affairs Laryngeal Cancer Study Group. *N Engl J Med*. 1991;**324**(24):1685–1690.

139 Hong WK, Lippman SM, Wolf GT. Recent advances in head and neck cancer–larynx preservation and cancer chemoprevention: the Seventeenth Annual Richard and Hinda Rosenthal Foundation Award Lecture. *Cancer Res*. 1993;**53**(21):5113–5120.

142 Hillman RE, Walsh MJ, Wolf GT, et al. Functional outcomes following treatment for advanced laryngeal cancer. Part I–Voice preservation in advanced laryngeal cancer. Part II--Laryngectomy rehabilitation: the state of the art in the VA System. Research Speech-Language Pathologists. Department of Veterans Affairs Laryngeal Cancer Study Group. *Ann Otol Rhinol Laryngol Suppl*. 1998;**172**:1–27.

192 Jensen AD, Nikoghosyan AV, Lossner K, et al. IMRT and carbon ion boost for malignant salivary gland tumors: interim analysis of the COSMIC trial. *BMC Cancer*. 2012;**12**:163.

194 Airoldi M, Garzaro M, Pedani F, et al. Cisplatin+Vinorelbine treatment of recurrent or metastatic salivary gland malignancies (RMSGM): a final report on 60 cases. *Am J Clin Oncol*. 2014;**40**(10):86–90.

199 Tchekmedyian V, Sherman EJ, Dunn L, et al. Phase II study of lenvatinib in patients with progressive, recurrent or metastatic adenoid cystic carcinoma. *J Clin Oncol*. 2019;**37**(18):1529–1537.

200 Ferrarotto R, Mitani Y, Diao L, et al. Activating NOTCH1 mutations define a distinct subgroup of patients with adenoid cystic carcinoma who have poor prognosis, propensity to bone and liver metastasis, and potential responsiveness to notch1 inhibitors. *J Clin Oncol*. 2017;**35**(3):352–360.

201 Ferrarotto R, Eckhardt G, Patnaik A, et al. A phase I dose-escalation and dose-expansion study of brontictuzumab in subjects with selected solid tumors. *Ann Oncol*. 2018;**29**(7):1561–1568.

202 Hotte SJ, Winquist EW, Lamont E, et al. Imatinib mesylate in patients with adenoid cystic cancers of the salivary glands expressing c-kit: a Princess Margaret Hospital phase II consortium study. *J Clin Oncol*. 2005;**23**(3):585–590.

209 Bernier J, Cooper JS, Pajak TF, et al. Defining risk levels in locally advanced head and neck cancers: a comparative analysis of concurrent postoperative radiation plus chemotherapy trials of the EORTC (#22931) and RTOG (# 9501). *Head Neck*. 2005;**27**(10):843–850.

210 Ang KK, Trotti A, Brown BW, et al. Randomized trial addressing risk features and time factors of surgery plus radiotherapy in advanced head-and-neck cancer. *Int J Radiat Oncol Biol Phys*. 2001;**51**(3):571–578.

243 Bernier J, Domenge C, Ozsahin M, et al. Postoperative irradiation with or without concomitant chemotherapy for locally advanced head and neck cancer. *N Engl J Med*. 2004;**350**(19):1945–1952.

272 Ferris RL, Blumenschein G Jr, Fayette J, et al. Nivolumab for recurrent squamous-cell carcinoma of the head and neck. *N Engl J Med*. 2016;**375**(19):1856–1867.

273 Burtness B, Harrington KJ, Greil R, et al. Pembrolizumab alone or with chemotherapy versus cetuximab with chemotherapy for recurrent or metastatic squamous cell carcinoma of the head and neck (KEYNOTE-048): a randomised, open-label, phase 3 study. *Lancet*. 2019;**394**(10212):1915–1928.

274 Vermorken JB, Mesia R, Rivera F, et al. Platinum-based chemotherapy plus cetuximab in head and neck cancer. *N Engl J Med*. 2008;**359**(11):1116–1127.

275 Cancer Genome Atlas Network. Comprehensive genomic characterization of head and neck squamous cell carcinomas. *Nature*. 2015;**517**(7536):576–582.

276 Haddad RI, Shin DM. Recent advances in head and neck cancer. *N Engl J Med*. 2008;**359**(11):1143–1154.

296 Khuri FR, Nemunaitis J, Ganly I, et al. A controlled trial of intratumoral ONYX-015, a selectively-replicating adenovirus, in combination with cisplatin and 5-fluorouracil in patients with recurrent head and neck cancer. *Nat Med*. 2000;**6**(8):879–885.

297 Brahmer JR, Tykodi SS, Chow LQ, et al. Safety and activity of anti-PD-L1 antibody in patients with advanced cancer. *N Engl J Med*. 2012;**366**(26):2455–2465.

300 Wieland A, Patel MR, Cardenas MA, et al. Defining HPV-specific B cell responses in patients with head and neck cancer. *Nature*. 2021;**597**:274–278. doi: 10.1038/s41586-020-2931-3.

302 Harrington KJ, Ferris RL, Blumenschein G Jr, et al. Nivolumab versus standard, single-agent therapy of investigator's choice in recurrent or metastatic squamous cell carcinoma of the head and neck (CheckMate 141): health-related quality-of-life results from a randomised, phase 3 trial. *Lancet Oncol*. 2017;**18**(8):1104–1115.

303 Haddad R, Concha-Benavente F, Blumenschein G Jr, et al. Nivolumab treatment beyond RECIST-defined progression in recurrent or metastatic squamous cell carcinoma of the head and neck in CheckMate 141: a subgroup analysis of a randomized phase 3 clinical trial. *Cancer*;**125**(18):3208–3218.

304 Saba NF, Blumenschein G Jr, Guigay J, et al. Nivolumab versus investigator's choice in patients with recurrent or metastatic squamous cell carcinoma of the head and neck: efficacy and safety in CheckMate 141 by age. *Oral Oncol*. 2019;**96**:7–14.

305 Bauml J, Seiwert TY, Pfister DG, et al. Pembrolizumab for platinum- and cetuximab-refractory head and neck cancer: results from a single-arm, phase II study. *J Clin Oncol*. 2017;**35**(14):1542–1549.

80 Cancer of the lung

Daniel Morgensztern, MD ■ Daniel Boffa, MD ■ Alexander Chen, MD ■ Andrew Dhanasopon, MD ■ Sarah B. Goldberg, MD ■ Roy H. Decker, MD, PhD ■ Siddhartha Devarakonda, MD ■ Jane P. Ko, MD ■ Luisa M. Solis Soto, MD ■ Saiama N. Waqar, MBBS, MSCI ■ Ignacio I. Wistuba, MD ■ Roy S. Herbst, MD, PhD

Overview

Lung cancer is the most common cause of death from cancer both worldwide and in the United States. There has been a remarkable progress in the treatment of lung cancer with an increasing number of highly effective targeted therapies and the incorporation of immune checkpoint inhibitors into the standard therapy of non-small-cell lung cancer, initially in patients with metastatic disease and more recently in earlier stages. These therapeutic advances in combination with reduced incidence of lung cancer associated with the decreased tobacco smoking have led to a sharp decrease in lung cancer mortality over the past few years.

Epidemiology and risk factors

Lung cancer is the most commonly diagnosed and the most common cause of death from cancer worldwide, with approximately 2.2 million new cases and 1.9 million deaths in 2017.[1] In the United States, the American Cancer Society estimated 247,270 new cases and 140,730 deaths for the year 2020, representing approximately 13.6% of the 1,806,590 cases and 23.2% of the 606,520 estimated deaths.[2] The mortality from lung cancer, however, has declined due to both decrease in the incidence and improvement in survival.[3]

Cigarette smoking is the leading cause of lung cancer, accounting for approximately 80–90% of cases.[4] Smoking increases the risk of lung cancer by approximately 20-fold when compared to never smokers and the risk remains elevated even after prolonged periods of abstinence. Both cigar and pipe smoking are also established risk factors for lung cancer although the risk is lower compared to cigarettes. Marijuana smoking is also considered a risk factor for lung cancer.[5,6] Passive smoking, also known as secondhand smoke, is a cause of lung cancer among nonsmokers, particularly among those who live with smokers, leading to an estimated 21,400 worldwide lung cancer deaths per year.[7] In a pooled analysis by the International Lung Cancer Consortium evaluating 18 case-control studies, the odds ratio for secondhand smoking compared to those never exposed was 1.31.[8]

Other environmental risk factors for lung cancer include residential radon from soil, which may accumulate to unsafe levels in the basements and lower building levels, ionizing radiation, asbestos exposure, and domestic fuel smoke such as the use of solid fuels for cooking or heating.[9,10] Previous lung diseases including chronic bronchitis, emphysema, pulmonary tuberculosis, and idiopathic pulmonary fibrosis have also been associated with increased risk for lung cancer.[4,11–13]

The fact that the vast majority of cigarette smokers do not develop lung cancer indicates the role for genetic susceptibility particularly with the increased risk in those with family history of lung cancer.[14,15] Initial genome-wide associated studies showed that alterations in some chromosome regions are associated with increased risk for lung cancer, including 5p15, 15q25, and 6p21.[16–18] Since then, several other cancer susceptibility loci have been identified with varying strength of evidence.[19]

Molecular pathogenesis

The rapidly developing technology of molecular biology has allowed the identification of multiple genes responsible for lung carcinogenesis. Interestingly, these genes are altered forms of genes normally present in eukaryotic cells. The plethora of genetic abnormalities and redundancy of altered pathways induced by tobacco and other carcinogens determines lung cancer heterogeneity, which is remarkable in comparison to that of other solid tumors. In this regard, it has to be remembered that individual tumors are characterized by specific genetic alternations and that there is a gradual accumulation of abnormalities in a given tumor, from normal epithelium to invasive carcinoma. Several genes have been implicated in carcinogenesis (Table 1).

Structural and genetic epithelial changes occur gradually, and invasive carcinoma develops 5–20 years after initial insult to the airways (Figure 1). In patients that develop lung cancer, the widespread injury of the tissue exposed to carcinogen, originates the appearance of foci of molecular damaged and histopathology altered lesions (field cancerization phenomenon).[20–22] Of note, molecular alterations that precede lung cancer have been documented not only in preneoplastic and invasive malignant tumors but also in normal-appearing lung tissue adjacent to lung cancer tumors. It is noteworthy that many of these changes are seen in histologically normal bronchial epithelium from smokers, but not nonsmokers, in which the field of damage is usually more restricted.[21,23,24]

In squamous cell carcinoma (SCC), genetic abnormalities have been seen in adjacent normal-appearing bronchial epithelium and augment with progression of histopathologic changes (dysplastic epithelium and *in situ* carcinoma) in a multistage manner. In lung adenocarcinoma, sequential premalignant changes are poorly documented. Adenomatous atypical hyperplasia (AAH) is the only sequence of morphology change identified and seems to be involved in the linear progression of cells of the terminal respiratory unit to adenocarcinoma *in situ* (AIS) and invasive

Table 1 Summary of molecular abnormalities associated with the NSCLC adenocarcinomas and squamous-cell carcinoma histologies.

Gene	Molecular change	Adenocarcinoma (%)	Squamous-cell carcinoma
EGFR	Mutation	10–40	Very rare
	Amplification/CNG[a]	15	40%
	IHC[b] overexpression	15–39	58%
KRAS	Mutation	10–30	Very rare
BRAF	Mutation	2	3%
EML4-ALK	Translocation	13	Very rare
R1	Translocation	1	Very rare
RET	Translocation	1	Very rare
LKB1	Mutation	80–30	0–5%
HER2	Mutation	2–4	Very rare
	Amplification	8	2%
	IHC[b]	35	1%
DDR2	Mutation	Rare (%)	4%
TP53	LOH[c]	50–70	60–70%
FGFR1	Amplification	1–3	8–22%
PIK3CA	Amplification/CNG[a]	2–6	33–35%
	Mutation	2	2%
AKT	Mutation	0	5%
MET	Exon 14 mutations	3–4	2%
	Amplification/CNG[a]	2–10	8%
	IHC[b] overexpression	35–72	38%
NTRK	Translocation	<1	Very rare
NRG1	Translocation	<1	Very rare
RET	Translocation	<1	Very rare

[a]CNG, copy number gains.
[b]IHC, immunohistochemistry.
[c]LOH, loss of heterozygosity.

lung adenocarcinoma. Studies conducted in AAH lesions have identified several alterations in AAH lesions including mutations in epidermal growth factor receptor (*EGFR*), *KRAS, BRAF, RBM10 TP53,* among others.[25–28] Small-cell lung carcinoma (SCLC) is not associated with histologically identifiable preneoplastic lesions. Normal-appearing tissue adjacent to SCLC shows a more widespread and molecular damage than non-small-cell lung cancer (NSCLC), indicating that in SCLC, a severely molecularly damaged epithelium develops rapidly into an invasive lesion with no histologically recognizable sequence of changes.[20,21,29]

Pathology of lung cancer

From histopathologic and biologic perspectives, lung cancer is a complex neoplasm. The current 2015 WHO classification, supported by a pathology panel of the International Association for the Study of Lung Cancer (IASLC), is based on the analysis of lung tumors by light microscopy with standard histology techniques and immunohistochemical analysis of proteins representing differentiation markers (Table 2).[30–32] The most common histologic types of lung cancer are NSCLCs (which include squamous cell carcinoma, adenocarcinoma, and large-cell carcinoma) and small SCLC.[32,33] Lung neoplasms are generally classified by the best-differentiated region of the tumor and graded by its most poorly differentiated portion.

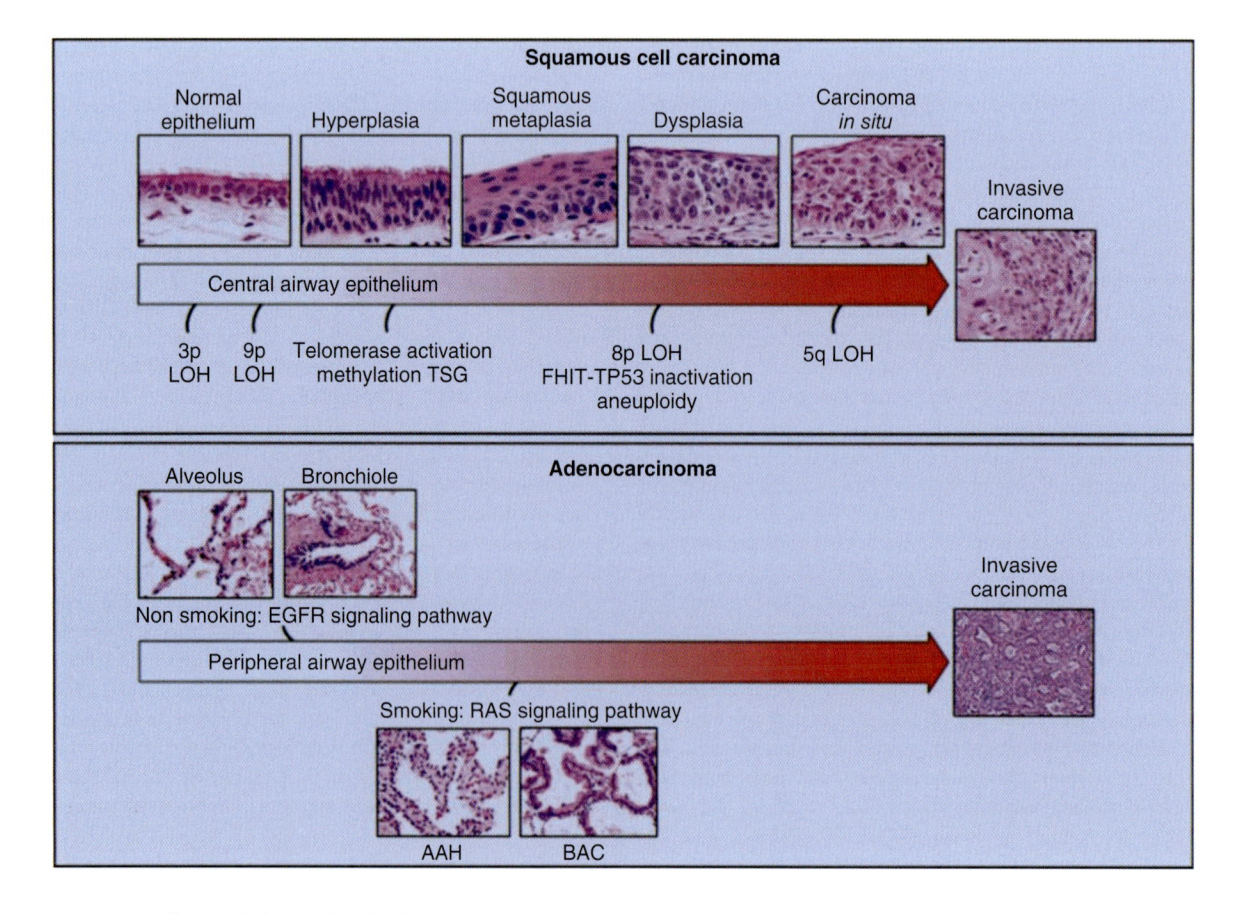

Figure 1 Summary of histopathologic and molecular changes involved in the pathogenesis of squamous cell carcinoma and adenocarcinoma of the lung.

Table 2 Histological classification of lung cancer.

(I) Epithelial tumors
    (a) Benign
        (i) Papillomas
            (a) Squamous-cell papilloma
            (b) Glandular papilloma
            (c) Mixed squamous-cell and glandular papilloma
        (ii) Adenomas
            (a) Sclerosing pneumocytoma
            (b) Alveolar adenoma
            (c) Papillary adenoma
            (d) Mucinous cystadenoma
            (e) Pneumocystic adenomyoepithelioma
            (f) Mucous gland adenoma
    (b) Preinvasive lesions
        1 Atypical alveolar hyperplasia (AAH)
        2 Adenocarcinoma *in situ* (AIS)
        3 Squamous dysplasia and carcinoma *in situ*
        4 Diffuse idiopathic pulmonary neuroendocrine cell hyperplasia
    (c) Malignant
        (i) Adenocarcinoma
            (a) Minimally invasive adenocarcinoma (MIA)
            (b) Invasive adenocarcinoma
            (c) Variants of invasive adenocarcinoma: mucinous, colloid, fetal, and enteric
        (ii) Squamous-cell carcinoma
            (a) Keratinizing
            (b) Nonkeratinizing
            (c) Basaloid carcinoma
        (iii) Adenosquamous carcinoma
        (iv) Sarcomatoid carcinoma
            (a) Pleomorphic
            (b) Spindle cell
            (c) Giant-cell carcinoma
            (d) Carcinosarcoma
            (e) Pulmonary blastoma
        (v) Large-cell carcinoma
        (vi) Neuroendocrine tumors
            (a) Typical carcinoid
            (b) Atypical carcinoid
            (c) Large-cell neuroendocrine carcinoma (LCNEC)
            (d) Small-cell carcinoma (SCLC)
        (vii) Other and unclassified carcinomas
            (a) Lymphoepithelioma-like carcinoma
            (b) NUT-carcinoma
        (viii) Salivary gland tumors
            (a) Mucoepidermoid carcinoma
            (b) Adenoid cystic carcinoma
            (c) Epithelial–myoepithelial carcinoma
            (d) Pleomorphic adenoma
(II) Mesenchymal tumors
(III) Lymphohistiocytic tumors
(IV) Tumors of ectopic origin
(V) Metastatic tumors

Precursor lesions

Lung cancers are believed to arise after the development of a series of progressive pathological changes (preneoplastic or precursor lesions) in the respiratory mucosa. The 2015 WHO histological classification of preinvasive lesions of the lung lists three main morphologic forms: (1) squamous dysplasia and carcinoma *in situ* (CIS); (2) AAH and AIS; and (3) diffuse idiopathic pulmonary neuroendocrine cell hyperplasia (DIPNECH), which has been associated with the development of carcinoid tumors of the lung.[30,31] While the sequential preneoplastic changes have been defined for centrally arising squamous carcinomas, they have been poorly documented for large-cell carcinomas, adenocarcinomas, and SCLCs.[20,21,34,35]

Invasive tumors

Minimally invasive adenocarcinoma (MIA)

This lesion is defined as a small (≤3 cm), solitary adenocarcinoma with a predominantly lepidic pattern and with ≤5 mm invasion area in greatest dimension.[30,32,36] MIA is usually composed of nonmucinous cells, but infrequently, it may be mucinous. The measurement of the invasive area should include the presence of histological subtypes other than a lepidic pattern (i.e., acinar, papillary, micropapillary, and/or solid), or the identification of malignant cells clearly infiltrating stroma.[30,32] If a tumor invades lymphatics, blood vessels or pleura, or contains tumor necrosis, it should be diagnosed as invasive adenocarcinoma.

Adenocarcinoma

This tumor type accounts for nearly 40% of all lung cancers (Figure 2a, b). Most adenocarcinomas are histologically heterogeneous, and according to the 2015 WHO classification, adenocarcinoma can be subclassified based on the predominant histological pattern present into acinar, papillary, solid with mucin production, micropapillary, and lepidic.[30,32] When tumor cells grow in a purely lepidic fashion without evidence of invasion, they are regarded as AIS.[30] The solid adenocarcinoma pattern is, by definition, poorly differentiated, and these poorly differentiated tumors usually demonstrate mucus production as shown by mucicarmine or periodic acid-Schiff staining. Lung adenocarcinomas typically immunostain for thyroid transcription factor-1, Napsin A, and cytokeratin 7. The IASLC recommends to perform TTF-1 for the differential diagnosis of adenocarcinoma, while Napsin A is recommended to distinguish adenocarcinoma from large-cell neuroendocrine carcinoma (LCNEC) or SCLC. Neuroendocrine markers such as chromogranin, synaptophysin, and CD56 should be performed only when neuroendocrine features are present.[37] While adenocarcinomas of the lung spread primarily by lymphatic and hematogenous routes, aerogeneous dissemination often occurs in mucinous tumors and is characterized by spread of tumor cells through the airways forming lesions separate from the main mass.[32,38]

Squamous cell carcinoma

Squamous cell carcinoma accounts for approximately 30% of all lung cancers. Intercellular bridges, squamous pearl formation, and individual cell keratinization characterize squamous differentiation in this tumor type (Figure 2c). While all these features are very apparent in well-differentiated squamous cell carcinomas, they are difficult to find in poorly differentiated tumors. The histologic subtypes included in the 2015 WHO classification include keratinizing, nonkeratinizing, and basaloid.[32,39] In tumors with keratinizing features, there is no need for immunohistochemistry (IHC) analysis. The nonkeratinizing tumors necessitate IHC examination to distinguish these tumors from poorly differentiated adenocarcinoma, large-cell carcinoma with a null immunophenotype in surgical resections, or other types of poorly differentiated NSCLCs. The recommendation of the IASLC for subtyping of NSCLC is to perform IHC for TTF-1 and p40. Negative TTF-1, absence of mucin, and more than 50% of p40 expression confirm their squamous phenotype and classification as a nonkeratinizing squamous cell carcinoma. In more difficult cases, p63 and CK5/6 could be used as an alternative.[37] Approximately 70% of squamous cell carcinomas of the lung present as central tumors.[40] The tumor may grow to a large size and central cavitation secondary to necrosis is a common gross finding.[41]

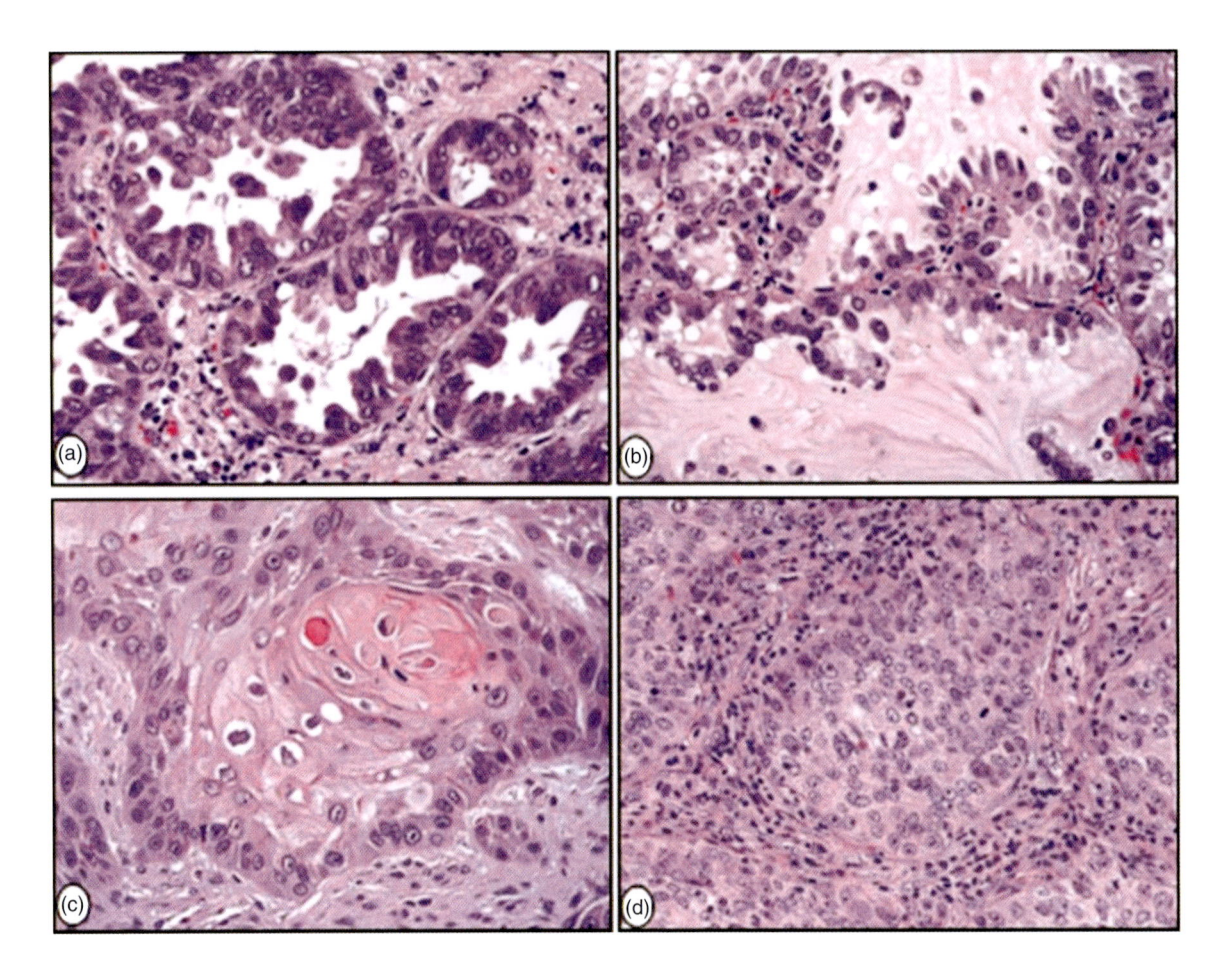

Figure 2 Histopathologic characteristics of the major forms of NSCLC: (a) invasive adenocarcinoma with acinar pattern, (b) adenocarcinoma with lepidic (noninvasive) pattern, (c) keratinizing squamous-cell carcinoma, and (d) large-cell carcinoma.

Adenosquamous carcinoma

Adenosquamous carcinoma of the lung is characterized by the presence of squamous cell carcinoma and adenocarcinoma with each comprising at least 10% of the tumor.[32,42] They account for 0.4–4% of lung cancers and are usually located in the periphery of the lung and may contain a central scar. The routes of dissemination and metastasis are similar to other NSCLCs.

Sarcomatoid carcinomas

Sarcomatoid carcinomas of the lung are a group of poorly differentiated NSCLCs that contain a component of sarcoma or sarcoma-like (spindle and/or giant cell) differentiation.[32,43] Currently, there are five variants identified: pleomorphic carcinoma, spindle cell carcinoma, giant cell carcinoma, carcinosarcoma, and pulmonary blastoma.[32,43,44] Sarcomatoid carcinomas are rare tumors (0.3–1.3% of lung tumors).[43,45] IHC and molecular biomarkers play a key role to distinguish them from their mimics such as sarcomatoid mesothelioma, sarcomas, or melanoma. TTF-1 and p40 are frequently negative, a panel of carcinoma markers is useful to demonstrate epithelial differentiation, and GATA3 is a useful biomarker to exclude a sarcomatoid mesothelioma.

Large-cell carcinoma

Large-cell carcinoma is defined as an undifferentiated NSCLC that lacks the cytological, architectural, and immunohistochemical features of squamous cell carcinoma, adenocarcinoma, or SCLC. Thus, it is a diagnosis of exclusion. Large-cell carcinomas account for approximately 10% of all lung cancers, and they represent a spectrum of morphology, most consisting of large cells with abundant cytoplasm and large nuclei with prominent nucleoli (Figure 2d).[41] The 2004 WHO classification listed five histological variants of large-cell carcinoma: LCNEC, basaloid carcinoma, lymphoepithelioma-like carcinoma, clear cell carcinoma, and large-cell carcinoma with rhabdoid phenotype. However, in the 2015 WHO classification, LCNEC was reclassified into a new category (neuroendocrine carcinoma), and basaloid carcinoma is included as a variant of squamous cell carcinoma. Pure large-cell carcinoma with clear cells or rhabdoid phenotype is extremely uncommon. If these components are detected in a large-cell carcinoma, their presence should be added in the description of the tumor.

Neuroendocrine tumors

Lung neuroendocrine tumors account for approximately 15% of lung cancers. They are composed of malignant cells showing neuroendocrine differentiation and representing a wide spectrum of tumors. Typical and atypical carcinoids are classified as low and intermediate-grade carcinoma, respectively, and LCNEC and SCLC, are classified as high-grade neuroendocrine carcinoma in the current 2015 WHO classification of lung tumors (Figure 3a–c).[32]

Carcinoid tumors

Carcinoid tumors are characterized by organoid growth pattern, uniform cytologic features, and immunohistochemical

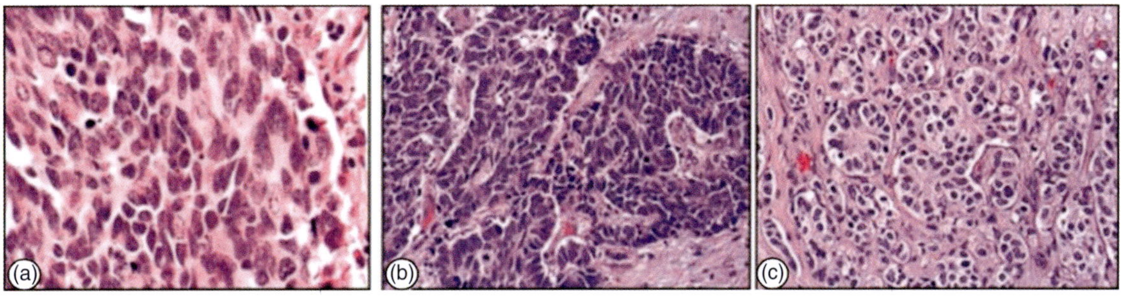

Figure 3 Neuroendocrine tumor of the lung: (a) SCLC, (b) LNEC, and (c) typical carcinoid.

expression of neuroendocrine markers, such as chromogranin, synaptophysin, CD56, and insulinoma-associated protein 1 (INSM1) (Figure 3c).[46–48] Carcinoid tumors have been divided into two categories, typical and atypical types, based on the clinical behavior and pathologic features, with atypical carcinoids having more malignant histologic and clinical features.[49] Histologically, typical carcinoids show fewer than 2 mitoses per 2 mm^2 field and lack necrosis, while atypical carcinoids show 2–10 mitosis per 2 mm^2 field and/or foci of necrosis.[32,46,48,50] Typical carcinoids are uniformly distributed throughout the lungs, whereas atypical carcinoids are more commonly peripheral tumors.[51] Compared to typical carcinoids, atypical carcinoids have larger tumor sizes, higher rate of metastases, and worse survival.[51] At presentation, approximately 10–15% of typical and 40–50% of atypical carcinoids demonstrate regional lymph node metastases.[46] In contrast to neuroendocrine tumors from other sites, IHC for Ki67 is not recommended for the classification of neuroendocrine tumors; however, it is useful in small or crushed biopsies or cytological specimens to distinguish these tumors from high-grade neuroendocrine tumors.[37,52]

Large-cell neuroendocrine carcinoma (LCNEC)
This tumor type is defined by the presence of large undifferentiated cells with prominent nucleoli, neuroendocrine pattern of growth, high mitotic rate, and neuroendocrine differentiation demonstrated by IHC (Figure 3b).[32,53] They are usually peripheral, nodular masses, with necrosis. LCNEC is considered an aggressive malignancy with a prognosis similar to SCLC.[53] The term combined LCNEC is used for tumors associated with other better-differentiated types of NSCLC, mostly adenocarcinomas.

Small-cell lung carcinoma (SCLC)
This tumor type accounts for approximately 15% of all lung cancers.[32,39] They characteristically consist of small epithelial tumor cells with finely granular chromatin and absent or inconspicuous nucleoli (Figure 3a). Necrosis is frequent and extensive and the mitotic count is high. Although there is not a precise upper limit for cell size to be defined as small cell, it has been suggested that the cells should measure approximately the diameter of two to three small mature lymphocytes.[54] While SCLC represents a light microscopic diagnosis, electron microscopy shows neuroendocrine granules in at least two-thirds of cases, and the IHC for neuroendocrine markers (chromogranin, synaptophysin, CD56, and insulinoma-associated protein1 (INSM1)) is positive in approximately 90% of cases.[47,54,55] Less than 10% of SCLCs demonstrate a mixture with NSCLC histologic types, usually adenocarcinoma, squamous cell carcinoma or large-cell carcinoma, and they are termed combined SCLCs.[29] Of note, some NSCLCs with acquired resistance to EGFR tyrosine kinase inhibitor (TKI) therapy show genotypic and histological evolution to SCLC.[56–58] Small-cell carcinomas are characterized for a very large number of genetic alterations including deletion in chromosome 3 (p14–p23), and inactivation of *TP53* and *RB1*.[29,59] Current understanding of SCLC biology based in recent progress in the genomic, epigenomic, and transcriptome profile of these tumors is leading to the development of a better biological classification of SCLC. This classification, which is based on the differential expression of the key transcriptional regulators achaete-scute homologue 1 (ASCL1), neurogenic differentiation factor 1 (NeuroD1), yes-associated protein 1 (YAP1), and POU class 2 homeobox 3 (POU2F3), is an area of active investigation and has unveiled differences among these tumor types that were typically regarded as homogeneous, and may guide to define better approaches for targeted therapy.[29,59–61]

NSCLC histological classification applied to small biopsies and cytology specimens
In small biopsies or cytology tumor samples, the NSCLC diagnosis has been lumped together without attention to more specific histologic typing. The 2015 WHO classification established standardized criteria and terminology for pathologic diagnosis of lung cancer in small biopsies and cytology.[62] In addition to the criteria and terminology, there is a paradigm shift for pathologists in tumor classification and management of specimens which indicates the need to perform IHC to further classify tumors formerly diagnosed as NSCLC not otherwise specified (NOS). Currently, if a NSCLC does not show clear glandular or squamous morphology in a small biopsy or cytology specimen, it is classified as NSCLC-NOS. Tumors with this morphology should be further evaluated with limited special immunohistochemical markers to classify them further. The current recommendations of the IASLC are to use TTF-1 or mucin as adenocarcinoma makers, p40 as a squamous marker.[37,62] Tumors that are positive for an adenocarcinoma marker or mucin are classified as NSCLC, favor adenocarcinoma. Tumors that are positive for a squamous marker with negative adenocarcinoma markers and are classified as NSCLC, favor squamous cell carcinoma. Cytology is also a powerful diagnostic tool that can accurately subtype NSCLC in most cases, and IHC is readily available if cell blocks are prepared for the cytology samples. Current IASLC recommendation indicates that all cytological preparations including ethanol-fixed and air-dried slides can be used for IHC. Cytological specimens can also be used to detect molecular abnormalities such as *EGFR* mutation or other targetable alteration, validation of the assay in cytological samples must follow rigorous protocol for optimization, validation, and quality control.[63]

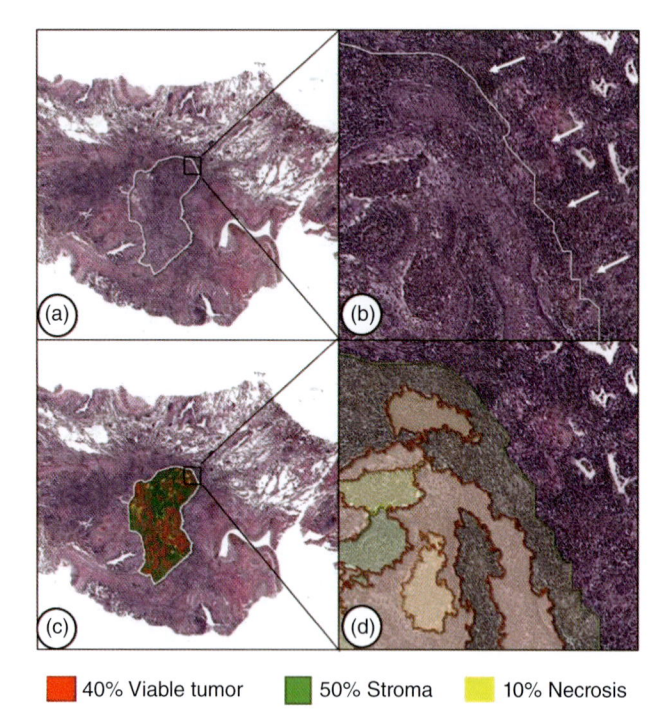

Figure 4 Pathological assessment of a lung cancer resected specimens after neoadjuvant therapy. (a) Low magnification (2×) and (b) High magnification microphotographs (20×) of a whole section H&E slide with a surgically resected non-small-cell lung carcinoma, after neoadjuvant therapy. White border delineates the border of the tumor bed; surrounding lung tissue shows reactive changes and inflammatory response. (c) and (d) show marked-up images from the same microphotographs with a color representation of the histopathological components of the tumor bed: viable tumor, stroma (including fibrosis and inflammation), and necrosis.

Pathological assessment of neoadjuvant therapies in NSCLC

Considering the increasing use of neoadjuvant systemic therapy in NSCLC, the IASLC has recently provided with detailed guidelines for the pathological evaluation of lung cancer tumors surgically resected after chemotherapy, chemoradiation, molecular, and immune targeted therapy. The purpose of these recommendations is to better assess major pathological response (MPR) and complete pathological response (CPR) in clinical trials and as good practice outside of clinical trials to improve consistency in the assessment of pathological response. The recommendations include correct, gross and microscopic, identification of the "tumor bed," defined as the location of the pretreated tumor as well as the pathological assessment of the percentages of viable tumor, necrotic areas and stroma, including fibrosis and inflammation (Figure 4). The term MPR has been coined to assess NSCLC response to neoadjuvant systemic therapy, and it has been defined as ≤10% of residual viable tumor cells. However, recent observations suggest that optimal cutoff for predicting survival varies among histologic types.[64,65] CPR is defined as lack of any viable tumor cells on review of slides after complete evaluation of the resected lung cancer specimen including all sampled regional lymph nodes.[64,66]

Immune biomarkers in lung cancer

Understanding the mechanisms of immune evasion in lung cancer had progressed in the last years. The immune evasion mechanisms include regulatory immune cells, defective antigen presentation, immunosuppressive cytokines, and expression of immune checkpoints.[67] The advances in this area have led to the development of immune therapies with a great impact in the management of lung cancer.[68,69] Currently, the immune checkpoint inhibitors (ICIs) that target the PD-1 (programmed cell death protein 1) and PD-L1 (programmed death ligand 1) axis are indicated in NSCLC and SCLC with advanced or metastatic disease.[69–71] Among the biomarkers that have been evaluated to predict response of therapy are PD-L1, tumor mutational burden, and tumor inflammation (Figure 5).

PD-L1, a type 1 transmembrane protein (B7-H1) that belongs to the B7 ligand family, can be expressed by tumor cells and immune cells. Several PD-L1 IHC assays are approved by the US Food and Drug administration as companion or complementary diagnosis (Table 3). There is a high concordance among PD-L1 clones for PD-L1 expression in tumor cells, except for SP142 which shows lower sensitivity, and low concordance for the evaluation of PD-L1 in immune cells.[72] The IHC expression of PD-L1 is evaluated in histological samples by a pathologist using standard microscopy, the percentage of tumor cells with complete circumferential or partial linear membrane expression is reported and several cutoffs are used

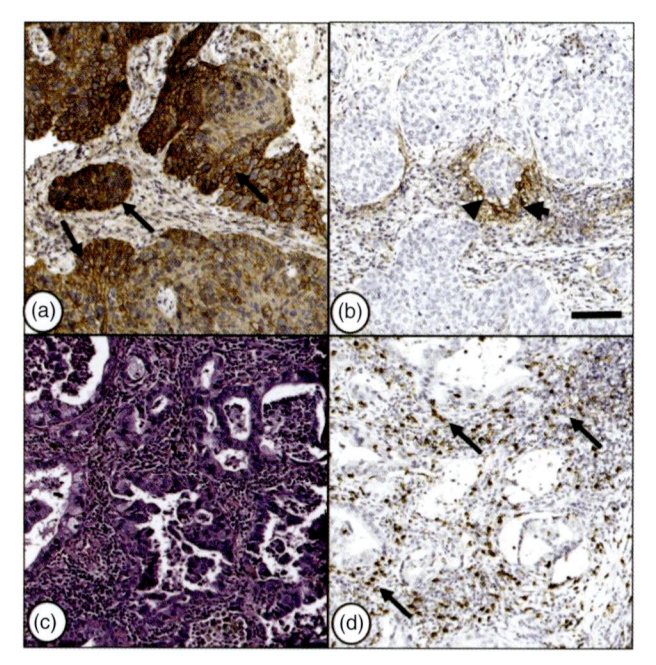

Figure 5 Immune biomarkers in lung cancer. (a) Squamous-cell carcinoma with immunohistochemical expression of PD-L1 (clone 28-8) in tumor cells (arrows). (b) Squamous-cell carcinoma with immune cells positive for PD-L1 (head arrows) in the tumor stroma. (c) Lung adenocarcinoma with tumor-infiltrating lymphocytes in the tumor stroma. (d) Lung adenocarcinoma with immune cells positive for CD8 (cytotoxic T-cells). Magnification 20×. Scale bar, 100 μm.

Table 3 FDA-approved PD-L1 Immunohistochemistry assays information.

PD-L1 clone	Vendor	Drug	Scoring	FDA approval
22C3	Dako	Pembrolizumab	Tumor cells	Companion
28-8	Dako	Nivolumab	Tumor cells	Complementary
SP263	Ventana	Durvalumab	Tumor cells	Complementary
SP142	Ventana	Atezolizumab	Tumor cells and immune cells	Complementary

depending on the drug and the assay. For clone SP142, PD-L1 in immune cells is also assessed as percentage of the tumor area with PD-L1 positive (membrane or cytoplasmic) immune cells. These assays require minimal number of tumor cells in histological samples, 100 cells for 22C3, 28-8, and SP263 clones, and 50 tumoral cells with associated stroma for SP142. Evaluation of PD-L1 has several limitations such as preanalytical factors, tumor heterogeneity, and its applications on cytological samples.[72,73]

Clinical manifestations

Some patients present with an asymptomatic lesion discovered incidentally on chest radiograph. The majority of lung cancers, however, are discovered because of the development of new or worsening clinical symptoms or signs. Signs or symptoms from lung cancer may be divided into four categories: (1) symptoms local tumor growth and intrathoracic spread, (2) symptoms from distant metastases, (3) nonspecific systemic symptoms, and (4) paraneoplastic syndromes.

Signs and symptoms referable to the primary tumor vary depending on location and size of the tumor (Table 4). Centrally located tumors produce cough, localized wheeze, hemoptysis, symptoms, and signs of airway obstruction and postobstructive pneumonitis such as dyspnea, fever, and productive cough. Peripheral tumors are more likely to be asymptomatic when they are small and confined within the lung.

Intrathoracic spread of lung cancer, either by direct extension or by lymphatic metastasis, is associated with a variety of symptom. Mediastinal invasion may be manifested as vague, poorly localized chest pain in association with other findings of nerve entrapment, vascular obstruction, and/or compression or invasion of the esophagus. One of the most common neurologic disorders arising from mediastinal involvement is hoarseness due to entrapment of the recurrent laryngeal nerve. Because of its longer intrathoracic course, the left recurrent laryngeal nerve is more likely to be the source of hoarseness than the right recurrent laryngeal nerve.[74] Compression of the esophagus by the tumor may lead to dysphagia. The formation of a tracheoesophageal or bronchoesophageal fistula can be manifested by vigorous cough, especially on swallowing, and recurrent aspiration pneumonia.[75] The principal vascular syndrome associated with the extension of lung cancer into the mediastinum is the superior vena cava (SVC) syndrome, most commonly caused by invasion of the vein and extrinsic compression by the tumor but also by intraluminal thrombosis.[76] Lung cancer accounts for 65–90% of all cases of SVC syndrome, and in approximately 85% of these cases, the primary lung tumor is on the right, primarily in the right upper lobe or right mainstem bronchus. Establishment of a histologic diagnosis is important before initiating treatment, because the SVC syndrome is no longer considered a radiotherapeutic emergency.

With apical tumors, the classic Pancoast's syndrome consisting of lower brachial plexopathy, Horner's syndrome, and shoulder pain, occurs due to local invasion of the lower brachial plexus (C8 and T1 nerve roots), satellite ganglion, and chest wall.[77] The tumor may cause symptoms through involvement of the first or second rib or vertebrae and other nerve roots.

Approximately 15% of patients with lung cancer have pleural involvement at initial presentation, and 50% of patients with disseminated lung cancer develop pleural effusion during the course of their illness. Pleural effusion may cause dyspnea, cough, or chest pain.[78] Pericardial involvement arises from direct extension of the tumor or as a result of retrograde spread through mediastinal and epicardial lymphatics. Lung cancer is the most frequent source of pericardial metastases.[79] Clinical findings include cardiac dysrhythmias, enlargement of the cardiac silhouette, and, infrequently, cardiac tamponade.

Systemic, nonspecific signs and symptoms are common in both SCLC and NSCLC (Table 5). The 30% rate of anorexia is probably underreported. Weight lost, which is usually but not always accompanied by anorexia, occurs in approximately one-half of the patients and generalized weakness in one-third. Fever and anemia occur in fewer than 20% of the patients.

Although lung cancer can metastasize to virtually any organ site, the most common sites of hematogenous spread that are clinically apparent are the central nervous system (CNS), bones, liver, and adrenal glands. Some of these patients have symptoms that can be attributed to a specific distant site, while others have no associated symptoms.

Paraneoplastic syndromes

Paraneoplastic syndromes are disorders caused by systemic effects away from the primary tumor or its metastasis.[80,81] Several of the paraneoplastic neurologic syndromes occur predominantly in patients with SCLC including limbic encephalitis, paraneoplastic cerebellar degeneration, and Lambert–Eaton myasthenia syndrome. Among the paraneoplastic endocrine syndromes, the syndrome of inappropriate antidiuretic hormone secretion and Cushing syndrome may occur in SCLC whereas hypercalcemia is more common in squamous cell lung cancer. Other paraneoplastic syndromes that may occur in patients with lung cancer include dermatomyositis, polymyalgia rheumatic, hypertrophic osteoarthropathy, neutrophilia, and thrombocytosis.

Table 5 Clinical manifestations caused by systemic effect at presentation.

Clinical manifestation	Frequency (%)	
	SCLC	NSCLC
Anorexia	50–76	40
Weight loss (≥10 lb)	34–40	30–40
Fatigue	35–36	25–40
Fever	15–23	15–35
Anemia	21–25	13–24

Table 4 Clinical manifestations of lung cancer caused by local tumor growth and intrathoracic spread at presentation.

Clinical manifestation	Frequency (%)	
	SCLC	NSCLC
Cough	50–76	40
Dyspnea	34–40	30–40
Chest pain	35–36	25–40
Hemoptysis	15–23	15–35
Pneumonitis	21–25	13–24
SVC syndrome	12	<10
Pleural effusion	10–15	15
Pancoast syndrome	Rare	3
Pericardial effusion	Uncommon	Rare

NSCLC, nonsmall-cell lung cancer; SCLC, small-cell lung cancer; SVC, superior vena cava.

Work-up and staging

Staging is the determination of the extent of disease, with the intent of grouping patients with similar levels of disease for analytical, therapeutic, and prognostic purposes. The staging of lung cancer provides a scale of relative disease, which can be assigned to all patients with primary lung malignancies. Accurate staging of lung cancer is essential for defining operability, for selecting treatment regimens, for predicting survival, and for reporting comparable end results.

Accurate staging of a patient with a suspected or confirmed lung cancer diagnosis is critical to determine an appropriate treatment plan. Staging studies can be noninvasive or invasive. Noninvasive studies include computed tomography (CT) scanning, positron emission tomography (PET) (usually PET-CT) scanning, and magnetic resonance imaging (MRI). Invasive procedures include bronchoscopy, CT or ultrasound (US)-guided fine needle aspiration (FNA) or biopsy, and surgical (open) biopsy using mediastinoscopy or thoracoscopy. Patients who present with clinical or radiographic evidence of advanced disease usually require the least invasive procedure to establish both the diagnosis and disease stage.

The current eighth edition of the AJCC lung cancer staging system (AJCC8) was updated in 2018 and is based on approximately 95,000 cases treated from 1999 to 2010, derived from more than 16 countries.[82] This staging system takes into account tumor characteristics (T), the presence of lymph node involvement (N), and the presence of metastases (M) to provide a stage from I to IV (Tables 6 and 7).

In some circumstances, when a clinical stage I malignancy is suspected, invasive diagnostic studies can be waived, and the patient can undergo resection for diagnosis and treatment. If a resection beyond a lobectomy is required or if the patient is a

Table 6 TNM descriptors.

T	Primary tumor
Tx	Primary tumor cannot be accessed
T0	No evidence of primary tumor
Tis	Carcinoma in situ
T1	Tumor ≤3 cm surrounded by lung or visceral pleura without invasion of the main bronchus
	T1mi (minimally invasive, T1a (≤1 cm), T1b (>1 cm but ≤2 cm), T1c (>2 cm but ≤3 cm
T2	Tumor >3 cm but ≤5 cm or involvement of the main bronchus, visceral pleura or atelectasis or obstructive pneumonitis extending into the hilar region (T2a = >3–4 cm), T2b = >4 cm to ≤5cm)
T3	Tumor >5 cm but ≤7 cm or associated with separate nodule(s) in the same lobe as the primary tumor, or direct invasion of chest wall, phrenic nerve, or parietal pericardium
T4	Tumor >7 cm or associated with separate nodule(s) in different ipsilateral lobes or invasion of: diaphragm, mediastinum, heart, great vessels, trachea, recurrent laryngeal nerve, esophagus, vertebral body, or carina
N	Regional lymph node involvement
NX	Regional lymph nodes cannot be accessed
N0	No regional lymph node metastases
N1	Metastasis in ipsilateral peribronchial, hilar, or intrapulmonary lymph nodes including direct extension
N2	Metastasis to ipsilateral mediastinal or subcarinal lymph nodes
N3	Metastasis to contralateral mediastinal or hilar lymph nodes, or ipsilateral or contralateral scalene or supraclavicular lymph nodes
M	Distant metastases
M0	No distant metastases
M1a	Separate nodule(s) in a contralateral lobe, pleural or pericardial nodule(s), or malignant pleural or pericardial effusion
M1b	Single extrathoracic metastasis including single distant (nonregional) lymph node
M1c	Multiple extrathoracic metastases in one or more organs

Table 7 Stage descriptors.

	T	N	M
Occult carcinoma	Tx	N0	M0
0	Tis	N0	M0
IA	T1	N0	M0
IA1	T1mi or T1a	N0	M0
IA2	T1b	N0	M0
IA3	T1c	N0	M0
IB	T2a	N0	M0
IIA	T2b	N0	M0
IIB	T1 or T2	N1	M0
	T3	N0	M0
IIIA	T1 or T2	N2	M0
	T3	N1	M0
	T4	N0 or N1	M0
IIIB	T1 or T2	N3	M0
	T3 or T4	N2	M0
IIIC	T3 or T4	N3	M0
IVA	Any	Any	M1a or M1b
IVB	Any	Any	M1c

high surgical risk, it is best to attempt preoperative diagnosis of the lesion. Patients with chest CT scan evidence of nodal involvement typically undergo further imaging and invasive staging with nodal biopsy. It is common practice to obtain a PET-CT in patients with at least clinical stage II NSCLC. Invasive mediastinal staging is used for patients with clinical stage II disease as the risk of occult mediastinal node involvement is approximately 25%.[83] Lymph node sampling is essential for patients with clinical stage III disease to confirm the stage prior to treatment. Any pathologic-appearing lymph nodes (>1 cm diameter in short-axis, or the with FDG avidity on PET imaging) should be biopsied. Mediastinal nodes are typically evaluated either by bronchoscopy or transcervical mediastinoscopy. Imaging of the brain is recommended for patients with stage III disease to rule out occult metastatic disease. MRI with and without gadolinium contrast is preferred, although CT with contrast is acceptable if MRI is not possible. When distant disease is suspected based on imaging, biopsy of a metastatic site is preferred when possible to establish both the diagnosis and confirm the advanced stage. This includes consideration of a thoracentesis or pericardiocentesis when an effusion is present. Patients with evidence of widespread metastatic disease who already have tissue confirmation of lung cancer from the primary site of disease may not require further biopsy if imaging is conclusive as to the presence of metastases. PET-CT or bone scan should be used to assess for bone involvement which may be missed on CT imaging. Brain imaging preferably using MRI with gadolinium is important given the high risk of brain metastases even in asymptomatic patients.

Noninvasive studies

Imaging

Lung cancer is generally first imaged and detected by chest radiography or CT of the lung PET/CT scan, and occasionally MRI are used to characterize nodules and to stage a known or suspected lung cancer and monitor response to therapy.

Chest radiography

Posterior–anterior and lateral chest radiographs remain the simplest method for identifying patients with lung cancer. Chest radiograph is widely available, has low cost, and low radiation dose. Although standard chest radiograph can detect a lesion as small as 3 mm in diameter, unsuspected nodules generally are not seen unless larger than 5 mm in diameter. Associated atelectasis, postobstructive pneumonitis, abscess, bronchiolitis, pleural reaction, rib erosion, pleural effusion, or bulky mediastinal lymphadenopathy may be identified on radiographs, raising suspicions of a primary lung malignancy.

Chest radiography may identify abnormal pulmonary nodules. There are no absolute criteria to confirm a benign lesion on the basis of its radiographic appearance, but stability of size for 2 years and the presence of specific patterns of calcification can be helpful. On chest radiography, a nodule can appear as homogeneously calcified, containing central calcification that occupies a majority of a nodule, or having laminated "bull's eye" appearance, which are considered indicators of benign lesions and have been described in granulomatous disease. Large chunky, clustered calcification has been described with hamartomas. However, some tumors such as carcinoids, metastatic disease, and lung cancer can contain calcification. Calcifications that are stippled, eccentric, or not occupying a majority of the nodule are indeterminate and can be seen in in cancer and benign diseases. A calcification pattern can be further investigated with chest CT. Some tumors such as typical carcinoids occasionally appear to be stable for 2 or more years, and hamartomas can demonstrate indolent growth.[84]

Lung cancer presents on chest radiography as a nodule (when less than 3 cm) or mass (when 3 cm or larger). In advanced stages, lung cancer can be associated with collapse of lobes, pleural effusions, hilar and mediastinal adenopathy, and destructive lesions. Tumor located centrally near the hilum and obstructing either upper lobe airways can result in collapse, forming the radiographic signs of the "S sign of Golden" if affecting the left upper lobe, or "reverse S sign of golden" if obstructing the right upper lobe (Figure 6). In these signs, a large round hilar contour representing mass or adenopathy is associated with a superior arc-like contour and upper lobe opacity, representing the displaced fissure and upper lobe atelectasis. Adenopathy leads to a lobulated contour of the typically smooth pulmonary arteries.

CT scan

As a single comprehensive study, CT scan remains the most effective noninvasive technique evaluating suspected or staging known lung cancer, which may have associated locoregional or distant metastatic disease.

Nodules are difficult to characterize on imaging from a single timepoint, as cancer and benign entities have overlapping imaging appearances. Nodule size, attenuation, and growth are major features that guide management. When lacking features that indicate a benign etiology, indeterminate nodules may be further investigated by follow-up chest CT surveillance, with PET/CT or tissue sampling. Given that nodules <8 mm are difficult to assess by PET/CT and sampling due to their size, chest CT surveillance has a major role in nodule management. Guidelines exist in terms of timing follow-up chest CTs, such as from the Fleischner Society and the American College of Chest Physicians.[85,86] Chest CT follow-up interval in these guidelines varies according to the risk of lung cancer for the nodule(s) in question. Nodule size is a major determinant, along with patient risk factors such as smoking history, family history of cancer, and occupational exposure. Nodule growth or progression on surveillance CT can be detected and is an indicator of malignancy. Nodule attenuation is a factor for nodule management, and differing recommendations exist for two categories of solid or sub-solid nodule attenuation. Solid nodules are soft tissue density, the same attenuation as vessels in the lungs. On CT, sub-solid nodules contain ground-glass opacity that is less dense than soft tissue yet higher than the lung parenchyma. Sub-solid nodules may be pure ground-glass attenuation (pGGN) (Figure 7) or part-solid (PSN) (Figure 8) in which soft tissue in addition to ground-glass opacity is present in the nodule.

Lung cancer most often appears as a solid attenuation lesion on CT. Suspicious features are spiculated and lobulated margins, although overlap with benign entities can occur. Additionally, pleural tags or linear soft tissue opacities that extend from the

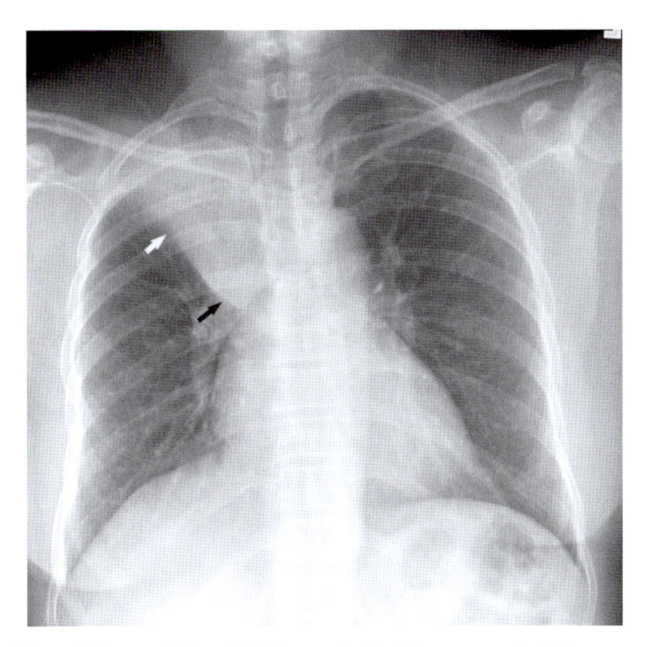

Figure 6 Reverse S sign of Golden created by hilar mass and right upper lobe atelectasis. On chest radiograph, a right hilar mass (arrow) is rounded inferiorly, and the smooth upper arc was created by atelectasis in the right upper lobe.

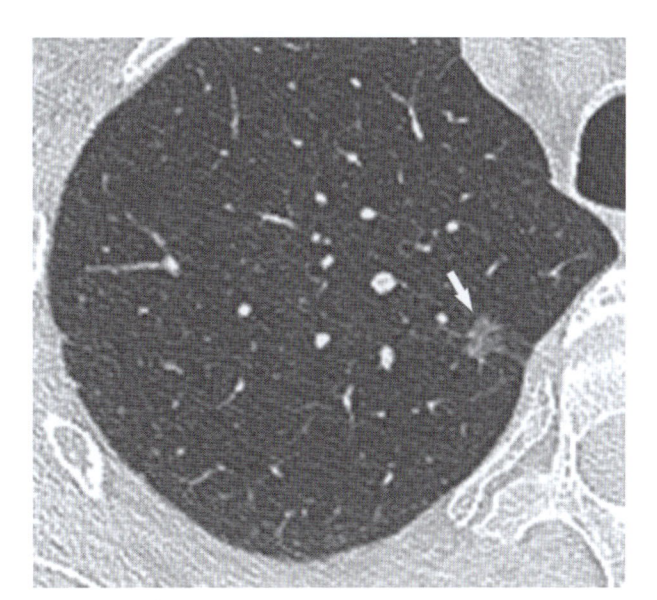

Figure 7 Pure ground-glass nodule on chest CT. On axial chest CT lung image, a 9 mm pure ground-glass nodule in the right upper lobe that was resected. Pathology revealed a lepidic-predominant lesion with 2 mm focus of acinar carcinoma that was not visible on the CT. This lesion descriptor was T1mi.

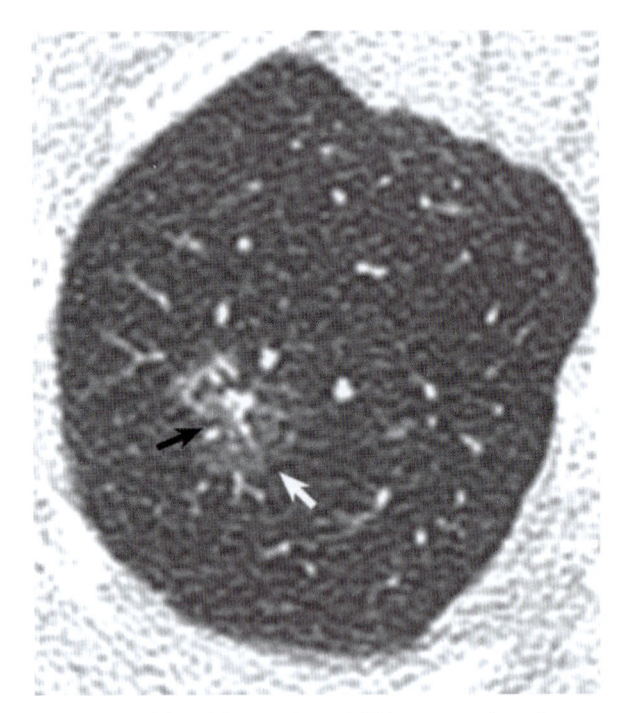

Figure 8 **Part-solid nodule on CT.** Axial CT lung image showed a 17 mm right upper lobe subsolid nodule comped predominantly of ground-glass opacity with a very small solid component. Pathology revealed LPA with a 7 mm focus of acinar invasion in the right upper lobe and was designated a pT1a lesion.

smaller, often well circumscribed, faint, and round.[30] AIS, another preinvasive lesion is comprised of lepidic tumor growth, lacks any invasive features, and measures up to 3 cm. The AIS diagnosis is rendered only upon full specimen evaluation therefore. AIS appears as a pGGN on CT, typically larger than 5 mm and less than 3 cm. MIA has foci of invasion, the largest focus being 5 mm maximally, and the overall lesion size is 3 cm maximally. These most commonly appear as PSN with a small solid component, although can range from a pGGN to a PSN with soft tissue greater than expected due to accompanying fibrosis. Lepidic-predominant adenocarcinoma (LPA) is considered a low-grade form, with an invasive component greater than 5 mm for the largest foci yet predominantly with lepidic growth. On chest CT, LPAs are typically PSNs containing soft tissue components larger than what would be seen in MIA on chest CT, although when the invasive components are small, LPAs may appear as containing only ground-glass opacity on CT.

Sub-solid nodules, however, can represent inflammatory or transient entities, and approximately one- to two-thirds of subsolid nodules seen on an initial baseline CT or developing between two CTs have been shown to resolve such as from lung cancer screening and other investigations.[87,88] These regressing nodules probably relate to organizing pneumonia, focal interstitial fibrosis, eosinophilic, and infectious causes.[89] Solid lung cancers typically have volume doubling times (VDT) between 30 and 400 days. In contrast, pGGNs proven to represent lung cancer are associated with slower growth on the order of 2–3 years.[90–92] PSNs are reported to have intermediate VDTs. Nodule growth typically presents as an increase in size whereas sub-solid nodules can increase in total size or increase in any solid component, representing invasion and fibrosis.

Chest CT assesses the central involvement and invasion of the mediastinum and chest wall. Given the significance of the solid component in sub-solid nodules, the sub-solid nodule has been added to the AJCC8 classification system for NSLC.[93]

The accuracy of CT scan in identifying metastatic disease in mediastinal lymph nodes is highly variable.[94–98] There are 14 nodal stations according to the IASLC (Figure 10). Sensitivity of chest CT ranges from 51% to 94%.[99] Such a wide range in accuracy is secondary to variations in the criteria for nodal abnormality, which are based on size and shape of a lymph node, CT scanner differences, and variability in nodal station categorization. A lymph node size ≥1 cm in short-axis diameter has been generally accepted

nodule to the pleura have been described. Cavitary areas can be seen in lung cancer, particularly squamous cell cancers (Figure 9). Additionally, squamous cell tumors tend to be central, while adenocarcinoma is described to be often peripheral. Sub-solid nodules, when persistent, correlate frequently with lung adenocarcinoma and its precursors. Ground-glass areas within adenocarcinomas have been associated with lepidic tumor or growth around the alveoli that lacks invasion.[30] Also, in PSNs, soft tissue areas are correlative with invasive areas and fibrosis.

Adenocarcinoma lesions that range from preinvasive to invasive pathologic entities correlate with the spectrum of appearances ranging from pGGN to solid lesions on chest CT. AAH is considered a preinvasive lesion according to the IASLC. On chest CT, AAH most often appears as a small pGGN that is 5 mm or

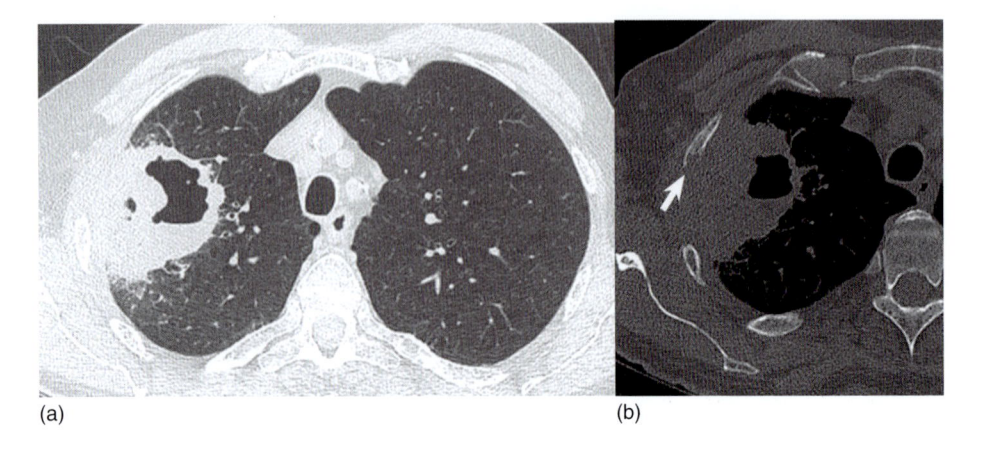

(a) (b)

Figure 9 **Chest wall invasion and cavitation in squamous cell carcinoma.** (a) Axial chest CT lung window showed a large rounded mass larger than 7 cm denoting T4 descriptor, with cavitation which has been described in squamous cell carcinoma. (b) Axial bone window image demonstrated erosion of adjacent rib (would denote T3 descriptor), consistent with chest wall invasion.

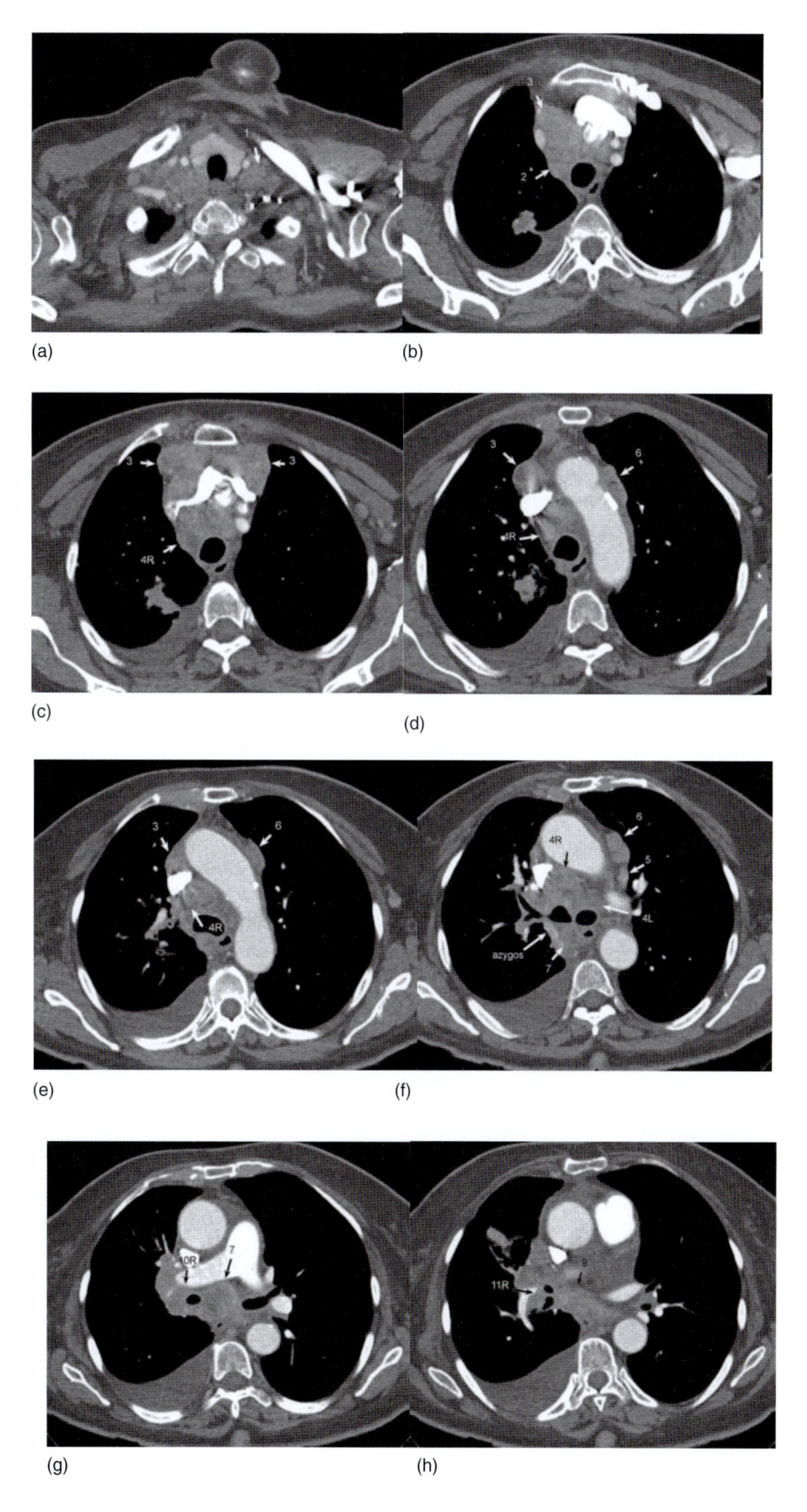

Figure 10 **Nodal stations**. (a–h) Axial chest CT images demonstrate adenopathy in nodal stations. Station 1, lower cervical, supraclavicular, and sternal notch nodes; station 2, upper paratracheal nodes; station 3a, prevascular nodes; station 3p, retrotracheal nodes (above level of carina); station 4, lower paratracheal nodes; station 5, subaortic nodes; station 6, para-aortic nodes (ascending aortic or phrenic); station 7, subcarinal nodes; station 8, para-esophageal nodes (below the level of carina); station 9, pulmonary ligament; station 10 hilar nodes; station 11, interlobar nodes; stations 12, 13, 14 lobar, segmental, and subsegmental lobes, respectively.

as the criterion of abnormal nodal enlargement. Approximately 8–15% of patients considered to have a negative CT scan for mediastinal nodal enlargement, with lymph nodes ≤1 cm, will ultimately be found to have mediastinal nodal involvement at the time of operation. Mediastinal lymph nodes that are ≥2 cm in diameter contain metastatic disease in over 90% of cases. Lymph nodes that are 1.5–2 cm in size contain disease in over 50% of cases. Lymph nodes that are 1–1.5 cm in size harbor metastatic disease in 15–30% of cases. The negative predictive accuracy of CT scan is 85–92% for mediastinal lymph node metastases.

Distant metastatic disease can be detected on CT and includes destructive bone lesions, soft tissue metastases to abdominal organs such as adrenal gland, liver, brain, and contralateral lung. Pleural and pericardial involvement, which indicates M1 disease, is suggested by a nodular or smooth thickening of the pleura or pericardium.[100,101]

MRI
Although MRI is not used for the routine evaluation of thoracic involvement in patients with lung cancer, it has specific advantages over CT scan. Because of its heightened ability related to high-contrast resolution to discern neurologic and vascular structures, tumors that reside in close proximity to neurovascular structures may be more accurately assessed by MRI than by CT scan. MRI is most useful in evaluating patients with superior sulcus tumors, in which brachial plexus involvement and relationship of tumor to the subclavian artery affect decisions as whether to pursue resection and, if so, surgical approach undertaken.[102,103] MRI can also be used to evaluate for brain metastases and is considered superior to noncontrast CT in sensitivity and comparable to or superior to contrast-enhanced CT.[104,105]

PET and integrated PET/CT
Over the past several years, PET scanning with 2-[^{18}F]fluoro-2-deoxy-D-gluce (FDG-PET) has been increasingly used in the diagnosis, staging, and therapeutic monitoring of lung cancer. This test identifies areas of increased glucose metabolism, which is a common trait in pulmonary tumors. Since commercial PET scanners provide nominal spatial resolution of 4.5–6.0 mm in the center of the axial field of view, even lesions that are ≤1 cm in diameter can be detected on the basis of an increased uptake of FDG. Although initially heralded as a reliable noninvasive method of characterizing pulmonary lesions as neoplasms, a number of limitations have become apparent. Many inflammatory processes such as abscesses and active granulomatous diseases. False-negative results have occurred primarily in tumors with low glucose metabolism such as carcinoid tumor, AIS, and MIA, and in small tumors, due to the limited spatial resolution of current PET scanners.[106] Combined PET/CT imaging has a major role in the initial evaluation and staging for patients with lung cancer, particularly in the preoperative assessment since it may potentially avoid unnecessary lung surgery by detecting metastases to the adrenals, liver, bone, and soft tissue.[107]

For tumor recurrence evaluation, PET/CT is not useful immediately after surgery or radiotherapy due to inflammation leading to abnormal uptake. Treatment-induced hypermetabolic inflammatory changes also may lead to difficulty differentiating between treatment effects and the of the residual tumor. Therefore, PET/CT utility is greatest when performed 6 months after radiotherapy, surgery, and minimally invasive ablative therapies such as cryoablation.[108] The development of new or increasing metabolic activity in regions that have prior therapy changes and previously had low-FDG uptake raises suspicion of neoplasm. In these cases, PET/CT information can be used direct any sampling approaches when recurrent disease suspected within posttreatment changes.

Sputum cytology
Cytologic evaluation of sputum, bronchial washings, bronchial brushings, and FNA specimens have high diagnostic yield, but the positive and negative predictive values of each and their accuracy of diagnosis certainly are dependent on sampling error, tissue preservation, processing quality, and observer experience. Sputum cytology is a simple test with a specificity rate of 99%. However, the sensitivity rate is approximately 70% for central tumors and less than 50% for peripheral lesions. To increase the yield, 3 specimens are usually collected. In practice, more invasive measures to obtain a diagnosis are used in most cases.

Invasive studies

Tissue is collected for histopathological diagnosis, molecular studies, and genetic testing. In most cases, FNA for cytological assessment does not suffice and core biopsies are recommended. Endobronchial and centrally located tumors are usually diagnosed with bronchoscopy, whereas peripheral lesions with image-guided biopsies such as CT or US. In many cases, the biopsy is targeted to a lesion that would determine the diagnosis and the stage of the disease.

FNA and core biopsy
Transthoracic percutaneous needle aspiration biopsy (TPNAB) and core needle biopsy have significantly heightened the ability to diagnose intrathoracic pathologic processes. With CT or US guidance, tissue samples can be obtained from poorly accessible sites in the lung, mediastinum, abdomen, and retroperitoneum. The procedure is performed under local anesthesia or conscious sedation using a small-gauge needle or core biopsy device to obtain either an aspirate or core biopsy sample, respectively. Aspiration and core biopsy material are immediately processed with optimal procedural coordination. Many centers use an on-site cytopathologist for interpretation. In case of inadequate material, a repeat aspiration can be performed. Multiple samples can be obtained for molecular testing if needed, often core samples.[109,110] TPNAB has been shown to be over 90% effective in establishing a final diagnosis. The false-positive rate is low (1%) and the false-negative rate ranges from 23% to 29%.[111] TPNAB can also be performed on sub-solid lesions.[112,113] Despite the high diagnostic yield of transthoracic percutaneous needle biopsy, the potential benefits of the procedure must be balanced with the risks. Pneumothorax occurs in approximately 10% of patients undergoing the procedure, and patients with significant emphysema and more centrally located lesions may be at increased risk.[114]

Fiberoptic bronchoscopy (FOB)
FOB is an essential and standard technique for the evaluation of patients with pulmonary neoplasms. FOB permits careful survey of the supraglottic, glottic, tracheal, and bronchial regions to the level of most subsegments. Tumor (T) status can be defined by measuring tumor proximity to the carina and various bronchi and by identifying unsuspected occult lesions that indicate multiplicity of disease. For lesions that are visible by endoscopy, an accurate histologic diagnosis can be achieved in over 90% of cases. For central lesions, cytologic studies via needle aspiration, washings,

and brushings, coupled with biopsy, heighten the diagnostic yield to over 95%. Peripheral lesions not visible endoscopically may be approached by cytologic studies of brushings and bronchioloalveolar lavage (BAL), which yield a diagnosis in 50–60% of patients. Cytologic studies, coupled with transbronchial FNA (TBNA), greatly enhance diagnostic yield.

TBNA biopsy has been used most widely to sample endobronchial and peripheral lesions, and significantly improves the diagnostic yield when coupled with standard diagnostic measures (washings, brushings, and biopsies).[115] TBNA is best performed in a suite that is equipped with fluoroscopy to enhance localization of the lesion. One of the most important applications of TBNA is the evaluation of mediastinal lymphadenopathy. The sensitivity and specificity of TBNA appear to range from 14% to 50% and 96% to 100%, respectively.

Endobronchial US-guided transbronchial needle aspiration (EBUS-TBNA) was developed to improve the diagnostic yield of TBNA for centrally located lesions, including lymphadenopathy. This technology incorporates an US transducer to the end of a bronchoscope, thereby allowing the bronchoscopist to have real-time, continuous visualization of TBNA within the targeted lesion. EBUS-TBNA has demonstrated diagnostic yield greater than 90% for NSCLC as well as for SCLC and has become the recommended procedure of first choice for pathologic staging due to its safety profile as well as ability to reach mediastinal and hilar lymph node stations using a minimally invasive approach.[116]

Advances in peripheral bronchoscopy

Conventional bronchoscopic approaches using fluoroscopy alone for the diagnosis of peripheral pulmonary lesions have largely yielded suboptimal results when compared to transthoracic approaches. Image guidance has been developed to improve the diagnostic yield of peripheral bronchoscopy. Electromagnetic navigational (EMN) systems and virtual bronchoscopic navigation (VBN) utilize thin-slice CT images to generate virtual airway reconstructions that the bronchoscopist utilizes to locate targeted peripheral lesions. ENB systems also include a sensor that is tracked during procedures to facilitate gaining proximity to peripheral lesions prior to biopsy.[64] Radial probe endobronchial ultrasound (r-EBUS) utilizes a radial scanning US probe advanced into the lung periphery through the bronchoscope to confirm lesion location in real-time prior to performing biopsies.[117] Additional advancements in peripheral bronchoscopy include thin and ultrathin bronchoscopes designed to augment reach into the lung periphery and even robotic bronchoscopic platforms, although these methods remain in early phases of investigation and validation.[118,119]

Mediastinoscopy

Transcervical mediastinoscopy is the best method for invasive evaluation of the middle mediastinum to include the peritracheal and subcarinal lymph nodes. The main indication is the preoperative mediastinal nodal assessment in patients with CT scan evidence of cross-sectional lymph node enlargement of ≥1 cm. In such patients who are proven to have lung cancer, the chance that these nodes contain metastasis is over 7%. If the nodes are enlarged to 1.5–2 cm or more, the risk of having metastatic involvement is over 30%. The accuracy of cervical mediastinoscopy ranges from 80% to 90%, and the false-negative rate ranges from 10% to 12%. The lymph node station most commonly missampled is the subcarinal region, which is difficult to access in some patients. The subaortic and aortopulmonary window regions are inaccessible by standard cervical mediastinoscopy.[120] Extended cervical mediastinoscopy, a variation of standard mediastinoscopy, has been useful for staging lesions in the left upper lobe. Anterior mediastinostomy allows a direct visual access to the anterior mediastinum through the second, third, or fourth anterior interspace, with or without removal of a short portion of the adjacent cartilage. For right-sided lesions, the procedure provides access to the proximal pulmonary artery and SVC.

Thoracoscopy

Thoracoscopy and video-assisted thoracoscopy (VATS) are used in a broader range of applications, including resectional techniques. The VATS approach is used in many thoracic conditions, and its role continues to evolve regarding the evaluation and management of lung cancer. It is currently considered for the evaluation and treatment of pleural tumors and effusions and in the diagnosis of indeterminate pulmonary nodules and has a complementary role to standard mediastinoscopy in the staging of mediastinal lymph nodes. It has also become an accepted approach for resection of peripheral early-stage lung cancer in many centers.[121]

Treatment of NSCLC

Treatment of patients with operable NSCLC

Surgery
For early-stage lung cancer, surgical resection has been the cornerstone of local treatment for the past several decades. Elimination of the primary tumor offers effective local control provided that the tumor is completely resected with microscopically negative margins (R0). Incompletely resected NSCLC patients with microscopic (R1) or macroscopic (R2) residual disease are at higher risk of early death, regardless of stage.[122] To fully realize the benefit of surgery, it is imperative to carefully select patients who could tolerate surgery, specifically in the context of comorbidities and the extent of lung resection required.

Patients being considered for lung cancer surgery should be evaluated and treated by a thoracic surgeon specializing in lung cancer surgery as a prominent part of their practice. Surgical candidacy is based on a thorough evaluation including age, frailty or performance status, preoperative pulmonary function testing (PFT), extent of lung resection required, and comorbidities especially cardiovascular. Risk assessment must reflect a global impression of the patient's health, and no single factor automatically disqualifies a patient for surgery. However, compounding high-risk patient characteristics such as advanced age, poor performance status, and cardiac disease would make it less likely the patient would survive the perioperative period, or preserve their quality of life enough to realize the benefit of surgical treatment.

PFT is critical to determining surgical candidacy. This outpatient noninvasive test measures spirometry values including lung volume, capacity, and flow rates, as well as gas exchange, requiring effort and cooperation by the patient. The parameters that surgeons often reference for surgical risk determination are forced expiratory volume after 1 second (FEV1) and diffusing capacity of the lung for carbon monoxide (DLCO). For comparative purposes, the FEV1 and DLCO are typically considered as a "percentage of predicted," with the predicted values calculated using reference values based on age, height, gender, and race. Recognizing that different pulmonary resections may impact pulmonary function to varying degrees, based on extent of resection and tumor location, many surgeons estimate the postoperative pulmonary function. The residual lung function after surgery can be estimated by multiplying the preoperative values by the fraction of residual lung segments following surgery (19 segments minus the number of segments removed divided by 19 segments). Postoperative FEV1 and DLCO of more than 40% of predicted is generally considered to be safe assuming that all segments contribute equally to lung function although this may not always be the case. A perfusion scan provides an estimate of the relative contribution of right and left lungs and may be particularly helpful in patients with prior treatment including surgery and radiation therapy.

Lung cancer surgery can be performed either minimally invasively or via thoracotomy. The decision about the approach is based on tumor size, location, relationship to critical structures, patient comorbidities, and surgeon experience. Minimally invasive approaches include VATS or robotic-assisted thoracic surgery (RATS). In addition, due to decreased pain with minimally invasive approaches, the postoperative recovery and length of stay are shortened, as well as reduced postoperative complications such as postoperative air leaks, pneumonia, and atrial fibrillation. The advent of robotic technology for the RATS approach continues to gain popularity and appears to be as safe, as oncologically sound, and with similar benefits of improved perioperative recovery as VATS, but comparative analyses of outcomes and costs are still ongoing.[123]

The extent of surgical resection refers to the amount of lung parenchyma that is taken during the procedure. In theory, failure to take sufficient lung parenchyma could expose a patient to higher risk of local failure, while removing too much could have implications for perioperative complications and long-term lung function. The determination of the optimal extent of resection is further complicated by need to consider the stage of the tumor, the histology, the perceived or observed natural history, and the patient's health.

Lobectomy has been the oncologic standard and is the most common type of resection performed for lung cancer, with a R0 lobectomy offering optimal local control by removing the primary tumor along with its lymphatic basins. Pneumonectomies are generally indicated for central tumors that either span across multiple pulmonary lobes, or are inseparable from bronchovascular structures servicing the uninvolved lobes. Right-sided pneumonectomy is the highest risk pulmonary procedure, with morbidities such as pneumonia, acute respiratory distress syndrome, bronchopleural fistula occurring at a higher rate and with significantly reduced stage-specific 5-year survival than left pneumonectomy.[124]

Sublobar resections involve the removal of less lung parenchyma than lobectomies and can either be anatomically based, by dividing the smaller bronchovasculature to the segment (a segmentectomy), or nonanatomic by simply pulling the lung tissue into a stapler without attempting to dissect out the airways and vessels (wedge resections). Currently, segmentectomy is indicated in patients where pulmonary function precludes lobectomy. Patients with tumors <2 cm in size who undergo segmentectomy appear to have similar oncologic outcomes as lobectomy, although trials are still ongoing.[125] Wedge resection, in contrast, is typically performed for peripheral lesions requiring diagnosis. Wedge resection as a therapeutic option is currently reserved for patients with particularly poor lung function, benign histology, indolent courses such as carcinoid tumors or potentially lesions lacking a solid component on imaging.[126]

Radiation therapy

Patients with early-stage NSCLC who are deemed high risk for surgical complications may be offered local control with nonsurgical treatments such as stereotactic body radiotherapy (SBRT). There is a substantial evidence that SBRT achieves comparable local control in patients who are unfit for surgery. Several randomized trials were launched to compare surgery to SBRT in patients who were operative candidates but ultimately closed secondary to poor accrual. While case series for SBRT in operable patients are encouraging, observational data consistently favors surgery although it is difficult to mitigate the health-related bias against SBRT in observational studies.[127] Overall, in patients who are surgical candidates, there is insufficient evidence to support SBRT as being equivalent to surgery, and surgery is currently the standard of care for patients felt to be reasonable candidates.

Adjuvant and neoadjuvant therapy

The standard of care for patients with completely resected NSCLC stage IB to IIA according to the AJCC sixth edition (AJCC6) is to administer four cycles of cisplatin-based adjuvant chemotherapy, which according to the lung adjuvant cisplatin evaluation (LACE) pooled analysis, increases the 5-year overall survival (OS) from 64% to 67% in stage IB, 39% to 49% in stage II and 26% to 39% in stage IIIA.[128,129] Although the role for adjuvant chemotherapy has been well established for patients with stage II or III according to the AJCC6 staging classification, the LACE analyses showed no benefit in OS or disease-free survival (DFS) for adjuvant chemotherapy in patients with stage IB disease and was detrimental for the with stage IA.[128] Nevertheless, in the exploratory analysis of the Cancer and Leukemia Group B (CALGB) 9633 study, which randomized patients with resected stage IB NSCLC to adjuvant chemotherapy with carboplatin plus paclitaxel or observation, there was a survival improvement for adjuvant therapy in the with tumors ≥4 cm with median OS of 99 months in the treatment group versus 77 in the control group (hazard ratio [HR] 0.69; 95% confidence interval [CI] 0.48–0.99, $p = 0.043$).[130] In a subsequent analysis of patients with stage IB enrolled into the JBR-10 trial, where patients with completely resected NSCLC were randomized to adjuvant chemotherapy with cisplatin plus vinorelbine or observation, there was no benefit from adjuvant chemotherapy although the 5-year OS was numerically higher for the with tumors ≥4 cm receiving chemotherapy (79% vs 59%; HR 0.66; 95% CI 0.39–1.14, $p = 0.13$).[131] This cutoff in tumor size for stage IB was subsequently used the ECOG-1505, which randomized patients with resected NSCLC stages IB ≥4 cm to IIIA according to the AJCC6, to cisplatin-based chemotherapy doublets with or without bevacizumab.[132] The trial showed that the addition of bevacizumab did not improve the OS compared to chemotherapy alone and, although it was not designed to compare the chemotherapy regimens, there were no clear differences among the four chemotherapy regimens used, which included cisplatin (75 mg/m^2 on day 1) plus docetaxel (75 mg/m^2 on day 1), gemcitabine (1200 mg/m^2 on days 1 and 8), vinorelbine (30 mg/m^2 on days 1 and 8), or pemetrexed (500 mg/m^2 on day 1) every 21 days.

In patients with resectable NSCLC, although no direct comparisons have been made between preoperative (neoadjuvant) and adjuvant chemotherapy, there appear to be no differences in benefit over observation regarding the timing of the chemotherapy. In the Southwest Oncology Group Trial 9900, patients with stage IB to IIIA NSCLC were randomized to surgery alone or preceded by three cycles of neoadjuvant carboplatin plus paclitaxel.[133] The trial started accrual in 1999 and was closed prematurely in 2004 due to compelling evidence for the benefit of adjuvant chemotherapy. Among the 354 enrolled patients, the median OS was 62 months and 41 months, respectively, in the neoadjuvant and surgery alone arms (HR 0.79; 95% CI 0.60–1.06, $p = 0.11$). In an indirect comparison meta-analysis involving 32 randomized trials with more than 10,000 patients, there was no evidence of a difference in OS or DFS between neoadjuvant and adjuvant chemotherapy.[134]

The role of adjuvant radiation therapy for patients with completely resected NSCLC is still unclear. Database studies have shown a benefit from postoperative radiation therapy (PORT) in patients with N2 disease[135,136] and the subset analysis of the Adjuvant Navelbine International Trialist Association (ANITA) showed improved 5-year OS from PORT compared to no radiation therapy in both patients treated with adjuvant chemotherapy (47.4% vs 34%) and in the randomized to observation (21.3% vs 16.6%).[137] Nevertheless, the LUNG ART trial which randomized patients with completely resected NSCLC with N2 involvement to PORT or observation, there were no significant differences with median DFS and 3-year DFS of 30.5 months and 47.1%, respectively in the PORT arm and 22.8 months and 43.8%, respectively for the control arm (HR 0.85; 95% CI 0.67–1.07, $p = 0.16$).[138]

More recently, both neoadjuvant and adjuvant trials have been focused on the use of targeted therapies or ICIs. For patients with completely resected NSCLC harboring *EGFR* exon 19 deletion or L858R mutation, adjuvant treatment with EGFR TKI, either gefitinib or erlotinib, showed improved DFS compared to chemotherapy.[139,140] Similarly, results were found in the ADAURA, where patients with completely resected stage II or III NSCLC harboring sensitizing *EGFR* mutations were randomized to osimertinib or placebo for 3 years.[141] The percentage of patients that were alive and disease-free at 24 months was 90% in the osimertinib group and 44% in the placebo group (HR 0.17; $p < 0.001$). Neoadjuvant treatment with ICI provides a theoretical benefit over adjuvant treatment since the higher levels of endogenous tumor antigens present in the primary tumor may enhance T-cell priming.[142,143] In patients with NSCLC, neoadjuvant treatment with ICI has shown promising results in multiple nonrandomized phase 2 studies including ICI alone or in combination with chemotherapy.[144–149] Several other studies including randomized trials comparing neoadjuvant chemotherapy plus ICI to chemotherapy alone or ICI alone are currently ongoing and may define the new standard of care for patients with resectable disease.[150]

Treatment of patients with inoperable locally advanced NSCLC

Radiation therapy
The majority of patients with lung cancer will receive radiotherapy at some point in their disease, either for initial treatment of localized disease, for palliation, or increasingly for aggressive treatment of limited metastatic sites.[151] Many of these patients will receive combined modality therapy, and increasingly their treatment will rely on advances in radiation technology that have offered incremental improvements in outcome over the past decade or more. Over the past two decades, radiation planning has evolved from two-dimensional (generous fields based on bony anatomic landmarks) to three-dimensional (requiring contouring of tumor and normal tissue volumes on CT datasets). The incorporation of 3D anatomy significantly reduces the exposure of normal tissue to unnecessary radiation, and as a result, significantly decreases the toxicity associated with treatment. Over the past 10 years, the increasing use of four-dimensional CT (4DCT) technology has allowed the capture of the movement of tumor and organs with respiration, further improving accuracy. The use of intensity-modulated radiation therapy (IMRT), volumetric-modulated arc therapy (VMAT), and proton therapy for treatment planning and delivery improve the conformality of the dose distribution to the tumor target.

The International Commission on Radiation Units and Measurements defines a number of volumes for radiation treatment planning.[152] The clinically macroscopic disease, as typically identified on any imaging modality, is defined as the gross tumor volume (GTV). The GTV in the lung cancer patient is derived from a treatment planning CT, often a four-dimensional CT that captures the motion of the tumor with respiration. These images are combined with pathologic staging information and PET/CT imaging. The clinical target volume (CTV) represents an expansion of the GTV in order to encompass microscopic disease. For the primary tumor and nodal disease, pathologically derived correlative data can be used to estimate the expansion required to account for microscopic extension beyond what is radiographically visible. This can be further informed by analysis of established patterns of tumor spread and the use of consensus radiographic atlases of nodal stations. The internal target volume (ITV) and internal gross tumor volume (IGTV) are defined as an expansion of a CTV or a GTV respectively to account for tumor motion that may occur with respiration. This is commonly generated from a four-dimensional CT, which captures the position of the tumor and surrounding organs at risk at various points throughout the respiratory cycle. The planning target volume (PTV) is a volumetric expansion of the CTV to account for daily variations in patient setup. Modern linear accelerators include cone-beam CT and other imaging modalities so that imaging can be obtained immediately before and during each fraction of radiation. The use of image-guided radiation therapy (IGRT) allows for increased accuracy, reducing the setup uncertainty and decreasing the expansion required for the PTV.

Normal tissue organs at risk are routinely defined for avoidance during radiation planning. For thoracic cases, the bilateral lungs, esophagus, heart, brachial plexus are included, with the addition of other organs such as upper abdominal structures for appropriate cases. Normal tissue dose limits are reasonably well established and should be considered in balance with adequate coverage of the target volume.[153] The risk of radiation pneumonitis is directly related to the volume of lung exposed to radiation, specifically to doses of 20 Gy or higher, and this frequently limits or even precludes treatment of large or extensive locally advanced tumors.[154] The mean radiation dose to the esophagus is highly correlated to esophagitis, the dose-limiting toxicity for combined modality therapy. Recent data demonstrate that radiation dose to the heart is predictive of late treatment-related cardiac events and mortality.

The overall goal of radiation treatment planning is to optimize the therapeutic ratio, that is, to maximize the dose to the target, while minimizing dose to surrounding normal organs. As described above, target and organ-at-risk volumes are defined based on imaging studies, established patterns of tumor spread, and pathologic staging information. Three-dimensional conformal radiotherapy (3D-CRT) indicates that the tumor targets and organs at risk have been defined (contoured) on CT image datasets, so that optimal beam angles can be determined. An essential part of 3D-CRT is the generation of a dose-volume histogram, which reports the incremental accumulated dose to partial volumes of targets and normal structures. This allows design of plans that can meet prespecified dose/volume limits. IMRT is a technically complex method of treatment planning in which radiation is delivered using a large number of beam angles or dynamic arcs, relying on computer algorithms to plan and deliver highly modulated beams. The use of IMRT or VMAT (an IMRT technique using rotational arcs) allows more conformal "painting" of dose around target volumes and normal tissues. Because of the potential for highly conformal plans using these techniques, a higher degree of accuracy is required. IMRT and VMAT for thoracic tumors typically require the use of IGRT and information on respiratory motion from 4D datasets.

SBRT allows precise targeting and delivery of high doses of radiation therapy. For lung cancer, SBRT can deliver highly conformal radiation to a discrete thoracic target such as an early primary lung cancer or metastatic pulmonary lesion. The technique requires multiple beam angles and/or arcs, and high-precision localization. This achieves significantly higher dose to the target when compared to fractionated techniques, with relatively low exposure of surrounding organs. For tumors that can be approached in this manner, the result is significantly improved control and survival, with lower toxicity, when compared with conventional fractionated radiation.[155] The use of SBRT is limited to discrete targets which are not immediately adjacent to mediastinal structures, so it is not routinely useful for the potentially curative treatment of locally advanced disease.

Due to their physical properties and method of interaction with matter, particle beams, such as protons, have the potential to offer improved dose profiles when compared with the more common photon beam radiation. In patients with lung cancer, proton therapy offers the promise of delivering therapeutic radiation doses to extensive or complex targets while sparing the surrounding dose-limiting structures such as lungs, heart, and esophagus. Initial studies demonstrate the ability to use photons to treat challenging tumors that are otherwise untreatable with standard photon radiation. A large randomized trial is in locally advanced NSCLC is ongoing (NCT01993810). Until its completion, the value of proton radiation for lung cancer, and the patient characteristics that would suggest a clinical benefit, remains unclear.

Combined modality therapy for inoperable stage III NSCLC

Historically, patients with unresectable stage III NSCLC were treated with fractionated radiation alone. The optimal radiation dose of 60 Gy in 30 fractions was established in the four-arm RTOG 7301 study, but outcomes were suboptimal including a 2-year OS of 25%, with high rates of both local and distant failure.[156] In an effort to improve outcomes, chemotherapy was added to radiation, first sequentially and ultimately concurrently. In the seminal CALGB 8433 study, two cycles of cisplatin and vinblastine sequentially prior to radiation improved the 5-year OS from 7% to 19% compared to radiation therapy alone.[157] Similarly, the addition of daily or weekly cisplatin concurrently with radiation improved both local control and survival compared to radiation alone[158] as did the concurrent delivery of mitomycin, vindesine, and cisplatin.[159] Finally, the RTOG 9410 compared concurrent cisplatin-based chemoradiotherapy to sequential treatment and demonstrated that concurrent therapy improved OS compared to sequential treatment (5-year OS 16% versus 10%).[160]

Recurrence within the radiation field remains one of the predominant patterns of failure after 60 Gy, with locoregional failure rates of approximately 40% despite the incorporation of concurrent chemotherapy.[160] A number of efforts were undertaken to increase the radiation dose, leveraging improvement in radiation technology to improve control rates without increasing toxicity. The phase III RTOG 0617 compared conventional (60 Gy) versus escalated (74 Gy) thoracic radiation with concurrent weekly paclitaxel and carboplatin with or without cetuximab in patients with stage IIIA or B NSCLC.[161] Surprisingly, the high-dose arms closed early due to futility, with an OS that was worse than conventional radiation therapy (median 20.3 vs 28.7 months), and with more treatment-related deaths. Subsequent analysis found that radiation dose to the normal tissue structures including the heart were predictive of an increased risk of death, a finding that has been corroborated with other datasets.[162] Intriguingly, the use of IMRT, which was optional in this study, was associated with significantly reduced dose to heart and lungs, and decreased toxicity, despite the fact that it was used predominantly in larger tumors.[163] Therefore, while results of the 0617 affirmed 60 Gy as the standard dose for thoracic radiation, there remains enduring interest in selectively escalating dose in an effort to reduce local failure, with attention to limiting normal tissue exposure with the use of advanced radiation technology. Strategies being examined to accomplish this include the use of proton therapy (NCT01993810) and adaptive treatment based on initial response (NCT01507428).

The optimal chemotherapy backbone has not been defined since no regimen has emerged as the most effective during concurrent use of thoracic radiation. Therefore, there are several acceptable options available (Table 8). In the PROCLAIM study, 598 patients with unresectable stage III NSCLC were randomized to cisplatin plus pemetrexed or cisplatin plus etoposide.[164] The study showed no significant differences in the median progression-free survival (PFS) (11.4 months vs 9.8 months; HR 0.86; 95% CI 0.71–1.04, $p = 0.13$) or 3-year OS (40% vs 37%). In the CALGB 30407 study, the addition of cetuximab to carboplatin plus pemetrexed did not improve the primary endpoint of 18-month OS compared to chemotherapy alone (58% vs 54%).[167] Nevertheless, the 18-month OS of 58% with the concurrent chemoradiotherapy arm including carboplatin plus pemetrexed met the prespecified criteria for further studies. In the PACIFIC trial, 709 patients with stage III NSCLC who did not have tumor progression after completion of concurrent chemoradiotherapy were randomized in a 2:1 ratio to receive durvalumab 10 mg/kg every 2 weeks for 12 months or placebo.[168,169] The co-primary endpoints were PFS and OS from the time of randomization. After a median follow-up of 25.2 months, durvalumab was associated with a significant improvement in both median PFS (17.2 months vs 5.6 months, HR 0.51, 95% CI 0.41–0.63) and 24-month (66.3% vs 55.6%, HR 0.68, 95% CI 0.47–0.99, $p = 0.002$). OS Pneumonitis occurred in 33.9% of patients treated with durvalumab (3.4% grade 3 or 4) and 24.8% in the placebo arm (2.6% grade 3 or 4). In the subsequent analysis with a median follow-up of 33.3 months, the median OS was 29.1 months with placebo and had not been reached with durvalumab.[170] The 36-month OS was 55.3% for durvalumab and 43.5% for the placebo arms (HR 0.68, 95% CI 0.53–0.87).

Table 8 Selected randomized trials in patients with locally advanced NSCLC.

Study	Regimen (N)	Median PFS (months)	Median OS (months)
PROCLAIM[164]	Cisplatin plus pemetrexed[165]	11.4	26.8
	Cisplatin plus etoposide[166]	9.8	25
CALGB 30407[167]	Carboplatin plus pemetrexed[48]	12.6	21.2
	Carboplatin plus pemetrexed and cetuximab[53]	12.3	25.2
PACIFIC[168,169]	Consolidation durvalumab	17.2	Not reached
	Placebo	5.6	29.1

Treatment of patients with stage IV NSCLC
The treatment of patients with stage IV NSCLC is dictated by the performance status, comorbidities, histology, molecular markers, and PD-L1 status. In general, patients with actionable gene alterations should receive a targeted agent as the initial treatment regardless of PD-L1 score.

Treatment of patients with stage IV non-small-cell lung cancer without driver alterations
The current treatment of patients with stage IV NSCLC without driver alterations or contraindications for the use of immunotherapy includes an ICI with or without a platinum-based chemotherapy doublet, with the choice depending on the PD-L1 expression and histology.[171]

Multiple randomized clinical trials have shown improved survival for first-line platinum-based combination chemotherapy over supportive care[172,173] and single-agent cisplatin.[174,175] The results from studies comparing platinum doublets to single-agent nonplatinum drugs, however, showed increased response rate and time to progression for cisplatin plus docetaxel or carboplatin plus paclitaxel compared to taxane alone but without a significant improvement in the median OS.[176,177] Nevertheless, platinum doublets were recommended as the standard of care by the American Society of Clinical Oncology (ASCO) guidelines based on the results from meta-analyses showing a benefit compared to single-agent chemotherapy.[178-180] Two meta-analyses comparing chemotherapy doublets including cisplatin or carboplatin showed increased toxicity for the former with increased response rates and a modest improvement in median OS.[181,182] Randomized clinical trials did not reveal the best platinum-based combination, with no significant differences in OS among the treatment arms.[183-185] The role for histology was initially observed in a subset analysis of the large randomized trial comparing cisplatin plus pemetrexed or gemcitabine.[186] Although the median OS was identical at 10.3 months, the cisplatin plus pemetrexed arm was associated with improved median OS in patients with nonsquamous histology (11.8 vs 10.4 months; HR 0.67; $p = 0.005$) and worse median OS in the with squamous histology (9.4 vs 10.8 months; HR 1.23; $p = 0.05$). In another large randomized trial comparing carboplatin plus *nab*-paclitaxel or paclitaxel, there were no significant differences in PFS or OS. Nevertheless, *nab*-paclitaxel was associated with a significant improvement in the objective response rate (33% vs 25%, $p = 0.005$), in an effect that was observed in patients with squamous histology (41% vs 24%, $p < 0.01$) but not in those with nonsquamous histology (26% vs 25%, $p = 0.9$).

The addition of bevacizumab to the chemotherapy double was associated with improved median PFS compared to chemotherapy alone in two randomized studies, although only one showed improvement in the median OS.[187,188] Of note, neither trial allowed patients with squamous cell histology due to the increased incidence of life-threatening hemoptysis observed in the phase II study.[189] The addition of cetuximab, a monoclonal antibody against EGFR, to cisplatin plus vinorelbine was associated with improved survival compared to chemotherapy alone.[190] Nevertheless, the survival was not improved with the addition of cetuximab to carboplatin plus paclitaxel.[191] The addition of necitumumab, a second-generation EGFR monoclonal antibody, to cisplatin plus gemcitabine, was associated with a significant improvement in the median OS compared to chemotherapy alone (11.5 vs 9.9 months, HR 0.84, $p = 0.01$) in patients with squamous cell carcinoma.[192] The improvement in the median OS, however, was not observed when necitumumab was added to cisplatin plus pemetrexed in patients with nonsquamous histology (11.3 vs 11.5 months; HR 1.01, $p = 0.96$).[193]

Following the initial four cycles of platinum-based chemotherapy, patients have been offered maintenance therapy with the same nonplatinum drug used during the initial regimen, a monoclonal antibody against EGFR or VEGF or both. Since neither pemetrexed nor bevacizumab have been used in patients with squamous cell carcinoma due to decreased efficacy and increased risk for toxicity respectively, recent studies on maintenance chemotherapy have been restricted to patients with nonsquamous histology.[194-197] In the ECOG-ACRIN 5508 trial, 1516 patients were treated with carboplatin plus paclitaxel and bevacizumab, with 874 subsequently randomized to maintenance therapy with pemetrexed, bevacizumab, or both.[198] Although the median PFS was higher in the combination arm (7.5 months vs 4.1 months for pemetrexed and 5.1 months for BCP), there was no significant improvement in the median OS (16.4 months vs 15.9 months with pemetrexed and 14.4 months with BCP) and the combination was associated with increased toxicity. In a randomized study comparing maintenance *nab*-paclitaxel to best supportive care after completion of four cycles of carboplatin plus *nab*-paclitaxel in patients with squamous cell lung cancer, the primary endpoint of PFS was not met (3.1 months vs 2.6 months; HR 0.85, $p = 0.36$), although there was a significant improvement in the median OS (17.7 months vs 12.1 months; HR 0.68; 95% CI 0.47–0.98, $p = 0.03$).[199]

ICIs in the treatment of lung cancer were initially evaluated in previously treated patients with advanced-stage NSCLC. In the CheckMate 003 phase I trial, 296 patients with solid tumors including NSCLC, melanoma, castration-resistant prostate cancer, renal cell, or colorectal cancer were treated with nivolumab from 0.1 to 10 mg/kg every 2 weeks for a maximum of 2 years.[200] Among the 129 patients with NSCLC treated with nivolumab doses of 1, 3, or 10 mg/kg, the objective response rate was 17% with an unprecedented estimated 5-year OS of 16%.[201] Promising initial results were also observed with pembrolizumab, particularly in patients with PD-L1 expression of at least 50%, and atezolizumab.[202,203] Subsequent randomized studies have shown that immune checkpoint inhibition with nivolumab, pembrolizumab, or ACP was more effective than docetaxel, leading to the approval of all three drugs in patients with previously treated stage IV NSCLC.[204-207]

The transition of ICIs to the first-line setting started with the landmark KEYNOTE-024 trial, where 305 patients with previously untreated NSCLC with PD-L1 expression of at least 50% and no *EGFR* mutation or *ALK* rearrangement were randomized to single-agent pembrolizumab or four to six cycles of a platinum-based chemotherapy.[208] The primary endpoint of median PFS was met with an increase from 6 months in the chemotherapy arm to 10.3 months with pembrolizumab (HR 0.50; 95% CI 0.37–0.68, $p < 0.001$). Pembrolizumab was also associated with increased response rate (44.8% vs 27.8%) and decreased treatment-related adverse events of any grade (73% vs 90% of patients) or grades 3–5 (26.6% vs 53.3%). In an updated analysis of the study, the median OS was significantly higher in the pembrolizumab arm (30.0 months vs 14.2 months; HR 0.63; 95% CI 0.47–0.86, $p = 0.002$).[209] Since then, several studies have evaluated the use of immune checkpoint blockers either alone or in combination with chemotherapy in the first-line setting (Table 9). The KEYNOTE-042 was a similar study, which randomized previously untreated patients with advanced-stage NSCLC to pembrolizumab or chemotherapy.[216] Unlike the KEYNOTE-24, however, patients with PD-L1 expression between 1% and 49% were also eligible and crossover from the chemotherapy to pembrolizumab was not allowed. The study showed that the median

Table 9 Selected randomized clinical trials involving first-line immune checkpoint inhibitors.

Trial	Treatment	Patients	Response rate (%)	Median PFS (months)	Median OS (months)
KEYNOTE-024[208,209]	Pembrolizumab	154	44.8	10.3	30.0
	Platinum doublet	151	27.8	6.0	14.2
IMpower-110[210]	Atezolizumab	107[a]	38.3	8.1	20.2
	Platinum doublet	98[a]	28.6	5.0	13.1
KEYNOTE-189[211,212]	Plat-Peme-Pembrolizumab	410	48	9	22
	Plat-Peme	206	19.4	4.9	10.7
KEYNOTE-407[213]	Plat-tax-pembrolizumab	278	62.6	8.0	17.1
	Plat-tax	281	38.4	5.1	11.6
IMpower-130[214]	Carb-nabPac-Atezolizumab	451	49.2	7.0	18.6
	Carb-nabPac	228	31.9	5.5	13.9
CheckMate-227 (PD-L1 ≥ 1%)[215]	Nivolumab plus ipilimumab	396	35.9	5.1	17.1
	Platinum doublet	397	30.0	5.6	14.9
CheckMate-227 (PD-L1 < 1%)[215]	Nivolumab plus ipilimumab	185	27.3	5.1	17.2
	Platinum doublet	387	23.1	4.7	12.2

KEYNOTE-024 included only patients with PD-L1 ≥ 50%.
KEYNOTE-189 and IMpower-130 included only patients with nonsquamous histology.
KEYNOTE-407 included only patients with squamous histology.
Carb, Carboplatin; nabPac, nab-paclitaxel; Peme, Pemetrexed; Plat, Platinum (carboplatin or cisplatin); Tax, Taxane (paclitaxel or nab-paclitaxel).
[a]Patients with PD-L1 ≥ 50%.

OS was significantly higher with pembrolizumab compared to chemotherapy among patients with PD-L1 ≥ 1%, ≥20%, or ≥50%. Nevertheless, in the important population of patients with PD-L1 between 1% and 49%, which was included only in a prespecified exploratory subset analysis, there was no improvement in the median compared to chemotherapy (13.4 months vs 12.1 months), suggesting that the benefit from pembrolizumab observed in the study was driven by the patients with PD-L1 ≥ 50%, which represented 47% of the total number of patients enrolled. In a similar study, the IMpower-110, first-line atezolizumab was associated with a significant improvement in the median OS compared to chemotherapy alone (20.2 months vs 13.1 months; HR 0.59, $p = 0.01$), with the benefit observed only in the high PD-L1 expression, leading to its approval in this setting.[210] The CheckMate-026 study, however, showed no improvement in either PFS or OS for first-line nivolumab compared to chemotherapy in patients with previously untreated NSCLC and PD-L1 expression ≥ 5%.[217] In the CheckMate-227, the combination of nivolumab and ipilimumab was associated with improved median OS compared to chemotherapy in patients with both PD-L1 ≥ 1% (17.1 months vs 14.9 months; HR 0.79, 95% CI 0.65–0.96, $p = 0.007$) and < 1% (17.2 months vs 12.2 months; HR 0.62; 95% CI 0.49–0.79).[215]

In addition to the chemotherapy-free regimens including single-agent pembrolizumab, atezolizumab or the combination of nivolumab plus ipilimumab, several studies have shown the benefit from the combination of chemotherapy with ICI in the first-line setting. In the KEYNOTE-021 study, 123 patients were randomized to chemotherapy plus pembrolizumab or chemotherapy alone.[218] The study showed an improvement in both objective response (55% vs 29%, $p = 0.0016$), the primary endpoint, and median PFS (13 months vs 8.9 months; HR 0.53, $p = 0.01$). The promising results from this trial led to two randomized trials comparing chemotherapy with or without pembrolizumab in patients with advanced stage, previously untreated NSCLC. In the KEYNOTE-189, 616 patients with metastatic nonsquamous NSCLC without sensitizing EGFR or ALK alterations were randomized to pemetrexed plus platinum followed by pemetrexed maintenance with or without pembrolizumab.[211] After a median follow-up of 10.5 months, the pembrolizumab arm was associated with increased median PFS (8.8 months vs 4.9 months; 0.52; 95% CI 0.43–0.64, $p < 0.001$) and estimated 12-month OS (69.2% vs 49.4%; HR 0.49; 95% CI 0.38–0.64, $p < 0.001$). The benefit was observed regardless of the platinum used and the PD-1 score. The response rates were 47.6% in the pembrolizumab combination and 18.9% in the chemotherapy alone arms ($p < 0.001$). The percentage of adverse advents of any cause were similar between the two groups for both any grade (99.8% vs 99%) and grades 3–5 (67.2% vs 65.8%). Similarly, the incidence of immune-mediated adverse events was not higher in the pembrolizumab combination than what had been previously observed with ICI alone. In the updated analysis, the median OS was 22 months in the pembrolizumab combination and 10.7 months for the chemotherapy alone arm (HR 0.56, 95% CI 0.45–0.70), with estimated 24-month OS of 45.5% and 29.9%, respectively.[212] The KEYNOTE-407 had a similar design and enrolled patients with squamous histology, which were treated with carboplatin plus a taxane (paclitaxel or nab-paclitaxel), with or without pembrolizumab.[213] After a median follow-up of 7.8 months, the pembrolizumab combination was associated with an increase in both median PFS (6.4 months vs 4.8 months; HR 0.56; 95% CI 0.45–0.70, $p < 0.001$) and median OS (15.9 months vs 11.2 months; HR 0.64; 95% CI 0.49–0.85, $p < 0.001$). The benefits from the addition of pembrolizumab were observed regardless of the taxane used and for both PD-L1 < 1% and ≥1%. There were no significant differences in the percentage of adverse events of any grade (98.2% vs 97.9%) or grade 3–5 (69.8% vs 68.2%). In the IMpower-130, 724 patients with advanced stage NSCLC without EGFR or ALK alterations, were randomized 2:1 to carboplatin plus nab-paclitaxel with or without atezolizumab.[214] The atezolizumab combination was associated with a significant improvement in the median PFS (7.0 months vs 5.5 months; 0.64; 95% CI 0.54–0.77, $p < 0.001$) and median OS (18.6 months vs 13.9 months; HR 0.79; 95% CI 0.64–0.98, $p = 0.03$). The atezolizumab combination had an acceptable toxicity profile, with adverse events occurring in 96% of patients, compared to 93% of the treated with chemotherapy alone. In contrast, the IMpower-131, which used the same design and evaluated the addition of atezolizumab to the same chemotherapy combination in patients with squamous histology, showed an improvement in median PFS (6.3 vs 5.6 months; $p = 0.0001$) but not median OS (14.2 months vs 13.5 months; $p = 0.16$) with the atezolizumab combination.[219] The IMpower-150 was a randomized trial where 356 patients with previously untreated patients with metastatic nonsquamous NSCLC

Table 10 Selected trials with targeted therapy in advanced-stage non-small-cell lung cancer.

Trial	Target	Setting	Treatment (N)	RR (%)	Median PFS (months)	Median OS (months)
FLAURA[223]	EGFR	1L	Osimertinib[224]	80	18.9	38.6
			Erl or Gef[225]	76	10.2	31.8
ALEX[226,227]	ALK	1L	Alectinib[152]	82.9	34.8	Not reached
			Crizotinib[151]	75.5	10.9	57.4
ALTA-1L[228]	ALK	1L	Brigatinib[137]	74	24	Not reached
			Crizotinib[138]	62	11	Not reached
PROFILE-1[229]	R1	1L+	Crizotinib[53]	72	19.3	51.4
ALKA/STARTRK[230]	R1	1L+	Entrectinib[53]	77	19	Not reached
Planchard[231]	BRAF (V600E)	1L	Dabrafenib plus Trametinib[36]	64	10.9	24.6
GEOMETRY[232]	MET exon 14	2L+1L	Capmatinib[69]	41	5.4	Not reported
			Capmatinib[28]	68	12.4	Not reported
VISION[233]	MET exon 14	1L+	Tepotinib[152]	56	8.5	Not reported
Hong[234]	KRAS G12C	2L+	Sotorasib[59]	32.2	6.3	Not reported
LIBRETTO-001[235]	RET	1L	Selpercatinib[39]	85	Not reached	Not reported
		2L+	Selpercatinib[105]	64	16.5	Not reported

Erl, Erlotinib; Gef, Gefitinib; 1L, first-line; 1L+, first-line and beyond; 2L+, second-line and beyond; RR, response rate.

were randomized to carboplatin plus paclitaxel in combination with atezolizumab (ACP), bevacizumab (BCP) or atezolizumab plus bevacizumab (ABCP).[220] When compared to BCP, ABCP was associated with increased median PFS (8.3 months vs 6.8 months; HR 0.62; 95% CI 0.52–0.74, $p < 0.001$) and median OS (19.2 months vs 14.7 months; HR 0.78; 95% CI 0.64–0.96, $p = 0.02$). Since the study included patients with *EGFR* mutations or *ALK* rearrangements it allowed the subgroup analysis in this setting. Among patients with sensitizing *EGFR* mutations, there was an improvement in median OS with ABCP compared to BCP but not with ACP compared to BCP.[221] In the MYSTIC study, 1118 patients with metastatic NSCLC were randomized to first-line durvalumab, durvalumab plus tremelimumab, or chemotherapy.[222] The primary endpoint of median OS in patients with PD-L1 ≥ 25% was not met for durvalumab or durvalumab plus tremelimumab versus chemotherapy.

Targeted therapy

The identification of targetable gene alterations has transformed the treatment of lung cancer, allowing the use of personalized therapy with increased activity and better toxicity profile compared to standard chemotherapy (Table 10).

EGFR

Successful targeting of tumors harboring *EGFR* mutations using TKIs has been a major therapeutic advance in the treatment of advanced NSCLC. Mutations in the *EGFR* tyrosine kinase domain that are associated with response to treatment include exon 19 deletions (45%) and exon 21 L858R mutations (40–45%). *EGFR* exon 20 mutations including T790M are associated with resistance to first-generation EGFR TKIs.[236]

The first-generation reversible EGFR TKIs include gefitinib, erlotinib, and icotinib. Gefitinib was the first EGFR TKI tested in patients with advanced NSCLC. The Iressa Pan Asia Study (IPASS) included patients with NSCLC who were enriched for *EGFR* mutations based on clinical characteristics including adenocarcinoma histology, former light or never-smokers, and randomized patients to receive gefitinib 250 mg orally once daily or chemotherapy with carboplatin and paclitaxel.[237] This study demonstrated that in patients with *EGFR* wild-type tumors, PFS was improved with chemotherapy compared to gefitinib (HR 2.85; 95% CI 2.05–3.98), while in patients with *EGFR* mutated NSCLC PFS was superior for gefitinib over chemotherapy (HR 0.48; 95% CI 0.36–0.64). Response rate to gefitinib was 71.2% in patients with *EGFR* mutated tumors but only 1.1% in patients with *EGFR* wild-type tumors. Interestingly, the response rate for chemotherapy in patients with *EGFR* mutated NSCLC was higher (47.3%) than response rate in *EGFR* wild-type patients (23.5%). Subsequent studies including NEJSG002 (10.8 months vs 5.4 months) and WJTOG3405 (9.2 months vs 6.3 months) showed improved PFS with gefitinib compared to chemotherapy.[238,239] Erlotinib, another first-generation EGFR TKI was similarly studied in the first-line setting and compared to first-line platinum-based chemotherapy and was found to improve PFS over standard platinum-based chemotherapy in both the OPTIMAL (13.1 months vs 4.6 months) and EURTAC (9.7 months vs 5.2 months) trials.[240,241] The phase 2 ACCRU study examined the role of adding bevacizumab to erlotinib, compared to erlotinib alone in the first-line setting. This study did not meet its endpoint of improved PFS with the erlotinib and bevacizumab combination.[242] However, the phase 3 NEJ026 study did show improved PFS with erlotinib and bevacizumab (median PFS 16.9 months) compared to erlotinib alone (median PFS 13.3 months).[243] The phase 3 RELAY study examined the combination of erlotinib and the VEGF receptor inhibitor, ramucirumab.[244] This study showed improved PFS for ramucirumab and erlotinib (median PFS 19.4 months) compared to erlotinib alone (median PFS 12.4 months).

The second-generation EGFR inhibitors afatinib and dacomitinib are irreversible EGFR inhibitors that inhibit wild-type and mutant *EGFR*. In addition, they also target ERBB2 and ERBB4. First-line afatinib was shown to improve median PFS over cisplatin and pemetrexed in patients with previously untreated metastatic NSCLC harboring *EGFR* exon 19 deletion or L858R mutations in the LUX-3 study (13.6 months vs 6.9 months).[245] The LUX-6 study also compared first-line afatinib to chemotherapy, using a regimen of cisplatin and gemcitabine, in patients with NSCLC harboring classic or rare *EGFR* mutations and showed improved PFS for the randomized to afatinib (11 months vs 5.6 months).[246] The phase 3 ARCHER study compared first-line dacomitinib to erlotinib and showed improved PFS with dacomitinib compared to erlotinib (14.7 months vs 9.2 months), although the former was associated with increased toxicities related to wild type EGFR inhibition including diarrhea and mouth sores.[247]

Despite the initial responses to EGFR-TKI therapy and prolonged median PFS compared to standard chemotherapy, virtually all *EGFR* mutant patients eventually developed acquired resistance to therapy.[248] The most common cause of acquired resistance to EGFR TKIs is the development of a secondary *EGFR* mutation in exon 20 (T790M).[249] Other potential causes include *MET* amplification, *PIK3CA* mutations, *HER-2* amplification, *BRAF* mutations, and SCLC transformation.[58,250] Third-generation EGFR TKIs are potent inhibitors of T790M tumors, with little wild type EGFR inhibition. Osimertinib is a third-generation EGFR TKI associated with an ORR of 61% in patients with *EGFR* T790M positive tumors.[251] The phase 3 AURA3 study demonstrated that first-line osimertinib improved median PFS compared to platinum and pemetrexed combination (10.1 months vs 4.4 months) in patients with *EGFR* T790M positive tumors.[252] Patients with asymptomatic stable brain metastases were allowed on this study, and the intracranial response rate to osimertinib was 70% compared to 31% with platinum pemetrexed. The phase 3 FLAURA study defined the new standard of care for *EGFR* mutant NSCLC.[223] This study randomized 556 patients with *EGFR* exon 19 del or L858R mutated NSCLC to receive osimertinib 80 mg orally once daily or standard therapy with erlotinib or gefitinib (standard EGFR TKI therapy). The primary endpoint was investigator-assessed PFS. The FLAURA study met its primary endpoint of improved PFS with osimertinib compared to standard EGFR TKI therapy (18.9 vs 10.2 months). Furthermore, objective response rate was numerically higher for osimertinib (80% vs 76%) while grade 3 or higher toxicities were less commonly observed in the osimertinib group (34% vs 45% for standard EGFR TKI therapy). Mechanisms of resistance to osimertinib include EGFR amplification, tertiary *EGFR* mutation (C797S), *MET* or *HER2* amplification, or mutations in *BRAF* or *KRAS*.[253]

ALK

ALK fusions with EML4, KIF5B, TFG, and KLC1, among others, result in constitutive activation of ALK and its downstream signaling pathways.[254] *ALK* fusions occur in approximately 5% of patients with NSCLC, especially in younger individuals who are light or never-smokers and with signet-ring subtype of adenocarcinoma.[255,256]

Crizotinib is an oral ATP-competitive inhibitor of ALK, MET, and ROS1 tyrosine kinases. The expansion cohort of the initial phase I study included 82 patients with ALK rearrangements, where 41% of patients had 3 more prior therapies.[257] The objective response rate was 57% with an additional 33% of patients achieving stable disease (SD). At the time of cutoff, the median PFS was not reached with the estimated probability of PFS at 6 months of 72%. The PROFILE 1007 showed improved PFS for crizotinib compared to second-line pemetrexed or docetaxel (7.7 months vs 3 months).[258] The PROFILE 1014 compared first-line crizotinib to platinum-pemetrexed chemotherapy in patients with ALK-positive NSCLC, with the primary endpoint of PFS.[259] First-line crizotinib was associated with improved median PFS compared to platinum plus pemetrexed (10.7 months vs 7 months; HR 0.45, 95% CI 0.35–0.60, $p < 0.001$), although there were no differences in OS, likely due to cross-over being allowed on this study.[259]

Several second-generation ALK inhibitors have been developed to treat patients with *ALK*-positive disease, including ceritinib, alectinib, and brigatinib. In the dose-escalation part of a phase 1 study, ceritinib was associated with a 58% response rate and a median PFS of 7 months, ranging from 6.9 months in patients previously treated with crizotinib to 10.4 months in the who had not received previous ALK directed therapy.[260] First-line ceritinib 750 mg orally once daily was compared to platinum plus pemetrexed chemotherapy in the ASCEND-4 study, where crossover to ceritinib was permitted upon progression in the chemotherapy arm.[261] The median PFS (16.6 months vs 8.1 months), 2-year OS (70.6% vs 58.2%) and objective response rate (72.5% vs 26.7%) were all superior for the ceritinib arm, which also was associated with increased adverse events compared to chemotherapy (grade 3–4 adverse events 65% vs 40%).[261] The J-ALEX study compared another ALK inhibitor, alectinib at a dose of 300 mg orally twice daily to crizotinib 250 mg orally twice daily in ALK inhibitor-naïve Japanese patients with *ALK*-positive metastatic NSCLC, which included both treatment naïve patients, as well as the that who had failed one previous chemotherapy regimen.[262] The median PFS was not reached in the alectinib arm and 10.2 months in the crizotinib arm, with grade 3–4 adverse event rates lower for the alectinib arm (26.2%) compared to crizotinib (51.9%).[262] The global ALEX study confirmed the benefit of first-line alectinib at a higher dose of 600 mg orally twice daily compared to crizotinib in treatment naïve patients with *ALK*-positive NSCLC. At the time of initial publication, median PFS was not reached for alectinib, but in the update with 34.8 months on follow-up, the median PFS was 11.1 months for crizotinib.[226,227] The cumulative incidence of intracranial progression was also lower for alectinib versus crizotinib (12-month cumulative incidence 9.4% vs 41.4%) showing its intracranial activity.[226] The ALTA study similarly compared brigatinib to crizotinib in the first-line setting and showed improved PFS with brigatinib (median PFS not reached for brigatinib and 9.8 months for crizotinib).[228] Due to the 3% incidence of pneumonitis or interstitial lung disease within the first 14 days of therapy with brigatinib, the recommended treatment is with an induction phase with 90 mg once daily for 7 days, escalated to 180 mg orally daily thereafter.

Secondary *ALK* resistance mutations are seen on 20–30% of patients treated with crizotinib, with only 10% of these mutations being G1202R.[263] Conversely in patients treated with second-generation ALK TKI inhibitors, the resistance mechanism is predominantly from ALK mutations, most commonly G1202R.[263] The only ALK inhibitor with activity against the G1202R mutation is lorlatinib, which also has excellent intracranial penetration. Lorlatinib has been associated with responses in previously treated patients including those who had received 2 or more prior ALK TKI therapies, with objective response rate of 39% and intracranial objective response rate of 49%, while the objective response rate in treatment naïve patients was 90%.[264]

Other targets

Several potentially targetable gene abnormalities have been described in NSCLC and are currently being investigated in clinical trials.[265]

ROS1 gene fusions lead to constitutive kinase activation and are seen most commonly in never smokers with adenocarcinoma. Patients with *ROS1* rearrangements have been successfully treated with crizotinib, with response rates and median PFS of approximately 75% and 19 months respectively.[229,230] Ceritinib and lorlatinib are also active in TKI inhibitor naïve patients, with objective response rate of 62% and 62%, respectively, and median PFS of 19–20 months.[266,267] Lorlatinib and repotrectinib were recently found to be active even in TKI pretreated patients, with objective response rate of 27% for lorlatinib and 55% for repotrectinib.[267,268]

Selpercatinib (LOXO-292), a potent and selective RET inhibitor, was approved for the treatment of *RET* positive NSCLC based on results of the LIBRETTO-001 study where the overall response in 105 patients with *RET* fusion-positive NSCLC previously treated with platinum-based chemotherapy was 64% whereas the response among 39 previously untreated patients was 85%, with median PFS of 16.5 months in the former and not reached in the later.[235] A second approved RET inhibitor is praseltinib (BLU-667), which was associated with broad and durable tumor activity across several solid tumor types including NSCLC.[269]

MET exon 14 skip alterations occur in 3% of nonsquamous NSCLC and result in truncated MET receptor lacking the Y1003 residue which is the binding site for CBL E3 ubiquitin ligase, leading to decreased ubiquitination and degradation of the MET protein with sustained MET activation.[270] The MET inhibitor capmatinib was FDA approved for the treatment of patients with *MET* exon 14 mutations based on the GEOMETRY phase 2 study, in which it was associated with response rates of 41% in patients with previously treated and 61% in those without previous treatment.[232] In a phase 2 study involving 152 patients with *MET* exon 14 mutations, the MET inhibitor tepotinib was associated with a response rate of 56% and median PFS of 8.5 months.[233]

BRAF V600E mutations have also been successfully targeted in NSCLC. In a basket study evaluating vemurafenib, a BRAF inhibitor, in multiple BRAF V600E tumors including NSCLC, a response rate of 42% was observed.[271] Dabrafenib was studied as a single agent, as well as in combination with the MEK inhibitor trametinib in *BRAF* V600E mutant NSCLC. The overall response rate with dabrafenib alone or in combination with dabrafenib was 33% and 63%, respectively.[272,273] In the first-line setting, the combination of dabrafenib and trametinib was associated with an overall response in 64% of patients, with median PFS and OS of 10.9 and 24.6 months, respectively.[231]

TRK fusions between one of the neurotrophic receptor tyrosine kinase genes (*NTRK1*, *NTRK2*, and *NTRK3*) and a 5 partner gene arise from intrachromosomal or interchromosomal rearrangements. Larotrectinib and entrectinib both have activity in patients with these alterations, including NSCLC, with response rates of 79% with larotrectinib and clinical benefit in all patients with NSCLC treated with entrectinib, two of whom had complete response.[274,275]

KRAS G12C mutations occur in approximately 13% of patients with NSCLC. In a phase 1 trial involving 129 patients with *KRAS* G12C mutations treated with the small irreversible KRAS inhibitor sotorasib (AMG-510), the response rate in the 59 patients with NSCLC was 32.2% with median PFS of 6.3 months.[234] Several other KRAS G12C inhibitors have been developed, including MRTX849, LY3499446, and JNJ-74699157.[276]

Treatment of SCLC

SCLC differs from NSCLC in its rapid growth rate, propensity for early systemic spread, and short natural history. With the general acceptance of SCLC as a systemic disorder and recognition of the superiority of multimodal regimens over local therapy alone, chemotherapy became the cornerstone of SCLC management.[277]

Surgery

Surgery followed by adjuvant chemotherapy is indicated in the less than 5% of patients who present with stage I SCLC.[278,279] Nevertheless, even in the presence of a small peripheral lesion, patients considered for surgical resection of SCLC should undergo complete staging to rule out mediastinal or distant metastases.

In a propensity-matched analysis of survival comparing surgery to chemoradiotherapy in patients with nonmetastatic SCLC from the National Cancer Database (NCDB), surgery was associated with a significantly longer survival for stage I (median 38.6 months vs. 22.9 months, HR 0.62, 95%CI 0.57–0.69, $p < 0.0001$).[280] Although there are no randomized studies comparing adjuvant chemotherapy to observation in patients with resected SCLC data from cancer registries suggest a benefit from adjuvant therapy. In a large NCDB study including 954 patients with completely resected stage I SCLC, adjuvant chemotherapy, with or without radiation, was associated with a significant increase in median OS (66.0 months vs 42.1 months) and 5-year (52.7% vs 40.4%) compared to observation.[225]

Radiation therapy

The standard primary therapy for the majority of patients with stage I–III SCLC, also known as limited-stage SCLC, is a combination of chemotherapy with platinum plus etoposide and thoracic radiation. The role of thoracic radiation therapy was established by several clinical trials and meta-analyses.[278] In a meta-analysis including 2140 patients with limited-stage SCLC enrolled into 13 trials the combination of chemotherapy with thoracic radiation therapy was associated with an increase in 3-year OS survival compared to chemotherapy alone (14.3% vs 8.9%, $p = 0.001$), with the greatest benefit found in patients younger than 55 years.[281] In another large meta-analysis involving 11 phase 3 trials, the addition of thoracic radiation increased the 2-year OS survival by 5.4% compared to chemotherapy alone.[224] Once the role for thoracic radiation was established, several other issues had to be addressed, including the timing and fractionation.

In a systematic review evaluating the timing of thoracic radiation therapy in combination with chemotherapy in patients with limited-stage SCLC, early radiation therapy was defined as starting before 9 weeks after the first dose of chemotherapy and prior to cycle 3 of chemotherapy, whereas late radiation was defined as starting after 9 weeks or cycle 3.[282] The study showed a statistically significant 5% absolute improvement in survival for early radiation therapy at 2 years (risk ratio [RR] 1.17, 95% CI 1.02–1.35, $p = 0.03$) and a nonsignificant improvement of 2% at 3 years (RR 1.13, 95% CI 0.92–1.39, $p = 0.23$). Subset analyses showed a significant survival improvement at both 2 and 3 years with the use of platinum-based chemotherapy or twice-daily radiation therapy. Other meta-analyses showed similar findings with improved survival with the use of early radiation therapy.[283–285]

Conventional radiotherapy fractionation can be modified by the use of hyperfractionation (radiation therapy more than once per day), acceleration (shortening the overall treatment time) or both.[286] Phase II trials evaluating hyperfractionated chemoradiotherapy in limited-stage SCLC showed promising results compared to historical controls using conventionally fractionated radiation.[287,288] In the pivotal Intergroup-0096 (INT-0096) trial, 417 patients with limited-stage SCLC were randomized to standard daily fractionation (1.8 Gy per fraction x 25 fractions in 5 weeks) or hyperfractionation (1.5 Gy twice daily x 30 fractions in 3 weeks).[289] The total dose of radiation therapy was 45 Gy in both arms and concurrent chemotherapy consisted of cisplatin 60 mg/m^2 IV on day 1 plus etoposide 120 mg/m^2 IV on days 1–3 for four cycles. The twice-daily radiation therapy arm was associated with a significant improvement in median OS (23 months vs 19 months) and 5-year OS (26% vs 16%, $p = 0.04$). Twice-daily radiation, however, was associated with increased incidence of grade 3 esophagitis (27% vs 11%). Despite the INT-0096 trial results, twice-daily radiation has not been widely adopted in the community, possibly because of the difficulty of scheduling and the increased rate of esophagitis.[290] Furthermore, the radiation dose used in the control arm was considered low. To address these issues, a new randomized trial was conducted. In the CONVERT trial, 547 patients with limited-stage SCLC were randomized to either 45 Gy in 30 twice-daily fractions of 1.5 Gy over 19 days or 66 Gy in 33 daily fractions of 2 Gy over 45 days, with radiation administered for five consecutive days per week in both arms.[291] Chemotherapy in both arms consisted of four to six cycles of etoposide 100 mg/m^2 on days 1 to 3 plus cisplatin at either 75 mg/m^2 on day 1 or 25 mg/m^2 on days 1 to 3, with the first cycle starting before the radiotherapy. There were no significant differences in outcomes, with median OS of 30 months in the twice daily and 25 months in the once daily arm (HR, 1.18; 95%CI, 0.95–1.45; $p = 0.14$). The 5-year OS was 34% in the twice-daily group and 31% in the once-daily group and there were no differences in the median PFS (15.4 months in the twice-daily group vs 14.3 months in the once-daily group, HR 1.12, 95% CI 0.92–1.38, $p = 0.26$). Similarly, there were no significant differences in toxicity, including esophagitis, with the only exception being grade 4 neutropenia which was observed more commonly in the twice-daily radiation group (49% vs 38%, $p = 0.05$).

Prophylactic cranial irradiation

Brain metastases are diagnosed in approximately 24% of patients with newly diagnosed SCLC undergoing brain MRI during staging.[292] During the course of disease, more than 50% of patients will eventually develop intracranial metastases, which are also common in the with limited-stage disease. Therefore, prophylactic cranial irradiation (PCI) was introduced in an attempt to eradicate undetectable brain metastases. Early trials evaluating the role of PCI in SCLC showed decreased brain metastases but no conclusive data on survival benefit, which was addressed in a meta-analysis including 929 patients from 17 clinical trials.[293] The study included patients with either limited or extensive-stage SCLC who had achieved complete remission after chemotherapy. PCI was associated with a significant decrease in the incidence of brain metastases at 3 years (33.3% vs 58.6%, $p < 0.001$) and 3-year OS (20.7% vs 15.3%, $p < 0.001$). In the EORTC trial, 286 patients with extensive-stage SCLC who achieve any response after four to six cycles of chemotherapy were randomized to PCI or observation, with the primary endpoint being the time for development of symptomatic brain metastases.[294] PCI was associated with reduced risk for symptomatic brain metastases (HR, 0.27, $p < 0.001$), cumulative risk for brain metastases within one year (14.6% vs 40.4%) and median OS (6.7 months vs 5.4 months, HR 0.68, $p = 0.003$). In a large multicenter Japanese trial, 224 patients with any response to chemotherapy were randomized to PCI or observation.[295] Patients in both arms underwent brain MRI every 3 months up to 12 months followed by repeated MRI at 18 months and 24 months after enrollment. The trial was terminated early for futility with no benefit from PCI on median OS (11.6 months vs 13.7 months). A possible explanation for the discrepancy between the trials was the lack of brain MRI at the completion of chemotherapy in the EORTC trial. Therefore, the survival improvement for PCI in the EORTC trial could have resulted from the early treatment of asymptomatic brain metastases that were present prior to randomization. Following completion of chemotherapy in patients with extensive-stage SCLC, both surveillance with brain every 3 months and PCI represent acceptable options.

Since most patients with extensive-stage SCLC who undergo chemotherapy and PCI have persistent intrathoracic disease which progresses within 1 year in 90% of cases, consolidation thoracic radiotherapy could potentially improve the outcomes. The CREST trial randomized 489 patients with extensive-stage SCLC treated who responded to chemotherapy to PCI with or without thoracic radiation.[296] The primary endpoint of OS at 1 year was not met with 33% and 28% of patients alive in the thoracic radiation and control groups respectively (HR 0.84, 95% CI 0.69–1.01, $p = 0.06$). In a secondary analysis, the 2-year OS was improved with thoracic radiation (13% vs 3%, $p = 0.004$).

Systemic therapy

SCLC is very sensitive to first-line chemotherapy, with the majority of patients achieving tumor reduction when treated with combination therapy. Cisplatin plus etoposide emerged as the standard of care for patients with metastatic disease, also known as extensive stage, following a randomized study where it was found to be as effective as cyclophosphamide plus doxorubicin and vincristine (CAV) with less toxicity.[297] However, due to the median OS of 8.6 months with cisplatin plus etoposide, it was clear that further improvements were needed. The Japanese Clinical Oncology Group (JCOG) 9511 randomized 154 patients to cisplatin (80 mg/m^2 on day 1) plus etoposide (100 mg/m^2 on days 1 to 3) every 3 weeks or cisplatin (60 mg/m^2 on day 1) plus irinotecan (60 mg/m^2 on days 1, 8, and 15) every 4 weeks.[298] The irinotecan regimen was associated with increased overall response rate (84.4% vs 67.5%, $p = 0.02$), median PFS (6.9 months vs 4.8 months, $p = 0.003$) and median OS (12.8 months vs 9.4 months, $p = 0.002$) compared to etoposide. Cisplatin plus irinotecan was associated with higher frequency of diarrhea whereas cisplatin plus etoposide was associated with higher frequency of hematologic toxicities including neutropenia and thrombocytopenia. Two subsequent studies conducted in the United States failed to show a benefit from cisplatin plus irinotecan compared to cisplatin plus etoposide.[166,299] In a subsequent analysis of JCOG-9511 and one of the US trials, the SWOG-0124, the outcomes for cisplatin pus etoposide were similar between the two studies, with median PFS and median OS of 4.7 months and 9.4 months, respectively, in the JCOG-9511 and 5.2 months and 9.1 months, respectively, in the SWOG-0124.[300] In contrast, despite the identical chemotherapy regimen and design, cisplatin plus irinotecan was more effective in the JCO-9511 study, with increased response rate (87% vs 60%, $p < 0.001$) and median OS (12.8 months vs 9.9 months, $p < 0.001$), suggesting inherent genetic differences in the genes involved in the irinotecan drug disposition between the patient populations.

Due to the toxicities observed with cisplatin, several studies have evaluated the use of chemotherapy regimens including carboplatin.[165,301,302] In the COCIS meta-analysis, which included 663 patients with both limited and extensive-stage SCLC enrolled into four randomized clinical trials, there were no differences in outcomes with cisplatin associated with a numerically higher response rate (67.1% vs 66%), median PFS (5.5 months vs 5.3 months), and median OS (9.6 months vs 9.4 months) without reaching statistical significance.[303] Carboplatin was associated with increased rates of myelosuppression whereas cisplatin was associated with increased rate of nausea, vomiting, neurotoxicity, and renal toxicity. Therefore, the combination of etoposide with either cisplatin or carboplatin can be considered the standard backbone chemotherapy for SCLC.

The most important recent development in the treatment of extensive-stage SCLC has been the incorporation of ICI in the first-line setting. In the IMpower 133 study, 201 patients with extensive-stage SCLC were randomized to four cycles of carboplatin plus etoposide with or without atezolizumab, with the latter followed by maintenance atezolizumab.[304] During the maintenance phase, patients were allowed to receive PCI but not thoracic radiotherapy. PCI was administered to 11% of patients in each arm. The addition of atezolizumab was associated with a significant improvement in the median OS (12.3 months vs 10.3 months, HR 0.70, 95% CI 0.54–0.91, $p = 0.007$) and median PFS (5.3 months vs 4.3 months, HR 0.77, 95% CI 0.62–0.96, $p = 0.02$). In the CASPIAN trial, 805 patients with extensive-stage SCLC were randomized to etoposide plus a platinum (carboplatin or cisplatin) alone plus durvalumab or plus durvalumab and tremelimumab.[305] Patients in the experimental arms received up to four cycles of chemotherapy whereas the control arm could receive up to six cycles. PCI was allowed only in the control arm and consolidation thoracic radiation was not allowed in the study. The addition of durvalumab was associated with a significant improvement in the median OS (13.0 months vs 10.3 months, HR 0.73, 95% CI 0.59–0.91, $p = 0.0047$). In contrast, there was no survival benefit from the combination of durvalumab and tremelimumab.[306] In the Keynote-604 trial, patients with extensive-stage SCLC were randomized to platinum plus etoposide with or without pembrolizumab.[307] PCI was allowed in the study. The addition of pembrolizumab was associated with increased median PFS but not OS. Since none of the trials allowed consolidation radiation therapy, its role in patients treated with the combination of chemotherapy and ICI remains unclear.

Despite the initial response to first-line therapy in SCLC, virtually all patients eventually develop tumor progression which is often resistant to chemotherapy. Based on the interval from the completion of the last cycle of chemotherapy to the detection of relapse beyond 3 months and within 3 months, tumors have been classified as chemotherapy-sensitive or chemotherapy-resistant, respectively. Topotecan was the initially approved for previously treated SCLC patients based on a randomized clinical trial where in comparison to CAV, it showed similar median OS (25 weeks vs 24.7 weeks) but with greater symptomatic improvement including dyspnea, hoarseness, and fatigue.[308] An oral formulation topotecan was also approved based on similar outcomes when compared to the standard intravenous regimen.[309] Despite the promising initial results with amrubicin, there was no improvement in median PFS or OS when compared to topotecan in a large randomized trial.[310] In a phase 2 study evaluating lurbinectedin 3.2 mg/m^2 every 3 weeks in 105 patients with previously treated SCLC, the overall response rate was 35.2% with a median PFS of 3.5 months in the overall population, 4.6 months in the chemotherapy-sensitive population, and 2.6 months in patients with chemotherapy-resistant disease.[311] The ongoing ATLANTIS is a stage III study where patient with previously treated SCLC are randomized to lurbinectedin or a control arm with topotecan or CAV.[312]

Both nivolumab and pembrolizumab have shown activity in patients with previously treated SCLC.[313,314] In the randomized cohort of CheckMate 032 comparing the combination of nivolumab 1 mg/kg plus ipilimumab 3 mg/kg every 3 weeks to single-agent nivolumab 3 mg/kg every 2 weeks, the combination arm was associated with improved objective response rate (21.9% vs 11.6%, $p = 0.03$) but not median OS (5.7 months vs 4.7 months) or median PFS (1.5 months vs 1.4 months).[315] With the lack of survival improvement and increased toxicity, the combination of nivolumab plus ipilimumab is not currently indicated for the treatment of SCLC.

Other options for patients with previously treated SCLC include irinotecan, paclitaxel, docetaxel, temozolomide, and ICI if not previously used in the first-line setting.[279]

Conclusions

Lung cancer is the leading cause of cancer death and the mortality has decreased in the United States mostly due to decreased incidence and improved survival due to the use of targeted therapies and ICI. For patients with NSCLC and early-stage disease, the standard therapy is surgical resection followed by adjuvant chemotherapy in tumors with lymph node involvement or measuring at least 4 cm. Patients with inoperable locally advanced disease and good performance status should be treated with platinum-based chemotherapy and concurrent thoracic radiotherapy, followed by durvalumab. The treatment for patients with metastatic disease depends on the molecular profile, with targeted therapy usually indicated in the with actionable gene alterations, whereas ICI with or without chemotherapy is recommended as the first-line therapy in the without actionable alterations. The next step in the treatment of NSCLC is the incorporation of both targeted therapy and ICI in patients with operable disease, with promising trials using neoadjuvant immunotherapy and adjuvant EGFR TKI. Although the progress in the treatment of SCLC has been slower, recent randomized trials showed improved survival with the addition of ICI to first-line platinum plus etoposide and there are several studies with new drugs in previously treated patients.

Key references

The complete reference list can be found on Vital Source version of this title, see inside front cover.

1. Global Burden of Disease Cancer C, Fitzmaurice C, Abate D, et al. Global, regional, and national cancer incidence, mortality, years of life lost, years lived with disability, and disability-adjusted life-years for 29 cancer groups, 1990 to 2017: a systematic analysis for the global burden of disease study. *JAMA Oncol.* 2019;**5**(12):1749–1768.
2. Siegel RL, Miller KD, Jemal A. Cancer statistics, 2020. *CA Cancer J Clin.* 2020;**70**(1):7–30.
3. Howlader N, Forjaz G, Mooradian MJ, et al. The effect of advances in lung-cancer treatment on population mortality. *N Engl J Med.* 2020;**383**(7):640–649.
24. Wistuba II, Lam S, Behrens C, et al. Molecular damage in the bronchial epithelium of current and former smokers. *J Natl Cancer Inst.* 1997;**89**(18):1366–1373.
32. Travis WD, Brambilla E, Nicholson AG, et al. The 2015 World Health Organization Classification of lung tumors impact of genetic, clinical and radiologic advances since the 2004 classification. *J Thorac Oncol.* 2015;**10**(9):1243–1260.
59. Rudin CM, Poirier JT, Byers LA, et al. Molecular subtypes of small cell lung cancer: a synthesis of human and mouse model data. *Nat Rev Cancer.* 2019;**19**(5):289–297.
64. Travis WD, Dacic S, Wistuba I, et al. IASLC multidisciplinary recommendations for pathologic assessment of lung cancer resection specimens after neoadjuvant therapy. *J Thoracic Oncol.* 2020;**15**(5):709–740.
72. Tsao MS, Kerr KM, Kockx M, et al. PD-L1 immunohistochemistry comparability study in real-life clinical samples: results of blueprint phase 2 project. *J Thoracic Oncol.* 2018;**13**(9):1302–1311.
82. Detterbeck FC, Boffa DJ, Kim AW, Tanoue LT. The eighth edition lung cancer stage classification. *Chest.* 2017;**151**(1):193–203.
86. MacMahon H, Naidich DP, Goo JM, et al. Guidelines for management of incidental pulmonary nodules detected on CT images: from the fleischner society 2017. *Radiology.* 2017;**284**(1):228–243.
93. Travis WD, Asamura H, Bankier AA, et al. The IASLC lung cancer staging project: proposals for coding T categories for subsolid nodules and assessment of tumor size in part-solid tumors in the forthcoming eighth edition of the TNM classification of lung cancer. *J Thoracic Oncol.* 2016;**11**(8):1204–1223.
128. Pignon JP, Tribodet H, Scagliotti GV, et al. Lung adjuvant cisplatin evaluation: a pooled analysis by the LACE Collaborative Group. *J Clin Oncol.* 2008;**26**(21):3552–3559.
129. Kris MG, Gaspar LE, Chaft JE, et al. Adjuvant systemic therapy and adjuvant radiation therapy for stage I to IIIA completely resected non-small-cell lung cancers: American Society of Clinical Oncology/Cancer Care Ontario Clinical Practice Guideline Update. *J Clin Oncol.* 2017;**35**(25):2960–2974.
132. Wakelee HA, Dahlberg SE, Keller SM, et al. Adjuvant chemotherapy with or without bevacizumab in patients with resected non-small-cell lung cancer (E1505): an open-label, multicentre, randomised, phase 3 trial. *Lancet Oncol.* 2017;**18**(12):1610–1623.

134. Lim E, Harris G, Patel A, et al. Preoperative versus postoperative chemotherapy in patients with resectable non-small cell lung cancer: systematic review and indirect comparison meta-analysis of randomized trials. *J Thoracic Oncol*. 2009;**4**(11):1380–1388.
138. Le Pechoux C, Pourel N, Barlesi F, et al. An international randomized trial, comparing post-operative conformal radiotherapy (PORT) to no PORT, in patients with completely resected non-small cell lung cancer (NSCLC) and mediastinal N2 involvement: primary end-point analysis of LungART (IFCT-0503, UK NCRI, SAKK) NCT00410683. *Ann Oncol*. 2020;**31**:S1178-S.
141. Wu YL, Tsuboi M, He J, et al. Osimertinib in resected EGFR-mutated non-small-cell lung cancer. *N Engl J Med*. 2020;**383**(18):1711–1723.
145. Forde PM, Chaft JE, Smith KN, et al. Neoadjuvant PD-1 blockade in resectable lung cancer. *N Engl J Med*. 2018;**378**(21):1976–1986.
153. Bentzen SM, Constine LS, Deasy JO, et al. Quantitative analyses of normal tissue effects in the clinic (QUANTEC): an introduction to the scientific issues. *Int J Radiat Oncol Biol Phys*. 2010;**76**(3 Suppl):S3–S9.
161. Bradley JD, Hu C, Komaki RR, et al. Long-term results of NRG oncology RTOG 0617: standard- versus high-dose chemoradiotherapy with or without cetuximab for unresectable stage III non-small-cell lung cancer. *J Clin Oncol*. 2020;**38**(7):706–714.
164. Senan S, Brade A, Wang LH, et al. PROCLAIM: randomized phase III trial of pemetrexed-cisplatin or etoposide-cisplatin plus thoracic radiation therapy followed by consolidation chemotherapy in locally advanced nonsquamous non-small-cell lung cancer. *J Clin Oncol*. 2016;**34**(9):953–962.
169. Antonia SJ, Villegas A, Daniel D, et al. Overall survival with durvalumab after chemoradiotherapy in stage III NSCLC. *N Engl J Med*. 2018;**379**(24):2342–2350.
171. Hanna NH, Schneider BJ, Temin S, et al. Therapy for stage IV non-small-cell lung cancer without driver alterations: ASCO and OH (CCO) joint guideline update. *J Clin Oncol*. 2020;**38**(14):1608–1632.
182. Ardizzoni A, Boni L, Tiseo M, et al. Cisplatin- versus carboplatin-based chemotherapy in first-line treatment of advanced non-small-cell lung cancer: an individual patient data meta-analysis. *J Natl Cancer Inst*. 2007;**99**(11):847–857.
183. Schiller JH, Harrington D, Belani CP, et al. Comparison of four chemotherapy regimens for advanced non-small-cell lung cancer. *N Engl J Med*. 2002;**346**(2):92–98.
187. Sandler A, Gray R, Perry MC, et al. Paclitaxel-carboplatin alone or with bevacizumab for non-small-cell lung cancer. *N Engl J Med*. 2006;**355**(24):2542–2550.
198. Ramalingam SS, Dahlberg SE, Belani CP, et al. Pemetrexed, bevacizumab, or the combination as maintenance therapy for advanced nonsquamous non-small-cell lung cancer: ECOG-ACRIN 5508. *J Clin Oncol*. 2019;**37**(26):2360–2367.
200. Topalian SL, Hodi FS, Brahmer JR, et al. Safety, activity, and immune correlates of anti-PD-1 antibody in cancer. *N Engl J Med*. 2012;**366**(26):2443–2454.
201. Gettinger S, Horn L, Jackman D, et al. Five-year follow-up of nivolumab in previously treated advanced non-small-cell lung cancer: results from the CA209-003 study. *J Clin Oncol*. 2018;**36**(17):1675–1684.
208. Reck M, Rodriguez-Abreu D, Robinson AG, et al. Pembrolizumab versus chemotherapy for PD-L1-positive non-small-cell lung cancer. *N Engl J Med*. 2016;**375**(19):1823–1833.
210. Herbst RS, Giaccone G, de Marinis F, et al. Atezolizumab for first-line treatment of PD-L1-selected patients with NSCLC. *N Engl J Med*. 2020;**383**(14):1328–1339.
211. Gandhi L, Rodriguez-Abreu D, Gadgeel S, et al. Pembrolizumab plus chemotherapy in metastatic non-small-cell lung cancer. *N Engl J Med*. 2018;**378**(22):2078–2092.
213. Paz-Ares L, Luft A, Vicente D, et al. Pembrolizumab plus chemotherapy for squamous non-small-cell lung cancer. *N Engl J Med*. 2018;**379**(21):2040–2051.
214. West H, McCleod M, Hussein M, et al. Atezolizumab in combination with carboplatin plus nab-paclitaxel chemotherapy compared with chemotherapy alone as first-line treatment for metastatic non-squamous non-small-cell lung cancer (IMpower130): a multicentre, randomised, open-label, phase 3 trial. *Lancet Oncol*. 2019;**20**(7):924–937.
215. Hellmann MD, Paz-Ares L, Bernabe Caro R, et al. Nivolumab plus ipilimumab in advanced non-small-cell lung cancer. *N Engl J Med*. 2019;**381**(21):2020–2031.
220. Socinski MA, Jotte RM, Cappuzzo F, et al. Atezolizumab for first-line treatment of metastatic nonsquamous NSCLC. *N Engl J Med*. 2018;**378**(24):2288–2301.
223. Soria JC, Ohe Y, Vansteenkiste J, et al. Osimertinib in untreated EGFR-mutated advanced non-small-cell lung cancer. *N Engl J Med*. 2018;**378**(2):113–125.
226. Peters S, Camidge DR, Shaw AT, et al. Alectinib versus crizotinib in untreated ALK-positive non-small-cell lung cancer. *N Engl J Med*. 2017;**377**(9):829–838.
228. Camidge DR, Kim HR, Ahn MJ, et al. Brigatinib versus crizotinib in ALK-positive non-small-cell lung cancer. *N Engl J Med*. 2018;**379**(21):2027–2039.
229. Shaw AT, Ou SH, Bang YJ, et al. Crizotinib in ROS1-rearranged non-small-cell lung cancer. *N Engl J Med*. 2014;**371**(21):1963–1971.
231. Planchard D, Smit EF, Groen HJM, et al. Dabrafenib plus trametinib in patients with previously untreated BRAF(V600E)-mutant metastatic non-small-cell lung cancer: an open-label, phase 2 trial. *Lancet Oncol*. 2017;**18**(10):1307–1316.
232. Wolf J, Seto T, Han JY, et al. Capmatinib in MET exon 14-mutated or MET-amplified non-small-cell lung cancer. *N Engl J Med*. 2020;**383**(10):944–957.
234. Hong DS, Fakih MG, Strickler JH, et al. KRAS(G12C) inhibition with sotorasib in advanced solid tumors. *N Engl J Med*. 2020;**383**(13):1207–1217.
235. Drilon A, Oxnard GR, Tan DSW, et al. Efficacy of selpercatinib in RET fusion-positive non-small-cell lung cancer. *N Engl J Med*. 2020;**383**(9):813–824.
248. Jackman D, Pao W, Riely GJ, et al. Clinical definition of acquired resistance to epidermal growth factor receptor tyrosine kinase inhibitors in non-small-cell lung cancer. *J Clin Oncol*. 2010;**28**(2):357–360.
259. Solomon BJ, Mok T, Kim DW, et al. First-line crizotinib versus chemotherapy in ALK-positive lung cancer. *N Engl J Med*. 2014;**371**(23):2167–2177.
269. Gainor JF, Curigliano G, Kim DW, et al. Registrational dataset from the phase I/II ARROW trial of pralsetinib (BLU-667) in patients (pts) with advanced RET fusion plus non-small cell lung cancer (NSCLC). *J Clin Oncol*. 2020;**38**(15).
281. Pignon JP, Arriagada R, Ihde DC, et al. A meta-analysis of thoracic radiotherapy for small-cell lung cancer. *N Engl J Med*. 1992;**327**(23):1618–1624.
289. Turrisi AT 3rd, Kim K, Blum R, et al. Twice-daily compared with once-daily thoracic radiotherapy in limited small-cell lung cancer treated concurrently with cisplatin and etoposide. *N Engl J Med*. 1999;**340**(4):265–271.
291. Faivre-Finn C, Snee M, Ashcroft L, et al. Concurrent once-daily versus twice-daily chemoradiotherapy in patients with limited-stage small-cell lung cancer (CONVERT): an open-label, phase 3, randomised, superiority trial. *Lancet Oncol*. 2017;**18**(8):1116–1125.
294. Slotman B, Faivre-Finn C, Kramer G, et al. Prophylactic cranial irradiation in extensive small-cell lung cancer. *N Engl J Med*. 2007;**357**(7):664–672.
295. Takahashi T, Yamanaka T, Seto T, et al. Prophylactic cranial irradiation versus observation in patients with extensive-disease small-cell lung cancer: a multicentre, randomised, open-label, phase 3 trial. *Lancet Oncol*. 2017;**18**(5):663–671.
296. Slotman BJ, van Tinteren H, Praag JO, et al. Use of thoracic radiotherapy for extensive stage small-cell lung cancer: a phase 3 randomised controlled trial. *Lancet*. 2015;**385**(9962):36–42.
304. Horn L, Mansfield AS, Szczesna A, et al. First-line atezolizumab plus chemotherapy in extensive-stage small-cell lung cancer. *N Engl J Med*. 2018;**379**(23):2220–2229.
305. Paz-Ares L, Dvorkin M, Chen Y, et al. Durvalumab plus platinum-etoposide versus platinum-etoposide in first-line treatment of extensive-stage small-cell lung cancer (CASPIAN): a randomised, controlled, open-label, phase 3 trial. *Lancet*. 2019.
308. von Pawel J, Schiller JH, Shepherd FA, et al. Topotecan versus cyclophosphamide, doxorubicin, and vincristine for the treatment of recurrent small-cell lung cancer. *J Clin Oncol*. 1999;**17**(2):658–667.
315. Ready NE, Ott PA, Hellmann MD, et al. Nivolumab monotherapy and nivolumab plus ipilimumab in recurrent small cell lung cancer: results from the CheckMate 032 randomized cohort. *J Thoracic Oncol*. 2020;**15**(3):426–435.

81 Malignant pleural mesothelioma

Michele Carbone, MD, PhD ■ Daniel R. Gomez, MD, MBA ■ Anne S. Tsao, MD ■ Haining Yang, PhD ■ Harvey I. Pass, MD

Overview

Malignant pleural mesothelioma is an aggressive malignancy with an incidence that may be peaking worldwide. While the majority of patients do ultimately die of this disease, there have been substantial treatment and diagnostic shifts over the past decade that may improve long-term outcomes. These changes include worldwide interest in defining early detection biomarkers for the disease, a debate as to the optimal surgical approach (extrapleural pneumonectomy vs lung-sparing methods such as pleurectomy/decortication), further refinement of radiation techniques that allow for conformal treatment fields and the delivery of radiation with the involved lung intact, and the emergence of systemic therapies that are targeted in nature and allow for the increased individualization of care. Indeed, prospective clinical trials assessing the safety and efficacy of novel treatment approaches will be essential to the standardization of paradigms that improve outcomes. It is hoped that the maturation of these efforts will lead to an optimal approach in which earlier stage patients will benefit from multiple modalities that will provide synergistic control while limiting toxicity, thereby increasing the number of long-term survivors over the next one to two decades.

Mesotheliomas are malignancies of the mesothelial cells that constitute the pleura and the peritoneum. Rarely, mesothelioma can originate in the pericardium and in the tunica vaginalis. Between 1994 and 2008, age-adjusted mesothelioma mortality rates increased by 5.37% per year worldwide with the highest age-standardized incidence rates observed in the United States, Australia, Russia, Western Europe, Turkey, South Africa, and Argentina.[1,2] Mesothelioma mortality rates among males but not females have decreased in in Australia, New Zealand, and the United Kingdom due to asbestos regulatory legislation,[3] and as more countries place restrictions on asbestos use, mesothelioma rates globally should decrease in the future. Approximately 3200 mesotheliomas are registered each year in the United States,[1] and the incidence varies between 1 and 2 cases/million in states with no asbestos industry, to 10–20 cases/million in states with an asbestos industry.[4] There is little doubt that a significant number of mesotheliomas are not properly coded, thus underestimating the incidence in the United States.

With a latency period of 30–50 years, malignant pleural mesothelioma (MPM) is a disease of elderly males for the most part, with a mean age of death being 73 years and a male to female ratio of 4.2:1 in the United States.[2] The disease can occur at any age, including in childhood.[5] Mesothelioma cases reported from South America are younger, have a higher percentage of females, and have median survivals longer than that seen in the United States,[6] and it is unknown whether the differences are due to incorrect diagnosis or genetic predisposition. In autopsy studies, the frequency of malignant mesothelioma varies from 0.02% to 0.7%, with a rate of 0.2% in the largest series.[7] In most hospital series, the pleura is more often involved than the peritoneum, with a predominance of the right side over the left.[7] In some epidemiologic studies monitoring cohorts of asbestos workers, however, the peritoneal form is more common than the pleural.

Etiology

Household or neighborhood exposure to asbestos increases the odds ratio for pleural mesothelioma five to sevenfold,[8] and this relationship is dependent on the type of fiber. Amphiboles such as crocidolite, amosite, and erionite have a higher association with mesothelioma incidence than serpentine fibers such as chrysotile,[8] and fiber length may influence pathogenicity. In the absence of lung content analyses, the combination of a history of occupational exposure and radiological evidence of exposure, such as bilateral, calcified pleural plaques, and/or histological evidence of several asbestos fibers in lung tissue can be used to establish asbestos exposure with a certain level of reliability at the individual level.[2] The role of pleural plaques and their association with mesothelioma has been debated for several years. One recent study addressed this issue through a screening program in France and there was a significant association between pleural plaques, with a hazard ratio of 8.9. The authors concluded that the presence of pleural plaques appeared to be an "independent risk factor for mesothelioma."[9] While asbestos exposure and cigarette smoking act synergistically to produce lung cancer, smoking is not an established risk factor for mesothelioma, although an association between cigarettes using "micronite" filters has been postulated.[10] Other less common causative agents include radiation therapy (RT), as has been observed in young adults who have received RT for Wilms tumor or for mediastinal lymphoma.[11] In the 1990s, a relationship between the DNA virus SV40 and mesothelioma was pursued based on findings that SV40 could transform mesothelial cells and also promote the development of mesotheliomas in hamsters. Moreover, early polio vaccines were contaminated with SV40 until 1963.[12] Despite the demonstration of SV40 genetic components in human mesothelioma tumors, the US National Academy of Medicine concluded there was inadequate epidemiologic evidence to prove causality of the vaccines to mesothelioma.[2]

There has been renewed interest in talc as a possible cause of mesothelioma due to contamination with asbestos fibers, but the verdict on whether contaminated cosmetic talc is associated with mesothelioma remains controversial. Various studies point to no conclusive epidemiologic evidence to support this hypothesis[13,14] while others document amphibole fibers in talc users without other asbestos exposure.[15,16]

Molecular biology of mesothelioma

High Mobility Group Box 1 Protein (HMGB1), tumor necrosis factor-alpha (TNF-α), and Nuclear Factor Kappa B (NF-κB) signaling play an important role in the survival and malignant transformation of genetically damaged mesothelial cells.[17] HMGB1 is a typical DAMP (damage-associated molecular patterns)[18,19] and a key mediator of inflammation.[20] Moreover, it is a critical regulator in the initiation of asbestos-mediated inflammation leading to the release of TNF-α and subsequent NF-κB signaling.[21] Phagocytic macrophages at sites of inflammation internalize asbestos and release mutagenic reactive oxygen species and numerous cytokines including TNF-α and interleukin (IL)-1β, which have been linked to asbestos-related carcinogenesis.[17,22] HMGB1 is also released by reactive macrophages, other inflammatory cells, and human mesothelial cells (HMCs) upon exposure to asbestos.[21] Carcinogenic mineral fibers such as asbestos and erionite fibers induce programmed necrosis in most exposed HMC. During programmed necrosis, HMGB1 is released and then binds several proinflammatory molecules and triggers the inflammatory responses that distinguish this type of cell death from apoptosis. Moreover, it has been recently discovered that autophagy was up-regulated in HMC via HMGB1 after asbestos exposure. The autophagy activation serves as a surviving mechanism that protects HMC from dying.[23] Extracellular HMGB1 stimulates Advanced Glycosylation End-Product Specific Receptor (RAGE) and TLR4 (the two main HMGB1 receptors) expressed on neighboring inflammatory cells such as macrophages and induces the release of TNF-α and IL-1β. Asbestos-mediated TNF-α signaling then induces the activation of NF-κB-dependent mechanisms, further promoting the survival of HMCs after asbestos exposure,[21] and thus allowing HMCs with accumulated asbestos-induced genetic damage to survive, divide, and propagate genetic aberrations in premalignant cells that can give rise to a malignant clone. In addition, HMGB1 enhances the activity of NF-κB, which promotes tumor formation, progression, and metastasis[24] (Figure 1).

The serum levels of HMGB1 increase progressively in mice upon injection of crocidolite, a type of asbestos characterized by its biopersistence. Instead, chrysotile, a type of asbestos that is less biopersistent and rapidly degraded by inflammatory cells, induces a transient increase in serum HMGB1.[25] Continuous chrysotile administration results in sustained HMGB1 levels similar to those caused by crocidolite.[25] These findings demonstrate a clear causative effect between asbestos exposure and increased HMGB1 serum levels. High serum levels of HMGB1 have also been detected in the serum of individuals exposed to asbestos and in patients with mesothelioma.[21,26,27] Noncarcinogenic fibers such as palygorskite do not induce HMGB1 secretion.[28] Moreover, targeting HMGB1 using HMGB1 antagonists significantly inhibits HMC transformation and mesothelioma progression.[23,26,29,30] The findings support a contributory pathogenic role of HMGB1 in asbestos carcinogenesis and mesothelioma.[2,31]

Genomic abnormalities

Mesothelioma has a very large number of genomic alterations, including deletions, recombinations, etc. of several chromosomes.[32,33] However, most of these alterations are random as they are different in different tumors and among different biopsies of the same tumor, and only few genetic alterations have been identified as driver mutations which are associated with the growth and progression of mesothelioma.[34,35] Karyotyping studies, as well as comparative genomic hybridization (CGH), reveal that genomic loss in mesothelioma carcinogenesis is much more frequent than gain of function alterations. Losses in chromosome regions 1p, 3p, 6q, 9p, 13q, 15q, and 22q are common in mesothelioma and frequent genetic alterations in these losses include inactivating mutations of NF2 (neurofibromatosis 2), CDKN2A (cyclin-dependent kinases 2A), *BAP1* (BRCA-1 associated protein 1), and TP53 tumor suppressor genes.[32-34] BAP1 is the most commonly mutated gene, as about 60% of mesotheliomas carry acquired BAP1 mutations.[36] Initial studies, including our own,[37] underestimated the true number of BAP1 mutations in mesothelioma because these studies used Sanger sequencing and next-generation sequencing (NGS)[37-39] techniques designed to identify point mutations. Instead, over 50% of somatic BAP1 mutations in mesotheliomas consist of small deletions of 300–3000 kb, which are easily detected by multiplex ligation-dependent probe amplification (MLPA) and high-density array CGH but are missed by Sanger and NGS sequencing.[36,40] The critical driver role of BAP1 mutations in mesothelioma is discussed in more detail in the following section. Homozygous chromosomal loss and focal deletions of the 22q12 locus inactivate the **NF2** gene, resulting in low or absent expression of Merlin. This tumor suppressor protein regulates signal transduction of the epidermal growth factor receptor, PI3K (phosphoinositide 3-kinase), mTORC1/2 (mTOR complex 1/2), Hippo (Salvador-Warts-Hippo), Rac, Ras GTPase, and FAK (focal adhesion kinase) pathways. Loss of Merlin results in increased motility, migration, and invasion.[41] Deletions and point mutations of the **LATS2** gene often co-occur with *NF2* inactivation. *LATS2* loss results in abnormal control of the Hippo pathway, and can be associated with dysregulated immunoregulation.[42,43] Deletions of the **CDKN2A** (cyclin-dependent kinase inhibitor 2A) 9p21 locus occurs in about half of mesothelioma cases.[44,45] *CDKN2A* encodes p16INK4A and *CDKN2B* produces p14ARF, which influences cell cycle progression and apoptosis.[46] Moreover, p16INK4A and p15INK4B inhibit CDK4/6 activity, causing hypophosphorylation and functional activation of pRb (the retinoblastoma tumor suppressor protein), thereby preventing cell cycle progression and proliferation.[35,47] Co-deletion of *CDKN2A* and *CDKN2B* genes is associated with a shorter overall survival (OS) rate in mesothelioma.[34,41,48] **TP53** mutations are less common in mesothelioma but are associated with decreased survival.[49] Moreover, an unusual mesothelioma phenotype described from the Cancer Genome Atlas (TCGA, see below) includes young females with aggressive tumors who have *TP53* co mutations with **SETDB1**[50] and near haploidization. The **SETD2** tumor suppressor gene regulates genes controlling epigenetic modifications which influence active transcription and is frequently inactivated in MPM through gene fusions, splice alterations, and nonsynonymous mutations.[39] Others have described mutations in the telomerase reverse transcriptase (*TERT*) promoter in MPM and that their presence is associated with a poor survival and nonepithelioid histology.[49]

NGS and other metatranscriptomic studies

There have been several comprehensive, multi-platform, genomic studies of pleural mesothelioma[35,39,44,49] which have not only defined the genomic landscape of the disease but have been able to integrate analyses to define dominant molecular pathways, and their association with clinical, histologic, and prognostic features. The most important findings have defined a key role for *BAP1* in the pathogenesis of the disease (see below) as well as the ability to perform integrated multiplatform analyses defining prognostic clusters. Data from Bueno et al. and TCGA originally

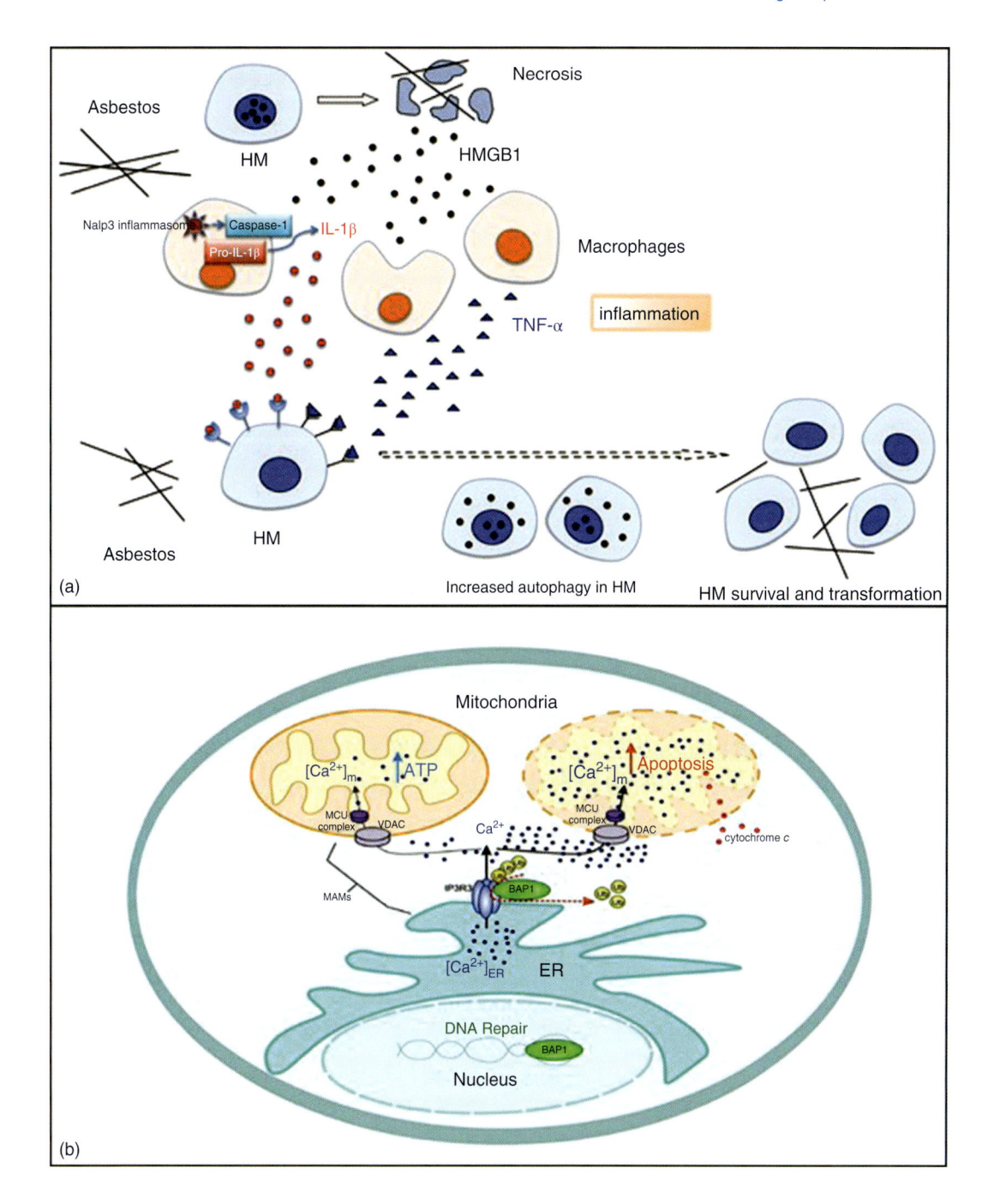

Figure 1 (a) Working hypothesis of asbestos carcinogenesis and HM transformation. Asbestos causes necrotic HM death that leads to the release of HMGB1 into the extracellular space. HMGB1 elicits macrophage accumulation, triggers the inflammatory response, and induces the secretion of inflammatory factors such as TNF α and IL-1-β which increases the survival of asbestos-damaged HM. In the meantime, asbestos also induces the autophagy levels in HM that further increase HM survival. This allows key genetic alterations to accumulate within HM that sustain asbestos-induced DNA damage that leads to the initiation of mesothelioma. (b) BAP1 controls distinct cellular activities by modulating DNA repair and Ca^{2+} intracellular levels. In the nucleus, BRCA1-associated protein 1 (BAP1) regulates DNA repair. Increased DNA damage is observed in BAP1-mutant cells after exposure to asbestos, ultraviolet light, radiation, and chemotherapy. Source: Based on Carbone et al.[2]

defined four clusters with different survival characteristics and differences in immune cell infiltrates without correlation to clinical variables.[39,44] The cluster with the *best prognosis* had a greater proportion of epithelial histology, lower somatic copy number alterations, relatively few CDKN2A homozygous deletions (11%), a high level of methylation, and *BAP1* alterations. A novel finding was that V-domain Ig suppressor of T cell activation (VISTA), an immune checkpoint inhibitor, was found to be highly expressed in the good prognosis cluster and was inversely correlated with epithelial-mesenchymal transition (EMT). VISTA is present on the surface of antigen-presenting cells (APC) which includes the normal mesothelium and inhibits early-stage T-cell activation.[51] The *poor prognosis cluster* was characterized by EMT, mesothelin promoter methylation, and low expression of mesothelin which was associated with poorly differentiated sarcomatoid and biphasic mesotheliomas, *LATS2* mutations, and *CDKN2A* homozygous deletions.[44] Poor prognosis signaling pathways include PI3K-mTOR and RAS-MAPK as well as a Th2 cell signature, which regulates cytokines involved in asbestos carcinogenesis. The TCGA integrative prognostic cluster was validated from the transcriptomic data performed by Bueno et al.[39] and also in reports by Blum et al.[52] and Quetel et al.[49] Mate-pair sequencing analyses[53,54] and target NGS in combination with high-density array CGH[40,55] have revealed many more genomic aberrancies than standard NGS. Yoshikawa et al.[40] discovered that chromothripsis (i.e., chromosome shattering followed by random chromosomal rearrangement) causes some of the genetic alterations in mesothelioma, a finding independently confirmed by Mansfield et al.[53,54] Moreover, these genetic alterations may be responsible for neo-antigens production, offering new immunotherapeutic discovery approaches in mesothelioma.

Genetic predisposition to mesothelioma: the role of BAP1

The genetic susceptibility to mesothelioma was first discovered in Cappadocia Turkey, where high mesothelioma incidence (>50%) in some families was associated with a clear pattern of autosomal dominance inheritance.[56] This study, together with additional genetic studies with two American families, eventually led to the discovery of germline heterozygous mutation on the *BAP1* gene that contributed mesothelioma to predisposition and caused the high incidence of mesothelioma in those families even without occupational asbestos exposure.[37] Animal studies performed using *Bap1*$^{+/-}$ heterozygous mice demonstrated that animals developed mesothelioma when exposed to 10-fold lower doses of asbestos fibers that barely caused any mesothelioma in wild type *Bap1* mice.[57] The individuals with germline mutated *BAP1* were also susceptible to other types of cancer, including uveal melanoma, cutaneous melanoma, and clear cell renal carcinoma among others, leading to the identification of the "BAP1 Cancer Syndrome."[58,59] More than 200 families carrying germline *BAP1* mutations have been identified so far, including some large kindred dating back to the eighteenth century with high incidence of mesothelioma, uveal melanoma, and other cancers.[60] Recent studies noted that mesothelioma patients with germline *BAP1* mutations have significantly improved survival compared to sporadic mesothelioma patients without germline mutations.[61-63] The discovery of the BAP1 Cancer Syndrome underscores the importance of genotyping familial mesothelioma patients for genetic alterations in germline DNA to determine the presence of genetic mutations which may influence treatment response and prognosis.[64]

The function of BAP1 has been studied intensively following the discovery of BAP1 Cancer Syndrome (Figure 1b). *BAP1* is located at the 3p21, a region frequently deleted in MPM, and encodes for a deubiquitinase enzyme that plays multiple important functions in cells. In the nucleus, BAP1 is critical for normal DNA replication and DNA repair.[65-67] In the cytoplasm, BAP1 commonly localizes in the endoplasmic reticulum (ER), where it deubiquitylates and stabilizes the type 3 inositol-1,4,5-trisphosphate receptor (IP3R3), a Ca^{2+} channel that modulates the release of Ca^{2+} from ER into the mitochondria and regulates apoptosis and cell death.[68] In heterozygous *BAP1*$^{+/-}$ conditions, as in the individuals of the families with the BAP1 Cancer Syndrome, the reduced BAP1 dosage impairs the DNA repair, accumulating DNA damage, and the apoptotic response, which contributes to the malignant transformation and tumor development.[2,68,69] Moreover, reduced BAP1 level induces the Warburg effect, a shift of cell metabolism from oxidative phosphorylation (Krebs cycle) to aerobic glycolysis, a hallmark of cancer cells, which also favors malignant growth.[70] Additionally, BAP1 binds ASXL2 and this complex binds and deubiquitylates histone H2A. This complex regulates cell proliferation and is disrupted in cancer cells carrying BAP1 mutations.[71] Finally, the high frequency of *BAP1* alterations (around 60%) found in somatic mesotheliomas[36,38-40,44] further highlights the importance of BAP1 in mesothelioma pathogenesis, and related pathways may provide possible novel targets for therapeutic approaches in the future. One of these associated pathways may involve inhibition of EZH2 methyltransferase with tazemetostat, since BAP1 loss is associated with EZH2-dependent transformation.[72]

Diagnosing and staging the patient with possible mesothelioma

Symptoms and signs

The onset of mesothelioma is associated with chest pain, dyspnea, or cough (Figure 2). Progressive invasion of the chest wall often leads to intractable pain. Pleural effusion is present initially in up to 95% of cases. Later, tumor growth usually results in complete obliteration of the pleural space and encasement of the lung. Late symptoms of bulky mesotheliomas include mediastinal invasion with dysphagia, phrenic nerve paralysis, pericardial effusion, and superior vena cava syndrome.[73] Peritoneal involvement by mesothelioma is characterized by ascites and intestinal compromise leading to cachexia.

Laboratory evaluation

There are several laboratory abnormalities associated with mesothelioma. Of these, the presence of thrombocytosis with platelet counts greater than 400,000 is probably the most common.[74] Others include hypergammaglobulinemia, eosinophilia, anemia of chronic disease, elevated homocysteine levels, folic acid deficiency, and vitamins B12 and B6 deficiency.[73]

Histologic subtypes

A pathologist experienced with diagnosing mesothelioma should confirm all diagnoses since concordance amongst expert panels for the diagnosis of pleural mesothelioma is only 69%.[75] The three primary types of mesothelioma are epithelial type (50–70%), the fibrous morphology type, also called sarcomatoid type (10%), and the rest are a combination called biphasic or mixed type. Epithelioid mesotheliomas are the least aggressive, while biphasic mesotheliomas usually behave similarly to the sarcomatoid type. Among epithelioid mesotheliomas, some sub-types have a better prognosis (trabecular and tubular-papillary sub-types) than others (solid and micropapillary sub-types). A recent Euracan/IASLC proposal for updating mesothelioma pathologic classification has suggested updating to include architectural patterns and stromal and cytologic features that might improve prognosis, and permit early treatment and/or avoid misdiagnosis.[76] These architectural epithelioid patterns include tubulopapillary, trabecular, adenomatoid, microcystic, solid, micropapillary, transitional pattern, and pleomorphic. Likewise, for sarcomatoid mesothelioma, patterns that are desmoplastic, lymphohistiocytoid, transition, or pleomorphic should be described and quantitated. Biphasic malignant mesothelioma should represent any combination of patterns of epithelioid and sarcomatoid mesothelioma with at least 10% of each component. Moreover, grading of epithelioid

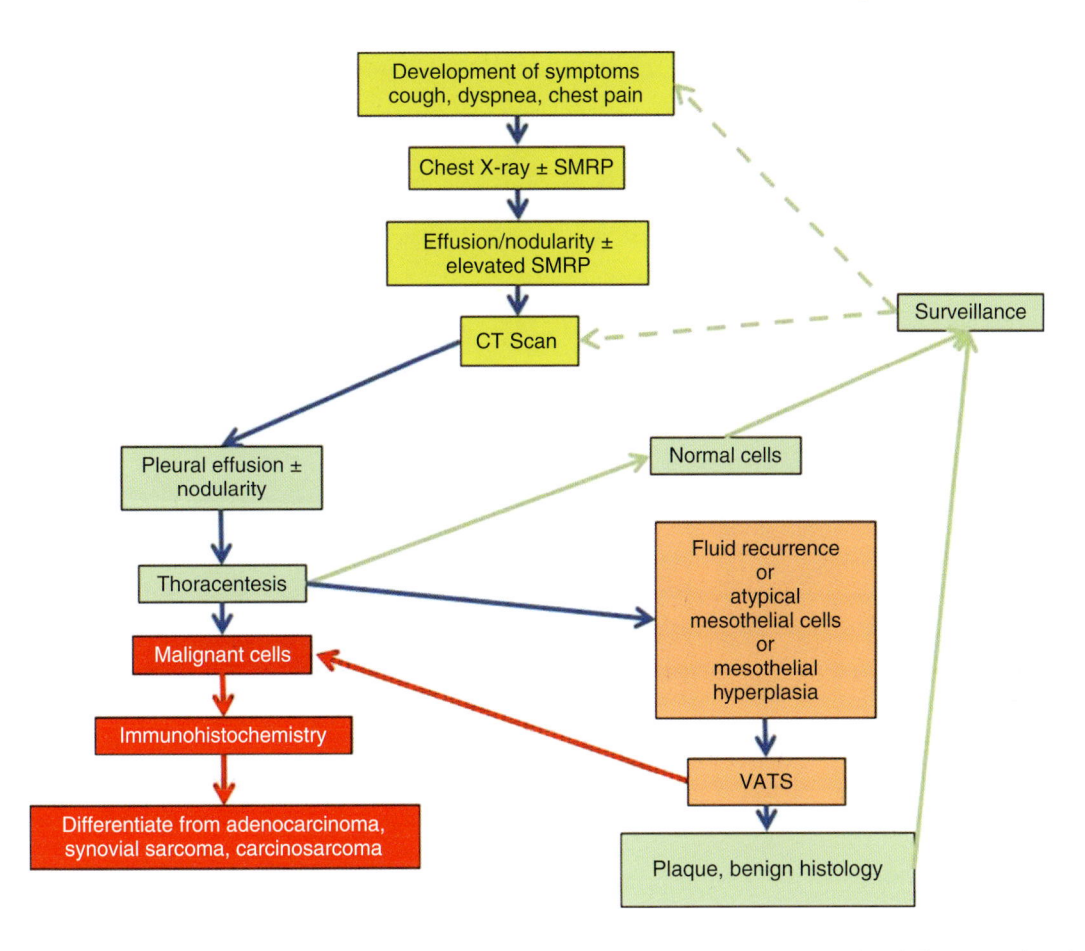

Figure 2 Algorithm for the workup of the asbestos-exposed individual who presents with new symptoms. Any new pleural effusion must have thoracentesis and immunohistochemical analyses. If atypical mesothelial cells are seen, thoracoscopy should be performed for histologic confirmation of malignancy or inflammatory disease.

mesothelioma based on nuclear atypia, mitotic count, and necrosis was recommended.[76]

Immunohistochemistry (IHC) is the standard for classification, and diagnosis. These markers include positive pankeratin (usually CAM5.2), keratin 5/6, calretinin, and WT-1 as well as negative markers including CEA, CD15, Ber-EP4, Moc-31, TTF-1, and B72.3.[77] One must consider, however, that 50% of sarcomatoid mesotheliomas will stain with calretinin or WT1 antibodies, while close to 100% of them will stain with Cam5.2. Cam 5.2 immunostaining is also seen with carcinosarcomas.[78] BAP1 IHC has entered the routine of most pathology laboratories, improving the ability to diagnose mesothelioma.[36,79,80] BAP1 wild-type (*BAP1*WT) protein is found in the nucleus and the cytoplasm, resulting in strong nuclear staining and less intense cytoplasmic staining.[36] *BAP1* mutations and deletions nearly always result either in complete absence of staining or in cytoplasmic staining without nuclear staining and as detailed above, approximately 2/3 of epithelial and 50% of sarcomatoid mesotheliomas contain somatic *BAP1* mutations, resulting in absence of *BAP1* nuclear staining.[36,81,82] Because benign cells always show *BAP1* nuclear staining, the absence of *BAP1* nuclear staining is a specific and reliable marker to distinguish mesothelioma from atypical mesothelial hyperplasia at its earliest stages of development.

Cytopathology is usually not helpful for patients with sarcomatoid mesothelioma since they seldom exfoliate cells. In general, suspicious cytologic examinations revealing atypical mesothelial cells in three-dimensional structures or as mesothelial hyperplasia should be confirmed by direct pleural biopsy.

Tumor markers

Despite a multitude of studies in the literature, there are no validated blood-based biomarkers for either the diagnosis or prognosis of mesothelioma except for soluble mesothelin-related peptides (SMRP) or mesothelin. SMRP has consistent sensitivities and specificities of 40% and 98%, respectively, and a large meta-analysis has confirmed that the sensitivity and specificity of SMRP are similar in many studies.[83] Serum SMRP levels are higher in MPM patients than in lung cancer patients, as are the SMRP levels in MPM pleural fluid when compared to other nonMPM pleural effusions. Indeed, prior studies have suggested that the accuracy of detection is superior in pleural fluid than in serum, though serum analysis is more convenient measure. SMRP is not ideal for mesothelioma screening in an asbestos-exposed population. While some studies show a rise in SMRP levels in the year prior to diagnosis, SMRP level lacks adequate sensitivity to serve as a reliable stand-alone screening test and current evidence collectively suggests that it lacks sufficient sensitivity to be used for screening in high-risk populations.[83–85] SMRP is useful, however, for the monitoring of disease after or during treatment.[86] SMRP is elevated in the majority of epithelioid mesotheliomas and a portion of biphasic but cannot be detected in sarcomatoid tumors. The use of fibulin 3 to diagnose mesothelioma remains controversial, but levels are generally elevated in all types of mesothelioma.[87,88] There are no validated data on using microRNAs in serum or plasma to predict types of tumor, and the use of immuno-oncologic methods to diagnose MPM using transcriptional panels is in its infancy.[87] Most recently, serum levels of calretinin measured by

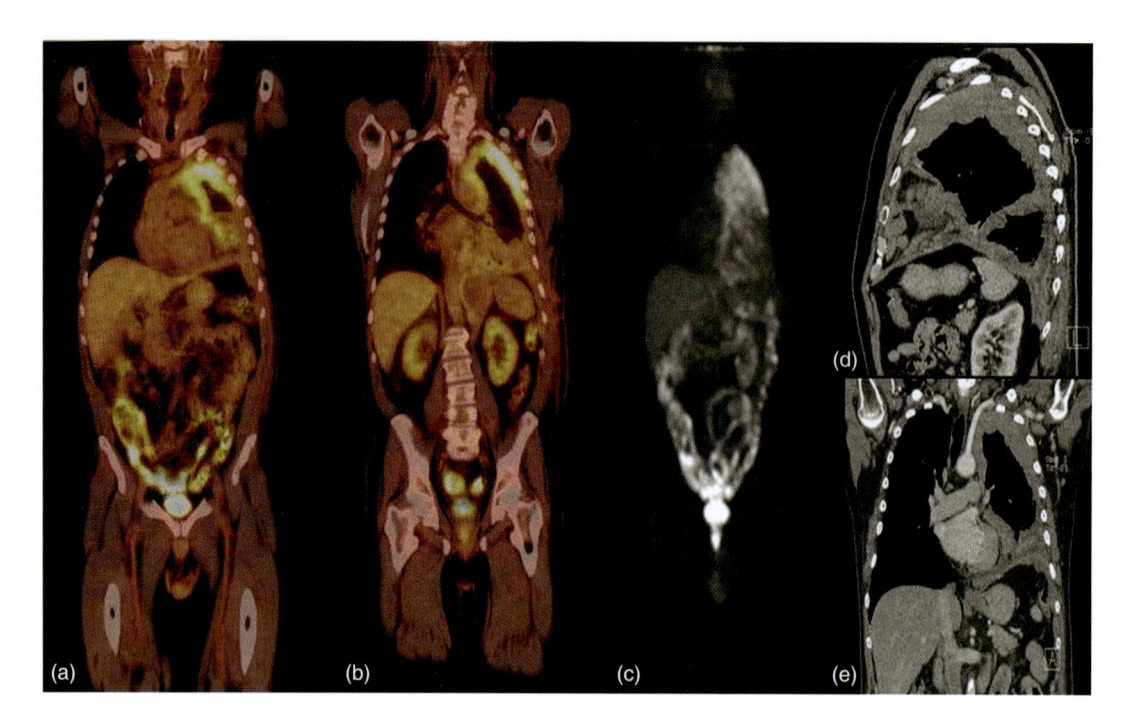

Figure 3 PET-CT and pleural mesothelioma. (a, b) Posterior and anterior views of the left chest reveal a bulky hypermetabolic tumor. (c) Maximum intensity projection (MIP) view confirming no disease outside the chest. (d) Sagittal view of CT image reveals bulky disease in the fissures. (e) Coronal view reveals abutment of the subclavian artery and possible diaphragmatic involvement.

enzyme-linked immunosorbent assay in males with mesothelioma have been able to differentiate MPM types in a case-control study: differences between sarcomatoid ($n = 28$) and epithelioid ($n = 103$) ($p < 0.0041$) as well as sarcomatoid and biphasic ($n = 44$) ($p < 0.0001$) were statistically significant.[89]

Imaging

Computerized tomographic (CT) chest scanning, preferably performed with intravenous contrast and with slices of 3 mm or less in thickness, is very useful for mesothelioma diagnosis and disease assessment. Findings on CT scan include a pleural effusion, pleural nodularity, and concentric pleural thickening. Nevertheless, investigators from Oxford recently estimated the positive and negative predictive value of CT scans in approximately 400 patients prior to thoracoscopy for diagnosis. The positive predictive value of a CT scan that demonstrated "malignant" findings was 80%, while the negative predictive value was 65%. Thus, CT scans alone appear to be insufficient to determine which patients should undergo invasive pleural biopsies.[90]

Additional imaging modalities for mesothelioma include magnetic resonance imaging (MRI) and positron emission tomography (PET) scanning. MRI is not frequently used but may be of additional benefit to detect diaphragm invasion, involvement of the endothoracic fascia, or an isolated area of chest wall involvement in patients who may be candidates for surgical resection. MRI also has been reported to be superior to CT for detecting involvement of bone, interlobar fissures, diaphragm (particularly transmural involvement and extension through the diaphragm), and endothoracic fascia. Diffusion-weighted MRI may provide information on MPM tumor histology, and perfusion CT and MRI also have been explored for the enhancement of diagnostic accuracy and for assessment of response to therapy.[91,92]

PET/CT imaging is now recommended for staging by the National Comprehensive Cancer Network (NCCN) guidelines Version 1.2020 for patients who are being considered for surgical resection (Figure 3). The chief benefit of fluoro deoxy glucose (FDG)-PET/CT is its ability to detect distant and occult metastatic lesions that would not be apparent by other modalities and that, when present, contraindicate surgery. Additional sites of disease not seen on CT have been described in approximately 10% of patients.[93] In a study of 29 MPM patients, integrated PET/CT correctly assigned the overall stage in 72% of cases, showed increased sensitivity for T4 disease in 67% of patients compared to 9% for PET alone, recognized 7 patients with extrathoracic disease missed by conventional radiographic studies, and identified 12 patients who would have been precluded from surgical resection based on conventional studies.[94] In early MPM, the effusion tends to lack avidity, especially if there is no associated pleural thickening or nodularity and if possible the PET/CT should be obtained before any type of pleurodesis.[95] Investigators from Memorial Sloan-Kettering Cancer Center examined the accuracy of PET scan in detecting histologic subtype. In 100 patients with MPM who underwent preoperative PET scans, they found that the mixed subtype of epithelioid mesothelioma had higher standard uptake values (SUVs) than patients with the nonpleomorphic subtype, thus supporting the conclusion that higher SUVs are correlated with aggressive disease.[96] Metabolic response after neoadjuvant chemotherapy has also been correlated with OS.[97]

Invasive staging

Whether invasive staging is performed for mesothelioma depends on institutional guidelines. Invasive staging techniques including mediastinoscopy and endobronchial ultrasound (EBUS) should confirm the presence of lymph node metastases suspected on CT or PET CT. Unfortunately, however, half of involved mediastinal lymph nodes are located in areas not accessible with these procedures, including the anterior mediastinum, pericardial fat pad, and peridiaphragmatic and posterior intercostal regions.

While some institutions routinely perform mediastinoscopy or EBUS/EUS for staging, others use these procedures selectively, depending on findings from imaging studies and the overall plans for multimodality treatment. Laparoscopy can clarify whether transdiaphragmatic tumor invasion is present. Bulky tumor in the lower hemithorax often involves and depresses the hemidiaphragm, making it difficult to determine whether T4 or M1 disease is present. Laparoscopy can identify tumor directly extending through the diaphragm (T4) or peritoneal metastases. While some institutions routinely perform staging laparoscopy, most use it selectively to supplement information available from imaging studies.[98]

Staging and prognosis

There have been a variety of staging systems for pleural mesothelioma. The American Joint Commission on Cancer/The Union for International Cancer Control (AJCC/UICC) has accepted staging proposals from the International Association for the Study of Lung Cancer staging committee through an international database which includes over 3519 cases.[99] The present version of the staging system is the Eighth Edition (Figure 4), and there were some notable changes from the Seventh Edition. Survival by T category was examined for T categories according to the current seventh edition staging system to make new recommendations. None of the Seventh Edition T descriptors were shifted or eliminated. Additionally in an exploratory evaluation, tumor thickness and nodular or rindlike morphology were significantly associated with survival. There was clear separation between all clinically staged categories except for T1a versus T1b and these were collapsed into a single T1 category.[101] For the N descriptor, no separation in survival was noted between clinical N0–N2. For pathologically staged tumors, patients with pN1 or pN2 tumors had worse survival than those with pN0 tumors but no survival difference was noted between those with pN1 and pN2 tumors. The eighth edition N categories were therefore revised to collapse both clinical and pN1 and pN2 categories into a single N category comprising ipsilateral, intrathoracic nodal metastases (N1), and nodes previously categorized as N3 have been reclassified as N2.[102] For the M category, only 84 cases were clinical M1. Median OS for cM1 cases was 9.7 versus 13.4 months ($p = 0.0013$) for the locally advanced (T4 or N3) cM0 cases, supporting inclusion of only cM1 in the stage IV group. For stage grouping, the final recommendations for the eighth edition were stage IA (T1N0), stage IB (T2-3N0), stage II (T1-2N1), stage IIIA (T3N1), stage IIIB

Stage	Definition
Primary tumor (T)	
TX	Primary tumor cannot be assessed
T0	No evidence of primary tumor
T1	Tumor limited to the ipsilateral parietal ± visceral ± mediastinal ± diaphragmatic pleura
T2	Tumor involving each of the ipsilateral pleural surfaces (parietal, mediastinal, diaphragmatic, and visceral pleura) with at least one of the following features: • involvement of diaphragmatic muscle • extension of tumor from visceral pleura into the underlying pulmonary parenchyma
T3	Describes locally advanced but *potentially resectable* tumor. Tumor involving all of the ipsilateral pleural surfaces (parietal, mediastinal, diaphragmatic, and visceral pleura) with at least one of the following features: • involvement of the endothoracic fascia • extension into the mediastinal fat • solitary, completely resectable focus of tumor extending into the soft tissues of the chest wall • nontransmural involvement of the pericardium
T4	Describes locally advanced *technically unresectable* tumor. Tumor involving all of the ipsilateral pleural surfaces (parietal, mediastinal, diaphragmatic, and visceral pleura) with at least one of the following features: • diffuse extension or multifocal masses of tumor in the chest wall, with or without associated rib destruction • direct transdiaphragmatic extension of tumor to the peritoneum • direct extension of tumor to the contralateral pleura • direct extension of tumor to mediastinal organs • direct extension of tumor into the spine • tumor extending through to the internal surface of the pericardium with or without a pericardial effusion, or tumor involving the myocardium
Regional lymph nodes (N)	
NX	Regional lymph nodes cannot be assessed
N0	No regional lymph node metastases
N1	Metastases in the ipsilateral bronchopulmonary, hilar, or mediastinal (including the internal mammary, peridiaphragmatic, pericardial fat pad, or intercostal lymph nodes) lymph nodes
N2	Metastases in the contralateral mediastinal, ipsilateral, or contralateral supraclavicular lymph nodes
Distant metastasis (M)	
M0	No distant metastasis
M1	Distant metastasis present

	N0		N1/N2		N1		N3		N2	
Stage	Seventh edition	Eighth edition	Seventh edition	Eighth edition	Seventh edition	Eighth edition	Seventh edition	Eighth edition	Seventh edition	Eighth edition
T1	I (A, B)	IA	III		II		IV			IIIB
T2	II	IB	III		II		IV			IIIB
T3	II	IB	III		IIIA		IV			IIIB
T4	IV	IIIB	IV		IIIB		IV			IIIB
M1	IV	IV	IV		IV		IV			IV

Figure 4 IASLC/AJCC Eight Edition of Mesothelioma Staging from Ref. 100. Abbreviations: T, primary tumor; T1, limited to ipsilateral pleura only (parietal pleura, visceral pleura); T2, superficial local invasion (diaphragm, endothoracic fascia, ipsilateral lung, fissures); T3, deep local invasion (chest wall beyond endothoracic fascia); T4, extensive direct invasion (opposite pleura, peritoneum, retroperitoneum); N, lymph nodes; N0, no positive lymph node; N1, positive ipsilateral hilar nodes; N2, positive mediastinal nodes; N3, positive contralateral hilar nodes; M, metastases; M0, no metastases; M1, metastases; blood-borne or lymphatic. Source: Modified from de Perrot et al.[100]

(T1-3N2 or any T4), and stage IV (any M1).[99] The IASLC/IMIG Mesothelioma Registry also has reported that histology, age, sex, and white blood cell and platelet counts stratified survival for 906 patients.[74] Future staging will build not only on these studies but also on preoperative quantitation imaging studies including CT volumetrics which have been associated with prognosis[103] and lymph node involvement[104] or linear measurements at three levels[101] or of diaphragm thickness.[100]

Surgery

There is little consensus amongst mesothelioma physicians regarding the role of resection in pleural mesothelioma and whether surgery actually extends survival. In fact, most of the patients having resection are referred to tertiary centers for "definitive" surgical therapy and are thought to have minimal disease. For the most part, however, the preoperative studies underestimate the extent of disease and also are poor in predicting whether there is extensive invasion of the mediastinum, diaphragm, visceral pleura, or chest wall. Surgery is sometimes essential for the accurate diagnosis of the disease either by video-assisted thoracic surgery or open pleural biopsy for cases in which the pleural cavity is frozen by tumor.

The goal of cytoreductive surgery in MPM should be the removal of all visible or palpable tumor (R0 or R1) or a "macroscopic complete resection" (MCR) regardless of whether that involves extrapleural pneumonectomy (EPP) (Figure 5) or a lung-preserving operation (Figure 6). In order to standardize the terminology of MCR techniques, the Mesothelioma Domain of the International Association for the Study of Lung Cancer has recommended the following as uniform nomenclature for pleural mesothelioma resections.[105] *EPP*: en bloc resection of the parietal and visceral pleura with the ipsilateral lung, pericardium, and diaphragm. In cases where the pericardium and/or diaphragm are not involved by tumor, these structures may be left intact. *Extended P/D*: parietal and visceral pleurectomy to remove all gross tumor with resection of the diaphragm and/or pericardium. *P/D*: parietal and visceral pleurectomy to remove all gross tumor without diaphragm or pericardial resection. *Partial pleurectomy*: partial removal of parietal and/or visceral pleura for diagnostic or palliative purposes but leaving gross tumor behind.

Considering the high morbidity rate from MCRs, the operations should be performed only by experienced mesothelioma surgical specialists, and the candidacy for surgery will depend on the cardiopulmonary/functional status of the patient, and patient/tumor demographics at presentation. Patients with compromised performance status or who have limiting cardiac reserve either with nonreversible myocardial ischemia or compromised ventricular function (ejection fraction <50%) are usually not candidates for cytoreductive procedures. Moreover, patients with compromised pulmonary function testing who are not felt to be candidates for pneumonectomy must still be carefully evaluated for extended P/D so that the operation will not compromise existing lung function but may recruit trapped lung and possibly improve dyspnea. Unfortunately, it is not possible to predict with certainty which patients are actually going to benefit from surgical therapy of mesothelioma despite the litany of studies which have tried to predict preoperative prognostic factors. Certainly epithelial

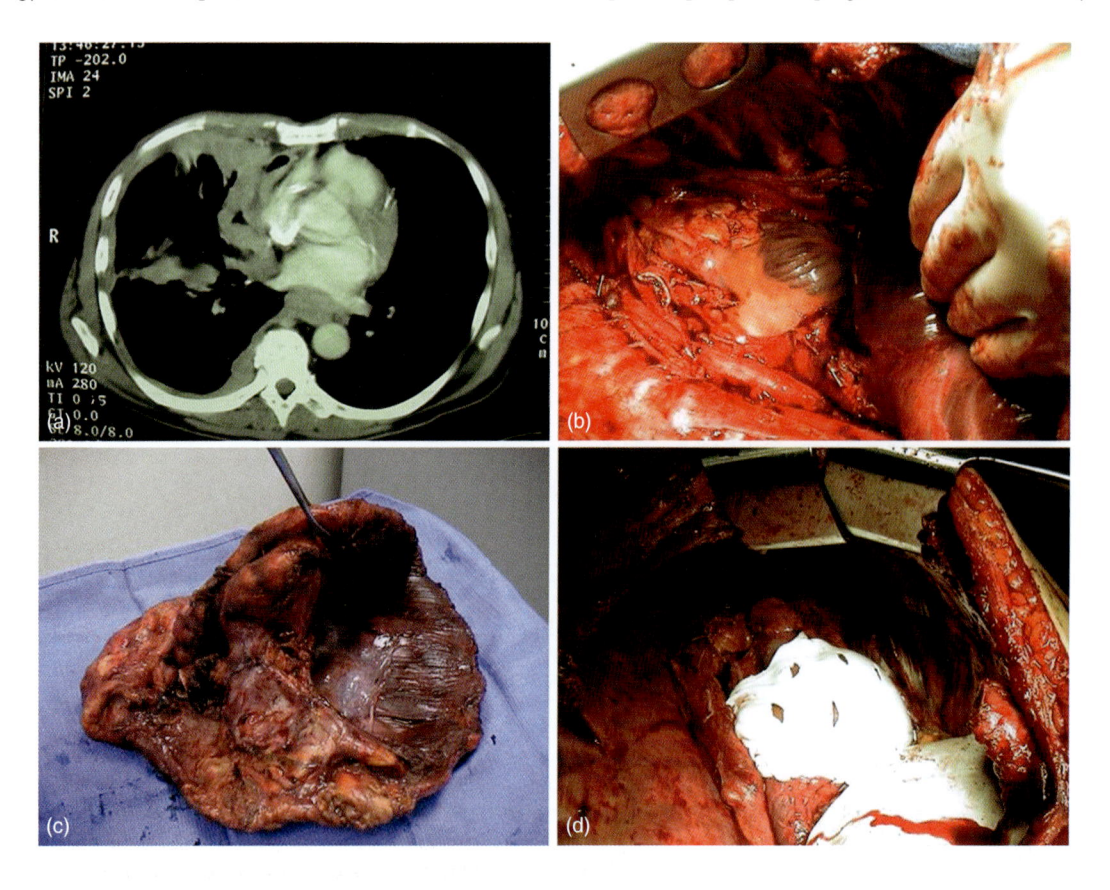

Figure 5 Extrapleural pneumonectomy for mesothelioma: (a) Computer tomography reveals thickened pleura, pericardium, and disease in the fissures. (b) Intraoperative view after the resection with hand on the liver. Stapled bronchial stump, right atrium, and extent of pericardiotomy are seen. (c) Operative specimen reveals diaphragmatic resection to the right and thickened pleura encasing the lung. (d) Reconstruction of the diaphragm and pericardium with Gore-Tex patches.

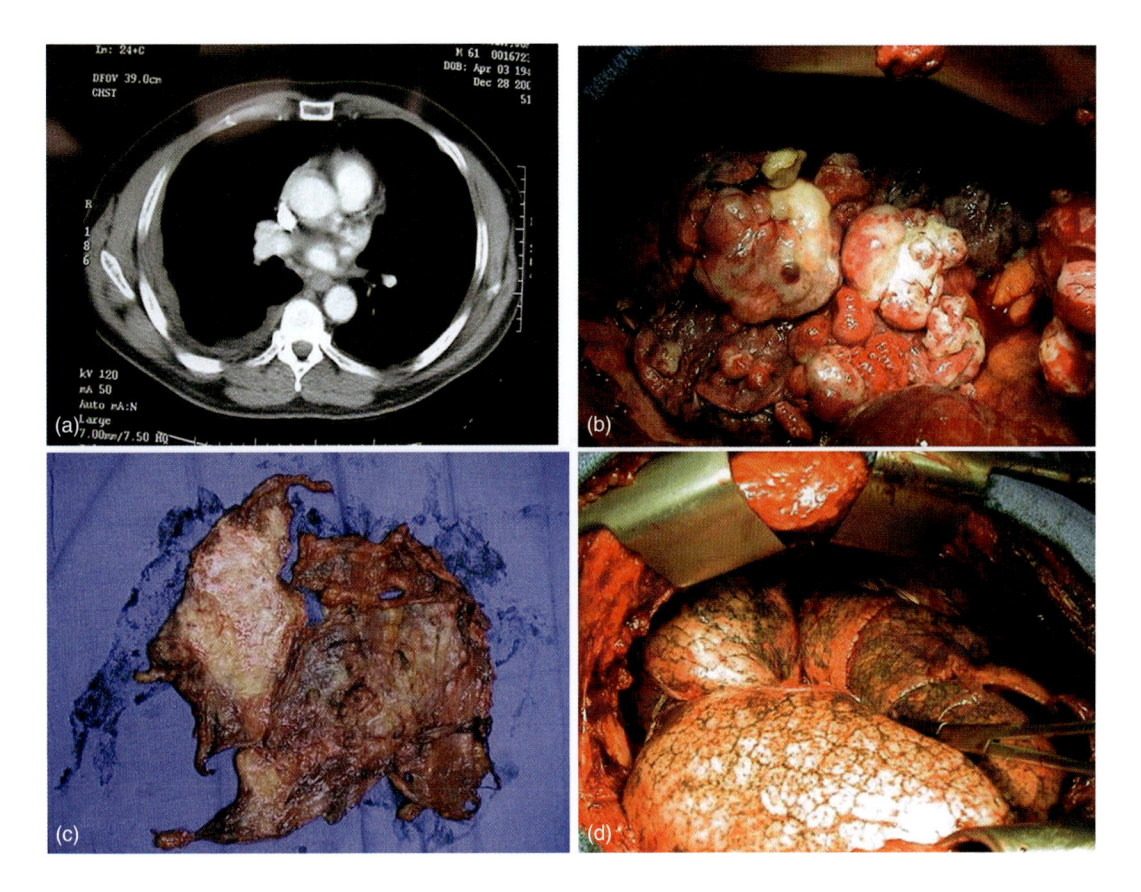

Figure 6 Pleurectomy for mesothelioma: (a) typical computer tomogram reveals thickened pleura; (b) operative view reveals disease primarily on the parietal pleura; (c) operative specimen; (d) completion of satisfactory cytoreduction with sparing and decortication of the lung.

histology, female gender, and low volume of disease seem to be seen in patients who survive the longest after an MCR.[74]

The addition of adjuvant therapy is crucial in all patients having surgical resection of mesothelioma, as many studies have revealed that surgery alone is inferior to surgery and adjuvant or neoadjuvant therapy (see section titled "Systemic Therapy for Mesothelioma" for a discussion of neoadjuvant and adjuvant therapies). With the advent of pemetrexed and cisplatin as the standard of care for mesothelioma chemotherapy[106] and the use of hemithoracic intensity modulated radiation therapy (IMRT) after EPP[107] (see section titled "Radiation therapy for mesothelioma," induction trials were popular with the surgical procedure being EPP. Neoadjuvant chemotherapy has the potential to adversely delay surgical resection or induce complications prior to resection. Also, significant response rates with tumor shrinkage ranging 29–44% with cisplatin-pemetrexed were recorded. It is estimated from clinical trials that in 42–84% of cases, an EPP after neoadjuvant chemotherapy will be able to be completed.[108–114] However, as reviewed by Optiz, these studies were associated with major morbidities in 30–80% of participants, mortality of 2.2–8%, and median survival times of 10–59 months.[115]

A number of factors led to the shift in philosophy to lung-sparing approaches instead of EPP for MCR. The mesothelioma and radical surgery (MARS) trial deflated much optimism for the EPP trimodality approach when it not only failed to show an added benefit of surgery when combined with induction therapy but actually reported worse survival among patients who underwent EPP compared to patients treated with chemotherapy alone.[116] Despite the small size of the MARS trial and its extraordinary 19% operative mortality, pessimism for EPP, and surgery in general, has persisted. The modern-day 30-day or in-hospital mortality after EPP is reported to be 5–7%, and 90-day mortality rates as high as 11% at high-volume mesothelioma centers.[2] Most mesothelioma surgeons now advocate for extended pleurectomy decortication (EPD), which involves extensive parietal and visceral decortication with lung-sparing, and diaphragmatic/pericardial resection if needed. Equal survival rates, lower morbidity, and lower mortality rates have been recorded by a number of single-center studies comparing EPP versus EPD either as retrospective comparisons with or without propensity matching.[2] An important prospective randomized trial, MARS2, in the United Kingdom which could determine whether P/D or EPD after induction chemotherapy leads to superior outcomes compared with chemotherapy has almost completed accrual at this writing.[117] When all the data from surgical studies of mesothelioma are reviewed, the median survival after EPD hovers around 20 months with the majority of patients recurring in the ipsilateral chest.[118] For this reason, some thoracic surgeons and medical oncologists feel that better prediction of mesothelioma biology by metatranscriptomic/immunological clustering of individual mesothelioma patients should guide whether potentially morbid surgery should be performed.[119]

Novel experimental surgical approaches have included preoperative hemithoracic radiation followed by EPP (SMART, surgery for mesothelioma after radiation therapy). Data *in vivo* demonstrate specific activation of the immune system against mesothelioma using this approach with the development of an *in situ* vaccination, which is maintained through memory T cells directed against the tumor.[120,121] The most recent long-term data in 69 patients from the University of Toronto reveals a median survival of 34.4 months in patients with epithelioid MPM treated with SMART compared with 21.6 months in patients with epithelioid MPM treated with induction chemotherapy and EPP, and survival was influenced by histology and CD8+ tumor-infiltrating lymphocytes (TILs). Preoperative immunotherapy studies followed by surgery are also underway.

Radiation therapy for mesothelioma

With the exception of the SMART approach described above, RT is typically delivered in the adjuvant setting for MPM. The RT approach and risks are primarily determinant on the type of surgical resection involved and can be divided into two categories: RT after EPP and RT after P/D or no surgery.

Adjuvant radiation therapy after extrapleural pneumonectomy

Attempts to control mesothelioma microscopic disease with RT have typically included treating the entire hemithorax, specifically the entire pleura +/− the ipsilateral lung and pericardium. Historically, hemithoracic radiation has been given using two-dimensional, or "conventional" techniques. These approaches utilize a limited number of fields and nonconformal methods. As a result, a great deal of dose heterogeneity typically occurs, with the target volume being underdosed and surrounding normal tissue, such as the esophagus, lung, heart, and spinal cord, receiving increased dose, or "hot spots." However, in the past decade, the conformal technique of intensity-modulated radiation therapy, or IMRT, has been advanced and applied to this clinical context (Figure 7). Several institutions have reported their outcomes with this approach. An early study from MD Anderson Cancer Center treated 28 patients with hemithoracic IMRT after EPP to doses of 45–50 Gy.[122] Results have been updated twice[123,124] and again in 2013,[125] with the most recent report demonstrating 90% OS at 1 year and 71% at 2 years in this selected group of patients. Grade 3 toxicity dermatitis and gastrointestinal side effects were generally less than 20%.[126]

Conformality with IMRT comes with the tradeoff of a "low dose radiation bath" to the remaining lung that needs to be closely monitored when performing RT planning. Adhering to dose constraints is essential to minimize the risk of high-grade and potentially fatal toxicity. In one report by investigators from the Dana Farber Cancer Institute,[126] 6 of 13 patients receiving IMRT after EPP experienced fatal pneumonitis. Notably, 11 of 13 patients also received intraoperative cisplatin, and the dose threshold to the remaining lung was a V20 (volume of lung receiving 20 Gy or more) of 20%. In order to minimize this risk going forward, the V20 dose constraint is typically 7–8%.

One recent publication also questioned the utility of delivering hemithoracic radiation therapy in the post-EPP setting. In the Swiss Group for Clinical Cancer Research (SAKK) 17/04 Phase 2 randomized study, 54 patients who received induction chemotherapy followed by EPP were randomized to hemithoracic RT with 3D conformal radiation or IMRT versus no RT. The investigators found no difference in median locoregional relapse-free survival between the two groups, thus leading the authors to conclude that there is no role for the "routine" use of hemithoracic radiotherapy for mesothelioma.[127] However, there were several critiques of this study, including the low statistical power, the higher than expected rate of radiation toxicities, and the lack of central review for radiation plans.[128] Therefore, while the data presented by the SAKK trial is provocative, given its substantial limitations it is not definitive and radiation therapy should still be considered in this context, individualized based on factors such as performance

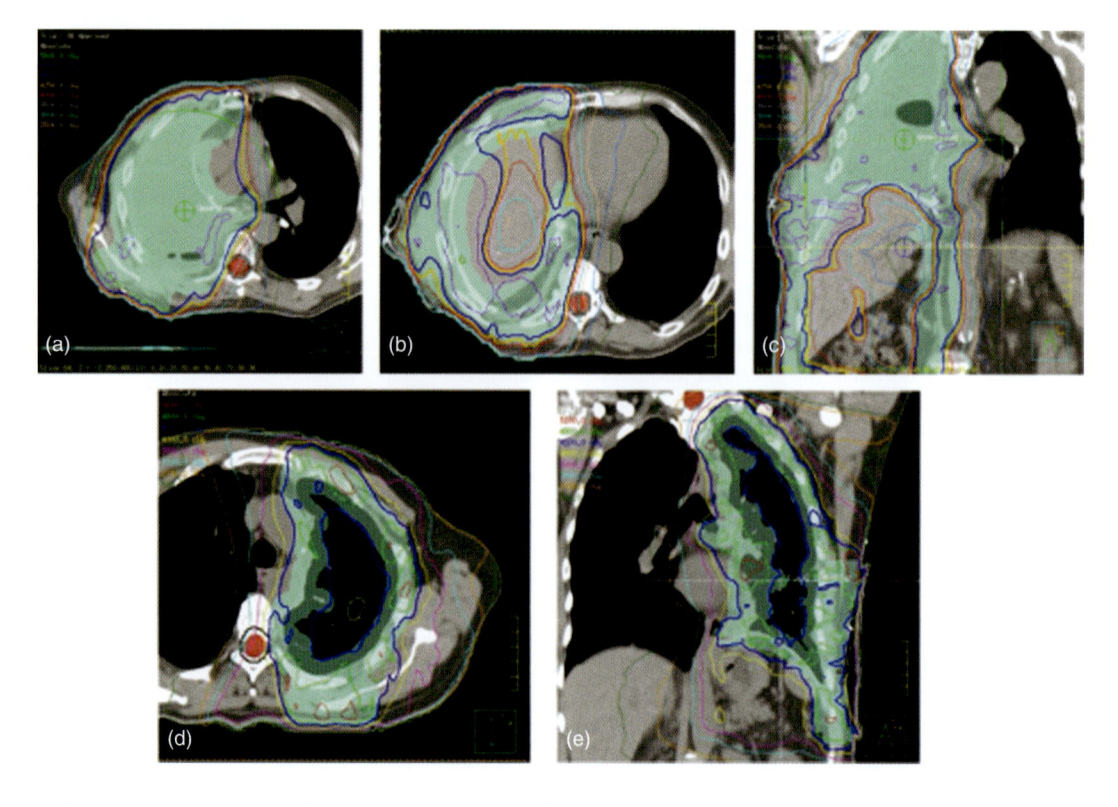

Figure 7 (a–c) Two axial slices and a coronal view of IMRT after extrapleural pneumonectomy. IMRT offers improved conformality and better dose homogeneity to both the target volume and critical normal structures. (d, e) An axial and a coronal view of a patient treated with IMRT after pleurectomy/decortication. A "rind" is created to attempt to spare the inner portion of the lung, though full sparing of the ipsilateral lung is typically not feasible.

status, disease extent, institutional experience, and the capability to meet radiation dose constraints.

Radiation therapy after pleurectomy/decortication (P/D) or unresectable disease

The role of radiation therapy after P/D is not yet established. Indeed, there are several reasons why hemithoracic radiation is more challenging when patients do not undergo an EPP. First, treating with a hemithoracic approach in the setting of an intact lung increases the risk of radiation pneumonitis by increasing radiation exposure to that lung. Second, it has been postulated that by treating a substantial portion of the ipsilateral lung and rendering it nonfunctional, a "shunting" effect can be produced whereby perfusion continues yet very little air exchange occurs. Initial studies examining this approach demonstrated suboptimal outcomes.

However, as in the post-EPP setting, the use of IMRT has provided much better results. Figure 7 demonstrates a patient that has received hemithoracic RT after P/D, with attempted sparing of the ipsilateral lung through the creation of a "rind" in treatment volume delineation.[129] When comparing this approach to historical controls treated with EPP and adjuvant IMRT, no differences were found in high-grade toxicity, and both median OS (28.4 vs 14.2 months, $p = 0.04$) and progression-free survival (PFS) (16.4 vs 8.2 months) favored P/D.[130] A multi-institutional Phase II trial examined the safety and efficacy of hemithoracic intensity-modulated pleural radiation therapy (IMPRINT) in this setting. Forty-five patients were enrolled, of which 27 were evaluable, 21 of which underwent at least a partial P/D. No Grade 4 or 5 toxicities were observed, with promising median PFS and OS rates of 12.4 and 23.7 months.[131] As a result of these outcomes, a national Phase III randomized trial (NRG-LU006) is now comparing patients who undergo P/D with chemotherapy, +/− the IMPRINT technique, with a primary endpoint of OS. This trial began accruing in 2020, with an accrual target of 150.

Alternative radiation therapy approaches

Several radiation approaches to treating mesothelioma have been explored in the past several years. First, a Phase III randomized trial examined the role of prophylactic radiotherapy for the prevention of procedure-tract metastases (PTMs) after pleural procedures, the rationale being that this technique could provide a palliative benefit in local control and palliation without the toxicity of including the lung. The primary intervention was the incidence of PTMs within 7 cm of the site of pleural intervention, within 12 months from randomization. A total of 203 patients were randomized between 2011 and 2014, and no significant difference was found in PTMs.[132] Therefore, this technique is not routinely recommended in patients with mesothelioma.

Proton therapy has been reported in small studies in the context of mesothelioma, both after EPP[133] and after lung-sparing surgery.[134] In a recent consensus statement by the Proton Therapy Cooperative Group, it was concluded that proton therapy had been promised in this setting with respect to reducing normal tissue toxicity, but that further studies are needed and that given the complexities of this treatment it should be reserved for highly experienced centers.[135]

Summary recommendations on radiation therapy in mesothelioma

An expert panel convened at the National Cancer Institute in 2019 to formulate recommendations on the use of radiation therapy in the context of mesothelioma. In a follow-up manuscript, the authors highlighted indications for use and treatment parameters in three settings: (1) post-EPP, (2) post-lung-sparing surgery, and (3) the palliative setting.[136] The details of these aggregate recommendations, which are beyond the scope of this chapter, include guidance on radiation simulation, dosimetric constraints, and evidence supporting their approach. However, the panel concluded that it was appropriate to offer patients radiation in the palliative setting and, in experienced centers, hemithoracic radiation after EPP. Hemithoracic radiation with lung intact, using the SMART approach described above, or with proton therapy, should not be offered routinely in the community. These treatments should be reserved for the context of a clinical trial or at highly experienced centers that have gained experience with these specific approaches and after discussion with the multidisciplinary team.

Systemic chemotherapy for mesothelioma

As detailed in the section titled "Surgery," the standard practice in the United States for the treatment of resectable MPM is to consider trimodality therapy that includes four cycles of either neoadjuvant or adjuvant cisplatin-pemetrexed. However, several issues regarding the optimal sequence of trimodality therapy and the choice of systemic regimen remain unclear.

Newer neoadjuvant or adjuvant systemic therapy choices

Several investigational approaches to neoadjuvant therapy with novel agents have been performed in the resectable MPM population. An exploratory window of opportunity trial with neoadjuvant dasatinib was performed at the University of Texas M.D. Anderson Cancer Center. MPM cell lines and tumor cells have overexpression of activated Src kinase and preclinical studies demonstrated antitumor efficacy of dasatinib.[137] This study demonstrated that Src kinase^{Tyr419} was a pharmacodynamic marker and higher baseline levels were predictive of a metabolic response by PET/CT to neoadjuvant dasatinib therapy. In addition, distinct patterns of PDGFRα and β expression by IHC were predictive of sensitivity or resistance to dasatinib treatment.

Memorial Sloan Kettering has pioneered the use of an adjuvant WT-1 (Wilm's Tumor-1) vaccine in a Department of Defense-sponsored clinical trial.[138] The peptide vaccine, galinpepimut-S, delivered in the trial stimulates host T cells to identify and eliminate WT-1 expressing cells. Eligible patients were required to express WT-1 by IHC on their mesothelioma tumor cells. In normal cells, WT-1 is a transcription factor that is present in young children but is lost once adulthood is reached. In this trial, 41 resected MPM patients were randomized to adjuvant galinpepimut-S or placebo. There was no clinically significant toxicity noted but since there was a prespecified futility analysis to be applied to either arm, the trial ended up closing early due to the control arm having more than 10 patients develop progression. At 1-year, the PFS rate was 33% in the control arm and 45% in the vaccine arm. The vaccine arm had a higher median PFS (10.1 vs 7.4 months) and higher median OS (22.8 vs 18.3 months).[138] Additional studies using galinpepimut-S and possibly in combination with immunotherapy are underway.

Currently, immunotherapy neoadjuvant studies are under exploration but there are no published results yet (https://clinicaltrials.gov/ct2/home). The premise is that adding in immunotherapy with neoadjuvant treatment will activate T cells against any microscopic systemic disease. The Southwest Oncology Group (SWOG) 1619 trial (NCT03228537) is ongoing and is evaluating the combination of neoadjuvant cisplatin-pemetrexed-atezolizumab (checkpoint inhibitor of PD-L1) for four cycles followed by resection (EPP or P/D) than 1 year of atezolizumab. This study has recently completed accrual and results are pending. Translational studies will include PD-1/PD-L1 IHC expression in tumor cells, serum cytokine analysis, and gene expression profiling of plasma. There are three window-of-opportunity trials (https://clinicaltrials.gov/ct2/home) using pembrolizumab (NCT02707666), a Phase II study of durvalumab with and without tremelimumab (NCT02592551), and a window-of-opportunity trial of nivolumab with and without ipilimumab (NCT 03918252).

Intrapleural strategies

There has been significant research on intrapleural administration of chemotherapies for MPM. However, it is not standard of care and it is recommended to only perform intrapleural therapy within a well-designed clinical trial. The premise behind the use of intrapleural treatment is to bring the agent into direct tumor cell contact and deliver high concentrations of the drug. In the past, intracavitary platinum-based regimens have been used with median PFS ranging between 7.5 and 13.6 months and median OS 11.5–18.3 months.[139–141] The most significant adverse event identified in these studies was renal failure from systemic absorption of cisplatin. Hyperthermic intrapleural therapy administered after P/D yields median OS ranges of 9–13 months.[142–145]

Intrapleural gene therapy using adenovirus vectors containing the herpes virus thymidine kinase (Ad-HSVtk) suicide gene and an adenoviral vector containing an immune stimulant, interferon (Ad.hu.IFN)[130] have also been explored with some preliminary positive results for successful gene transfer into patient tumor cells.[146–149] However, this strategy appears to primarily benefit patients with less bulky disease. A Phase 3 gene therapy clinical trial evaluating the efficacy and safety of intrapleural administration of adenovirus-delivered interferon alpha-2b (rAd-IFN) in combination with celecoxib and gemcitabine in patients with MPM is underway.

Systemic therapies for unresectable mesothelioma

In the front-line metastatic setting, cisplatin-pemetrexed is the Food and Drug Administration (FDA)-approved regimen in the United States.[106] Vogelzang et al. conducted a study in 456 patients randomized to cisplatin (75 mg/m^2 intravenous every 3 weeks) monotherapy or cisplatin (75 mg/m^2) and pemetrexed (500 mg/m^2) given intravenously every 3 weeks for a maximum of six cycles. The cisplatin-pemetrexed regimen improved response rate (41.3% vs 16.7%, $p < 0.001$), time to progression (5.7 vs 3.9 months, $p < 0.001$), and median OS (12.1 vs 9.3 months, $p = 0.02$). The main grade 3/4 side effects experienced with the combination regimen in over 10% of patients were neutropenia, nausea/vomiting, and fatigue. Pemetrexed usage must be accompanied by vitamin B12 and folic acid supplementation. Also, use of corticosteroids during pemetrexed administration is necessary. In the unresectable setting, carboplatin is a very reasonable alternative to cisplatin and has demonstrated equivalent survival.[150,151] Other platinum antifolate regimens (raltitrexed)[152] or platinum-gemcitabine[153,154] have been investigated and would be reasonable alternatives if a patient is unable to receive pemetrexed. In patients who cannot tolerate platinum, single-agent pemetrexed can be given.[155]

The MAPS trial[156] performed by the French Cooperative Thoracic Intergroup (IFCT), randomized 448 patients to carboplatin-pemetrexed with and without bevacizumab. The triplet regimen with bevacizumab improved median OS (18.8 vs 16.1 months, HR 0.77, $p = 0.0167$). The bevacizumab arm had a higher rate of grade 3 hypertension (23% vs 0%) and thrombotic events (6% vs 1%) compared to chemotherapy.[156] Although this large Phase III trial showed a higher survival benefit, it did not lead to regulatory approval. Current guidelines do include the regimen of carboplatin-pemetrexed-bevacizumab followed by bevacizumab maintenance as an option for frontline therapy. Other trials of frontline small molecule tyrosine kinase inhibitor antiangiogenic therapy showed preliminary efficacy in Phase II studies,[157] but not in subsequent Phase III trials.[158]

Maintenance therapy for mesothelioma

Recently, a randomized clinical trial of maintenance therapy was reported; but this study was closed early due to poor accrual.[159] A total of 49 eligible patients (22 observation arm, 27 maintenance pemetrexed) were evaluated. The pemetrexed maintenance arm did not have significantly different median PFS (3.4 vs 3 months; HR 0.99, $p = 0.9733$) but had a numerically higher OS (16.3 vs 11.8 months, HR 0.86, $p = 0.6737$). This trial was unable to enroll sufficient participants as many patients in the community were receiving maintenance pemetrexed or bevacizumab based on extrapolations from NSCLC trials.

Salvage chemotherapy for mesothelioma

In the salvage setting for mesothelioma, patients are encouraged to enroll in clinical trials with novel agents and immunotherapy (see below). However, off-protocol, the agents that are most commonly prescribed include gemcitabine, vinorelbine, or the combination of gemcitabine-vinorelbine. Gemcitabine (1250 mg/m^2 intravenous on days 1, 8, and 15 of a 28-day cycle) has been reported to have a response rate of 7% and median OS 8 months in the chemo-naïve setting.[144] Gemcitabine-vinorelbine (1000 mg/m^2 gemcitabine and 25 mg/m^2 vinorelbine on days 1 and 8 every 3 weeks for up to six cycles) has been reported to have minor efficacy with a response rate of 7.4% and median time to progression of 2.8 months.[145,160] A Phase II trial of single-agent vinorelbine ($n = 63$) reported a response rate of 16% and OS of 9.6 months.[161] A retrospective analysis[162] of 60 salvage mesothelioma patients conducted at Memorial Sloan Kettering treated in the second and third-line setting reported minimal response rates to either gemcitabine or vinorelbine but significant stabilization of disease. There was no significant gain in OS benefit. Gemcitabine ($n = 27$) had a median PFS of 1.6 months and median OS 4.9 months, while vinorelbine ($n = 45$) had a median PFS of 1.7 months and median OS 5.4 months.

First-line immunotherapy for mesothelioma

The DREAM (DuRvalumab with first-line chEmotherApy in Mesothelioma) trial[163] sponsored by the Australasian Lung Cancer Trials Group and NHMRC Clinical Trials Centre, was a single-arm Phase II trial of durvalumab with cisplatin/pemetrexed in patients with MPM. Unresectable MPM patients (PD-L1 IHC was not an eligibility criteria) were given six cycles of cisplatin-pemetrexed with durvalumab (1125 mg Q3 weeks) followed by up to 1 year of maintenance durvalumab (17 cycles). In the trial, 54 eligible patients had a 57% 6-month PFS rate with a median PFS of 6.9 months by modified RECIST and 7 months by iRECIST. The overall response rate was 48%, but two additional reports of pseudoprogression were documented. There were grade 3–4 toxicities seen with neutropenia, nausea, and anemia. Five patient deaths were noted but not attributed to study therapy. A Phase III trial is in planning to evaluate this regimen further. There are other ongoing studies looking at triplet immunotherapy combinations for MPM, including pembrolizumab plus chemotherapy (NCT 2784171. https://clinicaltrials.gov/ct2/home), as well as a PrECOG0505 study of cisplatin/pemetrexed and durvalumab (NCT02899195). Results from these trials are eagerly anticipated to further define the role of chemotherapy with immunotherapy in MPM.

In addition to combination chemotherapy-immunotherapy regimens, the CheckMate743 (NCT 02899299) randomized 600 treatment-naïve MPM patients to nivolumab-ipilimumab (until progression or unacceptable toxicity) or platinum-pemetrexed for six cycles of therapy. This trial collected tumor tissue for PD-L1 IHC and additional analysis. The results of this study demonstrated a 26% reduction in risk of death when patients were treated with ipilimumab–nivolumab. The median OS with the dual immunotherapies was 18.1 months compared to 14.1 months for platinum-pemetrexed (HR 0.74, $p = 0.002$). Patients with nonepithelioid MPM had a larger magnitude of benefit with dual immunotherapies (median OS 18.1 vs 8.8 months, HR 0.46).[164] This combination was approved by the FDA on 2 October 2020, only the second FDA-approved systemic therapy for mesothelioma in 16 years (https://www.fda.gov/news-events/press-announcements/fda-approves-drug-combination-treating-mesothelioma).

Salvage immunotherapies

At this time, immunotherapies in the salvage setting of MPM have lagged behind in global regulatory approval. In 2018, Japan became the first country to grant regulatory approval for the salvage use of nivolumab based on the MERIT trial,[165] but other countries have not followed suit. In the United States, the NCCN salvage guidelines for mesothelioma have been updated to include nivolumab with or without ipilimumab or pembrolizumab in PD-L1 positive MPM patients. Unfortunately, as there is still no global regulatory approval, it remains difficult in most countries to obtain insurance coverage for immunotherapies for mesothelioma patients. The following section describes the latest data for specific immunotherapy agents.

Nivolumab (anti-PD-1) The Phase II MERIT study[165] treated 34 MPM patients (treatment naïve or pretreated) with nivolumab 240 mg IV every 2 weeks. The overall response rate (ORR) was 29% and disease control rate (DCR) was 67%. Fifty-nine percent of patients had PD-L1 IHC >1%. When comparing outcomes by PD-L1 IHC, patients with positive PD-L1 IHC had a higher ORR (40% vs 8.3%), median PFS (7.2 vs 2.9 months), and median OS (17.3 vs 11.6 months) compared to patients who were PD-L1 IHC negative. Based on these results, Japan approved nivolumab for unresectable MPM patients who progressed on prior chemotherapy in August 2018.

In the Netherlands, a single-arm Phase 2 trial[166] treated 34 patients with nivolumab 3 mg/kg IV every 2 weeks. The majority of patients were treatment naïve and had epithelioid disease. At 12 weeks, the DCR was 47% and overall response rate was 23.5%. Three cases of potential pseudoprogression were seen. The median PFS was 2.6 months and median OS was 11.8 months. PD-L1 IHC expression was not predictive for a response. Several randomized Phase 2 and 3 studies of single-agent PD-1 pathway blockade after prior chemotherapy for mesothelioma are ongoing including the placebo-controlled CONFIRM study of nivolumab in the United Kingdom (NCT03063450).

Pembrolizumab (anti-PD-1) KEYNOTE-028[167] enrolled 25 MPM patients (PD-L1 IHC positive patients >1%) and treated them with pembrolizumab (10 mg/kg every 2 weeks). The ORR was 20% ($n = 5$) with a median duration of response of 12 months. Subsequent trials have had similar response rates[168]; however, PD-L1 IHC expression has had variable predictive capability.

Avelumab (anti-PD-L1)
The JAVELIN trial[169] was a Phase 1b trial that enrolled 53 unresectable MPM patients that progressed after platinum-pemetrexed and treated patients with avelumab 10 mg/kg every 2 weeks. Close to half the patients enrolled had three or more prior lines of therapy. The ORR was 9% with a median duration of response of 15.2 months. Patients who had PD-L1 IHC >5% had a higher ORR of 19% compared to 7% in PD-L1 IHC negative patients. The median PFS was 4.1 months and median OS was 10.7 months.

Tremelimumab (anti-CTLA-4) Unfortunately, single-agent trials evaluating anti-CTLA-4 therapies have not shown survival benefits. The Phase II DETERMINE study[170] randomized second and third line mesothelioma patients to tremelimumab to placebo. There was no survival difference from this trial and further single-agent development was halted.

Salvage combination checkpoint inhibitor therapies

Several trials have assessed the combination of checkpoint inhibitors with anti-CTLA-4 therapies. The Phase II NIBIT-MESO-1 trial (NCT02588131)[171] enrolled treatment naïve and second-line therapy mesothelioma patients to treatment with tremelimumab (1 mg/kg) with durvalumab (20 mg/kg) every 4 weeks for four cycles, followed by maintenance durvalumab for nine doses. The ORR was 27.5% with a median duration of response of 16.1 months. The DCR was 65%, median PFS 8 months, and median OS 16.6 months. There was no correlation of clinical outcome with PD-L1 IHC expression. The Phase II IFCT MAPS2 trial (NCT02716272),[172] enrolled 125 pretreated MPM patients and randomized them to 2 cohorts, nivolumab (3 mg/kg/2 weeks) alone or combined with ipilimumab (1 mg/kg/6 weeks) for up to 2 year. Stratification factors included histology, number of prior therapies, and chemosensitivity. The dual immunotherapy combination had an ORR of 25.9% and DCR of 50%. The nivolumab alone arm had an ORR of 18.5% and DCR 44.4. The median survival was 11.9 months in the nivolumab cohort and 15.9 months for the nivolumab–ipilimumab cohort. This study evaluated PD-L1 IHC expression and did report a correlation with response with high expressors, but this did not translate into an OS benefit. The INITIATE trial (NCT03048474)[173] enrolled 34 eligible pretreated MPM patients and treated them with nivolumab (240 mg/kg Q2 weeks) with ipilimumab (1 mg/kg/6 weeks for up to four times). The study reported a 29% ORR and 68% DCR and also confirmed that positive PD-L1 IHC expression correlated with better response rates.

Based on the growing body of literature supporting the use of immunotherapies in MPM, the dual immunotherapy combinations are currently included in the US NCCN guidelines as a salvage treatment option.[174] It is anticipated that regulatory approvals will follow eventually in both the unresectable salvage and treatment-naïve space. Earlier stage trials are underway to evaluate biomarkers and provide valuable information on the biology of the disease.

Key references

The complete reference list can be found on Vital Source version of this title, see inside front cover.

2. Carbone M, Adusumilli PS, Alexander HR Jr, et al. Mesothelioma: scientific clues for prevention, diagnosis, and therapy. *CA Cancer J Clin*. 2019;69(5):402–429.
4. Carbone M, Amelio I, Affar EB, et al. Consensus report of the 8 and 9th Weinman Symposia on Gene x Environment Interaction in carcinogenesis: novel opportunities for precision medicine. *Cell Death Differ*. 2018;25(11):1885–1904.
15. Roggli VL, Carney JM, Sporn TA, Pavlisko EN. Talc and mesothelioma: mineral fiber analysis of 65 cases with clinicopathological correlation. *Ultrastruct Pathol*. 2020;44(2):211–218.
17. Yang H, Bocchetta M, Kroczynska B, et al. TNF-alpha inhibits asbestos-induced cytotoxicity via a NF-kappaB-dependent pathway, a possible mechanism for asbestos-induced oncogenesis. *Proc Natl Acad Sci U S A*. 2006;103(27):10397–10402.
21. Yang H, Rivera Z, Jube S, et al. Programmed necrosis induced by asbestos in human mesothelial cells causes high-mobility group box 1 protein release and resultant inflammation. *Proc Natl Acad Sci U S A*. 2010;107(28):12611–12616.
26. Jube S, Rivera ZS, Bianchi ME, et al. Cancer cell secretion of the DAMP protein HMGB1 supports progression in malignant mesothelioma. *Cancer Res*. 2012;72(13):3290–3301.
27. Chen Z, Gaudino G, Pass HI, et al. Diagnostic and prognostic biomarkers for malignant mesothelioma: an update. *Transl Lung Cancer Res*. 2017;6(3):259–269.
35. Guo G, Chmielecki J, Goparaju C, et al. Whole-exome sequencing reveals frequent genetic alterations in BAP1, NF2, CDKN2A, and CUL1 in malignant pleural mesothelioma. *Cancer Res*. 2015;75(2):264–269.
36. Nasu M, Emi M, Pastorino S, et al. High Incidence of Somatic BAP1 alterations in sporadic malignant mesothelioma. *J Thorac Oncol*. 2015;10(4):565–576.
37. Testa JR, Cheung M, Pei J, et al. Germline BAP1 mutations predispose to malignant mesothelioma. *Nat Genet*. 2011;43(10):1022–1025.
39. Bueno R, Stawiski EW, Goldstein LD, et al. Comprehensive genomic analysis of malignant pleural mesothelioma identifies recurrent mutations, gene fusions and splicing alterations. *Nat Genet*. 2016;48(4):407–416.
47. Sekido Y. Molecular pathogenesis of malignant mesothelioma. *Carcinogenesis*. 2013;34(7):1413–1419.
52. Blum Y, Meiller C, Quetel L, et al. Dissecting heterogeneity in malignant pleural mesothelioma through histo-molecular gradients for clinical applications. *Nat Commun*. 2019;10(1):1333.
54. Mansfield AS, Peikert T, Vasmatzis G. Chromosomal rearrangements and their neoantigenic potential in mesothelioma. *Transl Lung Cancer Res*. 2020;9(Suppl 1):S92–S99.
57. Napolitano A, Pellegrini L, Dey A, et al. Minimal asbestos exposure in germline BAP1 heterozygous mice is associated with deregulated inflammatory response and increased risk of mesothelioma. *Oncogene*. 2016;35(15):1996–2002.
59. Carbone M, Yang H, Pass HI, et al. BAP1 and cancer. *Nat Rev Cancer*. 2013;13(3):153–159.
62. Pastorino S, Yoshikawa Y, Pass HI, et al. A subset of mesotheliomas with improved survival occurring in carriers of BAP1 and other germline mutations. *J Clin Oncol*. 2018;36(35):Jco2018790352.
69. Carbone M, Harbour JW, Brugarolas J, et al. Biological mechanisms and clinical significance of BAP1 mutations in human cancer. *Cancer Discov*. 2020;10(8):1103–1120.
74. Pass HI, Giroux D, Kennedy C, et al. Supplementary prognostic variables for pleural mesothelioma: a report from the IASLC staging committee. *J Thorac Oncol*. 2014;9(6):856–864.
83. Hollevoet K, Reitsma JB, Creaney J, et al. Serum mesothelin for diagnosing malignant pleural mesothelioma: an individual patient data meta-analysis. *J Clin Oncol*. 2012;30(13):1541–1549.
87. Pass HI, Alimi M, Carbone M, et al. Mesothelioma biomarkers: a review highlighting contributions from the early detection research network. *Cancer Epidemiol Biomarkers Prev*. 2020;29:2524–2540.
89. Johnen G, Burek K, Raiko I, et al. Prediagnostic detection of mesothelioma by circulating calretinin and mesothelin - a case-control comparison nested into a prospective cohort of asbestos-exposed workers. *Sci Rep*. 2018;8(1):14321.
92. Armato SG 3rd, Francis RJ, Katz SI, et al. Imaging in pleural mesothelioma: a review of the 14th International Conference of the International Mesothelioma Interest Group. *Lung Cancer (Amsterdam, Netherlands)*. 2019;130:108–114.
99. Rusch VW, Chansky K, Kindler HL, et al. The IASLC mesothelioma staging project: proposals for the M descriptors and for revision of the TNM stage groupings in the forthcoming (Eighth) edition of the TNM classification for mesothelioma. *J Thorac Oncol*. 2016;11(12):2112–2119.
103. Rusch VW, Gill R, Mitchell A, et al. A multicenter study of volumetric computed tomography for staging malignant pleural mesothelioma. *Ann Thorac Surg*. 2016;102(4):1059–1066.
105. Rice D, Rusch V, Pass H, et al. Recommendations for uniform definitions of surgical techniques for malignant pleural mesothelioma: a consensus report of the international association for the study of lung cancer international staging committee and the international mesothelioma interest group. *J Thorac Oncol*. 2011;6(8):1304–1312.
106. Vogelzang NJ, Rusthoven JJ, Symanowski J, et al. Phase III study of pemetrexed in combination with cisplatin versus cisplatin alone in patients with malignant pleural mesothelioma. *J Clin Oncol*. 2003;21(14):2636–2644.
110. Krug LM, Pass HI, Rusch VW, et al. Multicenter phase II trial of neoadjuvant pemetrexed plus cisplatin followed by extrapleural pneumonectomy and radiation for malignant pleural mesothelioma. *J Clin Oncol*. 2009;27(18):3007–3013.
116. Treasure T, Lang-Lazdunski L, Waller D, et al. Extra-pleural pneumonectomy versus no extra-pleural pneumonectomy for patients with malignant pleural mesothelioma: clinical outcomes of the Mesothelioma and Radical Surgery (MARS) randomised feasibility study. *Lancet Oncol*. 2011;12(8):763–772.
127. Stahel RA, Riesterer O, Xyrafas A, et al. Neoadjuvant chemotherapy and extrapleural pneumonectomy of malignant pleural mesothelioma with or without hemithoracic radiotherapy (SAKK 17/04): a randomised, international, multicentre phase 2 trial. *Lancet Oncol*. 2015;16(16):1651–1658.
136. Gomez DR, Rimner A, Simone CB 2nd, et al. The use of radiation therapy for the treatment of malignant pleural mesothelioma: expert opinion from the National Cancer Institute Thoracic Malignancy Steering Committee, International Association for the Study of Lung Cancer, and Mesothelioma Applied Research Foundation. *J Thorac Oncol*. 2019;14(7):1172–1183.
145. Sugarbaker DJ, Gill RR, Yeap BY, et al. Hyperthermic intraoperative pleural cisplatin chemotherapy extends interval to recurrence and survival among low-risk patients with malignant pleural mesothelioma undergoing surgical macroscopic complete resection. *J Thorac Cardiovasc Surg*. 2013;145(4):955–963.
148. Sterman DH, Recio A, Vachani A, et al. Long-term follow-up of patients with malignant pleural mesothelioma receiving high-dose adenovirus herpes simplex thymidine kinase/ganciclovir suicide gene therapy. *Clin Cancer Res*. 2005;11(20):7444–7453.
156. Zalcman G, Mazieres J, Margery J, et al. Bevacizumab for newly diagnosed pleural mesothelioma in the Mesothelioma Avastin Cisplatin Pemetrexed Study (MAPS): a randomised, controlled, open-label, phase 3 trial. *Lancet*. 2016;387(10026):1405–1414.
159. Dudek AZ, Wang X, Gu L, et al. Randomized study of maintenance pemetrexed versus observation for treatment of malignant pleural mesothelioma: CALGB 30901. *Clin Lung Cancer*. 2020;21:553–561.e1.
163. Nowak AK, Lesterhuis WJ, Kok PS, et al. Durvalumab with first-line chemotherapy in previously untreated malignant pleural mesothelioma (DREAM): a multicentre, single-arm, phase 2 trial with a safety run-in. *Lancet Oncol*. 2020;21(9):1213–1223.
164. Baas P, Scherpereel A, Nowak, A. et al. *First-line Nivolumab + Ipilimumab vs Chemotherapy in Unresectable Malignant Pleural Mesothelioma: CheckMate 743*. VPS2020 – WCLC 2020 – Virtual Presidential Symposium, 2020.
169. Hassan R, Thomas A, Nemunaitis JJ, et al. Efficacy and safety of avelumab treatment in patients with advanced unresectable mesothelioma: phase 1b results from the JAVELIN solid tumor trial. *JAMA Oncol*. 2019;5(3):351–357.
172. Scherpereel A, Mazieres J, Greillier L, et al. Nivolumab or nivolumab plus ipilimumab in patients with relapsed malignant pleural mesothelioma (IFCT-1501 MAPS2): a multicentre, open-label, randomised, non-comparative, phase 2 trial. *Lancet Oncol*. 2019;20(2):239–253.
173. Disselhorst MJ, Quispel-Janssen J, Lalezari F, et al. Ipilimumab and nivolumab in the treatment of recurrent malignant pleural mesothelioma (INITIATE): results of a prospective, single-arm, phase 2 trial. *Lancet Respir Med*. 2019;7(3):260–270.

82 Thymomas and thymic tumors

Mayur D. Mody, MD ■ Gabriel L. Sica, MD, PhD ■ Suresh S. Ramalingam, MD, FACP, FASCO ■
Dong M. Shin, MD, FACP, FAAAS

Overview

Malignancies of the thymus gland comprise a group of uncommon but heterogeneous diseases with variable clinical behavior. Recent collaborative efforts have helped to create consensus histopathological and staging criteria. Furthermore, developments in molecular and gene signature technology have helped us to better understand the pathogenesis of thymic tumors. Diagnosis and treatment frequently require a multidisciplinary approach, with surgery, radiation, and systemic therapy all having a synergistically important role. While there are several chemotherapy regimens available for first-line treatment for advanced-stage or recurrent disease, numerous novel chemotherapeutics, immunotherapeutics, and targeted therapies are being evaluated. In this article, we provide a comprehensive overview of the histopathology, diagnosis, and management of most intriguing tumors.

Introduction

Thymic tumors are a group of rare and heterogeneous diseases in which malignant cells form in the thymus. The World Health Organization (WHO) histological classification distinguishes thymomas (types A, AB, B1, B2, and B3) from thymic carcinomas (type C) based upon the morphology of epithelial tumor cells, the proportion of lymphocytic involvement, and resemblance to normal thymic tissue. It is becoming more apparent that type A, AB, B1, B2, B3 thymoma, and thymic carcinomas have distinct molecular features that may be clinically relevant with aggressive clinical behavior.[1]

Thymic malignancies are rare and comprise 0.2–1.5% of all solid tumors or 0.13 per 100,000 person years in the United States.[2] As a result, traditional clinical research has been challenging in these tumors. A number of obstacles have also hindered our progress over the last few decades. One of the most significant has been the overall lack of an international consensus surrounding appropriate histopathological and staging criteria. At least 15 different stage classifications have been proposed and used.[3] This variability has hampered clinical research and made it difficult to collaborate on an international level. A recent step in the right direction has been the collaborative effort of the International Thymic Malignancies Interest Group (ITMIG) and the International Association for the Study of Lung Cancer (IASLC) to develop a tumor, node, metastasis (TNM) based staging system for thymic malignancies that have been recognized by the American Joint Committee on Cancer (AJCC) and the Union for International Cancer Control (UICC) as an official, universally accepted stage classification system.[4]

Surgical resection continues to be the cornerstone of therapy for early-stage disease while a multidisciplinary approach incorporating surgery, radiation, and chemotherapy is recommended in advanced or recurrent disease. Additionally, intense interest is now focused on targeting the immune system. Thymomas are known to be associated with a variety of autoimmune disorders, such as myasthenia gravis, which have been linked to T-cell mediated autoimmunity. Processes such as failure of positive and negative selection of T lymphocytes and defects in the autoimmune regulator gene (AIRE) have been proposed as theories underlying autoimmunity but additional research is required. Studies utilizing checkpoint inhibitors, for example, PD-1 inhibitors, are ongoing as immunotherapeutic strategies and may hold promise for those patients with chemo-resistant disease. Additionally, the actively recruiting National Cancer Institute-Molecular Analysis for Therapy Choice (NCI-MATCH) and Targeted Agent and Profiling Utilization Registry (TAPUR) clinical trials are evaluating treatments targeting specific genetic changes found in primarily rare or uncommon cancers, including thymomas and thymic carcinomas, through genomic sequencing, and may provide important precision medicine therapeutic strategies.

This article discusses the new histological and staging systems that are being developed and highlights some of the molecular biology breakthroughs that are improving our understanding of these rare tumors. In addition, we discuss the updated treatment of thymic malignancies focusing on surgery, radiotherapy (RT), and systemic therapy. Recent clinical trials involving chemotherapy and targeted therapeutics are emphasized and future targets are explored.

Incidence and epidemiology

Although thymic malignancies are relatively rare, they are among the most common mediastinal primary tumors, comprising up to 50% of anterior mediastinal masses.[5] Males have a slightly higher risk of developing thymomas than females, and the risk rises with age, reaching a peak in the seventh decade of life.[6] Compared with controls, patients with thymoma are more likely to have an autoimmune disease at some point during their lives (32.7% vs 2.4%; $P < 0.001$), most frequently myasthenia gravis (24.5%), systemic lupus erythematosus (2.4%), or red cell aplasia (1.2%).[7] Thymoma incidence in the United States is higher in African Americans and especially Asian/Pacific Islanders than among whites or Hispanics, although the exact causes of such differences have not been well understood. Ethnic variations in terms of higher incidence rates and younger age at diagnosis suggest a role for genetic factors. The distribution of alleles at the human leukocyte antigen (HLA) locus on chromosome 6 varies markedly across racial groups.[6] Both class I and class II HLA proteins are highly expressed on thymic epithelial cells.[8] Further research is needed to

---

Holland-Frei Cancer Medicine, Tenth Edition. Edited by Robert C. Bast, John C. Byrd, Carlo M. Croce, Ernest Hawk, Fadlo R. Khuri, Raphael E. Pollock, Apostolia M. Tsimberidou, Christopher G. Willett, and Cheryl L. Willman.
© 2023 John Wiley & Sons, Inc. Published 2023 by John Wiley & Sons, Inc.

understand whether particular genetic variants (at HLA or other loci) predispose to thymoma.

Anatomic pathogenesis

Embryology and anatomy
The thymus is embryologically derived from the endodermal epithelium of the third pharyngeal pouches (which also give rise to the lower pair of parathyroid glands) and, less consistently, the fourth also.[9,10] The right and left thymic anlagen migrate downward into the anterosuperior mediastinum, joining together without complete fusion to form a bilobate organ. Although most thymic tumors are located in the anterior mediastinum, variations in migration account for the findings of gross or microscopic thymic tissue anywhere between the hyoid bone superiorly and the diaphragm inferiorly. The absolute weight of the thymus reaches its peak in the pubertal years (mean 34 ± 15 g between age 10 and 15 years) and then gradually decreases. The thymus plays a critical role in the maturation of bone marrow-derived lymphocytes into T cells and, as such, in cell-mediated immunity.

Thymic neoplasms
The thymus can develop a variety of epithelial, germ cell, lymphoid, mesenchymal, and other neoplasms listed in Table 1.[9]

Pathology of thymic epithelial neoplasms
Thymic epithelial neoplasms include low-grade malignant lesions, designated as thymomas, and malignant lesions of moderate to high-grade malignant potential classified as thymic carcinomas.[9,11,12]

Pathology of thymomas
Thymomas present often as single or multiple neoplasms that range in size from microscopic lesions to large tumors that compress and invade the adjacent intrathoracic structures. Thymomas can be well encapsulated and limited to the thymic gland (Figure 1), while locally invasive thymomas can invade through a capsule (Figure 2) and into mediastinal soft tissues, lung, superior vena cava (SVC), and other vascular structures, lymph nodes, pleura, pericardium, trachea, and/or other intrathoracic structures adjacent to the thymus (Figure 3). On section, thymomas exhibit a distinctive fibrous capsule and multiple fibrous septa that divide the lesion into a characteristic lobulated appearance (Figure 4). They are usually solid tumors but can undergo cystic degeneration.[9,13–17]

Microscopically, the epithelial and lymphoid cells of thymomas are arranged in solid sheets usually divided by fibrous septa in a somewhat lobulated appearance that can be observed at low power microscopy in most thymomas (Figure 4). Other histologic features of thymomas include perivascular spaces (Figure 5), medullary areas (Figure 6), pseudo-rosettes, gland-like structures, Hassall's corpuscles, areas of cystic degeneration, and less frequently hemorrhagic and/or calcified areas. Mitoses, cellular atypia, and necrosis are unusual in thymomas and should raise the suspicion of a B3 thymoma and thymic carcinoma.[13–17]

Table 1 Thymic neoplasms overview.

Thymoma (see Table 2 for subtypes)
Thymic carcinoma (see Table 3 for subtypes)
Thymic neuroendocrine tumors
  Carcinoid tumors
    Typical carcinoid
    Atypical carcinoid
  Large cell neuroendocrine carcinoma
    Combined large cell neuroendocrine carcinoma
  Small cell carcinoma
    Combined small cell carcinoma
  Combined thymic carcinoma
Germ cell tumors of the mediastinum
  Seminoma
  Embryonal carcinoma
  Yolk sac tumor
  Choriocarcinoma
  Teratoma—mature and immature
  Mixed germ cell tumor
  Germ cell tumor with somatic-type solid malignancy
  Germ cell tumor with associated hematologic malignancy
Lymphomas of the mediastinum
  Primary mediastinal B-cell lymphoma
  Extranodal marginal zone lymphoma of mucosa-associated lymphoid tissue (MALT)
  Other mature B-cell lymphoma
  T lymphoblastic leukemia/lymphoma
  Anaplastic large cell lymphoma (ALCL) and other rare mature T- and NK-cell lymphomas
    ALCL, ALK+
    ALCL, ALK−
  Hodgkin lymphoma
Histiocytic and dendritic cell neoplasms of the mediastinum
  Langerhans cell lesions
    Thymic Langerhans cell histiocytosis
    Langerhans cell sarcoma
  Histiocytic sarcoma
  Follicular dendritic cell sarcoma
  Interdigitating dendritic cell sarcoma
  Fibroblastic reticular cell tumor
  Indeterminate dendritic cell tumor
Myeloid sarcoma and extramedullary acute myeloid leukemia
Soft tissue tumors of the mediastinum
  Thymolipoma
  Lipoma
  Liposarcoma
  Solitary fibrous tumor
  Synovial sarcoma
Vascular Neoplasms
  Lymphangioma
  Hemangioma
  Epithelioid hemangioendothelioma
  Angiosarcoma
Neurogenic tumors
  Tumor of the peripheral nerve
  Ganglioneuroma
  Ganglioneuroblastoma
  Neuroblastoma
Ectopic tumors of the thymus
  Others
Histiocytic and dendritic cell tumors
Myeloid sarcoma
Mesenchymal tumors
  Thymolipoma
  Solitary fibrous tumor
  Sarcoma
  Other

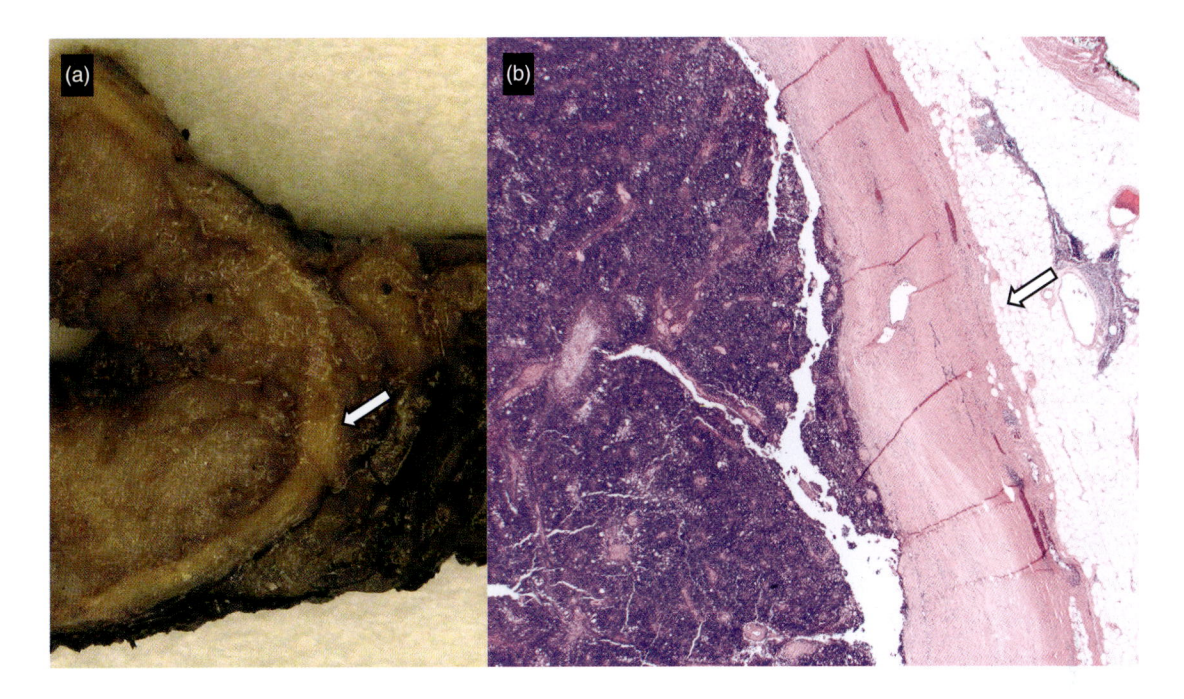

Figure 1 Encapsulated Thymoma. WHO type B1 thymoma with thick fibrous capsule (arrows), gross photograph (a), and H & E stained slide photomicrograph (b) (×200).

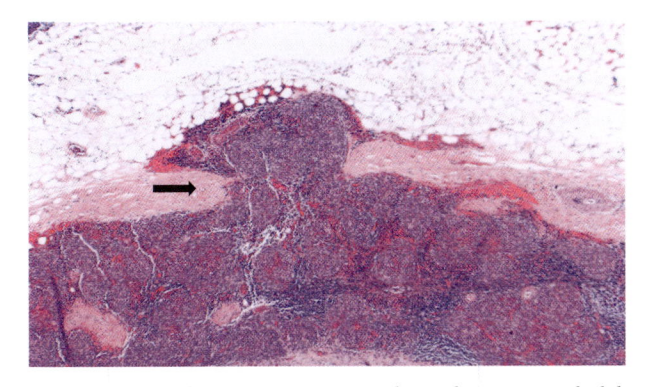

Figure 2 Transcapsular Invasion. Hematoxylin and eosin-stained slide showing thymoma invading into and through the capsule (arrow) into the adipose tissue of nonneoplastic thymic gland tissue (×400).

Table 2 2015 World Health Organization classification of thymomas and selected morphological features of the neoplasms.

Type A (Spindle cells, paucity or absence of immature (TdT+) T cells)
Atypical Type A Variant (Spindle cells with comedo-type necrosis, increased mitotic count, nuclear crowding)
Type AB (Mixed spindle and polygonal cells, abundance of immature (TdT+) T cells)
Type B1 (Lymphocyte-rich, scattered polygonal cells)
Type B2 (Lymphocyte-rich with higher density of polygonal epithelial cells and focal, minimal atypia)
Type B3 (Lymphocyte poor, polygonal cells with mild atypia)
Rare thymomas
Micronodular thymoma
Metaplastic thymoma
Microscopic thymoma
Sclerosing thymoma
Lipofibroadenoma

World Health Organization classification of thymomas

Different classification schema have been proposed for the categorization of thymic epithelial neoplasms but the most widely used classification scheme was proposed by the WHO in 1999 and has been modified in 2004 and 2015 (Table 2).[18]

Type A thymomas are composed predominantly of spindle epithelial cells with minimal numbers of lymphocytes (Figures 7 and 8).[18] Patients with thymoma A have a lower incidence of myasthenia gravis than those with other thymoma histologic types and a greater incidence of aplastic anemia.[19] In the 2015 edition, the WHO added an "atypical type A thymoma variant" of the conventional type A thymomas. This new classification includes a rare pattern of hypercellularity, increased mitotic activity, and necrosis. Type B thymomas are composed of polygonal epithelial cells and further subclassified into B1, B2, and B3. B1 thymomas are composed of inconspicuous polygonal epithelial cells admixed with a large number of mature lymphocytes. These lesions characteristically have scattered round, hypochromatic areas designated as medullary areas and have been described in the past as lymphocyte-predominant thymomas (Figure 6) because of the sparsity of visible epithelial cells. B2 thymomas are composed of polygonal cells that are more conspicuous than those seen in B1 lesions and frequently exhibit slight nuclear variability and focally prominent nucleoli (Figure 4). B3 thymomas, classified in other schema as "atypical thymoma" are composed of polygonal or spindled epithelial cells that exhibit moderate variability in cell size and shape (anisocytosis), focal nuclear hyperchromasia, and cytologic atypia (Figure 9). B3 thymomas characteristically have fewer lymphocytes than seen in B1 and B2 thymomas and can be difficult to distinguish from low-grade thymic squamous cell carcinomas. Type AB thymomas are similar to type A thymomas in that they contain bland-looking spindle epithelial cells (that may be optionally accompanied by oval or polygonal tumor cells) and are distinguished from each other by a high and low content of immature T cells, respectively (Figure 10). Specifically, any lymphocyte-dense area of more than 10% tumor area with a

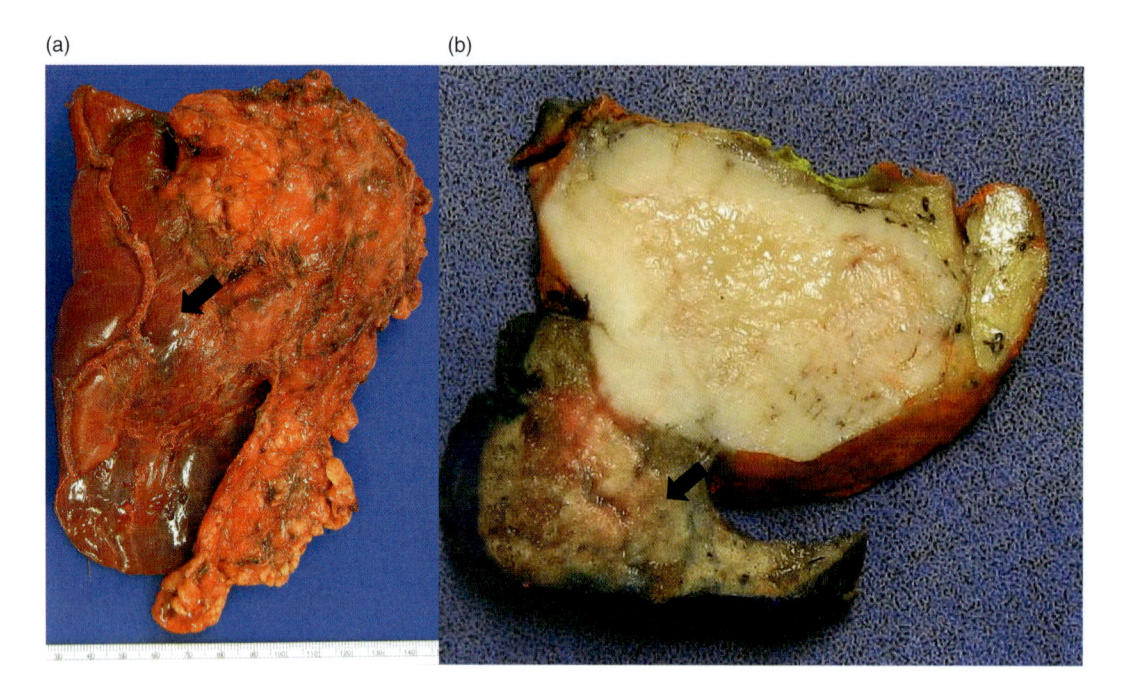

Figure 3 Gross photograph of an en bloc resection of an invasive thymoma, outer surface (a) and cut surface (b) with attached lung wedge (arrows). Thymoma invades into the lung.

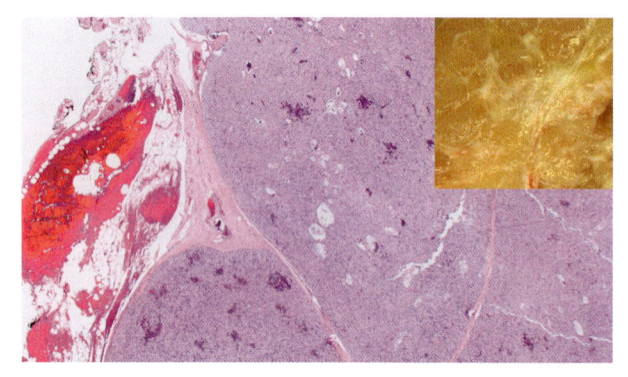

Figure 4 WHO type B2 thymoma showing fibrous septa and lobular architecture. The type B2 thymoma in this hematoxylin and eosin-stained slide is more eosinophilic in color than a B1 thymoma (×200). Gross picture (inset) of the cut surface of the thymoma shows the lobular architecture of the tumor with lobules bounded by tan fibrous septa.

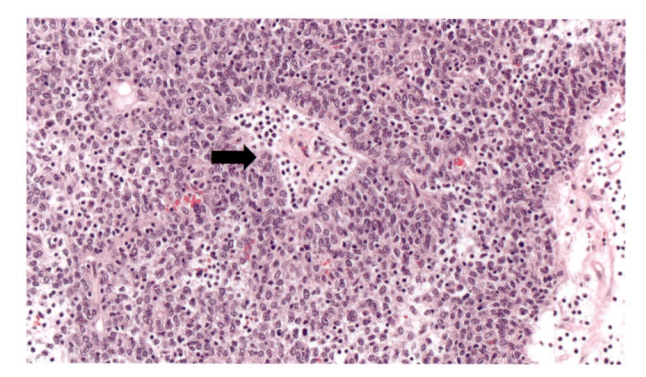

Figure 5 Perivascular space in a thymoma (arrow). Central, hyalinized blood vessel surrounded with serous fluid containing lymphocytes in a B2 thymoma. H & E stained slide (×200).

moderate infiltrate of immature T cells should indicate a type AB thymoma classification.[18,20]

Immunohistochemistry

The epithelial cells of thymomas exhibit cytoplasmic immunoreactivity to keratin AE1/AE3, a feature that is generally very helpful to confirm the diagnosis of thymoma on needle biopsies and other pathologic materials (Figure 6). A variety of other epitopes have been shown in the different WHO histologic types of thymomas, such as CD5, CD57, laminin, collagen IV, metallothionein, PE-53, cytokeratins such as CAM 5.2, CK7, CK14, and CK18, among others. CD5 is usually negative in thymomas other than thymic carcinoma. Foxn1, CD205, and desmoglein-3 are novel markers of thymic epithelial cells that may be useful to distinguish different thymomas and thymic carcinoma.

Histologic prognostic features in thymomas

All thymomas are low-grade malignant neoplasms.[20–23] Type A thymomas (spindle cell thymomas) have been considered benign lesions in the past, but these lesions can recur or metastasize in a small number of patients. Patients with thymomas A, AB, and B1 appear to have the best prognosis, while those with thymomas B3 generally have more frequent recurrences and metastases as well as a shorter survival.

Overview of selected thymic neoplasms

Thymic carcinomas

Thymic carcinomas are unusual epithelial tumors comprising approximately 0.06% of thymic neoplasms and composed of epithelial cells that exhibit cytological features characteristic of malignancy, such as considerable pleomorphism, hyperchromasia, prominent nucleoli, increased mitotic activity, and/or necrosis.[24–32] A variety of histologic variants, summarized in Table 3, have been described. Squamous cell carcinomas are probably the most frequent variant of these neoplasms (Figure 11). Lymphoepithelioma of the thymus is a particularly interesting variant of thymic

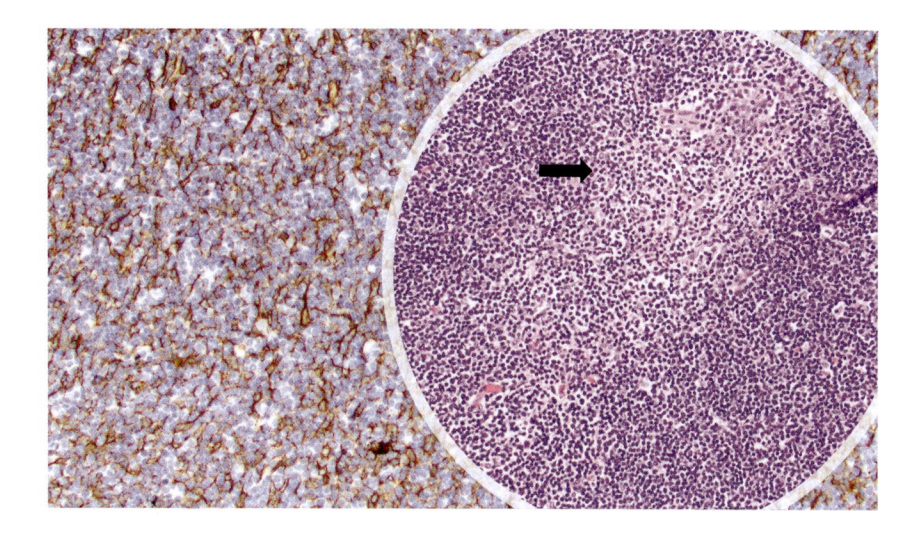

Figure 6 WHO type B1 thymoma. Background shows immunohistochemical stain for cytokeratin (AE1/AE3) that highlights in brown the meshwork of thymic epithelial cells. Inset shows corresponding hematoxylin and eosin-stained slide which illustrates how difficult it is to visualize the thymic epithelial cells in a sea of lymphocytes. The lighter area (arrow) in the H & E stained slide shows a medullary island.

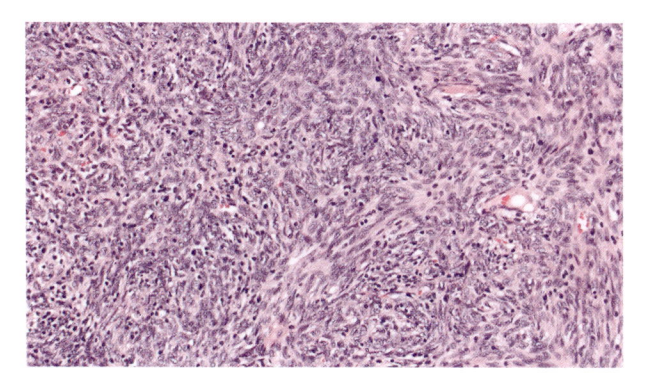

Figure 7 WHO type A thymoma. Type A thymoma with spindle cells (elongated nuclei) and scattered lymphocytes (no necrosis or increased mitoses seen). H & E stained slide (×200).

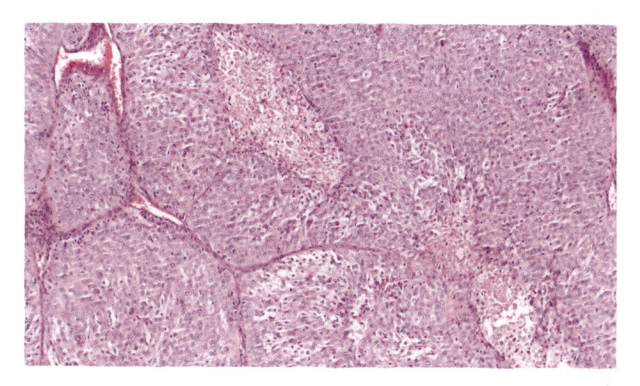

Figure 9 WHO type B3 thymoma. This thymoma has thin fibrous septa surrounding lobules of epithelial cells. There are foci of central necrosis, scattered hyperchromatic nuclei, mild pleomorphism, and minimal accompanying lymphoid cell population. H & E stained slide (×100).

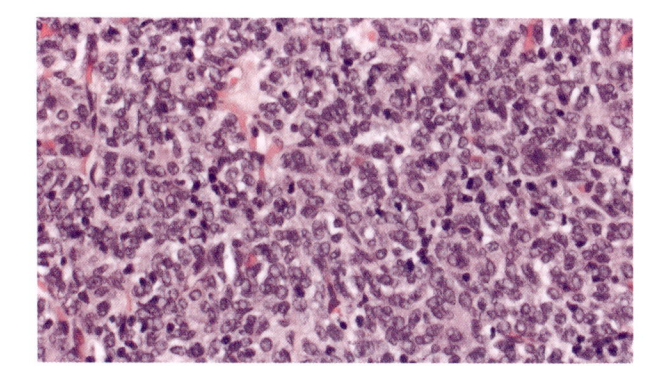

Figure 8 WHO type A thymoma. Ovoid tumor cells without significant atypia, necrosis, or mitotic activity. There are some scattered lymphocytes. H & E stained slide (×400).

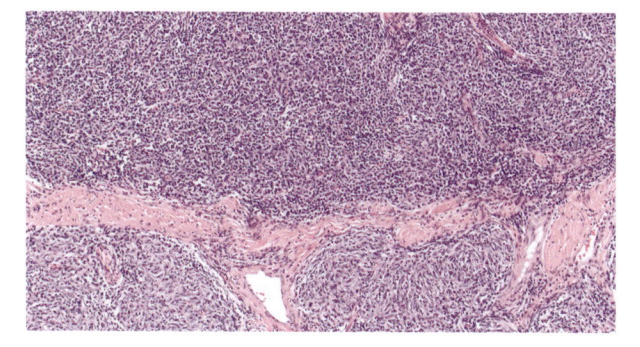

Figure 10 Thymoma, WHO type AB. AB thymoma with A and B component separated by a fibrous septa. The B component (top) resembles a B1 thymoma while the A component (lower) appears spindled. H & E stained slide (×400).

carcinoma that is frequently associated with Epstein–Barr virus (EBV) expression and exhibits similar histopathologic features to those seen in the head and neck area.[12] Carcinoma with NUT (nuclear protein in testis), t(15;19) translocation is a recently described aggressive variant of thymic carcinomas that affects children and young adults.[25]

Thymic carcinoid and neuroendocrine tumors

Carcinoid tumors and other neuroendocrine neoplasms shown in Table 1 can arise in the thymus.[33–38] They are more aggressive than their counterparts in the lung and other organs and present with metastases at diagnosis in 30–40% of cases.[11] The association with

Table 3 Thymic carcinomas.

Squamous cell carcinoma
Basaloid carcinoma
Mucoepidermoid carcinoma
Lymphoepithelioma-like carcinoma
Clear cell carcinoma
Sarcomatoid carcinoma
Adenocarcinoma—several subtypes present
NUT carcinoma
Undifferentiated carcinoma
Other rare thymic carcinoma

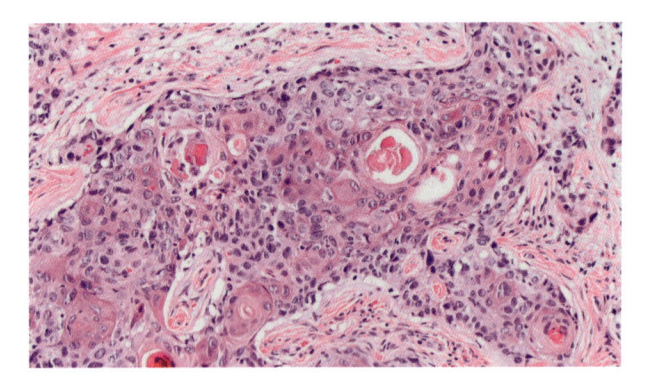

Figure 11 Thymic carcinoma. Nests of squamous cell carcinoma showing nuclear pleomorphism, keratinization, and stromal reaction to invasion. H & E stained slide (×200).

Cushing syndrome with ectopic adrenocorticotropin (ACTH) production occurs in 30% of patients with thymic carcinoid tumor but not in patients with thymoma. Other paraneoplastic syndromes, such as osteoarthropathy and Eaton–Lambert syndrome, and an association with multiple endocrine neoplasia (type I or II) have been described.[37,38]

Thymic lymphomas

Lymphomas are, with thymomas, the most common tumors of the thymus.[9,24,39–41] Although the thymus is a T-cell organ, the most frequent lymphomas of the thymus in adult patients are Hodgkin lymphoma and B-cell lymphomas (Table 1).

Germ cell tumors of the thymus

The thymus is a classic site of extragonadal primary germ cell tumors (Table 1). The most common ones are seminomas and teratomas (mature or immature). Embryonal carcinomas, yolk sac tumors, teratocarcinomas, and choriocarcinomas have also been described (Figure 12).

Other thymic tumors

Other thymic tumors include thymolipomas, which may become quite large, thymic cysts, metastases to the thymus, and other neoplasms listed in Table 1.

Molecular abnormalities of thymoma and thymic carcinoma

Molecular differences between thymomas and thymic carcinomas

Until recently, we have had limited information of the genomic changes that occur in thymic epithelial tumors. A significant

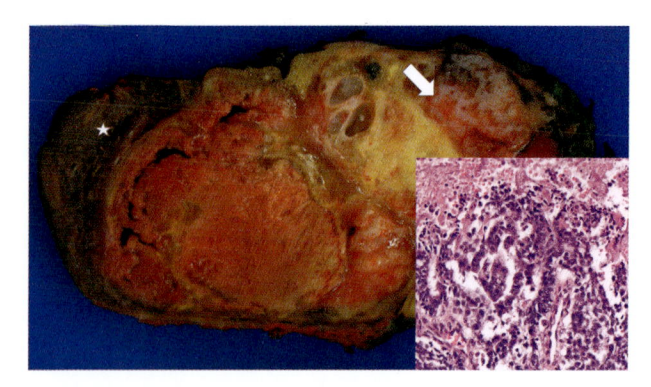

Figure 12 Gross photograph of a mediastinal mixed germ cell tumor (yolk sac and teratoma) status post neoadjuvant therapy with necrosis, invading the attached lung wedge (star). Teratomatous area with cystic change and cartilage (arrow). Inset shows the yolk sac component with foci of necrosis (top of the panel, H & E stained slide (×200).

challenge has been that types AB, B1, and B2 contain a significant number of nonneoplastic thymocytes which outnumber the malignant epithelial cells, making comparative genomic hybridization (CGH) and fluorescence *in situ* hybridization (FISH) analyses challenging. Thanks to newer techniques such as next-generation sequencing and expression array analysis, our knowledge of the tumor biology underlying different phenotypes between thymomas and thymic carcinomas has significantly improved in recent years. Genomic profiling distinguishes type B3 and thymic carcinoma from type A and B2 thymomas. In addition, type B3 tends to have a more distinct lymphocytic component and thymic carcinomas are C-Kit positive.

The most frequent genetic alterations occur on chromosome 6p21.3 (MHC locus) and 6q25.2–25.3.[1,42,43] Cytogenetic studies have demonstrated chromosomal abnormalities in all histological subtypes including the t(15;19)(q13:p13.1) translocation which generates the BRD4-NUT fusion gene which can occur in thymic carcinoma.[44] Additional data from CGH analysis performed on thymic carcinomas has demonstrated frequent copy number gains of 17q and 18 and loss of 3p, 16q, and 17p.[1,45] Further aberrations that have been described include multiple losses of genetic material and microsatellite instability (MSI) in different chromosomes (3p22–24.3, 3p14.2 (FHIT gene locus), 5q21 (APC gene), 6p21, 6p21–22.1, 7p21–22, 8q11.21–23, 13q14 (RB gene), and 17p13.1 (p53 gene).[45,46] The most frequent loss of heterozygocities (LOHs) (48.6%) occurred in region 6q25.2. Another hot spot showing LOH in 32.4% of tumors was located on 6q25.2–25.3. The third hot spot (30%) showing LOH appeared in region 6p21.31 including the major histocompatibility complex (MHC) locus and the fourth (26.3%) was detected on 6q14.1–14.3. MSI has also been described on chromosome 6 in 10% of thymomas, most commonly in type B thymoma. The 6p23 region encompasses the FOXC1 tumor suppressor gene and chromosomal loss is correlated with lower protein expression. Patients with FOXC1 negative tumors have a shorter time to tumor progression and shorter disease-related survival.[47,48]

Gene signatures to potentially determine prognosis in thymic tumors

The main prognostic indicators in thymic malignancies are tumor stage, histologic subtype, and the extent of surgical resection. As our understanding of the underlying molecular biology improves, gene signatures are seen as a next step in helping the oncologist move beyond clinical and morphological features to determine prognosis, aggressiveness of treatment, and extent of surveillance imaging. In an elegant study, genomic expression was performed and the authors correlated their findings with outcomes in 34 patients with thymoma.[49] Unsupervised clustering of gene expression data identified four clusters of thymic tumors that showed significant correlation with histological classification ($P = 0.002$). In addition, the authors identified a number of other genes associated with potential clinical behavior of thymic tumors including aldo-keto reductase family 1 B10 (*AKR1B10*), junctophilin-1 (*JPH1*), hedgehog target gene, *COL11A1*, *AKR1B10*, and *JPH1*. The authors also developed 9-gene and 12-gene signatures that can be used to identify patients at high or low risk for developing metastases from thymomas and thymic carcinomas, respectively. In these rare tumors with limited scope for randomized studies, an improved understanding of prognosis indicators based on the gene signatures would be of tremendous benefit in the future clinical trials.

IASLC/ITMIG staging system for thymic epithelial neoplasms

Staging guidelines for thymic epithelial neoplasms were not included in the AJCC staging manual until the development of the International Association for the Study of Lung Cancer/International Thymic Malignancy Interest Group (IASLC/ITMIG) Staging System for Thymic Epithelial Neoplasms in 2017, which has since been included in the eighth edition of the AJCC staging manual (Table 4).[4,50,51] Prior to this, in the last 4 decades at least 15 different stage classification systems have been proposed and used. Of these different classification systems, the most widely used has been the Masaoka-Koga staging system shown in Table 5.

The IASLC/ITMIG staging system contains nomenclature that describes the anatomic extent of the disease only, is applicable to all types of thymic tumors, and conforms to the TNM reporting structure. The T component is divided into four categories of levels of involvement. T1a involves a tumor that is encapsulated or not with or without extension into the mediastinal fat. T1b includes invasion of mediastinal pleura. Pathologically proven involvement of the pericardium is designated as T2 and several different structures are included in the T3 category including lung, brachiocephalic vein, SVC, chest wall, phrenic nerve, hilar, and pulmonary vessels. T4 tumors include several structures that indicate more extensive local involvement, for example, aorta, pulmonary artery, myocardium, trachea, and esophagus. Lymph node status "N" is assigned into two groups according to their proximity to the thymus with N1 indicating anterior (peri-thymic) involvement and N2 disease indicating deep cervical or thoracic nodes. Finally, metastatic disease is categorized as M1a, indicating separate pleural or pericardial nodule(s), and M1b indicating a pulmonary intra-parenchymal nodule or distant organ metastasis. The IASLC/ITMIG staging system has been accepted by both the AJCC and UICC and hopefully will allow for more accurate clinical staging, guide the formulation of effective treatment strategies.

Diagnosis of anterior mediastinal mass

The diagnosis of an anterior mediastinal mass is guided by the clinical suspicion of its etiology. Age and gender are the two most important features to consider from the outset as specific lesions tend to occur more commonly in certain demographic groups.

Table 5 Masaoka-Koga staging of thymomas.

Stage	Extent of disease
I	Totally encapsulated
II	Microscopic (IIa) or macroscopic (IIb) transcapsular invasion into surrounding fat or mediastinal pleura
III	Invasion of surrounding organs (pericardium, lung, great vessels)
IV	(A) Pleural or pericardial implants
	(B) Embolic metastasis

Table 4 IASLC/ITMIG staging system for thymic epithelial neoplasms (with AJCC prognostic groups).

Primary tumor (T)	
T1a	Tumor encapsulated or extending into the mediastinal fat; no mediastinal pleura involvement
T1b	Tumor encapsulated or extending into the mediastinal fat; direct invasion of mediastinal pleura
T2	Tumor with direct invasion of the pericardium (either partial or full thickness)
T3	Tumor with direct invasion into any of the following: lung, brachiocephalic vein, superior vena cava, phrenic nerve, chest wall, or extrapericardial pulmonary artery or veins
T4	Tumor with invasion into any of the following: aorta (ascending, arch, or descending) arch vessels, intrapericardial pulmonary artery, myocardium, trachea, esophagus
Regional lymph nodes (N)	
N0	No regional lymph node metastasis
N1	Metastasis in anterior (perithymic) lymph nodes
N2	Metastasis in deep intrathoracic or cervical lymph nodes
Distant metastasis (M)	
M0	No pleural, pericardial, or distant metastasis
M1a	Separate pleural or pericardial nodule(s)
M1b	Pulmonary intraparenchymal nodule or distant organ metastasis

AJCC prognostic groups			
Stage I	T1a,b	N0	M0
Stage II	T2	N0	M0
Stage IIIA	T3a	N0	M0
Stage IIIB	T3b	N0	M0
Stage IVA	Any T	N1	M0
	Any T	N0-N1	M1a
Stage IVB	Any T	N2	M0-M1a
	Any T	Any N	M1b

Table 6 Paraneoplastic/autoimmune syndromes associated with thymomas.

Condition	Findings	Treatments
Myasthenia gravis	Fatigable weakness with variable extension (from ocular to generalized)	Steroids, pyridostigmine, immunosuppression, IVIG, plasmapheresis
Pure red cell aplasia	Anemia	Steroids, immunosuppression
Hypogammaglobulinemia	Recurrent, severe infections	IVIG
Lambert Eaton syndrome	Fatigable weakness, autonomic symptoms	3,4-Diaminopyridine steroids, IVIG, plasmapheresis
Myositis	Muscle pain, weakness, elevated CK	Steroids
Acquired neuromyotonia	Diffuse fasciculations, cramps, hyperhydrosis	Sodium channel blockers (phenytoin), IVIG, plasmapheresis, steroids
Encephalitis	Memory impairment, behavioral changes, hallucinations, seizures, altered level of consciousness	Steroids, IVIG, rituximab, cyclophosphamide
Morvan's syndrome	Neuromyotonia and encephalitis, often with sleep disorder	Steroids, IVIG, rituximab, cyclophosphamide
Autoimmune Autonomic Neuropathy	Orthostatic hypotension, dry mouth, impaired pupillary responses, sexual dysfunction, urinary retention	Pyridostigmine, symptomatic therapies, IVIG, plasmapheresis, steroids, immunosuppression
Paraneoplastic cerebellar degeneration	Nystagmus, vertigo, dysarthria, ataxia	Steroids, IVIG, rituximab, cyclophosphamide

Laboratory investigations include alpha-fetoprotein, beta-human chorionic gonadotrophin, and lactate dehydrogenase. The causes include a wide variety of entities, the most common of which include the following approximations: thymic malignancy 35%, lymphoma 25% (Hodgkin's lymphoma 13% and non-Hodgkin's lymphoma 12%), thyroid and other endocrine tumors 15%, benign teratoma 10%, malignant germ cell tumors 10% (seminoma 4%, nonseminoma 6%), and benign thymic lesions 5%. Invasive incisional biopsy techniques, with mediastinoscopy or mediastinotomy for thymoma, carry the risk of violating the tumor capsule and disseminating tumor cells.[52] Otherwise, percutaneous fine-needle aspiration or core biopsy under fluoroscopic or computed tomography (CT) guidance is generally considered safe and effective. Combined with special stains and electron microscopy, if necessary, it has a sensitivity of 80% and specificity greater than 90%.[53]

Clinical features of thymomas

Most tumor-related symptoms are nonspecific (cough, dyspnea, chest pain) or secondary to local and regional mediastinal spread (pleural effusion, SVC syndrome, or pericardial effusion) and therefore, often indicate invasiveness. Occasionally, thymomas may present as diffuse pleural tumors and simulate malignant mesothelioma, particularly in recurrent thymoma.[54] About half of thymomas occur in asymptomatic persons and are discovered fortuitously on a chest radiograph, presenting as a retrosternal mass in the anterosuperior mediastinum forming a bulge in the cardiovascular silhouette. CT is invaluable for detecting small thymomas and assessing potential invasion of surrounding structures, such as the mediastinum, pleura, and pericardium.[53] The presence of a fat plane all around the tumor is a good sign of noninvasiveness, but, conversely, fibrous adherence to surrounding structures may simulate invasion. Thymomas show increased T1- and T2-weighted image signal intensity by magnetic resonance imaging (MRI), but the role of that technique in detecting possible capsular and vascular invasion, compared with CT, needs to be further defined.[55] The use of positron emission tomography (PET) with 18-flurodeoxyglucose (FDG) to distinguish malignant from benign mediastinal tumors has been evaluated and found to be useful. Thymic carcinomas and invasive thymomas show high FDG uptake, whereas noninvasive thymomas show moderate uptake. Teratomas and various benign cysts, on the other hand, show low FDG uptake.[56] It should be emphasized, however, that surgical exploration and pathologic evaluation remain the most reliable means to assess the invasiveness of thymomas.

Associated paraneoplastic syndromes

A number of paraneoplastic syndromes are associated with thymomas. They are mostly related to autoimmune mechanisms and are dominated by three characteristic entities (Table 6).

Myasthenia gravis

Myasthenia gravis occurs in approximately 33–50% of patients with thymoma, and approximately 10% of patients who have myasthenia gravis have a thymoma.[57] Myasthenia gravis is an autoimmune disorder that is characterized by the presence of antibodies to the acetylcholine receptors of the neuromuscular junction.[55] Myoid cells in the normal thymus raise the possibility of *in situ* sensitization.[58] Serum striational antibodies directed against elements of the sarcomere, such as titin, are found on average in 20–40% of thymoma patients, but in up to 80% of thymoma patients with myasthenia gravis.[55]

For patients with a thymoma and myasthenia gravis, total thymectomy, including removal of thymoma, is often indicated. Total thymectomy is also indicated in patients with myasthenia gravis without a thymoma, as the thymus has a key role in inducing acetylcholine receptor antibody production in patients with myasthenia gravis.[59] These benefits were recently confirmed in an international, randomized controlled trial published in 2016.[60] Patients with myasthenia gravis associated with thymoma tend to have more severe disease. Symptomatic therapy typically includes acetylcholinesterase inhibition. The presence of striational antibodies is an indication for immunosuppression and these patients have a particularly favorable response to rituximab (monoclonal antibody that binds specifically to the CD20 surface antigen on B lymphocytes).[61]

Red cell hypoplasia

Also called pure red cell aplasia (PRCA), red cell hypoplasia is an autoimmune disorder that is characterized by an acquired anemia with markedly decreased blood reticulocytes and a virtual absence of erythroblasts in the bone marrow.[62,63] There are often changes (an increase or a decrease) in white blood cell and/or platelet counts. PRCA is seen in approximately 5% of patients with thymoma, but 50% of patients with PRCA have a thymoma, which is of the spindle cell type in two-thirds of these patients.[62] Thymectomy produces remission of anemia in approximately 30% of cases.[63] Corticosteroids and immunosuppressive agents are also effective. A prolonged complete remission (with tumor regression) was described in one case with the combination of octreotide and prednisone.[64]

Hypogammaglobulinemia

First reported by Good in 1954, this acquired syndrome results in extreme susceptibility to recurrent, and often serious, infections.[65] It occurs in approximately 5–10% of patients with thymoma, and a thymoma is found in 10% of patients with acquired hypogammaglobulinemia.[53,62] There is a decrease in all major immunoglobulins (Igs), particularly IgG and IgA. Thymectomy does not result in any improvement of hypogammaglobulinemia; replacement therapy with Igs is indicated.[66]

A number of other paraneoplastic syndromes or associated disorders have been described in patients with thymoma (Table 6). It is noteworthy that Cushing syndrome with ectopic ACTH production is a typical feature of thymic carcinoids, not thymomas.[36]

Therapeutic approaches

Surgery

As indicated in the 2015 WHO classification revision, all major thymoma subtypes can behave in a clinically aggressive fashion, and should be considered potentially malignant.[18] Total thymectomy (complete surgical removal of thymus gland including tumor), rather than thymomectomy (resection of thymoma alone), is the procedure of choice, even for stage I encapsulated tumors.[53] It is also the procedure indicated for patients with myasthenia gravis, with or without thymoma. The usual approach is by median sternotomy, although additional thoracic or cervical incisions may be necessary, and some surgeons advocate for maximal thymectomy with exploration of all of the possible areas in which ectopic thymic tissue might be found.[67] There is a need for the surgeon to carefully explore the mediastinum for evidence of local invasion, which is the most reliable indication of malignancy and the most important prognostic factor. The tumor capsule should not be breached. Systematic microscopic examination is necessary to search for capsular invasion and to distinguish it from simple adhesions. Following total thymectomy, the recurrence rate is usually low (about 2%) for stage I encapsulated thymomas.[68] Recently, minimally invasive surgical techniques, including video-assisted and robot-assisted approaches, have been utilized for early-stage disease and shown to yield similar oncological results while being helpful in minimizing surgical trauma, improving postoperative recovery, and reducing incisional pain.[69] A systemic review and meta-analysis protocol has been established to further evaluate and compare these surgical modalities.[70]

Local invasion is seen in approximately 30–40% of thymomas at surgery, but the slow-growing nature of the tumor and the rarity of distant metastases justify attempts at radical surgery.[71–73] Identification of the phrenic, recurrent laryngeal, and vagus nerves is of major importance.[67] Extended resections—including one lung, one phrenic nerve, pericardium, and even resection and repair of great vessels, such as the innominate vein or SVC—have been performed. They should be undertaken only if they lead to complete tumor resection. With modern techniques of peri- and postsurgical care, surgical mortality is low (0–5%), even in patients with myasthenia gravis.[67,71,72]

In four large series with a total of 744 patients, the 5- and 10-year survival rates were 75–85% and 63–80%, respectively, for patients with noninvasive encapsulated thymomas.[71–73] Survival figures for patients with invasive thymomas were 50–67% at 5 years and 30–53% at 10 years. Whereas invasiveness is the major prognostic factor in patients with thymoma, most series also report a better prognosis for spindle cell thymomas and those with a higher ratio of lymphocytes and epithelial cells. Local recurrences and/or metastases (often intrathoracic) may also be amenable to surgical resection.

Radiotherapy

Thymomas are radiosensitive, and the efficacy of RT has been emphasized in many reports.[74] The role of RT is best discussed according to stage. For stage I disease following total surgical resection, postoperative RT is not indicated in view of the very low relapse rates. For stage II and III disease, the use of postoperative RT is recommended even after total surgical resection.[53,72,73,75] In a review of the literature, as well as their own experience, Curran and colleagues reported a 28% intrathoracic relapse rate after complete surgical resection without RT, as opposed to 5% when postoperative RT was given.[76] The latter figure may be unusual, however, because others have reported no such differences in favor of RT after complete surgical resection.[77] The routine use of RT after complete resection has been recently questioned particularly in stage II patients, but the small number of cases and the retrospective nature of the collected data do not allow a definitive conclusion in the absence of prospective randomized trials. The irradiated volume should include the mediastinum with adjacent areas and probably the supraclavicular areas, which are potential sites of relapse.[74] The total dose is approximately 45 Gy, with appropriate protection of the spinal cord, although doses of 50 Gy and higher have been given.[74,76] Radiation pneumonitis, mediastinitis, pericarditis, coronary artery fibrosis, and hypothyroidism as well as secondary cancers are potential complications.

RT is also given to patients with residual disease, following biopsy only or incomplete surgical resection for stage III disease. In 20 such cases, Curran and colleagues observed 4 mediastinal recurrences and 5 others outside the mediastinum, whereas no local relapse was seen when RT was given after total surgical resection for stage II or III disease.[76] Partial tumor debulking by surgery prior to RT in patients with stage III or IV disease does not appear to be beneficial. The 5-year survival rate for such patients was 45% overall, including 61% for stage III and 23% for stage IV disease after RT.[78] Collaboration between the surgeon and the radiation oncologist is essential to delineate areas of tumor involvement by radiopaque clips and to plan the treatment.

Systemic therapy

Chemotherapy

Chemotherapy has activity in both the operable and metastatic setting (Table 7). Platinum-based combination chemotherapy remains the standard of care in advanced-stage disease for both thymomas and thymic carcinomas. A four-drug regimen of doxorubicin, cisplatin, vincristine, and cyclophosphamide (ADOC) was considered the standard of care for many years with reported overall response rate of 92% and a median survival of 15 months.[80] An intergroup trial, however, demonstrated the benefits of the three-drug combination of cisplatin, doxorubicin, and cyclophosphamide (PAC) with an overall response rate of 50% and a median survival of 38 months.[79] Various regimens include corticosteroids, which have been shown to decrease tumor bulk in all histologic subtypes. A second three-drug regimen that is commonly used consists of cisplatin, doxorubicin, and methylprednisone (CAMP). This regimen was administered in the neoadjuvant setting and demonstrated a response rate of 93% with a 5 year overall survival (OS) of 81% in a small Phase II trial consisting of 17 patients.[86]

Table 7 Selected studies of chemotherapy regimens used in thymic malignancies.

Regimen	Stage	CR + PR (%)
PAC[79]	IV	50
ADOC[80]	III/IV	90
PE[81]	IV	56
VIP[82]	III/IV	32
Carbo-Px[83]	IV	35
Pemetrexed[84]	IV	17
CAPPR[85]	III/IV	81

PAC, cisplatin, doxorubicin, cyclophosphamide; ADOC, doxorubicin, cisplatin, vincristine, cyclophosphamide; PE, cisplatin, etoposide; VIP, etoposide, ifosfamide, cisplatin; Carbo-Px, carboplatin, paclitaxel; CAPPR, cyclophosphamide, doxorubicin, cisplatin, prednisone.

Table 8 Selected studies of targeted therapies in thymic malignancies.

Drug	Number of patients	Number of thymoma (T)	Number of thymic Ca (TC)	Response rate (%)
Geftinib[92]	26	19	7	4
Erlotinib + Bevacizumab[93]	18	11	7	0
Imatinib[94]	15	12	3	0
Belinostat[95]	40	24	16	5
Cixutumumab[96]	49	37	12	10
Everolimus[97]	51	32	19	12
Sunitinib[98]	41	16	25	26 (TC)

A retrospective study analyzed 87 patients with malignant thymoma treated with multimodality approach. The study concluded that because thymoma is a chemosensitive tumor but frequently recurs in patients with Stage II or greater disease, chemotherapy carries a potential survival benefit and should be incorporated into the multimodality approach to prolong disease-free survival.[87] Following this analysis, a single institution Phase II trial evaluated a multidisciplinary approach in 22 patients with unresectable thymomas, using induction chemotherapy followed by surgical resection, radiation therapy, and consolidation chemotherapy.[85] This sequential approach involved a 4-drug regimen of cyclophosphamide, doxorubicin, cisplatin, and prednisone (CAPPr) given for both induction and consolidation. With a median follow-up of 50.3 months, 18 of the 19 patients (95%) who completed the multidisciplinary approach were disease-free.[85]

Given higher toxicity rates in the multi-drug regimens, two-drug regimens have also been evaluated. The European Organization for Research and Treatment of Cancer (EORTC) investigated the combination of cisplatin and etoposide in 16 patients and demonstrated a response rate of 56% and a median survival of 4.3 years.[81] The addition of ifosfamide to this combination (VIP) demonstrated a partial response rate of 32% and an OS of 32 months, albeit with higher toxicities.[82] A Phase II trial by Lemma and colleagues investigated carboplatin AUC 5 and paclitaxel 225 mg/m^2 every 3 weeks up to a maximum of six cycles. An overall response rate of 33% and a progression-free survival (PFS) of 19.8 months for thymomas and 6.2 months for thymic carcinomas in 34 treatment naïve patients was reported and this was very well tolerated.[83] A second multicenter trial investigated the efficacy of carboplatin/paclitaxel in 40 Japanese patients with newly diagnosed thymic carcinoma. An overall response rate of 36% (95% CI, 21–53%; $P = 0.031$) and a median PFS of 8.1 months was seen with 1-year and 2-year survival rates of 85% and 71%, respectively.[88] The combination of carboplatin/paclitaxel is an effective regimen and if an anthracycline cannot be used, this combination is a good choice in the first-line setting for thymic carcinoma.

Multiple chemotherapeutic agents have been studied in the second-line therapy setting, with some showing efficacy. A Phase II study evaluated single-agent pemetrexed at a dosage of 500 mg/m^2 every 3 weeks in 27 patients with previously treated unresectable stage IVA ($n = 16$) or stage IVB ($n = 11$) recurrent thymic malignancies. The median number of cycles administered was 6 (range 1–6). In 23 fully evaluable patients, two complete and three partial responses (RECIST) were noted. Four responding patients had stage IVA thymoma, and one patient with a partial response had stage IVA thymic carcinoma.[84] Oral etoposide similarly may have some activity in pretreated patients with an overall response rate of 15% being reported.[89] Amrubicin in previously treated patients at a dosage of 35–40 mg/m^2 days 1–3 repeated every 3 weeks was evaluated in 33 patients in a recently published Phase II trial. Objective response rate was 18%, with median PFS of 7.7 months and median OS of 29.7 months.[90] Combination regimens, such as capecitabine and gemcitabine, have also shown activity in pretreated patients with thymic epithelial malignancies.[91]

Targeted therapy

Although large randomized Phase III trials are not possible in thymic malignancies, a number of small Phase II studies and case reports (Table 8) have highlighted benefits of targeted therapy for a subset of patients who have progressed on first-line therapy. Receptor tyrosine kinase (KIT) is frequently overexpressed in thymic carcinomas with protein overexpression observed in up to 73–86% of tumors; however, in thymomas, only 2% demonstrate overexpression.[99,100] Unfortunately, despite the high frequency of KIT expression in thymic carcinomas the rate of KIT mutations remains low at less than 10%. Case reports have identified that the type of KIT mutation determines the sensitivity to tyrosine kinase inhibitors. A number of mutations have been described, for example, V560 deletion and L576P substitution both found in exon 11, D820E mutation in exon 17 and the H697Y mutation found in exon 14.[45,101–103] V560 is highly sensitive to both sunitinib and imatinib, L576P has moderate sensitivity to sunitinib and low sensitivity to imatinib whereas D820E is resistant to both TKIs indicating that "one size does not fit all" when it comes to mutation testing in thymic tumors. The rarity and the sensitivity of mutations explains the disappointing results of a small Phase II trial that evaluated imatinib in patients with either type B3 thymoma or thymic carcinoma, as no treatment responses were seen in the trial.[94]

Epidermal growth factor receptor (EGFR) is similarly overexpressed (70% of thymomas and 50% of thymic carcinomas) in thymic malignancies, but somatic activating EGFR mutations are extremely rare.[99,103–105] There is no correlation between EGFR staining and histological subtype. EGFR gene amplification by FISH occurs in approximately 20% of thymic malignancies, most notably in type B3 thymomas and thymic carcinomas, and is associated with more advanced stage and capsule invasion.[106] Not unexpectedly, there was no anticancer activity in a study that evaluated the efficacy of gefitinib 250 mg or the combination of erlotinib and bevacizumab for patients with progressive malignant thymic tumors.[92,93] Similarly, the EGFR monoclonal antibody cetuximab has limited efficacy.[107,108] At the present time, the evidence from the literature suggests that both EGFR tyrosine kinase inhibitors and monoclonal antibodies cannot be recommended to treat patients with thymic malignancies. Similarly, no cases of HER2 gene amplification by FISH have been detected and there is no data to recommend HER2 targeted therapies in this disease setting.[109]

Targeting angiogenesis, which is thought to play an important role in thymomagenesis, may be a more successful strategy. Vascular endothelial growth factor A (VEGF-A) and its receptors VEGFR-1, -2 are overexpressed in both thymomas and thymic carcinomas.[110,111] Although low response rates have been observed with bevacizumab, case reports involving sorafenib and sunitinib have highlighted the activity of these multi-kinase inhibitors predominantly in thymic carcinomas. Activity has been reported in a patient receiving sorafenib who had a missense mutation in exon 17 (D820E) of the c-KIT gene and a second patient had prolonged stable disease (>9 months) in a nonmutated but high protein-expressing tumor for KIT, p53, and VEGF.[101,112] The multi-kinase inhibitor sunitinib has been evaluated in a Phase II clinical trial involving 23 patients with thymic carcinoma. An impressive response rate compared to historical data of 26% and a disease control rate of 91% was reported.[98]

Other targets that have been evaluated include the insulin-like growth factor-1 (IGF-1)/IGF-1 receptor (IGF-1R) which has been identified as a poor prognostic indicator in thymic malignancies.[113,114] Expression of IGF-1R does differ between thymomas (4%) and thymic carcinomas (37%) indicating a possible difference in tumor biology which may be targetable.[114] A Phase II study of cixutumumab, an IGF-1R monoclonal antibody, in 49 patients with previously treated advanced thymic tumors demonstrated a modest 14% response rate in thymomas; there was no efficacy in thymic carcinoma.[96]

In vitro studies have shown the inhibitory effect of octreotide, an octapeptide somatostatin analog, on thymic epithelial cells through blockage or inhibition of the insulin-like growth factor and epidermal growth factor.[115] Subsequent to this discovery, an Eastern Cooperative Oncology Group (ECOG) Phase II trial by Loehrer and colleagues evaluated octreotide with and without prednisone in patients with unresectable, advanced thymic malignancies in whom the pretreatment octreotide scan was positive. Of the 38 patients that were fully assessable, two complete and ten partial responses were observed. The 1- and 2- year survival rates were 86.6% and 75.7%, respectively.[116] While further trials are warranted, octreotide with or without prednisone is considered a potential second-line therapy in patients with octreotide-avid disease.

Moreover, studies targeting the mTOR pathway inhibitors are ongoing. Thus far, a recently reported multicenter Phase II study enrolled 51 patients with advanced/recurrent thymoma or thymic carcinoma who progressed after platinum-based chemotherapy. Patients received oral everolimus 10 mg/day and results indicated a disease control rate of 88% with a median follow-up of 25.7 months. The study population had a high rate of drug-related adverse events, and three patients died of pneumonitis while enrolled in the study.[97]

As outlined above, the results of targeted therapies in thymic malignancies have been somewhat disappointing given the rarity of these tumors and the fact that it is extremely challenging to preselect patients based on a certain molecular phenotype. It is hoped that future molecular profiling "basket studies" enrolling multiple tumor types with selected oncogenic driver mutations will identify patients with thymic malignancies that have significant sensitivities to targeted therapy. The actively recruiting NCI-MATCH and TAPUR trials are examples of these precision medicine cancer treatment trials evaluating targetable genetic changes identified in thymus tumors and other malignancies through genomic sequencing.[117]

Immunotherapy
Several Phase II studies targeting the PD-1/PD-L1 axis are ongoing at this time. High PD-L1 expression has been reported in approximately 30–80% of cases across the spectrum of thymic malignancies, with higher percentages seen in more aggressive tumor types (e.g., type B3 thymomas and thymic carcinomas).[118-120] This data indicates that the use of checkpoint inhibitors may prove more successful than targeting individual genetic alterations. However, concerns of exacerbating autoimmune phenomenon mandate investigation in type B3/thymic carcinomas first, prior to expanding to the other thymic malignancies. A high risk for immune-related adverse events was partly confirmed in a recent Phase I, dose-escalation trial that evaluated the anti-PD-L1 antibody avelumab in eight patients with thymic epithelial malignancies. Two patients with thymoma had a confirmed partial response by RECIST, another two had an unconfirmed partial response and three patients had stable disease. All responders, however, developed immune-related adverse events that resolved with immunosuppressive therapy.[121] Further evaluation of immunotherapy in thymic malignancies is pending data from ongoing trials.

Conclusions

Thymic tumors are a rare and heterogeneous group of malignancies that we continue to learn about and management. Incremental improvements in our understanding of molecular biology along with the recent developments of internationally accepted stage (IASLC/ITMIG) and histology (WHO) classification systems will provide a uniform nomenclature and pathway towards larger collaborative efforts. Surgical resection continues to be the cornerstone of therapy for early-stage disease, while a multidisciplinary

Table 9 Selected ongoing intergroup clinical trials involving treatment of thymic malignancies.

Name	Sponsor	Primary investigator	Therapy
Single-arm, multicentre, Phase II study of immunotherapy in patients with type B3 thymoma and thymic carcinoma previously treated with chemotherapy	EORTC	Nicolas Girad Solange Peters	Immunotherapy
A multicenter, Phase II trial of pembrolizumab and sunitinib in refractory advanced thymic carcinoma	NCI	Dwight Owen	Immunotherapy/targeted therapy
A pilot study to investigate the safety and clinical activity of avelumab in thymoma and thymic carcinoma after progression on platinum-based chemotherapy	NCI	Arun Rajan	Immunotherapy
A randomized Phase II trial of carboplatin-paclitaxel with or without ramucirumab in patients with unresectable locally advanced, recurrent, or metastatic thymic carcinoma	Southwest Oncology Group, NCI	Anne S Tsao	Chemotherapy/targeted therapy

http://Clinicaltrials.gov

approach is recommended in advanced stages or recurrent disease. Gene expression profiling and genomic clustering data indicating that the sub-classifications of thymic epithelial malignancies have different molecular features may allow for subset-specific therapeutics. It is hoped that molecular classification may be more useful to clinicians in the future than current classification systems. Future strategies using prognostic and predictive biomarkers or gene signatures may allow us to preselect or recurrent patients for the most appropriate treatment. Additionally, the association of thymic tumors with a wide variety of disorders secondary to T-cell mediated autoimmunity allied to high PD-L1 expression indicates that checkpoint inhibitors targeting PD-1 may hold promise for patients with chemo-resistant disease. Table 9 highlights currently active clinical trials in thymoma treatment.

Key references

The complete reference list can be found on Vital Source version of this title, see inside front cover.

1. Zettl A, Strobel P, Wagner K, et al. Recurrent genetic aberrations in thymoma and thymic carcinoma. *Am J Pathol*. 2000;**157**(1):257–266. doi: 10.1016/s0002-9440(10)64536-1.
3. Filosso PL, Ruffini E, Lausi PO, et al. Historical perspectives: the evolution of the thymic epithelial tumors staging system. *Lung Cancer*. 2014;**83**(2):126–132. doi: 10.1016/j.lungcan.2013.09.013.
4. Carter BW, Benveniste MF, Madan R, et al. IASLC/ITMIG staging system and lymph node map for thymic epithelial neoplasms. *Radiographics*. 2017;**37**(3):758–776. doi: 10.1148/rg.2017160096.
6. Engels EA, Pfeiffer RM. Malignant thymoma in the United States: demographic patterns in incidence and associations with subsequent malignancies. *Int J Cancer*. 2003;**105**(4):546–551. doi: 10.1002/ijc.11099.
12. Marx A, Strobel P, Badve SS, et al. ITMIG consensus statement on the use of the WHO histological classification of thymoma and thymic carcinoma: refined definitions, histological criteria, and reporting. *J Thorac Oncol*. 2014;**9**(5):596–611. doi: 10.1097/jto.0000000000000154.
16. Suster S, Moran CA. Thymoma classification: current status and future trends. *Am J Clin Pathol*. 2006;**125**(4):542–554. doi: 10.1309/CAV8-RNU5-TKNA-CKNC.
18. Marx A, Chan JK, Coindre JM, et al. The 2015 World Health Organization classification of tumors of the thymus: continuity and changes. *J Thorac Oncol*. 2015;**10**(10):1383–1395. doi: 10.1097/jto.0000000000000654.
22. Marchevsky AM, Gupta R, Casadio C, et al. World Health Organization classification of thymomas provides significant prognostic information for selected stage III patients: evidence from an international thymoma study group. *Hum Pathol*. 2010;**41**(10):1413–1421. doi: 10.1016/j.humpath.2010.02.012.
26. Hosaka Y, Tsuchida M, Toyabe S, et al. Masaoka stage and histologic grade predict prognosis in patients with thymic carcinoma. *Ann Thorac Surg*. 2010;**89**(3):912–917. doi: 10.1016/j.athoracsur.2009.11.057.
29. Moser B, Scharitzer M, Hacker S, et al. Thymomas and thymic carcinomas: prognostic factors and multimodal management. *Thorac Cardiovasc Surg*. 2014;**62**(2):153–160. doi: 10.1055/s-0032-1322611.
43. Inoue M, Starostik P, Zettl A, et al. Correlating genetic aberrations with World Health Organization-defined histology and stage across the spectrum of thymomas. *Cancer Res*. 2003;**63**(13):3708–3715.
45. Girard N, Shen R, Guo T, et al. Comprehensive genomic analysis reveals clinically relevant molecular distinctions between thymic carcinomas and thymomas. *Clin Cancer Res*. 2009;**15**(22):6790–6799. doi: 10.1158/1078-0432.CCR-09-0644.
46. Kelly RJ, Petrini I, Rajan A, et al. Thymic malignancies: from clinical management to targeted therapies. *J Clin Oncol*. 2011;**29**(36):4820–4827. doi: 10.1200/JCO.2011.36.0487.
48. Radovich M, Solzak JP, Hancock BA, et al. P2.13. A large microRNA cluster on chromosome 19 indentified by RNA-sequencing is a transcriptional hallmark of WHO type A and AB thymomas. *British J Cancer*. 2016;**114**(4):477–484.
49. Badve S, Goswami C, Gokmen-Polar Y, et al. Molecular analysis of thymoma. *PLoS One*. 2012;**7**(8):e42669. doi: 10.1371/journal.pone.0042669.
50. Detterbeck FC, Asamura H, Crowley J, et al. The IASLC/ITMIG thymic malignancies staging project: development of a stage classification for thymic malignancies. *J Thorac Oncol*. 2013;**8**(12):1467–1473. doi: 10.1097/JTO.0000000000000017.
53. Rosenberg JC, DVJ N, Hellman S, Rosenberg SA (eds). *Cancer. Principles and Practice of Oncology*, 4th ed. Philadelphia: Lippincott; 1993:759.
56. Kubota K, Yamada S, Kondo T, et al. PET imaging of primary mediastinal tumours. *Br J Cancer*. 1996;**73**(7):882–886.
58. Drachman DB. Myasthenia gravis. *N Engl J Med*. 1994;**330**(25):1797–1810. doi: 10.1056/NEJM199406233302507.
60. Wolfe GI, Kaminski HJ, Sonnett JR, et al. Randomized trial of thymectomy in myasthenia gravis. *J Thorac Dis*. 2016;**8**(12):E1782-e3. doi: 10.21037/jtd.2016.12.80.
64. Palmieri G, Lastoria S, Colao A, et al. Successful treatment of a patient with a thymoma and pure red-cell aplasia with octreotide and prednisone. *N Engl J Med*. 1997;**336**(4):263–265. doi: 10.1056/NEJM199701233360405.
66. Siegal FP. Immunodeficiency diseases and thymoma. In: Givel JC, Merlini M, Clarke DB, Dusmet M, eds. *Surgery of the Thymus. Pathology, Associated Disorders and Surgical Technique*. Berlin: Springer-Verlag; 1990:109.
69. Zhang X, Gu Z, Fang W. Minimally invasive surgery in thymic malignancies: the new standard of care. *J Thorac Dis*. 2018;**10**(Suppl 14):S1666–S1670. doi: 10.21037/jtd.2018.05.168.
76. Curran WJ Jr, Kornstein MJ, Brooks JJ, Turrisi AT 3rd., Invasive thymoma: the role of mediastinal irradiation following complete or incomplete surgical resection. *J Clin Oncol*. 1988;**6**(11):1722–1727.
79. Loehrer PJ Sr, Kim K, Aisner SC, et al. Cisplatin plus doxorubicin plus cyclophosphamide in metastatic or recurrent thymoma: final results of an intergroup trial. The Eastern Cooperative Oncology Group, Southwest Oncology Group, and Southeastern Cancer Study Group. *J Clin Oncol*. 1994;**12**(6):1164–1168.
82. Loehrer PJ Sr, Jiroutek M, Aisner S, et al. Combined etoposide, ifosfamide, and cisplatin in the treatment of patients with advanced thymoma and thymic carcinoma: an intergroup trial. *Cancer*. 2001;**91**(11):2010–2015.
85. Kim ES, Putnam JB, Komaki R, et al. Phase II study of a multidisciplinary approach with induction chemotherapy, followed by surgical resection, radiation therapy, and consolidation chemotherapy for unresectable malignant thymomas: final report. *Lung Cancer*. 2004;**44**(3):369–379. doi: 10.1016/j.lungcan.2003.12.010.
87. Park HS, Shin DM, Lee JS, et al. Thymoma. A retrospective study of 87 cases. *Cancer*. 1994;**73**(10):2491–2498. doi: 10.1002/1097-0142(19940515)73:10<2491::aid-cncr2820731007>3.0.co;2-6.
92. Kurup A, Burns M, Dropcho S, et al. Phase II study of gefitinib treatment in advanced thymic malignancies. *J Clin Oncol*. 2005;**23**(16_suppl):7068.
93. Bedano PM, Perkins S, Burns M, et al. A phase II trial of erlotinib plus bevacizumab in patients with recurrent thymoma or thymic carcinoma. *J Clin Oncol*. 2008;**26**(15_suppl):19087.
96. Rajan A, Carter CA, Berman A, et al. Cixutumumab for patients with recurrent or refractory advanced thymic epithelial tumours: a multicentre, open-label, phase 2 trial. *Lancet Oncol*. 2014;**15**(2):191–200. doi: 10.1016/S1470-2045(13)70596-5.
97. Zucali PA, De Pas T, Palmieri G, et al. Phase II study of everolimus in patients with thymoma and thymic carcinoma previously treated with cisplatin-based chemotherapy. *J Clin Oncol*. 2018;**36**(4):342–349. doi: 10.1200/jco.2017.74.4078.
101. Bisagni G, Rossi G, Cavazza A, et al. Long lasting response to the multikinase inhibitor bay 43-9006 (Sorafenib) in a heavily pretreated metastatic thymic carcinoma. *J Thorac Oncol*. 2009;**4**(6):773–775. doi: 10.1097/JTO.0b013e3181a52e25.
102. Strobel P, Hartmann M, Jakob A, et al. Thymic carcinoma with overexpression of mutated KIT and the response to imatinib. *N Engl J Med*. 2004;**350**(25):2625–2626. doi: 10.1056/NEJM200406173502523.
103. Yoh K, Nishiwaki Y, Ishii G, et al. Mutational status of EGFR and KIT in thymoma and thymic carcinoma. *Lung Cancer*. 2008;**62**(3):316–320. doi: 10.1016/j.lungcan.2008.03.013.
106. Ionescu DN, Sasatomi E, Cieply K, et al. Protein expression and gene amplification of epidermal growth factor receptor in thymomas. *Cancer*. 2005;**103**(3):630–636. doi: 10.1002/cncr.20811.
114. Zucali PA, Petrini I, Lorenzi E, et al. Insulin-like growth factor-1 receptor and phosphorylated AKT-serine 473 expression in 132 resected thymomas and thymic carcinomas. *Cancer*. 2010;**116**(20):4686–4695. doi: 10.1002/cncr.25367.
116. Loehrer PJ Sr, Wang W, Johnson DH, et al. Octreotide alone or with prednisone in patients with advanced thymoma and thymic carcinoma: an Eastern Cooperative Oncology Group Phase II Trial. *J Clin Oncol*. 2004;**22**(2):293–299. doi: 10.1200/jco.2004.02.047.
118. Chen Y, Zhang Y, Chai X, et al. Correlation between the expression of PD-L1 and clinicopathological features in patients with thymic epithelial tumors. *Biomed Res Int*. 2018;**2018**:5830547. doi: 10.1155/2018/5830547.
120. Wei YF, Chu CY, Chang CC, et al. Different pattern of PD-L1, IDO, and FOXP3 Tregs expression with survival in thymoma and thymic carcinoma. *Lung Cancer*. 2018;**125**:35–42. doi: 10.1016/j.lungcan.2018.09.002.

83 Tumors of the heart and great vessels

Moritz C. Wyler von Ballmoos, MD, PhD ■ Michael J. Reardon, MD

Overview

The most common neoplasms of the heart and great vessels are metastatic from other primary tumors, followed by benign primary cardiac tumors and then malignant primary tumors of the heart and great vessels. Cardiac-specific symptoms are due to mass effect, disruption of normal conduction, and embolic events. Echocardiography is the most commonly used and widely available imaging modality, while cardiac MRI provides more detailed resolution, tissue characteristics, and functional assessment that help with differential diagnosis, staging, and surgical planning. Most benign and malignant tumor benefit from surgical resection, when amenable, but overall prognosis for malignant neoplasm is poor with limited or no other options for treatment.

Introduction

Cardio-oncology is relatively new field at the intersection of neoplastic disorders and heart disease, including the primary cardiac neoplasms, metastatic disease to the heart and great vessels, and cardiovascular complications resulting from tumors or the treatment thereof. It recognized the complexity of these disease processes and the need to involve a multi-disciplinary team to achieve outcomes that are in line with the current standard of care and the patient goals of care. Tumors of the heart and great vessels are 20–30-times more commonly metastatic, than primary. And 10-times more commonly benign than malignant (Figure 1). The prevalence of cardiac metastatic disease is 0.7–3.5% in autopsy studies of the general population and around 15% in patients with known, advanced-stage cancer and metastasis.[1-5] Melanoma, breast- and lung carcinoma as well as lymphoma are frequently the primary malignancy. Primary cardiac tumors are much less common, with a prevalence of <0.1% to 0.3% based on autopsy series.[1,2,6,7] More than 75% of primary cardiac tumors are benign (Table 1), with papillary fibroelastoma and myxomas being the most common type.[9,10] Malignant primary cardiac tumors are most commonly undifferentiated sarcomas and angiosarcomas, which carry a poor prognosis despite treatment relying primarily on surgical resection.[11,12]

Clinical presentation of cardiac tumors

The clinical manifestations of cardiac tumors frequently reflect the cardiac structure involved, tumor size, and the friability of the tumor rather than its histology alone.[13] Cardiac specific symptoms originate from either a mass-effect on the cardiac chambers or an obstruction (atria, ventricles, valves), arrhythmias due to irritation or conduction disturbance, or embolic events as a result of a tumor protruding into the cardiac chambers and creating a nidus for thrombus formation or tumor fragmentation with subsequent embolization. Malignant tumors can also infiltrate the myocardium more diffusely or result in necrosis, intramyocardial hemorrhage, or pericardial effusions resulting in heart failure.

Both benign and malignant right atrial tumors can lead to tricuspid valve obstruction and symptoms of right heart failure (i.e., fatigue, peripheral edema, ascites, hepatomegaly, jugular vein distention). Similarly, benign and malignant left atrial tumors tend to cause symptoms by obstructing blood flow and typically present with left heart failure symptoms (i.e., dyspnea, orthopnea, pulmonary edema, or hemoptysis). Myocardial invasion is a feature of malignant tumors (such as sarcoma and lymphoma) presenting as arrhythmia, conduction abnormalities, systolic dysfunction, or diastolic dysfunction. Rarely, complete cavitary obstruction may lead to sudden death. Primary or secondary pericardial involvement can present as pleuritic chest pain or with cardiac tamponade. Hemopericardium is highly indicative of malignant tumors. Tumors with a high surface-to-volume area and friable tissue such as some myxomas and papillary fibroelastomas may present with evidence of pulmonary, cerebral, coronary, visceral, or peripheral emboli. Less specific symptoms include fever, weight loss, myalgias, arthralgias, fatigue, and weakness.

Many of the benign primary cardiac tumors are now diagnosed incidentally during a cardiac workup that is obtained for other reasons. With increasing resolution and availability of different imaging modalities (echocardiography, cardiac computed tomography, cardiac MRI), the incidence of cardiac tumors has also increased. Metastatic disease of the heart and great vessels is often found during the staging process or surveillance for the primary neoplasm. Malignant primary cardiac tumors tend to have more severe clinical presentations, although they can be quite nonspecific resulting in missed or delayed diagnosis. Occasionally, physical examination may disclose a murmur, either systolic or diastolic, that varies with body position if the tumor is mobile. The characteristic "tumor plop" of a mobile tumor such as a myxoma is heard in diastole following the second heart sound and is thought to be due to the tension on the tumor stalk as the mass prolapses from atrium to ventricle or to the tumor striking the myocardium.[4] The tumor plop may be mistaken for a third heart sound or mitral opening snap. Electrocardiograms are typically nonspecific and may show ST-T abnormalities that are present in all leads and not consistent with a specific coronary territory, atrial or ventricular arrhythmias, bundle branch block, or low voltage QRS complexes in the case of pericardial effusion. Chest X-ray findings include cardiomegaly and tumor calcification but is generally nondiagnostic.

Imaging for cardiac tumors

Multiple cardiac imaging techniques are available for evaluation of patients with suspected cardiac masses. Two-dimensional

---

Holland-Frei Cancer Medicine, Tenth Edition. Edited by Robert C. Bast, John C. Byrd, Carlo M. Croce, Ernest Hawk, Fadlo R. Khuri, Raphael E. Pollock, Apostolia M. Tsimberidou, Christopher G. Willett, and Cheryl L. Willman.
© 2023 John Wiley & Sons, Inc. Published 2023 by John Wiley & Sons, Inc.

Heart and great vessels neoplasms

- Metastatic
- Primary: benign
- Primary: malignant

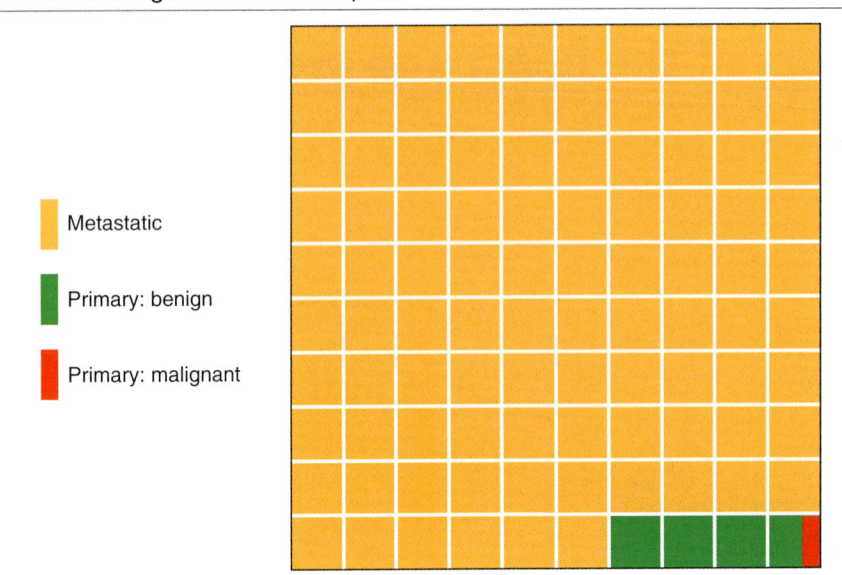

Figure 1 Relative incidence of cardiac neoplasms. The vast majority of neoplasms involving the heart and great vessels are metastatic in nature (originating from melanoma, breast, lung cancer etc.), followed by benign neoplams (such as myxoma or fibroelastoma). Malignant primary cardiac neoplasms are extremely rare.

transthoracic echocardiography (TTE) generally provides good spatial and excellent temporal resolution of cardiac masses. It is often the initial imaging modality of choice as it is widely available and inexpensive.[14] However, TTE can be limited by poor acoustic windows and lack of tissue characterization. Furthermore, right-sided structures (tricuspid valve, RV, RVOT, and proximal PA) are difficult to visualize with TTE. Transesophageal echocardiography (TEE) allows for better tumor localization and characterization as well as assessment of intra- and extracardiac invasion. It also provides better definition of lesions involving the valves and lesions in the RV and PA. The use of contrast echocardiography may help to improve echocardiographic resolution and provide information on tumor vascularity.[15] Real-time three-dimensional echocardiography can offer incremental value over two-dimensional echocardiography by providing an accurate assessment of size and shape of the mass and enabling better localization of attachment point.[16]

The quality and availability of cardiac computed tomography (CCT) and CCT magnetic resonance tomography (CMR) have increased significantly over the last decade. Both CCT and CMR provide full, three-dimensional volumes and allow multiplanar reconstruction of both cardiac and adjacent structures, providing substantially more information than echocardiography. Both modalities are able to depict intra- and extracardiac masses, as well as degree of myocardial or pericardial involvement, without limitations due to body habitus or poor acoustic windows. Cardiac CT has excellent spatial resolution but is limited by temporal resolution due to the rotation of the gantry. EKG-gating is used to time and collate images obtain over multiple cardiac cycles. With the advent of structural heart interventions heavily relying on CCT for planning purposes, CCT has become more widely available and images are obtained relatively quickly. Tissue characterization is limited to assessment of tissue density (hypo- and hyperdensity) with and without contrast. Functional assessment of the heart is also limited. There has been significant reduction in radiation dose with newer scanners and protocols, but radiation exposure and nephrotoxicity of contrast agents remain disadvantages of CCT.[17] Cardiac MRI provides the highest degree of soft-tissue contrast of any imaging modality and combines outstanding tumor localization, visualization of adjacent structures in combination with a comprehensive functional assessment of the heart and great vessels (Figure 2).[18–20] In addition, tailored imaging sequences allow more specific characterization of particular tumors.[19] Tissue characteristics of the cardiac mass can be evaluated using T1- and T2-weighted images, as well as enhancement with gadolinium contrast.[21] Some neoplasms have a specific features on CMR that help with making a diagnosis (Table 2). When a cardiac mass is discovered on an imaging study, the differential diagnosis includes thrombus and vegetation, in addition to primary or secondary tumors.[22,23] Thrombi are usually seen in the context of underlying heart disease including arrhythmia (e.g., atrial fibrillation or atrial flutter), cardiomyopathy, or myocardial infarction. Normal anatomic variants, such as a prominent Eustachian valve or Chiari network, may also mimic cardiac tumors.[24] Various CMR sequences, as well as imaging with and without contrast, facilitate the distinction between thrombus, vegetation, and neoplasm, which can be difficult with other imaging modalities but is often an important consideration during the workup. Therefore, CMR is the most useful imaging modality for neoplasms of uncertain etiology, when atypical findings are present on other imaging modalities, and for malignant tumors of the heat and great vessels. Positron emission tomography (PET) is used less commonly but can also help to identify cardiac involvement in patients with malignant tumors.[25]

Cardiac tumors

Benign primary cardiac tumors

Papillary fibroelastomas
Papillary fibroelastomas (PFE) are the most common primary tumor of the cardiac valves and are composed of papillary fronds similar to normal chordae tendinae.[6] They usually (88%) arise

Table 1 Primary cardiac neoplasms.[a]

	Age	Location	Genetic drivers
Benign neoplasms			
Papillary fibroelastoma	Adult	Valves	KRAS
Myxoma	Adult	Atria	PRKAR1A
Rhabdomyoma	Pediatric	Ventricles	TSC1, TSC2
Fibroma	Pediatric	Ventricles	PTCH1
Lipomatous hypertrophy of atrial septum	Adult	Atria	HMGA2
Lipoma	Adult	Pericardium	HMGA2, TSC1, TSC2
Hemangioma	Adult	Ventricles	–
Germ cell tumor	Pediatric	Pericardium	–
Histiocytoid cardiomyopathy	Pediatric	Ventricles	MT-CYB
Inflammatory myofibroblastic tumor	Pediatric	Ventricles, valves	–
Paraganglioma	Adult	Atria	RET, VHL, SDH
Granular cell tumor	Adult	Ventricles	–
Epithelioid hemangioendothelioma	Adult	Ventricles	WWTR1-CAMTA1
Hamartoma of mature cardiac myocytes	Adult	Ventricles	–
Schwannoma	Adult	Atria	–
Malignant neoplasms			
Undifferentiated pleomorphic sarcoma	Adult	Atria	MDM2
Angiosarcoma	Adult	Atria	Complex cytogenetics
Mesothelioma	Adult	Pericardium	–
Lymphoma	Adult	Pericardium	–
Synovial sarcoma	Adult	Pericardium	SS18-SSX
Rhabdomyosarcoma	Pediatric	Ventricles	–
Liposarcoma	Adult	Ventricles	–
Leiomyosarcoma	Adult	Vasculature	TP53[b]
Osteosarcoma	Adult	Atria	TP53[b]
Myxofibrosarcoma	Adult	Atria	TP53[b]
Solitary fibrous tumor	Adult	Pericardium	STAT6

[a] Source: Maleszewski et al.[8]
[b] Association with Li-Fraumeni syndrome.

from the valvular endocardium, most commonly the aortic valve, and occur over a wide range of ages.[26,27] They are typically small (<1 cm), have a central fibrous stalk, and present as multiple lesions in roughly 21% of patients.[7] About 80% of PFE have a rKRAS mutation, suggesting these are true neoplasms, although some studies have suggested they may also be associated with previous cardiac instrumentation.[9] Fibroelastomas commonly are asymptomatic and found incidentally during a cardiac workup for other reasons, or they may present with embolic events including transient ischemic attack, stroke, pulmonary embolism, or heart failure, angina, myocardial infarction, and rarely sudden cardiac death. It is unclear whether SCD is associate with PFE or rather leads to increased detection due to autopsies being done. Surgical resection is recommended for patients with prior embolic events, as well as patients with large (≥1 cm) and mobile masses at high risk for embolization. Surgical resection can usually be done using a minimally invasive approach, including robotic-assisted techniques, with very low morbidity and mortality.

Myxomas

Myxomas represent the second most common primary cardiac tumor in the adult population.[10] Histologically, these soft gelatinous tumors are thought to arise from the subendocardial mesenchyme and contain polygonal to stellate myxoma cells ("lepidic cells"), often around vascular channels in an eosinophilic matrix, with various areas of hemorrhage.[9] The cells are positive for factor VIII and can also express neuron-specific enolase and S-100 protein.[28] Most myxomas arise in the left atrium and are usually attached to the fossa ovalis. In a meta-analysis of 32 reports encompassing 1029 patients, 83% of myxomas were found to occur in the left atrium.[29] The remainder are found in the right atrium, or uncommonly, in the right or left ventricles. They often present as mobile masses attached to the endocardial surface.[30] Myxomas tend to be bigger than PFE but can vary in size from 1 to 15 cm. The mean age is 50 years at presentation, and more women are affected than men (2:1).[29] On cardiac imaging myxomas present as well-defined, smooth lesions within cardiac chambers, that may feature cysts, fibrosis, and calcifications. The classic clinical presentation includes a triad of constitutional symptoms, valvular obstruction, and embolization and is seen in roughly a third of all patients with myxomas. The constitutional symptoms are believed to be secondary to IL-6 over-expression. Embolic phenomena, seen in 30–40% of patients, are more prevalent with smaller-sized myxomas that also tend to have a more irregular surface (polypoid or myxoid) and more friable tissue.[13] Surgery is generally recommended at the time of diagnosis due to the risk of embolization or other cardiac complications and involves en bloc resection along with margins of normal tissue. Recurrence is rare but can occur in 2–5% of patients and is associated with incomplete resection. As with PFE, surgical resection and reconstruction of the inter-atrial septum if needed can easily be accomplished with minimally invasive surgery which has a shorter recovery and lower morbidity at experienced centers. Long-term follow-up is necessary and imaging is recommended at one and 5 years after surgery.[31–33]

Although most myxomas are sporadic, familial syndromes have been described. The Carney complex is an autosomal dominant multiple endocrine neoplasia syndrome that includes cardiac, endocrine, neural, and cutaneous tumors in addition to skin and mucosal pigmentation. The diagnostic criteria are shown in Table 2. Two disease manifestations and one genetic criterion are necessary for the diagnosis. Mutations in *PRKAR1A*, a gene located on chromosome 17q22-24, which encodes a regulatory subunit of cyclic-AMP dependent protein kinase A, have been identified in approximately one-half of affected patients. A variant associated with distal arthrogryposis has been linked to a missense mutation in the myosin heavy-chain gene on 17p12-p13.1. Familial myxomas present at a younger age, are more likely to be multiple and are more likely to recur after resection than sporadic myxomas. Identification of first-degree relatives facilitates the identification of myxomas at risk for embolization. After surgical resection, yearly follow-up and surveillance are recommended for patients with Carney complex.

Other benign tumors

Rhabdomyomas occur almost exclusively in children and are described below. Lipomatous septal hypertrophy is an exaggeration of the normal accumulation of fat within the atrial septum and present in 1–8% of the general population with increasing incidence above 75 years. The lipomas consist of both mature adipose tissue, cardiomyocytes, and brown fat, resulting in PET positivity due to the high metabolic rate.[11,12] There is usually no role for surgical resection of lipomatous septal hypertrophy in the absence of symptoms such as vena cava obstruction, atrial arrhythmia, or congestive heart failure.[30] Cardiac hemangiomas may be found anywhere in the heart and are more common in children. Hemangiomas are typically asymptomatic but can be associated

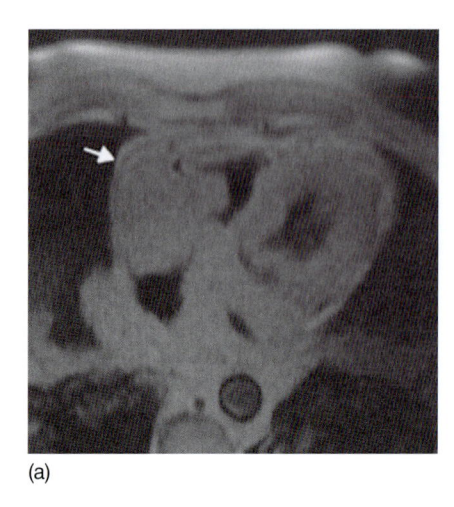

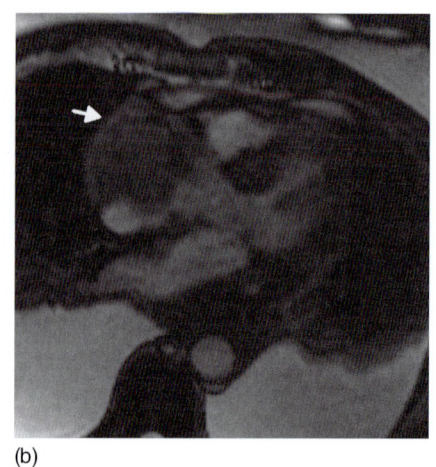

Figure 2 Cardiac MRI of a 69-year-old man with lymphoma demonstrating a large homogeneous mass (*arrows*) occupying most of the right atrium and extending into the right ventricle and posterior mediastinum. The image on the left is a dark-blood image in the four-chamber view obtained using T2-weighted half-Fourier acquisition single-shot turbo spin-echo. The image on the right is a bright-blood image in the four-chamber view obtained using steady-state free precession; note the large bilateral pleural effusions.

Table 2 Imaging characteristics of cardiac tumors on CMR.

Melanoma	Intrinsic T1-hyperintensity
Highly cellular metastasis (e.g., CA)	Restricted diffusion
Blood-vessel rich metastasis (e.g., renal CA)	Strong contrast enhancement
PFE (avascular)	No enhancement; T2 hyperintensity (connective tissue/MPS matrix) (smaller in size)
Myxoma (high H$_2$O content)	No enhancement; T2 hyperintensity (smooth surface; larger in size)
Cardiac lipomas	T1 hyperintensity; loss of signal with fat suppression; no significant enhancement (PET positive due to brown fat)
Cardiac hemangioma	T2 hyperintensity; gradual contrast enhancement pattern; isoattenuation with blood on delayed imaging
Sarcoma	Nonspecific (due to undifferentiated nature of tumor)
Angiosarcoma	T2 hyperintensity; enhancement variable (necrosis/hemorrhage)
Mesothelioma	Pericardial inflammation and thickening, nodular enhancement not specific (DD other reasons for pericarditis)

with Kasabach–Merritt syndrome consisting of hemangiomas, thrombocytopenia, and coagulopathy.[3] Histologically they consist of mature and immature blood vessels in a capillary, cavernous or arteriovenous configuration. Surgical resection can be quite complex due to the vascularity and is indicated only for symptomatic hemangiomas. Preoperative endovascular coil embolization of the feeding vessels can facilitate surgical resection. Fibromas primarily arise in the interventricular septum and more commonly affect the left ventricle. Pericardial cysts are most common in the right costophrenic angle, and bronchogenic cysts can be found in the myocardium.[9]

Malignant primary cardiac tumors

Sarcomas

Undifferentiated, high-grade pleomorphic sarcomas are the most common primary malignant neoplasm of the heart. The incidence is higher in women than men, and the typical age at presentation is between 40 and 50 years of age. Over 80% arise from the left atrial wall, but contrary to myxomas, commonly originate from the posterior wall.[4] Angiosarcomas usually arise in the right atrium and near the atrioventricular groove, although other chambers may be involved, and are associated with areas of hemorrhage, pericardial invasion, and effusion. Angiosarcomas most commonly present between 20 and 50 years of age, with a two- to threefold male predominance.[9] The clinical presentation of both tumor types may include palpitations, dyspnea, and chest pain (pleuritic and/or pericardial), or signs and symptoms related to congestive heart failure, thromboembolism, or arrhythmias. The relationship between cardiac angiosarcoma and Kaposi's sarcoma, in which cardiac involvement has been described, requires further investigation. Rhabdomyosarcomas are the second most common malignant neoplasm of the heart, and equally affect the right and left-sided heart chambers. Other types of endomyocardial-based sarcomas, often with smooth muscle or myofibroblastic differentiation, are rare tumors usually located in the left atrium and consist of multiple subtypes, including osteosarcoma, leiomyosarcoma, fibrosarcoma, and myxofibrosarcoma. The preferred imaging modality for all these tumors is CMR, which allows a detailed assessment, staging, and surgical planning if indicated. Unfortunately, the presenting symptoms of congestive heart failure and arrhythmias can also make acquisition of good imaging by CMR difficult and patients may tolerate lying flat for a prolonged period of time poorly.

The overall prognosis of cardiac sarcomas is poor, and aggressive local growth and metastatic spread are common. The median survival ranges from 6 to 12 months. Complete surgical resection of cardiac sarcomas is the treatment of choice, although many patients develop recurrent disease. In general, the response of these tumors to chemotherapy and radiation is poor. There has been some success with newer chemotherapy regiments and an approach using (neo)-adjuvant chemotherapy in combination with radical surgical resection in select patients.[5,13,14] A multidisciplinary tumor board is key to successful management of these patients.[15]

Neoplasms involving the right atrium, ventricle, and outflow tract can be accessed, resected, and reconstructed using a sternotomy approach and standard surgical technique. However, more complex lesions and those involving predominantly left-sided structure are often more difficult to access. Surgical procedures consisting of a cardiectomy, followed by resection of the tumor, reconstruction of the resected structures and autotransplantation is then often necessary to achieve complete resection.[16,17] In cases of lung involvement, the preferred surgical strategy is often a staged approach consisting of a radical resection of the tumor involving the heart and great vessels followed by a pneumonectomy the following day.[18] Orthotopic heart transplantation, at times combined with bilateral lung transplantation, has been described in a few small series and case reports. In most cases, heart transplantation followed by chemotherapy does not affect long-term outcome, however, selected patients may have good outcomes with transplantation.

Lymphomas
Primary cardiac lymphomas are extremely rare accounting for only 1% to 2% cardiac neoplasms and should be distinguished from systemic lymphoma with secondary cardiac involvement.[12] The typical sites are the right atrium and ventricle, where infiltration of the wall is frequent, as well as the pericardium. Cardiac lymphoma may be seen in immunocompetent patients but is also associated with acquired immune deficiency syndrome and organ transplant-related immunosuppression. Most are diffuse B-cell lymphomas.[19] Symptoms are due to mass effect, embolism, or diffuse infiltration of the myocardium leading to arrhythmias and heart failure. Unlike other cardiac tumors, the mainstay of treatment is chemotherapy, alone or in combination with radiation therapy, and occasionally autologous stem cell transplantation.

Mesothelioma
Primary cardiac mesothelioma as exceedingly rare, but accounts for 50% of all pericardial tumors.[20] Patients often present with a pericardial effusion, tamponade physiology, or constrictive pericarditis in more advanced cases. Hemopericardium should raise suspicion for mesothelioma, especially in combination with imaging studies showing features of inflammatory pericarditis, diffuse pericardial thickening, nodular enhancement. Pericardial biopsy with sufficient tissue is necessary to confirm the diagnosis, which carries a poor prognosis with less than 6 months median survival. Surgical drainage and pericardiectomy are predominantly palliative measures to alleviate symptoms of constriction or compression.

Metastatic cardiac tumors
Secondary tumors of the heart are 20–30 times more common than primary cardiac tumors (Figure 1). Mechanisms of metastasis include direct extension from nearby organs (lung), hematogenous spread (melanoma and lymphoma), lymphatic spread (retrograde from breast), and cavo-atrial or pulmonary vein extension (renal carcinoma). The pericardium is the most common location for cardiac metastasis, followed by the epicardium and myocardium. Malignancies likely to metastasize to the heart are shown in Table 3.[30] In a recent postmortem review of 7289 cases with malignant neoplasms, the incidence of cardiac metastasis was 9.1%.[5] The frequency of heart metastases was, in decreasing order, mesothelioma (48.4%), melanoma (27.8%), lung adenocarcinoma (21%), poorly differentiated lung carcinoma (19.5%), squamous cell lung carcinoma (18.2%), and breast carcinoma (15.5%). Almost any cancer, however, can metastasize to the heart. A high frequency of cardiac metastasis and/or invasion can be seen in patients with malignant pleural mesothelioma. In 19 autopsies, cardiac invasion was found in 14 (74%), with more than half involving the pericardium and more than one-quarter the myocardium. Treatment is generally palliative.

Table 3 Diagnostic criteria for the carney complex.[a]

Disease manifestations
Spotty skin pigmentation, distribution typically involving conjunctiva, lips, canthi, vaginal or penile mucosa
Cutaneous or mucosal myxoma
Cardiac myxoma
Breast myxomatosis (or suggestive magnetic resonance findings)
Primary pigmented nodular adrenocortical disease or Liddle's test with paradoxical positive response of urinary glucocorticosteroids to administration of dexamethasone
Acromegaly from growth hormone-producing adenoma
Large cell calcifying Sertoli cell tumor or characteristic calcification on testicular ultrasonography
Thyroid carcinoma or multiple ultrasonographically demonstrated nodules in a young patient
Psammomatous melanotic schwannoma
Multiple blue nevi
Multiple ductal adenomas of the breast
Osteochondromyxoma
Supplemental criteria
First-degree relative with the Carney complex
Inactivating mutation of the *PRKAR1A* gene

[a]Source: Based on Pinede et al.[32]

Pediatric tumors
In contrast to adults, metastases to the heart are rarely observed in the pediatric population. Many cardiac neoplasms in children occur in the context of familial syndromes (see section on the Carney Complex, above). The majority are hamartomas. Rhabdomyomas account for roughly 60% of pediatric cardiac tumors and are associated with tuberous sclerosis, an autosomal dominant disorder characterized by benign neoplasms of the heart, kidneys, brain, lungs, and skin. They occur most commonly in the left atrium and ventricle and, in the context of familial syndromes, often regress spontaneously; surgical resection is usually necessary only if symptoms such as obstruction or arrhythmias are present. Cardiac fibromas are mainly found in the ventricular septum and can grow to be quite large, often with areas of central calcification. Fibromas occur in a minority of patients with Gorlin syndrome, which is an autosomal dominant disorder presenting with multiple neoplasms, including basal cell carcinomas and medulloblastomas as well as odontogenic keratocysts and skeletal abnormalities. Neurofibromas are found in patients with von Recklinghausen's disease.[30]

Tumors of the great vessels
Primary tumors involving the aorta, pulmonary artery, and vena cavae are rare, appearing in the literature mainly as case reports or in small retrospective case series. Risk factors for the development of tumors of the great vessels remain poorly defined. Prior radiation exposure has been postulated as a possible causative factor. Plastic polymers, such as Dacron, have been linked to aortic tumors in animal studies; nonetheless, aortic tumors arising around a Dacron graft in humans, although reported, are extremely rare. Tumors of the great vessels typically present with thromboembolic events or an obstructive syndrome. MRI is particularly useful in differentiating tumors of the great vessels from intraluminal thrombus, mediastinal lymphadenopathy, or adjacent lung tumors.

Benign tumors of the aorta include endothelial papillary fibroelastomas arising in the aortic sinuses, which may present with intermittent prolapse into a coronary artery or with emboli to the heart or brain. Intra-aortic myxomas have also been described, presenting with recurrent arterial emboli.

Table 4 Tumors likely to metastasize to the heart.

Melanoma
Malignant germ cell tumor
Leukemia and lymphoma
Breast carcinoma
Lung carcinoma
Hepatocellular carcinoma
Renal cell carcinoma
Sarcoma
Esophageal and gastric carcinoma
Mesothelioma (may be primary to pericardium or metastatic)

Malignant tumors of the aorta and pulmonary artery are often aggressive, poorly differentiated sarcomas arising from intimal cells and showing myofibroblastic differentiation ("intimal type"). Rarely, malignant tumors of the great vessels are identified as angiosarcomas, leiomyosarcomas, hemangioendotheliomas, schwannomas, and fibrous histiocytomas. Sarcomas of the inferior vena cava tend to be well-differentiated leiomyosarcomas. Whereas sarcomas of the aorta present at a mean age of 62 years, sarcomas of the pulmonary artery present at a younger age. In a review of 60 cases of sarcoma involving the pulmonary trunk, the median age was 52 years, with a male-to-female ratio of 1:2 and a median duration of symptoms of 10 months. The clinical picture was suggestive of pulmonary embolism, with dyspnea (70%), chest pain (48%), cough (34%), hemoptysis (30%), and syncope (25%). Metastases to lung (67%) and lymph node (20%) were common (Table 4).

Although patients with tumors of the great vessels tend to present with advanced disease and prognosis is poor, a minority respond to resection and chemotherapy. The cornerstone of therapy is complete surgical excision. The use of various grafts has been advocated, along with postoperative radiation and chemotherapy, often with an anthracycline-based regimen. Although mean survival for patients with tumors of the great vessels is only 10 months, patients with sarcoma of the pulmonary artery may have a better prognosis compared with sarcoma of the aorta (23 vs 5 months). Prolonged survival is extremely rare but has been reported. For patients with unresectable disease, endovascular stent grafting may improve quality of life.

References

1 Bruce CJ. Cardiac tumours: diagnosis and management. *Heart*. 2011;**97**:151–160.
2 Lam KY, Dickens P, Chan AC. Tumors of the heart. A 20-year experience with a review of 12,485 consecutive autopsies. *Arch Pathol Lab Med*. 1993;**117**:1027–1031.
3 Silvestri F, Bussani R, Pavletic N, et al. Metastases of the heart and pericardium. *G Ital Cardiol*. 1997;**27**:1252–1255.
4 Paraskevaidis IA, Michalakeas CA, Papadopoulos CH, et al. Cardiac tumors. *ISRN Oncol*. 2011;**2011**:208929.
5 Bussani R, De-Giorgio F, Abbate A, et al. Cardiac metastases. *J Clin Pathol*. 2007;**60**:27–34.
6 Heath D. Pathology of cardiac tumors. *Am J Cardiol*. 1968;**21**:315–327.
7 Reynen K. Frequency of primary tumors of the heart. *Am J Cardiol*. 1996;**77**:107.
8 Maleszewski JJ, Bois MC, Bois JP, et al. Neoplasia and the heart. *J Am Coll Cardiol*. 2018;**72**(2):202–227. doi: 10.1016/j.jacc.2018.05.026.
9 McAllister HA, Fenoglio JJ. *Tumors of the Cardiovascular System*. Washington: Armed Forces Institute of Pathology; 1978.
10 Perchinsky MJ, Lichtenstein SV, Tyers GF. Primary cardiac tumors: forty years' experience with 71 patients. *Cancer*. 1997;**79**:1809–1815.
11 Donsbeck AV, Ranchere D, Coindre JM, et al. Primary cardiac sarcomas: an immunohistochemical and grading study with long-term follow-up of 24 cases. *Histopathology*. 1999;**34**:295–304.
12 Ikeda H, Nakamura S, Nishimaki H, et al. Primary lymphoma of the heart: case report and literature review. *Pathol Int*. 2004;**54**:187–195.
13 Burke A, Jeudy J Jr, Virmani R. Cardiac tumours: an update: cardiac tumours. *Heart*. 2008;**94**:117–123.
14 Auger D, Pressacco J, Marcotte F, et al. Cardiac masses: an integrative approach using echocardiography and other imaging modalities. *Heart*. 2011;**97**:1101–1109.
15 Mulvagh SL, Rakowski H, Vannan MA, et al. American society of echocardiography consensus statement on the clinical applications of ultrasonic contrast agents in echocardiography. *J Am Soc Echocardiogr*. 2008;**21**:1179–1201; quiz 1281.
16 Zaragoza-Macias E, Chen MA, Gill EA. Real time three-dimensional echocardiography evaluation of intracardiac masses. *Echocardiography*. 2012;**29**:207–219.
17 Araoz PA, Eklund HE, Welch TJ, et al. CT and MR imaging of primary cardiac malignancies. *Radiographics*. 1999;**19**:1421–1434.
18 Kaminaga T, Takeshita T, Kimura I. Role of magnetic resonance imaging for evaluation of tumors in the cardiac region. *Eur Radiol*. 2003;**13**(Suppl 6):L1–L10.
19 Grizzard JD, Ang GB. Magnetic resonance imaging of pericardial disease and cardiac masses. *Cardiol Clin*. 2007;**25**:111–140, vi.
20 Fussen S, De Boeck BW, Zellweger MJ, et al. Cardiovascular magnetic resonance imaging for diagnosis and clinical management of suspected cardiac masses and tumours. *Eur Heart J*. 2011;**32**:1551–1560.
21 Hoey ET, Mankad K, Puppala S, et al. MRI and CT appearances of cardiac tumours in adults. *Clin Radiol*. 2009;**64**:1214–1230.
22 Zee-Cheng CS, Gibbs HR, Johnson KP, et al. Giant vegetation due to *Staphylococcus aureus* endocarditis simulating left atrial myxoma. *Am Heart J*. 1986;**111**:414–417.
23 Auriti A, Chieffi M, Cianfrocca C, et al. Giant vegetation of the mitral valve simulating primary cardiac tumor. *Echocardiography*. 2004;**21**:183–185.
24 Kim MJ, Jung HO. Anatomic variants mimicking pathology on echocardiography: differential diagnosis. *J Cardiovasc Ultrasound*. 2013;**21**:103–112.
25 Rahbar K, Seifarth H, Schafers M, et al. Differentiation of malignant and benign cardiac tumors using 18F-FDG PET/CT. *J Nucl Med*. 2012;**53**:856–863.
26 Gowda RM, Khan IA. Clinical perspectives of primary cardiac lymphoma. *Angiology*. 2003;**54**(5):599–604.
27 Gowda RM, Khan IA, Nair CK, et al. Cardiac papillary fibroelastoma: a comprehensive analysis of 725 cases. *Am Heart J*. 2003;**146**(3):404–410.
28 Allard MFTG, Wilson JE, McManus BM. *Atlas of Heart Diseases*, Vol. III. St. Louis: Mosby; 1995:15.1–16.5.
29 Kuon E, Kreplin M, Weiss W, et al. The challenge presented by right atrial myxoma. *Herz*. 2004;**29**:702–709.
30 Burke AVR. *Tumors of the Heart and Great Vessels, Atlas of Tumor Pathology*. Washington, DC: Armed Forces Institute of Pathology; 1996.
31 Attum AA, Johnson GS, Masri Z, et al. Malignant clinical behavior of cardiac myxomas and "myxoid imitators". *Ann Thorac Surg*. 1987;**44**:217–222.
32 Pinede L, Duhaut P, Loire R. Clinical presentation of left atrial cardiac myxoma. A series of 112 consecutive cases. *Medicine (Baltimore)*. 2001;**80**:159–172.
33 D'Alfonso A, Catania S, Pierri MD, et al. Atrial myxoma: a 25-year single-institutional follow-up study. *J Cardiovasc Med (Hagerstown)*. 2008;**9**:178–181.

84 Primary germ cell tumors of the thorax

John D. Hainsworth, MD ■ Frank A. Greco, MD

Overview

Primary germ cell tumors (GCT) of the thorax are rare but potentially curable. Benign teratomas, which account for approximately 60–70% and usually appear in young adults, are curable with surgical resection. Malignant mediastinal GCT usually occur in young men and can be divided histologically into pure seminoma (about 52% of cases) and various nonseminoma histologies. Pure seminomas are highly sensitive to chemotherapy; treatment with three cycles of a standard cisplatin-based testicular GCT regimen is curative in more than 80%. Selected patients with small (<6 cm) localized seminomas have high cure rates with radiation therapy alone. Nonseminomatous mediastinal GCT are associated with Klinefelter syndrome (5–10% of cases) and are also associated with various acute leukemias. Optimal treatment includes four cycles of a standard cisplatin-based testicular GCT regimen, followed by resection of residual mediastinal masses. Since most patients require surgical resection following chemotherapy, use of a bleomycin-containing first-line regimen should be avoided if possible. The cure rate for these relatively poor prognosis GCT is approximately 45%.

Mediastinal germ cell tumors (GCT), although rare, are of particular interest because they usually affect young males and because curative therapy is now available for many patients.

Benign teratomas of the mediastinum

Although benign teratomas of the mediastinum (mature cystic teratomas or dermoid tumors) account for only 3–12% of mediastinal tumors, they comprise 60–70% of all mediastinal GCT.[1,2] These tumors have been described in patients with ages ranging from 7 months to 65 years; however, most occur in young adults, with an approximately equal incidence in males and females.[2,3]

Benign mediastinal teratomas have a histologic appearance identical to that of benign teratomas arising in the more common ovarian location. On histologic examination, mature tissue from ectodermal, mesodermal, and endodermal germ cell layers is typically present. Mature tissue that recapitulates the histology of any human organ can be found in these tumors. However, the ectodermal component (i.e., skin, sebaceous tissue, neural tissue) usually predominates.[3]

Approximately 95% of benign teratomas arise in the anterior mediastinum; the remainder arise in the posterior mediastinum.[2,3] These tumors are slow growing, and 50–60% of patients are asymptomatic at the time of diagnosis by routine chest radiography.[3] When symptoms are present, dyspnea and substernal chest pain are the most common. Spontaneous rupture of the teratoma into the lung, tracheobronchial tree, pleura, or pericardium can cause an acute onset of symptoms, but these events occur late in the disease course. Cough productive of hair or sebum, caused by rupture into the tracheobronchial tree, is pathognomonic of a benign mediastinal teratoma but occurs rarely. Superior vena cava syndrome is also rare and is a late manifestation. Serum levels of human chorionic gonadotropin (HCG) and alpha-fetoprotein are always normal in patients with benign teratoma.

Surgical excision is the treatment of choice for benign teratoma of the mediastinum. Surgical removal is sometimes difficult because of the large size and involvement of adjacent structures. Approximately 10–15% of patients require additional procedures (e.g., lobectomy, pericardiectomy) for complete tumor resection. Benign teratomas are resistant to radiation and cytotoxic drugs, and these modalities have no role in their treatment.

Tumor recurrence is rare following complete surgical resection.[2-4] Prolonged survival has been reported following subtotal resection of tumors involving vital mediastinal structures.

Malignant GCT

Etiology

Mediastinal GCT were initially thought to represent isolated metastases from an inapparent gonadal primary site. However, there is now abundant clinical evidence to substantiate the extragonadal origin of these tumors.[1,5]

Epidemiology

Malignant mediastinal GCT represent only 3–10% of tumors originating in the mediastinum and only 1–5% of all germ cell neoplasms.[6] The great majority of mediastinal malignant GCT occurs in males between 20 and 35 years of age. In the rare occurrences reported in females, mediastinal malignant GCT appear histologically and biologically identical to those occurring in males.

Patients with nonseminomatous extragonadal GCT have a subsequent increased risk of developing testicular cancer (approximately 10% at 10 years), strengthening the concept of a precursor abnormality in the germ cells of these patients.[7]

Histopathology

Mediastinal GCT appear to be histologically identical to GCT arising in the testis and contain the same range of histologic subtypes. However, the frequency of yolk sac tumor and teratocarcinoma is higher in mediastinal GCT, while embryonal carcinoma is less common. In a review of 229 malignant mediastinal GCT, pure seminoma was the most common histology, accounting for 52% of cases.[8] Nonseminomatous histologies included teratocarcinoma

(20%), yolk sac tumor (17%), choriocarcinoma (3.4%), embryonal carcinoma (2.6%), and mixed nonseminomatous tumors (5.2%).

Clinical characteristics

Malignant mediastinal GCT are usually symptomatic at the time of diagnosis. Most mediastinal GCT are large and cause symptoms by compressing or invading adjacent structures, including the lungs, pleura, pericardium, and chest wall. Pure seminomas are somewhat slower growing and have less potential for early metastasis than do tumors with nonseminomatous elements. Pure seminomas and tumors with nonseminomatous elements are therefore discussed separately, although substantial overlap exists in their clinical characteristics.

Seminoma

Seminomas grow relatively slowly and often become very large before causing symptoms. Tumors 20–30 cm in diameter can exist with minimal symptomatology. Approximately 20–30% of seminomas are detected by routine chest radiography while still asymptomatic.[9] The most common initial symptom is a sensation of pressure or dull retrosternal chest pain. Additional symptoms include exertional dyspnea, cough, dysphagia, and hoarseness. Superior vena cava syndrome develops in approximately 10% of patients. Systemic symptoms related to metastatic lesions are uncommon.

In order to be classified as a seminoma (or dysgerminoma in women), a mediastinal GCT must have no other histologic elements present. Tumors consisting of a mixture of seminoma and nonseminoma elements should be approached as nonseminomatous GCT.

At the time of diagnosis, only 30–40% of patients with mediastinal seminoma have localized disease; the remainder have one or more sites of distant metastases.[10] The regional lymph nodes (cervical, upper abdominal) are the most common metastatic sites; lung and bone are the most common visceral sites.[11]

Elevated serum levels of HCG are detected in up to 40% of mediastinal seminomas.[11] However, most of these are low-level elevations (2–10 ng/mL); levels of HCG exceeding 100 ng/mL are unusual and suggest the presence of nonseminomatous elements. The serum alpha-fetoprotein level is always normal in pure mediastinal seminoma, and any elevation of this tumor marker indicates the presence of nonseminomatous elements.

Nonseminomatous GCT

These rapidly growing neoplasms cause symptoms by compressing or invading local mediastinal structures, as seen in patients with mediastinal seminoma. Symptoms caused by metastases are much more common, since 85–95% of these patients have at least one metastatic site at the time of diagnosis.[12–14] Common metastatic sites include the lungs, pleura, lymph nodes (particularly supraclavicular and retroperitoneal), and liver. High levels of HCG are sometimes associated with gynecomastia. Constitutional symptoms are more common in these patients than in those with pure seminoma.

The serum tumor markers HCG and alpha-fetoprotein are usually abnormal in patients with mediastinal nonseminomatous GCT. Alpha-fetoprotein is elevated in 74–90% of patients, and elevation of HCG occurs in 30–38%.[15–17]

Approximately 5–10% of patients with mediastinal nonseminomatous GCT have Klinefelter syndrome.[18–20] The explanation for this association is unknown, but underlying germ cell defects related to the XXY chromosomal abnormality are likely to play a role.[21] The association of Klinefelter syndrome and mediastinal nonseminomatous GCT is specific; gonadal GCT show no association.[18,19]

Mediastinal nonseminomatous GCT are also associated with a variety of hematologic neoplasms including acute myeloid leukemia, acute nonlymphocytic leukemia, acute lymphocytic leukemia, erythroleukemia, acute megakaryocytic leukemia, myelodysplastic syndrome, and malignant histiocytosis.[22–28] Hematologic neoplasms in this setting are not treatment-related, but rather arise from clones of malignant lymphoblasts, myeloblasts, or progenitor cells contained within the GCT.[25–27]

Poorly differentiated neoplasm or carcinoma

In the large majority of patients, an extragonadal GCT can be diagnosed by histology, IHC stains, molecular testing, or elevated serum tumor markers. In rare instances, these features do not allow definitive exclusion of other nongerm cell cancers (e.g., lymphoma, thymic carcinoma, other metastatic carcinomas). In these rare patients, a trial of therapy for extragonadal GCT is appropriate.[29–31]

Pretreatment evaluation and staging

The diagnosis of a mediastinal GCT should be considered in all young males with a mediastinal mass. In addition to physical examination and routine laboratory studies, initial evaluation should include CT of the chest and abdomen and determination of serum levels of HCG and alpha-fetoprotein. Any symptoms suggestive of distant metastases should be appropriately evaluated with radiologic studies.

In patients with suspected mediastinal GCT, a histologic diagnosis should be made using the least invasive approach because rapid initiation of definitive systemic therapy is important. Because these neoplasms are poorly differentiated, specimens obtained by fine-needle aspiration biopsy are sometimes insufficient for a definitive diagnosis. In such patients, surgical biopsy via median sternotomy or limited thoracotomy is indicated. Attempts at complete surgical resection of these mediastinal neoplasms are not indicated because curative results with other treatment modalities are superior.

Treatment of seminoma

Pure mediastinal seminomas are curable in the large majority of patients, even when metastatic at the time of diagnosis. These tumors are highly sensitive to radiation therapy and to combination chemotherapy, and the selection of treatment, therefore, depends on tumor stage and size, as well as the anticipated short- and long-term toxicity of treatment.

Chemotherapy

Cisplatin-based combination chemotherapy, as used in patients with advanced testicular cancer, is highly effective treatment for mediastinal seminoma. Patients who have no extrapulmonary visceral metastases are classified as good risk GCTs by the International Germ Cell Consensus Classification,[32] and require first-line treatment with three cycles of combination chemotherapy. The most widely used combination regimen is BEP (bleomycin, etoposide, cisplatin).[33] For patients with underlying pulmonary disease, or those who have had previous radiation therapy, bleomycin should be avoided; four cycles of etoposide/cisplatin are preferred. Patients with mediastinal seminoma and metastases to extrapulmonary sites have intermediate risk, and therefore require four cycles of BEP. In this category, patients at risk for bleomycin toxicity should receive four courses of the etoposide, ifosfamide, cisplatin (VIP) regimen.[34]

Cure rates higher than 80% have been reported in all series of patients treated with modern cisplatin-based regimens.[10–12,14,33,35–39] In the largest retrospective analysis, 47 of 51 patients achieved complete remission, with subsequent relapses in only 14%.[11]

Radiation therapy

Radiation therapy is also potentially curative for patients with mediastinal seminoma.[4,10,40,41] When localized tumors are <6 cm in diameter, the cure rate is high with radiation therapy or chemotherapy, and the choice of treatment should be individualized. For young patients without contraindications, curative treatment with chemotherapy avoids potential long-term consequences of mediastinal irradiation (e.g., coronary artery disease, valvular disease, constrictive pericarditis, second cancers), and is, therefore, the treatment of choice.[42,43] Patients with tumors <6 cm in diameter who are poor candidates for chemotherapy should have radiation therapy (35–50 Gy) using a field that includes the mediastinum and bilateral supraclavicular fossae. Patients who relapse after radiation therapy have a high salvage rate with chemotherapy.[12,33]

Residual mass

Following completion of chemotherapy, CT scans frequently show a residual mediastinal mass. In most published experience, residual masses <3 cm contain only fibrosis and necrotic tumor, whereas residual masses >3 cm have up to a 30% chance of containing residual viable cancer.[44,45] Therefore, careful follow-up without resection is recommended for patients with residual masses <3 cm. Larger residual masses that are negative on positron emission tomography (PET) scan can also be followed.[46,47] Follow-up includes CT scans every 3 months during the first year, and every 6 months during the second year or until normal. This approach avoids a potentially difficult surgical procedure in most patients; intervention is necessary only if enlargement of masses is evident on serial scans.[44] Resection is recommended for residual masses >3 cm. Patients with residual seminoma in the resected mass should have additional salvage chemotherapy or, in selected instances, radiation therapy to the mediastinum.

Treatment of nonseminomatous GCT

Most patients with mediastinal nonseminomatous GCT currently receive multimodality therapy, utilizing combination chemotherapy followed by surgical resection of residual mediastinal masses.

Chemotherapy

The use of cisplatin-based chemotherapy developed for the treatment of advanced nonseminomatous testicular neoplasms has improved the previously dismal outlook in patients with mediastinal nonseminomatous GCT. However, cure rates remain between 40% and 50%, lower than those achieved in the treatment of testicular cancer.[12–17,35,36,39,48–51] Comparable long-term survival rates have been reported when testicular GCT with far advanced, bulky metastases are treated with similar cisplatin-based regimens.[32] However, inherent biologic differences between mediastinal and testicular GCT also play a role in determining the relatively low cure rate.[52]

All patients with mediastinal nonseminomatous GCT have poor risk tumors; therefore, first-line treatment should include four courses of a standard cisplatin-based testicular GCT regimen. If possible, bleomycin should be avoided by using the VIP or paclitaxel, ifosfamide, cisplatin (TIP) regimen, since postchemotherapy surgical resection of residual intrathoracic masses is frequently required, and operative risks are increased after bleomycin.[53] Following the completion of therapy, patients should be restaged with serum tumor markers and CT scans of the chest and abdomen.

Subsequent management is determined by the response to initial chemotherapy (Figure 1). Approximately 20% of patients have normal CT scans and tumor marker levels[17]; these patients require no further therapy. Standard follow-up of these patients includes monthly physical examination, chest radiography, and serum tumor marker determinations during the first year and similar evaluations every 2 months during the second year following therapy. However, about 20% of these patients will subsequently relapse, with almost all relapses occurring during the first 2 years after completion of therapy.

Residual mass

Most patients have residual radiographic abnormalities in the mediastinum after completion of chemotherapy.[16] In these patients, surgical resection of residual masses should be performed if technically feasible. Persistent elevation of serum tumor markers is not a contraindication to surgical resection in this setting.[54,55] Residual GCT is found in the resected specimen in a substantial proportion of patients (25–66%).[56–59] A few patients have residual cancer of various nongerm cell histologies (e.g., sarcoma, adenocarcinoma, neuroendocrine carcinoma).[58] The remainder of patients have either benign teratoma, necrosis, or fibrosis without active carcinoma.

Complete surgical resection is curative for a substantial proportion of patients. Patients with no malignant tumor remaining (i.e., necrotic tumor, fibrosis, and/or benign teratoma only) have a low risk of subsequent relapse (approximately 20%).[56,58] Patients with resection of residual GCT have a high risk of future relapse; however, surgical resection is curative in 20–30%.[57,58] In these patients, two additional courses of chemotherapy postoperatively may reduce the recurrence rate. Most patients with residual nongerm cell histologies do poorly even with complete resection, although occasional long-term survivors have been reported.[58] Further systemic treatment following resection in these patients has been ineffective.

Recurrent/progressive disease

The prognosis is poor for patients in whom complete surgical resection is not feasible, as well as in those who relapse after surgical resection. Standard second-line cisplatin-based regimens and high-dose chemotherapy regimens with autologous bone marrow transplant are curative in 20–50% of patients with recurrent testicular cancer but are effective in only 11% of patients with mediastinal nonseminomatous GCT.[54,55,60] Two doses of high dose chemotherapy with autologous peripheral stem cell transplantation appear more effective, improving the rate of durable complete response to 25% in patients with mediastinal GCT.[61,62]

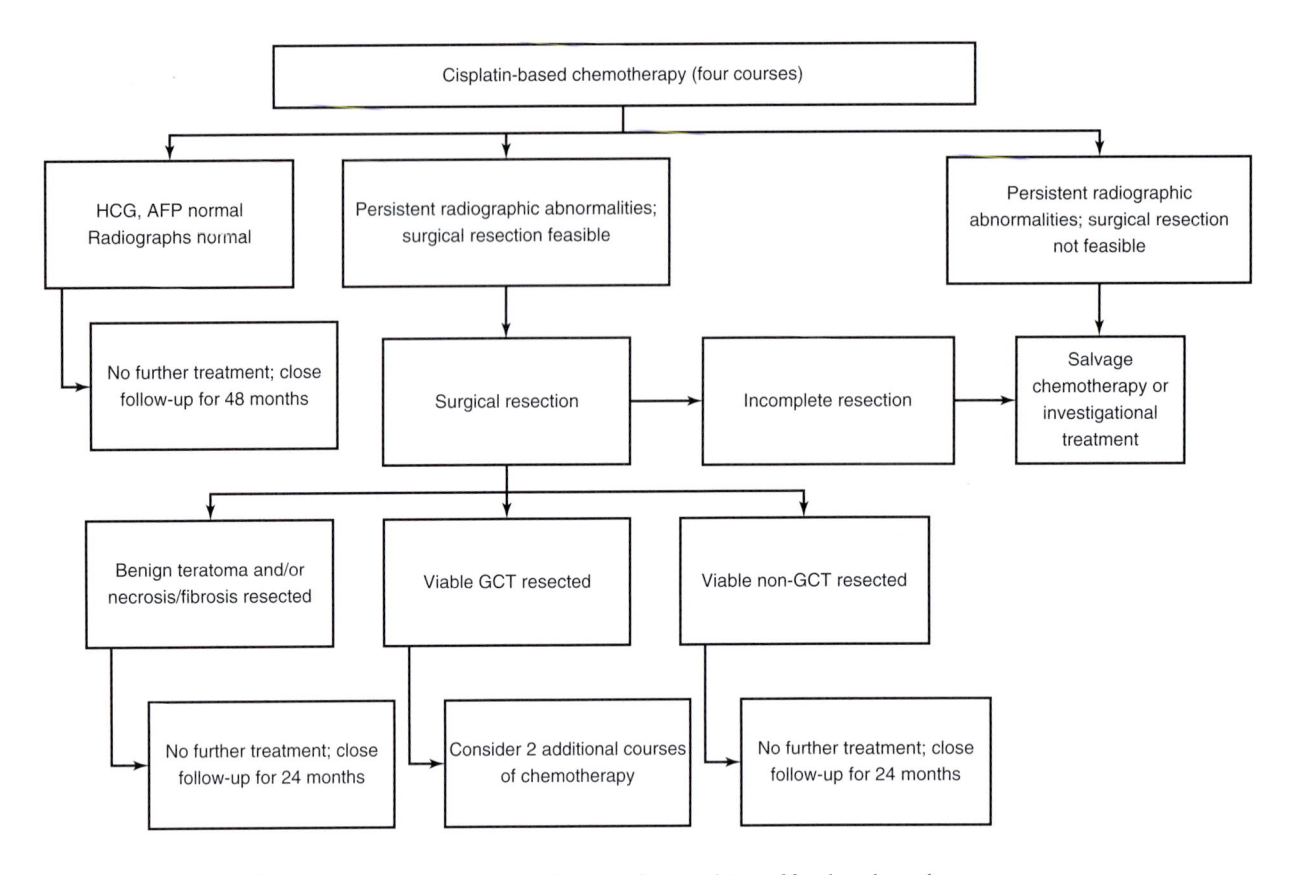

Figure 1 Management of mediastinal nonseminomatous germ cell tumors after completion of first-line chemotherapy.

Key references

The complete reference list can be found on Vital Source version of this title, see inside front cover.

2 Wychulis AR, Payne WS, Clagett OT, et al. Surgical treatment of mediastinal tumors: a 40 year experience. *J Thorac Cardiovasc Surg.* 1971;**62**(3):379–392.

3 Lewis BD, Hurt RD, Payne WS, et al. Benign teratomas of the mediastinum. *J Thorac Crdiovasc Surg.* 1983;**86**(5):727–731.

7 Hartmann JT, Fossa SD, Nichols CR, et al. Incidence of metachronous testicular cancer in patients with extragonadal germ cell tumors. *J Natl Cancer Inst.* 2001;**93**(22):1733–1738.

8 Moran CA, Suster S. Primary germ cell tumors of the mediastinum: I. Analysis of 322 cases with special emphasis on teratomatous lesions and a proposal for histopathologic classification and clinical staging. *Cancer.* 1997;**80**(4):681–690.

16 Ganjoo KN, Rieger KM, Kesler KA, et al. Results of modern therapy for patients with mediastinal nonseminomatous germ cell tumors. *Cancer.* 2000;**88**(5):1051–1056.

17 Bokemeyer C, Nichols CR, Droz JP, et al. Extragonadal germ cell tumors of the mediastinum and retroperitoneum: results from an international analysis. *J Clin Oncol.* 2002;**20**(7):1864–1873.

20 Nichols CR, Heerema NA, Palmer C, et al. Klinefelter's syndrome associated with mediastinal germ cell neoplasms. *J Clin Oncol.* 1987;**5**(8):1290–1294.

23 Nichols CR, Roth BJ, Heerema N, et al. Hematologic neoplasia associated with primary mediastinal germ-cell tumors. *N Engl J Med.* 1990;**322**(20):1425–1429.

28 Hartmann JT, Nichols CR, Droz JP, et al. Hematologic disorders associated with primary mediastinal nonseminomatous germ cell tumors. *J Natl Cancer Inst.* 2000;**92**(1):54–61.

38 Mencel PJ, Motzer RJ, Mazumdar M, et al. Advanced seminoma: treatment results, survival, and prognostic factors in 142 patients. *J Clin Oncol.* 1994;**12**(1):120–126.

39 Gerl A, Clemm C, Lamerz R, et al. Cisplatin-based chemotherapy of primary extragonadal germ cell tumors. A single institution experience. *Cancer.* 1996;**77**(3):526–532.

44 Schultz SM, Einhorn LH, Conces DJ Jr, et al. Management of postchemotherapy residual mass in patients with advanced seminoma: Indiana University experience. *J Clin Oncol.* 1989;**7**(10):1497–1503.

45 Puc HS, Heelan R, Mazumdar M, et al. Management of residual mass in advanced seminoma: results and recommendations from the Memorial Sloan-Kettering Cancer Center. *J Clin Oncol.* 1996;**14**(2):454–460.

47 Hinz S, Schrader M, Kempkensteffen C, et al. The role of positron emission tomography in the evaluation of residual masses after chemotherapy for advanced stage seminoma. *J Urol.* 2008;**179**(3):936–940.

50 Hidalgo M, Paz-Ares L, Rivera F, et al. Mediastinal non-seminomatous germ cell tumours (MNSGCT) treated with cisplatin-based combination chemotherapy. *Ann Oncol.* 1997;**8**(6):555–559.

51 Fizazi K, Culine S, Droz JP, et al. Primary mediastinal nonseminomatous germ cell tumors: results of modern therapy including cisplatin-based chemotherapy. *J Clin Oncol.* 1998;**16**(2):725–732.

53 Kesler KA, Rieger KM, Hammoud ZT, et al. A 25-year single institution experience with surgery for primary mediastinal nonseminomatous germ cell tuors. *Ann Thorac Surg.* 2008;**85**:371–378.

55 Hartmann JT, Einhorn L, Nichols CR, et al. Second-line chemotherapy in patients with relapsed extragonadal nonseminomatous germ cell tumors: results of an international multicenter analysis. *J Clin Oncol.* 2001;**19**(6):1641–1648.

56 Kesler KA, Rieger KM, Ganjoo KN, et al. Primary mediastinal nonseminomatous germ cell tumors: the influence of postchemotherapy pathology on long-term survival after surgery. *J Thorac Cardiovasc Surg.* 1999;**118**(4):692–700.

58 Schneider BP, Kesler KA, Brooks JA, et al. Outcome of patients with residual germ cell or non-germ cell malignancy after resection of primary mediastinal nonseminomatous germ cell cancer. *J Clin Oncol.* 2004;**22**(7):1195–1200.

59 Radaideh SM, Cook VC, Kesler KA, et al. Outcome following resection for patients with primary mediastinal nonseminomatous germ-cell tumors and rising serum tumor markers post-chemotherapy. *Ann Oncol.* 2010;**21**(4):804–807.

60 Broun ER, Nichols CR, Einhorn LH, GJK T. Salvage therapy with high-dose chemotherapy and autologous bone marrow support in the treatment of primary nonseminomatous mediastinal germ cell tumors. *Cancer.* 1991;**68**(7):1513–1515.

61 Feldman DR, Sheinfeld J, Motzer RJ. TI-CE high-dose chemotherapy for patients with previously treated germ cell tumor: results and prognostic factor analysis. *J Clin Oncol.* 2010;**28**:1706–1713.

62 Adra N, Abonour R, Althouse SK, et al. High-dose chemotherapy and autologous peripheral-blood stem-cell transplantation for relapsed metastatic germ cell tumors: the Indiana University experience. *J Clin Oncol.* 2016;**35**:1096–1102.

85 Neoplasms of the esophagus

Max W. Sung, MD ■ Virginia R. Litle, MD

> **Overview**
>
> Esophageal cancer, the sixth leading cause of cancer deaths worldwide, has benefitted from advances in therapeutic interventions, including noninvasive endoscopic mucosal resection for early-stage disease, and minimally invasive robotic-assisted surgical techniques for resection. For intermediate stage disease, multi-modality approaches with the addition of neoadjuvant chemoradiation to resection are the standard of care. For advanced disease, the addition of hormonal, targeted, and immunomodulatory approaches have extended the benefits from systemic chemotherapy. The increased incidence in esophagogastric adenocarcinoma compared esophageal squamous cell carcinoma, particularly in North America and in Europe, in the past three decades has led to changes in classification and therapeutic modalities for esophageal neoplasms.

Historical perspectives

Esophageal cancer was recognized as early as the twelfth century, with pathologic descriptions reported in the sixteenth and seventeenth centuries.[1] Initial attempts to treat the tumor included resection of a cervical esophageal cancer in 1877 and an intrathoracic cancer in 1913.[2,3] Surgical resection became the mainstay of therapy beginning in the 1940s. Radiotherapy was initially used in the 1920s, but it was not until the development of megavoltage techniques in the 1950s that this modality was used with any frequency. Active systemic therapeutic agents were first identified in the 1960s and have been incorporated into the treatment of advanced as well as intermediate-stage tumors.

Anatomy and histology

The esophagus is a muscular organ that extends from the cricopharyngeus muscle at its cephalad margin to the esophagogastric junction (EGJ). It is divided into regions on the basis of both anatomy and the proclivity for certain neoplasms to develop in specific regions (Figure 1). The cervical esophagus extends from the cricopharyngeus muscle to the thoracic inlet (15–18 cm from incisors). The upper third of the thoracic esophagus extends from the thoracic inlet to the tracheal bifurcation, just below the level of the aortic arch (18–24 cm). The middle thoracic esophagus extends from the tracheal bifurcation to a point midway between the carina and the EGJ (24–32 cm). The lower thoracic esophagus extends from this midway point to the EGJ (32–40 cm). Tumors of the EGJ and gastric cardia have often been included in discussions of esophageal cancer because of their pathophysiologic similarities to adenocarcinomas of the distal esophagus.[4] Classifications of EGJ tumors have developed that define the different types of tumors according to the epicenter of the mass (i.e., type I, >1 cm above EGJ; type II, 1 cm above to 2 cm below EGJ; type III, >2–5 cm below EGJ).[5]

The muscle tissues of the esophagus are arranged in an outer longitudinal layer and an inner circular layer. The proximal one-third to one-half of the muscularis propria is derived from the bronchial arches, making it principally skeletal (striated) muscle and giving it the potential to develop rhabdomyosarcomas (Table 1). The remainder of the esophageal musculature comprises smooth muscle, as does the rest of the foregut, in which leiomyomas or leiomyosarcomas may occur. Fibrous, fatty, and connective tissues interspersed in the wall of the esophagus may also give rise to sarcomas.

The esophagus is lined over most of its length with squamous epithelium, which can give rise to squamous cell carcinoma (SCC) and is the most common neoplasm of the esophagus in most of the world. These cancers occur most often in the cervical esophagus and in the upper and middle thoracic esophagus. Carcinosarcomas and spindle cell carcinomas, which are subtypes of squamous cell cancer, infrequently occur in these regions. The distal 2–3 cm of the esophagus and the cardia are lined by columnar epithelium, in which adenocarcinomas may occur.[5] The development of intestinal metaplasia, known as Barrett's esophagus, more proximally because of gastroesophageal reflux and other factors allows the development of adenocarcinomas in the middle and upper thoracic esophagus in isolated instances. Other cellular elements in the mucosa, submucosal glands, and muscularis propria may give rise to unusual neoplasms, such as small cell cancer, malignant melanoma, granular cell tumors, mucoepidermoid carcinoma, and adenoid cystic carcinoma.[6,7] The histologic types of benign and malignant tumors of the esophagus are shown in Table 1.

Etiology

In most of the world, dietary and nutritional factors are the most common etiologic agents and are associated with the development of predominantly SCCs. Among the most frequently cited carcinogens are nitrosamines, which have been found to be in high concentrations in foods in endemic areas of esophageal cancer in northern China.[8] Contamination of food by fungi that reduce nitrate to nitrite may further aggravate this situation. Mechanical factors that have been cited include drinking beverages at excessively high temperatures and consumption of foods containing silica or other substances, such as crushed seeds, that directly irritate the esophagus.[8,9] Deficiencies of folic acid, vitamins A and C, and riboflavin, molybdenum, and selenium also have been implicated in the development of esophageal neoplasms.[10–12] Higher intake of fruits and vegetables, on the other hand, has been reported in a meta-analysis of observational studies to be associated with a reduced risk of esophageal SCC.[13]

In the western hemisphere, social factors figure more prominently in the development of esophageal cancer. Heavy

---

Holland-Frei Cancer Medicine, Tenth Edition. Edited by Robert C. Bast, John C. Byrd, Carlo M. Croce, Ernest Hawk, Fadlo R. Khuri, Raphael E. Pollock, Apostolia M. Tsimberidou, Christopher G. Willett, and Cheryl L. Willman.
© 2023 John Wiley & Sons, Inc. Published 2023 by John Wiley & Sons, Inc.

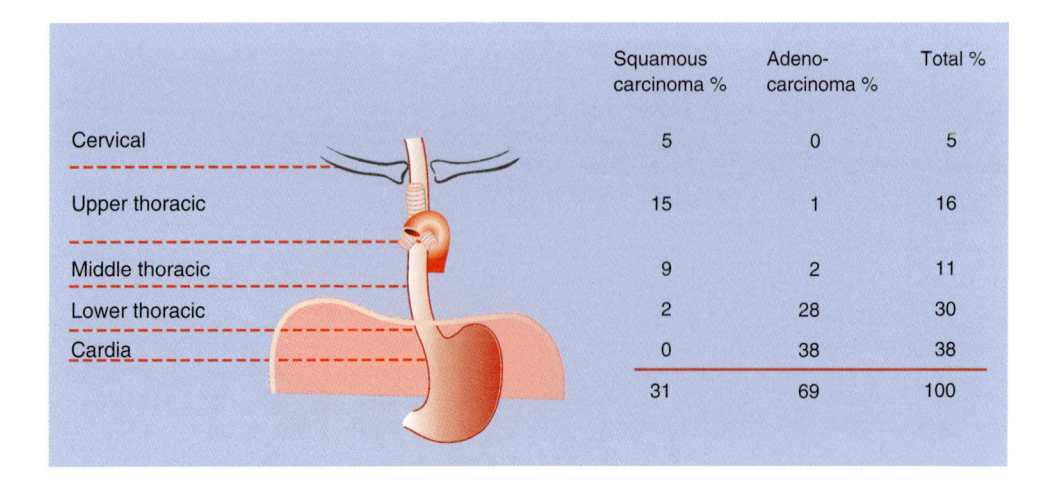

	Squamous carcinoma %	Adeno-carcinoma %	Total %
Cervical	5	0	5
Upper thoracic	15	1	16
Middle thoracic	9	2	11
Lower thoracic	2	28	30
Cardia	0	38	38
	31	69	100

Figure 1 The distribution of malignant neoplasms of the esophagus according to cell type and site of occurrence.

Table 1 Neoplasms of the esophagus.

Epithelial
- Squamous cell carcinoma
  - Spindle cell carcinoma
  - Carcinosarcoma
- Adenocarcinoma
- Adenosquamous carcinoma
- Mucoepidermoid carcinoma
- Adenoid cystic carcinoma
- Small cell carcinoma

Nonepithelial
- Leiomyoma
- Leiomyosarcoma
- Malignant melanoma
- Rhabdomyoma
- Rhabdomyosarcoma
- Granular cell tumors
- Malignant lymphoma

alcohol consumption increases the risk of cancer 10–25 times, depending on the concentration of alcohol in the beverage.[14] Cigarette smoking has been linked to the development of both squamous cell cancers and adenocarcinomas.[15] The combined exposure to low levels of tobacco and alcohol increases the risk of esophageal cancer by a factor of 10–20, whereas the synergistic effect of exposure to high levels of both alcohol and tobacco increases the risk by a factor of over 100.[16] Chronic esophageal injury due to gastroesophageal reflux has also been shown to be a risk factor for the development of adenocarcinoma, with severe, long-standing reflux symptoms increasing the risk of cancer by a factor of 40.[17] Chronic gastroesophageal reflux is believed to be etiologically related to the development of Barrett's esophagus, which occurs primarily in white males and is associated with a 40-fold increase in the risk of adenocarcinoma of the esophagus.[18] A relationship between reflux and the development of squamous cell cancers has also been suggested in patients who consume a diet high in linoleic acid.[19] The lifetime risk of squamous cell cancer of the esophagus is 5–10% in patients with esophageal achalasia, a 15-fold increase in incidence that is likely due to chronic irritation from retained food.[20–22]

Race and gender are associated with varying incidences of cancer of the esophagus in the western hemisphere. Men are more commonly affected than are women, blacks develop squamous cell cancers more often than do whites, and white males develop adenocarcinomas more often than do females or individuals of other race groups.[22] However, none of these increased frequencies has yet been linked to genetic factors, and most have been explained by variations in socioeconomic status and the attendant social habits described earlier. Mutations in the RHBDF2 gene, inherited in an autosomal dominant pattern, have been associated with a form of palmoplantar keratoderma (tylosisA) with a lifetime risk of SCC of the esophagus.[23] An autosomal recessive mutation in the BLM gene (Bloom syndrome) has been associated with heritable higher risk of SCC of the esophagus, as well as with acute leukemias and lymphomas. A number of genetic alterations are associated with neoplasms of the esophagus, including allelic losses at chromosomes 3p, 5q, 9p, 9q, 13q, 17p, 17q, and 18q. Abnormalities of TP53, Rb, cyclin D1, and c-myc have also been associated with esophageal cancer development.[24]

Infectious agents, including human papillomavirus (HPV), have been implicated in the development of neoplasms of the esophagus. Transforming proteins from high-risk HPV subtypes 16, 18 cause loss of function of the tumor suppressor genes TP53 and Rb, resulting in abnormal proliferative states.[25] HPV has been documented in up to 50% of patients with squamous cell cancers of the esophagus and appears to be more common in areas in which esophageal cancer is endemic.[26] These findings have not been universally reproducible, however.[27] A systematic review and meta-analysis of 66 case-control studies suggest an association between HPV infection and esophageal SCC.[28] There is significant variation and lack of consistency between studies; the International Agency for Research on Cancer (IARC) has concluded the epidemiologic evidence of the association is inconclusive.[29]

Epidemiology

The most common esophageal neoplasm worldwide is SCC (90%); in the United States and Europe, the incidence of adenocarcinoma has been rising and has surpassed SCC (Figure 2). The incidence of esophageal cancer varies more worldwide than any other cancer. In the United States, the incidence of esophageal cancer is approximately seven cases per 100,000 people, whereas in high-risk areas in China, Iran, and Russia, it can be more than 100 per 100,000 people.[31] In rural Linxian, China, esophageal cancer is the leading cause of death.[32,33] These geographical variations imply a strong role for local environmental carcinogens in esophageal carcinogenesis. The long-term survival rate for patients with esophageal cancer, regardless of histology, is less than 10%, which is due, in large

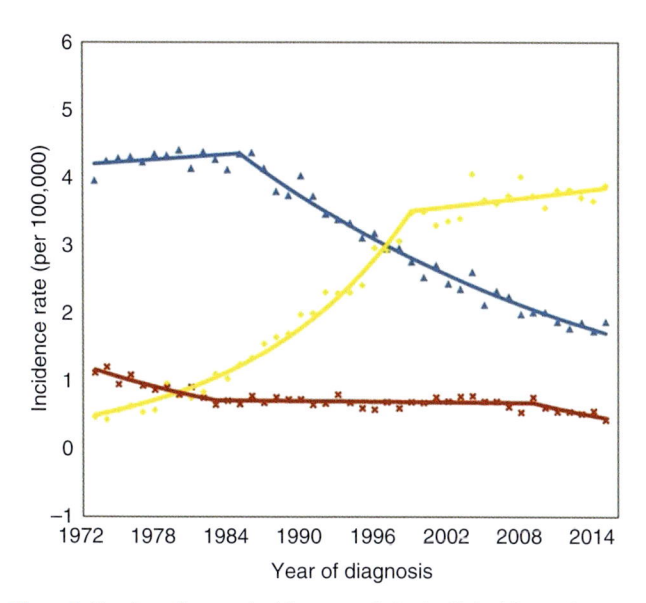

Figure 2 Esophageal cancer incidence trends in the United States. Source: From He et al.[30]

part, to the advanced stage at which these cancers are detected. Worldwide, the incidence and mortality for esophageal cancer are estimated for 2018 to be 572,034 and 508,585, respectively.[34] For the United States, incidence and mortality for 2020 (excluding EGJ tumors) were estimated at 18,440 and 16,170, respectively.[35] The age-adjusted mortality rate from esophageal cancer in the United States has increased overall by 3% between 1975 and 2017.[36]

Besides geographical differences, there are other important differences that have been described in the Western hemisphere. Esophageal carcinoma is more common in men than women regardless of the histologic subtype, and squamous cell cancers tend to occur more frequently in blacks than in whites. Since 1970, the incidence of SCC of the esophagus worldwide has continued to decrease, but in recent years has increased in women in some countries (Japan, Netherlands, New Zealand, Norway, Switzerland).[37] In the United States, incidence of esophageal SCC has decreased from 4.3 per 100,000 in 1984 to 2.0 per 100,000 in 2015; in the subgroup of black men and women, from 18 per 100,000 to 4 per 100,000 in the same time period.[38] Adenocarcinoma of the esophagus, on the other hand, has continued to increase in the United States, from 1.8 per 100,000 in 1975 to 2.3 per 100,000 in 1997; since then the increase has leveled off to 2.7 per 100,000 in 2010 (Figure 2).[30,39–41] The reasons for these changes in the United States and the Western hemisphere are not clear but may include increased Barrett's esophagus, gastroesophageal reflux, obesity, and over-the-counter medications as well as changing habits in smoking and alcohol use.[16] In other areas of the world (outside Europe and North America), SCC of the esophagus continues to predominate and adenocarcinoma has not increased.

Patients usually present because of complaints of dysphagia, which requires either the involvement of the entire circumference of the esophagus by the neoplasm or the growth of a large, polypoid obstructing mass. Dysphagia first develops in response to dense solid foods and progresses to result in difficulties with soft foods and then liquids. Accompanying vomiting and regurgitation are common. Symptoms of heartburn or gastroesophageal reflux (40%) are often associated and occur more frequently in patients with adenocarcinoma.[42] The most common symptom in the absence of dysphagia is pain (25% of cases).[42] It may be related to swallowing (odynophagia) or local extension of the tumor into adjacent structures such as the vertebral bodies, pleura, or mediastinum. In some instances, it may be due to bony metastases from systemic spread. Weight loss is noted in more than 70% of patients and is due to the inability to swallow or to systemic manifestations of the disease.[42] Patients with weight loss have a significantly worse prognosis in many series.[43,44]

The histology of the tumor depends in large part on its location. Adenocarcinoma is located predominantly in the lower esophagus, whereas SCC predominates in the cervical, upper, and middle esophagus (Figure 1). Unfortunately, because of the distensible nature of the esophagus, these symptoms often do not occur until the tumors are quite large and no longer localized to the esophagus.

In contrast to patients who present because of symptoms of dysphagia, a smaller subset of earlier stage adenocarcinoma patients are increasingly being identified in North America and Europe with endoscopic abnormalities noted during endoscopic surveillance for gastroesophageal reflux symptoms or Barrett's esophagus. These patients tend to present with smaller, earlier-stage tumors that are more likely to be localized and amenable to treatment. In addition, in some areas of China where squamous cell cancer is endemic, routine cytologic screening is performed, and if results are diagnostic or suspicious, follow-up endoscopy is performed. These mass screening efforts have led to early diagnosis in many areas of China, with 5-year survivals of more than 90%.[33] The low incidence of esophageal cancer in most areas of the world, however, makes this type of mass screening impractical and cost-ineffective from a public health standpoint.

Treatment overview

Patients who present with suspected esophageal cancer, either because of the abovementioned symptoms or mass screening efforts, initially require pathologic confirmation of malignancy (see section titled "Diagnosis"). Once the pathologic diagnosis has been obtained, patients are assessed for therapy by determining the clinical stage (see section titled "Presentation and staging evaluation") of the tumor and the physiologic status of the patient (see section titled "Pretreatment assessment"). With this information, an informed decision about treatment can be made that optimizes the chance to cure or palliate the disease while minimizing the treatment-related morbidity (see section titled "Therapy") (Figure 3).

Diagnosis

Symptomatic patients or patients in whom an esophageal mass is diagnosed by screening require endoscopy to enable biopsy for histologic examination and/or brushing for cytologic examination. The overall accuracy of histologic diagnosis of esophageal cancer using flexible endoscopy with biopsy is about 80%.[45,46] Endoscopically directed cytologic brushings have a diagnostic accuracy in excess of 90%. Combining these techniques yields an overall diagnostic accuracy of 98%.[45] In selected patients who have symptoms or findings on physical examination suggestive of metastatic disease, biopsy of the suspected metastatic site provides both a tissue diagnosis and a confirmation of stage.

Pretreatment assessment

In addition to a careful history and physical examination, the overall assessment of a patient with esophageal cancer focuses on specific concerns. Factors that are associated with treatment-related morbidity and mortality include patient age, continued alcohol or tobacco use disorder, >10% body weight loss,

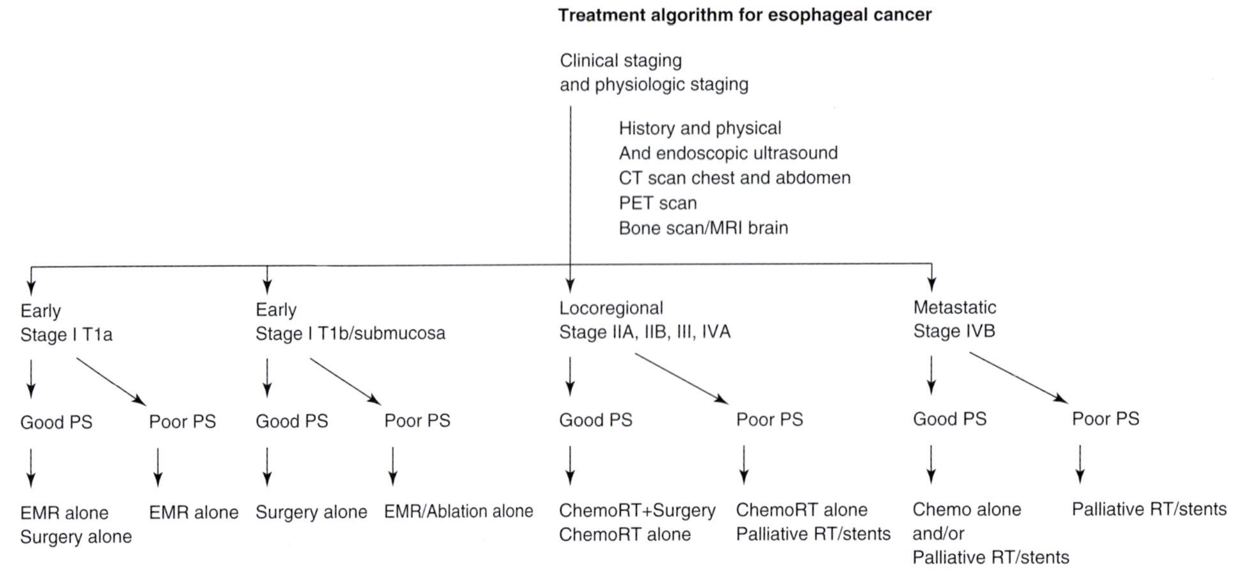

Treatment algorithm for esophageal cancer

Clinical staging and physiologic staging
- History and physical
- And endoscopic ultrasound
- CT scan chest and abdomen
- PET scan
- Bone scan/MRI brain

- Early Stage I T1a
  - Good PS → EMR alone / Surgery alone
  - Poor PS → EMR alone
- Early Stage I T1b/submucosa
  - Good PS → Surgery alone
  - Poor PS → EMR/Ablation alone
- Locoregional Stage IIA, IIB, III, IVA
  - Good PS → ChemoRT+Surgery / ChemoRT alone
  - Poor PS → ChemoRT alone / Palliative RT/stents
- Metastatic Stage IVB
  - Good PS → Chemo alone and/or Palliative RT/stents
  - Poor PS → Palliative RT/stents

Figure 3 Current treatment recommendations for esophageal cancer based on performance status and clinical stage. *Abbreviations:* Chemo, chemotherapy; CT, computed tomography; MRI, magnetic resonance imaging; PET, positron emission tomography; RT, radiotherapy.

malnutritional status, performance status, cardiopulmonary or hepatic dysfunction. Specific preoperative risk factors have been identified for esophageal resection and are, therefore, included in the physiologic assessment. Pulmonary complications are predicted by age, active smoking, and decreased pulmonary function tests.[47] Operative mortality is predicted by age, history of smoking, performance status, and the frequency with which the operation is performed in an institution.[47,48] Any symptoms of cardiac disease necessitate careful evaluation with electrocardiography (ECG), echocardiography, stress tests, and coronary arteriography as indicated. Patients with significant coronary artery disease are at increased risk of morbidity and mortality. Cardiac intervention may be warranted prior to surgical treatment.

Over the past 20 years, Enhanced Recovery After Surgery (ERAS) programs have been more widely applied to surgical patients perioperatively and those undergoing esophagectomy are no exception. Society guidelines have been developed and the primary goals are to improve complication rates and length of stay as well as reduce narcotic use and healthcare costs.[49] In addition to ERAS protocols, prehabilitation programs can improve the performance status of esophageal cancer patients many of whom have received potentially debilitating neoadjuvant therapy, so they may tolerate the physiologic insults of an esophagectomy.[50]

Presentation and staging evaluation

Assessment of stage permits medical practitioners to discuss the status of individual patients with accuracy, allows informed recommendations about therapy, and gives patients and their families necessary information about prognosis. The typical assessment for most patients often includes barium swallow, upper gastrointestinal endoscopy, endoscopic ultrasonography (EUS), and positron emission tomography-computed tomography (PET-CT) with dedicated chest and abdominal imaging. Other examinations are selected on the basis of specific findings in individual patients, such as neurologic symptoms including headaches [magnetic resonance imaging (MRI) of brain] or supraclavicular nodes (neck ultrasonography-guided fine-needle aspiration). Staging techniques allow patients to be accurately placed into groups in which risk can be assessed as well as the optimum type of therapy selected.

Presentation

Contrast radiography
A barium swallow is often the initial diagnostic examination obtained in patients with dysphagia. It allows confirmation of mucosal irregularity and serves as guide for subsequent endoscopy. It also allows evaluation of the esophagus and stomach distal to an area of stenosis, which cannot always be assessed by endoscopy if tight strictures exist.

Endoscopy
Upper gastrointestinal endoscopy with biopsy allows a pathologic diagnosis to be obtained in the majority of patients. The gross appearance of the tumor can be categorized as advanced or superficial, and the extent of the tumor including gastric involvement for distal tumors can be accurately determined.

Staging

Endoscopic mucosal resection
Over the past 20 years, endoscopic mucosal resection (EMR) has become not only the standard modality for staging superficial mucosal cancers but also the intervention of choice for treating these early cancers.[51] EMR essentially involves excising the lesion endoscopically so the pathologist may determine the depth of the tumor and whether it is restricted to the mucosal layer and thus a T1a lesion with a 0–7% likelihood of nodal metastases.[52-54] For T1b tumors, nodal involvement increases significantly, ranging from 21% to 50%[54]; thus, surgical resection is indicated. If the muscularis propria is involved, the suction technique EMR cannot be completed, and thus the tumor is staged as at least a T2. Additional staging information of tumor grade is provided with endoscopic biopsy or mucosal resection.

Endoscopic ultrasonography

EUS improves the staging accuracy of primary tumors and regional and some nonregional lymph nodes. It has become an essential tool to help identify patients with early-stage carcinoma who may not need multimodality treatment (Figure 3); however, if the patient has undergone an EMR for staging then EUS cannot provide tumor stage classification EUS depicts the normal esophagus as five alternating hyperechoic and hypoechoic layers representing the mucosa and lamina propria, muscularis mucosa, submucosa, muscularis propria, and adventitia. Depth of tumor invasion is determined by assessing the level to which the tumor extends. EUS is also useful for assessing whether there is involvement of the aorta, but airway invasion is not accurately determined because of interference of the ultrasound signal with the intratracheal air column. The accuracy of EUS determination of primary tumor stage is related to the pathologic tumor stage, being more accurate for more advanced stages of disease, with an overall accuracy of about 80%.[55-57] EUS is substantially less accurate in staging primary tumors after chemoradiotherapy is administered, primarily because of over-staging. The technique is not able to distinguish between treatment-induced fibrosis and residual tumor, leading to a mean overall accuracy in this setting of 45%.[58,59]

In assessing lymph nodes with EUS, three criteria are used: size, border characteristics, and internal architecture. Lymph nodes that are enlarged, have a well-defined external border, and are characterized by relatively uniform, hypoechoic internal architecture are more likely to be malignant. Using these criteria, the overall accuracy of lymph node staging by EUS is about 75%.[56,60] After chemoradiotherapy, the accuracy of EUS for staging lymph nodes decreases to just over 50%.[58] Development of fine-needle aspiration techniques has allowed pathologic confirmation of enlarged lymph nodes in both regional and nonregional sites.[57-61]

CT of the chest and abdomen

CT has become a standard technique for esophageal cancer staging since its inception in the late 1970s because it has allowed better identification of patients with metastatic (M1) and locally invasive tumors (T4). CT is not very accurate for determining the depth of the primary tumor (T) status, but it is helpful in identifying patients who might have direct invasion of local structures, such as the aorta, vertebral body, or major airways (T4b), either of which precludes surgical intervention.[55] Aortic invasion is suspected when more than 25% of the aortic circumference is effaced by an esophageal cancer.

CT does not accurately determine lymph node (N) status since normal lymph nodes often vary in size according to their location in the mediastinum and abdomen, and a single size limit for nodes is not possible to establish. In addition, lymph nodes involved by metastatic spread are often not enlarged.[62-65] The sensitivity for CT detection of involved lymph nodes is, therefore, poor (30–60%), and the overall accuracy of nodal detection by CT is less than 60%.[66-68]

CT is most useful for detecting distant often unsuspected metastatic (M) disease. The most common sites for metastatic spread, aside from nonregional lymph nodes, are (in decreasing order of frequency) the liver, lung, peritoneum, adrenal gland, bone, and kidney. CT of the thorax and abdomen evaluates almost all these regions. Accuracy of the CT detection of liver metastases is in excess of 90%.[62,67,69,70]

Bronchoscopy

Flexible bronchoscopy should be performed for all patients who are candidates for surgical therapy and whose tumors are adjacent to the trachea or mainstem bronchi, which typically are the mid-esophageal SCCs. This permits direct assessment of tumor invasion into the airway lumen or submucosa, which would be a contra-indication to surgical resection.

Magnetic resonance imaging

As a method for routine staging of esophageal neoplasms, MRI offers no advantages compared with CT and is therefore seldom used since it is a more difficult and expensive test to obtain. Both techniques have similar specificities, sensitivities, and overall accuracy for determining resectability with regard to direct invasion of the aorta and airway.[63,64,67] Neither test provides much useful information about regional or metastatic lymph nodes, and MRI offers no improvements over CT in evaluating the liver for metastatic disease. Whether advances in MRI technology will offer improved staging capabilities remains to be seen.

Positron emission tomography

PET scanning to detect involved lymph nodes and sites of metastatic disease through increased metabolism with 18F-fluorodeoxyglucose was introduced as an investigational staging technique for esophageal cancer in the mid-1990s. With the advent of PET-CT more than 15 years ago,[71-73] this modality has replaced PET alone at most institutions. PET-CT can identify second primaries more often than CT alone but it also provides three-dimensional imaging.[70]

PET-CT is most useful in helping identify patients with unsuspected metastatic disease. Given the possibility of false-positive results on PET, confirmatory biopsies of suspected advanced disease are still indicated. The PET scan often serves as a guide to help identify suspected areas of metastatic disease for confirmatory biopsy. Another potential role for PET may be in determining response to chemotherapy and radiation therapy although false positives induced by chemotherapy and radiation-induced inflammation remain a problem.[71,74,75]

Bone scintigraphy

Bone scans have been used for decades for staging patients with esophageal neoplasms, however, PET-CT scan has essentially replaced bone scans in the work-up of esophageal cancer. In patients without bone pain or other evidence for metastatic disease, the overall likelihood of identifying skeletal metastases is less than 5%.[76]

Neck ultrasonography

Cervical and supraclavicular lymph nodes are affected by metastatic spread in up to 30% of patients with neoplasms of the thoracic esophagus, and most are not detectable on physical examination. The use of routine ultrasound examination of the neck in patients without palpable lymph nodes yields unsuspected nodal metastases in over 10% of patients.[77] The overall accuracy of cervical and supraclavicular nodal assessment with ultrasonography is about 90%.[78,79] The addition of routine needle aspiration under ultrasound guidance for cytology may improve the yield of this potentially valuable technique.[79] At the present time, however, this is not a commonly used screening technique and is reserved for cases where nodes are palpable to confirm metastatic disease.

Minimally invasive surgical staging

Laparoscopy has been used since the early 1980s, and thoracoscopy has been used since the early 1990s in an effort to improve staging of esophageal neoplasms. Video-assisted thoracoscopic surgery (VATS) staging was studied in a Cancer and Leukemia Group B (CALGB) study in 1995 and was found to be feasible and 88% accurate.[80,81] With the current standard and accurate staging modalities of PET-CT and EUS, surgical staging is not routinely done except in conjunction with placement of a laparoscopic jejunostomy tube for nutritional support prior to chemoradiation therapy.

Biologic staging

A variety of biologic markers have been investigated for their utility in estimating prognosis in patients with esophageal neoplasms. These include growth factors [epidermal growth factor (EGF), transforming growth factor (TGF)-β, platelet-derived growth factor (PDGF)], oncogenes (*c-myc, int-2, hst-1, cyclin D, EGFR, HER-2/neu, h-ras*), tumor suppressor genes (*Rb, TP53, p73, APC, MCC, p27*), the cell adhesion molecule E-cadherin, the oncodevelopmental marker carcinoembyronic antigen (CEA), and deoxyribonucleic acid (DNA) content and ploidy.[82–84] To date, biomarker staging is not used routinely for patients with potentially curable disease.

TNM (tumor, node, metastasis) staging system

These pretreatment staging evaluations allow patients to be clinically staged by a cTNM staging system that can help determine the optimum therapy (Figure 3). The current staging system for esophageal cancer includes epithelial tumors of the cervical, thoracic, and intraabdominal esophagus, as well as of the EGJ extending to not more than 2 cm into gastric cardia (Table 2).[85,86] Tumors are staged according to clinical findings from noninvasive tests (cTNM) and pathologic findings resulting from any invasive

Table 2 TNM staging system for esophageal neoplasms.

Primary tumor (T)	
TX	Primary tumor cannot be assessed
T0	No evidence of primary tumor
Tis	High-grade dysplasia
T1	Tumor invades lamina propria, muscularis mucosae, or submucosa
T1a	Tumor invades lamina propria of muscularis mucosae
T1b	Tumor invades submucosa
T2	Tumor invades muscularis propria
T3	Tumor invades adventitia
T4	Tumor invades adjacent structures
T4a	Resectable cancer invades adjacent structures such as pleura, pericardium, diaphragm
T4b	Unresectable cancer invades adjacent structures such as aorta, vertebral body, trachea
Regional lymph nodes (N)	
Any periesophageal lymph node from cervical nodes to celiac nodes	
NX	Regional lymph nodes cannot be assessed
N0	No regional lymph node metastases
N1	1–2 positive regional lymph nodes
N2	3–6 positive regional lymph nodes
N3	≥7 positive regional lymph nodes
Distant metastasis (M)	
MX	Distant metastasis cannot be assessed
M0	No distant metastasis
M1	Distant metastasis
Additions of nonanatomic cancer characteristics	
Histopathologic cell type	
Adenocarcinoma	
Squamous-cell carcinoma	
Histologic grade	
GX	Grade cannot be assessed
G1	Well differentiated
G2	Moderately differentiated
G3	Poorly differentiated
G4	Undifferentiated
Cancer location	
Upper thoracic	>20–25 cm from incisors
Middle thoracic	25–30 cm from incisors
Lower thoracic	>30–40 cm from incisors
Esophagogastric junction	Includes cancers whose epicenter is in the distal thoracic esophagus, esophagogastric junction, or within the proximal 2 cm of the stomach (cardia) that extend into the esophagogastric junction or distal thoracic esophagus (Siewert II). These stomach cancers are stage grouped similarly to adenocarcinoma of the esophagus
Pathologic (p) staging squamous cell carcinoma esophagus	
Pathologic (p) staging adenocarcinoma esophagus	
Clinical (c) staging squamous cell carcinoma esophagus	
Clinical (c) staging adenocarcinoma esophagus	
Postneoadjuvant pathologic (yp) staging squamous cell carcinoma/ adenocarcinoma esophagus	

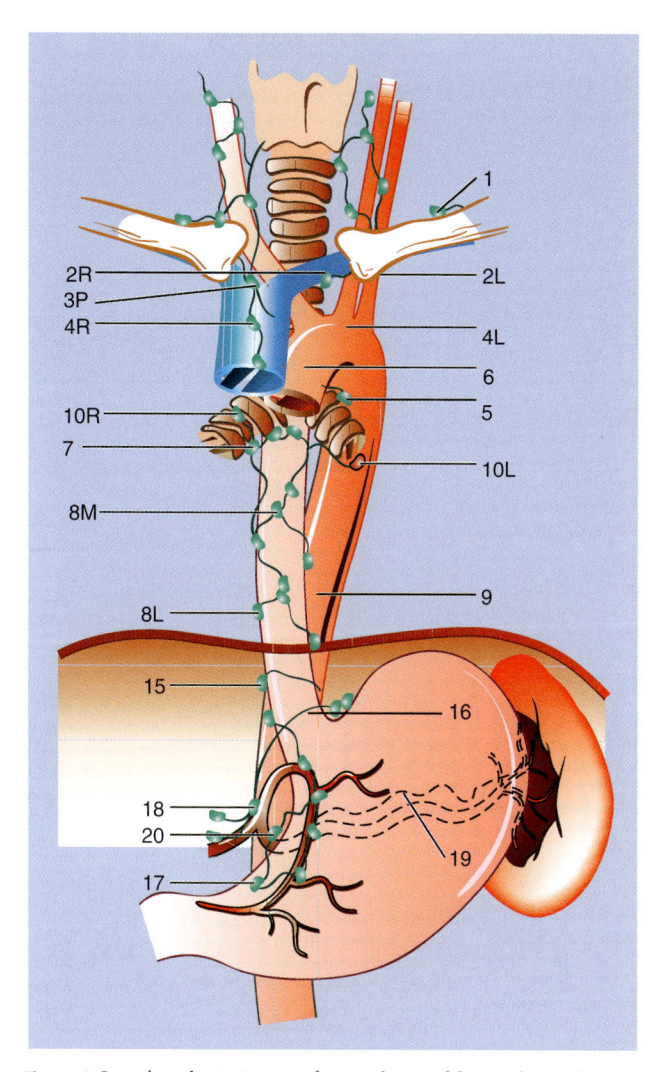

Figure 4 Lymph node staging map for neoplasms of the esophagus. Source: From Ferguson.[87]

staging procedures (pTNM, ypTNM if postneoadjuvant therapy). Lymph node locations are specified during biopsy and resection because their location determines whether they are considered regional nodes or nonregional metastatic nodal disease (Figure 4). The prognosis of patients with esophageal cancer is determined by the depth of penetration of the primary tumor (transmural vs nontransmural), whether there is lymph node involvement, the relative number of lymph nodes involved, and whether distant metastases are present.[85–95] Nonanatomic classifications have been added, including histopathologic cell type (adenocarcinoma, SCC), histologic grade (G1-4), and cancer location. The long-term survival in patients with esophageal neoplasms correlates well with the pathologic stage and histopathologic cell type (Figure 5).[88,94] Postneoadjuvant pathologic staging has been added to take into account different survival profiles. The ability of the clinical cTNM staging system to accurately predict the pTNM/ypTNM status has improved with time as the use of endoscopic ultrasound, CT of the chest and abdomen, and PET scan has increased.[95]

Therapy

Standard curative treatment options for esophageal cancer include surgical resection, external beam radiotherapy, chemotherapy, or combinations of two or three of these options. The selection of appropriate therapy is often challenging because few comparisons of these options have been performed in prospective, randomized fashion. In addition, these trials have often been performed over a long time period with an inadequate number of patients during which significant changes in histology and types of treatment have occurred (i.e., different radiation equipment, dosages and fields, and different surgical techniques and chemotherapy agents). Clinical staging techniques have also evolved over time, leading to stage migration and poor correlation with pathologic stage, especially from studies prior to CT scan, endoscopic ultrasound, and PET. These problems make comparisons between different trials or treatment arms difficult. Treatment strategies have therefore evolved over time based on regional experiences and biases. In an effort, to guide current treatment strategies, we have included an esophageal treatment algorithm that incorporates different treatment strategies based on the physiologic status and clinical stage of the patient (Figure 3). This algorithm reflects the treatment biases of the authors and is meant only to give some guidance in an otherwise confusing therapeutic arena (Figure 3).

In esophageal cancer, local control of the disease, as well as cure, are the primary objectives of therapy because of the debilitating effects of dysphagia caused by progressive tumor growth and esophageal obstruction. Treatment of superficial Tis and T1aN0 tumors are treated with EMR as outlined for staging above, while T1bN0 is treated with upfront esophagectomy. cT2N0 is a controversial area given the ~50% probability of occult nodal involvement and patients may be offered upfront surgical resection or neoadjuvant therapy after a multidisciplinary discussion and review of tumor characteristics including grade and lymphovascular invasion. Patients with at least clinical T3 and/or N1 tumors and good performance status are offered multimodality therapy with perioperative chemotherapy and resection or neoadjuvant chemoradiation followed by restaging, then esophagectomy. For patients who are initially recognized to be in advanced (metastatic) stages of disease, chemotherapy with or without palliative radiotherapy has been the mainstay of treatment (Table 3). The development of endoesophageal stents, cryotherapy, and occasionally photodynamic therapy (PDT) where available has provided additional locoregional palliation and has limited the need for palliative surgical bypass even in patients with tracheoesophageal fistulas (Figure 3).

Surgery

Esophagectomy remains the mainstay of treatment for locally or regionally advanced neoplasms of the esophagus. As previously mentioned the major paradigm shift in the 15 years has been management of superficial (clinical T1aN0) esophageal carcinomas in which EMR is used to stage and treat these intramucosal lesions. Numerous groups have concluded that EMR and ablation of the preneoplastic field of Barrett's esophagus is the standard of care for treatment of early cancers with eradication and 5-year survival rates reaching 80–90%.[106–109] Although mortality rates after esophagectomy have improved over the past 10–15 years with the increasing use of less invasive approaches and the evolving area of prehabilitation, the morbidity and 90-day mortality rates still can reach 59% and 4.5%, respectively.[49,50]

Surgery, however, remains an integral element in multimodality therapy for regionally advanced cancers because patients who undergo preoperative (neoadjuvant) therapy have a 75% incidence of residual local disease amenable to resection, although some

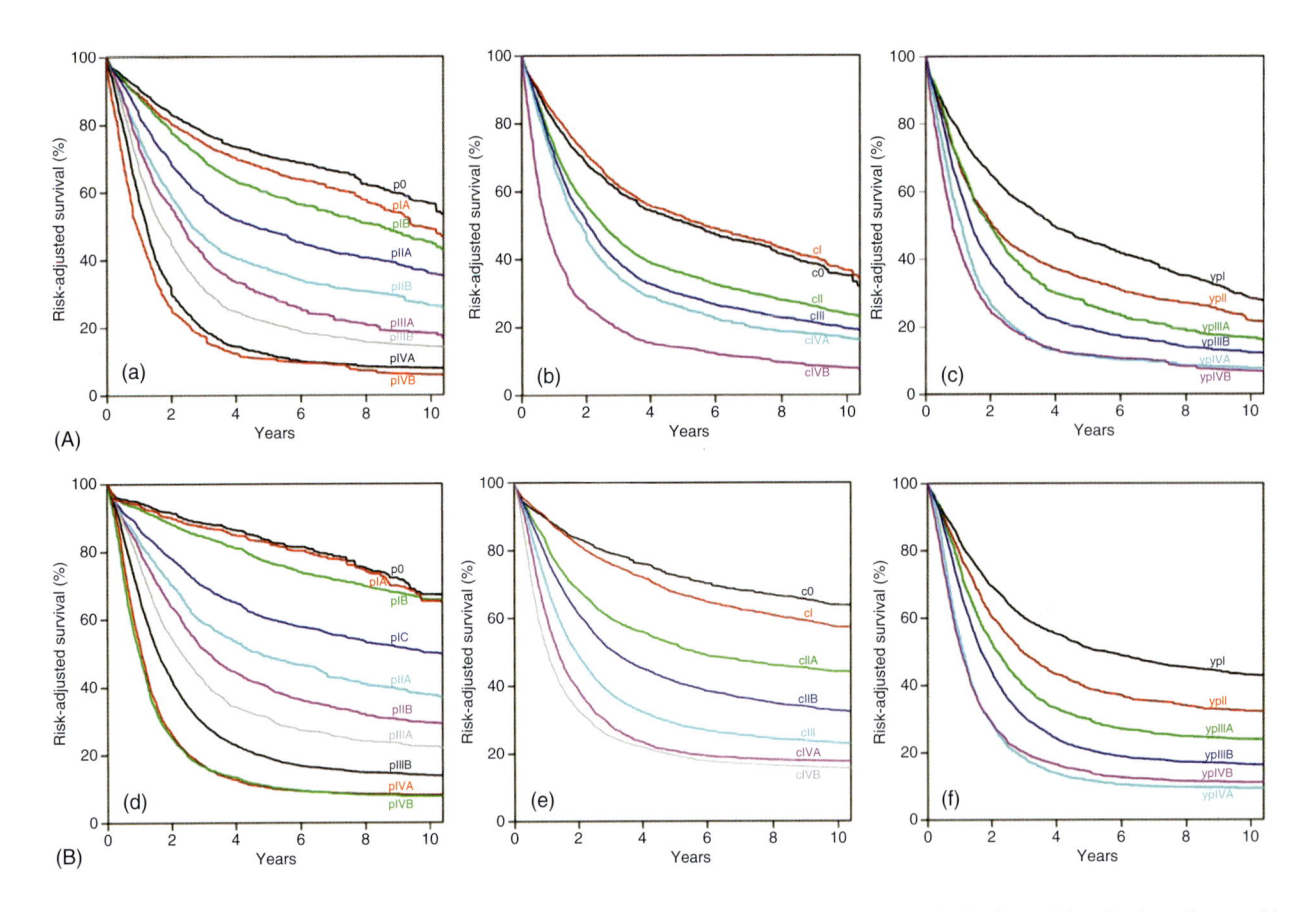

Figure 5 (A) Risk-adjusted survival for squamous cell carcinoma according to the AJCC Cancer Staging Manual, 8th edition. (B) Risk-adjusted survival for adenocarcinoma according to the AJCC Cancer Staging Manual, 8th edition. Source: Rice et al.[88]

Table 3 Results of randomized trials of definitive chemoradiotherapy for locoregionally advanced esophageal cancer.

Author	Year	Treatment	Technique	Histology	Patients	Median survival	p-Value
Chemo/RT versus RT alone							
Roussel et al.[96]	1989	Methotrexate + 56 Gy	C/RT	S	77	9 mo	NS
		56 Gy			73	8 mo	
Araujo et al.[97]	1991	5-FU, bleomycin, mito + 50 Gy	C/RT	S	28	18 mo	NS
		50 Gy			31	16 mo	
Hatlevoll et al.[98]	1992	Cisplatin, bleomycin + 53 Gy	C/RT	S	46	6 mo	NS
		53 Gy			51	6 mo	
Slabber et al.[99]	1998	Cisplatin, 5-FU + 40 Gy	C/RT	S	34	6 mo	NS
		40 Gy			36	5 mo	
Smith et al.[100]	1998	Mitomycin, 5-FU + 40 Gy	C/RT	S > A	60	15 mo	0.04
		40 Gy			59	9 mo	
Cooper et al.[101]	1999	Cisplatin, 5-FU + 50 Gy	C/RT	S > A	61	13 mo	0.01
		64 Gy			62	9 m0	
Minsky et al.[102]	2002	Cisplatin, 5FU + 50.4 Gy	C/RT	S > A	109	13.0 mo	NS
		Cisplatin, 5-FU + 64.8 Gy			109	18.1 mo	
Chemo/RT/surgery versus chemo/RT alone							
Stahl et al.[103]	2005	Cis, 5-FU, Etop.~Cis, Etop. + 40 Gy ~ Surgery	C~C/RT~S	S	86	16.4 mo	NS
		Cis, 5-FU, Etop.~Cis, Etop. + 65 Gy	C~C/RT		86	14.9 mo	
Bedenne et al.[104]	2007	Cis, 5-FU, + 46 Gy ~ Surgery	C/RT~S	S > A	129	17.7 mo	NS
		Cis, 5-FU, 66 Gy	CRT		130	19.3 mo	
Chemo/RT (5-FU) versus chemo/RT (no 5-FU)							
Ajani et al.[105]	2008	Cis, 5-FU, Paclitaxel ~ 5-FU, Paclitaxel + 50.4 Gy	C~RT	S > A	41	28.2 mo	NS
		Cis + Paclitaxel ~ Cis + Paclitaxel + 50.4 Gy	C~RT		43	14.9 mo	

oncologists argue that surgery should be reserved only for patients who relapse with locoregional disease. This idea of a salvage esophagectomy reserving resection only for those with recurrent disease after definitive chemoradiation therapy has been gaining traction, in particular, for SCCs given the higher response rates to chemoradiation as well as the often frailty of the patients. Still associated with higher perioperative mortality rates outside of experienced centers, salvage esophagectomy for adenocarcinomas continues to evolve as a component of the treatment algorithm as nonoperative therapies are refined as well.[110,111]

Approaches to resection

Surgical approaches to resection include a transthoracic operation, mobilization of the esophagus via a transhiatal route, and thoracoscopic (VATS)/laparoscopic resection (Table 4; Figure 6). The use of a surgical robot to assist with the esophagectomy should be considered an adjunct to the minimally invasive approaches with VATS and/or laparoscopy. All approaches are deemed acceptable by current NCCN guidelines (https://www.nccn.org/professionals/physician_gls/pdf/esophageal.pdf Accessed 6/28/2020).

Transthoracic approaches provide the ability to perform a more complete dissection of the primary tumor and lymph nodes than is possible using a transhiatal approach; however, the pulmonary complication rate, in particular, is higher when a thoracic dissection is involved. In the mid-1990s, as laparoscopic approaches were advancing for benign disease, a minimally invasive approach was introduced for oncologic procedures as well. The laparoscopic transhiatal approach was reported as a technically feasible procedure for nine patients in the late 1990s.[112] This was followed by advances in total thoracoscopic and laparoscopic approaches first as being feasible, then as associated with shorter length of stay and mortality rates less than 2%.[113] Additional studies demonstrated morbidity rates dropping from 60% to 44% with a significant reduction in pulmonary complications as compared with the open approaches.[114] The minimally invasive esophagectomy (MIE) has evolved from a three-hole modified McKeown to the Ivor Lewis approach with an intrathoracic component in particular for the distal esophageal and gastroesophageal junction carcinomas. The

Table 4 Operative approaches to resection for esophageal cancer.

Transthoracic
- Ivor Lewis (laparotomy, right thoracotomy, high intrathoracic anastomosis)
- McKeown modification of Ivor Lewis (cervical anastomosis)
- Left thoracotomy with intrathoracic anastomosis
- Left thoracotomy with cervical anastomosis
- Thoracoabdominal incision

Transhiatal

Minimally invasive
- Thoracoscopically assisted
- Laparoscopically assisted
- Thoracoscopic/laparoscopic

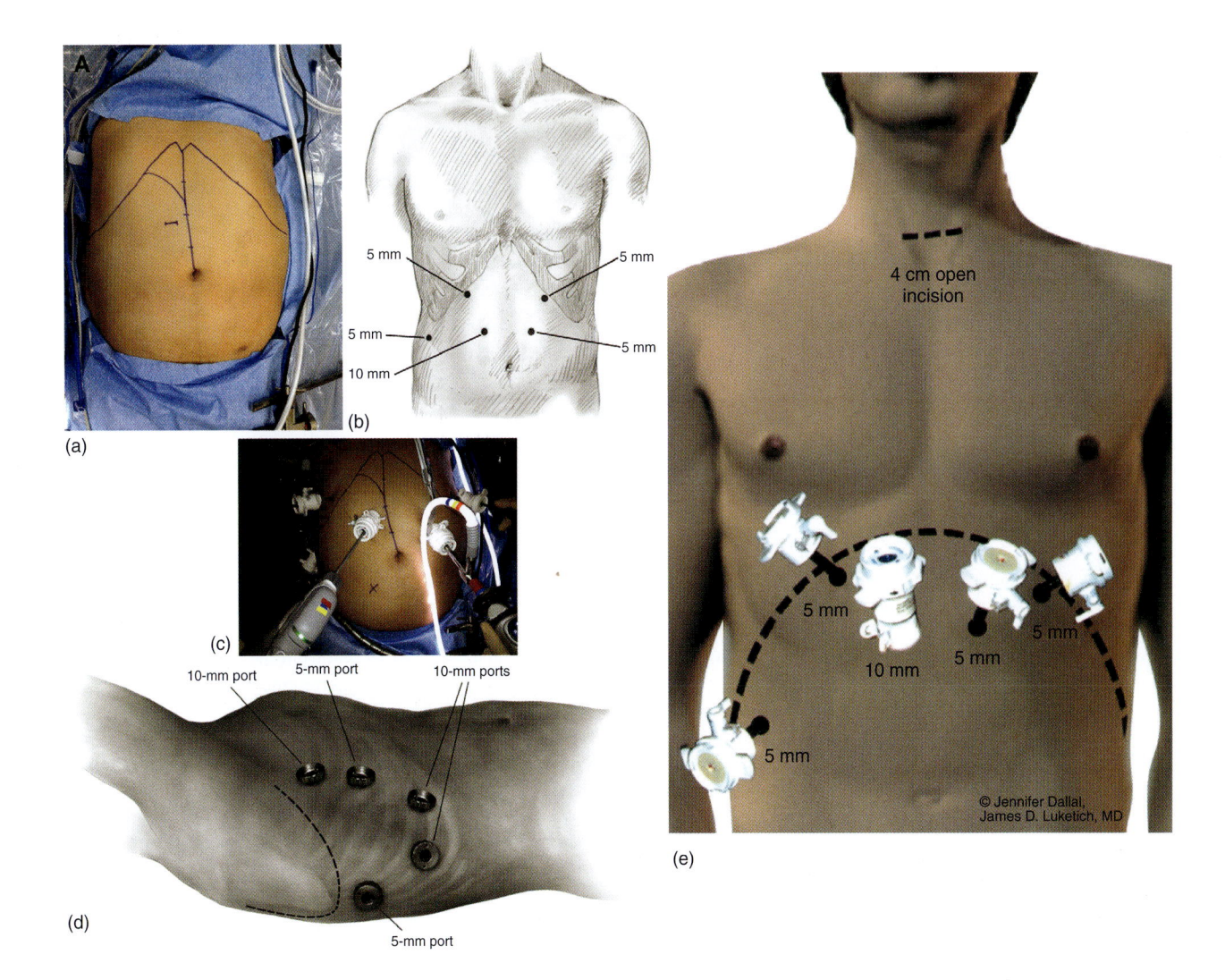

Figure 6 Approaches for esophagectomy. (a) Right thoracotomy and laparotomy with intrathoracic (Ivor Lewis operation) or cervical anastomosis (McKeown modification of Ivor Lewis esophagectomy). (b) Left thoracotomy, accessing the abdomen through a peripheral incision in the diaphragm, with intrathoracic or cervical anastomosis. (c) Transhiatal esophagectomy with cervical anastomosis. (d) Thoracoscopic esophagectomy: Port placement (MIE Ivor-Lewis). (e) Laparoscopic esophagectomy: Port placement.

benefit of this evolution was avoidance of recurrent laryngeal nerve injury and reduction in anastomotic leak rates.

The question of oncologic soundness with an MIE has been substantiated with longer follow-up. With the goal of retrieving more than 15 lymph nodes to adequately stage a patient with the current AJCC staging system, the median number of nodes is not diminished by a minimally invasive approach.[114,115] Three-year survival rates after MIE now approach 60% in experienced hands as reported in the intergroup study of 95 patients with locoregional recurrence rates as low as 7%,[116] and in a meta-analysis, open and minimally invasive esophagectomies had similar overall survival rates for cancer.[117]

The selection of an operative approach is dependent, in part, on tumor location and surgeon preference. Squamous cell cancers are most often located in the middle and upper thoracic esophagus and are approached with open or minimally invasive abdominal and transthoracic approaches with subsequent cervical anastomosis. In contrast, adenocarcinomas, which most often arise in the distal esophagus or cardia, are easily amenable to transthoracic and transhiatal approaches. Squamous cell cancers are multifocal in nearly 20% of patients, and near-total esophagectomy is recommended to minimize the risk of performing an incomplete resection.[118] This usually necessitates a cervical anastomosis for reconstruction. In contrast, adenocarcinomas usually are not multifocal but tend to spread submucosally. When negative proximal and distal margins are obtained on frozen section at the time of operation, the extent of the esophageal resection is theoretically satisfactory.

Results from 44 published reports of transthoracic or transhiatal esophagectomy for cancer demonstrate a higher incidence of anastomotic complications in the latter group, but otherwise no important differences in operative morbidity or mortality and similar 5-year survival rates.[119–124] Currently, the choice of the open versus minimally invasive approach to esophageal resection depends largely on the training, experience, and personal preference of the surgeon. The robot-assisted thoracoscopic esophagectomy (RATE or RAMIE) is also performed by a few surgical groups with varying reports of improved length of stay, overall morbidity, and number of nodes harvested compared with other approaches.[125,126] This approach continues to increase in popularity albeit at centers with dedicated robotic teams.

Effects of preoperative therapy
The use of preoperative therapy before surgery has the potential of increasing perioperative morbidity and mortality. One prospective randomized study reported that septic complications, respiratory complications, and operative mortality were higher in patients who underwent preoperative chemotherapy compared with surgery alone. However, several other studies assessing neoadjuvant chemotherapy or chemoradiotherapy have shown no important differences in postoperative complications or operative mortality.[43,127–131] The complexity of esophageal surgery supports that the procedure be performed at a high-volume referral center to minimize operative morbidity and mortality.[48] This morbidity and mortality may be even further increased when preoperative therapy is used. At less experienced centers, the morbidity and mortality of the procedure may be greater than the potential benefit, especially when considering the low likelihood of cure in locoregionally advanced patients.

Surgery for cervical esophageal cancer
Neoplasms of the cervical esophagus pose special problems with regard to surgical therapy. To obtain adequate surgical margins in tumors that extend to the cricopharyngeus muscle or invade the proximal trachea, it is necessary to include a laryngectomy as part of the resection, which adds substantial long-term morbidity to what is often a palliative not curative procedure. As a result, a higher percentage of patients with cervical esophageal cancer are treated nonsurgically than is the case for patients with cancers in other locations. Resection could provide good palliation for dysphagia but does not substantially influence long-term survival and the morbidity has led most people to recommend chemoradiation in this subset of patients.[132–135]

Reconstruction after esophagectomy
Reestablishing alimentary tract continuity after esophageal resection in a manner that permits ingestion of a normal diet is an important component of surgery for esophageal cancer. Options for reconstruction include using the stomach as a substitute or interposing a segment of colon or jejunum between the proximal esophageal remnant and the stomach (or duodenum after total gastrectomy). The use of the stomach for reconstruction is by far the most common technique because the stomach has the most reliable blood supply among any of the reconstructive options and because only a single anastomosis is required, compared with the three anastomoses necessary for bowel interposition. Cervical anastomoses are favored by some surgeons because they decrease the incidence of acid reflux into the esophageal remnant and because anastomotic leaks are usually easily managed by simple cervical drainage. The disadvantages of cervical anastomoses are a higher incidence of recurrent laryngeal nerve injury and more frequent anastomotic leaks. Whether the additional tumor-free proximal margin provided by a cervical anastomosis offers a survival advantage has not been proven.[136] Use of the posterior mediastinum (esophageal bed) for reconstruction optimizes emptying of the reconstructive organ but may predispose to tumor infiltration if a complete resection is not performed.[137]

Radiation therapy
Radiotherapy has been used for decades in the management of neoplasms of the esophagus and as with surgery targets the locoregional tumor rather than the systemic disease. The primary roles of radiotherapy, as with surgery, are as a potentially curative single modality for localized disease and as a palliative therapy for advanced tumors. Results of both uses have been disappointing because of a lack of complete response of the primary tumor and the development of radiation-induced strictures that limit its palliative benefits.

Treatment is planned to uniformly irradiate gross tumor and margins suspected of harboring microscopic disease, while minimizing injury to adjacent normal tissues, such as the lung, heart, and spinal cord. Regional nodal basins are usually included, typically cervical and supraclavicular nodes for cervical cancers, supraclavicular and subcarinal lymph nodes for upper thoracic cancers, and celiac axis nodes for lower thoracic and cardiac cancers. Initial treatment is to opposed, anterior-posterior and posterior-anterior fields using high-energy (6–24 MV) photons. In patients receiving potentially curative high-dose therapy, the final treatments are delivered at an oblique angle to minimize the total dose to the spinal cord. Daily treatments of 1.8–2 Gy to a total of 60–70 Gy were formerly used for curative intent, although this has been modified since recent trials have demonstrated equal efficacy and less toxicity with the lower dose (50.4 Gy).[102] Palliative doses tend to be even lower to further reduce this morbidity (30–40 Gy).

The use of radiation therapy as a single modality for esophageal cancer is sometimes indicated as a potentially curative therapy in patients who are unable to tolerate (or who refuse) resection or combined definitive chemoradiotherapy. Radiation therapy alone achieves 5-year survival rates of 0–20% in patients without distant metastatic disease, with the majority of survival rates being less than 10%. Although low, these survival rates may be biased by patient selection since good performance status patients are usually treated with surgery while radiation is often reserved for the poor performance status group. Treatment of unresectable but localized esophageal cancer with radiotherapy yields results similar to those reported for potentially resectable cancers, with survival rates at 5 years of less than 10%.[96–101,138,139] One small randomized study has demonstrated increased survival with surgery alone versus radiation therapy alone, although the authors focused more on endpoints of quality of life.[140]

In an effort to obtain better local control of disease, radiotherapy has been used both preoperatively and postoperatively as an adjunct to resection (Table 5).[141–143,145,149] The interval between completion of radiotherapy and resection is typically 3–5 weeks (1 week/10 Gy), which is felt to minimize perioperative complications from bleeding and radiation-induced fibrosis. In the proper setting, postoperative complication and mortality rates are not increased by the administration of preoperative radiotherapy, although this may be contingent on performing the surgical procedure in a high-volume center.[48] Most randomized, controlled studies have not demonstrated a survival advantage compared with surgery alone although these studies were often performed with outdated radiation therapy techniques.[132–136] Meta-analysis of the combined data from all randomized studies that have been published do not demonstrate improved survival with preoperative radiotherapy.[150]

The use of radiotherapy postoperatively enables the administration of higher radiation doses than are feasible with preoperative radiotherapy although this treatment has been associated with increases in the incidence of anastomotic strictures and prolonged recovery from surgery, adversely affecting the quality of life.[144,147,148] There is also some evidence that median survival is worse in patients who undergo postoperative radiotherapy, compared with resection only, as a result of an earlier appearance of distant metastatic disease and because of irradiation-induced deaths, although selection bias may also play a role.[138] Postoperative irradiation appears to decrease the local recurrence rate but overall has no proven influence on long-term survival.

Single modality radiation therapy has in recent years been supplanted by combined modality treatment with systemic chemotherapy added to radiation, Randomized trials have shown combined modality treatment to be superior for both definitive or neoadjuvant treatment of esophageal cancer when compared to single modality radiation therapy (see section titled "Combined Modality Therapy").

Intraluminal brachytherapy has been added in some centers to curative or palliative external beam radiotherapy in an effort to improve local control of disease. Doses of 10–20 Gy are added after completion of external beam treatment in one or more fractions using Iridium-192. In patients with potentially curable disease, the addition of intraluminal brachytherapy appears to enhance locoregional control, compared with external beam radiotherapy alone but is associated with a higher incidence of radiation-induced esophageal strictures.[146,151,152] Reducing the dose per fraction of intraluminal brachytherapy may in the future limit the incidence and severity of these local complications.[153] The use of brachytherapy in patients with unresectable or recurrent esophageal cancer is still under investigation but may provide better symptomatic relief than other modalities, such as chemotherapy, laser therapy, and stenting.[154–157]

Systemic therapy

There have been major advances in the systemic chemotherapy for esophageal cancer in the past 50 years (Table 6). In the 1970s, when chemotherapy drugs were beginning to be tested in clinical trials, esophageal cancer was predominantly SCC histology and localized mostly in the upper two-thirds of the esophagus. Chemotherapy agents found to be effective were therefore not surprisingly ones that were also active for head and neck SCC.

In the past two decades, in the United States and other developed countries in the West, esophageal cancer has shifted to primarily adenocarcinoma histology and localized mainly in the distal third of the esophagus, the EGJ extending into the gastric cardia. Chemotherapy regimens tested to be effective are also active against gastric adenocarcinoma, which also led to the development of targeted therapy against the Her-2-neu receptor (trastuzumab) and the vascular endothelial growth receptor (bevacizumab, ramucirumab). SCC still remains the predominant histology for

Table 5 Results of randomized trials of pre- and postoperative radiotherapy for locoregionally advanced esophageal cancer.

Authors	Year	Treatment	Histology	Patients (No.)	5-Year survival	p-Value
Preoperative RT versus surgery alone						
Launois et al.[141]	1981	Surgery alone	S	57	11.5%	NS
		Surgery + 40 Gy		67	7.5%	
Gignoux et al.[142]	1988	Surgery alone	S	106	10%	NS
		Surgery + 33 Gy		102	9%	
Wang et al.[143]	1989	Surgery alone	S	102	30%	NS
		Surgery + 40 Gy		104	35%	
Arnott et al.[144]	1992	Surgery alone	S	86	17%	NS
		Surgery + 20 Gy		90	9%	
Nygaard et al.[145]	1992	Surgery alone	S	41	4%	.08
		Surgery + 35 Gy		48	18%	
Postoperative RT versus surgery alone						
FUASR[146]	1991	Surgery alone	S	119	18%	NS
		Surgery + 45–55 Gy		102	20%	
Fok et al.[147]	1993	Surgery alone	S	65	11% (4 yr)	NS
		Surgery + 49–52.5 Gy		65	11% (4 yr)	
Ziernan[148]	1995	Surgery alone	S	35	20% (3 yr)	NS
		Surgery + 56 Gy		33	23% (3 yr)	

Table 6 Results of randomized trials of systemic therapy for advanced esophageal cancer.

Author (Ref)	Year	Treatment	Histology	Patients (No.)	Response rate	Median servival (mo)	p-Value
El-Rayes et al.[168]	2004	Paclitaxel-carboplatin (Phase 2)	S/A	35	43%	9	
Ilson et al.[170]	1998	Paclitaxel-5FU-cisplatin (Phase 2)	S/A	61	48%	10.8	
Ilson et al.[169]	1999	Irinotecan-cisplatin (Phase 2)	S/A	35	57%	14.6	
Kang et al.[165]	2009	Capecitabine-cisplatin	A (gastric)	160	46%	10.5	0.008
		5FU-cisplatin		156	34%	9.3	
Ross et al.[171]	2002	Mitomycin-cisplatin-5FU	S/A	290	42.40%	8.7	0.315
		Epirubicin-cisplatin-5FU	S/A	290	44.10%	9.4	
Cunningham et al.[172]	2008	Epirubicin-cisplatin-5FU	S/A	263	40.70%	9.9	0.36
		Epirubicin-cisplatin-capecitabine	S/A	250	46.40%	9.9	
		Epirubicin-oxaliplatin-5FU	S/A	245	42.40%	9.3	0.35
		Epirubicin-oxaliplatin-capecitabine	S/A	244	47.90%	11.2	
Enzinger et al.[173] CALGB 80403	2017	Epirubicin-cisplatin-5FU-cetuximab	S/A	63	S/A 67/60%	S/A 10.6/11.6	
		Irinotecan-cisplatin-cetuximab	S/A	71	S/A 12/45%	S/A 6.5/8.6	
		FOLFOX-cetuximab	S/A	66		S/A 12.4/11.4	
Bang et al.[174] (ToGA)	2010	5FU/capecitabine-cisplatin- trastuzumab	A	296	47%	13.8	0.0046
		5FU/capecitabine-cisplatin ToGA	A	298	35%	11.1	
Tabernero et al.[175] (JACOB)	2018	Chemo-trastuzumab-pertuzumab	A	780		17.5	0.057
		Chemo-trastuzumab JACOB	A	780		14.2	
Fuchs et al.[177] (REGARD)	2014	Ramucirumab (previously treated)	A	238		5.2	0.047
		Placebo (previously treated)	A	117		3.8	
Wilke et al.[178] (RAINBOW)	2014	Paclitaxel-ramucirumab (previously treated)	A	330	28%	9.6	0.017
		Paclitaxel-placebo (previously treated)	A	335	16%	6.4	
Ohtsu et al.[179]	2011	5FU/Capecitabine-cisplatin-bevacizumab	A	387	46.00%	12.1	0.1002
		5FU/Capecitabine-cisplatin-placebo	A	387	37.40%	10.1	
Lordick et al.[180] (EXPAND)	2013	5FU/Capecitabine-cisplatin-cetuximab	A	455		PFS 4.4	0.032
		5FU/Capecitabine-cisplatin	A	449		5.6	
Waddell et al.[181] (REAL3)	2013	Epirubicin-oxaliplatin-capecitabine panitumumab	A	278		8.8	0.013
		Epirubicin-oxaliplatin-capecitabine	A	275		11.3	
Kato et al.[182] (ATTRACTION-03)	2019	Nivolumab (previously treated)	S	210	19.30%	10.9	0.0189
		Paclitaxel/docetaxel (previously treated)	S	209	21.50%	8.4	
Kojima et al.[185] (KEYNOTE-181)	2019	Pembrolizumab (previously treated)	S PDL1>10	85	22%	10.3	0.0074
		Chemotherapy (previously treated)	S	82	7%	6.7	
Shitara et al.[176] (DESTINY-Gastric01)	2020	Trastuzumab deruxtecan (previously treated)	A	125	51%	12.5	0.01
		Chemotherapy (previously treated)	A	62	14%	8.4	
Kato et al.[186] (KEYNOTE-590)	2020	Pembrolizumab-chemotherapy	S/A	373	45%	12.4	<0.0001
		Placebo-chemotherapy	S/A	376	29%	9.8	
Janjigian et al.[183] (CheckMate 649)	2021	Nivolumab-chemotherapy	S/A CPS all	1581		13.8	0.0002
		Chemotherapy	S/A	792		11.1	
Janjigian et al.[187] (KEYNOTE-811)	2021	Pembrolizumab-trastuzumab-chemotherapy	A	133	74.40%		<0.0001
		Placebo-trastuzumab-chemotherapy	A	131	52%		
Kelly et al.[184] (CheckMate 577)	2021	Adjuvant nivolumab up to one year	S/A	532		DFS 22.4	<0.001
		Adjuvant placebo	S/A	262		11	

Abbreviations: A, adenocarcinoma; NS, not significant; S, squamous cell; 5FU, 5-fluorouracil.

esophageal cancer in non-Western countries, including those in the esophageal cancer belt in central Asia, and in Africa and Southeast Asia.

In the past 5 years, immunomodulatory therapies such as immune checkpoint inhibition have been tested and found to be effective in inducing tumor responses and prolonging survival for both SCC and adenocarcinoma of the esophagus.

Single-agent chemotherapy

Previous Phase II trials have identified a number of chemotherapy drugs with 15–30% response rates when administered as single agent for esophageal cancer. These drugs included cisplatin, mitomycin, 5-FU, capecitabine, S1, paclitaxel, and vindesine. Although responses up to 40% have been reported with single agents, median survival remains limited and rarely exceeds 9 months. Single-agent paclitaxel in a weekly schedule has shown response rates of 15% for both SCC and adenocarcinoma of the esophagus; median overall survival was 9 months.[163] S1, an oral combination of the prodrug ftorafur and oteracil, inhibits dihydropyrimidine dehydrogenase and delays degradation of 5FU, has pharmacokinetic advantages, but randomized trials have failed to shown superiority over oral capecitabine.[164] Nevertheless, single-agent chemotherapy is generally well tolerated and may be considered for patients with comorbidities precluding multi-agent chemotherapy.

Multiagent chemotherapy

Doublet combinations

Standard treatment for esophageal cancer has for many years been the combination of infusional 5FU with cisplatin. The substitution of capecitabine for 5FU in combination with cisplatin was evaluated in two randomized trials and shown to have higher response rates and overall survival.[165,166]

The paclitaxel-cisplatin combination without 5FU has also been found to be active for both SCC and adenocarcinoma in a Phase II trial with response rates of 40% with clinical benefit (relief of dysphagia, weight gain) achieved in 70% of patients.[167] The combination of paclitaxel-carboplatin in a Phase II trial showed response rates of 43%, median duration of response 2.8 months, and median survival 9 months. One-year survival was 43%. The combination was well tolerated with no treatment-related deaths.[168]

The combination of irinotecan-cisplatin in a weekly regimen has been reported in a Phase II trial to be active in esophageal cancer with response rates of 57%, median duration of response 4.2 months, median actuarial survival 14.6 months. Similar response rates were observed for adenocarcinoma (52%) and SCC (66%).[169]

Triplet combinations

The addition of paclitaxel to the 5FU-cisplatin backbone in a Phase II trial has been reported with response rates of 48% with a median duration of response of 5.7 months and median survival of 10.8 months. It was further noted that response rates were comparable for SCC (50%) and for adenocarcinoma (46%).[170]

Epirubicin-cisplatin-5FU (ECF) has been previously shown to be an active regimen for gastric adenocarcinoma. Its activity in esophagogastric cancer (SCC/adenocarcinoma) was demonstrated in a Phase III trial versus mitomycin-cisplatin-5FU with reported similar efficacy (response rates of 44.1% vs 42.4%, median survival of 9.4 vs 8.7 months).[171] The substitution of cisplatin and 5FU with oxaliplatin and oral capecitabine (EOX) was evaluated in a Phase III trial (REAL-2) in 964 evaluable patients in a two-by-two design showed improved overall survival in the EOX group as compared to the ECF group, while progression-free survival and response rates were similar between the two groups.[172]

ECF was compared to irinotecan-cisplatin and FOLFOX in the CALGB 80403 randomized Phase 2 trial. Response rates, progression-free survival, and median overall survival were comparable between the two groups. It should be noted that cetuximab was added to all three arms in this trial.[173] This and other clinical trials suggest that there is no additional benefit to adding epirubicin to 5FU-cisplatin and that FOLFOX or CAPOX is better tolerated without compromise in efficacy.

The combination of docetaxel to 5FU-oxaliplatin (FLOT) has shown efficacy with complete pathological responses when given as neoadjuvant therapy for esophagogastric adenocarcinoma (see section titled "Combined Modality Therapy").

Targeted therapy

Trastuzumab, a monoclonal antibody directed against the Her-2-neu receptor, has been tested in the Phase III ToGA trial of 5FU/capecitabine-cisplatin with and without trastuzumab.[174] Patients with gastric or esophagogastric adenocarcinoma were eligible if their tumors were positive for positive Her-2-neu expression by immunohistochemistry (IHC) (1 to 3+) or fluorescence *in situ* hybridization (FISH). Response rates were higher with trastuzumab (47% vs 35%) as was median survival (13.8 vs 11.1 months). Further studies showed that trastuzumab was most effective for IHC 3+ tumors. The addition for pertuzumab to trastuzumab-chemotherapy was studied in the Phase 3 JACOB trial in patients with gastroesophageal and gastric adenocarcinoma. Median overall survival was 17.5 versus 14.2 months in favor of the pertuzumab added arm, but did not reach statistical significance.[175]

Trastuzumab deruxtecan is an antibody drug conjugate bound to a cytotoxic topoisomerase I inhibitor by a tetrapeptide-based linker and can deliver drug payload in tumor cells. Trastuzumab deruxtecan was tested in a randomized Phase II trial (DESTINY-Gastric01) versus chemotherapy in patients with HER2-positive gastroesophageal junction or gastric adenocarcinoma who had progressed after prior trastuzumab and chemotherapy regimens. Objective responses were 51% versus 14%, and overall survival was 12.5 versus 8.4 months in favor of trastuzumab deruxtecan.[176]

Ramucirumab, a monoclonal antibody which inhibits the VEGF-2 receptor, has been tested in the Phase III REGARD trial versus placebo in previously treated gastric or esophagogastric adenocarcinoma.[177] The study showed in favor of ramucirumab with median progression-free survival was 2.1 versus 1.3 month, overall survival 5.2 versus 3.8 months, response rates 8% versus 3%. Disease control rates (responses plus stable disease) were 49% for ramucirumab versus 23% for the placebo group. A survival benefit was seen for the combination of ramucirumab in combination with paclitaxel in the Phase III RAINBOW trial versus paclitaxel plus placebo in previously treated metastatic gastric or esophagogastric adenocarcinoma.[178] The ramucirumab-paclitaxel combination was superior in median overall survival (9.6 vs 7.4 months), progression-free survival (4.4 vs 2.9 months), and response rates (28% vs 16%).

Bevacizumab, a monoclonal antibody directed against soluble VEGF, has been tested in combination with capecitabine-cisplatin in the Phase III AVAGAST trial versus placebo plus capecitabine-cisplatin in patients with previously untreated gastric or esophagogastric adenocarcinoma. Although response rates and median progression-free survival were higher in the bevacizumab group (46% vs 37%, 6.7 vs 5.3 months), no significant survival benefit was demonstrated (12.1 vs 10.1 months).[179]

Similarly, no survival benefit could be demonstrated in Phase III trials of adding an anti-EGFR agent to chemotherapy in patients with gastric or esophagogastric adenocarcinoma. The Phase III EXPAND trial of capecitabine-cisplatin with and without cetuximab showed median progression-free survival of 4.4 versus 5.6 months for the control arm.[180] In the Phase III REAL3 trial, patients with esophagogastric adenocarcinoma were randomized to epirubicin–oxaliplatin–capecitabine with or without panitumumab.[181] Median overall survival in an interim analysis was 8.8 versus 11.3 months in favor of the control arm and the study was halted.

Immunomodulatory therapy

Binding of the programmed death 1 (PD1) protein on T-lymphocytes to the programmed death-ligand 1 (PD-L1) protein on tumor cells has been shown in immune studies to promote immune tolerance. By inhibiting this binding using monoclonal antibodies targeted to the PD1 or PD-L1 proteins, the immune tolerance to tumor cells can be lifted, resulting in T-cell mediated cytotoxicity against tumor cells. PD1 inhibitors, such as the monoclonal antibodies nivolumab and pembrolizumab, or PD-L1 inhibitors such as atezolizumab and durvulumab, have been shown to induce tumor regression and prolong survival in a wide variety of tumor types. Certain tumor types exhibit characteristics which may predict for efficacy of these immune checkpoint inhibitors. Colorectal cancers with deficiency of mismatch repair proteins (microsatellite unstable) and lung cancers with enhanced expression of PD1 or PD-L1 proteins have been shown to predict for tumor regression and survival prolongation following treatment with immune checkpoint inhibitors.

For esophageal cancer, nivolumab was tested in a Phase III trial (ATTRACTION-03) versus chemotherapy in patients with esophageal SCC who were refractory or intolerant to at least one fluoropyrimidine and platinum-based regimen, Overall survival was superior in the nivolumab arm (10.9 vs 8.4 months), regardless of PD-L1 expression.[182]

Nivolumab was tested as first line therapy in combination with chemotherapy versus, chemotherapy alone in unresectable or metastatic SCC or esophageal adenocarcinoma (CheckMate 649). Overall survival was superior in the nivolumab arm, 13.8 versus 11.1 months, irrespective of PD-L1 expression.[183]

For esophageal SCC or adenocarcinoma patients with residual pathologic disease after neoadjuvant chemoradiation and resection, adjuvant treatment with nivolumab for up to one year was tested in a Phase III trial versus placebo (CheckMate 577). Disease free survival benefit 22.4 versus 11 months was shown in favor of the nivolumab arm.[184]

Pembrolizumab, in the Phase III KEYNOTE-181 trial versus chemotherapy in previously treated patients with esophageal SCC, showed overall survival benefit 10.3 versus 6.7 months, in patients with PD-L1 expression > CPS 10.[185]

Pembrolizumab was tested as first line therapy in combination with chemotherapy in unresectable or metastatic esophageal SCC or adenocarcinoma (Phase III KEYNOTE-590) versus placebo plus chemotherapy alone. Overall survival was superior in the pembrolizumab arm, 12.4 versus 9.8 months, irrespective of PD-L1 expression. Response rates were 45% versus 29% in favor of the pembrolizumab arm.[186]

For patients with HER2 positive gastroesophageal or gastric adenocarcinoma, pembrolizumab in combination with trastuzumab and chemotherapy as first-line treatment was superior to the control placebo-trastuzumab-chemotherapy arm. An interim analysis of the randomized KEYNOTE-811 trial reported response rates 74.4% versus 51.9% in favor of the pembrolizumab arm.[187]

Combined modality therapy

In locoregionally advanced esophageal cancer, combination chemotherapy has been investigated in combination with radiation or surgery to try to reduce the high rate of systemic relapse noted when surgery or radiation therapy alone is used. Attempts to use chemotherapy with surgery have included preoperative and postoperative strategies usually with cisplatin-based multiagent regimens (Table 7). The randomized trials with preoperative chemotherapy usually consist of two or three chemotherapy cycles followed by resection. Some studies have also added postoperative chemotherapy to the regimen. There is no clear increase in perioperative complications noted with preoperative chemotherapy when the surgery is performed at an experienced center. As Table 7 demonstrates, recent randomized trials have demonstrated a survival benefit with preoperative chemotherapy especially when larger number of patients are randomized.[44,128,131,132,189,190,193] The reasons for the failure of the majority of trials may be due in part to the small numbers of patient in each study. Meta-analyses have suggested with larger number of patients that there is a significant benefit to preoperative chemotherapy especially in patients with adenocarcinoma.[194]

Postoperative chemotherapy (cisplatin, 5-FU) for patients after esophagectomy has not demonstrated to date a survival advantage compared with surgery alone and has been associated with increased treatment-related complications.[158] Even in meta-analyses there has not been a clear benefit demonstrated with postoperative chemotherapy.[195]

The combination of epirubicin-cisplatin-5FU (ECF) has been tested in the MAGIC trial for survival benefit when administered in the perioperative setting for esophageal adenocarcinoma. In this trial, patients were randomized to receive three cycles of ECF pre- and postresection versus resection alone. Five-year overall survival was 36% versus 23% in favor of the perioperative chemotherapy group.[191] More recently, the perioperative ECF was compared to the FLOT regimen (fluorouracil, leucovorin, oxaliplatin, and docetaxel) also administered perioperatively in the FLOT 4 trial for esophagogastric adenocarcinoma. Median overall survival was 50 versus 35 months in favor of the perioperative FLOT group, heralding a new standard for the perioperative treatment of esophageal adenocarcinoma.[192]

Definitive chemoradiotherapy with selective surgery has also been evaluated as a strategy to improve survival in locoregionally advanced esophageal cancer. These studies have used both sequential and concurrent treatment strategies. The concurrent use of chemotherapy and radiotherapy is theoretically appealing

Table 7 Results of randomized trials of pre- or postoperative chemotherapy for locoregionally advanced esophageal cancer.

Author (Ref.)	Year	Treatment	Histology	Patients (No.)	Resectability	Operative mortality	Median survival (mo)	p-Value
Preoperative chemotherapy								
Roth et al.[44]	1988	Cisplatin, bleomycin, vindesine + surgery	S > A	19	—	10%	9	NS
		Surgery alone		20	—	0%	9	
Nygaard et al.[145]	1992	Cisplatin, bleomycin + surgery	S	50	58%	10	NS	
		Surgery alone		41	69%	13%	7	
Schlag et al.[127]	1992	Cisplatin, 5-FU + surgery	S	21	69%	—	6	NS
		Surgery alone		24	79%	—	8	
Maipang et al.[188]	1994	Cisplatin, bleomycin, vinblastine + surgery	S	24	—	—	17	NS
		Surgery alone		22	—	—	17	
Ancona et al.[189]	1995	Cisplatin, 5-FU + Surgery	S	35	78%	7%	—	NS
		Surgery alone		43	86%	5%	—	
Law et al.[130]	1997	Cisplatin, 5-FU + surgery	S	73	95%	9%	13	NS
		Surgery alone		74	89%	8%	17	
Kelsen et al.[131]	1998	Cisplatin, 5-FU + surgery	A > S	213	76%	7%	15	NS
		Surgery alone		227	89%	6%	16	
Medical Research Council[190]	2002	Cisplatin, 5-FU + surgery	A > S	400	78%	10%	17	<0.05
		Surgery alone		402	70%	10%	13	
Cunningham et al.[191]	2006	Epirubicin, cisplatin, 5-FU + surgery	A	250	69%	6%	23	<0.01
		Surgery alone		253	66%	6%	20	
Salah-Eddin et al.[192]	2019	5-FU-LV-oxaliplatin-docetaxel + surgery	A	356			50	HR 0.77
		Epirubicin, cisplatin, 5-FU/capecitabine + surgery	A	360			35	
Postoperative chemotherapy								
Ando et al.[150]	1997	Cisplatin, vindesine + surgery	S	105	—	—	58	NS
		Surgery alone		100	—	—	47	

Abbreviations: A, adenocarcinoma; NS, not significant; S, squamous cell; 5-FU, 5-fluorouracil.

Table 8 Results of randomized trials of preoperative chemoradiotherapy for locoregionally advanced esophageal cancer.

Author (Ref)	Year	Treatment	Histology	Patients (No.)	Technique	Operative mortality	Medial survival (mo)	p-Value
Le Prise et al.[158]	1994	Cisplatin, 5-FU + 20 Gy + surgery	S	41	Sequential	9%	10	NS
		Surgery alone		45		7%	10	
Walsh et al.[128]	1996	Cisplatin, 5-FU + 40 Gy + surgery	A	58	Concurrent	12%	17	0.01
		Surgery alone		55		3%	12	
Bosset et al.[129]	1997	Cisplatin + 37 Gy + surgery	S	143	Concurrent	12%	19	NS
		Surgery alone		139		4%	19	
Urba et al.[159]	2001	Cisplatin, 5-FU + 45 Gy + surgery	A	50	Concurrent	4%	18	0.15
		Surgery alone		50		2%	17	
Burmeister et al.[160]	2005	Cisplatin, 5-FU + 35 Gy + surgery	A,S	128	Concurrent	5%	22	NS
		Surgery alone		128		5%	19	
Tepper et al.[161]	2008	Cisplatin, 5-FU + 50.4 Gy + surgery	A > S	30	Concurrent	0%	54	0.002
		Surgery alone		26		4%	22	
Van Hagen et al.[199]	2012	Paclitaxel, carboplatin + 41.4 Gy + surgery	A,S	178	Concurrent	4%	49	0.003
		Surgery alone		188		4%	24	
Mariette et al.[162]	2014	Cisplatin, 5FU + 45 Gy + surgery	A,S	98	Concurrent	11%	32	0.99
		Surgery alone		97		3%	41	

Abbreviations: A, adenocarcinoma; NS, not significant; S, squamous cell; 5-FU, 5-fluorouracil.

because, in addition to the systemic effects of chemotherapy, certain agents behave as radiosensitizers. Randomized studies with a concurrent strategy demonstrate an advantage to combined treatment versus radiation therapy alone (Table 4).[122,124,125,128–131,148] Definitive chemoradiotherapy strategies with surgery used only as salvage appear most effective in SCC and less effective in adenocarcinoma where long-term survival is lower.[115] Two trials have been performed in Europe randomizing SCC patients to definitive chemoradiation or preoperative chemoradiotherapy and surgery.[103,104] These studies demonstrated similar survivals between groups and suggest that definitive chemoradiation may be an acceptable strategy for SCC of the upper and middle esophagus. The optimum dose for definitive chemoradiotherapy is currently 50.4 Gy as suggested by a randomized trial in which increased doses of radiation were associated with increased treatment-related mortality without a survival advantage.[102] Interestingly, the higher dose had no impact on local failure or continued persistent disease. Both arms of the trial report roughly 50% local failure after 24 months of cumulative follow-up.

For the definitive treatment of locally advanced esophageal cancer, combined chemotherapy and radiotherapy have been shown to be superior to single modality radiation therapy. In the RTOC 85-01, Phase 3 trial of radiation therapy with concurrent 5-fluorouracil and cisplatin compared to radiation therapy alone, 5-year survival was 26% versus 0% in favor of the chemoradiation group.[101,196,197] Local control in the chemoradiation group was 46%. The total radiation doses used in that trial were 50 Gy for both arms. The question as to whether higher RT doses in chemoradiation confers additional survival benefit was addressed in the INT-0123 Phase 3 trial where patients were randomized to receive 50.4 Gy compared to 64.8 Gy, both combined with chemotherapy. There was no difference in overall survival at 2 years.[102]

Preoperative chemoradiotherapy has also been investigated in locoregionally advanced esophageal cancer as a strategy in an attempt to reduce both the high locoregional and systemic relapse rate noted with surgery alone or preoperative chemotherapy and surgery. The theoretical advantages to preoperative as opposed to postoperative chemoradiation therapy include (1) the ability to control subclinical systemic metastases prior to the immune suppression that results from surgery; (2) downstaging locoregional disease to increase the likelihood of a complete resection at surgery; and (3) the ability to administer full doses of chemoradiation that would not be possible to administer postoperatively because of perioperative debility. As Table 8 demonstrates, the results are not consistent, although sequential chemoradiation does not appear to be beneficial.[103,128,129,158–160] There have been several trials that have been encouraging for concurrent preoperative chemoradiation in locoregionally advanced esophageal cancer especially in adenocarcinoma, but statistical significance has not been achieved in all trials. Meta analyses with larger numbers of patients have suggested that preoperative chemoradiation and preoperative chemotherapy have survival advantages compared with other strategies, although these studies are limited by different preclinical staging techniques and heterogenous patient populations.[197] A survival benefit for combined therapy is evident in most studies in patients who are found to have a complete pathologic response in the surgical specimen and have provided strong incentives to continue the investigations of this strategy. In addition, since surgery alone or radiation therapy alone has such poor outcomes, many oncologists currently use definitive chemoradiotherapy alone or preoperative chemoradiation and surgery for nonmetastatic, locoregionally advanced esophageal cancer (Figure 3). Two randomized trials from Europe have been reported comparing definitive chemoradiation versus preoperative chemoradiation and surgery in SCC.[103,104] Preliminary results demonstrated improved locoregional control with surgery but no survival advantages. Although operative mortality was higher than expected these trials suggest definitive chemoradiation may be an acceptable strategy in SCC of the upper and middle esophagus especially in institutions where trimodality treatment-related mortality is high.[103,104] The impact of neoadjuvant chemoradiotherapy on pathologic complete response and overall survival has been debated due to lack of a survival benefit in most randomized trials. Most of these trials have been criticized for the poor design and lack of power to detect an overall survival benefit. A recent and updated meta-analysis of 12 Surgery +/− neoadjuvant chemoradiotherapy encompassing 1854 patients demonstrated that the hazard ratio for all-cause mortality was improved for neoadjuvant chemoradiotherapy (0.78, 95% CI 0.70–0.88; $p < 0.0001$).[200] The benefit was seen for both the squamous (0.80, CI 0.68–0.93; $p = 0.004$) and for adenocarcinoma (0.75, CI 0.59–0.95; $p = 0.02$) histologies. While increased postoperative morbidity and mortality were seen in this analysis, the impact on survival remained.

In an effort to decrease the operative mortality and maintain high rates of R0 resections, a Phase 2 trial using paclitaxel and carboplatin with radiotherapy demonstrated low morbidity and 100% complete resection rates.[198] In the definitive Phase 3 trial, Chemoradiotherapy for Oesophageal Cancer Followed by Surgery Study (CROSS), patients with clinical stage T1N1, M0 or T2-3N0-1, M0 were randomized to this regimen against surgery alone.[199] Of the 366 patients randomized, 75% were adenocarcinoma. Complete (R0) resection was obtained in 92% of the chemoradiotherapy arm versus 69% in the surgery alone arm ($p < 0.001$). Postoperative complications did not significantly differ between the arms. Pathological complete remission was seen in 29% of patients in the chemoradiation group. Locoregional recurrence rate was 14% versus 34% in favor of the chemoradiotherapy arm. With a median follow-up of 45 months, median overall survival was 49.4 months in the chemoradiotherapy arm versus 24 months in the surgery alone arm ($p = 0.003$). Overall 5-year survival was 47% versus 34%. In this trial, the total RT dose was 41.4 Gy in 23 fractions, which is lower than the 50.8 Gy total dose used in the definitive chemoradiation RTOG 85-01 study. The benefit in OS was maintained in both the squamous and the adenocarcinoma histologies.

For patients with early-stage esophageal carcinoma (Stage I or II), a randomized trial from Europe comparing neoadjuvant chemoradiotherapy (4500 cGY plus 5FU-cisplatin) following by surgery versus surgery alone reported interim analysis which showed that 3-year overall survival was similar between the two groups: 47.5% versus 53.0% (HR 0.99). R0 resection rates were similar 93.8% versus 92.1% ($p = 0.749$). but postoperative mortality was higher in the neoadjuvant chemoradiotherapy group, 11.1% versus 3.4% ($p = 0.049$).[162]

Meta-analysis studies comparing chemoradiation versus chemotherapy alone in the neoadjuvant treatment of locally advanced esophageal cancer suggest chemoradiation group to be superior.[200] In the Preoperative Chemotherapy or Radiochemotherapy in Esophagogastric Adenocarcinoma Trial (POET), there was no advantage to patients receiving chemoRT versus chemotherapy alone for neoadjuvant treatment followed by resection, although the dose of RT was lower, at 30 Gy in 15 fractions than in the CROSS trial.[201] Currently, the neoadjuvant chemoradiotherapy CROSS regimen is being tested against perioperative chemotherapy (ECF or FLOT) without RT (Neo-AEGIS and ESOPEC trials).

For patients with residual pathologic disease at time of resection following combined modality therapy with neoadjuvant chemoradiation, the addition of post-operative treatment with the immune checkpoint inhibitor nivolumab for up to one year had been reported to show statistically significant improvement in disease free survival (CheckMate 577). In this Phase 3 trial, median disease free survival was reported to be 22.4 months in the nivolumab arm compared to 11.0 months in the placebo arm.[184]

Recommendations for therapy

As our treatment algorithm suggests (Figure 3), good performance patients with localized, early-stage disease should undergo endoscopic resection or esophagectomy depending on tumor depth whereas poor performance patients or patients refusing surgery can be treated with definitive chemoradiation or radiation alone. Locoregionally advanced esophageal cancer patients with good performance status are seldom cured with surgery or radiation therapy alone, and may therefore be candidates for investigational trials, definitive chemoradiation, or preoperative chemoradiation and surgery. Poor performance patients with locoregionally advanced esophageal cancer should be treated with chemoradiation or palliative radiation therapy and/or stents. Metastatic esophageal cancer patients who are good performance status may be offered chemotherapy alone with the addition of palliative radiation and/or stents for locoregional control. Chemotherapy should not be used if the patients have a poor performance status since the focus should be on palliation.

Palliative therapy of esophageal obstruction

In patients with advanced esophageal cancer not amenable to potentially curative therapy, a primary goal of treatment is relief of dysphagia.[202] This can be accomplished with palliative resection, but high operative morbidity and mortality rates as well as the prolonged period of recovery that is necessary preclude meaningful palliation and most oncologists currently recommend nonsurgical means for palliation. External beam radiotherapy, as an isolated modality or in combination with chemotherapy, is noninvasive but requires considerable time to complete and results in strictures in up to 30% of patients. Intraluminal brachytherapy is another option that is considered in some centers.[203,204] Photocoagulative laser therapy is another option that is usually performed with an Nd:YAG laser, with an initial improvement in dysphagia in 85% of patients and a mean duration of response of less than 1 month. PDT offers a similar initial efficacy but provides a more enduring response, although skin photosensitivity is an undesirable side effect.[205]

The development of endoesophageal stents has offered another therapeutic option in these difficult patients. Endoesophageal stent placement has led to rapid and enduring improvement in swallowing for many patients with advanced disease who are obstructed locoregionally. The introduction of self-expanding wire mesh stents has greatly simplified stent placement and associated complications and has improved palliation of dysphagia, compared with plastic prostheses.[206,207] These measures have provided a much less invasive mechanism to palliate these patients and have replaced surgical bypass as the primary modality to relieve dysphagia.

Malignant esophagorespiratory (tracheoesophageal) fistulas pose a special problem in patients with esophageal cancer. These patients were previously treated with surgical bypass although the high morbidity and short life expectancy of these patients was a significant problem.[208] The introduction of coated wire mesh stents offers a better option for the treatment of such fistulas because they palliate dysphagia while occluding the fistula without requiring an extensive surgical procedure in an often debilitated and poor performance status patient.[209,210]

Key references

The complete reference list can be found on Vital Source version of this title, see inside front cover.

14 Kjaerheim K, Gaard M, Andersen A. The role of alcohol, tobacco, and dietary factors in upper aerodigestive tract cancers: a prospective study of 10,900 Norwegian men. *Cancer Causes Control*. 1998;**9**:99–108.

15 Yu MC, Garabrant DH, Peters JM, et al. Tobacco, alcohol, diet, occupation, and carcinoma of the esophagus. *Cancer Res*. 1988;**48**:3843–3848.

28 Li X, Gao C, Tang T, et al. Systematic review with meta-analysis: the association between human papillomavirus infection and oesophageal cancer. *Aliment Pharmaceut Ther*. 2014;**39**:270.

30 He H, Chen N, Hou Y, et al. Trends in the incidence and survival of patients with esophageal cancer: a SEER database analysis. *Thorac Cancer*. 2020;**11**:1121–1128.

34 Bray F, Ferlay J, Soerjomataram I, et al. Global cancer statistics 2018: GLOBOCAN estimates of incidence and mortality worldwide for 36 cancers in 185 countries. *CA Cancer J Clin*. 2018;**68**:394–424.

40. Pera M, Cameron AJ, Trastek VF, et al. Increasing incidence of adenocarcinoma of the esophagus and esophagogastric junction. *Gastroenterology*. 1993;**104**:510–513.
49. Low DE, Allum W, De Manzoni G, et al. Guidelines for perioperative care in esophagectomy: enhanced recovery after surgery (ERAS®) society recommendations. *World J Surg*. 2019;**43**:299–330.
50. Minnella EM, Rashami A, Sarah-Eve L, et al. Effect of exercise and nutrition prehabilitation on functional capacity in esophagogastric cancer surgery: a randomized clinical trial. *JAMA Surg*. 2018;**153**(12):1081–1089.
85. Rice TW, Kelsen DP, Blackstone EH, et al. Esophagus and esophagogastric junction. In: Amin MB, Edge SB, Greene FL, *et al.*, eds. *AJCC Cancer Staging Manual*, 8th ed. New York: Springer; 2017:185–202.
86. Rice TW, Patil DT, Blackstone EH. 8th Edition ANCC/UICC staging of cancers of the esophagus and esophagogastric junction: application to clinical practice. *Ann Cardiothorac Surg*. 2017;**6**:119–130.
87. Ferguson MK. Carcinoma of the Esophagus and Cardia. *Surgery of the Alimentary Tract*. 5th ed., vol. 1: The Esophagus. Elsevier.
88. Ricc TW, Gress DM, Patil DT, et al. Cancer of the esophagus and esophagogasric junction – major changes in the American Joint Committee on Cancer eighth edition cancer staging manual. *CA Cancer J Clin*. 2017;**2017**(67):304–317.
89. Baba M, Aikou T, Yoshinaka H, et al. Long-term results of subtotal esophagectomy with three-field lymphadenectomy for carcinoma of the thoracic esophagus. *Ann Surg*. 1994;**219**:310–316.
94. Kamarajh SK, Navidi M, Wahed S, et al. Significance of neoadjuvant downstaging in carcinoma of esophagus and gastroesophageal junction. *Ann Surg Oncol*. 2020, 2020. doi: 10.1245/s10434-020-08358-0.
107. Ell C, May A, Gossner L, et al. Endoscopic mucosal resection of early cancer and high-rage dysplasia in Barrett's esophagus. *Gastroenterology*. 2000;**118**:670–677.
110. Hofstetter WL. Salvage esophagectomy. *J Thorac Dis*. 2014;**6**:S341–S349.
111. Levinsky NC et al. Outcome of delayed versus timely esophagectomy after chemoradiation for esophageal adenocarcinoma. *JTCVS*. 2020 June;**159**(6):2555–2566.
112. Swanstrom LL, Hansen P. Laparoscopic total esophagectomy. *Arch Surg*. 1997;**132**:943–947.
115. Luketich JD, Pennathur A, Awais O, et al. Outcomes after minimally invasive esophagectomy: review of over 1000 patients. *Ann Surg*. 2012;**256**:95–103.
116. Luketich JD, Pennathur A, Franchetti Y, et al. Minimally invasive esophagectomy: results of a prospective phase II multicenter trial – the Eastern cooperative Oncology Group (E2202) study. *Ann Surg*. 2015;**261**:702–707.
117. Gottlieb-Vedi E, Kauppila JH, Malietzis G, et al. Longterm survival in esophageal cancer after minimally invasive compared to open esophagectomy: a systematic review and meta-analysis. *Ann Surg*. 2019;**270**:1005–1017.
125. Sarkaria IS, Rizk NP, Finley DJ, et al. Combined thoracoscopic and laparoscopic robotic-assisted minimally invasive esophagectomy using a four-arm platform: experience, technique and cautions during early procedure development. *Eur J Cardiothorac Surg*. 2013;**43**:e107–e115.
144. Arnott SJ, Duncan W, Gignoux M, et al. Preoperative radiotherapy in esophageal carcinoma: a meta-analysis using individual patients data (Oesophageal Cancer Collaborative Group). *Int J Radiat Oncol Biol Phys*. 1998;**41**:579–583.
161. Tepper J, Krasna MJ, Niedzwiecki D, et al. Phase III trial of trimodality therapy with cisplatin fluorouracil, radiotherapy, and surgery compared with surgery alone for esophageal cancer; CALGB 9781. *J Clin Oncol*. 2008;**26**:1086–1092.
168. El-Rayes BF, Shields A, Zalupski M, et al. A phase II study of carboplatin and paclitaxel in esophageal cancer. *Ann Oncol*. 2004;**15**:960–965.
169. Ilson DH, Saltz L, Enzinger P, et al. Phase II trial of weekly irinotecan plus cisplatin in advanced esophageal cancer. *J Clin Oncol*. 1999;**17**:3270–3275.
172. Cunningham D, Starling N, Rao S, et al. Capecitabine and oxaliplatin for advanced esophagogastric cancer. *New Engl J Med*. 2008;**350**:36–46.
174. Bang YJ, van Cutsem E, Feyereislova A. Trastuzumab in combination with chemotherapy versus chemotherapy alpone for treatment of HER2-positive advanced gastric of gastrooesophageal junction cancer (ToGA): a phase 3, open-label randomized controlled trial. *Lancet*. 2010;**376**:687–697.
176. Shitara K, Bang Y-J, Iwasa S, et al. Trastuzumab deruxtecan in previousy treated HER2-positive gastric cancer. *N Engl J Med*. 2020;**382**:2419–2430.
177. Fuchs CS, Tomasek J, Yong CJ, et al. Ramucirumab monotherapy for previously treated advanced gastgric or gastro-esophageal junction adenocarcionoma (REGARD): an international randomised, multicenter, placebo-controlled, phase 3 trial. *Lancet*. 2014;**383**:31–39.
178. Wilke H, Muro K, Van Cutsem E, et al. Ramucirumab plus paclitaxel versus placebo plus paclitaxel in opatients with previously treated advanced gastric or gastro-oesophageal junction adenocarcinoma (RAINBOW): a double-blind randomized trial. *Lancet Oncol*. 2014;**15**:1224–1235.
181. Waddell T, Chau I, Cunningham D, et al. Epirubicin, oxaplliplatin and capecitabine with or without panitumumab for patients with previously untreated advanced oesophagogastric cancer (REAL3): a randomized, open-label phase 3 trial. *Lancet Oncol*. 2013;**14**:481–489.
183. Janjigian YY, Shitara K, Moehler M, et al. First-line nivolumab plus chemotherapy versus chemotherapy alone for advanced gastric, gatro-oesophageal junction and oesophageal adenocarcinoma. *Lancet*. 2021;**398**:27–40.
184. Kelly RJ, Adjani JA, Kuzdza J, et al. Adjuvant nivolumab in resected esophageal or gastroesophageal junction cancer. *N Engl J Med*. 2021;**384**:1191–1203.
186. Kato K, Sun J, Shah MA, et al. Pembrolizumab plus chemotherapy versus chemotherapy as first-line therapy in patients with advanced esophageal cancer: the phase 3 KEYNOTE-590 study. *Ann Oncol*. 2020;**31**(suppl 4):S142–S1215.
187. Janjigian YY, Kawazoe A, Yanez PE, et al. Pembrolizumab plus trastuzumab and chemotherapy for HER2+ metastatic gastric or gastroesophageal junction cancer: initial findings of the global phase 3 KEYNOTE-811 study. *J Clin Oncol*. 2021;**39**(suppl 15):4013.
191. Cunningham D, Allum WH, Stenning SP, et al. Perioperative chemotherapy versus surgery alone for resectable gastroesophageal cancer. *New Engl J Med*. 2006;**355**:11–20.
192. Salah-Eddin AB, Homann N, Paulijk C, et al. Perioperative chemotherapy with fluorouracil plus leucovorin, oxaliplatin, and docetaxel versus fluorouracil or capecitabine plus cisplatin and epirubicin for locally advanced, resectable gastric or gastro-oesophageal junction adenocarcinoma (FLOT4): a randomised, phase 2/3 trial. *Lancet*. 2019;**393**:1948–1957.
197. Cooper JS, Guo MD, Heskovic A, et al. Chemoradiotherapy of locally advanced esophageal cancer: long term follow-up of a prospective randomized trial (RTOC 85-01). *JAMA*. 1999;**281**:1623–1627.
199. Van Hagen P, Hulshof MC, van Lanschotg JJ, et al. Preoperative chemoradiotherapy for esophageal or junctional cancer. *New Engl J Med*. 2012;**366**:2074–2084.

86 Carcinoma of the stomach

Carl Schmidt, MD, FACS ■ Nour Daboul, MD ■ Carly Likar, PA-C ■ Joshua Weir, DO, MBA, MS

Overview

Gastric cancer is the fifth most common cancer and third most common cause of cancer-related death worldwide. Risk factors include chronic *Helicobacter pylori* infection, smoking, autoimmune gastritis, obesity, and other causes. Some countries with higher incidence have established screening programs but methodology and eligibility remain controversial. Despite knowledge of risk factors and screening for high-risk populations, identification of earlier stage potentially curable disease remains a challenge.

Multiple genetic mutations are involved in gastric cancer pathogenesis, and mutations in the cellular adhesion protein E-cadherin result in familial diffuse gastric cancer. Certain patterns of metastatic disease have been associated with particular molecular alterations. Increasing understanding of molecular pathways involved in gastric cancer allows efficacious use of targeted biologic therapies with cytotoxic chemotherapy in the advanced setting, such as trastuzumab in patients with gastric cancer and *HER2/neu* overexpression.

Surgical resection is the primary potentially curative therapy in those without metastatic disease. Type of resection, extent of lymphadenectomy, and use of laparoscopic or robotic surgery are variable emphasizing the need for best practice standards. Chemotherapy and radiation play an important role in the adjuvant setting. Choice and timing of these therapies require accurate staging by thorough evaluation with endoscopy, cross-sectional imaging, and in some cases endoscopic ultrasound (EUS) or positron emission tomography.

Palliative therapy is important for patients with symptoms in the metastatic setting and after recurrence since cure is not possible in either situation. Results of recent clinical trials are encouraging including hope that immunotherapy will add to the collective therapies available. Ultimately, most people diagnosed with gastric cancer in the world will die. Research is ongoing in all areas from epidemiology to screening to diagnosis to staging and therapy.

Incidence and epidemiology

The incidence of gastric cancer continues to decline particularly in Western nations due to several factors including improved hygiene, food standards, and possibly *Helicobacter pylori* suppression (NCCN 1-4). Despite this, it is the fifth most common cancer and third most common cause of cancer-related death. Gastric cancer occurs more frequently in China (accounting for 42% of cases worldwide), South America, Eastern Europe, Japan, and Korea, where it is the most common malignancy.[1] There are nearly one million cases of gastric cancer each year in the world and over 700,000 deaths.[2] There are no established screening programs for early detection in many countries, so the majority of gastric cancers present with advanced disease (positive lymph nodes or distant metastases) and have low chance for cure. In patients with advanced disease, poor performance status is a risk factor for worse outcomes.[3]

Risk factors and genetics

Environmental insults to the gastric mucosa may eventually lead to atrophic gastritis resulting in metaplasia, a precursor condition for some gastric cancers.[4] Other factors associated with increased risk include low serum ferritin levels, pernicious anemia, history of distal gastrectomy for peptic ulcer disease, and endemic *H. pylori* infection.[5–7] While some evidence is suggestive, it remains unknown whether eradicating *H. pylori* infection reduces the incidence of gastric cancer.[8] Behavioral associations with gastric cancer have long been thought to include dietary exposure to nitrates, nitrites, and bacterial or fungal contamination of food given decreasing incidence with the advent of refrigeration.[9] Studies have also documented increased incidence of proximal gastric cancer with obesity and a protective effect of physical activity on overall rates of gastric cancer.[10,11] Red meat consumption is associated with increased risk of gastric cancer based on multiple observational studies.[12,13] Some studies suggest a dose–response relationship between amount of red meat consumption and risk lending further support to this possibility. Consumption of fruit conversely may reduce the risk of gastric cancer.[14]

The majority of gastric cancers are sporadic, but familial clustering occurs in approximately 10%. Table 1 summarizes gastric cancer-predisposing syndromes.[15] Germline mutations account for only a small portion of these cases. Hereditary diffuse gastric cancer (HDGC) results from germline mutations of the E-cadherin gene (*CDH1*). E-cadherin mutation otherwise accounts for only a small percentage of families with a history of gastric cancer, approximately 1–3%. The E-cadherin gene is involved in cellular adhesion, and defects in this gene are associated with increased breast cancer risk and potentially colon cancer (data emerging).[16] Affected individuals with gastric cancer inherit one copy of the defective E-cadherin gene. Somatic mutation, deletion, or promoter methylation inactivates the other copy. Gastric cancers attributable to *CDH1* pathogenic mutations follow an autosomal dominant inheritance pattern with high penetrance. The lifetime risk of developing gastric cancer by age 80 in those patients with *CDH1* mutation is 67% for men and 83% for women, in addition to an earlier age of onset (average age between 38 and 40 years).[17]

Genetic counseling is important for people with suspected HDGC. If the diagnosis is established, those affected by HDGC face the decision whether to undergo prophylactic, or risk-reducing, total gastrectomy (without extended lymphadenectomy). Timing of operation is variable and greatly influenced by physical and psychosocial factors as well as degree of penetrance and age range of cancer onset in each family. Multifocal early gastric cancers are nearly always found in the resected specimens after prophylactic gastrectomy.[18] In those patients who carry *CDH1* pathogenic mutations and nonetheless decline prophylactic total gastrectomy, frequent surveillance is encouraged with upper endoscopy and multiple random biopsies. There is a paucity of long-term outcome data for prophylactic gastrectomy. Worster and colleagues studied

Holland-Frei Cancer Medicine, Tenth Edition. Edited by Robert C. Bast, John C. Byrd, Carlo M. Croce, Ernest Hawk, Fadlo R. Khuri, Raphael E. Pollock, Apostolia M. Tsimberidou, Christopher G. Willett, and Cheryl L. Willman.
© 2023 John Wiley & Sons, Inc. Published 2023 by John Wiley & Sons, Inc.

Table 1 Gastric cancer-predisposing syndromes.[a]

Syndrome	Genes	Cases associated with mutation (%)	Inheritance	Gastric cancer risk
Hereditary diffuse gastric cancer syndrome	CDH1	45	Autosomal dominant	56–70
Gastric adenocarcinoma and proximal polyposis syndrome	Implicated gene unknown	Not determined	Autosomal dominant	Not determined
Hereditary nonpolyposis colon cancer	MLH1, MSH2, MSH6, PMS2	MLH1 ~60 MLH2 ~30 others ~10	Autosomal dominant	2–30
Peutz-Jeghers syndrome	STK11	70	Autosomal dominant	29
Juvenile polyposis	SMAD4, BMPR1A	SMAD4 4-20 BMPR1A 20-25	Autosomal dominant	21
Familial breast cancer	BRCA1, BRCA2	—	Autosomal dominant	5.5 2.6
Li-Fraumeni syndrome	TP53	70	Autosomal dominant	3.1–4.9
Familial adenomatous polyposis	APC	≤90	Autosomal dominant	2.1–4.2
MYH-associated polyposis	MYH	~99	Autosomal recessive	Very low

The rare familial intestinal gastric cancer, ataxia telangiectasia, and xeroderma pigmentosum are not included in this table.
[a]Source: Setia et al.[15]

the impact of prophylactic total gastrectomy on health-related quality of life (HRQOL).[19] The study sample size was small comparing HRQOL for 32 patients after total gastrectomy to 28 patients at risk for HDGC who did not undergo total gastrectomy. While physical and mental function returned to baseline by 12 months after operation, symptoms persist specifically loose stools (70%), fatigue (63%), discomfort when eating (81%), reflux (63%), eating restrictions (45%), and body image (44%).

Gastric adenomatous polyps occur in approximately 10% of patients with familial adenomatous polyposis (FAP).[20,21] Whereas fundic gastric polyps are usually hamartomas, foveolar dysplasia, and invasive adenocarcinoma are possible. The lifetime risk of gastric cancer in patients with FAP approaches 0.6%. Hereditary nonpolyposis colorectal cancer (HNPCC), or Lynch Syndrome, is a genetic disorder characterized by germline mutations in a group of mismatch repair genes including MSH2, MLH1, MSH6, PMS2, and EPCAM. Defects in these genes result in genomic (microsatellite) instability. Although colorectal and endometrial cancers are the most common manifestations of HNPCC, gastric carcinoma occurs in up to 13%. This risk may be much lower in North American and Western European populations than in parts of Asia.[22] Other hereditary autosomal dominant conditions associated with an increased risk of gastric cancer include juvenile polyposis syndrome (JPS) and Peutz-Jeghers syndrome (PJS). One typical feature of JPS is multiple juvenile polyps throughout the gastrointestinal tract, and patients with JPS and SMAD4 pathogenic mutations have a risk of gastric cancer up to 30%. PJS includes characteristic hamartomatous polyps of the gastrointestinal tract and mucocutaneous pigmentation and arises from mutations in the STK11 gene. It carries a 29% risk of developing gastric cancer, among others. Of the two main types of gastric cancer, diffuse and intestinal, the intestinal subtype is associated with HNPCC, FAP, and PJS. The diffuse subtype is a hallmark of the HDGC syndrome.[23]

> **Box 1**
>
> - Gastric cancer is the third leading cause of cancer-related death worldwide
> - Risk factors include autoimmune gastritis, H. pylori infection, and obesity
> - Germline mutations in the CDH1 (E-cadherin) gene are associated with hereditary diffuse gastric cancer

Pathology

Adenocarcinoma is the dominant histology in gastric cancer. The Lauren and World Health Organization (WHO) classifications are the two major systems used. The Lauren's system classifies cancer as intestinal, diffuse, or mixed.[24] The simplicity of this system has resulted in widespread use. Intestinal-type gastric cancer, also called epidemic-type gastric cancer, features a retained glandular structure and cellular polarity. Grossly, it usually has a sharp margin. It arises from the gastric mucosa and is associated with chronic gastritis, gastric atrophy, and intestinal metaplasia. The diffuse-type histology is associated with an invasive growth pattern. Scattered clusters of uniform-sized malignant cells frequently infiltrate the submucosa with little glandular formation and mucin production is common (Figure 1).

Studies of gastrectomy specimens obtained from patients without clinical disease have shown early diffuse-type gastric cancer arising below normal-appearing epithelium.[18] Tumor cells in this type appear to arise from the superficial layer of the lamina propria. An infiltrative growth pattern in diffuse-type gastric cancer often results in the absence of a mass. The cancer may be difficult to identify using endoscopy, but thickened gastric folds and a difficult to distend stomach are hallmarks of diffuse gastric cancer. Malignant cells can infiltrate well beyond the apparent tumor margin. In advanced cases, this leads to the condition known as linitis plastic ("leather-bottle-like stomach") characterized by involvement of the entire stomach, rapid progression, resistance to therapy, and poor prognosis.

Pathogenesis and natural history

Molecular alterations

Multiple molecular alterations are important in the pathogenesis of gastric cancer. Epigenetic phenomena likely involved in early carcinogenesis include hypermethylation of promoter regions for genes including CDH1, hMLH1, and p16.[25–31] Further, microsatellite instability (MSI) caused by mutations in deoxyribonucleic acid (DNA) repair genes has been reported in up to 39% of gastric cancers.[32] Tumor suppressor genes such as p53, APC, MCC, and DCC are also mutated in gastric cancer, and the incidence often varies with histology and stage.[33–35]

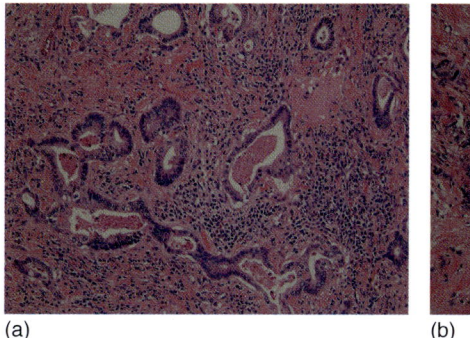

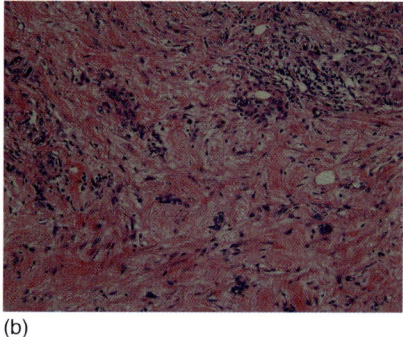

Figure 1 Histologic sections from intestinal (a) and diffuse (b) type gastric cancers.

Loss of normal cellular adhesion is an important feature of human cancer development and prevalent in genetic alterations of gastric cancer. Aberrant cellular adhesion with a pattern of infiltrative growth by a small cluster of or single tumor cells characterizes diffuse-type gastric cancer. The cadherin–catenin complex at the cell surface plays a critical role in cell adhesion and polarity. Up to 90% of gastric cancers have an abnormality in at least one component of the complex including E-cadherin, α-, and γ-catenin.[36,37] The *CD44* transmembrane glycoprotein, expressed in 31–72% of gastric cancers, may modulate invasion and metastasis.[38]

Similar to other adenocarcinomas, alterations in cellular signaling pathways occur in gastric cancer and provide potential targets for biologic therapies. *HER2/neu*, a tyrosine kinase receptor in the *erbB* family, is overexpressed in 10–38% of gastric cancers. *HER2/neu* expression is associated with intestinal-type distal cancer and worse prognosis.[34,39] Expression of other cellular receptors in gastric cancer correlates with oncogenic behavior, such as associations between the transmembrane receptor *EGFR* (epidermal growth factor receptor) with invasion and *c-Met* with peritoneal metastasis.[40] Angiogenesis appears essential for growth of gastric cancer and other solid tumors, and increased angiogenesis in gastric tumor specimens portends an unfavorable prognosis.[41] *VEGF* (vascular endothelial growth factor) and *bFGF* (basic fibroblast growth factor) are major regulators of angiogenesis, have prognostic value, and are potential targets for antiangiogenic therapy in patients with gastric cancer.[42,43] Expression of multiple transcription factors by gastric cancer cells, such as *Sp1* and *mTOR* promote abnormal cell growth, survival, and angiogenesis.[44,45]

Progression and patterns of metastasis

Gastric cancer may invade adjacent organs by direct extension including liver, diaphragm, pancreas, spleen, and colon (or its mesentery). Gastric cancers have a high tendency to spread through the lymphatic system to regional and distant nodes. The liver is a common site for hematogenous metastatic disease. Peritoneal metastatic disease is also common and may result in abdominal pain, bowel obstruction, cachexia, or all three. Japanese investigators have noted that histology and patient age may affect the pattern of spread of gastric cancer. In an autopsy study of 173 cases, they found diffuse histology to be associated with peritoneal metastasis and intestinal histology to be associated with hepatic metastasis.[46] They also found peritoneal metastasis to be more common in younger patients. In another study, case records of 216 patients with synchronous peritoneal or hepatic metastasis found at surgical exploration more commonly had poorly differentiated histology associated with peritoneal metastases and well to moderately differentiated histology associated with hepatic metastases.[47]

On a molecular level, expression of *VEGF* and its receptor *KDR* has been associated with liver metastasis.[41,48] Expression of *VEGF-C*, which can cause neogenesis of lymphatic vessels, is associated with lymph node metastasis.[49,50] In addition, dysregulation of cellular adhesion is likely central to the development of peritoneal metastasis. *CD44H* has been linked with increased gastric cancer cell adhesion to mesothelial cells and increased peritoneal metastasis in animal models.[51] As stated, *C-met* amplification increases the risk of peritoneal metastasis.[40,52] Further translational research of the molecular biology of metastasis may improve our ability to predict sites of failure and refine therapeutic strategies.

> **BOX 2**
>
> - Molecular alterations of many genes and cellular pathways promote the pathogenesis of gastric cancer including methylation of promoters, microsatellite instability, cellular adhesion, growth factors, and angiogenesis
> - Metastatic involvement of regional lymph nodes is very common
> - Peritoneal surfaces and liver are other common sites of metastasis

Screening

Several countries with a high incidence of gastric cancer, including Japan, Korea, Venezuela, and Chile, have large-scale screening programs. Available screening tests include, among others, upper gastrointestinal endoscopy and radiologic studies using oral contrast agents like barium. The method for most efficacious screening remains controversial, and there is no uniformity in terms of recommended age, interval, or type of screening exam. Comparisons between screening methods by large controlled trials are lacking. Screening of asymptomatic people in countries with lower risk of gastric cancer is generally not feasible or cost-effective.

It is important to mention that symptoms of gastric cancer are often nonspecific, leading to potential delay in diagnosis. This is because both stomach and abdominal cavity are large and distensible. Early symptoms, such as vague discomfort, episodic nausea/vomiting, or anorexia are common in patients without cancer and have a long differential diagnosis. Thus, physicians may not attribute such symptoms to gastric cancer for many months. It is common for patients to undergo several months of therapy for presumptive peptic ulcer disease prior to a diagnosis of gastric cancer. As such, we need research to develop better methods of early detection even in countries with lower incidence.

Diagnosis

Common symptoms of gastric cancer at diagnosis include abdominal pain and weight loss. Although anemia is also a frequent finding, overt upper gastrointestinal bleeding is much less common. Dysphagia may occur predominantly in patients with proximal cancer whereas nausea and vomiting are more common in patients with nonproximal cancer. Early satiety can be especially prominent in patients with linitis plastica. Abnormal physical examination findings often indicate advanced disease, such as a palpable epigastric mass, which may indicate a large locally advanced tumor. Jaundice usually indicates hepatic metastasis or metastatic lymphadenopathy in the porta hepatis.

Appropriate clinical staging of gastric cancer requires a stepwise approach. Potentially helpful laboratory studies include complete blood count, electrolytes, blood urea nitrogen, creatinine, alkaline phosphatase, transaminases, and bilirubin. Evaluation of tumor markers CEA, CA19-9, and CA125 may be considered. At the time of referral to surgeon or oncologist, upper endoscopy has usually already made the diagnosis. The surgeon must review the endoscopy report and images for tumor size and location, especially for gastroesophageal junction (GEJ) tumors, often classified as distal esophageal cancers. Pathologic analysis of the initial diagnostic biopsy should specify intestinal or diffuse subtype, grade, and level of invasion when feasible. In cases of proven or suspected metastatic disease, molecular testing for *HER2/neu*, MSI, and programmed death-ligand 1 (PD-L1) expression are important due to implications for therapy options.

Computed tomography (CT) scan of the chest, abdomen, and pelvis provides further information about the primary tumor, potentially malignant lymphadenopathy, or metastatic disease. The finding of even a small amount of ascites may indicate peritoneal disease. EUS assesses T and N stage, however, overall accuracy is operator dependent and may be no better than 50–70%.[53] EUS-guided fine needle biopsy of suspicious perigastric nodes or left liver masses for cytology contributes to pretherapy clinical staging in some cases. EUS is not required when CT scan findings are highly suggestive of advanced cancer, such as bulky lymphadenopathy, ascites, or peritoneal carcinomatosis. EUS is quite useful for assessment of small masses amenable to endoscopic mucosal resection (EMR) or early-stage cancers for which operation without neoadjuvant therapy is considered. The role of 18-fluorodeoxyglucose positron emission tomography (FDG-PET) for gastric cancer is unclear. PET is potentially useful for evaluating response to therapy.[54] Combined CT/FDG-PET improves accuracy of clinical-stage compared to either CT or FDG-PET alone.[55] Staging laparoscopy is considered essential for complete staging of gastric cancers by many high volume centers who advocate its use before therapy.[56] Laparoscopy upstages 20–25% of patients, primarily through detection of peritoneal metastases not seen on CT scan.[57–59]

TNM stage classification

The most recent American Joint Committee on Cancer Staging Manual, 8th edition (Springer, New York 2017) has three variations for gastric cancer classification based on either clinical stage, pathologic stage, or postneoadjuvant therapy stage. Table 2 represents current pathologic stage groups for patients without metastatic disease. Of note, pathologic stage IV requires presence of metastatic (distant) disease whereas clinical-stage IVA denotes patients with primary gastric tumors directly invading adjacent structures or organs (T4b) such as spleen, colon, diaphragm, pancreas, abdominal wall, adrenal gland, kidney or small intestine.

Table 2 AJCC pathologic stage grouping for gastric cancer without distant metastatic disease.

T stage	Nodal stage			
	N0	N1	N2	N3a/N3b
Tis	0			
T1a/b	IA	IB	IIA	IIB/IIB
T2	IB	IIA	IIB	IIIA/IIIB
T3	IIA	IIB	IIIA	IIIB/IIIC
T4a	IIB	IIIA	IIIA	IIIB/III
T4b	IIIA	IIIB	IIIB	IIIC/IIIC

Invasion into adjacent duodenum or esophagus is not classified stage T4b in most cases. The 8th edition also further clarifies tumors of the GEJ. Specifically, tumors within the gastric cardia not involving the GEJ use gastric cancer staging as do tumors involving the GEJ with an epicenter more than 2 cm into the proximal stomach. Tumors involving the GEJ with an epicenter less than 2 cm into the proximal stomach use staging for esophageal cancer.

The following definitions classify T and N stage:

- Tis—intraepithelial tumor with no invasion into lamina propria, high-grade dysplasia
- T1a—tumor invades lamina propria or muscularis mucosae
- T1b—tumor invades submucosa
- T2—tumor invades muscularis propria
- T3—tumor penetrates subserosal connective tissue without serosal invasion
- T4a—tumor invades serosa
- T4b—tumor invades adjacent organ or structure

- N1—regional nodal metastases, 1–2 nodes
- N2—regional nodal metastases, 3–6 nodes
- N3a—regional nodal metastases, 7–15 nodes
- N3b—regional nodal metastases, 16 or more nodes

> **Box 3**
> - Early gastric cancer may be detected by screening in countries with such programs
> - Possible symptoms of gastric cancer include abdominal pain, bleeding, dysphagia, nausea, anorexia, weight loss, and early satiety
> - Clinical staging is based on upper endoscopy and cross-sectional imaging of the chest, abdomen, and pelvis (typically CT scan)
> - Other potentially useful staging studies include laparoscopy, EUS, and PET

Multidisciplinary care

For patients with small tumors and low histologic grade, EMR is gaining acceptance as the primary method for local therapy. Such therapy is predicated on these tumors having a very low incidence of node-positive disease.[60] The incidence of nodal positivity with T1 tumors is approximately 10%, and other features of the primary tumor delineate patients with even lower risk. Tumors confined to the mucosa have a 1–3% incidence of nodal positivity versus a tumor with submucosal invasion with an incidence of up to 15%.[61] Other factors which increase the incidence of nodal disease include poor differentiation, signet-ring cells, lymphatic invasion, and tumor size greater than 2 cm.[62] It is therefore reasonable to consider EMR for patients with small, well-differentiated tumors confined to the mucosa. However, specialists at some centers propose expanded criteria for use of newer techniques like endoscopic submucosal dissection (ESD).[63] Removal of larger even ulcerated masses is feasible by experienced endoscopists at higher volume centers. In our opinion, this more aggressive approach yet requires careful histological evaluation of the resected specimen. Pathologic analysis of any gastric cancer specimen removed by EMR or ESD must include assessment of lymphovascular invasion, grade, depth of tumor invasion, and margin status. Current National Comprehensive Cancer Network (NCCN) guidelines suggest EMR is appropriate for tumors limited to T1a (mucosal) depth of invasion but that surgical resection is the standard of care for T1b or greater disease.[64]

Surgery

The choice of operation for gastric cancer depends on tumor location, histologic type, and disease stage. Gastrectomy is the most widely used approach for invasive gastric cancer, and the most common techniques are total gastrectomy, distal subtotal, and proximal subtotal gastrectomy. Segmental resection is less common for invasive gastric cancer but is very common and appropriate for other gastric malignancies such as gastrointestinal stromal tumors. Prospective and randomized studies reveal no survival advantage of total gastrectomy for tumors of the distal stomach compared to distal subtotal gastrectomy when resection has adequate margins. Both techniques are associated with similar rates of mortality (1–3%), complications, and 5-year survival (around 60%).[65,66] In most series, the quality of life after subtotal gastrectomy is superior to that after total gastrectomy.[67,68]

Tumors of the proximal stomach and GEJ generally require more complex resection and reconstruction. Siewert's classification is very useful and commonly used to describe GEJ tumors.[69,70]:

- Type I: carcinoma of the distal esophagus and may infiltrate the GEJ from above
- Type II: true carcinoma of the cardia arising at the GEJ within 1 cm above and 2 cm below
- Type III: subcardial gastric carcinoma infiltrating the GEJ and distal esophagus from below

In patients with an advanced tumor involving the GEJ, site of origin (esophagus or stomach) may be unclear. Patients with type I tumors are often treated as distal esophagus cancers using preoperative therapy followed by surgical resection with esophagogastrectomy and reconstruction using gastric conduit with anastomosis in the neck or chest. Either total gastrectomy or proximal subtotal gastrectomy, often through a transabdominal approach depending on the local extent of the tumor, is best for Type II and III tumors.[71,72] Total gastrectomy is generally favored in the United States over proximal gastrectomy because reflux esophagitis is rare after Roux-en-Y esophagojejunostomy reconstruction compared to roughly one-third of patients who will have significant reflux after proximal subtotal resection.[67,73,74] Further, proximal subtotal gastrectomy may fail to remove enough nodal tissue from the lesser curvature, a common site of nodal metastasis. Some surgeons continue to advocate for proximal subtotal gastrectomy.[72]

The extent of lymph node dissection is one of the most controversial surgical topics in the management of gastric cancer. Radical lymph node dissection involves removal of lymph nodes beyond the usual field of gastrectomy. The Japanese Gastric Cancer Association defines extent of lymph node dissection using the designation "D."[75] Generally, D1 dissection includes perigastric lymph nodes. D2 dissection extends the lymphadenectomy to include nodes along the hepatic, left gastric, celiac, and splenic arteries (Figure 2). D3 dissection includes nodes along the porta hepatis and in the retropancreatic and periaortic regions.

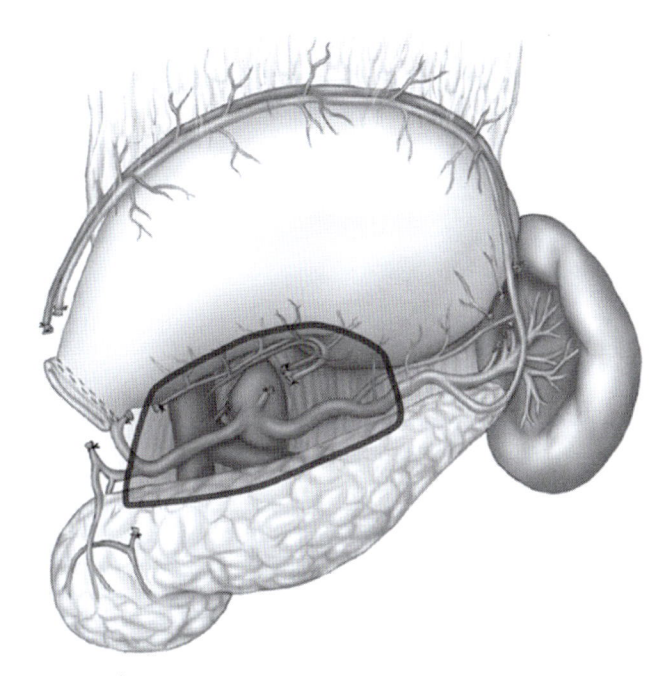

Figure 2 The major vasculature in the vicinity of the stomach is depicted. The shaded portion shows the area most important for modified D2 lymphadenectomy including celiac, hepatic, left gastric, and splenic artery lymph nodes.

The largest prospective study examining the potential benefit of extended lymphadenectomy is the Dutch D1D2 lymphadenectomy trial, which randomized more than 1000 patients (711 treated with curative intent) to D1 or D2 lymphadenectomy in the setting of gastrectomy for cancer, with surgical quality carefully controlled.[76,77] Operative morbidity and mortality rates were both significantly greater in the D2 group than in the D1 group (43% and 10%, respectively vs 25% and 4%). However, the increase in mortality rate was associated with either male patients undergoing D2 dissection or patients undergoing splenectomy and distal pancreatectomy for complete nodal dissection. Patients who underwent D2 dissection with preservation of the spleen/tail of the pancreas had operative mortality similar to that of patients who underwent D1 dissection. After median follow-up of 15.2 years, the D2 lymphadenectomy group had a higher disease-specific survival rate compared to the D1 group and lower rates of local (12% vs 22%) and regional (13% vs 19%) recurrence.[78]

A trial from the Italian Gastric Cancer Study Group evaluated the role of modified organ-preserving D2 lymphadenectomy.[79] Patients ($n = 267$) with potentially curable gastric cancer underwent randomization (intraoperative) to D1 or D2 dissection. Operation included partial pancreatectomy or splenectomy if suspected local invasion. Morbidity and mortality were 12% and 3%, respectively for the D1 group and 18% and 2% for the D2 group. Five-year disease-specific survival rates were 71% and 73% for the D1 and D2 groups; subgroup analysis revealed that in patients with node-positive disease the 5-year rate was 61% in the D2 group versus 46% in the D1 group. Further, in patients with T-stage 2–4 and positive lymph nodes, the 5-year survival was 59% in the D2 arm versus 38% in the D1 arm (Figure 3). The NCCN gastric cancer panel recommends D2 lymphadenectomy sparing distal pancreas and spleen with goal of pathologic examination of at least 16 nodes.[64]

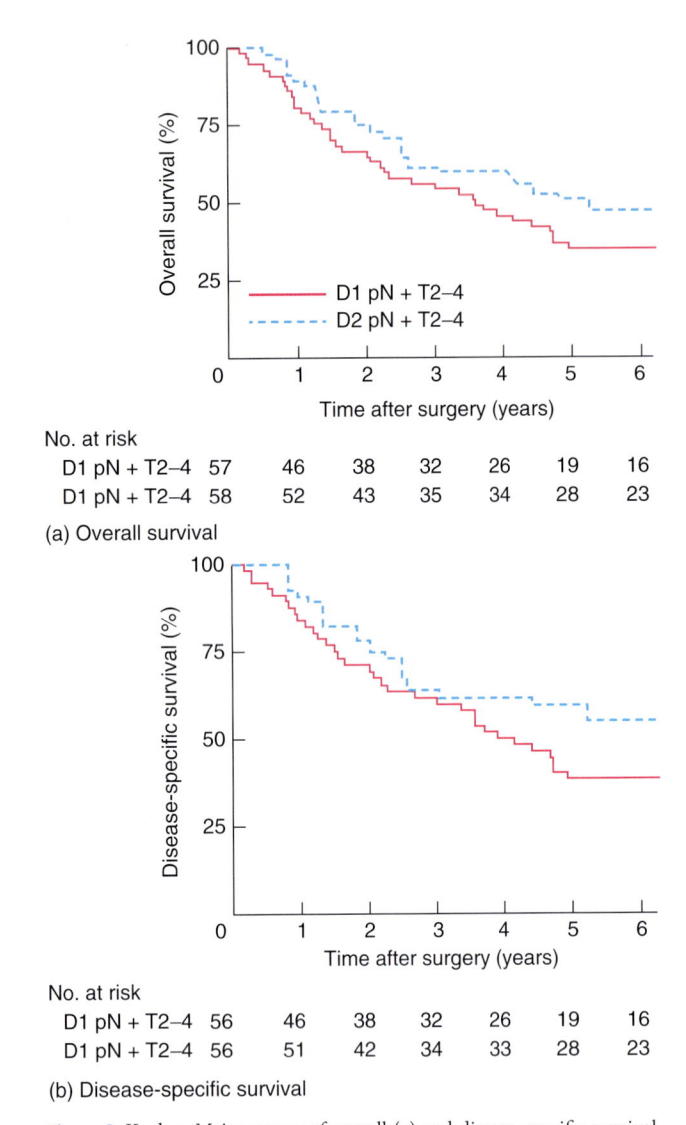

Figure 3 Kaplan–Meier curves of overall (a) and disease-specific survival (b) for patients with pathologic T2–4 and node-positive disease from the Italian Gastric Cancer Study Group D1D2 lymphadenectomy trial.[79] Source: Degiuli et al.[79]

achieving a margin negative resection may when primary tumor or grossly involved nodes invade. Investigators from Memorial Sloan-Kettering Cancer Center removed at least one additional organ about one-third of the time in a series of 800 patients who underwent R0 resection for gastric cancer over 15 years.[82,83] The operative mortality rate was 4% in these patients, similar to that reported in the Dutch trial for limited dissection and far lower than that for D2 dissection with adjacent organ resection. Interestingly, the likelihood of actual adjacent organ invasion was low (14%) after final pathological examination. The 5-year survival rate in these patients was 32% compared to 50% in patients who did not require multivisceral resection. These data support application of multivisceral resection when required to achieve R0 resection at centers where the operative mortality rate is low.

Minimally invasive approaches to the conduct of subtotal or total gastrectomy have increased in recent years using laparoscopy, computer-aided (robotic) surgery, or hybrid procedures. There are multiple retrospective studies comparing them, which suggest short and long-term patient outcomes are improved or not adversely affected by minimally invasive techniques.[84,85] Operating time and cost may increase with these approaches early in the surgeon's learning curve, offset by cost savings if shorter length of stay and more rapid overall recovery results. All studies without randomization are subject to patient selection bias and therefore require caution when interpreting. The Korean Laparoendoscopic Gastrointestinal Surgery Study (KLASS) Phase III multicenter randomized-controlled trial is underway comparing laparoscopic or open distal gastrectomy with D2 lymphadenectomy for cT2-T4a, N0-1 nonmetastatic gastric cancer. The primary endpoint is 3-year disease-free survival. An early report encouragingly shows less blood loss, less postoperative pain, lower complication rate, and shorter hospital stay in the laparoscopic group.[86] The CLASS-01 trial was a similarly designed study from 14 hospitals in China that randomized over 1000 patients to open or laparoscopic distal gastrectomy for cT2-T4a nonproximal gastric cancers without "bulky" nodes or metastatic disease. The 3-year disease-free survival rates were 77.8% and 76.5%, respectively with no difference in overall survival.[87]

> **Box 4**
>
> - Endoscopic mucosal resection (EMR) is considered for T1a gastric cancers without adverse pathologic features
> - Surgical resection is typically partial or total gastrectomy with upper abdominal (D2) lymphadenectomy
> - Removal of other organs, when needed due to local invasion, is appropriate
> - Use of the laparoscopic approach is safe and undergoing further study

Linitis plastica is an extremely virulent form of gastric cancer considered incurable by many. Some feel that patients with linitis plastica should never undergo gastrectomy since at best the 5-year survival is less than 10%.[80] One approach to patients with linitis plastica is to evaluate with staging laparoscopy and, in the absence of metastatic disease, treat first with neoadjuvant therapy in the hopes of selecting patients who do not develop metastatic disease for eventual gastrectomy. If a patient with linitis plastica has a positive margin of resection after operation, one should be cautious as to whether this deserves consideration or specific therapy given that isolated local recurrence is uncommon and rarely impacts survival compared to metastatic disease.

Evidence from the US Gastric Cancer Collaborative suggests the traditional necessity of wide >5 cm proximal margins for resection of distal cancers may not be necessary.[81] In their retrospective cohort study combining data from seven academic medical centers, the proximal margin distance was not associated with overall survival. Rather, T and N-stage were the primary associated factors, and a 3 cm margin was adequate in most patients. Routine lymphadenectomy does not require multivisceral organ resection, but

Radiation oncology

Radiation therapy is beneficial in the preoperative and postoperative settings for patients with resectable gastric cancer. Use of radiation in the postoperative setting is established based on results from the landmark Intergroup 0116 (INT 0116) trial.[88] Patients with moderate to high risk of locoregional failure (n = 556) were randomized to surgery followed by postoperative chemotherapy plus chemoradiation or surgery alone. Patients in the experimental arm received concurrent leucovorin and fluorouracil with external beam radiation to a dose of 45 Gray (Gy). The majority of patients had T3 or T4 tumors (69%) and node-positive disease (85%). At a median follow-up of five years, median survival for chemoradiation was 36 months compared to 27 months for surgery alone. Chemoradiation improved relapse-free survival (48% vs 31%) and local recurrence (19% vs 29%). There were increased gastrointestinal (33% grade 3/4) and hematologic (54% grade 3/4) side effects in the chemoradiation group, deemed acceptable given the magnitude of survival improvement. After 10 years of follow-up, survival remained improved in the chemoradiation group.[89] Comparison of adjuvant chemoradiation to chemotherapy alone by a meta-analysis of six trials found higher rate of disease-free survival and lower rate of local recurrence favoring chemoradiation.[90] Adjuvant chemoradiation remains the standard of care in patients with T3/T4 or node-positive gastric cancer treated first by potentially curative surgical resection.

Uncertainty remains on the value of preoperative radiation when incorporated into a neoadjuvant treatment approach for resectable gastric cancer. Some studies show sequential chemotherapy followed by chemoradiation and surgery is associated with favorable rates of tumor response and margin-negative resection. The Phase II RTOG 9904 study evaluated preoperative chemotherapy with fluorouracil, leucovorin, and cisplatin followed by concurrent chemoradiation with fluorouracil and paclitaxel. The pathologic complete response rate was 26% and R0 resection rate 77%.[91] Other studies have not shown an advantage to adding radiation to chemotherapy. The randomized Phase III CRITICS trial compared perioperative chemotherapy with preoperative chemotherapy followed by postoperative chemoradiation in patients with resectable gastric cancer. Patients in the chemotherapy arm received three preoperative and three postoperative cycles of modified epirubicin, capecitabine, and either cisplatin or oxaliplatin. The other group received preoperative chemotherapy and postoperative radiation of 45 Gy with capecitabine and cisplatin. Median survival was 43 and 37 months respectively, as such addition of radiation to perioperative chemotherapy did not improve the primary outcome. Poor patient compliance with postoperative treatment occurred in both treatment groups emphasizing the importance of optimal preoperative treatment.[92]

For radiation planning if intended prior to operation, diagnostic studies (EUS, EGD, CT, and PET/CT) delineate tumor and pertinent nodal volumes. Coverage of nodal areas is based on clinical circumstances and risk of toxicities. Relative risk of nodal metastases is dependent on site of origin, width, and depth of invasion. For postoperative planning, pretreatment diagnostic studies and possible use of fiducials, surgical clips or staple lines may identify tumor bed, anastomoses, duodenal stump, and pertinent nodal groups. Treatment to the remaining stomach or not is based on normal tissue tolerances and perceived risk for local relapse within stomach.

CT simulation and conformal planning are standard. Intensity-modulated radiation therapy (IMRT) is for clinical settings where dose to organs at risk can be reduced to limit toxicities. Immobilization devices allow reproducibility with patient setup. Planning with 4D-CT or other motion management is appropriate when organ motion is significant. Patients should avoid heavy meals for 3 h before simulation or treatment. Target volumes for tumors originating in the proximal one-third/fundus/cardia should encompass a 3–5 cm margin of the distal esophagus and include nodal areas at risk (perigastric, celiac, left gastric artery, splenic artery, splenic hilar, hepatic artery, and porta hepatic lymph nodes).[93] Target volumes for tumors originating in the middle one-third/body of stomach should include the aforementioned nodal areas at risk with the addition of suprapyloric, subpyloric, and pancreaticoduodenal lymph nodes. Target volumes for tumors originating from the distal one-third/antrum/pylorus should include the nodal areas at risk and a 3–5 cm margin of duodenum or duodenal stump. Dosing with radiation typically is in the range of 45–50 Gy with higher doses considered in cases of positive surgical margins.

Medical oncology

Preoperative chemotherapy

The Medical Research Council Adjuvant Gastric Infusional Chemotherapy (MAGIC) trial changed the landscape of treatment options for patients with gastric cancer.[94] This randomized Phase III trial compared surgery alone to surgery with three cycles of both preoperative and postoperative epirubicin, cisplatin, and 5-FU (ECF) chemotherapy. Among 503 patients accrued, ECF toxicity was manageable and the rates of postoperative morbidity and mortality were similar in the surgery alone and ECF groups. The resected tumors were smaller (3 vs 5 cm) with less advanced T and N stages in the ECF group. Most important, after median follow-up of four years, the ECF group had significantly better 5-year overall survival (36% vs 23%) and disease-free survival. This trial clearly established perioperative chemotherapy as a viable option for patients and, with the INT 0116 trial, that surgery alone is inadequate therapy for most nonmetastatic gastric cancers.

In 2017, the FLOT4 trial reported better overall survival using perioperative FLOT (four cycles of docetaxel, oxaliplatin, leucovorin, and fluorouracil before and after operation) compared to ECF/ECX (three cycles of epirubicin and cisplatin with either fluorouracil infusion or capecitabine orally) for patients with nonmetastatic ≥cT2 or cN+ gastric or GEJ cancer. Specifically, overall survival in the FLOT group was a median 50 months compared to 35 months for ECF/ECX; serious adverse events were similar at 27% for both groups.[95] Importantly, a higher proportion of people in the ECF/ECX group (13%) did not proceed to potentially curative surgery compared to the FLOT group (6%). While 90% or more patients completed all cycles of preoperative chemotherapy, less than half of patients in both groups completed all postoperative cycles of chemotherapy. This is similar to the MAGIC trial in which only 42% of patients in the perioperative chemotherapy group completed all cycles. Generally, oxaliplatin is now preferred over cisplatin due to lower toxicity, and FOLFOX (fluorouracil and oxaliplatin) is the preferred perioperative regimen for most patients.

The French Action Clinique Coordonnées en Cancérologie Digestive (ACCORD-07) study confirmed the use of preoperative chemotherapy for patients with GEJ cancers despite closing prematurely due to low enrollment.[96] A total of 224 patients with adenocarcinoma of the lower esophagus, GEJ, or stomach (25%) were randomized to 2–3 cycles of 5-FU/cisplatin followed by surgery followed by 3–4 cycles of the same chemotherapy versus surgery alone. The median follow-up was 5.7 years. Only 50% of patients received postoperative chemotherapy. Five-year survival rates were 38 % in the chemotherapy/surgery group versus 24% in the surgery alone group. In contrast, a study by the European Organization for Research and Treatment of Cancer (EORTC) randomized patients with locally advanced adenocarcinoma of the stomach or GEJ to preoperative chemotherapy with cisplatin, leucovorin, and 5-FU followed by surgery or surgery alone. This trial did not find a survival difference between these two strategies but was possibly underpowered due to poor accrual.[97]

Postoperative adjuvant chemotherapy

As stated, the INT 0116 trial established use of postoperative chemoradiation in patients with resected nonmetastatic gastric cancer. The MAGIC and FLOT trials further established use of the perioperative chemotherapy approach. The logical next question is which approach is best? The Adjuvant Chemoradiation Therapy in Stomach Cancer (ARTIST) trial compared postoperative treatment with chemotherapy versus chemoradiation in 459 patients after potentially curative resection of gastric cancer. Margin negative (R0) resection and D2 lymphadenectomy were required.[98] Patients were treated after operation with either six cycles of capecitabine and cisplatin or the same regimen for four cycles with five weeks of chemoradiation between cycles 2 and 3 (45 Gy with continuous capecitabine). Radiation targeted tumor bed, anastomosis, duodenal stump, regional nodes, and 2 cm beyond proximal and distal margins. Estimated 3-year disease-free survival rates were similar in both arms at 78.2% after chemoradiation and 74.2% after chemotherapy. Locoregional recurrence was also similar in both groups. Another study in node-positive patients found adding postoperative radiation to postoperative chemotherapy with S1 and oxaliplatin did not improve outcomes.[99] As both studies mandated D2 lymphadenectomy, it remains advisable to consider postoperative radiation as a component of overall adjuvant therapy if a patient has less than D2 lymph node dissection.

There are numerous other trials of systemic chemotherapy for gastric cancer in the adjuvant setting. Many early trials were underpowered, included improper control groups or used suboptimal methodology. These limitations along with heterogeneous inclusion criteria rendered much of their results unreproducible.[100] As such, the INT 0116, MAGIC, and FLOT trials define the most accepted standards of care for adjuvant therapy benefitting patients with nonmetastatic, T2-4, or node-positive gastric cancers. There is no established benefit for any adjuvant therapy in the setting of superficial (T1) or node-negative gastric cancer.

In Asian countries, the oral 5-FU prodrug S-1 shows promising results in the adjuvant setting. Investigators in one study randomly assigned 1059 patients with stage II or III gastric cancer after R0 gastrectomy and D2 or higher lymphadenectomy to surgery alone or surgery and postoperative S-1.[101] The 3-year survival rates were 80.1% in the S-1 group and 70.1% in the surgery alone group. The updated analysis after five years demonstrated 5-year survival of 71.7% in the S-1 group and 61.1% in the surgery-alone group. The safety profile of S-1 differs between Western and Asian patients due to differences in pharmacokinetics, and S-1 is currently not available in the United States.

Integration of multimodal care

Surgery is the cornerstone of potentially curative therapy for localized gastric cancer. Adjuvant therapy definitively improves the rate of cure of surgical resection alone for nonmetastatic gastric cancers other than very early stage (T1N0). Regardless of patient population, tumor location, or extent of lymph node dissection, surgery alone is not adequate for patients with more than early gastric cancer who are fit for adjuvant therapy. A direct comparison across studies is not advisable due to differences in study design, patient population, proportion of patients with node-positive disease, and extent of node dissection. However, it is interesting to note the magnitude of survival benefit for extended lymph node dissection and adjuvant therapy strategies are similar, typically around 10%.

We advise the following approach to therapy for patients with nonmetastatic gastric cancer. Diagnostic laparoscopy with cytologic washings is appropriate prior to choice of initial therapy. Laparoscopy or CT/PET or both add to staging studies if other imaging like CT suggests metastatic disease. Patients with adequate staging (CT and EUS) and apparent early disease (stage IA) should undergo surgical resection first as should patients with acute bleeding, obstruction, or other problem. Surgical resection should include D2 lymphadenectomy. Postoperative chemoradiation as in the INT 0116 study is given the final pathologic analysis confirms stage IB to IIIC. Patients with nonsuperficial gastric cancer should receive perioperative chemotherapy and surgical resection. For Asian patients, postoperative chemotherapy with S-1 is appropriate when available and indicated. Patients eligible for clinical trials should consider enrollment including nontherapeutic studies.

> **Box 5**
> - Adjuvant therapy has a proven benefit for most patients with gastric cancer and improves the rate of cure over surgical resection alone.
> - Multiple randomized clinical trials highly support use of perioperative chemotherapy.
> - Use of postoperative chemotherapy combined with chemoradiation remains an acceptable standard if surgical resection is needed first.

Monitoring for recurrence

The NCCN gastric cancer panel recommends surveillance for all patients after potentially curative therapy.[102] Suggested follow-up studies include only history and physical examination with laboratory studies as routine. Endoscopy and imaging are limited to evaluation of specific symptoms or concerns. The rationale for this approach is the limited benefit of therapy in the recurrent or metastatic setting. A Phase II randomized study compared clinical assessment after potentially curative resection for gastric and pancreas cancers to more intense surveillance including EUS and CT/PET. While the more intense regimen detected recurrence more often prior to symptoms, there was no difference in survival.[103] It is important to evaluate patients after gastrectomy for nutritional deficiencies particularly vitamin B_{12}, iron, and calcium.

Management of advanced disease

For patients with advanced, recurrent, or metastatic gastric cancer, therapy is mainly palliative. Poor performance status or multiple sites of metastases are associated with significantly worse outcomes. Despite advances in chemotherapy, survival rates show modest improvement only for patients with metastatic disease.[104] Many patients with metastatic disease can expect to liver less than 5 months, and enrollment in clinical trials may only increase survival range from 7 to 10 months.[105] Multiple trials confirm that palliative chemotherapy improves survival, quality of life, and symptom management compared to best supportive care (BSC).[106–109] Radiation therapy as a single modality has minimal benefit for patients with locally advanced unresectable tumors or poor surgical candidacy. Combination radiation and systemic chemotherapy in the palliative nonmetastatic setting may confer a survival advantage to chemotherapy alone.[110,111]

There are several viable options for first-line chemotherapy in the setting of advanced or metastatic gastric cancer. ECF was established in a pivotal trial over FAMTX (5-FU, Doxorubicin, and methotrexate).[112] In this Phase III trial of 274 patients, the response rate in the ECF group was 46% compared to 21% for FAMTX. Median survival duration was longer in the ECF arm (9 vs 6 months; $p < 0.01$).[113] REAL-2, a large study of over 1000 patients with gastric and gastroesophageal cancers, established treatment with ECF is equivalent to three other regimens, ECX (epirubicin and cisplatin plus capecitabine), EOF (epirubicin and oxaliplatin plus fluorouracil), and EOX (epirubicin and oxaliplatin plus capecitabine).[114] Response rates and median survival were around 41–48% and 9–11 months for all regimens. The addition of docetaxel to chemotherapy with 5-FU and cisplatin improves response rate (37% vs 25%) and survival by several weeks but at the cost of much higher toxicity.[115] S-1 also has efficacy in the advanced gastric cancer setting, and response rate and survival are improved when combined with cisplatin.[116] Irinotecan in combination with 5-FU is not superior to cisplatin and 5-FU in the first-line setting.[117] Irinotecan with oral S-1 is also no better than S-1 alone.[118] FOLFIRI is an acceptable regimen with equivalent outcomes to ECX in a large Phase III study.[119]

In the second-line setting, three agents improve survival over BSC. The Arbeitgemeinschaft Internistische Onkologie (AIO) study compared irinotecan with BSC to BSC alone in patients with advanced gastric or GEJ adenocarcinoma.[120] Irinotecan improved survival over BSC. In the COUGAR-02 study, 186 patients treated with docetaxel and BSC had improved survival of 5.2 months compared to 3.6 months with BSC alone.[121]

Molecularly targeted agents and immune therapy

Despite the incorporation of newer agents, survival of patients with advanced gastric cancer remains less than one year using cytotoxic chemotherapy. Molecularly targeted agents offer the hope of improving outcomes. Trastuzumab (a humanized mAb), when combined with chemotherapy in patients with advanced gastric cancer and *HER2/neu*-expressing tumors, prolongs survival from median 11.1–13.8 months.[122] The REGARD trial randomized treatment with ramucirumab, a human mAb binding VEGF-R2, versus placebo for patients with advanced, pretreated gastric cancer.[123] Ramucirumab improved survival over placebo (5.2 vs 3.8 months). The addition of paclitaxel to ramucirumab versus paclitaxel alone in the RAINBOW trial also found a survival advantage of 9.6 months compared to 7.4 months.[124] Some propose this combination as the new standard second-line treatment for patients with advanced gastric cancer.

As in other solid tumors, angiogenesis is an important part of gastric cancer progression. Bevacizumab, a *VEGF* inhibitor, improved median survival from 10.1 to 12.1 months in a study of 774 patients with advanced gastric or gastroesophageal cancer when combined with cisplatin and capecitabine compared to the same combination with placebo.[125] The PFS (6.7 vs 5.3 months) and response rate (46% vs 37%) were also better with bevacizumab. However, the study did not reach its primary endpoint. Further subgroup analysis revealed that North and Latin American patients appeared to have a survival benefit with the addition of bevacizumab (median 11.5 vs 6.8 months compared to placebo) whereas patients enrolled in Asia (90% from Japan and Korea) had no benefit. European patients had intermediate results.

Use of other targeted drugs has been disappointing. In the EXPAND trial, addition of cetuximab (a chimeric mAb against *EGFR*) to capecitabine and cisplatin (XP) provided no additional benefit over XP alone.[126] Furthermore, panitumumab (a fully humanized mAb against *EGFR*) resulted in worse survival of 8.8 months versus 11.3 months when added to epirubicin, oxaliplatin, and capecitabine (EOC) versus EOC alone.[127] The GRANITE-1 study randomized 656 patients to everolimus with BSC versus placebo with BSC.[128] Everolimus did not improve survival (median 5.4 months with everolimus and 4.3 months with placebo). Similarly, a study using lapatinib with paclitaxel versus paclitaxel alone in 420 patients with *HER2/neu* positive gastric cancer showed equivalent results.[129] Median survival was 11.0 months in the lapatinib and paclitaxel group versus 8.9 months in the paclitaxel alone group ($p = 0.21$).

Over the past decade, therapy with immune checkpoint inhibitors has been a major breakthrough in cancer treatment. Pembrolizumab is a mAb that binds programmed death 1 (PD-1), a negative costimulatory receptor expressed on the surface of activated T cells. Binding by pembrolizumab prevents interaction of PD-1 with ligands PD-L1 and PD-L2, and this helps to restore antitumor immunity. PD-1 overexpression in gastric cancer provides hope that immune checkpoint inhibition is an effective strategy. The KEYNOTE-61 trial randomized single-agent pembrolizumab versus paclitaxel as second-line therapy for patients with advanced gastric cancer. There was no difference in overall survival. Interestingly and supportive of continued efforts in personalized cancer care, the subgroup of patients with better performance status, higher expression of PD-L1, and high tumor MSI seemed to derive the most benefit from pembrolizumab monotherapy.[130] The CheckMate-032 study used nivolumab, another anti-PD-1 mAb, to treat patients with refractory metastatic gastric or esophageal cancers. Used alone or in combination with ipilimumab (targets cytotoxic T-lymphocyte-associated antigen 4), results were encouraging in that nearly one-third of patients experienced response and two-thirds had stable disease for three months or more.[131]

Further studies are ongoing to identify patients with gastric cancer more likely to benefit from immunotherapy or combination immunotherapy with other treatment (Figure 4). Using genomic mutation data and ribonucleic acid (RNA) transcription and proteomic expression profiles of gastric cancers, researchers proposed a novel classification system for gastric cancers that may aid further research into personalized therapies.[133] The study defined four basic molecular subtypes of gastric cancer: (1) EBV-positive tumors, (2) MSI tumors, (3) chromosomal instability tumors, and (4) genomically stable tumors.[132] NCCN guidelines for gastric cancer recommend testing for *HER2/neu*, PD-L1, and MSI for all patients with locally advanced unresectable, locally recurrent, or metastatic gastric cancer who are candidates for therapy.[64]

Supportive care

Patients with gastric cancer may present with symptoms including bleeding, obstruction, pain, early satiety, and weight loss. The intent of surgical resection is potential cure or palliation of symptoms or cancer-related problems. Severe symptoms in patients without metastatic disease may prompt the decision to proceed with gastrectomy first followed by adjuvant therapy. For 307 patients with gastric cancer who underwent noncurative resection at Memorial Sloan-Kettering Cancer Center, roughly half of the patients had a truly palliative resection, most commonly for bleeding (20%), obstruction (43%), or pain (29%).[134] In patients with metastatic disease, palliative gastrectomy is associated with high postoperative mortality (14%) and complications (27%).[135] In recent series, mortality has decreased to <5%, but caution remains important. Surgical bypass is also associated with high mortality in the palliative setting and frequently fails to achieve the desired benefit.[136,137]

When considering palliative resection, the surgeon should explicitly determine the degree of patient symptoms. For instance, while a patient with complete obstruction may only benefit from intervention such as resection, bypass, or endoscopic stenting, symptoms of incomplete obstruction may improve in up to 80% of patients with chemotherapy.[138] Therefore, obstruction may be a

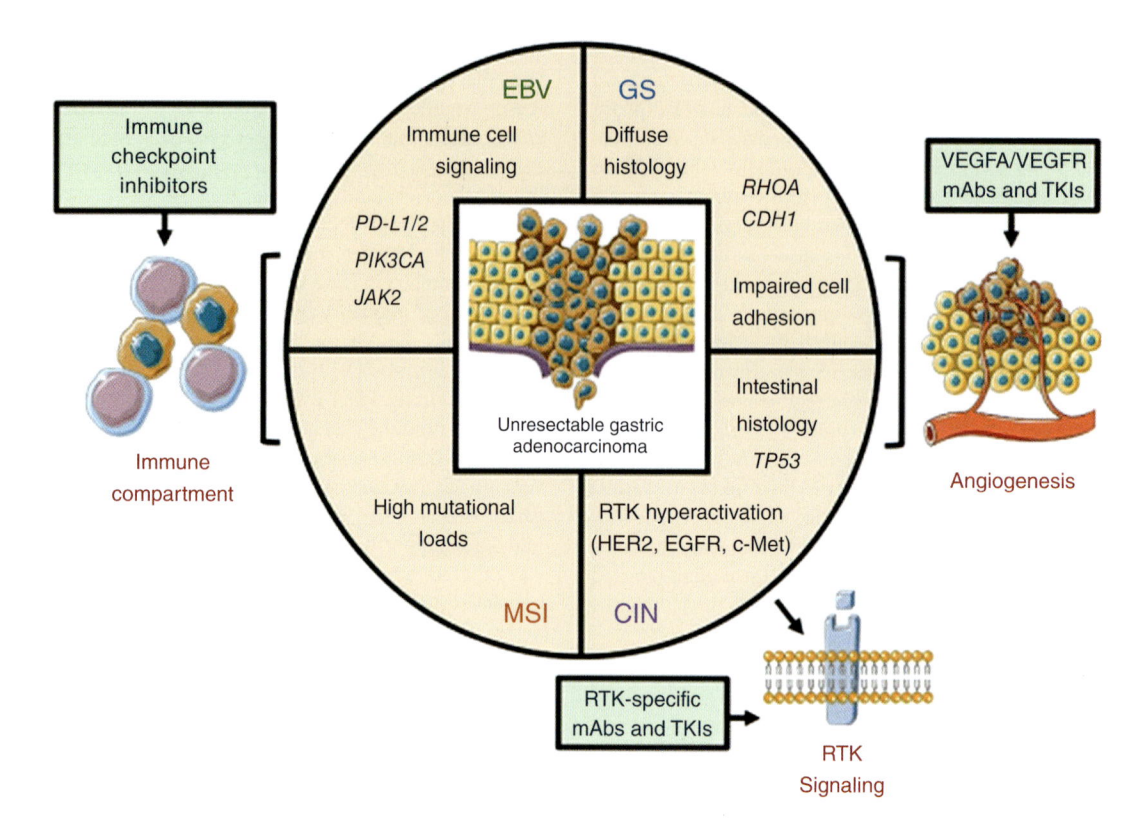

Figure 4 Four molecular subtypes of gastric cancer based on the Cancer Genome Atlas Project. Source: Duarte et al.[132]

relative indication for procedure rather than absolute. Invasion of the celiac plexus, intestinal obstruction, or bone metastases may all cause pain. Obstruction can further confound the problem of pain management. In the absence of obstruction, short and long-acting oral narcotics are appropriate for pain.

Massive life-threatening bleeding may require arterial embolization, endoscopic or surgical management. Patients with significant bleeding from gastric cancer undergoing resection without complete staging must be prepared that intraoperative findings of metastatic disease may change the intent of operation. In the metastatic setting, physicians must decide whether patients who are bleeding massively are surgical candidates and if not focus on BSC. Endoscopic and embolization maneuvers can occasionally allow the necessary time to have these often difficult discussions. For patients who are experiencing slow oozing and need a transfusion every 1–2 weeks, endoscopy may be successful. Several series have indicated that 50–75% of patients experience improvement of bleeding, gastric outlet obstruction, and pain with chemoradiation.[139,140]

The best interventions for obstruction are stenting, bypass, or resection. The technology of expandable stents has dramatically improved nonoperative options. Dormann reviewed 136 publications reporting the use of self-expanding metal stents for gastroduodenal malignancies in 32 case series and reported stent placement to be technically successful in over 90% of patients with no procedure-related mortality and a relatively low number of complications.[141] Relief of symptoms may be temporary; in 18% of cases, the stent became occluded secondary to tumor ingrowth. Generally, patients with malignant gastric outlet obstruction due to unresectable primary or metastatic cancers have poor survival (median around two months), but interventions such as endoscopic stenting or surgical bypass are associated with acceptable postprocedure quality of life.[142] In our opinion, surgical bypass is best for patients with high-performance status and longer life expectancy. Patients with short length, single sites of obstruction located in the pylorus or early duodenum are excellent candidates for endoscopic stenting. Patients with poor performance status, rapidly progressive cancer, carcinomatosis, malignant ascites, multiple sites of obstruction, and very short life expectancy should have percutaneous gastrostomy or no intervention.

One difficult and controversial area is therapy for nonevaluable disease in asymptomatic patients (such as those with low-volume abdominal carcinomatosis). Some advocate immediate use of chemotherapy, others advise observation. The rationale for observation is only 30–40% of patients have an objective response to any particular chemotherapeutic regimen. Delaying treatment until the appearance of early symptoms or evaluable disease may spare patients from unnecessary toxic effects and preserve quality of life. Medical history, physical examination, and CT scans may or may not be relevant while the patient is asymptomatic and choosing no therapy. Treatment may begin when evaluable disease is established or symptoms appear, though obstructive symptoms due to peritoneal disease sometimes eliminate the option for systemic therapy.

Unmet needs and future directions

There are many opportunities for clinicians and researchers to develop improved care for patients with gastric cancer. Exciting advances in care include intravenous lidocaine infusion to improve postoperative pain control,[143] sentinel node mapping,[144,145] early postoperative enteral immunonutrition,[146] and improved pathologic staging through use of surgical *ex vivo* dissection.[147] Further advancements must advance our collective understanding of molecular pathogenesis of gastric cancer. Clinical trials must expand therapies with realistic opportunities for cure or prolonged survival even in the metastatic setting. In the area of preventions and screening, several questions remain. Should we promote widespread efforts at H. pylori eradication? Should screening programs with upper endoscopy be developed for higher-risk patients in the West? In terms of operative management, laparoscopic and robotic resection are exciting new areas. However, we lack widely accepted standards for the conduct of procedures or public reporting of quality and long-term oncologic outcomes. Some decisions such as palliative gastrectomy will always require an individualized approach. Other considerations such as extent of lymphadenectomy or choice of adjuvant therapy require evidence to support rather than individual bias. For patients who do not respond or progress after preoperative chemotherapy, what therapy is best after operation, another chemotherapy regimen, or chemoradiation? Management of challenging postoperative symptoms such as delayed gastric emptying or poor stomach function are other areas ripe for novel research.

Conclusions

Fortunately, the incidence of gastric cancer is decreasing around the world. However, outcomes for many remain poor and overall cure rates low. Despite encouraging progress in all areas of the gastric cancer treatment (surgery, chemotherapy, and radiation), many patients with gastric cancer still suffer symptoms, decreased HRQOL, and will eventually die of disease despite best therapy. In the future, we must hope cost-effective screening programs and preventive measures will continue to decrease the incidence. As we enter the age of molecular targeted therapy and effective immunotherapy, we may see novel therapeutic strategies continue to push the needle. More options will allow more efforts at personalized medicine. The authors sincerely hope in our lifetime that people with locally advanced and metastatic gastric cancer will have even a small chance at curative therapy.

Key references

The complete reference list can be found on Vital Source version of this title, see inside front cover.

3 Chau I, Norman AR, Cunningham D, et al. Multivariate prognostic factor analysis in locally advanced and metastatic esophago-gastric cancer–pooled analysis from three multicenter, randomized, controlled trials using individual patient data. *J Clin Oncol*. 2004;**22**(12):2395–2403.
8 Ford AC, Forman D, Hunt RH, et al. *Helicobacter pylori* eradication therapy to prevent gastric cancer in healthy asymptomatic infected individuals: systematic review and meta-analysis of randomised controlled trials. *BMJ*. 2014;**348**:g3174.
10 Behrens G, Jochem C, Keimling M, et al. The association between physical activity and gastroesophageal cancer: systematic review and meta-analysis. *Eur J Epidemiol*. 2014;**29**(3):151–170.
11 Chen Y, Liu L, Wang X, et al. Body mass index and risk of gastric cancer: a meta-analysis of a population with more than ten million from 24 prospective studies. *Cancer Epidemiol Biomark Prev*. 2013;**22**(8):1395–1408.
18 Huntsman DG, Carneiro F, Lewis FR, et al. Early gastric cancer in young, asymptomatic carriers of germ-line E-cadherin mutation. *N Engl J Med*. 2001;**344**(25):1904–1909.
19 Worster E, Liu X, Richardson S, et al. The impact of prophylactic total gastrectomy on health-related quality of life: a prospective cohort study. *Ann Surg*. 2014;**260**(1):87–93.
23 Syngal S, Brand RE, Church JM, et al. ACG clinical guideline: genetic testing and management of hereditary gastrointestinal cancer syndromes. *Am J Gastroenterol*. 2015;**110**(2):223–262; quiz 63.
34 Wu MS, Shun CT, Wang HP, et al. Genetic alterations in gastric cancer: relation to histological subtypes, tumor stage, and *Helicobacter pylori* infection. *Gastroenterology*. 1997;**112**(5):1457–1465.
53 Spolverato G, Ejaz A, Kim Y, et al. Use of endoscopic ultrasound in the preoperative staging of gastric cancer: a multi-institutional study of the US gastric cancer collaborative. *J Am Coll Surg*. 2015;**220**(1):48–56.
54 Lordick F, Ott K, Krause BJ, et al. PET to assess early metabolic response and to guide treatment of adenocarcinoma of the oesophagogastric junction: the MUNICON phase II trial. *Lancet Oncol*. 2007;**8**(9):797–805.
56 De Andrade JP, Mezhir JJ. The critical role of peritoneal cytology in the staging of gastric cancer: an evidence-based review. *J Surg Oncol*. 2014;**110**(3):291–297.
63 Gotoda T. Endoscopic resection of early gastric cancer. *Gastric Cancer*. 2007;**10**(1):1–11.
65 Bozzetti F, Marubini E, Bonfanti G, et al. Subtotal versus total gastrectomy for gastric cancer. Five year survival rates in a multicenter randomized Italian trial. *Ann Surg*. 1999;**230**:170–178.
76 Bonenkamp JJ, Hermans J, Sasako M, van de Velde CJ. Extended lymph-node dissection for gastric cancer. *N Engl J Med*. 1999;**340**(12):908–914.
78 Songun I, Putter H, Kranenbarg EM, et al. Surgical treatment of gastric cancer: 15-year follow-up results of the randomised nationwide Dutch D1D2 trial. *Lancet Oncol*. 2010;**11**(5):439–449.
81 Squires MH 3rd, Kooby DA, Pawlik TM, et al. Utility of the proximal margin frozen section for resection of gastric adenocarcinoma: a 7-institution study of the US gastric cancer collaborative. *Ann Surg Oncol*. 2014;**21**(13):4202.
87 Yu J, Huang C, Sun Y, et al. Effect of laparoscopic vs open distal gastrectomy on 3-year disease-free survival in patients with locally advanced gastric cancer: The CLASS-01 randomized clinical trial. *JAMA*. 2019;**321**(20):1983–1992.
88 Macdonald JS, Smalley SR, Benedetti J, et al. Chemoradiotherapy after surgery compared with surgery alone for adenocarcinoma of the stomach or gastroesophageal junction. *N Engl J Med*. 2001;**345**(10):725–730.
89 Smalley SR, Benedetti JK, Haller DG, et al. Updated analysis of SWOG-directed intergroup study 0116: a phase III trial of adjuvant radiochemotherapy versus observation after curative gastric cancer resection. *J Clin Oncol*. 2012;**30**(19):2327–2333.
92 Cats A, Jansen EPM, van Grieken NCT, et al. Chemotherapy versus chemoradiotherapy after surgery and preoperative chemotherapy for resectable gastric cancer (CRITICS): an international, open-label, randomised phase 3 trial. *Lancet Oncol*. 2018;**19**(5):616–628.
94 Cunningham D, Allum WH, Stenning SP, et al. Perioperative chemotherapy versus surgery alone for resectable gastroesophageal cancer. *N Engl J Med*. 2006;**355**(1):11–20.
95 Al-Batran SE, Homann N, Pauligk C, et al. Perioperative chemotherapy with fluorouracil plus leucovorin, oxaliplatin, and docetaxel versus fluorouracil or capecitabine plus cisplatin and epirubicin for locally advanced, resectable gastric or gastro-oesophageal junction adenocarcinoma (FLOT4): a randomised, phase 2/3 trial. *Lancet*. 2019;**393**(10184):1948–1957.
98 Lee J, Lim DH, Kim S, et al. Phase III trial comparing capecitabine plus cisplatin versus capecitabine plus cisplatin with concurrent capecitabine radiotherapy in completely resected gastric cancer with D2 lymph node dissection: the ARTIST trial. *J Clin Oncol*. 2012;**30**(3):268–273.
101 Sakuramoto S, Sasako M, Yamaguchi T, et al. Adjuvant chemotherapy for gastric cancer with S-1, an oral fluoropyrimidine. *N Engl J Med*. 2007;**357**(18):1810–1820.
103 Bjerring OS, Fristrup CW, Pfeiffer P, et al. Phase II randomized clinical trial of endosonography and PET/CT versus clinical assessment only for follow-up after surgery for upper gastrointestinal cancer (EUFURO study). *Br J Surg*. 2019;**106**(13):1761–1768.
112 Waters JS, Norman A, Cunningham D, et al. Long-term survival after epirubicin, cisplatin and fluorouracil for gastric cancer: results of a randomized trial. *Br J Cancer*. 1999;**80**(1–2):269–272.
115 Van Cutsem E, Moiseyenko VM, Tjulandin S, et al. Phase III study of docetaxel and cisplatin plus fluorouracil compared with cisplatin and fluorouracil as first-line therapy for advanced gastric cancer: a report of the V325 study group. *J Clin Oncol*. 2006;**24**(31):4991–4997.
116 Koizumi W, Narahara H, Hara T, et al. S-1 plus cisplatin versus S-1 alone for first-line treatment of advanced gastric cancer (SPIRITS trial): a phase III trial. *Lancet Oncol*. 2008;**9**(3):215–221.
130 Shitara K, Özgüroğlu M, Bang YJ, et al. Pembrolizumab versus paclitaxel for previously treated, advanced gastric or gastro-oesophageal junction cancer (KEYNOTE-061): a randomised, open-label, controlled, phase 3 trial. *Lancet*. 2018;**392**(10142):123–133.
132 Duarte HO, Gomes J, Machado JC, Reis CA. Gastric cancer: basic aspects. *Helicobacter*. 2018;**23**(Suppl 1):e12523.
141 Dormann A, Meisner S, Verin N, Wenk Lang A. Self-expanding metal stents for gastroduodenal malignancies: systematic review of their clinical effectiveness. *Endoscopy*. 2004;**36**(6):543–550.
144 Kitagawa Y, Takeuchi H, Takagi Y, et al. Sentinel node mapping for gastric cancer: a prospective multicenter trial in Japan. *J Clin Oncol*. 2013;**31**(29):3704–3710.

87 Primary neoplasms of the liver

Hop S. Tran Cao, MD, FACS ■ Junichi Shindoh, MD, PhD ■ Jean-Nicolas Vauthey, MD

Overview

Primary liver cancer is the second leading cause of cancer death in men and the sixth leading cause among women worldwide. Its incidence in the United States has more than tripled since 1980. Hepatocellular carcinoma (HCC) constitutes three-fourths of primary hepatic neoplasms, followed by intrahepatic cholangiocarcinoma (ICC) (10–15%) and other less common hepatic malignancies (5%) such as hepatic angiosarcoma, epithelioid hemangioendothelioma, or hepatic lymphoma. Primary hepatic malignancies are generally associated with poor survival, and limited systemic therapy options are available. As such, prevention, screening (in the case of HCC), early diagnosis, and multidisciplinary management are key to maximizing outcomes. In addition, most primary hepatic neoplasms are associated with chronic liver disease or cirrhosis, such that the resultant decreased hepatic functional reserve often precludes aggressive treatment for tumors. Therefore, for treatment selection, one should consider two intrinsic conflicting factors: curability and safety of treatment. Currently, several clinical staging systems and treatment algorithms are available to adequately select therapeutic options for HCC. The choice of therapy is individualized based on the tumor burden, degree of underlying liver disease, patient performance status, and the overall possibility of side effects or complications, and must be balanced with the anticipated benefits. Selection of treatment should be determined in a multidisciplinary fashion with the available local expertise. For patients with HCC or ICC, treatment options with curative intent including surgical resection, ablation, and orthotopic liver transplantation (OLT) should be the first priority as long as these treatments are approved.

The liver is a unique organ through which all the visceral venous drainage passes before it reaches the heart. Because of this, it is the most common site of metastases from gastrointestinal malignancies. These secondary hepatic malignancies far outnumber tumors that originate from the cells within the liver and are termed primary hepatic neoplasms. Of these, hepatocellular carcinoma (HCC) is the most common, constituting 70–85% of primary liver cancers, followed by intrahepatic cholangiocarcinoma (ICC) (10–15%) and other less common hepatic malignancies (5%) such as hepatic angiosarcoma, epithelioid hemangioendothelioma or hemangiopericytoma, or hepatic lymphoma. Because primary hepatic malignancies are generally associated with poor survival, and systemic therapy options are limited, early diagnosis and multidisciplinary management are of most importance to achieve favorable long-term outcomes. This article will review and discuss the clinical features and current treatment approaches for HCC and ICC primarily, and will briefly touch upon some of the less common primary liver cancers.

Hepatocellular carcinoma

Incidence and epidemiology

HCC constitutes three-fourths of primary liver cancer. Nearly 85% of the cases occur in developing countries especially in sub-Saharan Africa and in East and Southeast Asia, with typical incidence rates of >20 per 100,000 individuals. Incidence rates are generally lowest in developed countries, with the exception of Japan where hepatitis C virus (HCV) infection is the most common cause of HCC.

Globally, the incidence of HCC is increasing in areas with historically low rates, including parts of Oceania, Central Europe, and North America.[1,2] A study reported in 2009 indicated that age-adjusted incidence rates of HCC tripled between 1975 and 2005 in the United States from 1.6 to 4.9 per 100,000 people.[1] In contrast, the incidence of HCC is decreasing in historically high-risk areas, such as China and Singapore, most likely due to reduction in hepatitis B virus (HBV) infection through improved public health.

The rates of HCC are more than twice as high in men as in women across geographic regions.[3] The incidence of HCC increases with age, though the age threshold varies among countries because of differences in predominant etiologies for HCC. The age threshold for HCC is generally younger when the predominant risk factor is vertical transmission of HBV (e.g., Southeast Asia and Africa), and older where acquired HCV infection during adulthood is the most common cause of HCC (e.g., Japan and the United States).

Risk factors

Cirrhosis is the main risk factor and is present in 80–90% of patients with HCC. It is hypothesized that chronic hepatocellular injury and inflammation from a variety of causes lead to cirrhosis and HCC as a result of hepatocyte regeneration and hyperplasia predisposing to mutations and malignant transformation.

Viral hepatitis (HBV and HCV)
It has been estimated that 75–80% of HCC are associated with chronic infections with HBV (50–55%) or HCV (25–30%).[4] Transmission of HBV occurs during delivery (vertical transmission), blood transfusions, sexual intercourse, or intravenous drug abuse. Transmission of HCV occurs via parenteral exposure primarily through blood transfusions and intravenous drug abuse.

HBV is a double-stranded DNA virus and chronic infection with HBV is the most common etiology for HCC, especially in China and Korea. Patients with positive hepatitis B surface antigen (HBsAg) are at high risk of developing cirrhosis and HCC. However, it has been reported that those who are positive for antihepatitis B core antibodies (HbcAb) are also at high risk for

Holland-Frei Cancer Medicine, Tenth Edition. Edited by Robert C. Bast, John C. Byrd, Carlo M. Croce, Ernest Hawk, Fadlo R. Khuri, Raphael E. Pollock, Apostolia M. Tsimberidou, Christopher G. Willett, and Cheryl L. Willman.
© 2023 John Wiley & Sons, Inc. Published 2023 by John Wiley & Sons, Inc.

HCC even when HBs-Ag is serologically negative.[5] In contrast to HCV-related HCC which usually arises in the liver with severe fibrosis or cirrhosis, approximately 20% of HBV-related HCC occurs in the absence of cirrhotic changes. A direct mutagenic effect that causes carcinogenesis has been postulated for HBV. Integration of HBV DNA in the host genome adjacent to cellular oncogenes or transactivating effect of the HBx protein on cellular gene expression may be attributable to the development of HCC without cirrhosis.[6–8] In fact, HBV-DNA integration has been detected in hepatocytes prior to tumor development among patients positive for HbsAg, which may enhance chromosomal instability and facilitate HCC development.[9,10]

HCV is a small, single-stranded RNA virus. The prevalence of HCV infection varies widely according to geographical areas. A meta-analysis of 21 case-control studies reported that HCC risk was 17 times higher among HCV-positive individuals as compared to HCV-negative individuals.[11] It has been suggested that oxidative stress is one of the mechanisms involved in inflammation-related carcinogenesis in patients infected with HCV.[12] In response to viral antigens, the activated macrophages and other recruited leukocytes release reactive oxygen species, causing areas of focal necrosis and compensatory cell division.[13] When these oxidants overwhelm the antioxidant defenses of neighboring cells, damages to biomolecules, particularly to oncogenes or tumor suppressor genes, may increase the carcinogenic potential of the underlying liver. HCV displays a high genetic variability. On the basis of nucleotide sequence homology, whole-sequenced HCV isolates are classified as genotype 1a, 1b, 2a, and 2b. The geographic distribution of these genotypes demonstrated that genotypes 1a, 1b, and 2a are predominant in Western countries and East Asia, whereas genotype 2b is predominant in the Middle East.[14] The HCV genotype 1b is reportedly more aggressive and more closely associated with advanced chronic liver diseases such as liver cirrhosis and HCC. However, these observations can be partially explained by the refractoriness to antiviral therapy and recent studies have reported that lower HCV viral load is correlated with improved survival outcomes after surgical resection of HCC irrespective of the genotypes of HCV.[15,16]

Alcohol
Excessive alcohol consumption is a major risk factor for chronic liver disease and HCC, causing various degrees of liver damage from simple fat accumulation to cirrhosis. Various studies have concluded that excessive alcohol intake is an important risk factor for HCC development. A US case-control study demonstrated approximately threefold increase in HCC risk among individuals with heavy alcohol consumption defined as more than 60 mL ethanol per day.[17] HCC rarely develops in the absence of cirrhosis, but the risk is increased with concurrent HBV or HCV infection.[18,19] A meta-analysis of 20 studies published between 1995 and 2004 that involved more than 15,000 patients with chronic HCV infection reported that the pooled relative risk of cirrhosis associated with heavy alcohol intake was 2.33, compared with no or low-quantity alcohol intake.[18] Therefore, alcohol consumption should be avoided among patients with viral hepatitis.

Aflatoxins
Aflatoxins (AFs) are potent hepatocarcinogens produced by *Aspergillus flavus* and *A. parasiticus* that grow readily on foods such as corn and peanuts stored in warm, damp conditions. There are four AF compounds: AFB_1, AFB_2, AFG_1, and AFG_2 and the most common and most toxic AF compound is AFB_1. When ingested, AFB_1 is metabolized to a highly active 8,9-epoxide metabolite, which can bind to and damage DNA. A consistent genetic mutation in codon 249 in the tumor suppressor p53 gene has been identified and positively correlated with aflatoxin exposure.[20,21] Although AFB_1 contributes to hepatocarcinogenesis, its role in pathogenesis of HCC is primarily mediated by its synergic effects on chronic hepatitis B because the areas where AFB_1 exposure is an environmental problem also have a high prevalence of chronic HBV infection. A prospective study from China showed that urinary excretion of aflatoxin metabolites was associated with increased risk for HCC up to fourfold, and HBV infection independently increased the risk sevenfold. However, the patients who excreted AFB_1 metabolites and had concomitant infection of HBV showed a 60-fold increase in risk of development of HCC.[22] These results suggest that prevention of HBV-related HCC would reduce the effects of AF on HCC risk.

Obesity
It is well established that obesity is associated with a wide spectrum of hepatobiliary diseases, including fatty liver diseases, steatosis, steatohepatitis, and cryptogenic cirrhosis.[23,24] In a large prospective cohort study of more than 900,000 individuals in the US followed up for a 16-year period, liver cancer mortality rates were five times greater among men with the greatest baseline body mass index (range 35–40) compared with those with a normal body mass index, while the risk of liver cancer was not as increased in women, with a relative risk of 1.68.[25] Two other population-based studies from Northern Europe have also shown that obesity is correlated with increased HCC risk.[26,27]

Nonalcoholic fatty liver disease (NAFLD) is the most common cause of chronic liver disease in the United States and strongly associated with obesity, diabetes, and metabolic syndrome.[28] The progressive subtype of NAFLD is termed as nonalcoholic steatohepatitis (NASH) that can result in progressive hepatic fibrosis, cirrhosis, and HCC.

Diabetes mellitus
Recently, diabetes has been recognized as a risk factor for chronic liver disease and HCC. Although adjustment of potential biases in cross-sectional and case-control studies is difficult, several studies have clearly demonstrated positive correlation between diabetes and HCC.[29–33] The postulated mechanisms for liver cell damage induced by type 2 diabetes mellitus involve insulin resistance and hyperinsulinemia.[34,35] Hyperinsulinemia reportedly reduces liver synthesis and blood levels of insulin growth factor binding protein-1 (IGFBP-1), which increases (1) bioavailability of insulin-like growth factor-1 (IGF-1), (2) promotion of cellular proliferation, and (3) inhibition of apoptosis.[36] Excessive insulin binds to insulin receptor and activates its intrinsic tyrosine kinase, leading to phosphorylation of insulin receptor substrate-1 (IRS-1),[37] and hyperinsulinemia is also associated with production of reactive oxygen species, which may cause damage to DNA. Overexpression of IRS-1 is associated with decreased apoptosis which is mediated by transforming growth factor β.[38] Given this evidence in basic research and pathologic observation that HCC tumor cells overexpress both IGF-1 and IRS-1,[39] diabetes mellitus seems to contribute to liver cell damage and development of HCC.

Hemochromatosis
Hemochromatosis is an autosomal recessive genetic disorder of iron metabolism, with a prevalence rate of 2–5 per 1000 in the

Caucasian population. In this inherited disorder, mutations have been documented in the *HFE* gene on chromosome 6 (Cys282Tyr [*C282Y*] and His63Asp [*H63D*]), the *HFR-2* gene on chromosome 1, and the *HFE-3* gene on chromosome 7. The *C282Y* mutation is the most commonly detected mutation and *C282Y* homozygotes or *C282Y*/*H63D* compound heterozygotes[40–42] are associated with increased absorption of dietary iron and accumulation in tissues such as the skin, heart, and liver, resulting in heart failure or liver cirrhosis.

There is growing evidence that even mild accumulation of iron is harmful to the liver, especially when other hepatotoxic factors such as chronic viral hepatitis or heavy alcohol intake are present. Iron enhances the pathogenicity of microorganisms, adversely affects the function of macrophages and lymphocytes, and enhances fibrogenic pathways.[43] A synergistic relationship between HCV infection and iron overload has been suggested[44] and iron depletion has been reported to improve liver function tests in patients with chronic hepatitis C.[45] Although the diagnosis of hemochromatosis can be difficult to establish, treatment with therapeutic phlebotomy or iron chelation therapy prior to onset of cirrhosis may be effective in preventing the development of cirrhosis and HCC in these patients.

α₁-Antitrypsin deficiency
α_1-Antitrypsin deficiency (AATD) is an autosomal dominant disorder with mutations in the serine protease inhibitor (Pi) gene. Over 75 different Pi alleles have been identified, most of which are not associated with the disease.[46] A relationship exists between Pi phenotypes and serum concentrations of α_1-antitrypsin. Typical clinical presentation of patients with AATD includes emphysema, hepatic necroinflammation, cirrhosis, and HCC. Because no effective medical treatment is available, liver transplantation is indicated for patients with decompensated cirrhosis to correct the underlying metabolic disorder.

Other potential risk factors
The higher incidence of HCC reported in men compared to women suggests the influence of hormonal factors on hepatocarcinogenesis. Long-term use of oral contraceptives has been thought to be a potential risk factors for HCC; however, a review of 12 case-control studies have yielded a nonsignificant overall adjusted odds ratio of 1.6 (95% CI, 0.9–2.5),[47] and the correlation between the oral contraceptives and risk for HCC remains inconclusive.

Hypothyroidism has also been reported to be a potential risk factor for HCC especially in women.[48,49] Patients with hypothyroidism may experience weight gain[50] and insulin resistance,[51,52] both of which are significant factors for nonalcoholic steatohepatitis. Although the actual mechanism is unclear and only limited clinical evidence is available, development of chronic liver disease and hepatocarcinogenesis might be influenced by these hormonal factors to some extent.

Prevention
Prevention of HCC is highly dependent on avoiding exposure to known risk factors, adequate treatment of the underlying chronic liver disease, and early diagnosis of precursor lesions. Because the most common cause of HCC is cirrhosis associated with viral hepatitis, prevention of infection to HBV/HCV and treatment of chronic hepatitis with antiviral therapy are of utmost importance in cancer prevention.

For hepatitis B, parenteral exposure is the most common cause of transmission in developing countries and improvements in hygiene conditions and public education are essential to avoid viral transmission. In addition, vaccination and effective antiviral therapy are currently available for HBV. After the initiation of HBV vaccination, significant declines in the incidence of HCC were documented in high-risk countries like Taiwan.[53] When HBV infection has been established, various effective antiviral agents are currently available and reduction of viral load has reportedly correlated with reduced risk of HCC and improved survival outcomes in patients with chronic hepatitis B.[54–56]

For hepatitis C, interferon (IFN)-based combination treatment has conventionally been the standard of care and reduction of HCC risk has been shown, especially in patients who achieved sustained viral response (SVR).[57–60] Recently, introduction of new direct-acting antiviral agents (DAAs) have dramatically improved virologic response rate and will likely contribute to the prevention of HCC among patients with chronic hepatitis C in the near future.[61–63]

Pathology
The malignant transformation of hepatocytes to HCC is thought to be a multistep process associated with genetic mutations, allelic losses, epigenetic alterations, and perturbation of molecular cellular pathways. However, the molecular process of carcinogenesis in HCC is poorly understood. The phenotypic expression of these potential multistep changes can be manifested by precursor lesions which can be distinguishable from surrounding regenerative nodules associated with cirrhosis with regard to size, color, texture, and degree of bulging of the cut surface. Changes in the tumor blood supply correspond to each step of the multistep process, from precursor lesions to classical HCC, and helps differential diagnosis on dynamic studies in CT or MRI (Figure 1).

Dysplastic nodules
It is commonly accepted that there is a stepwise progression from cirrhotic nodule to HCC. A unified nomenclature of such liver nodules has recently been reviewed by the International Working Party of the World Congress of Gastroenterology.[64] Dysplastic nodule (DN) is a distinct nodular lesion greater than 5 mm in diameter and subclassified into low-grade dysplastic nodule (LGDN) and high-grade dysplastic nodule (HGDN). LGDNs show only mild dysplasia without architectural atypia, while HGDNs are characterized by architectural and/or cytologic atypia, which is insufficient for a diagnosis of HCC. HGDNs often show increased cell density with an irregular trabecular pattern. Small cell change (small cell dysplasia) is the most frequently seen form of cytologic atypia in HGDNs.

Early HCC
Early HCCs are vaguely nodular tumors up to around 2 cm in diameter and are characterized by various combinations of the following major histologic features.[64]

1. increased cell density more than two times that of the surrounding tissue, with an increased nuclear/cytoplasm ratio and irregular thin-trabecular pattern
2. varying numbers of portal tracts within the nodule (intratumoral portal tracts)
3. pseudoglandular pattern
4. diffuse fatty change
5. varying numbers of unpaired arteries

Distinguishing early HCCs from HGDNs is an unresolved challenge. Stromal invasion, defined as the presence of tumor cells

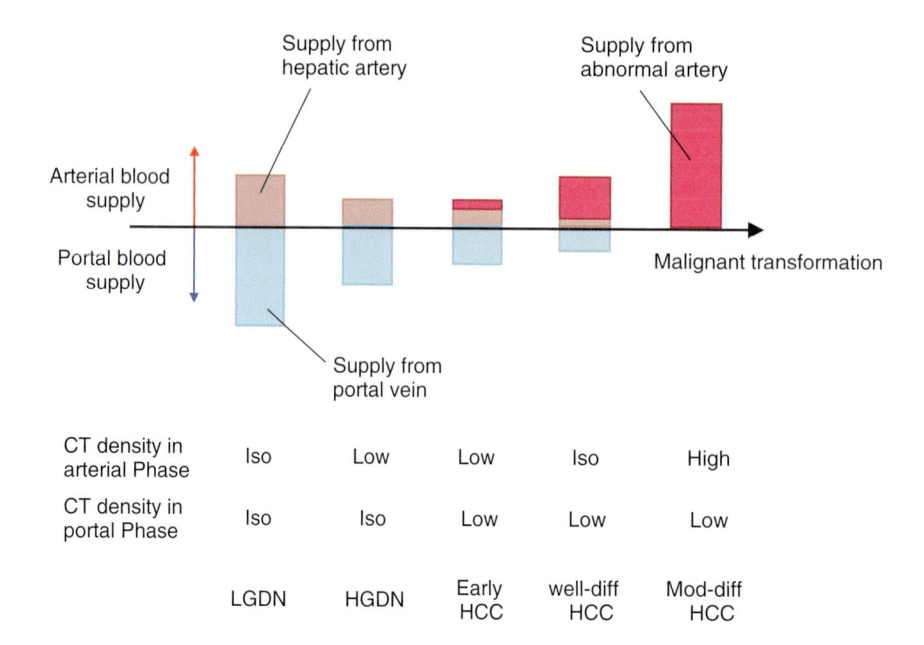

Figure 1 A model of dynamic changes in blood supply from precursor lesions to classical hepatocellular carcinoma. Dynamic changes in arterial and portal supply and exponential increase in abnormal arterial supply correlate with the typical patterns of enhancement in dynamic CT or MRI. *Abbreviations*: LGDN, low-grade dysplastic nodule; HGDN, high-grade dysplastic nodule; HCC, hepatocellular carcinoma; well-diff, well-differentiated; mod-diff, moderately differentiated.

invading into the portal tracts or fibrous septa, has been proposed as the most relevant feature discerning early HCC from HGDN. However, such features may be difficult to identify, especially on biopsy specimens. In that context, a panel of 3 immunohistochemical markers of malignant transformation: heat shock protein 70, glutamine synthetase, and glypican 3 has been used to distinguish HCCs from HGDNs as well as CK 7 immunostaining for recognition of stromal invasion in early HCC.[65,66]

Macroscopic presentation of HCC

HCC forms a soft mass with a heterogeneous macroscopic appearance, polychrome with foci of hemorrhage or necrosis (Figure 2). Grossly, three main growth patterns first described by Eggel in 1901 are observed.[67] The *nodular* type consists of well-circumscribed tumor nodules. *Massive* HCCs are circumscribed, huge tumor masses occupying most or all of a hepatic lobe. This type is commonly observed in patients without cirrhosis. The *diffuse* type is rare and characterized by innumerable indistinct small nodules studding the entire liver. The different patterns of growth are associated with various risks of spread, both intrahepatic and extrahepatic.[68] The Liver Cancer Study Group of Japan (LCSGJ) has proposed a modification, with the nodular category being divided into three subtypes: single nodular subtype, single nodular subtype with perinodular tumor growth, and confluent multinodular subtype.[69]

Multicentricity of tumor is noted in 16–74% of HCCs resected in cirrhotic livers.[68–72] Although it is sometimes difficult to distinguish intrahepatic metastases from HCCs generated by multicentric neocarcinogenesis, tumor nodules are considered intrahepatic metastases when (1) they show a portal vein tumor thrombus or grow contiguously with a thrombus, (2) multiple small satellite nodules surround a larger main tumor, or (3) a single lesion is adjacent to the main tumor but is significantly smaller in size and presents the same histology.[73]

Vascular invasion and formation of tumor thrombus are frequently observed especially in poorly differentiated HCC or large tumors. The portal vein is the most common site of vascular invasion, followed by hepatic veins, biliary tract, and hepatic arteries. The degree of tumor extension through the vascular structure is closely associated with prognosis. When a portal vein tumor thrombus extends up to the left or right portal pedicle (Vp3) or main portal trunk (Vp4), most patients develop recurrence and die within 2 years of surgery.[74]

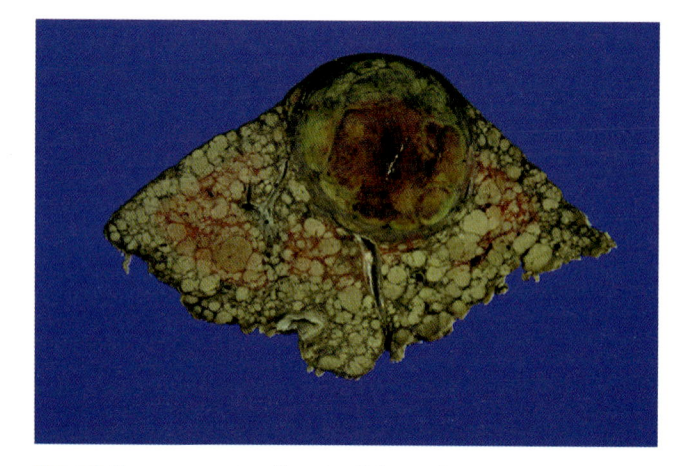

Figure 2 Gross appearance of hepatocellular carcinoma.

Microscopic presentation of HCC

Grading of HCC has relied on the Edmondson and Steiner classification for many years, which divided HCC into four grades from I to IV on the basis of histological differentiation.[75] Tumors with well-differentiated neoplastic hepatocytes arranged in thin trabeculae correspond to grade I. Larger and more atypical neoplastic cells are sometimes organized in an acinar pattern in grade II. Architectural and cytologic anaplasia are prominent in grade III, but the neoplastic cells are readily identified as hepatocytic in origin. When composed of markedly anaplastic neoplastic cells not readily identified as hepatocytic origin, the tumor is classified as grade IV.

Histologic variants of HCC

Fibrolamellar HCC
The fibrolamellar variant of HCC is a rare entity accounting for less than 1% of all cases of primary liver cancers. It is commonly encountered in young patients without chronic liver disease. Fibrolamellar HCCs are firm, sharply demarcated, and usually single tumors, ranging from 5 cm to over 20 cm. Histologically, it is characterized by the presence of lamellar stromal bands surrounding nests of large polygonal eosinophilic tumor cells with prominent nucleoli. Intensive surgical approaches have been reported to offer a chance at long-term survival even when extrahepatic recurrences occur for patients with fibrolamellar HCC.[76]

Combined HCC and cholangiocarcinoma
Combined HCC and cholangiocarcinoma (HCC-CC) contain unequivocal elements of both HCC and ICC. These tumors show variable combinations of characteristic features of HCC (e.g., bile production, intercellular bile canaliculi, or a trabecular growth) as well as ICC (e.g., glandular structures, intracellular mucin production, or immunoreactivity for MUC-1, CK7, and CK19).[77–79] Although the surgical outcomes of combined HCC-CC remain indeterminate, intermediate postoperative long-term survival between HCC and ICC has been reported in several studies.[80,81]

Pathogenesis and natural history
The pathogenesis of HCC in cirrhosis is a multistep de-differentiation process which progresses from regenerative nodule to dysplastic borderline nodule to frank HCC. Dysplastic nodules and early HCC are generally asymptomatic and are usually incidental findings on radiographic studies or detected as a result of screening procedures. Early HCC is a usually slow-growing lesion and remains indolent before acquiring oncological features of classical HCC. In stepwise sequence, small HCCs acquire progression ability with angiogenesis, increase in tumor size, invade into vascular structures, and metastasize within the liver. This microscopic cancer spread process can evolve toward macroscopic formation of vascular tumor thrombi or multiple tumor presentation. HCC is characterized by early development of such intrahepatic metastasis, whereas distant organs are usually involved late in this disease. HCCs usually remain asymptomatic until they stretch liver capsule, compress biliary structures, or rupture. In some cases, however, hyperbilirubinemia or hypercalcemia is observed without evidence of biliary obstruction or bone metastases as a paraneoplastic syndrome.

Extrahepatic metastases occur in later stages, primarily via the bloodstream to the lungs, bones, and brain. The prognosis for patients with extrahepatic disease is dismal with overall survival under 1 year depending on the extent of tumor involvement and other prognostic factors.

Screening and diagnosis
The primary objective of screening for HCC should be to diagnose the cancer as early as possible in patients who are at risk to improve survival in a cost-effective manner. Screening is not recommended for the general population, given the low incidence of HCC among individuals with no risk factors. Therefore, the first step in HCC screening should be the identification of patients at risk of HCC development. Traditionally, two methodologies have been employed in HCC screening for high-risk patients: tumor marker determination, specifically serum alpha-fetoprotein (AFP) concentration, and diagnostic imaging studies.

The American Association for the Study of Liver Disease (AASLD) has established guidelines regarding the use of these screening techniques based on the best existing evidence.[82] The AASLD currently recommends serial hepatic ultrasound and serum AFP measurement every 6 months in at-risk populations (e.g., any patient with cirrhosis or with chronic hepatitis B infection). Similarly, the Japanese Society of Hepatology has recommended hepatic ultrasound and serum AFP/plasma des-gamma carboxyprothrombin (DCP) every 3 to 4 months and dynamic CT or MRI every 6–12 months for very high-risk population (HBV-related cirrhosis or HCV-related cirrhosis) and hepatic ultrasound and tumor markers every 6 months for high-risk population (HBV-related chronic hepatitis, HCV-related chronic hepatitis, or cirrhosis with other etiologies) with or without dynamic CT or MRI every 6–12 months, as appropriate.[83] A randomized-controlled trial from China reported that the use of ultrasound and AFP enabled early detection of HCC and lowered HCC-related mortality by 37% in hepatitis B patients.[84] Various nonrandomized studies also confirmed prognostic improvement through regular surveillance programs among patients at high risk of HCC.[85–87] Regarding screening interval, a recent meta-analysis revealed that an interval of 6 months is significantly better than one of 12 months for the early detection of HCC. Santi et al.[88] reported that 70% of newly diagnosed HCC fell within Milan criteria (solitary tumor ≤ 5 cm or ≤3 tumors with each tumor ≤ 3 cm)[89] when at-risk patients were screened every 6 months or less, while the proportion of HCC within Milan criteria was 57%, and survival was inferior, for patients who were screened every 6–12 months. When a suspicious nodule was detected on screening ultrasound, a contrast-enhanced dynamic CT or MRI should be the next study obtained. Because HCC is mainly fed by arterial flow, early enhancement on the arterial phase and early washout of contrast on the delayed phase of the scan are typical findings suggestive of HCC (Figure 3). These enhancement characteristics increase the specificity of the scan to greater than 95%.[90]

An update of AASLD screening and diagnostic algorithm has been recently published (Figure 4).[82] These guidelines suggest that a liver mass detected on a radiographic study performed in an at-risk patient does not always need biopsy confirmation for the diagnosis of HCC as long as the liver lesion exhibits typical vascular enhancement patterns on dynamic imaging studies with CT scan or MRI for lesions greater than 1 cm in diameter. Lesions less than 1 cm in diameter should be followed with ultrasound every 3–6 months with or without screening for serum AFP level. If there is tumor growth or changes in character, further investigation is recommended according to size of tumor.

Staging
Because of the close association of HCC with underlying chronic liver disease, the prognosis of patients with HCC depends both on the extent of malignant involvement and the severity of the chronic liver disease. Thus, currently available staging systems for HCC are broadly divided into clinical and pathological staging systems. The clinical staging systems are particularly useful in guiding treatment selection, including the Okuda staging system,[91] the Cancer of the Liver Italian Program (CLIP) score,[92] and the Barcelona Clinic Liver Cancer (BCLC) staging system.[93] The pathologic staging systems are established based on the surgical outcomes and include the LCSGJ staging system,[94] the Japanese Integrated Staging (JIS)

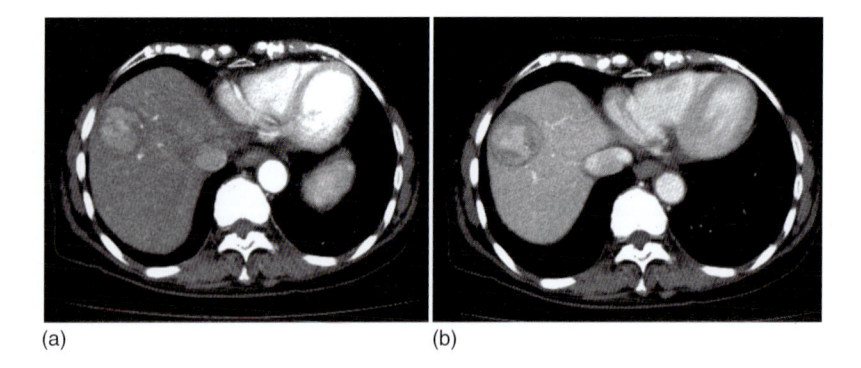

Figure 3 Typical enhancement pattern of hepatocellular carcinoma in dynamic CT scan. Early enhancement in the arterial phase (a) and washout in the late phase (b) are typically observed in moderately differentiated hepatocellular carcinoma.

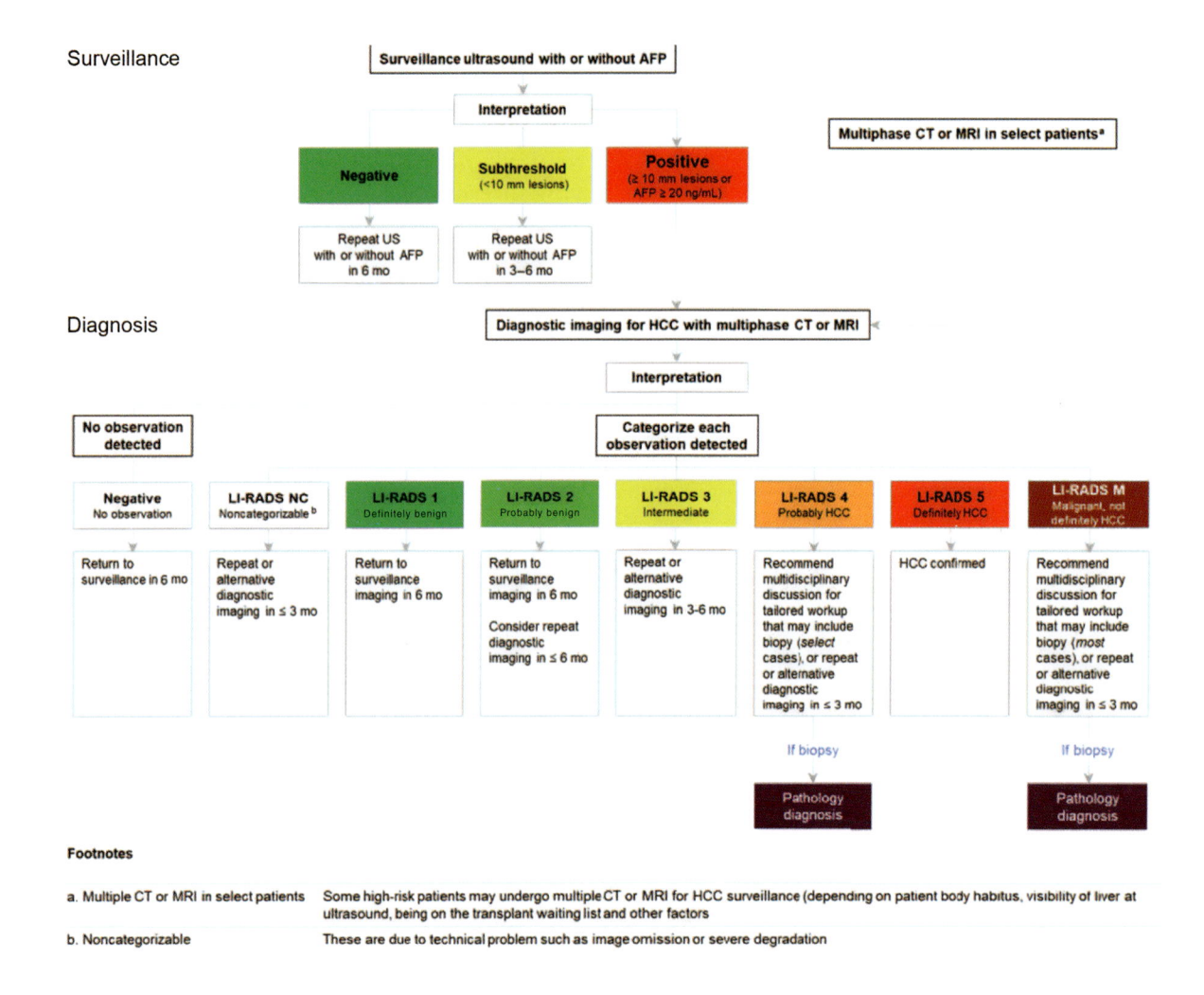

Figure 4 The American Association for the Study of Liver Disease (AASLD) diagnostic algorithm for suspected HCC.

score,[95] the Chinese University Prognostic Index (CUPI),[96] and the American Joint Committee on Cancer/International Union Against Cancer (AJCC/UICC) staging system.[97] Each staging system has strengths and weaknesses. However, combining cancer staging with treatment algorithm can be challenging and may result in being too conservative in some cases and too aggressive in other cases. Therefore, hepatic functional reserve and oncologic status of tumor should be classified separately.

Classically, the overall status of the hepatic functional reserve and risk of treatment are stratified by the Child-Turcotte-Pugh (CTP) score, which is calculated using five factors: presence and degree of encephalopathy, presence and degree of ascites, serum bilirubin concentration, serum albumin concentration, and prothrombin time (Table 1). CTP score is nowadays included in various treatment algorithms for hepatic neoplasms,[98–100] and liver resection is usually indicated for CTP class A patients or highly

Table 1 Child-turcotte-pugh (CTP) classification.

	Points		
	1	2	3
Albumin (g/dL)	>3.5	2.8–3.5	<2.8
Bilirubin (mg/dL)	<2.0	2.0–3.0	>3.0
Prothrombin time			
Seconds	<4	4–6	>6
International normalized ratio (INR)	<1.7	1.7–2.3	>2.3
Ascites	None	Moderate	Severe
Encephalopathy	None	Grade I–II	Grade III–VI
CTP class A	5–6 points		
CTP class B	7–9 points		
CTP class C	10–15 points		

Table 2 American Joint Committee on Cancer/International Union against Cancer (AJCC/UICC) 8th edition staging system for hepatocellular carcinoma.[a]

T classification	
T1a	Solitary ≤2 cm
T1b	Solitary >2 cm without vascular invasion
T2	Solitary >2 cm with vascular invasion or multifocal ≤5 cm
T3	Multiple tumors >5 cm
T4	Single tumor or multiple tumor of any size involving a major branch of the portal vein or hepatic vein, or tumor(s) with direct invasion of adjacent organs other than the gallbladder or with perforation of visceral peritoneum
Stage grouping	
Stage IA	T1aN0M0
Stage IB	T1bN0M0
Stage II	T2N0M0
Stage IIIA	T3N0M0
Stage IIIB	T4N0M0
Stage IVA	Any T N1M0
Stage IVB	Any T Any N M1

[a]Source: Edge et al.[96]

selected patients classified as CTP class B. Consensus exists that CTP class C patients should not undergo surgical resection due to high perioperative mortality rate.[99] In the field of liver transplantation, the Model for End-stage Liver Disease (MELD) has widely been adopted for graft allocation to minimize the mortality rate of potential recipients on the waiting list. The main advantage of the MELD score is that it contains objective parameters (i.e., bilirubin, creatinine, and international normalized ratio-INR) combined according to the following equation: $9.57 \times [\text{Ln creatinine (mg/dL)}] + 3.78 \times [\text{Ln bilirubin (mg/dL)}] + 11.2 \times \text{Ln INR} + 0.643$.[101] Although the MELD score is not routinely used for selection of treatment options in patients with preserved hepatic functional reserve, HCC patients with higher MELD scores may benefit more from liver transplantation than liver resection.[102]

The AJCC/UICC 8th edition TNM staging system (Table 2) is a modification of 6th and 7th editions, which were based on a study from the International Cooperative Study Group on HCC that included data from the United States, Japan, and France who all underwent surgical resection.[103] A major strength of the AJCC/UICC staging system was the use of centralized pathological review. Although the AJCC/UICC staging system was developed using a cohort dominated by hepatitis C-related HCC, it has also been independently validated in a Chinese cohort with a high prevalence of hepatitis B.[104] Modification in the 8th edition was based on the results of an international multicenter study reporting that microvascular invasion or tumor differentiation does not affect surgical outcomes in small HCC measuring up to 2 cm. This specific group of patients is now classified as a new subset of patients with favorable prognosis.[97,105]

Treatment

The choice of therapy for HCC is individualized based on the tumor burden, degree of underlying liver disease, patient performance status, and the overall possibility of side effects or complications. The BCLC staging system[93] is widely used to stratify patients into cohorts for whom specific therapies are best suited (Figure 5). However, the limitation of the BCLC algorithm is that it is fairly conservative with regard to the application of surgical therapy (Figure 5, red color). Patients with larger solitary tumors are not considered surgical candidates despite a growing experience with resection with acceptable outcomes (Figure 6) in this group.[105–108] Investigators have acknowledged that the BCLC algorithm limits resection criteria and a modified BCLC algorithm has been proposed in response to extend the indications for resection of HCC (Figure 7).[109] In the guidelines on liver cancer treatment proposed by the Japan Society of Hepatology,[100] surgical resection is currently indicated for CTP class A or class B patients with 3 or fewer HCC nodules, irrespective of the size of each tumor, while liver transplantation is limited only for CTP class C patients meeting the Milan criteria. Selection of treatment should be determined in a multidisciplinary approach considering the local expertise. However, the most effective treatment including surgical resection, ablation, and orthotopic liver transplantation (OLT) should be the first priority as long as such treatments are permitted.

Surgical resection

For liver resection, strict assessment of hepatic functional reserve is needed for patients with HCC because HCC usually develops in an injured liver, and accordingly, maximum extent of resection is needed to be estimated carefully. Functional investigations have been proposed to better evaluate the severity of chronic liver disease. The measurement of indocyanine green retention rate at 15 min (ICG-R15) is the most frequently used test. For patients with obstructive jaundice or congenital intolerance to indocyanine green, ^{99m}Tc-galactosyl human serum albumin (GSA) scintigraphy sensitively estimates the hepatic functional reserve.

Liver resection is indicated only for CTP class A or B patients with controllable ascites and serum total bilirubin level of <2.0 mg/dL, and the maximum extent of resection can be determined based on the measurement of ICG-R15.[110] At the University of Tokyo, the maximum extent of resection is set up to 67% (right hepatectomy or trisectionectomy) for patients with ICG-R15 <10%, up to 33% (left hepatectomy or left lateral sectorectomy) for those with ICG-R15 between 10% and 20%, segmentectomy for those with ICG-R15 between 20% and 30%, and only limited partial hepatectomy is indicated for patients with ICG-R15 greater than 30%. Following strictly this algorithm, no mortality due to hepatic insufficiency was reported in 1056 consecutive patients.[111] Recently, more sophisticated criteria based on the ICG disappearing rate and precise volumetry have shown that these conventional criteria can be expanded safely.[112,113] At MD Anderson Cancer Center, portal vein embolization (PVE) has been used to induce hypertrophy of the future liver remnant (FLR) and increase the candidacy of HCC patients for major hepatectomy and to improve postoperative outcomes and safety.[114] The procedure has shown to be safe and well tolerated with increased survival rates.[109] PVE has another major benefit in HCC: it is a test of the regenerative potential of the liver. Most patients with HCC have

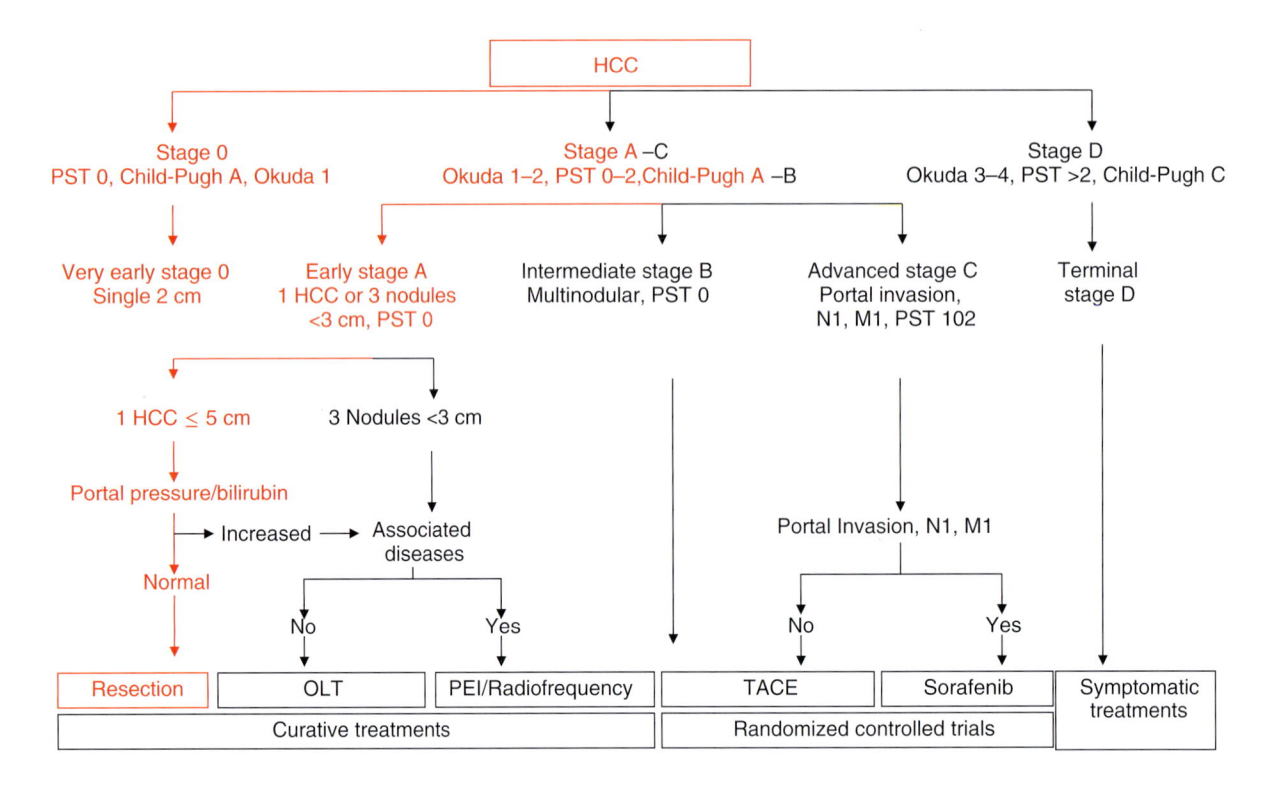

Figure 5 BCLC algorithm for treatment selection in patients with HCC. Red color indicates patients potentially candidates for resection according to the BCLC algorithm. Source: Llovet et al.[106]. Reproduced with permission of Elsevier.

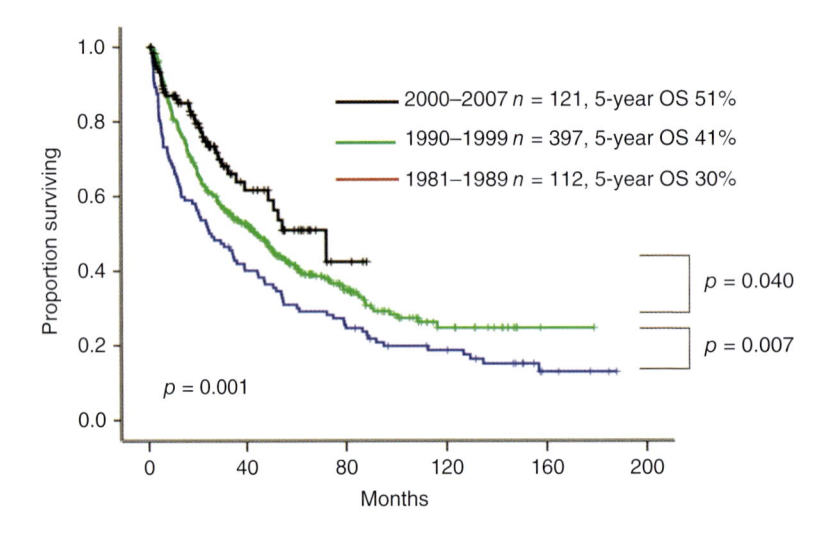

Figure 6 Kaplan–Meier plots of survival after resection of ≥4 segments in patients with HCC (n = 630) stratified by three different time periods. Source: Andreou et al.[107]

underlying cirrhosis, and it is clinically challenging to assess liver function and make validated treatment decisions, especially when a major liver resection is required. The degree of hypertrophy after PVE is inversely associated with the regenerative potential of the liver. Subsequently, the degree of hypertrophy provides valuable information of potentially missed liver injury: less than 5% hypertrophy after PVE is associated with increased mortality after liver resection.[115]

Orthotopic liver transplantation (OLT)
Unlike liver resection, liver transplantation addresses both the tumor and the underlying liver condition. Clinical outcomes of liver transplantation for HCC were poor in the early era. However, after the landmark study by Mazzaferro et al.[89] from which the Milan criteria were established, it is widely recognized that favorable survival outcomes can be expected in a selected population with a limited size and number of HCC. Selection criteria for transplantation used in this study were tumor diameter of 5 cm or less in patients with single HCC, or 3 cm or less if the patient had two or three lesions.[89] Nowadays, these criteria are extended with or without tumor markers or biopsy findings in several high-volume transplant centers.[116–127]

Locoregional ablation therapies
Image-guided ablation is accepted as the best therapeutic choice for patients with early-stage HCC when surgical options are precluded.

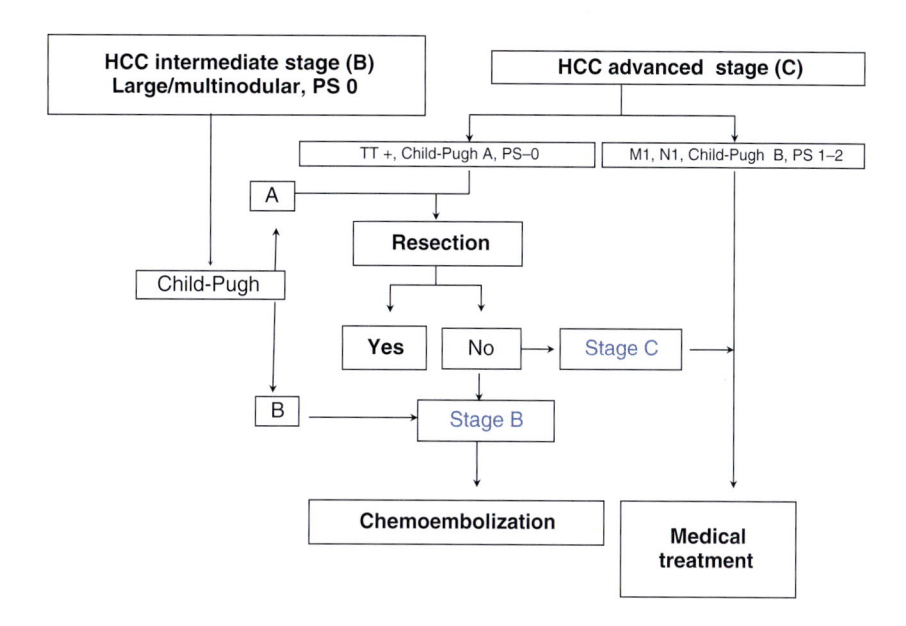

Figure 7 Modified BCLC algorithm extending resection indications in HCC. Source: Torzilli et al.[109]

Several methods for local tumor destruction have been developed and clinically used over the two decades. Radiofrequency ablation (RFA) has shown superior ablative effect and greater survival benefit compared to conventional percutaneous ethanol injection in meta-analyses of randomized controlled trials,[128–132] and is now established as the standard ablative modality. Currently, thermal or nonthermal ablation methods including microwave ablation and irreversible electroporation are under investigation as potential alternatives to RFA.

Transarterial chemoembolization (TACE)

The normal liver receives dual blood supply from the hepatic artery (25%) and the portal vein (75%). HCC exhibits intense neo-angiogenic activity during its progression and is mostly dependent on the hepatic arterial supply. This provides the rationale for using arterial obstruction with or without regional chemotherapy as an effective therapeutic option for HCC. Transarterial therapies are usually considered palliative and should be offered to patients with intermediate-stage disease without extra-hepatic metastases and sufficient hepatic functional reserve. The most commonly used agents for transarterial chemoembolization (TACE) are doxorubicin and cisplatin, followed by epirubicin. None was found superior to the others in RCTs.[133,134] Regarding the embolizing material, gelatin sponge (gelfoam) has conventionally been used. However, it could provide only short-term arterial occlusion up to 2 weeks. Currently, polyvinyl alcohol (PVA) particles are used in many centers, which offer permanent arterial occlusion and also achieves more distal embolization with its small particle size.[135] Drug-eluting beads have been recently developed to provide a combined local ischemic and cytotoxic effect. Although its superiority to conventional TACE remains debatable, equivalent efficacy and safety compared to conventional TACE have been reported in several studies.[136,137]

Currently, TACE is the only arterial therapy recommended for intermediate stage HCC in the AASLD guidelines.[82] However, recent studies comparing the safety and efficacy for TACE and transarterial radioembolization (TARE) using yttrium-90 (^{90}Y) microspheres for unresectable HCC have reported encouraging results in patients who underwent TARE,[138] and this could be a treatment option especially for patients with portal venous tumor thrombus, whereas TACE is not recommended for such patients. Further studies are needed to establish an optimal choice of directed arterial therapies for HCC.

Systemic treatment

Systemic chemotherapy may be the only option for patients with advanced and/or disseminated disease in patients with HCC. For decades, various systemic therapies have been explored for the treatment of advanced HCC. Nevertheless, no satisfactory results have been obtained in cytotoxic chemotherapy so far. Our group has previously shown that cisplatin/interferon α-2b/doxorubicin/5-fluorouracil (PIAF) combination therapy improves response, resectability, and patient survival in patients with initially unresectable HCC when limiting the indication only for patients with no hepatitis or cirrhosis.[139] This traditional regimen might provide an option for unresectable HCC developed in noncirrhotic patients (Figures 8 and 9).

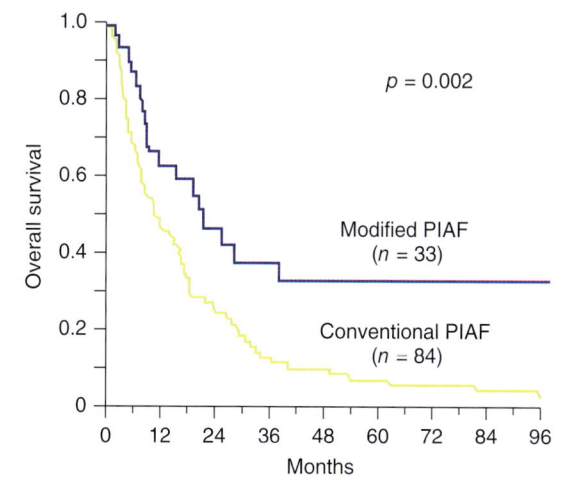

Figure 8 Kaplan–Meier plots of survival with initially unresectable HCC ($n = 117$) stratified on treatment with PIAF (cisplatin/interferon α2b/doxorubicin/5-fluorouracil regimen). Source: Kaseb et al.[139]

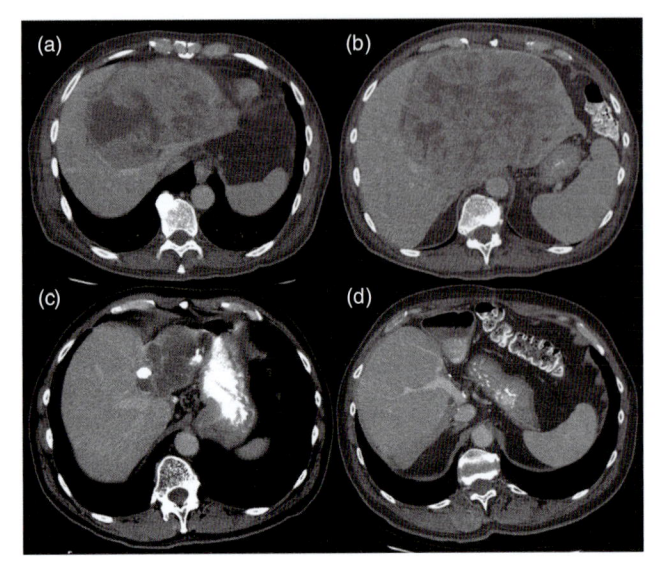

Figure 9 Computed tomography of a 60-year-old male with large HCC. (a, b) A 15 cm in diameter HCC involving left lobe, right anterior sector, and abutting the right hepatic vein. (c) After treatment with Platinum Interferon, Adriamycin, 5-fluorouracil, and transarterial chemoembolization. (d) After extended left hepatectomy including resection of the caudate lobe and the inferior vena cava. The patient is alive without evidence of disease 8 years after surgery.

Recently, various new biologic agents have been introduced and tested in the field of HCC. Sorafenib is a polyvalent molecule which has been shown in HCC cell line to inhibit the serine-threonine kinase Raf-1 and several receptor tyrosine kinases such as vascular endothelial growth factor receptor (VEGFR2), platelet-derived growth factor receptor (PDGFR), FLT3, Ret, and c-Kit. Two-Phase III studies, the SHARP trial[140] and the Asia-Pacific trial,[141] demonstrated a survival benefit with sorafenib in patients with HCC, and this has been only the systemic therapy agent approved for clinical use for HCC for decades. However, recently approved new agents such as lenvatinib (1st line),[142] regorafenib (2nd line),[143] cabozantinib (2nd line),[144] or ramucirumab (2nd line)[145] are changing the landscape of systemic therapy and are expected to improve survival outcomes of patients with HCC. Additionally, randomized Phase III trials investigating the efficacy of anti-PD-1/anti-PD-L1 + antiangiogenic agent combination regimens are ongoing. IMbrave150 has recently demonstrated significant improvement in both overall survival and progression-free survival for atezolizumab + bevacizumab (vs sorafenib) in patients with unresectable HCC who have not received prior systemic therapy.[146]

Intrahepatic cholangiocarcinoma

Incidence and epidemiology
ICC is the second most common primary hepatic malignancy after HCC. Among bile duct cancers, ICC are less common than extrahepatic (including perihilar) cholangiocarcinomas, although its incidence is rising rapidly, having nearly tripled in the past four decades in the United States. The number of new cases per 100,000 has increased from 0.44 in 1973 to 1.18 in 2012, with a steepening of the trend in the past decade.[147] This rise has been attributed to improvements in imaging capabilities, molecular diagnostics, and pathological evaluation. This last category stems from previous misclassification of these tumors as cancers of unknown primary (CUP) with adenocarcinoma features, which have seen a corresponding decline in incidence.[147] Throughout the world, there is considerable geographic variation in the incidence of ICC, with a greater incidence in East Asia.[148] The overall survival rate for unresectable tumor is dismal, with 5-year survival rate of 5% to 10%. Because systemic therapy for ICC has not yet been established, surgical resection offers the only chance for cure. However, the overall survival after curative-intent surgery is disappointing, with a 5-year survival rate of 20–35%.[149]

Risk factors
ICC is thought to derive from a common hepatic progenitor cell that may also give rise to HCC,[150] and combined hepatocellular-cholangiocarcinoma having histopathologic features of HCC and ICC is sometimes observed. Risk factors for ICC have not yet been well established, though chronic liver disease and cirrhosis are reportedly correlated with ICC. In particular, recent epidemiological studies suggest an association between ICC and chronic hepatitis C infection[151] and metabolic syndrome.[152]

Other predisposing conditions include infections that affect the biliary tract, such as *Opisthorchis viverini* or *Clonorchis sinensis*, sclerosing cholangitis, the presence of choledochal cysts, hepatolithiasis, tobacco, or other causes of cirrhosis.[153] Because common predisposing conditions are lacking and due to rarity of ICC, it is difficult to determine a clear target population for routine screening to facilitate early diagnosis.

Pathology
There are three morphologic subtypes of ICC that can be characterized on cross-sectional appearance: mass-forming, periductal-infiltrating, and intraductal-growing (Figure 10), with mass-forming being the most common subtype. Unlike HCC, ICC shows invasive tumor growth without a tumor capsule. Therefore, when a tumor is found to about a major vascular structure on imaging, microscopic invasion of the vascular wall should be suspected and en-bloc resection is usually needed.

Recent genomic profiling of cholangiocarcinomas has identified a number of promising potential therapeutic targets. In a comprehensive genetic profiling study of biliary tract cancers, the most commonly altered genes among 412 ICC were TP53 (27%), CDKN2A/B (27%), KRAS (22%), IDH1/2 (20%), ARID1A (18%), and FGFR1-3 (11%).[154] Targeted therapies against some of these molecular aberrations are currently being investigated in clinical trials in solid organ malignancies including ICC.[155]

Diagnosis
ICCs are often diagnosed incidentally on cross-sectional imaging performed for other reasons. Due to their location, ICC tend not to cause early symptoms and instead present at advanced stages, at which time vague, nonspecific abdominal pain and weight loss may be reported. Although blood work, including liver function tests, and tumor markers such as CEA, CA 19-9, and AFP are routinely drawn, none are specific for ICC. CA 19-9 may be elevated with pancreatobiliary malignancies, but can also be falsely elevated in benign conditions, including biliary obstruction. On the other hand, an elevated AFP should raise suspicion of a HCC or a combined HCC/ICC rather than a pure ICC, especially in the setting of cirrhosis.

Work-up and staging of ICC should include high-quality, multiphasic cross-sectional imaging of the chest, abdomen, and

Mass-forming type   Periductal infiltrating type   Intraductal growth type

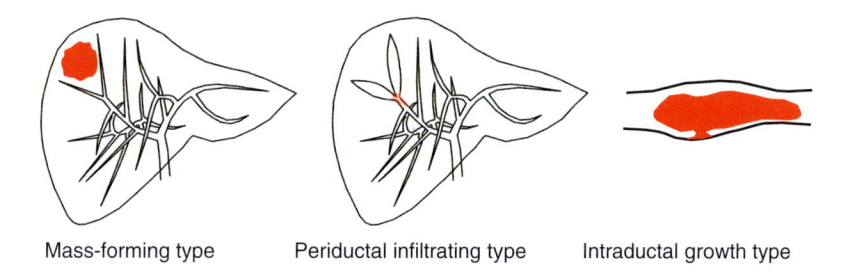

Figure 10 Gross classification of intrahepatic cholangiocarcinoma. Source: Adapted from Liver Cancer Study Group of Japan.

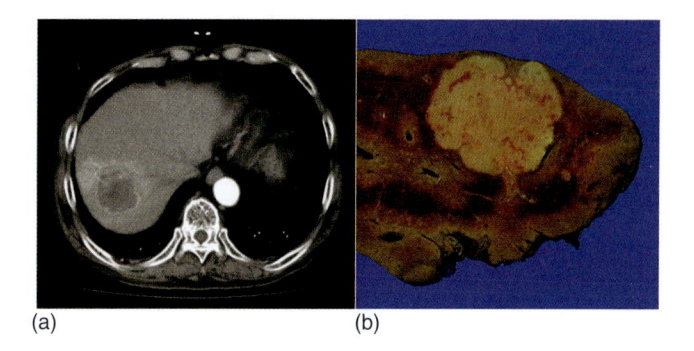

(a)   (b)

Figure 11 (a) Typical ring enhancement in enhanced CT scan and (b) gross appearance of intrahepatic cholangiocarcinoma.

pelvis. In the right context, upper and lower gastrointestinal endoscopies may be helpful to rule out a primary tumor, as a major differential for ICC is metastatic disease. On dynamic imaging studies, ICC tends to be hypo-enhancing due to its hypovascular nature. However, various degrees of enhancement may be observed surrounding the lesion, reflecting the fibrous connective tissue frequently observed around the tumor (Figure 11). Assessing the tumor's relationship to major vascular and biliary structures, the presence of satellitosis, metastatic disease, or nodal involvement will be key in determining resectability. MRCP is not routinely indicated in the evaluation of ICC unless the tumor encroaches onto second or third-order biliary radicals. The role of PET scan in the work-up of ICC remains unclear, although it may improve detection of nodal and metastatic disease.[156]

Staging

Through the 6th edition of the AJCC system, the staging of ICC was identical to that of HCC. However, based on survival outcomes for 598 patients who underwent liver resection for ICC from the SEER database that found multiple tumors, vascular invasion, and nodal involvement to be independent prognostic factors, the staging system for ICC was modified to be independent and separate from that of HCC in the 7th edition of the AJCC.[157] This revised staging system has been validated externally and independently by the French Surgical Association (AFC)-IHCC 2009 study group.[158] In the 8th, and most recent, edition of the AJCC staging system, two major changes took place, both with regards to T stages. For T1 tumors, which represent a single tumor without vascular invasion, a cutoff of 5 cm marks the difference between T1a and T1b tumors. T2 tumors are no longer separated into T2a (single tumor with vascular invasion) and T2b (multiple tumors with or without vascular invasion).[97]

Treatment

The management of ICC is complex and requires careful multidisciplinary review and planning. For ICC, only complete surgical resection offers a chance of cure because these are no established other curative treatment options. Surgical treatment for ICC involves margin-negative resection, which may require extrahepatic bile duct resection, in addition to systematic regional nodal dissection. R0 hepatectomy is associated with improved overall and recurrence-free survival.[159,160] Other independent predictors of survival include multifocal disease, vascular invasion, and nodal involvement.[147] Although some groups consider these features contraindications to resection, our group regards them instead as high-risk features for disease recurrence and early dissemination and will selectively use neoadjuvant therapy in this scenario before proceeding with surgery. The role of portal lymphadenectomy remains controversial. On the one hand, there appears to be no survival benefit to routine lymphadenectomy.[161] On the other, nodal involvement provides important prognostic information for ICC and has been reported in up to 30% of patients.[162] For this reason, we do recommend routine portal lymphadenectomy at the time of ICC resection. It should be noted that nodal disease beyond the porta hepatis represents metastatic disease, and surgery in this setting is associated with poor outcomes. As is the case for hepatectomy for other pathologies, ensuring an adequate FLR is critical to the safe performance of surgery. PVE may be employed to elicit hypertrophy of the FLR to avoid posthepatectomy liver failure when necessary.

The high rate of disease recurrence after resection of ICC has long generated a strong interest in adjuvant therapy. Yet, until recently, no level one data had been available to guide management in this regard for a number of reasons, including the relative rarity of this cancer and, by extension, the tendency of studies to lump ICC with other biliary tract cancers despite their differing biology. Still, one such study—the BILCAP trial—has provided the most convincing evidence to date to support adjuvant chemotherapy.[163] This Phase 3 trial of 447 patients with completely resected biliary tract cancers, including 84 cases of ICC, showed improved recurrence-free survival (HR 0.70, 95% CI 0.54–0.92) and overall survival (HR 0.75, 95% CI 0.58–0.97) with capecitabine compared to observation in the a priori determined per-protocol analysis.

The role of OLT in the management of ICC is much less well established than for HCC. The early experience had been disappointing, with reported 5-year survival rates of 23% and a median time to recurrence of 9 months.[164] More recently, our early experience with OLT for locally advanced ICC treated with neoadjuvant therapy has yielded more encouraging results. Among six patients who underwent OLT, OS was 100%, 83%, and 83% at 1, 3, and 5 years, respectively. Three patients developed recurrent disease at a median of 7.6 months. The key to careful selection of patients for OLT was demonstration of pretransplant disease stability on neoadjuvant therapy.[165]

For patients with advanced ICC, systemic chemotherapy has made some progress in the past decade. The response rate to single-agent 5-fluorouracil-based or gemcitabine-based systemic therapy is only about 10% to 30%.[166,167] In the ABC-02 Phase 3 randomized controlled trial, which studied 510 patients who had locally advanced or metastatic biliary tract cancer, the combination of gemcitabine plus cisplatin was associated with improved progression-free survival and overall survival (11.7 months vs 8.1 months) compared with gemcitabine alone.[168] On the heels of this study, this regimen became standard-of-care, first-line treatment for patients with advanced cancer of the bile ducts and gallbladder. Recently, the addition of nab-paclitaxel to this doublet was shown to improve median overall survival to 19.2 months for patients with advanced biliary tract cancers in a Phase 2 trial.[169] Other regimens to consider include FOLFIRINOX, which has been shown to represent a safe and effective salvage treatment in patients with advanced biliary tract cancers refractory to gemcitabine/cisplatin.[170] The two regimens are being investigated head-to-head as first-line therapy for locally advanced, nonresectable, or metastatic biliary tract cancer.[171] Improved understanding of the molecular carcinogenesis of biliary tract cancers has also led to growing interest in examining novel, targeted anticancer agents.[153,155] As such, routine molecular profiling of ICC should be undertaken to guide second-line treatment should standard chemotherapy fail because significant subsets of patients may derive a meaningful sustained response to targeted therapy against actionable molecular aberrations, including FGR fusion gene[172] or IDH1.[173] As is the case with HCC, locoregional therapy options including ablative options, TACE, transarterial radioembolization with yttrium-90, and radiation therapy may be considered for patients with unresectable ICC.

Hepatic angiosarcoma

Hepatic angiosarcoma is a rare tumor derived from the malignant transformation of hepatic endothelial cells, and close association with environmental carcinogens such as thorotrast (contrast agent used in the 1940s and 1950s), vinyl chloride, arsenicals, and androgenic-anabolic steroids has been reported. Because no clear etiology or association with chronic liver disease has been identified, hepatic angiosarcoma is usually advanced at the time of diagnosis. Although complete surgical resection or OLT may provide a chance of prolonged survival, prognosis is generally poor even after liver transplantation.[174] The efficacy of chemotherapy has not been well documented for this tumor.

Epithelioid hemangioendothelioma

Epithelioid hemangioendothelioma (EHE) is a very rare, low-grade malignant neoplasm of endothelial origin with a reported incidence of less than 0.1 per 100,000 people.[175] EHE presents heterogeneous clinical features, nonspecific radiological characteristics, and a variable natural history.[176] The management options for EHE include liver resection, OLT, chemotherapy, and radiotherapy. However, it is difficult to compare the clinical outcomes among these therapeutic options because of the rarity of the disease. Favorable outcomes have been reported after liver resection for EHE, with 1- and 5-year survival rates of 100% and 75%, respectively.[177] However, due to frequent diffuse presentation in the disease, liver resection is not possible in a majority of the cases. The result of OLT is also encouraging with 1- and 5-year survival rates of 96% and 54.5%. A recent study has also shown favorable long-term outcomes after OLT with 5- and 10-year survival rates of 83% and 74%, irrespective of the presence of nodal involvement or extrahepatic disease.[178] Due to the indolent nature of the disease, a recent study concluded that initial observation followed by resection or OLT in the patients who remained candidates for surgery could be beneficial to stratify treatment options.[179] However, because of the rarity of the disease, strong evidence-based management strategies are difficult to establish and large multicenter prospective trials may be necessary for improved understanding of EHE.

> **Summary**
>
> Primary liver cancer is the second leading cause of cancer death in men and the sixth leading cause among women worldwide. Hepatocellular carcinoma (HCC) constitutes 70–85% of primary hepatic neoplasms, followed by intrahepatic cholangiocarcinoma (ICC) (10–15%) and other less common hepatic malignancies (5%) such as hepatic angiosarcoma, epithelioid hemangioendothelioma, or hepatic lymphoma. Primary hepatic malignancies are generally associated with poor survival. In light of limited effective systemic therapy options, prevention, appropriate screening (in the case of HCC), early diagnosis, and multidisciplinary management are critical to maximizing outcomes. In addition, most primary hepatic neoplasms are associated with chronic liver disease or cirrhosis, such that the resultant decreased hepatic functional reserve often precludes aggressive treatment. Therefore, for treatment selection, one should consider two intrinsic conflicting factors: curability and safety of treatment. Currently, several clinical staging systems and treatment algorithms are available to adequately select therapeutic options for HCC. The choice of therapy is individualized based on the tumor burden, degree of underlying liver disease, patient performance status, and the overall possibility of side effects or complications, and must be balanced with the anticipated benefits. Selection of treatment should be determined in a multidisciplinary fashion with the local expertise. Curative treatment options including surgical resection, ablation, and orthotopic liver transplantation (OLT) should be the first priority as long as these treatments are approved.

Key references

The complete reference list can be found on Vital Source version of this title, see inside front cover.

9 Brechot C. Hepatitis B virus (HBV) and hepatocellular carcinoma. HBV DNA status and its implications. *J Hepatol.* 1987;**4**:269–279.
14 Dusheiko G, Schmilovitz-Weiss H, Brown D, et al. Hepatitis C virus genotypes: an investigation of type-specific differences in geographic origin and disease. *Hepatology.* 1994;**19**:13–18.
15 Shindoh J, Hasegawa K, Matsuyama Y, et al. Low hepatitis C viral load predicts better long-term outcomes in patients undergoing resection of hepatocellular

16. carcinoma irrespective of serologic eradication of hepatitis C virus. *J Clin Oncol.* 2013;**31**:766–773.
17. Hassan MM, Spitz MR, Thomas MB, et al. Effect of different types of smoking and synergism with hepatitis C virus on risk of hepatocellular carcinoma in American men and women: case-control study. *Int J Cancer* 2008;**123**:1883–1891.
19. Ikeda K, Saitoh S, Suzuki Y, et al. Disease progression and hepatocellular carcinogenesis in patients with chronic viral hepatitis: a prospective observation of 2215 patients. *J Hepatol.* 1998;**28**:930–938.
25. Calle EE, Rodriguez C, Walker-Thurmond K, Thun MJ. Overweight, obesity, and mortality from cancer in a prospectively studied cohort of U.S. adults. *N Engl J Med.* 2003;**348**:1625–1638.
28. Loomba R, Abraham M, Unalp A, et al. Association between diabetes, family history of diabetes, and risk of nonalcoholic steatohepatitis and fibrosis. *Hepatology.* 2012;**56**:943–951.
30. El-Serag HB, Tran T, Everhart JE. Diabetes increases the risk of chronic liver disease and hepatocellular carcinoma. *Gastroenterology.* 2004;**126**:460–468.
54. Tan ZM, Sun BC. Effects of antiviral therapy on preventing liver tumorigenesis and hepatocellular carcinoma recurrence. *World J Gastroenterol.* 2013;**19**:8895–8901.
58. Omata M, Yoshida H, Shiratori Y. Prevention of hepatocellular carcinoma and its recurrence in chronic hepatitis C patients by interferon therapy. *Clin Gastroenterol Hepatol.* 2005;**3**:S141–S143.
61. Kumada H, Suzuki Y, Ikeda K, et al. Daclatasvir plus asunaprevir for chronic HCV genotype 1b infection. *Hepatology.* 2014;**59**:2083–2091.
62. Lawitz E, Poordad FF, Pang PS, et al. Sofosbuvir and ledipasvir fixed-dose combination with and without ribavirin in treatment-naive and previously treated patients with genotype 1 hepatitis C virus infection (LONESTAR): an open-label, randomised, phase 2 trial. *Lancet.* 2014;**383**:515–523.
63. Lawitz E, Sulkowski MS, Ghalib R, et al. Simeprevir plus sofosbuvir, with or without ribavirin, to treat chronic infection with hepatitis C virus genotype 1 in non-responders to pegylated interferon and ribavirin and treatment-naive patients: the COSMOS randomised study. *Lancet.* 2014;**384**(9956):1756–1765.
64. International Consensus Group for Hepatocellular NeoplasiaThe International Consensus Group for Hepatocellular N. Pathologic diagnosis of early hepatocellular carcinoma: a report of the international consensus group for hepatocellular neoplasia. *Hepatology.* 2009;**49**:658–664.
69. Liver Cancer Study Group of Japan. *The General Rules for the Clinical and Pathological Study of Primary Liver Cancer*, 5th ed. Tokyo: Kanehara; 2008.
72. Imamura H, Matsuyama Y, Tanaka E, et al. Risk factors contributing to early and late phase intrahepatic recurrence of hepatocellular carcinoma after hepatectomy. *J Hepatol.* 2003;**38**:200–207.
73. Sakamoto M, Hirohashi S, Tsuda H, et al. Multicentric independent development of hepatocellular carcinoma revealed by analysis of hepatitis B virus integration pattern. *Am J Surg Pathol.* 1989;**13**:1064–1067.
74. Ikai I, Yamaoka Y, Yamamoto Y, et al. Surgical intervention for patients with stage IV-A hepatocellular carcinoma without lymph node metastasis: proposal as a standard therapy. *Ann Surg.* 1998;**227**:433–439.
82. Marrero JA, Kulik LM, Sirlin CB, et al. Diagnosis, staging, and management of hepatocellular carcinoma: 2018 practice guidance by the American association for the study of liver diseases. *Hepatology.* 2018;**68**:723–750.
87. Trevisani F, Cantarini MC, Labate AM, et al. Surveillance for hepatocellular carcinoma in elderly Italian patients with cirrhosis: effects on cancer staging and patient survival. *Am J Gastroenterol.* 2004;**99**:1470–1476.
88. Santi V, Trevisani F, Gramenzi A, et al. Semiannual surveillance is superior to annual surveillance for the detection of early hepatocellular carcinoma and patient survival. *J Hepatol.* 2010;**53**:291–297.
89. Mazzaferro V, Regalia E, Doci R, et al. Liver transplantation for the treatment of small hepatocellular carcinomas in patients with cirrhosis. *N Engl J Med.* 1996;**334**:693–699.
94. Makuuchi M, Belghiti J, Belli G, et al. IHPBA concordant classification of primary liver cancer: working group report. *J Hepatobiliary Pancreat Surg.* 2003;**10**:26–30.
97. Amin M, Edge S, Greene F, Byrd D. *AJCC Cancer Staging Manual*, 8th ed. Switzerland: Springer International Publishing; 2017.
98. Bruix J, Sherman M, Practice Guidelines Committee AAftSoLD. Management of hepatocellular carcinoma. *Hepatology.* 2005;**42**:1208–1236.
101. Malinchoc M, Kamath PS, Gordon FD, et al. A model to predict poor survival in patients undergoing transjugular intrahepatic portosystemic shunts. *Hepatology.* 2000;**31**:864–871.
105. Shindoh J, Andreou A, Aloia TA, et al. Microvascular invasion does not predict long-term survival in hepatocellular carcinoma up to 2 cm: reappraisal of the staging system for solitary tumors. *Ann Surg Oncol.* 2013;**20**:1223–1229.
106. Llovet JM, Burroughs A, Bruix J. Hepatocellular carcinoma. *Lancet.* 2003;**362**:1907–1917.
110. Makuuchi M, Kosuge T, Takayama T, et al. Surgery for small liver cancers. *Semin Surg Oncol.* 1993;**9**:298–304.
112. Kobayashi Y, Kiya Y, Nishioka Y, et al. Indocyanine green clearance of remnant liver (ICG-Krem) predicts postoperative subclinical hepatic insufficiency after resection of colorectal liver metastasis: theoretical validation for safe expansion of Makuuchi's criteria. *HPB (Oxford).* 2020;**22**:258–264.

88 Gallbladder and bile duct cancer

Mariam F. Eskander, MD, MPH ■ Christopher T. Aquina, MD, MPH ■ Timothy M. Pawlik, MD, MPH, PhD

Overview

Biliary tract malignancy, which includes gallbladder cancer and cholangiocarcinoma, is an aggressive disease that is often advanced at the time of diagnosis and thus associated with a poor prognosis. In this article, we will review the epidemiology, risk factors, pathology, clinical presentation, diagnostic imaging modalities, and current treatment recommendations for gallbladder adenocarcinoma and cholangiocarcinoma.

Gallbladder cancer

Adenocarcinoma of the gallbladder is the sixth most common digestive-system malignancy in the United States.[1] In Western countries such as the United States, where there is a low incidence of hepatocellular carcinoma (HCC), gallbladder cancer is relatively more common. The American Cancer Society estimates that about 12,360 new cases of gallbladder and extrahepatic bile duct cancer were diagnosed in 2019 in the United States. About 3960 people died of these cancers in 2019.[2] Of these new cases and deaths, about half are due to gallbladder cancer. Between 1980 and 1995, mortality rates from gallbladder cancer decreased in the United States, Canada, Australia, and the United Kingdom, while increasing in Japan, Italy, Spain, and Chile.[3] Unlike HCC and cholangiocarcinoma, gallbladder carcinoma has a higher incidence in females than males with an overall female-to-male ratio between 2:1 and 6:1.[1,3] The preponderance of this cancer in females is even greater in patients <40 years old, with a female-to-male ratio of 20:1.[4]

The incidence of gallbladder carcinoma increases with age and varies dramatically by geographic region. Rates are very high in South American and Asia, relatively high in several countries in eastern and central Europe, such as Hungary, Germany, and Poland, and low in the United States and Mediterranean European countries.[1] In Chile, gallbladder cancer is the number one cause of cancer mortality in women.[5] The geographic and population-based variation in the incidence of gallbladder cancer suggest that environmental risk factors, including carcinogens, infectious agents like *Salmonella typhi* and *Helicobacter pylori*, and diet, have a role in gallbladder tumorigenesis.[5,6]

In the United States, gallbladder cancer is more common in Southwest Native Americans than in the general American population. Incidence rates for U.S. white males, U.S. black males, and Native American males in New Mexico are 0.4, 0.6, and 3.8 cases per 100,000 per year, respectively. The corresponding rates for females are 1.0, 0.8, and 10.3.[3] Gallbladder carcinoma has been found in 6% of Southwest Native American undergoing biliary tract surgery.[7] Additionally, it is the second most common gastrointestinal malignancy in this population, and the youngest reported case of gallbladder carcinoma occurred in an 11-year-old Navajo girl.[8]

Causative factors

There are no apparent associations between gallbladder carcinoma and hepatitis B or C virus infection, cirrhosis, or mycotoxin exposure. Similarly, chemical hepatocarcinogens have not been clearly demonstrated to increase the risk of developing gallbladder carcinoma. However, there are suggestions that workers exposed to carcinogenic substances, such as methylcholanthrene and nitrosamines, have a higher incidence and earlier onset of gallbladder carcinoma when compared with control populations.[9] There is a significant association between gallstones and gallbladder cancer, with gallstones present in 74–92% of patients with gallbladder carcinoma.[10,11] The risk of developing gallbladder carcinoma increases directly with increasing gallstone size.[12] Patients with gallstones 2.0–2.9 cm in diameter have a 2.4 times higher relative risk of developing gallbladder carcinoma, whereas patients with gallstones greater than 3.0 cm in diameter have a 10.1 times higher risk. Patients with longstanding chronic cholecystitis can develop calcification of the gallbladder wall, also known as a porcelain gallbladder. It is possible that chronic inflammation and/or infection of the gallbladder increases the risk of developing gallbladder carcinoma because 22% of patients with calcified gallbladders have gallbladder cancer.[13] Furthermore, pathogenic bacteria are cultured from the gallbladders of patients with gallbladder cancer at a significantly greater frequency than from patients with simple cholelithiasis.[14] Cholelithiasis and cholecystitis are more common in females, which may in part explain the higher incidence of gallbladder carcinoma in females.[15]

There are two models of gallbladder carcinogenesis: the metaplasia–dysplasia–carcinoma sequence and the adenoma–carcinoma pathway.[16] The most common pathway is the metaplasia–dysplasia–carcinoma sequence. Epithelial dysplasia, atypical hyperplasia, and carcinoma *in situ* have been identified in the gallbladder mucosa of 83%, 13.5%, and 3.5%, respectively, of patients undergoing cholecystectomy for cholelithiasis or cholecystitis.[17] Areas of mucosal dysplasia can be observed in >90% of patients with invasive gallbladder carcinoma.[18] There is also evidence that adenomatous polyps arising from the gallbladder mucosa are premalignant lesions, especially in the presence of gallstones or primary sclerosing cholangitis.[19,20] For polyps larger than 1 cm, the incidence of carcinoma is between 43% and 77%.[21] For polyps larger than 2 cm, the incidence is 100%.[22] For this reason, it is generally recommended to perform cholecystectomy in patients with gallbladder polyps and gallstones or primary sclerosing cholangitis.

There appears to be an increased expression of epithelial growth factors and protooncogenes, particularly KRAS in the progression from chronic cholecystitis to dysplasia and then to invasive carcinoma.[23] In patients with anomalous pancreaticobiliary ductal union, a condition known to be associated with an increased risk of developing gallbladder cancer, chronic inflammation results in hyperplasia of the gallbladder epithelium.[24] KRAS mutations were noted in some of these patients with high-grade dysplasia, suggesting that mutations in this protooncogene may be an early event in gallbladder mucosal proliferation leading to carcinogenesis. Studies performed in patients with invasive gallbladder carcinoma have demonstrated that the majority have abnormal or mutated tumor suppressor (*p53* and *p16*), cell cycle regulation (cyclin E), and apoptosis regulation (Bcl-2) genes, as well as increased expression of angiogenesis factors (VEGF) and the HER-2/*neu* protooncogene.[16,25,26]

Pathology

The gross appearance of gallbladder carcinoma varies, depending on the stage of the disease and extent of spread. Early-stage lesions that have not infiltrated through all layers of the gallbladder wall may be indistinguishable from chronic cholecystitis. Occasionally, a sessile or pedunculated tumor is present and suggests the diagnosis of a gallbladder cancer. More advanced gallbladder carcinomas are grossly evident by infiltration into the liver or contiguous organs, such as the duodenum or stomach.[27]

Microscopically, >90% of gallbladder carcinomas are adenocarcinomas, with the remaining cases being adenosquamous, squamous, and anaplastic carcinomas, and, rarely, carcinoid tumors or embryonal rhabdomyosarcoma.[28] Carcinoma *in situ* is an early lesion, with the malignant cells involving only the mucosal layer of the gallbladder wall. Gallbladder adenocarcinomas generally have a predominant papillary or tubular arrangement of cells.[27] Papillary adenocarcinoma is characterized by an extended stroma covered by columnar cells. The tubular formations of tubular adenocarcinoma may be lined by tall columnar cells or by cuboidal epithelium. Mucin production and signet ring cells can be identified frequently in gallbladder adenocarcinomas. More poorly differentiated carcinomas have solid sheets or nests of small, scattered cells infiltrating into the stroma and destroying the normal gallbladder wall architecture. Vascular, lymphatic, and perineural invasion by the carcinoma can be demonstrated frequently.[27]

Advanced locoregional disease usually is present at the time of diagnosis of gallbladder carcinoma. Only 10% of patients with this disease have cancer confined to the gallbladder wall.[10] Direct extension of the carcinoma into the gallbladder fossa of the liver is present in 69–83% of patients.[27,29,30] Direct invasion of the liver usually indicates the presence of other regional disease because fewer than 12% of patients with liver involvement have no other sites of regional disease. Direct invasion of the extrahepatic biliary tract occurs in 57% of cases; the duodenum, stomach, or transverse colon is involved in 40%; and the pancreas is involved in 23%. The hepatic artery or portal vein is encased by tumor in 15% of patients. Regional lymph node metastases in the cystic, choledochal, or pancreaticoduodenal lymphatic drainage basins are present in 42–70% of patients.[27] More distant lymph node metastases occur along the aorta or inferior vena cava in approximately 25% of cases. Importantly, lymph node metastases can occur in the absence of liver or other contiguous organ involvement by the gallbladder carcinoma.

The pattern of lymph node metastases from gallbladder carcinoma is predictable on the basis of anatomic studies that have identified three pathways of lymphatic drainage of the gallbladder (Figure 1).[31] The main pathway is the cholecysto-retropancreatic pathway, with lymphatic vessels on the anterior and posterior surfaces of the gallbladder that converge at a large retroportal lymph node. This principal retroportal lymph node communicates with the choledochal and pancreaticoduodenal lymph nodes. The cholecysto-celiac pathway consists of lymphatics from the anterior and posterior walls of the gallbladder that run to the left in front of the portal vein and then communicate with groups of pancreaticoduodenal lymph nodes or aorticocaval lymph nodes lying near the left renal vein. The final pattern of spread of gallbladder carcinoma is related to vascular invasion.[31] Metastases can occur to any organ, including liver (most commonly segments IV and V), adrenal gland, kidney, spleen, brain, breast, thyroid, heart, uterus, and bone.[32,33]

The staging systems used for gallbladder carcinoma are based on the pathologic characteristics of local invasion by the tumor and lymph node metastases. Before the American Joint Cancer Committee (AJCC) developed a tumor-node-metastasis (TNM) staging schema for gallbladder carcinoma, the Nevin and colleagues staging system was used frequently.[34] Studies of gallbladder carcinoma performed in Japan had generally applied the staging system of the Japanese Society of Biliary Surgery.[35] Most recent studies stage patients according to the TNM criteria with the 8th edition of the *AJCC Cancer Staging Manual* released in 2017 (Table 1).[36]

Clinical presentation

The most common signs and symptoms in patients with gallbladder carcinoma are nonspecific. Right upper quadrant abdominal pain, which may or may not be exacerbated by eating a fatty meal, is the predominant presenting complaint in 75–97% of patients.[3,10,37] Right upper quadrant abdominal tenderness is present in a slightly smaller percentage of patients. These symptoms and signs usually

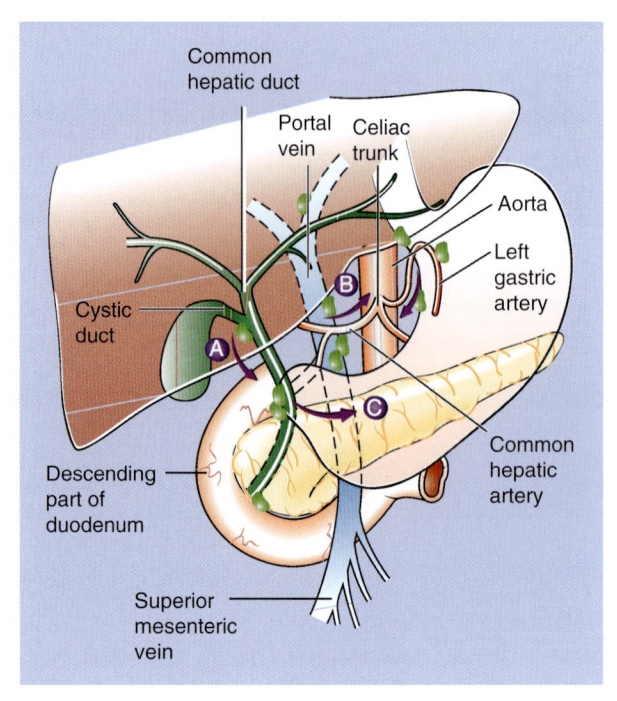

Figure 1 Patterns of lymphatic drainage from the gallbladder. (a) The main pathway of lymphatic drainage, and thus, lymph node metastasis from gallbladder cancer is to the cholecysto-retropancreatic nodes. This pathway drains from the gallbladder to nodes along the cystic duct and common bile duct and then to nodes posterior to the duodenum and pancreatic head. (b) The cholecysto-celiac pathway courses from the gallbladder through the gastrohepatic ligament to celiac nodes. (c) The third lymphatic drainage route is the cholecysto-mesenteric pathway, coursing from the gallbladder posterior to the pancreas to aortocaval lymph nodes.

Table 1 American Joint Cancer Committee (AJCC) TNM classification, 8th edition[a].

T category	T criteria
Tx	Primary tumor cannot be assessed
T0	No evidence of primary tumor
Tis	Carcinoma *in situ*
T1	Tumor invades the lamina propria or muscular layer
T1a	Tumor invades the lamina propria
T1b	Tumor invades the muscular layer
T2	Tumor invades the perimuscular connective tissue on the peritoneal side, without involvement of the serosa (visceral peritoneum) or tumor invades the perimuscular connective tissue on the hepatic side, with no extension into the liver
T2a	Tumor invades the perimuscular connective tissue on the peritoneal side, without involvement of the serosa (visceral peritoneum)
T2b	Tumor invades the perimuscular connective tissue on the hepatic side, with no extension into the liver
T3	Tumor perforates the serosa (visceral peritoneum) and/or directly invades the liver and/or one other adjacent organ or structure, such as the stomach, duodenum, colon, pancreas, omentum, or extrahepatic bile ducts
T4	Tumor invades the main portal vein or hepatic artery or invades two or more extrahepatic organs or structures
N category	N criteria
Nx	Regional lymph nodes cannot be assessed
N0	No regional lymph node metastasis
N1	Metastases to one to three regional lymph nodes
N2	Metastases to four or more regional lymph nodes
M category	M criteria
M0	No distant metastasis
M1	Distant metastasis

[a]Source: Amin.[36]

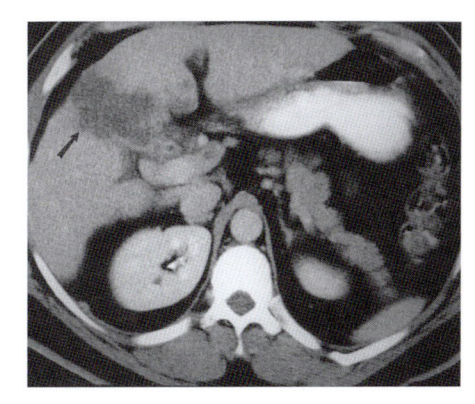

Figure 2 High-resolution, helical CT scan in a patient with gallbladder carcinoma. Direct tumor invasion into the hepatic parenchyma is evident.

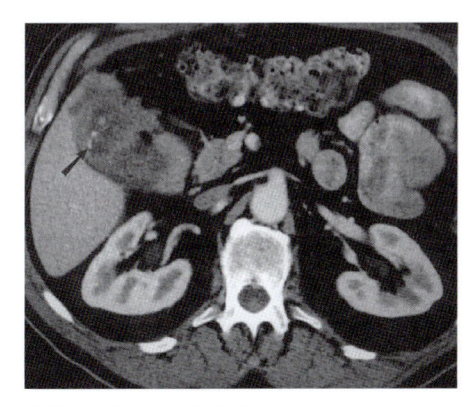

Figure 3 A high-resolution, helical CT scan in another patient with gallbladder cancer. A locally invasive tumor is again noted with areas of calcification (*arrow*) noted in the thickened gallbladder wall.

are ascribed to cholelithiasis or cholecystitis. Nausea, vomiting, and anorexia are present in 40–64% of patients, clinically evident jaundice is present in 45%, and weight loss of greater than 10% of normal body weight is noted in 37–77%.

Although 45% of patients obviously are jaundiced at presentation, 70% of patients present with a serum bilirubin elevated at least two times greater than normal.[37] Serum alkaline phosphatase levels are elevated in two-thirds of patients with gallbladder carcinoma. Alanine aminotransferase and aspartate aminotransferase levels are elevated in one-third of patients and are consistent with advanced hepatic invasion and metastases. Carcinoembryonic antigen (CEA) and carbohydrate antigen 19-9 (CA 19-9) are often elevated but lack sensitivity and specificity for gallbladder carcinoma.[38,39]

Diagnostic studies

Before ultrasonography and computed tomography (CT) became widely available, the preoperative diagnosis rate for gallbladder carcinoma was only 8.6–16.3%.[3] Ultrasonography is the primary imaging study for symptomatic patients with presumed cholelithiasis or choledocholithiasis. Ultrasound findings associated with gallbladder cancer are the presence of a solitary gallstone, displaced gallstone, intraluminal mass, gallbladder-replacing or invasive mass, and discontinuity of the mucosal echo.[40] Gallbladder wall thickening, mucosal plaque, and wall irregularity are nonspecific findings. In patients with locally advanced gallbladder carcinoma, ultrasonography can demonstrate extrahepatic and intrahepatic bile duct obstruction, porta hepatis lymphadenopathy, direct hepatic extension of tumor, and hepatic metastases. Preoperative ultrasonography may suggest the correct diagnosis in up to 75% of patients with gallbladder carcinoma.[41,42] However, ultrasonography does not accurately detect celiac or paraaortic lymphadenopathy or peritoneal dissemination of tumor.[43] Blood flow studies with color Doppler ultrasonography are also useful because gallbladder cancers have high-velocity arterial flow in 90% of cases, while benign lesions have minimal flow.[44] Recent advances in endoscopic ultrasonography, including the use of contrast-enhancing agents, may improve the diagnostic accuracy in assessing the T stage of the gallbladder cancer as well as detecting lymph node involvement in the porta hepatis or peripancreatic regions.[45]

Cross-sectional imaging with CT or magnetic resonance imaging (MRI) is performed less frequently in patients with presumed benign biliary tract disease. However, if gallbladder cancer is suspected, CT findings can predict correctly the diagnosis in 88–95% of patients.[46,47] The CT characteristics of gallbladder carcinoma include diffuse or focal gallbladder wall thickness of greater than 0.5 mm in 95% of patients, gallbladder wall contrast enhancement in 95%, intraluminal mass in 90%, direct liver invasion by tumor in 85% (Figure 2), regional lymphadenopathy in 65%, concomitant cholelithiasis in 52%, dilated intrahepatic or extrahepatic bile ducts in 50%, noncontiguous liver metastases in 12%, invasion of contiguous gastrointestinal tract organs in 8%, and intraluminal gallbladder gas in 4%.[46] CT can also demonstrate calcification of the gallbladder wall (Figure 3). In comparison to CT, MRI, and magnetic resonance cholangiopancreatography (MRCP) are more accurate in differentiating benign from malignant polyps and detecting tumor invasion into the hepatoduodenal ligament, encasement of the portal vein, and lymph node involvement.[47–49] CT abdomen/pelvis or MRI/MRCP is

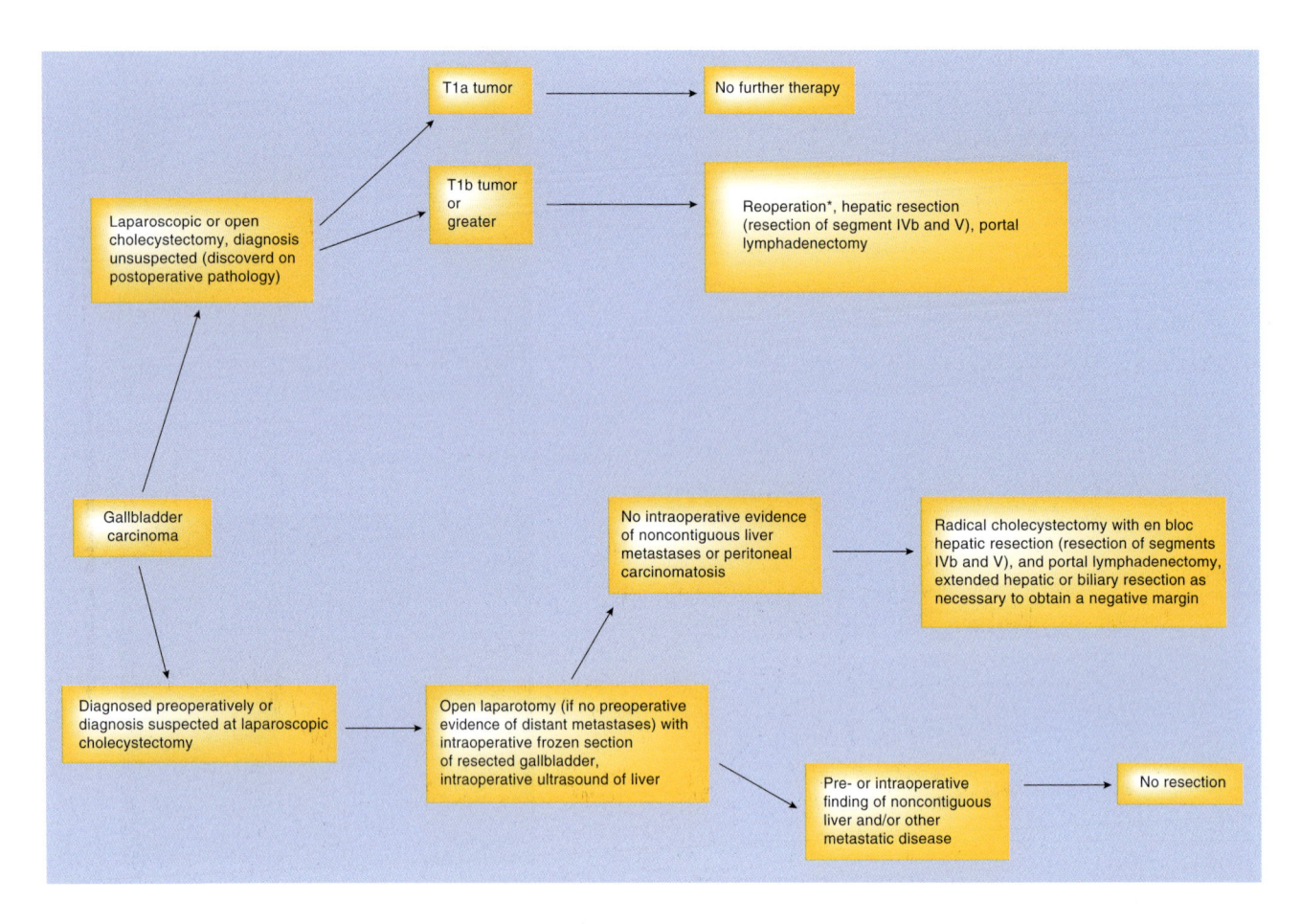

Figure 4 Algorithm to guide surgical decision-making for patients with gallbladder cancer. *Consider diagnostic laparoscopy for high-risk patients including T3 or higher tumors, poorly differentiated tumors, or margin-positive cholecystectomy.

recommended in cases in which gallbladder cancer is suspected preoperatively per the National Comprehensive Cancer Network (NCCN) and European Society of Medical Oncology (ESMO) guidelines.[50,51]

Treatment

Resection
The curative resection rates for gallbladder carcinoma range from 10% to 30%.[52] Only 15–47% of patients are candidates for curative resection because of extensive locoregional disease, noncontiguous liver metastases, and/or distant metastases.[53] Although the median overall survival following resection is 16 months, long-term survival can be achieved in some patients with resectable lesions.[54] However, the extent of resection remains a controversial issue.

Simple cholecystectomy is an adequate therapy for gallbladder carcinoma confined to the mucosa (T1aN0M0) if a negative cystic duct margin is obtained.[55] The 5-year survival rate for patients undergoing simple cholecystectomy for disease confined to the mucosa ranges from 57% to 100%.[56,57] However, there is not universal agreement on simple cholecystectomy as the sole therapy for patients with T1aN0M0 tumors as some authors recommend that extended cholecystectomy with wedge resection of the gallbladder fossa including a 3–5 cm margin of normal liver be performed to treat patients with these very early-stage lesions.[58] Given that major postoperative morbidity occurs in up to 30% of patients and postoperative mortality in as many as 16%, extended resection does not appear justified for T1aN0M0 tumors.[57,59,60]

There is a rationale for performing extended cholecystectomy with resection of the adjacent liver parenchyma and portal lymphadenectomy in patients with T1b tumors or AJCC-TNM stage II and III gallbladder carcinomas (Figure 4). Of patients with T1 gallbladder carcinomas, the incidence of regional lymph node metastasis is 1.8% for T1a carcinomas compared to 10.9% for T1b tumors.[55] Furthermore, a decision-analytic Markov model for T1b tumors demonstrated an improvement in 5-year survival from 61.3% to 87.5% with re-resection for incidentally found gallbladder cancer.[61] For T2, T3, and T4 tumors, the rates of lymph node metastases are 33%, 58%, and 69%, respectively, and the rate of peritoneal or liver metastases are 16%, 42%, and 79%, respectively.[62] For those with incidentally found gallbladder cancer, the incidence of residual disease at any site upon re-resection was 37.5% for T1, 56.7% for T2, and 77.3% for T3 tumors.[63] Evaluation of at least six lymph nodes is recommended to attain accurate staging.[64] Extrahepatic bile duct resection followed by Roux-en-Y hepaticojejunostomy is only necessary when the tumor extends into the common bile duct or a negative cystic duct margin cannot be obtained as there is no survival benefit associated with routine bile duct resection.[56,63,65] Similarly, major hepatectomy is associated with increased morbidity and has not demonstrated improved survival compared to R0 resection obtained through nonanatomic partial hepatectomy or formal segment IVb/V resection.[65]

With respect to the overall management of gallbladder cancer, the American Hepato-Pancreato-Biliary Association (AHPBA) released an expert consensus statement in 2015 to establish a set of practice guidelines.[66] The guidelines were constructed based

Table 2 AHPBA practice guidelines for the management of gallbladder cancer[a].

Consensus statements
Pathologic evaluation of routine cholecystectomy specimens and gallbladders with neoplastic changes and polyps
• Particularly in areas of high incidence, routine gallbladder specimens should be pathologically assessed and the minimum examination should include the microscopic evaluation of three sections and the cystic duct margin
• During the initial analysis, a finding of high-grade dysplasia, hyalinizing cholecystitis, and/or neoplastic polyps should prompt the complete sampling of the entire gallbladder specimen to accurately stage any associated invasive malignancy
• Gallbladder specimens with proven cancers should be extensively sampled and prognostic factors determined, including microscopic depth of tumor invasion, tumor involvement of the cystic duct margin, involvement of Rokitansky–Aschoff sinuses, and serosal versus hepatic surface involvement
• Provided the patient is medically fit for surgery, data support the resection of all gallbladder polyps of >1.0 cm in diameter and those with imaging evidence of vascular stalks
Evaluation and management of a gallbladder mass
• The minimum staging evaluation of patients with suspected or proven GBC includes contrasted cross-sectional imaging and diagnostic laparoscopy
• Adequate lymphadenectomy includes intraoperative assessment of any suspicious regional nodes, evaluation of the aortocaval nodal basin, and the recovery of at least six nodes. Patients with confirmed metastases to periaortic, pericaval, superior mesentery artery, and/or celiac artery nodal stations do not benefit from radical resection and should receive systemic and/or palliative treatment
• Primary resection of patients with early T-stage (T1b-2) disease should include en bloc resection of adjacent liver parenchyma. Resection of the common hepatic duct/common bile duct is only beneficial or required in cases of gross direct extension or microscopic involvement of the cystic duct margin
• In patients with locally advanced primary tumors, and particularly in those with jaundice, the risk:benefit ratio of radical surgery, to include major hepatectomy, vascular and/or adjacent organ resection, is marginal and these methods should only be considered in expert centers after multidisciplinary discussion
• Minimally invasive gallbladder cancer resections should be limited to early T-stage patients treated by expert surgeons who have demonstrated outcomes using this approach that are oncologically equivalent to those of open surgery
Evaluation and management of incidentally discovered gallbladder cancer
• Patients with incidentally identified T1b, T2, or T3 disease in a cholecystectomy specimen should undergo re-resection unless this is contraindicated by advanced disease or poor performance status
• Prior to re-resection, patients should undergo high-quality cross-sectional imaging with CT or MRI; PET should be used selectively to clarify features of concern identified on CT or MRI
• Staging laparoscopy should be considered prior to laparotomy, particularly in patients with T3 tumors and adverse pathologic characteristics. Routine port site excision is not indicated
• Re-resection should include portal lymphadenectomy and excision of all lymph nodes in the hepatoduodenal ligament. Extended lymph node dissection is not routinely indicated
• The goal of re-resection is an R0 resection. Major hepatectomy and/or bile duct resection is not routinely indicated unless these are required to achieve an R0 margin
Advances in neoadjuvant and adjuvant chemotherapy and radiation approaches
• Given their poor postoperative prognosis and elevated surgical morbidity, patients with preoperatively staged T3-4 N1 disease should be considered for clinical trials studying the efficacy of neoadjuvant chemotherapy
• Following R0 resection of stage T2 and higher N1 gallbladder cancer, patients should be considered for adjuvant systemic chemotherapy and/or chemoradiotherapy
• Patients with resected gallbladder cancer with positive margins should be considered for adjuvant chemoradiation therapy
• In patients with unresectable locally advanced and N2-positive gallbladder cancer, systemic chemotherapy with gemcitabine doublets can provide effective palliation and prolong survival

[a]Source: Based on Aloia et al.[66]

on a meeting of expert panelists that convened in January 2014 in which current evidence was reviewed. The consensus statements include recommendations regarding pathologic evaluation of the gallbladder when cancer is not suspected preoperatively, evaluation and management of a gallbladder polyp or mass, evaluation and management of incidentally found gallbladder cancer, and approaches to systemic therapy and radiation (Table 2).

Unfortunately, most series quote a long-term survival of 5–12% despite surgery with curative intent.[53] Regional lymph node metastases and/or direct tumor invasion of the hepatic parenchyma are indicators of poor prognosis, with significant reductions in 5-year overall survival rates associated with these pathologic findings.[67,68] Microscopically positive liver resection margins also have a negative impact on survival as these patients have a median survival of 8.9 months compared with 67.2 months for patients with tumor-free margins.[67]

Chemotherapy
There are currently little data available regarding neoadjuvant chemotherapy for advanced gallbladder cancer. In one systematic review that included 474 patients from eight cohort studies who received neoadjuvant chemotherapy +/− radiation, 30.6% of patients had progressive disease, 40.3% underwent surgery with curative intent, and 35.4% obtained an R0 resection.[69] The authors concluded that there is insufficient evidence to support the routine use of neoadjuvant therapy given that it only benefited a third of the entire cohort.

While there is also a paucity of data regarding adjuvant chemotherapy, there is enough evidence to support its use in the current NCCN guidelines, especially for those with positive regional lymph nodes or positive margins following resection.[70] While the recommendation is largely derived from retrospective studies, there was one randomized Phase III study conducted in Japan that demonstrated superior 5-year disease-free survival (20.3% vs 11.6%) and 5-year overall survival (26% vs 14.4%) for those who received adjuvant 5-fluorouracil and mitomycin C compared to controls.[71–73] The preferred regimen per the NCCN is capecitabine; other acceptable regimens include fluoropyrimidine-based or gemcitabine-based chemotherapy regimens or participation in a clinical trial.[70,73,74]

Radiation therapy
While 72% of patients with initial disease recurrence have distant metastasis, 28% of all gallbladder recurrences have a locoregional recurrence, and 15% develop locoregional recurrence alone.[75] Therefore, adjuvant radiotherapy is unlikely to have a significant

impact in the overall management of patients with gallbladder disease. This notion is further supported by a meta-analysis that demonstrated no survival benefit with radiation alone for gallbladder or bile duct tumors.[72] However, patients who have nodal disease or a positive margin following surgical resection or who experience locoregional recurrence may benefit from radiation therapy.[70,71,76] In an adjuvant setting using external beam therapy, target volumes should cover regional lymph nodes to 45 Gy at 1.8 Gy/fraction and the tumor bed to 50–60 Gy at 1.8–2 Gy/fraction depending on margin status. For locoregional recurrence, conventionally fractionated radiotherapy with 5-fluorouracil-chemotherapy is an acceptable regimen.[70]

Palliation
Unfortunately, most patients diagnosed with gallbladder cancer present with advanced disease that is either unresectable or metastatic. Median survival for these patients ranges between 4.5 and 9.5 months depending on if they receive systemic therapy.[77] Therefore, the primary goal for these patients is palliation to improve quality of life, which may include pain relief, resolution of obstructive jaundice, treatment of gastrointestinal obstruction, and possible increased life with chemotherapy.

Pain occurs in over 90% of patients with unresectable or metastatic gallbladder cancer and is best treated with multimodality therapy including opioids and nonnarcotics.[78] Celiac plexus neurolysis is an option for patients with pain refractory to medications. A meta-analysis demonstrated that a percutaneous approach is associated with decreased pain scores and a reduction in opioid usage.[79] In addition, involvement of palliative care services may be of benefit in managing doses and side effects of pain medications.

Obstructive jaundice occurs in up to 50% of patients with advanced gallbladder cancer.[78] While surgical biliary bypass is often feasible, it is associated with high rates of morbidity and mortality and should be avoided. Less invasive options include endoscopic biliary stenting and percutaneous transhepatic biliary drainage. While an endoscopic approach is associated with lower rates of hemorrhage and biliary leak and allows for internal drainage of bile, a randomized trial demonstrated that the rate of successful drainage is higher (89% vs 41%, $p < 0.001$) and the rate of cholangitis lower (11% vs 48%, $p = 0.002$) for percutaneous transhepatic drainage compared to endoscopic stenting for hilar obstructions due to gallbladder cancer.[80,81] However, endoscopic stent placement may be attempted at high-volume institutions and is the preferred modality in the setting of distal biliary obstruction.

Gastric outlet obstruction is another potential complication of advanced gallbladder cancer. Similar to surgical biliary bypass, gastrojejunostomy is associated with high morbidity and mortality and is not the modality of choice for relief of gastrointestinal obstruction in patients with a short life expectancy. Endoscopic or fluoroscopic-guided gastroduodenal self-expandable metal stent placement is preferred due to lower risk of complications. Another option is percutaneous endoscopic gastrostomy (PEG) tube placement when stent placement is not feasible in order to avoid the need for long-term nasogastric suction.

For patients with acceptable performance status, palliative chemotherapy is an appropriate option to potentially improve life expectancy. Gemcitabine-based combination therapy is the regimen of choice. This recommendation is based upon the results of the ABC-02 trial in which 410 patients with locally advanced or metastatic gallbladder cancer, cholangiocarcinoma, or ampullary cancer were randomized to either cisplatin followed by gemcitabine or gemcitabine alone. Cisplatin plus gemcitabine was associated with longer median overall survival (11.7 months vs 8.1 months, $p < 0.001$), longer median progression-free survival (8.0 months vs 5.0 months, $p < 0.001$), and higher rate of tumor control (81.4% vs 71.8%, $p = 0.049$) compared to gemcitabine alone.[74] Other acceptable chemotherapy regimens per current NCCN guidelines based on data from Phase II trials include other gemcitabine-based combination therapies, capecitabine-based combination therapy, 5-fluorouracil combination therapy, and the single agents gemcitabine, capecitabine, and 5-fluorouracil.[70] Clinical trial participation also should be encouraged. Finally, newer targeted therapies including larotrectinib and entrectinib for *NTRK* gene fusion-positive tumors and pembrolizumab for MSI-H/dMMR tumors are additional options.[70]

Bile duct cancer

Cholangiocarcinomas, accounting for 10–20% of primary liver tumors, are malignant tumors that arise from the epithelium of the intrahepatic or extrahepatic bile ducts.[82] Cholangiocarcinomas can arise at any site in the intra- or extrahepatic biliary system, but perihilar tumors comprise two-thirds of the cases of cholangiocarcinoma (Figure 5).[83] In 1890, Fardel first described a primary malignancy of the extrahepatic biliary tract. A report in 1957 described three patients with small adenocarcinomas involving the confluence of the left and right hepatic ducts.[84] Such primary cholangiocarcinomas arising at the bifurcation of the extrahepatic biliary tree are known commonly as Klatskin tumors, following his report in 1965 of a larger series of patients with these lesions.[85]

In the United States, approximately 8000 patients are diagnosed with cholangiocarcinoma of both the intra- or extrahepatic biliary system annually.[2] There is only a slight male preponderance of cases. The 5-year overall survival for cholangiocarcinoma remains poor: 8% for intrahepatic tumors and 10% for extrahepatic tumors.[2]

Causative factors

There are distinct differences between the factors associated with cholangiocarcinoma and those associated with HCC. Only 10–20% of cholangiocarcinomas occur in cirrhotic patients,

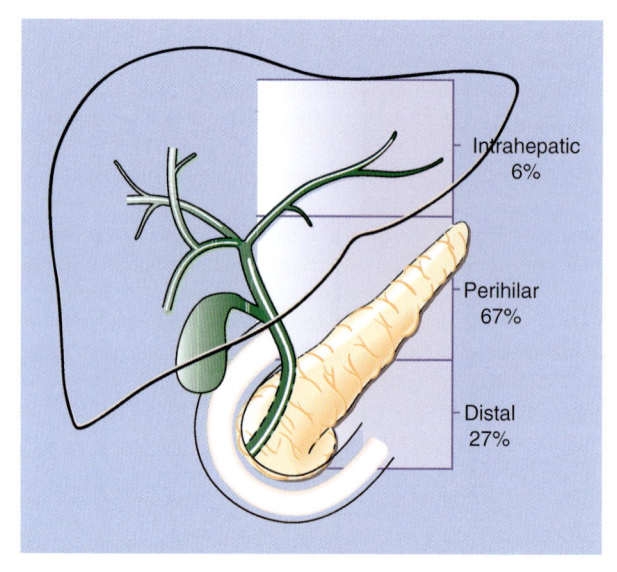

Figure 5 The distribution of 294 cholangiocarcinomas into intrahepatic, perihilar, and distal subgroups. Source: Nakeeb et al.[83]

compared with the 70–90% of HCCs that arise in cirrhotic livers.[86,87] A cohort study in Denmark of 11,605 patients with cirrhosis indicated a 60-fold increased risk of developing hepatocellular cancer and a 10-fold increased risk of cholangiocarcinoma.[86] Frequently, the cirrhosis associated with cholangiocarcinomas is a subacute secondary biliary type that results from the neoplastic obstruction of the bile ducts, indicating that, in some cases, cirrhosis in cholangiocarcinoma patients is the result of the tumor rather than its cause.

Cholangiocarcinoma is more prevalent in Southeast Asia than in other parts of the world. The higher incidence in this geographic region is related to parasitic infection with the liver flukes *Opisthorchis sinensis* and *Opisthorchis viverrini*.[88,89] Liver flukes induce hyperplasia, fibrosis, and adenomatous proliferation of human biliary epithelium and are associated with hepatolithiasis. The fluke infestation suggests a direct etiologic role in the subsequent development of cholangiocarcinoma, but this relationship is not established unequivocally.

Several disorders that can produce chronic inflammation of the bile ducts have been associated with an increased risk of developing cholangiocarcinoma. These include polycystic liver disease, choledochal cysts, congenital dilation of the intrahepatic bile ducts (Caroli syndrome), sclerosing cholangitis (occasionally in association with inflammatory bowel disease), hepatolithiasis, and cholelithiasis.[90–95] Hepatolithiasis is not a common disorder, and only 5–7% of patients with documented hepatic stones develop cholangiocarcinoma.[90,91] The reported incidence of cholangiocarcinoma developing in areas of congenital cystic dilation of the bile duct, including choledochal cysts and Caroli disease, ranges from 3% to 30%.[96,97] Patients with primary sclerosing cholangitis are also at increased risk to develop cholangiocarcinoma, with incidence rates ranging from 9% to 40%.[98–100] Patients with ulcerative colitis may also develop sclerosing cholangitis, but cholangiocarcinoma occurs in only 0.4–1.4% of individuals with ulcerative colitis.[99] In patients with sclerosing cholangitis, whether associated with ulcerative colitis or not, radiologic distinction between sclerosing cholangitis and cholangiocarcinoma is often impossible. One study showed that the serum tumor marker CA19-9 had an 89% sensitivity and 86% specificity in diagnosing cholangiocarcinoma in patients with sclerosing cholangitis.[101] Combining serum CA19-9 levels with serum CEA levels may further increase the diagnostic accuracy to detect cholangiocarcinoma in patients with sclerosing cholangitis.[102] Novel biomarkers and advanced techniques to aid with early detection are being studied.[103]

Patients who underwent diagnostic radiography with intravenous injection of Thorotrast (thorium dioxide) are at high risk of developing HCC, angiosarcoma, and cholangiocarcinoma.[104] Cholangiocarcinoma is the most frequent hepatic neoplasm reported in patients who have received Thorotrast. Exposure to several drugs or carcinogens has also been linked to an increased risk of the development of cholangiocarcinoma (Table 3). Because cholangiocarcinoma is a relatively rare neoplasm, it has been difficult to prove its pathogenesis related to any of these factors, but it is clear that chronic inflammation of the biliary tree by any cause is associated with an increased risk of developing cholangiocarcinoma.

Chronic inflammation of the biliary system or exposure to genotoxic agents concentrated in bile may produce damage to the DNA of biliary epithelial cells, leading to the development of cholangiocarcinoma. Mutations in the p53 tumor suppressor gene and in the K-ras protooncogene have been identified in cholangiocarcinoma patients.[105–107] There may be geographic and population-based differences in the mutation rates of these two genes, but alterations in p53 and K-ras are observed in significant proportions of patients with any of the identified factors (Table 3) that increase risk to develop cholangiocarcinoma. Overexpression of c-erbB-2, a protooncogene that encodes a transmembrane protein that is highly homologous to epidermal growth factor receptor (EGFR), has been confirmed in human cholangiocarcinoma cells and in benign proliferative biliary epithelium from patients with hepatolithiasis, primary sclerosing cholangitis, and liver fluke infestation.[108] Alterations in *c-erbB-2* expression may occur early in the chronic inflammation-induced proliferation of biliary epithelium leading to malignant transformation. Chronic inflammation may also produce the overexpression of the *Bcl-2* protooncogene observed in cholangiocarcinomas, which may promote tumorigenesis by inhibiting normal apoptotic processes.[109]

Table 3 Factors associated with increased risk of cholangiocarcinoma versus hepatocellular carcinoma.

Cholangiocarcinoma	Hepatocellular carcinoma
Liver fluke infection	Cirrhosis
Opisthorchis sinensis	Chronic hepatitis B virus infection
Opisthorchis viverrini	Chronic hepatitis C virus infection
Congenital/chronic cystic dilation	Aflatoxin B1 ingestion of the bile ducts
Choledochal cyst	Chronic ethanol ingestion
Caroli disease	Primary biliary cirrhosis
Hepatolithiasis	Hemochromatosis
Primary sclerosing cholangitis	α-1-Antitrypsin deficiency
Ulcerative colitis	Glycogen storage disease
Thorotrast exposure	Hypercitrullinemia
Cholelithiasis	Porphyrias
Asbestos	Hereditary tyrosinemia
Dioxin (agent orange)	Wilson disease
Polychlorinated diphenyls	Hepatotoxin exposure
Nitrosamines	Thorotrast
Isoniazid	Polyvinyl chloride
Methyldopa	Carbon tetrachloride

Clinical presentation

The clinical features of cholangiocarcinoma are nonspecific and depend on the location of the tumor. The usual clinical presentation of patients with hilar cholangiocarcinoma is painless jaundice. Patients may also report concomitant onset of fatigue, pruritus, fever, vague abdominal pain, and anorexia. Cholangiocarcinomas that arise in peripheral bile ducts within the hepatic parenchyma usually reach a large size before becoming clinically evident. Patients with these large peripheral hepatic tumors usually present with hepatomegaly and an upper abdominal mass, abdominal and back pain, and weight loss.[87] Jaundice and ascites are late and usually preterminal sequelae in patients with large intrahepatic cholangiocarcinomas. Jaundice associated with a large hepatic cholangiocarcinoma is caused by a combination of extension of the tumor to the bifurcation of the left and right hepatic ducts and by compression of contralateral bile ducts by the expanding tumor.

The serum liver function tests in patients with hilar cholangiocarcinoma commonly demonstrate obstructive jaundice. Serum alkaline phosphatase levels are elevated in >90% of patients.[87] Serum bilirubin also is elevated in the majority of cholangiocarcinoma patients, particularly in those with a tumor arising in the central portion of the liver or the extrahepatic hilar bile ducts.[110] In contrast to HCC, serum α-fetoprotein levels are abnormal in fewer than 5% of cholangiocarcinoma patients.[111] There is an increase in serum CEA levels in 40–60% of cholangiocarcinoma patients.[112] CA19-9 is elevated in >80% of patients.[112]

Pathology

Cholangiocarcinomas originating in the periphery of the hepatic parenchyma usually are solitary and large, but satellite nodules occasionally are present.[113] Gross tumor invasion of the large portal or hepatic veins occurs much less frequently than in HCC. The gross and microscopic appearance of intrahepatic cholangiocarcinomas may have prognostic significance because tumors with periductal infiltration have a higher incidence of lymph node and intrahepatic metastasis.[114] Metastases to the regional lymph nodes, lungs, and peritoneal cavity are more common in cholangiocarcinoma than in HCC. When the tumor causes longstanding biliary obstruction, the liver may show secondary biliary cirrhosis.

Microscopically, cholangiocarcinoma is characterized by low cuboidal cells that resemble the normal biliary epithelium. Varying degrees of pleomorphism, atypia, mitotic activity, hyperchromatic nuclei, and prominent nucleoli are noted from area to area in the same tumor. Morphologic variants include adenosquamous, sarcomatoid, mucoepidermoid, signet-ring cell, and squamous cell carcinoma.[115] Rarely, a clear cell variant of cholangiocarcinoma occurs, which must be distinguished from clear cell renal carcinoma with liver metastasis.[115] Cholangiocarcinomas are mucin-secreting adenocarcinomas, and intracellular and intraluminal mucin often can be demonstrated. The presence of mucin is useful in differentiating cholangiocarcinoma from HCC. The absence of bile production by cholangiocarcinoma can also be useful in distinguishing this tumor from a HCC. Immunohistochemical staining that is positive for epithelial membrane antigen and tissue polypeptide antigen may be useful in confirming a diagnosis of cholangiocarcinoma.[116,117] Immunohistochemical staining for cytokeratin subtypes can be helpful in differentiating cholangiocarcinoma from metastatic colorectal carcinoma.[118] Cholangiocarcinomas are usually locally invasive, spreading along nerves or in subepithelial layers of the bile ducts.

Diagnostic studies

Peripheral intrahepatic cholangiocarcinoma is often difficult to distinguish pathologically and radiographically from a deposit of metastatic adenocarcinoma within the liver. Although transabdominal ultrasonography can detect an intrahepatic malignant tumor greater than 2 cm in diameter, ultrasound findings do not differ between cholangiocarcinomas, liver metastases from extrahepatic adenocarcinomas, and multinodular HCC.[119] CT demonstrates a rounded, low attenuation mass with irregular or lobulated margins (Figure 6). Satellite lesions may be evident, particularly when using helical CT during the optimal period of hepatic contrast enhancement. Calcification within the tumor is present in 25% of cases, and a central scar is observed in 30%.[120] MRI shows a nonencapsulated mass with irregular margins that is hypointense compared with the normal liver on T1-weighted and hyperintense on T2-weighted images. The peripheral rim of the tumor usually enhances following MRI contrast administration. A hyperintense central scar is best seen on T2-weighted images, but the CT and MRI characteristics of intrahepatic cholangiocarcinomas may be present in other types of hepatic tumors.[120]

A diagnosis of hilar cholangiocarcinoma should be suspected in the patient with painless jaundice whose CT scan demonstrates dilated intrahepatic bile ducts with a normal gallbladder and extrahepatic biliary tree. High-resolution, helical CT scans can provide information on the location of an obstructing biliary tumor and may suggest the extent of involvement of the liver and porta hepatis structures by the tumor (Figure 7). Multiphasic helical CT scan correctly identifies the level of biliary obstruction by a hilar cholangiocarcinoma in 63–90% of patients.[121,122] Preoperative helical CT is also useful in demonstrating lobar or segmental liver atrophy caused by bile duct obstruction or portal vein occlusion (Figure 8).[122] However, helical CT is not accurate in assessing the resectability of hilar cholangiocarcinomas because of limited resolution in evaluating intraductal tumor spread and significant false-positive and false-negative rates in demonstrating portal vein or hepatic artery involvement by tumor.[121,122]

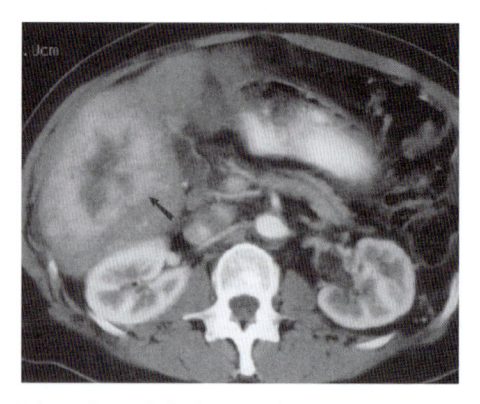

Figure 6 High-resolution, helical CT scan during the arterial contrast phase in a patient with an intrahepatic cholangiocarcinoma. The periphery of the tumor (*arrow*) has irregular margins and enhances with contrast. A relatively hypovascular area of scar and tumor necrosis is evident in the center of the tumor.

Like the CT scan, ultrasonography can demonstrate a nondilated gallbladder and common bile duct associated with dilated intrahepatic ducts. In addition, as grayscale ultrasonography has improved, the diagnosis of cholangiocarcinoma is supported by finding a hilar bile duct mass in 65–90% of patients.[123] Ultrasonography and CT scan may be used to demonstrate the presence of intrahepatic tumor due to direct extension or noncontiguous metastases and enlarged periportal lymph nodes, suggesting nodal metastases.[124] Even intraoperative ultrasonography is suboptimal for detecting intraductal spread by hilar cholangiocarcinoma, correctly demonstrating the extent of tumor spread away from the primary biliary tumor in only 18% of cases.[125] Intraoperative ultrasonography can be used to screen for noncontiguous liver metastases from the primary biliary cancer and can accurately detect direct tumor invasion of the portal vein and hepatic artery in 83.3% and 60% of cases, respectively.[125]

Similar to the intrahepatic variety, hilar cholangiocarcinoma usually shows hypointensity on T1- and hyperintensity on T2-weighted MRI. Dilated intrahepatic bile ducts are evident in patients with obstructing tumors, and lobar atrophy is seen in cases of portal venous occlusion. Fast low-angle shot (FLASH) MR with contrast-enhanced coronal imaging has been used to demonstrate intraluminal extension of tumor and to distinguish between blood vessels and bile ducts.[126] MRCP and MR virtual endoscopy can demonstrate hilar bile duct obstruction by tumor with dilated intrahepatic ducts.[126,127] The advantages of MRCP over direct cholangiography include noninvasiveness and possible visualization of isolated bile ducts.

Cholangiography can definitively demonstrate a lesion obstructing the left and right hepatic ducts at the hilar confluence (Figure 9), and percutaneous transhepatic cholangiography (PTC) and endoscopic retrograde cholangiopancreatography (ERCP) are both useful in assessing patients with extrahepatic biliary obstruction. A prospective, randomized comparison of PTC and ERCP in patients with jaundice concluded that the two techniques had

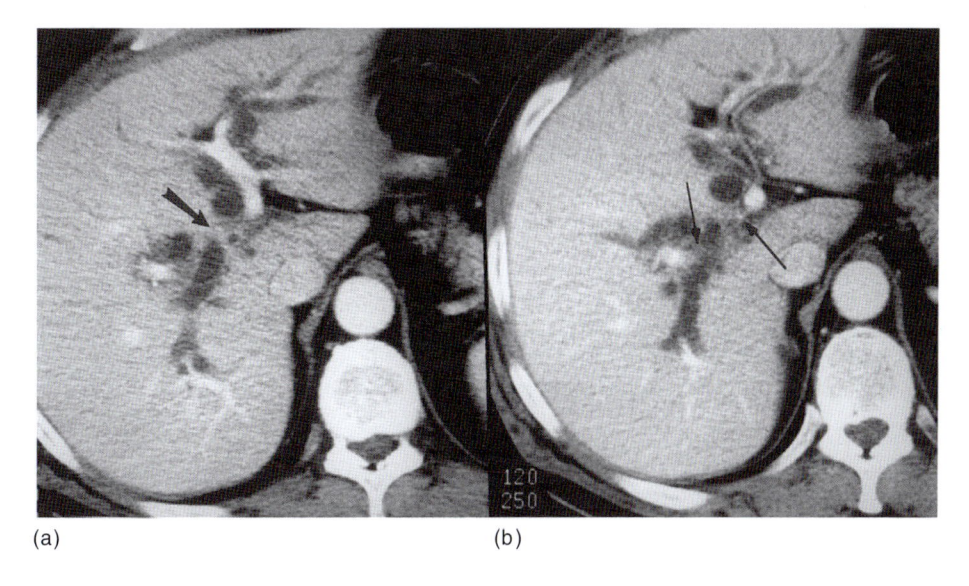

Figure 7 High-resolution, helical CT scan in another patient presenting with obstructive jaundice. The tumor mass (a), (*large arrow*) producing marked intrahepatic biliary duct dilatation is evident. Areas of tumor invasion of the portal vein (b), (*small arrows*) suggested on the CT scan were confirmed at the time of operation to be tumor invasion of the portal vein.

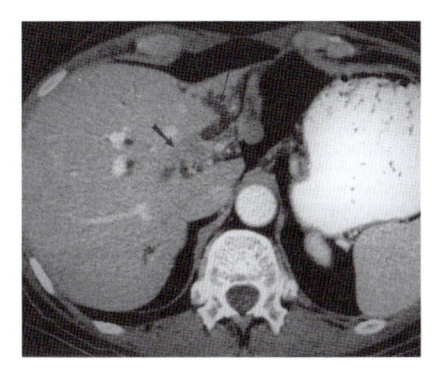

Figure 8 High-resolution, helical CT scan in a patient presenting with several months of increasing pruritus followed by the development of clinically evident jaundice. The relatively hypodense hilar cholangiocarcinoma (*large arrow*) is evident. Marked atrophy of the left hepatic lobe is noted with dilated intrahepatic bile ducts (*small arrow*), but little remaining hepatic parenchyma is evident.

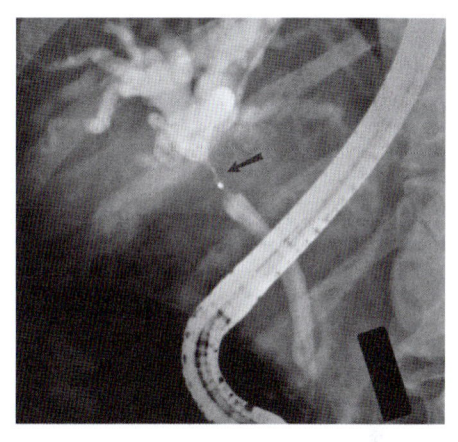

Figure 9 Endoscopic retrograde cholangiopancreatography showing a focal stricture of the proper hepatic bile duct (*arrow*) with marked dilatation of the intrahepatic bile ducts. This hilar cholangiocarcinoma was completely resected with Roux-en-Y hepaticojejunostomy reconstruction of biliary-enteric continuity.

similar diagnostic accuracy.[128] PTC was 100% accurate in demonstrating obstruction at the confluence of the left and right hepatic ducts, while ERCP had an accuracy of 92% in demonstrating these lesions. ERCP has the additional benefit of providing a pancreatogram. A normal pancreatogram helps to exclude a small carcinoma of the head of the pancreas as a cause of biliary obstruction. Cytologic specimens can be obtained at the time of PTC and ERCP. The presence of malignant cells in bile or bile duct brushings is confirmed in approximately 50% of patients undergoing PTC or ERCP.[129,130]

Drainage of the obstructed biliary tree with partial or complete relief of jaundice and associated symptoms can be achieved with PTC or ERCP. Internal–external catheters can be placed across the malignant obstruction into the duodenum to allow internal drainage, whereas distal bile duct obstruction can be relieved with endoscopic stents. It must be emphasized that providing symptomatic relief for patients by decompressing the biliary tract should not be the primary reason to place these stents. Prospective, randomized studies have failed to demonstrate a benefit in terms of a decrease in hospital morbidity or mortality by preoperative decompression of biliary obstruction.[131] In fact, biliary drainage can produce inflammation, increasing the risk of cholangitis and postoperative septic complications.[82] However, the catheters can be useful in identifying the hepatic duct bifurcation at the time of operation and aid in the reconstruction of the biliary tract following extirpation of the tumor.[132,133] Biliary drainage is especially important in patients eligible for major hepatic resections as it can improve the liver damage caused by obstructive jaundice; ideally, serum bilirubin should be less than 2 before undertaking a hepatectomy.[82] It is imperative that candidacy for liver transplantation be considered prior to placing a PTC, as this can exclude patients from transplant eligibility.[134]

Positron emission tomography (PET) has recently been used to aid in the diagnosis and staging of patients with bile duct cancer. PET assesses *in vivo* metabolism of positron-emitting radiolabeled tracers like [^{18}F] fluoro-2-deoxy-D-glucose (18FFDG), a glucose analog that accumulates in various malignant tumors because of their high glucose metabolic rates. It does not provide anatomic detail to assess the resectability of hilar cholangiocarcinomas or intrahepatic malignancies, but it may prove useful in detecting distant metastatic disease that would preclude a curative resection. In patients with primary sclerosing cholangitis, FDG-PET studies may be able to detect small hilar and intrahepatic cholangiocarcinomas and thus may be useful in therapeutic and transplant decision-making in these patients.[135] PET scan images correctly detected the primary cholangiocarcinoma in 24 of 26 patients (sensitivity 92.3%) and were true negative in eight patients with benign bile duct disease (adenoma, sclerosing cholangitis, Caroli disease). Distant metastatic disease was diagnosed correctly in 7 of 10 patients with histologically proven metastases, but regional lymph node metastases were identified in only 2 of 15 patients (13.3%).[136]

Staging laparoscopy can help patients with seemingly resectable tumors avoid an exploratory laparotomy when peritoneal tumor implants are found. In addition, patients at high risk of developing peritoneal carcinomatosis may be identified by positive cytologic specimens obtained from laparoscopic washings. A recent systematic review and meta-analysis of 12 studies showed a pooled sensitivity of 52.2% to detect unresectable disease, suggesting that one in four patients with potentially resectable hilar cholangiocarcinoma would benefit from staging laparoscopy.[137] Finally, laparoscopic ultrasonography can be used to exclude the presence of noncontiguous liver metastases or extensive hilar tumor infiltration in patients with extrahepatic bile duct cancers.[138]

Prognostic factors

The most important factor affecting prognosis is the resectability of the tumor. Patients who undergo curative resection (margin-negative) have 3-year survival rates from 40% to 87% and 5-year survival rates between 10% and 73%.[139] In one series in Japan, among 96 patients who underwent R0 (microscopically negative) resection for intrahepatic cholangiocarcinoma, the 5-year overall survival, and recurrence-free survival rates were 55% and 41.7%.[140]

Hilar cholangiocarcinomas have a poorer prognosis than do carcinomas arising in the middle or distal thirds of the extrahepatic bile duct, which is related directly to the presentation of hilar tumors at a more locally advanced stage with bilobar liver involvement by tumor and resultant lower rates of curative resection.[141]

Significant determinants of improved prognosis in patients undergoing curative resection include Eastern Cooperative Oncology Group (ECOG) performance status, total bilirubin, and tumor grade.[139] A meta-analysis assessing predictors of overall survival in patients who underwent curative-intent surgical treatment of intrahepatic found that older age, larger tumor size, presence of multiple tumors, lymph node metastasis, vascular invasion, and poor tumor differentiation were associated with shorter overall survival.[142] Large size of the primary tumor is an indicator of poor prognosis because of the increased frequency of vascular and lymphatic invasion by the tumor as well as growth along neighboring bile duct walls.[143] For distal cholangiocarcinoma, a study by the Dutch Pancreatic Cancer Group using the Netherlands Cancer Registry showed that increasing age, pT3/T4 stage, higher lymph node ratio, poor differentiation, and R1 resection were independent predictors of poor overall survival in resected patients.[144]

The status of regional lymph nodes is particularly important for prognosis. A study of 19 patients who underwent resection of intrahepatic cholangiocarcinoma demonstrated that patients with no porta hepatis lymph node metastases had a 3-year survival rate of 64% compared with 0% for patients with nodal metastases.[145] A larger cohort of 32 patients who underwent resection of intrahepatic cholangiocarcinomas confirmed the negative prognostic impact of regional lymph node metastases and large size (>5-cm diameter) of the primary tumor.[146] The presence of regional lymph node metastases reduces the 5-year overall survival rate following resection of middle or distal third bile duct cancer to 21% compared with the 65% survival rate in patients with node-negative disease.[147]

Pathologic features of the bile duct cancer are also predictors of outcome after resection. Prognosis is affected adversely if the tumor infiltrates the serosa of the bile duct, invades directly into the liver, demonstrates vascular invasion, or has metastasized to regional lymph nodes. Histologic type and grade are also important factors. Patients with the relatively unusual papillary bile duct adenocarcinoma have the most favorable prognosis, with 3-year survival rates up to 75%.[148] Patients with the more common nodular or sclerotic types of hilar cholangiocarcinoma have 3-year survival rates of <30%. A pathologic study that correlated gross tumor type with patterns of spread provides evidence that may explain the observed differences in survival outcomes. Papillary and superficial nodular tumors spread predominantly by mucosal extension, rarely invading the deeper layers of the bile duct wall or lymphatic channels, whereas nodular infiltrating or diffuse infiltrating tumors spread by direct or lymphatic extension in the submucosa.[149] The distance of mucosal or submucosal spread away from the gross tumor can be as great as 30 mm, but there were no local or anastomotic recurrences if at least a 5-mm tumor-free margin was attained.[149] In a series of 34 patients with resected carcinomas of the upper bile duct, those with well- or moderately differentiated carcinomas had a 3-year survival rate of up to 51%, whereas no patient with a poorly differentiated carcinoma survived longer than 2 years.[148]

Socioeconomic disparities based on race, geography, income, and insurance status have also been described.[150]

Treatment

Surgery
Resection of cholangiocarcinoma affords the patient the best chance for significant survival. However, most patients are unresectable at diagnosis, and additional 45% are unresectable upon exploration.[151–153]

For intrahepatic and hilar cancers, resection of the affected bile ducts and associated liver parenchyma is required. The caudate lobe must also be resected for hilar tumors.[154] Distal cholangiocarcinomas are treated with pancreaticoduodenectomy.[155] An understanding of the Bismuth-Corlette classification of hilar cholangiocarcinoma is useful in planning the extent and site of liver resection (Figure 10).[157] Long-term survival rates after resection of middle or distal common bile duct cholangiocarcinomas are generally higher compared with hilar tumors. This is most likely related to higher rates of margin-negative resection with middle or distal extrahepatic bile duct tumors and the absence of direct tumor extension into the liver.

Traditionally, the guidelines for resectability for cholangiocarcinoma include the absence of retropancreatic and paraceliac lymphadenopathy, the absence of portal vein or hepatic artery involvement, the absence of adjacent organ invasion, and the absence of metastatic disease.[155] For patients with a future liver remnant less than 30%, portal vein embolization can be utilized to induce lobar hypertrophy.[158] Resection of the portal vein or hepatic artery for locally advanced tumors is controversial.[159]

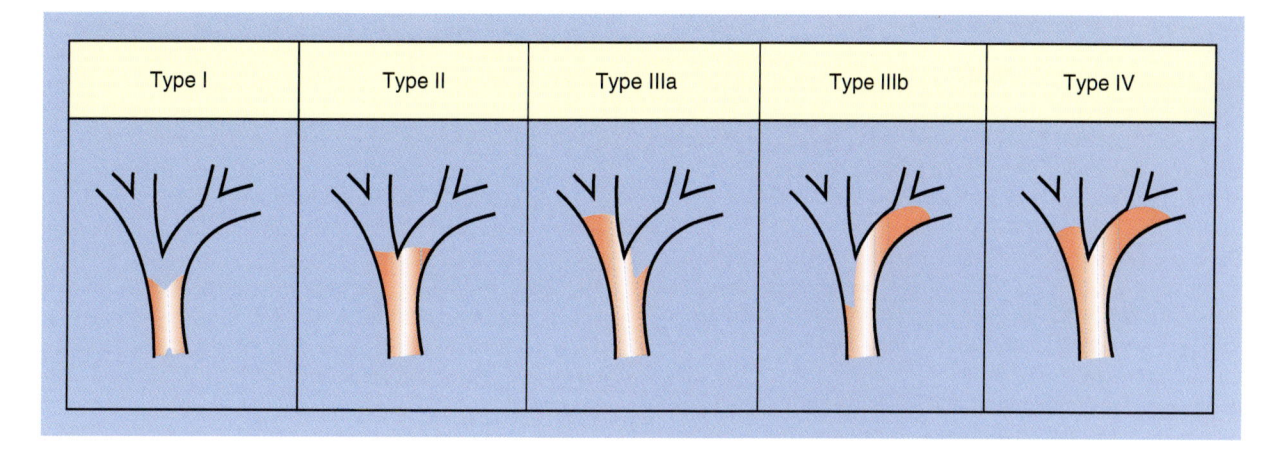

Figure 10 Bismuth-Corlette classification of hilar cholangiocarcinoma. Types 1 and 2 can be resected with excision of the extrahepatic bile duct with or without the hilar plate and caudate lobe. Types 3A and 3B can be resected with the addition of an en bloc right or left hepatic lobectomy, respectively. Type 4 is, by definition, unresectable.[156] Source: Based on Bengmark et al.[156]

Perioperative morbidity and mortality have decreased over time. One study of hilar cholangiocarcinoma showed a decrease in postoperative mortality from 11.1% before 1990 to 1.4%.[160] Thirty-day mortality differs by procedure performed: 11.9% for perihilar tumors managed with hepatectomy and biliary-enteric anastomosis and 1.2% for distal cholangiocarcinoma.[161] Surgical complications are reported in 25–45% of patients. Infectious complications are the most common postoperative problem, and preoperative placement of biliary stents with resultant contamination of the obstructed biliary tree increases the incidence of infection.[162]

Recurrence after resection is common. In one study of 402 patients with resected hilar cholangiocarcinoma (with an R0 resection rate of >80%), there was over a 50% rate of recurrence at 5 years. Initial recurrence was most commonly intrahepatic.[163]

For hilar cholangiocarcinomas, it is important that the caudate lobe is also removed. In a series of 25 patients undergoing surgery for hilar cholangiocarcinoma, direct invasion of hepatic parenchyma at the hilum was noted in 12 patients (46.2%), with 11 patients (42.3%) also having carcinoma extending into the bile ducts draining the caudate lobe or directly invading the caudate lobe parenchyma.[164] A study of 106 adult human cadavers showed that 97.2% had bile ducts draining the caudate lobe that entered directly into the main left hepatic duct, right hepatic duct, or both.[164] These caudate lobe bile ducts frequently enter the main left or right hepatic ducts within 1 cm of the proper hepatic duct. Thus, a carcinoma arising at the confluence of the right and left hepatic ducts need not be large to extend into the bile ducts draining the caudate lobe.

Liver transplantation

Total hepatectomy with immediate orthotopic liver transplantation is an option for early-stage but anatomically unresectable hilar cholangiocarcinoma without nodal or metastatic disease.[165] Liver transplant alone was associated with high rates of recurrence and poor survival leading to the development of the Mayo Clinic protocol which involves neoadjuvant high-dose radiotherapy followed by liver transplant.[166] The 5-year overall survival of patients with hilar cholangiocarcinoma undergoing liver transplant following neoadjuvant therapy is comparable to that of patients without nodal disease undergoing R0 resection.[165] However, patient selection is stringent and 25–31% of patients progress while awaiting transplant.[167]

Transplant for intrahepatic cholangiocarcinoma is currently not recommended outside of experimental studies. Retrospective studies of liver explants including several cirrhotic patients with incidental early intrahepatic cholangiocarcinoma showed a 5-year recurrence of 12% with patients with very early cancer compared to 77% among patients with cancers >2 cm or multinodularity; this corresponded to a 5-year overall survival of 65% compared with 45%.[168,169]

Systemic therapy

Given the high percentage of unresectable cholangiocarcinomas, various chemotherapy and radiation therapy regimens have been studied both in the neoadjuvant and adjuvant setting.

In the neoadjuvant setting, preoperative chemotherapy or chemoradiotherapy may be able to downstage locally advanced tumors into resectable tumors. In one study of patients with intrahepatic cholangiocarcinoma, 53% of 74 patients with locally advanced cancer underwent secondary resection after a median of six cycles of chemotherapy.[170] Of 91 patients with extrahepatic cholangiocarcinoma evaluated between 1983 and 1996 at MD Anderson Cancer Center, 51 (56%) presented with unresectable disease.[171] Nine patients, five with hilar and four with distal common duct cholangiocarcinoma, were treated with preoperative chemoradiation therapy (continuous intravenous infusion of 5-fluorouracil at 300 mg/m^2/day combined with external beam irradiation). Three of these nine patients had a pathologic complete response to chemoradiation treatment; the remaining six patients had varying degrees of histologic response to treatment. The rate of margin-negative resection was 100% for the preoperative chemoradiation group compared with 54% for the group not receiving preoperative treatment ($p < 0.01$). The patients treated with preoperative chemoradiation had no operative or postoperative complications related to treatment. Another study of extrahepatic cholangiocarcinoma compared 33 patients who underwent adjuvant chemoradiotherapy with 12 who were treated in the preoperative setting. Although the patients receiving neoadjuvant therapy had more advanced disease, they had a longer 5-year survival (53% vs 23%) with similar rates of grade 2–3 surgical complications.[172] Thus, it appears that neoadjuvant chemoradiation for extrahepatic bile duct cancer can be performed safely, produces significant antitumor response, and may improve the ability to achieve tumor-free resection margins. These results support a need for randomized trials for neoadjuvant therapy.

All patients with resected cholangiocarcinoma should undergo chemotherapy postoperatively. Patients with margin-positive or node-positive disease should also receive chemoradiation. The most active agents are gemcitabine, capecitabine, 5-FU, and oxaliplatin. There is no randomized data directly comparing gemcitabine-based with fluorouracil (FU)-based regimens. Conventional chemotherapy has been associated with a response rate of 10–40%.[173]

There are several studies evaluating the impact of adjuvant chemotherapy alone. One early study randomly assigned 90 patients with advanced pancreatic or biliary cancer ($n = 37$) to 5-FU-based systemic chemotherapy versus best supportive care alone and reported a median survival of 6 versus 2.5 months, respectively.[163] One randomized study from Japan compared postoperative chemotherapy (mitomycin C + infusional 5-FU followed by oral 5-FU until tumor progression) versus surgery alone in 508 patients with resected pancreaticobiliary malignancies (139 cholangiocarcinoma) showed that among the patients with bile duct cancer, there was no difference in 5-year overall survival between the groups.[73]

Several chemotherapy regimens were found to be active for locally advanced or metastatic cholangiocarcinoma. After a median of four cycles of single-agent gemcitabine in a 2005 study, 26.1% had a partial response, 34.8% had stable disease, and 39.1% had disease progression.[174] The ABC-2 trial studied gemcitabine alone or in combination with cisplatin in patients with biliary tract cancer. Cisplatin plus gemcitabine was associated with higher median overall survival (11.7 vs 8.1 months) and higher progression-free survival (8 vs 5 months), with similar rates of adverse events.[74] This established gemcitabine plus a platinum-based agent (cisplatin or oxaliplatin) as standard of care for advanced cholangiocarcinoma.[175] A study that also included patients with locally advanced or metastatic gallbladder cancer found that the addition of capecitabine to gemcitabine resulted in a disease control rate of 73% and a median overall survival of 14 months.[176] A 2007 pooled analysis of 104 trials of different chemotherapy regimens in advanced biliary cancer concluded that the gemcitabine/cisplatin combination offered the highest rates of objective response and of tumor control (objective response plus stable disease) compared to either gemcitabine-free or cisplatin-free regimens.[177]

More recently, there are studies of targeted agents in biliary tract cancers. One study of 42 patients suggested benefit from EGFR blockade by the oral tyrosine kinase inhibitor erlotinib in patients with biliary cancer. There were three partial responses, and seven patients remained progression-free at 6 months.[178] The combination of erlotinib and sorafenib has not shown promising clinical activity.[179]

Locoregional therapy

There are several options for locoregional therapy of unresectable tumors. Radiofrequency ablation (RFA) delivers high frequency alternating current with the aim of tissue coagulation and tumor destruction.[180] In a small study of unresectable intrahepatic cholangiocarcinoma, median survival after RFA was 38.5 months. Treatment failure occurred in patients with tumors larger than 5 cm.[181] Transarterial chemoembolization (using combinations of mitomycin C, doxorubicin, cisplatin, and gemcitabine) can result in favorable disease control for intrahepatic cholangiocarcinoma.[182–184]

External beam radiation therapy use is restricted to patients with small tumors, as a whole liver dose of more the 40 Gy of radiation can be associated with toxic side effects. The use of stereotactic body radiotherapy (SBRT) can allow for dose escalation up to 60 Gy. In a small study of 10 patients with primary or recurrent cholangiocarcinoma with 12 lesions, SBRT resulted in a complete response in 25% of lesions and a partial response in 42%. However, one patient developed biliary stenosis and another died of liver failure.[185] A systematic review of ten studies investigating SBRT for cholangiocarcinoma showed a pooled 1-year overall survival of 58.3% and 1-year rate of local control of 83.4%, with acceptable reported toxicities.[186]

Another option for patients with unresectable intrahepatic cholangiocarcinoma is radioembolization with yttrium-90 (Y90) which has been shown to reduce the size of unresectable tumors and in select cases, in combination with chemotherapy, allow for resection.[187]

Palliation

In general, curative surgical resection is possible in <30% of patients with hilar cholangiocarcinoma.[141] In patients deemed unresectable on the basis of the findings of diagnostic studies, laparotomy can be avoided by placing percutaneous external drains or endoscopically placed stents.[188,189] Expandable metal wall stents have improved long-term patency rates over plastic stents.[190,191] When unresectability is determined at the time of laparotomy, a decision must be made regarding surgical biliary-enteric bypass versus endoscopic stenting to provide drainage of the obstructed biliary tree. Both approaches provide for relief of jaundice in about 70% of patients.[192] Stenting has been associated with a higher re-admission and re-intervention rate.[193] However, one study found that median lifetime cost was less for endoscopic stenting as opposed to palliative surgical bypass for unresectable cholangiocarcinoma.[194]

Key references

The complete reference list can be found on Vital Source version of this title, see inside front cover.

1. Hundal R, Shaffer EA. Gallbladder cancer: epidemiology and outcome. *Clin Epidemiol*. 2014;**6**:99–109.
11. Khan ZR, Neugut AI, Ahsan H, Chabot JA. Risk factors for biliary tract cancers. *Am J Gastroenterol*. 1999;**94**(1):149–152.
12. Diehl AK. Gallstone size and the risk of gallbladder cancer. *JAMA*. 1983;**250**(17):2323–2326.
14. Csendes A, Becerra M, Burdiles P, et al. Bacteriological studies of bile from the gallbladder in patients with carcinoma of the gallbladder, cholelithiasis, common bile duct stones and no gallstones disease. *Eur J Surg*. 1994;**160**(6-7):363–367.
17. Albores-Saavedra J, Alcantra-Vazquez A, Cruz-Ortiz H, Herrera-Goepfert R. The precursor lesions of invasive gallbladder carcinoma. Hyperplasia, atypical hyperplasia and carcinoma in situ. *Cancer*. 1980;**45**(5):919–927.
23. Yukawa M, Fujimori T, Hirayama D, et al. Expression of oncogene products and growth factors in early gallbladder cancer, advanced gallbladder cancer, and chronic cholecystitis. *Hum Pathol*. 1993;**24**(1):37–40.
30. Shirai Y, Tsukada K, Ohtani T, et al. Hepatic metastases from carcinoma of the gallbladder. *Cancer*. 1995;**75**(8):2063–2068.
31. Ito M, Mishima Y, Sato T. An anatomical study of the lymphatic drainage of the gallbladder. *Surg Radiol Anat*. 1991;**13**(2):89–104.
35. Miyazaki M, Ohtsuka M, Miyakawa S, et al. Classification of biliary tract cancers established by the Japanese Society of Hepato-Biliary-Pancreatic Surgery: 3(rd) English edition. *J Hepatobiliary Pancreat Sci*. 2015;**22**(3):181–196.
37. Perpetuo MD, Valdivieso M, Heilbrun LK, et al. Natural history study of gallbladder cancer: a review of 36 years experience at M. D. Anderson Hospital and Tumor Institute. *Cancer*. 1978;**42**(1):330–335.
39. Ritts RE Jr, Nagorney DM, Jacobsen DJ, et al. Comparison of preoperative serum CA19-9 levels with results of diagnostic imaging modalities in patients undergoing laparotomy for suspected pancreatic or gallbladder disease. *Pancreas*. 1994;**9**(6):707–716.

40. Wibbenmeyer LA, Sharafuddin MJ, Wolverson MK, et al. Sonographic diagnosis of unsuspected gallbladder cancer: imaging findings in comparison with benign gallbladder conditions. *AJR Am J Roentgenol*. 1995;**165**(5):1169–1174.
45. Hirooka Y, Naitoh Y, Goto H, et al. Contrast-enhanced endoscopic ultrasonography in gallbladder diseases. *Gastrointest Endosc*. 1998;**48**(4):406–410.
46. Thorsen MK, Quiroz F, Lawson TL, et al. Primary biliary carcinoma: CT evaluation. *Radiology*. 1984;**152**(2):479–483.
48. Yoshimitsu K, Honda H, Kaneko K, et al. Dynamic MRI of the gallbladder lesions: differentiation of benign from malignant. *J Magn Reson Imaging*. 1997;**7**(4):696–701.
51. Valle JW, Borbath I, Khan SA, et al. Biliary cancer: ESMO Clinical Practice Guidelines for diagnosis, treatment and follow-up. *Ann Oncol*. 2016;**27**(suppl 5):v28–v37.
52. Kohya N, Miyazaki K. Hepatectomy of segment 4a and 5 combined with extra-hepatic bile duct resection for T2 and T3 gallbladder carcinoma. *J Surg Oncol*. 2008;**97**(6):498–502.
54. Margonis GA, Gani F, Buettner S, et al. Rates and patterns of recurrence after curative intent resection for gallbladder cancer: a multi-institution analysis from the US Extra-hepatic Biliary Malignancy Consortium. *HPB (Oxford)*. 2016;**18**(11):872–878.
55. Lee SE, Jang JY, Lim CS, et al. Systematic review on the surgical treatment for T1 gallbladder cancer. *World J Gastroenterol*. 2011;**17**(2):174–180.
56. Shih SP, Schulick RD, Cameron JL, et al. Gallbladder cancer: the role of laparoscopy and radical resection. *Ann Surg*. 2007;**245**(6):893–901.
63. Pawlik TM, Gleisner AL, Vigano L, et al. Incidence of finding residual disease for incidental gallbladder carcinoma: implications for re-resection. *J Gastrointest Surg*. 2007;**11**(11):1478–1486; discussion 1486–1477.
65. D'Angelica M, Dalal KM, DeMatteo RP, et al. Analysis of the extent of resection for adenocarcinoma of the gallbladder. *Ann Surg Oncol*. 2009;**16**(4):806–816.
69. Hakeem AR, Papoulas M, Menon KV. The role of neoadjuvant chemotherapy or chemoradiotherapy for advanced gallbladder cancer - a systematic review. *Eur J Surg Oncol*. 2019;**45**(2):83–91.
72. Horgan AM, Amir E, Walter T, Knox JJ. Adjuvant therapy in the treatment of biliary tract cancer: a systematic review and meta-analysis. *J Clin Oncol*. 2012;**30**(16):1934–1940.
73. Takada T, Amano H, Yasuda H, et al. Is postoperative adjuvant chemotherapy useful for gallbladder carcinoma? A phase III multicenter prospective randomized controlled trial in patients with resected pancreaticobiliary carcinoma. *Cancer*. 2002;**95**(8):1685–1695.
74. Valle J, Wasan H, Palmer DH, et al. Cisplatin plus gemcitabine versus gemcitabine for biliary tract cancer. *N Engl J Med*. 2010;**362**(14):1273–1281.
75. Jarnagin WR, Ruo L, Little SA, et al. Patterns of initial disease recurrence after resection of gallbladder carcinoma and hilar cholangiocarcinoma: implications for adjuvant therapeutic strategies. *Cancer*. 2003;**98**(8):1689–1700.
77. Sharma A, Dwary AD, Mohanti BK, et al. Best supportive care compared with chemotherapy for unresectable gall bladder cancer: a randomized controlled study. *J Clin Oncol*. 2010;**28**(30):4581–4586.
80. Speer AG, Cotton PB, Russell RC, et al. Randomised trial of endoscopic versus percutaneous stent insertion in malignant obstructive jaundice. *Lancet*. 1987;**2**(8550):57–62.
81. Saluja SS, Gulati M, Garg PK, et al. Endoscopic or percutaneous biliary drainage for gallbladder cancer: a randomized trial and quality of life assessment. *Clin Gastroenterol Hepatol*. 2008;**6**(8):944–950.e3.
99. Knechtle SJ, D'Alessandro AM, Harms BA, et al. Relationships between sclerosing cholangitis, inflammatory bowel disease, and cancer in patients undergoing liver transplantation. *Surgery*. 1995;**118**(4):615–620.
134. Rea DJ, Rosen CB, Nagorney DM, et al. Transplantation for cholangiocarcinoma: when and for whom? *Surg Oncol Clin N Am*. 2009;**18**(2):325–337.
139. Nagorney DM, Donohue JH, Farnell MB, et al. Outcomes after curative resections of cholangiocarcinoma. *Arch Surg*. 1993;**128**(8):871–879.
142. Mavros MN, Economopoulos KP, Alexiou VG, Pawlik TM. Treatment and prognosis for patients with intrahepatic cholangiocarcinoma: systematic review and meta-analysis. *JAMA Surg*. 2014;**149**(6):565–574.
155. Mansour JC, Aloia TA, Crane CH, et al. Hilar cholangiocarcinoma: expert consensus statement. *HPB*. 2015;**17**(8):691–699.
165. Zamora-Valdes D, Heimbach JK. Liver transplant for cholangiocarcinoma. *Gastroenterol Clin N Am*. 2018;**47**(2):267–280.
175. Malka D, Cervera P, Foulon S, et al. Gemcitabine and oxaliplatin with or without cetuximab in advanced biliary-tract cancer (BINGO): a randomised, open-label, non-comparative phase 2 trial. *Lancet Oncol*. 2014;**15**(8):819–828.
176. Knox JJ, Hedley D, Oza A, et al. Combining gemcitabine and capecitabine in patients with advanced biliary cancer: a phase II trial. *J Clinl Oncol*. 2005;**23**(10):2332–2338.
184. Vogl TJ, Naguib NNN, Nour-Eldin N-EA, et al. Transarterial chemoembolization in the treatment of patients with unresectable cholangiocarcinoma: results and prognostic factors governing treatment success. *Int J Cancer*. 2012;**131**(3):733–740.
192. Tocchi A, Costa G, Lepre L, et al. Non-resectable neoplasms of the biliary duct: palliative surgery vs non-surgical management. *G Chir*. 1996;**17**(8-9):408–412.

89 Neoplasms of the exocrine pancreas

Robert A. Wolff, MD ■ Donghui Li, PhD ■ Anirban Maitra, MBBS ■ Susan Tsai, MD ■ Eugene Koay, MD, PhD ■ Douglas B. Evans, MD

Overview

Pancreatic cancer is largely preventable with healthier lifestyle choices perhaps to include a predominantly plant-based diet. Currently, about 10% of patients have germline mutations putting them at increased risk for pancreatic cancer. Population-wide reductions in smoking, obesity, and diabetes will probably increase the proportion of patients with genetically driven disease, expanding the options for precision medicine. Pancreatic cancer is notorious for local invasion and metastatic dissemination and treatment paradigms must account for both. Surgical resection of localized disease provides the only meaningful chance for cure, with improvements in survival seen using both adjuvant and neoadjuvant approaches. Cytotoxic therapy is the mainstay of treatment for locally advanced and metastatic disease. The role of radiation is in evolution. Small subsets of patients are benefiting from precision medicine using targeted treatments and immunotherapy.

Introduction

Adenocarcinoma of the pancreas, better known as pancreatic cancer, is an increasing global burden characterized by late detection, resistance to current therapies, morbidity (tumor- and treatment-related), and high mortality. Its unique tumor microenvironment (TME) is tumor protective and immunosuppressive making it one of most challenging malignancies to treat. This article will review our current understanding of pancreatic cancer, with emphasis on its potential for prevention, expanding therapeutic options, and recent progress in precision medicine.

Epidemiology

Worldwide, pancreatic cancer is the 14th most common cancer and 6th leading cause of cancer-related death. In the United States (US), it is predicted that pancreatic cancer will become the 2nd leading cause of cancer death by 2030.[1] Risk of disease is low in the first few decades of life but increases sharply after age 50; most patients present between the ages of 60 and 80. Approximately 10% of patients are 50 or younger; they have a higher chance of harboring germline genetic mutations associated with pancreatic cancer.[2]

Etiologic factors

As with most other human cancers, pancreatic cancer etiology involves both genetic and nongenetic factors (Figure 1).

Hereditary risk factors

Inherited or familial pancreatic cancer (usually defined by two first-degree relatives with pancreatic cancer) represents approximately 5–10% of all cases.[3,4] Although the genetic mutations responsible for familial clustering of pancreatic cancer have not been fully elucidated, several gene mutations are now linked to known cancer syndromes or chronic inflammatory diseases which increase risk (Table 1).[3,5]

BRCA1 and BRCA2

Hereditary breast-ovarian cancer syndrome is associated with germline mutations in *BRCA1* or *BRCA2*. The risk of pancreatic cancer among *BRCA1* mutation carriers is lower than for *BRCA2*. Together they represent 10% of patients with familial pancreatic cancer and 7% of patients with sporadic pancreatic cancer.[6–8] Germline *BRCA2* mutations are the most common inherited mutations found in pancreatic cancer and pose a 10-fold greater risk of developing pancreatic cancer.[9]

PALB2 and ATM

Mutations in *PALB2* and *ATM* genes have also been discovered in familial pancreatic cancer cases.[10–12] The Palb2 protein binds with Brca2 to form a complex in the Fanconi anemia DNA repair pathway. *ATM* is an important regulator of cellular response to DNA damage. *PALB2* mutations account for 1–3% of the familial clustering of pancreatic cancer.[10,11] Germline mutations of *CDKN2A*, *TP53*, *MLH1*, *BRCA1*, *BRCA2*, and *ATM* genes have also been found in roughly 5% of patients with no family history of pancreatic cancer.[13]

CDKN2A (p16)

Germline mutations of the *CDKN2A (p16)* tumor suppressor gene are mostly related to familial atypical multiple-mole melanoma (FAMMM) syndrome and carriers have a 13- to 22-fold increased risk of developing pancreatic cancer.[14] Somatic mutations in *CDKN2A* are also frequent in sporadic pancreatic cancer.

HNPCC and FAP

Hereditary nonpolyposis colon cancer (HNPCC) is caused by germline mutations in several DNA mismatch repair (MMR) genes.[15] Families with HNPCC have an 8.6-fold increased risk of developing pancreatic cancer.[16] Germline testing or genomic analysis of tumor samples may reveal MMR deficiency or microsatellite instability (MSI)-high phenotype. These assays can identify patients whose disease may respond to immune checkpoint blockade.[17] Families with familial adenomatous polyposis (FAP) with mutations in the tumor suppressor gene *APC*, also have increased risk of pancreatic cancer.[18,19]

Holland-Frei Cancer Medicine, Tenth Edition. Edited by Robert C. Bast, John C. Byrd, Carlo M. Croce, Ernest Hawk, Fadlo R. Khuri, Raphael E. Pollock, Apostolia M. Tsimberidou, Christopher G. Willett, and Cheryl L. Willman.
© 2023 John Wiley & Sons, Inc. Published 2023 by John Wiley & Sons, Inc.

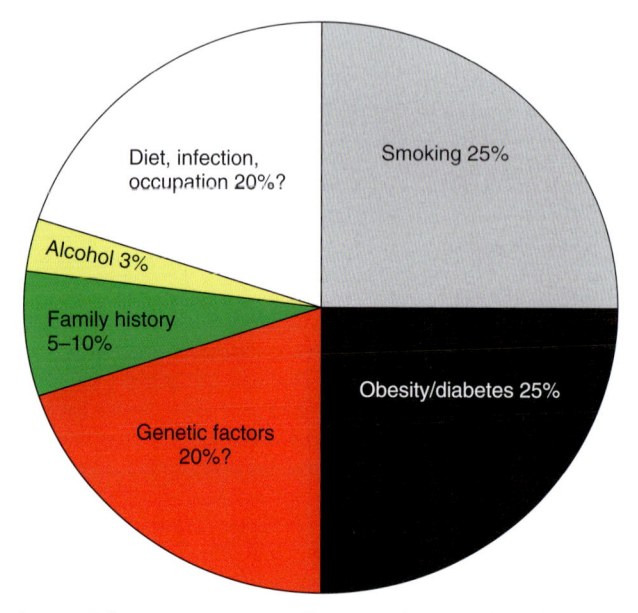

Figure 1 Schematic presentation of known and suspected risk factors for pancreatic cancer.

LKB1/STK11

Peutz–Jeghers syndrome is caused by mutations in the *LKB1/STK11* tumor suppressor gene. Patients with Peutz–Jeghers have significantly increased the risk of pancreatic cancer with relative risk (RR) ranging from 96 to 132 and a 36% lifetime risk.[19,20]

Hereditary pancreatitis

Germline mutations in *PRSS1* and *SPINK1* genes can result in hereditary pancreatitis. *PRSS1* encodes the cationic trypsinogen protein and its dysregulation can result in acute pancreatitis. *SPINK1* encodes a trypsin inhibitor with mutations causing chronic pancreatitis. Individuals with hereditary pancreatitis have a 53-fold increased risk for pancreatic cancer with a lifetime risk of 30–40%.[3]

Susceptibility variants

The polygenic theory for complex disease inheritance suggests that many disease-predisposing genetic loci have a small to moderate effect on risk.[21,22] Low-penetrance common-susceptibility loci have been identified for pancreatic cancer using genome-wide association studies (GWASs). Topping the list for Caucasians is an ABO gene variant. Individuals with A, AB, and B blood groups have an increased risk of pancreatic cancer and roughly 20% of pancreatic cancer may be attributable to non-O blood types.[23] Other top GWAS hits for pancreatic cancer include *NR5A2*, *PDX1*, and *HNF1B*, which code for transcription factors regulating the development, differentiation, and functions of the pancreas. A region on chr5p15.33 containing the *TERT* and *CLPTM1* genes; two loci on chr13q22.1 and 7q32.3, *BCAR1* and *ZNF3*, are all associated with increased risk.[24]

Acquired risk factors

Smoking

Cigarette smoking is an established risk factor for pancreatic cancer, contributing to approximately 25% of cases, increasing risk by about twofold.[25–28] Whether smokeless tobacco products increase pancreatic cancer risk remains controversial.[29]

Obesity

As the prevalence of cigarette smoking among US adults has dropped (13.7% in 2018 from >40% in 1960s), the prevalence of obesity has tripled to 42.4%.[30] This increase in obesity is likely responsible for the rising incidence of pancreatic cancer. Excess body weight contributes to roughly 25% of cases in the United States.[31] Beyond body mass index, excess abdominal fat also increases risk especially in women.[32,33] Obesity during adolescence or early adulthood likewise appears to increase risk.[34–36] Insulin resistance and inflammation are suspected mechanisms in carcinogenesis.[37]

Diabetes mellitus and antidiabetic medication

Diabetes mellitus may be an early manifestation of pancreatic cancer or a predisposing factor.[38–41] While type II DM is a risk factor, the tumor can also induce peripheral insulin resistance and type 3c (pancreatogenic) diabetes.[42,43] Hyperglycemia may occur up to two years before a diagnosis of pancreatic cancer with 1 in 125 new-onset diabetics developing pancreatic cancer within three years.[44,45] In the future, early detection among new-onset diabetics may be possible using biomarkers distinguishing type II diabetes mellitus from type 3c diabetes.[46,47]

The influence of antidiabetic therapy on risk of pancreatic cancer has also been investigated. Numerous studies have reported an association of metformin use and reduced risk of pancreatic cancer.[48] The value of metformin or other metabolic regulators as

Table 1 Susceptibility genes for pancreatic cancer.[a]

Gene	Syndrome	Chromosome location	Function
PRSS1	Hereditary pancreatitis	7q35	Trypsinogen, serine protease
SPINK1		5q32	Serine peptide (trypsin) inhibitor
CFTR	Cystic fibrosis	7q31.2	ABC transporter chloride channel
BRCA1	Hereditary breast-ovarian cancer	17q21	DNA damage repair
BRCA2		13q12.3	
CDKN2A/P16	Familial atypical multiple Mole melanoma	9p21	Cyclin-dependent kinase inhibitor
STK11/LKB1	Peutz–Jeghers syndrome	19p13.3	Serine/threonine kinase
MSH2, MLH1	Hereditary nonpolyposis colorectal cancer	2p21	DNA mismatch repair
PMS1/2, MGH6		3p21.3	
APC	Familial adenomatous polyposis	5q21	Negative regulator of β-catenin
PALB2	Breast and pancreatic cancer	16p12.2	Partner and localizer of BRCA2
ATM	Ataxia-Telangiectasia	11q22-q23	DNA damage response

[a]Source: Based on Klein[3] and Zhan et al.[5]

preventive or having therapeutic benefit in pancreatic cancer has not been established.[49,50]

Alcohol
Heavy alcohol consumption (30–40 g alcohol or ≥3 drinks/day) has been associated with an increased risk of pancreatic cancer.[51] In a meta-analysis, the RR of pancreatic cancer was 1.22 among heavy drinkers.[52]

Chronic pancreatitis
Nonhereditary chronic pancreatitis may develop with heavy alcohol consumption and cigarette smoking; this confounds a direct association between chronic pancreatitis and pancreatic cancer. Nevertheless, it is likely that patients with a history of chronic pancreatitis are at risk for pancreatic cancer.[53]

Infectious diseases
Helicobacter pylori may cause subclinical pancreatitis or increased gastrin levels, with resultant trophic effects on the pancreas. ABO genotype/phenotype status may also influence the behavior of *H. pylori*, modulating gastric and pancreatic secretory function and pancreatic carcinogenicity.[54] Hepatitis B likewise appears to be a risk factor for pancreatic cancer,[55] with subsequent reports providing additional support for HBV infection as increasing risk.[56]

Dietary factors
Generally, high dietary intake of fat or meat increases pancreatic cancer risk, whereas high intake of fruits, particularly citrus fruits, fiber, vegetables, and vitamin C reduces the risk.[57] Whether vitamin D is protective against pancreatic cancer is debatable.[58] Associations of dietary carbohydrates, refined sugars, and glycemic index or load with pancreatic cancer are inconsistent.[59]

Microbiota and microbiome
Recent research implicates specific microbial populations as promoting pancreatic carcinogenesis serving as potential biomarkers for early detection and refined treatment.[60] The gut microbiota is key to the development and modulation of the mucosal immune system and central to inflammatory signaling.[61] In animal models, the development of pancreatic cancer was associated with enrichment of specific strains of gut and intratumoral bacteria that induce an immunosuppressive microenvironment, facilitate cancer progression and resistance to immunotherapy.[62,63] Ablation of the microbiome with antibiotics remodels the TME, induces T-cell activation, improves immune surveillance, and increases sensitivity to immunotherapy.[64] Transfer of bacteria from tumor-bearing mice, but not controls, reverses the antitumor effects of antibiotics.[62,63] Microbes can also influence the metabolism and efficacy of chemotherapeutic drugs, such as gemcitabine.[65]

Fecal sample cultures demonstrate Proteobacteria, Synergistetes, and Euryarchaeota species are significantly more abundant in the patients with pancreatic cancer compared with healthy subjects.[63] Furthermore, investigators at the University of Texas MO Anderson Cancer Center found that microbiome diversity and composition influenced the survival of patients with pancreatic cancer.[66] Greater diversity in the tumor microbiome, and a specific microbiome signature predicted long-term survival.

When human fecal transplants were used in mouse models, tumor growth and immune profile were altered—suggesting the potential of bacteria to regulate tumors. Taken together, these studies highlight the growing appreciation for the role of microbes within the gut and tumors in carcinogenesis, therapeutic responses, and survival in pancreatic cancer.[67] Thus, rational modification of the microbiome could protect against oncogenesis, enhance chemosensitivity, reverse intratumoral immune tolerance, and enable immunotherapy in pancreatic cancer. In the future, artificial intelligence may refine risk stratification for pancreatic cancer using obesity, smoking, diabetes, diet, and microbiome analysis.[68]

Table 2 Interventions that may reduce pancreatic cancer risk.[a]

Lifestyle and nutritional factors
Cessation/avoidance of tobacco smoking and smokeless tobacco
Regular exercise
Weight control and weight reduction if needed to BMI <25 kg/m^2
Healthy diet high in fruits and vegetables
Potential chemopreventive agents
Metformin
Aspirin/celecoxib
Curcumin
Vitamins C, D, and E

[a]Source: Based on Stan et al.[70] and Fan et al.[71]

Summary
Modifiable risk factors (smoking, obesity, and diabetes) are responsible for up to 60% of pancreatic cancer cases and many may therefore be preventable.[69] Chemoprevention for pancreatic cancer, while not firmly established, may also have impact (Table 2).[70,71] Conversely, 10% of the pancreatic cancer cases are attributable to known inherited cancer syndromes or other germline mutations.[72] GWAS and other sequencing efforts have identified a number of susceptibility loci for pancreatic cancer. Identification of individuals with an increased risk of pancreatic cancer (those with a relevant family history, new-onset diabetes, or perhaps a specific microbiome signature) may provide target populations for better prevention and screening.[73]

Molecular events in human pancreatic carcinogenesis

Pancreatic cancer was one of the first human cancer types to undergo exome sequencing originally reported from 23 patient-derived cell lines and xenografts.[74] Using next-generation sequencing (NGS), the International Cancer Genome Consortium (ICGC), and The Cancer Genome Atlas (TCGA) comprehensively mapped the genomic landscape of pancreatic cancer across hundreds of tumors.[75,76] These efforts have identified the major recurrent alterations in pancreatic cancer and a significant number of less frequent mutations, many of which are actionable.[77,78] NGS panels have shown that about 25% of tumors may harbor potentially actionable mutations with results available in a feasible time frame.[79]

Oncogenes
Oncogenic mutations of *KRAS* are the defining genetic feature of pancreatic cancer, occurring in ~90% of cases.[76] Mutations of *KRAS* are present in the earliest precursor lesions of pancreatic cancer.[80] This oncogene orchestrates both pancreatic cancer initiation and maintenance as demonstrated in genetically engineered animal models.[81] Mutant Ras protein has profound growth-promoting effects on the cancer cells, activating downstream effector pathways such as mitogen-activated protein kinase

(MAPK), and reprogramming cellular metabolism for survival in a nutrient-depleted tumor milieu.[82,83] Beyond the autonomous effects on the cancer itself, the activated Ras protein also remodels the surrounding TME, through secretion of cytokines that attract immunosuppressive cells (e.g., myeloid cells), enabling the cancer to circumvent immune surveillance.[84,85]

KRAS mutations most commonly involve codon 12 and are usually either a glutamine to valine ($KRAS^{G12V}$) or glutamine to aspartic acid ($KRAS^{G12D}$) alteration. The uncommon $KRAS^{G12C}$ mutations are observed in only 1.5% of pancreatic cancers. This particular mutation may have clinical relevance with the development of small-molecule inhibitors that covalently bind the mutant protein, impeding its function.[86]

Despite the overarching importance of *KRAS* in pancreatic cancer pathogenesis, approximately ~10% of cases are wild type for this locus. In these cases, alternative driver mutations including *NRG1*, *ALK*, or *NTRK* fusions may be present.[73,87–89] The absence of *KRAS* mutation in pancreatic adenocarcinoma should, therefore, prompt interrogation for these alternative drivers preferably using RNA-based assays.[90,91] In addition to mutations and fusions, other mechanisms through which oncogenes are deregulated in pancreatic cancer include amplifications of chromosomal loci including *MYC*, *GATA6*, *EGFR*, or *KRAS*),[92,93] or by way of epigenetic alterations driving aberrant transcription.[94]

Tumor suppressor genes

Frequently altered tumor suppressor genes in pancreatic cancer are *TP53*, *CDKN2A/p16*, and *DPC4/SMAD4*.[76] *TP53* is the most commonly mutated gene in human cancer, and somatic alterations are present in ~75% of pancreatic cancers. Mutations of *TP53* are late events in the multistep progression of pancreatic carcinogenesis,[95] often occurring at the step of advanced precursor lesions. Nearly all pancreatic cancers harbor anomalies of the cyclin-dependent kinase inhibitor gene *CDKN2A/p16*, through a combination of mutation, genomic deletions, or promoter methylation. *CDKN2A/p16* is a cell cycle checkpoint protein that impedes the function of *CDK4/6*,[96] leading to investigation of small molecule *CDK4/6* antagonists in this cancer.[97,98] *DPC4/SMAD4* alterations occur in approximately 55% of pancreatic cancers, through a combination of mutations and genomic deletions. Amongst solid cancers, *DPC4/SMAD4* aberrations are somewhat specific for advanced pancreatic cancer,[99] and thus, immunohistochemical assessment for loss of SMAD4 protein may be a useful adjunct in carcinomas of unknown primary implicating a potential pancreatic origin. In autopsy series of patients with terminal pancreatic cancer, loss of *SMAD4* is associated with higher propensity for systemic dissemination, while retained *SMAD4* is usually observed in locally invasive or oligometastatic disease.[100] In resectable pancreatic cancers, loss of *SMAD4* is associated with higher risk of both local recurrence and distant failure.[101]

In addition, TCGA and ICGC analyses have identified other important classes of tumor suppressor genes in pancreatic cancer that are individually mutated at lower frequencies, but cumulatively, account for significant subsets. The most clinically relevant are genes encoding for proteins involved in DNA damage response and repair, including *BRCA2*, *BRCA1*, *PALB2*, *CHEK2*, *ATM*, *RAD51*, among others.[75,76] While germline mutations of these genes occur in the context of familial pancreatic cancer, approximately ~15% of cases harbor somatic loss of function mutations and these may be appropriate for DNA repair targeted therapies, such as poly(adenosine diphosphate-ribose) polymerase (PARP) inhibitors. As previously discussed, some pancreatic cancers (1%) harbor mutations in genes involved in DNA MMR, including *MLH1*, *MSH2*, *PMS2*, and *MSH6*; corresponding tumors have an exceptionally high tumor mutation burden (so-called "hypermutators").[75] Hypermutator tumors are susceptible to immune checkpoint inhibitor immunotherapy, which is approved for use in the first or second-line based on recent Food and Drug Administration (FDA) directives.[17] Of final note, a group of genes that encode for proteins involved in chromatin regulation such as *ARID1A*, *PBRM1*, *KDM6A*, and *MLL3* are cumulatively mutated in 15–25% of pancreatic cancers. Retrospective analyses and mouse models have shown that pancreatic cancers with chromatin regulatory gene mutations may be particularly aggressive.[102,103] However, there is emerging evidence from other solid tumors suggesting potential benefit using immunotherapy combinations in this context.[104,105]

Transcriptomic subtypes

While much of the focus within the translational landscape of pancreatic cancer has been on genomic alterations, RNA sequencing has also identified transcriptomic subtypes, with potential predictive and prognostic impact. In 2011, Collisson and colleagues proposed the first three-tier classification of pancreatic cancer based on RNA profiles: classical, quasimesenchymal, and exocrine-like),[106] with the quasimesenchymal subtype associated with a particularly aggressive natural history. Since then, other classifications have been proposed.[107] Currently, the most widely accepted classification scheme, proposed by Moffitt and colleagues[108] and embraced by the TCGA,[76] is dichotomous, subtyping pancreatic cancers into classical or basal-like. The classical phenotype is characterized by the expression of the endodermal transcription factors Gata6 and Hnf4a, both of which are absent in the basal-like tumors.[107,109] In contrast, basal-like, also described as the squamous subtype, is characterized by an aggressive natural history and mutations in genes encoding for chromatin regulatory factors.[93] Using refined RNA profiling techniques, admixtures of both subtypes may be observed within a single tumor.[110] Importantly, emerging data suggests that the "basal-like" tumors are resistant to treatment with folinic acid (leucovorin), fluorouracil (5FU), irinotecan and oxaliplatin (FOLFIRINOX),[108] and clinical trials that stratify choice of first-line therapy based on transcriptomic subtyping are ongoing.

Pancreatic cancer stroma

No discussion of the molecular pathology of pancreatic cancer is complete without alluding to the stroma and immune cell types that comprise its complex TME. First, the pancreatic cancer stroma is composed of a multitude of cell types and extracellular matrix proteins.[111] Second, the most common nonimmune cell type is the cancer-associated fibroblast (CAF), and single-cell RNA sequencing studies have identified at least three distinct types of CAFs,[112,113] with potentially distinct tumor-promoting versus tumor-suppressive roles. Previous strategies to target the pancreatic cancer CAFs (e.g., using small molecule inhibitors targeting the Hedgehog pathway) have been counter-productive,[105] underscoring the distinct roles played by CAF subpopulations in constraining or promoting the neoplastic process. Third, the pancreatic cancer TME is characterized by high interstitial pressure, attributable to the deposition of extracellular matrix proteins like hyaluronic acid and other glycosaminoglycans,[114] and implicated in reducing the delivery of systemic chemotherapy to the tumor milieu. Unfortunately, clinical efforts to degrade hyaluronic acid in the TME, theoretically enhancing cytotoxic therapy, have also been negative.[115,116]

Pathology

Pancreatic acinar cells account for approximately 80% of the gland. The ductal system, composed of single-layer, cuboidal epithelial cells comprise another 10–15% of the gland's structure with islet cells (1–2%) and a network of blood vessels, lymphatics, nerves, and collagenous stroma, creating the remainder. In carcinoma, this architecture is deranged and notable for a desmoplastic (fibrous) stroma, atrophic acini, preserved islet cell clusters, and a haphazard growth of malignant ducts (Figure 2). The diagnosis of ductal adenocarcinoma requires the identification of mitoses, nuclear and cellular pleomorphism, and evidence of perineural, vascular, or lymphatic invasion.[117] Furthermore, intra-ductal precursor lesions in the surrounding pancreatic parenchyma are common. There are two major subtypes of precursor lesions of ductal adenocarcinoma. The first, and by far most common, are the microscopic pancreatic intraepithelial neoplasia (PanIN) lesions. Roughly 90% of pancreatic cancers arise from these precursors. Histologically, PanIN lesions are graded as "low" and "high" grade with the latter harboring many of the genetic alterations found in frank carcinomas.[118] PanINs are not visible on radiological imaging, although the shadow of regional pancreatitis they create in the perilesional pancreas may be seen on endoscopic ultrasound (EUS), particularly in high-risk patients undergoing longitudinal surveillance.[119] In contrast, the macroscopic precursors of ductal adenocarcinomas are mucinous cysts of the pancreas, presenting either as intraductal papillary mucinous neoplasms (IPMNs) or mucinous cystic neoplasms (MCNs).[120] Analogous to PanINs, the cystic lesions also demonstrate low- and high-grade epithelial dysplasia, culminating in invasive neoplasia. Mucinous cysts of the pancreas can be followed radiologically for worrisome features indicating progression to carcinoma, and therefore present an opportunity for early detection in patients.

Almost all malignant neoplasms of pancreatic origin (95%) arise from the exocrine portion of the gland, of which ductal adenocarcinomas are the most common.[121] Pancreatic neuroendocrine tumors (PanNETs) arising from the islets of Langerhans (endocrine) cells are much more infrequent, and primary nonepithelial tumors (e.g., lymphomas or sarcomas) are extremely rare.

Summary

Pancreatic cancers often develop from microscopic precursor lesions described as PANins or arise from macroscopic IPMNs with main branch lesions at higher risk for malignant transformation. *KRAS* mutations are an early event in carcinogenesis with other relevant mutations *CDKN2A*, *p53*, and loss of Smad4 developing later. When *KRAS* is wild-type, other mutations are often responsible for driving tumorigenesis (*NRG1*, *ALK*, or *NTRK* fusions). The TME of pancreatic cancer is complex and comprised of intense desmoplastic stroma, and marrow-derived elements to include CAFs, macrophages, and immunosuppressive T-cells. Tumor cell metabolism is adapted to survive and thrive despite nutrient depletion.

Despite these complexities, some newly discovered vulnerabilities are facilitating early efforts in precision medicine for small subsets of patients. These include identification of DNA MMR deficient (MSI-high) tumors, a hallmark of HNPCC, amenable to immune checkpoint inhibition, tumors with *NTRK* fusions which are targetable with small molecule inhibitors, and mutations in the DNA repair genes *BRCA1* and *BRCA2* where clinical benefit can be provided by PARP inhibition.

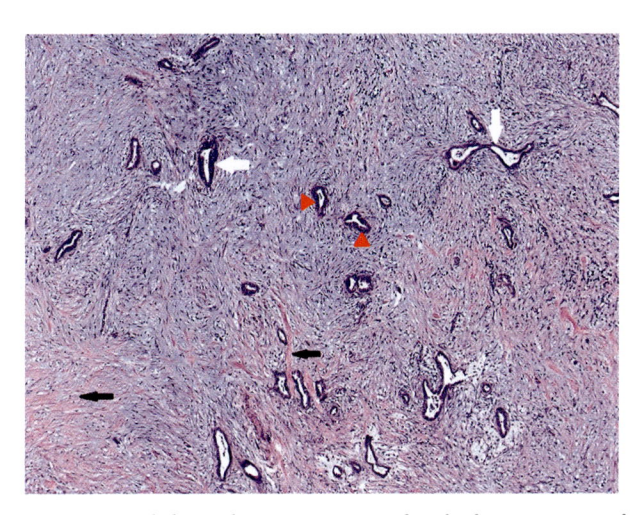

Figure 2 Stromal desmoplasia in pancreatic ductal adenocarcinoma of the pancreas. Infiltrating neoplastic glands (white arrows) are surrounded by a florid host response, comprised of spindle-shaped cancer-associated fibroblasts and myofibroblasts (red arrowheads) and extracellular matrix, including collagen 1 (black arrows).

Clinical management

Presentation, diagnosis, and staging

The clinical presentation of pancreatic cancer is primarily dependent on the location of the tumor within the pancreas. The majority (85%) develop within the pancreatic head with 10% located in the pancreatic body and 5% in the tail. Nonspecific, poorly localized, epigastric, or back pain is the most common initial presentation. Pain is often caused by invasion or compression of the celiac, splanchnic, or mesenteric plexi. Tumors in the head or neck typically cause pain in the epigastric area or right upper quadrant. Cancers of the body may cause severe, unremitting back pain, and tumors in the pancreatic tail may cause left upper quadrant pain. However, patients with tail lesions may remain asymptomatic until the development of signs or symptoms of metastatic disease.

Painless jaundice, another common presentation, is generally associated with tumors in the pancreatic head or uncinate process. If these head/neck tumors do not arise in proximity to the intra-pancreatic portion of the bile duct, they may be characterized by abdominal pain or back pain without jaundice, delaying diagnosis.

Acute pancreatitis, while uncommon, may result from a ductal adenocarcinoma in patients with no other reason for acute pancreatitis (lack of gallstones, no history of alcohol or precipitating drugs).[59]

The diagnostic work-up of patients ultimately found to have pancreatic cancer can be fragmented and inefficient. Surgeons or other specialists may be requested to evaluate a patient at any point in the diagnostic process to include assessment of abdominal pain, presence of a biliary stricture suspicious for malignancy, or biopsy-confirmed pancreatic cancer with or without complete staging. Information that may have important therapeutic implications can be obtained from a thorough history and physical examination and include careful estimation of performance status (PS), cardiopulmonary function, evaluation for left supraclavicular or periumbilical adenopathy, or evidence for venous thromboembolism (VTE).

Imaging

Imaging should be obtained prior to other interventions such as endoscopic retrograde cholangiopancreatography (ERCP) or EUS which may induce pancreatitis and compromise imaging reliability. The single most important imaging tool for the detection and staging of pancreatic cancer is dual-phase computed tomography (CT).[122] The first (arterial) phase is used for visualization of the primary tumor and optimal assessment of the tumor–arterial relationship. The second (venous) phase aids definition of the relationship of the tumor to the surrounding venous structures: superior mesenteric vein (SMV), portal vein (PV), and splenic vein. CT imaging may also uncover metastatic disease.

If a low-density mass is not seen on CT, the presence of biliary or pancreatic duct obstruction remains concerning for malignancy. Thus further imaging may be indicated and small pancreatic lesions (<2 cm) may be more conspicuous on magnetic resonance imaging (MRI) relative to CT.[123,124] Patients with a suspicion of pancreatic cancer, without radiographic evidence of a mass, should undergo EUS and when combined with target-guided fine needle aspirate (FNA) or core biopsy, may confirm malignancy. Rarely, patients may present with radiographic features concerning for pancreatic cancer without an identifiable mass on CT, MRI, or EUS. If the patient is jaundiced, an ERCP may provide additional radiographic information to include evidence for a double duct sign (dilated common bile duct and pancreatic duct) or smooth tapering of the common bile duct more suggestive of an inflammatory or autoimmune bile duct stricture. In these settings, biliary brushings can provide material for cytologic evaluation. Importantly, pancreatic cancer remains the major diagnostic consideration in patients (without a history of recurrent pancreatitis or alcohol abuse) who have a malignant-appearing stricture of the intrapancreatic portion of the common bile duct or evidence for pancreatic duct dilation without visualization of a mass. Repeat EUS should be considered, but if malignancy is not confirmed, attempt at resection should follow assuming that the patient is otherwise healthy with no contraindications for this surgery.

Classification of clinical stage

Using modern imaging techniques, objective radiologic criteria for staging can be applied. This can broadly partition patients into those with metastatic disease, locally advanced disease, or localized disease (borderline resectable and resectable). Most patients will present with metastatic disease, as evidenced by liver or lung metastases or ascites/peritoneal implants. In the absence of metastases, clinical stage is determined by the relationship of the primary tumor to adjacent vasculature as outlined in Table 3.

Radiographic findings of a potentially resectable pancreatic cancer (AJCC stages I or II) include (1) the absence of tumor–arterial abutment; and (2) <50% reduction in the transverse diameter of the SMV/PV due to tumor abutment/encasement (Figure 3). Some staging systems require the absence of venous abutment to define a resectable tumor. In general, any tumor abutment (defined as the tumor being inseparable from a vessel but with <180° tumor–vessel interface) or encasement (defined as >180° tumor–vessel interface) of the celiac axis, common hepatic artery, or superior mesenteric artery (SMA) or visible narrowing or distortion of the SMV-PV should be considered a contraindication to immediate surgery. Patients who have tumor abutment, without encasement, of the SMA or celiac axis, or short segment encasement of the hepatic artery are considered to have borderline resectable pancreatic cancer (Figure 4). In addition, tumors that cause >50% narrowing or short segment occlusion of the SMV/PV amenable to reconstruction are also defined as borderline resectable. With broader adoption of neoadjuvant therapy for operable pancreatic cancer, even subtle tumor–vein abutment may be classified as borderline resectable.

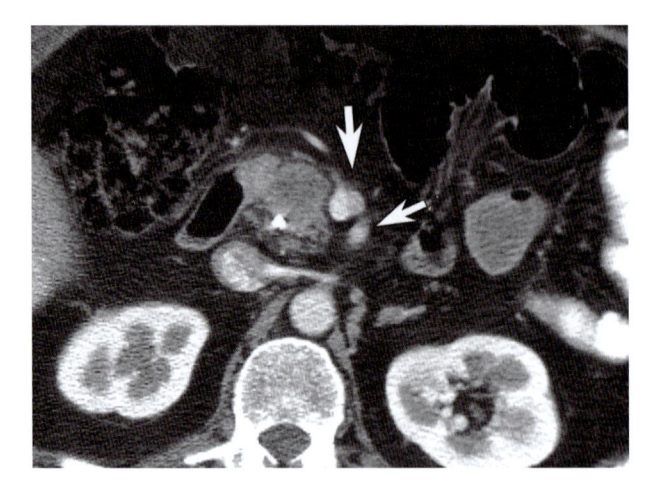

Figure 3 Contrast-enhanced computed tomography scan demonstrating a resectable adenocarcinoma of the pancreatic head. The low-density tumor is easily seen in the pancreatic head (T). Note the absence of tumor extension to the superior mesenteric artery (SMA); there is a normal fat plane between the low-density tumor and the SMA (right arrow). The upper arrow points to a narrow fat plane between tumor and the superior mesenteric vein (SMV). This patient may require venorrhaphy or venous resection and reconstruction at the time of pancreaticoduodenectomy. The critical margin for complete resection is the retroperitoneal (RP) margin (lower left arrow).

Table 3 Radiographic criteria for clinical staging of pancreatic cancer.

Resectable	
Tumor–artery relationship	No radiographic evidence of arterial abutment (celiac, SMA, or hepatic artery)
Tumor–vein relationship	Tumor-induced narrowing ≤50% of SMV, PV, or SMV-PV
Borderline resectable	
Artery	Tumor abutment (≤180°) of SMA or celiac artery. Tumor abutment or short segment encasement (>180°) of the hepatic artery
Vein	Tumor-induced narrowing of >50% of SMV, PV, or SMV-PV confluence. Short segment occlusion of SMV, PV, SMV-PV with suitable PV (above) and SMV (below) to allow for safe vascular reconstruction
Extrapancreatic disease	CT scan findings suspicious, but not diagnostic of, metastatic disease (e.g., small indeterminate liver lesions which are too small to characterize)
Locally advanced	
Artery	Tumor encasement (>180°) of SMA or celiac artery
Vein	Occlusion of SMV, PV, or SMV-PV *without* suitable vessels above and below the tumor to allow for reconstruction (no distal or proximal target for vascular reconstruction)
Extrapancreatic disease	No evidence of peritoneal, hepatic, extra-abdominal metastases
Metastatic	
Evidence of peritoneal or distant metastases	

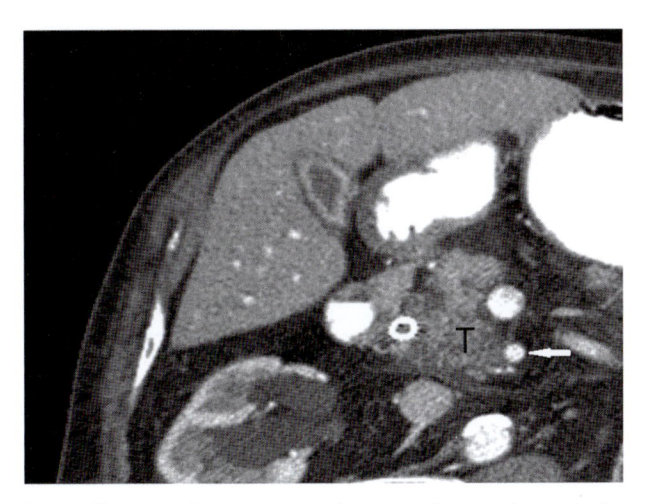

Figure 4 Contrast-enhanced computed tomography scan demonstrating a borderline resectable adenocarcinoma of the pancreatic head. The low-density tumor is seen in the pancreatic head (T). Note the tumor abutting the SMA for 180° of its circumference on the right.

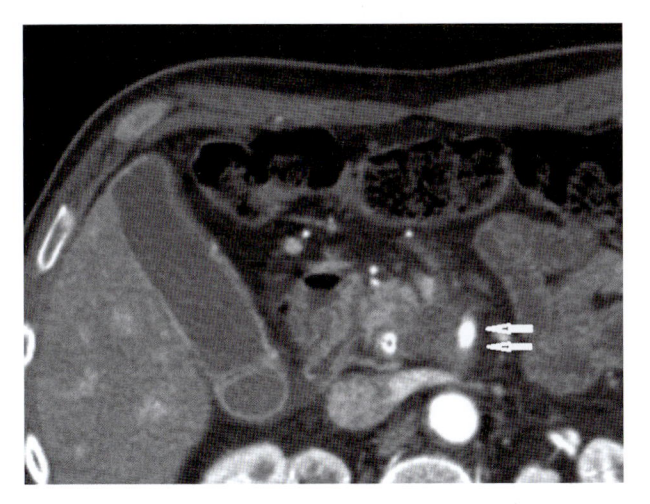

Figure 5 Contrast-enhanced computed tomography scan demonstrating an unresectable adenocarcinoma of the pancreatic head and uncinate process. The low-density tumor is encircled roughly 270° of the SMA with no tumor involvement of the remaining 90° (white arrows).

Locally advanced disease (AJCC stage III) is present when: (1) the tumor encases the SMA or celiac axis, or (2) occludes the superior mesenteric-portal vein (SMPV) confluence precluding any realistic chance for venous reconstruction, and (3) no metastatic disease is evident (Figure 5). Historically, locally advanced tumors were considered unresectable. However, improvements in neoadjuvant therapy, combined with innovations in surgery, are providing a larger proportion of patients with locally advanced pancreatic cancer an opportunity for resection with curative intent.

Tissue acquisition
In general, confirmation of malignancy is required in all patients with locally advanced or metastatic disease before initiation of anticancer treatment. With radiographic evidence of metastatic disease, image-guided percutaneous core needle biopsies of a metastasis are preferred to provide sufficient tissue for molecular profiling as recommended by the American Society of Clinical Oncology (ASCO) and the Pancreatic Cancer Guidelines Committee of the National Comprehensive Cancer Center Network (NCCN).[125,126] With localized disease potentially amenable to surgical resection, EUS-guided FNA or core needle biopsy is advised to minimize the risk of tumor seeding. When a negative cytology is obtained from an initial EUS-guided FNA, a 2nd EUS-guided biopsy improves diagnostic accuracy.[127] Given the emerging interest in biomarker interrogation of localized tumors, the safety and effectiveness of core needle biopsies with 22 or 25 gauge needles is being reported.[128]

Laparoscopic staging
When high-quality CT or MR imaging is employed, the role of staging laparoscopy is limited to patients with suspicion of metastatic disease based on imaging or high levels of serum carbohydrate antigen (CA) 19-9.[129] In addition, for marginal surgical candidates, a separate staging laparoscopy may be appropriate.

Biliary drainage
In patients with jaundice and localized pancreatic cancer, placement of endobiliary stents before surgery relieves the symptoms of biliary obstruction and facilitates the normalization of liver function. This is particularly important for patients to be treated with neoadjuvant therapy, as hyperbilirubinemia prevents the safe delivery of cytotoxic therapy. If neoadjuvant therapy is planned, biliary complications, including stent occlusion and cholangitis, can be minimized with insertion of a metal stent after biopsy confirmation of malignancy.[130] For patients with locally advanced or metastatic pancreatic cancer, self-expanding metal stents have superior long-term patency compared with plastic stents. However, without confirmation of malignancy, patients with symptomatic distal bile duct obstruction should generally undergo insertion of a plastic stent rather than a metal stent.

Treatment modalities in pancreatic cancer
Pancreatic cancer is notorious for being locally invasive with a striking propensity for early dissemination. For most patients, metastatic disease determines survival and systemic therapy is usually the sole treatment modality. Conversely, in the setting of localized disease, surgical resection aims to completely remove the primary tumor with systemic therapy delivered to eradicate microscopic metastatic disease. Radiation has a less precise role in localized and locally advanced disease. It is occasionally used as a component of adjuvant therapy, more often as part of neoadjuvant therapy, or to enhance local control in locally advanced, unresectable disease. At present, for patients with locally advanced disease, systemic therapy is the standard of care. However, in select patients, radiotherapy and even surgical resection may maximize local control and impact survival. As systemic therapy becomes more effective in eradicating low-volume metastatic disease, local modalities become increasingly relevant.

Until the last decade, gemcitabine was the mainstay of systemic therapy. Two newer cytotoxic combinations: FOLFIRINOX and gemcitabine plus nab-paclitaxel, are both superior to gemcitabine monotherapy in metastatic disease.[131,132] Furthermore, these two regimens are increasingly utilized in earlier stages of disease. In particular, FOLFIRINOX has proven superior to gemcitabine as adjuvant therapy (in select postoperative patients).

Surgical considerations
Surgical resection offers the only meaningful chance for cure in patients with localized pancreatic cancer. However, if the primary tumor cannot be resected completely (gross complete resection), surgery offers no survival advantage. Even microscopically positive

```
                    ┌─────────────────────────────────────┐
                    │ Cisplatin-based chemotherapy (four courses) │
                    └─────────────────────────────────────┘
```

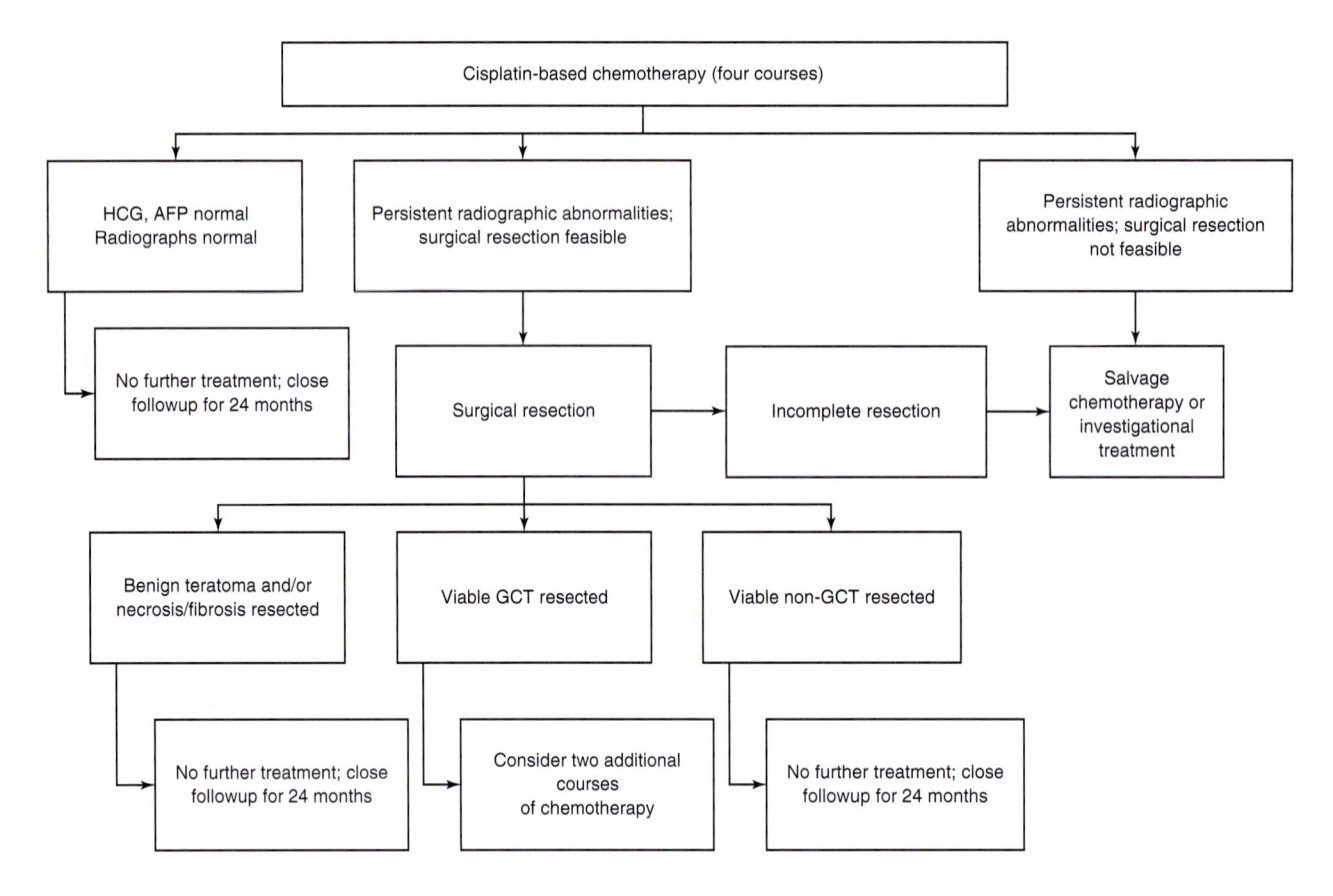

Figure 6 Six surgical steps of pancreaticoduodenectomy. Source: Evans et al.[136]

surgical margins have a negative impact on overall survival (OS) and the ability to obtain a margin negative resection should be considered necessary for long-term survival.[88] At present, for patients with potentially resectable disease, 2 distinct approaches to curative resection are being utilized: upfront surgery followed by adjuvant therapy or neoadjuvant therapy followed by resection.

Upfront surgery and adjuvant therapy
Many consider the standard of care for early-stage, resectable pancreatic cancer to be surgery followed by adjuvant therapy. High-quality surgery, anesthesia, and perioperative care yield 30-day mortality rates less than 2%. Higher hospital volume is associated with lower pancreatic cancer surgery-related mortality.[133,134] For those patients with adequate recovery from surgery, randomized trials have shown that upfront surgical resection, followed by six months of single-agent or combination chemotherapy, prolongs survival compared with surgery alone.

Pancreaticoduodenectomy
The standard surgical procedure for neoplasms of the pancreatic head and periampullary region is pancreaticoduodenectomy. The current technique of pancreaticoduodenectomy has evolved from the procedure first described by Whipple and colleagues in 1935.[135] Today's operation emphasizes the importance of removing all soft tissue to the right of the SMA as well as removing the perineural tissue surrounding the arteries at highest risk for harboring micrometastatic disease. The surgical resection is divided into six clearly defined steps (Figure 6); the most important oncologic aspect is Step 6, during which the pancreas is divided and the specimen is removed from the SMPV confluence and the right lateral border of the SMA.[136]

The high incidence of local recurrence after standard pancreaticoduodenectomy requires particular attention to the SMA or retroperitoneal (RP) margin, along its right lateral border proximally (Figures 3 and 7).[137] This margin must be identified for the pathologist and assessed histologically; the residual disease status ("R" factor) cannot be determined if the RP margin is not assessed histologically.[138,139]

Of note, vascular resection may be necessary to obtain an R0 resection, which requires complete removal of the tumor from the SMV/PV and exposure of the SMA to allow sharp dissection of the tumor off this artery. Venous resection and reconstruction should be performed for tumors adherent to the SMV or SMPV confluence or in the presence of short segment occlusion of the SMV/PV with no tumor encasement of the SMA or celiac axis (Figure 8).[136]

Pylorus preservation
Pylorus-preserving pancreaticoduodenectomy may be an attractive alternative to a conventional Whipple as it allows for more controlled gastric emptying. This may be of particular value in thin, older patients who may have difficulty maintaining postoperative weight. Randomized trials suggest no difference in perioperative factors or patient outcome between standard and pylorus-preserving pancreaticoduodenectomy.[140,141] Note pylorus preservation should not be performed in patients who have bulky tumors of the pancreatic head.

Minimally invasive pancreatectomy
Interest in applying minimally invasive surgery (MIS) to pancreatic resection stems from the hypothesis that open surgical resection is associated with substantial physiologic stress and morbidity. Rates

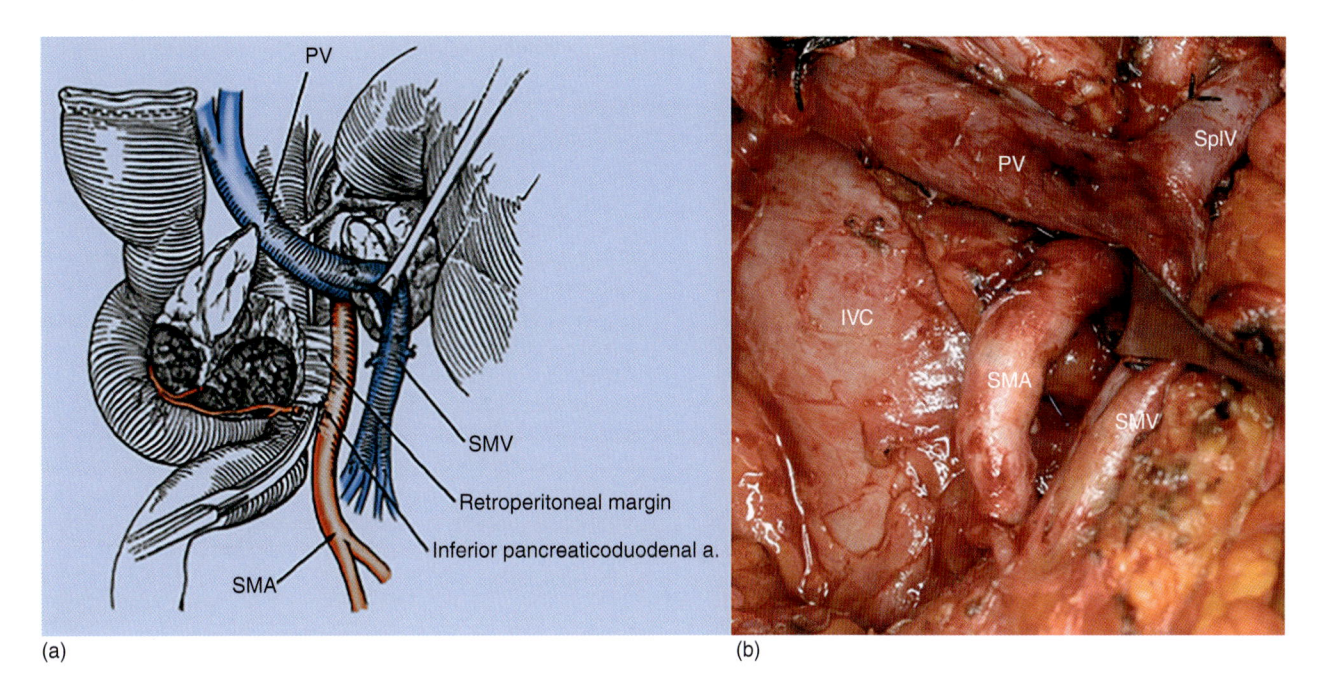

Figure 7 (a) Illustration of the retroperitoneal margin as defined at the time of tumor resection and (b) intraoperative photograph after the tumor has been removed. Medial retraction of the superior mesenteric vein (SMV) and SMV-portal vein (PV) confluence facilitates dissection of the soft tissues adjacent to the lateral wall of the proximal superior mesenteric artery (SMA); this site represents the SMA margin. Complete permanent-section analysis of the pancreaticoduodenectomy specimen requires that it be oriented for the pathologist to enable accurate assessment of the SMA margin of excision and other standard pathologic variables. The intraoperative photograph (b) shows complete skeletonization of the SMA which is not necessary for all patients but provides a very nice view of the relationship of the SMA to the SMV for purposes of this illustration. Source: Based on Raut et al.[137]

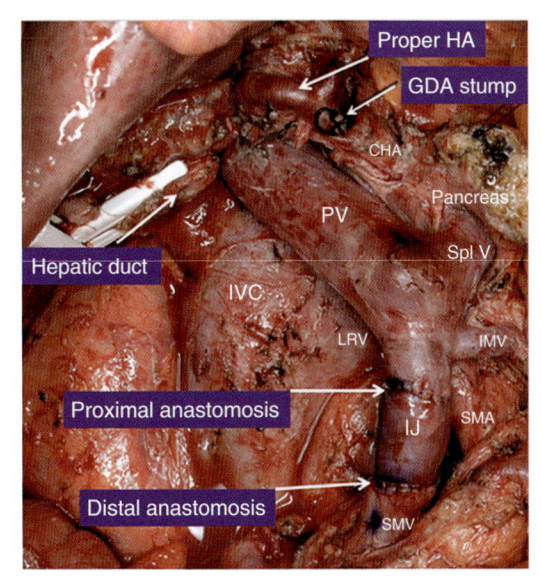

Figure 8 Segmental resection of the SMV with splenic vein (SplV) preservation adds significant complexity to this operation. GDA, Gastroduodenal artery; IVC, inferior vena cava; IMV, inferior mesenteric vein; LRV, left renal vein.

of minimally invasive pancreatectomy continue to increase.[142] MIS includes both laparoscopic and robotically assisted procedures.

Laparoscopic distal pancreatectomy is the most common MIS for pancreatic cancer as there is no requirement for anatomic reconstruction with tumor removal. Retrospective analysis and prospective trials have reported favorable perioperative outcomes with decreased blood loss, complications, and shorter hospital stays.[143,144] A recent propensity-matched analysis showed no differences in median OS comparing laparoscopic with open procedures.[145]

Laparoscopic pancreaticoduodenectomy has also been explored with early experience reporting conversion to an open procedure in 6–10% of patients.[146,147] The Dutch Pancreatic Cancer Group conducted (LEOPARD-2) to compare laparoscopic with open pancreaticoduodenectomy. Accrual to the trial was halted early because of an unexpectedly high 90-day mortality rate in the laparoscopic group (10% vs 2% for open cases).[148]

There is emerging interest in robotic pancreaticoduodenectomy; thus far, however, superior oncologic outcomes have yet to be established.[142,149,150] In one of the largest series of patients who underwent robotic resection for pancreatic cancer (226 robotic and 230 open), there was no difference in major complications, receipt of adjuvant therapy, or median OS.[151]

Pathologic staging and prognostic factors

The staging system of the American Joint Committee on Cancer (AJCC) and International Union Against Cancer is shown in Table 4. Recent modifications to the Tumor, Nodes, Metastasis (TNM) staging system rely on objective size criteria for T1–T3 tumors. T4 categorization is based on involvement of arterial structures with resectability removed from the definition. In addition to this refinement in the TNM system, which improves prognostic accuracy, R1 margin status, poorly differentiated tumors, and markedly elevated preoperative CA 19-9 levels have all been associated with decreased survival.[88,153,154]

Adjuvant (postoperative) therapy

A detailed history of adjuvant therapy in resected adenocarcinoma of the pancreas is beyond the scope of this text. Briefly, adjuvant therapy in pancreatic cancer began with the study of chemoradiation using fluorouracil (5FU) as a radiosensitizer. The

Table 4 TNM criteria for pancreatic adenocarcinoma TNM definitions.[a]

Tx	Primary tumor cannot be assessed
T0	No evidence of primary tumor
Tis	Carcinoma in situ
T1	Tumor <2 cm in greatest dimension
T1a	Tumor <0.5 cm in greatest dimension
T1b	Tumor >0.5 and <1.0 cm in greatest dimension
T1c	Tumor 1–2 cm in greatest dimension
T2	Tumor >2 and ≤4 cm in greatest dimension
T3	Tumor >4 cm in greatest dimension
T4	Tumor involves the celiac axis, hepatic artery, or superior mesenteric artery regardless of size
Nx	Regional lymph node status cannot be assessed
N0	No regional lymph node metastasis
N1	Metastasis in 1–3 regional lymph nodes
N2	Metastases in 4 or more regional lymph nodes
Mx	Distant metastasis cannot be assessed
M0	No distant metastasis
M1	Distant metastasis

Staging classification			
Stage	T	N	M
0	Tis	N0	M0
IA	T1	N0	M0
IB	T2	N0	M0
IIA	T3	N0	M0
IIB	T1–T3	N1	M0
III	T1–T4	N2	M0
IV	Any T	Any N	M1

[a]Source: Amin.[152]

earliest randomized trial demonstrated a clear benefit to adjuvant chemoradiation over surgery alone,[155] while a subsequent trial showed no benefit with chemoradiation.[156] Later, a 3rd trial concluded that chemoradiation was deleterious and inferior to treatment with chemotherapy alone.[157]

More recent randomized trials have focused on the delivery of chemotherapy as adjuvant therapy (Table 5). In a multinational randomized trial, six months of gemcitabine therapy was compared with observation after surgery.[158] Although the median survival advantage for patients randomized to gemcitabine was modest (22.8 months vs 20.2 months for observation, $p = 0.005$), the updated 3- and 5-year survival rates proved adjuvant gemcitabine to be superior to observation (26% vs 18% and 20% vs 9%, respectively).[159]

Since that time, three other randomized trials have compared combination chemotherapy with gemcitabine monotherapy. The European Society of Pancreatic Cancer (ESPAC) reported results from ESPAC-4 trial which randomized surgically resected patients to gemcitabine with or without capecitabine.[160] The chemotherapy doublet demonstrated an improvement in OS (28 compared to 25.5 months, $p = 0.032$). The PRODIGE-24/CCTG study provided yet another adjuvant regimen.[161] This trial compared six months of modified FOLFIRINOX with gemcitabine. The combination chemotherapy arm significantly improved disease-free survival from 12.8 to 21.6 months ($p < 0.001$) and median OS from 35 to 54.4 months ($p = 0.003$). Importantly, enrolled patients represented a very select cohort with a requirement for a postoperative CA 19-9 levels <180 U/mL and a World Health Organization PS 0–1. The most recent trial of adjuvant therapy for pancreatic cancer was the APACT trial. In this study, curatively resected patients were randomized to gemcitabine or to gemcitabine and nab-paclitaxel for six months. The primary endpoint was disease-free survival with no difference observed between the two arms.[162] At present, gemcitabine alone, gemcitabine/capecitabine, and modified FOLFIRINOX are considered acceptable adjuvant regimens after upfront surgery with curative intent.

Radiotherapy in adjuvant therapy for pancreatic cancer: Yes or no?
Despite years of investigation, controversy persists as to the benefit of radiotherapy as a component of adjuvant therapy. In an effort to definitely answer the question regarding the role of radiotherapy in adjuvant therapy, the Radiation Therapy Oncology Group (RTOG) has been conducting a large randomized trial (RTOG 0848), which delivers gemcitabine (with or without erlotinib) to all enrolled patients. For the subset of patients who do not develop metastatic disease after four months, a 2nd randomization assigns patients to either two more cycles of gemcitabine (± erlotinib) or one more cycle of gemcitabine followed by 5-FU-based chemoradiation. Based on a recent analysis, there is no survival benefit with the addition of erlotinib.[163] However, whether the addition of radiation after five cycles of gemcitabine provides a survival benefit has yet to be reported.

Stereotactic body radiation and adjuvant therapy
Stereotactic body radiation therapy (SBRT) has been investigated as a component of adjuvant therapy.[164–166] These data indicate that SBRT can be delivered safely. Two prospective studies are now evaluating SBRT in the adjuvant setting (NCT01357525 and NCT01595321).

Adjuvant therapy for resectable pancreatic cancer: Is this the right strategy?
By definition, efforts to advance adjuvant therapy rely on a surgery-first approach which has several significant drawbacks. First, even when the primary tumor appears technically resectable, positive surgical margins are common and associated with inferior survival compared with negative margins.[88,167] Second, pancreatic cancer can persist or relapse quickly after surgery. In the APACT trial comparing adjuvant gemcitabine monotherapy with gemcitabine and nab-paclitaxel, among 1226 patients screened for the trial, 200 (17%) were ineligible based on the presence of postoperative radiographic evidence of persistent or metastatic disease, or postoperative CA 19-9 level >100 U/mL. Third, pancreatic cancer surgery is associated with significant morbidity and significant postoperative complications precluded the delivery of adjuvant therapy. Furthermore, while 30-day operative mortality for pancreatic cancer resections is relatively low (3.7%), by 90 days, mortality rises to 7.4%.[168] Thus only 50–60% of patients who undergo surgery first for pancreatic cancer receive adjuvant therapy.[169] Upfront surgery puts patients at relatively high risk of an R1 resection, significant complications preventing adjuvant therapy, a 7% risk of death within 90 days, and early relapse for 15–20%. In this context, preoperative, or neoadjuvant therapy is gaining greater attention as a potentially superior approach to localized disease.

Rationale for preoperative (neoadjuvant) therapy
There are practical and theoretical advantages to preoperative treatment of patients with localized pancreatic cancer. Most compelling is the ability to provide immediate systemic therapy for a disease that is metastatic in virtually all patients at diagnosis. Furthermore, the delivery of neoadjuvant chemoradiation as a component of therapy may facilitate the achievement of negative surgical margins.[170] Another important advantage of neoadjuvant therapy is improved patient selection for pancreatic surgery. Using

Table 5 Results of recent randomized trials of adjuvant therapy in patients with resected pancreatic cancer.

Study year	Number of patients	Number of patients enrolled per site per year	R1 resection rate	Median survival (months)		p-Value
				Control arm	Experimental arm	
CONKO 001 2013	364	0.64	17	Observation 20.2	Gemcitabine 22.8	0.005
ESPAC 4 2017	730	1.32	60	Gemcitabine 25.5	Gemcitabine + capecitabine 28.0	0.032
PRODIGE 4/ACCORD 11/CCTG 2018	493	1.90	43	Gemcitabine 35.0	FOLFIRINOX 54.4	0.003
APACT 2019[a]	866[b]	Not stated	24	Gemcitabine 36.2	Gemcitabine + nab-paclitaxel 40.5	NR

Abbreviation: NR, not reported.
[a]The primary endpoint was independently assessed disease-free survival; overall survival was not the primary endpoint of this trial.
[b]1226 patients were screened for enrollment, 360 (29%) failed screening; of these, 200 (17%) failed based on presence of postoperative radiographic evidence of persistent or metastatic disease, or postoperative CA 19-9 level >100 U/mL.

a preoperative approach, patients with aggressive tumor biology experiencing interval metastases, or primary tumor progression, can be identified upon restaging prior to planned surgery. These patients will not benefit from surgical resection and have a prognosis similar to patients with locally advanced or metastatic disease.[171,172] Lastly, pancreatic cancer is frequently diagnosed in patients aged 60–80 years, many of whom may have obesity, diabetes, or are deconditioned on presentation. The delivery of neoadjuvant therapy provides an interval of time to both observe a patient's tolerance to anticancer therapy and optimize nutrition, activity level, and strength.[173]

Neoadjuvant therapy in resectable disease

Single-institution publications of neoadjuvant therapy in resectable pancreatic cancer report rates of completion of neoadjuvant therapy and surgery ranging from 83% to 87%. Patients who complete all intended therapy have a median OS ranging from 35 to 45 months.[174,175] This treatment sequencing approach has now been adopted in cooperative group trials.[176,177] The Southwest Oncology Group trial, S1505, investigated treatment with neoadjuvant FOLFIRINOX or gemcitabine/nab-paclitaxel among patients with resectable disease.[177] In this multi-institutional study, 77 of the 103 patients (76%) safely completed neoadjuvant therapy and underwent surgery; long-term results have yet to be reported. Neoadjuvant therapy for patients with resectable pancreatic cancer is now emerging as an acceptable alternative to upfront surgery. This is reflected in the most recent version of the National Comprehensive Cancer Network's algorithm for resectable pancreatic cancer.[178]

Neoadjuvant therapy in borderline resectable disease

With the application of quality cross-sectional imaging and a better understanding of the implications of positive surgical margins, tumors that are neither clearly resectable nor clearly unresectable are classified as borderline resectable. While definitions vary, borderline resectable tumors can broadly be defined as tumors which abut but do not encase critical arterial structures such as the SMA, or celiac axis, or tumors with varying degrees of abutment/encasement of the common hepatic artery, SMV, PV, and SMPV confluence.[179–181] As such, a borderline resectable tumor puts the patient at high risk for an R1 or even R2 resection. Prior experience using neoadjuvant chemoradiation in resectable disease led to relatively low R1 resection rates with evidence of treatment effect compared with upfront surgery.[171,172] Thus, neoadjuvant therapy has similarly become an attractive alternative to initial surgery in borderline resectable disease.[182] Recent reports of neoadjuvant chemotherapy and chemoradiation demonstrate that the majority of patients with borderline resectable disease can ultimately undergo surgical resection. In one high-volume pancreatic cancer center for those patients completing intended neoadjuvant therapy and surgery, the R0 resection rate was 96% with a median survival approaching four years.[175]

The neoadjuvant approach is further supported by a meta-analysis which compared a surgery-first approach to neoadjuvant therapy. The analysis included 3484 patients across 38 studies.[183] Neoadjuvant therapy was associated with higher R0 resection rates (81% vs. 66%, $p < 0.001$), decreased rates of positive lymph nodes (44% vs 65%), and an improved median OS (19 vs 15 months) by intention-to-treat analysis. Prospective data is now available from the Dutch Pancreatic Cancer Group. This group conducted a phase III trial (PREOPANC) comparing preoperative chemotherapy and chemoradiotherapy with immediate surgery followed by a similar regimen given postoperatively. Patients with resectable and borderline resectable pancreatic cancer were enrolled.[184] Neoadjuvant therapy led to higher rates of R0 resection compared with upfront surgery (71% vs 40%, $p < 0.001$), but this does not result in improved survival. However, in a preplanned subgroup analysis, neoadjuvant therapy was associated with improved OS in patients with borderline resectable disease. Lastly, results from ESPAC-5F provide additional support for preoperative therapy in borderline resectable disease.[185] This phase II study randomized patients with borderline resectable pancreatic cancer to upfront surgical resection versus neoadjuvant therapy with either FOLFIRINOX, gemcitabine/capecitabine, or capecitabine-based radiotherapy. The one-year OS rate was 40% and 77% for patients receiving surgery-first versus neoadjuvant treatment, respectively ($p < 0.001$). Given these lines of evidence, current practice guidelines recommend neoadjuvant treatment followed by eventual surgery for patients with borderline resectable pancreatic cancer.[126]

Defining the optimal neoadjuvant therapy and treatment endpoints

There is no consensus regarding the optimal neoadjuvant therapy for patients with pancreatic cancer in terms of systemic regimen used, duration of neoadjuvant chemotherapy, or the incorporation of radiotherapy. FOLFIRINOX and gemcitabine/nab-paclitaxel with or without chemoradiation have been the most popular regimens utilized in single-institution reports of neoadjuvant therapy.[186–188]

Table 6 Select trials of chemotherapy, radiation, and chemoradiation in patients with locally advanced pancreatic cancer.[a]

Study year	No. of patients	Median survival Control arm	Median survival (months) Experimental arm	p-Value
GITSG 1981	194	XRT 40 Gy (only) 5.5	5FU + XRT 40-60 Gy 10	< 0.01
FFCD/SFRO 2008	119	Gem alone 13.0	5FU/Cisplatin + XRT 60 Gy then gem 8.6	0.03
ECOG 4021 2011	74	Gem alone 9.2	Gemcitabine + XRT 50.4 Gy then gem 11.1	0.017
LAP07 2013	442 (269 in R2)	Induction gem ± erlotinib × 4 months if no progression then: gem × 2 mo 16.5	Induction gem ± erlotinib × 4 months if no progression then: capecitabine + XRT 54 Gy 15.3	0.83

Abbreviations: Gem, gemcitabine; XRT, radiation; Gy (gray).
[a]Source: Based on Chauffert et al.[197] and Loehrer et al.[198]

Whether chemoradiation is a necessary component of neoadjuvant therapy for borderline resectable disease is under investigation. In the United States, the ALLIANCE A021501 trial is comparing preoperative extended chemotherapy versus chemotherapy plus hypofractionated radiation therapy.[189] In Europe, based on the encouraging results from PREOPANC, PREOPANC 2 has been designed to compare treatment with mFOLFIRINOX alone with induction mFOLFIRINOX followed by chemoradiation.[184]

The criteria for surgical resection following neoadjuvant therapy have been difficult to establish. While imaging studies may identify local disease progression or interval metastases, the primary tumor may not significantly change following neoadjuvant therapy. However, longitudinal changes in tumor markers may predict long-term prognosis.[190–192] Significant declines in CA 19-9 levels during neoadjuvant therapy and normalization at completion appear prognostic. In one study, patients treated with neoadjuvant therapy who experienced normalization of CA19-9 prior to surgery had a significantly improved median OS compared with patients who did not experience normalization (46 vs 23 months, $p < 0.02$).[192]

The role of radiation in neoadjuvant therapy

In comparison with adjuvant therapy, radiotherapy may have a better-defined role in the preoperative treatment of potentially resectable and borderline resectable disease. Experience with neoadjuvant chemoradiation for localized pancreatic cancer has shown it can sterilize the periphery of the tumor and regional lymph nodes. For example, using neoadjuvant chemoradiation, R1 resection rates are reduced in comparison with upfront surgery and node-positive rates are also decreased.[193,194]

A common neoadjuvant approach uses induction FOLFIRINOX followed by chemoradiation. In a phase II trial from MD Anderson, this approach was used 45 patients with borderline resectable disease, median OS was 42 months for the subset of patients undergoing surgical resection, compared to 14 months for those who did not. This study also reported on imaging-based subtypes of disease identified on CT scans which demonstrated prognostic value.[195] In another study of FOLFIRINOX and individualized chemoradiation in 48 patients with borderline resectable disease, 32 underwent surgical resection (31 achieved an R0 resection). Median OS for resected patients was 37.7 months.[187]

Locally advanced pancreatic cancer

In the 1980s, when systemic therapy had little impact on OS, 5FU-based chemoradiation was the mainstay of therapy.[196] With the advent of gemcitabine, systemic therapy improved modestly and subsequent studies were conducted comparing systemic gemcitabine alone to chemoradiation, leading to conflicting results (Table 6).[197,198] Subsequently, some advocated for locally advanced pancreatic cancer patients to receive induction chemotherapy and in those without disease progression (after chemotherapy for three to four months), to then deliver chemoradiation.[199–201]

This approach was undermined by the result of the LAP 07 trial.[202] Using a 2 × 2 randomized design, 442 of 449 total patients received initial gemcitabine with or without erlotinib for four months and for the 269 patients who did not develop metastatic disease (51%), a second randomization assigned them to receive two additional months of systemic therapy or capecitabine-based chemoradiation (54 Gy). No difference in median OS was observed between the chemotherapy and chemoradiation arms (16.5 vs 15.2 months, respectively, $p = 0.83$). The addition of erlotinib also did not impact survival. Nevertheless, chemoradiotherapy was associated with decreased local progression (32% vs 46%, $p = 0.03$), a trend to improved progression-free survival (PFS) (9.9 vs 8.4 months), and no increase in grade 3–4 toxicity, except for nausea.

The results from LAP 07 has led to an overall decrease in the administration of chemoradiation in locally advanced disease. Nevertheless, there may be a subset of patients who benefit from follow-on chemoradiation after induction chemotherapy. For example, the LAPACT trial investigated gemcitabine plus nab-paclitaxel for 107 patients with locally advanced pancreatic cancer. Chemoradiation and surgery were not protocol-mandated but allowed at physician discretion; 17% of patients underwent subsequent chemoradiation and 16% underwent surgery. The median OS for the entire cohort was 18.8 months.[203]

Selecting patients for follow-on chemoradiation after induction chemotherapy

Similar to the delivery of preoperative therapy before surgical intervention, induction chemotherapy allows a mechanism to uncover unfavorable tumor biology manifest by local disease progression or interval metastases. Just as resectable patients who develop disease progression during neoadjuvant therapy will not benefit from surgery, patients with locally advanced disease that progresses on induction chemotherapy will not benefit from chemoradiation. While induction chemotherapy can distinguish patients with aggressive tumor biology from those with less aggressive disease, it does not identify the smaller group of patients who may benefit from subsequent chemoradiation. To date, neither imaging biomarker analysis nor other biomarkers have proven to be sufficiently predictive to enable selection of patients for consolidating radiotherapy.

Neoadjuvant therapy for locally advanced disease
A very select proportion of patients with locally advanced disease (as currently defined) may be considered for surgery (after neoadjuvant therapy).[204] A new classification of locally advanced disease has been developed to aid in the identification of the patients more apt to benefit from eventual resection.[205] Locally advanced type A patients have anatomic tumor–vessel relationships (Figure 5) which allow one to consider surgery after a period of treatment and locally advanced type B patients have disease where surgery would likely never be possible.

Surgical resection should only be considered when there is evidence of radiographic, biochemical (CA 19-9), and physiologic response (improved PS) to preoperative therapy. Importantly, it is unusual to see a change in critical tumor–vessel relationships after neoadjuvant therapy despite some evidence for a reduction in tumor size. Of note, however, while arterial abutment/encasement rarely changes, the contour and appearance of the SMV or PV may improve. In patients who respond well to induction chemotherapy, neoadjuvant chemoradiation is usually recommended. Surgical candidacy is re-assessed upon the completion of all intended neoadjuvant therapy. The most common operation performed for such patients has been a distal pancreatectomy, splenectomy, and en bloc resection of the celiac axis (Appleby procedure). In small series of patients where resection and arterial reconstruction have been performed, results have been encouraging.[206,207]

Radiation techniques for locally advanced pancreatic cancer
Patients with locally advanced tumors probably do not benefit from regional lymph node irradiation. Thus, radiotherapy fields should be confined to the gross tumor and generally dosed to 50.4 Gy. When there is a plan to deliver >60 Gy to the primary tumor, while sparing the duodenum, respiratory gating is recommended. In single-center reports, the use of higher-dose radiotherapy in locally advanced tumors has shown some encouraging results.[208,209]

SBRT is also capable of precisely delivering high doses of radiation to small tumor volumes. The feasibility of SBRT in locally advanced pancreatic cancer treatment was originally investigated using a single fraction of radiotherapy.[210,211] However, limited efficacy and significant toxicity, investigation of SBRT prompted a shift to five fractions. A multi-institutional trial evaluating SBRT (33 Gy in five fractions) demonstrated good tolerability with median OS comparable to chemoradiation at standard fractionation.[211] LAPC-1 was a phase 2 study of FOLFIRINOX followed by 40 Gy in five fractions.[144] The 1-year OS and PFS were 64% and 34%, respectively.

Irreversible electroporation
Irreversible electroporation (IRE) is a nonthermal locally ablative technique receiving increasing attention in oncology. The advantage of IRE over other ablative techniques is the absence of thermal injury to surrounding tissues, specifically vascular and ductal structures.[212] Results using IRE in locally advanced disease have historically been limited to single institutional experience.[213] Recently, in a multi-institutional phase II trial, percutaneous IRE (before or after induction chemotherapy) was applied to 40 patients and led to median survival of 17 months. Survival was worse for patients with larger tumors, pre-IRE CA 19-9 levels >2000, and those with less than a 50% drop in CA 19-9 three months after IRE. Randomized trials comparing IRE with chemoradiation are underway.[214]

Approach to the patient with locally advanced pancreatic cancer
When feasible, patients with locally advanced disease maintaining good PS should be treated in the context of a clinical trial. Outside of a trial, for patients with adequate PS, nutrition and biliary drainage, systemic therapy for three to four months is usually advised prior to considering local modalities. For those who remain on systemic therapy, a break from treatment after six months of stable or responding disease is reasonable.

Summary
Surgery remains the only curative strategy for nonmetastatic pancreatic cancer. MIS is increasingly utilized, but without evidence of superior oncologic outcomes to date. There is unequivocal evidence that adjuvant chemotherapy should follow upfront surgery. However, upfront surgery is associated with risk of margin positive tumor resection, early relapse in 15–20% of patients, and considerable morbidity and mortality. Surgical complications, early relapse, and postoperative death may preclude delivery of adjuvant treatment. Neoadjuvant therapy is increasingly utilized in resectable disease to facilitate identification of aggressive tumor biology and uncover patient frailty, contraindicating surgical intervention. Moreover, neoadjuvant therapy reduces the risk of an R1 resection in those with potentially resectable disease, allows for eventual surgery in most patients who present with borderline resectable disease, and provides an opportunity for resection for a small subset of patients with locally advanced disease.

The evolution of systemic therapy
Early trials of chemotherapy in advanced pancreatic cancer often utilized 5FU or 5FU-based combinations;[215] whether chemotherapy prolonged survival over best supportive care was debatable.[216] In the 1990s, the role of chemotherapy became clear with the development of gemcitabine, which proved superior to treatment with bolus 5FU in previously untreated patients with advanced disease.[217] Since then, efforts to build on gemcitabine monotherapy have been disappointing with some exceptions.

For example, gemcitabine combined with capecitabine demonstrated some modest improvement in response rate, PFS and OS compared with treatment using gemcitabine alone.[218] This doublet also proved superior in the adjuvant setting when compared with gemcitabine.[160] Second, gemcitabine and nab-paclitaxel also proved to be superior to gemcitabine as frontline therapy for metastatic disease. The Metastatic Pancreatic Adenocarcinoma Clinical Trial (MPACT) was a randomized trial comparing gemcitabine/nab-paclitaxel to gemcitabine as initial treatment for metastatic pancreatic cancer.[132] The doublet showed improvements in response rates (22% vs 10%), PFS (6 vs 4 months), and OS (8.5 vs 6.7 months, $p<0.001$) compared to gemcitabine (Table 7). However, unlike gemcitabine and capecitabine, when this combination was investigated in the adjuvant setting, no clear clinical benefit was observed compared with adjuvant gemcitabine.[162]

Ironically, even though gemcitabine supplanted 5FU therapy for advanced pancreatic cancer back in the late 1990s, 5FU-based FOLFIRINOX has now emerged as a new standard therapy for pancreatic cancer. This regimen was compared with gemcitabine as frontline treatment of metastatic pancreatic cancer in patients with ECOG PS 0–1. In this randomized phase III trial (aka PRODIGE 4/ACCORD 11), FOLFIRINOX led to better response rate (32% vs 9%), PFS (6 vs 4.5 months), and OS (11.6

Table 7 Summary of randomized trials of cytotoxic drugs or drug combinations changing the standard of care for advanced or metastatic PDAC.[a]

Treatment	Burris 1996		Conroy 2011 (ACCORD)		Von Hoff 2013 (MPACT)	
	Bolus 5FU	Gem	Gem	FOLFIRINOX	Gem	Gem/nab-P
PS	Karnovsky PS ≥ 50%		ECOG PS 0 or 1		Karnovsky PS ≥ 70%	
Patients with Met Dz	70%		100%		100%	
Response rate (%)	0	10	9	32	7	23
MS (months)	4.5	5.7	6.8	11.1	6.7	8.6
1-Year survival (%)	2	18	21	48	22	35
Neutropenia (%)	5	25	21	46	27	38
Fatigue (Grade 3–4)	NS	NS	18	24	1	17
Diarrhea (Grade 3–4)	6	2	2	13	1	6
Neuropathy	NS	NS	0	9	7	17

Abbreviations: PS, performance status; Gem, gemcitabine; nab-P, nanoparticle-albumin-bound paclitaxel; MS, median survival; NS, not stated.
[a]Source: Based on Von Hoff et al.[132]

vs 6 months, HR for death 0.75, $p = 0.003$). Based on the results from PRODIGE 4/ACCORD 11 and MPACT, both FOLFIRINOX and gemcitabine/nab-paclitaxel are frontline standards for the treatment of metastatic pancreatic cancer.

Importantly, the criteria for enrollment to MPACT and PRODIGE 4/ACCORD 11 were slightly different and clinically relevant. Patients were eligible for enrollment on MPACT with a Karnovsky PS≥70%, whereas enrollment in PRODIGE 4/ACCORD 11 required ECOG PS 0–1. Thus, in the real world, patients with PS 0–1 are often treated with frontline FOLFIRINOX. Alternatively, for patients with KPS 70–80% (ECOG 1–2), treatment with gemcitabine and nab-paclitaxel may be recommended. Thus, the availability of both regimens provides clinical oncologists with some flexibility in choosing frontline therapy for their patients. As shown in Table 7, there are differences in the toxicity profiles for these regimens with both regimens sharing a sizable risk for neutropenia.

Note that PS is a reliable predictor of OS. As early as 1985, PS was prognostic for all stages of pancreatic cancer.[219] This observation was subsequently supported by findings from CALGB 80803 and the MPACT trial. Patients with excellent PS experience a 3–4-fold longer survival than patients with PS 2 or KPS 70%.[220,221] Furthermore, in patients with compromised PS, aggressive combination therapy may be detrimental compared with delivery of gemcitabine monotherapy.[222]

Targeted drug therapy without predictive biomarkers in pancreatic cancer

The approval of gemcitabine coincided with the early era of molecular therapy in cancer treatment. Given its modest single-agent activity and favorable toxicity profile, there was enthusiasm for combining gemcitabine with a wide variety of targeted agents to include angiogenesis inhibitors, epidermal growth factor receptor (EGFR) inhibitors, farnesyl transferase inhibitors, and mitogen-activated protein (MAP)/extra cellular signal regulated kinase (MEK) inhibitors among others. Results using this "gemcitabine plus" approach were overwhelmingly negative. A meta-analysis of 27 randomized trials comparing a targeted drug in combination with gemcitabine-based chemotherapy with cytotoxic therapy alone found no significant survival benefit with the addition of a targeted agent.[223] Taken together, these trials enrolled over 8000 patients and of all the agents tested, only EGF-R inhibitors seemed to exert a small beneficial effect on survival (hazard ratio for death 0.88).

As mentioned previously, efforts to target the TME have likewise been disappointing. Hedgehog inhibitors and hyaluronidase were both intended to degrade the desmoplastic tumor stroma (albeit through different mechanisms). Both approaches failed to demonstrate any clinical benefit when combined with conventional cytotoxic therapy.[115,224] In one study, the addition of a pegylated hyaluronidase appeared to be detrimental when added to standard treatment.[116]

Table 8 New biomarker-driven precision medicines for patients with advanced pancreatic cancer.

Medication year of FDA approval	Indication and Biomarker
Pembrolizumab 2016	As second-line or later therapy advanced solid tumors (including pancreatic cancer) with mismatch repair deficiency
Olaparib 2019	As maintenance therapy after 4 months of platinum-based chemotherapy with germline BRCA 1 or 2 mutations
Larotrectinib 2018	As second- or later line therapy for patients with advanced solid tumors (including pancreatic cancer)with NTRK 1, 2, 3, or ROS1 fusions
Entrectinib 2019	As second- or later line therapy for patients with advanced solid tumors (including pancreatic cancer) with NTRK 1, 2, 3, or ROS1 fusions

The emergence of precision medicine in pancreatic cancer

Over the last five years, a growing number of molecular agents have been approved by the FDA for treatment of advanced pancreatic cancer. Three things have changed since the early efforts of the 1990–2000s. First, the newly approved agents all have a predictive biomarker as a prerequisite for use. Second, these drugs are administered as single agents, not in combination with cytotoxic therapy. Lastly, some of these drugs have a role in therapy for other solid tumors and FDA approval is described as "tumor agnostic" (Table 8).

Pembrolizumab

Preclinical studies and clinical experience showed that anti-PD1 therapy could lead to antitumor activity for MMR deficient tumors beyond colon cancer.[225] Pooled data from a few trials of noncolorectal cancer patients with MMR deficient tumors treated with pembrolizumab led to an overall response rate of 40% (78% of which lasted >6 months).[17] Based on these findings, the FDA-approved pembrolizumab as second-line therapy for patients with solid tumors harboring defects in MMR. Note that MMR deficiency is present in a very small subset of patients with pancreatic adenocarcinomas (1–2%).

Importantly, application of immunotherapy in pancreatic cancer beyond patients with MSI-high tumors has been disappointing.[226,227] Novel approaches currently under investigation include those designed to confer antigen specificity, enhance T cell effector function, and neutralize immunosuppressive elements within the TME.[228]

Maintenance olaparib
The POLO trial randomized 154 metastatic pancreatic cancer patients with germline BRCA1 or BRCA2 mutations whose disease had not progressed on at least 16 weeks of first-line platinum-based chemotherapy.[229] These patients were assigned to placebo or olaparib, a PARP inhibitor as maintenance therapy. The median PFS in the olaparib arm was significantly longer than for placebo (7.4 vs 3.8 months, HR: 0.53, $p=0.004$). To date, there has been no difference in OS between the groups. Nevertheless, olaparib was granted FDA approval as a maintenance therapy for this population.

Larotrectinib and entrectinib for NTRK 1, 2, or 3 fusion events
Fusion mutations in Neurotropic Tropomyosin-Related Kinase (NTRK) genes NTRK1, 2, or 3 are rare but clinically significant molecular events, occurring in up to 1% of patients with pancreatic cancer. These fusion proteins are targets for the Tropomyosin-Related Kinase (TRK) inhibitors larotrectinib and entrectanib; both of which have shown activity in advanced pancreatic cancer.[230,231]

Other potential biomarker-driven precision therapy

Platinum-containing regimens
Tumors deficient in DNA damage repair (DDR) proteins display heightened susceptibility to DNA-damaging agents, such as platinum therapy. Retrospective data reveal that for patients with a family history of breast, ovarian or pancreatic cancer, better survival is observed combining gemcitabine and a platinum agent over treatment with gemcitabine alone.[232] Supporting data comes from a recent randomized trial in patients with germline BRCA or PALB2 mutations. Patients received gemcitabine and cisplatin with or without velaparib, a PARP inhibitor.[233] While velaparib did not impact survival, the median OS of enrolled patients was impressive, ranging from 15.5 to 16.4 months. Thus, a strong family history of breast, ovarian, or pancreatic cancer, or a documented germline mutation in BRCA1/2 or PALB2 may serve as predictive biomarkers for combining gemcitabine with a platinum agent. Recent evidence suggests this may also apply to FOLFIRINOX.[234] Broader genetic testing will likely identify more patients who may benefit from platinum-containing regimens.

GATA6
Basal-like pancreatic cancers, which usually have loss of GATA6 are purported to be resistant to FOLFIRINOX.[107] In the future, intratumoral loss of GATA6 or other biomarkers may identify basal-like tumors that predict resistance to FOLFIRINOX.

Carboxylesterase 2
Carboxylesterase 2 (CES2), is the most efficient carboxyl esterase converting irinotecan to SN-38, the active moiety. In preclinical models, high intratumoral expression of CES2 predicted response to irinotecan. Furthermore, among patients undergoing neoadjuvant FOLFIRINOX, improved outcomes were observed for those with higher intratumoral CES2 expression.[235] If confirmed clinically, assays for intratumoral CES2 may inform decisions regarding systemic therapy options.

Clinical management of patients with metastatic pancreatic cancer

Patients with newly diagnosed metastatic disease should undergo a holistic evaluation to assess PS, adequacy of biliary drainage, pain control, and nutrition. For patients with good PS, enrollment on a frontline clinical trial should be encouraged. If not feasible, recommendations regarding frontline therapy should be dependent on careful assessment of PS. FOLFIRINOX is appropriate for patients with ECOG PS 0–1, whereas gemcitabine and nab-paclitaxel is a preferred combination for ECOG PS 1–2. After progression on frontline therapy, patients with preserved PS should be considered for a 2nd-line clinical trial. Outside that option, for patients previously treated with gemcitabine-based therapy, 5FU, leucovorin, and liposomal irinotecan is superior to 5FU and leucovorin.[236] Fluorouracil, leucovorin, and oxaliplatin or irinotecan (FOLFOX or FOLFIRI) are also a reasonable 2nd-line options.[237] In patients previously treated with FOLFIRINOX, gemcitabine and nab-paclitaxel have some demonstrated clinical benefit.[87]

Palliation
Metastatic pancreatic cancer is often accompanied by pain, fatigue, and anorexia. Palliation should be a priority and provided in multidisciplinary context. Addressing pain prior to initiation of systemic therapy is advised. Opioids are the mainstay of pain management and when prescribed, opioid-induced constipation should be actively managed. If pain is not adequately controlled with opioids or other analgesics, or if these are poorly tolerated, patients should undergo an evaluation with an interventional pain specialist to consider celiac or splanchnic plexus neurolysis. In addition to aggressive pain control efforts, other supportive measures to consider include appetite enhancers, pancreatic enzyme replacement, antidepressants, and central nervous system stimulants.

Whenever possible, biliary decompression using endobiliary stent deployment is preferred over surgical or percutaneous drainage. On occasion, percutaneous biliary drainage may be required. If gastric outlet obstruction occurs and life expectancy is greater than 12 weeks, a minimally invasive gastrojejunostomy is preferred. For patients at the end of life, deployment of an endoscopic duodenal stent is more appropriate. Large volume ascites, malignant or otherwise, requires repeated paracentesis or insertion of an indwelling peritoneal catheter for symptomatic relief.

> **Summary**
>
> Treatment for metastatic pancreatic cancer is usually limited to systemic therapy. These patients are dynamic and often suffer from high-symptom burden and palliative needs require frequent assessment. For most patients with adequate PS, cytotoxic therapy remains standard in the frontline and 2nd-line setting. NGS of tumor biopsies and genetic testing is recommended to identify specific subsets of patients who may benefit from platinum therapy, targeted therapy, or immunotherapy. Additional biomarkers for precision medicine in pancreatic cancer are certain to expand.

Key references

The complete reference list can be found on Vital Source version of this title, see inside front cover.

1. Rahib L, Smith BD, Aizenberg R, et al. Projecting cancer incidence and deaths to 2030: the unexpected burden of thyroid, liver, and pancreas cancers in the United States. *Cancer Res.* 2014;**74**:2913–2921.
4. Tersmette AC, Petersen GM, Offerhaus GJ, et al. Increased risk of incident pancreatic cancer among first-degree relatives of patients with familial pancreatic cancer. *Clin Cancer Res.* 2001;**7**:738–744.
13. Hu C, Hart SN, Polley EC, et al. Association between inherited germline mutations in cancer predisposition genes and risk of pancreatic cancer. *JAMA.* 2018;**319**:2401–2409.
16. Kastrinos F, Mukherjee B, Tayob N, et al. Risk of pancreatic cancer in families with Lynch syndrome. *JAMA.* 2009;**302**:1790–1795.
17. Marabelle A, Le DT, Ascierto PA, et al. Efficacy of pembrolizumab in patients with noncolorectal high microsatellite instability/mismatch repair-deficient cancer: results from the phase II KEYNOTE-158 study. *J Clin Oncol.* 2020;**38**:1–10.
23. Wolpin BM, Kraft P, Xu M, et al. Variant ABO blood group alleles, secretor status, and risk of pancreatic cancer: results from the pancreatic cancer cohort consortium. *Cancer Epidemiol Biomarkers Prev.* 2010;**19**:3140–3149.
27. Lynch SM, Vrieling A, Lubin JH, et al. Cigarette smoking and pancreatic cancer: a pooled analysis from the pancreatic cancer cohort consortium. *Am J Epidemiol.* 2009;**170**:403–413.
46. Pannala R, Basu A, Petersen GM, Chari ST. New-onset diabetes: a potential clue to the early diagnosis of pancreatic cancer. *Lancet Oncol.* 2009;**10**:88–95.
57. Pericleous M, Rossi RE, Mandair D, et al. Nutrition and pancreatic cancer. *Anticancer Res.* 2014;**34**:9–21.
63. Pushalkar S, Hundeyin M, Daley D, et al. The pancreatic cancer microbiome promotes oncogenesis by induction of innate and adaptive immune suppression. *Cancer Discov.* 2018;**8**:403–416.
66. Riquelme E, Zhang Y, Zhang L, et al. Tumor microbiome diversity and composition influence pancreatic cancer outcomes. *Cell.* 2019;**178**:795–806.
74. Jones S, Zhang X, Parsons DW, et al. Core signaling pathways in human pancreatic cancers revealed by global genomic analyses. *Science.* 2008;**321**:1801–1806.
76. Cancer Genome Atlas Research Network. Integrated genomic characterization of pancreatic ductal adenocarcinoma. *Cancer Cell.* 2017;**32**:185–203.
88. Ghaneh P, Kleeff J, Halloran CM, et al. The impact of positive resection margins on survival and recurrence following resection and adjuvant chemotherapy for pancreatic ductal adenocarcinoma. *Ann Surg.* 2019;**269**:520–529.
101. Klein AP, Wolpin BM, Risch HA, et al. Genome-wide meta-analysis identifies five new susceptibility loci for pancreatic cancer. *Nat Commun.* 2018;**9**:556.
106. Collisson EA, Sadanandam A, Olson P, et al. Subtypes of pancreatic ductal adenocarcinoma and their differing responses to therapy. *Nat Med.* 2011;**17**:500–503.
107. O'Kane GM, Grunwald BT, Jang GH, et al. GATA6 expression distinguishes classical and basal-like subtypes in advanced pancreatic cancer. *Clin Cancer Res.* 2020;**26**:4901–4910.
109. Brunton H, Caligiuri G, Cunningham R, et al. HNF4A and GATA6 loss reveals therapeutically actionable subtypes in pancreatic cancer. *Cell Rep.* 2020;**31**. doi: 10.1016/j.celrep.2020.107625.
115. Tempero MA, van Cutsem E, Sigal D, et al. HALO 109-301: a randomized, double-blind, placebo-controlled, phase 3 trial of pegvorhyaluronidase alfa (PEGPH2) + nab-paclitaxel/gemcitabine in patients with previously untreated hyaluronan-high metastatic pancreatic cancer. *J Clin Oncol.* 2020;**38**:3185–3194.
131. Conroy T, Desseigne F, Ychou M, et al. FOLFIRINOX versus gemcitabine for metastatic pancreatic cancer. *N Engl J Med.* 2011;**364**:1817–1825.
132. Von Hoff DD, Ervin T, Arena FP, et al. Increased survival in pancreatic cancer with nab-paclitaxel plus gemcitabine. *N Engl J Med.* 2013;**369**:1691–1703.
157. Neoptolemos JP, Stocken DD, Friess H, et al. A randomized trial of chemoradiotherapy and chemotherapy after resection of pancreatic cancer. *N Engl J Med.* 2004;**350**:1200–1210.
158. Oettle H, Post S, Neuhaus P, et al. Adjuvant chemotherapy with gemcitabine vs observation in patients undergoing curative-intent resection of pancreatic cancer: a randomized controlled trial. *JAMA.* 2007;**297**:267–277.
159. Oettle H, Neuhaus P, Hochhaus A, et al. Adjuvant chemotherapy with gemcitabine and long-term outcomes among patients with resected pancreatic cancer: the CONKO-001 randomized trial. *JAMA.* 2013;**310**:1473–1481.
160. Neoptolemos JP, Palmer DH, Ghaneh P, et al. Comparison of adjuvant gemcitabine and capecitabine with gemcitabine monotherapy in patients with resected pancreatic cancer (ESPAC-4): a multicentre, open-label, randomised, phase 3 trial. *Lancet.* 2017;**389**:1011–1024.
161. Conroy T, Hammel P, Hebbar M, et al. FOLFIRINOX or gemcitabine as adjuvant therapy for pancreatic cancer. *N Engl J Med.* 2018;**379**:2395–2406.
171. Evans DB, Varadhachary GR, Crane CH, et al. Preoperative gemcitabine-based chemoradiation for patients with resectable adenocarcinoma of the pancreatic head. *J Clin Oncol.* 2008;**26**:3496–3502.
172. Varadhachary GR, Wolff RA, Crane CH, et al. Preoperative gemcitabine and cisplatin followed by gemcitabine-based chemoradiation for resectable adenocarcinoma of the pancreatic head. *J Clin Oncol.* 2008;**26**:3487–3495.
178. National Comprehensive Cancer Network. *NCCN Clinical Practice Guidelines in Oncology: Pancreatic Adenocarcinoma 2020.* Version 1.2021, 2021; www.nccn.org/professionals/physician_gls/pdf/pancreatic.pdf (accessed 20 July 2021).
180. Varadhachary GR, Tamm EP, Abbruzzese JL, et al. Borderline resectable pancreatic cancer: definitions, management, and role of preoperative therapy. *Ann Surg Oncol.* 2006;**13**:1035–1046.
184. Versteijne E, Suker M, Groothuis K, et al. Preoperative chemoradiotherapy versus immediate surgery for resectable and borderline resectable pancreatic cancer: results of the dutch randomized phase III PREOPANC trial. *J Clin Oncol.* 2020;**38**:1763–1773.
192. Tsai S, George B, Wittmann D, et al. Importance of normalization of CA19-9 levels following neoadjuvant therapy in patients with localized pancreatic cancer. *Ann Surg.* 2020;**271**:740–747.
198. Loehrer PJ Sr, Feng Y, Cardenes H, et al. Gemcitabine alone versus gemcitabine plus radiotherapy in patients with locally advanced pancreatic cancer: an Eastern Cooperative Oncology Group trial. *J Clin Oncol.* 2011;**29**:4105–4112.
202. Hammel P, Huguet F, van Laethem JL, et al. Effect of chemoradiotherapy vs chemotherapy on survival in patients with locally advanced pancreatic cancer controlled after 4 months of gemcitabine with or without erlotinib: the LAP07 randomized clinical trial. *JAMA.* 2016;**315**:1844–1853.
217. Burris HA 3rd, Moore MJ, Andersen J, et al. Improvements in survival and clinical benefit with gemcitabine as first-line therapy for patients with advanced pancreas cancer: a randomized trial. *J Clin Oncol.* 1997;**15**:2403–2413.
225. Le DT, Uram JN, Wang H, et al. PD-1 blockade in tumors with mismatch-repair deficiency. *N Engl J Med.* 2015;**372**:2509–2520.
227. Brahmer JR, Tykodi SS, Chow LQ, et al. Safety and activity of anti-PD-L1 antibody in patients with advanced cancer. *N Engl J Med.* 2012;**366**:2455–2465.
229. Golan T, Hammel P, Reni M, et al. Maintenance olaparib for germline BRCA-mutated metastatic pancreatic cancer. *N Engl J Med.* 2019;**381**:317–327.
230. Drilon A, Laetsch TW, Kummar S, et al. Efficacy of larotrectinib in TRK fusion-positive cancers in adults and children. *N Engl J Med.* 2018;**378**:731–739.
233. O'Reilly EM, Lee JW, Zalupski M, et al. Randomized, multicenter, phase II trial of gemcitabine and cisplatin with or without veliparib in patients with pancreas adenocarcinoma and a germline BRCA/PALB2 mutation. *J Clin Oncol.* 2020;**38**:1378–1388.
236. Wang-Gillam A, Li CP, Bodoky G, et al. Nanoliposomal irinotecan with fluorouracil and folinic acid in metastatic pancreatic cancer after previous gemcitabine-based therapy (NAPOLI-1): a global, randomised, open-label, phase 3 trial. *Lancet.* 2016;**387**:545–557.

90 Neoplasms of the appendix and peritoneum

Annie Liu, MD, PhD ∎ *Diana Cardona, MD* ∎ *Dan Blazer, MD*

> **Overview**
>
> Neoplasms of the appendix, while rare, include a broad range of heterogenous malignancies. These are broadly divided into two subtypes: epithelial and nonepithelial. In this chapter, we detail the most recent classification guidelines, and describe clinical presentation, histology, and treatment options for these neoplasms.

Appendix

Neoplasms of the appendix are very rare, comprising only 1% of colorectal cancers. Appendiceal tumors are most often detected incidentally following appendectomy for acute appendicitis and are seen in only 0.2–3.7% of examined specimens.[1-8] Despite this low incidence, the heterogeneity of appendiceal neoplasms is quite varied and has historically led to confusion for treating clinicians regarding classification and best practices for management of these rare malignancies.

Consensus terminology and definitions for appendiceal neoplasms were established in 2016 by the Peritoneal Surface Oncology Group International (PSOGI) Modified Delphi Process[9] and further refined in the World Health Organization Classification of Digestive System Tumours 5th Edition from 2019.[10] Broadly, appendiceal neoplasms are divided into two subtypes: epithelial and nonepithelial neoplasms. Epithelial neoplasms include adenomas, serrated polyps, mucinous neoplasms (low grade and high grade), mucinous adenocarcinoma, mucinous adenocarcinoma with signet ring cells, mucinous signet ring cell carcinoma, nonmucinous adenocarcinoma, and neuroendocrine tumor. PSOGI guidelines originally classified neuroendocrine tumors as nonepithelial; however, updated WHO guidelines include neuroendocrine tumors in the epithelial category. Nonepithelial neoplasms include lymphoma and sarcoma. Treatment of appendiceal neoplasms is highly dependent on histologic subtype. Due to their rarity, there are no National Comprehensive Cancer Network guidelines for treatment of most types of appendiceal neoplasm, with the exception of neuroendocrine tumors.

Of note, true incidence of appendiceal neoplasms is difficult to ascertain, as these diseases are detected incidentally. Additionally, the classification and nomenclature of these lesions have changed over time.[9,11] For example, appendiceal adenocarcinoma is now divided into colonic-type and mucinous-type, the latter of which were previously described as malignant mucoceles in prior literature. Retrospective cohort analyses report the most common appendiceal neoplasm to be mucinous adenocarcinoma[1,7,8] or neuroendocrine.[2-6,12]

Clinical presentation

Appendiceal neoplasms are typically identified incidentally during abdominal imaging or, more commonly, following appendectomy for suspected acute appendicitis. Classic symptoms of acute appendicitis include right lower quadrant tenderness, migratory pain from periumbilical area to the right lower quadrant, anorexia, nausea, rebound pain, fever, leukocytosis, and left shift of white blood cell count.[13] There has been some effort to determine radiographic and clinical presentation differences between benign acute appendicitis and appendicitis secondary to malignancy.[14] One study found that patients with identification of appendiceal tumor on pathology following appendectomy were more likely to present without migratory right lower quadrant pain.[14] Radiographic features found to be associated with appendiceal neoplasms include increased soft tissue thickening and wall irregularities,[15] as well as focal dilatation, lack of periappendiceal fat stranding, mural calcification, and luminal diameter greater than 2 cm.[16] These studies are limited by the rarity of appendiceal neoplasms, making it difficult to validate models that predict appendiceal neoplasms in patients presenting with suspected acute appendicitis.

There is also an increase in incidence of appendiceal neoplasm in patients who present with perforated appendicitis and in patients treated with nonoperative management.[7,8,12,17] Given the evolving practice of managing perforated appendicitis nonoperatively with percutaneous drainage and antibiotics, further study is necessary to determine how to surveil and treat patients with an increased risk of primary appendiceal neoplasm.

Epithelial neoplasms of the appendix

As described above, the 2016 PSOGI consensus guidelines describe eight subtypes of epithelial-type appendiceal neoplasms: adenoma, serrated polyp, low-grade appendiceal mucinous neoplasm (LAMN), high grade appendiceal mucinous neoplasm, mucinous adenocarcinoma, poorly differentiated mucinous adenocarcinoma with signet ring cells, mucinous signet ring cell carcinoma, and adenocarcinoma.[9] Updated WHO classification also includes neuroendocrine tumors as epithelial neoplasms. The most common of these lesions are either LAMNs or neuroendocrine tumors. Figure 1 illustrates the histologic characteristics of LAMNs and invasive mucinous adenocarcinoma. Genetic profiling may help to further refine these classification criteria and delineate how these categories of neoplasms are related, which are likely to remain benign, and which represent precursor lesions. Several studies have identified that random mutations of KRAS, GNAS, and APC are commonly seen in LAMNs.[18,19]

Despite the heterogenous morphologic subtypes, epithelial appendiceal neoplasms can be broadly discussed in the context of their pathologic behavior. Adenomas, serrated polyps, and

Holland-Frei Cancer Medicine, Tenth Edition. Edited by Robert C. Bast, John C. Byrd, Carlo M. Croce, Ernest Hawk, Fadlo R. Khuri, Raphael E. Pollock, Apostolia M. Tsimberidou, Christopher G. Willett, and Cheryl L. Willman.
© 2023 John Wiley & Sons, Inc. Published 2023 by John Wiley & Sons, Inc.

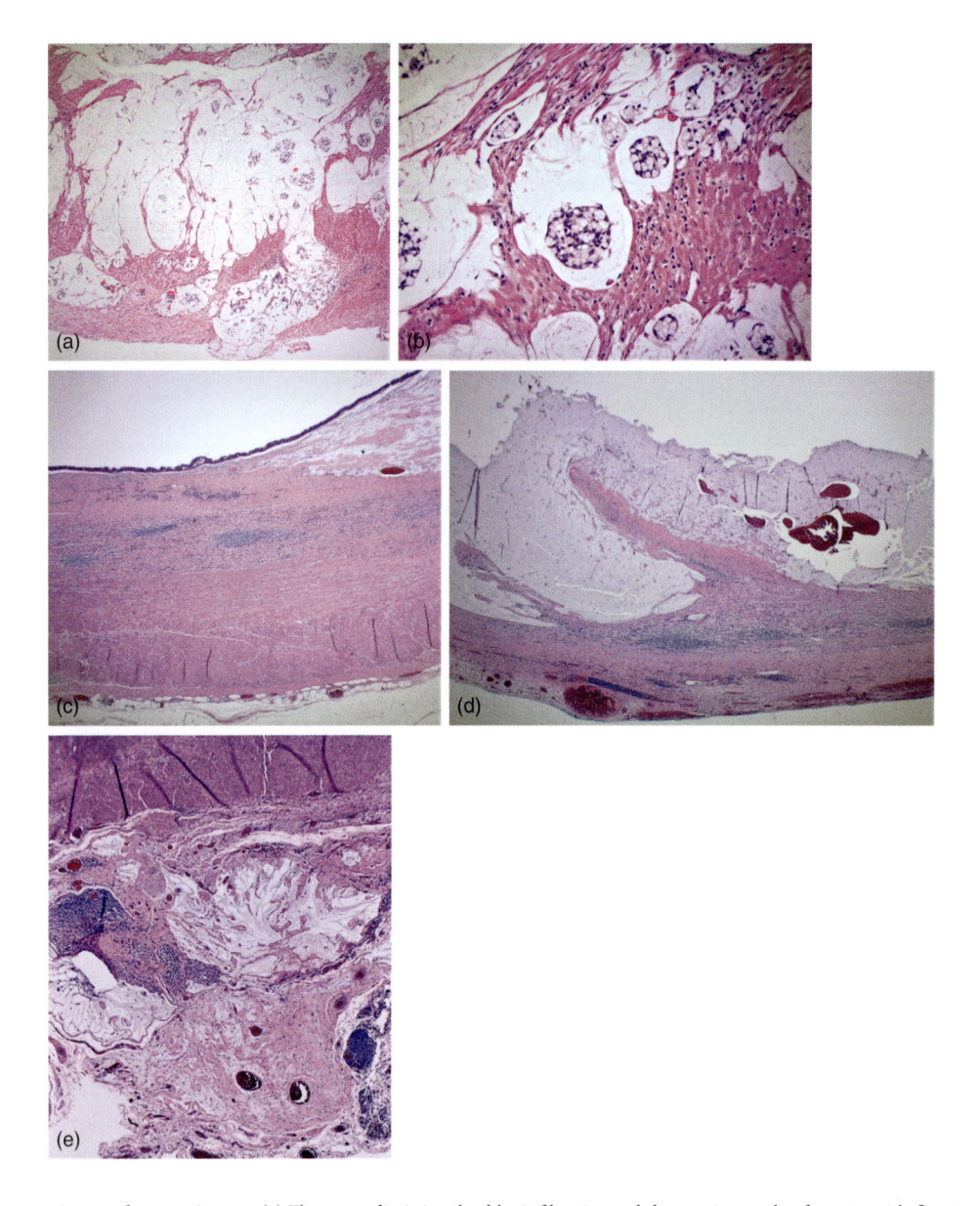

Figure 1 Invasive mucinous adenocarcinoma. (a) The appendix is involved by infiltrative and destructive pools of mucin with floating tumor cells that extend through the entire muscular wall and involve the serosal surface. (H&E, 40×) (b) The tumor cells are composed of epithelial cell clusters with large intracellular mucin deposits, reminiscent of signet rings. (H&E, 200×) **Low-grade appendiceal mucinous neoplasm (LAMN)** (c). Dilated appendix with flattened mucinous epithelium demonstrating low-grade dysplasia. There is complete loss of normal mucosal architecture and atrophy of underlying lymphoid tissue. Dissecting pools of mucin are seen within the wall of the appendix. (d) There were areas with complete loss of the epithelial lining and pools of mucin pushing into the wall. Atrophy of the lymphoid tissue and muscularis externa is noted. No invasive carcinoma is present. (e) Deposits of acellular mucin involving the serosa with an associated fibroinflammatory response. (H&E, 40×).

nonmucinous adenocarcinomas behave similarly to their colonic counterparts. Simple appendectomy remains appropriate for adenomas and serrated polyps, while nonmucinous adenocarcinoma on which pathology demonstrates infiltrative invasion, positive margins, or high-grade pathologic features require right hemicolectomy and complete staging.[20–23] Mucinous type lesions display the tendency to spread throughout the intraperitoneal cavity and lead to pseudomyxoma peritonei (PMP). Thus, when a mucinous appendiceal neoplasm is identified or suspected based on preoperative imaging, care must be taken to prevent perforation of the appendix during resection, which may cause inadvertent seeding of mucin-producing cells throughout the intraperitoneal cavity. Simple appendectomy rather than right hemicolectomy is the usual treatment for mucinous neoplasms without intraperitoneal spread.[21]

Neuroendocrine tumors of the appendix

Neuroendocrine tumors (NETs) of the appendix are typically asymptomatic and also found incidentally following appendectomy for presumed acute appendicitis.[24] There is a slight female predominance in patients with NETs compared to adenocarcinoma, and overall survival is better than for adenocarcinoma.[25] These tumors arise from the subepithelial neuroendocrine and Schwann cells located in the lamina propria of the appendix (Figure 2a–c).[26] Per the World Health Organization, grading is dependent on mitotic count and the Ki67 labeling index.[10,27]

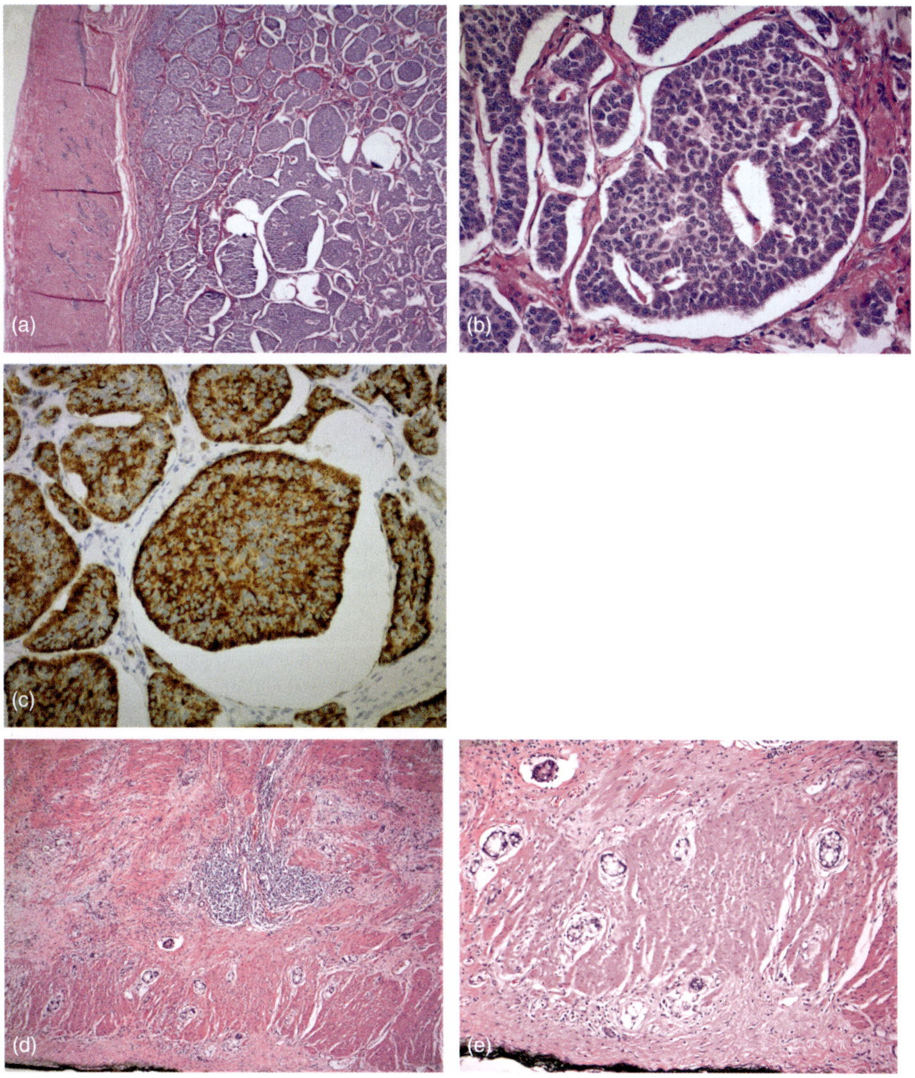

Figure 2 **Well-differentiated neuroendocrine neoplasm, low grade.** (a) Expanding the wall of the appendix are nests of cohesive cells that appear retracted from the surrounding stroma. Small clusters of tumor cells are seen infiltrating the muscularis externa. (H&E, 40×) (b) The tumor cells are uniform and bland. They have granular eosinophilic cytoplasm and round open nuclei with fine chromatin clumps. No increase in mitotic activity is present. (H&E, 200×). (c) Strong cytoplasmic expression of chromogranin. (200×) **Goblet cell adenocarcinoma.** (d) Infiltrative clusters of tumor cells composed of mucus-secreting cells and associated stromal fibrosis and chronic inflammation. (H&E, 40×) (e) Tumor clusters often demonstrate tubular architecture while individual cells are distended with mucin and also contain eosinophilic cytoplasm. (H&E, 100×).

Ki-67 index greater than 20% and a mitotic rate greater than 20 mitoses/2 mm² indicate a high-grade neoplasm.

NETs

With regards to NETs, there are significant differences in mortality based on tumor size; thus, treatment recommendations differ primarily based on size and location. About 90% of these tumors are located at the tip of the appendix. Based on a large study of the SEER database, 10-year survival rates are as follows: tumor size <1 cm with positive or negative lymph nodes—100%; tumor size between 1 and 2 cm with positive nodes—92% versus negative nodes—100%; tumor size >2 cm with positive nodes—91% versus negative nodes—100%.[28]

Surgical resection remains the primary treatment for appendiceal NETs, per National Comprehensive Cancer Network guidelines.[29] Tumors located at the distal 1/3 of the appendix and that are less than 2 cm in length can be treated with simple appendectomy. Following simple appendectomy, any incomplete resection, positive nodes, or positive margins necessitate re-exploration and possible right hemicolectomy. Tumors larger than 2 cm or tumors located at the base of the appendix require completion right hemicolectomy for accurate staging and prognosis. Additionally, as described by consensus guidelines from the North American Neuroendocrine Society (NANETS) and European Neuroendocrine Tumor Society (ENETS), the following features of tumors less than 2 cm also necessitate consideration of a right hemicolectomy: invasion at the base of the appendix or of the mesoappendix, mixed histology, mesenteric node involvement, or proliferative rate of the tumor as described by a Ki-67 index greater than 20%.[11,30–32]

Atypical NETs

Atypical neuroendocrine tumors comprise a subset of rare, more aggressive neoplasms and include goblet cell adenocarcinoma, mixed adenoneuroendocrine carcinomas (MANEC), and neuroendocrine carcinoma (NEC). Goblet cell adenocarcinoma (formerly known as goblet cell carcinoids) is an extremely rare appendiceal neoplasm that possesses features of both epithelial and nonepithelial subtypes but clinically behave like adenocarcinoma and should be treated as such (Figure 2d–e). 5-year overall survival of GCA is 76%. According to the Chicago Consensus on Peritoneal Surface Malignancies recommendations, GCAs confined to the appendix necessitate right hemicolectomy and consideration of systemic chemotherapy.[23] MANECs, also known as mixed exocrine–neuroendocrine carcinoma, are tumors that contain both adenocarcinoma and neuroendocrine histologic components, where each component comprises at least 30% of the tumor and 2 of the following neuroendocrine tumor markers are present: synaptophysin, chromogranin, CD56, or INSM1.[25,33,34] Given the rarity of MANECs, there are no clear treatment recommendations for these tumors. However, retrospective analyses demonstrate that these tumors are more aggressive than carcinoid lesions and may necessitate systemic therapy and right hemicolectomy rather than simple appendectomy.[35,36] NECs, also known as well-differentiated neuroendocrine carcinoma, are also extremely rare. These lesions are characterized by deep infiltration into the mesoappendix, size greater than 2.5 cm, and may have metastases. NECs may or may not be accompanied by carcinoid syndrome.[37]

Nonepithelial neoplasms of the appendix

Nonepithelial neoplasms of the appendix include lymphoma and sarcoma. Primary lymphomas and sarcomas of the appendix, including Burkitt's lymphoma, diffuse large B-cell, non-Hodgkin's lymphoma, and myeloid sarcoma, are extremely rare and tend to present as acute appendicitis, according to case reports.[38–44]

Peritoneum

Primary peritoneal neoplasms are extremely rare, with the peritoneum more commonly being the site of metastatic disease spread. Primary neoplasms include peritoneal mesothelioma and primary peritoneal serous carcinoma. Peritoneal carcinomatosis, the intraperitoneal spread of metastatic disease, results most commonly from ovarian, colorectal, pancreatic, and gastric cancers. Patients with peritoneal neoplasms typically present with vague abdominal symptoms including abdominal distension, pain, obstructive symptoms, and/or ascites. Treatment strategies for peritoneal malignancies include cytoreductive surgery (CRS), hyperthermic intraperitoneal chemotherapy (HIPEC), systemic chemotherapy, radiation, and palliative surgery for management of obstructive symptoms. This section will also describe pseudomyxoma peritonei (PMP), a rare condition defined by the PSOGI consensus as "the intraperitoneal accumulation of mucus due to mucinous neoplasia characterized by the redistribution phenomenon."[9] This disease is most often a sequela of epithelial-type appendiceal neoplasm and can very rarely be secondary to ovarian, uterine, or pancreatic origin, as described in case reports.[45–47]

Primary peritoneal mesothelioma

Malignant mesothelioma arising from the peritoneum (PPM) is the second most common type of malignant mesothelioma, the first being malignant pleural mesothelioma, and makes up 7–30% of mesothelioma cases worldwide.[48–51] Based on data from 2003 to 2008 in the National Program for Cancer Registries and the Surveillance, Epidemiology, and End Results (SEER) cancer registry, the incidence of primary peritoneal mesothelioma (PPM, also known as peritoneal malignant mesothelioma) was estimated to be 1.3 and 0.7 per million persons in the United States, for men and women, respectively.[52] Like malignant mesothelioma of the pleural cavity, it is correlated with prolonged asbestos exposure, smoking, and radiation exposure.[48,53,54] Due to incomplete data reporting, the worldwide incidence is unknown; however, there is evidence that industrialized countries with higher cumulative asbestos use also have the highest reported number of mesothelioma cases.[49–51]

Patients with PPM typically present with nonspecific abdominal symptoms, such as abdominal distension, pain, and serous ascites, with elevation of serum markers such as mesothelin-related protein, CA-125, CA 1503, hyaluronic acid, and osteopontin.[55,56] CT findings are heterogenous and nonspecific, and include ascites, irregular peritoneal thickening, extensive mesenteric, omental, or peritoneal involvement, and scalloped appearance of abdominal organs. Patients can present with either diffuse nodular disease with extensive intraabdominal involvement and encasement of the abdominal organs or, rarely, with a large tumor mass and diffuse peritoneal disease.[55–58] Definitive diagnosis requires confirmation with histology and immunohistochemistry, through tissue obtained via either imaging-guided core needle biopsy or laparoscopic biopsy. Because most MPM samples demonstrate multiple histologic patterns, immunohistochemistry is also necessary to determine MPM subtype. Ascites fluid and fine-needle aspiration are of lower yield, as these methods often do not yield an adequate cell concentration required for either histology or immunohistochemistry. MPM is categorized into three major histologic subtypes: epithelioid, sarcomatoid (fibrous), and biphasic (mixed) type. Epithelioid MPM is associated with a better prognosis than the other two subtypes and is characterized by proliferation of polygonal, cuboidal, or low columnar mesothelial tumor cells, arranged in a tubular, papillary, or sheet-like pattern (Figure 3).[59,60] Many subtypes of the epithelioid type have also been described further—tubular, tubulopapillary, papillary, micropapillary, solid, pleomorphic, tubular, and trabecular.[61] Sarcomatoid mesothelioma, which is characterized by proliferation of spindle cells, is more commonly described in cases of malignant pleural mesothelioma and is very rare subtype of MPM. Biphasic MPM demonstrates both epithelioid and sarcomatoid histologic patterns within the same tumor. While there is no single tumor marker specific for MPM, there are several markers that are useful in distinguishing MPM from other peritoneal neoplasms such as primary peritoneal serous carcinoma (PPSC) and reactive mesothelial hyperplasia (RMH). Positive staining for calretinin and negative staining for BerEP4 suggests MPM rather than PPSC. Loss of BRCA-associated protein 1 (BAP1) suggests MPM rather than RMH.[62–65]

With regards to management, aggressive CRS with HIPEC demonstrates the best outcomes for resectable disease.[66,67] The definition of "resectability" is not well defined and referral to centers with expertise in management of peritoneal surface malignancies is encouraged. The efficacy of systemic chemotherapy, radiation, and immunotherapy is currently unclear. CRS combined with HIPEC (with mitomycin c, cisplatin, and/or doxorubicin) has been demonstrated to improve median survival to 52 to 92 months, with a 5-year survival of 33–59%, compared to a median survival of 9–14 months with the treatment strategies of palliative surgery with or without systemic chemotherapy.[68–71] Extent of cytoreduction is highly correlated with survival. In one trial, median survival for patients with complete macroscopic resection (CC-0)

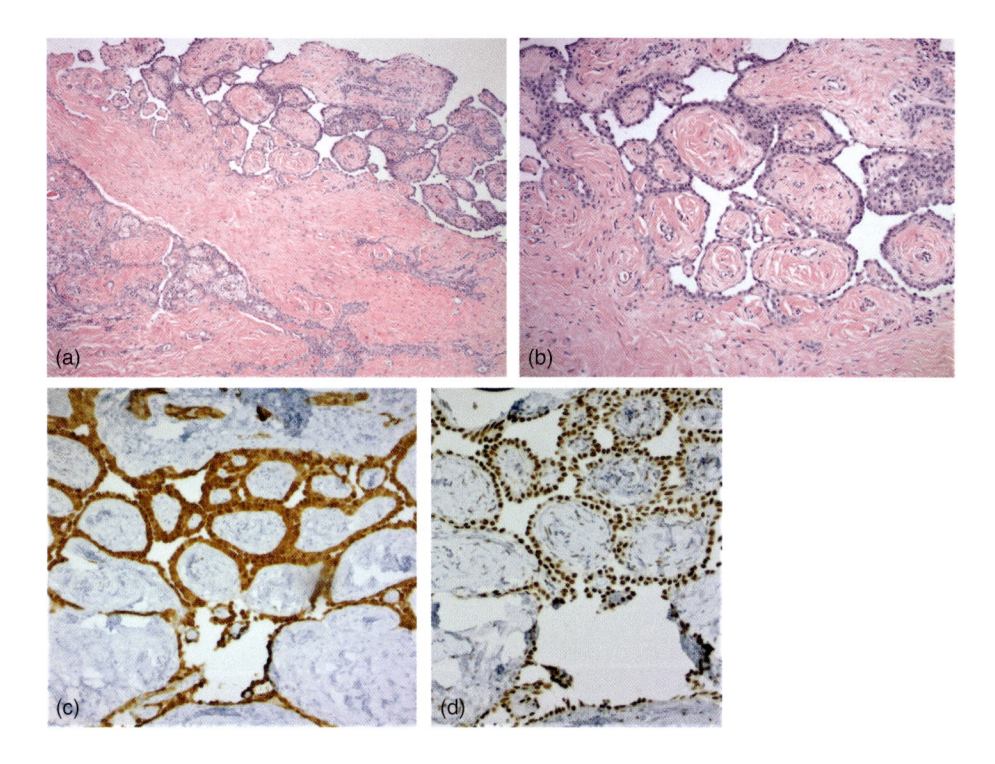

Figure 3 Malignant peritoneal mesothelioma, epithelioid variant, involving the abdominal peritoneum, diaphragm, bilateral ovaries, and uterine surfaces. (a) Serosal implant of tumor with a papillary architecture and infiltrative growth. (H&E, 100×) (b) Higher magnification highlights a monotonous proliferation of round, plump cells. (H&E, 200×) (c) Tumor cells were strongly and diffusely positive for calretinin and (d) WT1. (200×).

or no residual disease >2.5 mm (CC-1) was 37.8 months compared to 6.5 months for patients with less complete resections (CC-2, CC-3).[69] As stated previously, these patients should be evaluated at an experienced high volume center, managed by a multidisciplinary team, and enrolled in disease registries and clinical trials.[72]

Primary peritoneal serous carcinoma

Primary peritoneal serous carcinoma (also known as peritoneal papillary carcinoma or multiple focal extraovarian serous carcinoma) was first described in 1959 and has a very low incidence of 6.78 per million in the United States.[73] Patients present with abdominal distension and ascites. This disease has a number of features similar to epithelial ovarian carcinoma, including elevated serum CA125 and similar histologic features of high nuclear-cytoplasmic ratio and high mitotic index, with the important distinguishing feature being no ovarian involvement and no obvious primary disease origin site seen in primary peritoneal serous carcinoma.[74–77] Treatment consists of CRS followed by platinum-based chemotherapy, with similar outcomes as epithelial ovarian carcinoma.[75,78] One retrospective study of 36 patients demonstrated potential benefit of combining CRS with HIPEC.[79]

Pseudomyxoma peritonei

Pseudomyxoma peritonei is a rare disease with a yearly incidence of 1 per million.[80] It is characterized by the diffuse spread of mucin-producing tumor cells throughout the peritoneal cavity, resulting in mucinous ascites and numerous peritoneal implants. These patients present with progressive abdominal distension or obstructive symptoms as a result of the extensive disease.[81] CT imaging will demonstrate mucinous ascites seen as hypoattenuated fluid with omental haziness, as well as scalloping of the visceral surfaces, which result from pressure from mucinous implants of the visceral organs. PMP most commonly results from primary LAMNs, although the disease can also be secondary to ovarian, colon, gastric, and pancreatic neoplasms.[80] The disease process is thought to start when the appendix becomes filled with mucin-producing tumor cells, with progressive distension leading to perforation, thus allowing tumor cells to proliferate and spread throughout the peritoneal cavity. PMP can be classified based on histology into low-grade mucinous carcinoma peritonei (scant epithelial component with mild cytological atypia), high-grade mucinous carcinoma peritonei (more cellular with destructive invasion of adjacent tissue), and high-grade mucinous carcinoma peritonei with signet ring cells (any lesion with signet ring cells), which carry a worse prognosis than either low-grade or high-grade.[82]

Treatment centers around CRS and HIPEC.[81,83–85] Cytoreduction prioritizes the complete removal of all peritoneal implants and visible disease. Disease burden can be estimated intra-operatively using the peritoneal cancer index (PCI), which is a scoring system developed by Sugarbaker that divides the peritoneal cavity into 13 regions and assigns a lesion size score to each region, with a maximum possible score of 39.[86] This score can be used to determine prognosis. The completeness of cytoreduction score (CC) is used to determine prognosis after CRS: CC-0: no peritoneal seeding, CC-1: remaining nodules are <2.5 cm in size, CC-2: remaining nodules are 2.5–5 cm in size, CC-3: remaining nodules are greater than 5 cm. A score of CC-0 or CC-1 after surgery is considered complete cytoreduction, which is associated with higher survival.[86–89] Following cytoreduction, chemotherapy, cisplatin, and mitomycin-C are perfused through the closed abdominal cavity. The chemotherapy is heated during perfusing, which improves tissue penetration. For the right patient population, cytoreduction combined with HIPEC can improve survival, with a ∼60% 10-year survival rate.[90]

Peritoneal malignancy secondary to appendiceal neoplasm

Peritoneal carcinomatosis

Ovarian, colorectal, pancreatic, appendiceal, and gastric cancers can all result in peritoneal metastatic disease. Treatment recommendations differ based on extent of disease and the primary cancer but include the same treatment options as those for primary peritoneal neoplasms and pseudomyxoma peritonei, such as palliative surgery, debulking, HIPEC, and systemic chemotherapy. Preoperative detection of peritoneal disease is often difficult, as CT or MRI are unable to detect small volume disease. Diagnostic laparoscopy is often necessary to diagnose peritoneal disease with direct visualization of disease spread. For peritoneal carcinomatosis secondary to epithelial ovarian cancer and to gastric cancer, CRS combined with HIPEC may improve overall survival and progression-free survival, with extent of cytoreduction found to be related to outcome.[91,92] For gastric cancer, CRS combined with HIPEC improved median survival from 7.9 to 15 months.[93,94] The role of CRS with HIPEC in peritoneal carcinomatosis in colorectal cancer is currently under debate—the Prodige 7 trial demonstrated no benefit to overall survival with the addition of HIPEC with oxaliplatin to CRS.[95]

Conclusion

Appendiceal neoplasms comprise a rare but very heterogenous group of gastrointestinal cancer. The nomenclature and classification of these diseases have changed dramatically and are still not consistent within the current literature. They are most commonly found incidentally following appendectomy for acute appendicitis, and the mainstay for treatment of early disease remains surgical resection. However, advanced disease presenting as pseudomyxoma peritonei or peritoneal carcinomatosis may require surgical debulking in addition to intraperitoneal chemotherapy. Peritoneal neoplasms are also quite rare—the peritoneum is more often the site of metastatic disease spread rather than the origin of a primary neoplasm. Management centers around surgical debulking, systemic chemotherapy, intraperitoneal chemotherapy, and palliative surgery.

Key references

The complete reference list can be found on Vital Source version of this title, see inside front cover.

2 Kunduz E, Bektasoglu HK, Unver N, et al. Analysis of appendiceal neoplasms on 3544 appendectomy specimens for acute appendicitis: retrospective cohort study of a single institution. *Med Sci Monit Int Med J Exp Clin Res*. 2018;**24**:4421–4426.

3 Chandrasegaram MD, Rothwell LA, An EI, Miller RJ. Pathologies of the appendix: a 10-year review of 4670 appendicectomy specimens. *ANZ J Surg*. 2012;**82**:844–847.

4 Marudanayagam R, Williams GT, Rees BI. Review of the pathological results of 2660 appendicectomy specimens. *J Gastroenterol*. 2006;**41**:745–749.

5 Tchana-Sato V, Detry O, Polus M, et al. Carcinoid tumor of the appendix: a consecutive series from 1237 appendectomies. *World J Gastroenterol WJG*. 2006;**12**:6699–6701.

7 Furman MJ, Cahan M, Cohen P, Lambert LA. Increased risk of mucinous neoplasm of the appendix in adults undergoing interval appendectomy. *JAMA Surg*. 2013;**148**:703–706.

9 Carr N, Cecil T, Mohamed F, et al. A consensus for classification and pathologic reporting of pseudomyxoma peritonei and associated appendiceal neoplasia: the results of the peritoneal surface oncology group international (PSOGI) modified Delphi process. *Am J Surg Pathol*. 2016;**40**:14–26.

10 WHO Classification of Tumours Editorial Board. *Digestive System Tumours: WHO Classification of Tumours*, Vol. 1, 5th ed. WHO Classification of Tumours Editorial Board; 2019.

11 Pape U-F, Niederle B, Costa F, et al. ENETS consensus guidelines for neuroendocrine neoplasms of the appendix (excluding goblet cell carcinomas). *Neuroendocrinology*. 2016;**103**:144–152.

14 Loftus TJ, Raymond SL, Sarosi GA Jr, et al. Predicting appendiceal tumors among patients with appendicitis. *J Trauma Acute Care Surg*. 2017;**82**:771.

15 Wang H, Chen Y-Q, Wei R, et al. Appendiceal mucocele: a diagnostic dilemma in differentiating malignant from benign lesions with CT. *Am J Roentgenol*. 2013;**201**:W590–W595.

17 Sceats LA, Trickey AW, Morris AM, et al. Nonoperative management of uncomplicated appendicitis among privately insured patients. *JAMA Surg*. 2019;**154**:141.

18 Tsai JH, Yang C-Y, Yuan R-H, Jeng Y-M. Correlation of molecular and morphological features of appendiceal epithelial neoplasms. *Histopathology*. 2019;**75**:468–477.

21 Barrios P, Losa F, Gonzalez-Moreno S, et al. Recommendations in the management of epithelial appendiceal neoplasms and peritoneal dissemination from mucinous tumours (pseudomyxoma peritonei). *Clin Transl Oncol*. 2016;**18**:437–448.

23 Schuitevoerder D, Plana A, Izquierdo FJ, et al. The Chicago consensus on peritoneal surface malignancies: management of appendiceal neoplasms. *Ann Surg Oncol*. 2020;**27**:1753–1760.

25 Onyemkpa C, Davis A, McLeod M, Oyasiji T. Typical carcinoids, goblet cell carcinoids, mixed adenoneuroendocrine carcinomas, neuroendocrine carcinomas and adenocarcinomas of the appendix: a comparative analysis of survival profile and predictors. *J Gastrointest Oncol*. 2019;**10**:300–306.

28 Mullen JT, Savarese DMF. Carcinoid tumors of the appendix: a population-based study. *J Surg Oncol*. 2011;**104**:41–44.

29 Shah MH, Goldner WS, Benson AB, et al. NCCN clinical practice guidelines in oncology: neuroendocrine and adrenal tumors. *Natl Compr Cancer Netw*. 2020;**2**:1–141.

30 Boudreaux JP, Klimstra DS, Hassan MM, et al. The NANETS consensus guideline for the diagnosis and management of neuroendocrine tumors: well-differentiated neuroendocrine tumors of the Jejunum, Ileum, Appendix, and Cecum. *Pancreas*. 2010;**39**:753–766.

33 Rosenbaum JN, Guo Z, Baus RM, et al. INSM1: a novel immunohistochemical and molecular marker for neuroendocrine and neuroepithelial neoplasms. *Am J Clin Pathol*. 2015;**144**:579–591.

36 Brathwaite S, Yearsley MM, Bekaii-Saab T, et al. Appendiceal mixed adeno-neuroendocrine carcinoma: a population-based study of the surveillance, epidemiology, and end results registry. *Front Oncol*. 2016;**6**:148.

37 Klöppel G, Perren A, Heitz PU. The gastroenteropancreatic neuroendocrine cell system and its tumors: the WHO classification. *Ann N Y Acad Sci*. 2004;**1014**:13–27.

45 Baratti D, Kusamura S, Milione M, et al. Pseudomyxoma peritonei of extra-appendiceal origin: a comparative study. *Ann Surg Oncol*. 2016;**23**:4222–4230.

49 Abdel-Rahman O. Global trends in mortality from malignant mesothelioma: analysis of WHO mortality database (1994–2013). *Clin Respir J*. 2018;**12**:2090–2100.

52 Henley SJ, Larson TC, Wu M, et al. Mesothelioma incidence in 50 states and the District of Columbia, United States, 2003–2008. *Int J Occup Environ Health*. 2013;**19**:1–10.

56 Kebapci M, Vardareli E, Adapinar B, Acikalin M. CT findings and serum ca 125 levels in malignant peritoneal mesothelioma: report of 11 new cases and review of the literature. *Eur Radiol*. 2003;**13**:2620–2626.

60 Liu S, Staats P, Lee M, et al. Diffuse mesothelioma of the peritoneum: correlation between histological and clinical parameters and survival in 73 patients. *Pathology (Phila.)*. 2014;**46**:604–609.

67 Alexander HR, Bartlett DL, Pingpank JF, et al. Treatment factors associated with long-term survival following cytoreductive surgery and regional chemotherapy for patients with malignant peritoneal mesothelioma. *Surgery*. 2013;**153**:779–786.

69 Levine EA, Stewart JH, Shen P, et al. Cytoreductive surgery and hyperthermic intraperitoneal chemotherapy for peritoneal surface malignancy: experience with 1,000 patients. *J Am Coll Surg*. 2014;**218**:573–585.

70 Feldman AL, Libutti SK, Pingpank JF, et al. Analysis of factors associated with outcome in patients with malignant peritoneal mesothelioma undergoing surgical debulking and intraperitoneal chemotherapy. *J Clin Oncol*. 2003;**21**:4560–4567.

73 Goodman MT, Shvetsov YB. Incidence of ovarian, peritoneal, and fallopian tube carcinomas in the United States, 1995–2004. *Cancer Epidemiol Prev Biomark*. 2009;**18**:132–139.

77 Liu Q, Lin J, Shi Q, et al. Primary peritoneal serous papillary carcinoma: a clinical and pathological study. *Pathol Oncol Res*. 2011;**17**:713–719.

78 Roh SY, Hong SH, Ko YH, et al. Clinical characteristics of primary peritoneal carcinoma. *Cancer Res Treat*. 2007;**39**:65–68.

79 Bakrin N, Gilly FN, Baratti D, et al. Primary peritoneal serous carcinoma treated by cytoreductive surgery combined with hyperthermic intraperitoneal chemotherapy. A multi-institutional study of 36 patients. *Eur J Surg Oncol*. 2013;**39**:742–747.

80 Smeenk RM, Van Velthuysen MLF, Verwaal VJ, Zoetmulder FAN. Appendiceal neoplasms and pseudomyxoma peritonei: a population based study. *Eur J Surg Oncol EJSO*. 2008;**34**:196–201.

81 Baratti D, Kusamura S, Nonaka D, et al. Pseudomyxoma peritonei: clinical pathological and biological prognostic factors in patients treated with cytoreductive surgery and hyperthermic intraperitoneal chemotherapy (HIPEC). *Ann Surg Oncol*. 2008;**15**:526–534.

82 Carr NJ, Bibeau F, Bradley RF, et al. The histopathological classification, diagnosis and differential diagnosis of mucinous appendiceal neoplasms, appendiceal adenocarcinomas and pseudomyxoma peritonei. *Histopathology*. 2017;**71**:847–858.

85 Stewart JH, Shen P, Russell G, et al. A phase I trial of oxaliplatin for intraperitoneal hyperthermic chemoperfusion for the treatment of peritoneal surface dissemination from colorectal and appendiceal cancers. *Ann Surg Oncol*. 2008;**15**:2137–2145.

90 Chua TC, Moran BJ, Sugarbaker PH, et al. Early-and long-term outcome data of patients with pseudomyxoma peritonei from appendiceal origin treated by a strategy of cytoreductive surgery and hyperthermic intraperitoneal chemotherapy. *J Clin Oncol*. 2012;**30**:2449–2456.

92 Huo YR, Richards A, Liauw W, Morris DL. Hyperthermic intraperitoneal chemotherapy (HIPEC) and cytoreductive surgery (CRS) in ovarian cancer: a systematic review and meta-analysis. *Eur J Surg Oncol*. 2015;**41**:1578–1589.

95 Quenet F, Elias D, Roca L, et al. A UNICANCER phase III trial of hyperthermic intra-peritoneal chemotherapy (HIPEC) for colorectal peritoneal carcinomatosis (PC): PRODIGE 7. *J Clin Oncol*. 2018;**36**:LBA3503–LBA3503.

91 Carcinoma of the colon and rectum

Yota Suzuki, MD ■ Douglas S. Tyler, MD ■ Uma R. Phatak, MD

> **Overview**
>
> Colorectal cancer is the third most common malignant tumor and the second most common cause of cancer death worldwide. Improvements in education and performance of screening have led to a decrease in mortality and improvements in outcomes. Comprehensive management of colorectal cancer requires a multidisciplinary approach involving specialists in genetics, gastroenterology, radiology, radiation oncology, surgery, pathology, and medical oncology. New developments in cancer biology, medical therapeutics, and surgical techniques have also led to improvements in outcomes. Emerging concepts, such as total neoadjuvant therapy and watch-and-wait strategy for rectal cancer, are also changing treatment paradigms. This article will provide a comprehensive review of the current management and treatment of colorectal cancer.

Epidemiology

Colorectal cancer (CRC) is the third most commonly diagnosed cancer in males and the second in females globally, with 1.8 million new cases and 881,000 deaths in 2018 according to the World Health Organization.[1] CRC is most common in developed nations. In the United States alone, approximately 147,950 new cases of CRC are diagnosed annually, 104,610 of which are colon cancer and the remainder are rectal cancer.[2] Approximately 53,200 Americans die of CRC annually, accounting for approximately 8% of all cancer deaths.[2]

There are disparities in CRC incidence and mortality among genders, races, and ethnic groups. CRC incidence is approximately 25% higher in men than in women.[3] Right-sided/proximal colon cancers are more common among women, while distal tumors are more common in men.[1] Moreover, mortality is approximately one-third higher in men.[4] African-Americans have the highest rates of both incidence and mortality when compared to the White, Asian American, American Indian, and Hispanic populations.[5] In addition, some have shown that African-Americans who present at younger ages also have worse survival than whites.[6,7] The reasons for these disparities are not entirely known; however, it has been also postulated that differences in access to high-quality regular screening, timely diagnosis and treatment, dietary and lifestyle factors, and socioeconomic status could play a role.[5,8] On the other hand, studies comparing African-Americans to white CRC patients demonstrated differences in gene expression profiles, polymorphisms, and epigenetic phenomena.[9,10] African-Americans are more frequently diagnosed with microsatellite stable tumors in the proximal colon, and patients with proximal colon cancer tend to have higher mortality and poorer outcomes.[11,12] One study about survival with adjuvant therapy for colon cancer revealed worse overall survival with African-American compared to white despite receiving the same treatment.[13]

Despite the high prevalence of CRC in the United States, both the incidence and overall mortality from CRC have been declining over several decades. In the United States, CRC incidence rates have been declining by approximately 2% per year.[2] Mortality rates from CRC have declined since the mid-1980s. Studies have shown that increased screening and detection can reduce the chance of developing or dying from CRC by 10–75%, depending on which screening tests are used and how often they are performed.[14] This increased screening could also be a reason for the shift in anatomic distribution of CRC from rectum and left-sided cancers to more right-sided cancers. Data from the National Cancer Data Base from the years 1988 and 1993 show an increase from 51% to 55% of all CRC to be proximal to the splenic flexure.[15] Multiple studies have confirmed a higher rate of proximal colon cancer rates compared to distal colon or rectal carcinoma rates, both in the United States and globally.[15–18] Though the overall incidence in CRC is decreasing, there is a trend towards increased incidence in those aged 50 years and younger.[19]

Risk factors

Age and racial background

Age is a known risk factor for CRC. Most cases of CRC occur in people over age 50, with incidence continuing to increase thereafter.[14] In a recent report from surveillance, epidemiology, and end results (SEER), about 90% cases are diagnosed in patient older than 50 though CRC incidence among adults aged <50 years increased by 22% from 2000 to 2013.[20] To note, these increases are driven predominantly by left-sided cancers in general and rectal cancer in particular,[21] and the reason for this trend is unclear. Similar to incidence patterns as stated above, CRC death rates decreased by 34% among individuals aged >50 years during 2000 through 2014 but increased by 13% in those aged <50 years.[20] As discussed previously, African-American individuals have a higher incidence and mortality rate of CRC compared to other racial and ethnic populations.[5,14,15]

Personal or family history

Patients with a personal history of adenomatous polyps or previous CRC have an increased risk of developing colon cancer in the future. Size, number, and histology of polyps are important prognostic factors, with size >1 cm, villous or tubulovillous histology, and multiple polyps conferring a greater risk for CRC. In patients with previous CRC, the incidence of metachronous CRC is 6% and the incidence of metachronous adenomas is 25%.[22]

Family history of CRC in a first-degree relative increases the risk of developing CRC two- to three-fold, while cancer in a second-degree relative increases the risk of CRC by 25–50%.[23,24]

Holland-Frei Cancer Medicine, Tenth Edition. Edited by Robert C. Bast, John C. Byrd, Carlo M. Croce, Ernest Hawk, Fadlo R. Khuri, Raphael E. Pollock, Apostolia M. Tsimberidou, Christopher G. Willett, and Cheryl L. Willman.
© 2023 John Wiley & Sons, Inc. Published 2023 by John Wiley & Sons, Inc.

In addition, risk increases if there are more than one first-degree relative with colon cancer or if they are diagnosed before age 55.[25] Family history of colonic adenoma also increases the risk of CRC, especially if the adenoma is diagnosed early.

Inflammatory bowel disease

Ulcerative colitis (UC) and Crohn's disease are well-known risk factors for colorectal carcinoma. For UC, the extent of disease and the duration of disease are the primary prognostic factors. Patients with pancolitis have a 5- to 15-fold increased risk of developing CRC compared to a threefold increased risk with colitis limited to the left colon.[26] The risk also increases the longer the disease is present.[27] Similar characteristics and incidence of CRC have been reported in Crohn's disease.[28–30]

Diet and lifestyle

Westernized dietary habits—namely having a high-fat low fiber diet—are associated with CRC. There is conflicting evidence regarding the effect of diets high in fruits and vegetables, but the consensus is that while there may not be a protection associated with increased consumption, very low consumption does increase risk of developing CRC.[31–33] A high-fat diet containing mixed lipids and saturated fat has been shown to promote colon carcinogenesis.[34,35] Alternatively, high intake of poultry and fish appears to be protective.[36]

Obesity has been associated with an increased risk of CRC in both men and women, and people with a BMI ≥ 30 kg/m² appear to have nearly a 20% increased risk of CRC compared to nonobese patients.[37,38] In contrast, physical activity and exercise are correlated with a decreased risk of CRC.[39]

Diabetes mellitus and hyperinsulinemia

There is increasing evidence that diabetes mellitus and/or insulin resistance are risk factors for CRC. A meta-analysis of 15 studies found the estimated risk of CRC in diabetics was 30% higher than nondiabetics.[40,41] A possible explanation is the hyperinsulinemia associated with diabetes or even chronic insulin treatment for diabetes, resulting in growth signals to colonic mucosal cells via insulin-like growth factor 1.[41,42]

Alcohol and tobacco

Heavy alcohol consumption is correlated with a moderately increased risk of CRC. The association is dose-dependent and is irrespective of the type of alcoholic beverage consumed.[43,44] The association between smoking and CRC is not as straightforward, and cigarette smoking may have a greater impact depending on specific somatic polymorphisms.[45]

Protective effect of NSAID and aspirin

Multiple observational and interventional trials suggest aspirin and nonsteroidal anti-inflammatory drugs (NSAIDs) are protective against CRC. Systematic reviews for both aspirin and NSAIDs have shown that regular use of aspirin or NSAIDs is associated with a 20–40% reduction in the risk of colonic adenomas and CRC in individuals at average risk.[46,47] Although the mechanism of the protective effect is unclear, proposed explanations are increased apoptosis and impairment of tumor cell growth by inhibition of cyclooxygenase-2. The minimum dose and duration as well as subgroup who benefit from the chemoprevention are not clear at this point.

Genetics

Depending on the origin of the mutation, colorectal carcinomas can be classified as sporadic (70%), inherited (5%), and familial (25%).[48] Inherited CRCs are caused by inherited mutations that affect one of the alleles of the mutated gene. On the other hand, familial CRCs are caused by inherited mutations, although they are not classified as inherited cancers per se since they are not consistent with any known inherited syndromes.

CRC develops from a multistep gene mutation sequence termed loss of heterozygosity (LOH) that can be observed in inherited and sporadic CRC. Fearon and Vogelstein first postulated in 1990 that at least five genes had to be mutated in order to progress in the adenoma to carcinoma sequence[49] (Figure 1).

Three molecular pathways are known for colorectal carcinogenesis: the chromosomal instability (CIN) pathway, the mutator-phenotype/DNA mismatch repair pathway; and the hypermethylation phenotype pathway. The CIN pathway results in activation of oncogenes or deactivation of tumor suppressor genes. The DNA mismatch repair pathway results in accumulated errors due to loss of DNA mismatch repair. The hypermethylation pathway does not result in DNA damage but hypermethylation can result in changes to protein expression. Among these pathways, three major categories of genes have been implicated in the development of CRC: oncogenes, tumor-suppressor genes, and the mismatch repair genes (Table 1).

APC gene

The *APC* gene is located on the long arm of chromosome 5 (5q). It is mutated in familial adenomatous polyposis (FAP) and Gardner syndrome and in most cases of Turcot syndrome. A mutated *APC* gene is detected in 63% of adenoma and carcinoma, but not in the surrounding tissues, indicating that this is a somatic mutation. Because *APC* is a tumor suppressor gene, inactivation of the second allele must occur for the cell to lose the tumor-suppressing activity of the APC protein. There is considerable evidence that *APC* mutations occur early and may be the first event in sporadic colorectal mutagenesis.

DCC gene

The *DCC* gene is located on the long arm of chromosome 18 (18q). The gene product is involved in cell–cell adhesion and cell–matrix interactions, which may be important in preventing tumor growth, invasion, and metastasis. In sporadic CRC, *DCC* seems to play a critical role in the ability of a tumor to metastasize.

p53 gene

The *p53* is located on the short arm of chromosome 17 (17p). p53 seems to be the most important determinant of malignancy during colorectal tumorigenesis. As a tetramer, *p53* binds sequences of DNA in the promoter region of other genes to enhance their transcription.[51] Most genes activated by *p53* are thought to be involved in the inhibition of growth. Mutations of *p53* can be found in more than half of all human cancers.[52]

K-ras proto-oncogene

K-*ras* is an oncogene, which acts in a classic dominant fashion and is located on the short arm of chromosome 12 (12p). Mutations of K-ras result in unchecked cell growth leading to tumor formation. In sporadic colorectal tumors, K-*ras* mutations have been found in approximately 50% of carcinomas and large adenomas.[53] The presence of a RAS mutation in CRC is significantly associated with the absence of response to agents targeting the epidermal growth factor receptor (EGFR) such as cetuximab.

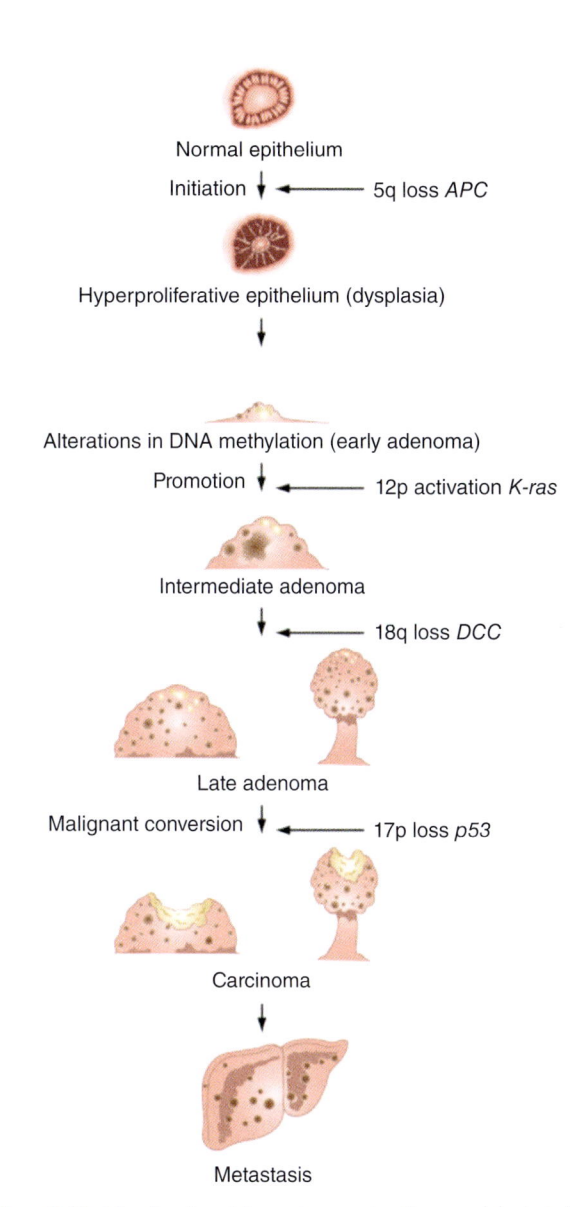

Figure 1 Model of colorectal carcinogenesis. Source: Adapted from Corman.[50]

Normal epithelium
Initiation ← 5q loss *APC*
Hyperproliferative epithelium (dysplasia)
Alterations in DNA methylation (early adenoma)
Promotion ← 12p activation *K-ras*
Intermediate adenoma
← 18q loss *DCC*
Late adenoma
Malignant conversion ← 17p loss *p53*
Carcinoma
Metastasis

Table 1 List of gene mutation causing colorectal cancer.

Type of gene	Gene
Oncogene	RAS, SRC, MYC, BRAF, HER2
Tumor-suppressor gene	APC, p53, DCC, SMAD4, SMAD2
Mismatch repair gene	hMSH2, hMLH1, hPMS1, hPMS2, hMSH3, hMSH6

hMSH, human mutS homolog; *hMLH1*, human mutL homolog 1; *hPMS*, human postmeiotic segregation; *DCC*, deleted in colorectal carcinoma; *HER2*, human epidermal growth factor receptor 2.

BRAF gene

BRAF is a member of the RAS/RAF family of kinases and is located on chromosome 7 (7q). Activating mutations in the BRAF gene (mostly V600E) is almost exclusively seen in MSI-H, CIMP+ CRC and is particularly prevalent in smokers with sporadic CRC. EGFR-targeted agents are unlikely effective in patients whose tumors harbor BRAF V600E mutations, even if they are RAS wild type.

Table 2 Inherited syndrome.[a]

	Inherited syndrome	Responsible gene
Polyposis		
Adenomatous polyposis syndromes	Familial adenomatous polyposis (FAP)	APC
	Attenuated familial adenomatous polyposis (AFAP)	APC
	MutY homologue (MYH)-associated polyposis	MYH
Hamartomatous polyposis syndromes	Peutz–Jeghers syndrome	STK11
	Juvenile polyposis syndrome	SMAD4 and BMPR1A
	Cowden syndrome	PTEN
Nonpolyposis	Hereditary nonpolyposis colorectal cancer (HNPCC: lynch syndrome)	MSH2, MLH1, MLH6, PMS1, PMS2

[a]Source: Modified from Syngal et al.[54]

Inherited syndromes

Even though most cases of CRC are sporadic rather than inherited or familial, inherited susceptibility results in a dramatic increase in risk of developing CRC. The genetic syndromes are typically inherited in an autosomal dominant fashion and are associated with a very high risk of developing CRC[54] (Table 2).

FAP is an autosomal dominant process characterized by numerous colonic adenomas which appear during childhood. This syndrome has penetrance approaching 100% with the onset of symptoms and diagnosis generally around age 15 years.[55] If left untreated, FAP will invariably become CRC with a mean age of diagnosis and death of 39 and 42 years, respectively.[56] An attenuated form of APC (AAPC) is a milder variant of FAP with a similar risk for developing CRC. AAPC is characterized by fewer adenomatous polyps and an older average age of diagnosis (usually in the early 50s). Both FAP and AAPC are caused by different germline mutations in the *APC* gene.[57]

Hereditary nonpolyposis colorectal cancer (HNPCC) is another autosomal dominant inherited syndrome which accounts for 1–5% of all colorectal carcinomas. Also known as Lynch syndrome, this disease is characterized by an early age of onset (some patients can present in their 20s, while the mean age of diagnosis is 48 years), right-sided predominance, multiple synchronous or metachronous colonic tumors, and extracolonic manifestations. The extracolonic neoplasms can include endometrial cancer, renal pelvis and ureter cancer, bladder cancer, small bowel cancer, and skin lesions.[58] As described above, HNPCC is caused by a mutation in one of the mismatch repair genes.[59]

MYH-associated polyposis (MAP) is an autosomal recessive polyposis syndrome associated with a somewhat attenuated phenotype compared to other familial polyposis syndromes.[60] Mutations in *MYH*, a base excision repair gene, are associated with an increased risk of multiple adenomas or polyposis coli.[61] In patients where no *APC* gene mutation is found, especially in those patients with 10–15 or more adenomas, work-up for an *MYH* gene mutation is indicated for diagnosis.[61,62] In addition, these patients are at high risk for synchronous gastrointestinal cancers.

Peutz–Jeghers syndrome (PJ) is an inherited hamartomatous polyposis syndrome that predisposes to CRC. The two major manifestations of PJ are pigmented mucocutaneous lesions and multiple colonic polyps which have the ability to undergo malignant transformation. PJ is associated with an increased risk of both GI and non-GI malignancies including ovarian, breast, pancreatic, uterine, Sertoli cell, and cervical neoplasms.[63–65] Juvenile polyposis (JP) is another inherited hamartomatous polyposis syndrome that can predispose to CRC. Patients with JP are also at increased risk for gastric, duodenal, and pancreatic cancers.[66,67]

Polymorphisms

Numerous genetic polymorphisms (normal variations in genes) have been found to be associated with developing CRC. Changes in genes such as carcinogen metabolism genes, methylation genes, and tumor-suppressor genes can lead to either an increase or decrease in cancer risk. Cytochrome P450 genes,[68,69] Glutathione-S transferase genes,[68] N-acetyltransferase genes,[68,70] and tumor suppressor genes such as APC gene[71,72] have all been implicated in CRC. On the other hand, some polymorphisms have been shown to be protective against CRC. Patients who eat a low-fat diet and who are homozygous for a variant APC gene at codon 1822 have a reduced risk of colon cancer.[73] In addition, variations in a methylation gene for methylenetetrahydrofolate reductase (MTHFR) have been shown to reduce CRC risk.[74]

Presentation

The presentation of large-bowel malignancy generally falls into three categories: insidious onset of chronic symptoms, acute onset of intestinal obstruction, or acute perforation. The most common presentation is that of an insidious onset of chronic symptoms (77–92%), followed by obstruction (6–16%), and then perforation (2–7%).[75–77]

Bleeding is the most common symptom of colorectal malignancy.[78] Unfortunately, patient and physician alike often attribute the bleeding to benign conditions. Bleeding may be occult, or it may be seen as stool that is black, maroon, or bright red depending on the location of the malignancy.

Change in bowel habits is the second most common complaint, with patients noting either diarrhea or constipation.[78,79] Constipation is more often associated with left-sided lesions because the diameter of the colon is smaller and the stool is more formed than on the right side. Patients may report a gradual change in the caliber of the stool or may have diarrhea if the narrowing has progressed sufficiently to cause obstruction. Carcinomas of the right side of the colon do not typically present with changes in bowel habits, but large amounts of mucus generated by a tumor may cause diarrhea, and large right-sided lesions or lesions involving the ileocecal valve may cause obstruction.

Abdominal pain is as common a presentation as change in bowel habits.[80] Left-sided obstructing lesions may present with cramping abdominal pain, associated with nausea and vomiting, and relieved with bowel movements. Right-sided malignancies may result in vague pain that is difficult to localize. Rectal lesions may present with tenesmus, but pelvic pain is generally associated with advanced disease after the tumor has involved the sacral or sciatic nerves. Less common symptoms include weight loss, malaise, fever, abdominal mass, and symptoms of urinary tract involvement. Bacteremia with *Streptococcus bovis* is highly suggestive of colorectal malignancy.[81,82]

Perforation occurs in 12–19% of patients with obstruction due to CRC.[83,84] When the perforation occurs proximal to the obstructing lesion, the patients present with diffuse peritonitis and sepsis. Perforation may result in localized or generalized peritonitis or, if walled off, it may present with obstruction or fistula to an adjacent structure such as the bladder. Emergent surgical intervention after adequate fluid resuscitation is usually indicated. Perforated colon cancer may be confused with alternative diagnoses such as appendicitis, diverticulitis, or Crohn's disease.

Table 3 Screening recommendations, National Comprehensive Cancer Network. National Comprehensive Cancer Network® (NCCN®): Colorectal Cancer Screening.[a][85]

Risk category	Screening and surveillance recommendations
Average risk: Age 45 or greater; no history of adenoma, sessile serrated polyp, or colorectal cancer, no history of inflammatory bowel disease, negative family history of colorectal cancer, or confirmed advanced adenoma	Starting at age 45, colonoscopy every 10 years OR flexible sigmoidoscopy every 5–10 years OR CT colonography every 5 years OR yearly stool-based testing (guaiac- or fecal immunochemical [FIT]-) OR multitargeted stool-DNA (mt-DNA)-based testing every 3 years
Increased risk without personal history: First-degree relative with CRC at any age	Colonoscopy begins at age of 40 or 10 years before earliest diagnosis of CRC. Repeat every 5 years
First-degree relative with confirmed advanced adenoma (high-grade dysplasia, greater than or equal to 1 cm in size, villous or tubulovillous histology, or an advanced sessile serrated polyp)	Colonoscopy beginning at age of 40 or at age of onset of adenoma in relative, whichever first. Repeat every 5–10 years

[a]Source: Adapted with permission from the NCCN Clinical Practice Guidelines in Oncology (NCCN Guidelines®) for Colorectal Cancer Screening Version 2.2021. © 2021 National Comprehensive Cancer Network, Inc. All rights reserved. The NCCN Guidelines® and illustrations herein may not be reproduced in any form for any purpose without the express written permission of NCCN. To view the most recent and complete version of the NCCN Guidelines, go online to NCCN.org. The NCCN Guidelines are a work in progress that may be refined as often as new significant data becomes available.

Screening

Various screening and surveillance modalities are available to detect colorectal cancers and adenomatous polyps. Screening guidelines are undergoing frequent change of recommendation and there is no uniform consensus yet. Current screening recommendations by the National Comprehensive Cancer Network® (NCCN®) are listed in Table 3 as an example,[85] but there is an ongoing debate on the starting age of screening (see the section "Colonoscopy").

Stool-Based screening methods

The advantage of fecal occult blood testing includes availability, convenience, and low cost. Limitations include low sensitivity, low specificity, low compliance, and inability to detect adenomas. In five large controlled studies including more than 300,000 patients, an increased detection of CRC at earlier stages was demonstrated with the proper use of stool-based screening,[86,87] and testing was also associated with a significant reduction in mortality.[86–89]

Stool-based screening techniques include high-sensitivity guaiac-based testing, immunochemical-based testing, and stool DNA tests, which are all recommended by guidelines.[90–92] Guiac-based testing needs three days of stool samples annually. As well, while doing guiac-based testing it is advised to not eat red meat for 3 days and to avoid ingesting large amounts of Vitamin C. Annual immunochemical-based testing does not need dietary restriction. In addition to this, immunochemical-based testing needs only one sample, which may result in higher adherence. Based on one meta-analysis, immunochemical-based testing was superior to guiac-based testing for detection of both CRC (RR 1.96, 95% CI 1.2–3.2) and advanced neoplasia (RR 2.28, 95% CI

1.68–3.10) with no loss of specificity.[93] DNA testing is relatively new diagnostic procedure which detects the presence genomic alterations that are known to occur in CRC oncogenesis; the best tests have demonstrated sensitivities as high as 95%.[94] Although the optimal interval is truly unknown, the guideline recommends testing every 3 years, which is potentially more convenient as a screening modality. Any abnormal test requires follow-up invasive screening, usually colonoscopy. Stool-based screening is a particularly good option for those who refuse more invasive options.[95]

Colonoscopy

Examination of the entire colon by colonoscopy is the gold standard screening method and is recommended by many expert groups. When performed by trained endoscopists, colonoscopy with polypectomy is a safe procedure with a perforation incidence of 0.1%, hemorrhage incidence of 0.3%, and a mortality of 0.01–0.03%. The cecum is visualized in up to 98.6% of patients and a CT colonography may be performed when the cecum is not reached.[96-100] Studies have shown that detecting and removing polyps reduces the incidence of colorectal malignancy, that detecting earlier lesions decreases disease-related mortality, and that fewer carcinomas develop in patients who have colonoscopy and polypectomy.[101,102] Furthermore, a tissue diagnosis or therapeutic intervention may be made at the time of initial evaluation. Colonoscopy also compares favorably with sigmoidoscopy because the entire colon may be directly visualized. In one study, a prevalence of 24% of new adenomas was found when 226 patients underwent colonoscopy within 1 year of flexible sigmoidoscopy. Advanced lesions proximal to the descending colon were found in 6% of these patients.[103]

The latest version of NCCN Guidelines® in 2021 has updated the recommendation on colonoscopy, starting at age 45 years in average-risk adult which was lowered from 50 years old in the previous version.[85] There is an epidemiologic report that CRC incidence is rising in young adults, with nearly half of patients who present with early-onset CRC are younger than 45 years old.[20,85] Given statistically predicted benefits based on those data, the American Cancer Society issued a qualified recommendation in 2018 to begin screening persons at average risk at age 45 years regardless of race.[104] There is a trend to start screening at younger age but the evidence supporting this practice is weak at present day as noted in the NCCN Guidelines®.[85] Further evidence is needed to make a stronger consensus for this topic.

CT colonography

CT colonography (virtual colonoscopy) is a relatively new technique which is now recommended as an option for CRC screening by expert groups including the NCCN.[85] This technique needs bowel preparation as well as colon insufflation by introducing air or carbon dioxide into the rectum via catheter. Multiple studies report high sensitivity of CT colonography for the detection of cancers and adenomas ≥10 mm, between 67% and 94%, with specificity of 96–98%.[105] CT colonography is particularly useful in the setting of incomplete colonography although it lacks tissue diagnosis. Current NCCN screening recommendations are for a virtual colonoscopy every 5 years with subsequent colonoscopy if a lesion is found.[85] The major limitations include need for full bowel preparation, radiation exposure, and follow-up colonoscopy for tissue diagnosis of radiographic abnormalities. As well, incidental radiologic finding with other organs is an issue. It is unclear if detection of such incidental findings improves health outcomes or only results in additional harms and costs.

Flexible sigmoidoscopy

Flexible sigmoidoscopies are inexpensive, require no conscious sedation, and afford direct visualization and biopsy of polyps and cancers.[106] The disadvantage of sigmoidoscopy is that the entire colon is not visualized, and lesions may be missed in the proximal colon. Current National Comprehensive Cancer Network and American Cancer Society Guidelines recommend sigmoidoscopy without stool-based screening every 5 years as an option, with subsequent full colonoscopy if adenomatous disease is found.[85] However, whereas studies suggest flexible sigmoidoscopy alone may serve as a substitute,[107,108] most physicians in the United States only reserve it for selected population who is not able to tolerate full colonoscopy or has financial issue.

Preoperative work-up and staging

The general physical examination remains a cornerstone in assessing a patient preoperatively to determine the extent of local disease, disclosing distant metastases, and appraising the general operative risk. Special interest should be paid to weight loss, pallor as a sign of anemia, and signs of portal hypertension. In addition, a complete workup should include laboratory work, colonoscopy, CT of the chest, abdomen and pelvis, and transrectal ultrasound (TRUS) or rectal protocol magnetic resonance imaging (MRI) for those with rectal cancer.

Laboratory work

A complete blood count (CBC) may reveal the presence of anemia. Liver function tests (LFTs) may be abnormal in the case of liver metastases. However, it needs to be noted that abnormal LFTs are present in only 15% of patients with liver metastases and may be elevated without liver metastases in up to 40%.[109] Carcinoembryonic antigen (CEA) levels should be obtained as a baseline against which further values may be compared. Metastatic disease to the liver is often accompanied with very high levels of CEA, and levels surpassing 10–20 ng/mL are associated with increased chances of treatment failure.[110] Thus NCCN guideline recommends obtaining serum CEA levels preoperatively to aid in surgical treatment planning and posttreatment follow-up.[111,112]

Colonoscopy

Colonoscopy remains the single most important investigation in the evaluation of colonic diseases because it allows for tissue sampling. It also allows assessment of tumor size localization in the colon and evaluation for synchronous tumors or polyps. Synchronous carcinomas occur in 2–7% of patients and synchronous polyps 29.7% of the time.[113] It has been suggested that preoperative colonoscopy alters the operative procedure in 30% of patients.[109] With increasing utilization of laparoscopic-assisted surgery it is important for all tumors to be tattooed at the time of colonoscopy. This is crucial for planned minimally invasive resections because the surgeon cannot palpate the colon intraoperatively. In case of stricture which prevents passage of the scope, CT colonography can be utilized.

Staging

The most common areas of distant spread for CRC are the liver, the lungs, and the peritoneum.[114] Therefore, once the diagnosis of CRC is confirmed, CT chest, abdomen, and pelvis should be obtained as a part of staging workup. Preoperative abdominal and pelvic CT scans can demonstrate regional tumor extension, regional lymphatic metastasis, and distant metastases, especially to the liver. Chest CT has replaced chest X-ray to detect pulmonary metastasis due to its high sensitivity. For those with suspected liver metastases seen on CT, further workup with liver MRI may be necessary.

Positron emission tomography (PET) scan is a study using the glucose analog fluorodeoxyglucose as a tracer, visualizing metabolically active tissues. PET has been investigated as a potential important imaging modality for CRC. However, several studies showed its small impact to alter surgical management,[115,116] and its routine use as the initial staging workup is currently not recommended.[111,112] The role of preoperative PET is not yet established but could be a useful diagnostic tool for selected high-risk patients; such as a patient with isolated liver metastasis which is potentially resectable, to rule out other metastasis.[111,112]

The staging of rectal cancer differs slightly from colon cancer in that assessment of locoregional extent of the disease is used to guide preoperative treatment and for operative planning. Rectal cancer protocol MRI or TRUS is recommended to stage the pelvis in patients with rectal cancer. The depth of invasion and lymph node status is important if local excision is considered to determine the treatment strategy. Today, for most patients with rectal cancer, MRI is the preferred imaging modality for evaluating the extent of the primary tumor as it will be able to provide information on the depth of transmural tumor invasion, the presence of suspicious regional nodes, the status of the circumferential resection margin (CRM), and invasion of other organs and structures. MRI has advantages to other modalities in evaluation of locoregional extent of rectal cancer, including superior soft-tissue contrast, a wider field of view for nodal evaluation, and the ability to assess soft tissue features. The results of a compilation of data from seven systematic reviews showed high accuracy of MRI for T stage (T1/T2 vs T3/T4) (sensitivity of 87% and the specificity of 75%), for lymph node involvement (sensitivity of 77% and the specificity of 71%), and for CRM status (sensitivity of 77% and the specificity of 94%).[117]

One of the current important roles of MRI is to assess preoperative status of the CRM. The MERCURY study utilized preoperative MRI to access the relationship of the primary rectal tumor to the mesorectal fascia, choosing a distance of less than 1 mm to signify potentially involved margins.[118] Patients with potentially involved margins were found to have substantially shorter 5-year OS, DFS, and likelihood of developing local recurrence following resection. In fact, preoperative MRI evaluation of the CRM was found to have superior prognostic ability compared to AJCC TNM staging. Thus, tumors in close proximity (1 mm) to the CRM on imaging are referred as "threatened" CRM. Because of the higher risk for locoregional recurrence, patients with an involved or threatened CRM are considered appropriate candidates for neoadjuvant chemoradiotherapy per NCCN guideline.[112]

Although largely replaced by MRI, TRUS remains an important tool for locoregional staging. The layers of the rectal wall can be identified and the depth of penetration determined. Perirectal lymph nodes also can be visualized. TRUS has superior spatial resolution compared with MRI, particularly useful in distinguishing T2 from early T3 tumors, which can be indistinguishable on MRI. On the other hand, TRUS has some limitations compared with MRI including operator dependency, limited field of view for assessing nodal status, and difficulty assess CRM especially for posterior or posterolateral tumor. For these reasons, the NCCN guidelines state a preference for MRI over TRUS for pretreatment staging of rectal cancer unless MRI is contraindicated.[112] However, the information obtained with TRUS and MRI may be complementary and both procedures may be needed. Fine-needle aspiration (FNA) biopsy of suspicious perirectal lymph nodes could be a potential advantage of TRUS over MRI but studies have failed to reveal an advantage in staging.[119,120]

Staging system

In 1932, Dukes proposed a classification based on the degree of direct extension along with the presence or absence of regional lymphatic metastases for the staging of rectal cancer. However, current TNM classification was proposed by the American College of Surgeons' Commission on Cancer to incorporate findings at laparotomy, and over multiple iterations, it has largely replaced Dukes' classification in clinical use.

The TNM staging system of the combined American Joint Committee on Cancer (AJCC)/Union for International Cancer Control (UICC) is most recently updated in 2017 (eighth edition)[121] (Table 4). The AJCC/UICC 8th edition TNM staging system also acknowledges following clinical factors as prognostic factors recommended for clinical care; CEA, lymphovascular and perineural invasion, the status of CRM, tumor regression score, microsatellite instability, and mutation status of KRAS, NRAS, and BRAF. Tumor regression score assesses residual tumor for surgical specimens after preoperative radiotherapy or chemoradiotherapy, which has become more important with increased application for neoadjuvant treatment. Prognosis has been reported to be correlated with tumor regression grade[122] but its clinical significance to modify the postoperative treatment strategy is not clear.

Surgical management of colorectal cancer

Bowel preparation

The use of bowel preparation before colorectal surgery has been a popular topic of debate. Although its effectiveness was questioned once, the most recent evidence has shown benefit of mechanical bowel preparation in combination with oral antibiotics. In the largest retrospective study, including 45,724 elective colectomies with anastomosis, the combination of mechanical bowel preparation and oral antibiotics was associated with lower rates of surgical site infection, anastomotic leaks, overall complications, and 30-day mortality.[123] Mechanical cleansing may be accomplished by laxatives along with repeated enemas. An oral lavage with a polyethylene glycol hypertonic electrolyte solution such as GoLYTELY has been commonly used. More recently, oral phospho-soda preparations have become increasingly popular but their use can be associated with fluid and electrolyte abnormalities and should be used with caution in at-risk patients.

Perioperative antibiotics can be delivered both orally and intravenously. Oral antibiotics have traditionally been used for two purposes: to act as a cathartic alongside mechanical bowel preparation, and to eradicate potentially pathologic intraluminal bacteria. Most commonly used regimen is either neomycin + erythromycin or neomycin + metronidazole, three repeated doses over a period of approximately 10 h.[124] Oral antibiotics preparation was shown to be effective to reduce SSI even solely delivered without mechanical bowel preparation.[125] However, as stated above, more recent studies have shown better outcome in combination with mechanical bowel preparation.[123,125,126] Current guideline from the American Society of Colon and Rectal Surgeons (ASCRS) and Society of American Gastrointestinal and Endoscopic Surgeons (SAGES) recommends the combination of mechanical bowel preparation and oral antibiotics prior to colorectal surgery.[127]

Table 4 Colorectal cancer TNM staging AJCC UICC 8th edition.[a]

Primary tumor (T)	
T category	T criteria
TX	Primary tumor cannot be assessed
T0	No evidence of primary tumor
Tis	Carcinoma in situ, intramucosal carcinoma (involvement of lamina propria with no extension through muscularis mucosae)
T1	Tumor invades the submucosa (through the muscularis mucosa but not into the muscularis propria)
T2	Tumor invades the muscularis propria
T3	Tumor invades through the muscularis propria into pericolorectal tissues
T4	Tumor invades[b] the visceral peritoneum or invades or adheres[c] to adjacent organ or structure
T4a	Tumor invades[b,a] through the visceral peritoneum (including gross perforation of the bowel through tumor and continuous invasion of tumor through areas of inflammation to the surface of the visceral peritoneum)
T4b	Tumor directly invades[b] or adheres[c] to adjacent organs or structures

Regional lymph nodes (N)	
N category	N criteria
NX	Regional lymph nodes cannot be assessed
N0	No regional lymph node metastasis
N1	One to three regional lymph nodes are positive (tumor in lymph nodes measuring ≥0.2 mm), or any number of tumor deposits are present and all identifiable lymph nodes are negative
N1a	One regional lymph node is positive
N1b	Two or three regional lymph nodes are positive
N1c	No regional lymph nodes are positive, but there are tumor deposits in the: • Subserosa • Mesentery • Nonperitonealized pericolic, or perirectal/mesorectal tissues
N2	Four or more regional nodes are positive
N2a	Four to six regional lymph nodes are positive
N2b	Seven or more regional lymph nodes are positive

Distant metastasis (M)	
M category	M criteria
M0	No distant metastasis by imaging, etc.; no evidence of tumor in distant sites or organs. (This category is not assigned by pathologists.)
M1	Metastasis to one or more distant sites or organs or peritoneal metastasis is identified
M1a	Metastasis to one site or organ is identified without peritoneal metastasis
M1b	Metastasis to two or more sites or organs is identified without peritoneal metastasis
M1c	Metastasis to the peritoneal surface is identified alone or with other site or organ metastases

Prognostic stage groups

When T is...	And N is...	And M is...	Then the stage group is...
Tis	N0	M0	0
T1, T2	N0	M0	I
T3	N0	M0	IIA
T4a	N0	M0	IIB
T4b	N0	M0	IIC
T1–T2	N1/N1c	M0	IIIA
T1	N2a	M0	IIIA
T3–T4a	N1/N1c	M0	IIIB
T2–T3	N2a	M0	IIIB
T1–T2	N2b	M0	IIIB
T4a	N2a	M0	IIIC
T3–T4a	N2b	M0	IIIC
T4b	N1–N2	M0	IIIC
Any T	Any N	M1a	IVA
Any T	Any N	M1b	IVB
Any T	Any N	M1c	IVC

[a]Source: Jessup et al.[121]
[b]Direct invasion in T4 includes invasion of other organs or other segments of the colorectum as a result of direct extension through the serosa, as confirmed on microscopic examination (e.g., invasion of the sigmoid colon by a carcinoma of the cecum) or, for cancers in a retroperitoneal or subperitoneal location, direct invasion of other organs or structures by virtue of extension beyond the muscularis propria (i.e., respectively, a tumor on the posterior wall of the descending colon invading the left kidney or lateral abdominal wall; or a mid or distal rectal cancer with invasion of prostate, seminal vesicles, cervix, or vagina).
[c]Tumor that is adherent to other organs or structures, grossly, is classified cT4b. However, if no tumor is present in the adhesion, microscopically, the classification should be pT1-4a depending on the anatomical depth of wall invasion. The V and L classification should be used to identify the presence or absence of vascular or lymphatic invasion whereas the PN prognostic factor should be used for perineural invasion.

Antibiotic administration

Intravenous antibiotics are utilized to prevent surgical site infections, which are particularly common among patients undergoing colorectal surgery. Intravenous antimicrobial prophylaxis significantly reduces SSI rates and mortality rates; one pooled analysis of 26 trials noted SSI rates of 4.5 versus 11.2 for treatment and control groups, respectively.[128] Although the exact antibiotic regimen remains debated, it should cover both aerobic and anaerobic bacteria. The enhanced recovery after surgery (ERAS) Group recommends a single dose of antibiotics within one hour of surgery, and there is level 1 evidence to support this guideline.[129] While an initial single dose provides equivalent prophylaxis compared to multidose regimens, subsequent dosing may be required in prolonged cases.[129]

Management of carcinoma in a polyp

Colon cancers that appear to be confined to an adenomatous polyp ("malignant polyps") have their invasion limited to the submucosa. Their propensity for lymph node metastasis appears to be related to a number of histopathologic features, including grade, presence of perineural/perivascular invasion, and overall gross morphology (i.e., sessile versus pedunculated).

The Haggitt classification system is used to define the depth of involvement of carcinoma into a pedunculated polyp (Table 5). The risk of lymph node metastasis in Haggitt level 1, 2, and 3 lesions is less than 1%, and these lesions can usually be managed with complete endoscopic excision and India ink tattooing of the polypectomy site. In these cases, careful colonoscopic surveillance of the polypectomy site is recommended. However, lymphovascular invasion, poor differentiation, or cancer close to the polypectomy resection margin (less than 2 mm) is usually an indication for a colectomy because of the increased risk of lymph node metastasis. Haggit level 4 lesions have an increased incidence of lymph node metastasis (12–25%) and should be managed with a colectomy.[130]

For sessile lesions, depth of submucosal invasion can be classified using the Kikuchi level system[131] (Table 6). Reported risks of lymph node metastasis are 0–3% for sm1 invasion, 8–10% for sm2, and 23–25% for sm3.[132] This classification may be difficult to apply when lesions have been resected endoscopically, as the muscularis propria is not included. As a result, a measurement of the distance of invasion from the muscularis mucosa is also commonly used. The results from a systematic review and meta-analysis demonstrated that a depth of submucosal invasion >1 mm was significantly associated with lymph node metastasis.[133]

Table 5 Haggitt classification of malignant polyps.

Haggit level	Characteristics
0	Carcinoma in situ
1	Carcinoma invading into submucosa but limited to head of polyp
2	Carcinoma invading level of neck of polyp
3	Carcinoma invading stalk
4	Carcinoma invading submucosa below the stalk (above the muscularis propria)

Table 6 Kikuchi classification of malignant polyps.

Kikuchi level	Characteristics
Sm1	Tumor invasion of the upper third of the submucosa
Sm2	Tumor invasion of the middle third of the submucosa
Sm3	Tumor invasion of the lower third of the submucosa

Most polyps throughout the colon can be removed through the colonoscope using the snare polypectomy technique. The polyp is visualized through the colonoscope, the snare wire is looped around the polyp and gently tightened while the electric current is applied. Whenever possible the polyp is retrieved for histology. When performed by trained endoscopists, colonoscopy with polypectomy is a safe procedure, with a perforation incidence of 0.3–1% and a hemorrhage incidence of 0.7–2.5%.[134]

Right-sided colon cancers

Cancers of the right colon account for up to 30% of primary CRCs.[135] Patients with adenocarcinoma involving the cecum or ascending colon who do not have HNPCC or other synchronous lesions should be treated with a right hemicolectomy (Figure 2a). The ileocolic, right colic, and right branch of the middle colic vessels should be ligated near their origins to assure adequate lymphadenectomy. Approximately 5–10 cm of distal small intestine should be resected in continuity with the right colon to assure adequate blood supply at the stapled edge of the small intestine.

Transverse colon cancers

Transverse colon cancers are relatively uncommon, accounting for only 10% of colorectal primaries.[135] Lesions of the proximal and mid-transverse colon are usually best managed with an extended right hemicolectomy involving ligation of the ileocolic, right colic, and middle colic vessels (Figure 2b). The ascending colon, hepatic flexure, transverse colon, and splenic flexures are removed with anastomosis of the ileum to the descending colon. It is advisable to avoid an anastomosis between the hepatic and splenic flexure because of concerns over adequacy of blood supply and tension at the anastomosis.

Left-sided colon cancers

Lesions of the splenic flexure and descending colon are also uncommon, accounting for 15% of colorectal primaries.[135] Splenic flexure cancers may be managed with an extended right or left hemicolectomy (Figure 2c). Cancers in the descending colon may be managed with a left hemicolectomy involving division of the left colic artery, preservation of the left branch of the middle colic artery, and anastomosis of the distal transverse colon to the distal sigmoid colon. Alternatively, a left hemicolectomy may be performed with ligation of the inferior mesenteric vessels and an anastomosis between the transverse colon and the upper rectum.

Sigmoid colon cancers

Tumors of the sigmoid colon account for 25% of colorectal primaries.[135] These tumors are usually removed by means of an anterior sigmoid colectomy, which usually involves division of the inferior mesenteric artery either above or below the left colic artery and the superior rectal arteries within the upper mesorectum with anastomosis of the descending colon to the upper rectum (Figure 2d). Large, bulky sigmoid cancers located above the peritoneal reflection but at the level of the pelvic inlet present a unique challenge as their posterolateral borders abut the ureters, hypogastric nerves, and iliac vessels. Proper preoperative planning based on optimal imaging and consideration of ureteral stent placement is essential.

Subtotal colectomy

This resection involves the removal of the entire colon to the rectum with an ileorectal anastomosis (IRA). This procedure is indicated for multiple synchronous colonic tumors that are not

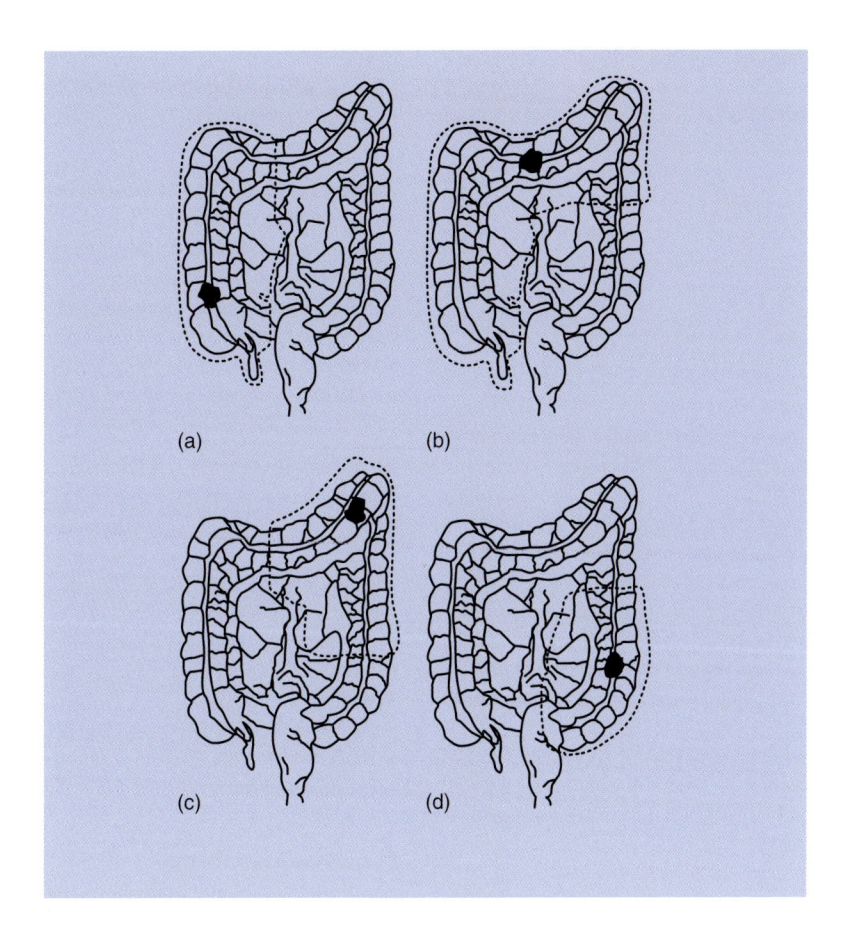

Figure 2 Extent of resection for colon carcinoma: (a) cecal or ascending colon cancer; (b) transverse colon cancer; (c) splenic flexure colon cancer; and (d) sigmoid colon cancer. *Abbreviations*: ICA, ileocolic artery; IMA, inferior mesenteric artery; LCA, left colic artery; MCA, middle colic artery; RCA, right colic artery; SA, sigmoidal arteries; SHA, superior hemorrhoidal (rectal) artery.

confined to a single anatomical distribution, for selected patients with FAP with minimal rectal involvement (discussed below), or for selected patients with HNPCC and colon cancer.

Total proctocolectomy

The surgical treatment of FAP depends on the age of the patient, and the polyp density in the rectum. Surgical options include proctocolectomy with Brooke ileostomy, total abdominal colectomy with IRA, or restorative proctocolectomy with ileal-pouch anal anastomosis (IPAA). Proctocolectomy with continent ileostomy is rarely performed today. Total abdominal colectomy with IRA has a low complication rate, provides good functional results, and is a viable option for patients with fewer than 20 adenomas in the rectum. These patients must be observed with 6-month proctoscopic examinations to remove polyps and detect signs of cancer. If rectal polyps become too numerous, completion proctectomy, when technically possible, is warranted. The Cleveland Clinic has evaluated its registry of patients with FAP who were treated with IRA or IPAA. Prior to the use of IPAA for patients with high rectal polyp burdens, the risk of cancer in the retained rectum was 12.9% at a median follow-up of over 17 years.[136] Alternatively, for patients treated with IPAA or the selected use of IRA (for those with small rectal polyp burdens), none developed rectal cancer in the remaining rectum at a median follow-up of 5 years. Restorative proctocolectomy with IPAA has the advantage of removing all or nearly all large intestine mucosa at risk of cancer, while preserving transanal defecation. Complication rates are low when the procedure is done in large centers, but morbidity includes incontinence, multiple loose stools, impotence, retrograde ejaculation, dyspareunia, and pouchitis. Approximately 7% of patients must be converted to permanent ileostomy due to complications from the procedure.[136]

Rectal cancers

The surgical approach to rectal tumors depends upon depth of invasion and distance from the anal verge. The three categories include transanal local excision, LAR with total mesorectal excision (TME), and APR.

Local excision

Local excision is best reserved for T1 rectal cancers within 15 cm of the anal verge, tumors less than 3 cm in diameter involving less than 30% of the circumference of the rectal wall, highly mobile exophytic tumors, and tumors of favorable histologic grade based upon biopsy which includes well- to moderately differentiated cancer and no lymphovascular or perineural invasion.[137] The decision to use local excision alone or to employ adjuvant therapy after local excision is based on the pathological characteristics of the primary cancer and the potential for micrometastases in draining lymph nodes.

Local excision of distal rectal cancers can be accomplished by transanal excision (TAE) or transanal endoscopic surgery (TES). TAE is the most straightforward approach and involves using the perirectal fat as the deep plane of dissection to achieve adequate circumferential margins of 1 cm. TES provides accessibility to tumors of the middle and upper rectum that would otherwise require a laparotomy or transsacral approach. It can be performed with one of three platforms, transanal endoscopic microsurgery (TEM), transanal endoscopic operation (TEO), or transanal minimally invasive surgery (TAMIS). These approaches can be used for selected lesions up to 15 cm from the anal verge. Compared with TAE, TES offers improved visualization, exposure, and access. As a result, TES was associated with lower rates of specimen fragmentation, positive margins, and local recurrences than TAE.[138]

T1 lesions have positive lymph nodes in up to 18% of cases, whereas the rate for T2 and T3 lesions is up to 38% and 70%, respectively. T2 tumors treated with local resection alone can have recurrence rates of 15–44%.[139] Thus local resection is generally not recommended for T2 tumors. For T1N0 tumors, local excision alone was associated with 8% local recurrence and 84% survival with long-term follow-up (7.1 years).[140] Survival outcomes in T2N0 tumors were comparable to T1N0 tumors (88% at 3 years) when patients are given preoperative chemoradiation therapy prior to local excision.[141] However, current guidelines do not support local excision for T2N0 rectal cancers and only should be done in patients who are unfit for or unwilling to undergo transabdominal surgery.

In addition to disease characteristics, patient characteristics are another consideration to determine suitability of local excision. The patient's ability to tolerate an abdominal surgery or capability to take care of stoma needs to be considered. Local excision is associated with lower perioperative mortality (RR 0.31, 95% CI 0.14–0.71), lower postop complications (RR 0.16, 95% CI 0.08–0.30), and decreased need for permanent ostomy (RR 0.17, 95% CI 0.09–0.30).[142] Therefore, for patients with more advanced stage rectal cancer who are poor operative candidates, local excision may be discussed in spite of increased risk of local and distant failure. Another group of patients who can be considered for local excision is those with good response to neoadjuvant therapy. The rate of lymph node metastasis in those found to have ypT0-1 rectal cancer after transabdominal resection was 3%.[143] Thus, a good response to preoperative therapy may be used as an indicator of low risk of spread to lymph nodes.

Low anterior resection with total mesorectal excision

The technique of TME, which involves resection of the rectum along with the mesorectum by dissecting outside the investing fascia of the mesorectum. TME optimizes the oncologic operation by not only removing draining lymph nodes but also maximizing CRM. The splenic flexure is routinely mobilized and the reconstruction is performed using the descending colon. The use of the sigmoid colon is discouraged, as the thickened and hypertrophic muscle of the sigmoid is less compliant than the descending colon. More recently, with significant advances in both surgical techniques and adjuvant therapy, a meta-analysis has shown patients whose distal margins were negative but less than 1 cm did not have higher local recurrence rates than those with greater distal margins.[144] In this study, however, patients who did not receive either TME or radiation therapy had higher local recurrence rates with less than 1 cm margin. Therefore, at least 1 cm distal margin is currently recommended, or else an APR was performed. The proximal margin should be at least 5 cm distal to remove draining lymphatics and assure an anastomosis to well-vascularized bowel. In addition, the CRMs are equally as important as the proximal and distal margin in rectal cancer surgery. A histologic CRM of greater than 1 mm is required. Neoadjuvant therapy in properly selected patients may be effective in converting probable APRs into sphincter-preserving operations.[145]

Abdominal perineal resection with total mesorectal excision

For patients who have rectal cancers that invade or abut the anal sphincter or who are incontinent of stool preoperatively, a combined approach of transabdominal and transperineal dissection is performed to remove the rectum and mesorectum. Once the rectal specimen is removed via the perineal opening or laparotomy, the perineum is sutured closed and a permanent colostomy is created.

Synchronous and metachronous lesions

The incidence of synchronous colon cancers ranges from 2% to 11% and incidence of synchronous adenomatous polyps may exceed 30%.[135] For lesions that are widely separated, preservation of colonic length via more than one anastomosis is desirable as long as the adequacy of the required individual cancer resections is not compromised. An alternative to multiple anastomoses is a subtotal colectomy with an ileorectal or ileosigmoid anastomosis. Metachronous colon cancers, defined as those detected more than 6 months following the management of the index lesion, may be managed with either partial or subtotal colectomy as dictated by the location of the lesions.

Lymphadenectomy

An appropriate lymph node dissection should extend to the origin of the primary vessel draining the portion of the colon incorporating the cancer. Resection of a lesion located near two major vessels should involve removal of the two major vessels along with the associated lymph nodes in an en bloc fashion. Apical lymph nodes at the origin of a primary vessel should be removed when feasible and tagged for pathologic analysis. Suspicious lymph nodes outside the field of resection should be sampled and resected when positive. Although not always feasible, efforts should be made by the pathologist to examine a minimum of 12 lymph nodes.[146,147] This allows for the most accurate staging, which can be used to appropriately select patients for adjuvant therapies.[148] In addition, the absolute number of lymph nodes examined has itself been shown to be associated with survival.[148]

Laparoscopic colectomy

Laparoscopic resection of the colon was first described in 1990.[149] The proposed benefits to laparoscopic colectomy include a shorter recovery time and less narcotic use than the traditional open procedure. The technique of a laparoscopically assisted colon resection consists of an intracorporal approach to explore the abdomen and mobilize the colon. The bowel is then exteriorized through a small incision for extracorporal resection and anastomosis. There was some initial concern regarding the ability to achieve an adequate oncologic resection and concern about the frequency of port-site recurrences using the laparoscopic technique for colon cancer.[150] However, the results of several large studies have provided solid evidence demonstrating laparoscopic colectomy in patients with colon cancer provides equivalent oncologic outcomes and superior short-term perioperative morbidity compared to open colectomy.

Four landmark prospective randomized trials, Australasian Laparoscopic Colon Cancer Study (ALCCaS), Clinical Outcomes of Surgical Therapy Study Group (COST), Conventional versus Laparoscopic-Assisted Surgery in Colorectal Cancer (CLASICC),

Table 7 Summary of large trials of laparoscopic colectomy.

Study name	Author, year	Sample size	Follow-up	Conclusion
COST	Weeks et al., 2002[151]	576	3-year	5-year OS, 5-year DFS, recurrence rates, and sites of first recurrence were similar between groups
	The Clinical Outcomes of Surgical Therapy Study Group, 2004[152]	872	5-year	
	Fleshman et al., 2007[153]			
CLASICC	Jayne et al., 2007[154]	794	3-year	No differences at 3 and 5 years in OS, DFS, or local recurrence
	Jayne et al., 2010[155]		5-year	
	Green et al., 2013[156]			
COLOR	Hazebroek et al., 2002[157]	859	5-year	Similar rates of positive surgical margins and number of regional lymph nodes retrieved, as well as equivalent DFS and OS
	Buunen et al., 2009[158]	1248	10-year	
	Deijen et al., 2017[159]	329 (Dutch only)	(Dutch only)	
ALCCaS	Hewett et al., 2008[160]	601	3-year	Similar rates of 5-year OS and RFS. Short-term gain in quality of life maintained at 2 months postsurgery.
	Bagshaw et al., 2012[161]	587	5-year	
	McCombie et al., 2018[162]	592		

and Colon Cancer Laparoscopic or Open Resection (COLOR) have reported long-term follow-up data on the equivalence of laparoscopic colectomy to open colectomy for colon cancer as summarized in Table 7. In those studies, hospital stay was shorter while operating time for laparoscopically assisted colectomy was longer. The length of ileus was significantly less with laparoscopic colectomy in both the CLASICC and COST trials while the COST trial also observed significantly less time of use of oral analgesics with laparoscopic colectomy.[152,163] In a meta-analysis of the four trials which included over 1500 patients, 3-year DFS and OS after laparoscopically assisted or open resection were similar, and disease-free OS rates for stages I, II, and III evaluated separately did not differ between the two treatments.[164] Laparoscopic-assisted colectomy when performed by experienced surgeons has proven to be an equivalent oncologic operation compared to open colectomy for patients with colon cancer.[165]

Surgical resection is an extremely important treatment modality for rectal cancer. The standard for middle and low rectal cancers is precise TME as described by Heald.[166] TME and adequacy of resection margins are associated with low recurrence and optimal survival.[167] Laparoscopic resection of rectal cancer must be able to achieve the same oncologic outcomes. The laparoscopic technique for rectal cancer involves transection of the proximal and distal bowel and mesorectum intracorporeally. An intracorporal end-to-end or end to side anastomosis is performed by using a circular stapler.[168,169]

There have been several prospective randomized trials comparing laparoscopic and open techniques for resection of rectal and rectosigmoid cancers. The Comparison of Open Versus Laparoscopic Surgery for mid and low Rectal Cancer after Neoadjuvant Chemoradiotherapy (COREAN) trial is a randomized trial to compare open surgery with laparoscopic surgery for mid or low rectal cancer after neoadjuvant chemoradiotherapy.[170,171] In this study involving 170 patients in each arm, there was no difference in the rate of CRM positivity, similar rates of completeness of mesorectal resection, and no difference in 3-year disease-free survival between two groups. In addition, the laparoscopic surgery group showed earlier recovery of bowel function than the open surgery group. The Laparoscopic Versus Open Surgery for Rectal Cancer (COLOR II) Trial was a multicenter, randomized, intention-to-treat based trial comparing laparoscopic and open resection for rectal cancers.[172–174] The trial included over 1100 patients, and demonstrated improvements in operative blood loss, return of bowel function, and hospital length of stay. As well, the two groups had similar rates of complete resection, including CRM positivity. The 3-year locoregional recurrence and survival rates were also comparable between surgical approaches. On the other hand, the Australasian Laparoscopic Cancer of the Rectum (ALaCaRT) trial, comparing laparoscopic and open resection failed to prove noninferiority of laparoscopic resection over the gold-standard open resections.[175] This randomized trial including 475 patients with T1–T3 rectal adenocarcinoma compared a composite of oncological factors indicating an adequate surgical resection. A successful resection was achieved in 194 patients (82%) in the laparoscopic surgery group and in 208 patients (89%) in the open surgery group (risk difference of −7.0%; $p=0.38$ for noninferiority). The most recent update for this topic is the result of a multicenter, noninferiority randomized trial to compare laparoscopic versus open rectal cancer surgery trial by the American College of Surgery Oncology Group (ACSOG-Z6051).[176,177] This trial compared a composite of CRM greater than 1 mm, distal margin without tumor, and completeness of TME but concluded that laparoscopic surgery for patients with stage II or III rectal cancer failed to demonstrate noninferiority for pathologic outcomes.[176] Subsequent 2-year follow-up revealed no statistically significant difference of disease-free survival and recurrence between the laparoscopic resection group and traditional open resections.[177]

Robotic colectomy

There are limited data regarding robotic colorectal surgery, either in comparison to laparoscopic or traditional open surgery. There have been limited number of relatively small RCT comparing robotic colectomy with laparoscopic colectomy,[178–180] which demonstrated equivalent lymph node harvest, margin positivity rate, and need for conversion to open surgery between the two groups. As of today, most other data have come from retrospective studies.

In comparison to laparoscopic colectomy, robotic resections have been associated with similar lymph node harvest, specimen length, and radial margins.[181,182] Robotic resections were associated lower conversion rate and shorter length of stay.[183–186] In the largest retrospective study by a review of the 2013 American College of Surgeons NSQIP database with 11,477 patients undergoing laparoscopic or robotic colorectal surgeries, robotic operations had a longer operative time and a statistically significant decreased length of stay (4.3 days compared with 5.3) and decreased conversion rates.[183] Even compared to laparoscopy, on the other hand, studies to date indicate that robotic colectomy is associated with increased operative room time and increased operating room costs.[181,186,187] These tendencies were also shown in recent meta-analysis in 2018 analyzing 11 articles, that robotic colectomy has been associated with lower rate of conversion to open compared with laparoscopic colectomy but also with longer operative time as well as increased costs of care.[188] The increase in OR time may be the result of more intracorporeal anastomoses being performed in robotic colectomies, as well as time associated with set-up of the laparoscopic system.[187]

Long-term survival data have yet to be reported. A Dutch group performed a nonrandomized prospective study comparing 378 patients undergoing robotic or laparoscopic resection for stage I–III CRC with a 15-month median follow-up, finding no statistically significant difference between the robotic and laparoscopic groups for locoregional recurrence rates.[182] A Korean group also reported no difference of 5-year disease-free survival comparing open, laparoscopic, and robotic approaches for right-sided colon cancer.[189] Only one of the RCTs followed long-term outcome.[190] In this article, there was no difference in 5-year DFS or OS reported. Therefore, the authors concluded there are no clinical benefits with robotic colon resection.[190]

Robotic rectal surgery has several theoretical advantages compared to both traditional open and laparoscopic techniques. In comparison to open surgery, these include a better morbidity profile, as well as improvements in short-term quality metrics such as hospital length of stay and readmission rates. In comparison to laparoscopic rectal resections, robotics may offer lower rates of conversion to open surgery. In a retrospective comparative-effectiveness study, robotic LAR has resulted in lower conversion rates and serious complication rates as compared to laparoscopic LAR.[179] Improvements were also appreciated in completeness of the TME. In a case-matched cohort study of robotic versus laparoscopic LAR, robotic technique resulted in shorter operative times and lower conversion rate.[191] In this study, overall survival and disease-free survival were shown comparable between two groups with a trend toward better disease-free survival in the robotic group. The robotic versus laparoscopic resection for rectal cancer (ROLARR) Trial is an international, multicenter, prospective, randomized controlled trial comparing robotic versus laparoscopic rectal resections which was published in 2017.[192] The primary outcome was conversion to open laparotomy, which was not significantly different between the groups. There was no statistically significant difference in secondary outcomes including intraoperative and postoperative complications, and CRM positivity. This initial result of ROLARR trial was analyzed using multilevel logistic regression to adjust for varying experience levels of the operating robotic surgeon.[193] Participating surgeons were experts in laparoscopic surgery, whereas some of these surgeons were still in the learning-curve phase of robotic surgery, which may have confounded the results of the ROLARR trial. Following the ROLARR trial, a subsequent systematic review compared outcomes in patients undergoing TME robotically versus laparoscopically.[194] This article analyzed one RCT (ROLARR) and 27 case-control study, showing comparable oncologic and perioperative outcomes. The authors concluded that the robotic approach is a feasible technique and oncologically safe but failed to demonstrate any superiority over laparoscopic approach. Longer-term end points of prospective randomized ROLARR trial at 3 years (local recurrence rates, disease-free survival, and overall survival) are still pending. In the interim, robotic rectal resections should be considered only a technique under investigation, best left to centers and surgeons with experience in advanced minimally invasive surgery.

Perforated colon cancers

Patients with perforated colon cancers often present with peritonitis. In this setting, the goals of surgical management are to remove the diseased segment of colon and prevent ongoing peritoneal contamination. Following resection and thorough irrigation of the peritoneal cavity, options for subsequent management include proximal diversion with creation of a mucous fistula/Hartmann pouch or primary anastomosis with proximal diversion via loop ileostomy. Perforated colon cancer is associated with a high rate of local recurrence and low rate of OS.[195]

Obstructing colon cancers

Cancer is the most common cause of large-bowel obstruction.[196] Obstructing right and transverse colon cancers are generally managed with a right hemicolectomy and primary anastomosis. Left-sided colon cancers can be managed with either a single-stage operation or a two-stage procedure. The options for single-stage management include segmental resection or subtotal colectomy with IRA. Subtotal colectomy is attractive because it removes the remaining of the potentially compromised colon, but it is a more extensive operation and may be associated with five to six bowel movements per day. On-table lavage has been used in the setting of segmental resection for obstruction, but postoperative complication rates remain a concern. A two-stage procedure involves first, resection of the primary tumor with proximal diversion and creation of a mucous fistula or Hartmann's pouch. The second stage, performed at a later time, involves reanastomosis of the colon. An alternative two-stage approach in select patients with an obstructing left colon lesion is resection with primary anastomosis and proximal fecal diversion with a loop ileostomy.[196]

Colonic stenting has been an established option for patients with malignant colon obstruction. For patients who are not good candidates for surgery.[197,198] Although it does not represent a long-term solution to the malignant colonic obstruction, stenting is useful in those whose prognosis is limited by the presence of metastatic disease or comorbidities. Stenting has also been used to allow transient relief of obstruction and bowel preparation with or without colonoscopic evaluation of the proximal colon before planned resection. A meta-analysis of seven randomized trials regarding colonic stent resulted 77% successful rate of stent placement and those treated with stenting had higher rates of primary anastomosis and lower rates of permanent ostomy.[199] However, this article has shown that 7% of patients had colonic perforation at stent insertion and another 14% had "silent" perforation discovered in the colectomy specimen. With concern for decreased survival due to these silent perforations, the European Society of Gastrointestinal Endoscopy (ESGE) clinical guideline recommends against its use for prophylactic purpose or bridge to elective surgery in curable patients who are good surgical candidates.[200]

Synchronous distant metastases

The liver is the most common site for colon cancer metastasis and approximately 17% of patients will present with synchronous liver metastasis.[135] Concomitant resection of colon and liver lesions may be undertaken safely in selected patients. Alternatively, management of liver metastasis may be dealt with at a subsequent operation. Systemic chemotherapy is also an essential component of therapy in these patients and will be discussed below.

Surveillance following resection

The goal of postoperative surveillance following resection of colon adenocarcinoma is identification of asymptomatic recurrences or new primaries that will allow for subsequent early treatment and lead to an improvement in survival. National Comprehensive Cancer Network (NCCN) guideline outlines recommendation for postsurgical surveillance (Table 8).[111,112] Colonoscopy is

Table 8 NCCN guidelines for surveillance following resection of stage II/III colorectal cancer.

Test	Recommendation
History and physical	Every 3–6 months for 2 years then every 6 months for a total of 5 years
Serum CEA	Every 3–6 months for 2 years then every 6 months for a total of 5 years
Colonoscopy	Colonoscopy in 1 year after surgery except if no preoperative colonoscopy due to obstructing lesion, colonoscopy in 3–6 months • If advanced adenoma, repeat in 1 year • If no advanced adenoma, repeat in 3 years, then every 5 years
Computed tomography	Chest/abdominal/pelvic CT every 6–12 months (category 2B for frequency <12 mo) for a total of 5 years

recommended for all stages at 1 year after surgery unless preoperative colonoscopy could not be performed due to obstructing lesion; in this case, colonoscopy should be performed in 3–6 months. For stage II and higher, serial CEA measurement and CT scan, as well as clinical examination, are recommended to assess distant metastasis. With these guidelines in mind, surveillance should be individualized depending on factors unique to a given case, including comorbidities and patient anxiety.

Local recurrence

Local recurrence following resection of colonic adenocarcinoma occurs in approximately 4% of cases with the highest rates in advanced-stage tumors.[201] Although these patients generally have a poor survival, surgical resection of locoregional recurrence can result in long-term survival in up to 15% of patients.[201] Best results are obtained in patients with isolated small recurrences (less than 5 cm) that can be resected with negative margins.

Adjuvant therapy for colorectal cancer

5-Fluorouracil-based regimens

The antifolate 5-FU has been the cornerstone of chemotherapy for CRC since the 1960s. A metabolite of 5-FU, fluorodeoxyuridine monophosphate (FdUMP), inhibits thymidylate synthase (TS) and thus interferes with DNA synthesis.[202] 5-FU is also incorporated into RNA, which disrupts protein synthesis. Studies, however, did not show a survival advantage for adjuvant 5-FU until it was combined with a biomodulator. Leucovorin (folinic acid), levamisole (an antihelminthic agent), and methotrexate were all explored as modulators of 5-FU.[203–207] Leucovorin (LV) has been accepted as the standard biomodulator and increases cytotoxicity by stabilizing the FdUMP/TS complex and increasing the intracellular pool of reduced folate.

Multiple prospective trials have shown the clinical benefit of postoperative 5-FU in combination with either leucovorin or levamisole.[203–206] The National Surgical Adjuvant Breast and Bowel Project C-03 trial showed that 6 months of 5-FU and LV were superior to combination therapy with methyl 1-[2-chloroethyl-3-(4methyl-cyclohexyl)] (CCNU), vincristine, and 5-FU.[207] The incremental increases in DFS from 64% to 73% and in OS from 77% to 84% were proportionally similar to other randomized trials with 5-FU and LV.[207]

The convenience of oral therapy and the prospect of avoiding long-term intravenous access complications, such as thrombosis and infection, have stimulated development of oral fluoropyrimidines. Capecitabine is a fluoropyrimidine carbamate that is converted to 5-FU in a three-step enzymatic cascade. Preclinical studies showed that capecitabine exhibits selectivity for neoplastic cells because the final enzymatic conversion involves thymidine phosphorylase, which is preferentially expressed in tumor as opposed to normal tissues.[208,209] Twice-daily oral administration simulates continuous infusion of 5-FU without the costs and inconvenience of a pump.

The X-ACT trial showed that capecitabine was at least equivalent to bolus 5-FU in the adjuvant setting.[208] This noninferiority trial randomized 1987 patients with resected stage III colon cancer to 6 months of adjuvant capecitabine twice daily for 2 weeks of a 3-week schedule or to bolus 5-FU daily days 1 through 5 of a 28-day cycle. The 3-year DFS was 64.2% in the capecitabine arm compared with 60.6% in the bolus 5-FU arm. With a hazard ratio of 0.87% and a $p < 0.001$, this study met its primary endpoint of equivalent DFS. The side effect profiles are slightly different, with capecitabine having an increased risk for hand-foot syndrome but markedly improved reductions in neutropenia and stomatitis seen in the bolus regimen.[208]

Oxaliplatin-based regimens

Oxaliplatin is a third-generation platinum compound that crosslinks DNA and induces apoptosis. Oxaliplatin has properties that are distinct from other platinum compounds such as cisplatin and carboplatin. The preclinical models showed both activity in cisplatin-resistant CRC cell lines and synergism when combined with 5-FU.[210] Oxaliplatin causes little nephrotoxicity, ototoxicity, and alopecia, but shares bone marrow suppressive properties and has its own sensory neuropathy that is typically reversible, cumulative, and exacerbated by exposure to cold.[210–213]

Oxaliplatin was quickly moved to the adjuvant setting after initial studies showed its efficacy in the metastatic setting. The MOSAIC trial randomized 2246 stage II (node-negative) and stage III patients to receive either oxaliplatin, folinic acid, and 5-FU (FOLFOX-4) combination or infusional 5-FU/LV.[210,212,213] FOLFOX-4 included the same regimen of 5-FU/LV with addition of oxaliplatin.[210] The probability of being free of disease at 3 years was 78.2% in the FOLFOX-4 arm compared with 72.9% in the infusional 5-FU/LV arm. Subgroup analysis revealed that stage III patients derived more benefit as evidenced by 3-year DFS (72% receiving FOLFOX-4 vs 65% receiving 5-FU/LV, $p = 0.0002$) than stage II patients (87% receiving FOLFOX-4 vs 84% receiving 5-FU/LV, $p =$ ns). Oxaliplatin regimens are still restricted by their dose-limiting toxicity of neuropathy, which seriously affected 12% of patients during the trial but the percentage of patients affected dropped to 0.5% after 18 months.[210,212] In 2009, long-term results from the MOSAIC trial were published, which demonstrated statistically significant improvements in 5-year DFS (73.3% vs 67.4%).[214] Among patients with stage III disease, there was a corresponding improvement in 6-year OS (72.9% vs 68.7%); however, there was no statistically significant difference in OS for patients with stage II disease. Furthermore, a subgroup analysis of the MOSAIC trial demonstrated that elderly patients (70–75 years old) with both stage II and III disease did not benefit from the addition of oxaliplatin to 5-FU/LV (Hazard ratio 1.1 for OS).[215] The benefit of oxaliplatin does not appear to be dependent on the schedule of 5-FU/LV. NSABP C-07 randomized 2407 patients with stage II/III colon cancer to bolus weekly 5-FU/LV (Roswell Park Regimen) or to FLOX (the same 5-FU/LV regimen with biweekly oxaliplatin).[211] The improvement in the hazard ratios and DFS was similar to that seen in the MOSAIC trial. The probability of being alive and free of disease at 3 years was 76.5% in the oxaliplatin arm compared with 71.6% in the control arm.[367] Although the efficacy of FLOX looked similar to the infusional 5-FU used in the MOSAIC trial, it does appear to be slightly more toxic, with increased diarrhea and dehydration. Modified FOLFOX-6 has been accepted as the preferred dosing schedule for the FOLFOX regimen.[216]

Regimen with capecitabine, instead of 5-FU/LV, is also proven effective and offers increased convenience The combination of capecitabine plus oxaliplatin infusion, a regimen termed XELOX was directly compared with standard intravenous bolus FU/LV.[217] In this Phase III trial involving 1886 patients with stage III colon cancer, after a median follow-up of 74 months, significantly superior DFS (7-year DFS 63% vs 56%) and overall survival (7-year overall survival 73% vs 67%) with XELOX were reported.

Irinotecan-based regimens
Irinotecan is a camptothecin derivative that inhibits topoisomerase I by stabilizing DNA breaks that arise in DNA uncoiling for transcription and replication.[218] Irinotecan is hydrolyzed in the liver to its active metabolite, SN-38, which in turn is glucuronidated to an inactive form by uridine diphosphate glucuronosyltransferase isoform 1A1 (UGT1A1).[218] The adverse events associated with irinotecan, including diarrhea, bone marrow suppression, and nausea or vomiting, have been shown in retrospective studies to correlate with polymorphisms of UGT1A1.

Two randomized controlled trials showed improved survival in patients receiving irinotecan along with 5-FU/LV, compared with 5-FU/LV alone, as first-line therapy in metastatic disease.[219,220] Despite the proven benefit in advanced disease, results from three large trials do not support the use of irinotecan in the adjuvant setting. CALGB C89803 compared a bolus version of irinotecan with 5-FU/LV (IFL) with 5-FU/LV alone and found an increase in grade III-IV toxicities (neutropenia, neutropenic fever, and death on treatment) without an improvement in DFS.[221] PETACC-3 and Accord02/FFCD9802 compared the addition of irinotecan with infusional 5-FU and also found increased toxicities in the experimental arm with no improvement in DFS in patients with stage III cancer.[222,223] On the basis of these trials, irinotecan-based regimens are not recommended in the adjuvant setting.

Biologic agents
The two most recent FDA-approved therapies in metastatic colon cancer are "targeted," "biologic" agents rather than standard cytotoxic drugs. Both agents are monoclonal antibodies. Bevacizumab targets the vascular endothelial growth factor (VEGF) pathway and cetuximab is directed against the EGFR pathway.

Bevacizumab is a humanized recombinant monoclonal antibody directed against VEGF. By binding ligand and preventing signaling of the VEGF receptor, bevacizumab is thought to interfere with the recruitment and growth of tumor-feeding blood vessels. Two Phase III trials have shown an improvement in both DFS and OS after the addition of bevacizumab to 5-FU-based regimens combined with either oxaliplatin or irinotecan in the metastatic setting.[224,225] Side effects seen in these trials thought to be due to the addition of bevacizumab included reversible hypertension and proteinuria, as well as rare serious, but not statistically significant, side effects including gastrointestinal perforation, wound dehiscence, bleeding, and clotting.[224,225] The AVANT trial compared FOLFOX-4, FOLFOX-4 plus bevacizumab, and XELOX plus bevacizumab in patients with stage III or high-risk stage II colon cancers.[226] This trial found that the addition of bevacizumab to oxaliplatin-based adjuvant chemotherapy did not improve DFS, and suggested that its addition may in fact result in decreased OS. The NSABP C-08 trial compared the addition of bevacizumab to modified FOLFOX-6 versus modified FOLFOX-6 alone in patients with resected stage II and III colon cancers and also found that the addition of bevacizumab did not increase 3-year DFS.[227]

Cetuximab is a monoclonal antibody directed against EGFR, which is involved with multiple growth signaling pathways. Cetuximab received FDA approval for treatment of irinotecan-resistant metastatic disease in 2004. In irinotecan refractory disease, a 22% response rate was reached in patients treated with cetuximab/irinotecan compared with an 11% response rate with cetuximab as a single agent in a randomized Phase II trial.[228] The side effects of cetuximab are relatively mild, with an acneiform rash over the face, chest, and back occurring in most patients.[228] Allergic reactions also occur as cetuximab, unlike bevacizumab, is not fully humanized.[228] The US Intergroup N0147 trial comparing FOLFOX-4 with and without cetuximab for patients with resected stage III colon cancer found no difference in 3-year DFS for either patients with wild-type or mutant KRAS.[229] Moreover, grade 3 adverse events and failure to complete 12 cycles of therapy were significantly higher in patients treated with cetuximab.

Summary recommendations
The magnitude of benefit from adjuvant therapy appears to be proportional to the risk of relapse based on pathologic stage. For stage III (node-positive) patients, the evidence supports the use of adjuvant chemotherapy for 6 months following resection.[111] FOLFOX or XELOX has the most convincing efficacy data but is associated with increased toxicities compared with 5-FU/LV alone. Capecitabine is a reasonable alternative to intravenous 5-FU/LV. Irinotecan-based regimens cannot be recommended in the adjuvant setting, nor can the addition of bevacizumab and cetuximab to established adjuvant regimens. For stage II (node-negative) patients, the absolute benefit appears to be real but much smaller. Following the NCCN practice guidelines, combination regimen with FOLFOX or XELOX, or single-agent regimen with 5-FU or capecitabine is often considered if the pathology displays high-risk features such as T4, poor differentiation, lymphatic or vascular invasion, bowel obstruction, inadequate staging (<12 lymph nodes removed), perineural invasion, perforation, or close/indeterminate/positive margins.[111] For stage II patients with no high-risk features, observation or single-agent regimen with 5-FU or capecitabine is recommended.[111]

The role of adjuvant chemotherapy in older patients remains controversial, particularly regarding the addition of oxaliplatin to 5-FU based therapies. While the MOSAIC trial failed to demonstrate a benefit in adding oxaliplatin to 5-FU/LV,[215] pooled analysis of three randomized clinical trials suggested that efficacy of adjuvant 5-FU-based chemotherapy was maintained in the elderly (defined as 70 years of age and older), and that toxicity was similar to younger patients except for an increase in leucopenia in one study.[230,231]

Neoadjuvant and adjuvant therapy for rectal cancer
As in colon cancer, surgical resection remains the cornerstone of the curative approach for rectal cancer. However, unlike colon cancer, there is significant tendency for local failure after potentially

curative resection. Improvements in the initial surgical procedure by performing a TME have reduced but not eliminated the risk of local recurrence. Salvage surgical procedures are technically difficult, often unsuccessful, and fraught with morbidity. Therefore the major difference in the treatment paradigm for rectal as compared with colon cancer is the addition of radiation therapy to reduce the risk of local failure.

Neoadjuvant chemotherapy and radiation

The neoadjuvant approach is particularly attractive in rectal cancer because downstaging may increase ease and rates of resectability, allow potential sphincter preservation, and increase compliance by avoiding long postoperative recoveries. The Swedish Rectal Cancer Trial was the first to show that a short-term regimen of high-dose preoperative radiotherapy decreased the rate of local recurrence and improved survival compared with surgery alone.[232] The German Phase III EORTC 22921 study was the first study to complete accrual in comparing neoadjuvant therapy with combined 5-FU/radiation to postoperative adjuvant 5-FU/radiation.[145] Patients with tumor extending through the muscle wall (T3) or with positive nodes (N1) were randomized to preoperative or postoperative chemoradiation. In both arms, the radiation (5040 GY in 28 fractions) was combined with 5-FU. All patients received additional systemic 5-FU for 4 months. The study failed to see an improvement in OS, but preoperative therapy was associated with an improved rate of local control at 5 years (6% failure compared to 13%), reduced acute and chronic toxicity, increased compliance, and an increased rate of sphincter preservation in patients with low-ling tumors.[145] Interestingly, posttreatment pathology results proved to be highly prognostic with patients who showed marked regression or negative nodes having improved DFS.[145] In 2012, long-term results from the German trial became available. At 10 years, preoperative chemoradiation therapy was associated with improved local control compared to postoperative therapy; however, there remained no difference in OS.[233] There are several theoretical benefits of neoadjuvant as opposed to adjuvant chemoradiation therapy. First, there is the increased possibility of ultimately performing a sphincter-sparing resection. While two studies have demonstrated higher rates of sphincter preservation,[145,234] other large meta-analyses have disputed these findings.[235,236] During resection, adhesions can result in bowel that becomes fixed in the pelvis. By administering radiation in the preoperative versus postoperative period, daily radiation to the same segment of fixed bowel can be avoided. A third hypothetical benefit is the presence of intact vasculature prior to resection, which may result in greater tissue oxygenation and better response to radiation.

Short-course radiation

Short-course radiation (e.g., Swedish or European approach) refers to 25 Gy of radiation without chemotherapy over a 5-day time period. Initially, the Swedish Rectal Cancer Trial demonstrated improved rates of local recurrence and OS for short-course preoperative radiotherapy compared to surgery alone.[232] However, a later analysis of this study population demonstrated that patients treated with short-course radiation had higher rates of gastrointestinal morbidity following surgery, most notably, bowel obstructions.[237] In a large randomized trial of more than 1300 patients, short-course preoperative radiation without any adjuvant therapy was compared to postoperative chemoradiation therapy in patients with a positive circumferential margin.[238] Short-course radiation was associated with improved local recurrence rates and DFS, although there was no detectable difference in OS. More recently, the TME trial comparing patients treated with short-course radiation to patients who underwent TME alone demonstrated improvements in local recurrence (5% vs 11%) without a corresponding increase in OS.[239] While OS was significantly improved among stage III patients treated with short-course RT who had a negative circumferential margin, among node-negative patients with negative margins the improvement in CRC-specific mortality was countered by an increase in other causes of death. Only one randomized trial has directly compared short-course high-dose radiotherapy to conventional preoperative chemoradiation, which showed no improvement in local recurrence, RFS, or OS.[240] Short-course radiation therapy appears to result in equivalent local control compared with traditional long-course chemoradiation therapy; however, improvements in OS have not been appreciated, and concerns about increased perioperative toxicity remain.

Indication

At present, T3–T4 tumor is the only definitive indication for neoadjuvant therapy supported by randomized trials. Among T3 tumors, a number of studies have shown that tumors with >5 mm extramural invasion have a higher rate of nodal involvement and worse prognosis.[241] Although this is not yet validated and incorporated into TNM staging, the European Society for Medical Oncology (ESMO) guidelines suggest that patients with a depth of invasion beyond the muscularis propria that is 5 mm or less are appropriate candidates for upfront surgery rather than neoadjuvant chemoradiotherapy, even if they are node positive.[242] In addition to clinical T3–T4 tumor, there are relative indications for neoadjuvant chemoradiotherapy, which includes T1/2 tumor with nodal involvement, or a tumor that appears to invade or "threaten" CRM. Neoadjuvant therapy for a distal cT1N0 or cT2N0 rectal cancer to avoid APR is controversial and not yet an accepted standard of care. Traditionally, the interval between completion of conventional neoadjuvant chemoradiotherapy and surgery has been 6 weeks as this was the duration used in the German Rectal Cancer Study Group trial. However, it was suggested the tumor regression takes time more than 6 weeks and multiple trials have been conducted to assess an adequate interval. A meta-analysis of data from randomized trials and nonrandomized series revealed a minimum 8-week interval is associated with greater odds of a pCR (OR 1.41, 95% CI 1.30–1.52) and tumor downstaging (OR 1.33, 95% CI 1.04–1.72) compared with a standard 6–8-week interval.[243] At present, the NCCN guidelines recommend an interval of 5–12 weeks.[112]

Total neoadjuvant therapy

Total neoadjuvant therapy (TNT) is a new approach to locally advanced rectal cancer owing to its high efficacy of neoadjuvant therapy. With this approach, preoperative systemic chemotherapy, such as FOLFOX, is given in combination with radiation compared with the traditional preoperative chemoradiation and postoperative adjuvant chemotherapy. It is reported higher rates of resectability and pCR can be achieved with this approach.[244] Improved compliance is also expected. Although there are no Phase III trials comparing this approach with neoadjuvant chemoradiotherapy alone, Phase II trials suggest good long-term outcomes with TNT.[245–247] Based on these results, current NCCN guidelines suggest TNT as a viable treatment strategy for patients with T3 tumors with an involved CRM, T4 tumors, or N1/2 disease, or for locally unresectable or medically inoperable patients with rectal cancer.[112] Long-term follow-up is needed to determine this approach leads to improved OS.

Watch and wait nonoperative management

The management of patients with clinical complete response (cCR) is an evolving topic. It is reported that conventional preoperative chemoradiotherapy can achieve pathological complete response (pCR) in about 20% patients.[248] Compared with patients who did not achieve a pCR, a pCR was associated with fewer local recurrences, less frequent distant failure, and a greater likelihood of being alive at 5 years.[249] With these favorable results, a nonoperative treatment strategy after cCR is emerging and under investigation. In one propensity-score-matched cohort analysis, 129 patients were offered a watch and wait approach after cCR with neoadjuvant chemotherapy.[250] Of the 129 patients managed with the watch and wait approach, 44 (34%) had local regrowth. Of the 41 patients with nonmetastatic local regrowth, 36 (88%) were salvaged by surgical resection. There was no significant difference in 3-year nonregrowth DFS (88% with watch and wait vs 78% with surgical resection) or 3-year overall survival (96% vs 87%).[250] However, the patients in the watch and wait group had a significantly higher rate of 3-year colostomy-free survival than those undergoing initial surgery (74% vs 47%).[250] The noninferior overall survival and disease-specific survival with the watch and wait strategy was also reported in a systematic review of 23 retrospective studies though poorer DFS is noted due to the intraluminal local regrowth.[251] Although there is no prospective randomized study performed, the NCCN guidelines suggest a "watch and wait" nonoperative management approach may be considered in centers with experienced multidisciplinary teams in patients who achieve a complete clinical response with no evidence of residual disease.[112] Currently, several prospective randomized trials of nonoperative therapy in complete responders to induction therapy are underway.

Adjuvant chemotherapy and radiation

Studies in the 1980s and 1990s solidified the superiority of postoperative chemoradiation over surgery alone and surgery followed by radiation without chemotherapy. A trial in 2012 comparing capecitabine-based chemoradiotherapy with 5-FU-based radiotherapy in patients with stage II–III rectal cancer found that capecitabine was noninferior to 5-FU in terms of 5-year OS, 3-year DFS, and local recurrence.[252] Distant metastasis was less common in the capecitabine group. Adverse reactions differed between the two arms, with leukopenia more common in patients receiving 5-FU, and hand-food skin reactions, fatigue, and proctitis more common in the capecitabine group. Capecitabine is thus a reasonable alternative to 5-FU in adjuvant chemoradiation regimens. In general, adjuvant therapy is recommended for any tumor that is T3 or greater or is node positive. Radiation therapy should be directed at the tumor bed, including a 2–5 cm margin as well as the presacral nodes and the internal iliac nodes. If an APR was performed, the perineal wound should be included in the radiation field.[112]

Summary recommendations

Neoadjuvant chemoradiation therapy has been shown to result in tumor downstaging in approximately half of patients, with a pathologic complete response in up to 20%.[248] Given that it is associated with a superior overall compliance rate, an improved rate of local control, reduced toxicity, improved function, and perhaps an increased rate of sphincter preservation in patients with low-lying tumors, although no survival benefit has been proven with preoperative compared to postoperative chemoradiotherapy, it is suggested that preoperative chemoradiotherapy be the preferred treatment for patients with locally advanced rectal cancer.[253] Although no trial has demonstrated conclusively that additional postoperative adjuvant 5-FU-based chemotherapy improves outcomes in patients who have undergone neoadjuvant chemoradiotherapy, the NCCN guidelines recommend that all such patients receive 5-FU-containing chemotherapy (FOLFOX, XELOX, 5-FU/LV, or capecitabine) even if they have a pathologic complete response to neoadjuvant therapy.[112]

Chemotherapy for hepatic metastasis

Conversion therapy

Selected patients with initially unresectable liver metastases may become eligible for resection if the response to chemotherapy is sufficient. This approach has been termed "conversion therapy" to distinguish it from "neoadjuvant therapy" which applies to preoperative chemotherapy given to patients who present upfront with apparently resectable disease. The key parameter for selecting the specific regimen in this scenario is not survival or improved quality of life (QOL), but instead, response rate. The NCCN currently recommends any chemotherapeutic regimen that is active in the metastatic setting, as the goal of conversion therapy is not to treat occult disease, but rather to obtain the tumor regression necessary to convert unresectable metastases to a resectable state.[111] Regimens studied include FOLFIRI,[254] FOLFOX,[255] FOLFOXIRI.[256,257] Between 12% and 40% of patients with isolated but initially unresectable CRC liver metastases have a sufficient downstaging response to permit a subsequent complete resection.[254–257] Following resection, 5-year survival rates average 30–35%, results that are substantially better than expected using chemotherapy alone. In the largest study, 138 (12.5%) of 1104 patients with initially unresectable CRC liver metastases were able to undergo resection after induction chemotherapy that consisted mainly of 5-FU/LV combined with either oxaliplatin (70%), irinotecan (7%), or both (4%).[258] Overall 5- and 10-year survival was 33% and 23%, respectively. Targeted and biologic agents have been tested in combination with established chemotherapy regimens in the conversion setting. Although not fully proven, it is usually said the addition a biologic agent to chemotherapy regimen may increase the number of patients potentially eligible for resection and improve outcomes. Cetuximab and panitumumab are EGFR blockers effective for individuals with RAS and BRAF wild-type tumors. The CRYSTAL and OPUS trials are two randomized trials, showed improved resection rates from 3.7% to 7% and from 2.4% to 4.7%, respectively, by adding cetuximab to an irinotecan- or oxaliplatin-based regimen.[259,260] The NCCN guideline recommends to add those agents to either FOLFOX, FOLFILI, or FOLFOXILI for patients with wild-type RAS/BRAF and left-sided tumors.[111,112] Bevacizumab, a VEGF blocker, has also been tested in combination with established chemotherapies in the setting of unresectable disease.[261] While there may be an improvement in conversion rates using bevacizumab, clinicians need to be cautious for its potential adverse effect especially in preoperative setting. This includes stroke and arterial thromboembolic events, bowel perforation, and bleeding, which could interfere subsequent surgical intervention. In addition, impaired wound healing and possibly impaired hepatic regeneration are of concern, particularly if performed too soon after bevacizumab administration. Thus, although its use in combination with established regimens is recommended, the NCCN guidelines warned an interval at least a

6-week between the last dose of bevacizumab and elective surgery, given the long half-life of bevacizumab (20 days).[111,112] To note chemotherapy alone is not curative in this setting with the majority of radiographic completely responding lesions containing viable tumor. Thus, even in the setting of a complete clinical response, resection is still needed.

Neoadjuvant therapy for hepatic metastasis

There is evidence that perioperative chemotherapy improves both progression-free survival and disease-free survival among patients with initially resectable hepatic metastases; however, its effect on overall survival remains unproven.[262] Whether patients benefit most from pre- or postoperative therapy remains unclear. The theoretical benefits of neoadjuvant chemotherapy for patients with resectable hepatic metastases include the guarantee that these patients will receive systemic therapy (versus patients who are unable to tolerate postoperative therapy), as well as an earlier initiation of systemic therapy compared to those who receive adjuvant chemotherapy. The EORTC trial randomly assigned 364 patients with up to four metastases without prior exposure to oxaliplatin to liver resection with or without perioperative FOLFOX-4 chemotherapy.[263] Six cycles of chemotherapy were administered prior to surgery, and six cycles were administered postoperatively. Sixty-seven of the 182 patients assigned to chemotherapy had an objective response, while 11 progressed, eight of whom were no longer considered resectable. Overall, 83% of patients were successfully resected, similar to the number who were successfully resected in the surgery alone group, 84%. The postoperative complication rate, however, was significantly higher in the chemotherapy group (25% vs 16%). Patients receiving perioperative chemotherapy had higher rates of hepatic failure, biliary fistulas, and intraabdominal infection. Postoperative mortality was similar between groups. There is increasing evidence that for patients with resectable hepatic metastases, the use of preoperative chemotherapy is associated with hepatic steatosis, vascular injury, and nodular regenerative hyperplasia, particularly among patients treated with irinotecan or oxaliplatin-containing regimens.[258,264,265] Moreover, there is evidence that among patients who have complete radiographic responses to neoadjuvant therapy, most sites of metastasis nonetheless harbor viable cancer cells.[424] Therefore, the NCCN guidelines recommend initial resection is preferred over neoadjuvant therapy. In case of neoadjuvant therapy is desirable, the NCCN recommends neoadjuvant therapy for 2–3 months with either FOLFOX, XELOX, FOLFIRI, or FOLFOXIRI followed by synchronous or staged colectomy and resection of metastatic disease.

Adjuvant therapy after hepatic resection

Adjuvant chemotherapy is commonly recommended following resection of hepatic colorectal metastasis despite the lack of data to support its use.[111,112] There are many unknowns, including the timing of resection, optimal drug combination, schedule, and duration of therapy. Although data is limited, FOLFOX or XELOX is currently recommended as the preferred regimens for six months in total with preoperative treatment. Irinotecan-based regimen is generally avoided in this setting with the lack of proven benefit. Because of the same reason, biologic therapy is only appropriate for continuation of favorable neoadjuvant response.

Summary recommendations

There are no widely accepted guidelines for determining which patients with CRC liver metastases should undergo immediate surgery and when neoadjuvant chemotherapy is indicated. However, the increasing reports of liver injury following neoadjuvant chemotherapy have prompted most physicians to recommend initial surgery for low risk (medically fit with four or fewer lesions), potentially resectable patients, followed by adjuvant chemotherapy.[266] On the other hand, neoadjuvant chemotherapy is reasonable for those who are higher risk or have borderline resectable or unresectable liver metastases. However, the duration should be limited, radiographic response assessment performed frequently, and surgery undertaken as soon as the metastases become clearly resectable.

Metastatic colorectal cancer

The last two decades have seen unprecedented advances in the treatment of metastatic CRC. In the era when 5-FU was the sole active agent, OS was approximately 11–12 months. Currently, the average median survival duration has doubled, with patients routinely living longer than 2 years. The average median survival duration is now approaching 3 years, and 5-year survival rates as high as 20% are reported in some trials of patients treated with chemotherapy alone.[267] This increase has been mainly driven by the availability of new active agents. There are now three different classes of primary chemotherapies with significant antitumor activity (fluoropyrimidines, irinotecan, and oxaliplatin), as well as multiple targeted and biologic therapies with an emerging role in the treatment of CRC (e.g., cetuximab, bevacizumab, and panitumumab). For most patients, the goal of treatment will be palliative and not curative, with the treatment goals being to prolong OS and maintain QOL for as long as possible. For most patients with noncurable metastatic CRC, rationally designed combinations, such as FOLFOX (folinic acid, 5-FU, oxaliplatin) or FOLFIRI (folinic acid, 5-FU, irinotecan) should be considered the standard chemotherapy backbone for first-line palliative therapy. These regimens have well-documented activity and a tolerable toxicity profile. Other appropriate therapies include XELOX, 5-FU/LV, capecitabine, and FOLFOXIRI. Commonly used combination regimens are shown in Table 9.

It is to be noted that the proportion of patients exposed to all three drug classes, fluoropyrimidines, irinotecan, and oxaliplatin, during the course of therapy correlates strongly with median survival.[272] In view of this observation, combination chemotherapy with a doublet, or even with a triplet if tolerable, is recommended as a backbone of initial therapy as this strategy increases the likelihood of exposure to all three drugs.[273,274]

FOLFOX

The first large size, randomized Phase III trial comparing 5-FU and leucovorin versus FOLFOX-4 included 420 patients.[213] Patients allocated to receive FOLFOX-4 had significantly longer PFS (median 9.0 vs 6.2 months; $p = 0.0003$) and better response rate (50.7% vs 22.3%; $p = 0.0001$) when compared with the control arm. However, although a trend could be seen, the improvement in OS did not reach statistical significance (median, 16.2 vs 14.7 months, $p = 0.12$).[213] The lack of survival benefit in this European trial delayed FOLFOX acceptance in the United States. Shortly after, the NCCTG and the American intergroup conducted the N9741, a Phase III trial with three arms.[270] The control arm received IFL regimen, and oxaliplatin was included in the two experimental arms. It was combined with irinotecan in the irinotecan and oxaliplatin (IROX) regimen, or with 5-FU and leucovorin, following the FOLFOX-4 regimen.[270] The final results showed a median

Table 9 Commonly used combination chemotherapy regimens.

Regimen		Doses	Schedule
5-FU/LV[268]		Leucovorin (LV) 200 mg/m^2 over 2 h day 1; Fluorouracil (5-FU) 400 mg/m^2 bolus day 1, 600 mg/m^2 over 22 h, days 1 and 2 (de Gramont schedule)	Every 2 weeks
IFL[269]		Irinotecan 125 mg/m^2 day 1; LV 20 mg/m^2; 5-FU 500 mg/m^2	Weekly for 4 weeks followed by 2-week rest in a 6-week cycle
IROX[270]		Irinotecan 200 mg/m^2 day 1; Oxaliplatin 85 mg/m^2 day 1	Every 3 weeks
FOLFILI[216]		Irinotecan 180 mg/m^2 day 1; LV 400 mg/m^2 over 2 h day 1; 5-FU 400 mg/m^2 bolus day 1, followed by 2400–3000 mg/m^2 over 46 h, continuous infusion	Every 2 weeks
FOLFOX	FOLFOX-4[270]	Oxaliplatin 85 mg/m^2 day 1; LV 400 mg/m^2 over 2 h days 1 and 2 before fluorouracil; 5-FU 400 mg/m^2 bolus, then 600 mg/m^2 over 22 h days 1 and 2	Every 2 weeks
	FOLFOX-6[216]	Oxaliplatin 100 mg/m^2 day 1; LV 400 mg/m^2 over 2 h day 1; 5-FU 400 mg/m^2 bolus day 1, followed by 2000–3600 mg/m over 46 h, continuous infusion	Every 2 weeks
	mFOLFOX-6[271]	Oxaliplatin 85 mg/m^2 day 1; LV 350 mg total dose over 2 h day 1; 5-FU 400 mg/m^2 bolus day 1, followed by 2400 mg/m^2 over 46 h	Every 2 weeks
XELOX[271]		Oxaliplatin 130 mg/m^2 day 1; Capecitabine 1000 mg/m^2 orally twice per day on days 1–14	Every 3 weeks
FOLFOXILI[256]		Irinotecan 165 mg/m^2 day 1; Oxaliplatin 85 mg/m^2 day 1; Leucovorin 400 mg/m^2 leucovorin over 2 h day 1; 5-FU 3200 mg/m^2 over 48 h	Every 2 weeks

time to progression of 8.7 months, response rate of 45%, and median survival time of 19.5 months for those patients assigned to FOLFOX-4. These results were significantly superior to those observed for IFL (6.9 months, 31%, and 15.0 months, respectively) or for IROX (6.5 months, 35%, and 1.4 months, respectively).[270] FOLFOX-4 was generally well tolerated but it was associated with a significantly higher rate of sensory neuropathy as described above. In the United States, modified FOLFOX-6 (mFOLFOX-6) is currently most commonly used as the preferred dosing schedule for the FOLFOX regimen because it does not require a day 2 bolus of leucovorin.[216]

Capecitabine/XELOX

Capecitabine, an orally active fluoropyrimidine, allows for the attractiveness of oral dosing, and the potential for eliminating the need for a central venous catheter and ambulatory infusion pump. At least five randomized Phase III trials have directly compared XELOX (capecitabine, oxaliplatin) versus FOLFOX for first-line or second-line chemotherapy in metastatic CRC.[275,276] None showed that XELOX was inferior to FOLFOX-type regimens in terms of response rate, PFS, or OS. However, in nearly all cases, the PFS and OS curves for XELOX trailed beneath the curves for FOLFOX. In no case was this effect statistically significant or clinically meaningful. Thus, the available evidence supports the view that XELOX can be considered as a noninferior substitute for FOLFOX in palliative therapy.

FOLFIRI

The effectiveness of irinotecan was initially demonstrated in a randomized Phase III trial conducted to evaluate irinotecan with or without standard bolus 5-FU and leucovorin versus a standard regimen of bolus 5-FU and leucovorin.[220] The combination regimen became known as the IFL regimen and included 5-FU, leucovorin, and irinotecan given weekly for 4 weeks every 6 weeks. Irinotecan alone was given at 125 mg/m^2 weekly for 4 weeks every 6 weeks, and the 5-FU/LV was given using the standard Mayo Regimen as described above.[220] The three-drug regimen was superior to either 5-FU and leucovorin or to irinotecan alone, and the latter produced similar results as the 5-FU/LV regimen. In a comparison of IFL and the Mayo regimens, the median PFS improved from 4.3 months to 7.0 months, and the median OS improved from 12.6 months to 14.8 months.[220] FOLFIRI is a variation of IFL using infusional 5-FU, leucovorin, and irinotecan. A European trial compared the use of FOLFIRI versus FOLFOX as a first-line therapy for metastatic CRC.[216] Although it has been criticized for its relatively small size, this trial was important because it showed similar response rates and median survivals for FOLFOX and FOLFIRI. These data are supported further by the 2005 multicenter trial from the Gruppo Oncologico Dell'Italia Meridionale, in which 360 patients were randomized to FOLFIRI versus FOLFOX4.[277] There were no differences in response rates, time to progression, duration of response, or overall survival between arms. A Phase III trial from Japan also confirmed noninferiority for PFS with FOLFIRI plus bevacizumab compared with mFOLFOX6 plus bevacizumab.[278]

While XELOX may be regarded as a valid substitute for FOLFOX, the situation is different for combinations of capecitabine with irinotecan (XELIRI) as an alternative to FOLFIRI. Capecitabine and irinotecan have partially overlapping toxicity profiles, particularly with regard to diarrhea. The potential for greater toxicity reduces the therapeutic advantage of an irinotecan/capecitabine combination and makes the selection of appropriate doses and schedules for this combination difficult.[248]

FOLFOXIRI

There have been four trials comparing FOLFOXIRI to a doublet regimen among patients with metastatic CRC.[256,279–281] The first trial randomized 244 treatment-naïve patients with metastatic, unresectable CRC to receive either FOLFOXIRI or FOLFIRI.[256] Partial response rates were higher in the FOLFIRI arm (44% vs 66%); however, there was no difference in complete response. Patients in the FOLFOXIRI arm were more likely to undergo a complete resection of their hepatic metastases (12% vs 36%). Most importantly, both PFS and OS were significantly improved in the FOLFOXIRI arm (7 vs 10 months and 17 vs 23 months, respectively).[256] The TRIBE trial showed similar high rates of objective response and significantly better median overall survival with FOLFOXIRI plus bevacizumab as compared with FOLFIRI plus bevacizumab (29.8 vs 25.8 months).[280] On the other hand, it was also reported that grade 3–4 toxic effects were more common with FOLFOXIRI including diarrhea, stomatitis, neutropenia, and peripheral neuropathy. The HORG trial also compared FOLFOXIRI to FOLFIRI, although the FOLFOXIRI dosing regimen was slightly different.[279] In this trial, no differences in overall survival, time to disease progression, or response rates were appreciated between groups while FOLFOXIRI was associated with a higher rate of treatment toxicity, including alopecia, diarrhea, and neurotoxicity. The TRIBE2 trial is the most recent update that compared FOLFOXIRI with a preplanned sequential strategy of exposure to the same agents in two subsequent lines of therapy.[281] This study resulted in significantly prolonged progression-free survival with FOLFOXILI (19.2 vs 16.4 months) at the cost of significantly more grade 3 or 4 diarrhea and neutropenia. With these results, the NCCN guidelines currently recommend to consider FOLFOXIRI for patients with excellent performance status over a regimen with a doublet as a backbone of initial therapy.[111,112]

Bevacizumab

CRC was the first malignancy for which clear evidence for efficacy of an anti-VEGF strategy was obtained in randomized trials. In a pivotal early trial, the addition of bevacizumab to the bolus IFL regimen significantly improved response rates from 35% to 45%; PFS was extended from 7.1 to 10.4 months, and more importantly, the OS improved from 15.6 to 20.3 months.[224] The adverse events in this trial were similar among the treatment with some notable exceptions. Patients receiving bevacizumab had an 11% incidence of grade 3 hypertension and a 1.5% incidence of bowel perforations. No patients in the IFL arm presented with such problems.[224] The ECOG 3200 trial compared the use of FOLFOX to combination therapy of bevacizumab and FOLFOX.[225] The median survival for combination therapy was 12.5 versus 10.7 months for FOLFOX alone. This confirmed that bevacizumab does significantly add potency to oxaliplatin-based regimens. Since 2004, the majority of patients with metastatic CRC have received bevacizumab as a component of first-line therapy regardless of the specific regimen chosen for chemotherapy backbone (FOLFOX, XELOX, and FOLFIRI). With regard to the addition of bevacizumab to established regimens in the advanced setting, FOLFOXIRI/bevacizumab appears to have increased progression-free survival and response rates compared to FOLFIRI/bevacizumab among patients who have not received prior adjuvant therapy.[282] FOLFOXIRI/bevacizumab was also found to be superior to FOLFOX/bevacizumab in the conversion setting for patients with hepatic metastases (rate of R0 resection 49% vs 23%).[283]

Anti-EGFR monoclonal antibodies

The benefit of cetuximab added to first-line or second-line irinotecan-containing therapy has been addressed in the CRYSTAL trial and CALGB 80203.[284,285] In the CRYSTAL trial, 1198 previously untreated patients were randomly assigned to FOLFIRI with or without cetuximab.[285] Although the addition of cetuximab significantly improved PFS, the incremental gain was only 0.9 months. The addition of cetuximab also improved the response rate, but only by 8%.[285] Early results from the Phase II CALGB 80203 trial, which randomly assigned 283 patients to FOLFOX or FOLFIRI with or without cetuximab as first-line therapy, provided confirmatory data supporting the results of the CRYSTAL trial.[284] In a preliminary report, there was a clear demonstration of increased response rate with cetuximab in conjunction with both FOLFOX and FOLFIRI, while the impact on PFS was inconclusive.[284] Furthermore, a retrospective analysis of the CRYSTAL trial investigating the role of KRAS mutation status on PFS and response rate showed that in the KRAS wild-type population, the 1 year PFS rate for those who received cetuximab and FOLFIRI was 43% versus 25% for those who received FOLFIRI alone and the risk of progression was decreased by 32% in the combination treatment arm.[286] In the KRAS mutant population, however, there was no difference in PFS between the two arms. A meta-analysis of 14 trials comparing standard therapies with or without the use of anti-EGFR monoclonal antibodies was performed, which found an increase in progression-free survival only among patients with wild-type KRAS.[287] In this analysis, patients with KRAS mutations demonstrated no clinical benefit from anti-EGFR therapies. More recently, it has turned out that resistance to anti-EGFR therapies can also be mediated by mutations in NRAS, and exclusion of patients with all RAS mutations identifies a population that is more likely to benefit from an anti-EGFR agent.[288,289] As well, evidence increasingly suggests that response to EGFR-targeted agents is unlikely in patients whose tumors harbor BRAF V600E mutations, even if they are RAS wild type.[290,291] In addition to those genetic consideration, recent evidence suggests that patients with tumors originating on the right side of the colon (hepatic flexure through cecum) are unlikely respond to cetuximab and panitumumab in first-line therapy for metastatic disease.[292] Therefore, the NCCN guidelines also recommend anti-EGFR therapy for KRAS/NRAS/BRAF wildtype and left-sided tumors (splenic flexure to rectum).[111,112]

Finally, two large randomized trials have compared the addition of bevacizumab versus anti-EGFR therapy to established chemotherapies among patients with metastatic wildtype KRAS CRC.[293,294] In a subsequent meta-analysis of these two trials and a third randomized Phase II trial, patients with RAS wild-type left-sided colorectal tumors had a significantly greater survival benefit from anti-EGFR therapy compared with bevacizumab when added to standard chemotherapy (HR 0.71, 95% CI 0.58–0.85).[295] To note, Bevacizumab is usually the preferred biologic agent when combined with FOLFOXILI even for left-sided tumors, because there is no available data for EGFR therapy in combination with FOLFOXILI

Summary recommendations

Initial combination therapy is preferred for patients with nonoperable metastatic CRC, in whom the palliative treatment strategy should aim to maximize the number of patients exposed to all active agents. This is best achieved by using well-established combination doublets (i.e., FOLFOX, XELOX, or FOLFIRI) as the chemotherapy backbone, which would then only require one additional step to have all three active agents included in the treatment algorithm for second-line therapy (e.g., FOLFOX followed by FOLFIRI, or FOLFIRI followed by FOLFOX, or FOLFOXIRI). Bevacizumab should be considered a component of first-line therapy regardless of which regimen is chosen. Cetuximab in patients with KRAS/NRAS/BRAF wildtype and left-sided tumors is a better alternative to bevacizumab in combination with established chemotherapy regimens.

Conclusion

CRC is a common cancer affecting a large number of patients globally as well as in the United States. There has been a huge progress in multidisciplinary approach over two decades, which has improved the prognosis significantly. Given increasing complexity of the management, understanding entire aspects of CRC such as genetics, prevention, screening, surgery, and chemotherapy has become essential for the physician who leads multidisciplinary oncology team to provide with the best management.

Key references

The complete reference list can be found on Vital Source version of this title, see inside front cover.

1. Bray F, Ferlay J, Soerjomataram I, et al. Global cancer statistics 2018: GLOBOCAN estimates of incidence and mortality worldwide for 36 cancers in 185 countries. *CA Cancer J Clin*. 2018;**68**(6):394–424. doi: 10.3322/caac.21492.
2. Siegel RL, Miller KD, Jemal A. Cancer statistics, 2020. *CA Cancer J Clin*. 2020;**70**(1):7–30. doi: 10.3322/caac.21590.
6. Holowatyj AN, Ruterbusch JJ, Rozek LS, et al. Racial/ethnic disparities in survival among patients with young-onset colorectal cancer. *J Clin Oncol*. 2016;**34**(18):2148–2156. doi: 10.1200/JCO.2015.65.0994.
7. Phatak UR, Kao LS, Millas SG, et al. Interaction between age and race alters predicted survival in colorectal cancer. *Ann Surg Oncol*. 2013;**20**(11):3363–3369. doi: 10.1245/s10434-013-3045-z.
12. Innocenti F, Ou F-S, Qu X, et al. Mutational analysis of patients with colorectal cancer in CALGB/SWOG 80405 identifies new roles of microsatellite instability and tumor mutational burden for patient outcome. *J Clin Oncol*. 2019;**37**(14):1217–1227. doi: 10.1200/JCO.18.01798.
19. Brenner DR, Heer E, Sutherland RL, et al. National trends in colorectal cancer incidence among older and younger adults in Canada. *JAMA Netw Open*. 2019;**2**(7):e198090. doi: 10.1001/jamanetworkopen.2019.8090.
20. Siegel RL, Miller KD, Fedewa SA, et al. Colorectal cancer statistics, 2017: Colorectal Cancer Statistics, 2017. *CA Cancer J Clin*. 2017;**67**(3):177–193. doi: 10.3322/caac.21395.
48. Mármol I, Sánchez-de-Diego C, Pradilla Dieste A, et al. Colorectal carcinoma: a general overview and future perspectives in colorectal cancer. *Int J Mol Sci*. 2017;**18**(1):197. doi: 10.3390/ijms18010197.
54. Syngal S, Brand RE, Church JM, et al. ACG clinical guideline: Genetic testing and management of hereditary gastrointestinal cancer syndromes. *Am J Gastroenterol*. 2015;**110**(2):223–262; quiz 263. doi: 10.1038/ajg.2014.435.
85. National Comprehensive Cancer Network. *NCCN Clinical Practice Guidelines in Oncology (NCCN Guidelines®): Colorectal Cancer Screening. Version 2.2021*. https://www.nccn.org/professionals/physician_gls/pdf/colorectal_screening.pdf. (accessed 13 April 2021). Referenced with permission from the NCCN Clinical Practice Guidelines in Oncology (NCCN Guidelines®) for Colorectal Cancer Screening Version 2.2021. ©National Comprehensive Cancer Network, Inc. 2021. All rights reserved. Accessed on July 21, 2021. To view the most recent and complete version of the guideline, go online to NCCN.org. NCCN makes no warranties of any kind whatsoever regarding their content, use or application and disclaims any responsibility for their application or use in any way.
91. Rex DK, Boland CR, Dominitz JA, et al. Colorectal cancer screening: recommendations for physicians and patients from the U.S. Multi-Society Task Force on Colorectal Cancer. *Am J Gastroenterol*. 2017;**112**(7):1016–1030. doi: 10.1038/ajg.2017.174.
92. Qaseem A, Crandall CJ, Mustafa RA, et al. Physicians CGC of the AC of screening for colorectal cancer in asymptomatic average-risk adults: a guidance statement from the American College of Physicians. *Ann Intern Med*. 2019;**171**(9):643–654. doi: 10.7326/M19-0642.
104. Wolf AMD, Fontham ETH, Church TR, et al. Colorectal cancer screening for average-risk adults: 2018 guideline update from the American Cancer Society: ACS Colorectal Cancer Screening Guideline. *CA Cancer J Clin*. 2018;**68**(4):250–281. doi: 10.3322/caac.21457.
111. National Comprehensive Cancer Network. *NCCN Clinical Practice Guidelines in Oncology (NCCN Guidelines®): Colon Cancer. Version 4*. 2020. https://www.nccn.org/professionals/physician_gls/pdf/colon.pdf (accessed 15 June 2020).
112. National Comprehensive Cancer Network *NCCN Clinical Practice Guidelines in Oncology (NCCN Guidelines®): Rectal Cancer. Version 6.2020*. https://www.nccn.org/professionals/physician_gls/pdf/rectal.pdf (accessed 25 June 2020).
117. Bruening W, Sullivan N, Paulson EC, et al. *Imaging Tests for the Staging of Colorectal Cancer*. Rockville, MD: Agency for Healthcare Research and Quality (US); 2014 http://www.ncbi.nlm.nih.gov/books/NBK248261/.
118. Taylor FGM, Quirke P, Heald RJ, et al. Preoperative magnetic resonance imaging assessment of circumferential resection margin predicts disease-free survival and local recurrence: 5-year follow-up results of the MERCURY study. *J Clin Oncol*. 2014;**32**(1):34–43. doi: 10.1200/JCO.2012.45.3258.
120. Dumonceau J-M, Polkowski M, Larghi A, et al. Indications, results, and clinical impact of endoscopic ultrasound (EUS)-guided sampling in gastroenterology: European Society of Gastrointestinal Endoscopy (ESGE) Clinical Guideline. *Endoscopy*. 2011;**43**(10):897–912. doi: 10.1055/s-0030-1256754.
121. Jessup J, Goldberg R, Asare E. Colon and rectum. In: Amin MB, ed. *AJCC Cancer Staging Manual*, 8th ed. Chicago: AJCC; 2017.
122. Fokas E, Liersch T, Fietkau R, et al. Tumor regression grading after preoperative chemoradiotherapy for locally advanced rectal carcinoma revisited: updated results of the CAO/ARO/AIO-94 trial. *J Clin Oncol*. 2014;**32**(15):1554–1562. doi: 10.1200/JCO.2013.54.3769.
126. Chen M, Song X, Chen L-Z, et al. Comparing mechanical bowel preparation with both oral and systemic antibiotics versus mechanical bowel preparation and systemic antibiotics alone for the prevention of surgical site infection after elective colorectal surgery: a meta-analysis of randomize. *Dis Colon Rectum*. 2016;**59**(1):70–78. doi: 10.1097/DCR.0000000000000524.
127. Carmichael JC, Keller DS, Baldini G, et al. Clinical practice guideline for enhanced recovery after colon and rectal surgery from the American Society of Colon and Rectal Surgeons (ASCRS) and Society of American Gastrointestinal and Endoscopic Surgeons (SAGES). *Surg Endosc*. 2017;**31**(9):3412–3436. doi: 10.1007/s00464-017-5722-7.
138. de Graaf EJR, Burger JWA, van Ijsseldijk ALA, et al. Transanal endoscopic microsurgery is superior to transanal excision of rectal adenomas. *Color Dis*. 2011;**13**(7):762–767. doi: 10.1111/j.1463-1318.2010.02269.x.
141. Garcia-Aguilar J, Renfro LA, Chow OS, et al. Organ preservation for clinical T2N0 distal rectal cancer using neoadjuvant chemoradiotherapy and local excision (ACOSOG Z6041): results of an open-label, single-arm, multi-institutional, phase 2 trial. *Lancet Oncol*. 2015;**16**(15):1537–1546. doi: 10.1016/S1470-2045(15)00215-6.
145. Sauer R, Becker H, Hohenberger W, et al. Preoperative versus postoperative chemoradiotherapy for rectal cancer. *N Engl J Med*. 2004;**351**(17):1731–1740. doi: 10.1056/NEJMoa040694.
156. Green BL, Marshall HC, Collinson F, et al. Long-term follow-up of the Medical Research Council CLASICC trial of conventional *versus* laparoscopically assisted resection in colorectal cancer: conventional *versus* laparoscopically assisted surgery for colonic and rectal cancer. *Br J Surg*. 2013;**100**(1):75–82. doi: 10.1002/bjs.8945.
159. Deijen CL, Vasmel JE, de Lange-de Klerk ESM, et al. Ten-year outcomes of a randomised trial of laparoscopic versus open surgery for colon cancer. *Surg Endosc*. 2017;**31**(6):2607–2615. doi: 10.1007/s00464-016-5270-6.
162. McCombie AM, Frizelle F, Bagshaw PF, et al. The ALCCaS trial: a randomized controlled trial comparing quality of life following laparoscopic versus open colectomy for colon cancer. *Dis Colon Rectum*. 2018;**61**(10):1156–1162. doi: 10.1097/DCR.0000000000001165.
164. Bonjer HJ, Hop WCJ, Nelson H, et al. Laparoscopically assisted vs open colectomy for colon cancer: a meta-analysis. *Arch Surg*. 2007;**142**(3):298–303. doi: 10.1001/archsurg.142.3.298.
183. Bhama AR, Obias V, Welch KB, et al. A comparison of laparoscopic and robotic colorectal surgery outcomes using the American College of Surgeons National Surgical Quality Improvement Program (ACS NSQIP) database. *Surg Endosc*. 2016;**30**(4):1576–1584. doi: 10.1007/s00464-015-4381-9.
189. Kang J, Park YA, Baik SH, et al. A comparison of open, laparoscopic, and robotic surgery in the treatment of right-sided colon cancer. *Surg Laparosc Endosc Percutan Tech*. 2016;**26**(6):497–502. doi: 10.1097/SLE.0000000000000331.
190. Park JS, Kang H, Park SY, et al. Long-term oncologic after robotic versus laparoscopic right colectomy: a prospective randomized study. *Surg Endosc*. 2019;**33**(9):2975–2981. doi: 10.1007/s00464-018-6563-8.
192. Jayne D, Pigazzi A, Marshall H, et al. Effect of robotic-assisted vs conventional laparoscopic surgery on risk of conversion to open laparotomy among patients undergoing resection for rectal cancer: the ROLARR Randomized Clinical Trial. *JAMA*. 2017;**318**(16):1569. doi: 10.1001/jama.2017.7219.
194. Jones K, Qassem MG, Sains P, et al. Robotic total meso-rectal excision for rectal cancer: a systematic review following the publication of the ROLARR trial. *World J Gastrointest Oncol*. 2018;**10**(11):449–464. doi: 10.4251/wjgo.v10.i11.449.
216. Tournigand C, André T, Achille E, et al. FOLFIRI followed by FOLFOX6 or the reverse sequence in advanced colorectal cancer: a randomized GERCOR study. *J Clin Oncol*. 2004;**22**(2):229–237. doi: 10.1200/JCO.2004.05.113.
217. Schmoll H-J, Tabernero J, Maroun J, et al. Capecitabine plus oxaliplatin compared with fluorouracil/folinic acid as adjuvant therapy for stage III colon cancer: final results of the NO16968 randomized controlled phase III trial. *J Clin Oncol*. 2015;**33**(32):3733–3740. doi: 10.1200/JCO.2015.09.9107.
232. Swedish Rectal Cancer Trial, Cedermark B, Dahlberg M, et al. Improved survival with preoperative radiotherapy in resectable rectal cancer. *N Engl J Med*. 1997;**336**(14):980–987. doi: 10.1056/NEJM199704033361402.
240. Ngan SY, Burmeister B, Fisher RJ, et al. Randomized trial of short-course radiotherapy versus long-course chemoradiation comparing rates of local recurrence in patients with T3 rectal cancer: trans-tasman radiation oncology group trial 01.04. *J Clin Oncol*. 2012;**30**(31):3827–3833. doi: 10.1200/JCO.2012.42.9597.
242. Glynne-Jones R, Wyrwicz L, Tiret E, et al. Rectal cancer: ESMO Clinical Practice Guidelines for diagnosis, treatment and follow-up. *Ann Oncol*. 2017;**28**: iv22–iv40. doi: 10.1093/annonc/mdx224.
243. Ryan ÉJ, O'Sullivan DP, Kelly ME, et al. Meta-analysis of the effect of extending the interval after long-course chemoradiotherapy before surgery in locally advanced rectal cancer. *Br J Surg*. 2019;**106**(10):1298–1310. doi: 10.1002/bjs.11220.

244 Garcia-Aguilar J, Chow OS, Smith DD, et al. Effect of adding mFOLFOX6 after neoadjuvant chemoradiation in locally advanced rectal cancer: a multicentre, phase 2 trial. *Lancet Oncol.* 2015;**16**(8):957–966. doi: 10.1016/S1470-2045(15)00004-2.

245 Cercek A, Roxburgh CSD, Strombom P, et al. Adoption of total neoadjuvant therapy for locally advanced rectal cancer. *JAMA Oncol.* 2018;**4**(6):e180071. doi: 10.1001/jamaoncol.2018.0071.

246 Fernandez-Martos C, Garcia-Albeniz X, Pericay C, et al. Chemoradiation, surgery and adjuvant chemotherapy versus induction chemotherapy followed by chemoradiation and surgery: long-term results of the Spanish GCR-3 phase II randomized trial. *Ann Oncol.* 2015;**26**(8):1722–1728. doi: 10.1093/annonc/mdv223.

248 Das P, Skibber JM, Rodriguez-Bigas MA, et al. Predictors of tumor response and downstaging in patients who receive preoperative chemoradiation for rectal cancer. *Cancer.* 2007;**109**(9):1750–1755. doi: 10.1002/cncr.22625.

250 Renehan AG, Malcomson L, Emsley R, et al. Watch-and-wait approach versus surgical resection after chemoradiotherapy for patients with rectal cancer (the OnCoRe project): a propensity-score matched cohort analysis. *Lancet Oncol.* 2016;**17**(2):174–183. doi: 10.1016/S1470-2045(15)00467-2.

251 Dossa F, Chesney TR, Acuna SA, Baxter NN. A watch-and-wait approach for locally advanced rectal cancer after a clinical complete response following neoadjuvant chemoradiation: a systematic review and meta-analysis. *Lancet Gastroenterol Hepatol.* 2017;**2**(7):501–513. doi: 10.1016/S2468-1253(17)30074-2.

252 Hofheinz R-D, Wenz F, Post S, et al. Chemoradiotherapy with capecitabine versus fluorouracil for locally advanced rectal cancer: a randomised, multicentre, non-inferiority, phase 3 trial. *Lancet Oncol.* 2012;**13**(6):579–588. doi: 10.1016/S1470-2045(12)70116-X.

267 Heinemann V, von Weikersthal LF, Decker T, et al. FOLFIRI plus cetuximab versus FOLFIRI plus bevacizumab as first-line treatment for patients with metastatic colorectal cancer (FIRE-3): a randomised, open-label, phase 3 trial. *Lancet Oncol.* 2014;**15**(10):1065–1075. doi: 10.1016/S1470-2045(14)70330-4.

280 Cremolini C, Loupakis F, Antoniotti C, et al. FOLFOXIRI plus bevacizumab versus FOLFIRI plus bevacizumab as first-line treatment of patients with metastatic colorectal cancer: updated overall survival and molecular subgroup analyses of the open-label, phase 3 TRIBE study. *Lancet Oncol.* 2015;**16**(13):1306–1315. doi: 10.1016/S1470-2045(15)00122-9.

282 Falcone A, Cremolini C, Masi G, et al. FOLFOXIRI/bevacizumab (bev) versus FOLFIRI/bev as first-line treatment in unresectable metastatic colorectal cancer (mCRC) patients (pts): results of the phase III TRIBE trial by GONO group. *J Clin Oncol.* 2013;**31**(15_suppl):3505. doi: 10.1200/jco.2013.31.15_suppl.3505.

283 Gruenberger T, Bridgewater JA, Chau I, et al. Randomized, phase II study of bevacizumab with mFOLFOX6 or FOLFOXIRI in patients with initially unresectable liver metastases from colorectal cancer: resectability and safety in OLIVIA. *J Clin Oncol.* 2013;**31**(15_suppl):3619. doi: 10.1200/jco.2013.31.15_suppl.3619.

284 Venook A, Niedzwiecki D, Hollis D, et al. Phase III study of irinotecan/5FU/LV (FOLFIRI) or oxaliplatin/5FU/LV (FOLFOX) ± cetuximab for patients (pts) with untreated metastatic adenocarcinoma of the colon or rectum (MCRC): CALGB 80203 preliminary results. *J Clin Oncol.* 2006;**24**(18_suppl):3509. doi: 10.1200/jco.2006.24.18_suppl.3509.

285 Van Cutsem E, Nowacki M, Lang I, et al. Randomized phase III study of irinotecan and 5-FU/FA with or without cetuximab in the first-line treatment of patients with metastatic colorectal cancer (mCRC): the CRYSTAL trial. *J Clin Oncol.* 2007;**25**(18_suppl):4000. doi: 10.1200/jco.2007.25.18_suppl.4000.

286 Lièvre A, Bachet J-B, Boige V, et al. *KRAS* mutations as an independent prognostic factor in patients with advanced colorectal cancer treated with cetuximab. *J Clin Oncol.* 2008;**26**(3):374–379. doi: 10.1200/JCO.2007.12.5906.

288 Douillard J-Y, Oliner KS, Siena S, et al. Panitumumab-FOLFOX4 treatment and RAS mutations in colorectal cancer. *N Engl J Med.* 2013;**369**(11):1023–1034. doi: 10.1056/NEJMoa1305275.

291 Rowland A, Dias MM, Wiese MD, et al. Meta-analysis of BRAF mutation as a predictive biomarker of benefit from anti-EGFR monoclonal antibody therapy for RAS wild-type metastatic colorectal cancer. *Br J Cancer.* 2015;**112**(12):1888–1894. doi: 10.1038/bjc.2015.173.

293 Stintzing S, Modest DP, Rossius L, et al. FOLFIRI plus cetuximab versus FOLFIRI plus bevacizumab for metastatic colorectal cancer (FIRE-3): a post-hoc analysis of tumour dynamics in the final RAS wild-type subgroup of this randomised open-label phase 3 trial. *Lancet Oncol.* 2016;**17**(10):1426–1434. doi: 10.1016/S1470-2045(16)30269-8.

294 Venook AP, Niedzwiecki D, Lenz H-J, et al. Effect of first-line chemotherapy combined with cetuximab or bevacizumab on overall survival in patients with *KRAS* wild-type advanced or metastatic colorectal cancer: a randomized clinical trial. *JAMA.* 2017;**317**(23):2392. doi: 10.1001/jama.2017.7105.

295 Holch JW, Ricard I, Stintzing S, et al. The relevance of primary tumour location in patients with metastatic colorectal cancer: a meta-analysis of first-line clinical trials. *Eur J Cancer.* 2017;**70**:87–98. doi: 10.1016/j.ejca.2016.10.007.

92 Neoplasms of the anus

Alexandre A. A. Jácome, MD, PhD ■ Cathy Eng, MD, FACP, FASCO

> **Overview**
>
> Squamous cell carcinoma of the anal canal (SCCA) is a rare human papillomavirus (HPV)-related malignancy, but with rising incidence in the last decade. Chemoradiotherapy (CRT) remains the cornerstone of the treatment of non-metastatic disease, characterized by remarkable response rates of 90% and 5-year overall survival (OS) of 80%. Nevertheless, despite the high efficacy observed with combined modality treatment, almost half of the patients with locally advanced disease have high-risk features (T3, T4, or node-positive disease) for treatment failure. The management of unresectable recurrences or metastatic disease is an unmet clinical need, marked by poor clinical outcomes. Immune checkpoint inhibitors and immunotherapeutic approaches have been demonstrating promising results in the management of advanced disease in the past few years, but big steps forward will only be taken when the underutilized HPV vaccination becomes more widely accepted for use.

Gross anatomy

In the past decades, there have been no consensus about the anatomic boundaries of the anus, which led to various definitions of the anal canal and the anal margin, impairing the comprehension of the natural history and the epidemiological data of the cancers originating in each region. To clarify this issue, the American Joint Committee on Cancer (AJCC) and the Union International Cancer Control (UICC) formed a consensus that the anal canal begins where the rectum enters the puborectalis sling at the apex of the anal sphincter complex (palpable as the anorectal ring on digital rectal examination and approximately 1–2 cm proximal to the dentate line) and ends with the squamous mucosa blending with the perianal skin, totalizing 3–4 cm long.[1-3] These two organizations agree that anal margin tumors behave in a similar fashion to skin cancers and therefore are classified and treated as skin tumors.

There are three regions where anal cancers occur: the lower rectum, the anal canal, and the perianal skin or anal margin. There is an extensive lymphatic system for the anus with many connections. The three main pathways include (1) superiorly from the rectum along the superior hemorrhoidal vessels to the inferior mesenteric lymph nodes, (2) from the upper anal canal and superior to the dentate line along the inferior and middle hemorrhoid vessels to the hypogastric lymph nodes, and (3) inferior from the anal canal and the anal margin to the superficial inguinal lymph nodes.

Epidemiology

Worldwide, it is expected anal cancer will be diagnosed in 1 per 100,000 individuals. Globally, 27 000 will be diagnosed per year. In the United States, cancers of the anal region account for 1–2% of all large bowel cancers and 4% of all anorectal carcinomas. Since 1997, the incidence of carcinoma *in situ* (CIS) and squamous cell cancer [Squamous cell carcinoma of the anal canal (SCCA)] of the anus have dramatically increased. Women are the most affected population, but CIS are more likely to be diagnosed in men.[4] A total of 8590 cases of cancers of the anal region are estimated to occur in the United States in 2020, including 5900 women and 2690 men.[5] It is estimated that there will be 1350 deaths.

Etiology and pathogenesis

HPV infection

Human papillomavirus (HPV) infection is the main risk factor for the development of anal cancers. Worldwide, it is estimated that approximately 88% of all SCCA cases are associated to the viral infection.[6] The types 16 and 18 are the most commonly found, representing 73% and 5% of all HPV-positive tumors, respectively.[7] The causal relationship with the HPV infection is reinforced by the presence of the viral DNA in more than 90% of the precancerous anal lesions, such as anal intraepithelial neoplasia 1 (AIN1) and AIN2/3.[7] Once infected by a high-risk HPV type, the transformation of a normal epithelial cell of the anal canal into a malignant cell seems to follow similar molecular steps that occur in cervical cancer. The two parts (the early (E) region and the late (L) region) of the viral genome will express the proteins responsible for the interaction with the host cell (E proteins) and for the structure of the viral capsid (L proteins). The LCR region is located between E- and L-regions, and it does not have gene-encoding regions, but contains promoter and enhancer DNA sequences critical to the regulation of the viral gene transcription.[8]

The two viral proteins E6 and E7 are continuously expressed in anogenital tumors and their activity contributes directly to the maintenance of the malignant phenotype of the host cell.[8,9] E6 and E7 interact with two well-known proteins in cell homeostasis: p53 and RB, respectively.[10-12] Ultimately, the interaction of the viral proteins with p53 and RB will lead to stimulation of mitotic activity in infected cells, with unchecked cell growth in the presence of genomic instability.[11,13,14] These HPV-induced molecular alterations may result in a pre-malignant phenotype in the host cell called squamous intraepithelial lesions (SIL), which can be divided in low-grade intraepithelial lesions (LSIL) and high-grade intraepithelial lesions (HSIL).[15] Such lesions represent a morphologic continuum that can be demonstrated as a spectrum, from lower grade lesions like condyloma and AIN grade 1 to higher grade lesions, such as AIN grades 2 and 3. Observational studies suggest that invasive cancer originates from HSIL.[16,17] The factors that determine this final transformation are not well known, but

---

Holland-Frei Cancer Medicine, Tenth Edition. Edited by Robert C. Bast, John C. Byrd, Carlo M. Croce, Ernest Hawk, Fadlo R. Khuri, Raphael E. Pollock, Apostolia M. Tsimberidou, Christopher G. Willett, and Cheryl L. Willman.
© 2023 John Wiley & Sons, Inc. Published 2023 by John Wiley & Sons, Inc.

it seems that immunosuppression is a contributing factor, since human immunodeficiency virus (HIV)-infected patients and organ transplant patients present higher probability to progress from HSIL to invasive cancer.[18]

AIN is rare in women and heterosexual men, while the incidence is 5–30% in men who have sex with men (MSM), even if HIV-negative. It is also common in immunosuppressed patients, especially those who are HIV-positive.[19,20] Meta-analysis of 53 studies examining the relationship of HPV infection in MSM revealed a pooled prevalence of HPV-16 of 35% in HIV-positive versus 13% in HIV-negative patients.[21] Another study of 90 MSM with an abnormal examination of the anal canal, 89% had HPV-associated lesions.[22]

Population-based case-control studies have demonstrated the link between sexual activity and anal cancer. One of the strongest risk factors for anal cancer in women [relative risk (RR) 4.5] and in heterosexual men (RR: 2.5) were 10 or more lifetime sexual partners. The risk of the disease was also increased (RR: 12.4–50.0) in MSM, mainly with a history a receptive anal intercourse (RR: 33.1).[23,24] The history of genital warts was also strongly associated with the occurrence of anal cancer, both in women (RR 4.6–32.5) and in men (RR 26.9). In addition, the risk of anal cancer was higher in patients infected with sexually transmitted diseases (STDs), such as herpes simplex 2 (RR: 4.1), *Chlamydia trachomatis* (RR: 2.3), and gonorrhea (RR 3.3).[23,24]

HIV (human immunodeficiency virus) infection

There is a clear association between HIV and anal cancer. Cross-referencing US databases for AIDS with those for cancer, the RR of anal cancer in MSM compared to men in the general population at the time of or after AIDS diagnosis was 84.1.[25] The RR of anal cancer for up to 5 years before AIDS diagnosis was 13.9.

Anal canal carcinoma and AIN are associated with condylomata.[20] However, HPV infection alone may be insufficient for malignant transformation, as many patients with HPV-positive cytology do not develop either AIN or anal cancer.[26] The immunosuppression associated with the HIV co-infection seems to increase the probability of the evolution of HPV-related pre-malignant alterations to overt malignant phenotype.[18]

Other factors

Cigarette smoking is a substantial risk factor in both women (RR 7.7) and men (RR 9.4).[24] The relationship between anal cancer and fistulas is conflicting. In one study, 41% of anal canal carcinomas were preceded by benign anorectal disease for at least 5 years.[27] However, two studies reveal only a temporal relationship but no evidence of causation.[28,29] In a separate study, MSM with a history of anal fissure or fistula had an elevated risk of anorectal squamous cell carcinoma (RR 9.1).[23] Overall, the incidence of anal canal cancers in patients with Crohn's disease is low.[30] Immunosuppressed renal transplant patients have a 100-fold increase in anogenital tumors compared with the general population.[31] In a series of 3595 patients undergoing a solid organ transplant, the incidence of anal cancer was 0.11%.[32]

Molecular characterization of the SCCA

The identification of the molecular alterations associated with SCCA is crucial for the development of novel therapeutic strategies. There are genetic alterations common to all HPV-related

Table 1 Frequency of the most commonly affected genes in SCCA.

Gene	Frequency (%)
PIK3CA	29–40
MLL3	32
MLL2	22
EP300	22
p53	15–20
FBXW7	13–14
PTEN	2–14
BRCA1	1–12
BRCA2	3–12
AKT1	3–7
EGFR	0–5
BRAF	0–5
KRAS	0–4
NRAS	0–2

malignancies, but the description of the molecular portrait specific to anal cancer will provide insights for the design of clinical trials evaluating targeted therapies and genome-guided personalized therapy (Table 1).

Comprehensive genomic profiling studies have consistently demonstrated that *PIK3CA* gene mutation is the most frequent genetic abnormality in SCCA.[33–36] A study that performed whole exome sequencing, copy number assessment, and gene expression profiling on tumor-normal pairs from 24 patients with metastatic SCCA found that 88% of the tumors had an activating mutation and/or gene amplification of PIK3CA.[35] Another study evaluating tumor samples from 70 patients with SCCA stages II–IV identified PIK3CA mutation in 40% of cases, while a third one identified 32% in a population of 199 patients using next generation sequencing or Sanger sequencing.[33]

MLL3 and *MLL2*, genes important in histone modification, were also found frequently mutated, as well as genes important to cell cycle dysregulation (CNTRL), DNA damage repair (p53, ATM, HUWE1, BRCA 1, BRCA 2), chromatin remodeling (EP300, SMARCB1, SMARCA4), cell differentiation (FLG, PTK2), and activation of Wnt/β-catenin signaling (FAM123B).[33] These studies also suggest that SCCA has a low tumor mutational burden (TMB), with a mean number of 2.5–3.5 somatic mutations/Mb, similar to those identified in other HPV-related malignancies, such as cervical cancer and HPV-positive head and neck cancer.[35] It seems that TMB is low even in the uncommon HPV-negative SCCA, which is associated with a higher probability of p53 mutation.[35] Interestingly, well-known clinically relevant genomic alterations such as KRAS, NRAS, BRAF, EGFR, and HER2 are infrequent (<5%) in SCCA.[37]

Comprehensive genomic profiling did not find association between genomic alterations and disease stage.[33] Nevertheless, it seems that there are different patterns of DNA methylation according to tumor volume. Analysis of DNA methylation status of 121 patients with nonmetastatic SCCA showed that 16 CpG loci were differentially methylated (14 increased and 2 decreased) in locally advanced disease compared to early-stage disease.[34] This finding generates the hypothesis of the potential role of epigenetic events in the progression of the disease.

Pathology

A variety of histologic cell types may occur in the anal area. The majority of these (75–80%) are SCC and 15% are adenocarcinomas (Table 2).[39] Squamous cell tumors are divided into those with

Table 2 Histologic types of anal cancer.[a]

Type	%
Squamous cell	87
Adenocarcinoma	7
Basal cell	2
Melanoma	2
Paget's disease	2

[a]Source: Modified from Peters and Mack.[38]

and without keratinization,[40] and nonkeratinizing tumors are further subdivided into basosquamous, basaloid, and cloacogenic carcinomas. Other rare histologic entities can arise, such as small cell carcinomas[41] and lymphomas. Melanomas constitute 1–2% of all anal cancers.[42]

Squamous tumors may arise from the entire length of the anal canal as well as from the anal margin. Basaloid carcinomas, which are a variant of squamous carcinoma are commonly referred to as cloacogenic carcinomas. Adenocarcinomas arise from the glands at the dentate line. Small cell carcinomas have neuroendocrine origin and are rare. Tumors of the anal margin include squamous carcinoma, basal cell carcinoma, Bowen's disease (squamous CIS), Paget's disease (adenocarcinoma in situ), verrucous carcinoma, and Kaposi's sarcoma. Malignant melanomas may arise from either location, but more commonly from below the dentate line.

Natural history

The most common route of spread is by local extension proximally to involve other organs in the pelvis. Hematogenous spread occurs more often from tumors that arise at or above the dentate line.[43] This pattern of spread allows tumor cells into the portal system resulting in liver and lung metastases in 5–8% of patients[43] and bone in 2%.[44] Distant metastases occur with equal frequency independent of the histologic cell type involved. Distant metastases are rarely seen with anal margin tumors. Lymphatic spread is common and involves the inguinal, pelvic, and mesenteric nodes. Inguinal lymph nodes are positive in 15–63% of cases.[45,46] The incidence of synchronous positive inguinal nodes is 15%.[43,47] In a series of 96 patients, metachronous positive inguinal nodes appeared in 25% with a median time to presentation of 12 months. Pelvic nodes are less commonly involved and mesenteric nodes are more likely to be involved if the tumors are proximal (50%) than distal (14%).[48] Positive mesenteric nodes in anal margin tumors are rare.

Historically, surgical series report overall survival (OS) rates of 0–20% following lymph node dissection with synchronous positive nodes.[49,50] Modern chemoradiotherapy (CRT) has substantially improved this. Patients who undergo lymph node dissection for metachronous lesions have more favorable survivals with rates as high as 83%.[49,51] The majority of these recurrences occur by 2 years but may present as late as 8 years.[48]

Diagnosis

The initial and most common symptom is anorectal bleeding, which occurs in over 50% of patients. Other common symptoms include pain, tenesmus, pruritus, change in bowel habits, abnormal discharge, and less commonly, inguinal lymphadenopathy.[48,52,53] Most of these symptoms are associated with benign conditions of the anus including hemorrhoids, fissure, pruritus, and anal condyloma. Benign perianal conditions may coexist in 60% of anal margin tumors and in 6% of anal canal tumors.[54]

The most common physical finding is an intraluminal mass which is often misdiagnosed as a hemorrhoid.[44,45] Endoscopically, the tumors may appear as flat or slightly raised lesions, as raised lesions with indurated borders, or as polypoid lesions. An incisional biopsy is recommended for diagnosis. Excisional biopsies should be limited to small superficial lesions <1 cm). Clinically palpable inguinal lymphadenopathy should be considered for cytological examination. A formal inguinal lymph node dissection is not recommended due to the associated morbidity, failure to have an impact on outcome, and the high control rates with CRT. In a study with 46 HIV+ patients, anal brush cytology was more sensitive and specific for external compared with internal lesions.[55] High-resolution anoscopy is helpful in detecting both high-grade intraepithelial as well as invasive lesions in HIV+[56] and HIV− patients.[57]

Staging

A common staging system was developed in 1997 by the AJCC and the UICC. This staging system accounts for the fact that anal canal carcinoma is primarily treated by CRT and abdominoperineal resection (APR) is reserved for treatment failure. The TNM classification is clinical. The primary tumor is assessed for size and for invasion of local structures such as the vagina, urethra, or bladder. The eighth edition of the AJCC staging system is seen in Table 3.[58]

The use of transrectal ultrasound has fallen out of favor. A diagnostic imaging work-up includes computed tomography (CT) of the chest, abdomen, and pelvis to evaluate the primary tumor and to exclude distant metastases. Some studies reveal a benefit of positron emission tomography (PET) for staging but are small, single institution studies.[59-62] In a series of 41 patients, [18]flourodeoxyuridine glucose positron emission tomography ([18]FDG-PET) detected 91% of non-excised primaries compared with 59% with CT alone.[63] In addition, 17% of inguinal nodes negative by CT and physical exam were positive by PET. In a retrospective analysis with 28 patients, PET/CT upstaged disease in 14% and changed the treatment plan in 17% compared to transrectal ultrasound.[61] Compared with either PET or CT alone, radiation field design was changed in 23% of patients who underwent a combined PET–CT.[64] Hence, a PET/CT scan is commonly offered to assist in guiding the radiation fields.

Prognostic factors

As with most gastrointestinal cancers, the most important prognostic factors in anal cancer are T and N stage. In patients treated with radiation with or without chemotherapy, the most striking difference in results is seen when comparing T1–2 primary cancers (≤5 cm) versus T3–4 primary cancers (>5 cm). The local failure rates with T3–4 primary cancers are approximately 50% following CRT. When a complete response (CR) is achieved, the local failure rate is 25%. An increase in local failure rate is associated with T-stage (T1: 11%, T2: 24%, T3: 45%, and T4: 43%) and a corresponding decrease in 5-year OS (T1: 94%, T2: 79%, T3: 53%, and T4: 19%).[65] A similar decrease in 5-year colostomy-free survival (CFS) with T1–2 tumors versus T3–4 tumors has been reported (T1: 83% and T2: 89% vs T3: 50% and T4: 54%).[66]

Table 3 AJCC TNM staging system for anal canal cancer (8th edition).

T category	T criteria
TX	Primary tumor not assessed
T0	No evidence of primary tumor
Tis	High-grade squamous intraepithelial lesion (previously termed carcinoma in situ, Bowen disease, anal intraepithelial neoplasia II–III, high-grade anal intraepithelial neoplasia)
T1	Tumor ≤2 cm
T2	Tumor >2 cm but ≤5 cm
T3	Tumor >5 cm
T4	Tumor of any size invading adjacent organ(s), such as the vagina, urethra, or bladder
N category	N criteria
NX	Regional lymph nodes cannot be assessed
N0	No regional lymph nodes metastasis
N1	Metastasis in inguinal, mesorectal, internal iliac, or external iliac nodes
N1a	Metastasis in inguinal, mesorectal, or internal iliac lymph nodes
N1b	Metastasis in external iliac lymph nodes
N1c	Metastasis in external iliac with any N1a nodes
M category	M criteria
M0	No distant metastasis
M1	Distant metastasis
Histologic grade	
G	G definition
GX	Grade cannot be determined
G1	Well differentiated (low grade)
G2	Moderately differentiated (low grade)
G3	Poorly differentiated (high grade)
G4	Undifferentiated (high grade)

AJCC prognostic stage groups			
Stage	T	N	M
0	Tis	N0	M0
I	T1	N0	M0
IIA	T2	N0	M0
IIB	T3	N0	M0
IIIA	T1–2	N1	M0
IIIB	T4	N0	M0
IIIC	T3–4	N1	M0
IV	Any T	Any N	M1

Note: Anal margin cancers are classified as skin cancers.

In contrast to T stage, the impact of positive lymph nodes is less clear. Unlike rectal cancer, inguinal lymph nodes in anal cancer are considered nodal (N) metastasis rather than distant (M) metastasis and patients should be treated in a potentially curative fashion. Patients with negative nodes who received CRT had a higher 5-year disease-specific survival compared with those with positive nodes (81% vs 57%).[67]

The RTOG 87-04 trial (Table 4) reported a higher colostomy rate (which is an indirect measurement of local failure) in N1 versus N0 patients (28% vs 13%).[67] In node-negative and, possibly, node-positive patients, the addition of mitomycin-C decreased the overall colostomy rates. The EORTC randomized trial (Table 4) of 45 Gy ± 5-FU/mitomycin-C also reported that patients with positive nodes experienced significantly higher local failure ($p = 0.035$) and lower OS ($p = 0.038$) rates compared to those with negative nodes.[68]

In the EORTC randomized trial, multivariate analysis identified that positive nodes, skin ulceration, and male gender were independent negative prognostic factors for local control and OS.[68] Retrospective series also suggested that women had a more favorable outcome than men.[69] In retrospective study with 167 patients, a multivariate analysis revealed that higher T and N stage correlated with increased local failure; N stage and basaloid histology were associated with distant failure, and N stage and HIV+ predicted for lower OS.[70] In the Intergroup RTOG 98-11 trial (Table 4), multivariate analysis revealed that male gender ($p = 0.04$), clinically N+ ($p < 0.0001$), and tumor size >5 cm (0.005) were independent prognostic factors for disease-free survival (DFS).[71]

The histologic cell type for squamous cancers of the anal canal (squamous vs cloacogenic) has not been found to be of major prognostic significance. In some series, cloacogenic carcinomas have been considered to have a slightly better prognosis.[72,73] However, in a series of 243 patients with resectable anal canal tumors, there was a worse prognosis for nonkeratinizing and basaloid carcinoma versus keratinizing lesions.[74] Small cell carcinomas of the anus are rare and, similar to extra-pulmonary small cell cancers in other parts of the body, appear to have a worse prognosis and a high incidence of metastatic disease.[41,75] In a separate study, tumor grade was a significant prognostic factor, with low-grade tumors resulting in a 5-year OS of 75% compared with only 24% for high-grade tumors.[76] Three studies have examined DNA content (diploid vs non-diploid). Two found no prognostic impact of this factor,[76,77] while in one multivariate analysis of 184 patients,[75] DNA ploidy was an independent prognostic factor for survival.

Treatment for primary disease

General principles

Local excision
Local excision has been used in select patients with tumors that are <2 cm, well-differentiated, or tumors found incidentally at the time of hemorrhoidectomy. Of 188 patients with anal canal carcinoma treated at the Mayo Clinic, a subset of 19 were treated with local excision.[41] For the 12 patients with tumors confined to the epithelium and subepithelial connective tissues, 11 had tumors <2 cm and 1 patient had two lesions. The OS was 100%. One of 12 patients recurred, and this patient had no evidence of disease 5 years after salvage APR. Patients with positive margins can be considered for re-excision or ideally combined CRT.

In summary, local excision alone is reasonable for small cancers excised with negative margins found incidentally following hemorrhoidectomy for T1 tumors, while maintaining sphincter continence. These require close follow-up and local recurrences can subsequently be treated with CRT.

Brachytherapy
In contrast with treatment programs in North America, where patients receive CRT, patients treated in selected European centers, most commonly France, receive external beam radiation therapy (EBRT) alone, with or without brachytherapy. Non-randomized data suggest that the results of radiation therapy alone are comparable to CRT; however, the radiation-related toxicity is higher.[78] Brachytherapy techniques commonly involve afterloading ^{192}Ir. A frequent treatment approach is EBRT for the first 45 Gy followed by an additional 15–20 Gy with a perineal boost or brachytherapy. Retrospective study evaluated the efficacy of brachytherapy with or without small field EBRT in 66 patients with T1/Tis tumors.[79] With a median follow-up of 50 months, there were only six local failures, of which four occurred outside of the radiation field.

Abdominoperineal resection (APR)
APR is reserved for salvage in patients who have failed radiation or in patients who have received prior pelvic radiation therapy. The results will be discussed later.

Table 4 Randomized trials of combined modality therapy for anal cancer.

Trial	N	Initial treatment	Assessment/treatment of residual		Arm	% CR	% Colostomy	% Local control		% Survival	
			Residual	Boost				Crude	Actuarial	CFS	Overall
Intergroup RTOG8704 ECOG1289	291	45 Gy + 5FU	Positive[a]	9Gy + 5FU/CDDP	RT + 5FU	85	22[b]	—	—	59[b]	70 (4 yr)
		45 Gy + 5FU/MMC	Negative	Observe	RT + 5FU/MMC	92	9	—	—	71	75 (4 yr)
ACT I	585	45 Gy	>50% CR[a]	15–20 Gy EBRT or brachytherapy	RT	—	—	41[b]	34 (5 yr)[b]	20	33 (5 yr)
		45 Gy + 5FU/MMC	<50% CR	Salvage surgery	RT + 5FU/MMC	—	—	64	59 (5 yr)	30	28 (5 yr)
EORTC	110	45 Gy	PR/CR[a]	15–20 Gy EBRT or brachytherapy	RT	54	—	55[b]	50 (5 yr)[b]	40 (5 yr)[b]	52 (5 yr)
		45 Gy + 5FU/MMC	<PR	Salvage surgery	RT + 5FU/MMC	80	—	73	68 (5 yr)	72 (5 yr)	57 (5 yr)
Intergroup RTOG 98-11 ECOG 1289	598	45 Gy 5FU/CDDP	Positive[c]	10–14 Gy 5FU/CDDP or MMC	5FU/CDDP	—	20	26	20	65 (5 yr)[b]	71 (5 yr)
		45 Gy 5FU/MMC	Negative	Observe	5FU/MMC	—	10	33	26	74 (5 yr)	78 (5 yr)
ACT II	940	50.4 Gy 5FU/CDDP ± maintenance 5FU/MMC	—	—	5FU/CDDP	90	—	—	—	—	72 PFS (3 yr)
		50.4 Gy 5FU/MMC ± maintenance 5FU/MMC	—	—	5FU/MMC	91	—	—	—	—	73 PFS (3 yr)

Abbreviations: CFS, colostomy free survival; MMC, mitomycin-C; CDDP, cisplatin; LN+, lymph node positive; CR, complete response; PFS, progression free survival; EBRT, external beam radiation therapy. The ACT I trial included 23% anal margin cancers.
[a]Biopsy at 6 weeks.
[b]Statistically significant ($p \leq 0.05$).
[c]Biopsy at 8 weeks.

Chemoradiation therapy
The conventional treatment for anal canal cancer was APR until the late 1970s. This standard was challenged by Nigro et al.[80] in his initial report of three patients with SCC of the anal canal, who following pre-operative treatment with 30 Gy plus concurrent 5-FU and mitomycin-C, were found to have a pathologic CR at the time of surgery. Since that time, many single-arm phase II studies have indicated that initial CRT yields 80–90% CR rates, with APR reserved for salvage. Even in patients with large ($\geq$5 cm) primary cancers, although the CR rates are lower (50–75%), most patients may be spared from colostomy and have an excellent OS.

Chemotherapy
Results of two randomized trials (Table 4) from Europe of CRT versus radiation alone (EORTC[68] and UKCCCR ACT I[81]) support the use of CRT. With a 13-year follow-up of the UKCCCR ACT I trial, patients who received CRT versus radiation alone had a significant improvement in both local control (59% vs 34%), and CFS (30% vs 20%). However, the improvement in OS (33% vs 28%) did not reach statistical significance.[81] In the EORTC trial, CRT resulted in higher rates of CR (80% vs 54%), 5-year actuarial local control (68% vs 50%), and CFS (72% vs 40%), but no significant difference in OS (57% vs 52%).[68] Although neither trial revealed a significant OS advantage, given the improvement in local control and CFS, they helped to establish CRT as the standard of care.

Results and controversies
In the North America, CRT has been well established, and randomized trials have focused on defining the ideal regimen. The role of mitomycin-C as a necessary component of CRT was confirmed by the Intergroup trial RTOG 87-04.[82] Patients were randomized to 45 Gy plus infusional 5-FU, with or without mitomycin-C. At 6 weeks following the completion of treatment, patients with less than a CR had an additional 9 Gy to the primary tumor plus concurrent 5-FU/cisplatin as salvage therapy. If there was still less than a CR 6 weeks after the completion of this salvage therapy, APR was performed. Patients who received mitomycin-C had a higher CR rate (92% vs 85%), significantly lower colostomy rate (9% vs 22%), and a corresponding significant increase in CFS (71% vs 59%) (Table 4). There was little difference in 4-year OS (75% vs 70%). Early grade 4+ toxicity was significantly increased in the mitomycin-C arm (23% vs 7%). Although OS was not significantly increased, given the advantage in CFS, mitomycin-C is considered a necessary component of CRT.

Mitomycin-C versus cisplatin
For patients who receive mitomycin-C-based regimens, rates of CR, local control, and 5-year OS are 84% (81–87%), 73% (64–86%), and 77% (66–92%), respectively. For patients with T1–2 disease, CR rates are >90%, with ultimate local control rates of 80–90% following surgical salvage. In patients with T3–4 disease, approximately 50% of patients will require a salvage APR. If they achieve CR following the completion of CRT, then only 25% will require salvage APR. Although the results of 5-FU, mitomycin-C, and concurrent 45 Gy are impressive, combined modality therapy can be improved, especially in patients with T3–4 disease. A variety of treatment approaches have been tested. These include the use of 5-FU and cisplatin (as induction therapy and/or concurrently with radiation) and intensifying the radiation dose beyond 45 Gy using EBRT or brachytherapy. The combination of 5-FU plus cisplatin is an attractive regimen: (1) patients who have failed 5-FU/mitomycin-C still respond to 5-FU/cisplatin, and (2) cisplatin is a radiation sensitizer.

The Intergroup randomized trial RTOG 98-11 was developed to compare conventional CRT with 5-FU/mitomycin-C versus induction 5-FU/cisplatin chemotherapy followed by CRT with 5-FU/cisplatin (Table 4).[83] A total of 682 patients with stages T2–4 squamous (86%), basaloid, or cloacogenic carcinoma of the anal canal were randomized. Patients were stratified by gender, clinical node status, and tumor size. The primary endpoint was DFS. Overall, 27% had tumors >5 cm, 35% had T3–4 tumors, and 26% were clinically node-positive. Treatment details by arm were as follows. Conventional CRT arm: 5-FU (1000 mg/m^2 days 1–4 and 29–32) plus mitomycin-C (10 mg/m^2 days 1 and 29) and radiation (45–59 Gy). Induction arm: 5-FU (1000 mg/m^2 days 1–4, 29–32, 57–60, and 85–88) plus cisplatin (75 mg/m^2 on days 1, 29, 57, and 85) and radiation (45–59 Gy beginning day 57). Radiation doses and techniques were the same for both arms. The whole pelvis received 30.6 Gy (1.8 Gy/fx) followed by a 14.4 Gy cone down to the true pelvis. For N0 patients, the inguinal nodes were excluded after 36 Gy. For patients with T3–4 and/or N+ disease, or for those T2 lesions with residual disease after 45 Gy, a second cone down of 10–14 Gy to the gross disease or nodal disease was performed. Palpable inguinal nodes were biopsied prior to treatment and a full thickness biopsy was optional 8 weeks following completion of CRT, if any palpable residual abnormality was present in the inguinal node region. Local regional failure was defined as the persistence of disease in the radiation field at the 8-week follow-up.

With long-term follow-up, patients who received mitomycin-C-based treatment had a significant improvement in 5-year DFS (68% vs 58%, $p = 0.006$), 5-year CFS (72% vs 65%, $p = 0.05$), and OS (78% vs 71%, $p = 0.026$). Although local-regional failure was lower (20% vs 26%), it did not reach statistical significance. There was no difference in Grade 3+ long-term toxicity (13% vs 11%). Consistent with other reports, a separate analysis revealed that higher T and N category had a significant negative impact on outcomes, including local regional failure, distant metastasis, CFS, DFS, and OS. What is difficult to differentiate in this trial is the role of induction versus the consideration of a cisplatin-based regimen. Regardless, it is agreed that the delay in initiation of chemoradiation therapy is likely the reason for the control arm to remain superior.[84]

To date, the largest phase III trial was the UKCCR ACT II trial. This four-arm trial compared cisplatin versus mitomycin-C-based CRT (50.4 Gy), with a secondary randomization to maintenance 5-FU/cisplatin versus observation (Figure 1).[85] The primary endpoint was superiority of 5-FU/cisplatin versus 5-FU/MMC for CR at 26 weeks and acute toxic effects (for chemoradiation), and progression-free survival (for maintenance). A total of 940 patients (81% anal canal, 15% anal margin, 43% T3–4, 62% N+) were randomized. Compared with mitomycin-C-based CRT, patients who received cisplatin-based CRT had no significant difference in the CR rate at 6 months (90% vs 91%), grade 3+ toxicity (72% vs 71%), and 3-year PFS, as well as there were no difference between maintenance (72% vs 73%) and no maintenance chemotherapy arms (74% vs 73%). In summary, mitomycin-C-based conventional CRT remains the standard of care due to the lack of superiority. Despite these results, a number of investigators still advocate the use of cisplatin-based CRT based on single-institution series due to the lack of hematological toxicity which may be best suited for the elderly and immunosuppressed patients.[86] It is important to keep in mind the majority of previously conducted clinical trials did not allow a history of HIV+. New CRT approaches including the use of cytotoxic agents, such as capecitabine, oxaliplatin, and

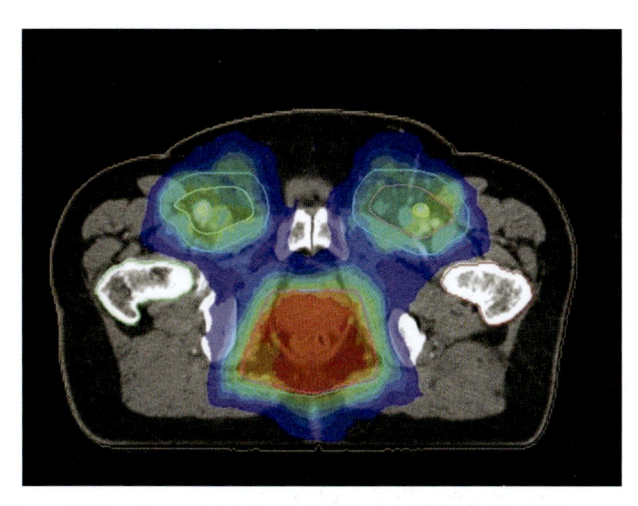

Figure 1 Intensity-modulated radiation therapy (IMRT) plan for the treatment of anal cancer. The fields include the primary tumor, pelvic, and inguinal lymph nodes.

cetuximab have been investigated.[87,88] To date, these approaches, as well as the use of triplet regimens,[89] have not shown superiority compared with 5-FU/mitomycin-C-based CRT.

Dose intensification

Conventional EBRT
In an attempt to improve local control and survival, two parallel pilot trials of radiation dose intensification were performed. In both trials, patients received 36 Gy to the pelvis (30.6 whole pelvis plus 5.4 Gy to the true pelvis), and following a 2-week break, received an additional 23.4 Gy to the primary tumor with a 2–3 cm margin for a total dose of 59.4 Gy. The main differences between the two trials was the type of chemotherapy. The RTOG 9208 trial used 5-FU and mitomycin-C,[90] whereas the ECOG 4292 trial (2297) used 5-FU and cisplatin.[91]

The RTOG 9208 trial reported similar results to the standard regimen of 45 Gy plus 5-FU/mitomycin-C used in RTOG 87-04, except for a higher 2-year colostomy rate (30% vs 7%). Likewise, the ECOG 4292 trial did not reveal a benefit compared with conventional treatment. Long-term follow-up of the ECOG 4292 trial revealed a 5-year PFS of 55% and a 5-year OS of 69%, which is consistent with other cisplatin-based trials.[92] One retrospective series revealed improved local control and survival with doses >60 Gy.[93] The RTOG 98-11 trial allowed a boost of 10–14 Gy; however, a dose response analysis has not been presented.[94]

The four-arm UNICANCER ACCORD-03 randomized trial examined the role of both induction chemotherapy and dose escalation. A total of 307 patients received 5-FU/cisplatin concurrently with 45 Gy, with or without induction 5-FU/cisplatin. This was followed by a brachytherapy or external beam boost of either 15 or 25 Gy.[95] Neither induction chemotherapy (77% vs 75%) nor the boost (78% vs 74%) had a significant improvement in 5-year CFS.

Brachytherapy
Brachytherapy is an ideal method by which to deliver conformal radiation while sparing the surrounding normal structures. In most series, patients received 30–55 Gy of pelvic radiation with or without chemotherapy, followed by a 15–25 Gy boost with Ir[192] afterloading catheters. Most used low dose rate, but some investigators have advocated high dose rate.[96–98]

Combining the series, the mean results include CR, local control, and 5-year OS rates of 83% (73–91%), 81% (73–89%), and 70% (60–84%), respectively. The primary concern is anal necrosis, and reports vary from 2% to as high as 76%,[97] with an average of 5–15%. Although a retrospective analysis revealed an improvement in local control with brachytherapy versus external beam boost,[99] and another series from France revealed a toxicity benefit from a brachytherapy boost versus no boost,[100] the randomized UNICANCER ACCORD-03 trial discussed above did not confirm a local control benefit.[95]

Intensity-modulated radiation therapy (IMRT)
Intensity-modulated radiation therapy (IMRT) is a method to deliver pelvic radiation therapy with lower acute and long-term toxicity. By identification of the dose limiting tissues surrounding the primary tumor and pelvic nodes, and using multiple radiation fields to avoid them, IMRT allows for dose escalation with less toxicity. Retrospective study with 53 anal cancer patients evaluated the efficacy and safety of IMRT-based CRT.[101] Patients received 45 Gy in whole pelvis followed by a boost to a median of 51.5 Gy. Acute grade 3 toxicities were 15% gastrointestinal and 28% skin. Acute grade 4 toxicities included 30% leucopenia and 34% neutropenia. Eighteen-month freedom from local and distant failure were 84% and 93%, respectively, and CFS was 84%, whereas OS was 93%. Other investigators have reported similar reductions in acute toxicity.[102–104]

The RTOG 0529 phase II trial examined IMRT in a cooperative group setting.[105] A total of 63 patients were treated with 5-FU/mitomycin-C plus IMRT based on stage (T2N0: 50.4 Gy primary PTV and 42 Gy nodal PTV, T3–4N0–3: 54 Gy primary PTV and 45 Gy nodal PTV). Compared with RTOG 98-11, patients who received IMRT had fewer treatment breaks (49% vs 62%), and lower acute toxicity [grade 2+ heme (73% vs 85%, $p = 0.032$), grade 3+ GI (21% vs 36%, $p = 0.0082$), and grade 3+ skin (23% vs 49%, $p < 0.0001$)]. Another finding was the steep learning curve for IMRT planning. Although institutions were required to be IMRT certified, 81% of the plans required initial modification and 46% required a second revision. Contouring guides are now routinely available.[106] Based on both single institution and RTOG data, IMRT has become the standard of care for combined modality treatment of anal cancer.

Response evaluation
As we have mentioned, SCCA is markedly sensitive to CRT, with high rates of CRs. However, it may regress slowly. ACT II trial, which randomized 940 patients to mitomycin-C or cisplatin concurrently with radiation therapy, and thereafter to a second randomization to maintenance chemotherapy or observation, proposed response assessments at 11 and 18 weeks (DRE, with or without examination under anesthesia) and at 26 weeks after the start of CRT (DRE, examination under anesthesia, abdomen and pelvis CT, and chest X-ray).[107] The CR rate increased over time in both CRT groups (52%, 71%, and 78% at 11, 18, and 26 weeks, respectively). Notably, 72% of the patients who had not reached CR at 11 weeks achieved it at 26 weeks. There was a strong correlation between response status (CR vs non-CR) at 26 weeks and outcomes (5-year PFS 80% vs 33% HR 0.16, 95% CI 0.12–0.21; and 5-year OS 87% vs 46%, HR 0.17, 95% CI 0.12–0.23). Patients have

not been submitted to biopsy during the first 26 weeks. These data from ACT II trial support the recommendation to not pursue APR before 26 weeks after the start of CRT, apart from patients who present progressive disease along this time interval. At 26 weeks, response evaluation will be classified in CR, persistent disease, and progressive disease. Patients who present progressive disease at any time, and those with persistent disease after 26 weeks should be biopsied, and once confirmed, must be referred to salvage surgery. The value of MRI in the response evaluation is uncertain.[108] Before 26 weeks, assessments are based on clinical examination (DRE and inguinal node palpation). After 26 weeks, once CR is reached, CT and/or MRI will be performed in the follow-up, as we will discuss in the next sections.

Treatment of the HIV-positive patient

In general, HIV-positive patients have historically received lower doses of radiation and chemotherapy due to a concern that standard therapy may not be tolerated.[25] With a better understanding of the immunological deficiencies seen in HIV-positive patients, more recent reports have recommended therapy based on clinical and immunological parameters, such as a history of prior opportunistic infections and CD4 counts.[109-111] Patients with a CD4 count >200 μL who receive effective doses of antiviral therapy have outcomes similar to non-HIV patients and should be treated as non-HIV+ patients.[112] CRT can result in prolonged decreased CD4 counts. One series reports an increase in late deaths,[113] whereas another series report no increased HIV-related morbidity up to 6 years following CRT.[114] Patients with a CD4 count <200 μL or who have signs or symptoms of other HIV-related diseases, may not tolerate full-dose therapy or mitomycin-C, and may require dose adjustments or chemotherapy regimens without mitomycin-C.

Toxicity of treatment

As seen with other cancer therapies, pelvic radiation is associated with acute and long-term toxicity. The acute toxicity is due to a combination of chemotherapy and radiation therapy. These include leukopenia, thrombocytopenia, proctitis, diarrhea, cystitis, and perineal erythema. Long-term toxicity is primarily increased, characterized by urgency and fecal incontinence.[115,116] This is due to both the impact of radiation on the sphincter as well as the fact that when the tumor responds, it is replaced by fibrotic tissue rather than new sphincter muscle. Acute toxicity is lower with IMRT versus conventional 3D radiation.[101-105,117]

There are limited reports of functional outcome in the anal cancer literature. One series reports that full function was maintained in 93% of patients,[118] and a second series, which used anorectal manometry, reported complete continence in 56%.[119] Another study reported good to excellent function in 93% of patients with a minimum of 1-year follow-up.[120]

Treatment of anal margin cancer

Anal margin cancers are considered to be skin cancers. In brief, a reasonable approach is to recommend a local excision for smaller tumors (≤4 cm) which are not in direct contact with the anal verge. If the patient would require an APR due to anatomic constraints, or if a local excision would compromise sphincter function, or if the tumor is >4 cm and/or node positive, then non-operative treatment is an appropriate alternative. Based on the randomized trial from the UKCCCR (which included 23% of patients with anal margin cancers),[81] CRT is recommended. In a long-term results of 101 patients, 5-year CFS (69%) and OS (54%) rates of anal margin tumors treated with CRT were lower than anal canal tumors.[121] However, this may have been due to the higher T stages.

Locally recurrent anal margin cancers are more successfully controlled by local excision than are recurrences of anal canal cancer.[122,123] A series of recurrent tumors included 16 of 48 patients who, following a local excision, recurred locally,[124] in the inguinal nodes,[125] or both.[126] There were no visceral failures. The median time to recurrence was 26 months. Ten of the patients with local recurrences underwent repeated local excision, and only one required APR. Nine of these patients survived more than 5 years. All four patients with inguinal node recurrences had inguinal lymphadenectomies, and two were long-term survivors. Although there is little reported experience with radiation therapy or CRT for patients with local recurrence after a local excision, it is a reasonable option for those who would otherwise require APR, dependent on prior radiation dose, if any.

Follow-up after treatment

Patients treated for anal cancer need to be followed carefully, especially the high-risk patients with $T > 4$ cm and node-positive disease, since those with local failure are amenable to salvage APR and can achieve long-term survival. After 26 weeks elapsed from the start of CRT, once CR is reached, patients should be examined by DRE and inguinal node palpation every 3–6 months for 5 years, anoscopy every 6–12 months for 3 years, and chest/abdominal/pelvic CT with contrast or chest CT without contrast and abdominal/pelvic MRI with contrast annually for 3 years. When failure of CRT occurs, 95% of the time it occurs within 3 years.[127]

Management of inguinal nodes

When examining the impact of positive inguinal lymph nodes on local control and survival, it is important to identify the site of nodal disease as well as to differentiate synchronous versus metachronous nodal disease. Unfortunately, most series do not separate N1 versus N2 versus N3 disease. However, there are data examining synchronous versus metachronous nodal disease.

There are conflicting reports as to the prognosis of patients with synchronous nodal disease who are treated with CRT. Compared with node-negative patients, it is observed a higher rate of local failure (N1–3: 36% vs N0: 19%),[128] and a higher colostomy rate (N1: 28% vs N0: 13%).[65] Although prospective study with 192 patients reported a local failure rate of only 13% in node-positive patients, 5-year disease-specific survival was lower (N1–3: 57% vs N0: 81%).[67] By multivariate analysis, the EORTC randomized trial reported that positive nodes were an independent negative prognostic factor for local failure and survival.[68]

In contrast, in a series evaluating CRT plus brachytherapy, patients with N1 versus N0 disease had similar 5-year disease-specific and OS rates.[66] Likewise, CR rates in the primary tumor are not affected by the presence of nodal disease. It was reported similar rates in patients receiving cisplatin-based therapy (N1–3: 92% vs N0: 100%).[129] In a separate series of patients receiving mitomycin-C-based therapy, all eight patients with N1–3 disease achieved CR.[130] Overall, EBRT alone can control positive nodes in 65% of patients,[131,132] and CRT can achieve nodal control in approximately 90%.[68,82,133]

Patients with T2N0 disease should receive radiation in inguinal nodes. In a retrospective review of patients with stages T1N0 and T2N0 disease in whom the inguinal nodes were excluded from the radiation field, the inguinal failure rate was 2% and 13%, respectively.[134]

The current treatment recommendations for patients with suspicious positive inguinal nodes include needle aspiration or, at the most, limited surgical sampling for confirmation of cancer, followed by CRT with a boost of 45–50.4 Gy to the involved groin. Although inguinal node dissection should not be performed as part of the initial therapy, it may be done for isolated inguinal recurrence in carefully selected patients since the morbidity from such an approach is significant.

The development of unilateral metachronous inguinal lymph nodes is not associated with an ominous prognosis. After therapeutic groin dissection, the 5- to 7-year survival rates exceed 50% in two series,[47] but there were no long-term survivors in a small series reported from the Mayo Clinic.[135] The use of systemic therapy and/or radiation therapy after formal groin dissection may be considered in patients with metachronous isolated inguinal node metastases after CRT. The use of radiation in this setting depends on prior dose and fields.

Treatment of metastatic disease

Approximately 15% of the anal cancer patients have metastatic disease at presentation.[39] In addition, despite the high response rates of CRT, it is estimated that approximately 10–20% of the patients submitted to combined modality therapy will present local recurrence not amenable to salvage surgery and/or distant recurrence.[68,85,133] Lungs, liver, lymph nodes, and bones are the most commonly affected sites.[136,137] Systemic chemotherapy is the cornerstone of the treatment of the metastatic disease, which is characterized by poor clinical outcomes, with 5-year OS estimated in 18%.[138]

Based on the high efficacy of the combined modality therapy with chemotherapeutic regimens composed of 5-FU with either mitomycin-C or cisplatin in localized disease, both regimens have been the preferred options as first-line therapy of metastatic disease.[139] Retrospective studies report meaningful response rates with the combination of 5-FU plus cisplatin (34–55%), but with dismal PFS and OS.[139–141] Recent non-randomized phase II trial reported results of 69 patients with metastatic disease or unresectable local recurrence who were submitted to the standard DCF (75 mg/m^2 docetaxel and 75 mg/m^2 cisplatin on day 1 and 750 mg/m^2 per day of fluorouracil for 5 days, every 3 weeks) or modified DCF (40 mg/m^2 docetaxel and 40 mg/m^2 cisplatin on day 1 and 1200 mg/m^2 per day of fluorouracil for 2 days, every 2 weeks).[142] PFS, the primary endpoint, and OS at 12 months were 47.0% and 83.1%, respectively. In the overall population, the median PFS was 11.0 months and objective response rate was 86%. There were no significant differences in the efficacy of both regimens. Nevertheless, grade 3–4 adverse events occurred in 83% of the standard DCF patients compared to 53% of the modified DCF counterparts, with neutropenia as the most common. Based on this findings, modified DCF has become a therapeutic option for metastatic anal cancer patients, but it should be restricted to patients with performance status 0–1, given its high rates of treatment-related adverse events.

InterACCT (*International Multicenter Study in Advanced Anal Cancer Comparing Cisplatin Plus 5FU vs Carboplatin Plus Weekly Paclitaxel*) was the first completed randomized clinical trial in advanced anal cancer.[143] Phase II study which randomized 91 patients with inoperable locally recurrent or metastatic treatment-naïve anal cancer to receive cisplatin at 60 mg/m^2 on D1 of a 21-day cycle plus 5-FU at 1000 mg/m^2 over 24 h on D1, four times during the cycle, or to be treated with carboplatin at AUC 5 on D1 every 28 days and paclitaxel at 80 mg/m^2 on days 1, 8, 15 every 28 days. The response rate to treatment, the primary endpoint, was 57.1% with cisplatin/5-FU compared to 59.0% with carboplatin/paclitaxel. However, survival was prolonged with carboplatin/paclitaxel. Median PFS was 5.7 months for cisplatin/5-FU versus 8.1 months for carboplatin/paclitaxel ($p = 0.375$) and median OS with the respective treatments was 12.3 months versus 20.0 months, hazard ratio HR 2.0 ($p = 0.014$). Grade ≥3 toxicity was reported in 32 (76%) patients on cisplatin/5-FU and 30 (71%) patients on carboplatin/paclitaxel. The incidence of serious adverse events (SAEs) was lower with carboplatin/paclitaxel. SAEs were reported in 62% of cisplatin/5-FU patients compared with 36% of patients receiving carboplatin/paclitaxel ($p = 0.016$). The findings of the InterACCT trial have established carboplatin/paclitaxel as the new standard of care of treatment-naïve advanced anal cancer patients.

There are no randomized clinical trials addressing the management of advanced anal cancer patients who have failed first-line therapy. The efficacy of immune checkpoint inhibitors in anal cancer was first evaluated in NCI9673, a multicenter phase II single-arm trial involving 37 patients with treatment-refractory metastatic disease.[137] Nivolumab, an anti-PD-1 monoclonal antibody, was given intravenously every 2 weeks at a dose of 3 mg/kg. The primary endpoint was response rate according to response evaluation criteria in solid tumors (RECIST) version 1.1. The median lines of previous therapy were 2 [interquartile range (IQR) 1–2.5]. Thirty-two (86%) of 37 patients had received a platinum-based regimen for metastatic disease and 31 patients (84%) had previously received radiation to the primary tumor. Two patients were HIV-positive. The median follow-up time was 10.1 months (95% CI 9.4–12.2). Patients received a median of six doses of nivolumab (IQR 3–10). Nine patients (24%) presented objective responses (seven partial and two CRs) and 17 patients (47%) had stable disease. One of the two HIV-positive patients had a partial response. Median reduction in target lesions for the responders from baseline (depth of response) was 70% (IQR 57–90). Median PFS was 4.1 months (95% CI 3.0–7.9), with a 6-month PFS of 38% (95% CI 24–60). Median OS was 11.5 months (95% CI 7.1–not estimable), with an estimated 1-year OS of 48% (32–74). The most common adverse events were anemia (70%), fatigue (68%), and rash (30%). No grade 3 or 4 adverse events occurred in the HIV-positive patients. Nine patients (four responders, five non-responders) had adequate fresh tissue from the pretreatment biopsy to analyze by flow cytometry. Flow cytometry analysis of fresh tumors specimens showed that PD-1 expression on CD8+ T cells was higher for responders than for non-responders at baseline, as were LAG-3 and TIM-3. CD45+ leucocytes had higher baseline expression of PD-L1 in responding patients than in non-responding patients. Among the CD8+ T cells, responders had higher dual expression of PD-1 and LAG-3 and of PD-1 and TIM-3 compared with non-responders.

Pembrolizumab, another anti-PD-1 antibody, has also been evaluated in advanced anal cancer population. KEYNOTE-158 (NCT02628067) is an open-label, phase II, multicohort study that evaluated antitumor activity and safety of pembrolizumab in patients with previously treated advanced cancer. Results from the anal cancer cohort were recently presented at the 2020 Gastrointestinal Cancers Symposium.[144] Metastatic or unresectable patients with prior treatment failure on or intolerance to standard first-line therapy were included. Patients received pembrolizumab 200 mg every 3 weeks until disease progression, unacceptable toxicity, or completion of 35 cycles. The primary endpoint was response rate per RECIST v1.1. Thirteen (11.6%) of 112 patients included presented objective response rate (eight partial and five CRs). Two or more prior therapies had been completed in 73.2% of the patients. Median follow-up was 12.0 months. Median duration of response was not reached (range, 6.0+ to 29.1+ months). Responses occurred in 11 (14.7%) of 75 patients with PD-L1 combined positive score (CPS) ≥1 and 2 (6.7%) of 30 patients with PD-L1 CPS < 1. Median PFS was 2.0 months (95% CI, 2.0–2.1) and median OS was 12.0 months (95% CI, 9.1–15.4). Treatment-related adverse events occurred in 68 (60.7%) patients, including 21 (18.8%) who had grade 3–4 events. Twenty-seven patients (24.1%) had immune-mediated adverse events or infusion reactions.

Anti-PD-1 inhibitors have been intensively investigated in SCCA, with many ongoing clinical trials evaluating its efficacy in monotherapy, and in combination with anti-CTLA-4 antibodies, chemotherapy, and anti-angiogenic therapy:

- *ECOG 2165*. A randomized phase-II study of nivolumab after combined modality in high-risk anal cancer (NCT03233711)
- *NCI9673 (Part B)*. A randomized phase-II ETCTN study of nivolumab plus or minus ipilimumab for refractory surgically unresectable or metastatic anal cancer
- Phase-II study of atezolizumab and bevacizumab in rare solid tumors including an HPV-malignancies arm (NCT03074513)
- A multicenter phase-II clinical trial of pembrolizumab in refractory metastatic anal cancer (NCT02919969)
- A phase-I study of ipilimumab and nivolumab in advanced HIV-associated solid tumors with expansion cohorts in HIV-associated solid tumors and a cohort of HIV-associated classical Hodgkin lymphoma (NCT02408861)
- A study of mDCF in combination or not with atezolizumab in advanced squamous cell anal carcinoma (SCARCE) (NCT03519295).

Immunotherapeutic vaccines

Immunotherapeutic vaccines using bacterial vectors have been widely evaluated in HPV-associated malignancies, primarily in cervical cancer. The bacterial vector most commonly used is *Listeria monocytogenes* (Lm), because of its immunological advantages. Following infection of the host cells, Lm can activate both the innate and adaptive immune responses. Lm-listeriolysin O (LLO) immunotherapies have been reported to present with multiple simultaneous mechanisms of action that contribute to generation of a therapeutic response. Axalimogene filolisbac (ADXS11-001; AXAL) is based on the irreversibly attenuated Lm fused to the nonhemolytic fragment of LLO, and has been developed to secrete the Lm-LLO-E7 fusion protein targeting HPV-positive tumors.

AXAL has been investigated in combination with standard of care RT and concurrent 5-FU and mitomycin-C in a phase-I study in patients with high-risk locally advanced SCCA (BrUOG 276).[145] Nine out of 11 patients had complete remission with a well-tolerated safety profile. Phase II trial evaluated the efficacy and safety of AXAL in patients with surgically unresectable or metastatic SCCA.[146] Thirty-six patients were treated, of which 29 patients were evaluable for response. One patient had a prolonged partial response (3.4% ORR). The 6-month PFS rate was 15.5%. Grade 3 adverse event were noted in 10 patients, with the majority being cytokine-release symptoms. Despite being safe and well-tolerated, ADXS11-001 study did not meet either primary endpoint (ORR ≥ 10% or 6-month PFS rate ≥ 20%) to proceed to the second stage of the study.

MEDI0457 is an investigational T-cell activation immunotherapy that targets cancers caused by HPV types 16 and 18, and it has been investigated in combination with durvalumab in patients with recurrent or metastatic HPV-associated cancers (NCT03439085).

Adoptive T-cell therapy

Phase I/II clinical trial of T cells genetically engineered to express a TCR that targets an HLA-A*02:01-restricted epitope of E6 (E6 TCR T Cells) for patients with metastatic HPV16-positive carcinoma evaluated 16 patients, of which four were anal cancer patients.[147] Two patients with anal cancer showed partial responses lasting 3 and 6 months after treatment. The patient with a 6-month response had complete regression of one tumor and partial regression of two tumors that were resected upon progression. Another clinical trial exploring the role of TCR-engineered T cells in SCCA is ongoing (NCT03247309).

Other histologies

Melanoma

Anorectal melanomas are relatively rare, accounting for less than 1% of all anal canal tumors.[148] The presenting stage, defined by the tumor thickness and nodal status, is the primary determinant of survival.[149,150] Distant metastases are common.[149,151–153] Despite a better local control rate with APR, most series have not shown a clear survival advantage for patients who have had APR compared with patients having wide local excision.[150,151,154–156] A retrospective analysis of the SEER database of 126 patients treated from 1973 to 2001 with a variety of therapies reported the 5-year survival based on disease status at presentation: local, 32%, local/regional, 17%, and distant, 0%.[157]

The inability to show a survival benefit for APR compared with wide local excision can be attributed to the small numbers of patients involved in the studies, selection bias, and the lack of randomized data. Any relative advantage of adjuvant immunotherapies, chemotherapy, and radiation therapy is similarly obscured and difficult to interpret. A histological margin of at least 3 mm should be obtained if local excision is to be used. In view of possible higher local control rates, APR is still a reasonable option.[149,151–153,158,159]

Adenocarcinoma

Primary adenocarcinoma of the anal canal arising from the anal glands is rare. Most adenocarcinomas in the canal represent rectal cancer with distal spread. In general, they should be treated like adenocarcinomas of the rectum. If T3 and or N+, then preoperative CRT followed by surgery and 4 months of postoperative adjuvant therapy is appropriate. However, the radiation fields should include the inguinal nodes. In a series of 34 patients, 13 (46%) were treated with local excision followed by RT or CRT.[86]

Fifteen patients (54%) underwent radical surgery and preoperative or postoperative CRT. Median DFS was 13 months after local excision and 32 months after radical surgery ($p = 0.055$). 5-year OS was 43% for patients treated with local excision and 63% for patients treated with radical surgery ($p = 0.3$). Tumor grade was predictive of OS ($p = 0.04$) and recurrence ($p = 0.046$). On multivariate analysis, the type of surgical treatment was an important predictor of OS ($p = 0.045$) and DFS ($p = 0.004$). Another series of 13 patients, the combination of CRT and APR associated with a 2-year actuarial survival of 62%.[160] Adenosquamous cancers of the anus are also rare and have a poor prognosis.[161]

Sarcoma

Few cases of leiomyosarcoma of the anus have been reported. The optimal treatment for this neoplasm is not known. The standard surgical approach is APR. Using a technique well established for management of sarcomas of the extremities, one approach is local excision and Iridium-192 brachytherapy in an attempt to preserve the anal sphincter.[162–164] This technique may be an alternative to APR in selected patients.

Others

Bowen's disease, Paget's disease and Kaposi's sarcoma are commonly treated with surgery if localized. In settings where this could compromise sphincter function, there are rare reports of treatment with radiation therapy.[165]

Key references

The complete reference list can be found on Vital Source version of this title, see inside front cover.

3. Ryan DP, Compton CC, Mayer RJ. Carcinoma of the anal canal. *N Engl J Med*. 2000;**342**(11):792–800.
5. Siegel RL, Miller KD, Jemal A. Cancer statistics, 2020. *CA Cancer J Clin*. 2020;**70**(1):7–30.
8. Palefsky JM, Holly EA. Molecular virology and epidemiology of human papillomavirus and cervical cancer. *Cancer Epidemiol Biomark Prev*. 1995;**4**(4):415–428.
15. Darragh TM, Colgan TJ, Thomas Cox J, et al. The Lower Anogenital Squamous Terminology Standardization project for HPV-associated lesions: background and consensus recommendations from the College of American Pathologists and the American Society for Colposcopy and Cervical Pathology. *Int J Gynecol Pathol*. 2013;**32**(1):76–115.
21. Machalek DA, Poynten M, Jin F, et al. Anal human papillomavirus infection and associated neoplastic lesions in men who have sex with men: a systematic review and meta-analysis. *Lancet Oncol*. 2012;**13**(5):487–500.
24. Daling JR, Weiss NS, Hislop TG, et al. Sexual practices, sexually transmitted diseases, and the incidence of anal cancer. *N Engl J Med*. 1987;**317**(16):973–977.
25. Melbye M, Coté TR, Kessler L, et al. High incidence of anal cancer among AIDS patients. The AIDS/Cancer Working Group. *Lancet*. 1994;**343**(8898):636–639.
33. Chung JH, Sanford E, Johnson A, et al. Comprehensive genomic profiling of anal squamous cell carcinoma reveals distinct genomically defined classes. *Ann Oncol*. 2016;**27**(7):1336–1341.
34. Siegel EM, Eschrich S, Winter K, et al. Epigenomic characterization of locally advanced anal cancer: a radiation therapy oncology group 98-11 specimen study. *Dis Colon Rectum*. 2014;**57**(8):941–957.
35. Morris V, Rao X, Pickering C, et al. Comprehensive genomic profiling of metastatic squamous cell carcinoma of the anal canal. *Mol Cancer Res*. 2017;**15**(11):1542–1550.
36. Smaglo BG, Tesfaye A, Halfdanarson TR, et al. Comprehensive multiplatform biomarker analysis of 199 anal squamous cell carcinomas. *Oncotarget*. 2015;**6**(41):43594–43604.
39. Myerson RJ, Karnell LH, Menck HR. The National Cancer Data Base report on carcinoma of the anus. *Cancer*. 1997;**80**(4):805–815.
65. Peiffert D, Bey P, Pernot M, et al. Conservative treatment by irradiation of epidermoid cancers of the anal canal: prognostic factors of tumoral control and complications. *Int J Radiat Oncol Biol Phys*. 1997;**37**(2):313–324.
66. Gerard JP, Ayzac L, Hun D, et al. Treatment of anal canal carcinoma with high dose radiation therapy and concomitant fluorouracil-cisplatinum. Long-term results in 95 patients. *Radiother Oncol*. 1998;**46**(3):249–256.
67. Cummings BJ, Keane TJ, O'Sullivan B, et al. Epidermoid anal cancer: treatment by radiation alone or by radiation and 5-fluorouracil with and without mitomycin C. *Int J Radiat Oncol Biol Phys*. 1991;**21**(5):1115–1125.
68. Bartelink H, Roelofsen F, Eschwege F, et al. Concomitant radiotherapy and chemotherapy is superior to radiotherapy alone in the treatment of locally advanced anal cancer: results of a phase III randomized trial of the European Organization for Research and Treatment of Cancer Radiotherapy and Gastrointestinal Cooperative Groups. *J Clin Oncol*. 1997;**15**(5):2040–2049.
69. Goldman S, Glimelius B, Glas U, et al. Management of anal epidermoid carcinoma–an evaluation of treatment results in two population-based series. *Int J Color Dis*. 1989;**4**(4):234–243.
70. Das P, Bhatia S, Eng C, et al. Predictors and patterns of recurrence after definitive chemoradiation for anal cancer. *Int J Radiat Oncol Biol Phys*. 2007;**68**(3):794–800.
71. Ajani JA, Winter KA, Gunderson LL, et al. Prognostic factors derived from a prospective database dictate clinical biology of anal cancer: the intergroup trial (RTOG 98-11). *Cancer*. 2010;**116**(17):4007–4013.
80. Nigro ND, Vaitkevicius VK, Considine B. Combined therapy for cancer of the anal canal: a preliminary report. *Dis Colon Rectum*. 1974;**17**(3):354–356.
81. Northover J, Glynne-Jones R, Sebag-Montefiore D, et al. Chemoradiation for the treatment of epidermoid anal cancer: 13-year follow-up of the first randomised UKCCCR Anal Cancer Trial (ACT I). *Br J Cancer*. 2010;**102**(7):1123–1128.
82. Flam M, John M, Pajak TF, et al. Role of mitomycin in combination with fluorouracil and radiotherapy, and of salvage chemoradiation in the definitive nonsurgical treatment of epidermoid carcinoma of the anal canal: results of a phase III randomized intergroup study. *J Clin Oncol*. 1996;**14**(9):2527–2539.
83. Gunderson LL, Winter KA, Ajani JA, et al. Long-term update of US GI intergroup RTOG 98-11 phase III trial for anal carcinoma: survival, relapse, and colostomy failure with concurrent chemoradiation involving fluorouracil/mitomycin versus fluorouracil/cisplatin. *J Clin Oncol*. 2012;**30**(35):4344–4351.
84. Gunderson LL, Moughan J, Ajani JA, et al. Anal carcinoma: impact of TN category of disease on survival, disease relapse, and colostomy failure in US Gastrointestinal Intergroup RTOG 98-11 phase 3 trial. *Int J Radiat Oncol Biol Phys*. 2013;**87**(4):638–645.
85. James RD, Glynne-Jones R, Meadows HM, et al. Mitomycin or cisplatin chemoradiation with or without maintenance chemotherapy for treatment of squamous-cell carcinoma of the anus (ACT II): a randomised, phase 3, open-label, 2 × 2 factorial trial. *Lancet Oncol*. 2013;**14**(6):516–524.
86. Chang GJ, Gonzalez RJ, Skibber JM, et al. A twenty-year experience with adenocarcinoma of the anal canal. *Dis Colon Rectum*. 2009;**52**(8):1375–1380.
87. Eng C, Jácome AA, Das P, et al. A phase II study of capecitabine/oxaliplatin with concurrent radiotherapy in locally advanced squamous cell carcinoma of the anal canal. *Clin Colorectal Cancer*. 2019;**18**(4):301–306.
88. Deutsch E, Lemanski C, Pignon JP, et al. Unexpected toxicity of cetuximab combined with conventional chemoradiotherapy in patients with locally advanced anal cancer: results of the UNICANCER ACCORD 16 phase II trial. *Ann Oncol*. 2013;**24**(11):2834–2838.
90. John M, Pajak T, Flam M, et al. Dose escalation in chemoradiation for anal cancer: preliminary results of RTOG 92-08. *Cancer J Sci Am*. 1996;**2**(4):205–211.
91. Martenson JA, Lipsitz SR, Wagner H, et al. Initial results of a phase II trial of high dose radiation therapy, 5-fluorouracil, and cisplatin for patients with anal cancer (E4292): an Eastern Cooperative Oncology Group study. *Int J Radiat Oncol Biol Phys*. 1996;**35**(4):745–749.
92. Chakravarthy AB, Catalano PJ, Martenson JA, et al. Long-term follow-up of a phase II trial of high-dose radiation with concurrent 5-fluorouracil and cisplatin in patients with anal cancer (ECOG E4292). *Int J Radiat Oncol Biol Phys*. 2011;**81**(4):e607–e613.
94. Ajani JA, Winter KA, Gunderson LL, et al. Fluorouracil, mitomycin, and radiotherapy vs fluorouracil, cisplatin, and radiotherapy for carcinoma of the anal canal: a randomized controlled trial. *JAMA*. 2008;**299**(16):1914–1921.
95. Peiffert D, Tournier-Rangeard L, Gérard JP, et al. Induction chemotherapy and dose intensification of the radiation boost in locally advanced anal canal carcinoma: final analysis of the randomized UNICANCER ACCORD 03 trial. *J Clin Oncol*. 2012;**30**(16):1941–1948.
105. Kachnic LA, Winter K, Myerson RJ, et al. RTOG 0529: a phase 2 evaluation of dose-painted intensity modulated radiation therapy in combination with 5-fluorouracil and mitomycin-C for the reduction of acute morbidity in carcinoma of the anal canal. *Int J Radiat Oncol Biol Phys*. 2013;**86**(1):27–33.
107. Glynne-Jones R, Sebag-Montefiore D, Meadows HM, et al. Best time to assess complete clinical response after chemoradiotherapy in squamous cell carcinoma of the anus (ACT II): a post-hoc analysis of randomised controlled phase 3 trial. *Lancet Oncol*. 2017;**18**(3):347–356.
112. Fraunholz I, Rabeneck D, Gerstein J, et al. Concurrent chemoradiotherapy with 5-fluorouracil and mitomycin C for anal carcinoma: are there differences

137 Morris VK, Salem ME, Nimeiri H, et al. Nivolumab for previously treated unresectable metastatic anal cancer (NCI9673): a multicentre, single-arm, phase 2 study. *Lancet Oncol.* 2017;**18**(4):446–453.

142 Kim S, François E, André T, et al. Docetaxel, cisplatin, and fluorouracil chemotherapy for metastatic or unresectable locally recurrent anal squamous cell carcinoma (Epitopes-HPV02): a multicentre, single-arm, phase 2 study. *Lancet Oncol.* 2018;**19**(8):1094–1106.

143 Rao S, Sclafani F, Eng C, et al. International rare cancers initiative multicenter randomized phase II trial of cisplatin and fluorouracil versus carboplatin and paclitaxel in advanced anal cancer: InterAAct. *J Clin Oncol.* 2020;**38**(22):2510–2518.

144 Marabelle A, Cassier PA, Fakih M, et al. *Pembrolizumab for Advanced anal Squamous Cell Carcinoma (ASCC): Results from the Multicohort, Phase II KEYNOTE-158 Study*. American Society of Clinical Oncology; 2020.

(The reference list begins with text continuing from a previous page: "between HIV-positive and HIV-negative patients in the era of highly active antiretroviral therapy? *Radiother Oncol.* 2011;**98**(1):99–104.")

93 Renal cell carcinoma

Claude M. Grigg, MD ■ Earle F. Burgess, MD ■ Stephen B. Riggs, MD, MBA, FACS ■ Jason Zhu, MD ■ Derek Raghavan, MD, PhD, FACP, FRACP, FASCO, FAAAS

Overview

Renal cell carcinoma occurs in 73,000 patients each year in the United States and results in almost 15,000 deaths. For localized disease, cure is achieved by nephrectomy. Meticulous surgical staging is crucial. With improved imaging techniques, active surveillance has become an option for small, asymptomatic renal masses. Modifications in surgical technique, including laparoscopic and robotic approaches, have contributed to reduced morbidity. In advanced clear cell carcinoma, cytotoxic chemotherapy has negligible activity but targeted therapies, such as tyrosine kinase and mammalian target of rapamycin inhibitors, can cause dramatic regressions. Immune checkpoint inhibitors, which stimulate the immune system to eradicate cancer cells, can also achieve substantial and durable tumor reductions. Other cancers of the kidney are rare, and optimal management beyond aggressive surgical resection has not been defined.

Introduction

The incidence of renal cell carcinoma (RCC) is estimated at approximately 73,000 cases with 15,000 deaths in the United States annually.[1] The reported incidence of RCC has increased over time, largely but not entirely owing to an increase in the number of asymptomatic tumors incidentally detected with abdominal imaging obtained for other indications.[2]

The management of RCC has evolved substantially. Treatment for renal masses now emphasizes less invasive approaches including nephron-sparing surgery and active surveillance. As the biology of RCC has been elucidated, agents targeting relevant biologic pathways have demonstrated robust clinical effect in the metastatic setting. This article details these advances.

Epidemiology

RCC commonly presents in the sixth to seventh decade of life and develops in men twice as frequently as in women. Tobacco exposure is an established two-to-three-fold risk factor.[3] Other risk factors include obesity (although specific dietary associations are not well defined),[4] hypertension, but not likely antihypertensive medicine,[5] acquired polycystic disease,[6] and various autosomal dominant syndromes that predispose patients to various RCC histologic subtypes that are detailed subsequently. Analgesic abuse is also associated with RCC, although more commonly this association is found for cancer of the renal pelvis.[7]

Clinical presentation

In contemporary series, more than 50% of RCC patients present as a result of abdominal CT scans or ultrasounds performed for an unrelated indication.[8] By comparison, in the 1970s, only 10% of RCCs were discovered incidentally.[9]

The most common local symptoms of RCC include hematuria, flank pain, and a palpable mass, although today this classic triad is observed infrequently. Left scrotal varicoceles occur in up to 11% of men because of obstruction of the gonadal vein by tumor in the left renal vein to which it directly empties. Venous involvement can also cause lower extremity edema, ascites, hepatic dysfunction, and pulmonary emboli. Pain or dysfunction of specific organs may be the presenting feature of the patient with metastatic disease.

Paraneoplastic syndromes, such as hypercalcemia, manifest in 13–20% of patients. Hypercalcemia is mediated by tumor production of parathyroid hormone (PTH) or PTH-related peptide. Polycythemia occurs in 1–8% of cases and may be mediated by elevated erythropoietin levels; anemia is far more common and can be severe. Stauffer's syndrome is hepatic dysfunction in the setting of RCC without liver metastases. Corticosteroid-insensitive polymyalgia rheumatica can occasionally occur and often resolves following nephrectomy. Endocrine abnormalities including elevated human chorionic gonadotrophin (HCG) and adreno cortico trophic hormone (ACTH) have also been reported uncommonly. Other constitutional symptoms such as fever, weight loss, and fatigue are common.

Pathophysiology

The World Health Organization classification of renal neoplasms was updated in 2016 to account for unique morphological, molecular, and genetic features of both common and rare subtypes of renal neoplasms.[10] The most common RCC histology remains the conventional clear cell subtype (ccRCC) accounting for 75–90% of all RCCs. Other previously recognized histologies include papillary (10–15%), chromophobe (5–10%), medullary (<1%), and collecting duct carcinomas (CDC) (<1%).

ccRCC arises from the proximal convoluted tubule and has clear cytoplasm on routine microscopic sections. Loss of chromosome 3p, which encompasses the four tumor suppressor genes VHL, PBRM1, BAP1, and SETD2, occurs in up to 91% of cases.[11] Additional genomic aberrations were outlined by The Cancer Genome Atlas (TCGA) involving the PI3K/Akt pathway and chromatin remodeling genes, implicating epigenetic dysregulation in ccRCC tumorigenesis.[11] Noninherited ccRCC tends to present with larger, unilateral tumors. The inherited von Hippel Lindau syndrome

(1/36,000 births) is a highly penetrant autosomal dominant disorder in which patients inherit a VHL gene defect on chromosome 3p25 and develop ccRCC and/or a constellation of cysts and tumors in the central nervous system and abdominal viscera.[12] CNS lesions include retinal hemangioblastomas, endolymphatic sac tumors, and craniospinal hemangioblastomas. The visceral lesions in these patients include ccRCCs, pheochromocytomas, pancreatic neuroendocrine tumors, epididymal cystadenomas, and broad ligament cystadenomas. Up to 14% of patients harbor a germline mutation known to elevate cancer risk, including CHEK2, MUTYH, APC, and BAP1, and routine germline testing has been implemented in some institutions.[13]

Papillary RCCs arise from the distal convoluted tubule and are composed of tubulopapillary structures with hemosiderin deposition and foamy histiocytes within the fibrovascular cores. They are subdivided into type 1 and type 2 papillary RCCs based on the morphology of the tumor cells lining the papillary structures.[10] Type 1 papillary carcinomas do not have VHL gene inactivation but have trisomy of chromosomes 7, 17 and loss of Y chromosome as the most frequent genetic alterations. Mutations in the MET oncogene occur in 10–20% of type 1 tumors, while type 2 tumors are associated with loss of CDKN2A and mutations in SETD2, PBRM1, and BAP1 similar to ccRCC.[14] Papillary tumors tend to have a multifocal nature and may present with bilateral kidney involvement. Hereditary papillary renal carcinoma (HRPC) is characterized by c-Met proto-oncogene activation (chromosome 7q31-34) and the development of type 1 papillary RCC. Hereditary leiomyomatosis renal cell carcinoma (HLRCC) involves abnormalities of the fumarate hydratase gene (chromosome 1q42-43) and development of type 2 papillary RCC, leiomyomas of skin, and uterine leiomyomas and leiomyosarcomas.[15]

Chromophobe RCC arises from the intercalated cells of the kidney and is characterized by large solid sheets of cells with pale or eosinophilic cytoplasm, a thick and distinct cell membrane, and pleomorphic nuclei with an irregular nuclear membrane and perinuclear clearing.[10] The most frequent genetic alterations are a combination of loss of heterozygosity in chromosomes 1, 2, 6, 10, 13, 17, 21, and hypodiploidy. Patients with chromophobe histology tend to present with early-stage disease with <5% of patients presenting with metastases.[16,17] Patients with Birt–Hogg–Dube syndrome have a high proportion of RCCs with chromophobe-predominant histology. They possess loss of function mutations in the BHD gene on chromosome 17p, have prominent cutaneous manifestations (fibrofolliculomas), and are predisposed to pneumothoraces from rupture of pulmonary cysts.[17,18] Comprehensive whole-genome analysis has identified prevalent genomic rearrangements within the promoter region of the TERT gene, the catalytic subunit of telomerase, leading to increased TERT expression.[19] Thus, enhanced telomerase expression via structural promoter rearrangements may be an early pathogenic event in the development of chromophobe RCC.

The newest WHO classification added several rare RCC subtypes including MiT family translocation RCC involving chromosomal arms Xp11 (TFE3) or 6p21 (TFEB), HLRCC syndrome-associated RCC, succinate dehydrogenase–deficient RCC, tubulocystic RCC, acquired cystic disease-associated RCC, and clear cell papillary RCC. While a review of these subtypes is beyond the scope of this article, clear cell papillary RCC is important in that it shows indolent behavior with no reported recurrences or metastases and was previously classified as ccRCC.[10] Unlike ccRCC, they are CK7 positive and show a cup-shaped staining pattern with CA-IX. They occur in 5% of resections and are associated with acquired cystic renal disease.[10]

Prognostic features

Grade
In patients with localized RCC, nuclear Fuhrman grade and TNM stage are consistently the most important prognostic factors.[20] The Fuhrman grading system scores the nuclear grade of RCCs on a scale of 1–4 (most aggressive) based on nuclear and nucleolar size, shape, and content.[21] Higher nuclear grade is associated with a worse 5-year overall survival. Five-year cancer-specific survival rates for localized grade 1, grade 2, and grade 3 or 4 tumors after nephrectomy are 89%, 65%, and 46%, respectively.[20] Fuhrman grading is not useful for chromophobe RCC.[21] Inter-observer variation has led to a modification, still with four grades, but with degree of nucleolar prominence assessed to define grades 1–3 and the presence of atypical pleomorphic cells and/or sarcomatoid or rhabdoid patterns defining grade 4. Grade is assigned according to the highest grade rather than the most prominent pattern.[10]

Staging
In a patient with a suspected RCC, staging investigations including a CT or MRI of the chest, abdomen, and pelvis are required to define the extent of the disease. The most common sites of metastases include the lungs, abdominal and mediastinal lymph nodes, liver, and bone. Without relevant symptoms, initial bone and brain imaging tend to produce relatively low yield.

The 2018 American Joint Committee on Cancer (AJCC) TNM staging system reflects the extent of tumor (T), lymph node involvement (N), and presence of metastases (M).[22] There have been some changes since the 2010 classification, including the description of pT3a disease with elimination of "grossly extends into" from description of renal vein involvement, change from "muscle containing" to "invasion into segmental veins," and addition of invasion of the pelvicalyceal system. In addition, increased rigor of tissue sampling has been specified, with greater consideration of molecular diagnostics.

Treatment of localized RCC
Management options for small (<4 cm) renal masses include surgical excision, radiofrequency ablation (RFA) or cryotherapy, or active surveillance with or without delayed intervention in very select populations. Surgical resection remains the cornerstone of the treatment of localized stage I and II RCC and usually obviates the need for a renal biopsy. Partial nephrectomy is preferred whenever feasible, especially in a patient with limited renal function, bilateral tumors, and/or a patient with a solitary kidney. Although nephron sparing is currently recommended as treatment for small renal masses, its absolute benefit compared to radical nephrectomy (in the elective setting) has come into question.[23,24] Laparoscopic partial nephrectomy is less invasive and has similar outcomes to that of an open approach. Robotic laparoscopic surgery has expanded the use of laparoscopy for partial nephrectomy by overcoming inherent limitations to traditional laparoscopy while improving outcomes.[25,26]

The preferred treatment of large tumors (>7 cm) and locally advanced tumors is a radical nephrectomy, either with a laparoscopic or open procedure. This involves ligation of the renal vasculature, excision of the kidney, Gerota's fascia, and the ipsilateral adrenal gland if it appears involved by tumor on preoperative imaging. Laparoscopic radical nephrectomy has decreased postoperative pain with shorter hospitalization and quicker recovery.

Long-term follow-up of cryoablation and RFA, when used for highly selected patients, suggests that these therapies may result in similar local recurrence-free survival as compared to partial nephrectomy for cT1a tumors.[27] However, there are no randomized trial results to prove this.

Partial nephrectomy has the perceived advantage of complete pathologic evaluation as well as reduced need for radiologic follow-up. In general, percutaneous ablation is favored in patients with smaller tumors (<4 cm) desiring an option other than surgery or who are not candidates for invasive operations.

Active surveillance is an emerging approach to small renal masses since 50–60% will be indolent, based on size and grade. Mean growth rate is around 0.3 cm per year with a 1–3% metastatic rate.[28] Increasing support for this approach is seen as studies with longer follow-up suggest low rates of progression and metastatic disease.[29] Importantly, utilization of percutaneous renal biopsies is evolving. Historically fraught with inconclusive results, more contemporary studies suggest nondiagnostic biopsies to occur less than 10% of the time. Unfortunately, grade accuracy remains intermediate (50–70%).[30]

Stage III disease involves perinephric tissues, lymph nodes, and/or invasion of the renal vein or inferior vena cava. The procedure of choice for these individuals is an open radical nephrectomy for curative intent. Lymph node dissection should be carried out in patients with evidence of enlarged lymph nodes. In patients with no suspected nodal metastases, the use of a routinely extended lymph node dissection remains controversial.[31]

Although preoperative treatment with targeted molecular therapies may be safe, a role for these agents in the nonmetastatic setting remains controversial. Initially, retrospective case series suggested that use of targeted agents before nephrectomy did not result in frequent down-sizing of primary tumors,[32] and exposed patients to the risk of progression and increased complexity of ensuing surgical management.[33] More contemporary case series and Phase II trials have found that preoperative targeted agents result in at least modest decreases in tumor volume in over 80% of tumors, with carefully selected patients experiencing surgical downstaging.[34] In patients with inferior vena cava tumor thrombi, neoadjuvant-targeted therapies have failed to show the same degree of cytoreductive effect on tumor thrombus burden and should not be routinely utilized to influence surgical decision making.[35,36]

Targeted agents, specifically tyrosine kinase inhibitors (TKIs), have been studied more extensively in the adjuvant setting after resection of tumors at high risk for recurrence (Table 1). High risk has been variably defined as high grade (Fuhrman grade 3 or 4), pathologic stage T3 or greater, or node positivity. Three large Phase III trials, ASSURE, PROTECT, and ATLAS, failed to demonstrate a benefit from prescription of adjuvant sunitinib, sorafenib, pazopanib, or axitinib for 1–3 years following resection of high-risk RCC.[37,39] In a fourth Phase III study called S-TRAC, one year of adjuvant sunitinib improved the median disease-free survival (DFS) by 1.2 years.[40] There was significant toxicity associated with treatment, and overall survival (OS) was not improved. The positive findings in this study, unlike in previous studies, may have been due to enrollment of a higher risk population limited to pT3 or higher disease (see Table 1). A post hoc analysis of similar patients enrolled in ASSURE did not find any such improvements in DFS or OS, while a similar analysis from ATLAS did identify an improvement in DFS in the higher risk subgroup.[37,43] A late analysis of the ASSURE trial suggested that local recurrence was a function of tumor biology rather than the surgery employed (partial vs radical) or surgical modality (open vs laparoscopic).[44] Sunitinib was approved by the FDA for adjuvant treatment of adult patients at high risk of recurrence following nephrectomy. In practice, however, adjuvant sunitinib is infrequently used due to its considerable toxicity and uncertain impact on overall survival. Because overall survival has not been improved (and DFS improvement might be expected with any effective treatment), consensus guidelines do not currently support routine use of adjuvant TKI therapies, despite the FDA imprimatur.[43]

While the experience with TKIs in the adjuvant setting has been disappointing, there is renewed hope that immune checkpoint inhibitors (ICIs) may be more effective given their success in the adjuvant setting for melanoma and lung cancer. Multiple Phase 3 trials of ICIs for resected ccRCC have completed accrual with results anticipated in 1–2 years.

Table 1 Adjuvant clinical trials of TKIs for renal cell carcinoma.

Clinical trial	Inclusion criteria	Agent	N (pts)	DFS	OS
ASSURE[37,38] Total cohort	Any RCC except medullary/collecting duct subtypes	Sunitinib	647	Median: 5.8 y	5 y OS: 77.9%
	pT1b + grade 3–4 or ≥pT2 or pN1	Sorafenib	649	6.1 y	80.5%
		Placebo	647	6.6 yNS	80.3%NS
ASSURE[37,38] High risk subgroup	Clear cell RCC ≥pT3 or pN1	Sunitinib	358	5 y DFS: 47.7%	5 y OS: 75.2%
		Sorafenib	355	49.9%	80.2%
		Placebo	356	50.0%NS	76.5%NS
PROTECT[39]	Clear-cell RCC pT2 + grade 3–4 or ≥pT3 or pN1	Pazopanib	571	Median: 30.4m	Median: NR
		Placebo	564	30.7mNS	NRNS
S-TRAC[40,41]	Clear-cell RCC ≥pT3 or pN1	Sunitinib	309	Median: 6.8 y	Median: NR
		Placebo	306	5.6 ySS	NRNS
ATLAS[42]	Clear-cell RCC ≥pT2 or pN1	Axitinib	363	HR = 0.870NS	HR = 1.026 NS
		Placebo	361		

Abbreviations: DFS, disease-free survival; OS, overall survival; T and N stages according to American Joint Committee on Cancer staging system; m, months; y, years; NR, median not reached; NS, not statistically significant; SS, statistically significant; HR, hazard ratio.
NS, Difference not statistically significant.
SS, Difference statistically significant with a p value 0.03 based on a HR 0.76, 95% confidence interval 0.59–0.98.

Therapeutic intervention for local and/or oligometastatic recurrences may improve patient outcomes, supporting the importance of detecting recurrences early. An ideal surveillance strategy following definitive management of primary renal tumors should balance the risk of recurrence against the desire to avoid unnecessary diagnostic testing. Individual risk-based surveillance guidelines have been proposed, although an optimal surveillance strategy remains to be defined.[45,46]

Metastatic disease

Prognostic factors

The most widely used prognostic factors for metastatic renal cell carcinoma (mRCC) were developed in the era when patients with mRCC were treated primarily with IL-2 and interferon. The Memorial Sloan Kettering Cancer Center (MSKCC) criteria consist of a clinical scoring system that classifies patients into favorable, intermediate, and poor prognosis categories based on the number of adverse risk features present.[47] In patients treated with IFN only, the median overall survival for each prognostic category was 30, 14, and 5 months, respectively (Table 2).[48]

A newer prognostic model has been developed for patients treated with molecular-targeted therapy. Prognostic factors were identified from a retrospective, multicenter analysis of 645 patients with mRCC treated with sunitinib, sorafenib, or bevacizumab, and the revised prognostic model consisted of three risk groups (Table 2).[50] External validation by an international mRCC database consortium (IMDC) supports the routine use of this prognostic model with current standard therapies and illustrates the survival improvements that have resulted from treatment advances.[49] IMDC risk stratification also has prognostic value in patients with metastatic non-ccRCC[51] and may facilitate decision making regarding cytoreductive nephrectomy[52] as discussed in the following section.

Table 2 Prognostic criteria for metastatic RCC.[a]

Memorial Sloan Kettering Cancer Center (MSKCC) criteria[48]
Adverse prognostic factors
- Karnofsky performance status < 80%
- Diagnosis to treatment interval < 1 year
- Hemoglobin < lower limit of normal
- Serum corrected calcium > 10 g/dL
- LDH > 1.5× upper limit of normal

Risk categories and clinical outcome:
- 0 prognostic factors (good risk): PFS: 8.3 m OS: 30 m
- 1–2 prognostic factors (intermediate risk): PFS: 5.1 m OS: 14 m
- 3–5 prognostic factors (poor risk): PFS: 2.5 m OS: 5 m

International Metastatic Renal Cell Carcinoma Database Consortium (IMDC) criteria[49]
Adverse prognostic factors
- Karnofsky performance status <80%
- Diagnosis to treatment interval <1 year
- Hemoglobin < lower limit of normal
- Serum corrected calcium > upper limit of normal
- Neutrophil count > upper limit of normal
- Platelet count > upper limit of normal

Risk categories and clinical outcome
- 0 prognostic factors (favorable risk): OS: 43 m
- 1–2 prognostic factors (intermediate risk): OS: 23 m
- 3–6 prognostic factors (poor risk): OS: 8 m

Abbreviations: OS, overall survival; PFS, progression-free survival.
[a]Source: Based on Motzer et al.[48]; Heng et al.[50]

Surgery in patients with metastatic disease

Radical cytoreductive nephrectomy to remove the primary renal mass when metastatic disease is present is controversial but remains indicated in carefully selected patients with ccRCC. Results from two Phase III studies completed in the early 2000s demonstrated that cytoreductive nephrectomy before IFN improved overall survival. In a combined analysis of these trials, median survival was 7.8 months in patients treated with interferon-alpha alone versus 13.6 months for patients who underwent cytoreductive nephrectomy initially.[53,54] A greater survival advantage was observed in patients with better performance status. The role for cytoreductive nephrectomy in patients with nonclear cell mRCC remains unproven.[55]

The cytoreductive paradigm has a less certain role in the modern era as more effective systemic therapies have been approved. A retrospective analysis of a cohort of 1658 patients treated with targeted therapies suggested that cytoreductive nephrectomy may benefit patients with at least a 12-month anticipated life expectancy and less than four IMDC risk factors.[52] However, a subsequent randomized Phase III trial, CARMENA, found that oral TKI therapy with sunitinib alone was noninferior to cytoreductive nephrectomy before sunitinib.[56] In fact, the median OS was numerically shorter in the surgical arm (13.9 vs 18.4 months for sunitinib alone), suggesting possible harm from surgery. This study enrolled a high proportion (over 40%) of patients with poor-risk mRCC, a population previously considered poor candidates for up-front surgery. Thus, the results may not be generalizable to patients with low volume, indolent, and favorable-risk disease.

A second Phase III trial, SURTIME, compared initial cytoreductive nephrectomy to 18 weeks of sunitinib before surgery.[57] The trial did not complete accrual; however, the progression-free rate at 28 weeks was similar between arms (42% vs 43%, respectively) and OS favored deferral of nephrectomy (median OS 32.4 vs 15.0 months, HR 0.57, $p = 0.03$). Nearly 30% of patients in the deferral arm never underwent nephrectomy due to cancer progression.

The results of CARMENA and SURTIME highlight the importance of careful patient selection before considering cytoreductive nephrectomy; it is not curative and should not be performed indiscriminately. Most patients should undergo a trial of systemic therapy prior to nephrectomy. Patients who are most likely to benefit from cytoreduction include those with (1) substantial tumor burden (e.g., >75%) in the involved kidney, (2) good performance status, (3) no central nervous system or liver metastases (with rare exceptions), and (4) 0–1 IMDC risk factors. Other considerations pertain to surgical resectability, particularly, the potential for morbidity if there is proximity to vital structures, encasement of the renal hilum, or other complicating factors.

Patients with mRCC with solitary metastases may be considered for metastasectomy, although they represent only 2–3% of cases. Favorable prognostic factors include a long interval between initial diagnosis and development of metastases, solitary metastatic site, and ability to achieve a complete resection of known metastatic disease. Patients with favorable features can anticipate up to a 40% 5-year survival with metastasectomy, and thus surgical resection of metastases can be considered in highly selected RCC patients. Although we are not aware of any randomized trials addressing these issues, a systematic review of 56 retrospective studies concluded that highly selected patients can experience long-term survival after metastasectomy without the use of systemic therapy, especially if complete resection is achieved. The number of metastases, performance status, and pulmonary site was important prognostic determinants.[58] However, the literature is dominated by highly selected nonrandomized studies; in this type of study, it has been postulated that complete surgical metastasectomy is associated with improved outcome in the postcytokine era, but it is likely that this observation is a function of careful case selection rather than biology or therapeutic impact per se.[59]

Systemic therapy for metastatic disease

Targeted therapy

New treatment approaches have resulted from a better understanding of the biology and genetics of RCC. This is such a rapidly changing field that we have had to alter this manuscript several times during its gestation because of the updated, peer-reviewed reporting of several randomized trials in 2019–2021. As noted previously, most ccRCCs demonstrate an abnormality of the VHL gene (Figure 1). Once inactivated, the VHL gene product cannot regulate the degradation of the transcription factor hypoxia-inducible factor (HIF) alpha, thus resulting in the transcription of numerous hypoxia-regulated genes including vascular endothelial growth factor (VEGF) and platelet-derived growth factor (PDGF). These growth factors promote angiogenesis and tumor growth through binding with their respective receptor tyrosine kinases (RTKs).[15] Activation of RTKs can induce signaling through the PI3K/Akt pathway and further downstream through the mammalian target of rapamycin (mTOR) pathway promoting cell proliferation and survival through regulation of mRNA translation. These intricate pathways have been identified as key therapeutic targets for the treatment of mRCC (Table 3).[60–71]

VEGF ligand-directed therapy

Bevacizumab is a recombinant monoclonal antibody that binds and neutralizes circulating VEGF. Addition of bevacizumab to interferon was associated with improved PFS in two Phase III trials but has not been proven to prolog OS.[71,72] Common toxicities include hypertension and proteinuria with rare but serious toxicity including bowel perforation, arterial ischemic events, and bleeding. Combined use with mTOR inhibition does not improve efficacy,[73] whereas concurrent use with additional VEGF targeted agents is associated with unacceptable risk of thrombotic microangiopathy.[74] The Phase 3 IMmotion151 trial found that bevacizumab plus the ICI atezolizumab improved PFS but not OS compared with sunitinib.[75] A trend towards improved OS was noted among tumors with PD-L1 expression ≥1%, and further follow-up may confirm this finding. At present, however, the role for bevacizumab in mRCC remains limited.

VEGF receptor tyrosine kinase inhibitors

RTKs play an integral role in the signaling cascade of VEGF and PDGF. RTKs have an extracellular domain that binds their respective ligand, which activates oncogenic intracellular signaling cascades through protein phosphorylation events regulated by a cytoplasmic kinase domain. Targeting RTKs with small-molecule TKIs has proven to be an effective therapeutic strategy in mRCC and has led to regulatory approval of multiple agents in this class as detailed below.

Sorafenib, the first TKI approved for use in mRCC, inhibits a broad repertoire of kinases including BRAF, CRAF, VEGFR-2, -3, PDGFB, Flt-3, p38, and c-kit. Sorafenib prolonged PFS compared to placebo (5.5 vs 2.8 months, $p < 0.01$), but not interferon, in patients with favorable and intermediate-risk disease.[64,65,76] Objective responses are uncommon with this agent, and its clinical role has been largely replaced by more effective TKIs.

Sunitinib is another oral multikinase inhibitor that blocks VEGFR-1, -2, -3, PDGFR-B, and related RTKs. A pivotal Phase III trial in untreated mRCC patients compared first-line sunitinib (50 mg daily 4 out of 6 weeks) with interferon and demonstrated a significant advantage in ORR (47% vs 12%; $p < 0.001$), PFS (11 vs 5 months, HR = 0.54; $p < 0.001$), and OS (26.4 vs 21.8 months, HR = 0.82; $p = 0.051$).[60,61] Most patients enrolled

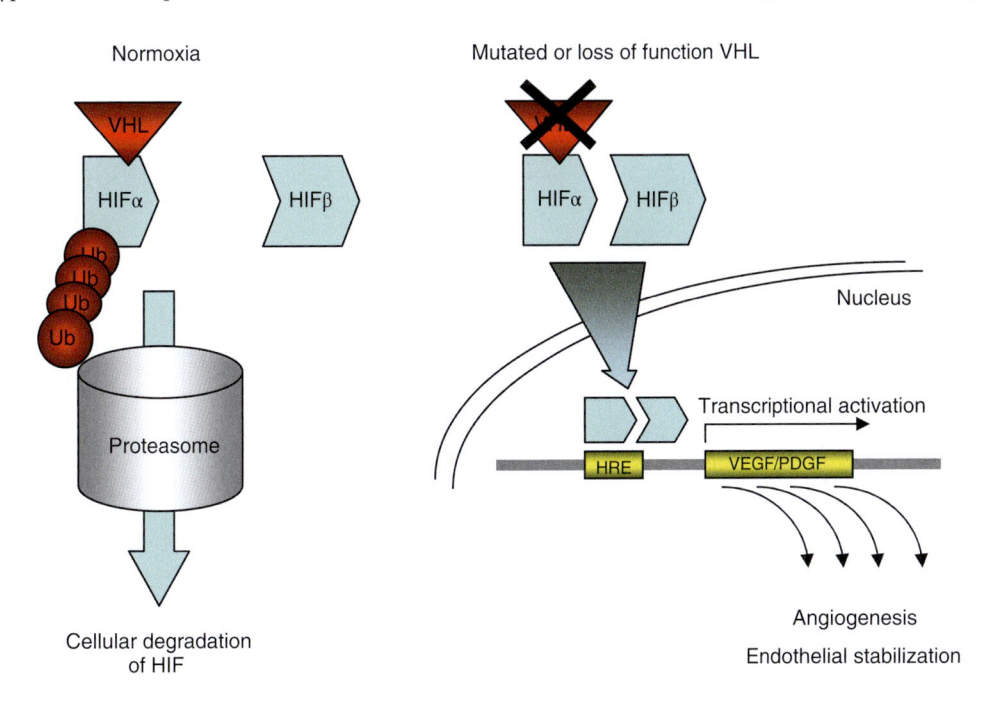

Figure 1 Normal function of VHL in the normoxic state compared to the aberrant VHL state/hypoxia. Under normal conditions, VHL binds to HIFα and polyubiquinates it to mark it for destruction in the cellular proteasome. In conditions of hypoxia or when VHL function is lost, HIFα binds HIFβ and then translocates into the nucleus to activate HIF responsive elements (HRE). This results in transcriptional activation of genes important in angiogenesis and endothelial stabilization such as VEGF and PDGF.

Table 3 Selected clinical trials of targeted single agents in metastatic renal cell carcinoma.[a]

Agent	Mechanism	Efficacy			
		Population and trial arms	RR	PFS (months)	OS (months)
Sunitinib[60,61]	Tyrosine kinase inhibitor of VEGF and related receptors	First-line sunitinib versus IFN	47%	11	26.4
			12%	5	21.8
			$p<0.001$	$p<0.001$	$p=0.051$
Pazopanib[62,63]	Tyrosine kinase inhibitor of VEGF and related receptors	First-line pazopanib versus sunitinib	31%	8.4	28.3
			25%	9.5	29.1
			$p=0.03$		NS
Sorafenib[64,65]	Tyrosine kinase inhibitor of VEGF and related receptors	Treatment refractory, second-line sorafenib versus placebo	10%	5.5	17.8
			2%	2.8	15.2
			$p<0.001$	$p<0.01$	$p=0.146$
Axitinib[66]	Tyrosine kinase inhibitor of VEGF and related receptors	Treatment refractory, second-line axitinib versus sorafenib	19%	8.3	20.1
			11%	5.7	19.2
			$p=0.0007$	$p<0.0001$	NS
Cabozantinib[67]	Tyrosine kinase inhibitor of VEGF and related receptors	First-line cabozantinib versus sunitinib	33%	8.2	30.3
			12%	5.6	21.8
				$p=0.0008$	NS
Lenvatinib[68]	Tyrosine kinase inhibitor of VEGF and related receptors	Treatment refractory lenvatinib plus everolimus versus lenvatinib versus everolimus	43%	14.6	25.5
			27%	7.4	18.4
			6%	5.5[b]	17.5
			$p<0.01$		NS
Temsirolimus[69]	mTOR inhibitor	Poor risk, first-line temsirolimus versus IFN	8.6%	N/A	10.9
			4.8%	N/A	7.3
			NS		$p<0.008$
Everolimus[70]	mTOR inhibitor	Treatment refractory, second-line everolimus versus placebo	1.8%	4.9	14.8
			0%	1.9	14.4
				$p<0.001$	NS
Bevacizumab[71,72,c]	VEGF ligand-binding antibody	First-line bevacizumab + IFN vs placebo + IFN	31%, 25%	10.2, 8.5	23.3, 18.3
			13%, 13%	5.4, 5.2	21.3, 17.4
			$p<0.0001$	$p<0.0001$	NS

Abbreviations: IFN, interferon; N/A, not available or data not yet mature; NS, not statistically significant; *p* values for PFS are based on hazard ratios.
[a]Source: Based on Motzer et al.[60–63,66,68,70]; Escudier et al.[64,65,71]; Choueiri et al.[67]; Hudes et al.[69]
[b]Lenvatinib + everolimus versus everolimus: $p=0.0005$; versus lenvatinib: $p=0.66$; lenvatinib versus everolimus: $p=0.048$.
[c]The results of two Phase III bevacizumab trials are shown.

(94%) had favorable or intermediate risk MSKCC prognostic criteria. Common toxicities included fatigue, hand-foot syndrome, diarrhea, mucositis, and hypertension. Until recently, this agent has remained a standard of care for the first-line treatment of mRCC based on these results. Efforts to improve the toxicity profile by altering dose and schedule of administration have had mixed success, with an abbreviated schedule of 50 mg daily for two out of three weeks demonstrating the best tolerability profile and similar efficacy.[77]

Pazopanib inhibits VEGFR-1, -2, and -3, PDGFR-A and -B, and c-kit.[78] A randomized Phase III trial comparing pazopanib to placebo in patients with mRCC demonstrated that pazopanib improved PFS (9.2 vs 4.2 months, HR = 0.46; $p<0.0001$) and ORR (30% vs 3%, $p<0.001$).[79] In COMPARZ, a noninferiority randomized Phase III trial for patients with untreated ccRCC, pazopanib resulted in a similar PFS to sunitinib (8.4 vs 9.5 months, HR = 1.05; 95% CI 0.90–1.22), higher ORR (31% vs 25%, $p=0.03$), and similar OS (28.3 vs 29.1 months, $p=0.24$).[62,63] Patients receiving pazopanib reported better quality of life scores including fatigue and hand-foot syndrome. Hepatic toxicity, however, is more common with this agent than with other TKIs and may be associated with UGT1A1 gene polymorphisms.[80]

Axitinib is a high potency inhibitor of VEGFR-1, -2, and -3 with fewer off-target effects.[81] In the AXIS trial, over 700 patients previously treated with one prior line of systemic therapy [cytokines (35%), sunitinib (54%), bevacizumab (8%), or temsirolimus (3%)] were randomized to receive axitinib (5 mg twice daily) or sorafenib (400 mg twice daily).[82] Notably, one-third of enrolled patients had MSKCC poor risk criteria. Median PFS favored the axitinib group (8.3 vs 5.7 months, $p<0.0001$), although OS (20.1 vs 19.2 months, $p=0.3744$) and patient-reported outcomes were similar between arms.[66] On the basis of these results, axitinib became a standard second or later line option. Axitinib has not been proven superior to sorafenib in the first-line setting.[82]

Resistance to first-generation TKIs is thought to occur by activation of alternative growth signaling pathways. Two newer TKIs, cabozantinib and lenvatinib, target a broad range of RTKs thought to mediate this resistance. Cabozantinib inhibits VEGFR-1, -2, and -3, KIT, TRKB, FLT-3, AXL, RET, MET, and TIE-2, with MET and AXL thought to be most involved in mRCC progression.[83] Cabozantinib was superior to everolimus in METEOR, a randomized Phase III trial that included 658 patients with mRCC previously treated with at least one TKI.[84] All efficacy outcomes favored cabozantinib including ORR (21% vs 5%, $p < 0.001$), PFS (median 7.4 vs 3.8 months, $p < 0.001$), and OS (median 21.4 vs 17.1 months, $p < 0.001$).[85] This benefit included subjects who had received prior pazopanib or sunitinib.[86] Drug tolerance at the studied dose (60 mg/day) is a concern, as nearly three-quarters of patients experienced grade 3 or 4 adverse events and 60% of patients required a dose reduction.

Cabozantinib was subsequently tested in the first line against sunitinib in the randomized Phase II trial CABOSUN.[67] This study enrolled only patients with intermediate (81%) and poor (19%) risk clear cell mRCC. Treatment with cabozantinib was associated with significantly improved PFS (Table 3). The trial was not powered to detect a difference in OS, which was longer in the cabozantinib arm.

Lenvatinib is a potent inhibitor of VEGFR-1, -2, and -3, FGFR-1, -2, -3, and -4, PDGFR-A, KIT, and RET.[68,87] This drug was approved for second or later line use in combination with everolimus based on the results of a Phase II trial which randomized 153 pretreated patients to lenvatinib, everolimus, or their combination.[68] PFS was improved for the combination (median 14.6 months, $p = 0.0005$) and lenvatinib arms (7.4 months, $p = 0.048$) compared with everolimus monotherapy (5.5 months). We are not aware of peer-reviewed data comparing lenvatinib with any other TKI, although randomized trials comparing Lenvatinib versus immunotherapy are in progress.

Another emerging focus of importance is the cost-effectiveness and absolute cost of these agents for patients and payers, particularly in an era in which health insurance companies are increasingly shifting costs via co-pays to patients. This remains an area with lack of clarity, although some preliminary data are available, against a background of shifting charges associated with competition between pharmaceutical companies. For example, a recent Canadian comparison of pazopanib versus sunitinib for mRCC, using data from COMPARZ and other secondary sources, suggested that costs associated with pazopanib were lower than for sunitinib.[88] Others have suggested that attenuated dose schedules of sunitinib due to toxicity yield similar cost profiles to pazopanib.[89] In the United Kingdom, modeling studies have suggested that cabozantinib is more effective than axitinib or everolimus, but associated with higher costs, and that cabozantinib has nominally higher efficacy and lower costs than nivolumab.[90] A range of sophisticated modeling techniques may provide useful guidance regarding cost-effectiveness; however, the larger network meta-analyses are likely to miss important nuances of case selection bias when rank ordering the clinical utility of agents without considering the substantial impact of case selection bias.[91] This is of significant concern if politicians and payers use these artificial data comparisons to influence health policy and reimbursement patterns. More prospective data, from randomized and well-structure real-world studies, will be required to resolve this vexed issue definitively.

mTOR inhibition
The "mTOR" kinase is activated by a signaling cascade consisting of VEGFR, Akt, and PI3 Kinase, and promotes tumor growth and proliferation through regulation of mRNA translation. Temsirolimus is an FDA-approved mTOR inhibitor that binds to FKBP-12 to create a complex that directly inhibits mTOR. Temsirolimus monotherapy improved OS compared to interferon-alpha (10.9 vs 7.3 months, $p = 0.008$) in a poor risk population with clear and nonclear cell mRCC.[69] However, temsirolimus is inferior to sorafenib and its clinical utility remains limited.[92]

Everolimus is an oral mTOR inhibitor with US FDA approval for use in patients with mRCC after TKI failure based on results from the RECORD-1 randomized Phase III trial comparing everolimus to placebo.[70,93] Everolimus improved PFS (4.9 vs 1.9 months, $p < 0.001$) but not OS, owing in part to the high cross-over rate of patients from the placebo arm. Everolimus is generally administered in combination with lenvatinib (vide supra) or as monotherapy after multiple TKI failures given its inferiority to both sunitinib and cabozantinib in Phase III trials.[84,94]

Immunotherapy
Decades of clinical trials employing chemotherapy against renal cell carcinoma did not produce any significant benefit, often at the cost of substantial toxicity,[95] and this treatment modality is rarely employed for RCC today. Immunotherapy, which harnesses the innate immune response has long been a standard of care for mRCC. While cytokine therapy with interferon and high-dose interleukin-2 produced response rates of around 10–20%, dramatic and durable complete responses sometimes occurred.[96] Toxicity with these agents was high, including capillary leak syndrome, which usually necessitated intensive monitoring and vasopressor support.

ICIs have largely supplanted cytokine therapies for the treatment of mRCC. These include therapeutic monoclonal antibodies which bind the cell surface proteins programmed death 1 (PD-1), programmed death-ligand 1 (PD-L1), and cytotoxic T-lymphocyte-associated protein 4 (CTLA-4). They function by suppressing inhibitory signaling programs in lymphocytes, particularly cytotoxic T-cells, and result in lymphocyte activation.[97] Nivolumab (anti-PD-1) was the first ICI approved for mRCC based on results from CHECKMATE-025, a randomized Phase III trial comparing nivolumab versus everolimus in pretreated patients.[98] Nivolumab was associated with improved OS (median 25.0 vs 19.6 months, HR 0.73, 95% CI 0.57–0.93) and ORR (25% vs 5%), but not PFS possibly due to delayed and/or mixed response kinetics commonly observed with immunotherapies. Nivolumab was quite well tolerated with just 19% of patients experiencing treatment-related grade 3 or 4 adverse events, although 8% of patients did experience severe autoimmune side effects such as pneumonitis or colitis resulting in drug discontinuation. Nivolumab is now considered a standard second-line treatment option.

In the front-line, nivolumab was tested in combination with ipilimumab (anti-CTLA-4) against sunitinib in the randomized, Phase III trial CHECKMATE-214.[99] In melanoma, this combination had previously been shown to be more effective than nivolumab alone. 847 patients with IMDC intermediate- or poor-risk mRCC were enrolled. Both PFS (median 11.6 versus 8.4 months, $p = 0.03$) and OS (HR 0.63, 95% CI 0.44–0.89, $p < 0.001$) were longer with ipilimumab plus nivolumab. The ORR was 42% with the combination versus 27% with sunitinib ($p < 0.001$). ICIs can induce durable responses lasting years in some cases, a consistent finding across studies in different tumor types. In CHECKMATE-214, after a minimum follow-up of 30 months, 59% of treatment responses were ongoing (compared with 35% for sunitinib).[100] Biomarkers of response, such as PD-L1 expression on tumor cells, were studied but remain investigational. A substudy enrolled 249 patients with IMDC favorable-risk disease and found potentially worse outcomes in the immunotherapy arm, and thus front-line ipilimumab plus nivolumab should only be considered for intermediate- and poor-risk patients.

Toxicities remain a concern with ipilimumab plus nivolumab and are more severe than for sunitinib or for nivolumab monotherapy. In CHECKMATE-214, there was a 22% drug discontinuation rate (versus 12% for sunitinib) and 29% of patients required high-dose steroids to alleviate autoimmune toxicity. Eight (1.5%) deaths occurred because of treatment. Thus, patients must be carefully selected for performance status, pattern of co-morbidities, and reliability and also counseled carefully before starting this therapy.

ICIs have also been tested in combination with TKIs in the front-line setting. In KEYNOTE-426, 861 patients were randomized to receive pembrolizumab (anti-PD-1) plus axitinib versus sunitinib.[101] The combination was associated with both improved PFS (0.69, 95% CI 0.57–0.84; $p < 0.001$) and OS (0.53; 95% CI 0.38–0.74; $p < 0.0001$), and results were consistent across IMDC risk categories including favorable risk. A similar Phase III trial, the JAVELIN Renal 101, compared avelumab (anti-PD-L1) plus axitinib versus sunitinib.[102] This combination was also associated with an improvement in PFS (HR 0.69, 95% CI 0.56–0.84; $p < 0.001$) although mature OS results have yet to be reported. An updated analysis of 866 patients confirmed an ongoing statistically significant difference in PFS, but OS data were still immature; interestingly the PFS difference applied to both PD-L1 positive patients and the overall population.[103] Nonetheless, both regimens are highly active with ORR 55–60%, and both have been approved by regulatory agencies in the United States and Europe.

As expected, adverse events on these regimens include both autoimmune and TKI-related toxicities. Overlapping toxicities, like diarrhea, rash, and fatigue, may require a trial-and-error approach at management that includes sequential dose reductions, drug cessation, and steroids. Phase III studies combining ICIs with lenvatinib or cabozantinib are also ongoing.

Currently, the standard of care for most patients with new mRCC is dual therapy with either ipilimumab plus nivolumab (intermediate- and poor-risk mRCC) or an ICI plus TKI (all IMDC risk groups). These regimens have not been directly compared in clinical trials, and the optimal choice of treatment will vary depending on patient preferences and comorbidities, drug access, and cost. Other commonly cited reasons for choosing each treatment include higher response rates (ICI plus TKI), higher complete response rates, and proven durability (ipilimumab plus nivolumab). A summary of approved treatments for mRCC and their recommended sequencing are described in Table 4.

Table 4 Preferred therapies for mRCC.[a]

	First line	Second or later line	Less commonly used agents
Clear cell, favorable risk	Axitinib + pembrolizumab/ avelumab	Cabozantinib	Bevacizumab
	Sunitinib	Nivolumab	Sorafenib
	Pazopanib	Ipilimumab + Nivolumab	Temsirolimus
Clear cell, intermediate- or poor-risk	Ipilimumab + Nivolumab	Axitinib	Interleukin-2
	Axitinib + pembrolizumab/ avelumab	Lenvatinib + Everolimus	Interferon alfa-2b
	Cabozantinib	Everolimus	
Nonclear cell	Sunitinib	Any other ccRCC approved regimen	
	Cabozantinib	Bevacizumab + erlotinib (for HLRCC-associated Type 2 papillary)	
	Ipilimumab + Nivolumab		

[a]Source: Adapted from NCCN Guidelines[104]; Bedke et al.[105]

Uncommon cancers of the kidney

A detailed discussion of the biology and management of nonclear cell variants is beyond the scope of this article, in accordance with editorial directions, but has been covered in detail elsewhere.[106,107] In brief, nonclear cell RCC such as papillary and chromophobe histologies are treated in a similar manner as clear cell RCC, with surgery remaining the most important therapeutic modality. In the metastatic setting, observational studies suggest that TKIs and ICIs are active in these variants but have less robust antitumor activity compared with ccRCC.[108,109] Randomized trials comparing ipilimumab plus nivolumab (NCT03075423) or cabozantinib (NCT02761057) versus sunitinib are ongoing.

Collecting duct carcinoma (CDC) is an extremely rare medullary kidney cancer representing less than 1% of kidney cancers, although its incidence is increasing.[110,111] Often surrounded by desmoplastic stroma, CDC has a variable tubular-papillary pattern of growth, with high-grade nuclei and high mitotic activity. Mucin and sarcomatoid changes may be seen. Clinically, CDC is an aggressive tumor that often presents at an advanced stage.[106,110,111] Most reports of treatment of metastatic disease have involved the use of cisplatin-based chemotherapy, sometimes accompanied by gemcitabine or bevacizumab, and anecdotal responses to ICIs have also been reported.[106,110,111] Unfortunately, most remissions are of short duration. Collecting duct carcinoma is detailed here merely as an example of the importance of focusing on uncommon malignancies, and referring such cases to centers of excellence to facilitate optimal treatment, when known, and to lead to the acquisition of structured case experience.[107] Extensive anecdotal experience is now reported routinely online, but caution should be exercised in applying such recommendations, given the uncertainties of pathological and radiological review, and the variability of isolated case experience.

Conclusion

RCC incidence is increasing worldwide. Surgery remains a mainstay of treatment for localized tumors and is sometimes part of multimodality therapy in the metastatic setting. An enhanced understanding of the biology of RCC has led to the clinical development of targeted therapies and immunotherapies that have substantially altered the therapeutic landscape. Future investigative endeavors include refinement of the approach to the small renal mass, better understanding of the biology of response and resistance to systemic therapy, and optimizing sequencing of systemic therapies.

Key references

The complete reference list can be found on Vital Source version of this title, see inside front cover.

9 Nguyen MM, Gill IS, Ellison LM. The evolving presentation of renal carcinoma in the United States: trends from the Surveillance, Epidemiology, and End Results program. *J Urol.* 2006;**176**(6Pt 1):2397–2400; discussion 2400.

11 Cancer Genome Atlas Research Network. Comprehensive molecular characterization of clear cell renal cell carcinoma. *Nature.* 2013;**499**(7456):43–49.

13 Carlo MI, Mukherjee S, Mandelker D, et al. Prevalence of germline mutations in cancer susceptibility genes in patients with advanced renal cell carcinoma. *JAMA Oncol.* 2018;**4**(9):1228–1235.

16 Cheville JC, Lohse CM, Zincke H, et al. Comparisons of outcome and prognostic features among histologic subtypes of renal cell carcinoma. *Am J Surg Pathol.* 2003;**27**(5):612–624.

17 Patard JJ, Leray E, Rioux-Leclercq N, et al. Prognostic value of histologic subtypes in renal cell carcinoma: a multicenter experience. *J Clin Oncol.* 2005;**23**(12):2763–2771.

20. Tsui KH, Shvarts O, Smith RB, et al. Prognostic indicators for renal cell carcinoma: a multivariate analysis of 643 patients using the revised 1997 TNM staging criteria. *J Urol*. 2000;**163**(4):1090–1095; quiz 1295.
22. Amin MB, Edge S, Greene F, et al. (eds). *AJCC Staging Manual*, 8th ed. New York: Springer; 2017.
23. Van Poppel H, Da Pozzo L, Albrecht W, et al. A prospective, randomised EORTC intergroup phase 3 study comparing the oncologic outcome of elective nephron-sparing surgery and radical nephrectomy for low-stage renal cell carcinoma. *Eur Urol*. 2011;**59**(4):543–552.
24. Gershman B, Thompson RH, Boorjian SA, et al. Radical versus partial nephrectomy for cT1 renal cell carcinoma. *Eur Urol*. 2018;**74**:825–832.
26. Jeong IG, Khandwala YS, Kim JH, et al. Association of robotic-assisted vs laparoscopic radical nephrectomy with perioperative outcomes and health care costs, 2003 to 2015. *JAMA*. 2017;**318**(16):1561–1568.
27. Andrews JR, Atwell T, Schmit G, et al. Oncologic outcomes following partial nephrectomy and percutaneous ablation for cT1 renal masses. *Eur Urol*. 2019;**76**(2):244–251.
31. Blom JH, van Poppel H, Marechal JM, et al. Radical nephrectomy with and without lymph-node dissection: final results of European Organization for Research and Treatment of Cancer (EORTC) randomized phase 3 trial 30881. *Eur Urol*. 2009;**55**(1):28–34.
32. Abel EJ, Culp SH, Tannir NM, et al. Primary tumor response to targeted agents in patients with metastatic renal cell carcinoma. *Eur Urol*. 2011;**59**(1):10–15.
33. Lane BR, Derweesh IH, Kim HL, et al. Presurgical sunitinib reduces tumor size and may facilitate partial nephrectomy in patients with renal cell carcinoma. *Urol Oncol*. 2015;**33**(3):112.e15–112.e21.
37. Haas NB, Manola J, Dutcher JP, et al. Adjuvant treatment for high-risk clear cell renal cancer: updated results of a high-risk subset of the ASSURE randomized trial. *JAMA Oncol*. 2017;**3**(9):1249–1252.
39. Motzer RJ, Haas NB, Donskov F, et al. Randomized phase III trial of adjuvant pazopanib versus placebo after nephrectomy in patients with localized or locally advanced renal cell carcinoma. *J Clin Oncol*. 2017;**35**(35):3916–3923.
42. Gross-Goupil M, Kwon TG, Eto M, et al. Axitinib versus placebo as an adjuvant treatment of renal cell carcinoma: results from the phase III, randomized ATLAS trial. *Ann Oncol*. 2018;**29**(12):2371–2378.
43. Karakiewicz PI, Zaffuto E, Kapoor A, et al. Kidney cancer research network of Canada consensus statement on the role of adjuvant therapy after nephrectomy for high-risk non-metastatic renal cell carcinoma: a comprehensive analysis of the literature and meta-analysis of randomized controlled trials. *Can Urol Assoc J*. 2018;**12**:173–180.
44. Lee Z, Jegede OA, Haas NB, et al. Local recurrence following resection of intermediate-high risk nonmetastatic renal cell carcinoma: an anatomical classification and analysis of the ASSURE (ECOG-ACRIN E2805) adjuvant trial. *J Urol*. 2020;**203**:684–689.
49. Heng DY, Xie W, Regan MM, et al. External validation and comparison with other models of the International Metastatic Renal-Cell Carcinoma Database Consortium prognostic model: a population-based study. *Lancet Oncol*. 2013;**14**(2):141–148.
53. Flanigan RC, Mickisch G, Sylvester R, et al. Cytoreductive nephrectomy in patients with metastatic renal cancer: a combined analysis. *J Urol*. 2004;**171**(3):1071–1076.
56. Mejean A, Ravaud A, Thezenas S, et al. Sunitinib alone or after nephrectomy in metastatic renal-cell carcinoma. *N Engl J Med*. 2018;**379**(5):417–427.
59. Lyon TD, Thompson RH, Shah PH, et al. Complete surgical metastasectomy of renal cell carcinoma in the post-cytokine era. *J Urol*. 2020;**203**:275–282.
66. Motzer RJ, Escudier B, Tomczak P, et al. Axitinib versus sorafenib as second-line treatment for advanced renal cell carcinoma: overall survival analysis and updated results from a randomised phase 3 trial. *Lancet Oncol*. 2013;**14**(6):552–562.
67. Choueiri TK, Halabi S, Sanford BL, et al. Cabozantinib versus sunitinib as initial targeted therapy for patients with metastatic renal cell carcinoma of poor or intermediate risk: the alliance A031203 CABOSUN trial. *J Clin Oncol*. 2017;**35**(6):591–597.
75. Rini BI, Powles T, Atkins MB, et al. Atezolizumab plus bevacizumab versus sunitinib in patients with previously untreated metastatic renal cell carcinoma (IMmotion151): a multicentre, open-label, phase 3, randomised controlled trial. *Lancet*. 2019;**393**(10189):2404–2415.
77. Motzer RJ, Hutson TE, Olsen MR, et al. Randomized phase II trial of sunitinib on an intermittent versus continuous dosing schedule as first-line therapy for advanced renal cell carcinoma. *J Clin Oncol*. 2012;**30**(12):1371–1377.
79. Sternberg CN, Davis ID, Mardiak J, et al. Pazopanib in locally advanced or metastatic renal cell carcinoma: results of a randomized phase III trial. *J Clin Oncol*. 2010;**28**(6):1061–1068.
83. Zhou L, Liu XD, Sun M, et al. Targeting MET and AXL overcomes resistance to sunitinib therapy in renal cell carcinoma. *Oncogene*. 2016;**35**(21):2687–2697.
86. Powles T, Motzer RJ, Escudier B, et al. Outcomes based on prior therapy in the phase 3 METEOR trial of cabozantinib versus everolimus in advanced renal cell carcinoma. *Br J Cancer*. 2018;**119**(6):663–669.
90. Meng J, Lister J, Vataire AL, et al. Cost-effectiveness comparision of cabozantinib with everolimus, axitinib, and nivolumab in the treatment of advanced renal cell carcinoma following the failure of prior therapy in England. *Clinicoecon Outcomes Res*. 2018;**10**:243–250.
91. Heo JH, Park C, Ghosh S, et al. A network meta-analysis of efficacy and safety of first-line and second line therapies for the management of metastatic renal cell carcinoma. *J Clin Pharm Ther*. 2021;**46**(1):35–49. doi: 10.1111/jcpt.13282.
98. Motzer RJ, Escudier B, McDermott DF, et al. Nivolumab versus everolimus in advanced renal-cell carcinoma. *N Engl J Med*. 2015;**373**(19):1803–1813.
101. Rini BI, Plimack ER, Stus V, et al. Pembrolizumab plus axitinib versus sunitinib for advanced renal-cell carcinoma. *N Engl J Med*. 2019;**380**(12):1116–1127.
102. Motzer RJ, Penkov K, Haanen J, et al. Avelumab plus axitinib versus sunitinib for advanced renal-cell carcinoma. *N Engl J Med*. 2019;**380**(12):1103–1115.
103. Choueiri TK, Motzer RJ, Rini BI, et al. Updated efficacy results from the JAVELIN Renal 101 trial: first=line avelumab plus axitinib versus sunitinib in patients with advanced renal cell carcinoma. *Ann Oncol*. 2020;**31**:P1030–P1039. doi: 10/1016/j.annonc.2020.04.010.
106. DeVelasco G, Signoretti S, Rini BI, Choueiri T. Uncommon tumors of the kidney. In: Raghavan D, Ahluwalia MS, Blanke CD, et al., eds. *Textbook of Uncommon Cancers*, 5th ed. Hoboken: Wiley Blackwell; 2017:19–40.
107. Raghavan D. A structured approach to uncommon cancers: what should a clinician do? *Ann Oncol*. 2013;**24**(12):2932–2934.
109. Dason S, Allard C, Sheridan-Jonah A, et al. Management of renal collecting duct carcinoma: a systematic review and the McMaster experience. *Curr Oncol*. 2013;**20**(3):e223–e232.
111. McGregor BA, McKay RR, Braun DA, et al. Results of a multicenter phase II study of atezolizumab and bevacizumab for patients with metastatic renal cell carcinoma with variant histology and/or sarcomatoid features. *J Clin Oncol*. 2020;**38**:63–70.

94 Urothelial cancer

Derek Raghavan, MD, PhD, FACP, FRACP, FASCO, FAAAS ■ Richard Cote, MD, FRCPath, FCAP ■ Earle F. Burgess, MD ■ Derek McHaffie, MD ■ Peter E. Clark, MD

Overview

Urothelial malignancy is one of the commonest cancers in Western society and involves the bladder, urethra, ureters, and renal calyces. It is associated with smoking, industrial dyes, schistosomiasis, radiation exposure, and certain geographical locations. Well-defined molecular prognosticators and predictors have been identified, and in combination with improved staging techniques, have led to improved outcomes. Patients with nonmuscle invasive urothelial malignancy are best managed by surgical resection, often in combination with intravesical immunotherapy or chemotherapy. Muscle invasive disease is best managed by neoadjuvant cisplatin-based chemotherapy followed by cystectomy; less robust patients are often effectively treated by chemoradiation. Patients with metastatic disease achieve response rates of up to 70% with MVAC or GC combination chemotherapy but are infrequently cured. The major innovation in the past decade has been the introduction of targeted therapies, in particular directed to the PD1/PD-L1 interface, which have shown substantial activity in first-line and salvage treatment of early-stage and metastatic disease, but with a new spectrum of side effects.

Introduction and epidemiology

Bladder cancer is one of the most common malignancies in Western society, with an annual incidence of about 16 cases/100,000 males per year and 5 cases/100,000 females, and additional cases are found throughout the urothelial tract.[1] This is one of the malignancies for which the incidence and mortality figures have not changed greatly in the past 50 years,[1,2] although it is possible that the incidence figures in males are beginning to plateau, reflecting the reduction in cigarette smoking. This is predominantly a disease of older-aged males, with a median age at presentation of 60–65 years. There are geographical variations in incidence with increased rates in the Great Lakes region of the United States, in the littoral basin of the Middle East, and in regions with an increased incidence of schistosomiasis (most often squamous carcinoma). In the Balkan region, endemic familial interstitial nephropathy is associated with a 100- to 200-fold increase in upper tract tumors. Urothelial cancer occurs more often in Caucasians than in other populations.[2]

The etiology is well defined, causes including cigarette smoking, exposure to dyes and industrial reagents, motor exhaust, reduced intake of fluids (controversial), prior alkylating agent chemotherapy, family history, and analgesic (phenacetin) abuse.[1,2]

Pathobiology and molecular determinants

Bladder cancer consists predominantly of urothelial carcinoma (UC), formerly known as transitional cell cancer.[1,3] This type of cancer can occur anywhere along the urothelial tract and may be multifocal in origin, with identical tumor histology irrespective of site of origin. About 90% of incident cases are UC, with about 5–10% being squamous cell carcinoma, 4–5% being adenocarcinoma, and the remainder consisting of rare cancers, such as small cell anaplastic cancer, sarcoma, melanoma, or lymphoma. Occasionally other tumors metastasize to the bladder.

It is increasingly believed that bladder cancer arises from cancer stem cells[4] and that the cancer stem cells have the ability to differentiate along different pathways. It is, therefore, not surprising that intermixed histological patterns will be found, although usually, UC predominates in such situations. These tumors are associated with a field defect of the urinary mucosa, probably carcinogen-induced, and can occur at multiple sites.

Urothelial carcinoma presents as either noninvasive or invasive disease. Two distinct noninvasive histological subtypes are known, papillary and flat carcinoma *in situ* (CIS). Noninvasive papillary carcinoma is the most common presentation for bladder cancer, more than 60% of incident cases. This can be classified according to grade of disease, ranging from tumors generally considered benign (papilloma) to high-grade tumors with a high risk of developing invasion (grades 3 and 4). Grading systems are generally restricted to noninvasive papillary neoplasms, as CIS is high grade by definition, and virtually all invasive tumors are high grade as well.[3] The latest WHO nomenclature combines tumor differentiation into only low and high grades, based on the finding that tumor behavior is more accurately reflected in a dichotomized system.[3,5] Although the bladder is heavily invested by fat and muscle, this is not the case in the upper tracts, and thus the barriers to spread, and patterns of spread, are somewhat different.

Because the different morphologic subtypes of bladder cancer have long been recognized to have different biologic behavior, these subtypes became the focus of molecular analysis.[5–9] The earliest cytogenetic studies in bladder cancer demonstrated alterations in chromosomes 9, 11, and 17, reflecting the possible presence of tumor suppressor genes in these areas.[5–9] On the basis of consistent and frequent genetic defects in bladder tumors, it has become clear that there are at least two distinct molecular pathways involved in bladder cancer tumorigenesis and progression (Figure 1), as reviewed elsewhere.[5–9] Low-grade papillary tumors frequently show constitutive activation of the receptor tyrosine kinase-RAS pathway, exhibiting activating mutations in the HRAS

Holland-Frei Cancer Medicine, Tenth Edition. Edited by Robert C. Bast, John C. Byrd, Carlo M. Croce, Ernest Hawk, Fadlo R. Khuri, Raphael E. Pollock, Apostolia M. Tsimberidou, Christopher G. Willett, and Cheryl L. Willman.
© 2023 John Wiley & Sons, Inc. Published 2023 by John Wiley & Sons, Inc.

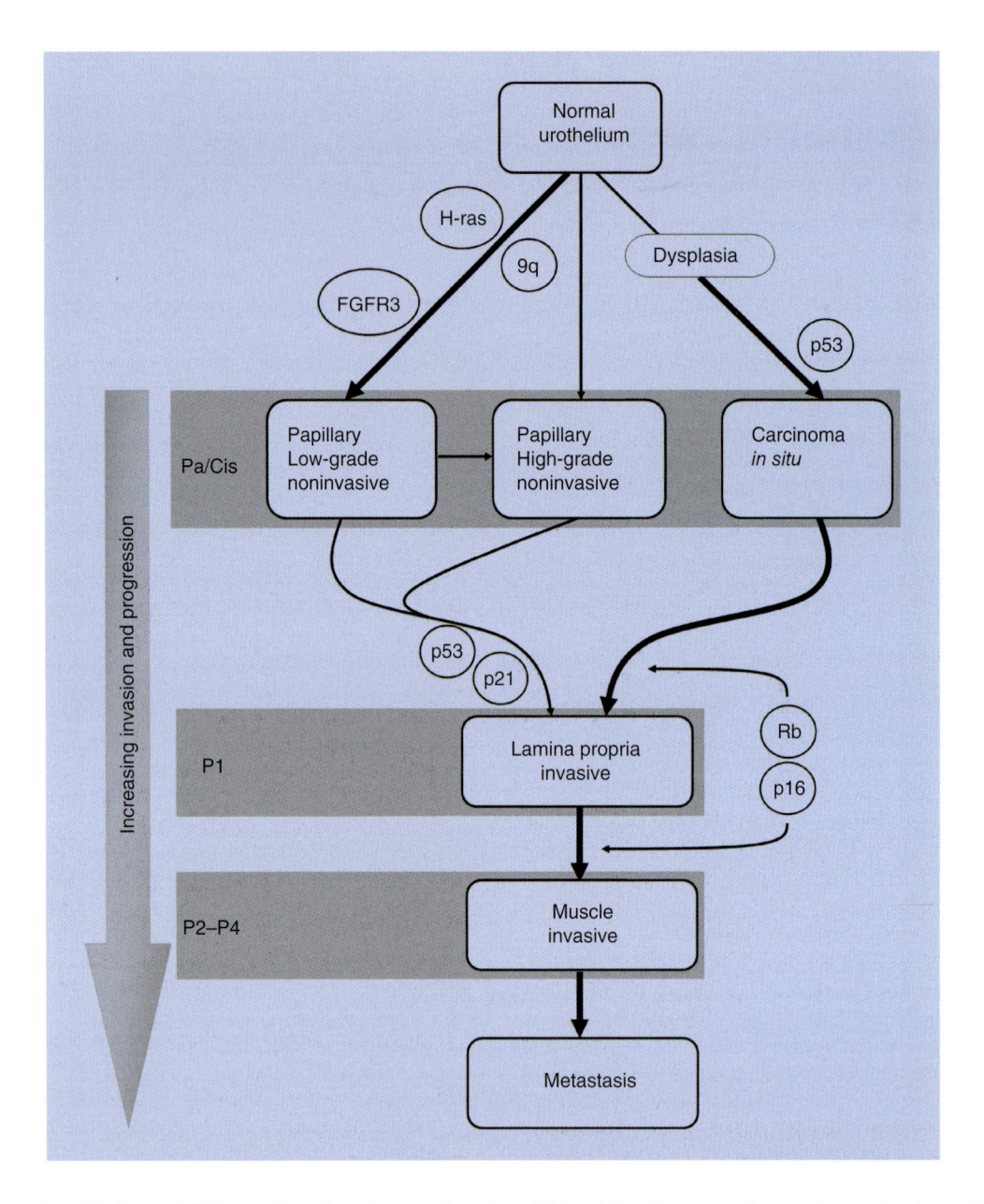

Figure 1 Proposed model for urothelial tumorigenesis and progression. Superficial and invasive tumors have unique molecular profiles and arise from distinct pathways. The locations of molecules indicate events that pose a risk for progression of a particular phenotype. The rare papillary carcinomas that invade are more likely to have genetic alterations at crucial loci. The thickness of arrows represents the relative frequency of occurrence. Source: From Seisen et al.[10]

and fibroblast growth factor receptor 3 (FGFR3) genes. High-grade papillary tumors frequently show alterations in chromosome 9, particularly at the INK4a/p16 locus, and much lower frequency of FGFR3 mutations. Flat CIS and invasive tumors frequently show alterations in cell cycle regulation, especially p53 gene and protein (TP53) and in the retinoblastoma (RB) gene.[5] Similar molecular changes are found in upper tract tumors, and added abnormalities in chromosomes 5q, 1p, 14q, and 8p have been identified.

The RAS-MAPK signal transduction pathway is also important in noninvasive papillary tumors. Most noninvasive papillary UC's show activation of this pathway, generally through the activation of FGFR3, and potentially presenting a target for novel therapies. Other receptor tyrosine kinases are also involved, such as epidermal growth factor receptor (EGFR) and Her2-neu, as reviewed previously.[5] Interestingly, an uncommon and aggressive histologic variant, micropapillary UC, has been shown to frequently overexpress the HER2 gene and protein, making it a potentially interesting therapeutic target in this subtype.[6]

Gene expression profiling has been used to study UC, resulting in proposed subtypes of muscle-invasive disease with genetic features similar to breast cancer molecular subtypes (basal, luminal, p53-like).[7] Additionally, integrated multiplatform and multiplex analyses of mRNA, miRNA, long noncoding RNA (lncRNA), DNA methylation, copy number, protein expression, and whole-genome and whole-exome sequencing by The Cancer Genome Atlas Research Network stratified muscle-invasive disease into five subtypes (luminal, luminal-papillary, luminal-infiltrated, basal/squamous, and neuronal), with associated potential treatment strategies for each subtype.[8] The Bladder Cancer Molecular Taxonomy Group has identified a set of six molecular classes of muscle-invasive bladder cancer: luminal

Table 1 Molecular pathway alterations in urothelial carcinoma.

Pathway	Factors	Potential outcome
Cell cycle regulation	p53, p21, RB, Mdm2	Increased tumor suppression
Apoptosis	Caspase-3, Survivin, Bcl-2	Programmed cell death
Cell signaling and gene regulation	FGFR, MAPK, sex hormone receptors, Janus kinase, MRE11	Interference with dysregulated cell proliferation
Inflammation and immune modulation	IL-6, MF-KB, CRP, PDL-1	Checkpoint inhibition with activation of immunity
Angiogenesis	VEGf, uPA, TSP-1	Interference with tumor vasculature
Cancer cell invasion	Cadherins, MMP, ICAM1, CA 19-9, CEA	Reduction of invasion and metastasis

papillary, luminal-nonspecified, luminal-unstable, stroma-rich, basal/squamous, and neuroendocrine-like.[9] These classes are characterized by unique oncogenic mechanisms, infiltration by immune and stromal cells, histologic and clinical characteristics, and outcomes. Alterations in specific molecular pathways are increasingly described, and may lend themselves to future therapeutic intervention, as summarized in Table 1 and reviewed in detail elsewhere.

Clinical presentation

The presentation of bladder cancer usually reflects the extent of disease, with somewhat different patterns associated with non-muscle-invasive tumor, invasive disease, metastases, and the nonmetastatic manifestations of malignancy.[1] Patients with noninvasive tumors may present with asymptomatic hematuria (diagnosed on urinalysis), visible hematuria, frequency, dysuria, burning, or nocturia. Invasive tumors have a similar pattern of presentation, although more advanced tumors may be associated with pelvic pain, slowing of urinary stream, dyspareunia, and occasionally pneumaturia or fecal incontinence. Occasionally tumors involving the trigone will cause obstruction of ureter(s), with concomitant flank pain. Flank pain or more generalized abdominal pain occasionally reflects the presence of an upper tract tumor, although usually these symptoms are associated with more advanced local disease with associated retroperitoneal lymphadenopathy or ureteric obstruction.

The presenting features of metastatic disease usually reflect the site(s) of involvement. Common sites include distant lymph nodes, lung, liver, and bone, and less commonly brain, skin, and other viscera. Metastases will sometimes be detected upon routine follow-up scans. Pulmonary involvement will classically be associated with cough and dyspnea, and occasionally with hemoptysis or chest pain. Liver involvement may present with right upper quadrant pain or shoulder tip pain, and occasionally disruption of function, most commonly manifested by jaundice. Osseous metastases are often associated with bone pain, and less commonly with pathologic fracture, with common sites of involvement including spine, ribs, pelvis, and skull. Brain metastases may be suggested by the development of headache, confusion, or other motor features. A CT or MRI brain scan is usually diagnostic, but a spinal tap would be required to diagnose carcinomatous meningitis in a patient with headache and a normal scan. Skin metastases are uncommon but usually are manifest by an infiltrative pattern or isolated cutaneous or subcutaneous nodules. Constitutional features, such as anorexia, weight loss, cachexia, and fatigue may be harbingers of these presentations.

Nonmetastatic manifestations of malignancy consist predominantly of serological syndromes, although patients may present with the thrombo-emboli. Bladder cancer is occasionally associated with the production of granulocyte-macrophage colony-stimulating factors or other cytokines, and an associated high white blood cell. Squamous cell tumors with squamous differentiation may be associated with hypercalcemia, due to excess production of immunoreactive parathyroid hormone (PTH)-like substance.

Investigation and staging

The presentation will usually govern the choice of the investigations. Hematuria or other urinary symptoms will usually lead to urinalysis and assessment of possible infection or urinary calculi. The absence of these conditions or the presence of sterile pyuria leads to urinary cytology and/or cystoscopy. To improve upon the sensitivity of urine cytology, and to reduce the need for periodic cystoscopy in the follow-up of patients with non-muscle-invasive bladder cancer, biomarker dipstick assays have been developed, based on soluble bladder tumor antigens or cell-based markers (NMP22, BTA-TRAK, BLCA-4, Immunocyt). Molecular analysis (Urovysion) allows detection of aneuploidy reflecting changes in chromosomes 3, 7, and 17, which are associated with high-grade tumors, and loss of the 9p21 site that is characteristic of low-grade disease. UroVysion and NMP-22 have been approved by the US Food and Drug Administration (FDA) for use in screening and in combination with cystoscopy for the diagnosis of recurrence. False positives can occur in cystitis, urolithiasis, bowel interposition, or in the presence of foreign bodies. Urinary cytology is said to be more than 95% specific, and a positive reading mandates further investigation but negative findings are less definitive. In a systematic review and meta-analysis, Sathianathen et al.[11] noted that CxBladder, NMP22, UroVysion, and uCyt+ have sensitivity of 0.67 to 0.95 and specificity of 0.68 to 0.93, and thus may have superior sensitivity but inferior specificity to cytology. The technology of endoscopic examination has improved in recent years with the introduction of more sophisticated endoscopic cameras, high-resolution videography, fluorescence cystoscopy, and narrow banding imaging cystoscopy, leading to improved specificity and sensitivity.[12] This has also facilitated instrumentation of the upper tracts.

There is no specific serological workup for bladder cancer. Routine hematological and biochemical testing may reveal anemia of chronic disease or from blood loss, an elevated white cell count in association with infection or colony stimulating factor (CSF) production by the tumor, renal dysfunction (from obstruction or the underlying cause of the cancer), and occasionally evidence of metastases, such as raised alkaline phosphatase or liver function tests. No tumor markers have been shown to be specific to bladder cancer, although occasional elevation of HCG, CEA, CA 19-9, or CA125 will be seen, the latter particularly in the presence of elements of adenocarcinoma. Raised chromogranin or neuron-specific enolase may be present with small cell bladder cancer.

Imaging of the urinary tract may be carried out before or after cystoscopy. A relatively standard approach is to obtain CT urography to delineate the anatomy of the urinary tract, including the presence of tumors of the bladder and upper tracts or hydronephrosis. CT urography is more commonly used in the current era, based on its ability to evaluate the renal parenchyma in addition to the urothelium, and it is performed more rapidly than excretory urography. MRI imaging may also be helpful to define the local anatomy and the extent of an invasive tumor, while also providing staging information about lymph node and distant sites of involvement. However, it should be emphasized that the sensitivity and specificity of non-muscle-invasive pelvic imaging are somewhat limited. CT and MRI scans performed soon after transurethral resection of bladder tumor (TURBT) may suffer from the artifact of apparently increased depth and invasion due to a post-resection inflammatory infiltrate. Positron emission tomography (PET) has been used increasingly in recent years, especially linked to CT or MR scanning, improving the positive predictive rates. Negative PET scans do not rule out the possibility of active cancer. Improved technology has led to increased sensitivity for nodal detection from 30% to around 90% and specificity of greater than 90%.

Definitive investigation involves transurethral resection with the usual goals of complete local tumor eradication, where possible, and accurate staging. Bimanual examination at the time of transurethral resection (TUR) may assist in assessment of tumor stage and the presence of significant extravesical disease, although this technique is notoriously inaccurate. In the setting of high-grade cancer, it is important to determine the existence of muscularis propria invasion. Unless cystectomy is planned, repeat TUR (in patients with non-muscle invasive disease) within 4–6 weeks, for those with high-grade disease and lamina propria invasion, shows upstaging in 30% of patients with muscle identified in the original specimen, and 60% of patients in whom no muscle was present initially.

Prognosis

The prognosis of primary bladder cancer reflects factors already discussed, including stage and grade of the tumor, multifocality, presence of lymphovascular invasion, association with CIS, morphology, gene mutations, aneuploidy, presence of anemia, and hydronephrosis. Similar factors govern the prognosis of upper tract tumors.[1,13]

The AJCC Staging Classification[13] generally correlates well with outcome and has recently been updated with further subtle changes to T, N, and M categorization. The bladder is heavily invested by fat and muscle, but this is not the case in the upper tracts, and thus the physical barriers to spread, and patterns of metastasis in upper-track tumors are somewhat different from tumors in the bladder.

Algorithms for estimating risk and prognosis for patients with advanced disease have evolved, focused on the presence of visceral metastases, performance status, and anemia[14] and have intermittently been modified to improve precision. Several modifications have been studied, including prognostic criteria for second-line and salvage chemotherapy[15] but have not led to improved survival figures, although they may have avoided futile chemotherapy. As outlined below, expression of PD-1/PD-L1 is increasingly being used as a predictor of response to immune-oncology agents but does not yet have a defined role as a prognostic predictor.

Management of non-muscle-invasive bladder cancer

The key to effective management of non-muscle-invasive bladder cancer involves cystoscopy and resection of visible bladder tumor(s),[16,17] sometimes followed by postoperative use of intravesical therapy (immunological or cytotoxic reagents) to reduce the risk of recurrence.[16,17] As bladder cancer is associated with a field defect, multiple random biopsies of apparently normal urothelium should be performed to identify occult CIS if urine cytology is positive or in the presence of high-grade disease when bladder conservation is contemplated. Usually, endoscopic resection is repeated within 4 weeks of the initial resection in patients with high-grade disease and/or T1 tumors, as up to 50% will have evidence of invasive bladder cancer into muscularis propria on re-biopsy.[16–18]

The grade and stage of the tumor will dictate subsequent management. Patients with non-muscle-invasive, low-grade papillary bladder cancer are at low risk of progression to invasive disease, although the risk of recurrence may be as high as 60–80%. Patients at increased risk for recurrence on the basis of tumor size, multifocal tumors, or prior recurrent tumors are often given adjuvant intravesical therapy (usually weekly instillations for 6–8 weeks) following resection, mostly with bacillus Calmette Guerin (BCG), which reduces the risk of recurrence by up to around 40%.[16,17] The mechanism of action of BCG is based on local immunological stimulation, perhaps with alteration of suppressor-helper T cell ratios. Effectively, such treatment allows the bladder to "reject" implantation and recurrence of bladder cancer. This may be a harbinger of the apparent utility of PD-1 targeting, which releases the brake on T cell function, for invasive and metastatic disease.

Randomized trials suggest that BCG is superior to other intravesical agents at preventing tumor progression,[16,17] and an initial bladder preservation strategy involving intravesical BCG is associated with long-term outcomes similar to those with early cystectomy for low-grade tumors.[17] Maintenance BCG is associated with a reduction in tumor recurrence and reduced requirement for cystectomy, compared to a single 6-week induction regimen. The optimal schedule of BCG administration has not been defined, and similarly, the optimal commercial preparations and the ideal duration of administration remain controversial.

The side effects of all the intravesical agents in common use include irritative symptoms and hematuria. BCG may also cause a flu-like syndrome and, because it is an attenuated mycobacterium, it can produce local, regional, and systemic TB-like infections. Granulomatous infections can occur at extravesical sites, including the prostate, epididymis, testes, kidney, liver, and lungs. BCG sepsis is the most serious complication, and can be life-threatening, and should usually be treated with triple-antituberculous therapy.

In some centers, cytotoxic agents, such as mitomycin C, docetaxel, gemcitabine, or combination therapy,[18] are preferred because of purportedly reduced toxicity, although it is not yet certain that this is true. For patients who refuse cystectomy for relapsed non-muscle-invasive disease, several lines of immunological or cytotoxic intravesical therapy may be feasible and may delay recurrence and progression. For example, pembrolizumab was recently approved by the FDA for recurrent CIS after BCG failure.

After completion of treatment, patients should be monitored closely with periodic cystoscopy and selective urine cytology and/or tumor marker evaluation at 3–6 month intervals to detect recurrence early. Patients with high-risk non-muscle-invasive bladder cancer (high-grade Ta, T1, or CIS) have at least a 50%

risk of developing invasive bladder cancer and a 35% risk of dying from bladder cancer. Moreover, those with persistent or recurrent high-grade disease after one or two salvage courses of intravesical therapy will develop muscle invasion and progression in 80% of cases. Thus, we advocate timely radical cystectomy with urinary diversion for relapsed high-risk disease, particularly for patients with long life expectancy.[18,19] Cure rates approach 90% in this setting, and when cystectomy is delayed, deeply invasive disease may develop and is associated with diminished survival.[18] In the recent COVID-19 pandemic, there has been variable delay in moving to radical surgery, but it is too early to assess the impact of this change in practice.

Management of invasive bladder cancer

Definitive surgery

In the past decades, radical cystectomy with bilateral pelvic lymphadenectomy has been widely viewed as the standard treatment for clinically localized, invasive bladder cancer.[1,19,20] This traditionally requires the en bloc removal of the anterior pelvic organs, which include the bladder, prostate, and seminal vesicles in men and the bladder, urethra, uterus, ovaries, and vaginal cuff plus anterior vaginal wall in women.[19] A urinary diversion is formed by the connection of the ureters to a urinary conduit or detubularized intestinal reservoir. Continent reservoirs, such as the Indiana pouch and orthotopic neobladder, are now standard as they offer improved continence without an external collecting bag. The orthotopic neobladder is an intestinal reservoir which is attached to the urethra and enables the patient to void normally, usually without self-catheterization.

Radical cystectomy, without adjuvant therapy, is curative in up to 60% of patients with invasive bladder cancer,[19,20] depending on stage and other prognostic factors. The 5-year overall survival rates in large series of patients with T2–T3 disease range from 40% to 65%. Relapse rates reflect stage, grade, presence of lymphovascular invasion, and expression of adverse molecular prognosticators. Radical cystectomy alone has been reported to be curative in 20–40% of patients with regional metastasis to pelvic lymph nodes, and the outcome is influenced by the primary tumor stage, number of involved lymph nodes, and the presence of extranodal extension.[1,20,21] Extended template node dissection may improve cure rates.[20] However, this may reflect the case selection bias, surgical skill or support, and salvage techniques available in centers of excellence.

Advances in instrumentation

Laparoscopic radical cystectomy, with or without robotic assistance, has been reported in modest series from centers experienced in laparoscopic surgery.[22,23] The cystectomy and lymph node dissection are commonly performed laparoscopically and the urinary diversion is carried out through a midline incision smaller than is usual for conventional surgery. The potential advantages include reduced blood loss, less postoperative pain, and shorter convalescence, although most of the data have been derived from nonrandomized series, carried out by technically superb surgeons, with careful case selection and relatively short follow-up. In an underpowered randomized trial of only 118 cases, Bochner et al. reported no major differences in outcome between open and robotic-assisted surgery but noted an increase in metastatic sites for those undergoing open surgery and an increase in local/intra-abdominal recurrence in those treated via robot-assisted surgery.[22] Similarly, the RAZOR trial, carried out in 15 US centers, randomized 350 patients with T1-4, N0-1, M0 tumors to robot-assisted or open radical cystectomy, and showed no significant difference in outcomes, both with 2-year PFS around 72%.[23]

Role of radiotherapy

For patients with invasive, clinically nonmetastatic bladder cancer who are not surgical candidates, either by their choice, technical considerations, or physical fitness, combined modality therapy consisting of maximal TURBT and chemoradiation is the preferred treatment.[24,25] All previous attempts at well-designed, randomized trials comparing bladder preservation with cystectomy were closed due to poor accrual. We have not generally favored post hoc "real world" studies that compare outcomes in groups of irradiated and surgical cases because of their inadequate attention to occult biases of case selection and other variables and have thus not addressed them here. However, a contemporary Swedish national study of 3309 patients, published with appropriate caveats, noted that cases selected for radiotherapy were older with more comorbid conditions, had a worse survival than those selected for radical cystectomy, but emphasized that confounding selection variables precluded a true comparison.[26]

The optimal technique of dose delivery, either conformal or IMRT, and fractionation schedules remain controversial.[27] Favorable prognostic features for use of radiotherapy include small, localized, T2 tumors, absence of hydronephrosis, normal renal function, maximum debulking by transurethral resection, and absence of anemia.[1,24]

A relatively standard radiotherapy approach is to deliver more than 64–66 Gy over 6–7 weeks, with 40 Gy delivered to the bladder, and the highest doses confined to the tumor plus a reasonable margin, as defined by diagnostic scans. Although controversial, second-look cystoscopy can be performed after the initial phase of radiation to document CR/extensive PR before committing to the final boost.[24] A pooled analysis of the RTOG experience with chemoradiation for bladder preservation, including 468 patients from 6 prospective trials, reported 5- and 10-year disease-specific survival of 71% and 65%, respectively.[24] Among 5-year survivors, 80% had an intact bladder.

In the United Kingdom, a randomized trial of chemoradiation with 5-fluorouracil and mitomycin C versus radiation alone showed a significant increase in local control and a strong trend towards a survival benefit from the combination.[25] There was also a strong statistical trend ($p = 0.07$) in the long-term follow-up of an earlier international randomized trial that compared neoadjuvant CMV plus radiotherapy versus radiotherapy alone.[28]

Toxicities of radiation include cutaneous inflammation, proctitis occasionally complicated by bleeding and/or obstruction, cystitis or bladder fibrosis, impotence, incontinence, and development of secondary malignancies in the region surrounding the radiation field. Of importance, if radiotherapy fails, salvage surgery is much more complex because of the formation of fibrosis in the irradiated field, emphasizing the importance of cystoscopic surveillance and early identification of incomplete response, allowing for early salvage surgery. It is important to emphasize that the local toxicity of radiotherapy is worse in patients who have undergone multiple TURB's, due to inflammation and contraction of the bladder prior to radiotherapy.

Several innovations in radiation planning and treatment have been introduced in recent years to maximize the conformality of dose distribution. These include devices for tracking physiological movement of the tumor, dynamic shaping of the radiation beam, and intra-fraction patient monitoring systems. The role of particle therapy, such as proton beam, remains unclear for invasive bladder cancer.

Combined modality strategies

Neoadjuvant (preemptive) cytotoxic chemotherapy
We first studied preemptive or neoadjuvant systemic chemotherapy plus local treatment almost 40 years ago,[29] based on the rationale that chemotherapy might reduce the extent of local tumor while controlling occult metastases. Our preliminary studies showed that this can shrink primary bladder cancers, and result in downstaging, sometimes achieving a complete clinical and pathological remission.[29] However, initial randomized trials did not confirm a survival benefit for single-agent regimens. The introduction of multidrug chemotherapy regimens, such as the methotrexate, vinblastine, doxorubicin, and cisplatin (MVAC) and cisplatin, methotrexate, and vinblastine (CMV), adapted from use in metastatic disease, into neoadjuvant protocols yielded survival benefit, confirmed by randomized clinical trials, and became the standard of care (Table 2).[28,30,31]

The consensus is that neoadjuvant MVAC or equivalent chemotherapy affords an absolute increase in cure rate of 7–8%, with an increase in median survival of up to 3 years, when added to radical cystectomy. A statistically significant survival benefit has not been proven when the primary treatment is radiotherapy, despite a strong trend favoring the combination modality. However, national surveys of patterns of practice have indicated that more than 60% of eligible patients still do not receive neoadjuvant chemotherapy, suggesting that change has come slowly in this area, predicated largely on the choices of urologists, the gatekeepers of this domain.[32]

To date, no multidrug cytotoxic regimen has been shown to be superior, or even equivalent to the MVAC or CMV regimens for neoadjuvant chemotherapy. However, the newer, less toxic regimens, such as gemcitabine-cisplatin (GC) or gemcitabine-carboplatin are increasingly being used for neoadjuvant therapy. This may be reasonable for the older or frail patients but may lead to a greater risk of death from cancer for the more robust patient without intercurrent medical disorders.

The importance of dose-dense (dd) MVAC, as initially developed and tested by the EORTC in the metastatic setting, remains unclear and somewhat controversial, although it appears that common practice is increasingly to use this approach as neoadjuvant therapy when the MVAC regimen is applied; while this is reasonable, it remains unsupported by level 1 evidence. It does appear that toxicity may be reduced by this approach, but it is unclear whether long-term results are equivalent, despite the imprimatur of the NCCN guidelines. The European "VESPER" trial has compared (dd) MVAC to GC, and a preliminary report noted greater down-staging and toxicity from ddMVAC, but survival has not yet been reported.[33]

Neoadjuvant (preemptive) targeted therapies
Consequent upon the demonstrated utility of PD1/PD-L1 inhibitors for metastatic bladder cancer, several early phase clinical trials have assessed the utility of these agents as neoadjuvant therapy for invasive bladder cancer. Powles et al reported a pathological CR rate of 31% (95% CI 21–41%) after two cycles of atezolizumab before cystectomy.[34] Necchi et al. administered three cycles of 200 mg pembrolizumab prior to radical cystectomy for 114 patients with T2–T4a disease (including 30% with variant histology) and noted pT0 in 37% (95% CI 28–46%), with comparable figures for variant histology.[35] Tumor mutational burden and PD-L1 expression appeared to be predictors of response. These data are preliminary and there are no level 1 comparisons of targeted immune-oncology agents versus cytotoxics in this context.

Adjuvant chemotherapy
Chemotherapy administered after radical cystectomy for patients with T3–T4 tumors and/or lymph node involvement improves disease-free survival, as one would expect for any effective chemotherapy.[36,37] However, in the randomized trials reported to date, most of which have been flawed by poor design, a disease-free statistical target, or inadequate sample size, a statistically significant improvement in total survival has never been demonstrated.[38] It should not be forgotten that an Italian group tested the use of adjuvant GC and demonstrated a statistically nonsignificant inferior survival in the adjuvant chemotherapy arm.[39] An attempt was made to address these problems in the EORTC international randomized trial that had been in progress for several years, which suffered from poor accrual, leading to premature closure. This study confirmed a disease-free survival benefit, the largest benefit (counter-intuitively in patients without node metastases) but no overall survival benefit.[40] This may have suggested that the adjuvant chemotherapy may have compensated for inadequate definitive surgery.

Although meta-analysis can sometimes help to resolve the failure of small trials to resolve an issue, we believe that the published

Table 2 Results of clinical randomized trials of neoadjuvant chemotherapy for invasive bladder cancer, stages T1–T4.

Series	Neoadjuvant regimen	Definitive therapy	Median survival with/without neoadjuvant therapy (months)	Actuarial long-term survival with/without neoadjuvant therapy
Neoadjuvant				
MRC-EORTC	CMV	RT/cystectomy	44/37.5	35%/30% at 10 y
Intergroup	MVDC	Cystectomy	77/46	42%/35% at 10 y
Nordic 1 trial	DC	Cystectomy	Not reached/72	59%/51% at 5 y
Adjuvant				
EORTC	MVDC	Cystectomy	81/55	44%/39% at 5 y
Stanford	CMV	Cystectomy	63/36	42%/38% at 5 y
USC	CDCy	Cystectomy	52/30	44%/39% at 5 y
Cognetti	GC	Cystectomy	38/58	44%/44% at 6.5 y

Abbreviations: C, cisplatin; D, doxorubicin; M, methotrexate; Cy, Cyclophosphamide; V, vinblastine; G: gemcitabine; MRC-EORTC, Medical Research Council/European Organization for Research and Treatment of Cancer; RT, radiotherapy.

meta-analyses are flawed by grouping a heterogeneous set of small trials that were either poorly designed, poorly executed, or which did not actually compare adjuvant chemotherapy with chemotherapy at relapse. Despite limitations of historical controls and poorly executed randomized trials, it is still possible that there is a survival benefit from adjuvant chemotherapy, and it is unlikely that there would be a survival deficit, and thus we sometimes offer this approach to carefully selected otherwise healthy, postcystectomy patients with high-risk disease.

Recently several adjuvant studies of PD1-PDL1 targeted immune-oncology agents have been conducted in the adjuvant setting. While the outcomes of many remain undisclosed, it is noteworthy that Hussain et al.[41] reported another negative study of adjuvant therapy, using atezolizumab at the 2020 Annual Scientific Meeting of the American Society of Clinical Oncology; while a peer-reviewed publication has not yet been released, these data add no support to the use of adjuvant systemic therapy for invasive bladder cancer.

Metastatic bladder cancer

Cytotoxic chemotherapy

For decades, systemic chemotherapy has been the first-line treatment of choice for patients with metastatic bladder cancer. The combination of methotrexate, vinblastine, and cisplatin, with[42] or without[43] doxorubicin first produced objective responses in more than 60% of cases, with a median survival of 1 year. The utility of the MVAC regimen was proved in a randomized trial against single-agent cisplatin, which confirmed that the benefit persisted with a median follow-up beyond 6 years.[44] The major limitation of the MVAC regimen was substantial toxicity, including grade 3–4 GI effects, stomatitis, and myelosuppression, as well as occasional cases of renal dysfunction and cardiotoxicity.[42,44] Attempts were made to improve the regimen, and Sternberg et al. demonstrated that a dose-intense variant of MVAC yielded higher response rates and reduced toxicity compared to the original regimen, but without achieving a major increment in median survival or 5-year survival.[45]

Single-agent response rates of around 20–30% have been reported for paclitaxel, gemcitabine, docetaxel, ifosfamide, and pemetrexed. The combination of these agents with other standard or investigational drugs has resulted in response rates of 50–80%, sometimes with less toxicity than the conventional-combination MVAC regimen, but median survival figures have remained in the range of 12–20 months, and remissions longer than 3 years for patients with visceral metastases have not exceeded 10–15%. After initial studies of GC revealed apparently equivalent response rates and substantially less toxicity than the MVAC regimen,[46] a randomized trial confirmed similar survival but less toxicity from G-C.[47] The addition of paclitaxel to this doublet did not improve survival significantly. No other conventional chemotherapy regimens have yielded a greater survival benefit.

Stage migration has occurred in the management of advanced bladder cancer, largely due to the increased use of aggressive postsurgical imaging via CT, MRI, and PET scans, and there has been increased use of systemic chemotherapy to treat patients with small volume, asymptomatic metastases, and this should be remembered to set context on more recent regimens with reportedly improved outcomes.

Targeted agents and other innovative approaches

Alternative approaches have been intensively investigated. Agents that modulate the function of EGFR and other tyrosine kinase inhibitors have been studied as monotherapy and in combination with chemotherapy. The ability to identify expression of the HER-2/neu oncogene or EGFR may allow some tailoring of treatment, but a recent systematic review of 11 reported trials was unable to demonstrate major specific anticancer effect in bladder cancer.[48] However, this may be explained by the observation that there is substantial intratumoral heterogeneity of expression of HER-2/neu in urothelial tumors, and that expression seen in the primary tumors is often lost in metastatic deposits, particularly associated with heterogeneity of expression. This may well explain these puzzling results as many trials using HER-2/neu targeted therapy are predicated on biopsies of primary tumors only.[49]

By contrast, in a series of 99 patients with locally advanced or metastatic disease, erdafitinib, a tyrosine kinase inhibitor of fibroblast growth factor receptor (FGFR) 1–4 had antitumor effect against bladder cancers that express FGFR alterations.[50] In this phase 2 study of chemotherapy-treated relapsed cases, 40% showed confirmed responses, with a median overall survival of 13.8 months. Grade 3–4 toxicities included hyponatremia and stomatitis, with occasional patients discontinuing because of retinal detachment, hand-foot syndrome, and cutaneous events; hyperphosphatemia occurred in most patients. Several other FGFR inhibitors, as well as combination regimens, are in clinical development, all with similar spectra of activity and toxicity, but an optimal drug has not yet been defined.[51]

Another targeted agent with substantial activity against urothelial malignancy is enfortumab vedotin, an antibody that targets the cell adhesion molecule nectin-4, which is linked to a microtubule inhibitor conjugate. In an open-label phase II trial, 125 patients who had previously received platinum complexes and PD1/PD-L1 inhibition, were treated with this agent, and achieved a CR rate of 12% and overall response rate of 44%.[52] The median overall survival was reported as 12 months, although this was an early report and longer follow-up will be required to set true context. The more severe toxicities included neutropenia, anemia, and fatigue, and common side effects were peripheral neuropathy, ocular toxicity, rash, and hyperglycemia.

Several other agents are in development, with FDA assessment pending, and several early phase trials are assessing combination targeted regimens and combinations of cytotoxic-targeted therapies, but it is too early to define an evidence-based algorithm for first-line use or even the optimal sequence for salvage therapy.

There is substantial expression of PD-1 and PDL-1 in urothelial malignancy, and remarkable activity was demonstrated in phases I and II studies in heavily pretreated patients,[53-55] and then as first-line treatment in patients deemed unsuitable for cisplatin-based therapy.[56] With minimum follow-up of 2 years, for cisplatin-ineligible patients with bladder cancer, the median duration of response was 30 months, median survival was 11.3 months, and 2-year overall survival was 31%.[56] In platinum-treated patients, pembrolizumab confers a survival benefit with less toxicity over salvage chemotherapy and we usually prefer it to second-line chemotherapy in this setting.[54]

For this brief review, a detailed assessment of the pattern of toxicity of the immune-oncology agents is not appropriate, but they are well documented and include colitis, hypophysitis, bone marrow suppression, renal and hepatic dysfunction, and a range of impacts of immunologic self-activation and targeting. It is important to emphasize that these agents require proactive and informed management, and it can be dangerous for the clinician inexperienced in their use to apply them without consultation. An important issue that has been troubling is the frequent disconnect between expression of PD1/PDL-1 and outcome of treatment with targeted agents. This may be explained by our observation of substantial differences in expression of PD1/PDL-1 between primary tumors and metastatic deposits,[57] a similar observation to what we have observed with expression of HER-2/neu. This has clinical importance as predictive analysis is often derived from biopsies only of the primary tumor.

An unexpected and potentially important innovation has been the recent demonstration in a randomized trial that adjuvant atezolizumab, delivered as adjuvant therapy upon completion of definitive cytotoxic management may improve survival.[58] This has not been shown by studies of other targeted agents, and will require validation by time; it remains possible that differences in subsequent salvage therapy between the two arms or occult differences in patterns of practice in the large number of investigator sites could explain some of the difference in outcome.

Several targeted agents are clearly very active against urothelial malignancy, and first- and second-line response rates and survival figures are surprisingly similar to those achieved by treatment with MVAC and GC, but with a different spectrum of toxicity. There are no level 1 data to allow us to rank order which regimen is superior, nor which sequence of use is optimal, either regarding increased activity or reduced toxicity. To date, two monoclonal antibodies targeting PD-1 (pembrolizumab, nivolumab) and three targeting PD-L1 (atezolizumab, avelumab, durvalumab) have received FDA approval for second-line treatment after platinum therapy, and atezolizumab and pembrolizumab are approved for use in cisplatin-ineligible patients.

One point of considerable importance is that some physicians have fallen into the trap of forgetting cytotoxics completely; in our quaternary referral practice, we sometimes have to remind clinicians who believe that a patient is at the end of the line, that they have not tried cytotoxic chemotherapy! What is absolutely clear is that the introduction of immune-oncology agents into the care of urothelial malignancy is a game changer and will potentially improve long-term survival from metastatic disease.

Another approach that is being tested is the use of surgery to consolidate remissions achieved from chemotherapy,[59] supported by the 33% incidence of viable cancer found within resected specimens after complete clinical response. Five-year survival rates, as high as 30–40%, have been reported in patients following complete resection of metastatic sites after cisplatin-based chemotherapy, but it should be noted that these represent very heavily selected cases, dominated by single metastases. A study of 16,382 patients with metastatic bladder cancer from the National Cancer Database suggested that only 6.6% had undergone metastatectomy, with a median survival of only 7 months; greater survival benefit was seen for patients in whom lung and brain metastases were resected.[60]

Uncommon histologic variants
A detailed discussion of the management of rare cancers of the bladder is beyond the scope of this chapter and has been detailed elsewhere.[61] The general principles include all of the uncommon variants tend to be more resistant to cytotoxic chemotherapy than are the pure UCs, and thus a greater emphasis is placed on surgical resection or definitive radiotherapy when possible; it is important to ensure that the diagnosis is confirmed by an expert tumor pathologist and to exclude the diagnosis of a metastatic second primary cancer; referral to a center of excellence at least for confirmation of the diagnosis and a second opinion regarding management should be implemented when possible.[62] With the introduction of targeted therapies focused on immunological function, there are emerging data to suggest that some variants of urothelial malignancy show response rates more akin to the pure UCs, and this domain of treatment will continue to evolve.

The prognosis of metastatic tumors of nontransitional type reflects the sites of involvement, growth characteristics, and bulk of disease. As the yield from chemotherapy is less impressive than for urothelial cancer,[44,61] it is important to consider context (age, anticipated active life expectancy, intercurrent disease, sites of metastases) when planning the approach to treatment of advanced disease.[62]

Squamous carcinomas are sensitive to combinations that include a platinum complex, paclitaxel, and gemcitabine, and occasional responses have been reported after treatment with methotrexate, bleomycin, and ifosfamide. We have previously shown that the MVAC regimen is not especially useful for squamous carcinoma of the bladder.[44] Adenocarcinomas tend to respond transiently to regimens used for cancers of the GI tract, such as combinations involving oxaliplatin, irinotecan, and fluoropyrimidines.

For small cell undifferentiated bladder cancer, the most useful regimens resemble those used for small cell cancers of the lung and generally involve combinations that include a platinum complex, etoposide, doxorubicin, a taxane, and/or an oxazophorine. These tumors are more resistant to chemotherapy than are bronchogenic variants, and there is thus a greater emphasis on surgery for the primary tumor. In the metastatic setting, this is less relevant. In addition, there is good level-2 evidence that chemotherapy adds to the survival impact of surgical resection for clinically nonmetastatic disease.[61] There is also emerging evidence, predominantly case reports to date, of the activity of PD-1/PD-L1 inhibitors in this disease.

Upper tract tumors
The approach to upper tract urothelial cancers is very similar to that employed for cancers of the bladder, with the caveat that the extent of surrounding fat and muscle is less, thus constituting less obstruction to metastasis. In addition, the phenomenon of "drop metastasis" may occur, in which tumor deposits from the upper tract(s) may seed to the urothelium of the bladder; whether this is the only mechanism of metachronous tumors, or whether it reflects the presence of field defect remains unclear. What is important is that a recent study has shown substantial differences in gene expression overall between bladder tumors and upper tract tumors, with the latter having increased expression of FGFR3, but also that there is clonal identity when lower tract and upper tract tumors coexist in individual patients.[63] Details regarding etiology, epidemiology, clinical presentation, and investigation have been addressed in the relevant sections above and elsewhere.[64]

Surgical treatment
The surgical approach to upper tract tumors is quite different from that employed for the bladder.[65,66] The standard treatment for localized upper tract urothelial carcinoma is radical nephroureterectomy, with complete removal of the kidney, surrounding fat, and Gerota's fascia, removal of the affected ureter, as well as the en bloc resection of a bladder cuff. We believe that ipsilateral node dissection or extensive sampling should be performed for prognostication purposes, although there is no level 1 evidence to prove a therapeutic impact from the procedure.

Laparoscopic radical nephroureterectomy is increasingly being considered as a reasonable alternative to open surgery, although long-term outcome equivalence not been proven in randomized studies. Nonrandomized series appear to indicate that the results are comparable with respect to tumor control, and probably with less operative morbidity,[65–68] although these studies suffer from small numbers and modest follow-up.

Nephron-sparing surgery is considered for settings such as bilateral disease, solitary kidney, impaired renal function, or significant comorbid medical conditions. This can be achieved by partial ureterectomy, partial resection of renal pelvis, and percutaneous resection of a renal pelvic tumor. The decision to take this approach is essentially a cost-effective choice, and which must take into consideration the likely outcome of tumor management versus the morbidity of treatment and its impact on the comorbid state. Low-grade tumors may be treated safely and effectively by endoscopic means or perhaps by a reverse thermal gel (see below). Case selection is of critical importance, and recurrence rates reflect surgical experience and technique, instrumentation employed and the prognostic determinants of the tumors being treated.

Radiotherapy and chemotherapy

There is remarkably scanty level 1–2 information to support the use of radiotherapy for upper tract tumors, beyond palliation for inoperable cases. Dosing is limited by the sensitivity of the normal tissues to the impact of radiotherapy. Furthermore, those tumors with sufficiently poor prognosis to require consideration of radiotherapy for local control actually have a high chance of synchronous or metachronous distant nodal or metastatic involvement, thus vitiating the true role of radiotherapy. In structured trials, adjuvant radiotherapy has not been shown to have a major survival impact for upper tract tumors.[69,70]

The efficacy of intravesical therapy for bladder cancer led investigators to use these agents in upper urinary tract tumors. The most common approach has been to place bilateral ureteral stents followed by instillation of cytotoxic agents (mitomycin or doxorubicin) or BCG via a urinary catheter,[71] as for bladder cancer; however, uncertainty remains as to how well the agents are being delivered upstream. Alternatively, there have been reports of transcutaneous insertion of flexible catheters into the ureters, followed by infusion of agents. Anecdotal data suggest that tumor regression occurs in response to topical delivery of chemotherapy or immunotherapy. These agents have also been delivered via nephrostomy tube after percutaneous treatment. The quality of the data, including length of follow-up, has been variable, but the overall consensus is that relapse and progression can be reduced by this type of treatment. More recently, a reverse thermal gel with mitomycin C (UGN-101 or Jelmyto®) was FDA approved for low-grade tumors of the upper tract.[10] Approximately 30% of patients with upper tract urothelial cancer will develop a recurrence in the bladder, thus requiring long-term cystoscopic surveillance of the bladder for patients with upper tract UC.[65,72]

The considerations for systemic chemotherapy for upper tract urothelial cancers are essentially identical to those pertaining to urothelial bladder cancer.[42–47] In the past, it had been suggested that upper tract tumors are less responsive than those arising in the bladder. However, there is little evidence to support this, and the international randomized study of MVAC versus cisplatin confirmed similar response rates and survival.[44] Thus systemic chemotherapy is covered in detail in the section above on chemotherapy for bladder cancer. In the perioperative setting for local disease, patients eligible for chemotherapy may be considered for adjuvant platinum-based chemotherapy on the basis of improved disease-free survival observed in one randomized study.[73] Whether these results can be applied to the neoadjuvant setting has not been defined. Due to the relatively high prevalence of FGFR3 aberrations in upper tract cancers,[63] a future role for adjuvant FGFR targeted therapy may also be established depending on the outcome of ongoing studies.

> **Summary**
>
> There has been significant progress in the management of bladder cancer in the past 30 years, with refinement of our understanding of the underlying biology, relevance of gene expression and stem cell function, molecular prognostication, and improvement in the nature of surgery, reduction in morbidity of surgery, and rationalization of the role of chemotherapy for advanced disease. There is also a place for bladder conservation via chemoradiation. Most patients with metastatic disease still die of their disease, and this has led to the search for new systemic therapies, with recent successes including immune-oncology agents targeting the PD1/PDL1 interface. Of importance, recent trials have shown similar activity of cytotoxic chemotherapy and agents targeted to the PD1/PD-L1 interface, and extensive phase III studies are underway to show optimal sequencing and combinations of the standard and targeted agents.

Key references

The complete reference list can be found on Vital Source version of this title, see inside front cover.

1. Raghavan D, Shipley WU, Garnick MB, et al. Biology and management of bladder cancer. *N Engl J Med*. 1990;**322**:1129–1138.
2. Fleshner N, Kondylis F. Demographics and epidemiology of urothelial cancer of the urinary bladder. In: Droller M, ed. *American Cancer Society Atlas of Clinical Oncology: Urothelial Tumors*. London, Hamilton: BC Decker; 2004:1–16.
3. Cote RJ, Mitra AP, Amin MB. Bladder and urethra. In: Weidner N, Cote RJ, Suster S, Weiss LM, eds. *Modern Surgical Pathology*, 2nd ed. Philadelphia, PA: Saunders; 2009, Chapter 31:1079ff.
4. Brown JL, Russell PJ, Philips J, et al. Clonal analysis of a bladder cancer cell line: an experimental model of tumor heterogeneity. *Br J Cancer*. 1990;**61**:369–376.
5. Cote RJ, Mitra AP. Molecular biology of bladder cancer. In: Post TW, ed. *UpToDate*. Waltham, MA: UpToDate Inc.; 2020 www.uptodate.com (accessed 5 November 2020).
9. Kamoun A, de Reyniès A, Allory Y, et al. A consensus molecular classification of muscle-invasive bladder cancer. *Eur Urol*. 2020;**77**:420–433.
13. Amin MB, Gress DM, Meyer Vega LR, et al. (eds). American joint committee on cancer: bladder cancer. In: *AJCC Cancer Staging Manual*, 8th ed. NY: Springer; 2018:757–765.
14. Bajorin DF, Dodd PM, Mazumdar M, et al. Long-term survival in metastatic transitional-cell carcinoma prognostic factors predicting outcome of therapy. *J Clin Oncol*. 1999;**17**:3173–3181.
15. Sonpavde G, Pond GR, Rosenberg JE, et al. Improved 5-factor prognostic classification of patients receiving salvage systemic therapy for advanced urothelial carcinoma. *J Urol*. 2016;**195**:277–282.
16. Woldu SL, Bagrodia A, Lotan Y. Guideline of guidelines: non-muscle-invasive bladder cancer. *BJU Int*. 2017;**119**:371–380.
18. Herr HW, Sogani PC. Does early cystectomy improve the survival of patients with high risk superficial bladder tumors? *J Urol*. 2001;**166**:1296–1299.
19. Stein JP, Lieskovsky G, Cote R, et al. Radical cystectomy in the treatment of invasive bladder cancer: long-term results in 1054 patients. *J Clin Oncol*. 2001;**19**:666–675.
21. Kader AK, Richards KA, Krane LS, et al. Robot-assisted laparoscopic vs open radical cystectomy: comparison of complications and perioperative oncological outcomes in 200 patients. *BJU Int*. 2013;**112**:E290–E294.
23. Parekh DJ, Reis IM, Castle EP, et al. Robot-assisted radical cystectomy versus open radical cystectomy in patients with bladder cancer (RAZOR): an open-label, randomized, phase 3, non-inferiority trial. *Lancet*. 2018;**391**:2525–2536.
24. Mak RH, Hunt D, Shipley WU, et al. Long-term outcomes in patients with muscle invasive bladder cancer after selective bladder-preserving combine modality

25 James ND, Hussain SA, Hall E, et al. Radiotherapy with or without chemotherapy in muscle-invasive bladder cancer. *New Engl J Med*. 2012;**366**:1477–1480.

29 Raghavan D, Pearson B, Duval P, et al. Initial intravenous cis-platinum therapy: improved management for invasive high-risk bladder cancer? *J Urol*. 1985;**133**:399–402.

30 Grossman HB, Natale RB, Tangen CM, et al. Neoadjuvant chemotherapy plus cystectomy compared with cystectomy alone for locally advanced bladder cancer. *N Engl J Med*. 2003;**349**:859–866.

32 Macleod LC, Yabes JG, Yu M, et al. Trends and appropriateness of perioperative chemotherapy for muscle-invasive bladder cancer. *Urol Oncol*. 2019;**37**:462–469.

36 Freiha F, Reese J, Torti FM. A randomized trial of radical cystectomy plus cisplatin, vinblastine and methotrexate chemotherapy for muscle invasive bladder cancer. *J Urol*. 1996;**155**:495–500.

38 Raghavan D, Bawtinhimer A, Mahoney J, et al. Adjuvant chemotherapy for bladder cancer – why does level 1 evidence not support it? *Ann Oncol*. 2014;**10**:1930–1934.

40 Sternberg CN, Skoneczna I, Kerst JM, et al. Immediate versus deferred chemotherapy after radical cystectomy in patients with pT3-pT4 or N+M0 urothelial carcinoma of the bladder (EORTC 30994): an intergroup, open-label, randomised phase 3 trial. *Lancet Oncol*. 2014;**16**(1):76–86.

41 Hussain MHA, Powles T, Albers P, et al. IMvigor010: primary analysis from a phase III randomized study of adjuvant atezolizumab (atezo) versus observation (obs) in high-risk muscle-invasive urothelial carcinoma (MIUC). *Proc Am Soc Clin Oncol, J Clin Oncol*. 2020;**38**:277s, abst 5000.

44 Saxman SB, Propert K, Einhorn LH, et al. Long-term follow up of phase III intergroup study of cisplatin alone or in combination with methotrexate, vinblastine, and doxorubicin in patients with metastatic urothelial carcinoma: a cooperative group study. *J Clin Oncol*. 1997;**15**:2564–2569.

47 von der Maase H, Sengelov L, Roberts JT, et al. Long-term survival results of a randomized trial comparing gemcitabine plus cisplatin, with methotrexate, vinblastine, doxorubicin, plus cisplatin in patients with bladder cancer. *J Clin Oncol*. 2005;**23**:4602–4608.

48 Koshkin VS, O'Donnell P, Yu EY, Grivas P. Systematic review: targeting HER2 in bladder cancer. *Bladder Cancer*. 2019;**5**:1–12.

50 Loriot Y, Necchi A, Park SH, et al. Erdafitinib in locally advanced or metastatic urothelial carcinoma. *N Engl J Med*. 2019;**381**:338–348.

52 Rosenberg JE, O'Donnell PH, Balar AV, et al. Pivotal trial of enfortumab vedotin in urothelial carcinoma after platinum and anti-programmed death 1/programmed death ligand 1 therapy. *J Clin Oncol*. 2019;**37**:2952–2600.

53 Powles T, Eder JP, Fine GD, et al. MPDL3280A (anti-PD-L1) treatment leads to clinical activity in metastatic bladder cancer. *Nature*. 2014;**515**:558–562.

54 Bellmunt J, de Wit R, Vaughn DJ, et al. Pembrolizumab as second line therapy for advanced urothelial carcinoma. *N Engl J Med*. 2017;**376**:1015–1026.

55 Powles T, Duran I, van der Heijden MS, et al. Atezolizumab versus chemotherapy in patients with platinum-treated locally advanced or metastatic urothelial carcinoma (IMvigor 211): a multicentre, open-label controlled trial. *Lancet*. 2018;**391**:748.

57 Burgess EF, Livasy C, Hartman A, et al. Discordance of high PD-L1 expression in primary and metastatic urothelial carcinoma lesions. *Urol Oncol*. 2019;**37**:299.e19–299.e25.

58 Powles T, Park SH, Voog E, et al. Avelumab maintenance therapy for advanced or metastatic urothelial carcinoma. *N Engl J Med*. 2020;**383**:1218–1230.

59 Lehmann J, Suttmann H, Albers P et al. Surgery for metastatic urothelial carcinoma with curative intent: the German experience (AUO AB 30/05). *Eur Urol*. 2009;**55**:1293–1299.

61 Al-Shamsi H, Hansel DE, Bellmunt J, et al. Uncommon cancers of the bladder. In: Raghavan D, Ahluwalia MS, Blanke CD, *et al*., eds. *Textbook of Uncommon Cancer*, 5th ed. Oxford, Hoboken: Wiley Blackwell; 2017:41–53.

62 Raghavan D. A structured approach to uncommon cancers: what should a clinician do? *Ann Oncol*. 2013;**24**:2932–2934.

65 Roupret M, Babjuk M, Burger M, et al. European association of urology guidelines on upper urinary tract urothelial carcinoma: 2020 update. *Eur Urol*. 2021;**79**(1):62–79. doi: 10.1016/j.eururo.2020.05.042.

67 Fairey AS. Comparison of oncological outcomes for open and laparoscopic radical nephroureterectomy: results from the Canadian upper tract collaboration. *BJU Int*. 2013;**112**:791–797.

71 Thalmann GN, Markwalder R, Walter B, et al. Long-term experience with bacillus Calmette-Guerin therapy of upper urinary tract transitional cell carcinoma in patients not eligible for surgery. *J Urol*. 2002;**168**:1381–1385.

73 Birtle A, Johnson M, Chester J, et al. Adjuvant chemotherapy in upper tract urothelial carcinoma (the POUT trial): a phase 3, open label, randomized controlled trial. *Lancet*. 2020;**395**:1268–1277.

95 Neoplasms of the prostate

Ana Aparicio, MD ■ Patrick Pilie, MD ■ Devaki S. Surasi, MBBS ■ Seungtaek Choi, MD ■ Brian F. Chapin, MD ■ Christopher J. Logothetis, MD ■ Paul G. Corn, MD, PhD

Overview

Cancer of the prostate is the most commonly diagnosed nonskin neoplasm and the second leading cause of cancer-related mortality in men in the United States. Considerable advances have been made in screening, diagnosis, and therapy options, particularly in advanced disease, but controversies about the diagnosis and management of prostate cancer, especially in the areas of screening and choice of therapy, continue to evolve. Research initiatives in advanced disease have shifted from prognostication to prediction, and current treatment considerations are focused on optimization of therapy sequence, development of rational combinations, biomarker-driven patient selection, determining the role of local disease control in patients with metastases, and bone targeting therapies. Despite progress, prostate cancer survival has not improved at the same pace as other cancer subtypes. It is anticipated that addressing knowledge gaps will lead to the development of novel agents with unique mechanisms of action and optimization of integrated strategies (surgical, radiation, and medical) to improve overall survival.

Prostate cancer awareness, clinical application of improved biopsy schemes, and advances in imaging combined with the widespread use of prostate-specific antigen (PSA) have resulted in increased detection of early prostate cancer. The question of whether PSA screening would reduce mortality from prostate cancer has now been tested in the European Randomized Study of Screening for Prostate Cancer (ERSPC) and the Prostate, Lung, Colorectal, and Ovarian (PLCO) Cancer Screening Trial first published in 2009. Though many of the apparent discrepancies between these trials can be accounted for by trial design and patient cross-contamination, they brought to the forefront the dilemma of overdiagnosis and overtreatment, as well as the heterogeneous nature of prostate cancer and the urgent need to improve the accuracy of identifying clinically significant early disease with lethal potential. It is hoped that enhancing the current morphologic and anatomic classification of prostate cancer with a better understanding of the molecular underpinnings of diverse disease states will lead to a more refined taxonomy of prostate cancer and ultimately improve outcomes while minimizing treatment-related morbidity.

Salient features that distinguish prostate cancer from other malignancies and frame the dilemmas surrounding it are its striking age-dependent incidence, with progressively increasing frequency with increasing age, a strong familial and hereditary component, the variable lethality of morphologically identical cancers, the central role of androgen signaling, the preponderance of bone-forming metastases, and metabolic derangements contributing to lethal progression. Important advances made in each of these areas will modify the approaches currently used to prevent, prognosticate, predict, and treat prostate cancer.

Biology of prostate cancer

Normal anatomic and histologic features of the prostate

The prostate gland sits in the pelvis, surrounded by the rectum posteriorly and the bladder superiorly, and it is anchored to the bladder pelvic floor; the urethra communicates between the bladder and the prostate into the penis (Figure 1). The prostate is composed of stromal, ductal, and luminal epithelial cells and is organized around branching ducts and individual glands lined with secretory epithelial cells and basal cells.[1] The secretory epithelial cell is the major cell type in the gland. These androgen-regulated cells produce prostate-specific antigen (PSA) and prostatic acid phosphatase (PAP). The central role of androgen signaling in prostate cancer biology likely accounts for the utility of PSA and PAP in determining disease status clinically. The vast majority of prostate cancers have cells that share properties with the secretory epithelial cells. Unlike the epithelial cells, the basal cell layer is not directly controlled by androgen signaling. Evidence has been shown for both basal cell population and luminal cell populations as being the preferred cells of origin for prostate cancer.[2,3]

As in other human tissues, cells belonging to the neuroendocrine system are also present within the prostate. Neuroendocrine cells contain secretory granules and extend dendrite-like processes between adjacent epithelial cells or toward the acinar or urethral lumina.[4,5] A variety of secretory products can be found within the granules, including serotonin, calcitonin, gastrin-releasing peptide, and somatostatin. Neuroendocrine cells are commonly identified immunohistochemically by the presence of markers such as chromogranin A or synaptophysin in the cytoplasm. They are terminally differentiated cells that are thought to regulate the growth, differentiation, and function of coexisting prostatic cells, but their exact role remains to be fully understood.

The view that the prostate has a lobar pattern has been challenged. McNeal et al. conducted detailed studies of the normal and pathologic anatomy of the prostate and introduced the transforming concept of anatomic zones rather than lobes to describe the gland.[6] There are four major zones within the normal prostate: peripheral, central, transition (constituting 70%, 20%, and 5% of the glandular tissue, respectively), and anterior fibromuscular stroma (Figure 2). The peripheral zone, which extends posterolaterally around the gland from the apex to the base, is the most common site for the development of prostate carcinomas. The central zone surrounds the ejaculatory duct apparatus and makes up

---

Holland-Frei Cancer Medicine, Tenth Edition. Edited by Robert C. Bast, John C. Byrd, Carlo M. Croce, Ernest Hawk, Fadlo R. Khuri, Raphael E. Pollock, Apostolia M. Tsimberidou, Christopher G. Willett, and Cheryl L. Willman.
© 2023 John Wiley & Sons, Inc. Published 2023 by John Wiley & Sons, Inc.

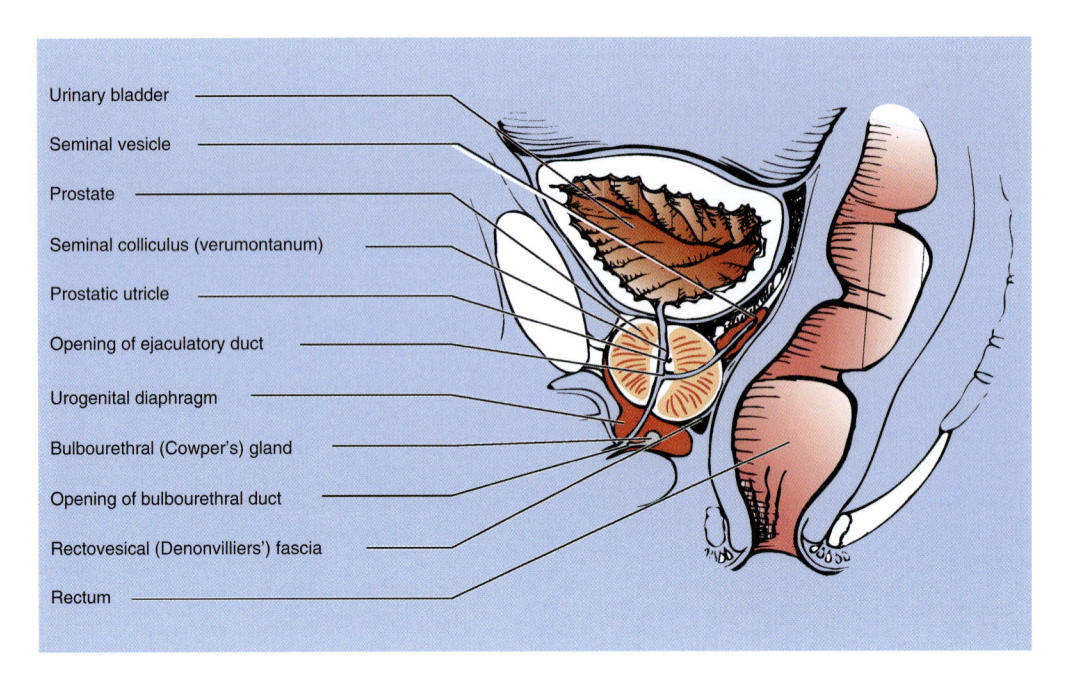

Figure 1 Normal prostate anatomy.

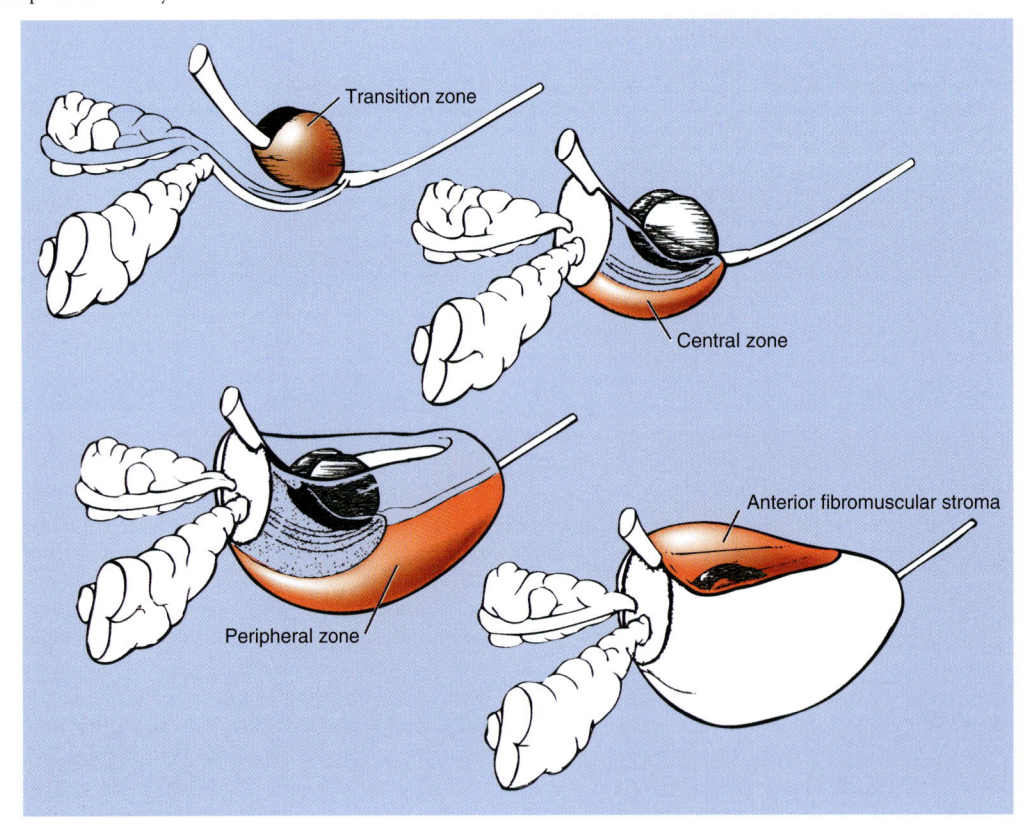

Figure 2 Zonal anatomy of the prostate: the three glandular zones of the prostate and the anterior fibromuscular stroma.

the majority of the prostatic base. The transition zone constitutes two small lobules that abut the prostatic urethra and is the region where benign prostatic hypertrophy (BPH) primarily originates. Some reports suggest that transition zone cancers have a lower malignant potential, but other studies report no difference in outcome compared with those originating in the peripheral zone when controlled for grade and stage.[7,8]

Surrounding the gland is stroma, which includes fibroblasts, smooth muscle, nerves, and lymphatic tissue. Stromal–epithelial interactions are fundamental in normal prostate development and physiology, with aberrant interactions contributing to the development of malignancy via various mechanisms. Stromal–epithelial interactions may exert both tumor-promoting as well as carcinogenesis-and progression-inhibitory effects. Furthermore, stromal–epithelial interacting pathways implicated in the development of the tumor microenvironment in prostate cancer progression may be those shared by the prostate and bone in their normal development and function.[9]

There are varying distinct anatomic barriers surrounding the prostate. The smooth muscle of the prostatic stroma gradually extends into fibrous tissue that ends in loose connective and adipose tissue. Of particular relevance is the absence of any semblance of a capsule at the gland's apex and anteriorly. This understanding of anatomic detail allows clinicians to determine the adequacy of prostate surgery by accurately defining the surgical margin with increasing confidence. It also allows the surgical delineation of disease as "organ-confined" or "specimen-confined." The organ-confined cancers do not extend beyond the confines of the prostate, whereas specimen-confined indicates that the cancer does not extend beyond the cut margins. The distinction between these two terms is important because they are used to determine the adequacy of surgery and the need for postoperative radiation therapy in selected patients.

A final note about the anatomy of the prostate is that Walsh and Donker described the presence of two neurovascular bundles that pass adjacent to the gland posterolaterally.[10] The neurovascular bundles are essential for normal erectile function and defining their presence outside of the posterior-lateral prostatic fascia allowed Walsh to develop a "nerve-sparing" radical retropubic prostatectomy procedure that improves the odds of preserving potency.[11]

Premalignant prostatic lesions

Paradigms that are used to explain the progression of other solid tumors may not apply to prostate cancer. Many clinicians accept that premalignant lesions in the prostate may precede the development of cancer by many years. However, since there is a lack of knowledge about the nature or rate of their progression, the morphologic identification of premalignant lesions on biopsy specimens only serves to provide rationale for close monitoring of patients. Prostate cancer is also a heterogeneous disease, and it is unlikely that all prostate cancers develop through a "linear progression model" as proposed by Fearon and Vogelstein for colorectal cancer and subsequently applied to conceptualize other solid tumors.[12]

Morphologically heterogeneous lesions are included under the single term "prostatic intraepithelial neoplasia" (PIN) (Figure 3).[13] PIN is defined by the presence of cytologically atypical or dysplastic epithelial cells within architecturally benign-appearing glands and acini. Although three different grades have been described, 1 (mild), 2 (moderate), and 3 (severe), grades 2 and 3 PIN are often combined as "high grade." PIN is presumed to be a premalignant lesion because it is commonly present adjacent to prostate adenocarcinomas.[14] Although the finding of PIN is associated with the existence of cancer in sites not sampled on biopsy and implies increased risk of developing a morphologic cancer, the risk of progression has not been established or quantified.

Small prospective studies have reinforced the hypothesis that PIN is a precursor lesion to prostate cancer. The data have suggested that the presence of high-grade PIN predicts the subsequent development of cancer through a multistep carcinogenesis process. However, close clinical follow-up rather than definitive local therapy remains the standard of care after diagnosis of high-grade PIN alone.

Another potential premalignant lesion is atypical adenomatous hyperplasia (AAH). The characteristic appearance with AAH is the fulfillment of the architectural criteria for malignancy, with disruption of the basal cell layer, mainly in the transition zone, but without the cytologic changes diagnostic of cancer.[15] Some authors have suggested that a prostatic lesion composed of focal areas of epithelial atrophy associated with chronic inflammation (called "proliferative inflammatory atrophy", or PIA) is a precursor of PIN and eventually prostate cancer.[16] Evidence for this hypothesis includes the observation that PIA often occurs adjacent to areas of PIN and prostate cancer and that somatic genetic abnormalities seen in PIA often resemble those seen in prostate carcinoma.[17,18] Of particular relevance is that PIA implicates inflammation in the progression of prostate cancer.[19] If this hypothesis is confirmed and causally implicated with greater confidence in prostate cancer progression, the detection of PIA may lead to more effective prevention strategies.

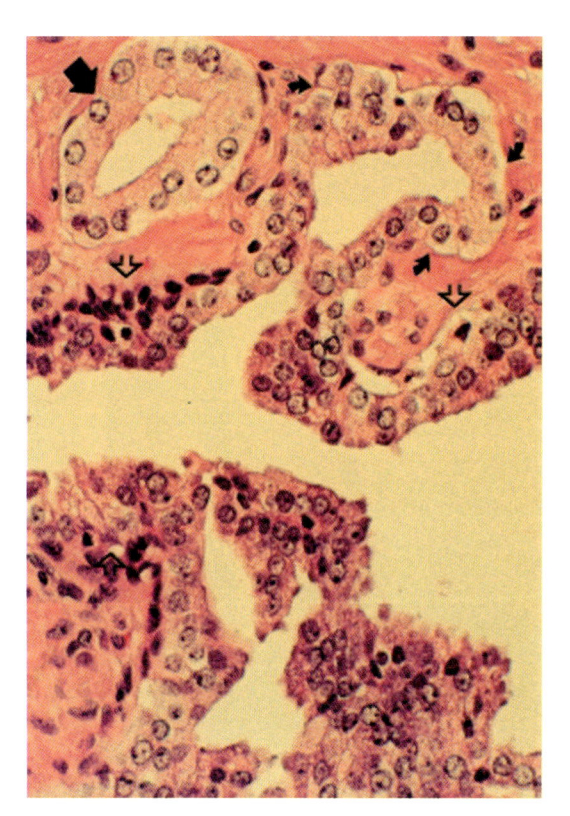

Figure 3 Photomicrograph of high-grade prostatic intraepithelial neoplasia (PIN) with basal cell layer (open arrows) with budding microacinus lacking basal cells (curved solid arrows). A microacinus of invasive Gleason pattern 3 adenocarcinoma is seen in the adjacent stroma (straight solid arrow). Hematoxylin and eosin × 160. Source: Courtesy of Thomas M. Wheeler, MD.

Histologic features of prostate cancer

Cancers that arise in the epithelium account for >95% of prostate cancers and acinar adenocarcinomas are by far the most common histology (Figure 4).[20] Prostate cancer variant histology will be discussed later in the article.

Studies have confirmed the prognostic importance of the degree of histologic differentiation of prostate adenocarcinoma. The degree of this differentiation is typically determined by patterns of gland formation and, less importantly, by cytologic detail. The most widely accepted grading scheme for adenocarcinoma of the prostate is that developed by Gleason (Figure 5).[21] Gleason created a system for classifying prostate tumors based on two levels of scoring that recognize the heterogeneous nature of prostate carcinomas. The primary pattern of differentiation is assigned a Gleason grade of 1–5 according to the dominant morphologic features of the specimen and its departure from normal appearance; the next most common pattern is also assigned a grade. This results in a two-digit score; for example, $3 + 4 = 7$. The Gleason system has been criticized for inadequately recognizing the

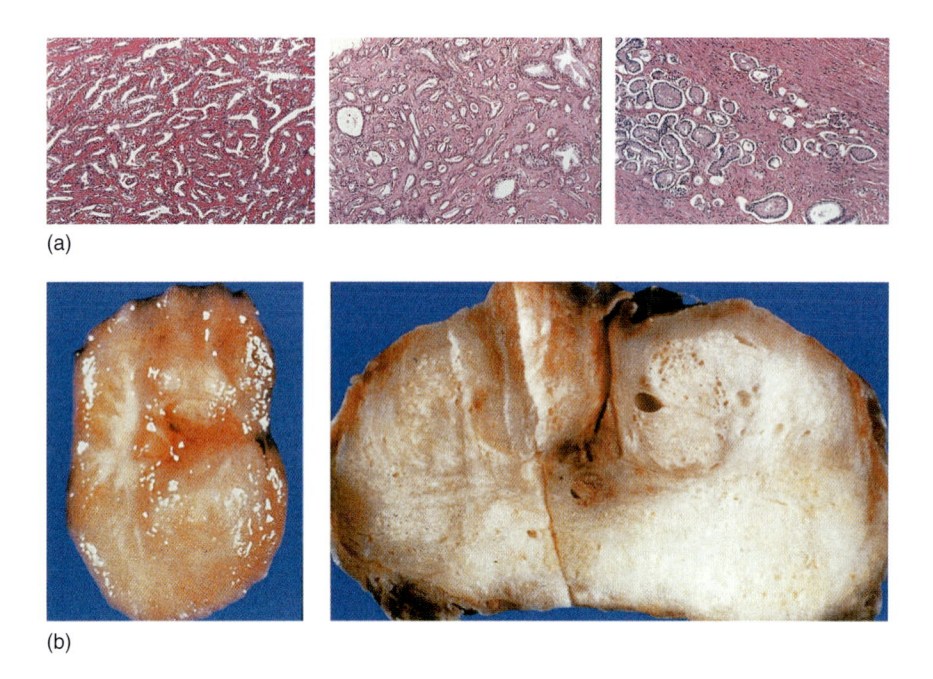

Figure 4 (a) Microscopic histologic appearance of prostate adenocarcinoma. (b) Gross histologic appearance of prostate adenocarcinoma.

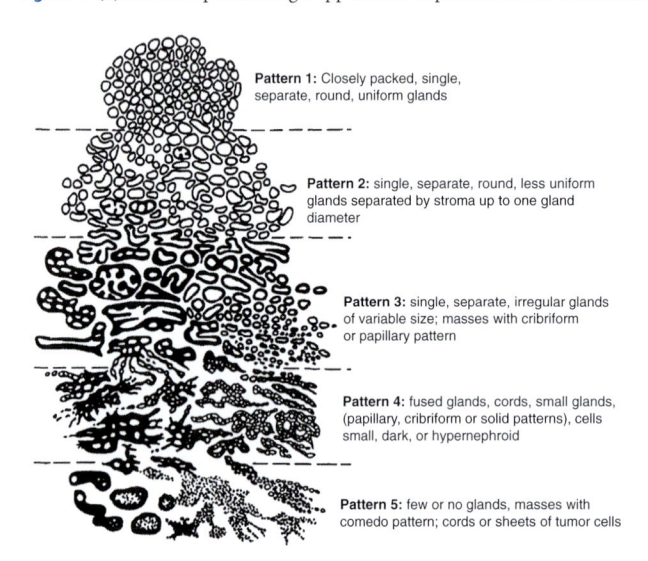

Figure 5 Histologic grading scheme for adenocarcinomas of the prostate. Source: Gleason.[23] Reproduced with permission from Elsevier.

Table 1 Grade group system.[a]

Grade group	Gleason score	Gleason pattern
1	≤6	≤3+3
2	7	3+4
3	7	4+3
4	8	4+4, 3+5, 5+3
5	9 or 10	4+5, 5+4, 5+5

[a] Source: NCCN Guidelines Version 2.2020.

proportion of the tumor that is composed of the secondary pattern as well as for lacking adequate distinction between good and poor prognoses in patients whose cancers have Gleason scores of 5–7 (most patients). However, the reproducibility and reliability of Gleason grading between pathologists are excellent. Gleason's original work demonstrated a clear association between a higher score and a higher mortality rate, which others have since confirmed.[22] While many other predictors of the clinical behavior of prostate cancer have been explored, the Gleason score remains the most broadly applicable and prognostically useful histologic grading system.

Since its inception, several limitations to the Gleason score system have been noted including: (1) two-digit combination scores of 2–5 are currently no longer assigned and certain patterns that Gleason originally defined as a score of 6 are now graded as 7, thus leading to contemporary Gleason score 6 cancers having a better prognosis than historic score 6 cancers; (2) the combination of Gleason scores into a 3-tier grouping (6, 7, 8–10) is used most frequently for prognostic and therapeutic purposes but 3+4=7 versus 4+3=7 and 8 versus 9–10 have very different prognoses, and (3) the lowest combination score now assigned is 6 but since the scale remains 2–10, patients may come to the logical yet incorrect assumption that their cancer is in the middle of the scale, compounding the fear of their cancer diagnosis with the belief that the cancer is serious and warrants treatment.

To address the above deficiencies, a new 5 Grade Group system was recently developed (Table 1).[24] Advantages of the new grading system include more accurate grade stratification, a simplified grading system of 5 (as opposed to multiple possible scores depending on various Gleason pattern combinations) and a lowest grade of 1 (as opposed to current practice of Gleason score 6) with the potential to reduce overtreatment of indolent prostate cancer. The new grading system, using the above terminology, has been accepted by the 2016 World Health Organization (WHO). However, to avoid confusion, the new grading system is being reported in conjunction with the Gleason system until it becomes more widely accepted and practiced [i.e., *Gleason score 3 + 3 = 6 (Grade Group 1)*].[24]

Genetic risk factors and molecular pathogenesis

Histopathologic characterization of prostate cancer remains the clinical standard for risk stratification and treatment algorithms.[22] However, it is increasingly evident that distinct subgroups of prostate cancer can be identified based on molecular aberrations at both the germline (hereditary) and/or somatic (tumor-specific) levels. Furthermore, identification of specific genetic defects now influences prostate cancer screening guidelines, disease monitoring, and treatment recommendations in daily clinical practice.

Prostate cancer remains one of the most hereditary forms of cancer, with the relative risk of prostate cancer increasing by 2- to 3-fold for men with a family history of prostate cancer in ≥1 first degree relative. This familial risk displays a dose-dependency whereby the greater number of impacted relatives results in even higher risk. Despite this strong heritable component, moderate or high penetrant mutations in cancer-related genes explain only a small fraction of hereditary or familial prostate cancer. The *HOXB13* G84E mutation, first identified as a prostate cancer susceptibility gene in 2012, is consistent with a founder allele and accounts for approximately 5% of all cases of hereditary prostate cancer in men of European descent.[25]

Multiple studies have consistently shown that mutations in select DNA damage response (DDR) genes involved in the hereditary breast and ovarian cancer (HBOC) syndrome can significantly increase a man's risk of developing prostate cancer and these germline mutations are enriched in patients with high-risk or metastatic disease. *BRCA2* is the gene most frequently found mutated in patients with prostate cancer and confers the highest risk in unaffected carriers. Unaffected carriers with deleterious variants in *BRCA2* display higher incidence of prostate cancer, are more likely to have clinically significant disease, and are diagnosed at a younger age compared to matched noncarriers.[26] In addition, men with prostate cancer and deleterious BRCA2 variants display worse metastasis-free survival and cause-specific survival.[27]

Germline mutations in other homologous recombination repair (HRR)-related genes, including *ATM, CHEK2,* and *PALB2* can also be seen in men with prostate cancer, with varying penetrance and less clear impact on phenotypic outcomes and targeted treatment selection, as discussed later in this article.[28] Mismatch repair (MMR) deficiency as seen in Lynch syndrome does confer an increased risk of prostate cancer and MMR deficiency can influence treatment selection in men with advanced prostate cancer as discussed later in this article. A recent study has shown that family history of hereditary prostate cancer conferred the highest risk of prostate cancer as compared to HBOC and Lynch Syndrome.[29] There are consensus guidelines recommending universal clinical germline genetic testing of *BRCA1/2* in men with metastatic prostate cancer, with consideration of inclusion for other DDR genes as well particularly in patients considering clinical trial participation. In addition, NCCN guidelines recommend universal germline testing in men with high-risk localized disease.

Prostate cancer also displays an array of somatic mutations that vary with the stage of the disease and phenotype. Alterations that affect the development and progression of prostate cancer include those in the hormonal and growth factor milieu, in growth factor receptors, in intracellular signaling pathways, in DDR and cell cycle regulation, and apoptosis.

Pathogenic or deleterious variants in the same DDR genes found mutated at the germline level are more commonly found at the somatic, or tumor-associated level. Compared to other solid tumors such as melanoma or urothelial cancers, advanced prostate cancer overall displays a relatively low tumor mutational burden (TMB), with rare exceptions including those tumors with MMR deficiency and/or subsequent high microsatellite instability (MSI-H). Defective MMR genes and/or MSI-H are seen in ~3–8% of prostate cancer, with the majority being of sporadic origin and with Lynch syndrome not displaying particularly high penetrance in prostate cancer as previously mentioned.[30–32]

The remainder of DDR defects seen in prostate cancer center mostly around the DNA double-strand break repair, replication stress signaling, and cell cycle regulation pathways. DDR gene alterations occur in ~25% of metastatic castration-resistant prostate cancer (mCRPC), with *BRCA2* being by far the most frequently altered gene in this pathway (with combined germline and somatic alterations seen in ~8–13% of men with metastatic prostate cancer), followed by *ATM*, and then to a lesser degree *BRCA1* and *CDK12*, with more rare deleterious variants found in multiple other HRR and cell cycle genes.[28,33] Alterations in *BRCA2* are found at significantly greater frequency in advanced prostate cancer overall compared to primary disease, and certain histologic subtypes like ductal and cribriform disease are enriched for deleterious variants in DDR genes (genes).[34,35]

Point mutations in the *SPOP* gene, an E3 ubiquitin ligase substrate-binding adaptor, commonly occur in prostate cancer and are more frequently seen in localized disease. Multiple studies have shown that patients with *SPOP* variants display a better prognosis and good response to androgen-targeted therapies. Mechanistic insight into why SPOP-variant prostate cancer displays this favorable phenotype and further prognostic and predictive biomarker applications of the SPOP-molecular subclass are areas of active investigation.[36]

Hormone and growth factor signaling

Androgen receptor (AR) signaling plays a central role in prostate cancer growth and progression, though its role in prostate cancer susceptibility is less clear. In early cancer, AR mutations are relatively uncommon, but germline variation (CAG repeats) in the *AR* gene has been shown to be a predictor of cancer aggressiveness and may play a role in the frequency and aggressiveness of prostate cancer in African-Americans.[37–39] AR mutations are more commonly seen in androgen-independent (castrate-resistant) prostate cancer, suggesting that the AR gene remains central in the growth and survival of prostate cancer even after the need for the ligand (androgens) has been mitigated.[37,40]

Several theoretical frameworks have been proposed for the development of androgen independence, most of which still postulate a cancer cell that depends on a functional *AR* but one that is amplified, oversensitive, promiscuous, or activated by upregulated coactivators or downregulated by corepressors.[41] For example, in LNCaP prostate cancer cells, an *AR* mutation, T877A, which is a substitution of alanine for threonine at position 877, results in an AR that is activated by other steroid hormones and by the androgen antagonist flutamide.[42] This *AR* mutation could help explain the "antiandrogen withdrawal syndrome." However, *AR* mutations occur too infrequently to account for the eventual evolution of most metastatic prostate cancers to a castrate-resistant state.

AR splice variants have been identified in prostate cancer.[43] AR splice variants lacking the ligand-binding domain (ARVs), originally isolated from prostate cancer cell lines derived from a single patient, are detected in normal and malignant human prostate tissue, with the highest levels observed in the late stage, castrate-resistant prostate cancer (CRPC). Approximately 20 AR splice variants have been identified to date, and they are not exclusively found in prostate tissue. The first AR splice variant was identified in the placenta. The most studied variant (called AR-V7 or AR3) activates AR reporter genes in the absence of ligand and therefore, could play a role in castration resistance. Correlative studies have associated the presence of ARV7 in prostate cancer-infiltrated bone marrow biopsies and circulating tumor cells from patients with mCRPC who have primary resistance to novel "second-generation" androgen signaling inhibitors abiraterone acetate (CYP17 inhibitor) and enzalutamide (antiandrogen).[44,45] Therefore, AR-V7 may serve as a predictive biomarker after progression on androgen signaling inhibition for resistance to abiraterone acetate and enzalutamide. However, AR-V7 positivity is very low (~3%) in men who have not received abiraterone, enzalutamide, or taxanes, and testing is not recommended in this treatment-naive setting.

Recent observations support the view that "intracrine" production of androgens acting in both an autocrine and paracrine fashion are implicated in the progression of prostate cancer.[46] Several lines of evidence support the concept that CYP17 lyase contributes to remodeling the prostate cancer tumor microenvironment: androgens in the microenvironment are at a higher concentration than they are in the serum, CYP17 expression occurs in stage-dependent cancer progression, and tumor regression occurs clinically in castrate-resistant cancers treated with CYP17 inhibitors (e.g., abiraterone). These data support the hypothesis that androgen signaling can be considered a stromal–epithelial interacting pathway.

True androgen independence is likely to arise from alternative stromal–epithelial interacting and/or other signaling pathways. Several bone and prostate developmental pathways are involved in prostate cancer progression and associated with higher-grade cancers.[47] This attractive hypothesis could account for the bone-homing and bone-forming phenotype of prostate cancer and its resistance to therapy in an organ-specific manner.

Molecules that alter intracellular signaling pathways also may be important in the pathogenesis and progression of prostate cancer to a castrate-resistant state. The clearest example to date is the tumor suppressor gene *PTEN*.[48] This gene encodes for a phosphatase that is important in modulating the signal generated by activated growth factor receptors. Loss of PTEN, which negatively regulates the PI3K–AKT–mTOR pathway, is strongly linked to advanced prostate cancer progression and poor clinical outcome. One study documented a 60% rate of *PTEN* mutations, with most in cell lines from metastatic disease, although mutations were also seen in primary cancers.[49] In fact, another group demonstrated higher rates of *PTEN* loss or mutation in tumors of advanced stage and grade.[50] Another pathway that may be aberrantly activated in prostate cancer is the hedgehog pathway. Normal hedgehog signaling is important in early development and patterning of the prostate epithelium. Work by Karhadkar et al. demonstrated that activation of the hedgehog pathway distinguishes prostate cancer from normal prostate cells and, further, metastatic prostate cancer from localized cancer.[51] Moreover, they demonstrated that hedgehog pathway inhibition results in PC3 xenograft regression. Both the PTEN and hedgehog pathways are being explored as targets for drug development.

African-American men are at an increased risk of developing prostate cancer and more likely to die from prostate cancer. The potential contributions to this disparity are multifactorial, including access to high-quality care, socioeconomic barriers, environmental exposures, and potential biological differences.[52] While African-American men with metastatic prostate cancer are at the same risk of harboring hereditary (germline) variants in cancer-related genes as white men, recent genomic profiling has revealed certain mutations that occur at a higher frequency in primary prostate tumors from black men, such as mutations in *FOXA1*.[53] Furthermore, genomic profiles of metastatic prostate cancers have shown that black men are more likely to have actionable mutations than white men, including high frequency of DDR gene mutations.[53] Crucial studies are needed to explore the different facets of prostate cancer outcome disparities to guide better-targeted prevention and treatment strategies.

While AR-signaling is the master regulator of prostate cancer, other growth factors have been implicated in the development and progression of the disease. For example, several lines of evidence suggest that insulin-like growth factor I (IGF-I) is important in prostate cancer growth. First, several prostate cancer cell lines and prostate xenograft models express both IGFs I and II and their receptors.[54,55] Second, Chan et al. reported on the relationship between plasma IGF-I concentration and prostate cancer, citing a relative risk of 4.3 for men in the highest quartile, compared with men in the lowest quartile.[56] Moreover, a higher incidence of prostate cancer has been noted in patients who had relatively high IGF-I concentrations in plasma samples that had been obtained 5 years prior to the cancer diagnosis, supporting the concept that IGF-I may be important early in the development of prostate cancer.[57] Although this observation has yet to be confirmed, it does implicate IGF-I signaling in prostate cancer progression.

Other growth factors and stromal–epithelial interacting pathways likely cooperate in prostate cancer development and progression. These include epidermal growth factor, vascular endothelial growth factor (VEGF), platelet-derived growth factor (PDGF), and transforming growth factor-beta (TGF-β) (Table 2).[57–59] Therapeutic strategies to inhibit stromal–epithelial interacting pathways are under development and will be discussed later in this article.

Table 2 Growth factors implicated in prostate cancer.[a]

Transforming growth factor beta
Fibroblast growth factor
Epidermal growth factor
Insulin-like growth factor
Platelet-derived growth factor
Vascular endothelial growth factor
Neurotensin
Endothelins
Colony-stimulating factors

[a]Source: Based on Stattin et al.[57]; Ware[58]; Corn.[59]

Early detection of prostate cancer

Early detection of prostate cancer, when it remains confined to the prostate, challenges patients and their physicians with the controversial question of how localized disease is best managed. More specifically, how patients with nonlethal disease can avoid overtreatment and preserve quality of life while patients with lethal disease receive treatment with curative intent.

Prostate cancer screening and early detection are controversial because for every 18 cases detected, only 3 will result in death. The cost of radical prostatectomy, which removes the threat of disease if there is no metastasis, may be the risk of impotence and urinary incontinence, which might affect disease-specific quality-of-life.[60] To determine whether screening for prostate cancer and three other cancers reduces mortality, the National Cancer Institute's (NCI's) Division of Cancer Prevention undertook the randomized, controlled Prostate, Lung, Colorectal, and Ovarian PLCO Screening Trial at 10 sites in 1993. The prostate screening arms have been published with commentary.[61,62] Participants underwent annual PSA screening examinations for 6 years and follow-up of 13 years for the latter publication.[63,64]

With a sample size of 76,685 men allocated to intervention (38,340) or control (38,345), the extended follow-up diagnosed 4250 cancers in the intervention arm and 3815 in the control. These events corresponded to 158 deaths in the intervention arm and 145 in the controls. The key conclusion was that PSA screening increased detection but did not affect mortality. A common critique of this study was significant contamination in the arms in the form of noncompliant screening in the intervention arm and opportunistic screening in the control arm.

Also launched in the 1990s was the European Randomized Study Prostate Cancer, which is also testing whether screening saves lives. It was published along with the PLCO trial in 2009. Updated results at 11 years and at 13 years have been published.[63,65] In this trial, there was significantly less contamination of the arms. The ERSPC's results showed a significant relative reduction in prostate cancer mortality by 21% and 29% after adjustment for noncompliance.[66] To prevent one death, the number needed to be screened was 1055 and to detect was 37. The additional follow-up time improved the screening metrics as expected. The authors cautioned that all-cause mortality was not affected and that overdetection and overtreatment remains a problem with PSA screening. The trial is often criticized as its design was not a unified multicenter study but rather a merger of several screening studies with differences in methodology and outcomes.

As a result, the US Preventive Services Task Force (USPSTF) initially issued a "D" rating for PSA screening (which discourages the use of this service). The USPSTF later changed the rating to a "C" in 2017 which recommends the test for selected patients depending on individual circumstances.[67]

Men who are carriers of a pathogenic *BRCA2* variant should start prostate cancer screening at age 40 years or 10 years before the youngest prostate cancer diagnosis in a family, with consideration for the same screening in men with *HOXB13, BRCA1, ATM,* and/or MMR germline variants.[68]

Identifying early disease

Strategies to manage the diagnosis of localized prostate cancer including active surveillance (AS), radical prostatectomy, and radiotherapy will result in superior recurrence-free outcomes if applied at earlier disease stages. The goal to detect early prostate cancer has led to a debate centered around using absolute PSA cutoffs versus prostate-specific antigen velocity (PSAV) or PSA isomers. The PSAV, one measure used in monitoring patients with localized disease, has been scrutinized as a tool for use in the diagnosis and prediction of outcomes. It is calculated using the log slope of at least three PSA values calculated over at least 2 years with no less than 6 months between measures.[69] Conceived as a way to capture the variability of prostate cancer or its progression, PSAV measures are used preoperatively and postoperatively. Researchers sometimes rely on measures taken closer together, consider fewer than three measures, and reduce the longitudinal period to less than 2 years.

Prostate cancer screening can be oversimplified into an algorithm in which all patients with a certain threshold of PSA (e.g., 2.5 or 4.0 ng/mL) or abnormal digital rectal exam (DRE) findings are referred to a urologist for evaluation and possible biopsy. However, patients' overall interests are better served if a more comprehensive evaluation takes place that considers whether they are at increased risk of having prostate cancer because of ethnicity (e.g., African-Americans are at increased risk), age, and/or family history and whether a prostate cancer diagnosis would be likely to affect their overall survival (OS) because of a younger age and fewer competing comorbid conditions. A comprehensive PSA history may be beneficial for calculating PSAV, and the complexed PSA test may be useful as a frontline screening tool because it has slightly better specificity than total PSA in the total PSA range of 2.5–4.0 ng/mL.[70]

The PSA blood test has been described as a test that "neither excludes benign disease nor wholly predicts meaningful malignancies."[69] Ian Thompson, principal investigator of the Prostate Cancer Prevention Trial (PCPT), and his colleagues studied 8575 men from the study's placebo group to estimate the receiver operating characteristic (ROC) curve for PSA and concluded that no absolute cutoff value had the high degree of sensitivity and specificity simultaneously required for identification of a risk-free value.[71] Instead, they endorsed viewing all PSA values as a continuum of risk for prostate cancer.

More widely investigated have been measures of PSAV, a calculation of rising PSA level that was introduced in the early 1990s as a marker of prostate cancer development, a means to reduce unnecessary biopsies, and a way to improve the specificity of PSA testing. However, current standards that shorten the minimum longitudinal monitoring period for calculating PSAV and push ever lower the levels of PSAV considered worrisome (0.35 ng/mL/year for PSA values <4 ng/mL and 0.75 ng/mL/year for patients with total PSA values >4 ng/mL) actually increase the likelihood of biopsy.[72–74] Cautious investigators argue that to use PSAV to monitor men with a PSA <4 ng/mL, it is necessary to have evidence that such measures ensure that enough cases will be detected within the "window of curability" to make them worthwhile and that the financial and emotional costs of overdiagnosis will not undermine other advances.[74]

An early study on the PSAV was one of men enrolled in a geriatric trial. Carter et al. concluded that in men with PSA values <4 ng/mL, a PSAV <0.75 μg/mL/year indicated absence of prostate cancer, and a PSAV >0.75 μg/mL/year indicated its presence.[72] In a work published 15 years later, Krejcarek et al. reported that in the undiagnosed patients they studied who had PSAV values <1.0 ng/mL/year, only 6% of those younger than 70 years with cT1c disease had high-grade cancer; however, they found that a median PSAV value of 2.71 ng/mL/year, age, and clinical T stage were significantly related to clinical significant disease (Gleason score 4 + 3).[75] Because these subjects had undergone radiotherapy, the findings were not generalizable to patients treated with other therapeutic modalities. The study by Krejcarek et al. was a retrospective evaluation in 358 men to identify those at higher risk, so they could improve outcomes by adding androgen-suppression therapy to radiotherapy and by improving the selection of radiotherapy fields.

A prospective trial conducted at the Royal Marsden Hospital and reported in 2008 studied 237 patients enrolled in an AS trial who had a median PSA level of 6.5 ng/mL at the outset and a median pretreatment PSAV of 0.44 ng/mL/year.[76] The investigators determined that PSA density was a statistically significant independent determinant of PSAV in untreated patients: those with a PSA density measure >0.185 ng/mL had a median PSAV of 0.92 ng/mL/year, and those with a PSA density measure <0.185 ng/mL had a median PSAV of 0.35 ng/mL/year. Because PSA density is a measure available at the outset of diagnosis and does not require longitudinal data collection, it will be a more efficient marker than PSAV is if others confirm this finding.

However, despite these data, a commentary by Vickers et al. questions the use of PSAV in prostate cancer early detection and management of clinically localized disease. The main arguments against PSAV clinical utility are that it does not add to established predictors of prostate cancer diagnosis, methodologic variability, and it being a poor prognosticator for mortality after conservative management and after prostatectomy.[77]

More recently, additional markers have been developed for patients with clinical suspicion of prostate cancer who are being considered for a prostate biopsy. These include prostate health index (PHI), 4K score, prostate cancer gene 3 (PCA3), select MDX, and confirm MDX.[78] These noninvasive tests are intended to predict the likelihood that the biopsy will reveal clinically significant disease [e.g., Gleason ≥7 (4 + 3)]. These tests may be especially salient in men with a negative DRE and/or initial negative biopsy who warrant continued monitoring.

Staging of prostate cancer

The initial staging of prostate cancer, which is integral to the treatment decisions that follow, comprises clinical results from digital palpation of the prostate, laboratory studies, imaging studies (which for patients at low and intermediate risk are sometimes omitted), and needle biopsy results. Physicians can combine the clinical stage as assessed by DRE with two other significant prognostic factors, the Gleason score and the preoperative PSA value, to classify the case according to the D'Amico system as low, intermediate, or high risk.[79] This system was first described in 1998 in the report of a retrospective study in which D'Amico et al. evaluated 1872 men with prostate cancer who had been treated with radical prostatectomy, external beam radiotherapy, or radioactive implant with or without neoadjuvant androgen-deprivation therapy. In that study, clinical staging was based on DRE findings alone (American Joint Committee on Cancer tumor stage).[80] The researchers found that with that system, men who had been classified as having low or intermediate-risk disease had outcomes that were not statistically significantly different from others within their subgroup. Most of this reliability is attributable to the Gleason score and the PSA level.

In the staging of prostate cancer, physicians rely on the tumor, node, and metastasis (TNM) system of the American Joint Committee on Cancer to classify cases (Table 3).[81] It reports the extent of the tumor(T), the presence or absence of disease in the regional lymph nodes (N), and the extent of metastasis (M). In a second step of the staging process, the Gleason Grade Group is combined with the TNM classification, and cases are identified as stage I, II, III, or IV, progressively representing advances in the extent of disease (Table 4).[80]

Prostate cancer is the most commonly diagnosed cancer in US men, with the exception of skin cancers and in situ cancers.[82] About

Table 3 TNM clinical and pathologic staging of prostate cancer.[a]

	Clinical stage		Pathologic stage
Primary tumor			
TX	Primary tumor cannot be assessed		
T0	No evidence of primary tumor		
T1	Clinically inapparent tumor neither palpable nor visible by imaging		
T1a	Tumor incidental histologic finding in 5% or less of tissue resected		
T1b	Tumor incidental histologic finding in more than 5% of tissue resected		
T1c	Tumor identified by needle biopsy (e.g., because of elevated PSA)		
T2	Tumor palpable and confined within prostate[b]	pT2	Organ confined
T2a	Tumor involves one half of one lobe or less	pT2a	Unilateral, involving one-half of one lobe or less
T2b	Tumor involves more than one-half of one lobe but not both lobes	pT2b[c]	Unilateral, involving more than one-half of one lobe but not both lobes
T2c	Tumor involves both lobes	pT2c	Bilateral disease
T3	Tumor extends through the prostate capsule[d]	pT3	Extraprostatic extension
T3a	Extracapsular extension (unilateral or bilateral)	pT3a[e]	Extraprostatic extension[e]
T3b	Tumor invades seminal vesicle(s)	pT3b	Seminal vesicle invasion
T4	Tumor is fixed or invades adjacent structures other than seminal vesicles: bladder neck, external sphincter, rectum, levator muscles, and/or pelvic wall	pT4	Invasion of bladder, rectum
Regional lymph nodes			
NX	Regional lymph nodes were not assessed	pNX	Regional nodes not sampled
N0	No regional lymph node metastasis	pN0	No positive regional nodes
N1	Metastasis in regional lymph node(s)	pN1	Metastasis in regional nodes
Distant metastasis			
MX	Distant metastasis cannot be assessed (not evaluated by any modality)		
M0	No distant metastasis		
M1	Distant metastasis[f]		
M1a	Nonregional lymph nodes		
M1b	Bone(s)		
M1c	Other site(s) with or without bone disease		

[a]Source: Edge.[81]
[b]Tumor found in one or both lobes by needle biopsy, but not palpable or reliably visible by imaging, is classified as T1c.
[c]There is no pathologic T1 classification.
[d]Invasion into the prostatic apex or into (but not beyond) the prostatic capsule is classified not as T3 but as T2.
[e]Positive surgical margin should be indicated by an R1 descriptor (residual microscopic disease).
[f]When more than one site of metastasis is present, the most advanced category (pM1c) is used.

Table 4 Prostate cancer stages.[a]

Group	T	N	M	PSA	Grade group
Stage 1	cT1a–c	N0	M0	PSA < 10	1
	cT2a	N0	M0	PSA < 10	1
	pT2	N0	M0	PSA < 10	1
Stage IIA	cT1a–c	N0	M0	PSA ≥ 10 < 2	1
	cT2a	N0	M0	0	1
	pT2	N0	M0	PSA ≥ 10 < 2	1
	cT2b	N0	M0	0	1
	cT2c	N0	M0	PSA ≥ 10 < 20	1
				PSA < 20	
				PSA < 20	
Stage IIB	T1–2	N0	M0	PSA < 20	2
Stage IIC	T1–2	N0	M0	PSA < 20	3
	T1–2	N0	M0	PSA < 20	4
Stage IIIA	T1–2	N0	M0	PSA ≥ 20	1–4
Stage IIIB	T3–4	N0	M0	Any PSA	1–4
Stage IIIC	Any T	N0	M0	Any PSA	5
Stage IVA	Any T	N1	M0	Any PSA	Any
Stage IVB	Any T	Any N	M1	Any PSA	Any

[a]Source: NCCN Guidelines Version 2.2020.

Table 5 Risk stratification for localized prostate cancer.[a]

Risk level	PSA level (ng/mL)		Gleason score		Clinical stage
Low	≤10	and	≤6	and	T1c or T2a
Intermediate	>10–20	or	7	or	T2b but not qualifying for high risk
High	>20	or	8–10	or	T2c

[a]Source: Thompson et al.[84]

Historically, the American Urological Association has characterized localized disease into three risk categories (Table 5).[84] Low-risk disease is generally characterized by a PSA value ≤ 10 ng/mL, a Gleason score ≤ 6, a lack of symptoms, and absence of both diseases in the lymph nodes and metastases (i.e., clinical stage T1c or T2). Disease is nonpalpable on DRE, but evidence of tumor may be detected by a transurethral resection of the prostate (TURP) performed because of what was thought to be BPH or by needle biopsy prompted by a high PSA level. PSA values >10 ng/mL but ≤20 ng/mL and/or a Gleason score of 7 (3 + 4 or 4 + 3) are associated with intermediate risk. PSA values >20 ng/mL and/or Gleason scores of 8–10 indicate high-risk cases.

Following the recent introduction of the grade group system to complement Gleason score, the NCCN has proposed a more contemporary risk stratification for localized disease (Table 6).

Staging is meant to refine the risk of oncologic end points and can be augmented with commercialized genomic prognostic biomarkers taken from biopsy specimens. Cuzick et al. reported a panel of cell cycle progression (CCP) genes known from breast cancer studies and validated them in a cohort of patients managed

3/4 of US men report having been screened at least once, and early prostate cancer, because it has no symptoms, is often diagnosed in outpatient settings. Distinguishing between clinically insignificant and potentially lethal variations of localized prostate cancer, maximizing disease control and survival, and avoiding overtreatment, especially in men likely to die of other comorbidities, are challenges physicians who treat these men face daily.[83]

Table 6 Contemporary risk stratification for localized prostate cancer.[a]

Risk group	Clinical/pathologic features			
Very low	Has all of the following: • T1c • Grade group 1 • PSA < 10 ng/mL • Fewer than 3 prostate biopsy fragments/cores positive, ≤50% cancer in each fragment/core • PSA density < 0.15 ng/mL/g			
Low	Has all the following but does not qualify for very low risk: • T1–T2a • Grade Group 1 • PSA < 10 ng/mL			

Intermediate	Has all of the following:
	• No high-risk group features
	• No very-high-risk group features
	• Has one or more intermediate risk factors (IRF):
	  ○ T2b–T2c
	  ○ Grade Group 2 or 3
	  ○ PSA 10–20 ng/mL
		Favorable
		Intermediate
		
		Unfavorable
		Intermediate
				Has all of the following:
				• 1 RF
				• Grade Group 1 or 2
				• <50% biopsy cores positive
				Has one or more of the following:
				• 2 or 3 IRFs
				• Grade Group 3
				• ≥50% biopsy cores positive

High	Has no very-high-risk-feature and has at least one high-risk feature: • T2a OR • Grade Group 4 or Grade Group 5 OR • PSA >20 ng/mL			
Very high	Has at least one of the following: • T3b–T4 • Primary Gleason pattern 5 • 2 or 3 high-risk features • >4 cores with Grade Group 4 or 5			

[a]Source: NCCN Guidelines Version 2.2020.

conservatively.[85] The CCP score, a numerical representation of average CCP gene expression compared to a housekeeping gene panel, was statistically superior in predicting 10-year mortality rates compared to clinical features. Another panel of genes was validated by Klein et al. that mixed several pathways (stromal response, androgen signaling, proliferation, and organization) and linked elements in a small sample of a prostate biopsy with long-term radical prostatectomy outcomes.[86] The development and validation efforts have created a genomic score that estimates adverse pathology (Gleason ≥ 4 + 3 and/or pT3 stage) at radical prostatectomy, from patients with favorable biopsy findings (Gleason 3 + 3 to 3 + 4). Both biomarkers have strong statistical validation but need additional studies on clinical utility impact such as changing recommendations between active surveillance (AS) and immediate treatment and correlating such decisions with superior oncologic and quality-of-life outcomes.

The theme of disease prognosis from genomics can continue into the postradical prostatectomy space, with CCP score in this setting predicting for biochemical recurrence rates along with clinical features, and another genomic classifier (commercialized as Decipher, GenomeDx, San Diego, CA) specifically estimates early metastatic progression from patients with known high-risk pathology. Table 7 compares key clinical end points, clinical utility, and cost.

Imaging of prostate cancer

Although bone and CT scans remain standard to establish metastatic disease, imaging approaches are rapidly evolving and herein we describe incorporation of "state of the art" imaging modalities including MRI and PET imaging into the evaluation and treatment of prostate cancer across different disease states.

Initial staging

Primary tumor

The imaging modality of choice for prostate carcinoma is multiparametric magnetic resonance imaging (mpMRI) which combines anatomical imaging using T1-weighted and T2-weighted sequences along with one or more functional imaging methods like diffusion-weighted images (DWI) or dynamic contrast-enhanced (DCE) imaging. It is usually performed and reported as per the prostate imaging reporting and data system (PIRADS) standard which was designed to standardize image acquisition techniques and interpretation of prostate MRI and thereby improve detection, localization, characterization, and risk stratification in patients with suspected cancer in treatment naïve prostate glands. The current version is termed PI-RADS v 2.1 which uses a five-point scale from 1 to 5 (1—very low; 2—low; 3—intermediate; 4—high; 5—very high) based on the probability that a combination of mpMRI findings on T2, DWI, and DCE correlates with the presence of a clinically significant cancer for each lesion in the prostate gland.[88]

The role of MR imaging has evolved from staging patients with biopsy-proven prostate cancer to detecting, characterizing, and guiding the biopsy of suspected prostate cancer. The PROMIS trial (diagnostic accuracy of mpMRI and TRUS biopsy in prostate cancer) was a multicenter trial in which patients underwent mpMRI followed by both TRUS-biopsy (standard test) and template prostate mapping biopsy (reference test). This study showed that mpMRI has significantly better sensitivity and negative predictive value for clinically important prostate cancer compared with TRUS-biopsy enabling mpMRI to be used as a triage test before first biopsy to allow one-quarter of men at risk to avoid biopsy.[89]

A multicenter randomized trial (PRECISION) suggested the use of risk assessment with MRI prebiopsy detecting clinically significant cancer in 38% of patients in the MRI-targeted biopsy group as compared 26% in the standard transrectal ultrasonography-guided biopsy group in men at clinical risk for prostate cancer who had not undergone biopsy previously.[90] However, MRI-fusion biopsy can also miss clinically significant prostate cancer as demonstrated by the MRI-FIRST study.[91] A meta-analysis determining the predictive factors of missed clinically significant prostate cancer with negative MRI concluded that a PSA density less than 0.15 ng/mL/mL was the most useful factor in identifying men without clinically significant prostate cancer who could avoid biopsy.[92] In men with a previously negative biopsy and rising PSA levels, if a repeat biopsy is recommended and there is availability of a high-quality MRI examination and interpretation, prostate MRI and subsequent MRI targeted cores facilitate the detection of clinically significant disease over standardized repeat biopsy.[93] The role of MRI in AS is well accepted as stable findings on mp-MRI are associated with Gleason score stability and MRI findings provide additional useful information to existing clinicopathologic scoring systems of prostate cancer to guide treatment decisions.[94-96]

Locoregional staging performed using mpMRI includes assessment of extraprostatic extension (EPE) and seminal vesicle invasion (SVI) (Figure 6). Overall staging accuracy of mpMRI for EPE was 73.8%, with sensitivity, specificity, positive predictive value, and negative predictive value of 58.2%, 89.1%, 84.1%, and 68.3%, respectively.[97] MRI has a high sensitivity and specificity of 83% and 99%, respectively, for detecting SVI.[98] Though there still exists variation in study acquisition, image quality, and radiologists' interpretation based on their experience, prostate MRI has undergone tremendous improvements in the last decade and an increasing number of urological practices are incorporating prostate MRI into routine clinical care.

Table 7 Comparison of key features of three commercialized genomic tests for prostate cancer.[a]

	Decipher	Oncotype DX	Prolaris
Tissues tested	RP for high risk—pT3, positive margin, PSA rise	Biopsy—for NCCN very low to intermediate risk	Biopsy or RP
Clinical end points	Early regional nodes or bone metastasis	Risk of unfavorable pathology—pT3 and/or ≥Gleason 4 + 3	Biopsy—10-year mortality with conservative management
			RP—biochemical recurrence risk
Clinical utility	Adjuvant/salvage therapy	Active surveillance or immediate therapy	Biopsy—active surveillance or immediate therapy
			RP—adjuvant/salvage therapy

Abbreviations: RP, radical prostatectomy; pT3, pathologic stage with extraprostatic extension and/or seminal vesicle invasion; PSA, prostate-specific antigen; NCCN, National Comprehensive Cancer Network; USD, United States Dollar equivalent.
[a] Source: Davis.[87]

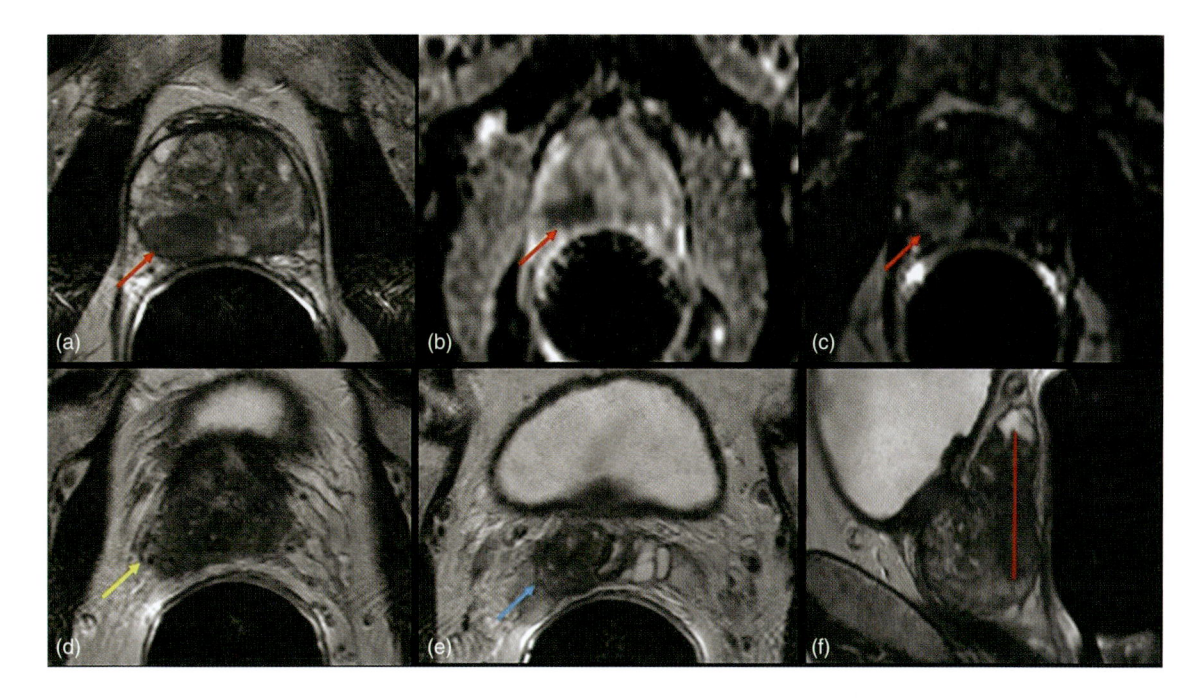

Figure 6 65-Year-old male with adenocarcinoma of prostate. Axial T2 weighted image (a) demonstrates a PIRADS 5 dominant lesion in the right peripheral zone (red arrow) extending from the apex to base with corresponding restricted diffusion on the axial apparent diffusion coefficient map from diffusion-weighted image (b) and enhancement on the axial dynamic contrast-enhanced image (c). Axial T2 weighted image (d) at the level of the right posterolateral base demonstrates extracapsular extension and neurovascular bundle involvement (yellow arrow). Axial T2 weighted image (e) shows involvement of the right seminal vesicle (blue arrow). Sagittal T2 weighted image (f) demonstrates the entire extent of the lesion from apex to base with involvement of right seminal vesicle (red line).

Lymph node evaluation
Surgical lymph node dissection with histopathologic examination is the traditional way of determining nodal metastases. However, it is invasive and there is a risk of missing nodes outside the normal resection template. In patients with intermediate and high-risk prostate cancer with a predicted risk of >10% lymph node involvement, the National Comprehensive Cancer Network (NCCN) guidelines recommend pelvic imaging with or without abdominal imaging. CT and MRI have been commonly used; however, they often underestimate nodal involvement as they are based on size thresholds. Among 4264 patients who underwent CT and pelvic dissection, CT detected disease in only 2.5% of the patients while 15.3% of the patients had pathologically proved lymphadenopathy. Median estimated CT sensitivity, specificity, negative predictive value, and positive predictive value were 7%, 100%, 85%, and 100%, respectively.[99] The pooled sensitivity and specificity were 42% and 82% for CT and 39% and 82% for MRI demonstrating an equally poor performance in detecting nodal disease from prostate cancer in a meta-analysis including 24 studies.[100] Though MRI is better than CT by allowing for better node characterization, it is still limited.

Molecular imaging using positron emission tomography (PET) is being used increasingly with the development of agents specific for prostate cancer imaging. The well-established radiotracer, ^{18}F-FDG (fluorodeoxyglucose), has not proven useful for prostate cancer until late in the course of the disease.[101] The prostate-specific membrane antigen (PSMA) is overexpressed in more aggressive prostate cancers and has therefore become a popular target. Multiple prostate cancer-specific PET tracers have been developed and tested. The PET agents are particularly used to assess early biochemical recurrence and metastatic disease; however, the utility of PSMA PET tracers in the initial staging of high-risk prostate cancer is promising. The proPSMA trial is a prospective, multicenter study in which patients with untreated high-risk prostate cancer were randomized to gallium-68-PSMA-11 PET/CT versus conventional imaging, consisting of CT of the abdomen/pelvis and bone scintigraphy.[102] PSMA PET-CT had a 27% greater accuracy than that of conventional imaging with consequent management changes and fewer equivocal results. Though not widely used, the utility of Ga-68 PSMA PET/CT has been studied for primary lymph node staging. In a prospective study, patient-based analysis showed that the sensitivity and specificity for detecting nodal metastases were 39% and 100% with ^{68}Ga-PSMA PET/CT, 8% and 100% with MRI/CT, and 36% and 83% with DW-MRI, respectively.[103]

Most of the available literature on PSMA PET is on PET/CT; however, there is significant interest in the simultaneous acquisition of PET/MRI in prostate cancer. In primary tumors, the pooled sensitivity of PET/MRI for the patient-based analysis was 94.9% and the pooled detection rate at restaging was 80.9%.[104] ^{68}Ga-PSMA-11 PET/MRI improves diagnostic accuracy for cancer localization in the prostate when compared with multiparametric MRI.[105–107] PSMA PET/MRI combines the high-resolution anatomical and the metabolic information serving as a "single stop" imaging which increases patient convenience. Another benefit of PET/MRI is the increased PET acquisition time which acquiring MRI sequences concurrently that are typically time limiting. This can result in increased rates of nodal detection.[108]

Bone evaluation
Evaluation for osseous metastases is usually performed using Technetium 99m-Methyl Diphosphonate Bone scan (Tc-99mMDP) with or without single-photon emission computed tomography (SPECT). Detection of metastases on bone scan is based on PSA

levels. In a systematic review including 23 studies, bone scan metastases were detected in 2.3%, 5.3%, and 16.2% of patients with PSA levels less than 10, 10.1–19.9, and 20–49.9 ng/mL, respectively with detection rates as high as 30% in men with Gleason score ≥8 prostate cancer.[99] Fluorine 18-Sodium fluoride Positron Emission Tomography (F-18 NaF PET/CT) can also be performed, but it is not commonly used due to reimbursement issues. In comparison to Tc-99m MDP, F-18 NaF has two-fold higher bone uptake, decreased uptake time, faster blood clearance, higher target to background ratio, superior spatial resolution, and higher specificity leading to its higher accuracy.[109–112]

The diagnostic performance of ^{68}Ga-PSMA PET compared to ^{99m}Tc-MDP Bone scan for the detection of osseous metastases in a mixed cohort of patients with initial diagnosis, recurrent disease, and advanced mCRPC was performed in a retrospective study of 126 patients by Pyka et al.[113] Patient-based sensitivities and specificities were 98.7–100% and 88.2–100%, respectively, for PSMA PET and 86.7–89.3% and 60.8–96.1%, respectively, for bone scans. In the subgroup analysis, PSMA PET outperformed BS specifically in the primary staging cohort (sensitivity, 100% vs 57.1%)

Imaging of biochemical recurrence

Though biochemical recurrence is not consistent with the presence of clinical disease, it provides an opportunity for early initiation of salvage therapy. Imaging plays an important role in assessing for the presence and distribution of recurrent disease which in turn has profound implications in the treatment decision-making process. The most common site of local recurrence after radical prostatectomy is the vesicourethral anastomosis and precise localization of recurrent disease is a key factor in treatment planning. mpMRI is the most widely used imaging technique for the detection of local recurrence after definitive therapy. A meta-analysis assessing the performance of mpMRI for the detection of local recurrence demonstrated pooled sensitivities and specificities of 82% and 87%, respectively after radical prostatectomy and 82% and 74%, respectively after radiation therapy.[114]

Posttreatment changes cause distortion of anatomy and MRI may be limited due to artifacts associated with radiation therapy seeds. PET imaging can also play a significant role in detecting disease. Various PET agents are available that depend on the biology of choline, upregulation of amino acid transport, and expression of PSMA. Other emerging PET radiotracers include the bombesin group targeting the gastrin-releasing peptide receptor (GRPR), and ^{18}F-fluoro-5α-dihydrotestosterone (^{18}F-FDHT) that binds to AR. Of these, Choline, Fluciclovine, and PMSA were FDA approved in 2012, 2016, and 2020 respectively in the setting of biochemical recurrence.

Imaging with either ^{11}C- or ^{18}F-labeled choline is based on an increased uptake and turnover of phosphatidylcholine in cancer cells, which is an essential part of the phospholipids in the cellular membrane.[115] A meta-analysis evaluating the diagnostic performance of ^{18}F-choline and ^{11}C-choline PET or PET/CT in detection of locoregional or distant metastases in prostate cancer provided a pooled sensitivity of 85.6% (95% CI: 82.9–88.1%) and pooled specificity of 92.6% (95% CI: 90.1–94.6%) for all sites of disease (prostatic fossa, lymph nodes, and bone).[116] In a study of 358 patients with biochemical recurrence evaluated with ^{11}C-choline PET/CT, the percentage of positive disease at PET/CT increased with increasing PSA level, with a positive disease percentage of 19% in those with PSA level of 0.2–1 ng/mL, 46% in those with PSA level of 1–3 ng/mL, and 82% in those with PSA level higher than 3 ng/mL.[117] Limitations of Choline tracers include short half-life of C11, need for an onsite cyclotron, nonspecific prostate uptake, and overall low sensitivity in comparison to other tracers.

FACBC (*anti*-1-amino-3-^{18}F-fluorocyclobutane-1-carboxylic acid) also known as Fluciclovine (Axumin), is an analog of L-leucine that is transported into the cell by upregulated cell membrane amino acid transporters (LAT1 and ASCT2).[118] This was FDA approved for detection of biochemical recurrence of prostate cancer in 2016. A multicenter prospective, multicenter (LOCATE) trial reported that ^{18}F-fluciclovine PET/CT tumor detection was broadly proportional to the prescan PSA, detecting lesions in 31%, 50%, 66%, and 84% of patients, with PSA 0–0.5 ng/mL, >0.5–1.0 ng/mL, PSA > 1.0–2.0 ng/mL, and >2.0 ng/mL, respectively, in a per-patient basis. This study also assessed the impact of ^{18}F-fluciclovine on management plans for patients with BCR prostate cancer after curative-intent primary therapy. Overall, 59% of the patients had a change in management after the scan, with 78% of these being major changes, that is, change from salvage or noncurative systemic therapy to watchful waiting (25%), or from noncurative systemic therapy to salvage therapy (24%) or from salvage therapy to noncurative systemic therapy (9%).[119] Figure 7 shows a case of biochemical recurrence after prostatectomy.

PSMA also known as glutamate carboxypeptidase II or folate hydrolase I is a type II transmembrane glycoprotein with an extensive extracellular domain providing an excellent target for imaging, a transmembrane domain, and an intracellular domain. PSMA expression is 100–1000-fold higher in prostate cancer than in other tissues. Radiolabeled small molecules that bind to the extracellular domain have emerged as a new diagnostic standard for prostate cancer, resulting in images with high tumor-to-background contrast.[120] It should be noted that despite the term "prostate specific", PSMA is expressed in a range of normal tissues and in other benign and nonprostate malignant processes. Thus, a good knowledge of its physiologic distribution and other causes of uptake is vital to minimize false-positive imaging findings. The most widely used PSMA compound in clinical studies (PSMA-HBED-CC) is labeled with ^{68}Ga and is known as ^{68}Ga-PSMA-11. PSMA can be labeled with other tracers like ^{68}Ga, ^{18}F, ^{111}In, and ^{99m}Tc, such as ^{18}F-DCFBC/^{18}F-DCFPyL, ^{18}F-PSMA-1007, ^{18}F-rhPSMA, ^{68}Ga/^{111}In-PSMA-617, or 123I-MIP-1095 among others.[121]

The meta-analysis of ^{68}Ga-PSMA-11 at initial staging demonstrated a sensitivity and specificity of 74% and 96% respectively, using nodal pathology at prostatectomy as a gold standard. At biochemical recurrence, the PPV was 99%. The detection rate was 63% with a PSA of less than 2.0 and 94% with a PSA of more than 2.0.[122] However, PSMA is not yet FDA approved in the United States. A prospective head-to-head comparative imaging trial between ^{18}F-fluciclovine PET-CT and ^{68}Ga-PSMA-11 PET-CT for localizing BCR after radical prostatectomy in patients with PSA ≤ 2.0 ng/mL showed detection rates were significantly lower with ^{18}F-fluciclovine PET-CT than with PSMA PET-CT with an odds ratio (OR) of 4.8 (95% CI 1.6–19.2; $p = 0.0026$) at the patient level.[123] Another head to head comparison study comparing the two tracers showed better detection of local recurrence on Fluciclovine which is attributed to the negligible urinary activity of Fluciclovine.[124]

Imaging of mCRPC

Most patients with mCRPC develop bone metastases. A few studies have shown that the semiquantitative FDG PET parameters and number of bone lesions contribute independent prognostic information on OS in men with mCRPC.[125,126]

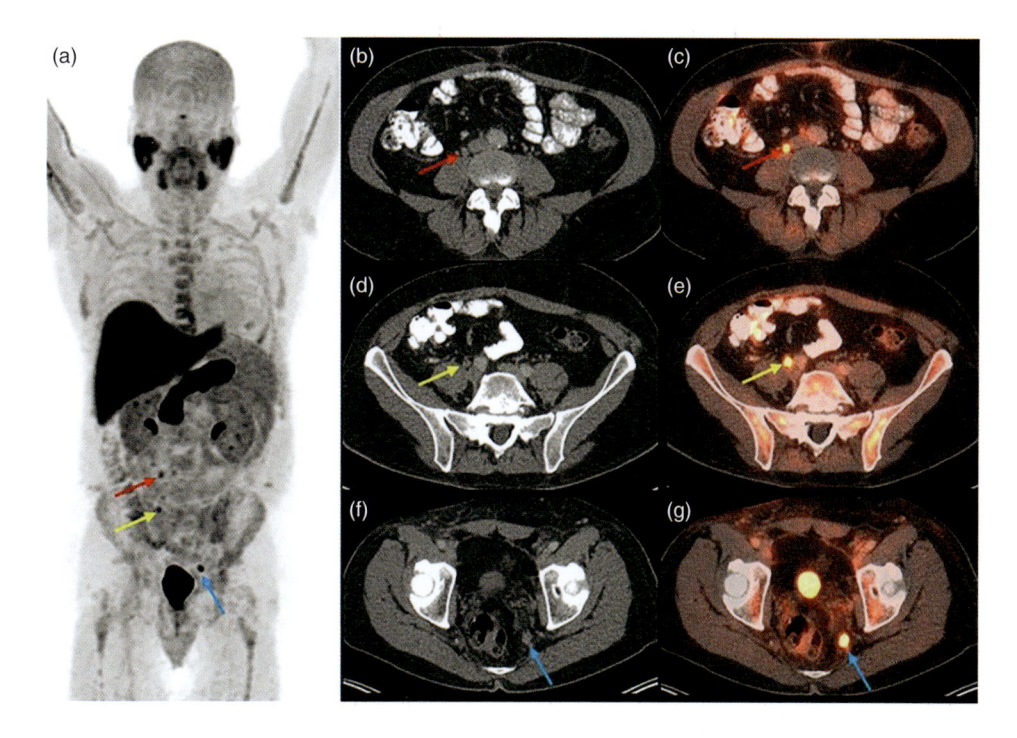

Figure 7 54-Year-old male with Gleason 9 (5 + 4) prostate adenocarcinoma status-post radical prostatectomy presenting with PSA of 3.9 ng/mL. ^{18}F-Fluciclovine Maximum intensity projection image (a) shows the typical distribution of Fluciclovine with multiple avid retroperitoneal and pelvic lymph node metastases. Axial CT (b) and Axial fused PET/CT (c) images show a right paracaval node (red arrow) with SUV 5.4. Axial CT (d) and Axial fused PET/CT (e) images show a right common iliac node (yellow arrow) with SUV 6.6. Axial CT (f) and Axial fused PET/CT (g) images show a left mesorectal node (blue arrow) with SUV 8.2.

Theranostics

PSMA is an excellent target not only for diagnostic imaging but also for therapy of prostate cancer. High expression in tumors, suitable binding affinity, and internalization of PSMA ligands allows selection of patients who may benefit from lutetium 177 (177Lu)–labeled PSMA peptide receptor radionuclide therapy (PRRT) in mCRPC. A meta-analysis on the therapeutic effects of 177Lu-PSMA-617 in patients with mCRPC included 10 eligible studies with 455 patients and showed that approximately two-thirds of any PSA decline and one-third of a greater than 50% PSA decline can be expected after the first cycle of 177Lu-PSMA-617 radioligand therapy in patients with mCRPC. Moreover, any PSA decline showed survival prolongation after the first cycle of the 177Lu-PSMA-617 radioligand therapy.[127]

TheraP is a randomized phase II trial comparing 177Lu-PSMA versus cabazitaxel in men with mCRPC progressing after docetaxel using both FDG and PSMA PET imaging.[128] The initial results showed that PSA response rate (defined by ≥ 50% reduction) is higher in LuPSMA group than cabazitaxel with relatively fewer Grade 3–4 adverse events and PSA–PFS (progression-free survival) favoring LuPSMA (ASCO 2020). The efficacy of PSMA radioligand therapy is currently being evaluated in an ongoing phase III VISION trial (ClinicalTrials.gov identifier NCT03511664) which will evaluate the outcomes of patients with mCRPC treated with 177Lu-PSMA-617 compared with the best standard care.[129]

Prevention of prostate cancer

The PCPT involved 18,882 men randomized to treatment with finasteride (a selective inhibitor of type 2 5α-reductase) or placebo.[130] PCPT ended more than a year earlier than planned because its Data Safety and Monitoring Committee determined that the trial had met its primary objective. Prostate cancer prevalence during the 7-year treatment period was 24.8% lower in men taking finasteride than in men taking placebo (95% CI 18.6–30.6; $P < 0.001$). This good news was tempered, however, by the finding that tumors detected in those taking finasteride were 1.67 times more likely to be of a higher grade (Gleason score 7–10) than were those in subjects taking placebo (37.0% of graded tumors vs 22.2%; $P < 0.001$).

Subsequent studies of the PCPT data eased concerns that finasteride caused more aggressive cancers in the treated group. However, the use of finasteride as a preventative agent is not widely in use in clinical practice, in part because after 18 years of follow-up, there was no significant between-group difference in the rates of OS or survival after the diagnosis of prostate cancer.[131] Studies of dutasteride (a selective inhibitor of both type 1 and type 2 5α-reductase) are ongoing but preliminary results from a placebo-controlled study suggest it can reduce the risk of incident prostate cancer detected on biopsy prostate cancer among men who are at increased risk for the disease. Eligible patients were men 50–75 years of age with a PSA level of 2.5–10.0 ng/mL, and who had one negative prostate biopsy (6–12 cores) within 6 months before enrollment. Men received dutasteride (0.5 mg daily) versus placebo and underwent a 10-core transrectal ultrasound-guided biopsy at 2 and 4 years. Among 6729 men who underwent a biopsy or prostate surgery, cancer was detected in 659 of the 3305 men in the dutasteride group, as compared with 858 of the 3424 men in the placebo group, representing a relative risk reduction with dutasteride of 22.8% (95% confidence interval, 15.2–29.8) over the 4-year study period ($P < 0.001$).[132]

Another important NCI-supported chemopreventive randomized, placebo-controlled trial is called Selenium and Vitamin E Cancer Prevention Trial (SELECT). The study evaluated the effects of selenium and vitamin E, separately and combined, against those of placebo in preventing prostate cancer.[133] Paradoxically, the investigators reported a statistically nonsignificant increase in prostate cancer risk in the vitamin E alone group in their first report, which became significant with longer follow-up and more prostate cancer events.[134,135] The serial collection of biospecimens from all SELECT study participants will enable the construction of risk models to help determine which men are most likely to develop prostate cancer and to help identify those most likely to benefit from selenium and vitamin E chemopreventive therapy.

Putative chemopreventive agents other than finasteride that have been studied include celecoxib, sulindac, toremifene, soy isoflavones, lycopene, and doxercalciferol. Additionally, novel preventive strategies such as immunotherapy and mechanistically based drug combinations are being explored.[136] Currently under way are molecular epidemiologic studies of diet and prostate cancer risk as well as basic research into the carcinogenicity of specific diet-derived compounds such as heterocyclic amines. Statins have also been of previous interest, with studies showing long-term use of lipid-lowering medications conferring a potentially lower risk of prostate cancer and a recent study showing significantly lower risk of PTEN-null prostate cancers with enrichment of immune pathways in normal tissue of men on statins.[137,138]

Therapy options for localized prostate cancer

Active surveillance (AS)
In the pre-PSA era, "watchful waiting" implied an alternative to active treatment and described a period when patients were monitored but not treated until the disease progressed and/or symptoms developed. With the advent of PSA testing, a paradigm shift occurred, in which we now diagnose considerably more early prostate cancers, including those destined to remain clinically insignificant. New strategies are needed for managing select cases of low-risk prostate cancer without imposing immediate therapy. Such an approach has been called different terms, including "watchful observation with selective delayed intervention" and "active surveillance."[139,140] This new strategy foregoes immediate treatment but closely follows patients with low-risk prostate cancer, pursuing early detection of tumor progression when the disease is still curable and initiating definitive therapy appropriately. For this strategy to fulfill its promise, two clinical tools are mandatory: a method of identifying a priori patients harboring small low-grade, indolent tumors and a surveillance strategy that reliably detects tumor progression when the disease is still curable.

Data supporting conservative management of cases with clinically localized prostate cancer can be gleaned from population-based studies and a meta-analysis.[141–143] These pre-PSA era studies had a preponderance of older patients and patients with clinically evident cancers; therefore, their results cannot be directly extrapolated to the PSA-screened population. Other problems included the way patients had been diagnosed—many had not undergone a full workup for metastasis, and for many, diagnosis was based on fine-needle biopsy results and the fact that the researchers did not centralize pathology review.[141,142] Despite their limitations, these observational studies showed that men with low-grade prostate cancer have a protracted course of indolent disease and a very small risk of disease-specific death, even after 20 years of follow-up.[144]

In contrast, the risk of death from disease progression is higher for men with Gleason scores of 7–10. Watchful waiting and prostatectomy were compared prospectively in an important study by Swedish investigators who followed up their initial report with further analyses 3 years later and an estimated 15-year results.[145–147] The researchers studied 695 men with T0d, T1b, T1c, or T2 disease who were randomly assigned to undergo radical prostatectomy ($n = 347$) or watchful waiting ($n = 348$). Two-thirds had palpable tumors, but fewer than half in each group—43.8% of those undergoing prostatectomy and 39.7% of those assigned to watchful waiting—had symptoms. In the recently reported extended 23.2 years of follow-up analysis, the investigators observed statistically significant differences at 18 years of follow-up between those who underwent prostatectomy and those in watchful waiting including use of androgen deprivation therapy [42.5% vs 67.4%, RR 0.49 (95% CI 0.39–0.60; $P < 0.001$)], development of distant metastasis [26% vs 38.3%, RR 0.57 (95% CI 0.44–0.75; $P < 0.001$)], and disease-specific mortality [17.7% vs 28.7%, RR 0.56 (95% CI 0.41–0.77; $P = 0.001$)].[148]

The benefit from prostatectomy was confined to men younger than 65 years of age. Also, it is important to note that a large proportion of men in the watchful waiting arm did not require any palliative treatment. Whether these findings would be replicable in a US study population is unknown because prostate cancer is typically diagnosed earlier here than it is in Sweden. The Prostate Cancer Intervention versus Observation Trial conducted in the United States compared prostatectomy with watchful waiting in 731 of mostly screened men with localized prostate cancer and life expectancy of at least 10 years.[149] At median follow-up of 10 years, there was no significant statistical difference in all-cause mortality and prostate cancer-specific mortality between the two groups. There was a trend toward lower prostate cancer-specific mortality with surgery among men with PSA levels >10 ng/mL and subgroups with higher-risk cancers. In fact, for men with low-risk prostate cancer, there was nonstatistically significant increase in prostate cancer-specific mortality by 15%.

Two of the longest-running prospective cohort studies have examined the feasibility of AS, or expectant management. Additionally, there are other large cohort prospective studies underway.[150] Carter et al. studied 81 men believed to have T1c low-volume prostate cancer for a median of 23 months (range 12–58 months).[151] Their median age was 65 years (range 52–73 years). At baseline, all men had a PSA density ≤0.15 ng/mL/cm^3 and a Gleason score of <7. Free PSA in the men was a median of 17% (range 4.3–37%). Every 6 months, subjects underwent PSA measurement (both free and total) and DRE. Every 12 months, patients underwent transrectal ultrasound-directed biopsy, including evaluation of at least 12 cores. After at least 1 year in the study, 56 (69%) of the men were free of progression and still on surveillance. The other 25 men (31%) met the criteria of progression, which were adverse findings on prostate needle biopsy, including a Gleason score ≥ 7, any Gleason pattern of 4 or 5, more than two cores with cancer involvement, or 50% cancer involvement in any core. Their median time to disease progression was 14 months (range 12–52 months). The researchers found that in men who experienced progression by their definition, the PSA density was statistically significantly higher and the free PSA value statistically significantly lower than those values in men who did not experience progression.

In a larger phase II study, Klotz reported findings on 299 men who at baseline had prostate cancer of grade T2b or lower, a PSA of <15 ng/mL, and a Gleason score ≤ 7.[152] All subjects were older than 70 years. Surveillance included PSA measures, serial bone scans, transrectal sonography (every 6 months for first 2 years and then annually thereafter), and biopsy within 1.5 or 2 years of entering the trial. Criteria for progression were that patients demonstrate PSA, clinical, and histologic disease progression. PSA progression was defined as having a PSA doubling time of <2 years (measured at least three times during a minimum of 6 months), a final PSA of >8 ng/mL, and a regression analysis of ln (PSA) on time $P < 0.05$. Clinical progression was defined as one of the following: doubling of the product of the maximum perpendicular diameters of the primary lesion (measured digitally), TURP necessitated by local progression, ureteral obstruction, or clinical or radiologic evidence of distant metastasis. Histologic progression was defined as a Gleason score ≥ 8 at subsequent biopsy. At 55 months, 60% remained on surveillance; at 96 months, disease-specific survival was 99%, and OS was 85%. Thirty-five percent had a PSA doubling time of >10 years (median doubling time 7.0 years). Reasons for abandoning surveillance included patient preference (16%), rapid biochemical progression (12%), clinical progression (8%), and histologic progression (4%). In a recently published update of the study with the median follow-up time of 6.4 years from the first biopsy (range 0.2–19.8 years), Klotz et al. reported the prostate cancer-specific mortality in AS of 1.5%.[153] The risk of dying of another cause was 9.2 times greater than the likelihood of dying from prostate cancer. As AS methods move toward integration of novel imaging and biomarkers, investigators are challenged with including more men with early prostate cancer, minimizing risk of cancer progression, and maximizing quality of life.

The Prostate Testing for Cancer and Treatment (ProtecT) compared AS, radical prostatectomy, and external-beam radiotherapy for the treatment of clinically localized prostate cancer.[154] Between 1999 and 2009, a total of 82,429 men 50–69 years of age received a PSA test; 2664 received a diagnosis of localized prostate cancer, and 1643 agreed to undergo randomization to active monitoring (545 men), surgery (553), or radiotherapy (545). At a median of 10 years, prostate-cancer-specific mortality was low irrespective of the treatment assigned, with no significant difference among treatments. Surgery and radiotherapy were associated with lower incidences of disease progression (8.9 events per 1000 person-years versus 9.0 events versus 22.9 events, respectively) and metastases (2.4 events per 1000 person-years vs 3.0 events vs 6.3 events, respectively) than was active monitoring. Results from this trial should help physicians and patients collaborate better in decision-making for localized disease detected through PSA screening.[155]

Curative therapy for localized disease: a discussion of the challenges of disease control and minimizing side effects

The patient with early disease has the option to pursue one of a number of definitive therapeutic options, each with its own variations in technique. Fundamentally, the options include a radical prostatectomy or dose-escalated radiation therapy. Both treatment categories aim to treat the entire gland by surgical removal or radiation-based destruction. Alternative treatments have also emerged, such as cryotherapy and high-intensity focused ultrasound, that treat all or a portion of the gland. All treatments are associated with a risk of disease recurrence and varying degrees of quality-of-life side effects specific to prostate cancer treatments including erectile dysfunction, urinary incontinence, urinary irritation and/or obstruction, and bowel dysfunction. The desire to diminish side effects and disease recurrence has left the field with numerous updates in technique, entirely new technologies, and numerous comparisons. For each question involving treatment efficacy and side effects, the patient and practitioner want to know both the average results expected and any contributing features that help predict whether an individual patient will experience the favorable or unfavorable end of the range of results. In addition, studies have shed light on whether a particular procedure is reproducible across the range of treatment centers.[156–158] Most patients diagnosed today are very much aware of the potential for side effects and the concept that a practitioner's experience may affect outcomes.

The selection of patients for treatment is often derived by considering the slow natural history of prostate cancer, the life expectancy of the aging man, and the personal wishes of the patient. The most commonly accepted recommendation is that a patient may benefit from treatment if he has 10 or more years of life expectancy. However, this estimation may be a moving target because death from cardiac disease is declining with better treatments. Men should not be denied treatment on the basis of age alone, but the study by Albertsen et al. demonstrated significantly reduced prostate cancer-related death when the disease was diagnosed at age 70 and higher, especially for men with Gleason scores <7.[142,159] The recent update of the Bill-Axelson study that randomized radical prostatectomy and watchful waiting has been highly beneficial in decision-making.[148] The majority of survival benefit in the radical prostatectomy cohort was observed in men < age 65. However, men ages 65–75 had secondary benefits in reduced hormonal therapy, palliative therapy, and metastatic progression.

Anatomy of the prostate gland: a model for the treatment dilemmas concerning surgical and radiation therapy approaches for localized prostate cancer

The challenges of treating early prostate cancer can be illustrated by an anatomic tour of a radical prostatectomy operation and by using the steps of the operation to highlight what the surgeon and radiation oncologist must consider in achieving cancer control with minimal side effects. Refer to Figure 8 as we narrate our way through the intricate anatomy surrounding the prostate gland.

The radical prostatectomy operation involves complete removal of the prostate gland, seminal vesicles, and distal vas deferens. Conceptually, the prostate gland can be thought of as a conical structure with open ends—the bladder neck and the urethra. The sides of the cone have a capsular structure (although not a true histologic capsule) and are surrounded by endopelvic fascia laterally and by Denonvilliers fascia posteriorly. At its apex, the prostate is surrounded by the rhabdosphincter muscle and the dorsal vein complex, which is narrow over the urethra and then spreads into an apron-like structure as it traverses over the midprostate, base of the prostate, and then over the bladder. Regardless of approach and technique, the removal of the prostate requires an intimate understanding of the intricate anatomic structures to be encountered, and a set of allowed surgical motions can be defined.

Access to the prostate

The prostate gland is among the more difficult structures to access for surgery. It is covered anteriorly by the pubic arch, distally by the dorsal vein complex and rhabdosphincter, inferiorly by the rectum, inferolaterally by the nerve bundles, and superiorly by the bladder. The prostate can be exposed with a lower midline abdominal incision from the pubic bone to the umbilicus, and the exposure progresses through extraperitoneal spaces. Alternative approaches include minilaparotomy, laparoscopic access via 5 or 6 ports in the lower abdomen (extraperitoneal or transperitoneal), and perineal access. The minilaparotomy incision is generally 8–10 cm rather than the 15–20 cm long needed for the standard laparotomy. Visualization of the prostate is similar in the two open

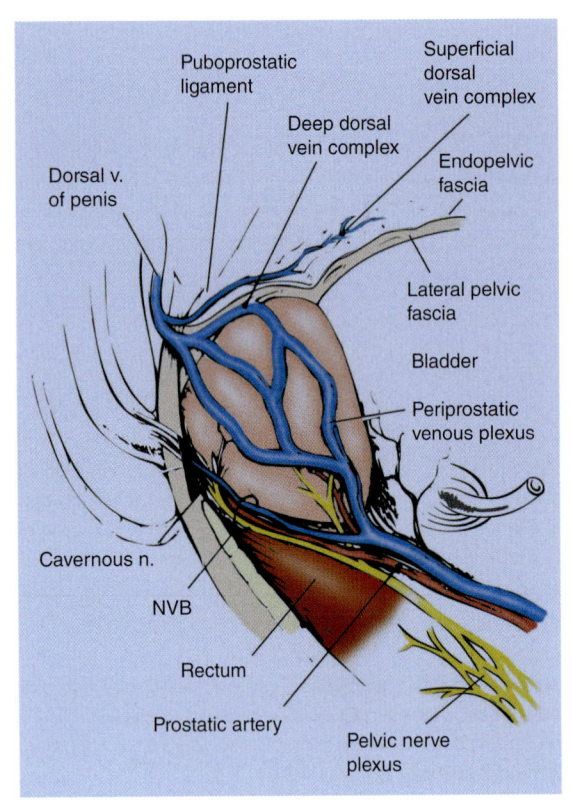

Figure 8 Surgical anatomy of the prostate in relationship to the deep dorsal vein complex, neurovascular bundle (NVB), and other surrounding periprostatic structures (lateral view).

abdominal approaches, but in the minilaparotomy, the surgeon will rely more on instrument dissection than on manual dissection. The laparoscopic approach has become increasingly popular with the availability of robotic surgical systems to increase the laparoscopic surgeon's dexterity with instruments, with seven degrees of motion and three-dimensional camera view.

The choice of surgical approach depends on both the surgeon's training and the patient's characteristics. The retropubic approach has been taught in most residency programs worldwide; it provides access to the prostate and lymph nodes and entails a familiar transabdominal orientation. The perineal approach may be associated with less pain, and the scar is certainly less visible. There may be an advantage to this procedure in the circumstances of morbid obesity. However, the lymph nodes are not as easily accessible, and this approach may be difficult for larger prostates, for example, those >60 g. The laparoscopic approach requires a steep learning curve of more than 100 cases, whereas the robot-assisted laparoscopic approach requires fewer.[160,161] Differences in postoperative pain and hospital discharge are not reliably seen between open retropubic and laparoscopic approaches but may be decreased with the perineal approach.[162–164] Both perineal and laparoscopic approaches are associated with less bleeding, but in expert hands, the transfusion rates are probably not significantly different.[165] Results from nonrandomized comparisons show increased transfusion rates in retropubic prostatectomy if the rates for this group are more than 10–15%.[166]

Moving forward with this discussion, we will discuss only the open retropubic and laparoscopic (both manual and robot-assisted types) operations. However, it is worth noting that although historic discussions on the perineal operation suggest that the outcomes may increase positive margin rates, decrease potency rates, and cause de novo rectal incontinence, several high-volume centers have published very competitive outcomes, and there is arguably a cost saving relative to the use of robotic approaches.[164,167–170]

Exposure and dissection of the apex

The anterior and lateral surfaces of the prostate are covered by endopelvic fascia. This fascia can be cut sharply or by using cautery, with care to avoid or ligate varying networks of veins that course along the prostate and often penetrate the apex at 11 and 1 o'clock. The pubovesical ligaments are cut by most surgeons to allow distal ligation of the dorsal vein complex. Mistakes in this region can cause significant blood loss in the open operation, although less so in the laparoscopic and/or robotic approaches because of the positive pressure of the CO_2 pneumoperitoneum.

The rhabdosphincter surrounds the urethra distally, and the apex of the prostate has no capsule-like structure. Therefore, there is tremendous potential for mistakes in this region, and this may be the step of the operation that improves the most with experience. In essence, the surgeon must control the dorsal vein complex with proximal and distal sutures and then make a tangential cut that is as close to the apex as possible to avoid damaging the rhabdosphincter complex yet avoid a positive apical margin. Numerous technique descriptions are available and cannot be fully cataloged, but the objectives of cancer control (i.e., negative surgical margins) and urinary control are strongly influenced by this step.

Exposure and dissection of the bladder neck

Dissection of the bladder neck is by comparison much easier than that of the apex in the open operation. The Foley catheter can be used as a guide, and electrocautery can be used safely. Care must be taken to preserve the posterior plate of the bladder neck and divide it away from the ureteral orifices. The bladder neck-sparing technique has been reported as possibly beneficial in avoiding urinary continence but is possibly associated with an increased incidence of positive margins.[171] A nonbladder neck-sparing plane can be reconstructed with sutures to match the urethral size for the anastomosis.

Alternatives to surgery must completely treat the base of the prostate while avoiding damage to the bladder. Modern radiation therapy techniques, including IMRT, proton therapy, and brachytherapy, effectively increase the dose to the prostate while holding down the dose to the bladder with combination of improved radiation dose shaping to the prostate and daily image guidance to make sure that the radiation therapy is given to the prostate. However, there is a rim of bladder tissue next to the prostate that receives the full radiation therapy dose, which can lead to urinary side effects such as irritation, increased frequency and urgency, and hematuria.

Exposure and dissection of the seminal vesicles

The seminal vesicles (SV) present their own surgical challenges. These structures lie immediately posterior to the bladder, with their tips coursing laterally. The vesicles are surrounded by several small arterial branches that must be controlled with clips or sutures. If uncontrolled, these branches may cause significant postoperative bleeding, which may require a second surgery. However, electrocautery must be avoided if possible because the tips of the vesicles lie immediately medial to the neurovascular bundles. Some researchers have reported the concept of leaving the tips intact to avoid nerve damage.[172] Laparoscopic surgeons may address this challenge by dissecting the seminal vesicles posterior to the bladder through the pouch of Douglas. For radiation therapy planning, inclusion of the seminal vesicles is usually based on the risk of involvement by cancer and possible involvement seen on MRI. Even when treated, only the proximal seminal vesicle may need to be included in the radiation therapy field to cover the area at risk for cancer spread for patients without evidence of SV involvement.[173] If the entire SV needs to be covered with the radiation therapy dose, external beam radiation therapy is preferred over brachytherapy. The proximal seminal vesicles (especially the intraprostatic portion of the SV) can sometimes be treated adequately with brachytherapy.

Neurovascular bundle dissection
The technique for neurovascular bundle dissections is usually retrograde (apex to base) for open surgery and anterograde (base to apex) for laparoscopic surgery. For the retrograde approach, the dorsal vein and urethral division steps are completed, and the plane posterior to the Denonvilliers fascia is developed with blunt finger dissection. The bundles on each side can then be palpated. Visually, the neurovascular bundles blend well into the sides of the prostate through a series of lateral fascial layers. A triangle of fascia exists, with its borders being the prostatic fascia medially, the endopelvic fascia laterally, and the Denonvilliers fascia posteriorly. Regardless of the technique, the nerve bundle must be released at two junctions: the anterolateral junction of the prostatic fascia and levator fascia and the medial posterior junction of the Denonvilliers fascia.

During the course of neurovascular bundle dissection, the use of electrocautery must be avoided as the thermal transmission may produce irreparable nerve damage. The portion of the bundle from middle to apex has mostly parallel vessels and a few perforating veins that can be controlled with clips or just transected and left to clot. In contrast, the portion of the bundles near the base gives off perforating arteries to the prostate that must be controlled with clips to avoid hemorrhage. Alternative coagulation devices have been described that produce less thermal discharge, but the nerve bundles are very sensitive to heat, and an athermal technique is preferable. Two different planes of nerve-sparing dissection have been described: intrafascial and interfascial. Surgeons must use judgment in this area because although the closer margin obtained from the intrafascial approach may improve postoperative potency, it moves the inked margin of the resection closer to the prostate gland.[174]

Surgeons may choose to sacrifice the nerve bundles depending on the estimated risk of extraprostatic extension, as determined from pretreatment parameters such as PSA, clinical stage, biopsy Gleason score, number of biopsies with cancer, and volume of cancer on biopsies, and possibly by imaging with sonography or endorectal coil MRI. Nomograms may assist with arriving at this estimate, but the surgeon's intuition and experience always play a role that is difficult to measure.[175–177] In general, most patients prefer to have a nerve-sparing operation as long as cancer control can be maintained.

The proximity of the nerve bundle and the prostate capsule also relates to radiotherapy planning. Radiation therapy is usually designed to give full dose 4–7 mm from the edge of the prostate to treat possible microscopic extension of the cancer. The addition of this margin means that some of the normal tissues, such as bladder, rectum, and the neurovascular bundles, receive radiation dose. Much work has been done to minimize the dose to the bladder and rectum to decrease the dose to these structures, including a recent development of insertion of a hydrogel into the space between the rectum and the prostate. In comparison, there has not been much work in trying to decrease the dose to the neurovascular bundles, especially as the most likely place for extracapsular extension is in the posterolateral direction.[178] Currently, there are studies beginning to look at the feasibility and safety of decreasing the radiation dose to the neurovascular bundles.

Urethral division
The urethra must be divided close to the prostate apex, essentially right near the verumontanum. The surrounding rhabdosphincter should be preserved, and excessive trauma from urethral dilators and catheters should be avoided.

Anastomosis
Both running and interrupted suture lines have been described, the latter more popular and feasible with the laparoscopic approaches. The objective is to approximate the bladder to the urethra so that the anastomosis is watertight and the mucosal surfaces are in contact. Excessively large urethral bites that may shorten the functional urethral length should be avoided. Anastomoses that leak or separate may lead to a higher rate of scarring and contracture.[179] Retzius space sparing (RSS) during laparoscopic robot-assisted radical prostatectomy (RALP) has been offered as an approach that reduces perioperative complications and enables faster gaining of full urinary continence due to bladder anatomy preservation.[180]

Technical modifications for high-risk disease
A shift has been observed toward selecting more surgical patients with higher-risk disease.[181] This requires additional surgical skill to obtain negative margins while maximizing feasible neurovascular bundle preservation and adding additional staging information with an extended pelvic lymph node dissection. As reviewed by Yuh et al., the incidence of nerve sparing in high risk varies, and positive lymph nodes may be observed in one-third of patients.[182]

Radiation therapy techniques

Intensity-modulated radiation therapy (IMRT)
The most commonly available radiation treatment is using X-rays (also known as "photons"). Generated by a linear accelerator, X-rays are shaped to the patient's anatomy with small metallic leaves ("collimators") to give a high dose of radiation therapy to the prostate, while minimizing radiation dose to the normal tissue such as the rectum and bladder. These X-rays are of much higher energy than the X-rays used for diagnostic imaging and are used due to their ability to deposit radiation dose deeper into tissues. IMRT uses multiple angles where the radiation beam comes into the prostate with multiple "beamlets/segments" to change the intensity of the beam to better shape the radiation therapy dose. The most modern form of IMRT is called volumetric arc therapy (VMAT), which uses an arc (instead of set angles) to deliver treatment. The benefits of VMAT over IMRT include a more conformal radiation therapy dose distribution (due to more angles of beam entry) and a decreased treatment time (which means that the patient does not have to lay still on the treatment table as long).

One of the newer techniques of radiation therapy delivery is stereotactic body radiation therapy (SBRT). Using either IMRT/VMAT on a conventional linear accelerator or a linac on a robotic arm (CyberKnife), SBRT can deliver a high dose of radiation therapy (usually 7.25–8 Gy per fraction, compared to 1.8–2.0 Gy per fraction for conventional treatment) over five treatments given over 1–1½ weeks.

Proton therapy
One of the issues with using X-rays for cancer treatment is that the X-ray beam does not stop inside the patient. This is why multiple angles or arcs are needed to concentrate the radiation dose inside the patient's body where the cancer is located. Using these multiple angles or arcs will therefore give a low radiation dose throughout the pelvis, which theoretically may lead to more complications. Proton beam radiation therapy is a type of radiation that will give all of its radiation dose at a certain in the body (known as the Bragg Peak) without any exit dose beyond that point. This allows patients to be treated to the prostate with one or two beams, with decreased dose to the rest of the pelvis. Because of this dosimetric advantage, the use of proton therapy has been increasing for treatment of all cancers, including prostate cancer. To date, there has been no randomized trial comparing protons to X-rays that has been published. The PartiQoL study is currently randomizing patients with either low or intermediate-risk prostate cancer to either protons or X-rays and using patient-reported outcomes to compare toxicity and sense of general well-being between the two treatment modalities. The COMPPARE trial is a prospective trial comparing proton to X-rays in a nonrandomized fashion. Although this trial allows patients to choose which treatment modality they can get, it will be a very large study (with an accrual goal of 3000 patients).

Image-guided radiation therapy (IGRT)
Whether the patient gets treated with IMRT/VMAT or proton therapy, patients undergoing modern radiation therapy undergo image guidance every day to make sure that the radiation therapy is being given accurately to the prostate. IGRT for prostate cancer is usually done by imaging fiducial markers in the prostate with daily diagnostic X-rays or imaging the prostate directly with a CT scan done by the X-ray imager on the linear accelerator (known as a "cone beam CT"). The image guidance not only makes sure that the prostate is treated properly every day (which should lead to higher probability of cure), it also means that the normal tissue such as the rectum and the bladder are not being overtreated (with less risk of side effects). Newer forms of IGRT are currently being developed are improved imaging with cone beam CT with improved hardware and image reconstruction algorithms and use of MR imaging during treatment with improving soft tissue contrast.

Brachytherapy
External beam radiation therapy (either with X-rays and protons) is also known as teletherapy. In contrast, brachytherapy uses radioactive sources placed in or near the cancer to give a high dose of radiation which is localized to that site. For prostate cancer, both low dose-rate (LDR) and high dose-rate (HDR) brachytherapy has been used for treatment. LDR brachytherapy consists of placing radioactive seeds (most commonly Iodine-125 or Palladium-103) in and around the prostate using a transperineal approach. Because of this approach, some patients may not be able to undergo brachytherapy due to the blockage of the approach by the pubic bone (also known as pubic arch interference). HDR brachytherapy consists of placing catheters in the prostate using ultrasound guidance. Once the catheters are placed, a single high activity radiation source (Iridium-192) is sent into the prostate (through the catheters). The radiation dose is given to the entire prostate by having the radioactive source move through the prostate (through the catheters) in a stepwise fashion giving dose. The dose given to any part of the prostate is defined for how long the source remains at that location (known as a "dwell position"). LDR and HDR brachytherapy can both be used as monotherapy (for low and intermediate-risk patients) and as a boost to external beam radiation therapy (usually for high-risk patients). Currently, the two types of brachytherapy are considered to be equivalent in terms of effectiveness.

Outcomes of treatment for localized disease

Cancer control
Most modern studies use PSA recurrence-free survival as an end point because the data can be collected in a 5- to 10-year time frame rather than the 15- to 20-year time frame needed for longer end points such as disease-specific and OS rates. However, as the AUA guidelines stress, PSA recurrence is inconsistently defined and does not directly correlate with longer survival.[84] The most commonly used definition of PSA failure for surgery is a PSA level >0.2 ng/mL, and for radiation, the updated American Society for Therapeutic Radiology and Oncology (ASTRO) recommendation is PSA nadir plus 2 ng/mL.[183] Definitions of risk stratification also vary in different studies. The AUA guidelines recommend the D'Amico criteria and the options for each[79]:

- Low risk: PSA ≤ 10 ng/mL, a Gleason score ≤ 6, and clinical-stage cT1c–cT2a.
- Intermediate risk: PSA > 10–20 ng/mL or a Gleason score ≤ 7or clinical stage T2b.
- High risk: PSA > 20 ng/mL or a Gleason score ≤ 8–10 or clinical stage T2c.

According to these risk groupings, the expected cancer control outcomes of brachytherapy, external beam radiotherapy, and radical prostatectomy in terms of PSA recurrence-free survival are seen in Figure 9.[79] For each modality, the 5-year range of outcomes are low risk, 75–95%; intermediate risk, 70–90%; and high risk, 30–80%. At 10 years, the ranges are low risk, 60–90%; intermediate risk, 40–80%; and high risk, 20–60%. On the basis of the limitations of lack of standardized reporting, different definitions of failure, and lack of head-to-head randomized controlled trials, the AUA panel stated that there are insufficient data to conclude that one treatment is superior to another. For patients choosing radiation therapy, the panel cited two randomized controlled clinical trials showing that higher-dose radiation may decrease the risk of a PSA recurrence.[184,185]

Androgen deprivation therapy (ADT) [most typically with luteinizing hormone-releasing hormone (LHRH) agonists, LHRH antagonists, or surgical orchiectomy] remains the principal "front-line" systemic treatment for prostate cancer. Randomized clinical trials of neoadjuvant ADT plus radical prostatectomy showed no benefit in terms of PSA recurrence-free survival.[186,187] The use of neoadjuvant ADT plus docetaxel chemotherapy was evaluated in CALGB 90203, a randomized controlled trial of neoadjuvant ADT plus docetaxel followed by radical prostatectomy compared to upfront radical prostatectomy for men with high-risk prostate cancer. The study did not meet its primary endpoint of biochemical recurrence-free survival at 3 years but did demonstrate a statistically significant improvement in overall biochemical progression-free survival, metastasis-free survival, in addition to an OS advantage in the docetaxel arm. Given that Grade 3 and 4 adverse events occurred in 26% and 19% in the docetaxel arm the authors caution against the routine use of neoadjuvant chemotherapy in the standard treatment of men with high-risk prostate cancer.[188]

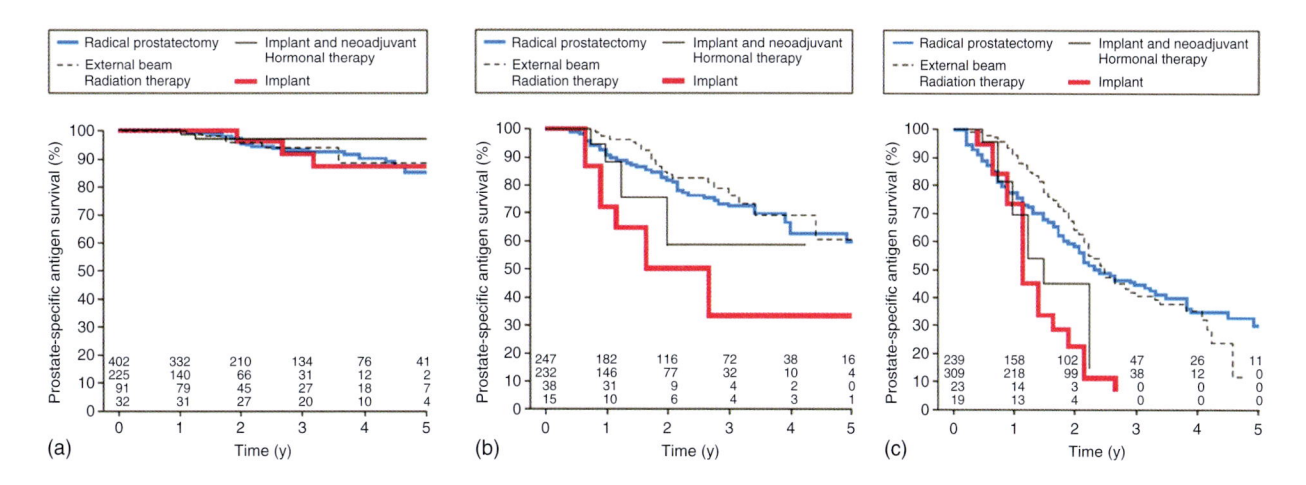

Figure 9 Prostate-specific antigen (PSA) recurrence-free survival in patients with low- (a), intermediate- (b), and high-risk (c) prostate cancer treated with radical prostatectomy, external beam radiotherapy, brachytherapy, or brachytherapy + hormonal therapy.[79] Source: With permission of the American Medical Association.

Recent studies at MDACC and the Dana-Farber Cancer Institute evaluated the impact of "androgen annihilation therapy" for 3 to 6 months prior to surgery in patients with high-risk disease.[189,190] At MDACC, patients were randomized to LHRH agonist treatment with or without abiraterone for 3 months prior to surgery. At the Dana Farber, patients were randomized to LHRH agonist treatment with or without abiraterone for 3 months and then all patients received an additional 3 months of LHRH agonist plus abiraterone prior to surgery. Collectively, data from these studies indicate that tissue androgens and AR-signaling are more potently suppressed with the addition of abiraterone. While complete responses were rare, cytoreduction and lower epithelial tumor volume were more pronounced with LHRH agonist plus abiraterone compared to LHRH agonist alone. Longer-term clinical outcomes (e.g., PSA and progression-free survival, cure rates) are pending but these studies inform a strategy to build on for future neoadjuvant approaches. A randomized Phase III trial of ADT ±apalutamide for 12 months with radical prostatectomy performed at 6 months (PROTEUS) is underway to address the question of benefit with this approach (ClinicalTrials.gov identifier NCT03767244).

In comparison, ADT has been shown to have benefit when added to radiation therapy in randomized clinical trials for both intermediate-risk and high-risk patients. RTOG 9408 showed that the addition of 4 months of ADT (given two months before and two months during radiation therapy) improved 10-year OS (62% vs 57%, $p = 0.03$), 10-year disease-specific mortality (4% vs 8%, $p = 0.001$), biochemical failure (26% vs 41%, $p < 0.001$), distant metastases (6% vs 8%, $p = 0.04$), and the rate of positive findings on repeat biopsy at 2 years in patients with intermediate-risk prostate cancer (20% vs 39%, $p < 0.001$).[191] D'Amico et al. randomized patients with intermediate-risk patients to either radiation therapy and 6 months of ADT (given 2 months before, during, and after radiation therapy) or radiation therapy alone.[192] Although reports of the trial at 5- and 8-years showed OS benefit with the addition of ADT, the most recent publication of the trial no longer shows that survival benefit.[193] Interestingly, patients with no or minimal comorbidities as defined by the Adult Comorbidity Evaluation-27 (ACE-27) index continue to have a survival benefit with the addition of ADT, while patients with moderate to severe comorbidities actually had worse survival with the addition of the ADT.[193] Although this worse outcome was not statistically significant (with a $p = 0.07$), it does question the need for ADT in all intermediate-risk patients, especially in the modern era with dose-escalated, image-guided radiation therapy. RTOG 0815, which randomizes intermediate-risk patients to 6 months of ADT or no ADT has finished accrual and may help answer that question in the era of modern radiation therapy.[194]

For high-risk patients, there are several trials showing the benefit of adding ADT to radiation therapy. RTOG 9202 randomized high-risk patients and locally advanced patients to either short-term ADT (STAD, 4 months total given 2 months before and during radiation therapy) or long-term ADT (LTAD, 28 months total with 2 months before and during and 24 months after).[195] The 20-year update showed that LTAD improved disease-free survival (29% relative reduction, $p < 0.0001$), local progression (46% relative reduction, $p = 0.02$), distant metastases (36% relative reduction, $p < 0.0001$), disease-specific survival (30% relative reduction, $p = 0.003$), and OS (12% relative reduction, $p = 0.03$).[195] Two additional trials, EORTC 22863 and EORTC 22961, showed benefit of 36 months of ADT compared to 0 and 6 months of ADT with radiation therapy, respectively.[196,197] However, long-term ADT can have significant side effects and negatively affected quality of life. Recent trials have looked at shortening the duration of ADT for high-risk patients.

The Prostate Cancer Study (PCS) IV showed that 36 months of ADT was not superior to 18 months in terms of 5-year OS (91% vs 86%, $p = 0.07$).[198] In addition, quality of life analysis showed a significant difference in 6 scales and 13 items favoring 18 months of ADT compared to 36 months ($p < 0.001$).[198] The ASCENDE-RT trial randomized patients with intermediate- and high-risk to either external beam radiation therapy with a brachytherapy boost with 12 months of ADT or external beam radiation therapy alone with 12 months of ADT.[199] There was improvement in the 7-year biochemical progression-free survival in the brachytherapy boost arm (86% vs 75%, $p < 0.001$) compared to the external beam radiation therapy alone arm. There was no significant difference in OS difference between the two arms. Although this study was designed to study the potential benefit of using a brachytherapy boost, it also demonstrated that 12 months of ADT may be adequate for some high-risk patients.[199]

Several large, phase III randomized trials underway studying the benefit of addition of second-generation androgen signaling inhibition to ADT to radiotherapy. To date, the only published study looking at this is the STAMPEDE trial.[200] This trial randomized patients with both nonmetastatic and metastatic disease to ADT alone or ADT with abiraterone and prednisone. Patients with nonmetastatic, locally advanced disease were mandated to have pelvic radiation therapy, while patients with lymph node positive, but nonmetastatic disease were "strongly encouraged" to have pelvic radiation therapy. As the study states that 41% in each arm received planned radiation therapy, it is somewhat difficult to know the exact characteristics of the patients receiving said radiation therapy. However, as 47% and 45% in the ADT alone and ADT with abiraterone arms had nonmetastatic disease, respectively, it is likely that more 80% of nonmetastatic patients in each arm received radiation therapy. The results of the study showed significant improvement in failure-free survival (FFS) and OS for all patients in the study receiving ADT and abiraterone. In the patients with nonmetastatic disease (who received radiation therapy), the addition of abiraterone to the ADT significantly improved FFS but not OS but not over ADT alone.[200] However, the benefit was so significant that many believe that OS benefit will be seen with longer follow-up in this patient population.

In summary, the AUA and NCCN guidelines list AS, brachytherapy, radiotherapy, and radical prostatectomy as treatment options for low-, intermediate-, and high-risk disease. For radiotherapy, randomized controlled trials are cited regarding dosages and androgen deprivation use. For the high-risk patient, it is noted that recurrence rates are high and that patients should consider clinical trials examining new forms of therapy, including combination therapies, with the goal of improved outcomes. It is also worth noting that the AUA panel concluded that first-line hormonal therapy is seldom indicated in the patients with localized prostate cancer.[201] This recommendation is based on two randomized trials comparing lifelong hormonal therapy alone vs lifelong hormonal therapy with radiation therapy in patients with locally advanced prostate cancer. Mason et al. showed that the addition of radiation therapy to the lifelong hormone therapy significantly improved OS (HR 0.70, 95% CI 0.57–0.85, $p < 0.001$).[202] Fossa et al. showed that that the addition of radiation therapy to the lifelong hormone therapy significantly improved the 15-year prostate cancer mortality (17% vs 34%, $p < 0.001$).[203] Compared to the hormonal therapy alone arm, the patients receiving hormonal therapy and radiation therapy had their median OS prolonged by 2.4 years.[203]

The European Association of Urology has also issued a guideline statement on prostate cancer, in which it cites many of the same randomized clinical trials regarding watchful waiting, surgery, and radiotherapy.[204]

Postprostatectomy radiation
Radiation therapy may be given after radical prostatectomy for two indications. The first, called adjuvant radiation therapy, is for prevention of recurrence of prostate cancer due to risk factors seen on pathology after the prostatectomy. Classically, these risk factors were positive margin(s), extracapsular extension, and seminal vesicle involvement. There is now data emerging that patients with positive lymph nodes may also benefit from adjuvant radiation therapy. The second, called salvage radiation therapy, is indicated for patients with either persistently elevated or rising PSA after prostatectomy or a clinical and/or radiologic recurrence of prostate cancer.

The results of three randomized trials have shown similar benefit for adjuvant radiation after prostatectomy for the indications of extracapsular extension, seminal vesicle involvement, and positive surgical margins, the latter being the most significant predictor of the benefit of radiation.[205–207] All three of these studies have now demonstrated a benefit of at least 20% points in PSA disease-free survival with 10 years of follow-up. The EORTC and the SWOG trials also a reported decrease in local recurrence rates and clinical progression. At a median follow-up of 11.5 years, the SWOG trial showed a statistically significant difference in metastasis-free survival, which was the primary study end point. At 15 years after treatment, 54% of the men treated with adjuvant radiation had developed metastatic disease or died, compared with 62% treated with prostatectomy alone; this is a hazard reduction of 25% in favor of the use of adjuvant radiation. Significant improvement in OS in the irradiated group was also seen.

Despite the evidence for showing the benefit of adjuvant radiation therapy, it was not widely adopted due to the worry about potential toxicity. Fortunately, recent randomized phase III clinical trials have shown that biochemical progression-free survival is similar for patients treated with adjuvant versus early salvage radiotherapy, and that adjuvant radiotherapy increases the risk of urinary morbidity.[208–210] Based on these data, early salvage is now the favored treatment for patients without persistently elevated PSA after prostatectomy with adverse pathologic features as mentioned above.

For salvage radiation therapy, the most common indication is for a rising PSA after prostatectomy. Most patients receiving salvage radiation therapy undergo staging with CT of the abdomen and pelvis and/or MRI of the pelvis and bone scan, which are often negative due to the low PSA values (usually less than 0.5 ng/mL) when the imaging is done. However, as multiple studies have shown the benefit of giving salvage radiation therapy at lower PSA's, radiation therapy is often given without identifying the area of recurrence.[211,212] Most likely, the advent of newer PET imaging technologies mentioned in this article will allow better localization of the recurrence so that the salvage radiation therapy can be better targeted.

ADT has been shown to be beneficial when added to radiation therapy in the salvage setting. There are now two published phase III that randomized patients to salvage radiation therapy alone versus salvage radiation therapy with hormone ablation therapy. Carrie et al. reported on the GETUG-AFU 16 study showed that 6 months of androgen suppression added to salvage radiation significantly reduced the risk of progression compared to salvage radiation alone (120-month progression-free survival 64% vs 49%, HR 0.54 [CI 0.43–0.68], $p < 0.0001$).[213] Shipley et al. showed that 24 months of 150 mg bicalutamide compared to placebo improved OS at 12 years (76.3% vs 71.3%, HR 0.77 [CI 0.59-0.99], $p < 0.04$), death from prostate cancer (5.8% vs 13.4%, $p < 0.001$), and incidence of metastatic disease (14.5% vs 23.0%, $p = 0.005$).[214] The benefit of ADT may be from patients having lymph node disease at the time of recurrence. There have been multiple retrospective studies showing the benefit of adding pelvic radiation therapy in the salvage setting. The NRG SPPORT/RTOG 0534 randomized patients to three arms: prostate fossa only radiation, prostate fossa radiation with 6 months of ADT, prostate fossa and pelvic radiation with 6 months of ADT. Although the study has not yet been published, report of the data showed that patients benefit from the addition of pelvic radiation therapy in addition to the hormone ablation therapy.

Complications of treatment for localized disease

General
In general, radical prostatectomy results in more urinary incontinence than radiotherapy, brachytherapy, or AS.[215] Brachytherapy and radiotherapy are associated with more irritative bladder symptoms with possible hematuria. Radiotherapy also has the

potential risk of bowel/rectal symptoms, although increased use of a hydrogel spacer between the rectum and the prostate has significantly decreased the risk of rectal side effects. All mentioned treatment options have the potential of sexual dysfunction, although the timing may differ. The pattern with radical prostatectomy is one of early loss with gradual improvement, while the pattern with brachytherapy or radiotherapy is one of more gradual and delayed loss of function. Younger age and better preexisting function predict for decreased risk of sexual dysfunction after these treatments.

However, there are numerous sources of bias and variability in comparisons, and there is no evidence that any one therapy "has a more significant cumulative overall risk of complications."[216] Although patients often request a single statistic, such as an incontinence rate or potency rate, it is accepted that more accurate quality-of-life research will result from the use of (1) validated instruments that ask multiple questions and offer a range of potential answers; (2) an instrument that is administered by someone other than the treating practitioner; (3) a prospective longitudinal design, including a pretreatment baseline measurement; and (4) an instrument that maintains response rates at >70% throughout the study period. The recent multicenter study by Ferrer et al. evaluated the three standard treatments (radical prostatectomy, brachytherapy, and radiotherapy) with such an ideal method (except for treatment randomization).[217] In the absence of comparisons of side effects in randomized controlled trials, various categories of studies can assist with our understanding of side effects: (1) results from multicenter community or academic series (i.e., voluntary reporting of what goes on in the community), (2) single-surgeon high-volume series (i.e., idealistic results), and (3) Medicare- or claims-based studies (i.e., involuntary outcome reporting).

Multicenter studies
Penson et al. reported the results from the Prostate Cancer Outcomes Study, which is a community-based cohort study conducted at six centers where men underwent radical prostatectomy in 1994 and 1995.[218] In this study, the only relevant predictive information was that the men underwent a radical prostatectomy in the community, that is, no description of technique or quality analysis of the surgeon and/or surgery was given. Among the 1288 patients studied, frequent urinary leakage occurred in 3% at baseline, in 19% at 6 months, in 13% at 1 year, in 9% at 2 years, and in 11% at 5 years. At 5 years, the urinary control level was described as having total control in 35%, occasional leakage in 51%, frequent leakage in 11%, and no control in 3%.

Additional data were presented regarding pad use, irritative symptoms, and bother. Urinary bother started as no problem in 87% at baseline; at 5 years, 45% reported no problem, 42% reported a slight problem, and 13% reported a moderate to great problem. The percentages of patients who reported experiencing erections sufficient for intercourse were 81% at baseline, 9% at 6 months, 17% at 1 year, 22% at 2 years, and 28% at 5 years. Although urinary function and bother scores improved between 2 and 5 years, the percentages of men with no sexual activity were 15% at baseline, 44% at 1 year, and 46% at 5 years. Bilateral nerve sparing predicted a better return of erections at 5 years: 40% for bilateral compared with 23% for unilateral and 23% for nonnerve sparing. Age was also a predictor: in the most favorable group, 61% of men 39–54 years old reported erections.

Sanda et al. reported on a multi-institutional cohort from nine university-affiliated centers, with surgery completed with open, laparoscopic, and robotic-assisted techniques. In theory, this group of surgeons has a high volume, but again, specific technique was not reported.[60] Using the 100-point Expanded Prostate Cancer Index Composite (EPIC) scale, patients who underwent radical prostatectomy had a baseline score for urinary continence of just 90; the score dropped to 50 at 2 months, improved to 70 at 6 months, and plateaued at 80 at 12–24 months.

However, as the results from these two large studies demonstrate, the literature contains varying definitions of incontinence. Sexual function was adversely affected by both radical prostatectomy and radiotherapy. Among patients who underwent radical prostatectomy, potency was better preserved with nerve-sparing techniques. Among patients who underwent radiotherapy, however, potency was better preserved in patients treated with monotherapy than in those given a combination with hormonal therapy (even after a short duration of 6 months). Bowel function was most affected by radiotherapy and brachytherapy even after 1 year—9% with distress related to bowel function.

The AUA guideline panel review reported a range of 3–74% for urinary incontinence and suggested that there are insufficient data to provide an overall assessment of urinary outcomes.[84] Those AUA guidelines also provide a large-scale review of published results of erectile dysfunction after radical prostatectomy without details of surgical technique and experience. Rates of erectile dysfunction after 1 year are as high as 90%, and nerve-sparing techniques are helpful.

Expert series
The nerve-sparing operation was initially described by Walsh et al. in the early 1980s, and it became increasingly popular and oncologically safe after the introduction of PSA screening.[219] As one can imagine, patient demand for Walsh's services and the services of other surgeons dedicated full time to this operation became quite high. Walsh et al. published a validated quality-of-life survey study that demonstrated the return of urinary control at 1 year in 93% of patients and a potency rate of 86% at 18 months.[220] A high-volume robot-assisted prostatectomy series also demonstrated excellent results: 1032 of 1110 patients (93%) wore one or no pads per day at 1 year, and potency was reported in 79.2%.[221] Although other studies have looked closely at factors affecting urinary control or potency rates, a recent trend has been to estimate the odds of achieving the "trifecta" of desired outcomes: cancer control, urinary control, and potency. The group from Memorial Sloan Kettering Cancer Center has published the concept as a nomogram.[222]

Expert comparisons have extended across technique choices. Touijer et al. performed a single-institution study involving two high-volume surgeons, one of whom performed laparoscopic and the other, open surgeries.[223] There was an unexpected finding of better return of continence (defined as patient reports of no leakage or not requiring a pad) in the open-surgery group: at 12 months, 75% versus 48%. Descriptions of the surgical techniques were cited, but the true difference that affected outcomes was not described. Those authors suspected the result was due to the apical dissection in the laparoscopic approach and stated that further prospective analysis is needed.

Thus, a clear need in outcomes research in early disease is to better link technique to outcome. An example is seen in the study by Masterson et al. which demonstrated that a specific technical improvement in nerve sparing can be described and the results measured.[224] In the standard technique, the apex is dissected starting with the dorsal vein complex, cutting the urethra, and then bluntly mobilizing the posterior plane before releasing the posterolateral neurovascular bundles. In the modified technique, the sequence starts with dissection of the entire neurovascular bundle off the lateral aspect of the prostate from apex to seminal vesicle before the urethra is cut and posterior dissection performed. This avoids excessive traction applied to the neurovascular bundles. The 6-month recovery of erections improved from 40% with the standard technique to 67% with the modification. Such analogies can be seen in the literature on brachytherapy, in which the D90 analysis of the implant quality is a significant predictor of long-term biochemical disease-free interval.[225]

Variations in outcomes and Medicare databases
In multicenter studies and expert series, researchers voluntarily submit their own results and therefore have the ability to decide whether to participate. In the case of other studies, accessible data are used without such a decision to participate from each physician. Even among expert surgeons, complications vary.[158] The Medicare database and the Surveillance, Epidemiology, and End Results (SEER) registries are common sources for data from studies such as these. The advantages of these studies include their large numbers of patients and the opportunity they offer for studying a more average community cohort of patients. Their limitations include sampling only patients over age 65 and that their data end points are designed for billing purposes more than for research and can be incomplete in their assessment of the outcomes.

Quality-of-life data seen in such databases appear quite different from those in expert series. Benoit et al. found urethral stricture in 19.5%, urinary incontinence in 21.7%, and erectile dysfunction in 21.5%.[226] Begg et al. looked at morbidity after radical prostatectomy in the SEER-Medicare Linked Database and found significant trends in the association between surgeon volume and complications and between hospital volume and complications.[227] Recently, Hu et al. analyzed a Medicare sample of patients who underwent minimally invasive radical prostatectomy versus open radical prostatectomy.[228] The trends demonstrated fewer perioperative complications and shorter hospital stay for those who had a minimally invasive radical prostatectomy, although they had higher rates of salvage therapy and anastomotic strictures. However, the unfavorable outcomes with the minimally invasive radical prostatectomy procedure decreased significantly with increasing surgeon volume.

PSAV as a predictor after diagnosis and radical prostatectomy
Researchers have also relied on PSAV to predict disease progression, relapse, and outcomes. In a retrospective study of 102 men who underwent radical prostatectomy, researchers found a statistically significant association between a PSAV of 2 ng/mL/year in the year before diagnosis and tumor volume, which was 2.55 cm^3 in men with biochemical recurrence and 0.94 cm^3 in men who were disease free 5 years postsurgery ($P<0.05$).[229] The median PSAV in the men who experienced relapse was almost twice that of men who did not (1.98 ng/mL/year vs 1.05 ng/mL/year). Although these results help identify those at high risk, they may also help physicians identify patients whose tumors are more likely eradicable.

The results of two studies published in 2005 revealed associations between PSAV and outcomes. D'Amico et al. studied PSAV in the year before diagnosis in 1095 men with localized prostate cancer to identify those most at risk of death from prostate cancer.[230] They determined that a PSAV of >2.0 ng/mL/year was related to a statistically significantly shorter time to death from prostate cancer ($P<0.001$) and to death from any cause ($P=0.01$); those outcomes were also influenced by PSA level, tumor stage, and Gleason score at diagnosis. Factors that predicted time to death from prostate cancer were a clinical tumor stage of T2; a Gleason score of 8, 9, or 10; and an increasing PSA level at diagnosis.

In an even larger study with a follow-up of more than 7 years, Sengupta et al. also found a significant association between increased risk of death from prostate cancer and both preoperative PSAV and PSA doubling time.[231] In 2290 men who underwent radical prostatectomy, 460 with a PSAV of >3.4 ng/mL/year had a greater than 6-fold increase in risk of prostate cancer death [hazard ratio (HR) 6.54; 95% CI 3.51–12.91] compared with those with lower PSAV values. In addition, the 506 men whose PSA doubling time was <18 months had a similar increased risk (HR 6.22; 95% CI 3.33–11.61) compared with those with lower PSA doubling times. The authors said that their findings that PSAV is a better predictor than PSA doubling time of biochemical progression while PSA doubling time is a better predictor than PSAV of clinical progression and death conform to the notion that prostate cancer growth follows an exponential rather than a linear model.[231]

In a study in a group of 379 men with prostate cancer who experienced biochemical recurrence after radical prostatectomy, Freedland et al. found that PSA doubling time along with pathologic Gleason score and time from surgery to recurrence were statistically significant risk factors for prostate cancer-specific mortality; in a separate study in a cohort with a PSA doubling time of <15 months, the same investigators found that 90% of deaths could be attributed to prostate cancer.[232,233] In studies of PSAV and PSA doubling time, those same investigators found no relationship between those variables and adverse pathologic findings or biochemical recurrence after radical prostatectomy.[234]

Furthermore, though African-American men are at higher risk for prostate cancer than men of other races, researchers found no relationship between PSAV or PSA doubling time and race among whites, blacks, Hispanics, and Asians. As might be predicted, no relationship was found between PSAV and prostate volume.[229]

Algorithm for therapy for patients with localized disease: future directions

Future studies will affect therapy most dramatically if they address limitations reported in current reviews of the literature. These studies must (1) use a randomized design, including an untreated control group, (2) use standard definitions of cancer control and quality-of-life outcomes, (3) link specific techniques to outcome, and (4) demonstrate that a specific technique can be reproduced by multiple practitioners and produce an effect that is similar across settings in the same way that prescribing a drug produces similar effects across patient groups in different settings. After scientific standards are met, the study design should incorporate measures that will make progress possible by resolving questions, both large and small, posed by other works or by producing data that eliminate potential explanations that could undercut conclusions.

Using current knowledge, investigators can outline an algorithm for patients with localized disease as follows: make a determination about treatment, follow an evidence-based guideline or enroll the patient in a clinical trial if treatment is the option of choice, and incorporate molecular signatures to address tumor heterogeneity. First, patients and their physicians must cooperatively decide whether to pursue treatment. As described earlier, expectant management, also called watchful waiting or AS, permits patients with localized disease to forgo treatment, and national organizations, including the National Comprehensive Cancer Network, have created guidelines for management; however, in some AS studies, as many as 75% of men electing expectant management have been found to pursue therapy within 5 years, mostly because of rising PSA values.[235] Advances in better identification of low-risk cases with refined arrays of prognostic factors, including molecular markers, and closer surveillance may change that trend.

Critical to efforts in the future to spare patients with localized disease the side effects of unnecessary definitive therapy will be better tools for differentiating aggressive from indolent disease. Such tools, some of which are in development, may take the form of nomograms such as those described earlier, of a combination of one or more molecular markers added to PSA values, of genetic variants, or of discriminating molecular signatures.[236,237] With these combinations, we may be inspecting findings not for one specific value but for patterns of values within each collection of factors, and we may be able to obtain this information not only preoperatively but also before biopsy. Furthermore, predictions achieved this way may encompass not only therapeutic response but also natural disease progression.

Locally advanced and N1M0 disease

Clinical presentation
Locally advanced prostate cancer is heralded by disease extension outside the prostate capsule (T3a), into the seminal vesicles (T3b), into adjacent structures (T4), or into regional lymph nodes (N1). The tumor may grow laterally into the pelvic sidewall, centrally into the urethra, superiorly into the bladder neck and trigone, interiorly into the base of the penis, or posteriorly into the rectum. Although patients may be relatively asymptomatic when they are first seen, complaints are related to the direction of spread.

Common symptoms can be similar to those seen with BPH and vesicle outlet obstruction, such as urinary urgency, frequency, and hesitancy, nocturia, dysuria, and decreased stream. Invasion of the bladder or urethra can produce hematuria, and ureteral obstruction can lead to renal impairment, hematospermia can be seen as well. Although Denonvilliers fascia is usually an effective barrier to tumor spread, rectal invasion produces symptoms similar to those seen in primary rectal cancer, such as hematochezia, constipation and obstruction, reduced stool caliber, and pelvic pain. Tumor extension inferiorly into the urogenital diaphragm or corporal bodies may result in perineal pain, priapism, or impotence.

In addition to DRE, the use of pelvic CT scanning or MRI, transrectal ultrasonography, cystoscopy, and rectosigmoidoscopy can help to better define the extent of disease and the adjacent organs involved. The PSA level is usually high in these patients, sometimes markedly so, although Gleason cancers, anaplastic tumors, and ductal variants may produce little PSA, and in these cases, the PSA level is disproportionately low compared to the amount of disease present. In PSA-producing tumors, the PSAV is an important consideration because it is a measure of the growth rate and aggressiveness of the disease. A PSAV >2 ng/mL/year before treatment (prostatectomy or radiation) has been shown to relate to a higher rate of cancer-specific death.[238] A rapid PSA doubling time can also be an early indication of metastatic disease. Laboratory work related to the local extent of the tumor may show a low red blood cell count secondary to chronic bleeding or elevated blood urea nitrogen and creatinine values secondary to ureteral obstruction and renal impairment.

To assess potential disease outside the pelvis, abdominal CT or MRI, bone scanning, and chest X-ray are also indicated.

Therapy options and applications for locally advanced and N1M0 disease
According to the results of a patient care evaluation completed by the American College of Surgeons in 1990, the most common treatment for locally advanced prostate cancer at that time was radiation or hormone therapy. Combination treatment was used in just 12% of patients.[239] Poor outcomes and subsequent reports of superior results achieved with the addition of radiation to androgen-deprivation therapy led to a planned multimodality approach as the mainstay of treatment for these patients.[240–245] Although surgery may be used selectively for locally advanced disease, it is usually combined with postoperative adjuvant radiation or with chemohormonal therapy or molecular targeting agents in a clinical trial.

Radiation and hormone therapy
Because radiation alone does not successfully eradicate the bulky local disease burden in patients with locally advanced disease (<50% chance) and this modality does not address the significant risk for metastasis in these patients, combined radiation and ADT has become the standard of care for high-risk disease as previously discussed and adjuvant or salvage radiotherapy for men with elevated PSA and/or concerning pathologic features following prostatectomy. The results of three randomized clinical trials—RTOG 8610, RTOG 9202, EORTC 22863—with 10 years of follow-up provide compelling supportive evidence for the use of combining ADT with radiation therapy. Patients with locally advanced tumors comprised the study group in the Radiation Therapy Oncology Group (RTOG) trials, and the European Organization for Research on the Treatment of Cancer (EORTC) trial patients had either T3 or T4 tumors or high-grade disease. The radiation dose in all of these trials was low by today's standards, 65–70 Gy. In all of those trials, the main drug was an LHRH agonist.

RTOG 86-10 compared the effects of 4 months of hormone therapy, started 2 months before radiation, with those of radiation therapy alone. Patients benefited more from the combined radiation and hormone therapy in the end points of biochemical failure, distant metastasis, and disease-free and disease-specific survival.[242,246] The latest report revealed that just 4 months of adjuvant androgen-deprivation therapy had a profound effect on disease-specific survival: one-third of the patients treated with radiation alone died as a result of prostate cancer within 9 years, whereas it took an additional 9 years for the same number of patients to die of their disease when hormone therapy had been added.[246] However, there still was no significant difference in the OS rate.

RTOG 92-02 was a randomized trial testing long-term (LT) adjuvant ADT after initial ADT with external-beam radiotherapy (RT) in patients with locally advanced prostate cancer (PC; T2c-4) and with PSA level less than 150 ng/mL.[243] Patients received a total of 4 months of goserelin and flutamide, 2 months before and 2 months during RT. A radiation dose of 65–70 Gy was given to the prostate and a dose of 44–50 Gy to the pelvic lymph nodes. Patients were randomly assigned to receive no additional therapy (short-term [ST]ADT-RT) or 24 months of goserelin (LTADT-RT); 1554 patients were entered onto the study. The LTAD-RT arm showed significant improvement in all efficacy end points except OS (80.0% vs 78.5% at 5 years, $P = 0.73$), compared with the STADT-RT arm. In a subset of patients not part of the original study design, with tumors assigned Gleason scores of 8 to 10 by the contributing institutions, the LTAD-RT arm had significantly better OS (81.0% vs 70.7%, $P = 0.044$).[243]

In EORTC 22863, men with T1–T3 (~10 ≤T2, ~80% T3, ~10% T4) were randomly assigned (1 : 1) to receive radiotherapy alone or radiotherapy plus immediate androgen suppression.[196] The LHRH agonist, goserelin acetate (3.6 mg subcutaneously every 4 weeks), was started on the first day of irradiation and continued for 3 years; cyproterone acetate (50 mg orally three times a day) was given for 1 month starting a week before the first goserelin injection. Patients were irradiated to a total dose of 50 Gy to the whole pelvis, with an additional 20 Gy to the prostate and seminal vesicles. Median follow-up was 9.1 years (IQR 5.1–12.6). 10-Year clinical disease-free survival was 22.7% (95% CI 16.3–29.7) in the radiotherapy-alone group and 47.7% (39.0–56.0) in the combined treatment group (hazard ratio [HR] 0.42, 95% CI 0.33–0.55, $p < 0.0001$). 10-Year OS was 39.8% (95% CI 31.9–47.5) in patients receiving radiotherapy alone and 58.1% (49.2–66.0) in those allocated combined treatment (HR 0.60, 95% CI 0.45–0.80, $p = 0.0004$), and 10-year prostate-cancer mortality was 30.4% (95% CI 23.2–37.5) and 10.3% (5.1–15.4), respectively (HR 0.38, 95% CI 0.24–0.60, $p < 0.0001$).[196]

Taken in conglomerate, the results from these studies and others suggest that a longer duration of hormone therapy in conjunction with radiation better addresses not only local disease but also distant dissemination in patients who have a significant local tumor burden, especially in patients with high Gleason scores.

In another randomized trial in men with locally advanced (T2b–T4) disease, that of the Trans Tasman Radiation Oncology Group (96.01), the addition of 6 months of total androgen blockade begun 5 months before radiation to a dose of 66 Gy significantly reduced biochemical, local, and distant failure and improved prostate cancer-specific survival.[247] The benefit of adding hormone therapy appeared to increase as the PSA and Gleason score became indicative of higher-risk disease. Although the current trend is to try to decrease the use of hormone therapy or at least limit its duration, because of the recent reports of cardiac morbidity, metabolic syndrome, and bone density effects, the ideal duration of hormone therapy has yet to be determined on the basis of a maximal therapeutic ratio.[248,249]

Analysis of the control arm of the STAMPEDE trial also suggests a benefit for radiation therapy to patients with locally advanced tumors. In the N0M0 and N + M0 cohorts receiving ADT, the addition of radiation therapy improved Failure Free Survival. In this study, lymph nodes status for the N + M0 cohort was determined radiographically and it is likely that many patients in the N0 cohort had microscopic involvement of lymph nodes. These nonrandomized data were consistent with previous trials that support routine use of RT with HT in patients with N0M0 disease and suggest that the benefits of RT extend to men with N + M0 disease.[250]

Radiation and chemotherapy
Because the results of combined hormone therapy and radiation leave ample room for improvement, combinations with chemotherapy have been tested in clinical trials. In RTOG 99-02, patients with high-risk disease were randomized to treatment with radiation plus 2 years of androgen ablation or to treatment with the same combination followed by treatment with paclitaxel, estramustine, and etoposide for four cycles beginning 8 weeks after radiation.[251] This study was closed prematurely because of excessive thromboembolic toxicity. A randomized phase III study, RTOG 05–21 assessed the addition of six cycles of adjuvant docetaxel chemotherapy to androgen suppression and radiotherapy, showing only a modest improvement in OS for the addition of chemotherapy (89% vs 93% (HR, 0.69; 90% CI, 0.49–0.97; one-sided $P = 0.034$).[252] Future analysis will give some indication as to the efficacy of these agents delivered adjuvantly with radiation. Similar to trials for metastatic disease, attention has turned to the newer targeted agents and the possible combination with radiation.

Radical prostatectomy
Although prostatectomy has been used to treat patients with locally advanced prostate cancer, the reported studies are usually qualified by including patients with less-extensive, resectable disease and lower-grade tumors than have been included in radiation trials. With prostatectomy, PSA disease-free outcome has been in the 50–60% range 5–10 years after treatment, and 60–80% of patients have required adjuvant and/or salvage radiation or hormone ablative therapy postoperatively.[253–256] Unlike the combined approach with radiation, the use of short-course ADT has not resulted in significant improvement in PSA disease-free progression when combined neoadjuvantly with prostatectomy.[187,257]

Castrate-resistant locally advanced disease
Bulky tumor located within the prostate is especially problematic in patients with castrate-resistant disease. An evaluation of men progressing to castrate-resistant disease identified patients with an untreated primary tumor as having a significantly increased risk of subsequent local symptoms (20% post-RP vs 46.7% EBRT vs 54.3% with an intact prostate).[258] In men with retained primaries, hormonal therapy will often not debulk the tumor to achieve the desired response with radiation. Additionally, preclinical and clinical data have shown that androgen deprivation is coupled to DNA repair gene expression and activity; and, thus tumors which demonstrate early androgen insensitivity may be less susceptible to radiation therapy.[259] In patients with metastatic disease, radiation alone can serve the purpose of palliation, relieving symptoms such as hematuria or recurrent urinary obstruction. In patients with greater expected longevity, chemotherapy may be used as a debulking agent prior to or in conjunction with radiation, although the duration and degree of response have not been well documented. Alternatively, prostatectomy may be feasible and will provide symptomatic relief in many of these patients.[260] However, late palliative local therapy is most often in the form of aggressive surgical procedures (cystoprostatectomy and pelvic exenteration) may provide relief but are often fraught with significant risk of complications and necessary reoperations making these late interventions less appealing.[261]

Algorithm for therapy for localized and locally advanced tumors: future directions
To apply the most appropriate treatment strategy, it is critical that physicians use diagnostic imaging, pathology review, PSA kinetics, and tumor markers to assess the tumor and individualize therapy. The current emphasis is on exploring combined therapies that will not only eradicate local disease but prevent or treat distant micrometastases as well. Ideally, in the future, molecular markers will enable more precise individualized therapy, predicting tumor growth and dissemination patterns (locoregional vs distant) so that treatment can be designed to achieve the best response. The molecular targets of new agents and their effects on tissue—both tumor and stroma—must be defined in detail so that therapy can be matched to the tumor's molecular characteristics. It is in this manner that an individualized, multidisciplinary approach will provide the best strategies for both local and distant disease controls as we move forward.

Biochemically recurrent prostate cancer

After therapy directed toward localized disease, the earliest presentation of *micrometastatic disease* is most commonly a rising PSA serum level. Given that approximately one-third of patients treated for localized prostate cancer will experience treatment failure, it has been estimated that nearly 70,000 men are diagnosed yearly with the *rising PSA disease state*, and the prevalence in the United States may be as high as 1 million.[262]

Biochemical recurrence of prostate cancer may be defined variably after surgery as time to PSA >0.2 ng/mL with the confirmatory value of ≥0.2 ng/mL, or after radiation therapy, as time to PSA nadir + 2 ng/mL.[263,264] Such working definitions can assist in annotating and harmonizing reportable outcomes from therapy. It is important to recognize that a rise in PSA is not an absolute indicator of malignancy, an absolute indication for therapy, or fully predictive of disease progression or disease-specific mortality. The reasons for this are as follows: (1) benign explanations for PSA rise include incomplete prostatectomy or PSA bounces after radiation therapy, (2) the biochemically recurrent disease is capable of exceptional indolence, (3) early therapy has no established efficacy in improving OS or quality of life, and (4) comorbidities are common in aging men (the median age at diagnosis of the rising PSA disease state is 70 years), and (5) alternative causes of death are incrementally dominant among lower-risk rising PSA disease states.

The *long natural history* of biochemically recurrent disease after radical prostatectomy for localized adenocarcinoma of the prostate has been described as a median time to metastases of 8 years and a median life expectancy of 13 years.[265]

Using PSA doubling time, time to biochemical failure from surgery, and the histologic Gleason grade, different metastasis-free, and OS outcomes can be estimated. For example, men with high-grade disease (Gleason score 8–10) and evidence of biochemical failure within 2 years of surgery have a 70% probability of developing metastases in 5 years, and those with PSA doubling times of <3 months have a probability of prostate cancer-specific mortality of nearly 50% within 5 years.[232,265] In contrast, men with very long PSA doubling times (≥ 15 months) have prostate cancer-specific mortality rates of no greater than 10% at 10 years.[232] The PSA doubling time is a useful tool to estimate time to meaningful progression and the knowledge deploy therapy in a "risk-adapted manner" and design clinical trials.

In men with biochemically recurrent disease, there is no evidence that the early application of hormonal therapy—before the emergence of metastases—improves OS or quality of life. The demonstration of improved survival with the integration of hormonal therapy and radiation therapy for high-risk localized disease likely relates to improved local control and a decrease in a late wave of metastases from the primary tumor rather than to the control of micrometastatic disease.[240,241,266] In contrast, in a small study of immediate adjuvant versus deferred hormonal therapy for node-positive disease after radical prostatectomy, poorer than expected outcomes with hormonal therapy in the deferred therapy arm suggested that as in the antecedent Medical Research Council trial of immediate versus deferred hormonal therapy in metastatic disease, late application of hormonal therapy results in inferior outcomes in some studies.[267,268] There is a critical dearth of high-quality studies examining the role of hormonal therapy in the high-risk postoperative adjuvant setting or the rising PSA disease state regarding OS and quality-of-life end points.

Nonetheless, hormonal therapy is often used in the recurrent nonmetastatic setting, with intermittent schedules regarded as being equally efficacious to continuous.[269,270] Eventually, nonmetastatic castration-resistant prostate cancer (nmCRPC) may arise. Retrospective studies have also shown wide variations in outcome, with shorter PSA doubling times significantly associated with shorter metastasis-free survival and OS.[271] Notably, in one 1238 patient study, those with PSA doubling times <9 months had prostate cancer-specific mortality as the predominant cause of death but in those with PSA doubling times ≥9 months, other cause mortality and prostate cancer-specific mortality were relatively equal competitors.[272] Other cause mortality was the predominant cause of death in men older than 80 years of age with a Charlson comorbidity index >3.

In men with a baseline PSA of ≥ 2 ng/mL and a PSA doubling time ≤10 months, phase III, placebo-controlled, randomized clinical trials have shown improvements in metastasis-free survival and OS with the addition of any one of the second-generation antiandrogens enzalutamide, apalutamide, and darolutamide to castration, with preservation of health-related quality of life.[273–280] In these studies, median metastasis-free survival ranged from approximately 15 to 18 months in the placebo arms and from approximately 37 to 40 months in the treatment arms. Median OS ranged from approximately 56 to 60 months in the placebo arms and 67 to 74 months in the treatment arms.

Metastatic prostate cancer

Among the leading causes of cancer-related deaths worldwide, metastases from adenocarcinoma of the prostate possess a highly conserved clinical phenotype, characterized by osteoblastic bone metastases. Although morbidity and mortality from advanced disease correlate with the volume of bone metastases, notable phenotypic variants observed in approximately 10% of patients include lymph node-dominant metastases, visceral-dominant (liver or lung) metastases, and locally advanced manifestations without bone metastases. Outgrowth of neuroendocrine or small-cell carcinoma is a particular phenomenon associated with prostate cancer at the initial visit or, more commonly, after lengthy periods of hormonal therapy.

Diagnosis

At the time of diagnosis of prostate cancer, overt radiologic evidence of metastatic disease varies from 10% to 15% of men from populations among which screening for the disease is commonplace to ≥70% of men from unscreened populations. A diagnosis of metastatic prostate cancer may be suspected with the emergence of symptoms or signs of the disease or with a rapidly rising and/or markedly elevated PSA concentration.

Symptoms and signs of metastatic disease
The emergence of bone pain is perhaps the most common symptom of metastatic prostate cancer. Correctly diagnosing the cause of the pain is critical. A change in the character, location, and severity of preexisting "arthritis" pain, for example, should arouse suspicion. Malignant bone pain is usually unremitting and worsens over time. Base-of-skull syndromes can manifest as occipital pain or cranial nerve palsy; the sixth and twelfth nerves are frequently affected. Mental neuropathy presents as chin numbness related to unilateral or bilateral mandibular infiltration and compression of the vulnerable inferior alveolar nerve. A concomitant finding of exquisite sternal tenderness caused by replacement of the bone marrow with high-volume disease is reminiscent of acute

leukemia. Referred pain from malignant nerve-root impingements can mimic benign disease; for example, L2 pain can be mistaken for degenerative disease of the hips and lower thoracic root impingement, as an acute abdomen. The Lhermitte sign may signal spinal cord impingement. Back pain can result from bulky retroperitoneal adenopathy rather than from spinal metastases. On bone scans, benign diseases such as vertebral compression fractures from osteoporosis, severe degenerative disease, and Paget's disease of the bone can mimic malignant progression.

The emergence of cough, shortness of breath, and interstitial perihilar infiltrates on chest X-ray suggests lymphangitic spread of disease; infection caused by *Pneumocystis carinii* is rare in men with prostate cancer, even those with long-term steroid exposure. Visceral metastases are rarely the sole manifestation of distant disease.[281] High-volume lung metastases, although unusual, should raise the suspicion of concomitant brain metastases. Liver metastases usually remain asymptomatic. High-volume liver metastases, lytic bone disease, and brain metastases can imply the presence of neuroendocrine or small-cell carcinoma.

Local progression in the intact or irradiated prostate may be the dominant manifestation of advancing disease, and DRE is a surprisingly neglected diagnostic tool. Late emergence of irritative or obstructive urinary symptoms after radiation, rectal urgency, a change in stool caliber, or perineal pain suggests failure of local control and invasion of local structures. Lymphedema results from infiltration of regional lymphatics and can be particularly debilitating. Invasion of the base of the bladder can result in obstruction of the bladder outlet or ureter (with resultant hydronephrosis and renal failure), hematuria, and recurrent infections. Penile and scrotal metastases are less common.

Radiologic studies
Radiologic studies that are most useful for staging metastatic disease include radionuclide bone scanning and CT of the abdomen and pelvis. A chest X-ray can identify less common pulmonary manifestations, and CT of the chest is occasionally useful to further characterize small pulmonary nodules, the presence of mediastinal lymphadenopathy, or lymphangitic disease. CT-guided needle biopsies are occasionally required to diagnose indeterminate lesions, but sampling errors and false negatives such as with small bone lesions remain a problem; follow-up is usually required to properly resolve the diagnostic question. MRI is useful for defining the presence of metastatic disease in bony lesions that are indeterminate on bone scans or plain X-rays, screening for suspected spinal cord compression or brain metastases, and evaluating the extent of infiltrative locally advanced disease in the pelvis. In addition, as discussed earlier in the article, PET imaging with different tracers (FDG, PMSA, fluciclovine) is quickly evolving into standard practice for the management of patients with metastatic disease.

Pathologic studies
Pathologic studies to confirm a diagnosis of metastatic disease may include immunohistochemical testing for PSA, PAP, prostein, and NKX3.1 expression. PSA expression is absent in small-cell prostate cancers may be lost over time in adenocarcinomas following treatment with ADT and second-generation AR-targeting agents. In the future, molecular evidence of characteristic fusion genes may help resolve indeterminate cases. Systemic therapy can be initiated in men who have a markedly elevated serum PSA concentration (e.g., >100 ng/mL) and a typical metastatic phenotype such as osteoblastic bone metastases at diagnosis in the absence of a biopsy to confirm the presence of metastatic disease.

Currently used therapies

Hormonal therapy
Since the discovery of the hormonal, androgen-driven biology of prostate cancer, hormonal therapy directed at androgen production and signaling has been the mainstay in the control of advanced disease.[282] Current therapies are directed toward lowering the concentrations of circulating androgens by surgical or medical castration therapy or by pharmacologic blockade of the binding of androgens to their receptor in target tissue (Figure 10).[283] In addition, a novel class of drugs referred to as "second-generation AR-targeting" (SART) agents have been developed the potently suppress endocrine as well as paracrine and autocrine sources of androgens implicated in castrate-resistance.[284] Examples of SARTs include CYP17 inhibitors and novel antiandrogens. Abiraterone is a steroidogenesis CYP17 inhibitor that selectively and potently inhibits adrenal androgen synthesis by inhibiting 17-α hydroxylase and C17,20 lyase.[285] Apalutamide, darolutamide, and enzalutamide are second-generation antiandrogens that display significantly higher binding affinity for the AR compared to the antiandrogen bicalutamide.

Metastatic castrate-sensitive prostate cancer
In patients with metastatic castrate-sensitive prostate cancer (mCSPC), abiraterone and prednisone plus ADT are approved in the front-line setting based on improved OS compared to ADT alone based on data from the phase III STAMPEDE and

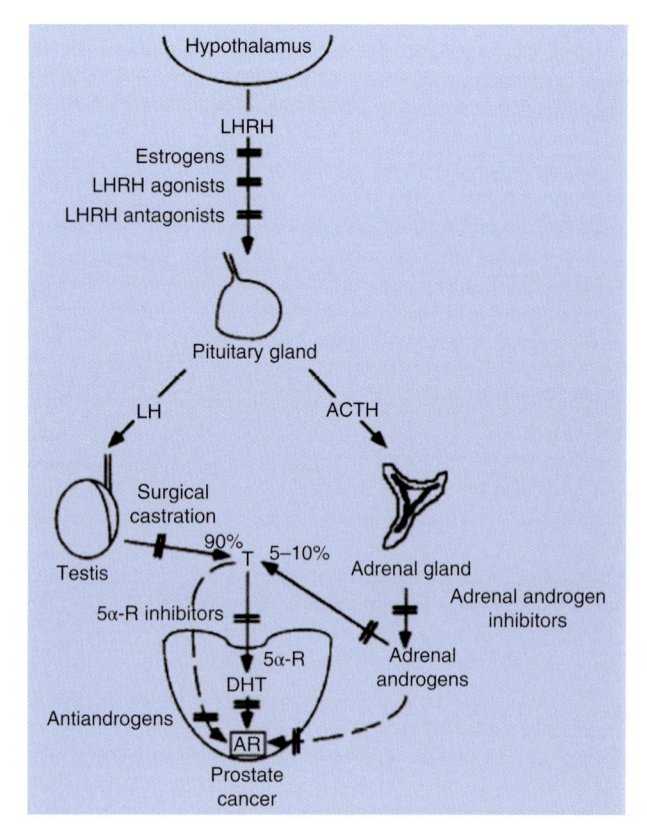

Figure 10 Hormonal axis and therapeutic agents in prostate cancer. Abbreviations: LHRH, luteinizing hormone-releasing hormone; LH, luteinizing hormone; ACTH, adrenocorticotropin; AR, androgen receptor; DHT, dihydrotestosterone; 5α-R, 5-alpha-reductase. Source: Miyamoto et al.[283] Reproduced with permission of John Wiley & Sons.

LATITUDE trials. Hypertension and hypokalemia that result from upstream accumulation of pregnenolone and adrenocorticotropic hormone as a result of the 17a hydroxylase inhibition are suppressed with prednisone supplementation. Apalutamide and enzalutamide also are approved as front-line therapy in mCSPC based on significantly improved PFS and OS seen in the phase III ENZAMET and TITAN trials, respectively.[286,287] Darolutamide does not yet have an approval in this space, with trials (e.g., ARASENS, EORTC-1532) ongoing. While these three inhibitors share the same antitumor mechanism, they display slightly different side effect profiles. The choice of which second-generation antiandrogen to utilize is a patient-by-patient decision that should factor in a patient's comorbid conditions, side effects of the medication, and cost toxicity.

Complications of hormonal therapy include hot flashes, weight gain, diminished libido and energy level, insomnia, mood and intellectual impairment, osteoporosis, sarcopenia, and acceleration of the metabolic syndrome or cardiovascular disease.[288] Some parts of these complications attributed to hormonal therapy, such as neurocognitive effects, may also relate to aging and the debilitating effects of advanced disease.[289] Monotherapy with nonsteroidal antiandrogens (e.g., high-dose bicalutamide) may yield survival outcomes equivalent to those produced by medical castration in low-risk disease but with lesser effects on bone mass, muscle strength, and libido.[290] Intermittent castration therapy with LHRH agonists reduces the cost and morbidity of therapy.

In a phase 3 study by SWOG, men with newly diagnosed, metastatic, castrate-sensitive prostate cancer received a luteinizing hormone-releasing hormone analogue and an antiandrogen agent for 7 months.[291] Patients in whom the PSA level fell to 4 ng per milliliter or lower were randomly assigned to continuous or intermittent androgen deprivation with OS as a primary endpoint. A total of 3040 patients were enrolled, of whom 1535 were included in the analysis: 765 randomly assigned to continuous androgen deprivation and 770 assigned to intermittent androgen deprivation. The median follow-up period was 9.8 years. Median survival was 5.8 years in the continuous-therapy group and 5.1 years in the intermittent-therapy group (hazard ratio for death with intermittent therapy, 1.10; 90% confidence interval, 0.99–1.23). Intermittent therapy was associated with better erectile function and mental health ($P < 0.001$ and $P = 0.003$, respectively) at month 3 but not thereafter. However, the findings were overall statistically inconclusive, leaving the use of intermittent schedules in patients with mCSPC controversial.[291]

In men with either the rising PSA disease state or metastatic disease, the decline in PSA with castration therapy yields a nadir value that may be prognostically useful.[292,293] A nadir PSA >4 ng/mL in men with metastatic disease after 7 months of hormonal therapy was associated with a median OS of 13 months in contrast to a median survival of 75 months with a nadir PSA of ≤0.2 ng/mL.[293] These data suggest that a lethal phenotype can be identified in this manner for early intervention with experimental strategies.

Chemotherapy in castrate-sensitive disease
Front-line docetaxel with ADT can be considered in men with metastatic prostate cancer given results from CHAARTED and STAMPEDE trials showing a significant OS benefit, with particular consideration for men with high-burden disease.[294–296] However, chemotherapy with docetaxel should not be used in men with M0 castration naïve prostate cancer.

Treatment of the primary in M1 castrate-sensitive disease

Several population-based studies have analyzed the effect of local therapy in the metastatic castrate-sensitive setting and have suggested improved survivals for those men receiving radiation or surgery to the primary.[297,298] This influence may be directly related to symptomatic local progression and subsequent complications, but more interestingly local therapy may disrupt the process of metastases and therefore alter tumor biology. The feasibility of radical prostatectomy in the metastatic setting was demonstrated by one study, which showed acceptable morbidity with surgery.[299] Two clinical trials evaluating the role of radiation therapy delivered within 3 months of starting systemic therapy in M1, castrate-sensitive patients have been reported: STAMPEDE arm H ($n = 2061$) and the HORRAD trial ($n = 446$).[300,301] Both failed to detect an OS improvement in the overall population. In the STAMPEDE arm H, a prespecified subgroup analysis in the 819 men with low volume disease (defined as NOT having visceral metastasis and/or ≥4 bone mets with ≥1 outside the vertebral bodies or pelvis) detected a survival benefit at a median follow-up of 37 months (HR 0.68, 95%CI 0.52–0.90; $p = 0.007$). It is noteworthy that patients on this trial received either a daily (55 Gy in 20 fractions over 4 weeks) or weekly (36 Gy in six fractions over 6 weeks), none received secondary hormonal therapies such as abiraterone or enzalutamide, and only 18% of the 2061 participants received upfront docetaxel.

A phase II trial out of M.D. Anderson Cancer Center assessed the addition of definitive treatment to the primary tumor (either surgery or radiation) after 6 months of best systemic therapy (to include upfront intensification of therapy) in men with *de novo* metastatic castrate-sensitive disease (ClinicalTrials.gov identifier NCT01751438) and has been expanded to the phase III international study SWOG1802 [(ClinicalTrials.gov identifier NCT03678025] accrual ongoing). While the concept of local therapy in metastatic disease is intriguing, widespread adoption of this practice should not occur until we have more definitive data. These trials will help to identify the subset of patients likely to benefit from an integrative strategy incorporating local therapy in the metastatic setting.

Treatment of oligometastatic castration-sensitive disease

Oligometastases refer to the detection of a relatively low volume of metastatic lesions visualized on scans. While variable definitions have been proposed, most limited to <3–5 lesions.[302] Oligometastatic disease was originally postulated by Hellman and Weichselbaum in 1995 to be a disease state in the continuum of systemic progression that would be amenable to site-directed local therapies creating a possibility of cure.[303] More recent articulations of the concept that site-directed local therapy may significantly improve radiographic progression-free survival and/or delay the use of the systemic therapies which may be associated with substantial side effects.[304] In a phase 2 study (STOMP), 62 patients were randomly assigned (1 : 1) to either surveillance or site-directed therapy to all detected lesions (surgery or stereotactic body radiotherapy) with a primary end point of ADT-free survival.[305] ADT-free survival was longer with site-directed therapies than with surveillance alone for oligorecurrent prostate cancer.

More recently, in the ORIOLE study, 54 men with oligo-recurrent castrate-sensitive prostate cancer following treatment to the local tumor (surgery or radiation) were randomized in a 2 : 1 fashion between stereotactic ablative radiotherapy (SABR) versus observation.[306] The primary outcome was progression at 6 months by PSA level increase, progression detected by conventional imaging, symptomatic progression, ADT initiation for any reason, or death. Progression at 6 months occurred in 7 of 36 patients (19%) receiving SABR and 11 of 18 patients (61%) undergoing observation ($P = 0.005$). Taken together, results from STOMP and ORIOLE support the idea that stereotactic ablative radiotherapy is a promising treatment approach for men with recurrent castrate-sensitive oligometastatic prostate cancer who wish to delay initiation of ADT.[306]

Further interest in this approach has spawned a number of clinical trials examining the potential of targeting oligometastatic disease as a single treatment modality and/or in combination with systemic treatments as part of an integrated therapeutic strategy to improve patient outcomes. In patients who present with de novo prostate cancer and oligometastases, one potential application of this strategy is to treat with systemic therapy and radiation to the primary tumor and oligo-metastases concurrently (ClinicalTrials.gov Identifier: NCT03599765).

Metastatic castrate-resistant disease (mCRPC)

Durations of hormonal control vary from 6 years in men without metastases to 18 months in men with metastatic disease with surgical or medical castration alone.[307,308] When evidence of progressive disease emerges in the context of low serum concentrations of testosterone, by consensus <50 ng/dL, the term *CRPC* may be preferable to "hormone-refractory" or "androgen-independent" prostate cancer.[309,310] These tumors are often responsive to alternative hormonal therapeutic agents and hence are not strictly hormone refractory. Because persistent signaling via a "supersensitive" AR may occur despite the serum levels of testosterone after castration, they are often not truly androgen independent, either.

Prognosis

The prognosis of men with mCRPC varies between symptomatic and asymptomatic[311–313] disease and ranges from 9 to 23 months, respectively. Several predictive nomograms incorporate a range of easily determined clinical and biochemical parameters to predict 12- and 24-month OS rates.[314–316] A model that incorporated PSA doubling time, time to PSA progression after initiation of castration therapy, and presence of metastatic disease at the time of CRPC transition defined three prognostic groups to predict clinical progression or event-free survival (EFS): (1) a low-risk group defined solely by a PSA doubling time of >10 months (median EFS 96 months); (2) an intermediate-risk group with a PSA doubling time of <10 months and a time to PSA progression of >13 months (median EFS 33 months); and (3) a high-risk group defined by a PSA doubling time of ≤10 months, the presence of metastatic disease at progression from androgen-dependent prostate cancer to CRPC transition, and a time to PSA progression of ≤13 months (median EFS 6 months).[316]

Given these evident variations in the natural history of mCRPC, there is clearly a need for reliable prognostic models both for routine clinical practice and for accrual stratification and reporting in clinical trials. Interpretations of differences in survival outcomes in clinical trials must take into account the potential effect of such variations, which may be incompletely accounted for by strategies of randomization and prognostic stratification.

Management of mCRPC

A key principle in the management of mCRPC is to balance the limitations of benefit of therapies and the variable threat of the disease. Current therapies can serve to control the disease by improving symptoms, reducing specific morbidity, and improving quality of life as well as OS time. The burden of androgen-deprivation syndrome, which can exacerbate already present medical comorbidities, influences therapeutic choices. The prevailing approach is to apply therapeutics sequentially based on prognostication and predicted tolerance. Future direction will be leveraging advances in biology to apply more effective combinations in select patient identified by predictive markers. Strides have been made in molecularly classifying patients likely to be androgen responsive or have aggressive variants.[44,45,317–319] These observation and associations are the foundational studies to transition from the prevailing prognostic model for allocation of therapies to a biologically based predictive model.[320,321]

Secondary hormonal therapy

Responses to secondary hormonal therapies are explained by the incompletely defined endocrine mechanisms that drive the progression of CRPC via the persistently expressed AR or AR bypass pathways. In general, the median duration of progression-free survival for an unselected population treated with secondary hormonal therapy is <6 months with first-generation androgen signaling inhibitors such as bicalutamide.[322,323] Men with short durations of primary hormonal control and with suboptimal PSA nadir response and rapid PSA doubling times are less likely to experience a prolonged response to secondary hormonal therapies. On a practical level, the choice of a secondary hormonal therapy in CRPC is influenced by details of prior hormonal therapy, comorbidity, and the risk of drug interactions.

A small but significant fraction of men with progressive CRPC given concurrent antiandrogen therapy will experience a 50% drop in PSA and objective regression of disease with *antiandrogen withdrawal* alone; this phenomenon has been described across the broad spectrum of steroidal and nonsteroidal antiandrogen agents. Estimates of the frequency and duration of the antiandrogen withdrawal response (AAWR) have varied, but the single largest prospective study of nonsteroidal antiandrogen agent (bicalutamide, flutamide, or nilutamide) withdrawal ($n = 132$) demonstrated a PSA decline by half in 11%, an objective response in 2%, and a median time to PSA progression of 6 months.[324]

On the whole, only modest benefit is seen and interest has been supplanted with modern "second-generation" AR-targeting agents including antiandrogens, (apalutamide, darolutamide, enzalutamide) or androgen biosynthesis inhibitors (abiraterone acetate). The finding points to the clinical relevance of the emerging knowledge of the alterations in AR alteration and androgen biosynthesis in prostate cancer progression.[325] Mutations of the AR were found in 10% of bone metastases, and these did not correlate with the AAWR.[326] Withdrawal responses have also been described with steroidal antiandrogens, including the progestins and glucocorticoids. These data suggest that the AAWR observation has yet to be fully elucidated and may be more complex than initially anticipated. Presence of AR splice variants and more specifically ARV7 has been strongly associated with primary resistance to novel androgen signaling inhibitors, namely, the irreversible inhibitor abiraterone acetate and the second-generation antiandrogen enzalutamide.[44,45,327]

Abiraterone acetate is currently indicated in mCRPC following two positive phase III studies in chemotreated and chemonaive mCRPC.[328,329] Enzalutamide is approved in mCRPC following two positive phase III studies in chemotherapy-treated and chemotherapy-naive mCRPC. Fatigue is the most common adverse events. In the chemotherapy-naive mCRPC trial

(PREVAIL), increased incidence of hypertension was reported.[330] Enzalutamide administration has been associated with rare events of seizure disorder. Recent data from the CARD trial show that treatment with either abiraterone acetate or enzalutamide following progression on docetaxel and one of these antiandrogen agents is inferior to the use of cabazitaxel as next line of therapy.[331] With multiple recent approvals moving up novel antiandrogens to earlier in the treatment course of patients with advanced prostate cancer, further experience and research are needed to determine the most appropriate treatment sequence that incorporates a patient's individual germline background and prostate cancer phenotype.

Alternative androgen signaling inhibitors
High doses of the azole antifungal agent *ketoconazole* (400 mg, 3 times daily) may function to enhance the effects of castration by ablating synthesis of adrenal androgens, themselves weak ligands of the AR but also a source of testosterone. Glucocorticoid replacement is required for ketoconazole-induced adrenal insufficiency. Adverse effects and complications include fatigue, nausea, hepatotoxicity, and drug interactions with agents metabolized by the cytochrome P450 system. This agent has largely been replaced by the more effective and less toxic irreversible CYP17 inhibitor abiraterone acetate.

Estrogens possess some activity in prostate cancer, due at least in part to their castration effects. In the control of advanced disease, DES has demonstrated efficacy equal to that of LHRH agonist therapy, but DES has come into disrepute because of its well-documented thrombotic and cardiac complications, particularly with daily doses >3 mg. The efficacy of oral DES 1–3 mg daily in mCRPC has been described without clear evidence of a dose–response relationship[332,333] The mechanism of action of DES has not been fully established. Thrombotic complications of DES persist even with low doses; concomitant therapy with low-dose warfarin and enteric-coated aspirin or low molecular weight heparin may offer prophylactic benefit. DES-related gynecomastia can be particularly troublesome, and prophylactic breast irradiation is recommended prior to initiation of therapy.

Glucocorticoids as single agents have modest activity in CRPC. The different glucocorticoids have not been compared directly, but low-dose dexamethasone has arguably the highest single-agent activity reported.[334] Many mechanisms may account for the effects of glucocorticoids such as suppression of the hypothalamic–pituitary axis, direct effects via steroid receptors, or modulation of the tumor microenvironment. Cushingoid side effects, weight gain, hyperglycemia, osteoporosis, sarcopenia, insomnia, and mood disturbance are all important considerations with prolonged use of glucocorticoids.

The rationale for *continued castration therapy* in men treated with an LHRH agonist is unsettled. Although select retrospective data suggest the potential for inferior survival outcomes without persistent castration, no randomized prospective data demonstrate an advantage to this approach.[335] A consensus statement from the PSA Working Group for the purpose of harmonizing the conduct of clinical trials in mCRPC recommended maintenance of a castrate level of testosterone of <50 ng/dL.[309] The role of more complete suppression of androgen signaling in prostate cancer progression is no longer debated given the efficacy of androgen signaling inhibition in the context of castrate-resistant progression.[328,329]

Serum testosterone levels of >50 ng/dL in men treated with optimal doses of LHRH agonist therapy or after orchiectomy are usually associated with low levels of free serum testosterone. However, rare instances of acquired LHRH agonist resistance have been described, likely related to immunologic mechanisms; these cases emphasize the need for periodic monitoring of serum testosterone concentration. Recent studies have applied methodologies that determine lower concentration of testosterone and establish the clinical relevance of "paracrine/intracrine" concentration of androgens (<50 ng/dL of testosterone).[46,336,337]

In contrast to these considerations, PSA decreases and objective responses to *testosterone therapy* in prostate cancer have been described, a further reminder that a deeper understanding of the steroid-regulated biology of prostate cancer is necessary.[338–340]

Chemotherapy in mCRPC
Although there has been long-standing for years there was significant nihilism with regard to the role of chemotherapy in mCRPC, in the last few years, the results of randomized controlled clinical trials have demonstrated the *overall-survival* and/or *quality-of-life* advantages of chemotherapy in men with mCRPC.[312,341–344]

Mitoxantrone plus prednisone (MP) therapy with 12 mg/m² of mitoxantrone at 3-week intervals and 5 mg of prednisone given twice daily was approved for use in the United States by the Food and Drug Association on the basis of greater pain relief with that regimen than with that achieved using prednisone monotherapy in symptomatic mCRPC; however, a survival advantage for MP therapy was not shown in this 160-patient randomized trial.[311,312] In a 770-patient study, the SWOG used treatment with 60 mg/m² of docetaxel given every 21 days plus 280 mg of estramustine given three times daily for five consecutive days and compared that regimen with treatment with MP; the results demonstrated an increase in progression-free survival from 3 to 6 months and an improvement in median survival by 2 months with the docetaxel–estramustine regimen.[342] However, the toxic effects attributed to estramustine were clinically significant, and the patients' quality of life was not improved.

In the multinational 1006-patient TAX 327 trial, a regimen of 10 mg of prednisone daily plus 30 mg/m² of docetaxel given weekly for 5 of 6 weeks and a regimen of 10 mg of prednisone daily plus 75 mg/m² of docetaxel given every 3 weeks were compared with a regimen of 10 mg of prednisone daily plus 12 mg of mitoxantrone given every 3 weeks.[343] A statistically significant improvement in median survival time similar to that in the SWOG trial (i.e., 2 months) was described for the every 3-week schedule of docetaxel compared with the MP regimen.[345] Similar improvement in PSA decline rates, pain response, and global quality of life were reported for the two dosing schedules of docetaxel compared with those resulting from the MP regimen; in contrast, objective responses were infrequent and no different in the three groups. Progression-free survival outcomes for the individual arms were not described. The results from these studies prompted the US Food and Drug Administration to approve a regimen of daily prednisone plus 75 mg/m² of docetaxel given every 3 weeks for the treatment of mCRPC.

Cabazitaxel, a novel tubulin-binding taxane with activity in preclinical models resistant to paclitaxel and docetaxel, was compared (in combination with 10 mg of prednisone daily) to MP for the treatment of men with mCRPC whose disease had progressed during or after treatment with a docetaxel-containing regimen.[344,346] In this 775-patient randomized clinical trial, 25 mg/m² of cabazitaxel given intravenously every 3 weeks resulted in an improvement of 2.4 months in median OS, compared to the MP regimen. Pain palliation was similar in both groups.[347] A 1200 patient phase III study confirmed the efficacy of cabazitaxel plus prednisone in postdocetaxel patients and demonstrated the noninferiority of a 20 mg/m² dose compared to a 25 mg/m² dose, although trends in favor of the higher dose were observed in patients with unfavorable features.[348] Fewer adverse events were observed with the lower dose. In another 1168 patient randomized study docetaxel 75 mg/m^2 was compared to cabazitaxel 25 mg/m^2 or 20 mg/m^2 in chemotherapy-naïve patients (all in combination with prednisone). No OS difference was observed between either dose of cabazitaxel and docetaxel.[349] Thus, cabazitaxel has remained as a second-line chemotherapy for the treatment of mCRPC, although it may be given in the first line if docetaxel was used upfront, in the hormone-naïve setting, or if comorbidities, such as peripheral neuropathy, contraindicate the use of docetaxel.

When should patients with mCRPC be offered chemotherapy?

The CARD study suggested that in patients who had previously received docetaxel and an androgen-signaling inhibitor (abiraterone or enzalutamide) in the castrate-sensitive setting, radiographic progression-free survival, and pain response were improved by cabazitaxel versus the alternative androgen-signaling inhibitor.[331] However, it should be noted that participants on this trial had to have progressed within 12 months of starting the previous androgen-signaling inhibitor and that approximately 70% had pain progression at trial entry. Thus, in patients that are asymptomatic, have low burdens of metastatic disease, and indolent PSA kinetics observation alone or an alternative androgen-signaling inhibitor may be considered.

The *optimal duration* of chemotherapy in mCRPC is also undetermined. Continued treatment to two cycles beyond the best response followed by observation is reasonable and commonly used because cumulative fatigue and peripheral neuropathy are common with docetaxel-based therapy. These toxicities have a significant detrimental effect on patients' quality of life. Intermittent chemotherapy with a view toward retaining control and providing interrupted therapy for quality-of-life purposes has been described, but the drug holidays become progressively shorter as drug resistance invariably emerges. In addition, the role of maintenance chemotherapy in patients with a stable response is uncertain, and its use must be balanced against emergent toxicity.[350]

The *limits of benefit* of chemotherapy are clear with docetaxel, cabazitaxel, and with all other cytotoxic agents reported to date. Improvements in survival are tangible, but though comparable to those obtained in breast cancer, they remain modest. Another limitation is that therapeutic agents can be expensive and toxic, and the disease is still incurable, with few long-term survivors beyond 5 years.

Third-line therapy, used after treatment with cabazitaxel failures, has not been standardized, and for such patients, participation in a clinical trial should be strongly considered.[351] When assessing therapeutic options for a patient whose disease is taxane resistant, unexplored secondary hormonal maneuvers should be considered.

Consistent with the data that the *microtubule* is an important target in mCRPC, *paclitaxel* has also demonstrated significant activity when given weekly as a single agent as well as in several estramustine-containing combinations.[352–354] MP therapy was considered the *de facto* standard after docetaxel failures, prior to the approval of cabazitaxel, but the results observed were discouraging, with 50% PSA decreases of approximately 20%.[355,356] Data for the role of MP following cabazitaxel have not been published to date. Oral cyclophosphamide given in chronic schedules has demonstrable activity in mCRPC and is an alkylator-based approach, distinct from the approaches with the taxanes and anthracyclines described to date.[357,358]

Carboplatin has also been evaluated in various combination regimens in phase II studies in mCRPC, more recently with an emphasis on the treatment of aggressive variants of the disease sharing clinical and phenotypic features with the small-cell neuroendocrine carcinomas of the prostate based on the hypothesis that the shared clinical features should predict for shared sensitivity to platinum-based chemotherapy.[354,359–366] Indeed, in a 160-patient phase II randomized study of cabazitaxel 25 mg/m^2 plus prednisone with or without carboplatin AUC 4 mg/mL, the benefit of adding carboplatin to cabazitaxel appeared restricted to patients with aggressive variant features.[367] A randomized phase III study is planned to confirm these findings.

Precision medicine approaches for prostate cancer therapy

The rapid proliferation and increasingly cheaper cost of next-generation sequencing (NGS) have ushered in precision medicine into daily clinical practice for the management of advanced prostate cancer. As previously mentioned, upwards of 25% of patients with advanced prostate cancer harbor either germline and/or somatic defects in DDR genes.

Currently, there are three FDA-approved therapies for advanced prostate cancer with associated DNA-based biomarkers for patient selection and those include the anti-PD1 immune checkpoint blockade, pembrolizumab, and two poly (ADP-ribose) polymerase (PARP) *inhibitors (PARPi), olaparib, and rucaparib*. Rucaparib was granted accelerated approval for men with mCRPC with deleterious variants in *BRCA1* or *BRCA2* only (somatic or germline origin) based on data from the ongoing TRITON2 study (ClinicalTrials.gov identifier NCT02952534) showing promising objective response rate (ORR) and duration of response (DOR) for rucaparib 600 mg BID, with a Phase III confirmatory trial pending.[368] Olaparib was approved for men with advanced prostate cancer based on the ongoing PROfound study.[369] In this trial, men who previously progressed on abiraterone or enzalutamide and had a deleterious HRR gene variant (somatic or germline) based on demonstrated a statistically significant improvement in radiographic progression-free survival (rPFS) compared to the alternative androgen-signaling directed agent, with statistically significant benefit in *overall survival* and ORR also seen in cohort A of the study which included men with *BRCA1*, *BRCA2*, and/or *ATM* variants.

However, multiple subgroup analyses of clinical trials and retrospective analyses of men with advanced prostate cancer treated with PARPi have shown that responses, and particularly meaningful radiographic responses, are predominantly driven by those men with *BRCA1/2* alterations. Meaningful responses have also been seen in other HRR genes, such as the closely related partner and localized of *BRCA2* (*PALB2*) gene, though patients with variants in *PALB2* are relatively rare in currently published studies. In converse, while there is a biological rationale for using PARPi in *ATM*-altered cancers and early phase in-human studies showed initial promise, relatively few meaningful responses to PARPi have been reported for men with *ATM* alterations from subsequent later stage studies and retrospective analyses, though some PSA response and reduction in CTCs have been seen in this patient population. Multiple clinical trials of combination therapy approach to extend the benefits of PARPi to a larger patient population are underway, as well as trials of novel DDR inhibitors targeting pathways outside of PARP, such as ATR and DNA-PK. Preclinical and limited early phase clinical data suggest that ATM-aberrant prostate cancers may respond better to ATR inhibitor-based therapy, but this is still under investigation.[370–372]

Pembrolizumab, a well-known immune checkpoint blockade therapy, was FDA-approved for treating advanced MMR deficient/MSI-high cancers, agnostic of tissue origin.[373] More recently, this tissue agnostic approval was extended to previously treated advanced solid cancers with a tumor mutational burden (TMB) ≥ 10 mut/mb utilizing the FoundationOne CDX as a companion diagnostic. It is important to note that MMR deficiency/MSI high is rarely seen in prostate cancer, and the newly established threshold of ≥10 mut/mb as predicting response to immune checkpoint blockade has not been prospectively evaluated in a prostate-specific manner. Recent studies of the combination of ipilimumab and nivolumab for men with mCRPC have also shown that men with DDR gene alterations, like BRCA1/2, display better response to immune therapy—which has been noted in other tumor types as well.[374] Prostate cancer that has alterations in *CDK12* gene display worse outcomes to androgen directed therapies and chemotherapy but may respond better to immune checkpoint blockade in the setting of bi-allelic loss.[375]

The frequent inactivation of the PTEN tumor suppressor in high-grade disease with activation of the *PI3-kinase/Akt signaling and downstream cell survival and proliferation pathways* is a dominant pathway in the lethal phenotype.[376] Clinical trial targeting androgen signaling with abiraterone acetate/prednisone and Akt signaling with ipatasertib in men with mCRPC showed the combination was superior to abiraterone acetate/prednisone alone, with greater benefit in men with PTEN-loss tumors.[377]

A high frequency of *novel gene fusions* in primary prostate cancer specimens was reported in 2005.[378] A 5′ untranslated region of a TMPRSS2 gene is fused to a 3′ ETS-1 family member in most specimens. The aberrant activation of the ERG oncogenic pathway due to the *TMPRSS2-ERG* gene fusion contributes to prostate cancer development. This fusion is commonly seen across all Gleason grades and displays a higher prevalence in men of European descent.[379] The fusions appear nonrandom and are largely exclusive within each individual tumor across all tumor foci. There are no currently approved therapies directed at ERG, with preclinical and clinical studies underway to better understand the downstream pathways that may guide targeted treatments.

Bone and stromal targeting therapies

The propensity of prostate cancer to metastasize to bone is one of the most striking examples of microenvironment-dependent tumor progression in human cancer. Bone metastases contribute to therapy resistance and represent the lethal progression of disease. In contrast to most other solid tumors that demonstrate osteolytic lesions (e.g., breast and lung), prostate cancer bone metastases are typically osteoblastic. The hallmark pathologic feature is prostate carcinoma cells nested in woven bone with adjacent functionally active osteoblasts. A principal reason for the osteoblastic phenotype is the secretion of soluble factors by prostate cancer epithelial cells. These factors act in a paracrine manner to stimulate osteoblast activity resulting in an imbalance with osteoclast activity. While the epithelial–osteoblast interaction remains a central focus of basic and clinical research, more recent efforts have expanded to include analysis of the effects of prostate cancer epithelial cells on other bone stromal elements including endothelial cells, fibroblasts, adipose cells, and immune cells. A major hypothesis driving this research is that elucidating the specific epithelial–stromal interactions that define the bone-predominant metastatic phenotype of prostate cancer will lead to the development of novel therapy strategies.[59,380]

Toward this goal, a number of epithelial–stromal pathways are implicated in tumor-associated bone formation including integrin signaling networks, bone development-related pathways, and angiogenesis. In the last decade, therapeutics that target these pathways have been tested in clinical trials in men with metastatic-castrate-resistant disease (Figure 11).[380] While most of these agents successfully modulated the bone microenvironment in a therapeutically favorable manner (e.g., eliciting a reduction in bone-specific alkaline phosphatase, a marker of osteoblast activity) and delayed disease progression, none tested in phase III trials demonstrated an improvement in OS. Examples of agents that were promising in phase 2 studies but failed in randomized, placebo controlled, phase III studies as single agents and/or combined with docetaxel include multi-tyrosine kinase inhibitors targeting Src (dasatinib), c-MET/VEGFR2 (cabozantinib) and VEGF (sunitinib), monoclonal antibodies targeting RANK Ligand (denosumab) and VEGF (bevacizumab), and an endothelin-receptor antagonist (atrasentan).[381–386] Potential reasons for this surprising outcome include the absence of predictive biomarkers for patient enrichment, drug resistance, the possibility that the therapeutic benefit of these agents would be enhanced in earlier disease states, and the probable necessity for combinatorial strategies to optimize their efficacy.

In contrast to the efforts described above, two classes of therapy that principally target the tumor microenvironment have recently demonstrated promising efficacy in patients with mCRPC. The first class is radiopharmaceuticals that principally target osteoblasts. Selective uptake in bone and prolonged retention of radiopharmaceutical agents at sites of increased bone mineral turnover guided initial studies of bone targeting in advanced prostate cancer. The natural affinity of β emitter radioisotopes *such as* strontium chloride Sr 89 (half-life 50 days) and samarium Sm 153 (half-life 1.9 days) for the bone, on the basis of their strong homology with calcium permits delivery of radiation to the tumor–bone matrix interface.[387] While β emitters offer a palliative option, and observations of a survival benefit in mCRPC with consolidative radioisotope therapy after the initial response to chemotherapy, their general use has been hindered by hematologic toxicity.[388,389]

A more effective radioisotope is radium-223 (RAD-223), an alpha-emitting and bone-homing radiopharmaceutical, with a shorter tissue range and higher linear energy transfer than β emitters, properties that permit delivery of a highly targeted effect with limited hematologic toxicity. In a phase III ALSYMPCA trial of patients with bone-mCRPC and no known visceral metastases, RAD-223 significantly extended *overall survival* [RAD-223, 14.9 months; placebo, 11.3 months; HR, 0.70 (95% CI 0.58–0.83), $P < 0.001$].[390] RAD-223 also provided clinically meaningful improvement in health-related quality of life and prolonged the time to first symptomatic skeletal event (SSE) and subsequent SSEs. Interestingly, the benefit of Rad-223 is linked to reductions in BAP without corresponding reductions in PSA, underscoring that osteoblasts, rather than prostate cancer epithelial cells, are the principal target of RAD-223.

To build on this result, an effort was made to rationally "co-target" prostate cancer cells and osteoblasts by combining abiraterone ± Rad-223 in a randomized, double-blind, placebo-controlled, phase III trial in patients with mCRPC with a primary endpoint of symptomatic skeletal event-free survival (SSEFS).[391] Notably, the addition of RAD-223 to abiraterone did not improve SSEFS and was associated with an increased frequency of bone fractures compared with placebo. However, since most fractures were outside sites of bone metastases and bone-strengthening agents (e.g., bisphosphonates and/or denosumab) were not mandated per protocol (~40% in both groups),

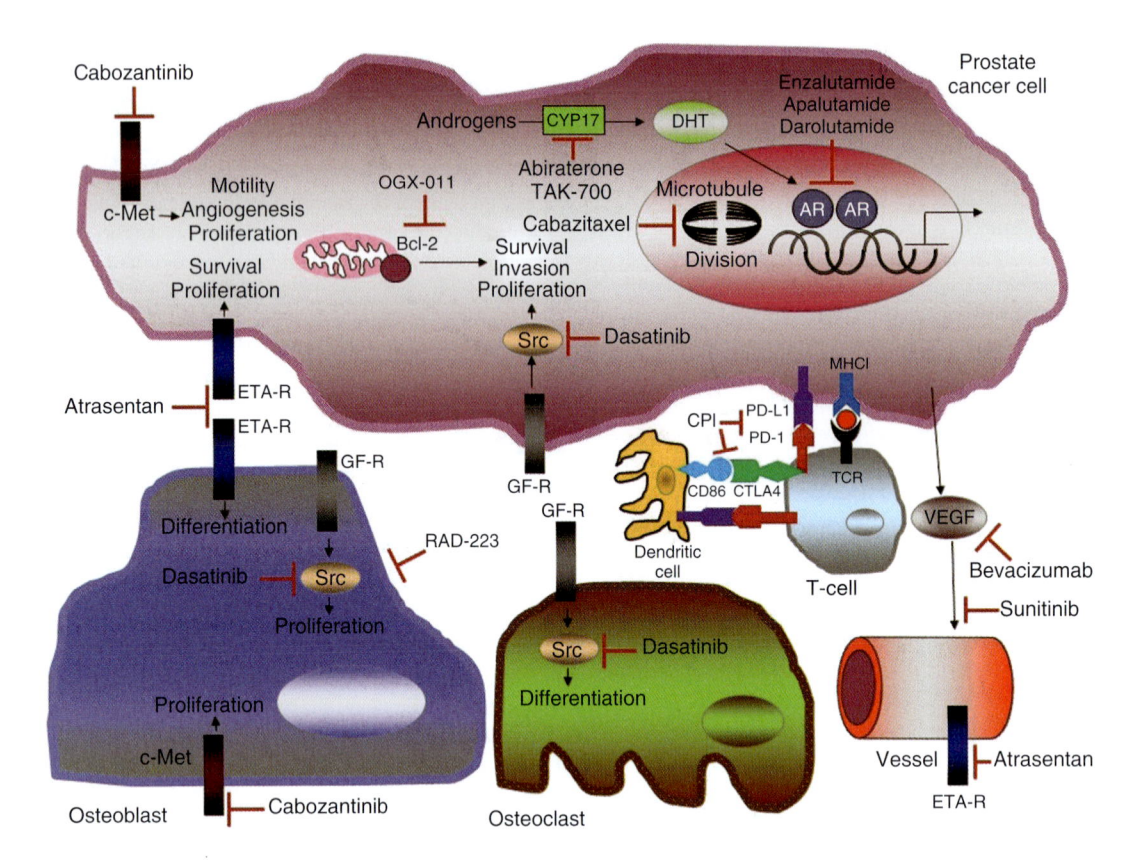

Figure 11 The two-compartment model in bone for novel therapeutics in metastatic castrate-resistant prostate cancer. The "epithelial compartment" contains the prostate cancer epithelial cell (top). The "stromal compartment" contains multiple different cell types including osteoblasts, osteoclasts, T-cells, and endothelial cells (bottom). Multiple autocrine and paracrine signaling pathways that contribute to prostate cancer progression are depicted. The different novel therapeutics that target these pathways are also shown. Please refer to the body of the text for additional details. AR = androgen receptor; ETA-R = endothelin type A receptor; VEGF = vascular endothelial growth factor; DHT = dihydrotestosterone; GF-R = growth factor receptor, CPI = checkpoint immunotherapy. Source: Based on Corn et al.[380] with permission from the author.

it is possible this strategy could be re-visited with more aggressive bone loss prevention measures.

The second class of therapy that principally targets the tumor microenvironment is immunotherapeutic approaches including vaccines and checkpoint immune inhibitors (CPI).[392] Although current vaccine approaches have not yielded major antitumor activity, the results of phase III trials indicate a survival advantage that led to the approval of Sipuleucel-T (Provenge), a prostate cancer vaccine.[392,393] The lengthening of OS was greatest in the subset with more favorable (less volume) cancers. The perplexing finding was lengthening of OS with no observed tumor regression, PSA response, or prolongation of progression-free survival. This outcome has made it difficult to identify the individual patients who derive benefit and hindered the development of predictive markers that can be used to apply vaccines with greater precision.

CPI are monoclonal antibodies that bind and block negative regulators of T-cell activation. Bone metastatic CRPC (BM-CRPC) is an immunologically "cold" tumor based on minimal T-cell infiltrates and resistance to CPI therapy. Reflecting this, ipilimumab (targeting CTLA-4) failed to improve OS in two phase 3 studies in patients with mCRPC (pre- and postdocetaxel, respectively) and nivolumab (targeting PD-1) has shown minimal activity in earlier phase trials that included cohorts of patients with mCRPC.[394–396] An important exception is the subset of mCRPC patients with microsatellite instability-high (MSI-H) or mismatch repair-deficient (dMMR) tumors (~3% of patients). These patients display high response rates to CPI and can receive pembrolizumab (targeting PD-1) based on accelerated approval by the Food and Drug Administration (FDA) for the treatment of MSI-H solid tumors.[373,397]

Based on this, therapeutic strategies to convert BM-CRPC into an immunologically "hot" tumor are of great interest. For example, Cabozantinib (CBZ), an oral small-molecule inhibitor of c-MET/VEGFR2 signaling, significantly potentiates CPI's antitumor activity in preclinical mouse models of mCRPC, has shown promising activity in early phase clinical trials in mCRPC combining CBZ and Atezolizumab (targeting PD-L1) and a phase 3 study is planned. In addition, mechanistic studies of ipilimumab-treated tumors showed that although ipilimumab increases tumor-infiltrating T cells, there were increased levels of the PD-L1 and VISTA inhibitory molecules on macrophages.[398] These findings suggest that the blockade of multiple immune checkpoints (e.g., PD-1/PD-L1 and CTLA-4) may be more effective in prostate cancer. In support of this hypothesis, preliminary results from phase II clinical trial combining ipilimumab and nivolumab in patients with mCRPC show overall response rates of 25% and 10% (including four with a complete response), median radiographic PFS of 5.5 and 3.8 months, and median OS of 19.0 and 15.2 months in pre- and postchemotherapy patients, respectively.[374] Mature data from this study and others that seek to potentiate CPI benefit in mCRPC (e.g., by targeting VISTA) are forthcoming.

Bone-health and skeletal-related complications
Evidence of increased markers of bone resorption in cases of CRPC with bone metastases has justified the study of osteoclast-inhibitory bisphosphonates.[399] A large randomized phase III trial evaluating zoledronic acid in men with mCRPC receiving concomitant chemotherapy demonstrated a reduction in bone pain and "skeletal-related events" with the use of this highly potent bisphosphonate.[400] The receptor activator of nuclear factor κB (RANK) ligand antibody denosumab has demonstrated promising activity in reducing bone lysis markers in men with progressive mCRPC treated with zoledronic acid. In a phase III study of 1904 patients comparing zoledronic acid and denosumab in mCRPC, denosumab was superior in preventing skeletal-related events.[401] A prospective study of denosumab in men with nonmetastatic CRPC did not meaningfully delay the onset of bone metastases in men at high risk for bone progression.[384,402] Denosumab is typically prescribed in prostate cancer patients to treat bone loss due to hormone ablative therapy in the castrate-sensitive or castrate-resistant states (administered every 6 months) and/or to prevent SREs in patients with mCRPC (administered up to every 4 weeks). Several ongoing studies suggest that when using denosumab to prevent SREs in mCRPC, administering every 12 weeks is equivalent to every 4 weeks.[403] A role for denosumab to prevent SREs in CSPC has not been established.

Future directions for treatment of advanced prostate cancer

Over the past five years, we have obtained a deeper understanding of the germline and somatic molecular profiles associated with localized, advanced, and lethal prostate cancer. However, prostate cancer remains a highly heterogeneous disease in terms of patients' response to therapy, morbidity, and long-term outcomes. Informed by the knowledge of how diverse genotypes influence prostate cancer phenotype, precision medicine is now integrated into daily clinical practice for men with advanced prostate cancer, including the aforementioned approvals of PARP inhibitors for men with DDR gene defects. However, next steps need to focus on using molecular data to guide rational therapy combinations or sequential therapy application to provide more durable, longer-lasting benefit to patients with prostate cancer. In addition, research that moves precision medicine approaches earlier in the course of the disease should produce proportionally greater benefit.

Current perspectives targeting the epithelial cell are centered on androgen-dependent pathways that may activate downstream androgen signaling independent of AR or entirely independent of the androgen signaling.[41] Evidence that tissue androgens exist and AR signaling occurs despite medical castration has justified continued AR targeting in castrate-resistant disease.[46,404] AR inactivation, whether by reducing or eliminating ligand synthesis, blocking the ligand–receptor interaction, enhancing degradation of the receptor, inhibiting AR nuclear translocation, or interfering with the interaction between the AR and androgen-response elements, may spare putative AR-negative stem cells that perpetuate the disease.[41] Autopsy series have demonstrated the heterogeneity of AR expression with 40% of metastatic sites expressing <10% AR by immunohistochemistry.[405]

In addition, recent advances in tumor biology reflect a growing appreciation for the role of the tumor microenvironment in promoting prostate cancer progression. Prostate cancer is no longer viewed predominantly as a disease of abnormally proliferating epithelial cells but rather as a disease of complex interactions between prostate cancer epithelial cells (epithelial compartment) and bone (stromal compartment) in which they reside. The bone microenvironment is rich in extracellular matrix proteins and stromal cells including hematopoietic cells, osteoblasts, osteoclasts, fibroblasts, endothelial cells, adipocytes, immune cells, and mesenchymal stem cells. Multiple signaling pathways provide crosstalk between the epithelial and the stromal compartments to enhance tumor growth, including AR signaling, tyrosine kinase receptor signaling, and immune surveillance. The rationale to disrupt this "two-compartment" crosstalk has led to the development of drugs that target tumor-stromal elements in addition to the cancer epithelial cell.

Summary perspectives

Advances in the understanding of the biology and heterogeneity of prostate cancer have increased dramatically. We now have access to technologies that allow us to characterize clinical prostate cancer in great detail, model systems that reflect the complexities of prostate cancer have been characterized, and multiple new therapies have been added to our clinical armamentarium as described above. These advances have created optimism and elevated the expectations of patients, physicians, and researchers. *The heterogeneity of virtually all known therapeutic targets* indicates that assessing biologic subsets with disproportionate benefit to specific interventions and understanding subsequent emergent resistance remain a preeminent challenge in experimental design. Prognostic and predictive biomarkers are crucial to maximally treat those men with ultimately lethal disease while sparing the morbidity of therapies in those men with more indolent phenotypes who are less likely to die from prostate cancer. Progress toward achieving these goals has been made. For example, predictors of benefit or resistance to androgen inhibition have been proposed, and the characterization of variants that may benefit most for chemotherapy, immunotherapy, and targeted therapy, such as PARP inhibitors, has been accomplished. These groupings may account for a majority of men with advanced prostate cancer and therefore serve as the solid foundation for the reclassification of prostate cancer. Acquisition of informative biomarkers is difficult, given the unique distribution of heterogeneous disease to bone; the phenotype of circulating tumor cells may vary substantially from those embedded in a metastatic environment under distinctive paracrine influences. The development of new methods to acquire relevant specimens and apply technologies to characterize them has demonstrated the potential of these strategies. These include enumeration or characterization of circulating tumor cells, bone marrow tumor cells, organoids, cytokine profile, and steroid metabolome amongst others. In addition, much progress has been made in the development of noninvasive methods of molecular monitoring, including liquid biopsies, single-cell analysis, and functional imaging.

Palliative care in mCRPC

At no time in the management of mCRPC is a focus on symptom control inappropriate. The selective and strategic use of external beam *radiation therapy* for palliation of bone pain, spinal cord compression, and prevention of fracture is critical in the management of mCRPC. Early in the course of mCRPC, external beam radiation or radioisotope therapy must be used sparingly, however, because bone marrow reserve critical for support of systemic therapy may be significantly compromised. *Palliative surgery* on the spine or long bones to prevent or manage pathologic fractures is less commonly required in mCRPC than in breast cancer or myeloma. However, minimally invasive (incisionless) procedures (e.g., kyphoplasty and vertebroplasty) are commonly used to treat painful compression fractures of the spine caused by cancer or osteoporosis. Surgical extirpation of progressive symptomatic localized CRPC can prevent the grievous burden of pelvic floor invasion. The services of a *palliative care specialist* skilled in analgesic pharmacy and the management of a range of symptoms of advanced disease such as anorexia, nausea, constipation, depression, weight loss, insomnia, and delirium can be very valuable. The rediscovery of methadone as an effective and inexpensive opioid with a well-defined safety margin has been influential on patterns of care, and it is the rare patient for whom indwelling devices such as epidural pumps are necessary for maintaining effective analgesia. Finally, facilitation of end-of-life discussions and transition to hospice care at the appropriate time is of major benefit for patients and their families.

Histologic variants of prostate cancer

Acinar adenocarcinomas are by far the most common histology encountered in prostate tumors. However, a number of histological variants of prostate adenocarcinoma with diverse courses and prognoses can also be encountered (Table 8). A review of the National Cancer Database using the International Classification of Diseases in Oncology diagnosis codes for the AJCC recognized variants determined that overall 0.38% of men diagnosed with prostate cancer presented with a rare variant between 2004 and 2015.[406] In this series, the frequency of metastatic disease at presentation was found to be highest in neuroendocrine carcinomas (63%), followed by sarcomatoid (33%), adenosquamous (31%), signet ring cell (10%), and ductal (10%) compared to 4% in typical acinar adenocarcinomas.[406] It is not uncommon for these histological variants to be found mixed, within the same tumor.[407]

Ductal adenocarcinomas

Of the epithelial tumor variants, the most common are the ductal adenocarcinomas, originally described by Melicow and Pachter as endometrial carcinoma of the prostatic utricle. Ductal adenocarcinomas are characterized by duct-like structures lined by single layer or pseudostratified tall columnar cells with abundant eosinophilic to amphophilic cytoplasm displaying a papillary, cribriform, solid, or glandular architecture.[408,409] Up to 20% present as pure ductal adenocarcinomas, but most cases are mixed with elements of acinar adenocarcinomas.[410–412] When mixed, the ductal and acinar components are frequently intermingled, suggesting a common origin. Moreover, while the *TMPRSS2-ERG* rearrangement appears to be less common in adenocarcinomas with ductal morphology, in most mixed cases there is concordance for its presence/absence, again supportive of a common origin and gene expression profiling of microdissected cell populations showed remarkable similarity between both components.[413,414] In addition to lower rates of *TMPRSS2-ERG* rearrangements, prostate carcinomas with ductal components appear to have higher rates of DNA damage repair gene alterations as shown by a study in which targeted next-generation sequencing of 262 genes in primary and metastatic samples from 51 patients with known ductal adenocarcinomas showed alterations in at least one DNA damage repair gene in 49% of cases, with 14% having evidence of MMR gene alterations with associated high tumor mutation burden.[34] On the other hand, similarly to acinar adenocarcinomas, ductal adenocarcinomas stain positively for PSA and PAP

Table 8 Principle prostate cancer tumor types.

Glandular neoplasms
Acinar adenocarcinoma
• Atrophic
• Pseudohyperplastic
• Microcystic
• Foamy gland
• Mucinous (colloid)
• Signet ring-like cell
• Pleomorphic giant cell
• Sarcomatoid
Prostate intraepithelial
• High grade
Intraductal carcinoma
Ductal adenocarcinoma
• Cribriform
• Papillary
• Solid
Squamous neoplasms
• Adenosquamous
• Squamous cell carcinoma
Basal cell carcinoma
Neuroendocrine tumor
• Adenocarcinoma with neuroendocrine differentiation
• Well-differentiated neuroendocrine tumor
• Small-cell neuroendocrine carcinoma
• Large cell neuroendocrine tumor
Mesenchymal tumors
• Stromal tumor of uncertain malignant potential
• Stromal sarcoma
• Leiomyosarcoma
• Rhabdomyosarcoma
• Angiosarcoma
• Synovial sarcoma
• Inflammatory myofibroblastic tumor
• Osteosarcoma
• Undifferentiated pleomorphic sarcoma
• Solitary fibrous tumor
• Hemangioma
• Granular cell tumor
Tumors of the seminal vesicles

although intensities may vary, and both primary and metastatic tumors that are negative for both have been reported.[415,416] They often express α-methylacyl coenzyme A racemase (AMACR) and occasionally carcinoembryonic antigen (CEA).[417–419] Approximately 30% of these tumors also demonstrate residual basal cells, as demonstrated by positive staining for high molecular weight cytokeratin (HMWCK or 34betaE12) and p63. Ductal adenocarcinomas should not be confused with intraductal carcinoma of the prostate, a new subtype of prostatic adenocarcinoma included in the 2016 WHO classification that is found in approximately 17% of radical prostatectomy cases and 2.8% of needle biopsies and is defined as an intra-acinar and/or intraductal neoplastic epithelial proliferation that is typically associated with high-grade, high-stage prostate carcinoma.[420]

Ductal adenocarcinomas are frequently located in the periurethral area and commonly manifest with symptoms of urinary obstruction and/or hematuria. Cystoscopic examination frequently reveals infiltration of the prostatic urethra and occasional polypoid or villous intraurethral projections arising at or near the verumontanum.[410,417] These tumors are typically high volume and locally advanced at diagnosis, with a 55–93% incidence of extraprostatic extension and a 20–47% incidence of positive margins reported in radical prostatectomy series.[411,412] In a recent series reporting on 435 men with a diagnosis of ductal adenocarcinoma treated at a single institution between 2005 and 2018,

25% had presented with de novo metastatic disease.[421] Of those that did not have metastases at the time of presentation, 17% went on to develop distant disease later in the course of their disease. Of note, the majority of men with de novo metastases presented with lower urinary tract symptoms and 27% of them had PSA <10 ng/mL. Patients who developed metastatic disease after treatment did so with a median PSA of 4.4 ng/mL consistent with previous reports that patients with ductal adenocarcinomas are more likely to present with distant disease and at lower PSA values than those with acinar prostate adenocarcinomas.[422–424] In addition, while the most common site of metastases was the bone, higher rates of lymph node and visceral metastases (lung and liver) were observed, as well as metastases to atypical sites such as the brain, penis, adrenal gland, peritoneum, and paraspinal muscles.[421,425]

The natural history of ductal adenocarcinomas and their responsiveness to systemic therapies are debated. Some series describe cases with indolent courses and prolonged survival, whereas others describe cases with aggressive courses and relatively low 5-year survival rates.[410–412,415,417,425,426] Some authors have proposed that the pure ductal adenocarcinomas have a more indolent behavior, and the prognosis of the more common mixed ductal adenocarcinomas is dictated by the acinar component, which is frequently high grade. Much like acinar adenocarcinomas, most ductal adenocarcinomas are sensitive to both radiation, hormone-deprivation therapies, and chemotherapies.[421,427] To date, no published data indicate that ductal adenocarcinomas should be treated any differently than acinar adenocarcinomas.

Neuroendocrine tumors

Neuroendocrine tumors in the 2016 WHO classification include adenocarcinomas with neuroendocrine differentiation, well-differentiated neuroendocrine tumors (carcinoid tumors), small-cell neuroendocrine carcinomas, and large cell neuroendocrine carcinomas.

Focal neuroendocrine differentiation, defined as immunohistochemical staining for neurosecretory products such as chromogranin A, serotonin, or synaptophysin, is encountered to some extent in almost all cases of acinar adenocarcinoma and appears to increase during treatment with androgen deprivation.[428–430] Most studies do not detect an effect of neuroendocrine differentiation on clinical outcomes and thus, there is no evidence that acinar adenocarcinomas with neuroendocrine differentiation should be treated any differently than typical acinar adenocarcinomas.[420,431] True carcinoids of the prostate are extremely rare and, although they tent to present with locally advanced disease, they have a favorable prognosis.[431]

Prostatic small-cell neuroendocrine carcinomas, in contrast, are extremely aggressive tumors with an atypical clinical behavior and distinct therapy response profiles. Small-cell carcinomas of the prostate are characterized by small round to spindle-shaped malignant cells displaying scanty cytoplasm, with hyperchromatic nuclei, coarse (salt-and-pepper) chromatin, nuclear molding, and absent or inconspicuous nucleoli. These cells are arranged in sheets with frequent necrosis and a high mitotic rate. Large cell neuroendocrine carcinomas are similar to small-cell neuroendocrine carcinomas, but are even less common, and are characterized by tumor cells with abundant cytoplasm, coarse nuclei with prominent nucleoli, and growth patterns of large nests, sheets, cords, and peripheral palisading.[432–434] As with other histological variants, small-cell carcinomas often harbor the *TMPRSS2:ERG* fusion, concordant with the mixed adenocarcinoma components and again, supporting a common origin.[435–437]

Most but not all small-cell carcinomas stain positively for cytokeratin AE1/AE3 and CAM 5.2 (with a characteristic cytoplasmic dot-like pattern), as well as for neuroendocrine markers such as synaptophysin, chromogranin A, neuron-specific enolase, bombesin, and CD56.[438–441] They are also often positive for TTF-1 and P504S and occasionally positive for CEA. Most small-cell prostate carcinomas lack markers of prostatic luminal differentiation such as AR, PSA, PSAP, PSMA, and p501s.[433,438,439,442,443] Instead, they often express markers that are characteristic of neural progenitor cells, including ASCL1, POU4F2, BRN2, FOXA2, and MYCN.[434,444–447] A decrease in the expression of RE-1-silencing transcription factor (REST), a master repressor of neuronal differentiation, has been proposed as a mechanism involved in this transdifferentiation.[448,449] In addition, small-cell prostate carcinomas are characterized by high Ki67 staining and high levels of expression of genes involved in cell cycle and mitosis, including AURKA, AURKB, PLK1, and UBE2C.[434,447,448] Small-cell prostate carcinomas have also been shown to bear frequent Tp53 mutations RB1 and PTEN losses, a high rate of copy number alterations, and distinct DNA methylation profiles.[450–456]

Only 0.5–2% of primary prostate tumors contain small-cell carcinoma elements, but 12–20% of cases in autopsy series have revealed small-cell carcinoma in the context of acinar adenocarcinoma.[405,457,458] Between 42% and 75% of the clinical cases are preceded by a diagnosis of acinar adenocarcinoma, and mixed elements of high-grade acinar adenocarcinoma are present in 33–74% of the cases. Small-cell carcinomas are described as "treatment-emergent" following AR-signaling inhibition of adenocarcinomas.[459] Most patients with primary small-cell carcinomas have advanced-stage disease at their first visit, with large primary masses leading to lower urinary tract symptoms, bladder outlet obstruction, pelvic pain, ureteral obstruction, and/or hematuria[460–462] Metastases are present in 75% of patients at the time of diagnosis of small-cell carcinoma. When preceded by a diagnosis of acinar adenocarcinoma of the prostate, the time between that original diagnosis and the diagnosis of small-cell carcinoma can range between 1.5 months and 10 years. Metastases are most often located in pelvic lymph nodes, liver, lungs, and bones, although bony metastases are often osteolytic instead of osteoblastic, as would be typical for acinar adenocarcinoma. Metastases to uncommon sites, such as the epididymis, subcutaneous tissue, pericardium, or omentum, have been described. Brain metastases occur in up to 20% of patients during the course of the disease, so MRI of the brain or contrast-enhanced CT should be performed as part of the staging workup. Serum PSA and PAP levels are often within normal ranges, but serum CEA and lactic acid dehydrogenase levels have been found to be higher than normal in 53–65% and 39–76% of patients, respectively. Elevated levels of circulating bombesin, calcitonin, adrenocorticotropic hormone, and somatostatin have also been observed.[463] As is the case for small-cell carcinomas of the lung, a number of paraneoplastic syndromes have been described in association with small-cell carcinomas of the prostate, including hypercalcemia, elevated adrenocorticotropic hormone, syndrome of inappropriate antidiuretic hormone, myasthenic syndrome, and hyperglucagonemia.[441,463–472]

Although chemotherapeutic agents are active in the treatment of small-cell carcinomas of the prostate, the prognosis remains poor, with reported median survival times ranging from 5 to 17.5 months. In an 83-patient retrospective series, patients with non-metastatic disease at their initial visit appeared to do slightly better (median disease-specific survival 17.1 months vs 12.5 months in patients with metastatic disease at the initial visit), although only 20% of the patients with nonmetastatic disease received local therapy in addition to systemic therapy.[440] Since these are radiosensitive tumors and at least one patient was apparently cured by surgical excision, it is clear that the role of local therapies deserves further investigation in this patient population. In a 21-patient series described by Amato et al., four of eight patients responded to a combination of vincristine, doxorubicin, and cyclophosphamide.[473] In a 38-patient phase II study of doxorubicin, etoposide, and cisplatin in patients with histologically proven small-cell carcinoma of the prostate (either pure or mixed with adenocarcinoma), the response rate in patients with measurable disease was 61%, and 84% of symptomatic patients experienced pain reduction.[366] However, there were no complete responses, and the median time to progression and median OS were short, at 5.8 months and 10.5 months, respectively. It was concluded that the addition of doxorubicin to the standard etoposide–cisplatin regimen increased the toxic effects without any apparent increase in efficacy. It is also noteworthy that none of the 13 patients subjected to antiandrogen withdrawal in this study responded to that maneuver. It should be noted that even though small-cell carcinomas do not appear to respond to androgen-deprivation therapies, a large proportion of cases have shown coexisting components of acinar adenocarcinoma, so it is recommended that hormonal therapy accompany chemotherapy in the treatment of this disease.

Mucinous adenocarcinomas

Mucinous (or colloid) adenocarcinomas of the prostate are defined by the presence of at least 25% of the tumor being composed of glands with extracellular mucin pools.[420] Patients can present with urinary obstructive and irritative symptoms, hematuria, and mucoid appearing prostatic secretions.[474,475] Early reports described a poor prognosis associated with these tumors, but more recent series indicate that their prognosis are similar to typical prostate acinar carcinoma.[474,476–478] A report of 47 patients diagnosed with mucinous adenocarcinoma of the prostate and treated with radical prostatectomy between 1991 and 2006 indicated that at a median follow up of 6 years, only one patient had PSA progression 3 years after his surgery, without evidence of local recurrence or distant metastasis.[479]

Signet ring cell

In contrast to mucinous adenocarcinomas of the prostate, signet ring cell adenocarcinomas of the prostate are associated with an aggressive course and poor survival.[480] Patients may present with obstructive urinary symptoms and hematuria but, in some series, up to a third presented with distant disease. These tumors are characterized by intracytoplasmic vacuoles that compress the nucleus into a crescent shape, and a majority stain positively for PSA and PSAP. The diagnosis of a signet ring cell adenocarcinoma of the prostate requires a negative gastrointestinal work-up. With less than 100 cases reported in the literature, the treatment of choice has not been defined, although multimodality therapy is recommended and occasional long-term responses to systemic therapies have been reported.[480–483]

Sarcomatoid carcinomas

Carcinomas of the prostate with spindle cell differentiation, also known as carcinosarcomas or sarcomatoid carcinomas, are rare tumors that are characterized by the presence of both malignant high-grade epithelial and mesenchymal components. The epithelial component consists most commonly of acinar adenocarcinoma but may consist of ductal adenocarcinoma or contain elements of small-cell or squamous cell carcinoma.[484–486] In approximately two-thirds of the cases, the mesenchymal component is a nonspecific malignant spindle cell proliferation, but in one-third, it displays specific mesenchymal elements such as those of osteosarcoma, chondrosarcoma, or rhabdomyosarcoma.[485] The adenocarcinoma components are positive for keratin, and the sarcomatoid elements are positive for vimentin. The adenocarcinoma components are also positive for PSA and NKX3-1 in most cases.[484] Most cases demonstrate immunoreactivity for at least one epithelial marker within the sarcomatoid component which together with loss-of-heterozygosity analyses and *ERG* fluorescence *in situ* hybridization studies support the notion that both components have a common origin.[484,487–491]

In approximately 50–80% of the reported cases of sarcomatoid carcinomas of the prostate, patients had a prior history of adenocarcinoma treated with ADT and/or radiation 2 months to 20 years before.[484,485,491,492] These tumors typically manifest as large prostatic masses with local invasion, resulting in pelvic or perineal pain, lower abdominal mass, and symptoms of urinary obstruction with low serum PSA levels.[484,493] Both the carcinomatous and sarcomatous elements can metastasize, and metastatic disease is often present at the time of diagnosis, with the most common sites of nonlymph node metastases being the lung, bone, and brain.[484]

The prognosis of prostatic sarcomatoid carcinomas is poor, regardless of the histologic type of the sarcomatous elements.[494] Case series report median *overall survival* of approximately 10 months, although those presenting with localized disease, amenable to treatment with surgery and/or radiation can have more prolonged disease-free survivals.[484,490,491] Androgen-deprivation therapy is usually administered to target the malignant epithelial component. Responses to traditional prostate cancer agents (docetaxel) as well as to carboplatin and etoposide, and to chemotherapy drugs typically administered for the treatment of sarcomas, such as ifosfamide and doxorubicin, have been reported, but when they occur, they last at best a few months. Given the morbidity caused by the local invasion of the primary tumors, palliative surgery (which often will need to involve anterior exenterations with urinary diversion) with or without adjuvant radiation may be appropriate. It is noteworthy that the only long-term survivor described by Dundore et al. was treated by pelvic exenteration and resection of lung metastases. Two other patients in their series, who survived 89 and 107 months, were treated with intratumoral iodine 125 (^{125}I) before dying of carcinosarcoma.[490]

Adenosquamous carcinomas

Adenosquamous carcinomas of the prostate are characterized by the presence of both glandular and squamous components. Most cases are preceded by a prior history of acinar adenocarcinoma treated with hormonal therapy and/or radiation therapy, and up to 20% present with distant disease. The prognosis is poor, even in patients presenting with localized disease, and the 5-year cancer-specific survival rate has been estimated at 30%.[406,495–497]

Algorithm for therapy: future directions for histologic variants

The main question about these histologic variants is whether they represent true biologic variants with different responses to standard treatments for prostate acinar adenocarcinomas that would require different therapeutic approaches, although differences in prognosis as treatment response profiles between the extremes of morphologic groupings (small-cell vs acinar adenocarcinoma) are obvious. However, these are rare subsets and are often insufficient discriminators to make decisions in the majority of patients. Aparicio et al. noted that a group of men with mCRPC and clinical features of small-cell cancers had heterogeneous morphologies but shared chemotherapy response profiles, prognosis, and shared biology in experimental model systems.[364,433,434] These clinicopathologically identified variant prostate cancers with virulent features have been dubbed 'aggressive variant prostate cancer' and shown to be characterized by combined defects in the tumor suppressors p53, RB1 and PTEN, and by unique sensitivity to platinum-based chemotherapies.[319,364,367] The report highlights to the inadequacy of morphological characterization in predicting benefit to specific therapies and the urgent need to add molecular classification that reflects "driver biology."

For all histological variants, the role of local therapies remains to be determined, and in the case of small-cell carcinoma, it is reasonable to ask whether prophylactic brain irradiation should be offered to patients whose systemic disease is otherwise controlled.

Key references

The complete reference list can be found on Vital Source version of this title, see inside front cover.

13. Häggman MJ, Macoska JA, Wojno KJ, Oesterling JE. The relationship between prostatic intraepithelial neoplasia and prostate cancer: critical issues. *J Urol.* 1997;**158**(1):12–22.
20. Bostwick DG. The pathology of early prostate cancer. *CA Cancer J Clin.* 1989;**39**(6):376–393.
28. Pritchard CC, Mateo J, Walsh MF, et al. Inherited DNA-repair gene mutations in men with metastatic prostate cancer. *N Engl J Med.* 2016;**375**(5):443–453.
33. Robinson D, Van Allen EM, Wu YM, et al. Integrative clinical genomics of advanced prostate cancer. *Cell.* 2015;**161**(5):1215–1228.
40. Taplin ME, Bubley GJ, Shuster TD, et al. Mutation of the androgen-receptor gene in metastatic androgen-independent prostate cancer. *N Engl J Med.* 1995;**332**(21):1393–1398.
45. Antonarakis ES, Lu C, Wang H, et al. AR-V7 and resistance to enzalutamide and abiraterone in prostate cancer. *N Engl J Med.* 2014;**371**(11):1028–1038.
79. D'Amico AV, Whittington R, Malkowicz SB, et al. Biochemical outcome after radical prostatectomy, external beam radiation therapy, or interstitial radiation therapy for clinically localized prostate cancer. *Jama.* 1998;**280**(11):969–974.
80. Greene FPD, Fleming I, et al. *AJCC Cancer Staging Manual*, 6th ed. New York: Springer; 2002.
81. Edge SBD, Compton CC, Fritz AG, et al. (eds). *AJCC Cancer Staging Manual*. New York: Springer; 2010.
84. Thompson I, Thrasher JB, Aus G, et al. Guideline for the management of clinically localized prostate cancer. 2007 update. *J Urol.* 2007;**177**(6):2106–2131.
87. Davis JW. Novel commercially available genomic tests for prostate cancer: a roadmap to understanding their clinical impact. *BJU Int.* 2014;**114**(3):320–322.
89. Ahmed HU, El-Shater Bosaily A, Brown LC, et al. Diagnostic accuracy of multi-parametric MRI and TRUS biopsy in prostate cancer (PROMIS): a paired validating confirmatory study. *Lancet.* 2017;**389**(10071):815–822.
90. Kasivisvanathan V, Rannikko AS, Borghi M, et al. MRI-targeted or standard biopsy for prostate-cancer diagnosis. *N Engl J Med.* 2018;**378**(19):1767–1777.
102. Hofman MS, Lawrentschuk N, Francis RJ, et al. Prostate-specific membrane antigen PET-CT in patients with high-risk prostate cancer before curative-intent surgery or radiotherapy (proPSMA): a prospective, randomised, multicentre study. *Lancet.* 2020;**395**(10231):1208–1216.
123. Calais J, Ceci F, Eiber M, et al. (18)F-fluciclovine PET-CT and (68)Ga-PSMA-11 PET-CT in patients with early biochemical recurrence after prostatectomy: a prospective, single-centre, single-arm, comparative imaging trial. *Lancet Oncol.* 2019;**20**(9):1286–1294.
148. Bill-Axelson A, Holmberg L, Garmo H, et al. Radical prostatectomy or watchful waiting in early prostate cancer. *N Engl J Med.* 2014;**370**(10):932–942.
188. Eastham JA, Heller G, Halabi S, et al. Cancer and leukemia group B 90203 (alliance): radical prostatectomy with or without neoadjuvant chemohormonal therapy in localized, high-risk prostate cancer. *J Clin Oncol.* 2020;**38**(26):3042–3050.
191. Jones CU, Hunt D, McGowan DG, et al. Radiotherapy and short-term androgen deprivation for localized prostate cancer. *N Engl J Med.* 2011;**365**(2):107–118.
197. Bolla M, de Reijke TM, Van Tienhoven G, et al. Duration of androgen suppression in the treatment of prostate cancer. *N Engl J Med.* 2009;**360**(24):2516–2527.
200. James ND, de Bono JS, Spears MR, et al. Abiraterone for prostate cancer not previously treated with hormone therapy. *N Engl J Med.* 2017;**377**(4):338–351.
210. Sargos P, Chabaud S, Latorzeff I, et al. Adjuvant radiotherapy versus early salvage radiotherapy plus short-term androgen deprivation therapy in men with localised prostate cancer after radical prostatectomy (GETUG-AFU 17): a randomised, phase 3 trial. *Lancet Oncol.* 2020;**21**(10):1341–1352.

96 Tumors of the penis and the urethra

Jad Chahoud, MD, MPH ■ Andrea Necchi, MD ■ Philippe E. Spiess, MD, MS

Overview

Penile cancer is predominantly of squamous histology, a proportion of those are related to human papillomavirus (HPV). Penile squamous cell carcinoma (PSCC) is rare in the developed world and among circumcised men. For patients with localized PSCC, early potentially less debilitating surgery can be curative. Other modalities are less robust. Metastasis presents initially with lymphatic local regional disease progression, also the lymph node metastatic extent remains the strongest prognostic indicator of clinical outcomes. Patients with bulky locally advanced disease may benefit from multimodal approach with neoadjuvant cisplatin-based chemotherapy followed by consolidative inguinal lymph node dissection.

Urethral cancer is a rare and histologically heterogenous carcinoma but can be aggressive depending on tumor histology. The prognosis and treatment approach depend on the gender, histology, location of the tumor within the urethra, and extent of disease.

Cancer of the penis

Squamous cell carcinoma (SCC) is the most common histologic subtype, accounting for over 95% of cases. Early recognition of tumor lesions correlates with lower staging and more effective treatment with better organ sparing and lower mortality. Penile squamous cell carcinoma (PSCC) is a rare disease in the United States (<2100/year) but is a major health problem in Africa, Asia, and South America. Another cancer involving the penis is verrucous carcinoma, alternatively known as giant condyloma or Buschke–Lowenstein tumor, a variant of squamous carcinoma which does not metastasize, but which spreads aggressively by local extension and destroys surrounding tissue.[1] Also, Epidemic Kaposi's sarcoma is associated with uncontrolled acquired immunodeficiency syndrome (AIDS), while melanoma and basal cell carcinoma very rarely involve the penis. A scaly red clearly demarked intraepithelial squamous carcinoma *in situ* (CIS) is denominated Bowen's disease when it involves the base of the penis and the scrotum. When CIS involves the glans or prepuce, it appears as shiny red velvet and is known as erythroplasia of Queyrat. Carcinomas *in situ* have the potential to develop into invasive squamous carcinoma in about 20% of cases. A biopsy is required to establish a diagnosis. Leukemias, lymphomas, or metastatic solid organ cancers can present as priapism (typically high flow nonischemic), and diagnosis and therapy for them are systemic. In this article, we will focus our detailed description of the epidemiology, diagnosis, and management of PSCC as it is the predominant histology of penis cancer.

Epidemiology and etiology

In 2020, the estimated number of new cases is 2200 in the United States, with 440 deaths related to PSCC.[1] On the other hand, the worldwide number of new cases in 2018 was estimated to be around 35,000.[2] In countries where infant circumcision is common, such as Israel and the United States, the incidence of squamous carcinoma of the penis tends to be lower. Circumcision later in life has not conferred protection, perhaps because it was performed after phimosis has already occurred. The increased risk associated with a lack of circumcision appears to be due to a history of phimosis among uncircumcised men. In fact, history of phimosis increased the risk of PSCC in comparison to uncircumcised men who did not report a history of phimosis (OR, 0.5; 95% CI, 0.1–2.5).[3] Proper hygiene is made difficult by phimosis, perpetuating chronic inflammation of the glans penis and preputial tissue. Other risk factors that have been associated with PSCC include HPV (30–50% of patients),[4–6] smoking (higher risk 3–4 times),[7–10] and phimosis or lack of circumcision (higher risk 7–10 times).[3,10] The presence of HPV in tumor tissue is established using numerous methods, also, p16INK4a expression has been used as a surrogate marker of transforming HPV infections.[11,12] The largest pooled meta-analysis of the prevalence of HPV infection in 4000 PSCC cases was 50.8% HPV DNA in the overall cohort with higher rates in cases with basaloid SCCs (84%) and warty-basaloid carcinoma (75.7%).[4] They report that HPV type 16 is by far the most common HPV type in both penile cancer and penile intraepithelial neoplasia.[4] Noteworthy, a large retrospective study provided preliminary insights into the role of HPV infection as a predictor of clinical outcome after particular therapeutic approaches, and in particular nodal radiotherapy (RT) in patients with locally advanced tumors.[13,14]

Diagnosis

PSCC first presents with a skin abnormality or painless palpable lesion on the penis.[15] Inguinal adenopathy can be present in around 50% of cases at the time of diagnosis,[16] whereas distant visceral or bone metastases are uncommon at the initial time of diagnosis.[16–18] Initial diagnosis requires a biopsy for tissue confirmation and pathological risk stratification with a physical examination to assess for any palpable lymph nodes. Well-differentiated tumors tend to metastasize infrequently, while more poorly differentiated tumors have a high propensity for early metastasis. Several studies have confirmed that higher tumor grade increases the likelihood of inguinal nodal metastases.[12,19]

Early penile invasive tumors may be small and largely unremarkable, sometimes resembling small abrasions or calloused thickenings of penile skin, which can cause delay in initial diagnosis. The initial lesion of squamous carcinoma most commonly presents on the glans or prepuce. It varies from a small, velvety, reddened, raised maculopapule to an ulcer, hyperkeratotic area, or exophytic papillary tumor. More advanced lesions may be exophytic or ulcerated, and very advanced cancers may destroy the penile shaft. Metastases to the inguinal lymph nodes (ILNs) may produce large ulcerations in the groin late in the course of the disease.

Invasive squamous carcinoma of the penis follows a predictable pattern of metastasis. Lesions of the glans, coronal sulcus, prepuce, and distal shaft spread to the deep inguinal nodes, while lesions of the proximal shaft and base of the penis spread to the more lateral and superficial inguinal nodes, subsequent spread to the external iliac, obturator, and iliac chains follows.[20–22] Metastases to distant sites are infrequent and occur late in the course of disease.

Tumor staging

Once the diagnosis of squamous carcinoma is established, complete staging is undertaken. Tumor grade, as well as stage, is important in assessing the risk of nodal metastases. Patients with grade I well-differentiated tumors that are limited to the skin and superficial tissues of the penis are unlikely to have tumor metastases to inguinal nodes. Patients with moderately or poorly differentiated lesions with any degree of invasion of the deeper penile structures are at significant risk of groin metastasis.[23]

Inguinal nodes are carefully palpated, in addition to the penile lesion evaluation of lymph nodes is also critical. The involvement of the ILNs, the number and location of positive nodes, and extracapsular nodal involvement provide the strongest prognostic factors of survival.[24] Additional studies should involve cross-sectional imaging of the abdomen, pelvis, and chest that may include computerized tomography (CT), magnetic resonance imaging (MRI), positron emission tomography (PET)–computed tomography, and/or chest X-ray. MRI provides good discrimination of penile structures and may identify corpora cavernosal or spongiosal invasion. This is especially helpful for patients with planned organ-sparing surgery, and this is supported by the current European Association of Urology (EAU) and National Comprehensive Cancer Network (NCCN) guidelines.[25,26]

The American Joint Committee on Cancer (AJCC) Tumor, Nodes, Metastases (TNM) system, eighth edition, is the accepted staging system for penile cancer in the United States since 2018 and outside of the United States starting in 2017, with major differences in comparison to the seventh edition.[27] A major difference in the current TNM staging system compared to the previous version is the presence of perineural invasion, which was added as another factor to separate T1a disease from T1b disease. Another difference is the nodal category of pN1, which is now defined as ≤2 unilateral inguinal metastases with no extranodal extension (ENE). Additionally, pN2 is now defined as ≥3 unilateral inguinal metastases or bilateral metastases and pN3 is defined as any ENE or pelvic lymph node metastasis without ENE.[28]

Surgical treatment

Treatment of penile cancer is based on the extent of the primary tumor and its tumor grade, established by biopsy of the lesion, also lymph node metastasis is assessed. Once the tissue diagnosis is confirmed, small superficial tumors (Tis, Ta, and T1a) may be treated successfully with local surgical excision, laser surgery, Mohs' micrographic surgery,[29] or topical therapy.[30,31] Larger tumors with invasion may sometimes be managed with organ-sparing surgery but deeply invasive cancers, particularly those that deform the glans or that involve the shaft structures, may not be amenable to conservative measures. These lesions, which involve the distal shaft or glans, are usually managed by partial penectomy providing that a 2-cm margin can be achieved and still leave enough penile length to allow voiding while standing and to permit intercourse.[32–34] More advanced cancers that involve the base of the penis are best managed by total penectomy with creation of a perineal urethrostomy. Extensive lesions that involve the base of the penis and the bulbar urethral portion may require cystoprostatectomy or even an anterior or total pelvic exenteration with urinary diversion.[32,33]

Inguinal or pelvic lymph node metastasis constitutes an important factor predicting survival in men with SCC of the penis. The superficial ILNs receive lymphatic drainage from the penile shaft and base.[24] The deep ILNs receive drainage from the glans, prepuce, and distal shaft. There is crossover of the lymphatic channels at the base of the penis so that a lesion on one side of the penis may metastasize to the contralateral inguinal nodes. The deep inguinal nodes drain to the external iliac and obturator chains and, subsequently, to the common iliac nodes and the retroperitoneal nodes surrounding the aorta and inferior vena cava.[35]

ILNs are palpable in 50–82% of patients at initial diagnosis, but only in about half of these cases is cancer found on lymph node dissection.[36] The management of patients with suspected clinical lymphadenopathy is usually to first confirm nodal disease and then to determine the extent of disease involvement via a clinical exam, imaging, and percutaneous biopsy. A meticulous inguinal node dissection is curative in 40–60% of cases. Traditional node dissection carries with it the likelihood of morbidity: flap necrosis, wound infection, chronic lymphangitis, lymphocele, and chronic lower limb edema. Lymphadenectomy alone can be curative and should be incorporated into the treatment planning for most patients. However, due to the morbidity of traditional lymphadenectomy, especially among those patients with clinically negative groins, contemporary controversial issues include the following: (1) the selection of patients for lymphadenectomy versus careful observation; (2) the types of procedures to correctly stage the inguinal region with low morbidity; and (3) multimodality strategies (e.g., neoadjuvant chemotherapy) to improve survival among patients with bulky inguinal metastases. Consideration must be given to whether the primary lesion showed any adverse prognostic factors. If one or more of these high-risk features is present, then pathologic ILN staging must be performed. Up to 25% of patients with nonpalpable lymph nodes harbor micrometastases. The EAU determined risk stratification groups for patients with nonpalpable ILNs, with the low-risk group defined as patients with Tis, Ta,G1–2 or T1,G1; the intermediate-risk group as those with T1,G2; and the high-risk group as those with T2 or G3.[37] Therefore, for patients in the high-risk group (T2 or G3) and intermediate-risk patients with lymphovascular invasion, it is recommended to perform a modified or radical inguinal lymphadenectomy. If positive nodes are present on the frozen section, then a superficial and deep inguinal lymphadenectomy should be performed (with consideration of a pelvic lymph node dissection).[38]

For patients with unilateral palpable nodes <4 cm and low-risk primary tumor, fine-needle aspiration of the lymph nodes is considered standard of care. A negative fine-needle aspiration biopsy should be confirmed with an excisional biopsy. Alternatively, active surveillance can be considered following a negative fine-needle aspiration. Positive findings from either procedure warrant an immediate inguinal lymph node dissection (ILND). On the other hand, in patients with high-risk feature on primary tumor, the procedure should be omitted to avoid delay of lymphadenectomy.

For patients with bulky ILNs or pelvic lymph nodes, A negative fine-needle aspiration biopsy should be confirmed with an excisional biopsy. Alternatively, careful surveillance may be considered following a negative fine-needle aspiration. Positive findings from either procedure warrant an immediate ILND. Once metastatic disease is confirmed, a multimodal approach is recommended with neoadjuvant chemotherapy followed by consolidative surgical lymphadenectomy in patients with tumor response.

Chemotherapy

Chemotherapy is used in treating penile cancer as a neoadjuvant or adjuvant setting to definitive surgical or as a radiosensitizer or palliative in the setting of recurrent or visceral metastasis. Neoadjuvant chemotherapy allows for timely delivery of systemic chemotherapy, results in potential volume reduction for enlarged lymphadenopathies, provides prognostic information, and facilitates subsequent surgical consolidation.[39,40] Patients with bulky, fixed, or bilateral inguinal lymphadenopathy typically will not benefit from upfront surgery alone.[41] Neoadjuvant systemic therapy for these patients is currently recommended as the preferred strategy by the NCCN and the EAU guidelines.[38,42] Unfortunately, there are currently no clinical or pathological factors that can accurately predict a patient's benefit from neoadjuvant chemotherapy.[43–45] The only predictor of better survival after neoadjuvant chemotherapy is achievement of a pathological complete response (pCR) at the time of consolidative surgery.[46]

The most relevant trial that established the approach of neoadjuvant chemotherapy followed by surgery as the standard of care is a Phase 2 clinical trial by Pagliaro et al.[46] The trial used neoadjuvant chemotherapy: paclitaxel 175 mg/m^2 administered over three hours on day 1; ifosfamide 1200 mg/m^2 on days 1–3; and cisplatin 25 mg/m^2 on days 1–3 every three weeks (TIP), with the goal of completing a total of four cycles before proceeding with consolidation surgery. The study showed that 15 patients (50.0%) had an objective response, with 3 CRs and 12 PRs, and 22 patients (73.3%) subsequently underwent consolidation surgery. The estimated median TTP was 8.1 months (95% CI, 5.4–50 months) and median overall survival (OS) was 17.1 months (95% CI, 10.3–60 months).[46,47] Additional retrospective studies confirmed that neoadjuvant chemotherapy in this setting resulted in an objective response rate of 50% and a pCR-rate in 10–15% of patients[48]. Unfortunately, the survival outcomes remained dismal despite the use of perioperative chemotherapy added to radical surgery, and less than 50% of the patients are alive at 10 years.

On the other hand, the role of adjuvant chemotherapy is less validated; only small retrospective studies have been reported, as well as large retrospective and multicenter case series. Like in the neoadjuvant setting, the use of combination chemotherapy that includes taxanes and cisplatin is supported by the literature data.[49] Recently, a large multicenter retrospective study assessed 141 patients with advanced pathological pelvic lymph node involvement and demonstrated a median OS improvement with the use of adjuvant chemotherapy.[50] This study does highlight a potential benefit of adjuvant chemotherapy use for patients with pelvic lymphadenopathy who did not receive neoadjuvant chemotherapy. NCCN guidelines recommend using adjuvant chemotherapy if neoadjuvant chemotherapy was not given, with level 2A evidence, for patients with high pathological risk features (pathological N2, N3, or ECE).[38] Similarly, there is level 2B evidence for adjuvant chemotherapy if neoadjuvant chemotherapy was not given in the current EAU guidelines, and this should be regarded as a treatment option only for patients with pathological N2 or N3 disease after lymphadenectomy.[42] As for patients with pathological N1 disease, the EAU guidelines recommend adjuvant therapy only in the setting of clinical trials.[42] Tumor biomarkers that could allow for better patient selection are desperately needed in this disease. Preliminary data from a single retrospective study pointed to the role of TP53 immunohistochemical expression as a potentially suitable tool to identify those case with TP53-expressing and a predicted poor outcome after adjuvant taxane, cisplatin, and 5FU.[51]

Radiotherapy

Primary RT of primary penile cancers is used more widely in Europe than in the United States but may be appropriate for small superficial lesions or for selected larger lesions when organ preservation is the goal, or when patients refuse surgery.[52–54] Tissue preservation may not be feasible in more advanced lesions, however. Randomized trials comparing RT to surgery have not been reported. In one study of clinically localized penile cancer, local regional relapse occurred in 56% of those treated with definitive primary radiation therapy compared to 13% of those treated by surgery. Of the RT failures, 73% were salvaged with surgery.[55]

RT with concurrent chemotherapy has become a standard management strategy for locally advanced head and neck, vulvar, and anal squamous cancers,[56–58] but its use in the perioperative setting in locally advanced PSCC is limited.[59] The EAU penile cancer guidelines group recently conducted a systematic review of the evidence and concluded that, because of the heterogeneous and limited evidence showing clinical benefit, a routine recommendation of adjuvant RT is not at this time warranted.[60] Further clinical trials evaluating the role of concurrent chemotherapy with radiation are needed in both the neoadjuvant and adjuvant setting. Nevertheless, the current standard of care for locally advanced PSCC with bulky lymph node metastasis is supported by limited data for neoadjuvant chemotherapy with TIP as the preferred regimen, followed by consolidation surgery.[46]

Acute radiation reactions—edema, tissue inflammation, skin irritation, tenderness, and dysuria—are common. Such symptoms usually subside promptly when therapy is completed. Long-term effects of radiation may include telangiectasia, hyperpigmentation, diminished sensation, scarring, and atrophy of the treated tissues. Fibrotic change and fistulization may occur in large lesions where significant tissue damage has occurred before the RT. Late recurrences in radiated sites may occur up to a decade after definitive treatment, affirming that close follow-up is essential.

Prognosis

Left untreated, squamous carcinoma of the penis is invariably lethal, killing most of those afflicted within three years. Outcome is directly related to the extent of the disease at diagnosis and the presence or absence of inguinal metastases.[24] A large European experience reports that the 5-year cancer-specific survival of patients with cN0 disease treated between 2001 and 2012 was 92%, significantly improved since 1994, the year dynamic sentinel node biopsy was introduced in Europe. It has been shown that ENE, number of tumor-positive nodes, and pelvic involvement in node-positive cases are associated with worse cancer-specific outcomes.[24] Therefore, the use of neoadjuvant chemotherapy for such cases is recommended. Most of these patients with bulky or advanced disease will have disease recurrence. Unfortunately, patients with disease recurrence after cisplatin-based chemotherapy and a surgical consolidation, have few treatment options with limited survival.[61]

Carcinoma of the urethra

Epidemiology and risk factors
A SEER database review found primary urethral carcinoma was identified in 1075 men and 540 women, with an annual age-adjusted incidence rate of 4.3 per million and 1.5 per million, respectively.[62] The annual incidence rate increased with age to a peak of 32 per million men and 9.5 per million women in the 75- to 84-year age group.[62] The rate was 5.0 per million and 2.5 per million for African Americans and whites, respectively. The histologic types were transitional cell carcinoma in 888 patients (55%), SCC in 348 (21.5%), and adenocarcinoma in 265 (16.4%).[62]

Although the etiology of urethral cancer is not well understood, the main risk factors that have been associated with urethral cancer include, chronic inflammation and HPV infection.[63–66]

Diagnosis and staging
The initial diagnosis should be confirmed with a required biopsy and review by a specialized pathologist followed by a physical examination and evaluation of the palpable portion of the urethra as well as the ILNs. A cystourethroscopy should be done to assess the extent of disease. Retrograde urethrography in men can help establish the exact location and extent of disease and urine cytology should be sent. It is important to know that the sensitivity of cytology is low, and the definitive diagnosis should be made with transurethral biopsies. Also, cross-sectional imaging using computed tomography or MRI with chest imaging should be performed for complete staging of the locoregional spread of cancer. The TNM staging system is used for staging carcinoma of the urethra. The eighth edition of this system (2017) is supported by both the AJCC and the Union for International Cancer Control (UICC). Staging is based on depth of invasion of the primary tumor and the presence or absence of regional lymph node involvement and distant metastasis. Staging will help guide the general treatment approach for this rare and heterogenous disease. The treatment approaches are based on the tumor location, extent and histology, and patient gender, according to retrospective case series and extrapolation from the management of other malignancies of the urinary tract. Generally, for patients with localized disease to the primary tumor only upfront surgery is preferred. On the other hand, for patients with locally advanced disease with lymph node metastasis, a multimodal approach is preferred with neoadjuvant chemotherapy or chemotherapy with radiation followed by surgical resection in patients with tumor regression. For patients with disease that is progressing after initial therapy or those with distant metastasis palliative intent systemic therapy is recommended.

According to an analysis made from the database of Foundation Medicine Inc. urothelial carcinoma and SCC subtypes were more common in men, while adenocarcinoma and clear cell were more prevalent in women. Looking deeper at the genomic signature specific genes were more prominently effect in specific histologies. As an example, *ERBB2* mutations were present in all subtypes, while *FGFR1-3* alterations were present in SCC and *BRAF* in adenocarcinoma. These alterations have known therapeutic targets and might help guide clinicians in clinical decision-making.[67] A potential for immunotherapy benefit associated with higher TMB and PD-L1 staining levels were seen in urothelial carcinoma and SCC subtypes compared to adenocarcinoma and clear-cell tumors.

Male urethral carcinoma
The male urethra averages some 18 cm in length and is subdivided into the penile urethra, the membranous urethra, and the prostatic urethra. Beginning distally, the penile urethra is composed of the meatus and fossa navicularis, which is lined with stratified squamous epithelium. The pendulous urethra extends from the proximal fossa navicularis to the suspensory ligament of the penis, where it then becomes the bulbar urethra between the ligament and the urogenital membrane. These areas are lined with stratified or pseudo-stratified columnar epithelium as is the short (1.5 cm) membranous urethra. This contains the external sphincter, which is composed of striated muscle fibers. The prostatic urethra passes through the prostate and is lined with transitional cell epithelium. From 50% to 75% of male urethral cancers arise in the bulbar urethra. The remainder occurs predominantly in the fossa navicularis. About 90% of male urethral tumors demonstrate SCC histology.[68] Stricture of the urethra is often a result of the cancer. Transitional cell or undifferentiated carcinomas usually predominate at the bladder neck and within the prostatic urethra. Poorly differentiated transitional cell carcinomas often exhibit squamous characteristics. Adenocarcinoma can arise in the glands of Littre or the prostatic utricle but are rare. Metastasis to the penis from other organ sites is also rare. Obstructive symptoms are common in proximal lesions, while urethral bleeding and a palpable mass characterize cancers of the penile urethra. In general, the more proximal a tumor, and the longer its delay in diagnosis, the higher the stage is. If the urethra is retained following cystectomy for bladder cancer, urethral tumors if they develop are usually transitional cell carcinomas. If urethrectomy is a component of cystectomy for bladder cancer, the entire structure, including the fossa navicularis, must be excised.[69] Lymphatic draining of the distal urethra is like that of PSCC. Tumors of the fossa and pendulous urethra drain to the superficial ILNs, whereas tumors of the bulbar, membranous, and prostatic urethral segments drain to the iliac obturator and presacral node groups. Crossover metastasis may occur at the prepubic lymphatic plexus.

Surgical management
Low-grade, low-stage tumors of the urethra are uncommon but can be managed by transurethral resection or laser fulguration. Biopsy is essential to establish histopathology and the depth of the neoplasm. Patients with noninvasive urothelial carcinomas of the prostate may be treated with transurethral resection in addition to adjuvant Bacillus Calmètte–Guerin (BCG) therapy, with reports showing 5-year recurrence-free survival rates of 90%.[70–72] Partial penectomy with at least a 2 cm margin may be adequate if the tumor does not involve the corpus spungiosum or the corpora cavernosa.[64,68,69] Advanced or more proximal lesions usually require total penectomy and creation of a perineal urethrostomy. Patients with locally advanced disease (T2 to T4) should be treated with multimodal therapy including histology-directed neoadjuvant chemotherapy or chemotherapy with radiation. In patients that have tumor response, extensive surgical resection will follow, to include penectomy and cystoprostatectomy with perineal reconstruction and anterior pelvic exenteration. Patients who have tumors abutting the inferior pubic ramus should undergo en bloc inferior pubectomy, and those with inguinal lymphadenopathy should undergo inguinal lymphadenectomy.

Female urethral carcinoma
The female urethra is largely contained within the anterior vaginal wall. In the adult, it is 2–4 cm in length. It is lined distally with stratified squamous epithelium changing to columnar epithelium proximally. At the bladder neck, transitional cell epithelium is found. A urethral diverticulum in the distal urethra may be a remnant of Wolffian or ectopic cloacal epithelium. The histopathology

of female urethral cancer depends on the cell of origin. Squamous carcinoma is the most frequent, comprising about 50% of tumors. Transitional cell carcinoma and adenocarcinoma are about 25% each. Tumor grade apparently does not influence metastasis and prognosis as much as in men. Mixed tumors, undifferentiated carcinomas, melanoma, cloacogenic carcinoma, and clear cell adenocarcinomas are rare but do occur. Urethral carcinomas spread first by local extension and then metastasize by lymphatic channels and hematogenously. Lymphatic drainage of the distal urethra and the labia leads to the superficial and deep inguinal nodes. Proximal urethral drainage leads to iliac, obturator, presacral, and preaortic nodes. Palpable adenopathy is present at presentation in up to half the patients and almost always represents metastatic cancer.[73] Adenocarcinomas more commonly metastasize to distant sites hematogenously, including liver, lung, brain, and skeleton.

Surgical management

Most urethral tumors in women present with bleeding or dysuria because of a urethral mass. Distal urethral lesions generally are diagnosed early at a low stage. Local excision, partial urethrectomy, RT, and laser ablation have all been employed with some success. Higher stage more extensive urethral carcinomas can be managed with cystourethrectomy and an ileal urinary diversion (i.e., ileal conduit or catheterizable stoma), or when bladder preservation is possible, interposition of the amputated vermiform appendix as a conduit to the surface (the Mitrofanoff procedure). Proximal lesions present later and at a higher stage than distal lesions. Obstructive symptomology is the hallmark of proximal urethral lesions. Extensive lesions that involve the bladder or the vaginal wall may necessitate cystectomy or even anterior exenteration with urinary diversion. Local recurrence is common. Positive inguinal nodes by clinical or imaging techniques may require neoadjuvant chemotherapy followed by extensive surgical resection to include anterior pelvic exenteration, including anterior vaginectomy. Patients who have tumors abutting the inferior pubic ramus should undergo en bloc inferior pubectomy.

Neoadjuvant and adjuvant therapy

Because most urethral cancers carry a poor prognosis from surgery alone, if they are not superficial and local, chemotherapeutic regimens appropriate for the tumor type have been used as adjuvant treatment.

Neoadjuvant therapy with chemotherapy or chemoradiotherapy can decrease tumor size and the extent of surgery required to treat a primary urethral carcinoma. The potential role of such perioperative therapy was shown by a multicenter retrospective study of 124 patients with primary urethral cancer in which only 39 received perioperative or adjuvant chemotherapy or chemoradiotherapy. The study had 12 with neoadjuvant chemotherapy, 6 with neoadjuvant chemotherapy plus RT, and 21 with adjuvant chemotherapy.[74,75] With a median follow up of 21 months, the 3-year OS rate for the eight patients who received neoadjuvant therapy was 100%, while 50% of those treated with surgery alone and 20% of those given surgery plus adjuvant chemotherapy were alive at three years.

The choice of chemotherapy regimen is based on histology, knowing the heterogenous pathology of this cancer. For patients with urothelial carcinoma, options include cisplatin, gemcitabine, with or without ifosfamide (GC or CGI); ifosfamide, paclitaxel, and cisplatin (TIP); or dose-dense methotrexate, vinblastine, doxorubicin, and cisplatin (ddMVAC). As for patients with SCC, they are treated with TIP if they can tolerate it.

Radiation therapy is also used as adjuvant therapy or as definitive therapy concurrently with systemic chemotherapy for patients that refuse surgery and offers potential for genital preservation. The largest, retrospective series included 25 patients with locally advanced SCC of the urethra treated with two cycles of 5-fluorouracil and mitomycin C with concurrent radiatiotherapy[76] This study reported a complete response rate to primary chemoradiotherapy of 79% with a 5-year OS and disease-specific survival of 52% and 68%, respectively.[76]

Key references

The complete reference list can be found on Vital Source version of this title, see inside front cover.

1. Siegel RL, Miller KD, Jemal A. Cancer statistics, 2020. *CA Cancer J Clin*. 2020;**70**(1):7–30. doi: 10.3322/caac.21590.
4. Olesen TB, Sand FL, Rasmussen CL, et al. Prevalence of human papillomavirus DNA and p16 INK4a in penile cancer and penile intraepithelial neoplasia: a systematic review and meta-analysis. *Lancet Oncol*. 2019;**20**(1):145–158.
11. Gunia S, Erbersdobler A, Hakenberg OW, et al. p16[INK4a] is a marker of good prognosis for primary invasive penile squamous cell carcinoma: a multi-institutional study. *J Urol*. 2012;**187**(3):899–907. doi: 10.1016/j.juro.2011.10.149.
12. Cubilla AL, Velazquez EF, Amin MB, et al. The World Health Organisation 2016 classification of penile carcinomas: a review and update from the International Society of Urological Pathology expert-driven recommendations. *Histopathology*. 2018;**72**(6):893–904. doi: 10.1111/his.13429.
13. Chahoud J, Pham R, Guo M, et al. p16INK4a expression and survival outcomes in patients with penile squamous cell carcinoma: The M.D. Anderson Cancer Center Experience. *J Clin Oncol*. 2020;**38**(6_suppl):5–5. doi: 10.1200/jco.2020.38.6_suppl.5.
16. Heyns CF, Mendoza-Valdés A, Pompeo ACL. Diagnosis and staging of penile cancer. *Urology*. 2010;**76**(2 Suppl 1):S15–S23.
23. Horenblas S, Van Tinteren H. Squamous cell carcinoma of the penis. IV. prognostic factors of survival: analysis of tumor, nodes and metastasis classification system. *J Urol*. 1994;**151**(5):1239–1243. doi: 10.1016/S0022-5347(17)35221-7.
26. NCCN. *Penile Cancer*. National Comprehensive Cancer Network; 2018.
28. Pettaway CA, Srigley JR, Brookland RK. Penis cancer. In: Amin MB, ed. *AJCC Cancer Staging Manual*, 8th ed. Springer International Publishing; 2017:701–715.
32. Agrawal A, Pal D, Ananthakrishnan N, et al. The histological extent of the local spread of carcinoma of the penis and its therapeutic implications. *BJU Int*. 2000;**85**(3):299–301. doi: 10.1046/j.1464-410X.2000.00413.x.
33. Minhas S, Kayes O, Hegarty P, et al. What surgical resection margins are required to achieve oncological control in men with primary penile cancer? *BJU Int*. 2005;**96**(7):1040–1043. doi: 10.1111/j.1464-410X.2005.05769.x.
38. Clark PE, Spiess PE, Agarwal N, et al. Penile cancer: clinical practice guidelines in oncology. *J Natl Compr Canc Netw*. 2013;**11**(5):594–615.
40. Necchi A. Systemic therapy for penile cancer. *Eur Urol Suppl*. 2018;**17**(6):160–163.
46. Pagliaro LC, Williams DL, Daliani D, et al. Neoadjuvant paclitaxel, ifosfamide, and cisplatin chemotherapy for metastatic penile cancer: a phase II study. *J Clin Oncol*. 2010;**28**(24):3851–3857.
48. Necchi A, Pond GR, Raggi D, et al. Clinical outcomes of perioperative chemotherapy in patients with locally advanced penile squamous-cell carcinoma: results of a multicenter analysis. *Clin Genitourin Cancer*. 2017;**15**(5):548–555.e3. doi: 10.1016/j.clgc.2017.02.002.
51. Necchi A, Lo Vullo S, Nicolai N, et al. Prognostic factors of adjuvant taxane, cisplatin, and 5-fluorouracil chemotherapy for patients with penile squamous cell carcinoma after regional lymphadenectomy. In: *Clinical Genitourinary Cancer*, Vol. 14. Elsevier Inc.; 2016:518–523. doi: 10.1016/j.clgc.2016.03.005.
54. Khalil MI, Wan F, Eltahawy E, et al. Survival following salvage surgery after failed radiotherapy for penile cancer: a SEER-based study. *Curr Urol*. 2019:142–146. doi: 10.1159/000489432.
59. Johnstone PAS, Boulware D, Djajadiningrat R, et al. Primary penile cancer: the role of adjuvant radiation therapy in the management of extranodal extension in lymph nodes. *Eur Urol Focus*. 2019;**5**(5):737–741.
61. Wang J, Pettaway CA, Pagliaro LC. Treatment for metastatic penile cancer after first-line chemotherapy failure: analysis of response and survival outcomes. *Urology*. 2015;**85**(5):1104–1110. doi: 10.1016/j.urology.2014.12.049.
67. Grivas P, Jacob JM, Shapiro O, et al. Comprehensive genomic profiling (CGP) of histologic subtypes of urethral carcinomas (UrthCa). *J Clin Oncol*. 2020;**38**(15_suppl):5087–5087. doi: 10.1200/jco.2020.38.15_suppl.5087.

97 Testis cancer

Michael Hawking, MD ■ Gladell Paner, MD ■ Scott Eggener, MD ■ Walter M. Stadler, MD

> **Overview**
>
> This chapter reviews the epidemiology, pathology, and standardized therapy for this group of malignancies.

Cancer of the testis is a relatively uncommon disease, accounting for approximately 1% of all cancers in males. However, it represents a highly curable neoplasm, and the incidence is highest in young patients with an extremely long estimated life expectancy. The goal of initial therapy is never palliation or prolongation of survival, but cure.

Epidemiology

Incidence
Age-related incidence of testicular cancer reveals a bimodal distribution. The major peak occurs between ages 15 and 35 years, owing almost exclusively to tumors of germ cell origin, which account for approximately 95% of all testicular cancer. Embryonal carcinoma represents the predominant histopathologic diagnosis up to the age of 35 years, after which seminoma is more common. From 2013 to 2017, the median age at diagnosis for cancer of the testis was 33.[1]

The incidence of testicular cancer varies based on geographic distribution. The incidence is highest in northern Europe and North America and lowest in Asia and Africa. There is also a long recognized striking influence of race, with the incidence among black and Hispanic males worldwide far less than their white counterparts.[2,3] In the United States, estimates of the incidence ratio between white and African–American patients ranges from 4 to 5 : 1. Testicular cancer appears to be increasing among young white males in the United States and Europe.[4] Standardized incidence rates increased annually 2–5%, with marginal differences between seminomas and nonseminomas. In the United States, the annual percentage change from 2008 to 2017 was 0.8%. It is estimated approximately 9500 cases of testicular cancer were diagnosed in the United States in 2020, with approximately 440 dying of the disease.[5]

Risk factors
Cryptorchidism is the major identifiable risk factor associated with the development of testicular cancer, with a risk ratio reported between 2.5 and 14 in case-control studies.[6] The location of the maldescended testicle appears to be an important cofactor, because those patients with intra-abdominal retention have a fourfold higher incidence of malignancy than if the testicle is retained in the inguinal canal. It seems unlikely maldescent alone represents the initiating event in the development of germ cell tumors: Only 10% of testicular tumors are associated with cryptorchidism, whereas 10–20% of the malignancies in patients with cryptorchidism occur in the contralateral, normally descended testicle; prepubertal orchiopexy fails to prevent the subsequent development of malignancy in the undescended testicle; and first-degree male relatives of patients with testicular cancer exhibit an increased incidence of cryptorchidism, hydroceles, and inguinal hernias, as well as testicular cancer.[7,8] These data suggest some genetic predisposition and/or in utero environmental event may result in several genitourinary developmental abnormalities, including maldescent and germ cell neoplasia. In fact, an increase in the frequency of cryptorchidism has been observed and appears to parallel the timing and magnitude of the increase in incidence of testicular cancer.

Notably, patients with a history of unilateral testicular cancer are at risk of developing cancer in the other testicle. For example, Fossa et al.[9] evaluated the risk of contralateral testicular cancer and survival in a large population-based cohort of men diagnosed with testicular cancer before age 55 years using surveillance, epidemiology, and end results (SEER) data. Among 29,515 testicular cancer cases from 1973 through 2001, a total of 175 men presented with synchronous contralateral testicular cancer and 287 men developed metachronous contralateral testicular cancer (observed/expected = 12.4 [95% CI = 11.0–13.9%]; 15-year cumulative risk = 1.9% [95% CI = 1.7–2.1%]). The low absolute cumulative risk of metachronous contralateral testicular cancer and favorable overall survival of patients diagnosed with metachronous contralateral testicular cancer is in accordance with the current US approach of not performing a biopsy nor routine radiographic/serologic screening of the contralateral testis, although self-examination is encouraged.

There is a familial component to testicular cancer. Brothers of men with testicular germ cell tumors have an 8-fold to 10-fold risk of developing TGCT, whereas the relative risk to fathers and sons is approximately fourfold. This familial relative risk is much higher than for most other types of cancer, with estimations of heritability as high as nearly 50% with at least 44 independent risk loci identified.[10,11] More specifically, there is evidence that alterations in the *CHEK2* gene (associated with a variety of other cancers), may predispose to TGCT via DNA repair deficiency.[12]

An additional predisposition is the association of mediastinal nonseminomatous germ cell tumors (NSGCT) with Klinefelter's syndrome, with an estimated 1 out of every 4000 Klinefelter patients diagnosed with mediastinal nonseminoma.[13] Testicular germ cell tumors, particularly seminomas, also occur at an increased rate in men with HIV/AIDS; although, this difference has greatly diminished in the era of effective antiretrovirals.[14]

Holland-Frei Cancer Medicine, Tenth Edition. Edited by Robert C. Bast, John C. Byrd, Carlo M. Croce, Ernest Hawk, Fadlo R. Khuri, Raphael E. Pollock, Apostolia M. Tsimberidou, Christopher G. Willett, and Cheryl L. Willman.
© 2023 John Wiley & Sons, Inc. Published 2023 by John Wiley & Sons, Inc.

Pathology

Origin and molecular genetics

Testicular tumors fall into several broad groups (Table 1). Classification of the germ cell tumors has been based on morphology, but recent molecular studies have yielded a more ontological scheme consisting of five distinct subtypes that differ in their proposed cell of origin.[15] Accordingly, teratomas and yolk sac tumors arising in neonates and young children are derived from primordial germ cells or very early gonocytes distributed along the gonadal ridge or in the testis/ovary. These tumors retain most of the genomic imprinting from both parental genomes. The teratomas remain diploid, while the yolk sac tumors show gains of chromosomes 1q, 12p13-14, and 20q, and losses of 1p, 4, and 6q.[15]

Spermatocytic tumor is a second, distinct subtype of germ cell tumor thought to derive from postpubertal spermatogonia/spermatocytes. Accordingly, these tumors have a paternal pattern of genomic imprinting and show variable ploidy.[16]

Two of the other five proposed subtypes of germ cell tumor do not occur in the testis. Dermoid cysts of the ovary, which are thought to arise from oogonia/oocytes, are diploid/tetraploid and show maternal genomic imprinting. Hydatidiform mole (gestational trophoblastic disease) is a placental-derived neoplasm that contains a purely paternal genome as a result of fertilization of an empty ovum.

The fifth subtype of germ cell tumor consists of seminoma and the NSGCT, accounting for 95% of primary testicular neoplasms (Table 1). Variants also occur/originate in the ovary (dysgerminoma), anterior mediastinum, retroperitoneum, dysgenic gonad, and midline brain (germinoma). It is suggested seminoma and NSGCT are derived from gonocytes that have lost their genomic imprinting as a result of being later in their development than those that give rise to infantile teratomas and yolk sac tumors. These gonocytes are polypoid (triploid or tetraploid), probably because of meiotic arrest. Depending on exactly when this arrest occurs during fetal development, the affected cells may be distributed to one or both testes, accounting for the bilateral germ cell tumors observed in 2–3% of patients.

Seminomas and NSGCT share a common precursor lesion previously called intratubular germ cell neoplasia, unclassified (ITGCNU) but 2016 World Health Organization (WHO) guidelines renamed it as germ cell neoplasia *in situ* (GCNIS).[17] Growing in situ within seminiferous tubules, GCNIS cells express markers shared with embryonic stem cells, including the transcription factors OCT3/4 and NANOG.[18,19] These factors are essential to the development of embryonic stem cells in mice but are not expressed in normal spermatogonia in mice or humans. Their presence in GCNIS supports the theory that a pluripotent gonocyte is the cell of origin for both seminoma and NSGCT. In addition, OCT3/4 serves as a specific immunohistochemical marker in the diagnosis of extra-TGCTs (Table 2).[19,20]

Table 1 Primary tumors of the testis.

Type	Relative frequency	Genotype/comments
Germ cell tumors		
Infants and children	~1% of all testis tumors	
Yolk sac tumor	65–80% of prepubertal	Aneuploid
Teratoma	20–35% of prepubertal	Diploid; mature elements; benign
Adolescents and adults	95% of all testis tumors	
GCNIS	>90% of postpubertal	Aneuploid (near triploid)
Seminoma	~55% of postpubertal	Aneuploid (near triploid); iso12p
Nonseminomatous (NSGCT)	~45% of postpubertal	Aneuploid (near triploid); iso12p
Embryonal carcinoma	~75% of NSGCT	
Yolk sac tumor	~50% of NSGCT	
Teratoma	~50% of NSGCT	Malignant (even mature elements)
Choriocarcinoma	~10% of NSGCT	
Adults (usually >50 yr)		
Spermatocytic seminoma	<1% of postpubertal	Variable ploidy; gain of chromosome 9
Spermatocytic seminoma with sarcoma	Very rare	
Sex-cord stromal tumors		
Leydig cell tumor	~3% of all testis tumors	7–10% metastasis (postpubertal)
Sertoli cell tumor	<1% of all testis tumors	
Granulosa cell tumor		
Adult type	Very rare	
Juvenile type	Uncommon	Infants <6 months
Mixed/indeterminate	Rare	
Mixed germ cell/sex-cord stromal tumors		
Gonadoblastoma	Very rare	

Table 2 Markers of testicular germ cell tumors.

Morphologic subtype	Serum	Immunohistochemistry	FISH
GCNIS		PLAP, KIT, OCT3/4	
Seminoma	HCG (10–15%)	PLAP, KIT, OCT3/4	Excess 12p
Embryonal carcinoma	HCG	PLAP, CD30, OCT3/4	Excess 12p
Yolk sac tumor	AFP	AFP, PLAP, Glypican 3	Excess 12p
Choriocarcinoma	HCG (typically high)	HCG	Excess 12p
Teratoma			Excess 12p

Abbreviations: AFP, α-fetoprotein; FISH, fluorescence *in situ* hybridization; HCG, human choriogonadotropin; PLAP, placental/germ cell alkaline phosphatase.

Progression of GCNIS to an invasive germ cell tumor is accompanied by a number of common events.[21] One is the acquisition of excess genetic material from the short arm of chromosome 12. In 80% of cases, this is accomplished through loss of 12q and reduplication of 12p (i12p), while in 20%, the additional 12p sequences are distributed among other derivative chromosomes. Interestingly, the embryonic stem cell gene NANOG is on 12p. Fluorescence *in situ* hybridization (FISH) for 12p is used in paraffin sections as a diagnostic marker for germ cell tumors and also for nongerm cell derivatives.

Additional events associated with malignant progression of GCNIS include loss of expression of the homeobox gene *NKX3.1*,[22] loss of the tumor suppressor PTEN,[23] and decreased expression of the cell cycle regulator p21.[24] Mutations of TP53 are rare in postpubertal germ cell tumors, but the effects of this important tumor suppressor may be through MDM2 overexpression,[24] or downregulation of LATS2 by micro-RNAs mi-R372 and mi-R373.[25]

Although seminoma and NSGCT share a common origin, they are clinicopathologically distinct cancers. Little is known of what determines their differences, but oncogenic mutations in KIT (a receptor tyrosine kinase) are found in 25% of seminomas and are essentially absent in NSGCT. These mutations may occur very early in seminoma tumorigenesis, as they are present in GCNIS, and in dysgerminoma/germinoma of the ovary, mediastinum, and brain. Based on studies in mice, *KIT* gene function is essential to the development of primordial germ cells and to normal spermatogenesis; therefore, constitutive activation of this kinase may favor the seminoma pathway. Unfortunately, KIT kinase inhibitors such as imatinib are of no benefit to seminoma patients harboring KIT-mutant tumors, because most of the published mutations are inherently resistant to the available drugs. It is thought that NSGCT develops after GCNIS and intratubular seminoma are reprogrammed to become an embryonal carcinoma cell, likened to a pluripotent embryonal stem cell capable of differentiating to other cell types, however, the exact mechanism is still unclear.

Seminoma

Seminomas are slightly more common than NSGCT, especially in cryptorchid testes, for which they constitute approximately 60% of the cases. On gross examination, such tumors are generally homogeneous and well demarcated. Distinct lobulation may be apparent, with the nodules separated by dense fibrous bands. Areas of necrosis and hemorrhage are usually discrete or absent. Microscopically, there is a monotonous distribution of uniform, rounded cells with large, centralized nuclei and nucleoli. The cytoplasm may be either clear or granular and will frequently stain for glycogen, lipid, and/or placental/germ cell alkaline phosphatase (PLAP). The seminoma cells are usually arranged in nests surrounded by fibrous septa with infiltrate rich in T-lymphocytes and containing occasional granulomas (Figure 1). Granulomatous reaction composed of epithelioid histiocytes may occur and if florid may mimic granulomatous orchitis.

Seminoma presents most commonly in the fourth and fifth decades, usually as an enlarging, painless testicular mass. Approximately 70% of patients present with stage I disease, 20% with stage II, and only rarely with visceral disease or above the diaphragm (stage III). Lymphatic spread is typically to the retroperitoneal lymph nodes then to the mediastinal or supraclavicular lymph nodes. Hematogenous dissemination to the lung, liver, bone, or adrenal is a late occurrence. Seminomas contain syncytiotrophoblastic giant cells that stain for human chorionic gonadotropin

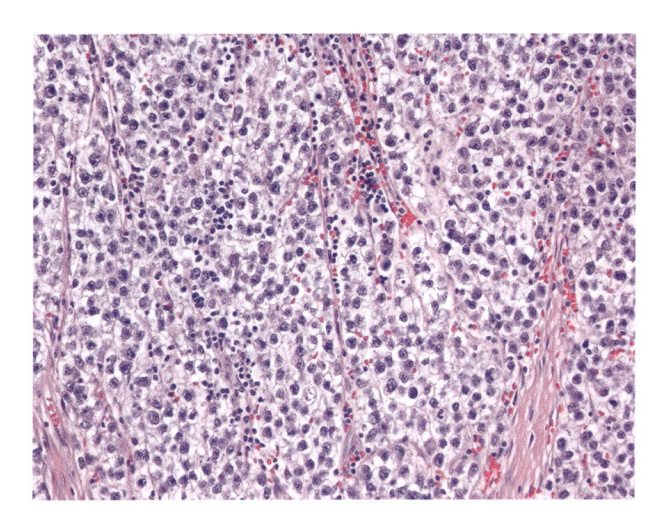

Figure 1 Small nests of seminoma cells with cytoplasmic clearing are separated by thin fibrous septa with lymphoid infiltrates.

(HCG). Low-level HCG elevation is seen in 5–10% of patients with pure seminoma and likely reflects syncytiotrophoblastic elements present within the tumor (Table 2). Seminoma does not secrete α-fetoprotein (AFP).

Nonseminomatous germ cell tumors

The most common postpubertal germ cell tumors of the testis are composed of one or more elements that are collectively known as "nonseminomatous." Four morphologic patterns, detailed below, are recognized among this group. In most cases, these patterns are intermixed in varying proportions (termed "mixed germ cell tumors"). Areas of seminoma may also be included but diagnosis and clinical management follow nonseminoma paradigms when there are any elements of nonseminoma. These germ cell tumors are more aggressive than pure seminomas and tend to present about one decade earlier, on average.

Embryonal carcinoma

Embryonal carcinoma is present in up to 90% of NSGCT cases. Macroscopically, it forms a soft, fleshy, inhomogeneous mass often with areas of necrosis and hemorrhage. Direct invasion of the spermatic cord, epididymis, and tunica albuginea can occur.

The microscopic appearance is extremely variable and may include papillary, solid, tubular, and glandular patterns, frequently interrupted by geographic necrosis (Figure 2). Large polygonal pleomorphic cells with indistinct cytoplasmic borders (unlike seminoma) are the rule, with pale granular cytoplasm, large nuclei, and one or more centrally placed nucleoli. Mitotic figures and multinucleated cells are common.

Yolk sac tumor

Yolk sac tumor, formerly called endodermal sinus tumor, is present in approximately half of NSGCT cases but is rare in pure form in the postpubertal patient.[26] The most readily recognized pattern consists of a cluster of tumor cells surrounding a small central blood vessel (Schiller–Duval body). The morphologic spectrum is broad, including microcystic (lacelike), micropapillary, solid, and hepatoid patterns (Figure 3). The tumor cell nuclei are smaller than those of embryonal carcinoma. Cytoplasmic globules are common and stain for AFP, which accounts for the serum elevations characteristically present in patients with this tumor (Table 2).

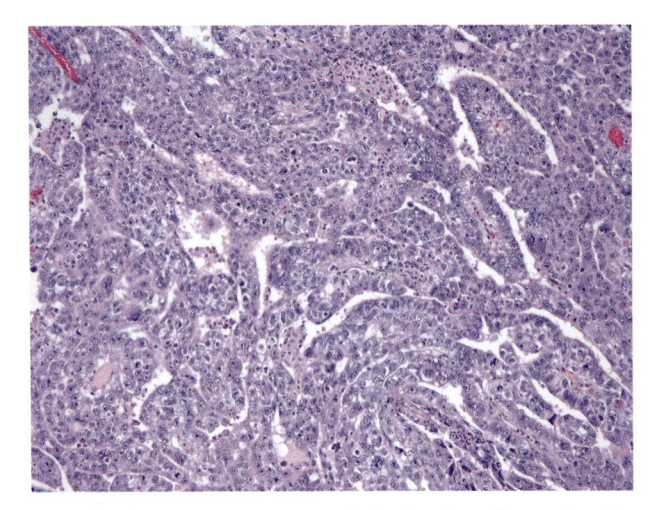

Figure 2 Embryonal carcinoma. Irregularly shaped papillae are lined by mitotically active pleomorphic cells with vesicular, crowded nuclei, and poorly defined cytoplasmic membranes.

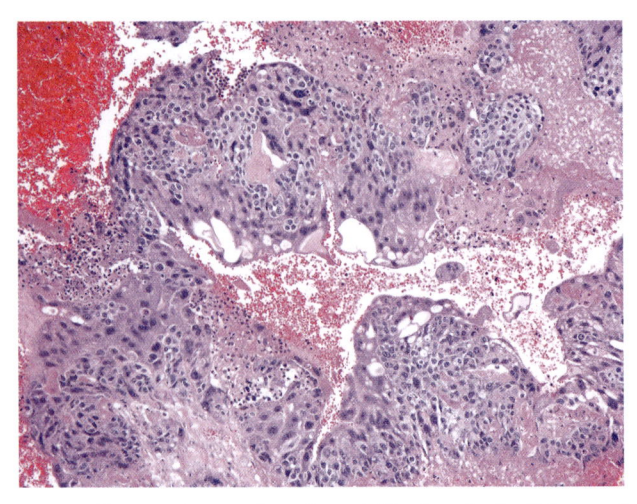

Figure 4 Choriocarcinoma. Syncytiotrophoblastic cells "cap" layers of mononucleated cytotrophoblast reminiscent of placental villi. Note the hemorrhagic background.

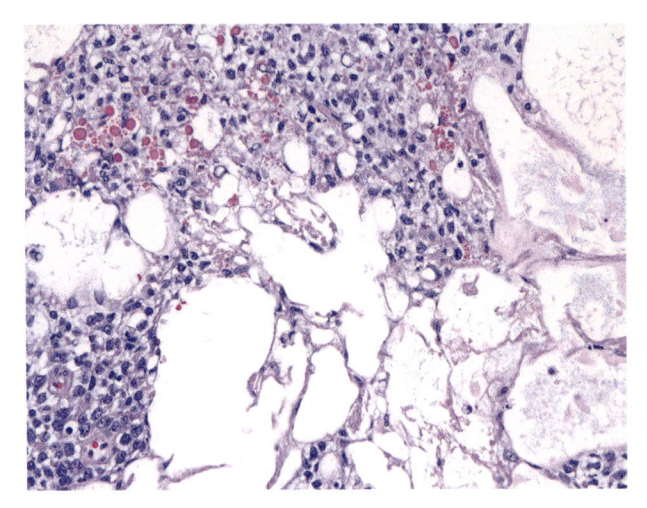

Figure 3 Yolk sac tumor-forming microcysts and solid growth with abundant cytoplasmic globules.

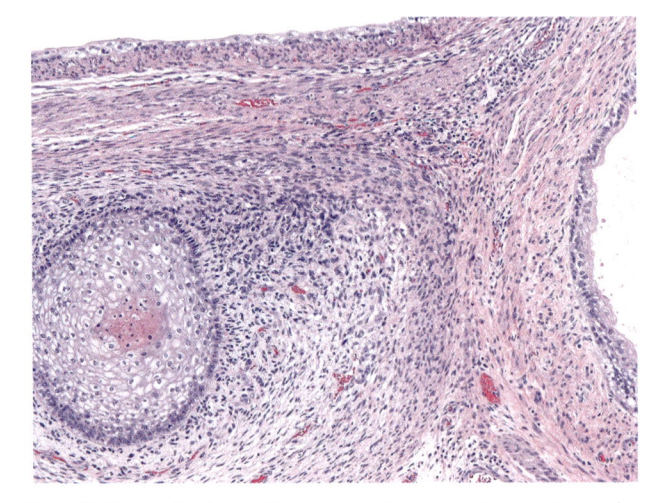

Figure 5 Mature teratoma. There are mature-appearing portions of a pilosebaceous unit, bundles of smooth muscle, and bronchial respiratory epithelium.

In its pure form, yolk sac tumor is the most common testicular neoplasm in infants and young children (Table 1). Despite morphologic similarity to the subtype observed in postpubertal NSGCT, the pediatric tumor is an oncogenetically distinct entity and carries a better prognosis.

Choriocarcinoma

Choriocarcinoma is an uncommon element in NSGCT (15%) and rare as a pure tumor.[27] On gross examination, areas of choriocarcinoma are characteristically hemorrhagic. Microscopically, the diagnosis requires a biphasic combination of cytotrophoblasts and syncytiotrophoblasts (Figure 4). Stroma is sparse but tends to be highly vascular. Choriocarcinoma of the testis represents the most aggressive subtype of NSGCT, often presenting with large-volume visceral metastases and/or brain metastases. Extreme elevations of serum HCG levels are characteristic.

Teratoma

Teratoma contains elements of all three germ layers (endodermal, mesodermal, ectodermal) and presents with varying degrees of differentiation. Teratomatous elements are recognized in approximately half of NSGCT cases but are not usually pure.

Macroscopically, teratomas tend to be large and have multiloculated cysts containing serosanguineous fluid with occasional cartilaginous solid areas. Microscopically, all manner of tissue elements may be present, including cysts with squamous, respiratory, or intestinal-type linings, mature cartilage, muscle, and fibroblastic stroma (Figure 5). Areas that are less well differentiated ("immature teratoma") are often intermixed (Figure 6). Regardless of the degree of differentiation, all teratomas in the postpubertal setting are regarded as potentially malignant. In postchemotherapy specimens, teratoma is the most common residual element.

A pure form of mature teratoma is common among pediatric patients under the age of 4 years. Although morphologically similar to mature areas of teratoma within NSGCT, these lesions arise through a different pathway and are essentially benign (Table 1). Rarely, a nonteratomatous element is identified and may give rise to metastases.

Somatic-type cancers arising from germ cell tumors

Given the pluripotent nature of the gonocytes from which seminomas and NSGCT are thought to arise, a nongerm cell or

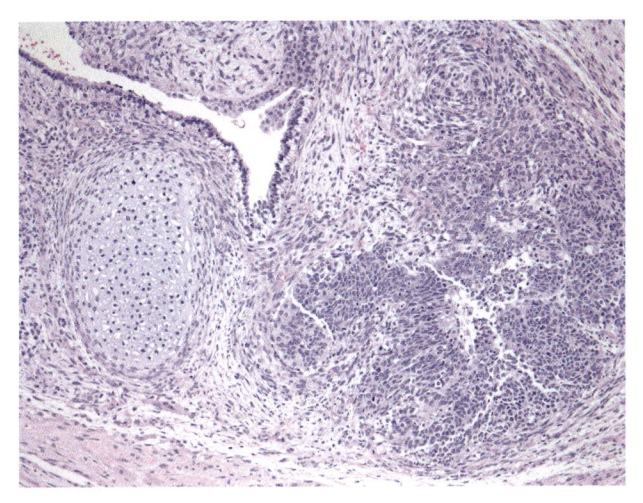

Figure 6 Immature teratoma. An island of immature neuroepithelium is present adjacent to a nodule of hyaline cartilage and glandular epithelium.

somatic-type cancer may emerge and become the dominant pattern in advanced cases of postpubertal testicular cancer. Among these are cancers morphologically resembling sarcoma such as embryonal rhabdomyosarcoma, or leiomyosarcoma, carcinoma such as adenocarcinoma, or squamous cell carcinoma, and primitive neuroectodermal tumor (PNET), all of which are associated with resistance to chemotherapy. The transformed somatic-type malignancy will also harbor 12p overexpression similar to its germ cell tumor origin.[28] Myelodysplasia and leukemia may also evolve from NSGCT, most commonly in the setting of mediastinal NSGCT.[29]

Spermatocytic tumor

Spermatocytic tumor (renamed from spermatocytic seminoma in the 2016 WHO classification scheme), accounts for 1–2% of TGCTs.[17] On gross examination, it has a grayish appearance and tends to be softer than classic seminoma. Microscopically, the hallmark is presence of polymorphous cells of highly variable size (small, intermediate, and giant cells) that bear resemblance to the cellular stages of normal spermatogenesis. The intermediate cells have characteristic filamentous (spireme) nuclear chromatin. In contrast to classic seminoma, stromal lymphocytic infiltration is not a feature of spermatocytic tumor. This tumor tends to occur over the age of 50, with a median age of 65 years. The prognosis following orchiectomy is excellent. As there are only anecdotal reports of metastases, surveillance is always recommended.[30]

Sex cord-stromal tumors

Tumors arising from stromal tissue account for <5% of all adult testicular tumors but represent almost 20% of childhood testicular tumors. These tumors are thought to arise from primitive gonadal mesenchyme and are subcategorized as Leydig cell tumor, Sertoli cell tumor, gonadoblastoma, granulosa cell tumor, and mixed/indeterminate types (Table 1).

Leydig cell tumor

Leydig cell tumors can infrequently present in children but tend to present in older men, at a median age 60 years. Histologically, they are typified by sheets of cells with abundant oncocytic cytoplasm and round, regular nuclei. Clinical symptoms are rare and usually related to the production of both androgens and/or estrogens by tumor cells, leading to precocious puberty in a child and gynecomastia in the adult. Approximately 10% of Leydig cell tumors metastasize, but this occurs only in the postpubertal patient. In patients with metastatic disease, treatment with radiation or chemotherapeutic agents have generally been ineffective. Retroperitoneal lymph node dissection (RPLND) should be considered in patients with clinical stage I tumors and high-risk features.

Sertoli cell tumor

Sertoli cell tumor shows no age predilection, presenting as a testicular mass that may be accompanied by gynecomastia or impotence secondary to estrogen production. Microscopically, these lesions are composed of rounded cells growing in tubules, cords, or sheets in a fibrous background. Therapy is primarily directed at resection of the primary lesion. RPLND is controversial in clinical stage I disease though can be considered if higher-risk features such as large primary tumors with frequent mitoses or necrosis are present.

Clinical presentation

Most patients seek medical attention because of a palpable abnormality on their testicle, although swelling, diffuse enlargement/firmness, "heaviness," or pain can be presenting signs or symptoms. Severe pain is rare, unless there is associated epididymitis or bleeding in the tumor. Because testicular cancer can be associated with low sperm counts, patients may present during an infertility work-up.

Approximately 25% of patients with disseminated disease present with symptoms from metastatic disease. Severe back pain from metastasis to the retroperitoneum is the most frequent and is often the presenting symptom in patients with primary retroperitoneal germ cell tumors. Shortness of breath, chest pain, or hemoptysis, are usually manifestations of advanced lung metastases. Primary mediastinal germ cell tumors are an exception, in that these tumors (if malignant) present with symptoms of mediastinal compression with pain, dysphagia, shortness of breath, and superior vena cava syndrome.

Diagnosis

Understanding the diagnosis and staging of TGCTs depends on understanding the anatomy of the vascular and lymphatic drainage of the testis as well as the likely sites of metastatic spread of the disease. The spermatic cord contains the lymphatic and vascular supply of the testis. The lymphatic and vascular supply diverges medially when the spermatic vessels cross ventral to the ureter. The most common landing zone for the lymphatic drainage of the right testis is the interaortocaval region below the renal vasculature although it can also metastasize to paracaval or retrocaval regions. Right-sided testicular tumors, when present in these area, can then progress to the left retroperitoneum (preaortic, retro-aortic, para-aortic). The most common landing zone for a left-sided primary tumor is the para-aortic or preaortic nodes below the left renal vessels. Regardless of laterality, ipsilateral common iliac nodes are uncommonly involved unless large-volume disease is present.

Unusual patterns of disease can be seen (or created) in patients who have had prior pelvic surgeries including herniorrhaphy, abdominal orchiopexy, or scrotal violations.[31] Accordingly, radical inguinal orchiectomy is the standard diagnostic and therapeutic surgery for suspicion of testicular cancer, rather than transscrotal procedures.

Tumors of the testis can present with a discrete nodular density or as diffuse infiltration of the entire testis (particularly seminoma and lymphoma). The other testis serves as a useful reference standard. If a testicular mass is suspected, transscrotal ultrasonography and serum tumor markers (STM) (discussed later) should be obtained. The typical appearance of a testicular neoplasm is a hypoechoic mass although many variations exist. Any retroperitoneal or mediastinal mass in a male under age 50 should prompt a scrotal examination and consideration of testicular ultrasound with STM's.

Extragonadal germ cell tumors (EGCTs) arising within the retroperitoneum or mediastinum require specialized management. A diagnosis may be made on the basis of significantly elevated tumor markers in a patient with a mass in the anterior mediastinum or retroperitoneum. If there is no marker elevation, tissue confirmation is required. Chemotherapy is the primary treatment; attempts at debulking or total removal of mediastinal germ cell tumors as initial management are inappropriate. Primary retroperitoneal germ cell tumors may be associated with an occult testicular primary. Such patients should have a thorough evaluation of the gonads, including the use of testicular ultrasonography. If a previously unsuspected testicular tumor is found, orchiectomy can serve as the diagnostic procedure. Otherwise, if STM's are normal, core biopsy of the abdominal mass or, rarely, exploratory laparotomy may be required. In addition, an i(12p) chromosomal abnormality is diagnostic for germ cell tumor in a patient who presents with undifferentiated cancer.

A transscrotal biopsy should never be performed. If a scrotal orchiectomy is performed and testicle is removed, subsequent removal of the inguinal portion of the spermatic cord should be strongly considered, although individual circumstances vary. If a testicular biopsy was performed, management of the hemiscrotum depends on the primary treatment modality. Patients who are receiving primary chemotherapy do not need hemiscrotectomy. Prophylactic inguinal lymphadenectomy, based on lymphatic drainage of the scrotum, is never performed.

Tumor markers

Serum HCG and AFP have significant value in the diagnosis, prognosis, and management of patients with germ cell tumors. AFP is derived from the yolk sac or rarely embryonal carcinoma elements of germ cell cancers. In germ cell cancers, syncytiotrophoblastic components elaborate on HCG. The protein comprises an alpha subunit and a beta subunit, each of which is antigenically distinct.

Serum HCG and/or AFP are elevated in 85% of patients with disseminated NSGCT. AFP alone is elevated in 40% of patients, and HCG alone is elevated in 50–60% of patients with disseminated nonseminomatous testicular cancer. Elevated lactic acid dehydrogenase (LDH) is less specific and mainly a correlate of disease bulk.

Pure seminoma is most frequently associated with normal AFP and HCG, but approximately 10% of all cases, and up to 30% of patients with advanced disease, may have mild elevations (usually <100 mIU/mL).[32] Any elevation of AFP in patients with seminoma must be viewed as evidence of nonseminomatous disease, and management should proceed accordingly.

AFP and HCG should be determined before and after orchiectomy. The postorchiectomy STM nadirs are essential for risk prognostication and appropriate management. The normal HCG half-life is approximately 24–36 h, while the AFP half-life is approximately 5–7 days. HCG half-life of >3 days or AFP half-life >7 days following chemotherapy are typically associated with persistent or progressive disease.

The presence of tumor markers also can lead to errors in clinical management. First, HCG determination can be nonspecific, and there is some cross-reactivity in the radioimmunoassay with luteinizing hormone. HCG determination should be repeated to ensure elevation is not a laboratory error. If the level is still high and discordant with the clinical picture, a testosterone suppression test can be considered. Testosterone should be given in a dose of 300 mg intramuscularly to suppress luteinizing hormone and rule out a spuriously elevated HCG. If the level remains increased, restaging procedures and investigation of sanctuary sites (brain and contralateral testis) are recommended.

False-positive elevation of AFP is quite rare. Differential considerations include laboratory error, other tumor types (such as hepatocellular carcinoma), and liver inflammation from cirrhosis or hepatitis. An occasional patient may have baseline elevation of AFP (usually <30 ng/mL) that remains static over time and does not reflect active disease. Some individuals have familial, hereditary, mildly elevated serum AFP levels in the range of 15–30 ng/mL. Patients with clinical stage I disease, normal imaging, normal contra-lateral testicle, and a minimally elevated AFP level (<25 ng/mL) should be observed and only be treated if there is a clear AFP increase and/or development of metastases.[33,34]

Work is ongoing to improve biomarker sensitivity and specificity in these tumors. Micro-RNA 371 is a highly sensitive and specific biomarker for seminomatous and NSGCT, outperforms HCG and AFP, and may make its way into clinical practice in the near future.[35]

Staging

Germ cell tumors are typically categorized as stage I, referring to tumors confined to the testis; stage II, indicating metastatic disease to the retroperitoneal lymph nodes without pulmonary or visceral involvement; and stage III, which denotes metastasis above the diaphragm or involving other viscera. Standard procedures to establish clinical-stage include physical examination, abdominal and chest imaging, and serum levels of AFP, β-HCG, ±LDH. The American Joint Committee on Cancer (AJCC) and WHO classification is the international standard (Table 3).[36]

Therapy for early-stage disease

Testicular cancer therapy is highly standardized and multiple guidelines and pathways exist. Practitioners are strongly urged to closely follow national or institutional standards.[37,38]

Stage I NSGCT

There is an ongoing controversy regarding the optimal management of patients with clinical stage I nonseminoma following radical orchiectomy. RPLND, adjuvant chemotherapy, or active surveillance are all considered legitimate approaches to treatment, each with advantages and disadvantages. In general, treatment decisions are driven by risk of recurrence. The two main risk factors for tumor recurrence are lymphovascular invasion (LVI) and embryonal carcinoma predominance; although, the independent prognostic value of the latter is less clear.[39–43] Higher risk individuals, should be imaged with shorter intervals, and should be considered for active adjuvant therapy.[37] We will begin with a summary of each approach and then further discuss risk-stratified decision-making and guideline recommendations below.

Table 3 AJCC staging.

TNM clinical classification	
T:	Primary tumor: The extent of the primary tumor is classified after radical orchiectomy (see pT). If no radical orchiectomy has been performed, TX is used
N:	Regional lymph nodes
cNX	Regional lymph nodes cannot be assessed
cN0	No regional lymph node metastasis
cN1	Metastasis with a lymph node mass ≤2 cm in greatest dimension or multiple lymph nodes, not >2 cm in greatest dimension
cN2	Metastasis with a lymph node mass 2–5 cm in greatest dimension, or multiple lymph nodes, 2–5 cm in greatest dimension
cN3	Metastasis with a lymph node mass >5 cm in greatest dimension
M:	Distant metastasis
MX	Distant metastasis cannot be assessed
M0	No distant metastasis
M1	Distant metastasis
M1a	Nonretroperitoneal lymph node or pulmonary metastasis
M1b	Distant visceral metastasis other than lungs
pTNM pathologic classification	
pT:	Primary tumor
pTX	Primary tumor cannot be assessed (if no radical orchiectomy has been performed TX is used)
pT0	No evidence of primary tumor (e.g., histologic scar in testis)
pTis	Germ cell neoplasia in situ
pT1	Tumor limited to testis (including rete testis invasion) without vascular/lymphatic invasion
pT1a	Tumor < 3 cm
pT1b	Tumor ≥ 3 cm
pT2	Tumor limited to testis and epididymis with vascular/lymphatic invasion, or tumor extending through tunica albuginea with/without vascular/lymphatic invasion
pT3	Tumor invades spermatic cord with or without vascular/lymphatic invasion
pT4	Tumor invades scrotum with or without vascular/lymphatic invasion
pN:	Regional lymph nodes
pNX	Regional lymph nodes cannot be assessed
pN0	No regional lymph node metastasis
pN1	Metastasis with a lymph node mass ≤2 cm in greatest dimension and ≤5 positive nodes, none >2 cm in greatest dimension
pN2	Metastasis with a lymph node mass >2 cm but not >5 cm in greatest dimension; or >5 nodes positive, non >5 cm; or evidence of extranodal tumor extension
pN3	Metastasis with a lymph node mass >5 cm in greatest dimension
pM:	Distant metastasis
	The pM category corresponds to the M category
S:	Serum tumor markers
SX	Serum marker studies not available or not performed
S0	Serum marker study levels within normal limits LDH HCG α-fetoprotein
S1	LDH <1.5xN and HCG <5000 and AFP <1000
S2	LDH 1.5–10xN or HCG 5000–50,000 or AFP 1000–10,000
S3	LDH >10xN or HCG >50,000 or AFP >10,000

RPLND

Based on a predictable lymphatic pattern of spread of testicular tumors, RPLND emerged as a treatment option for testicular cancer as early as 1907.[44–46] In the United States, primary RPLND became the conventional approach for patients with clinical stage I NSGCT.

Primary RPLND has the advantages of a very high cure rate, low rate of ever needing chemotherapy, removing potential teratoma, which is chemo-resistant, and virtually eliminating the risk of late relapse of teratoma.[47] The overall relapse rate following RPLND for clinical stage I is 5–10%, with the great majority of relapses occurring in the lungs; long-term cure rate is 99%.

In experienced hands, the classic, bilateral RPLND is associated with minimal perioperative morbidity and virtually no mortality. A classic bilateral RPLND is performed from the renal hilum superiorly, to the ureters laterally, to the anterior spinous ligament posteriorly (including all retrocaval and retroaortic tissue), and to the common iliac lymph nodes inferiorly.[48,49] An improved understanding of the nerves and pathways responsible for seminal emission and ejaculation along with meticulous anatomic studies of the distribution of right-sided and left-sided tumors led to modification of the original surgical "templates" for RPLND. Most common is prospective nerve-sparing with use of modified templates to preserve contralateral sympathetic nerves by eliminating dissection in regions with a low risk of metastases.[50–52] Although several modified templates exist, in general, dissection is minimized on the contralateral side particularly below the level of the inferior mesenteric artery (IMA). To minimize retroperitoneal recurrence, some advocate bilateral infrahilar dissections only sparing the contralateral nodes below the IMA.[53] Regardless of the specific template utilized, strict principles of thoroughly resecting all lymph nodes are necessary as is meticulous preservation of the postganglionic sympathetic fibers arising from the sympathetic chain and the hypogastric plexus. Results from multiple case series confirm uniformly high rates of preservation of ejaculatory function (96–100%) while maintaining a 99% cure rate.[50,54,55]

To further reduce the morbidity of surgery, laparoscopic/robotic techniques for RPLND have been used.[56] Advantages include smaller incisions, less pain, and quicker recovery. Among experienced surgeons, lymph node counts and cure rates are similar to those of open RPLND series although extended (>5–10 years) follow-up is lacking. Isolated reports of unique patterns of recurrence following laparoscopic surgery have stimulated debate whether this resulted from poor surgical technique from inexperienced surgeons or from the pneumoperitoneum itself.[57]

However, even in excellent centers, preoperative evaluations routinely fail to reliably identify the 50% percent of patients with high-risk features who are pathological stage I thus subjecting many patients to major surgery without therapeutic benefit, and a small percentage of those who do undergo surgery will still require chemotherapy.

Adjuvant chemotherapy

The definition of a high-risk group by vascular invasion and predominant embryonal cancer, the efficacy and safety of chemotherapy for good-risk metastatic disease, and the near-perfect results of two cycles of chemotherapy in the setting of fully resected stage II disease have prompted investigators to consider the use of primary chemotherapy in high-risk stage I disease.

The MRC designed a prospective study offering two cycles of BEP to patients with high-risk stage 1 NSGCT.[58] They observed limited toxicity and achieved near-universal cure in patients with stage I disease with relapse rates in various studies ranging from 0% to 2%. Whereas two cycles of BEP had previously been the standard adjuvant chemotherapy regimen, recent data suggest one cycle of BEP results in similar outcome and one cycle of BEP is now recommended as the adjuvant chemotherapy of choice.[59–61]

Adjuvant chemotherapy, in particular for high-risk disease, is considered the standard of care in many countries. While the recurrence rate is decreased to 2–4%, adjuvant chemotherapy, just like adjuvant RPLND, will also result in overtreatment in at least 50% of patients. All of these patients will experience hair loss, a significant disruption from work, school, and life, anxiety, and effects on fertility. Acutely, patients may develop myelosuppression with 1% incidence of grade 3 ear labyrinth disorders secondary to cisplatin.[60]

Active surveillance
The main rationale for active surveillance is that systemic chemotherapy is highly effective and thus, patients who are cured by orchiectomy alone can be spared the treatment-related toxicity of a primary RPLND or adjuvant chemotherapy. As such, only patients who relapse will receive treatment. Treatment of these patients will be more intense than adjuvant therapy, typically EP×4 or BEP ×3 (see below), but active surveillance completely spares 70–75% of all stage I patients the burden of any active treatment.

An early large prospective study of surveillance included 373 patients with a median follow-up of 5 years.[43] The recurrence rate was 27% and of these 80% recurred within the first year. Overall cure rate for the entire cohort of patients exceeded 98%. A large data set including 1139 stage I nonseminoma patients recently confirmed active surveillance as an excellent and safe management modality. With a recurrence rate of 19% (44% in LVI positive and 14% in negative patients) and a disease-specific survival of 99.7% on long-term follow-up, this series of surveillance underlines the efficacy of the approach.[41] Thus careful surveillance plus chemotherapy at the earliest sign of recurrence is an effective management approach to patients with stage 1 NSGCTT.

Concerns regarding the lack of compliance is an argument against surveillance, in particular in high-risk nonseminoma. However, there is no evidence that level of compliance across varying geographies materially impacts survival.[62-64] Survival rates consistently approach 100% even in series with reported "unsatisfactory" compliance. Educating patients is crucial and emphasizing that later identification of disease might well lead to more complicated and complex therapies is fully warranted. Concerns about the undissected retroperitoneum leading to a significant number of late refractory cancer or late recurrence of teratoma have not been realized.[59,62-64]

Comparative trials and a risk-stratified approach
Patients with stage 1 NSGCT, especially those at high risk of recurrence, have a choice of management options. Each option, when carried out meticulously, results in the same excellent long-term survival but each has unique merits and potential risks. The major prospective comparative study for these patients was conducted by the German Testicular Cancer Study Group. They reported that one cycle of BEP led to a 2-year recurrence-free survival of 99% compared to 92% for RPLND, suggesting BEP as a superior option.[59] Critics of this study highlight the 61 participating centers and 9 abdominal relapses in the RPLND arm, suggesting inadequate cancer operations and explaining the differences in recurrence-free survival.

In terms of guidelines, active surveillance has been adopted as the standard of care for patients with low-risk disease by the European and for both low-risk and high-risk by the Canadian Consensus Guidelines.[38] In the United States, National Comprehensive Cancer Network and AUA guidelines recommend surveillance for low-risk individuals. For individuals with risk factors, surveillance, surgery, or chemotherapy are considered options.[37] Consistent with these guidelines, in the United States, 70, 17, and 13% of patients with clinical stage 1A NSGCT received surveillance, RPLND, and chemotherapy, respectively. Surveillance increased in this group from 65% in 2004–2005 to 74% in 2012–2013 ($p = 0.004$). Of the 2580 men who had clinical stage IB NSGCT, 46, 20, and 34% received surveillance, RPLND, and chemotherapy, respectively, with little change over time.[65]

Stage II NSGCT

Clinical stage II disease
In clinical stage IIA disease, RPLND or primary chemotherapy are appropriate treatment options. The distinction between clinical stage I and IIA is often challenging in the setting of small equivocal retroperitoneal nodes within an expected landing zone; therefore, repeat imaging and STM's in 6–8 weeks is often preferred.[33]

In clinical stage IIB disease, RPLND is an option in select situations. Otherwise, primary chemotherapy is preferred. Tumor-marker-positive disease and/or large-volume abdominal disease (>3 cm on abdominal CT, multiple nodes, unexpected locations) should be treated with primary chemotherapy with BEP ×3 or EP ×4, as discussed below.

Pathologic stage II disease
After RPLND, pN0 disease should be followed with surveillance. In the setting of pN1 disease, surveillance is preferable with durable cure rates of 85–90% although adjuvant chemotherapy (EP ×2 or BEP ×2) is also acceptable. In the setting of pN2 disease, adjuvant chemotherapy is typically recommended although surveillance would be preferred in the rare setting of pure teratoma.[66] Presence of pN3 disease should be very rare with appropriate RPLND patient selection and should be treated as disseminated cancer, which is discussed in detail below.[37]

Stage I seminoma

Orchiectomy and postoperative radiation therapy constituted the standard of care for early-stage seminoma patients during most of the twentieth century given the known pattern of spread and seminomatous tissue's extreme radiosensitivity.[67,68] However, orchiectomy alone is highly effective for most patients as only ~20% will experience a relapse.

Adjuvant treatment
A large randomized trial by the EORTC/MRC randomly allocated patients with stage I seminoma to standard prophylactic radiation therapy (primarily PA radiation at 20–30 Gy) or treatment with single-course, single-agent, carboplatin (AUC 7).[69] With median 4-year follow-up, the 3-year relapse-free survival rate was 96% for radiation compared to 95% for carboplatin ($p = 0.31$). There were fewer new contralateral TGCTs with carboplatin.

Surveillance as preferred management
Stage I disease comprises 85% of all seminoma cases. Surveillance studies demonstrated orchiectomy is curative in 80–85%, establishing it as the preferred management strategy in most patients.[70,71] Regardless of the elected management method, disease-specific survival at 5 years is over 99% and treatment of relapsed treatment-naïve disease appears to be as curable as at initial presentation. The European consensus statement favors surveillance for all patients independent of the individual risk for relapse. The NCCN guidelines also favor surveillance, though acknowledge adjuvant radiation or carboplatin as acceptable alternatives.

The schedule for surveillance testing is in flux and previously intense schedules have been modified to be less onerous.[41] Many centers concentrate testing during the highest period of risk and use progressively fewer CT scans in follow-up. Many schedules recommend a 3–2–1 with 3 abdominal/pelvic CTs the first year, 2 the second, and 1 the third with no CTs thereafter. Although possible, it is rare to diagnose a recurrence with chest imaging or a new HCG elevation. As in the case of NSGCT, surveillance is a very attractive option but compliance is essential. Therefore, patients who cannot reliably participate in surveillance can be considered for adjuvant therapy.

Stage II seminoma

In stage II seminoma, nodal size plays a major role in treatment decisions, as the potential for supradiaphragmatic involvement increases with the size of the subdiaphragmatic disease. At most centers, the arbitrary cutoff for systemic chemotherapy is largest retroperitoneal node of 3–5 cm, while patients with nodal masses <3–5 cm are treated with radiation alone. The expected 5-year relapse-free survival is 89–95% for patients treated with radiation alone.[69,72] The overall survival remains around 97–99% because of the effectiveness of salvage therapy. For patients with stage II seminoma, the standard radiation field incorporates the PA and ipsilateral pelvic lymph nodes with dose-escalation to 30–36 Gy. The treatment of stage II seminoma with radiation has also evolved. Historically for a patient with stage II seminoma, radiation was delivered to the PA nodes, pelvic lymph nodes, and prophylactically to the mediastinum. This practice, although effective at limiting supradiaphragmatic failures, became associated with cardiac morbidity. Chemotherapy is now favored for patients who are at significant risk of supradiaphragmatic involvement. An ongoing trial is evaluating the potential role of RPLND for stage IIA seminoma.

Initial chemotherapy for disseminated disease

Historical context

A broad spectrum of chemotherapeutic agents was tested from 1952 to 1972 in disseminated germ cell tumors. In the early 1960s, the vinca alkaloids achieved short remissions in a small number of patients.[73] Several antitumor antibiotics were also found to have single-agent activity, including actinomycin D. An early combination regimen described in 1960, which contained methotrexate, actinomycin D, and chlorambucil, was reported to have an objective response rate of 52%, with more than half being complete responses.[74] In 1970, bleomycin was reported to induce complete remissions.[75] A further advance occurred when vinblastine and bleomycin were used in combination.[76] This regimen resulted in 65% of patients achieving a complete remission, including some durable responses.

The most important event in the development of curative therapy for disseminated disease was the 1965 report by Rosenberg et al.[77] of the antibacterial effect of platinum coordination compounds. Initially shown to induce testicular atrophy in the dog model, cisplatin was soon reported to be the single most active agent against testicular germ cell tumors, with response rates of 70% and complete remission rates of 50%.[78] Over four decades later, it remains the most active drug in this disease.

In 1977, investigators at Indiana University published studies using combination cisplatin, vinblastine, and bleomycin (PVB) in patients with disseminated testicular cancer.[79] This study incorporated principles of combination chemotherapy, as well as the concept of surgically resecting residual disease after the completion of chemotherapy, and remains a landmark study in modern oncology. Later studies supported lower vinblastine dosing and the elimination of maintenance therapy (which had been included in earlier regimens).[80,81]

Table 4 International germ cell consensus classification.

Good prognosis:
Nonseminoma testis or retroperitoneal primary and no nonpulmonary visceral metastases and α-fetoprotein <1000 ng/mL, βHCG <5000 IU/L, and LDH <1.5 upper limit of normal
Seminoma of any primary site and no nonpulmonary visceral metastases and normal α-fetoprotein, any βHCG, any LDH
Intermediate prognosis:
Nonseminoma testis or retroperitoneal primary and no nonpulmonary visceral metastases and α-fetoprotein >1000 ng/mL and <10,000 ng/mL or βHCG >5000 IU/L and <50,000 IU/L or LDH >1.5 normal and <10 normal
Seminoma of any primary site and nonpulmonary visceral metastases and normal α-fetoprotein, any βHCG, any LDH
Poor prognosis:
Nonseminoma with mediastinal primary, nonpulmonary visceral metastases or α-fetoprotein >10,000 ng/mL or βHCG >50,000 IU/L or LDH >10 upper limit of normal

Abbreviations: LDH, lactate dehydrogenase; βHCG, β human chorionic gonadotropin.

The next critical advance was a randomized trial comparing cisplatin plus bleomycin and either vinblastine (PVB) or etoposide (BEP).[82] Of those randomly allocated to BEP, 83% achieved a disease-free status, while 74% of those allocated to receive PVB attained a disease-free status. PVB patients also experienced significantly more paresthesias, myalgias, and abdominal cramping. As a result, the BEP regimen of bleomycin, etoposide, and cisplatin for four cycles became and remains a standard regimen.

Prognostic classifications

Therapeutic decisions for disseminated disease therapy are based on data from the International Germ Cell Cancer Collaborative Group (IGCCCG).[83] Independent predictors of outcome in univariate analysis are mediastinal primary site for nonseminomatous tumors, degree of AFP, HCG, and LDH elevation, and the presence of nonpulmonary visceral metastasis. Of note, marker elevation is based on postorchiectomy levels. Good, intermediate, and poor-risk groups are defined for nonseminomatous germ cell tumors. For seminoma, only good-risk and intermediate-risk groups are defined by the absence or presence of nonpulmonary visceral metastases (Table 4).

Treatment of good-risk disseminated germ cell tumors

Patients with good-risk disease constitute approximately 60% of patients presenting with disseminated disease. For IGCCCG, good-risk disease 90–95% of patients experience long-term disease-free survival. Because virtually all these patients achieve complete remission with standard chemotherapy, additional trials addressed the possibility of reducing the amount of chemotherapy (thus decreasing acute and chronic toxicity), while maintaining the excellent cure rate.

The Southeastern Cancer Study Group (SECSG) randomized good-risk disease patients to either three or four courses of BEP.[84] There was no difference in complete response rate or long-term disease-free rate, thus establishing BEP ×3 as a standard of care. ECOG conducted a trial randomizing patients with low or intermediate-risk disease to receive three courses of etoposide plus cisplatin (EP) with or without bleomycin to potentially eliminate the toxicity, especially pulmonary toxicity, of weekly bleomycin.[85] However, patients receiving bleomycin had superior failure-free and overall survival. Similarly, attempts at substituting carboplatin for cisplatin, to minimize neurotoxicity, nephrotoxicity, and need for prehydration, also demonstrated superior survival with standard cisplatin.[86,87]

Perhaps the most controversial approach to minimizing toxicity in good-risk disseminated germ cell tumors has been to utilize four cycles of etoposide/cisplatin (EP ×4) rather than three cycles of BEP in order to eliminate both short- and long-term toxicities of bleomycin (see also Survivorship below). One informative trial was conducted by the EORTC comparing EP ×4 with or without bleomycin.[88] Complete remission rate (95% vs 89%) favored the bleomycin-containing arm, but there was no difference in time to progression or relapse rates (4%). Of note, this trial utilized a total weekly etoposide dose of 360 mg rather than the now accepted dose of 500 mg weekly. The more direct comparison between BEP ×3 and EP ×4 was conducted by the Genito-Urinary Group of the French Federation of Cancer Centers.[89] The 4-year event-free survival rates in this 257 patient trial were 91% and 86%, in the BEP and EP arms, respectively ($p = 0.135$). The 4-year overall survival rates were not significantly different either with 5 versus 12 deaths, respectively ($p = 0.096$).

There subsequently have been multiple debates regarding whether EP ×4 is an appropriate standard for good risk disseminated disease, especially given consensus that it is not adequate for intermediate and poor-risk disease (see next), and incomplete data on comparative long-term toxicities. Currently, European and Canadian consensus statements endorse BEP × 3 as the standard regimen for IGCCCG good-risk disseminated disease, whereas the American NCCN guidelines consider either BEP ×3 or EP ×4 appropriate for this patient population.

Treatment of intermediate and poor-risk disseminated germ cell tumors

While outcomes for good risk disseminated disease are excellent, 5 year survival rates of intermediate and poor-risk disease are 79% and 48%.[83] Efforts here have thus focused on improving outcomes over that seen with BEP ×4. An early effort evaluated the use of high-dose cisplatin, which was not successful.[90] A more prominent approach has been to substitute ifosfamide for bleomycin based on its activity in refractory disease. This VIP ×4 (V = VePesid® = etoposide) regimen has been compared in two randomized trials.[91,92] Both trials demonstrated equivalent cancer outcomes with significantly greater toxicity, especially hematologic toxicity, with VIP.

There have been several additional efforts to utilize agents or combinations that have demonstrated activity in the refractory setting in the first line intermediate and poor-risk disease setting. This includes the addition of paclitaxel to BEP (T-BEP), a dose-dense approach with cisplatin, cyclophosphamide, doxorubicin, vinblastine, and bleomycin (CISCA-VB), and a combination of paclitaxel, ifosfamide, and cisplatin (TIP), none of which showed a survival benefit in randomized studies.[93–95]

Finally, several investigators have evaluated dose intensification. One such approach is based on the prognostic value of tumor marker decline after the first cycle of BEP chemotherapy.[96] In a study led by the French GETUG, patients with slower than predicted marker decline were randomized to either completing standard BEP or a dose-dense intensification regimen including bleomycin, paclitaxel, oxaliplatin, cisplatin, ifosfamide, and etoposide.[97] Three year progression-free survival was improved in the dose-dense group (59% vs 48%; $p = 0.05$), but this risk-stratified approach has not been routinely adopted. The use of high-dose chemotherapy (HDCT) and stem cell rescue has also been investigated. Two courses of standard therapy (BEP) followed by two cycles of high-dose carboplatin, etoposide, and cyclophosphamide were compared to standard BEP × 4.[98] No significant difference was seen between the two arms.

As such, and despite multiple attempts, BEP ×4 remains the standard of care for intermediate and high-risk disease with VIP ×4 considered a reasonable alternative in patients with a contraindication to bleomycin.

Postchemotherapy surgery

Introduction

Surgical resection of residual masses following chemotherapy for disseminated disease is a vital component of the multimodality treatment of testis cancer, particularly for nonseminomas. Twenty to fifty percent of patients who undergo induction chemotherapy for metastatic germ cell cancer have significant residual retroperitoneal disease requiring resection for cure. The presence of large residual masses around vital structures and the resultant postchemotherapy reaction often makes surgery challenging. These operations should ideally be performed by experienced surgeons in high-volume centers.

Indications for postchemotherapy RPLND (PC-RPLND)

Postchemotherapy surgery should be considered only if STMs have normalized or reached a plateau. Typically, PC-RPLND is indicated if there is radiographic evidence of residual disease postchemotherapy, although the indications are different for seminomas than nonseminomas. PC-RPLND should be performed 4–6 weeks following the last round of chemotherapy in order to allow patients to recover. Imaging must include CT scan of the chest, abdomen, and pelvis which should be performed reasonably close to time of surgery to ascertain persistence of residual disease in the retroperitoneum.

Nonseminoma

Although most authors advocate resection of "residual" masses following chemotherapy for NSGCT, there is no consensus on nodal size criteria. It is often difficult to measure the exact size of residual nodal tissue, since nodes are often matted together. The definition of a "normal" CT scan following chemotherapy for testis cancer varies, and has become even more problematic with modern scanners. Investigators have reported that up to one-third of small retroperitoneal postchemotherapy masses measuring ≤2 cm in diameter contain residual teratoma or viable germ cell tumor.[99] There are currently no reliable imaging techniques or prediction models to accurately identify patients who have residual teratoma or viable GCT postinduction chemotherapy.[100] 18-fluoro-deoxyglucose positron emission tomography (FDG-PET) scan is not recommended in the decision-making analysis of postchemotherapy residual masses in NSGCT since it cannot distinguish fibrosis from teratoma. As such, most experts agree that PC-RPLND is indicated when there are residual radiographically detectable lesions >1 cm following first-line chemotherapy, and should be considered even in patients with initial intermediate or poor-risk disease and radiographic complete response. Patients with initial good risk disease and a complete response can be safely observed with 15-year recurrence-free survival of ~95%.[101]

Patients with teratoma present in the orchiectomy specimen are at increased risk of residual teratoma in the retroperitoneum; however, this should rarely be a major factor in determining whether a PC-RPLND is indicated.[100] Patients who have a modestly increased serum AFP, teratoma in the primary tumor, and a postchemotherapy cystic mass in the retroperitoneum may also be candidates for PC-RPLND since these are often residual teratoma. Beck et al.[102] confirmed that cystic teratomas contain variably elevated levels of intra-cystic HCG and AFP and postulated a leak into the bloodstream could explain the elevated STMs in this situation. Teratomas can rarely invade the vena cava and present with a tumor thrombus, and this should not be mistaken for a deep venous thrombosis.

Seminoma
Following induction chemotherapy, CT scans often reveal a sheet-like distribution of tissue around the IVC and/or aorta that can resolve over a prolonged period.[103] Viable cancer is present in approximately 20% patients with residual masses >3 cm and almost no patients with residual masses <3 cm.[104] Since there is no concern about residual teratoma in pure seminomas, routine PC-RPLND for residual disease postchemotherapy will result in overtreatment in approximately 80% of patients. PC-RPLND in this setting is one of the most challenging surgical scenarios that urologists encounter and rates of adjunctive surgery and complications tend to be higher. To minimize the number of men needing surgery, investigators evaluated the role of FDG-PET. In a multicenter study ("SEMPET" trial), 56 PET scans were evaluated in 51 patients with CT-documented residual masses measuring 1–11 cm after adequate chemotherapy for bulky seminoma. The sensitivity, specificity, and positive predictive values of PET in determining residual viable disease were 80%, 100%, and 100%, respectively.[105] Other studies, however, have not confirmed the reliability of PET.[106] Resection of postchemotherapy masses and the value of FDG-PET for decision-making in seminoma thus remains controversial, and management should be individualized. In general, a markedly elevated SUV, interval growth, or positive biopsy should be present prior to recommending a PC-RPLND for seminoma.

Extent of surgery
PC-RPLND is a technically demanding operation. The boundaries of surgical resection remain controversial. Although modified, nerve-sparing templates may be appropriate for select patients with lower-stage disease, several investigators have demonstrated the presence of tumor outside these templates in advanced disease. For example, in a study of 50 PC-RPLND specimens, all low-volume left-sided primary tumors followed a predictable pattern of spread to a modified left-sided template, whereas right-sided primaries had about a 20% crossover rate. After a mean follow-up of 53 months, there were no infield recurrences.[107] On the other hand, Carver et al.[108] reviewed their experience with 532 patients who underwent PC-RPLND for metastatic NSGCT and found that 7–32% patients had evidence of extra-template retroperitoneal disease. Interestingly 2/24 (8%) patients with residual masses less than 1 cm had extra-template metastases. Therefore, it appears the most prudent approach is a full bilateral dissection in the postchemotherapy setting, although a limited template can be considered in low-volume left-sided primaries.

The surgical approach should be adapted to the size and location of the mass. Most masses can be accessed via a midline approach whereas larger masses and those requiring suprahilar dissections are best approached through a thoracoabdominal incision or a midline incision extended to the costochondral junction. Adjunctive surgery is required in about 20% of patients undergoing PC-RPLND. The most common adjunctive procedure includes a left nephrectomy and occasionally vena caval and/or aortic reconstruction, resection, or replacement.[109] Although simultaneous PC-RPLND and thoracic resections are feasible, more complex mediastinal masses are probably best approached in a staged manner to reduce complications. Findings of fibrosis in the retroperitoneal specimen should not automatically preclude thoracic resections since 10–20% of patients can have teratoma or viable cancer in the chest.[110]

Complication rates following PC-RPLND performed at high-volume centers are higher than for primary RPLND, ranging from 7% to 30% with a mortality rate of about 1%.[111] The most significant source of morbidity in this postchemotherapy group is pulmonary toxicity related to prior bleomycin. Ejaculatory dysfunction remains a significant problem; although, patients with smaller masses are candidates for nerve-sparing approaches with about an 80% probability of preservation of ejaculatory function.[111]

Pathology
The histopathologic findings in postchemotherapy surgical specimens determine the need for further treatment and surveillance protocol. The incidence of persistent cancer is decreasing, most likely due to optimized chemotherapy regimens and better selection of patients for surgery. Pathologic findings in patients with advanced NSGCT after induction therapy are approximately: necrosis in 40–50%; teratoma in 35–40% and; viable carcinoma in 10–15% of specimens.[112] RPLND following salvage chemotherapy reveals residual viable carcinoma in about 50% of patients. Patients with viable disease resected at postchemotherapy surgery following front-line chemotherapy are generally recommended to receive two postoperative cycles of cisplatin-based therapy, with two-thirds remaining disease-free in the long term.[113] Patients with unresectable disease, partial resection, or elevated tumor markers should be considered for full salvage chemotherapy.

Salvage chemotherapy
Twenty to thirty percent of germ cell tumor patients will not achieve durable complete remission with first-line therapy. These individuals, as well as those who relapse from complete remission, are candidates for salvage chemotherapy. The decreased efficacy and increased toxicity of second-line chemotherapy require the expertise of individuals well versed in the intricacies of and options for refractory testicular cancer.

Patient selection
There are several clinical situations that may mimic persistent, progressive, or recurrent disease. One involves the appearance of nodular lesions in the chest at the end of chemotherapy or soon after completion.[114] These nodules can represent bleomycin-induced pulmonary injury and are characteristically located in a subpleural region. This possibility should be considered in a patient who is otherwise responding serologically or radiographically and has new abnormalities in the lungs in separate sites from the original disease.

Another clinical situation frequently mistaken for progressive disease is growing teratoma.[115] Radiographically enlarging metastatic lesions during chemotherapy concurrently with normal or normalizing serologic markers often represent teratoma. Appropriate management is surgical resection of residual radiographic abnormalities rather than salvage chemotherapy.

A conservative policy is to reserve salvage therapy until there is a clear demonstration of rising markers on serial determinations. The vagaries of interpretation of low-level marker elevation make such a policy necessary to ensure that patients are not treated with intensive salvage chemotherapy on the basis of a false-positive marker elevation. As noted earlier, this is especially critical for modestly elevated AFP levels, which often do not reflect active disease.[34]

Occult central nervous system (CNS) metastasis should be considered in the setting of systemic sustained remission and elevation of STMs. CT scans or MRI should be performed. The CNS evaluation should proceed even in the absence of clinical signs or symptoms if the only evidence of progressive disease is a rising marker. Brain metastases are most common with choriocarcinoma and are at high risk of bleeding.

The other important sanctuary site from chemotherapy is the testis. In most settings, the primary in the testis has been removed in the initial diagnostic process. However, in some patients presenting with advanced disease, chemotherapy is initiated without a tissue diagnosis. In such cases, the testis must be removed at the completion of chemotherapy, even if the primary tumor is no longer evident. The possibility of a metachronous contralateral testicular primary should also be entertained.

Prognostic factors in the salvage situation

The importance of clinical prognostic factors in the second-line situation has been increasingly recognized. Outcomes in different studies are difficult to interpret based on the heterogeneity of this patient population. Patients with gonadal primary tumor sites, cisplatin sensitive disease, and relapse after complete response to first-line therapy are more likely to achieve a favorable treatment outcome than patients with cisplatin-refractory disease, an incomplete response to first-line therapy or a mediastinal primary tumor site. The International Prognostic Factor Study Group developed a prognostic classification for relapsed patients similar to the IGCCCG classification for treatment naïve patients, which included individual data from almost 2000 relapsed patients collected at high volume centers around the world.[116] Based on seven significant factors on multivariate analysis including histology (seminoma vs nonseminoma), primary tumor site (mediastinal vs retroperitoneal vs gonadal), response to first-line chemotherapy (CR vs PR vs other), progression-free interval following first-line chemotherapy, AFP and HCG level at diagnosis of relapse, and the presence of nonpulmonary visceral metastases the model is able to differentiate five distinct risk groups ranging from very-low to very-high, with a 3-year survival probability ranging between 6 and 77%.

Standard salvage therapy

During the three decades since the introduction of cisplatin, several agents including ifosfamide, paclitaxel, gemcitabine, and oxaliplatin have demonstrated activity in platinum-refractory patients. The rate of patients responding favorably to conventional salvage chemotherapy is approximately 50% and thus substantially lower than after first-line treatment. Nevertheless, long-term remissions are still achieved in 20–30% of patients.

The combination of vinblastine, ifosfamide, and cisplatin (VeIP) was the initial salvage therapy reported, with approximately 50% of patients experiencing a complete response.[117,118] Subsequently, investigators from Memorial Sloan-Kettering Cancer Center evaluated paclitaxel plus ifosfamide plus cisplatin (TIP).[119] Thirty-two of 46 patients (70%) achieved a complete response to chemotherapy alone. Similar results have been reported by others.[120] While no head-to-head phase III trial has compared VeIP and TIP, the outcomes appear to be better with the latter, and TIP has evolved into the most widely used standard conventional-dose salvage regimen.

High-dose chemotherapy as initial salvage therapy

HDCT with bone marrow or peripheral stem cell rescue has been studied by a variety of investigators utilizing a number of different specific regimens. Due to heterogeneity in patients enrolled, details of the chemotherapy administered, and advances in supportive care, comparisons amongst approaches and versus standard salvage chemotherapy are challenging. With those caveats, a large retrospective analysis was performed by the International Prognostic Factor Group and included 1594 patients treated with either conventional or HDCT. A significant advantage in favor of HDCT was seen across all subgroups.[121]

Thus, HDCT with peripheral stem cell rescue has become a standard of care for refractory testicular germ cell tumors. More importantly, its benefit versus standard salvage chemotherapy has not been definitively demonstrated and there is thus an ongoing international trial of standard salvage therapy with TIP versus paclitaxel-ifosfamide induction and stem cell harvest followed by three cycles of HDCT with etoposide plus carboplatin and stem cell rescue.[122]

Treatment of multiply recurrent germ cell cancer

Outcomes in patients with disseminated germ cell tumors following multiple prior therapies are generally poor. Guidelines recommend enrollment in a clinical trial, HDCT (when this has not already been utilized), or desperation surgery when technically possible.[37]

Salvage surgery

Some refractory patients are best approached with salvage surgery rather than chemotherapy. This is especially true for those who relapse late or for patients with relapsed disease confined to a single anatomic site. One of the initial reports of this approach in the modern era is a retrospective review from Indiana University.[123] Of 48 patients, the majority underwent isolated retroperitoneal lymphadenectomy (33). Of these, 38 (79%) were rendered free of gross disease by surgery, and 29 (60%) attained a serologic remission. Ten patients (21%) remain continuously free of disease with follow-up ranging from 31 to 89 months. Clinical benefit was obtained only in the group of completely resected patients with a solitary site of disease. Patients with multiple sites of metastasis, although resectable, were not cured. Albers et al.[124] also reported a high long-term disease-free rate after salvage surgery for patients with persistently elevated tumor markers. Such decisions about surgeries should be made at centers with significant experience in germ cell tumor management. In general, selection to attempt desperation surgery includes slowly increasing tumor markers after an initial complete response to either first-line or second-line chemotherapy, radiographically resectable residual disease in one or two sites, and exhaustion of all chemotherapy options.

Alternative chemotherapy regimens

Systemic therapy of highly refractory disease is generally palliative only, but a small number of patients are apparently cured, especially with the addition of subsequent surgical resection. A number of agents and combinations have been investigated, some of which such as paclitaxel and ifosfamide, have been incorporated into early salvage therapy. Four regimens for highly refractory disease deserve specific mention. Low dose daily etoposide is very well tolerated with a median progression-free survival on the order of 3 months.[125] The combination of paclitaxel and gemcitabine was evaluated by ECOG in 32 patients with refractory germ cell tumors.[126] The overall response rate was 31%, including six patients with complete remissions, four of whom were continuously disease-free. Oxaliplatin plus gemcitabine has been investigated with reported long-term survival rates on the order of 10%.[127,128] Finally, the combination of paclitaxel, oxaliplatin, and gemcitabine has been studied by the German Testicular Cancer Study Group.[129,130] In their most recent update, the overall response rate was 44%, the median progression-free and overall survival were 4.0 months (95% CI: 3.08–4.94) and 13.3 months (95% CI: 9.50–17.06), respectively, and long-term survival of greater than 2 years was achieved in 21%.

Notably, PD1 pathway checkpoint inhibitors have not been particularly useful in patients with refractory testicular germ cell tumors.[131,132]

Special situations

Late relapse

The majority of relapses in patients with disseminated testicular cancer who achieve a complete remission with chemotherapy occur within 2 years. A late relapse is generally considered a recurrence after a disease-free interval of more than 24 months after initial cisplatin-based chemotherapy. Late relapses following complete remission occur in 2–3% of cases, with recurrences as late as 32 years following complete remission. Those patients who have had recurrences with isolated mature teratoma, in general, have done well following excision, whereas those with marker positive carcinoma, disseminated disease, and/or transformation have a worse prognosis. Chemotherapy-naïve patients, for example, relapsing from active surveillance or from primary RPLND, have a very good prognosis with cisplatin-based chemotherapy even if they relapse beyond 3 years.[41]

Sharp and colleagues reviewed 75 patients for management of late relapse of germ cell tumor.[133] In this modern series, the median time to late relapse was 6.9 years (range, 2.1–37.7 years). Overall, 56 patients (75%) had recurrence in the retroperitoneum. The 5-year cancer-specific survival was 60% (95% CI, 46–71%). Patients who underwent complete surgical resection at time of late relapse (n = 45) had a 5-year cancer-specific survival of 79% versus 36% for patients without complete resection (n = 30; P < 0.0001). The 5-year cancer-specific survival for chemotherapy-naïve patients was significantly greater than patients with a prior history of chemotherapy as part of their initial management (5-year cancer-specific survival, 93% vs 49%, respectively). As this was a series of patients referred at the time of late relapse, it is unknown how representative these results are for the late relapsing population as a whole. Nonetheless, these and other data suggest patients can obtain long remissions or cures after late relapse. Patients who are chemotherapy naïve often are rendered disease-free with standard approaches including cisplatin-based chemotherapy coupled with postchemotherapy surgery. A consistent feature of such studies is that for patients with regional confined disease who have late presentations with atypical yolk sac findings, elevated AFP and prior chemotherapy are best served by aggressive primary surgery.

Survivorship

Since the mid-1970s, the majority of testicular cancer patients with disseminated disease have been cured with combination chemotherapy with or without adjunctive surgery or radiation. As such, long-term survivorship issues have become paramount, and information is now available on a significant number of patients with follow-up of more than 10 years.

Nephrotoxicity

The acute effects of cisplatin on both renal glomerular and tubular functions are well documented, with decreases in both glomerular filtration rate (GFR) and effective renal plasma flow (ERPF) accompanied by magnesium wasting and elevated levels of β2-microglobulin, indicative of proximal tubule dysfunction. Most investigators reported the acute decreases in GFR and ERPF do not deteriorate further during the months to years following completion of chemotherapy; however, long-term subclinical impairment is frequently found.[134]

Vascular toxicity

Raynaud's phenomenon is the most common vascular toxicity seen in patients following chemotherapy for testicular cancer. Although anecdotally reported after therapy with single-agent bleomycin, it is much more common following combination therapy. Vogelzang et al.[135] reported a 21% incidence in patients treated with vinblastine plus bleomycin, as compared with 41% when cisplatin was added to these two drugs. The incidence of Raynaud's also appears to be higher in patients treated with BEP as opposed to EP.[89] Studies employing provocative testing suggest that even asymptomatic individuals may exhibit an exaggerated vasospastic response to cold stimuli.[136] Symptoms persist indefinitely, with 49% of patients in one series reporting continued symptoms at a median of 8.5 years from completion of therapy. The vasospasm has, in general, been refractory to therapy, although some success has been reported with the calcium channel blocker nifedipine.[137]

The relationship of cisplatin-based chemotherapy to acute large-vessel ischemic events is less clear. There are case reports of myocardial ischemia and infarction, as well as cerebrovascular accidents, following vinblastine administration as a single agent or combined with bleomycin. Several anecdotal reports of major cardiovascular events in young men receiving chemotherapy for testicular cancer suggested a causal association between chemotherapeutic treatments and these events.[138] One population-based study did find increased cardiovascular disease mortality in the first year following testicular cancer patients treated with chemotherapy, but not in those treated with surgery alone.[139]

Population-based studies also highlight a substantial long-term increase in risk for cardiovascular disease particularly in patients who have received high cumulative doses of cisplatin. Fossa et al.,[140] for example, identified 38,907 patients, who were 1-year survivors of testicular cancer within 14 population-based cancer registries in North America and Europe. They calculated standardized mortality ratios (SMRs) for noncancer deaths and evaluated associations between histology, age at testicular cancer diagnosis, calendar year of diagnosis, and initial treatment and the risk of noncancer mortality. A total of 2942 deaths from all noncancer causes were reported after a median follow-up of 10 years, exceeding the expected number of deaths from all noncancer causes in the general population by 6% (SMR = 1.06, 95% CI = 1.02–1.10); the noncancer SMRs did not differ statistically significantly between patients diagnosed before and after 1975, when cisplatin-based chemotherapy came into widespread use. Mortality from all circulatory diseases was statistically significantly elevated in men diagnosed with testicular cancer before age 35 years (1.23, 95% CI = 1.09–1.39) but not in men diagnosed at older ages (SMR = 0.94; 95% CI = 0.89–1.00). Men treated with chemotherapy (with or without radiotherapy) specifically in 1975 or later had higher mortality from all noncancer causes (SMR = 1.34, 95% CI = 1.15–1.55), all circulatory diseases (SMR = 1.58, 95% CI = 1.25–2.01), all infections (SMR = 2.48, 95% CI = 1.70–3.50), and all respiratory diseases (SMR = 2.53, 95% CI = 1.26–4.53). Testicular cancer patients who were younger than 35 years at diagnosis and were treated with radiotherapy alone in 1975 or later had higher mortality from all circulatory diseases (SMR = 1.70, 95% CI = 1.21–2.31) compared with the general population. In longer follow-up, hypertension, glucose intolerance, unfavorable lipid profiles, and vascular events often arose. The development of metabolic syndrome is well described in association with testicular cancer and cisplatin-based chemotherapy.[141]

Patients with testicular cancer should be followed indefinitely. They benefit from weight reduction, smoking cessation, lipid profile monitoring, and appropriate blood pressure management. Patients and their treating physicians should remain cognizant of a persisting unfavorable cardiovascular risk profile in long-term survivors.[142,143]

Neurotoxicity

Peripheral neuropathy and ototoxicity observed in treated testicular cancer patients are attributable primarily to cisplatin, with a somewhat lesser contribution in older studies by vinblastine. The peripheral effects became manifest clinically as a distal sensory neuropathy, with paresthesias and dysesthesias, disturbances of position and vibratory sensation, and relative sparing of motor units.[144] Subjectively, these symptoms may be present for prolonged periods, with 43% of patients in one study reporting persistent symptoms 6–12 years after completion of therapy.[145] Objective studies confirmed the irreversibility of the neuropathy and suggest the dorsal root ganglion represents the primary target of cisplatin-induced damage.

The ototoxicity associated with cisplatin is primarily high-frequency hearing loss and is related to the cumulative dose of cisplatin.[146] Other risk factors for ototoxicity include a serum creatinine level higher than 1.5 mg/dL, increased age, and pre-existing hearing impairment. There is also emerging evidence that genetic factors make some individuals more susceptible to cisplatin toxicity.[147]

Second malignancies

Second primary cancers are a leading cause of death among men with testicular cancer.[148] For example, Travis et al. reviewed 14 population-based tumor registries in Europe and North America (1943–2001) and identified 40,576 patients, who were 1-year survivors. A total of 2285 second solid tumors were reported in the cohort. The relative risk and excess annual risk decreased with increasing age at testicular cancer diagnosis ($p < 0.001$); the excess annual risk increased with attained age ($p < 0.001$) but the excess relative risk decreased. Among 10-year survivors diagnosed with testicular cancer at age 35 years, the risk of developing a second solid tumor was increased (RR = 1.9, 95% CI = 1.8–2.1). Risk remained statistically significantly elevated for 35 years (RR = 1.7, 95% CI = 1.5–2.0; $P < 0.001$). Cancers of the lung (RR = 1.5, 95% CI = 1.2–1.7), colon (RR = 2.0, 95% CI = 1.7–2.5), bladder (RR = 2.7, 95% CI = 2.2–3.1), pancreas (RR = 3.6, 95% CI = 2.8–4.6), and stomach (RR = 4.0, 95% CI = 3.2–4.8) accounted for almost 60% of the total excess. Overall patterns were similar for seminoma and nonseminoma patients, with lower risks observed for nonseminoma patients treated after 1975. Statistically significantly increased risks of solid tumors were observed among patients treated with radiotherapy alone (RR = 2.0, 95% CI = 1.9–2.2), chemotherapy alone (RR = 1.8, 95% CI = 1.3–2.5), and both (RR = 2.9, 95% CI = 1.9–4.2). For patients diagnosed with seminomas or nonseminomatous tumors at age 35 years, cumulative risks of solid tumors 40 years later (i.e. to age 75 years) were 36% and 31%, respectively, compared with 23% for the general population and are also at increased risk of developing leukemia.

Fertility

Gonadal dysfunction is common in patients with a history of testicular cancer even when managed by orchiectomy alone. Before the effects of therapy on fertility are examined, it must be recognized that a significant proportion of testicular cancer patients may be oligospermic prior to the initiation of any therapy.[149] Although the etiology of this oligospermia is not fully understood, several mechanisms have been proposed, including an autoimmune process or a primary endocrine dysfunction resulting in impaired spermatogenesis.[150,151]

The chemotherapy administered for testicular cancer has acute effects on both spermatogenesis and Leydig cell function; most patients remain azoospermic with elevated serum gonadotropins for the first 12 months following therapy. These toxic effects are reversible in a significant number of patients, however, as approximately 50% will see a return of both spermatogenesis and Leydig cell function during the second year after completion of therapy.[149,151] Several factors decrease the likelihood of the return of spermatogenesis, including age over 30 years, treatment duration of more than 6 months, and prior abdominal radiotherapy. All men should be counseled on sperm cryopreservation prior to initiating chemotherapy.

Pulmonary toxicity

Pulmonary toxicity is most prominent with bleomycin and is related to cumulative dose, with a significant increase above 450 units. The earliest physical finding is an inspiratory lag and should prompt immediate discontinuation of the drug. Subsequent signs and symptoms include bibasilar rales, nonproductive cough, and exertional dyspnea. Laboratory abnormalities include decreases in diffusing capacity and late changes, including hypoxia and hypercapnia. Radiographic abnormalities include subpleural-based nodules, visible on the chest radiograph or chest CT scan.

The risk of developing symptomatic bleomycin-induced lung disease increases with age, prior or concomitant chest radiotherapy,[152] decreased renal function,[153] and high concentrations of inspired oxygen. Because the mortality for this condition approaches 50% and therapeutic interventions such as corticosteroids are ineffective, early diagnosis of asymptomatic patients and subsequent discontinuation of the drug are particularly important. High concentrations of inspired oxygen during postchemotherapy surgery should be avoided if possible in BEP-treated patients. The incidence of clinically significant bleomycin toxicity is negligible, however, with three cycles of BEP, with some evidence that with modern monitoring of pulmonary function, the 15-year cumulative risk of pulmonary disease in patients treated with BEP was comparable to those with stage I disease who were followed with surveillance when controlling for pulmonary surgery, pulmonary emboli, and initial prognosis.[154]

Toxicity of radiation

Acute

Acute radiation toxicity is dependent on what organs are irradiated, the radiation dose, and the volume. For example, the MRC TE10 trial randomized stage I seminoma patients to PA only or PA with an ipsilateral pelvic field (dogleg [DL]).[155] The acute toxicity of nausea/vomiting was similar but slightly higher in the DL arm and both groups experienced nausea requiring medication in 25–30% of patients. Since DL treats much more bone marrow, the rates of mild leukopenia were twice as high when compared with the PA field alone (19% vs 42%, $p < 0.0001$), but this is rarely clinically significant. Diarrhea was reported in 7% of the PA arm only, but 14% in the ipsilateral pelvic field arm ($p = 0.013$).

In regards to fertility, exposure of the remaining testis to internal radiation scatter from adjuvant radiotherapy to the PA or PA and ipsilateral pelvic nodes after orchiectomy may further impair fertility. The degree of fertility impairment is dose dependent, and temporary azoospermia may occur at dose levels as low as 40–50 cGy (0.4–0.5 Gy).[156,157] Permanent sterility occurs after 2–3.5 Gy. Testicular shielding dramatically reduces the dose to the testis. For patients treated with PA and DL or PA radiation fields with gonadal shielding, the average testicular dose per fraction is 1.48 and 0.65 cGy, respectively.[158] Hormonal changes require much higher doses and are not detectable based on testosterone. Subtle Leydig cell dysfunction, as measured by serum FSH and LH concentrations may occur, which are also dose and field dependent.[159]

Consequently, before adjuvant radiation, appropriate counseling, baseline fertility testing, and semen cryopreservation should be considered in patients considering having children in the future.

Chronic

The avoidance of chronic toxicity or permanent late effects has raised the profile of surveillance as a preferred treatment option for many young patients with seminoma. Because radiation for seminoma historically incorporated a mediastinal field, cardiac toxicity developed in many. At M. D. Anderson, of 477 men with stage I or II testicular seminoma treated between 1951 and 1999 with a median follow-up of 13.3 years, the cardiac-specific SMR was 1.61, while the cancer-specific SMR was 1.91.[160] Both toxicities were only evident after 15 years of follow-up. Fifteen years may represent the latency period for chronic toxicity to develop, but it may also demonstrate that radiation treatment doses and fields prior to 1990 are more toxic versus modern practices. Additional data on chronic vascular and mortality impact of radiation is discussed above.

Extragonadal germ cell tumors (EGCTs)

An important subset of germ cell tumors is extragonadal in origin. Overall, approximately 5% of all germ cell cancers arise in nongonadal sites, particularly in the mediastinum and retroperitoneum. EGCTs have also been described in the pineal region, sacrococcygeal region, and rarely in the prostate, vagina, orbits, liver, and gastrointestinal tract.

EGCTs were once thought to represent metastasis from an occult gonadal primary. Autopsy findings in 20 patients with extragonadal mediastinal germ cell tumors found only one case of a testicular primary and one patient with a testicular scar.[161] Both of these cases were associated with clinically occult lower retroperitoneal involvement. Primary retroperitoneal germ cell tumors are more commonly associated with an occult testicular primary site, especially when the tumor is not midline in origin. EGCTs more likely represent malignant transformation of germinal elements distributed to these sites without a testicular focus.

In adults, the mediastinum is the most common extragonadal site for the development of germ cell tumors. The most frequent symptoms at initial presentation include dyspnea, chest pain, and cough followed by fever, weight loss, vena cava occlusion syndrome, and fatigue/weakness. The presence of mature teratoma is suggested by a large circumscribed anterior mediastinal mass with normal serum HCG and AFP. Management of mature teratoma is surgical, and there is no role for chemotherapy or radiotherapy. Although these tumors histologically are benign, removal is often difficult.[162]

The principles of management of extragonadal NSGCT parallel those of testicular germ cell cancer. The diagnosis should be considered in any young person with a poorly differentiated cancer arising in midline structures. STMs should be obtained and, if the clinical condition is stable, a biopsy also should be obtained. In most settings, surgical debulking should not be considered part of primary management. Cisplatin-based chemotherapy followed by surgical resection of residual masses should be performed as with testicular germ cell cancer. However, cure rates for NSGCT of mediastinal origin are significantly inferior compared with those of testicular origin. An international analysis of 635 patients with EGCTs demonstrated an almost 90% chance of cure with pure seminoma irrespective of the primary site, but only 45% survival at 5 years for patients with mediastinal nonseminomatous tumors.[161]

Several important biologic associations have been specifically reported with mediastinal NSGCT, include a high frequency (up to 20%) of Klinefelter syndrome.[13] Additionally, approximately 10% of patients with mediastinal NSGCT develop associated malignant hematologic dyscrasias.[163] Careful clinical and cytogenetic analyses of these cases suggest they do not arise as a consequence of therapy for germ cell tumors but represent a unique and biologically important association between these disorders. Similar cases are not found among those patients with testicular or retroperitoneal germ cell cancer treated with identical chemotherapy. Most compelling, however, is the finding of the most common karyotypic abnormality of germ cell cancer, isochromosome 12p, in a mediastinal germ cell tumor and in the leukemic blasts of one of these patients. This implies the mediastinal germ cell tumor and the hematologic malignancy arose from a common progenitor cell.

Patients with EGCTs, particularly those with retroperitoneal or nonseminomatous tumors, are at an increased risk of metachronous testicular cancer.[164] The cumulative risk 10 years after a diagnosis of EGCT was approximately 14% for patients with retroperitoneal or nonseminomatous EGCTs.

Key references

The complete reference list can be found on Vital Source version of this title, see inside front cover.

1. SEER (2019) *U.S. Population Data - 1969-2018*, https://seer.cancer.gov/popdata/ (accessed 8 October 2020).
9. Fossa SD, Chen J, Schonfeld SJ, et al. Risk of contralateral testicular cancer: a population-based study of 29,515 U.S. men. *J Natl Cancer Inst*. 2005;**97**(14):1056–1066.
17. Paner GP, Stadler WM, Hansel DE, et al. Updates in the eighth edition of the tumor-node-metastasis staging classification for urologic cancers. *Eur Urol*. 2018;**73**(4):560–569.
28. Kum JB, Ulbright TM, Williamson SR, et al. Molecular genetic evidence supporting the origin of somatic-type malignancy and teratoma from the same progenitor cell. *Am J Surg Pathol*. 2012;**36**(12):1849–1856.
36. Amin MB, American Joint Committee on Cancer, American Cancer Society. In: Amin MB, Edge SB, Gress DM, et al., eds. *AJCC Cancer Staging Manual*, 8th ed. Chicago IL: American Joint Committee on Cancer, Springer; 2017:xvii, 1024.
37. National Comprehensive Cancer Network (2020) *Testicular Cancer. Version 2.20*, https://www.nccn.org/professionals/physician_gls/pdf/testicular.pdf (accessed 1 October 2020).
59. Albers P, Siener R, Krege S, et al. Randomized phase III trial comparing retroperitoneal lymph node dissection with one course of bleomycin and etoposide plus cisplatin chemotherapy in the adjuvant treatment of clinical stage I Nonseminomatous testicular germ cell tumors: AUO trial AH 01/94 by the German Testicular Cancer Study Group. *J Clin Oncol*. 2008;**26**(18):2966–2972.
60. Cullen M, Huddart R, Joffe J, et al. The 111 study: a single-arm, phase 3 trial evaluating one cycle of bleomycin, etoposide, and cisplatin as adjuvant chemotherapy in high-risk, stage 1 nonseminomatous or combined germ cell tumours of the testis. *Eur Urol*. 2020;**77**(3):344–351.
66. Motzer RJ, Sheinfeld J, Mazumdar M, et al. Etoposide and cisplatin adjuvant therapy for patients with pathologic stage II germ cell tumors. *J Clin Oncol*. 1995;**13**(11):2700–2704.
78. Higby DJ, Wallace HJ Jr, Albert DJ, et al. Diaminodichloroplatinum: a phase I study showing responses in testicular and other tumors. *Cancer*. 1974;**33**(5):1219–1225.
79. Einhorn LH, Donohue J. Cis-diamminedichloroplatinum, vinblastine, and bleomycin combination chemotherapy in disseminated testicular cancer. *Ann Intern Med*. 1977;**87**(3):293–298.
83. The International Germ Cell Collaborative Group. International germ cell consensus classification: a prognostic factor-based staging system for metastatic germ cell cancers. International Germ Cell Cancer Collaborative Group. *J Clin Oncol*. 1997;**15**(2):594–603.
85. Loehrer PJ Sr, Johnson D, Elson P, et al. Importance of bleomycin in favorable-prognosis disseminated germ cell tumors: an Eastern Cooperative Oncology Group trial. *J Clin Oncol*. 1995;**13**(2):470–476.
86. Bajorin DF, Sarosdy MF, Pfister DG, et al. Randomized trial of etoposide and cisplatin versus etoposide and carboplatin in patients with good-risk germ cell tumors: a multiinstitutional study. *J Clin Oncol*. 1993;**11**(4):598–606.
88. de Wit R, Stoter G, Kaye SB, et al. Importance of bleomycin in combination chemotherapy for good-prognosis testicular nonseminoma: a randomized study of the European Organization for Research and Treatment of Cancer Genitourinary Tract Cancer Cooperative Group. *J Clin Oncol*. 1997;**15**(5):1837–1843.
89. Culine S, Kerbrat P, Kramar A, et al. Refining the optimal chemotherapy regimen for good-risk metastatic nonseminomatous germ-cell tumors: a randomized trial of the Genito-Urinary Group of the French Federation of Cancer Centers (GETUG T93BP). *Ann Oncol*. 2007;**18**(5):917–924.
92. Nichols CR, Catalano PJ, Crawford ED, et al. Randomized comparison of cisplatin and etoposide and either bleomycin or ifosfamide in treatment of advanced disseminated germ cell tumors: an Eastern Cooperative Oncology Group, Southwest Oncology Group, and Cancer and Leukemia Group B Study. *J Clin Oncol*. 1998;**16**(4):1287–1293.
98. Motzer RJ, Nichols CJ, Margolin KA, et al. Phase III randomized trial of conventional-dose chemotherapy with or without high-dose chemotherapy and autologous hematopoietic stem-cell rescue as first-line treatment for patients with poor-prognosis metastatic germ cell tumors. *J Clin Oncol*. 2007;**25**(3):247–256.
101. Ehrlich Y, Brames MJ, Beck SD, et al. Long-term follow-up of cisplatin combination chemotherapy in patients with disseminated nonseminomatous germ cell tumors: is a postchemotherapy retroperitoneal lymph node dissection needed after complete remission? *J Clin Oncol*. 2010;**28**(4):531–536.
105. De Santis M, Becherer A, Bokemeyer C, et al. 2-18fluoro-deoxy-D-glucose positron emission tomography is a reliable predictor for viable tumor in postchemotherapy seminoma: an update of the prospective multicentric SEM-PET trial. *J Clin Oncol*. 2004;**22**(6):1034–1039.
112. Shayegan B, Carver BS, Stasi J, et al. Clinical outcome following post-chemotherapy retroperitoneal lymph node dissection in men with intermediate- and poor-risk nonseminomatous germ cell tumour. *BJU Int*. 2007;**99**(5):993–997.
119. Kondagunta GV, Bacik J, Donadio A, et al. Combination of paclitaxel, ifosfamide, and cisplatin is an effective second-line therapy for patients with relapsed testicular germ cell tumors. *J Clin Oncol*. 2005;**23**(27):6549–6555.
134. Fossa SD, Aass N, Winderen M, et al. Long-term renal function after treatment for malignant germ-cell tumours. *Ann Oncol*. 2002;**13**(2):222–228.
139. Fung C, Sesso HD, Williams AM, et al. Multi-institutional assessment of adverse health outcomes among North American testicular cancer survivors after modern cisplatin-based chemotherapy. *J Clin Oncol*. 2017;**35**(11):1211–1222.
140. Fossa SD, Gilbert E, Dores GM, et al. Noncancer causes of death in survivors of testicular cancer. *J Natl Cancer Inst*. 2007;**99**(7):533–544.
142. Strumberg D, Brugge S, Korn MW, et al. Evaluation of long-term toxicity in patients after cisplatin-based chemotherapy for non-seminomatous testicular cancer. *Ann Oncol*. 2002;**13**(2):229–236.
143. Meinardi MT, Gietema JA, van der Graaf WT, et al. Cardiovascular morbidity in long-term survivors of metastatic testicular cancer. *J Clin Oncol*. 2000;**18**(8):1725–1732.
147. Trendowski MR, El Charif O, Dinh PC Jr, et al. Genetic and modifiable risk factors contributing to cisplatin-induced toxicities. *Clin Cancer Res*. 2019;**25**(4):1147–1155.
148. Travis LB, Fossa SD, Schonfeld SJ, et al. Second cancers among 40,576 testicular cancer patients: focus on long-term survivors. *J Natl Cancer Inst*. 2005;**97**(18):1354–1365.
151. Huddart RA, Norman A, Moynihan C, et al. Fertility, gonadal and sexual function in survivors of testicular cancer. *Br J Cancer*. 2005;**93**(2):200–207.

98 Neoplasms of the vulva and vagina

Michael Frumovitz, MD, MPH ■ Summer B. Dewdney, MD

Overview

Vulvar and vaginal carcinomas are uncommon diseases that generally affect postmenopausal women, although 19% of vulvar carcinomas occur in women <50 years old. Risk factors for vulvar carcinoma include human papilloma virus and chronic inflammation. Vulvar intraepithelial neoplasia can often be managed with wide local excision, but several other modalities have been utilized. Most vulvar malignancies are squamous cell carcinomas that are managed by surgical excision and radiotherapy. Sentinel lymph node biopsy has been used to spare the morbidity observed after regional lymph node dissection. For more advanced lesions, chemo-radiotherapy with agents such as 5-FU, cisplatin, and mitomycin C is utilized. Other vulvar malignancies include Bartholin gland carcinomas, basal cell carcinomas, verrucous carcinomas, and melanomas. Carcinomas of the vagina are most frequently squamous cell, but clear cell adenocarcinomas have been seen in younger women. In the past, clear cell carcinomas were associated with pre-natal exposure to diethylstilbestrol. Vaginal melanomas can occur, as well as endodermal sinus tumors, rhabdomyosarcomas, and fibroepithelial vaginal polyps.

Cancer of the vulva

Incidence and epidemiology

Vulvar cancer accounts for about 4% of cancers in the female reproductive organs and 0.6% of all cancers in women. It is the fourth most frequent gynecologic cancer.[1] The American Cancer Society estimated that in 2020, about 6120 cancers of the vulva were diagnosed in the United States and about 1350 women die of this cancer.[2]

Risk factors include cigarette smoking, human papillomavirus (HPV), vulvar or cervical intraepithelial neoplasia, chronic immunosuppression, chronic vulvar inflammatory diseases (e.g., lichen sclerosis and lichen planus), and northern European ancestry.[3] Most vulvar carcinomas occur in older women, with more than 50% of the patients being 60–79 years of age. Kumar et al. found that younger patients with vulvar cancer are increasing with frequency, and through evaluation of the SEER database found that 19% of patients diagnosed with vulvar cancer are <50 years old. In addition, there is a striking survival difference between the younger and older women with squamous cell vulvar cancer (Figure 1).[4] This increased frequency in younger patients may be attributed to an increase in HPV, specifically HPV-related vulvar intraepithelial neoplasia (VIN) that progresses to cancer.

Vulvar cancer is thought to develop through two types of pathways, the first related to HPV infections and the second related to a chronic inflammatory process.[5] Several epidemiologic studies suggest a sexually transmitted origin for carcinoma of the vulva. Condyloma acuminatum associated with HPV has been noted in many patients with premalignant and malignant vulvar disease. It has been estimated that in the United States, over 1 million women each year develop perineal warts and that as many as 10% are infected with HPV.[6] Currently, HPV types 6 and 11 are most frequently found in benign vulvar warts, and HPV types 16, 18, 31, 33, and 45 are more frequently associated with intraepithelial neoplasia or invasive carcinoma.[6–8] HPV can be found in approximately 50% of vulvar carcinomas; the tumors are often multifocal and associated with vulvar dysplasias. HPV-negative tumors are often found in older women.[9,10] These can be associated with chronic inflammatory disease as seen with vulvar dystrophies.

Although epidemiologic evidence strongly suggests a viral cause, other associations have been implied as well. Factors such as granulomatous diseases of the vulva, diabetes, hypertension, and obesity also have been associated with vulvar carcinoma, but perhaps this is because of the usually advanced age of patients. A case-control study by Mabuchi et al.[11] found that domestic servants, or those working in laundry or cleaning plants, have an increased risk of vulvar carcinoma, thus suggesting an environmental component.

The association of carcinoma *in situ* (CIS) with invasive carcinoma of the vulva indicates a continuum from preinvasive to invasive carcinoma. Jones et al.[12] evaluated 405 cases of VIN 2–3, they found that 3.8% of patients that are treated will progress to cancer, and 10 patients who did not undergo treatment progressed in 3.9 years (mean). Progression, however, may differ between younger and older patients. Some authors suggest that the multifocal CIS of women in their thirties or forties are less likely to progress compared to older women.[13–15]

Vulvar intraepithelial neoplasias

In 2004, The International Society for the Study of Vulvar Disease developed the current classification system for VIN (Table 1). Previous classification included VIN 1, 2, and 3 according to the degree of abnormality. Currently, only high-grade disease is defined as VIN and hence would take that nomenclature. It has been shown that VIN 1 is not a cancer precursor and therefore is not described as VIN. In 2004, they developed two categories to describe VIN: VIN, usual type (includes former VIN 2 and 3 of warty or basaloid and mixed types), and VIN, differentiated type (associated with lichen sclerosus).[17] In addition, the College of American Pathologists and the ASCCP confirmed a two-tier system with the recent Lower Anogenital Squamous Terminology (LAST) terminology project.[18] ACOG-ASCCP issued a committee

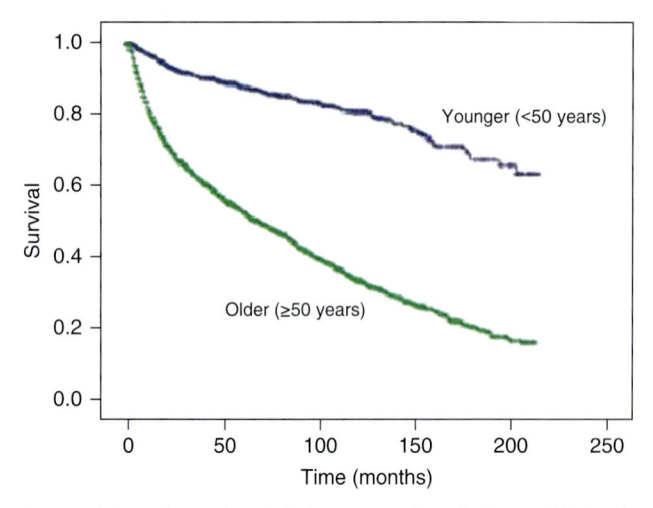

Figure 1 Comparison of survival of younger patients (<50 years; blue line) with that of older patients (≥50 years; green line) with squamous cell cancer of the vulva, 1988–2005. Log-rank $p = 0.001$. Source: Kumar et al.[4]

Table 1 Classifications of vulvar dysplasias.[a]

ISSVD 1986 (old classification)	ISSVD 2004 (new classification)	LAST (lower anogenital squamous terminology) 2012
VIN 1	Flat condyloma or HPV effect	LSIL
VIN 2 and VIN 3	VIN, usual type: 1. VIN, warty type 2. VIN, basaloid type 3. VIN, mixed	HSIL
Differentiated VIN	VIN, differentiated type	Differentiated VIN (dVIN)

Abbreviations: VIN, vulvar intraepithelial neoplasia; HPV, human papillomavirus; LSIL, low-grade squamous intraepithelial lesion; HSIL, high-grade squamous intraepithelial lesion.
[a]Source: Rogers and Cuello.[16]

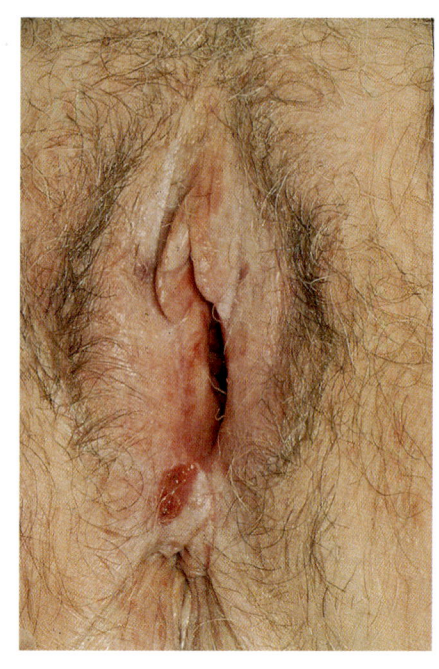

Figure 2 White, brittle paperlike appearance or lichen sclerosus of the vulva.

opinion on treatment of VIN cases given that there has been such an increase over the past 30 years, confirming agreement with ISVDD nomenclature of VIN differentiated type and usual type, and discussing treatment recommendations. Of note, many pathologists and practitioners still use the old classifications.

VIN can present with a variety of symptoms. The most common is irritation or itching; however, 20% of patients are asymptomatic.[19] Grossly, the lesions can be flat, raised (maculopapular), or verrucous. In color, they may be brown (hyperpigmented), red (erythroplastic), white, or discolored.

White lesions can appear to have a whitish, thickened keratin layer (leukoplakia) or a diffuse, white, brittle, paper-like appearance (lichen sclerosus) (Figure 2). Areas of squamous hyperplasia (hyperplastic dystrophy) and dysplasia can also have a white appearance. Unlike lichen sclerosus, however, the tissue often is thickened, and the process tends to be focal or multifocal rather than diffuse.[15] It is important to biopsy lichen sclerosus as there may be an underlying vulvar carcinoma.[20,21]

Microscopically, atypical changes in the vulvar epithelium consistent with preinvasive lesions usually are marked by loss of maturation of the squamous epithelium. There is increased mitotic activity and an increase in the nuclear-cytoplasmic ratio.

There is suggestion that there are two distinct causes of vulvar dysplasia leading to vulvar cancer. The first type is seen in younger patients and is related to HPV infection and smoking. This type presents itself as a "warty" dysplasia. The more common type is in elderly patients and is unrelated to smoking or HPV. This group is more related to lichen sclerosus adjacent to the tumor. Approximately 20% of vulvar cancer has been reported to have vulvar dysplasia.

The best method of establishing a diagnosis is a high index of suspicion and early biopsy. Several methods also can be used to help assess these lesions. Cytology, colposcopy, acetic acid, and toluidine blue O can be used cautiously before biopsy. In general, however, cytologic evaluation of the vulva has not been helpful as a screening examination because the vulvar skin often is thickened and keratinized. Colposcopic examination of the vulva is difficult because unlike cervical lesions, the changes are difficult to recognize. Therefore, colposcopic examination is not used for routine vulvar examination; rather, it is primarily employed for patients who are being evaluated or followed for vulvar atypia or intraepithelial malignancies. The toluidine blue O test is nonspecific and stains nuclei in the superficial part of the epithelium. Colposcopy is performed after applying a 1% aqueous solution of toluidine blue O to the vulva for 1 min and decolorizing the tissue with 1% acetic acid. Areas that retain the stain are biopsied. A positive test, however, does not always indicate a premalignant condition because 20% of benign areas on the vulva stain positively.[20]

To obtain the entire thickness of the skin for a definitive diagnosis, a biopsy of the vulva usually is done with a Keyes dermal punch. Occasionally, a larger biopsy is needed, in which case a larger field can be locally anesthetized with lidocaine and a small scalpel or cervical biopsy punch used to obtain a specimen.[22]

Once the correct diagnosis has been established by biopsy, appropriate therapy can be undertaken. For lichen sclerosis, local measures, for example, wearing cotton underclothes and avoiding strong soaps and detergents, often are used to diminish irritation. Topical fluorinated corticosteroids applied twice daily for 1–2 weeks are helpful in controlling pruritus, but prolonged use of these steroid preparations can lead to vulvar atrophy or contracture. If long-term therapy is needed, a nonfluorinated compound such as 1% hydrocortisone is used. Some patients with lichen sclerosis have severe contracture in the area of the posterior fourchette. Treating these areas surgically with plastic repair of the fourchette has been suggested.[23,24]

VIN can be treated by a variety of methods, and many authors have reported successful control of the disease by wide local excision.[10,23] Adequate margins must be obtained with wide excision; however, this often may be difficult because of the multifocal nature of the disease. Wallbillich et al.[25] found that positive margins increased recurrence from 11% to 32%, and recurrence was associated with smoking and a large lesion size.

Other modalities also have been reported in the treatment of VIN. Carbon dioxide laser vaporization and photodynamic therapy[26] of the vulva to a depth of 3 mm have been used, and current evidence indicates that laser therapy is as effective as surgical excision for the control of this disease. Before lasering the vulva, however, it is necessary to ascertain by histologic confirmation that invasive disease does not exist. Leuchter et al.[27] treated 142 patients with CIS of the vulva. Of those treated by laser, 17% had a recurrence, a result that is similar to that in lesions treated by local excision.

Imiquimod has been used also for conservative medical treatment. A systematic review that included two randomized control trials found a complete response rate of 51%.[28] 5-Fluorouracil (5-FU) cream has been used successfully to treat CIS of the vulva, and application of this has been reported to be successful in 75% of cases. With continuous application, however, this treatment causes edema and pain. Most recently, a multicenter, randomized, phase 2 trial between cidofovir and imiquimod for treatment of VIN3 showed a response rate of approximately 46% for both groups treated.[29]

Paget disease

Paget disease is a rare intraepithelial disorder of the vulvar skin that is seen in postmenopausal women.[30–32] Unlike VIN, the intraepithelial neoplastic cells are glandular rather than squamous. The lesion primarily occurs in Caucasians of an average age of 65 years. Grossly, it appears as a reddish, eczematoid lesion. Microscopically, this type of lesion is characterized by large pale cells that often occur in nests and infiltrate the epithelium. Once the diagnosis is made, it is important to rule out the presence of an underlying cancer. Invasive vulvar Paget disease occurs in approximately 10% of Paget disease.[21] If the anal area is involved, one needs to consider an anal carcinoma. A review by Lee et al.[31] reported a total of 75 cases of Paget disease of the vulva: 16 (22%) of the patients had underlying invasive carcinoma of the adnexal structures and 7 (9%) had adnexal CIS.

Paget disease of the vulva often spreads in an occult manner, with margins extending beyond the normal appearance of the lesion.[32] If there is no evidence of an underlying malignant neoplasm, a wide local excision or total vulvectomy usually is performed.[33] If a wide local excision is performed, a slightly deeper excision is needed to remove the epidermis down to the level of the underlying fat to ensure removal of adnexal skin structures. Because this lesion extends sub-epithelially, a frozen section in the operating room may assist in ensuring complete removal.

Onaiwu et al. reported on 89 patients with Paget disease of the vulva of which 74 (83%) underwent surgical excision.[34] In these patients, 87% had positive margins on the pathologic specimen demonstrating the difficulty in obtaining a complete resection. Recurrence of Paget disease is common with over half of patients requiring retreatment for disease. Margin status, however, does not seem to predict recurrence so we recommend simple vulvectomy with resection of disease attempting to get grossly negative margins. Utilizing Moh's surgery to achieve pathologically negative margins does not appear to reduce recurrent rates although studies utilizing this surgical approach are small.[34]

Nonsurgical treatments for Paget disease have also been explored. These include topical therapies such as 5-FU, bleomycin, and imiquimod. In small studies, imiquimod appears to show some promise while 5-FU and bleomycin have not proven effective.[35] Imiquimod cream is an immune response modulator that is FDA approved for the treatment of external anogenital warts, actinic keratosis, and basal cell carcinomas. In a study of 8 patients with recurrent Paget disease of the vulva, 6 had a complete response to therapy by 12 weeks.[36] Unfortunately the majority of patients recurred even after a complete response.

Invasive vulvar carcinomas

The International Federation of Gynecology and Obstetrics (FIGO) adopted a new surgical staging system in 2009 (Table 2). This surgical staging has been modified once prior, in 1995, after it became a surgically staged cancer in 1989. The most recent staging system addresses lack of predictive value seen in the previous stages with regard to the size of the lesion and number and size of lymph node metastasis.[37] Specifically, in the new system, there was an addition of three pathologic groupings within stage III (A, B, and C), this identifies the number of positive node, the size of each node, and extracapsular spread. In addition, many centers use the tumor, node, and metastasis (TNM) classification (Table 2).

Vulvar cancer can spread by direct extension, lymphatic embolization, or hematogenous dissemination. Metastasis to the femoral nodes without inguinal node involvement has been reported but is uncommon. The direct lymphatic pathways from the clitoris to the pelvic nodes have been described but are not of clinical significance. The overall incidence of lymph node metastasis is approximately 30%. Pelvic node metastasis is uncommon with an overall frequency of 9%. Approximately 20% of patients with positive groin nodes have positive pelvic nodes.[38,39]

Squamous cell carcinoma

Squamous cell carcinomas comprise approximately 90% of primary vulvar malignancies. Grossly, these carcinomas usually appear as ulcerated or polypoid masses on the vulva. Biopsy reveals the characteristic histologic appearance: the tumor appears in nests and cords of squamous cells infiltrating the stroma, often with islands of keratin. On physical examination, there is usually an ulcerated lesion or wart-like lesion. Recently, there has been an increased incidence of warty carcinomas accounting for 20% of all cases.

Different clinical results have been reported with this definition. Spread to regional lymph nodes has varied from 0% to 10% in tumors with less than a 5 mm depth of invasion.[40–45] For example, Hoffman et al.[43] reported no nodal metastases in 43 patients whose tumor invaded <2 mm. Lesions that were at risk of spreading to inguinal nodes included tumors with confluent tongues rather than those with individual tongues merely extending into the stroma. Depth of invasion of the stroma to ≤1 mm is associated with a risk of lymph nodes metastasis of <1%, hence no need for a patient with <1 mm stromal invasion to undergo a inguinal lymph node dissection. Tumors with a depth of invasion of 1.1–3.0 mm are associated with lymph node metastasis of 6–12%, and this rate increases to 15–20% with depth of invasion of 3.1–5 mm.[46]

The risk of nodal involvement may be decreased when CIS is present in the lesion. Rowley et al.[44] noted that only 1 of 35 cases with adjacent CIS had nodal metastases. By contrast, 5 of 27 had positive lymph nodes when superficial stage I lesions penetrating 2.1–5.0 mm did not have adjacent CIS.

Table 2 TNM classification and staging of vulvar carcinoma.[a]

TNM classification		
T		Primary tumor
TX		Primary tumor cannot be assessed
T0		No evidence of primary tumor
T1		Tumor confined to the vulva and/or perineum
		Multifocal lesions should be designated as such. The largest lesion or the lesion with the greatest depth of invasion will be the target lesion identified to address the highest pT stage
		Depth of invasion is defined as the measurement of the tumor from the epithelial-stromal junction of the adjacent most superficial dermal papilla to the deepest point of invasion
T1a		Lesions 2 cm or less, confined to the vulva and/or perineum, and with stromal invasion of 1 mm or less
T1b		Lesions more than 2 cm, or any size with stromal invasion of more than 1 mm, confined to the vulva and/or perineum
T2		Tumor of any size with extension to adjacent perineal structures (lower/distal third of the urethra, lower/distal third of the vagina, anal involvement)
T3		Tumor of any size with extension to any of the following—upper/proximal two-thirds of the urethra, upper/proximal two-thirds of the vagina, bladder mucosa, or rectal mucosa—or fixed to the pelvic bone
N		Regional lymph nodes
NX		Regional nodes cannot be assessed
N0		No regional lymph node metastasis
N0(i+)		Isolated tumor cells in regional lymph node(s) no greater than 0.2 mm
N1		Regional lymph node metastasis with one or two lymph node metastases each less than 5 mm, or one lymph node metastasis greater than or equal to 5 mm
N1a[b]		One or two lymph node metastases each less than 5 mm
N1b		One lymph node metastasis greater than or equal to 5 mm
N2		Regional lymph node metastasis with three or more lymph node metastases each less than 5 mm, or two or more lymph node metastases greater than or equal to 5 mm, or lymph node(s) with extranodal extension
N2a[b]		Three or more lymph node metastases each less than 5 mm
N2b		Two or more lymph node metastases greater than or equal to 5 mm
N2c		Lymph node(s) with extranodal extension
N3		Fixed or ulcerated regional lymph node metastasis
M		Distant metastases
M0		No distant metastasis (no pathological M0; use clinical M to complete stage group)
M1		Distant metastases (including pelvic lymph node metastases)
FIGO staging (2009)		
IA	T1a, N0, M0	Tumor confined to the vulva and/or perineum: 2 cm or less in greatest dimension, ≤1 mm stromal invasion, no nodal metastasis
IB	T1b, N0, M0	Tumor confined to the vulva and/or perineum: 2 cm or greater in greatest dimension, >1 mm stromal invasion, no nodal metastasis
II	T2, N0, M0	Tumor of any size with extension to adjacent perineal structures (1/3 lower urethra, 1/3 lower vagina, anus) with negative nodes
IIIA	T1 or T2, N1, M0	Tumor of any size with or without extension to adjacent perineal structures (1/3 lower urethra, 1/3 lower vagina, and anus) and positive inguinofemoral lymph node, (1) 1–2 lymph node metastasis (<5 mm) or (2) 1 lymph node metastasis ≥5 mm
IIIB	T1 or T2, N2a or N2b, M0	Tumor of any size with or without extension to adjacent perineal structures (1/3 lower urethra, 1/3 lower vagina, and anus) and positive inguinofemoral lymph node, (1) 3 or more lymph node metastasis (<5 mm) or (2) 2 or more lymph node metastasis ≥5 mm
IIIC	T1 or T2, N2c, M0	Positive node with extracapsular spread
IVA	T1 or T2, N3, M0 or T3, any N, M0	Tumor invades any of the following: upper urethra, bladder mucosa, rectal mucosa, pelvic bone, and/or bilateral regional node metastasis
IVB	Any T, Any N, M1	Any distant metastasis including pelvic lymph nodes

Abbreviations: FIGO, International Federation of Gynecology and Obstetrics; TNM, tumor, node, and metastasis.
Note: The site, size, and laterality of lymph node metastases should be recorded.
[a]Source: American College of Surgeons, Chicago, Illinois. The original source for this information is the AJCC Cancer Staging Manual, Eighth Edition (2017) published by Springer International Publishing. Corrected at 4th printing, 2018.
[b]Includes micrometastasis, N1mi and N2mi.

Sentinel inguinal lymph node biopsy

Sentinel lymph node biopsy (SLNB) has now become the standard of care for lymph node assessment in the surgical treatment of vulvar cancer. In patients with a clinically negative groin examination, a SLNB is the preferred alternative to inguinofemoral lymphadenectomy. SLNB results in less morbidity without compromising detection for lymph node metastases. The Gynecologic Oncology Group (GOG 173) compared SLNB to inguinofemoral lymphadenectomy in 452 women with squamous cell vulvar cancer, for tumors with a depth >1 mm, and size between 2 and 6 cm.[47] The sensitivity of the SLNB was 92%, and the negative predictive value is 96% in this study. Another multicenter observational study GROINSS-V analyzed 623 groin nodes from 403 patients.[48] In this study, all women with tumors <4 cm underwent a SLNB alone. If the sentinel node was negative, they were followed for 2 years. In these patients, the groin recurrence rate was 3% which was similar to historic controls after complete inguinofemoral lymphadenectomy. For patients who had a positive sentinel node, a complete inguinofemoral lymphadenectomy was performed and taken off study. When comparing those patients who underwent SLNB alone to those who had a complete inguinofemoral lymphadenectomy, patients undergoing a SLNB alone reported less treatment-related morbidity compared to inguinofemoral lymphadenectomy without compromising the overall quality of life.[49]

Treatment

Clinical stage IA
Tumors showing a depth of the stroma 1 mm or less have minimal risk for lymphatic dissemination. They do not require an inguinofemoral lymph node dissection because the risk of lymph node metastases in this setting is very low risk. These lesions are usually treated with a wide local excision. These patients do NOT have a high recurrence rate; however, surveillance is needed to rule out recurrence.

Clinical stage I/II
The recommendation for a clinical-stage I or II vulvar cancer is a wide radical excision with unilateral or bilateral SLNB versus an inguinal femoral lymphadenectomy (depending on size, location, and institution) for both staging and therapeutic purposes. Margins need to include at least a 2 cm margin lateral of normal tissue, with the deep margin to the deep perineal fascia. The laterality of the lesion determines the need for bilateral versus unilateral inguinofemoral lymph node dissection (or SLNB). A subanalysis of GOG 173 shows that a bilateral lymph node dissection is required except when the tumor is located more than 2 cm or greater from the midline. For both stages I and II, surgical resection usually leads to excellent long-term survival and local control.

The pattern of spread for this carcinoma relates to the intricate lymphatic drainage of the vulva (Figure 3). Tumors located in the middle of either labium initially drain to the ipsilateral inguinal femoral nodes, whereas midline perineal tumors can spread to either the left or right side. Using technetium-99m colloid, Iversen and Aas showed that when radioactivity was injected to one side of the vulva, 98% of it localized in the ipsilateral nodes and <2% in the contralateral nodes.[39] Tumors along the midline in the clitoral or urethral areas may spread to either groin. From the inguinal-femoral nodes, lymphatic spread continues to the deep pelvic iliac and obturator nodes. Although there has been concern in the past that tumors in the clitoral–urethral area could spread directly to the deep pelvic nodes, current evidence indicates that this is rare.

Stages I, II, and III invasive carcinoma
The prognosis of a patient with vulvar carcinoma relates to the stage of disease (Figure 4). The presence of carcinoma in the regional lymph nodes correlates with the size and thickness of the primary lesion, the degree of tumor differentiation, and the involvement of vascular spaces by the tumor as seen in Table 3, which comes from a classic study by Sedlis et al.[50] In 272 women with invasive vulvar carcinoma reported by the GOG, regional nodes were involved in 8.9% of stage I, 25.3% of stage II, and 31.1% of stage III lesions.[51,52] With larger lesions, 4 mm or greater in thickness, 31% of nodes were positive. Hacker et al.[53] reported an actuarial 5-year survival rate of 96% in those with negative nodes survival decreased to 94% with one positive node, 80% with two positive nodes, and 12% with three or more nodes involved by tumor.

Not only is the number of nodes important, but there also appears to be a correlation with the size of the metastases. Hoffman et al.[54] noted that 14 of 15 patients with inguinal lymph node metastases measuring <36 mm survived free of disease for 5 years compared with 12 of 29 patients whose tumor metastases measured >100 mm. No additional treatment may be advised if only one lymph node in the groin in microscopically positive;

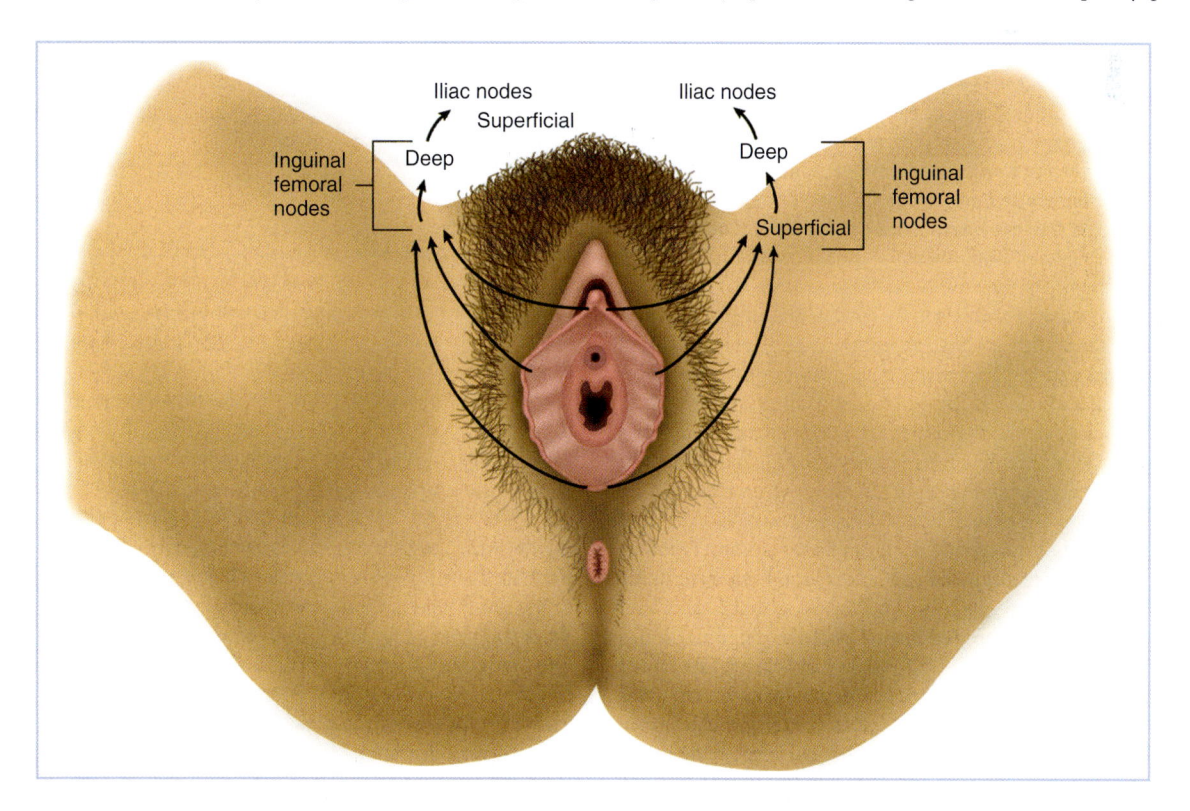

Figure 3 Lymphatic drainage of the vulva.

Percent of cases by stage

- Localized (59%) confined to primary site
- Regional (32%) spread to regional lymph nodes
- Distant (5%) cancer has metastasized
- Unknown (4%) unstaged

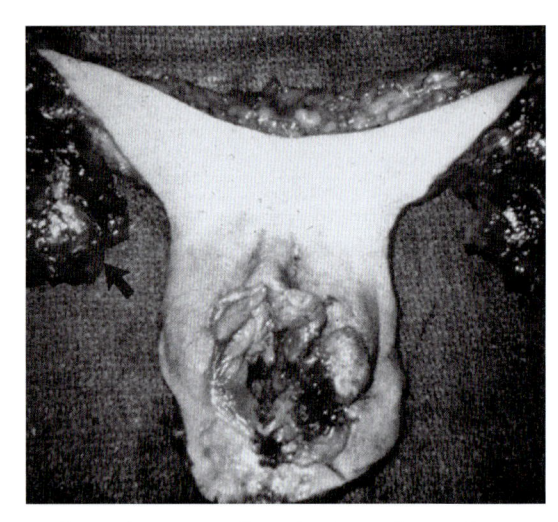

(a)

Five–year relative survival

- Localized: 85.7%
- Regional: 53.9%
- Distant: 15.9%
- Unstaged: 45.5%

(b)

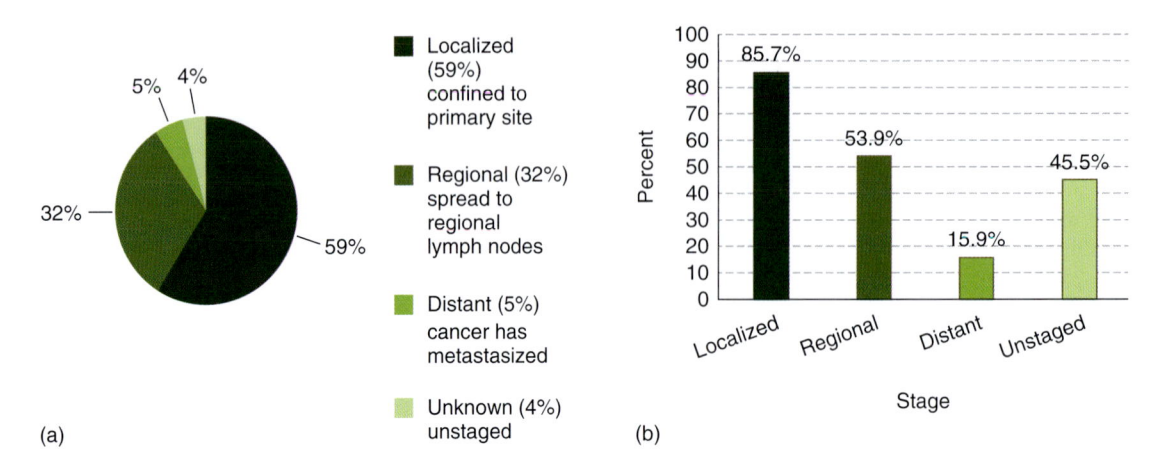

Figure 4 (a) Percent of cases and (b) 5-year relative survival by stage at diagnosis: vulvar cancer. Source: Modified from National Cancer Institute, Surveillance, Epidemiology, and End Results Program (SEER) 2011. Stat Fact Sheets: Vulvar Cancer.

Table 3 Prognostic factors of stage, grade, and tumor thickness associated with positive regional nodes.[a]

Stage	Positive nodes (%)	Grade	Positive nodes (%)	Tumor thickness (mm)	Positive nodes (%)
I	8.9	1	0	<1	3.1
II	25.3	2	8.0	2	8.9
III	31.1	3	24.6	3	18.6
IV	62.5	4	47.7	>4	31.0

[a]Source: Modified from Sedlis et al.[50]

Figure 5 Gross vulvectomy specimen showing a vulvar carcinoma.

however, this is controversial. Patients with stage 1 lesions did not have positive nodes, yet in patients with stage 4 lesions, 47.7% of nodes were positive. Vascular space involvement is prognostic with 72% vascular invasion showing regional node metastasis compared to 34% of those without vascular invasion. Nodal involvement also correlates with the location of the primary lesion.[55] Lesions on the labia are associated with 7.4% positive nodes, whereas clitoral lesions have a higher incidence of positive nodes (27.4%).[56] Boyce et al.[57] reported that six tumors under 1 cm in diameter had no metastases to regional nodes but that the fraction of tumors with positive nodes rose to 55% for 29 cases with lesions over 4 cm.

Therapy for stages I and II and early-stage III vulvar carcinoma is accomplished with radical vulvectomy and either bilateral inguinal femoral node dissection[58] or SLNB. In the past, en bloc of radical vulvectomy and bilateral dissection of the groin and pelvic nodes was standard treatment (specimen seen in Figure 5). Over the past 30 years, there has been modification of this surgical approach through triple incisions, decreasing the morbidity of the surgery. Since the disease can occur in younger women with small tumors, the morbidity associated with en bloc resection is of particular concern. The deep pelvic nodes are rarely removed unless the inguinal nodes are involved. Most oncologists now perform sentinel lymph node biopsy or remove only the inguinofemoral nodes at the time of operation and treat the deep pelvic nodes with external radiation if superficial nodes are involved with tumor.

A wide variety of management options of the primary lesion have been proposed. Management of patients with small lesions should be individualized. Since the early 1980s, radical local excision has been advocated in patients with small tumors. The literature indicates that the incidence of local invasive recurrence is similar with local excision and more radical approaches. Radical local excision is most appropriate for unilateral, isolated lesions. This approach has been used for risk factors such as large tumor sites, positive capillary-lymphatic space invasion, or surgical margins that are <8 mm.

Different surgical approaches to invasive vulvar carcinoma have been evaluated. Classically, an en bloc dissection has been performed. Radical vulvectomy and groin dissection have been carried out through a single suprapubic incision that extends between the left and right anterior iliac spines (Figure 5). This operation removed the entire vulva, including the clitoris, subcutaneous tissue, and inguinal femoral nodes. If the lesion involved the distal urethra, this has often been removed without the loss of urinary continence. In this procedure, the major complication has been wound breakdown and infection (occurring in 50% of the patients). Modifications have been introduced to decrease the incidence of wound breakdown. These modifications include performing the inguinal femoral node dissection through separate inguinal incisions and then completing the radical vulvectomy, which is the standard currently. Tumor recurrences rarely occur in the skin bridge when separate groin incisions are used.[52,59]

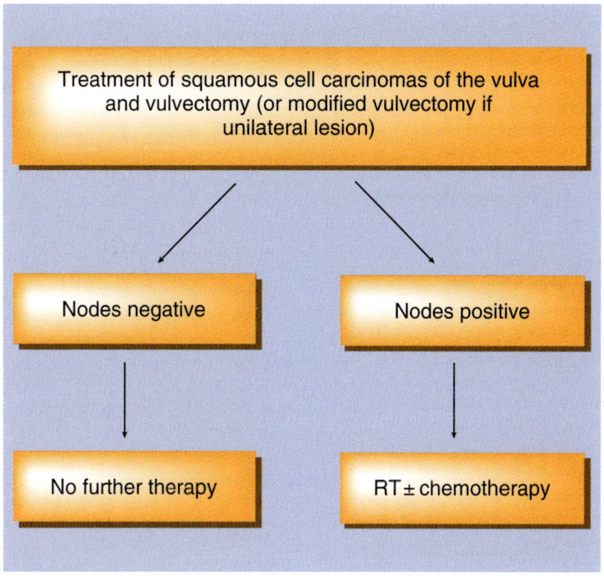

Figure 6 Treatment of squamous cell carcinomas of the vulva. RT, radiation therapy.

Modifying the approach for these early-stage lesions appears to be effective and is associated with less morbidity than the standard radical vulvectomy. If the nodes are free from tumor in stages I and II carcinomas of the vulva, no further therapy is required. If the nodes (especially the femoral nodes) are involved, pelvic irradiation is required. From a randomized study, Homesley et al.[51] reported an improved survival rate in 118 patients with positive lymph nodes who received 4500–5000 cGy of radiation (Figure 6).

Advanced vulvar tumor

Large tumors of the vulva encroaching on the anorectal area and the urethra require more extensive treatment than a radical vulvectomy. Depending on location and ability for resection, approaches can include a radical surgery, neoadjuvant chemoradiation followed by resection, or definitive chemoradiation with intent to cure. Radical surgery may leave larger defect that could require skin grafts such as gracilis myocutaneous grafts. If the nodes are negative, a 5-year survival rate of 50% has been reported.[55,60]

A combination of preoperative radiation and surgery is an option depending on location and need for extensive radical surgery. External radiation using techniques such as intensity-modulated radiotherapy (IMRT) often is given to reduce the size of the tumor before surgical removal by radical vulvectomy, with or without regional lymph node dissection. Approximately 4000–4500 cGy is delivered to the pelvis and inguinal nodes, the operation being performed 5 weeks after the completion of radiation. This approach may obviate a urinary or fecal diversion. Boronow et al.[61,62] reported a 5-year survival rate of 80% in 26 patients with primary carcinoma of the vagina and vulva who were treated with this technique. Rotmensch et al.[63] reported 16 patients with advanced vulvar lesions who were treated with preoperative radiation to the vulva and achieved an overall 5-year survival rate of 45%. Recurrences were more likely if the resection margins were within 1 cm of the tumor. Complications have included stenosis of the introitus and urethra as well as rectovaginal fistula.

The approach has been to not only administer preoperative radiation for advanced lesions but also add chemotherapy. Commonly, agents such as 5-FU, cisplatin, and mitomycin C have been used, producing up to 46% reduction in tumor with chemoradiation in previous studies, the most common toxicities were acute cutaneous and wound complications.[64] The GOG performed a phase II trial (GOG 101), which enrolled locally advanced (T3 or T4 tumors not amenable to surgical resection via radial vulvectomy), and treated them with radiation plus weekly cisplatin followed by surgical resection of residual tumor. They found a 64% completely response rate.[65] Because the vulvar skin is prone to radiation dermatitis, fibrosis, and ulceration, radiation as the sole therapy has been less than desirable. If the patient is inoperable because of medical conditions; however, radiation can be used as the primary treatment of a vulvar carcinoma.[66]

Definitive chemoradiation has also emerged as an option in treating locally advanced, surgically unresectable vulvar cancers. Rishi et al. reviewed the cases of 26 patients who underwent combined platinum-based chemotherapy and IMRT and found 81% achieved a complete response.[67] In a review of patients in the National Cancer Database (NCDB) who received chemoradiation alone for locally advanced squamous cell carcinoma of the vulva, Rao et al. found a 5 year overall survival rate of 50%.[68] This compared to only 27% for those who received radiation alone. Another NCDB study compared outcomes for patients who underwent chemoradiation therapy to those that received neoadjuvant radiation followed by surgery.[69] For patients who received a definitive dose of >55 Gy, there was no difference in survival compared to those who underwent neoadjuvant radiation followed by surgery (HR 1.14, 95% CI 0.97–1.34).

Recurrent vulvar cancer

Recurrences may be local or distant. More than 80% of recurrences occur in the first 2 years after therapy. The risk of recurrence of vulvar carcinoma increases as the stage of disease increases. In an analysis of 502 patients, the majority of recurrences were local; 53.4% were located in the perineal region.[70] Other areas included the inguinal regional, 19% and then distant recurrences in pelvis and beyond, 6% and 8%, respectively.

Different modalities have been used to treat local recurrences. Both radiation therapy and resection of local vulvar recurrence provide effective control and a 5-year survival rate of approximately 60% if local.[70] Local vulvar recurrences can be further excised. However, if recurrence is located in the inguinal region, survival drops dramatically, with a 5-year survival of 27%. The combination of chemotherapy and radiation therapy has been used to treat recurrent disease and some large primary vulvar carcinomas. Disseminated disease requires chemotherapy, but, unfortunately, no chemotherapy has been successful in this situation. There are no prospective trials in this patient population and much of the data that exists is extrapolated from metastatic cervical cancer. Therefore, most metastatic recurrences are treated with a platinum-based regimen plus bevacizumab, usually carboplatin, paclitaxel, and bevacizumab. Carboplatin is frequently chosen over cisplatin due to better tolerance. Palliative care is recommended for patients who cannot tolerate chemotherapy. Overall prognosis is poor for this population (Figure 7).

Bartholin gland carcinoma

Primary carcinoma of Bartholin gland accounts for 5% of all vulvar cancers, and over 200 cases have been reported[27]; approximately 50% of those tumors are nonepidermoid in nature. Bartholin gland carcinomas can be squamous if they originate near the orifice of the duct, or papillary if they arise from the transitional epithelium of the duct, or they can be adenocarcinomas if they arise from the gland itself. An enlargement of Bartholin gland in a postmenopausal female should raise the suspicion of malignancy.

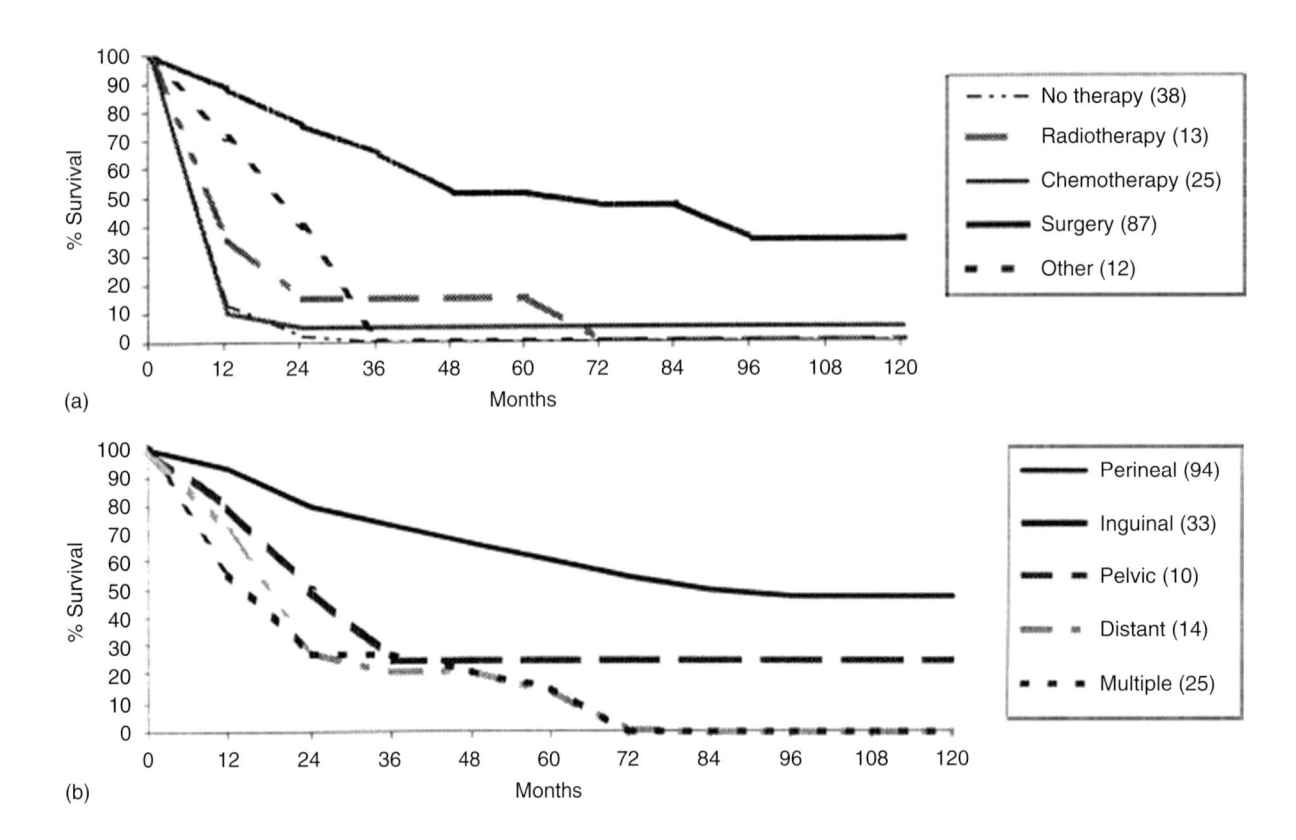

Figure 7 (a) Survival rate after vulvar carcinoma recurrence by type of therapy. The number of cases is shown in parentheses. There was a statistical difference between surgery and other forms of treatment (p, 0.000,001). (b) Survival rate of patients with disease recurrence according to the site of the recurrence the number of patients is shown in parentheses. Source: Maggino et al.[62] Reproduced by permission of John Wiley & Sons.

These tumors are treated similarly to primary squamous cell carcinomas of the vulva, by radical vulvectomy and bilateral inguinal femoral lymphadenectomy. The overall 5-year survival rate of approximately 70% is below that reported for all carcinomas of the vulva and probably relates to a delay in diagnosis. A Bartholin gland carcinoma of the vulva is classified if the tumor is in the correct anatomic position, deeply located in the labium majora, the underlying skin is intact, and there is some normal gland present.

The adenoid cystic variety of Bartholin gland carcinoma invades locally and rarely metastasizes. It is slow-growing with a tendency to recur locally and invade the perineum tissue. It usually requires only wide local excision for adequate therapy. Rosenberg et al.[71] reported five cases of adenocystic carcinoma of Bartholin's gland, with four patients alive and free of disease 28–57 months after treatment.

Basal cell carcinoma
Basal cell carcinoma is rarely encountered in the female genital tract. Such lesions are usually locally invasive, nonmetastatic tumors that are commonly found on the labium majus. Metastasis to the regional lymph nodes is uncommon. Therapy consists of wide local excision of the lesion. If the surgical margins are free of tumor, the disease is cured.

Verrucous carcinoma
Verrucous carcinoma of the vulva is a variant of epidermoid carcinoma. Clinically, it appears as large, condylomatous lesions. These cancers are locally aggressive, nonmetastatic, fungating tumors that gradually increase in size, pushing into rather than invading the underlying structures. Histologically, they consist of mature squamous cells with extensive keratinization. To establish the diagnosis, adequate biopsy is important because biopsy of a large verrucous carcinoma often can lead to an incorrect diagnosis of condyloma acuminatum.

These tumors tend to grow slowly and invade locally, rarely spreading to regional lymph nodes. In 24 cases of verrucous carcinoma, Japaze et al.[72] found no lymph node metastases. Depending on the size and location of the tumor, a wide local excision or simple vulvectomy is effective therapy; radical vulvectomy with inguinal node dissection or radiation therapy is not indicated as treatment for this entity. Radiation therapy is ineffective and can even worsen the prognosis, causing malignant changes within the tumor. The 17 cases treated surgically by Japaze et al. had an excellent 5-year survival rate of 94%. Close long-term follow-up is needed because disease can recur locally, especially if the tumor is large. If concurrent squamous cell carcinoma is found within the verrucous carcinoma, local excision is an inadequate therapy.[73]

Melanoma
Melanoma is the most frequent nonsquamous cell malignancy of the vulva and comprises approximately 5% of primary carcinomas of the vulva. The incidence in the United States is 0.136 cases per 100,000 women and the 5-year survival rate ranges from 10% to 63%.[74] Age at diagnosis has been found to be an independent risk factor for survival in multiple studies. Patients with malignant melanoma of the vulva vary widely in age, ranging from 10 to 96 years, with an average age of approximately 60 years and are most frequently seen in Caucasian women. These lesions most often affect the labia minora or the clitoris.[75]

For vulvar melanomas, the FIGO classification usually has been used. This classification is not, however, as good a prognostic indicator as is the depth of invasion. A system for vulvar melanoma

Table 4 Classification of melanomas of the vulva.

Clark level	
I	Intraepithelial
II	Extension to papillary dermes
III	Filling the dermal papillae
IV	Invasive of collagen in reticular dermis
V	Extension into subcutaneous fat
Breslow depth of invasion	
I	<0.75 mm from skin surface
II	0.76–1.4 mm from skin surface
III	>1.5 mm from skin surface

analogous to that used by Clark for cutaneous melanoma has been adopted (Table 4). New prognostic factors have been described to predict survival. These include the primary tumor thickness, ulceration, number of metastatic lymph nodes, micrometastatic disease in the sentinel lymph node, and the site of distant metastasis. Levels I–V have been identified based on the Clark classification. The level of invasion correlates with survival, which varies from 100% for level II to 83% for level IV and 28% for level V.[76]

Two varieties of melanoma have been described: nodular and superficial spreading melanoma.[77] The superficial spreading melanoma is more common and has a better prognosis, with a 5-year survival rate of 71%. Nodular melanoma has a worse prognosis, and this directly relates to its potential for vertical growth. The 5-year survival rate for nodular melanoma, which is more invasive, is only 38%.

The thickness of the tumor also may be useful in evaluating this lesion. Breslow[78] reported a classification using depth of invasion as measured from the skin surface. In his classification, Breslow reported the overall prognosis as excellent and the spread to regional nodes as unlikely for melanomas with a thickness of <0.76 mm, measured from the surface to the deepest point of penetration.

Wide local excision has been recommended for Clark level I and II disease when no palpable regional nodes are present.[79] In a report of 36 melanoma cases, Rose et al.[80] noted that wide excision was as effective as radical vulvectomy. Prognosis was better for younger patients, presumably because most had superficial spreading rather than nodular melanomas.

A reasonable approach is to excise a melanoma with a 2 cm margin and without node dissection for cases that are <2 mm thick. However, others would recommend a radical local excision with 1–2 cm margins from the primary lesions and an ipsilateral inguinofemoral lymphadenectomy or SLNB. This is based on a multi-institutional nonrandomized trial of elective lymph node dissection versus obstruction for intermediate thickness cutaneous melanoma. This study showed elective lymph node dissection had a significantly better 5-year survival rate than observation for melanomas 1–4 mm.

An excision with a 2–3 cm margin combined with node dissection could be performed for more advanced melanomas. An alternative approach for lesions that have extended to Clark levels III, IV, and V is radical vulvectomy with groin and pelvic lymphadenectomy.[81] Although the therapeutic benefit of a lymph node dissection in this population is controversial. The role for adjuvant chemotherapy in completely resected, node-negative vulvar melanoma is limited. There are no studies that have shown a survival benefit in these patients although no prospective studies have been performed.

It has been reported that melanoma of the vulva can metastasize to pelvic nodes, bypassing the inguinal and femoral nodes, but current evidence indicates that pelvic node involvement does not occur without prior inguinal node involvement. A further therapeutic consideration is that patients with melanoma whose pelvic nodes are involved with tumor usually do not survive their disease.

Long-term results generally are not available for large series of melanomas. Most series of malignant melanoma report an overall survival rate of approximately 50%.[82] For lesions that correspond to Clark level I or II (lesions 0.76 mm thick) and are treated by wide local excision, the 5-year survival rate is in the vicinity of 100%. Prognosis becomes poorer with melanomas more than 3 mm thick. If the regional nodes are negative, the survival rate is approximately 60%; if the regional nodes are involved with tumor, survival is only 30%.

Radiotherapy is used sparingly in patients with vulvar melanoma as there are limited responses documented for cutaneous and mucosal melanomas at all sites. The role of chemotherapy for distant metastasis has not been well established. Regressions, but not cures, have been reported with various multiagent cytotoxic programs, including chemotherapy and/or immunotherapy. These patients should be encouraged to enroll in clinical trials if available.

Sarcoma

Sarcomas of the vulva are rare. Leiomyosarcomas appear to be the most frequently encountered sarcomas in this group of patients[83] and surgical removal by wide local excision is the recommended initial treatment of choice. The 5-year survival rate is reported to be approximately 100%. Locally recurrent lesions are similarly treated. Chemotherapeutic considerations are the same as for those sarcomas in other sites of the female genital tract.[84]

Cancer of the vagina

Primary vaginal cancers are rare, constituting about 3% of all gynecologic malignancies.[2,85–87] It is estimated that 6230 cases of vaginal cancer will be diagnosed in the United States in 2020 and 1450 of those women will die of this cancer.

Carcinoma of the vagina is defined as a primary carcinoma arising in the vagina and not involving the external os of the cervix superiorly or the vulva inferiorly. The majority of vaginal tumors are secondary to metastasis from other sites. Approximately 30% of primary vaginal cancers have *in situ* or invasive cervical cancers previously treated.

The most common symptom of vaginal carcinoma is abnormal painless bleeding or discharge. With advanced tumors, pain or urinary frequency occasionally occurs, especially in cases of anterior wall tumors. Constipation or tenesmus has been seen with tumors involving the posterior vaginal wall. These tumors usually are diagnosed by direct biopsy of the tumor mass, and abnormal cytologic findings often will lead to diagnosis of a vaginal cancer.

The staging criteria for vaginal carcinomas according to the FIGO are given in Table 5.

Premalignant vaginal disease

Premalignant disease of the vagina is generally detected on cytologic screening. Once an abnormal cytology is obtained, a biopsy directed by colposcopic examination is required to verify the severity of the changes. Because vaginal intraepithelial neoplasia is often multifocal, it is necessary to inspect the entire vaginal canal.[88]

Most lesions occur at the vaginal apex. Audet-Lapointe et al.[89] noted that 61 of 66 cases of vaginal intraepithelial neoplasia occurred in the upper third of the vagina. These lesions usually can be excised locally. Other modalities often are preferred, however,

Table 5 FIGO staging classification for vaginal carcinoma.[a]

Stage	
I	The cancer has grown through the top layer of cells but it has not grown out of the vagina and into nearby structures. It has not spread to nearby lymph nodes or to distant sites
II	The cancer has spread to the connective tissues next to the vagina but has not spread to the wall of the pelvis or to other organs nearby. It has not spread to nearby lymph nodes or to distant sites
III	Either the cancer has spread to the wall of the pelvis and may—or may not—have spread to nearby lymph nodes, or the cancer is in the vagina and it may have grown into the connective tissue nearby and it has spread to lymph nodes nearby. It has not spread to distant sites
IV	Carcinoma extends beyond true pelvis or involves mucosa of bladder or rectum
	Stage IVA the cancer has grown out of the vagina to organs nearby (such as the bladder or rectum). It may or may not have spread to lymph nodes but it has not spread to distant sites. At **Stage IVB** the cancer has spread to distant organs such as the lungs

FIGO, International Federation of Gynecology and Obstetrics.
[a]Source: Adapted from Society of Gynecologic Oncology Vaginal Cancer Stages.

because of the multifocal nature of this disease or the necessity of excising large areas, requiring skin grafting.[90]

Nonsurgical approaches for treating these lesions include laser ablation and 5-FU cream for widespread multifocal disease. Carbon dioxide laser frequently has been used and, if carried to a depth of 2–4 mm, allows for vaporization of abnormal tissue. Preliminary results reported by Petrilli et al.[91] with this modality have shown a success rate of approximately 90%. Radiation currently is not recommended for the treatment of noninvasive disease because of the proximity of the bladder and rectum and the availability of newer modalities.

Another approach to treating vaginal intraepithelial neoplasia is the use of 5% 5-FU cream for approximately 7 days, repeated every 3–4 weeks if the vaginal intraepithelial neoplasia persists. Hyperkeratotic lesions appear to be less sensitive to treatment because of their thickness and parakeratosis. Krebs[92] reported on the use of 5% 5-FU daily for 10 days and noted that 17 of 20 patients with vaginal condylomas responded to this therapy. Petrilli et al.[91] and Ballon et al.[93] reported success rates of 80–90% for vaginal intraepithelial neoplasia after multiple cycles of therapy. Another approach is the use of imiquimod as described for treatment of vulvar dysplasias (as seen above in vulvar sections), there have been retrospective studies describing response, however, the use is considered off-label.

Invasive carcinomas of the vagina

Squamous cell carcinomas of the vagina may appear grossly as either ulcerated or fungating tumors or they may be exophytic and protrude through the vaginal canal. They are the most common vaginal malignancy and account for 90% of primary vaginal cancers. The disease occurs primarily in women over 50 years of age. Most squamous cell carcinomas occur in the upper third of the vagina. In examining the patient, it is important to visualize the entire vagina because lesions on the posterior wall can be concealed by the speculum.[94] Microscopically, these tumors have the classic findings of invasive squamous cell carcinoma. They have pleomorphic squamous cells with occasional keratin pearls.

The location of the tumor determines the areas of lymphatic spread (Figure 8).[95] The lymphatics of the middle and upper vagina communicate superiorly with the lymphatics of the cervix and drain into the pelvic nodes of the obturator, internal, and external iliac chains. The lymphatics of the distal third of the vagina drain to the inguinal and pelvic nodes, with a pattern of drainage similar to that of the vulva. Although tumors in most women will follow these traditional drainage routes, lymphatic mapping studies have shown variability with some apical tumors draining to the groin

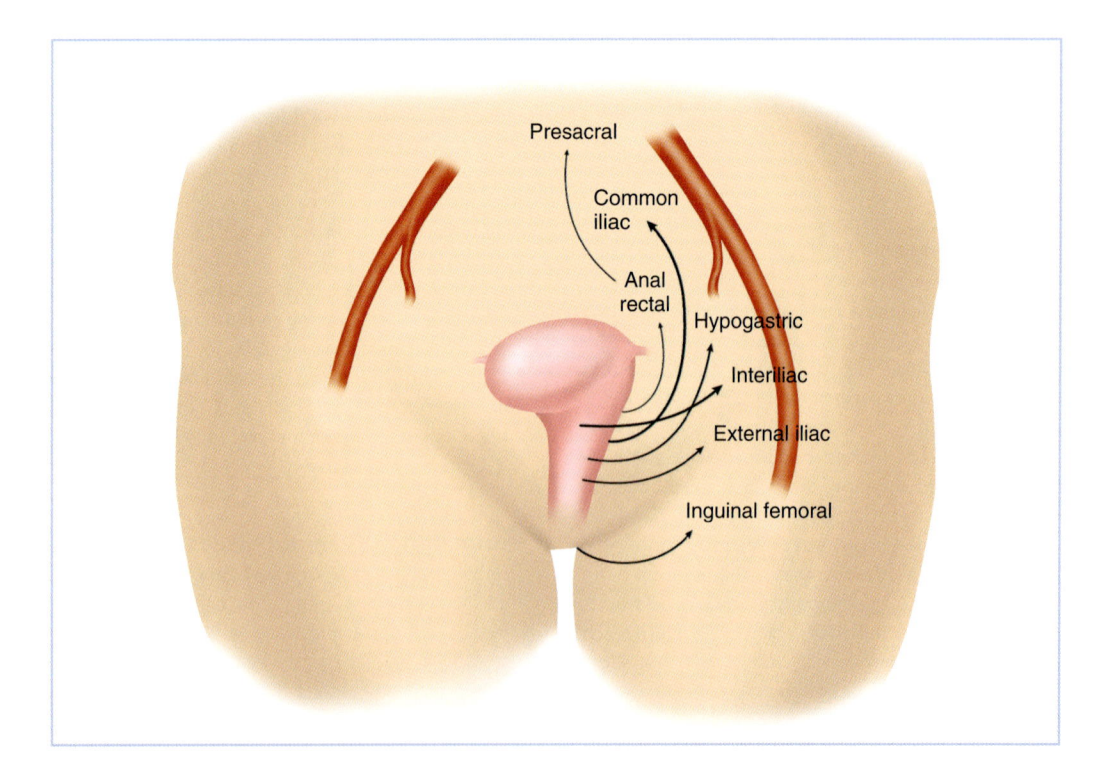

Figure 8 Lymphatic drainage of the vagina. Source: Plentl and Friedman.[95]

Table 6 Treatment scheme for vaginal carcinoma.[a]

Stage	External therapy (cGy)	Implant (interstitial) (cGy)
I		
∑, small tumors (<2 cm)	—	6000–7000
∑, all others	Whole pelvis (4000)	3000–4000 cGy
II	Whole pelvis (4000–5000)	3000–4000 cGy
III	Whole pelvis (5000)	2000
IV	Whole pelvis (5000; an additional 1000–2000 through reduced field if implant not possible)	2000 (if possible)

1 cGy = 1 rad.
[a]Source: Adapted from Nori et al.[97]

and some distal tumors draining to the pelvis.[96] The posterior wall lymphatics drain to the rectal lymphatic system. Positive inguinal nodes are present in 31.6% of disease in the lower vagina. The treatment for vaginal cancer is individualized.

Depending on the location, both radiation including high dose rate brachytherapy and surgery have been used effectively in treating these lesions (Table 6). Treatment is often individualized, depending on the size, stage, and location of the tumor.[93,98]

If the tumor is <2 cm thick, some investigators advocate using only local radiation.[99,100] If the carcinoma is <0.5 cm thick, intracavitary irradiation with a vaginal cylinder to deliver 8000 cGy to the mucosa will give over 90% tumor control.[97] Spirtos et al.[101] studied 23 stage I patients and noted only two local recurrences, and both of these had tumor doses of <7500 cGy. For larger lesions, external radiation is used, with a concomitant reduction in the local vaginal component of primary tumor treatment.[102] Implants, however, often cannot be used in patients with larger stage III or IV carcinomas. If such is the case, only external beam radiation is used, and a central boost is given after an initial whole-pelvis dose of 5000 cGy radiation.[103]

Small tumors located in the upper third of the vagina often can be excised.[104,105] In patients with these, a radical hysterectomy, partial vaginectomy, or pelvic lymphadenectomy usually is effective. Surgery has been preferred in younger patients.

If distant metastasis occurs, effective cis-platinum-based chemotherapy for recurrent squamous cell carcinoma of the vagina has not been developed.[106] For squamous cell carcinoma, a variety of regimens using multiagent chemotherapy similar to those for cervical carcinoma have been employed.

The overall survival rate for patients with primary carcinoma of the vagina is related to the stage of the disease.

Clear cell adenocarcinoma of the vagina

Clear cell adenocarcinomas have been seen more frequently in young women since 1970 because of the association with intrauterine exposure to diethylstilbestrol.[107,108] Three predominant histologic patterns are found with clear cell carcinoma; they have been described as tubulocystic, solid, and papillary patterns.[109,110] Most clear cell carcinomas of the vagina are polypoid or nodular, with a reddish color.

Clear cell carcinomas can spread locally and by the lymphatic and hematogenous routes. Metastases to regional pelvic nodes have been found in approximately one-sixth of stage I cases. Spread to regional pelvic nodes becomes more frequent in higher-stage tumors.

Clear cell adenocarcinomas are staged as other carcinomas of the vagina are by the FIGO. Some 80% have been diagnosed as stage I or II.

Several prognostic factors have been identified. Older patients (i.e., >19 years of age) have a more favorable prognosis than younger patients.[111] This difference has been associated with the presence of a more favorable tubulocystic pattern of clear cell adenocarcinoma, which is the most frequent histologic pattern found in older patients. In addition, smaller tumor diameter and superficial depth of invasion correlate with improved patient survival. Survival also depends on the stage of the disease. In 547 patients treated for clear cell adenocarcinoma of the vagina, the 5-year survival rate for those in stages I, II, III, and IV has been 93%, 83%, 37%, and 0%, respectively (Table 7).[101]

Because of the young age of these patients, surgery often is the primary therapy. For stage I and early stage II disease (Figure 9), radical hysterectomy, partial or complete vaginectomy, pelvic lymphadenectomy, and replacement of the vagina with a split-thickness skin graft have been the approaches most frequently used.[112]

In patients with small stage I tumors of the vagina, efforts have been made to preserve fertility. The tumor has been excised with retroperitoneal lymph node dissection, followed by local radiation. Senekjian et al.[112] reported that the survival rate of patients with

Table 7 Survival at 5 and 10 years for 547 patients with clear cell adenocarcinoma of the vagina and cervix.[a]

Stage	Survival (%)	
	5 years	10 years
I	93	87
IIA	80	66
IIB	58	49
II (vagina)	83	67
III	37	12
IV	0	0

[a]Source: Based on Spirtos et al.[101]

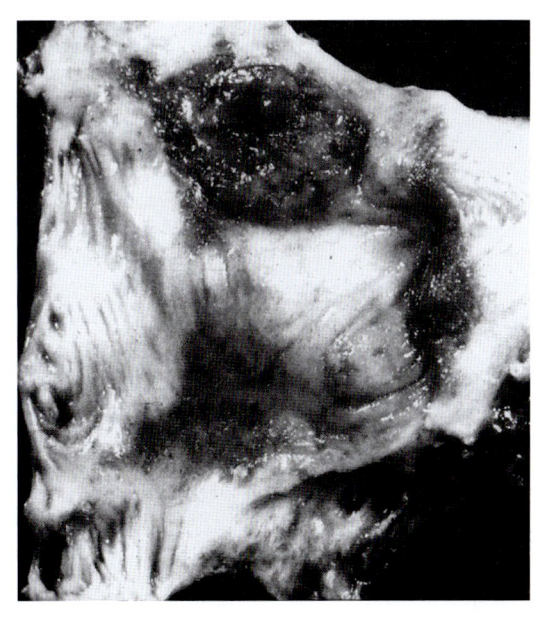

Figure 9 Clear cell adenocarcinoma of the anterior wall, with vaginal adenosis on the posterior wall at the edge of the tumor.

small vaginal tumors treated with such an approach compares favorably with that of patients treated with conventional therapy. In their series, eight pregnancies were reported in five patients who were treated locally.

Larger tumors have been treated with whole-pelvis radiation in addition to intracavitary implant. For tumors >2 cm, whole-pelvis radiation of 4000–5000 cGy has been given, with an additional implant of 3000–4000 cGy.[113] In a few instances, exenterative surgery has been performed for larger tumors; however, this procedure usually has been applied to central recurrences following primary radiation therapy.[114]

If there is a recurrence, therapy consists of additional radical surgery, often requiring exenteration or extensive radiation localized to the pelvis. Systemic chemotherapy has been used in cases of metastatic disease. Cisplatin (75–100 mg/m^2) with a continuous infusion of 5-FU (1 g/m^2 for 3–5 days every 3–4 weeks) is currently recommended. However, no single agent or combination of chemotherapeutic agents has emerged as the most effective.[115] Prolonged follow-up is necessary because recurrences, especially in the lungs and supraclavicular areas, have been reported as long as 19 years after primary therapy.

Vaginal melanomas

Malignant melanomas of the vagina are rare; they constitute <1% of all melanomas occurring in females. The age distribution of the neoplasm has ranged from 26 to 98 years, with a median age of 70 years. Most patients are postmenopausal and present with vaginal bleeding, discharge, or a mass. Tumors may vary from 0.5 to 7.5 cm in diameter, with approximately 30% being 2 cm or less in diameter. Most of these tumors develop in the distal third of the vagina, commonly on the anterior wall. Primary vaginal melanomas presumably arise from vaginal melanocytes that are present in approximately 3% of normal females. Histologically, this neoplasm is similar to other melanomas found elsewhere and tends to be deeply invasive in the vagina.

The prognosis is worse than that of vulvar melanomas. Chung et al.[116] reported a 5-year survival rate of only 21% in a series of 19 patients. Reid et al.[117] reported a 5-year survival rate of 17.4% in 15 cases, but the prognosis was improved for those tumors that were small and <3 cm in diameter. More recently, Borazjani et al.[118] reported improved survival for cases in which there were fewer than six mitoses/10 high-power fields. The best prognostic factor is the size of the lesion.

Optimal treatment has not been established. Treatment usually consists of radical surgery or wide excision of the vagina and dissection of the regional lymph nodes, depending on the location of the lesion. Recently, a more conservative approach has been used for wide local excision followed by pelvic radiation. Because of the poor prognosis, adjunctive radiation and chemotherapy have been used as local recurrences, and distant metastases with this disease are common. If possible, these patients should enroll in a clinical trial.

Rare vaginal tumors in young females

Endodermal sinus tumor is a rare germ cell malignancy that is usually found in the ovary.[119] This tumor secretes alpha-fetoprotein, which often is a useful tumor marker for monitoring patients with this neoplasm. It is usually found in infants and children under the age of 3.[120,121] Patients generally present with complaints of bleeding or spotting from the vagina. On physical examination, there is a friable red to pinkish-white polypoid tumor. This tumor is aggressive, and most patients have died. Therapy has involved surgery, radiation, and chemotherapy. Young and Scully[122] reported six patients who were disease free from 2 to 9 years after local therapy with operation, irradiation, or both, followed by systemic chemotherapy with vincristine, actinomycin D, and cyclophosphamide (VAC).[122] Copeland et al.[123] reported similar results using the combination of chemotherapy and excision, and Collins et al.[124] noted the regression of tumor with chemotherapy alone. In this report, a 5-month-old patient had regression of the tumor after VAC therapy.

Another rare tumor found in the vaginas of young females is sarcoma botryoides or embryonal rhabdomyosarcoma.[125] This tumor is usually found in children <8 years of age. As with endodermal sinus tumor, the most common symptom has been vaginal bleeding. In 58 cases, the average age at onset of symptoms was 38.3 months. This tumor resembles clusters of grapes and forms multiple polypoid masses that are believed to begin in the subepithelial layers of the vagina and to rapidly expand, filling the vagina. Histologically, these tumors are identified by the presence of rhabdomyoblasts that may contain cross-striations. Because of infiltration of the tumor under the vaginal epithelium, there is often a distinct subepithelial zone, called the cambium layer. The 5-year survival rate of these tumors in the past has ranged from 10% to 35%, and exenterative procedures have often been used.[126] Hilgers reviewed the literature on pelvic exenterations in 21 cases of embryonal rhabdomyosarcoma and found that this form of therapy was ineffective in curing these patients.[56] Effective control with less radical surgery has been achieved using multimodal treatment consisting of multiagent chemotherapy, VAC, combined with operation or radiation.

Hayes et al.[127] reported 21 patients with vaginal rhabdomyosarcoma who received chemotherapy. In their series, seven relapsed, with five of these seven having had residual disease following incomplete resection. In 17 of 21 patients who received chemotherapy before surgery, a subsequently delayed excision could be performed. Data regarding the long-term survival of a large number of patients are not available, but such a combined approach appears to result in effective therapy with less mutilating surgery.

A rare, benign, fibroepithelial vaginal polyp that resembles sarcoma botryoides can be found in the vaginas of infants or pregnant women.[128,129] Although large atypical cells are present microscopically, epithelial infiltration, a cambium layer, and strap cells are absent. Grossly, these polyps do not resemble the grape-like appearance of sarcoma botryoides. These hormonally stimulated hyperplastic lesions are called pseudo-sarcoma botryoides, and treatment by local excision is effective.

Key references

The complete reference list can be found on Vital Source version of this title, see inside front cover.

2 Siegel RL, Miller KD, Jemal A. Cancer statistics, 2020. *CA Cancer J Clin*. 2020; **70**(1):7–30.

4 Kumar S, Shah JP, Bryant CS, et al. A comparison of younger vs older women with vulvar cancer in the United States. *Am J Obstet Gynecol*. 2009;**200**:e52–e55.

5 de Koning MN, Quint WG, Pirog EC. Prevalence of mucosal and cutaneous human papillomaviruses in different histologic subtypes of vulvar carcinoma. *Mod Pathol*. 2008;**21**(3):334.

6 Sutton GP, Stehman FB, Ehrlich CE, Roman A. Human papilloma virus deoxyribonucleic acid in lesions of the female genital tract: evidence for types 6/11 in squamous carcinoma of the vulva. *Obstet Gynecol*. 1987;**70**:564.

10 Stroup AM. Demographic, clinical, and treatment trends among women diagnosed with vulvar cancer in the United States. *Gynecol Oncol*. 2008;**108**:577–583.

11. Mabuchi K, Bross DS, Kessler II. Epidemiology of cancer of the vulva: a case control study. *Cancer*. 1985;**55**:1843–1848.
12. Jones RW, Rowan DM, Stewart AW. Vulvar intraepithelial neoplasia: aspects of the natural history and outcome in 405 women. *Obstet Gynecol*. 2005;**106**(6):1319–1326.
16. Rogers LJ, Cuello MA. Cancer of the vulva. *Int J Gynaecol Obstet*. 2018;**143**(Suppl 2):4–13. doi: 10.1002/ijgo.12609.
17. Sideri M, Jones RW, Wilkinson EJ, et al. Squamous vulvar intraepithelial neoplasia: 2004 modified terminology, ISSVD vulvar oncology subcommittee. *J Reprod Med*. 2005;**50**:807–810.
18. Darragh TM, Colgan TJ, Cox JT, et al. The lower anogenital squamous terminology standardization project for HPV-associated lesions: background and consensus recommendations from the College of American Pathologists and the American Society for Colposcopy and Cervical Pathology. *Arch Pathol Lab Med*. 2012;**136**:1266–1297.
19. Hart WR, Norris HJ, Helwig ED. Relation of lichen sclerosis et atrophicus of the vulva to development of carcinoma. *Obstet Gynecol*. 1975;**45**:369.
22. Mulvany NJ, Allen DG. Differentiated intraepithelial neoplasia of the vulva. *Int J Gynecol Pathol*. 2008;**27**:125–135.
23. Rutledge F, Sinclair M. Treatment of intraepithelial neoplasia of the vulva by skin excision and graft. *Obstet Gynecol*. 1968;**102**:806.
24. Woodruff JD, Genadry R, Poliakoff S. Treatment of dyspareunia and vaginal outlet distortions by perineoplasty. *Obstet Gynecol*. 1981;**57**:750.
27. Leuchter RS, Hacker NF, Voet RL, et al. Primary carcinoma of the Bartholin gland: a report of 14 cases and review of the literature. *Obstet Gynecol*. 1982;**60**:361.
31. Lee SC, Roth LM, Ehrlich C, Hall JA. Extramammary Paget's disease of the vulva—a clinicopathologic study of 13 cases. *Cancer*. 1977;**39**:2540.
32. Friedrich EG Jr, Wilkinson EJ, Steingraeber PH, Lewis JD. Paget's disease of the vulva and carcinoma of the breast. *Obstet Gynecol*. 1975;**46**:130.
35. Lam C, Funaro D. Extramammary Paget's disease: summary of current knowledge. *Dermatol Clin*. 2010;**28**:807–826.
38. Rouzier R, Preti M, Sideri M, et al. A suggested modification to FIGO stage III vulvar cancer. *Cancer Res*. 2008;**110**:83–86.
44. Rowley KC, Gallion HH, Donalson ES, et al. Prognostic factors in early vulvar cancer. *Gynecol Oncol*. 1988;**31**:43.
46. Yoder BJ, Rufforny I, Massoll N, Wilkinson EJ. Stage IA vulvar squamous cell carcinoma. *Am J Surg Pathol*. 2008;**32**(5):765–772.
47. Levenback CF, Ali S, Coleman RL. Lymphatic mapping and sentinel lymph node biopsy in women with squamous cell carcinoma of the vulva: a gynecologic oncology group study. *J Clin Oncol*. 2012;**30**(31):3786–3791.
48. Van der Zee AG, Oonk MH, De Hullu JA, et al. Sentinel node dissection is safe in the treatment of early-stage vulvar cancer. *J Clin Oncol*. 2008;**26**(6):884–889.
49. Oonk MH, van Os MA, de Bock GH, et al. A comparison of quality of life between vulvar cancer patients after sentinel lymph node procedure only and inguinofemoral lymphadenectomy. *Gynecol Oncol*. 2009;**113**(3):301–305.
50. Sedlis A, Homesly H, Bundy BN, et al. Positive groin lymph nodes in superficial squamous vulvar cancer. *Am J Obstet Gynecol*. 1987;**156**:1159.
51. Homesley HD, Bundy BN, Sedlis A, Adcock L. A randomized study of radiation therapy versus pelvic node resection for patients with invasive squamous cell carcinoma of the vulva having positive groin nodes. *Obstet Gynecol*. 1986;**68**:733.
57. Boyce J, Fruchter RG, Kasambilides E, et al. Prognostic factors in carcinoma of the vulva. *Gynecol Oncol*. 1985;**20**:364.
60. Blotti F, Zullo MA, Angioli R. Incontinence after radical vulvectomy treated with Macroplastique implantation. *J Minim Invasive Gynecol*. 2008;**15**:113–115.
63. Rotmensch J, Rubin SJ, Sutton HG, et al. Preoperative radiotherapy followed by radical vulvectomy with inguinal lymphadenectomy for advanced vulvar cancer. *Gynecol Oncol*. 1990;**36**:181.
64. Moore DH, Thomas GM, Montana GS, et al. Preoperative chemoradiation for advanced vulvar cancer: a phase II study of the Gynecologic Oncology Group. *Int J Radiat Oncol Biol Phys*. 1998;**42**:1317–1323.
66. Farey RN, McKay PA, Benedet JL. Radiation treatment of carcinoma of the vulva 1950–1980. *Am J Obstet Gynecol*. 1985;**151**:591.
74. Boer FL, Ten Eikelder MLG, Kapiteijn EH, et al. Vulvar malignant melanoma: pathogenesis, clinical behaviour and management: review of the literature. *Cancer Treat Rev*. 2019;**73**:91–103.
77. Mitchell M, Talerman A, Sholl JS, et al. Pseudosarcoma botryoides in pregnancy: report of a case with ultra-structural observations. *Obstet Gynecol*. 1987;**70**:522.
78. Breslow A. Thickness, cross-sectional areas, and depth of invasion in the prognosis of cutaneous melanoma. *Ann Surg*. 1970;**172**:908.
80. Rose PG, Piver S, Tsukada Y, Lau T. Conservative therapy for melanoma of the vulva. *Am J Obstet Gynecol*. 1988;**159**:57.
90. Gallup DG, Morley GW. Carcinoma in situ of the vagina: a study and review. *Obstet Gynecol*. 1975;**46**:334.
95. Plentl AA, Friedman EA. *Lymphatic System of the Female Genitalia*. Philadelphia, PA: W.B. Saunders; 1971.
107. Herbst AL, Scully RE. Adenocarcinoma of the vagina in adolescence. *Cancer*. 1970;**25**:745.
115. Lacy J, Capra M, Allen L. Endodermal sinus tumor of the infant vagina treated exclusively with chemotherapy. *J Pediatr Hematol Oncol*. 2006;**28**:768–771.

99 Neoplasms of the cervix

Anuja Jhingran, MD

> **Overview**
>
> Cervical cancer is the third most common cancer among women worldwide and the fourth leading cause of female cancer deaths, with an estimated 529,800 new cases and 275,100 deaths in the year 2008. The incidence is declining in the United States with 13,800 new cases and 4290 deaths in 2015. Squamous cell carcinoma is the most common histology with the human papilloma virus being the most common etiology. Cervical cancer and precancer can be easily detected with pap smears and HPV testing and prevented with HPV vaccine. Early-stage cervix cancer can be treated with surgery including now fertility-sparing surgery and there are high cure rates. Locally advanced cervical cancer is treated with combination of chemotherapy and radiation therapy with high survival rates but there is room for improvement with advancing stage. Systemic chemotherapy can be used for treatment of both recurrent and metastatic disease, but careful attention should be paid to balancing benefit and toxicity. The key to improving overall outcomes will be translating the success seen in developed countries to areas of the world where advanced-stage invasive cervical cancer is most common.

Epidemiology

Incidence and mortality

Cervical cancer is the fourth most common cancer among women worldwide and the fourth leading cause of female cancer deaths, with an estimated 570,000 new cases and 311,000 deaths in the year 2018.[1] Approximately 84% of all cervical cancers and 88% of all deaths caused by cervical cancer occur in lower-resource countries (i.e., those with HDI <0.80).[1] In the United States, it is estimated that there will be 13,800 new cases of cervical cancer in 2020, with 4290 related deaths.[2] Cervical cancer is frequently seen in the Hispanic population (9.2% of all cases of cervical cancer) followed by American Indians (9.2%) African-Americans (9.2%), whites (7.1%), and Pacific Islanders/Asians (6.0%).[2]

In the last 40 years, primarily because of the introduction of screening with the Pap smear, the incidence and mortality rates for cervical cancer have declined in most developed countries.[3] In the United States; incidence rates have declined by nearly 70% during this period. In developing countries, however, cervical cancer continues to be a significant health problem due to suboptimal screening programs and a lack of therapy for precancerous conditions.

Risk factors for cervical neoplasia

Human papillomavirus and other sexually transmitted agents

Epidemiologic evidence has long suggested a sexually transmitted etiology for cervical neoplasia. Supporting this hypothesis, several measures of sexual behavior (including multiple sexual partners, early age at first sexual intercourse, and sexual habits of male partners) have consistently been associated with an increased risk of cervical neoplasia.[4] In the mid-1970s, the hypothesis of a causal relationship between human papillomavirus (HPV) and cervical neoplasia was first proposed.[5] Since then, a large body of experimental, clinical, and epidemiologic research has accumulated, supporting an etiologic role for some types of HPV.[6]

Of the more than 78 types of HPV that have been described, in excess of 35 types are associated with anogenital disease, and 30 or more are associated with cancer.[7] Similarly, HPV DNA has been detected by PCR in up to 94% of women with preinvasive lesions (cervical intraepithelial neoplasia [CIN]) and in up to 46% of women with cytologically normal tissue.[6,8]

HPV types classified as intermediate and high risk have been identified in about 77% of high-grade squamous intraepithelial lesions (HGSILs) (CIN 2 and 3) and in 84% of invasive lesions.[9] In the series studied by Bosch et al.,[10] HPV types 16, 18, 31, and 45 were detected in approximately 80% of cases. HPV 16 is by far the most prevalent HPV type in women with cervical neoplasia, present in up to 50% of HGSILs and invasive lesions, and is the most common HPV type identified in cytologically normal women.[9,11,12]

The association between cervical neoplasia and HPV is independent of the study population, study design, and HPV detection method.[10] Higher risk has been associated with specific HPV types (16, 18, 31, 33, 35, and 45), increasing viral load, and concurrent infection with multiple HPV types.[13,14] An increased risk of high-grade CIN ranging from 16- to 122-fold has been reported among women whose test results were positive for HPV of any type.[14] The percentage of cases of CIN attributed to HPV has been estimated to range from 60% to 92%.[8] In addition, adjustment for HPV status appears to account for most of the associations between cervical neoplasia and number of sexual partners and other characteristics of sexual behavior.[8,13,14]

Although a strong and consistent association between HPV and cervical neoplasia has been clearly established, the discrepancy between HPV prevalence and the incidence of cervical neoplasia suggests that other cofactors are necessary for the development and progression of the disease.

Numerous studies have addressed the association between HIV and cervical neoplasia.[4] The Centers for Disease Control and Prevention added invasive cervical cancer to the list of conditions related to AIDS in 1993.[12] HIV-positive women have been reported to have higher rates of cervical abnormalities, larger lesions, higher-grade histology, and higher recurrence rates than HIV-negative women. In addition, HIV-positive women have been reported to have higher HPV prevalence and HPV persistence rates than HIV-negative women. A meta-analysis by Mandelblatt and colleagues concluded that HIV is a cofactor in the association between HPV and cervical neoplasia,

---

Holland-Frei Cancer Medicine, Tenth Edition. Edited by Robert C. Bast, John C. Byrd, Carlo M. Croce, Ernest Hawk, Fadlo R. Khuri, Raphael E. Pollock, Apostolia M. Tsimberidou, Christopher G. Willett, and Cheryl L. Willman.
© 2023 John Wiley & Sons, Inc. Published 2023 by John Wiley & Sons, Inc.

and this association seems to vary with the level of immune function.[15]

Other molecular markers
Other specific genetic abnormalities may also play an important role in carcinogenesis and the aggressiveness of cervical tumors, although, to date, the role of most of these abnormalities in cervical cancer do not appear as important as the role of HPV. Most studies report a 32–34% incidence of *c-myc* activation in cervical cancers, predominantly through amplification.[16,17] Amplification has been related to tumor size and nodal status as well as a risk factor for relapse.[18] Mutations have been reported in the *K-ras* and *H-ras* genes in cervical cancer at a rate of only 10–15%.[19] One report found that increased ras p21 expression correlated with risk of lymph node metastasis.[20]

EGFR is expressed not only in a large proportion of cervical carcinomas but also in normal and premalignant epithelia. The prognostic role of EGFR in cervical carcinoma remains controversial, although two studies found EGFR prognostic for overall survival and disease-specific survival in patients with invasive cervical cancer.[21,22]

The apoptosis inhibitor Bcl2 prevents apoptosis. Two studies have shown that Bcl2 is overexpressed in 61–63% of all cervical cancer and correlates inversely with overall survival,[23,24] whereas other studies have found no correlation with survival.[25]

Angiogenesis is critical for the progression of most cancers. One angiogenic factor, VEGF, has recently been associated with cervical cancer,[26,27] but the precise role that angiogenic factors play in the development and progression of cervical cancer requires further elucidation.

Sexual behavior
Although previous studies report a strong and consistent association between cervical neoplasia and some characteristics of sexual behavior among women and their male sexual partners, a weaker association has been found in more recent studies in which HPV infection has been taken into account.[13,28] These, characteristics of sexual behavior may be only a proxy measurement for infection with HPV and other infectious agents that may be causally related to cervical neoplasia.

The association between early age at first sexual intercourse and increased risk has been less consistent. After controlling for HPV and other risk factors, a statistically significant association between age at first sexual intercourse and cervical neoplasia has remained in some studies, but in others, no association has been observed.[13,14,29] The association between cervical neoplasia and early age at sexual intercourse may indicate a period of higher susceptibility of the cervical tissue, a higher likelihood of exposure, or a longer period of exposure to carcinogenic factors. Establishing age at first sexual intercourse as an independent effect is, however, difficult because of its high correlation with number of sexual partners.

Reproductive factors
No consistent relationships have been established between cervical neoplasia and menstrual or reproductive characteristics, including age at menarche or menopause, number of spontaneous or induced abortions, age at first pregnancy, first live birth, or last birth, and number of vaginal deliveries or Cesarean sections. There is an association between increased risk of cervical neoplasia and higher parity, early age at first birth, higher number of live births, and vaginal deliveries.[13,14,30,31] Repeated trauma to the cervix during childbirth could be an etiologic factor.[31]

Smoking habits
Several epidemiologic studies have provided evidence supporting an approximately twofold increased risk among smokers and a dose–response relationship with duration and intensity of smoking.[32,33] Some support an independent effect of smoking, whereas others do not.[13,14,34] High levels of nicotine, cotinine, and tobacco-specific *N*-nitrosamines have been detected in the cervical mucus of active and passive smokers. DNA damage has been found in cervical tissue and exfoliated cells of women smokers. The local cell-mediated immune response is impaired in smokers. Furthermore, reduction of cervical lesion size has been documented among women participating in smoking cessation intervention.[35] Although the mechanism of smoking-induced carcinogenesis in cervical tissue is not fully understood, current biologic, epidemiologic, and clinical studies suggest that cigarette smoking may be a risk factor for cervical neoplasia.

Risk factors for cervical adenocarcinoma
Adenocarcinoma of the cervix accounts for more than 20% of all cervical cancers. However, in most developing countries the incidence is increasing, particularly among younger women. Between the early 1970s and mid-1980s, the incidence of adenocarcinoma more than doubled among women under 35 years of age.[36] Adenocarcinoma is associated with a higher likelihood of HPV-16 and HPV-18, which is present in more than 80% of cases. HPV-18 accounts for approximately 50% of adenocarcinomas of the cervix, but only 15% of squamous cell carcinomas.[37] Adenocarcinoma has been linked to several other risk factors more commonly associated with endometrial cancer, including obesity[38] and nulliparity.[39]

Summary

Cervical neoplasia continues to be a major health problem worldwide. Higher incidence and mortality rates are observed in developing countries. Among more developed countries, a significant decline in incidence and mortality has been observed in the last 50 years, which has been attributed to the introduction of screening programs. Current epidemiologic data support a strong role for HPV infection in the etiology of cervical neoplasia. This association satisfies all criteria for causality in epidemiologic research: strength, consistency, and specificity of the association; dose–response and temporal relationship; and biologic plausibility.[8] HPV infection appears to explain many of the established risk factors for cervical neoplasia, including sexual behavior and cigarette smoking. Nonetheless, the high prevalence of HPV infection in young healthy women compared with the low incidence of cervical neoplasia and the low progression rate of untreated CIN lesions support the existence of other cofactors in cervical carcinogenesis.[40] The role of viral factors such as HPV persistence and HPV variants in the progression of cervical neoplasia as well as of the determinant factors of HPV persistence will require further evaluation.[41] Similarly, the impact of recent trends in such environmental factors as smoking, exogenous hormones, and dietary factors deserves further attention.[4]

Histologic classification of epithelial tumors

The histologic classification of the World Health Organization (WHO) separates cancers of the uterine cervix into three main groups: squamous cell carcinomas, adenocarcinomas, and other epithelial tumors (Table 1).[42,43]

Table 1 Modification of the WHO histologic classification of epithelial tumors of the uterine cervix.[a]

Squamous cell carcinoma
   Microinvasive squamous cell carcinoma
   Invasive squamous cell carcinoma
   Verrucous carcinoma
   Warty (condylomatous) carcinoma
   Papillary squamous cell (transitional) carcinoma
   Lymphoepithelioma-like carcinoma
Adenocarcinoma
   Mucinous adenocarcinoma
      Endocervical type
      Intestinal type
      Signet-ring type
   Endometrioid adenocarcinoma
   Endometrioid adenocarcinoma with squamous metaplasia
   Clear cell adenocarcinoma
   Minimal-deviation adenocarcinoma
      Endocervical type (adenoma malignum)
      Endometrioid type
   Serous adenocarcinoma
   Mesonephric carcinoma
   Well-differentiated villoglandular adenocarcinoma
Other epithelial tumors
   Adenosquamous carcinoma
   Glassy cell carcinoma
   Mucoepidermoid carcinoma
   Adenoid cystic carcinoma
   Adenoid basal carcinoma
   Carcinoid-like tumor
   Small-cell carcinoma
   Undifferentiated carcinoma

[a]Source: Wright et al.[42]

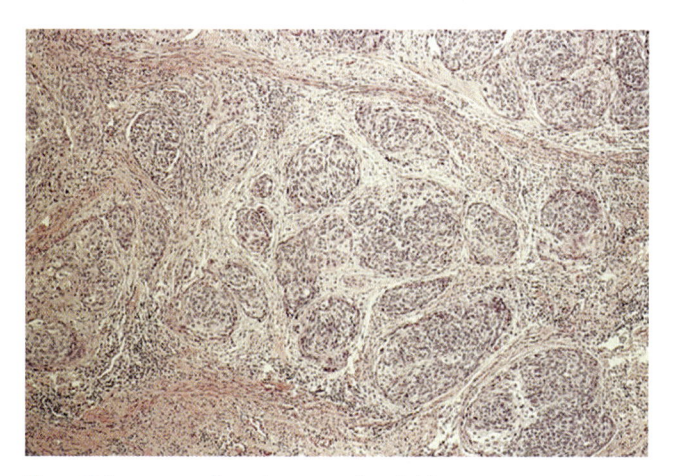

Figure 1 Squamous cell carcinoma, nonkeratinizing.

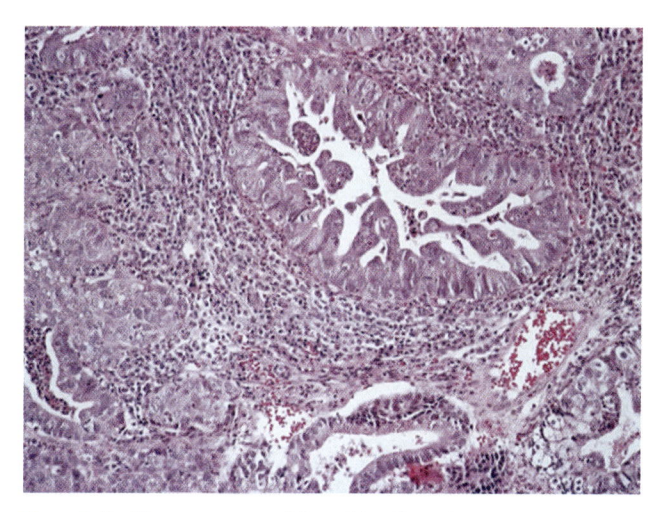

Figure 2 Papillary squamous cell (transitional) carcinoma.

Squamous cell carcinoma

The majority of cervical carcinomas are squamous cell carcinomas, which are classified as either large-cell nonkeratinizing or large-cell keratinizing. Nonkeratinizing carcinoma is characterized by squamous cells with somewhat hyperchromatic nuclei and a moderate amount of cytoplasm growing in discrete nests separated by stroma (Figure 1). In the center of some of the nests, the squamous cells appear to differentiate and degenerate. Keratinizing carcinoma is characterized by cells with very hyperchromatic nuclei and densely eosinophilic cytoplasm growing in irregular invasive nests. Many of these nests have central "pearls" that contain abundant keratin. The average age of patients with squamous cell carcinoma is 51.4 years. Selected variants of squamous cell carcinoma are described in the following paragraphs.

Verrucous carcinoma

Verrucous carcinomas are exophytic with frond-like papillae and macroscopically resemble condylomas. They rarely metastasize, but local invasion can be extensive. Death usually occurs because of ureteral obstruction, infection, or hemorrhage. This tumor rarely goes to the nodes, therefore, for early-stage disease, the treatment of choice is a type II modified radical hysterectomy without lymphadenectomy.

Papillary squamous cell carcinoma

Papillary squamous cell carcinomas of the uterine cervix with transitional or squamous differentiation often resemble transitional cell carcinomas of the urinary tract (Figure 2). Urinary tract transitional cell carcinomas have a cytokeratin profile strongly positive for cytokeratin 20, whereas primary genital tract transitional cell carcinomas stain positive for cytokeratin 7.[44] Invasive papillary transitional cell carcinomas of the uterine cervix are potentially aggressive carcinomas. It is important to distinguish these carcinomas from benign squamous papillomas and condyloma acuminata.[45] Biopsy material must include the underlying stroma to permit identification of invasion.

Lymphoepithelioma-like carcinoma

Lymphoepithelioma-like carcinomas are histologically similar to lymphoepitheliomas arising in the nasopharynx and salivary glands (Figure 3). These carcinomas are usually well circumscribed and composed of undifferentiated cells. The cancer cells are surrounded by inflammatory infiltrates composed of lymphocytes, plasma cells, and eosinophils.[46] Hasumi and colleagues reported 39 cases from the Cancer Institute Hospital in Tokyo. Their patients, 72% of whom were younger than 50 years of age, were treated with radical hysterectomy and pelvic lymphadenectomy. Two patients had positive lymph nodes. At the time of the report, 38 of the 39 patients were alive. The single death occurred 5 months after surgery and was due to hepatitis.

Adenocarcinoma

Adenocarcinomas represent 20–25% of cervical carcinomas today, whereas from 1950 to 1960 they represented only 5%.[47] This change in prevalence is a worldwide phenomenon.[48] The mean age at diagnosis for patients with invasive adenocarcinoma is between 47 and 53 years. Selected variants of adenocarcinoma are described in the following paragraphs.

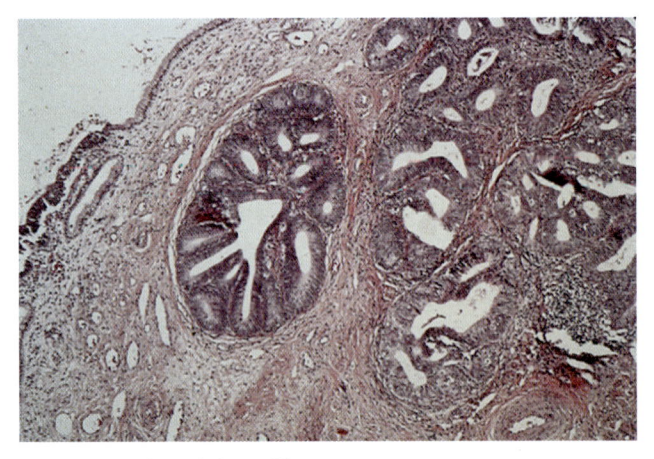

Figure 3 Lymphoepithelioma-like carcinoma.

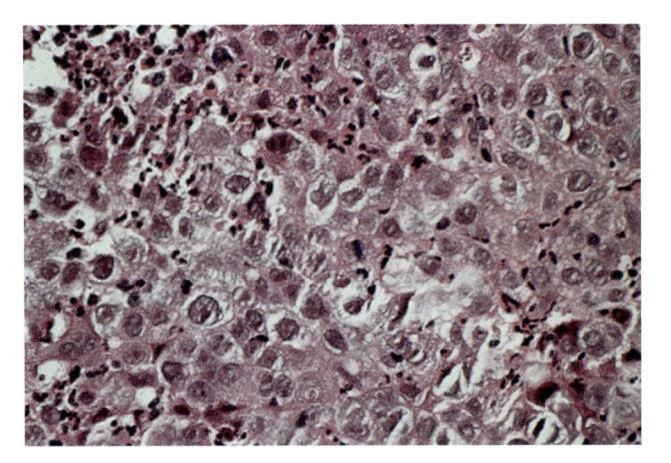

Figure 4 Mucinous adenocarcinoma, endocervical type.

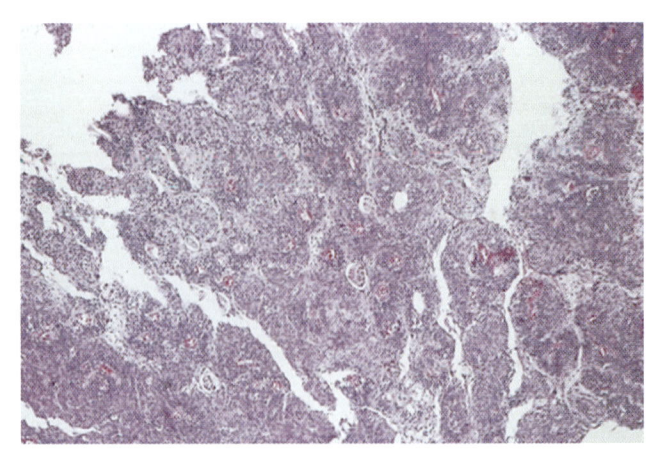

Figure 5 Endometrioid adenocarcinoma.

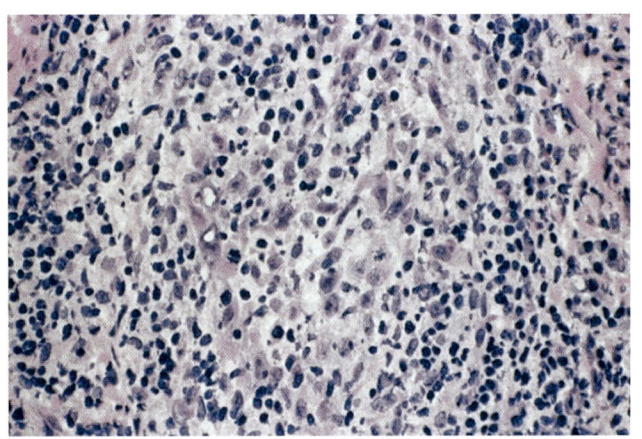

Figure 6 Mucinous adenocarcinoma, endocervical type (adenoma malignum).

Mucinous adenocarcinoma is the most common type of cervical adenocarcinoma.[49] In the WHO classification, the first type of mucinous adenocarcinoma is composed of cells that resemble the columnar cells of the normal endocervical mucosa and is referred to as the endocervical type (Figure 4). The second type is termed the intestinal type because it is composed of cells similar to those present in adenocarcinomas of the large intestine. A third type is composed of signet-ring cells and designated the signet-ring type. Frequently, mucinous adenocarcinomas are a mixture of these cell types.

Endometrioid adenocarcinoma is the second most common type of primary endocervical cancers, accounting for 30% of all primary endocervical cancers. Endometrioid adenocarcinomas resemble typical endometrioid adenocarcinomas arising from the endometrial cavity (Figure 5). Identification of the site of origin (i.e., whether the primary tumor is in the endocervix or endometrium) may be difficult, but proper identification is important as the site or origin significantly influences therapy.

Adenoma malignum is difficult to distinguish cytologically from normal endocervical glands (Figure 6) and is referred to as minimal-deviation adenocarcinoma. A distinguishing feature of adenoma malignum is a bizarre and irregular glandular branching pattern. These irregular glands invade deeply into the stroma, and diagnosis requires a large tissue specimen from a cone biopsy or hysterectomy specimen. Adenoma malignum is extremely rare and is sometimes associated with Peutz–Jegher syndrome.[50] The survival rate is poor if the well-differentiated pattern leads to undertreatment.

Other epithelial tumors

Adenosquamous carcinoma is defined as a cancer that contains an admixture of histologically malignant squamous and glandular cells.[51] Adenosquamous carcinomas account for 5–25% of the cervical carcinomas in some series.[52,53] These carcinomas are similar in their clinical presentation, epidemiology, and pattern of spread to squamous cell carcinomas and adenocarcinomas. The poorly differentiated form of adenosquamous carcinoma can be made up of large uniform polygonal cells with a finely granular cytoplasm of the ground-glass type, hence the term "glassy cells" (Figure 7). Similar to other undifferentiated tumors, glassy cell carcinomas spread early and are aggressive.[53] The mucoepidermoid carcinomas, also placed in this category, contain large-cell nonkeratinizing or focally keratinizing squamous carcinomas, which stain positive for mucin but lacks recognizable glands. The mucinous component includes goblet or signet-ring-type cells localized in a nest of squamous cells. These carcinomas represent 20% of the carcinomas in some series if mucin is measured.

Small-cell neuroendocrine carcinomas contain small anaplastic cells with scant cytoplasm (Figure 8). These highly aggressive cancers diffusely infiltrate the cervical stroma.[54] Staining reveals neuroendocrine markers in most cases. Women with small-cell carcinoma are likely to be 10 years younger than those with squamous cell carcinoma. Small-cell carcinomas are frequently associated with widespread metastasis to multiple sites, including bone, liver, skin, and brain. These tumors should not be confused with small squamous cell carcinomas, which are associated with

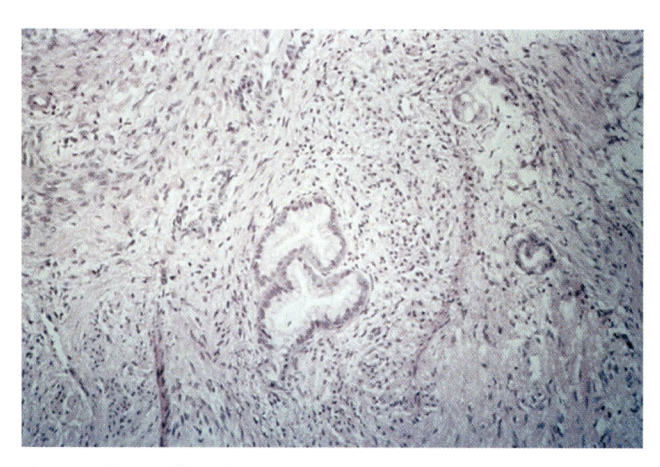

Figure 7 Glassy cell carcinoma.

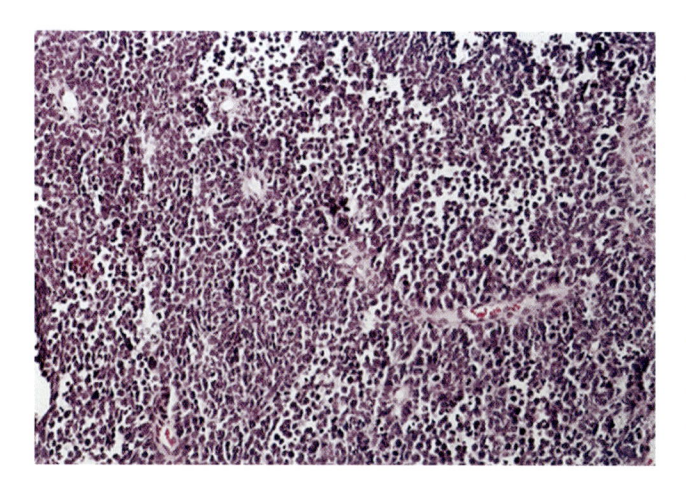

Figure 8 Small-cell carcinoma.

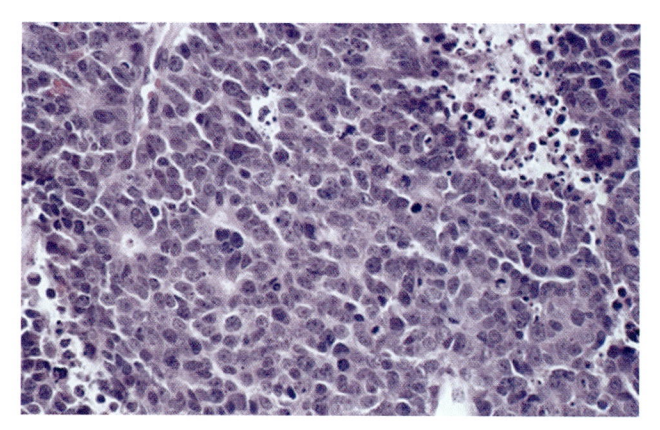

Figure 9 Non-small-cell neuroendocrine carcinoma.

a better prognosis. Efforts to treat these cancers with approaches typically used for small-cell carcinomas of the lung have had mixed results.

Non-small-cell neuroendocrine carcinoma
Non-small-cell neuroendocrine carcinomas of the cervix have been reported, but they are not listed in the current WHO classification of cervical tumors.[55] The tumors contain intermediate to large cells, high-grade nuclei, and eosinophilic cytoplasmic granules of the type seen in neuroendocrine cells. A trabecular pattern is frequently evident, with or without glandular differentiation (Figure 9). Tumors are usually immunoreactive for chromogranin. Reported survival rates for patients with these aggressive carcinomas are similar to those for patients with small-cell carcinoma.

Diagnosis and treatment of precancerous lesions

Screening and management of low-grade cytologic abnormalities

The most recent recommended guidelines for screening for cervical cancer are listed in Table 2.[56] Screening with cervical cytology alone, primary high-risk human papillomavirus (hrHPV) alone, or contesting can detect high-grade precancerous cervical lesion and cervical cancer.[56] Evidence from randomized control trials[40,57–59] indicate that (hrHPV) testing and co-testing can detect more cases of CIN3, but they also have higher false-positive rate compared with cytology alone leading to more colposcopies. However, based on data from these studies, the recommendation is screening every 3 years with cytology alone for age 21–29 years, every 5 years with hrHPV testing alone, or every 5 years with both test (contesting) in women aged 30–65 years.[56] In low-resource settings, pap smears are a challenge where there is poor organization, coverage, and lack of quality assurance.[60] In these settings, visual inspection with acetic acid (VIA) may be a better option and in some countries in Africa a single-visit approach is used with VIA screening, rapid diagnosis, and treatment.[61,62] Treatment of low-grade cytologic abnormalities are shown in (Figures 10–12).[63,64]

Management of high-grade cytologic abnormalities

Optimal management of HGSILs includes colposcopic evaluation and biopsy or in women older than 24 years of age to proceed to a loop electrosurgical excision procedure (LEEP) without performing colposcopic evaluation. The consensus is that HGSILs should be treated once diagnosed.[65] For biopsy-proven HGSILs with negative findings on endocervical curettage (ECC), a satisfactory colposcopy examination, and congruent Pap smear and biopsy results, ablation of the transformation zone has been the standard of care for several decades. Three outpatient therapies are used in the United States for treating these lesions: cryotherapy, laser ablation, and LEEP. For patients with unsatisfactory colposcopic examination findings, a Pap smear result more severe than the biopsy findings, presence of an adenomatous component, suspicion of invasive cancer, or positive findings on ECC, a cone biopsy is indicated. Cone biopsies (talked about later in this article) remove tissue to a depth of 20–30 mm and up to 30 mm in diameter, including the transformation zone.

The three outpatient therapies of cryotherapy, laser vaporization, and LEEP have been the focus of controversy. Safety, efficacy, and cost issues have dominated the debate. Cryotherapy, introduced in 1972, was the first outpatient treatment of CIN and remains a dependable treatment because of its reliability, low complication rate, ease of use, and low cost.[66] Another advantage of cryotherapy is that leaving a large dead viral HPV load within disrupted cells may improve the immune response to the causative agent of CIN. Major disadvantages include lack of ability to tailor treatment to the size of the lesion, lack of a tissue specimen, and the risk of treatment of undetected invasive lesions. Cryotherapy is

Table 2 Clinical summary: screening for cervical cancer.[a]

Population	Women aged 21–29 years	Women aged 30–65 years	Women younger than 21 years, women older than 65 years with adequate prior screening, and women who have had a hysterectomy
Recommendation	Screen for cervical cancer every 3 years with cytology alone	Screen for cervical cancer every 3 years with cytology alone, every 5 years with hrHPV testing alone, or every 5 years with co-testing	Do not screen for cervical cancer

[a]Source: Modified from Curry et al.[56]

Cytology every 3 y from ages 25–65 y

Abnormal test result	Recommended next steps
ASC-US	Cytology in 1 y *or* hrHPV test: hrHPV+ → Colposcopy; hrHPV− → Cytology in 3 y
LSIL or worse	Colposcopy

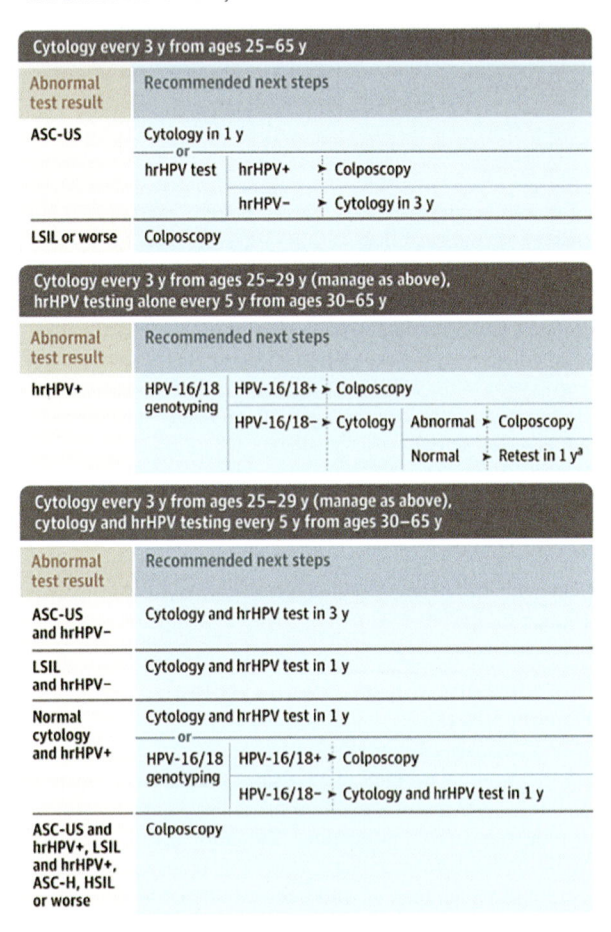

Cytology every 3 y from ages 25–29 y (manage as above), hrHPV testing alone every 5 y from ages 30–65 y

Abnormal test result	Recommended next steps
hrHPV+	HPV-16/18 genotyping: HPV-16/18+ → Colposcopy; HPV-16/18− → Cytology: Abnormal → Colposcopy; Normal → Retest in 1 y[a]

Cytology every 3 y from ages 25–29 y (manage as above), cytology and hrHPV testing every 5 y from ages 30–65 y

Abnormal test result	Recommended next steps
ASC-US and hrHPV−	Cytology and hrHPV test in 3 y
LSIL and hrHPV−	Cytology and hrHPV test in 1 y
Normal cytology and hrHPV+	Cytology and hrHPV test in 1 y *or* HPV-16/18 genotyping: HPV-16/18+ → Colposcopy; HPV-16/18− → Cytology and hrHPV test in 1 y
ASC-US and hrHPV+, LSIL and hrHPV+, ASC-H, HSIL or worse	Colposcopy

Figure 10 Screening guidelines for the early detection of cervical cancer. Source: Sawaya et al.[63]

appropriate for patients with satisfactory findings on colposcopic examination, negative findings on ECC, and small lesions (2.5–3.0 cm in diameter) that allow the entire lesion and transformation zone to be covered by the cryotherapy probe.

Laser vaporization was introduced in 1977. It has the advantage of being easily tailored to lesion size, but the cost of the equipment and the lack of a tissue specimen are major disadvantages.[66] In addition, laser vaporization requires more training and skills than the other two procedures and is associated with more serious safety issues (eye injuries and inadvertent burns). Candidates for this procedure are patients with large CIN lesions, young women with suspicious or invasive lesions or adenocarcinoma *in situ* in whom preservation of fertility is desired, and patients unwilling to undergo LEEP under local anesthesia.

LEEP was introduced in 1989, and it is currently the technique of choice for the treatment of HGSILs. LEEP is reliable and easy to use. It can be tailored to lesion size and provides a tissue specimen.[66] The advantage of this last characteristic is underscored by the finding of unsuspected adenocarcinoma *in situ* and microinvasive squamous cell carcinoma in 2–4% of LEEP specimens.[63,66] LEEP, however, has the potential to result in unintentional removal of excessive cervical stroma and removal of disease-free tissue (more frequent when LGSILs are treated). Other disadvantages include its high cost and the increased risk of bleeding and infection. Bleeding after LEEP has been reported in 2–7% of cases.[66] The high rates of overtreatment observed with LEEP have been related to misdiagnosis of abnormality and multiple punch biopsies of small lesions prior to treatment.[63] The use of LEEP in see-and-treat protocols has been shown to improve patient compliance with treatment when patient selection is adequate. This strategy has been suggested as having the greatest potential benefit for populations with poor treatment compliance.[63]

Prevention

Vaccine development

Papillomaviruses are epitheliotropic agents that induce benign papillomas of the skin and mucous membranes. In contrast to hepatitis B virus (HBV), there are more than 100 HPV genotypes (types). A subset of HPV types that are almost always transmitted sexually is the main cause of human cervical cancer. Infection with these HPV types is a strong risk factor for cervical cancer, and HPV DNA from one or more of these types is found in virtually all cervical tumors.[67,68] The virus encodes oncoproteins that appear to be required both for the induction and the maintenance of the cancer.

Three prophylactic HPV vaccines are currently available in many countries for use in females and males from the age of 9 years. All three vaccines are recombinant vaccines composed of virus-like particles and are not infectious since they do not contain viral DNA. The three vaccines include a quadrivalent vaccine targeting HPV 6, 11, 16, and 18,[69] a bivalent vaccine which targets HPV 16 and 18[70] and a nonvalent vaccine targeting HPV types 31, 33, 45, 52, and 58 in addition to HPV 6, 11, 16, and 18. The recommended schedule of vaccination presently includes two doses, but there are recent observational studies that have reported evidence for effectiveness in prevention high-risk HPV infections following a single dose and further long-term follow-up will clarify the role of one dose in preventing cervical neoplasms.[71,72]

A recent study examined the efficacy of the quadrivalent HPV vaccine in preventing invasive cancer in women in Sweden. They found an 88% lower incidence of invasive cancer in women who were vaccinated before the age of 17 years compared to women who never were vaccinated.[73] However, there are problems in widespread distribution of the vaccine, including price of the vaccines, accessibility of the vaccines in countries due to lack of immunization infrastructure, and opposition by conservative groups to the vaccination of young girls against what is perceived to be a sexually transmitted disease.[74]

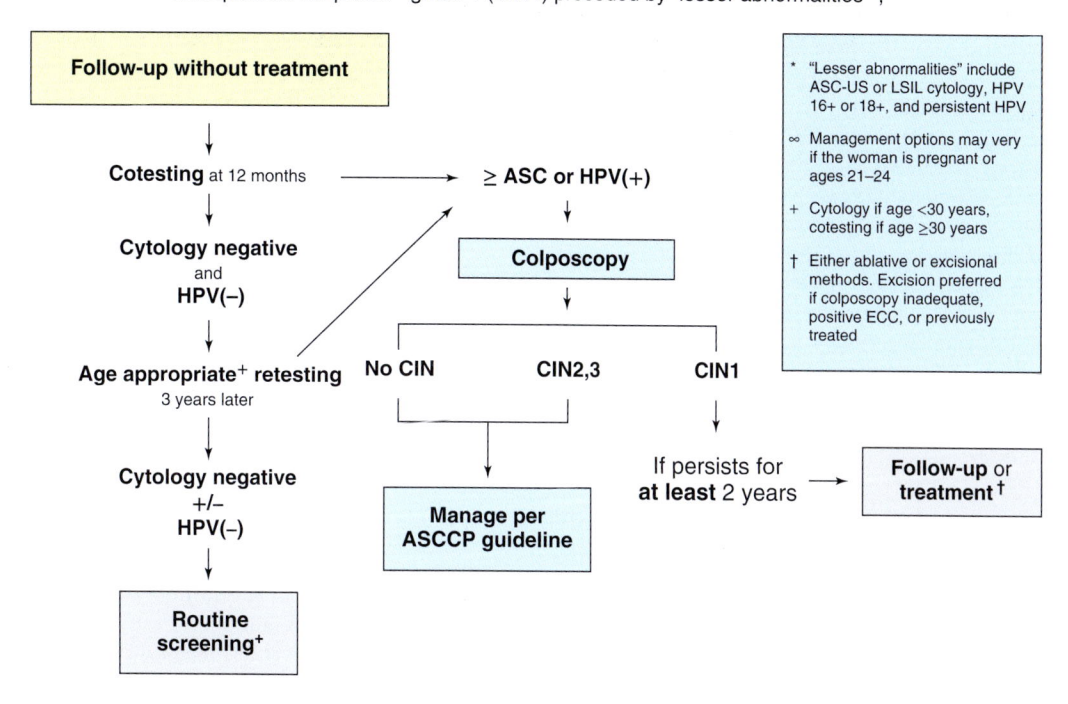

Figure 11 Management of women with biopsy-confirmed cervical intraepithelial neoplasia-grade 1 (CIN 1). Source: Massad et al.[64]

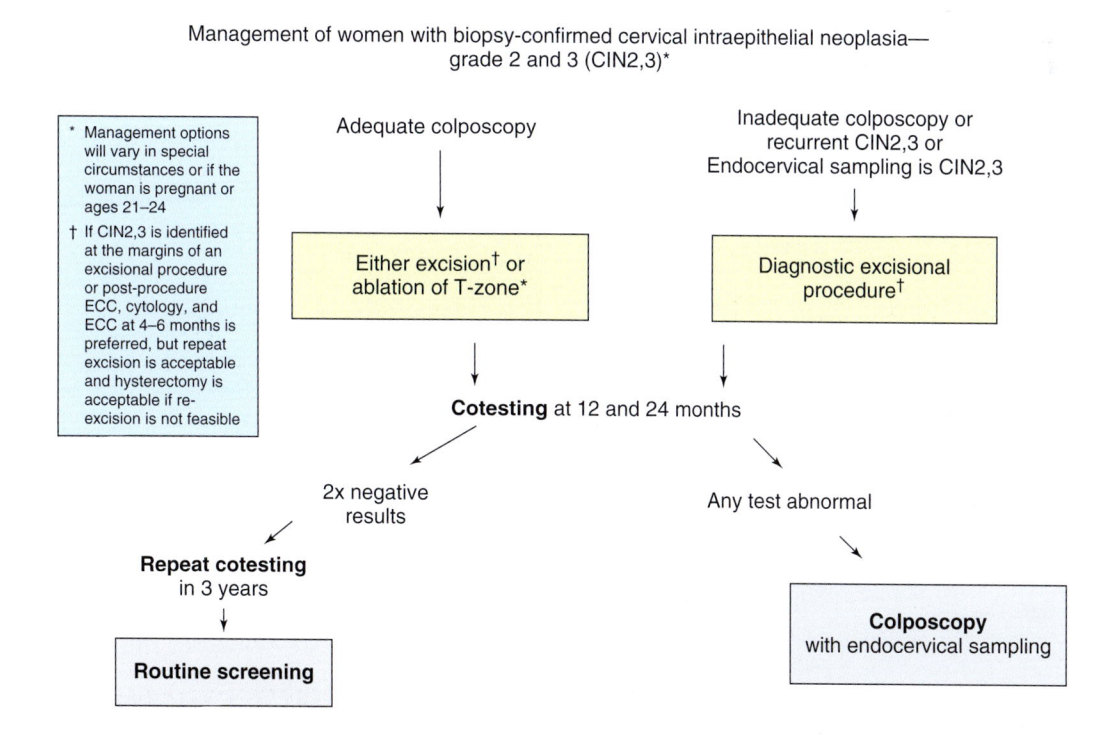

Figure 12 Management of women with biopsy-confirmed cervical intraepithelial neoplasia grades 2 and 3 (CIN 2,3). Source: Massad et al.[64]

Diagnosis and treatment of invasive lesions patterns of spread

During the transition from *in situ* to invasive carcinoma, tumor cells penetrate the epithelial basement membrane and enter the underlying cervical stroma. Once the cervical stroma is invaded, the lymphatics and blood vessels are accessible, and dissemination beyond the cervix is possible.

The cervical, vaginal, and uterine lymphatic channels coalesce to form major drainage pathways. The major lymphatic trunks are the utero-ovarian (infundibulopelvic), parametrial, and presacral, which drain into the paracervical, obturator, hypogastric, external iliac, common iliac, inferior gluteal, presacral, and lower aortic lymph nodes. A series studying the incidence and distribution pattern of retroperitoneal lymph node metastases in 208 patients with stages 1B, IIA, and IIB cervical carcinomas who underwent radical hysterectomy and systemic pelvic node dissection reported that 53 patients (25%) had node metastasis.[75] The obturator lymph nodes were the most frequently involved, with a rate of 19% (39 of 208), and the authors proposed them as sentinel nodes for cervical cancers.

Cervical cancers of similar size may have very different metastatic potentials, depending on their intrinsic aggressiveness and histologic cell type. Cervical carcinomas also invade directly. As the cancer grows, disease may extend to the lateral pelvic walls, into the bladder or rectum, or into the vagina.

The incidence of lymph node metastasis at diagnosis for each of the squamous cell carcinoma stages designated by the International Federation of Gynecology and Obstetrics (FIGO) has been well defined by surgical series.[76–78] Pelvic node involvement occurs in 10–25% of stage I carcinomas, 25–30% of stage II carcinomas, and 30–45% of stage III and IV carcinomas. Stage I carcinomas are more likely to metastasize to nodes once they reach 3 cm.[79,80] The incidence of positive nodes for poorly differentiated squamous cell carcinoma and for poorly differentiated adenocarcinoma is higher than that for the better-differentiated carcinomas.

Carcinoma of the cervix spreads in an orderly manner. Nodes adjacent to the cervix are usually the first to be involved, and "skip" metastases are uncommon. Patients with positive para-aortic nodes usually have positive pelvic nodes. The incidence of positive para-aortic nodes in 978 patients with stage IB and IIA carcinoma whose aortic nodes were sampled prior to radical hysterectomy was 4.7% and 8.4%, respectively. The incidence of positive nodes in patients with adenocarcinomas is probably equal to that in patients with squamous cell-carcinomas when cancer size, histologic differentiation, and extent of tumor or FIGO stage are similar. Many large series report poorer survival rates for patients with adenocarcinomas than for patients with squamous cell carcinomas, especially those who have bulky lesions.[81,82] Small-cell carcinoma and some of the carcinomas classified as other epithelial tumors are particularly aggressive. Carcinomas of the cervix, regardless of histology and size of the primary tumor, may contain highly malignant clones of cells that can prove unpredictable and spread extensively.

Clinical symptoms

The clinical symptoms of carcinoma of the cervix are vaginal bleeding, discharge, and pain. The growth pattern of the carcinoma plays a role in the development of symptoms. Exophytic carcinomas bleed earlier in a sexually active patient (because of contact) than lesions that expand the cervix. Lesions that expand the endocervix in a barrel-shaped configuration may leave the squamous epithelium of the exocervix intact until the lesions exceed 5 or 6 cm in transverse diameter; therefore, carcinomas with this growth pattern may be silent and grow large before the patient bleeds. Cytologic findings may be negative unless the endocervix is sampled with a brush device. Ulcerative lesions that destroy the exocervix bleed early, and necrosis and infection induced by the cancer's outgrowing its blood supply result in a foul-smelling vaginal discharge.

Severe pelvic pain experienced during the pelvic examination may indicate salpingitis. Tubal infections require management before radiation therapy. Patients with an adnexal mass need surgical treatment before radiation therapy is started.

Paracervical extension of a carcinoma may remain silent until fixation to the pelvic wall occurs. Fixation with or without nodal involvement may obstruct a ureter. Ureteral encroachment is usually a silent process. Patients may present with bilateral ureteral obstruction with impending renal failure and report no history of urinary system complaints. Direct invasion of branches of the sciatic nerve roots causes back pain, and encroachment on the pelvic wall veins and lymphatics causes edema of a lower extremity. The triad of back pain, leg edema, and a nonfunctioning kidney is evidence of an advanced carcinoma with extensive pelvic wall involvement.

The anatomic position of the bladder, so closely adjacent to the cervix, favors contiguous spread from the cervix to the bladder. Urinary frequency and urgency are early manifestations of such spread; patients with advanced disease may present with hematuria or incontinence, suggesting direct extension of tumor to the bladder. Cystoscopy and biopsy should confirm the cause of hematuria or incontinence.

In contrast, posterior extension to the rectum and disruption of the rectal mucosa is an unusual pattern of disease spread in untreated patients. The deep cul-de-sac provides anatomic separation of the rectum and cervix. In patients who present with rectal mucosal involvement, there is usually extensive involvement of the posterior vaginal wall with direct extension to the rectum. For staging and treatment planning, cystoscopy and sigmoidoscopy are essential.

Metastatic carcinoma in para-aortic nodes may extend through the node capsule and directly invade the vertebrae and adjacent nerve roots. Back pain owing to involvement of the lumbar vertebrae and psoas muscles may be a manifestation of massive nodal disease; however, hematogenous spread to the lumbar vertebrae and involvement of the psoas muscle without significant nodal disease may occur.

Diagnosis

The diagnosis of cervical carcinoma is made by pathologic examination of a tissue specimen. The endocervix should be curetted if no lesion is visible or if the cervix is enlarged, nodular, or hard. Older patients with adenocarcinoma require an endometrial biopsy. It may be difficult to distinguish an endocervical primary tumor from an endometrial primary tumor involving the lower uterine segment. Patients with an abnormal Pap smear and no visible lesion require colposcopy and biopsy. The tissue specimen may be a simple colposcopy-directed biopsy specimen, an endocervical specimen obtained with a curette, or a conization specimen.

Evaluation and staging

Successful therapy planning requires detailed evaluation of the patient's general medical condition and the size and extent of the carcinoma. Patients with anemia, which has been extensively studied, have a higher local relapse rate than patients with a

Table 3 Relapse rates for patients with stage IIB or III cervical cancer.[a]

Hemoglobin (gm/dL)	Patients (no.)	Relapse rate (%)		
		Local	Distant	Total
<10	29	46	18	49
10–11.9	319	29	24	47
12–13.9	578	20	16	33
≥14	129	20	18	33

[a]Source: Bush.[83]
Relapse rates for patients with stage IIB or III cancer of the cervix according to average hemoglobin level during radiation therapy. p Values: $p = 0.002$ (local), $p = 0.1$ (distant), $p = 0.0007$ (total).

normal hemoglobin (Table 3).[83,84] The patient's surgical history is important, and operative notes may describe the status of the abdominal organs as well as report abdominal and pelvic operations. Diagnoses of importance to therapy planning include ulcerative bowel disease, diverticulitis, and pelvic inflammatory disease. Such inflammatory conditions induce adhesions and fix loops of the intestines to each other, to adjacent organs, and to peritoneal surfaces.

Patients with small stage I carcinomas should undergo chest radiography, a complete blood count, urinalysis, and blood chemistry analysis before treatment. Patients with advanced carcinomas may require cystoscopy and proctoscopy. It is important to apply the FIGO rules for clinical staging (Table 4).[85] Prior to 2018, FIGO staging was based mainly on clinical examination with addition of certain procedure, however, the new 2018 FIGO staging allows for imaging and pathological findings.

The best radiologic imaging technique for detecting lymph node metastases is unclear. CT and MRI are good in identifying enlarged nodes; however, the accuracy of these techniques in the detection of positive nodes is compromised by their failure to detect small metastases, and many enlarged nodes are due not to metastases but to inflammation associated with advanced disease. The accuracy of MRI in the detection of lymph node metastases (72–93%) is similar to that of CT; however, when compared with surgical findings, MRI is superior to CT, clinical examination, and sonography in the evaluation of tumor location, tumor size, depth of stromal invasion, vaginal extension, and parametrial extension of cervical cancer.[86–89] Furthermore, studies suggest that MRI is a cost-effective method of evaluating cervical cancers.[89] Figure 13 shows an MRI of a patient with a cervical tumor.

PET or PET/CT is the rapidly expanding modality in oncologic imaging (Figure 14). In a study of 101 patients with carcinoma of the cervix, Grigsby and colleagues reported that CT demonstrated enlarged pelvic lymph nodes in 20% and enlarged para-aortic lymph nodes in 7%, while PET demonstrated abnormal FDG uptake in pelvic lymph nodes in 67%, abnormal FDG uptake in para-aortic lymph nodes in 21%, and abnormal FDG uptake in supraclavicular lymph nodes in 8%.[90] The 2-year progression-free survival rate (PFS), based solely on para-aortic lymph node status, was 64% in CT-normal and PET-normal patients, 18% in CT-normal and PET-abnormal patients, and 14% in CT-abnormal and PET-abnormal patients. The authors concluded that often than CT and that the findings on PET are a better predictor of survival than those on CT in patients with carcinoma of the cervix.

In some patients, surgical examination of the lymph nodes is warranted. The risk of occult para-aortic metastases is highest in patients with grossly involved pelvic nodes, and these patients may be the best candidates for operative exploration. These patients also may benefit from removal of the grossly enlarged nodes, which may be difficult to control with radiation alone.[91] Surgical staging of

Table 4 Modified FIGO staging.[a]

Stage	Description
I	The carcinoma is strictly confined to the cervix (extension to the corpus should be disregarded)
IA	Invasive cancer that can be diagnosed only by microscopy, with maximum depth of invasion <5 mm[b]
IA1	Measured invasion of stroma, 3 mm in depth
IA2	Measured invasion of stroma ≥3 mm and <5 mm in depth
IB	Invasive carcinoma with measured deepest invasion ≥5 mm (greater than stage IA), lesion limited to the cervix uteri[c]
IB1	Invasive carcinoma ≥5 mm depth of stromal invasion and <2 cm in greatest dimension
IB2	Invasive carcinoma ≥2 cm and <4 cm in greatest dimension
IB3	Invasive carcinoma ≥4 cm in greatest dimension
II	The carcinoma invades beyond the uterus but has not extended onto the pelvic wall or to the lower third of vagina
IIA	Involvement of up to the upper 2/3 of the vagina. No obvious parametrial involvement
IIA1	Clinical visible lesion <4 cm
IIA2	Clinical visible lesion ≥4 cm
IIB	Obvious parametrial involvement but not to the pelvic wall
III	The carcinoma involves the lower third of the vagina and/or extends to the pelvic wall and/or causes hydronephrosis or nonfunctioning kidney and/or involves pelvic and/or para-aortic lymph nodes
IIIA	No extension onto the pelvic wall but involvement of the lower third of the vagina
IIIB	Extension onto the pelvic wall and/or hydronephrosis or nonfunctioning kidney
IIIC	Involvement of pelvic and/or para-aortic lymph nodes, irrespective of tumor size and extent (with r and p notations)[d]
IIIC1	Pelvic lymph node metastasis only
IIIC2	Para-aortic lymph node metastasis
IV	The carcinoma has extended beyond the true pelvis or has clinically involved (biopsy proven) the mucosa of the bladder or rectum
IVA	Spread to adjacent organs
IVB	Spread to distant organs

Abbreviation: FIGO, International Federation of Gynecology and Obstetrics.
[a]Source: Bhatla et al.[85]
[b]Imaging and pathology can be used, where available, to supplement clinical findings with respect to tumor size and extent, in all stage.
[c]The involvement of vascular/lymphatic spaces does not change the staging. The lateral extent of the lesion is no longer considered.
[d]Adding notation of r (imaging) and p (pathology) to indicate the findings that are used to allocate the case to Stage IIIC. Example: if imaging indicates pelvic lymph node metastasis, the stage allocation would be Stage IIIC1r, and if confirmed by pathologic findings, it would be Stage IIIC1p. The type of imaging modality or pathology technique used should always be documented.

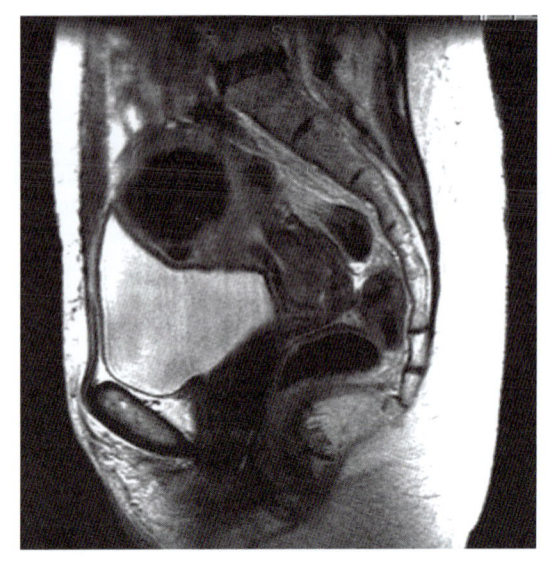

Figure 13 Magnetic resonance image of a patient with cervical tumor.

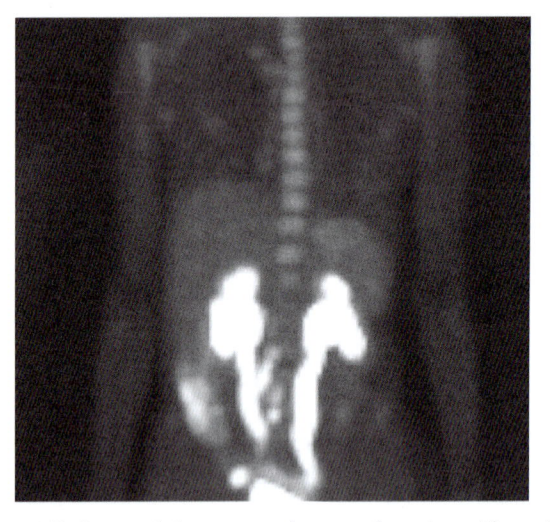

Figure 14 Positron emission tomography scan of a patient with cervical tumor showing positive nodes.

para-aortic lymph node involvement has been reported to have a better prognosis than radiographic exclusion alone.[92] When lymph node metastases are sought surgically, the extraperitoneal approach is currently the preferred technique.[93] Lymph node exploration and dissection may also be performed using a laparoscopic approach, which is associated with a shorter postoperative recovery time and probably less late radiation morbidity than open transperitoneal staging.[94]

Prognostic factors

FIGO stage correlates with survival and control of pelvic disease in patients with cervical cancer; however, prognosis is also influenced by other factors, including tumor characteristics and patient characteristics that are not included in the FIGO staging system.

Tumor size and local extent

Tumor size is one of the most important predictors of local recurrence and death in patients with cervical cancer treated with surgery or radiation therapy (Figure 15).[95] The FIGO staging classification for stage I–II disease was modified to include tumor diameter.[85] For patients with more advanced disease, other estimates of tumor bulk that correlate with prognosis include presence of medial versus lateral parametrial involvement in FIGO stage IIB disease and unilateral versus bilateral pelvic wall involvement in FIGO stage IIIB disease.[96,97]

In patients who have had a radical hysterectomy, histologic evidence of extra-cervical spread (>10 mm) and deep stromal invasion (>70% invasion) are associated with a poorer prognosis, as is parametrial extension, which is associated with higher rates of lymph node involvement, local recurrence, and death from cancer.[78,98–100] Uterine body involvement is associated with an increased rate of distant metastases in patients treated with radiation or surgery.[101]

Lymph node involvement

Lymph node metastasis is another important prognostic factor for survival and now the new revised 2018 FIGO staging includes nodal involvement. In several surgical series, after a radical hysterectomy, patients with positive pelvic lymph nodes had a 35–40% lower 5-year survival rate than patients with negative nodes.[76,78] However, recent studies suggest that postoperative chemoradiation improves these results.[102] Patients with positive para-aortic nodes have a survival rate that is about half that of patients with similar-stage disease and negative para-aortic nodes.[76,78,99,103,104] With extended-field radiation therapy, patients with early-stage disease and positive para-aortic nodes have a cure rate of approximately 40–50%.

There is a strong correlation between positive lymph nodes in patients with cervical neoplasms and positive lymph-vascular space invasion (LVSI) in the tumor specimen. However, LVSI may be an independent predictor of prognosis, as a number of large series of patients treated with radical hysterectomy have demonstrated.[98,99,105,106] Roman and colleagues reported a correlation between the percentage of histopathologic sections containing LVSI and the incidence of lymph node metastasis.[107] In patients with adenocarcinoma of the cervix, there is a strong correlation between LVSI and outcome.[108,109]

Histologic type

There is controversy regarding whether adenocarcinomas of the cervix are associated with outcome similar to that seen with squamous carcinomas of the cervix. In several retrospective studies, investigators found that patients with adenocarcinomas of the cervix had outcomes similar to those of patients with squamous carcinoma of the cervix treated with radiation therapy.[110,111] However, other investigators have come to an opposite conclusion. Among patients treated surgically, they found that patients with adenocarcinoma had unusually high relapse rates compared with the rates in patients with squamous cell carcinoma, and among patients treated with surgery or irradiation, they found that patients with adenocarcinoma had poorer survival rates than the rates seen in patients with squamous cell carcinoma.[95,112,113] Eifel and colleagues, in an analysis of 1767 patients treated with radiation for FIGO stage IB disease, reported that patients with adenocarcinoma had a significantly higher risk of recurrence and death from disease.[112] This finding was independent of age, tumor size, and tumor morphology. There was no difference in the rate of pelvic recurrence between patients with bulky adenocarcinoma (≥4 cm) and patients with squamous cell carcinoma; however, the rate of distant metastasis was almost twice as high in patients with adenocarcinoma as in patients with squamous cell carcinoma. Although the prognostic significance of histologic grade for squamous carcinomas has been disputed, there is a clear correlation

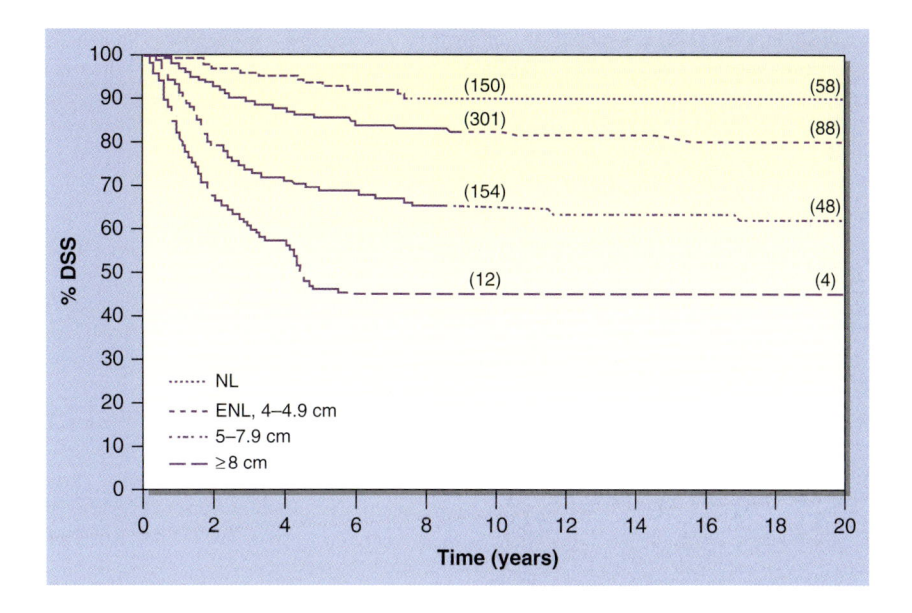

Figure 15 Disease-specific survival (DSS) is indicated for patients grouped according to size of cervix (NL, cervix of normal size; ENL, enlarged cervix, 4–4.9 cm). Source: Modified from Lai et al.[95]

between the degree of differentiation and the clinical behavior of adenocarcinomas.[108,109,114]

Other tumor factors

Pretreatment squamous cell carcinoma antigen (SCCAg) levels have correlated with tumor bulk, stage, histology, grade, type of tumor (i.e., exophytic vs infiltrative), microscopic depth of invasion, and risk of lymph node metastases in patients with early-stage disease.[115–117] The most important property of the pretreatment SCCAg level, however, is its ability to predict clinical outcome. Several authors have reported significantly lower survival rates in patients with very elevated values compared with patients with normal baseline levels, independent of stage.[117–120] Monitoring of tumor response using SCCAg needs further investigation, especially studies designed to determine how often SCCAg measurement should be done, the level of SCCAg that is significant, which patients would benefit from this monitoring and the cost-effectiveness of using SCCAg as a tool for monitoring patients after treatment.[121]

Several authors have reported a correlation between HPV subtype and prognosis.[122–124] In two studies of patients with histologically negative lymph nodes, investigators reported higher rates of disease recurrence when findings on PCR assay of the lymph nodes were strongly positive for HPV DNA.[125,126]

Other molecular markers that have recently been evaluated for predictive power in cervical carcinoma are epidermal growth factor receptor and cyclooxygenase-2.[127] Other biologic features that have been investigated for their predictive power, with variable results, include inflammatory response in cervical stroma, peritoneal cytology, tumor vascularity, and DNA ploidy or S-phase fraction.[128,129]

Patient factors

Several investigators have reported correlations between low hemoglobin level before or during treatment and poor prognosis.[96,130] It has been speculated that the poor prognosis of anemic patients is caused in part by hypoxia-induced radiation resistance. Other patient-related factors that have been shown to correlate with prognosis include age, platelet count, platelet-to-lymphocyte ratio,[131] socioeconomic status, and smoking.[80,132–136] Kucera et al.[135] reported that smokers with cervical cancer had a poorer 5-year survival rate than nonsmokers, and this relationship was statistically significant in patients with stage III disease (5-year survival rate 20.3% vs 33.9%, $p < 0.01$).

Surgical treatment options

Sentinel lymph nodes

A biopsy of sentinel lymph node was originally a process meant to simplify the surgical procedure and decrease morbidity by removing just one or a few nodes instead of systematic lymphadenectomy. However, the concept may have other advantages including a more reliable detection of key nodes in atypical localizations, detection of small metastasis, and intraoperative triage of patients, thanks to identification of key nodes for pathologic evaluation. The first large, multicenter study on sentinel lymph nodes for cervical cancer was published in 2008 and found a sensitivity of only 77% which was major set back for this procedure in cervical cancer.[137] However, there were multiple problems with this study including the size of tumors included, lack of surgeon proficiency assessment, and pathologic ultrastaging. Subsequent studies have shown a very high sensitivity in women with small tumors undergoing lymphatic mapping including a recent large French SENTICOL study that has reported a sensitivity of 92% and a negative predictive value of 98%.[138] Presently, sentinel lymph node biopsies are a useful intraoperative triage for patients with small tumors where the false-negative rate is lower. A large phase III trial, SENTICOL III is looking at sentinel lymph node biopsy and survival.

Cervical conization and LEEP

Cervical conization is a procedure that excises the transformation zone in a cone-shape or cylindrical wedge and can be diagnostic, therapeutic, or both. Patients requiring conization usually have one of the following: normal colposcopy findings and an abnormal Pap smear or positive ECC specimens; abnormal colposcopy findings in the form of failure to visualize the entire squamocolumnar junction or failure to define the extent of the lesion; microinvasive carcinoma in a biopsy specimen; adenocarcinoma *in situ* in a biopsy or ECC specimen; or a lack of correlation between cytologic (Pap smear), colposcopic, and histologic interpretations.

Another surgical technique that can be used for conization is LEEP. In LEEP, a thin wire loop electrode is used to excise the lesion in patients with HGSIL. LEEP is an outpatient procedure. Although destructive techniques (such as laser ablation and cryotherapy) can provide effective treatment of suspicious lesions; the preferred technique is one that provides an appropriate histologic specimen, such as cervical cold knife conization (CKC) LEEP, or laser conization. Recently, Linares and colleagues compared CKC, laser conization, and LEEP and found that LEEP was associated with fewer complications and a shorter operating time than the other two procedures.[139] The only drawback of the LEEP procedure was a slightly shorter cone depth and a slightly higher risk of lesion recurrence.[139]

Patient selection
Conization as sole treatment of early cervical cancers is a relatively recent concept. For women who have very limited risk of lymph node spread and who have a strong desire to maintain fertility, conization may be an option.[140,141]

Complications of CKC include hemorrhage, pelvic cellulitis, cervical stenosis, and incompetent cervix.[142] In addition, because this procedure requires general anesthesia, there is the additional burden of possible complications and cost of anesthesia.

Complications of LEEP are similar to but not the same as those of CKC: Infection, bleeding, burns to the vagina, cervical stenosis, cervical incompetence, and recurrence of dysplasia. With LEEP, however, stenosis is rare (occurring in 1% of patients) and is seen primarily in nulliparous, perimenopausal, or postmenopausal patients. Cervical incompetence is usually only a complication of multiple procedures. The other advantage of LEEP is that it does not require general anesthesia. As mentioned above, when three conization techniques (CKC, laser conization, and LEEP) were compared, LEEP was associated with fewer complication as well as decreased operative time.[139]

Radical trachelectomy
Recently, for early-stage disease, several groups have tried to preserve the uterus and child-bearing capability by treating patients with a radical vaginal trachelectomy. This technique involves a laparoscopic pelvic lymphadenectomy followed by vaginal resection of the cervix, the upper 1–2 cm of the vaginal cuff, and the medial portions of the cardinal and uterosacral ligaments. The cervix is transected at the lower uterine segment, and a prophylactic cerclage is placed at the time of surgery. Several investigators recommend that this procedure be limited to patients with a tumor not exceeding 2 cm.[143,144]

Extrafascial hysterectomy
The extrafascial technique permits removal of the intact uterine fundus and cervix, leaving the parametrial soft tissues and a portion of the upper vagina. Extrafascial hysterectomy can be accomplished through an abdominal incision, transvaginally, or by using a combination of laparoscopic and transvaginal techniques.

Simple extrafascial hysterectomy is the standard definitive treatment option for women with stage IA1 cervical cancers and is sometimes performed following radiation therapy for bulky endocervical carcinomas. For patients with stage IA2 disease, there is some controversy regarding the most appropriate surgical procedure. These patients have 3–5% incidence of lymph node metastases and a higher rate of vaginal recurrence than patients with IA1 disease. So, although some data suggest that these IA2 lesions can be effectively resected with extrafascial hysterectomy, many American gynecologic oncologists limit this operation to women with IA1 tumors.[145,146]

Radical hysterectomy
Radical hysterectomy involves the en bloc removal of the uterus, cervix, parametrial tissues, and upper vagina. Table 5[147] shows the different types of hysterectomies. A radical hysterectomy with pelvic lymphadenectomy is the standard treatment in the management of stage IA2-IIA tumors. The type II (modified radical) hysterectomy is a less extensive version of the type III (radical) hysterectomy. The primary indication for type II hysterectomy is early invasive carcinoma, tumors less than 2 cm diameter. The incidence of bladder and ureteral complications is lower with the type II operation than with a type III procedure. The type II hysterectomy can be performed with a modified or complete pelvic lymphadenectomy.

The type III (radical) hysterectomy is the classic Wertheim–Meigs radical hysterectomy. This operation is reserved for patients with stage IB and selected stage IIA carcinomas. The vaginal extension for stage IIA patients should be limited to no more than 1 cm. A large randomized study was done that compared minimally invasive surgery versus abdominal radical hysterectomy for patients with stage IA1-IB1 cervical cancer.[148] This study was closed early with finding of a lower rate of disease-free survival and overall survival in patients who were treated with minimally invasive surgery compared to patients treated with abdominal radical hysterectomy.[148] At the same time, a systematic review and meta-analysis found that among patients undergoing radical hysterectomy for early-stage cervical cancer, minimally invasive radical hysterectomy was associated with an elevated risk of recurrence and death compared to open surgery.[149] At this time, for patients with cervical cancer, open surgery is the recommendation but there are several trials ongoing looking at the question of minimally invasive surgery versus open surgery.

Intraoperative and immediate postoperative complications of radical hysterectomy include blood loss (average, 0.8 L), ureterovaginal fistula (occurring in 1–2% of patients), vesicovaginal fistula (<1%), pulmonary embolus (1–2%), small bowel obstruction (1–2%), and postoperative fever secondary to deep vein thrombosis, pulmonary infection, pelvic cellulitis, urinary tract infection, or wound infection (25–50%).[150] Subacute complications include lymphocyst formation and lower-extremity edema, the risk of which is related to the extent of the node dissection. Lymphocysts may obstruct a ureter, but hydronephrosis usually improves with drainage of the lymphocyst.[151] The risk of complications may be increased in patients who undergo preoperative or postoperative irradiation.

Although most patients have transiently decreased bladder sensation after radical hysterectomy, with appropriate management severe long-term bladder complications are infrequent. However, chronic bladder hypotonia or atony occurs in approximately 3–5% of patients despite careful postoperative bladder drainage.[152] Radical hysterectomy may be complicated by stress incontinence, but reported incidences vary widely and may be influenced by the addition of postoperative radiation therapy.[152] Patients may also experience constipation and, rarely, chronic obstipation after radical hysterectomy.

Criteria for selecting patients who are appropriate candidates for radical hysterectomy include factors affecting the patient's suitability for major surgery as well as tumor characteristics, including

Table 5 Types of radical hysterectomy.[a]

	Simple extrafascial hysterectomy	Modified radical hysterectomy	Radical hysterectomy
Piver and rutledge classification	Type I	Type II	Type III
Querleu and morrow classification	Type A	Type B	Type C
Indication	Stage IA1	Stage IA1 with LVSI, IA2	Stage IB1 and IB2,m selected IIA
Uterus and cervix	Removed	Removed	Removed
Ovaries	Optional removal	Optional removal	Optional removal
Vaginal margin	None	1–2 cm	Upper 1/4 to 1/3
Ureters	Not mobilized	Tunnel through broad ligament	Tunnel through broad ligament
Cardinal ligaments	Divided at cervical border	Divided where ureter transits broad ligaments	Divided at pelvic sidewall
Uterosacral ligaments	Divided at cervical border	Partially removed	Divided near sacral origin
Urinary bladder	Mobilized to base of bladder	Mobilized to upper vagina	Mobilized to middle vagina
Rectum	Not mobilized	Mobilized below cervix	Mobilized below cervix

[a]Source: Bhatla et al.[147]

Table 6 Five-year survival rates for stage IB-IIA cervical cancer patients after radical hysterectomy and bilateral pelvic lymphadenectomy.

First author (Ref.)	Stage	Year	n	Survival (%)
Sall[153]	IB-IIA	1979	219	90.0
Kenter[154]	IB-IIA	1989	213	87.3
Lee[155]	IB-IIA	1989	343	87.2
Ayhan[77]	IB-IIA	1991	270	80.7
Hopkins[114]	IB	1991	213	92.5
Alvarez[156]	IB	1991	401	85
Averette[76]	IIB-IIA	1993	726	90.1
Landoni[157]	IB-IIA	1997	172	83

Abbreviation: N, number of patients.

tumor volume and lymphatic involvement. Patient factors play a very important role in the selection of primary radical surgery versus primary radiation therapy in patients with early-stage disease. The ability to preserve ovarian function as well as a more pliable vagina is important to young women facing this decision. Just as important, for women with significant medical problems, including obesity, primary radiation therapy may be the better treatment option. Careful selection also should be made so patients do not receive multiple treatments that would increase their complications due to risk factors that will be discussed further in this article.

Outcomes after surgical treatment

Reported 5-year survival rates for women with stage IB cervical cancer treated with radical hysterectomy and pelvic lymphadenectomy are approximately 80–90% (Table 6).[76,77,114,153–157] Patients with positive surgical margins or positive lymph nodes are at the highest risk of recurrence and poor outcome. Delgado and colleagues, in a large prospective study, reported 3-year disease-specific survival rates of 85.6% in patients with negative nodes and 50–74% in patients with positive nodes.[78] In the group with positive nodes, increasing number of positive nodes and involvement of common iliac nodes correlated with decreased survival. A randomized study showed that postoperative chemoradiation improved survival in patients with positive lymph nodes, positive surgical margins, or tumor present in the parametrium.[102]

Radiation therapy

The management of invasive carcinoma of the cervix with primary radiation therapy involves a combination of external beam radiation therapy (EBRT) plus either low-dose-rate (LDR) or high-dose-rate (HDR) intracavitary irradiation. The goal of treatment is to balance these two elements in a way that optimizes the ratio of tumor control to treatment complications. The required dose varies according to the tumor burden in the cervix, paracervical sites, and regional nodes. Factors that influence the tolerable dose of radiation include the patient's vaginal and uterine anatomy, the degree of tumor-related tissue destruction and infection, and patient characteristics (e.g., body habitus, comorbid illnesses, and smoking habits).

Treatment options EBRT

EBRT is used as initial treatment in patients with bulky tumors. The usual plan is to give 40–45 Gy to the whole pelvis. This gives a homogeneous distribution to the central mass plus the regional lymph nodes. Such treatment reduces the primary tumor and any regional lymph nodes harboring disease, and it destroys microscopic foci in lymph-vascular spaces adjacent to the tumor. The shrinkage of the primary tumor allows better dose distribution from intracavitary irradiation.

High-energy photons (15–18 MV) are usually preferred for pelvic treatment because they spare superficial tissues that are unlikely to be involved with tumor. Simulation films, as well as CT, MRI, or PET scan guide the radiation oncologist in selecting boundaries for the portals. Typical radiation therapy fields are shown in Figure 16. A standard course of 40–45 Gy whole-pelvis EBRT. Patients with grossly positive pelvic nodes within the 40- to 45-Gy field require a boost with a small field (Figure 16). The dose to the boost area is 8–10 Gy. The total dose to the positive nodes, including a 1–2 cm margin, is 60–66 Gy, which includes the contributions from brachytherapy intracavitary systems.

Intensity-modulated radiation therapy (IMRT) is starting to replace standard three-dimensional radiation therapy in many parts of the world. Unlike standard treatment, IMRT allows one to dose paint tissues in the area of treatment, that is, allowing higher doses to tumor while giving less dose to normal tissues especially small bowel (Figure 17). NRG Oncology/RTOG 1203 randomized patient's postsurgery with cervical or endometrial cancer between IMRT and standard pelvic radiation. The conclusion from this study was that pelvic IMRT was associated with significantly less GI and urinary toxicity than standard RT from the patient's perspective and should be used as standard of treatment for patients postsurgery with cervical or endometrial cancer.[158] Three prospective randomized trials and one meta-analysis[159–162] have shown that IMRT decreases acute and late GI and urinary toxicities compared to 3D conformal in patients with locally advanced cervical cancer. EMBRACE I and now II are trials looking at the use of IMRT in patients with locally advanced cervical cancer.[159]

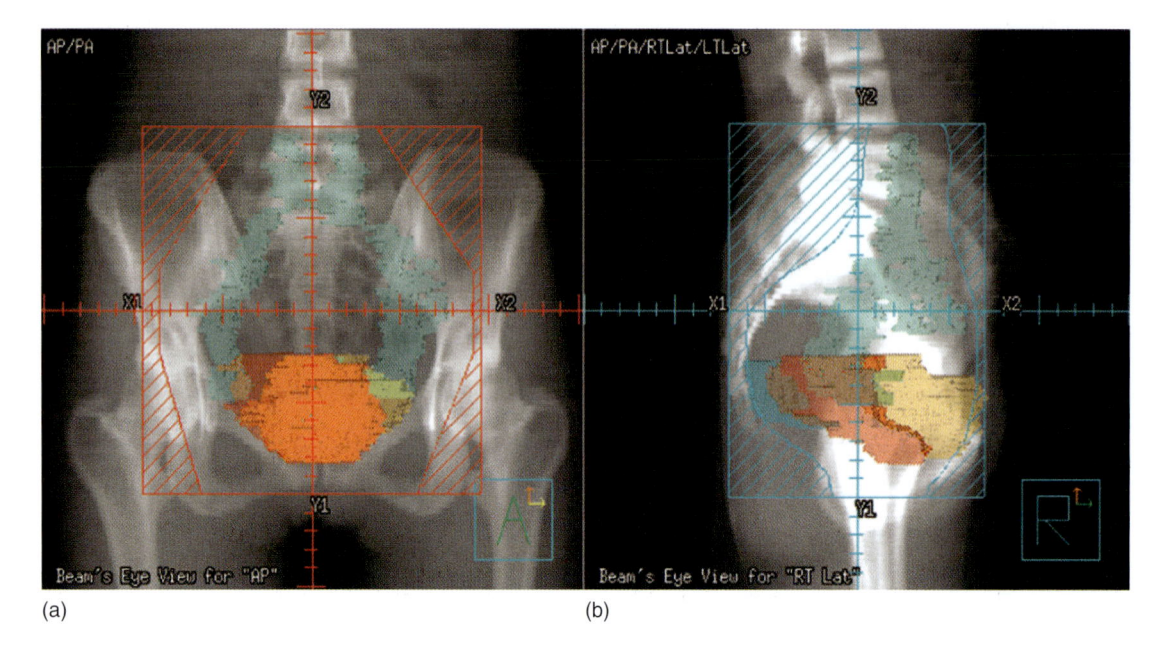

Figure 16 Typical radiation fields for a patient with cervical cancer. (a) Anterior field; (b) lateral field.

With the use of IMRT, the physician needs to take account of target motion during treatment with daily image guidance or the target may be missed.

Intracavitary radiation therapy (ICRT)

Brachytherapy plays an integral component in the definitive treatment of cervical cancer. In two large national database studies,[163,164] the use of brachytherapy was associated with improved survival compared with IMRT or SBRT as a boost. The omission of brachytherapy had a stronger effect on survival than the exclusion of chemotherapy.[164]

Brachytherapy is usually delivered using after-loading applicators that are placed in the uterine cavity and vagina. Ideal placement of the intrauterine tandem and vaginal ovoids produces a pear-shaped radiation distribution, delivering a high radiation dose to the cervix and paracervical tissues and a reduced dose to the rectum and bladder (Figure 18).

In the past, clinicians regarded the radiobiological advantages of low-dose rates (LDRs) intracavitary treatment (usually delivery of 40–60 cGy/h to point A) as a major factor contributing to the success of cervical cancer treatment. These low-dose rates permit repair of sublethal cellular injury, preferentially sparing normal tissues and optimizing the therapeutic ratio. During the past two decades, computer technology has made it possible to deliver brachytherapy at very high-dose rates (HDR, <100 cGy/min) using a high-activity cobalt 60 or iridium 192 source and remote after loading. HDR intracavitary therapy is now become the standard of care in most parts of the world. Clinicians have found this approach attractive because it does not require that patients be hospitalized and may be more convenient for the patient and the physician. Multiple randomized and nonrandomized studies have suggested that survival rates and complications rates with high-dose-rate treatment are similar to those with traditional low-dose-rate treatment.[165]

Prospective and retrospective data have shown that image-guided brachytherapy (MRI or CT) may improve local control as well as decrease both GI and GU toxicity compared to 2-D brachytherapy[166–168] and is emerging as standard practice in many centers (Figure 19). Standard tandem and ovoids/rings applicators may not always adequately cover the residual extent of disease at the time of brachytherapy and emerging data shows that the addition of interstitial needles may help optimize dose distribution by allowing higher doses to targets, while still meeting normal OAR constraints.[169]

Patient selection

For patients with IB1 tumors, the choice between surgery and radiation therapy is based primarily on patient preference, anesthetic and surgical risks, physician preference, and understanding of the nature and incidence of complications of radiation therapy and hysterectomy. In general, surgery is often chosen for younger patients in the hope of preserving ovarian function and hopefully reducing vaginal shortening, while radiation therapy is often selected for older postmenopausal women to avoid the morbidity of a major surgical procedure. Patients with stage IB2 disease can be treated with either surgery followed by radiation therapy or definitive radiation therapy. The biases are so large that the GOG could not complete trial randomizing patients with stage IB2 disease between surgery followed by chemoradiation therapy and definitive radiation therapy. Radiation therapy is the primary local therapy for most patients with stage IIB-IVA disease.

Outcomes

Stage IB-IIA disease
Radical radiation therapy achieves excellent survival and pelvic disease control rates in patients with stage IB-IIA cervical cancer. Dr. Eifel and colleagues reported 5-year disease-specific survival rates of 90%, 86%, and 67% in patients with stage IB tumors with cervical diameters of less than 4, 4–4.9, and greater than 5 cm, respectively.[170] The 5-year survival rates of patients with stage IIA disease range from 70% to 85% and, like survival rates in patients with stage IB disease, are strongly correlated with tumor size.[97,171,172] Studies suggest that results for patients with bulky tumors may be improved further by concurrent administration of chemotherapy.[173,174]

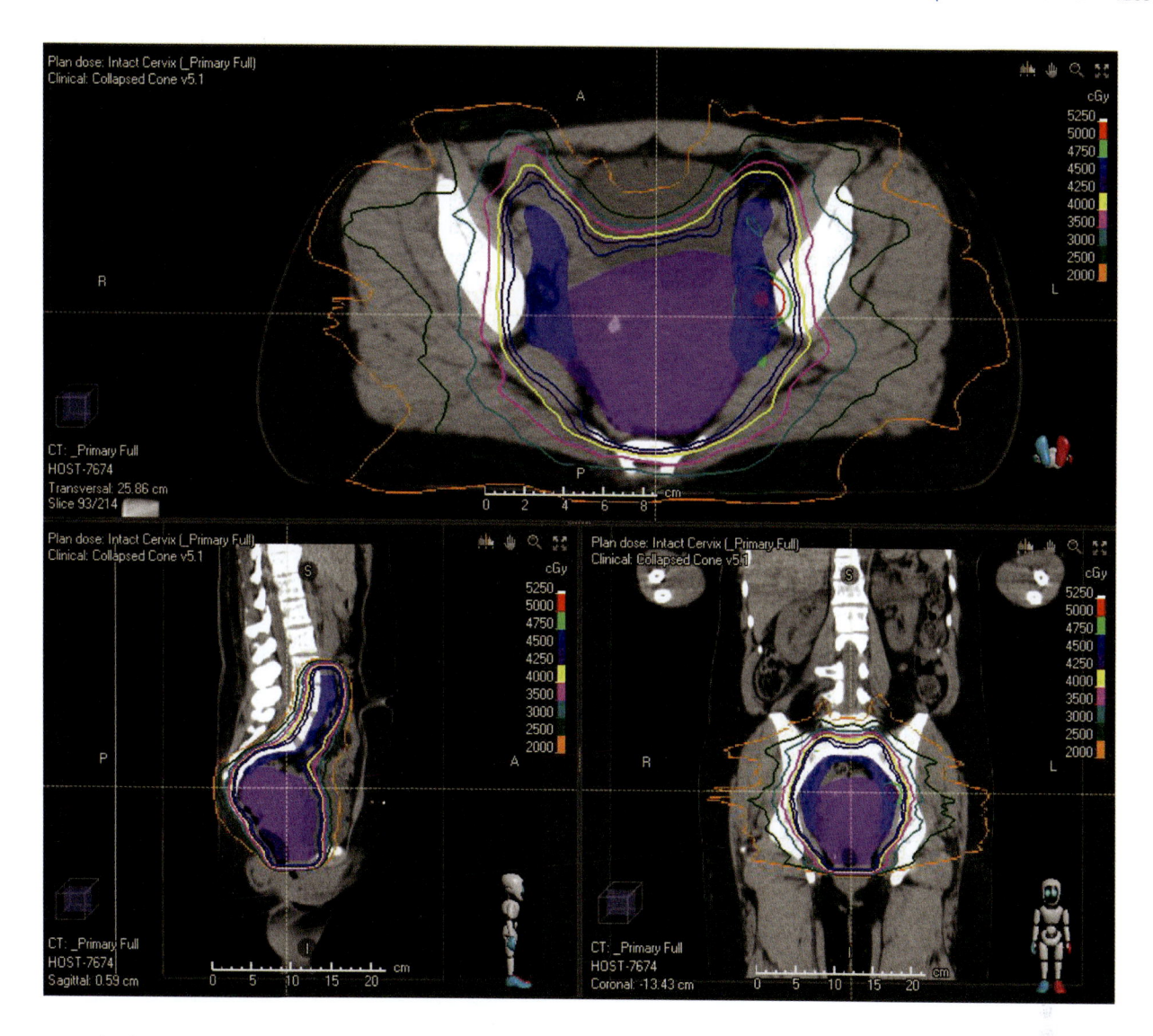

Figure 17 This shows a patient with cervical cancer being treated with radiation therapy. The areas that need to be covered are the nodes, cervix, and uterus. This is an IMRT plan that conforms to the area that needs to be covered while sparing the small bowel. The purple is the uterus and cervix, blue is the clinical negative nodes and red is the pet positive node. Everything is getting 45 Gy, except the pet positive node in red that is get 50 Gy all in 25 fractions. You can see that the anterior bowel is being spared as well as the entire spinal cord and a lot of the pelvic bones.

Stage IIB-IVA disease

Five-year survival rates of 65–75%, 35–50%, and 15–20% have been reported in patients who received radiation therapy alone for stage IIB, IIIB, and IV tumors, respectively (Table 7).[97] The addition of cisplatin-containing regimens may further improve local control and survival.[174–176]

Complications

Acute side effects

Acute side effects of pelvic irradiation include symptoms related to the bowel, bladder, rectum, and vagina. Most patients experience mild fatigue and mild to moderate diarrhea that usually is controllable with antidiarrheal medication and dietary modifications. Less frequently, patients may complain of bladder or urethral irritation. These symptoms may be treated with Pyridium or antispasmodics after urinalysis and urine culture have ruled out a urinary tract infection. Patients treated with extended-field radiation may have nausea, gastric irritation, and mild depression of peripheral blood cell counts. Acute symptoms may be increased in patients receiving concurrent chemotherapy. Unless the ovaries have been transposed, all premenopausal patients who receive pelvic radiation therapy experience ovarian failure by the completion of treatment.

Table 7 Pelvic disease control and survival rates.[a,b]

FIGO stage	Patients (n)	Control rate (%)	Survival rate (%)
I	229	93	89
IIA	315	88	85
IIB	314	80	62
IIIA	266	63	62
IIIB	216	57	50
IV	43	18	20

[a]Source: Barillot et al.[97]
[b]Pelvic disease control rates and survival rates of 1383 patients with carcinoma of the intact uterine cervix treated with irradiation alone, according to the Fletcher guidelines: a French cooperative study.[97]

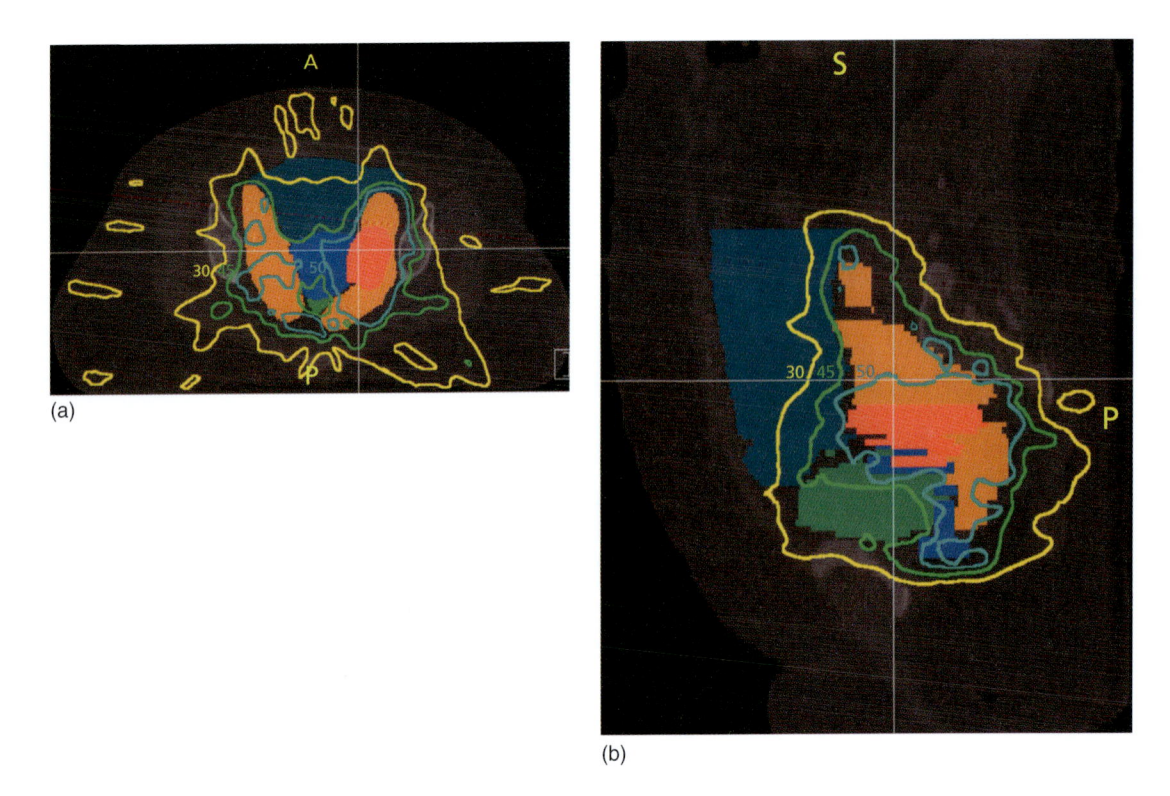

Figure 18 Dose distribution of a typical intracavitary system; it is important to note how quickly the dose falls off the further one gets from the system. (a) Anterior view and (b) lateral view.

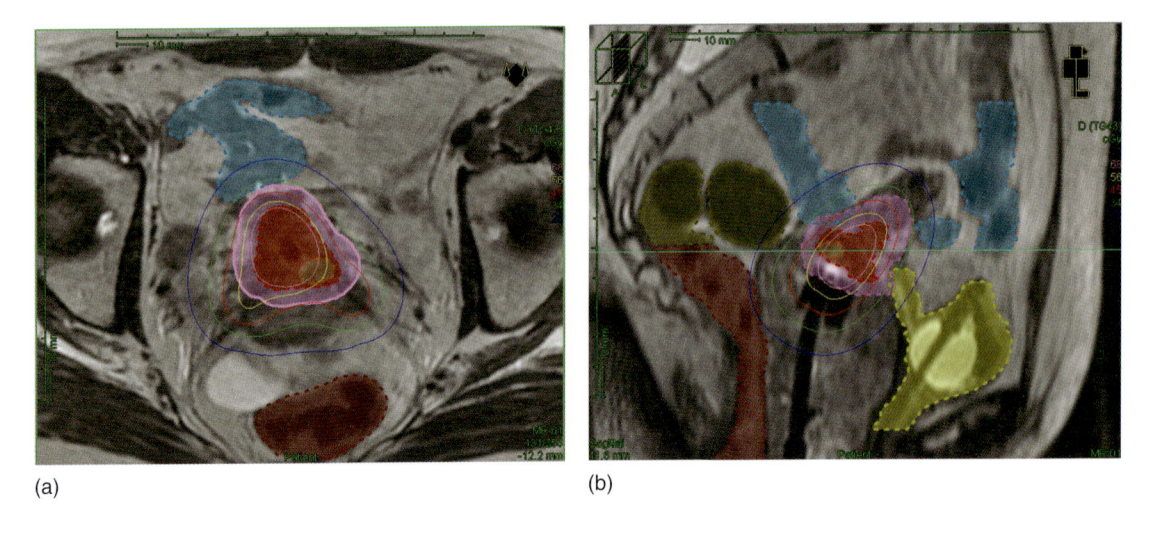

Figure 19 (a) Axial view of a brachytherapy procedure using MRI at time of the brachytherapy and (b) sagittal view of the same view. Yellow—bladder, dark red—rectum, mustard yellow—sigmoid, lite blue—small bowel, pink—intermediate-risk CTV (IRCTV), bright red—high-risk CTV (HrCTV—includes disease at time of brachytherapy procedure and entire cervix) and orange—GTV (gross disease on the MRI). The isodose lines include—red—100%, green—75%, blue—50%, yellow—120%, and pink—150%.

Fatal or life-threatening complications of intracavitary radiation therapy are rare. Thromboembolic events, uterine perforation, fever, vaginal laceration, and the usual risk of anesthesia are other less serious complications associated with intracavitary radiation therapy.[177]

Problems after therapy
For patients with cervical cancer, overall estimates of the risk of major complications of radiation therapy usually range between 5% and 15%.[178,179] The risk of experiencing a late complication is greatest within the first 3 years after treatment; however, major complications have been reported as late as 30 years or more after treatment. Most complications occurring after radiation involve the rectum, bladder, or small bowel. During the first 3 years after treatment, rectal complications are most common and include bleeding, stricture, ulceration, and fistula. The average onset of major urinary tract complications tends to be somewhat later than that of intestinal complication, with an actuarial risk of hematuria

requiring transfusion of 2.6% at 5 years.[178] The overall risk of developing a gastrointestinal or urinary tract fistula was 1.7% at 5 years with an increased risk of patients who underwent adjuvant hysterectomy or pretreatment transperitoneal lymphadenectomy. The risk of small bowel obstruction is strongly correlated with several patient characteristics and treatment factors including type of surgery, history of pelvic infection, history of smoking, and body habitus.[136,178,179]

Patients who are treated with radiation for cervical cancer tend to have varying degrees of atrophy, telangiectasia, or scarring of the upper third of the vagina. However, more severe shortening can occur. Changes may be greater in patients with very extensive tumors and in patients who are elderly, sexually inactive, or hypoestrogenic.[179,180] Regular intercourse and use of vaginal dilators may help prevent vaginal shortening.

Current practice by disease stage

Stage IA1 disease

Conization is accepted as the treatment of choice for patients with Stage IA1 cervical cancer.[181] In patients with LVSI, pelvic node dissection or sentinel lymph node mapping is recommended in addition to conization. This recommendation was reached after the finding from a large SEER database study that found women age ≤40 years with stage IA1 cervical cancer had no difference in 5-year survival between being treated with conization alone versus hysterectomy (98% vs 99%). It is important to have negative margin at the time of the conization. In women who have completed childbearing or elderly women, a total extrafascial hysterectomy may also be done. Patients can also be treated with radiation therapy alone, usually consisting of intracavitary therapy alone. The 10-year disease control rate with radiation therapy alone is 95–100%.[182]

Stage IA2 disease

Small lesions that invade 3–5 mm have an average risk of lymph node metastasis of about 5%. The standard treatment of patients with this stage of disease is type II (modified radical) hysterectomy and pelvic node dissection.

Recently, a number of studies have explored less radical surgical options for early-stage cervical cancer, including simple hysterectomy, simple trachelectomy, and cervical conization with or without sentinel lymph node biopsy and pelvic lymph node dissections especially in patients who wish to preserve fertility. Such options may be available for patients with low-risk early-stage cervical cancer including patients with any histology except neuroendocrine tumor, tumor size <2 cm, stromal invasion <10 mm, and no lymph-vascular space invasion. Presently, three international trials are underway looking at these options for patients with early-stage disease.

If surgery is contraindicated, these patients can be treated with radiation alone, usually with pelvic radiation therapy plus brachytherapy. However, in special situations, brachytherapy alone may be sufficient in controlling disease.

FIGO 2018 stage IB1 and small stage IIA1 (<2 cm) disease

Treatment of invasive carcinoma or carcinoma of FIGO stage IB or greater is determined on the basis of tumor size and the presence or absence of lymph node metastases. FIGO 2018 stage IB1 tumors and small IIA are considered low risk if they have the following criteria: largest tumor diameter <2 cm, cervical stromal invasion less than 50%, and no suspicious lymph nodes on imaging. The standard treatment for these patients is type 2 radical hysterectomy with lymph node dissection. In young patients desiring fertility sparing, a radical trachelectomy maybe an option if tumor measures ≤2 cm in largest diameter.[183] Two studies have evaluated the use of simple hysterectomy with lymph node dissection in the low-risk patients as described above. In both studies, the authors concluded a simple hysterectomy may be a feasible option in low-risk stage IB1 and stage IIA in women not desiring fertility sparing.[184,185]

FIGO 2018 stage IB2 and stage IIA1 disease

These tumors are less than 4 cm in size, and are considered small; however, they are associated with a significant risk of microscopic paracervical extension or lymph node metastasis. In a prospective study in patients treated with radical hysterectomy who had clinically estimated maximum tumor diameter less than 3 cm, the GOG reported that 16% of the patients (42 of 261) had lymph node metastases.[186] Landoni and colleagues found a 25% incidence of positive nodes (28 of 114 patients) in patients treated with radical hysterectomy for stage IB-IIA tumors that measured 4 cm or less on initial clinical examination.[157] Therefore, for patients with stage IB2 or small IIA (<4 cm diameter) disease, the treatment is either type III (radical) hysterectomy plus bilateral pelvic lymphadenectomy or radical radiation therapy.

Overall survival rates for patients with stage IB1 or small IIA disease treated with either surgery or radiation therapy are usually in the range of 80–90%, suggesting that the two treatments are equally effective. However, only one prospective randomized trial has compared the two treatments directly.[157] There was no significant differences in the rates of relapse or survival between the two arms, but the overall rate of grade 2 and 3 complications was greater for patients treated with hysterectomy. Therefore, for patients with stage IB1, the choice of treatment is based on patient preference, anesthetic and surgical risks, physician preference, and an understanding of the nature and incidence of complication with radiation therapy and hysterectomy.

The role of neoadjuvant chemotherapy (NACT) is being explored in this group of patients. Indications for NACT include reduction of the size of the tumor to help with surgical resection and to minimize prognostic factors associated with a poor response, thereby hopefully eliminating the need of postoperative radiation therapy.[187] NACT has been shown to reduce nodal metastases, parametrial infiltration, and tumor size making the case more feasible for fertility-sparing surgery in patients who desire fertility.[188] The timing of lymph node dissection is still up for discussion and a topic for further studies.

FIGO 2018 stage IB3 disease and IIA2

Patients with tumors greater than 4 cm in diameter whose para-aortic lymph nodes are found to be free of disease have excellent survival rates when treated with whole-pelvis EBRT plus brachytherapy. However, these tumors appear on clinical examination to be technically resectable and have equal survival to radiation and therefore the ideal management of these tumors is a subject of considerable controversy. Although radiation therapy is effective for many patients with stage IB2 disease, central disease recurrences occur in at least 8–10% of patients with bulky endocervical cancers.[157,171,172] The literature contains numerous reports on the use of an adjunctive hysterectomy for patients with bulky endocervical carcinomas treated with primary radiation therapy. However, in 1999 the GOG concluded from a study that evaluated adjunctive hysterectomy, that adjunctive hysterectomy did not improve local control or survival but did increase toxicity when added to chemo-radiation therapy in patients with stage IB2 disease.[173]

Several investigators recommend treating these tumors with initial surgery followed by postoperative radiation therapy or chemoradiation depending on the pathology findings. In a randomized trial by Landoni and colleagues, patients with stage IB2 tumors were randomized to initial surgery versus definitive radiation therapy.[157] In this trial, even though the survival was similar in both arms, 84% of the patients treated with initial surgery required postoperative radiation therapy, which contributed to a higher complication rate in that arm. This trial has been updated recently, confirming the original findings of equal efficacy of the two modalities but a higher incidence of complications when patients received both treatments.[189]

The role of pelvic radiation therapy after radical hysterectomy is still being defined. The GOG, in a prospective trial, randomized patients with intermediate risk of recurrence after radical hysterectomy for stage IB carcinoma to pelvic irradiation or no further treatment.[190] The preliminary analysis showed a 47% reduction in the risk of recurrence when postoperative irradiation was given (15% vs 28%, $p = 0.008$), An update of this study published in 2006 showed a statistically significant reduction in the risk of recurrence and progression-free survival, but no statistical difference in overall survival with the addition of postoperative radiation therapy. The conclusion by the authors was that pelvic radiation therapy after radical surgery significantly reduces the risk of recurrence and prolongs PFS in women with stage IB cervical cancer, particularly in patients with adenocarcinoma or adenosquamous histologies.[189] The Southwest Oncology Group reported the results of a randomized trial of patients treated with radical hysterectomy followed by radiation therapy versus radiation therapy plus cisplatin-based chemotherapy in patients with high-risk factors including pelvic lymph node metastases, parametrial involvement, and or positive margins. The authors found that patients who received radiation therapy plus chemotherapy had a significant improvement in survival compared with the survival of patients treated with radiation alone.[102]

Neoadjuvant chemotherapy is a very attractive option in this group of patients and a meta-analysis[191] as well as a GOG trial[192] reported reductions in the rate of nodal metastasis and parametrial infiltration as well as improvement in progression-free survival (PFS), but there was no difference in overall survival (OS). Two recent trials evaluated neoadjuvant chemotherapy (NCAT) followed by surgery compared to chemotherapy and radiation in patients with stage IB1-IIB cervical cancer. The first of these trials final results reported a superior 5-year DFS with chemoradiation therapy compared with NACT followed by surgery with similar OS.[193] Early reports from the EORTC trial suggest higher toxicity with the neoadjuvant arm but final results are pending. It appears with the data available, there is no benefit of NCAT followed by surgery over chemoradiation therapy if optimal chemoradiation therapy is available.[194]

Two prospective randomized trials[173,174] indicate that patients who are treated with radiation for bulky central disease benefit from concurrent administration of cisplatin-containing chemotherapy. Due to these studies and the data presented above, chemotherapy and radiation therapy is the standard treatment for patients with stage IB3 and Stage IIA2 cervical carcinoma.

Stage IIB-IVA disease

Radiation therapy is the primary local treatment of most patients with locoregionally advanced (stages IIIB-IVA) cervical carcinoma. The success of treatment depends on a careful balance between EBRT and brachytherapy that optimizes the dose to tumor and normal tissues and on the overall duration of treatment. In the French Cooperative Group study of 1875 patients treated with radiation therapy according to Fletcher guidelines, Barillot and colleagues reported 5-year survival rates of 70%, 45%, and 10% for patients with stage IIB, IIIB, and IVA tumors, respectively (Table 7).[97]

Local and distant disease recurrences continue to be a problem for patients with locally advanced disease. Since 1999, the standard treatment for patients with stage IIB-IVA is concomitant chemotherapy and radiation. The benefit of chemotherapy for FIGO stage IIIB-IVA is only about 3–4% as reported in an individual patient data meta-analysis.[195] Recently, the final results of a large randomized trial of 850 patients found an absolute benefit of 8.5% in DFS and 8% in OS at 5 years with the addition of chemotherapy to radiation therapy in patients with FIGO stage III B cervical cancer.[196] Neoadjuvant chemotherapy has produced excellent tumor responses; however, randomized trials have failed to demonstrate improvements in survival. Other approaches that have been used to try to improve outcome in these patients, including neutrons, hyperbaric oxygen, and hypoxic cell sensitizers, have also produced disappointing results.

Concurrent chemoradiation

In 1999, five prospective randomized trials involving patients with locoregionally advanced cervical cancer,[102,173–176] provided compelling evidence that the addition of concurrent cisplatin-containing chemotherapy to standard radiation therapy reduces the risk of disease recurrence by as much as 50%, and thereby improves the rates of pelvic disease control and survival (Table 8).[102,173–176,197–199]

Taken together, the randomized trials provide strong evidence that the addition of concurrent cisplatin-containing chemotherapy to pelvic radiation therapy benefits selected patients with locally advanced cervical cancer. A meta-analysis of 18 trials[200] with concurrent chemotherapy and radiation (4580 patients) in patients with cervical cancer concluded that concomitant chemotherapy and radiation therapy improved overall and PFS and reduced local and distant recurrence in selected patients with cervical cancer. Concomitant chemotherapy and radiation therapy produced a 12% absolute increase in survival with greater evidence of benefit in the trials using platinum-based chemotherapy than in those with nonplatinum-based chemotherapy.[200] More recently, a systematic review and meta-analysis based on individual patient data (IPD)[195] have documented a 7% absolute improvement in 5-year survival. The benefits were similar in the trials using platinum and nonplatinum chemo-radiation therapy.[195] In this analysis, there is a suggestion that the magnitude of benefit with chemo-radiation therapy varies according to stage, but not to other patient's characteristics, suggesting a greater benefit in patients with early-stage disease compared to stage III and IV disease.[195]

These studies raise other interesting questions that will undoubtedly be the subjects of future studies. One of the first questions raised is the optimal dose and dosing schedule of cisplatin. Results of a phase-II trial from Korea comparing weekly 40 mg/m^2 and tri-weekly 75 mg/m^2 cisplatin used concurrently showed superiority of tri-weekly cisplatin in terms of 5-year survival rate of 88.7% in comparison with 66.5% in the weekly regimen leading to a phase III trial that is comparing weekly cisplatin to tri-weekly cisplatin in

Table 8 Prospective randomized trials: role of concurrent radiotherapy and cisplatin-containing chemotherapy.[a]

First author (Ref.)	Eligibility	Patients (no.)	CT: investigational arm	CT: control arm	Relative risk of recurrence (90% CI)	p values
Rose[175]	FIGO IIB-IVA	526	Cisplatin 40 mg/m^2/wk (up to 6 cycles)	HU 3 g/m^2 (2×/wk)	0.57 (0.42–0.78)	<0.001
			Cisplatin 50 mg/m^2; 5-FU 4 g/m^2/96 h; HU 2 g/m^2 (2×/wk) (2 cycles)	HU 3 g/m^2 (2×/wk)	0.55 (0.40–0.75)	<0.001
Morris[174]	FIGO IB-IIA (≥5 cm); IIB-IVA or pelvic nodes involved	403	Cisplatin 75 mg/m^2; 5-FU 4 g/m^2/96 h (3 cycles)	None[a]	0.48 (0.35–0.66)	<0.001
Keys[173]	FIGO IB (≥4 cm)	369	Cisplatin 40 mg/m^2/wk (up to 6 cycles)	None[b]	0.51 (0.34–0.75)	0.001
Whitney[176]	FIGO IIB-IVA	368	Cisplatin 50 mg/m^2; 5-FU 4 g/m^2/96 h (2 cycles)	HU 3 g/m^2 (2×/wk)	0.79 (0.62–0.99)	0.03
Peters[102]	FIGO I-IIA after radical hysterectomy with nodes, margins, or parametrium positive	268	Cisplatin 50 mg/m^2; 5-FU 4 g/m^2/96 h (2 cycles)	None	0.50 (0.29–0.84)	0.01
Pearcey[197]	FIGO IB-IIA (≥5 cm), IIB-IVA or pelvic nodes involved	259	Cisplatin 40 mg/m^2/wk (up to 6 cycles)	None	0.91 (0.62–1.35)[c]	0.43
Wong[198]	FIGO IB-IIA (>4 cm), IIB-III	220	Epirubicin 60 mg/m^2, then 90 mg/m^2 q4 wks for five more cycles[d]	None	~0.65	0.02
Lorvidhaya[199][e]	FIGO IB-IVA	926	Mitomycin-C 10 mg/m^2 day 1 and 29 Oral 5-FU 300 mg/day days 1–14 and 29–42	None		0.001

Abbreviations: CI, confidence interval; FU, follow-up; HU, hydroxyurea; PA, para-aortic; RT, radiotherapy.
Results from prospective randomized trials that investigate the role of concurrent radiotherapy and cisplatin-containing chemotherapy for patients with locoregionally advanced cervical cancer.
[a]Patients in control arm had prophylactic para-aortic irradiation.
[b]All patients had extrafascial hysterectomy after radiotherapy.
[c]Survival.
[d]Chemotherapy was begun on day 1 and continued every 4 weeks throughout and after radiation therapy.
[e]This study had four arms: arm 1, conventional radiation therapy (RT); arm 2, conventional RT with adjuvant chemotherapy consisting of 5-FU orally at 200 mg/day given for three courses of 4 weeks, with a 2-week rest every 6 weeks; arm 3, conventional RT with concurrent chemotherapy; and arm 4, conventional RT with concurrent and adjuvant chemotherapy. The addition of adjuvant therapy did not affect recurrence, but there was a significant difference in the recurrence rate between the conventional RT and the conventional RT plus concurrent chemotherapy arms.

patients with locally advanced cervical cancer (TACO trial; Clinical Trials.gov identifiers: NCT01561586.) Another question regards the benefit of adjuvant chemotherapy after definitive chemoradiotherapy which is being addressed by the OUTBACK study (Clinical Trials.gov identifiers: NCT01414608) that is randomizing patients with locally advanced cervical cancer to chemoradiation versus chemoradiation plus adjuvant chemotherapy. This trial has finished accrual and the results should be presented at ASCO 2021.

Although North American studies have emphasized cisplatin-containing regimens, investigators in Southeast Asia have reported improved outcome when radiation was combined with epirubicin[198] or mitomycin and 5-FU.[199] Other drugs that are being studied for their radiosensitizing effects in patients with advanced disease are paclitaxel,[201] carboplatin,[202] nedaplatin,[203] topotecan,[204] gemcitabine,[205,206] and multiple biologic response modifiers. The RTOG conducted a phase II study that evaluated the combination of bevacizumab with cisplatin in combination with radiation therapy in 49 patients and found promising results with 3-year OS, DFS, and LRF of 81.3%, 68.7%, 23.3%, respectively.[207] Another potential pathway is the inhibition of ribonucleotide reductase (RNR). Elevated RNR levels are associated with an increased risk of an incomplete response to chemoradiation and an increased risk of disease recurrence.[208] Therefore, inhibitors of RNR may have potential value in combination with radiation therapy. One such agent, 3-aminopyridine-2-carboxaldehyde thiosemicarbazone has been evaluated in a single-institution phase 2 trial and with a median follow-up of 20 months; clinical responses were observed in 24 of 25 patients with suggested metabolic complete responses noted in 23 of 24 patients evaluated by PET/CT at 3 months.[209] These encouraging results have prompted a larger, multi-institutional, randomized phase II study as well as a possible phase III through NRG.

Neoadjuvant chemotherapy followed by chemoradiation is still an attractive option, especially in countries where there is a delay in starting radiation therapy. Results from a multi-institutional phase II trial evaluating neoadjuvant chemotherapy (NACT) before definitive CTRT observed 68% responders and 3-year OS and PFS of 67% and 68%, respectively.[210] This has led to an ongoing phase III that is randomizing patients with locally advanced cervical cancer to NACT followed by CTRT versus CTRT (INTERLACE study; clinicaltrials.gov identifiers: NCT01566240).

New directions with radiation therapy

In the last few years, the development of new therapeutics and a better understanding of the molecular characteristic as well as microenvironment has led to many new directions and agents that can be used with radiation to improve treatment results in patients with cervical cancer. The new agents can be considered in three general categories: (1) enhancement or alteration of the immune system; (2) disruption of DNA damage response mechanism; and (3) impediment of cellular pathways involved in processes such as signaling, growth, and angiogenesis.

Immunotherapy is emerging as a promising treatment for cervical cancer and more details will be discussed later in this article. Several trials are underway using immunotherapy with radiation therapy in the potentially curative setting as well as with recurrent disease. In the potentially curative setting, three trials are using concurrent and/or sequential anti-PD-1 with chemotherapy and radiation. Collectively, these trials all leverage the pro-inflammatory, immune, and neoantigen stimulating effects of radiation therapy in combination with immunotherapy checkpoint blockade. In the recurrent setting, immunotherapy is being used with a combination of drugs and stereotactic radiation in small phase I–II trials.

Other agents that are being used with radiation include PARP inhibitors, ATR inhibitors, and WEE1 inhibitors, as well as several agents that are targeting hypoxic cancer cells and angiogenesis. Thus, multiple agents can be combined with radiation therapy to improve survival in patients with locally advanced and recurrent cervical cancer.

Para-aortic metastasis

Metastatic cancer in the para-aortic lymph nodes can be confirmed with fine-needle aspiration, laparoscopy, or extra-peritoneal laparotomy. Laparoscopy and laparotomy, using the extra-peritoneal approach, allows the removal of positive nodes and sampling of other para-aortic nodes, which may enhance control with radiation therapy and help design the treatment field.

Patients with para-aortic lymph node involvement can be treated effectively with extended-field irradiation. Five-year survival rates range from 25% to 50%.[211,212] The value of prophylactic extended-field irradiation was tested in two randomized trials and both trials found no advantage in the use of prophylactic para-aortic radiation.[213,214]

The role of concurrent chemotherapy with extended-field irradiation has been evaluated in several phase II studies.[215] Although, side effects are greater when treatment fields are enlarged, combined therapy may be tolerable if careful consideration is given to the chemotherapy regimen, volume of tissue irradiated, and other factors that might increase the risk of serious toxicity. In conclusion, it is tempting to extrapolate from the results achieved with combinations of pelvic radiation and chemotherapy; however, patients need to be informed that the cost-benefit ratio of concurrent chemotherapy and extended-field irradiation has not been formally tested but this is where IMRT may be a benefit in reducing acute toxicity.

Unsuspected invasive cancer discovered after simple hysterectomy

Sometimes the pathologist discovers unsuspected invasive cervical carcinoma in the tissue specimen in patients who undergo hysterectomy for what is presumed to be a benign pelvic condition. Many factors can lead to such an event.[216]

Patients with unsuspected invasive cervical carcinoma detected after simple hysterectomy have fallen into five groups based on the amount of disease and presentation: (1) microinvasive cancer, (2) tumor confined to the cervix with negative surgical margins, (3) positive surgical margins but no gross residual tumor, (4) gross residual tumor by clinical examination documented by biopsy, and (5) patients referred for treatment more than 6 months after hysterectomy (usually for recurrent disease).[217] The therapy plan is based on the amount of residual disease. Patients with minimal invasion and no residual disease require at most brachytherapy to the vaginal apex. Patients with gross disease at the specimen margin require full-intensity therapy. Patients with minimal or no known gross residual disease (groups 1–3) have excellent 5-year survival rates (59–79%), whereas survival rates for patients with gross residual disease (groups 4 and 5) are poorer (in the range of only 41%).[218]

Recurrent disease

Prognostic factors
Various clinicopathologic features have been associated with adverse outcomes in patients with recurrent cervical carcinoma in the pelvis; however, the relatively small numbers of patients and the heterogeneity of clinical and treatment parameters in most series preclude detailed statistical analysis of these factors. Two clinical factors commonly correlate with the probability of the success of salvage therapy are the location (central vs sidewall involvement) and the size of the recurrent pelvic tumor.[219] The presence of nodal disease in conjunction with pelvic relapse portends a dismal outcome; other unfavorable clinical variables include nonsquamous histologies (particularly adenocarcinomas) and a higher FIGO stage at the time of diagnosis of the primary tumor.[220] Controversial factors include the interval between primary therapy and relapse and symptomatic versus asymptomatic pelvic failures.[155,220,221]

Radical hysterectomy
In rare, carefully selected patients initially treated with primary radiation therapy, radical hysterectomy for salvage may be a feasible alternative to exonerative surgery. Coleman and colleagues reported 50 patients who underwent radical hysterectomy for persistent or recurrent disease after definitive radiation therapy.[222] The 5-year and 10-year survival rates were 72% and 60%, respectively. Severe complications were noted in 64% of patients, and 42% of patients had permanent complications. The authors concluded that radical hysterectomy was an alternative to exenteration in patients with small, centrally recurrent cervical cancer, but that it should be used only in carefully selected patients.[222]

Pelvic exenteration
Pelvic exenteration is a potentially curative procedure for patients who, following radiation therapy, have a central pelvic recurrence or a new primary tumor in the irradiated field.[223–225] Advances in surgical technique, anesthesia, and postoperative care have decreased intraoperative and postoperative complications and thus have greatly reduced operative mortality.[216,224,225] Advances in ostomy appliances and care have given patients the opportunity to live a nearly normal life and to be able to meet their personal needs and responsibilities after surgery. The type of exenteration is determined by the anatomical site of the cancer (Figure 20).[223]

Anterior exenteration
Anterior exenteration encompasses the removal of the uterus, adnexa, bladder, urethra, and vagina. Patients selected for this

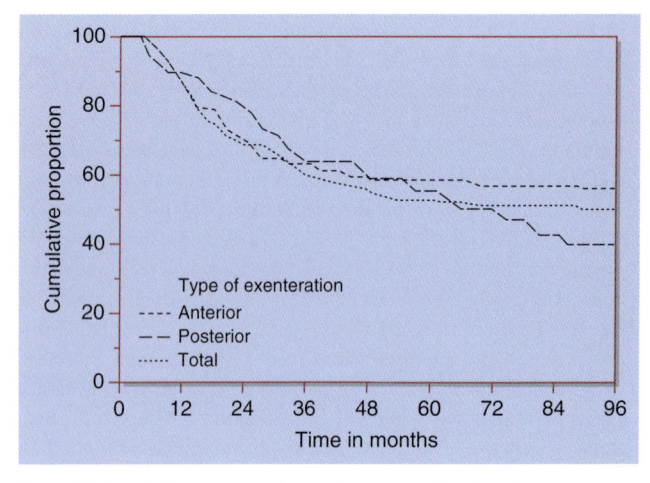

Figure 20 Survival curves are shown to compare the three types of exenterations performed in an MD Anderson series (1955–1984). Although the curves are similar, it should be noted that posterior exenteration is performed more frequently than the other procedures for vulvar and anorectal cancer and is associated with more local cancer recurrences. Source: Modified from Coleman et al.[222]

operation have cancers that are sufficiently anterior to allow clearance of the rectum and do not extend to involve the vaginal apex or the posterior vaginal wall. Vaginal reconstruction is performed as indicated.

Posterior exenteration
In posterior exenteration, the uterus, adnexa, anus, rectosigmoid colon, levator muscles, and vagina are removed. Many gynecologic oncologists leave a portion of the anterior vaginal wall to support the urethra, and this can lessen postoperative urinary incontinence. This procedure is performed in patients with lesions confined to the posterior vaginal wall and rectovaginal septum.

Total pelvic exenteration
In total pelvic exenteration, the uterus, adnexa, bladder and urethra, vagina, rectosigmoid colon, levatores, and anus are all removed. Patients treated with this procedure usually have lesions that are central or involve the upper half of the vagina. Contiguous extension to the base of the bladder and rectovaginal septum leaves no opportunity to perform a less extensive operation. Vaginal reconstruction is performed for functional purposes and to aid in the reconstruction of the pelvic floor. An omental pedicled graft is required to aid in reconstruction of the pelvic floor, and this technique for bringing in a new blood supply has been a major factor in reducing postoperative complications.[226] In both anterior and total pelvic exenteration, a continent urinary conduit can be constructed.

Total pelvic exenteration is widely used, and 5-year survival rates of 40–50% can be expected. At MD Anderson, a total of 448 exenterations were done from 1955 to 1984 and reported by Rutledge.[223] The 5-year survival rates for patients treated with exenteration are shown in (Figure 20).

Radiation therapy
Patients who have an isolated pelvic recurrence after initially being treated with a radical hysterectomy should be treated with radical radiation therapy. A literature review by Lanciano found disease-free survival rates ranging from 20% to 50% following radiation therapy for locoregional failures. More favorable outcomes were reported in patients with small-volume disease and a central pelvic relapse location.[219] In most patients, treatment consisted of EBRT with or without brachytherapy. Patients who have isolated central recurrences without pelvic wall fixation or regional metastasis can be cured in up to 60–70% of cases.[221] The prognosis is much poorer when the pelvic wall is involved (usually 10–20% of patients survive 5 years after radiation therapy).

With the recent advances in radiation therapy, especially image-guided therapy in general, re-radiation has become a feasible option in certain cases. Re-radiation using image-guided interstitial brachytherapy for central or pelvic wall recurrences is an effective treatment although it is associated with 20–25% severe late toxicity. Stereotactic radiation is another technique that can be used for re-radiation purposed for recurrent tumors in the radiated field.

Treatment of stage IVB or recurrent disease

Chemotherapy
Single-agent cisplatin is regarded as the most active agent in cancer of the cervix. The response rate is 17–21%.[227,228] Bonomi and colleagues[229] compared 50–100 mg/m^2 and noted that the higher dose was associated with a better partial response rate (31% vs 21%) and a slightly better complete response rate (13% vs 10%). Response duration, PFS, and survival measures failed to improve with the higher dose.[228] These response rates were seen in chemotherapy naïve patients and with the introduction of concurrent chemotherapy with radiation therapy in 1999, the response rates went down and led to trials look at other agents as well as combination with cisplatin. This underlines the need for improvement especially evaluating molecular targets.

Paclitaxel has consistently demonstrated clinical activity, even in patients who received prior platinum-based therapy with response rates of 17–31% and a median survival of about 7 months, including those patients with nonsquamous histology. The other three—topotecan, vinorelbine, and ifosfamide[230–236] have also shown substantial responses and are being used in combination therapy in phases II and III trials.

Several phase II/III trials showed superiority of combinations therapy over cisplatin alone including a GOG trial comparing cisplatin-topotecan to cisplatin alone.[237] The response rate was 13% in the cisplatin arm and 27% in the combination arm. There was also an improvement in median survival by 3 months as well as a slight improvement in quality of life as determined by the functional assessment of cancer therapy-cervical (FACT-CX). At the same time, other combinations showed promise as well including combinations of cisplatin and continuous infusion 5-FU,[238–240] cisplatin and paclitaxel,[241,242] cisplatin and vinorelbine,[243] and cisplatin and gemcitabine.[244,245]

This has led to the next GOG phase III trial that randomized patients to four arms: (1) paclitaxel and cisplatin (PC); (2) vinorelbine and cisplatin (VC); (3) gemcitabine and cisplatin (GC); and (4) topotecan and cisplatin (TC).[246] This study was closed early due to futility. The response rate (29.1%) and survival trends, both progression-free (5.82 months, 95% CI 4.53–7.59) and overall (12.87 months, 95% CI 10.02–16.76), favored the paclitaxel and cisplatin combination and that became the standard of care for patients with recurrent or stage IVB cervical cancer.[246] Prognostic factors were evaluated by Moore et al, and they found that race, performance status, pelvic disease, prior radiosensitizer, and time interval from diagnosis to the first recurrence <1 years were important and could help identify women who would not respond to cisplatin-based regimens.[247] Paclitaxel-carboplatin combination compared to paclitaxel-cisplatin was concluded to be noninferior in JCOG0505 trial. Paclitaxel-carboplatin combination proved itself noninferior in regard to progression-free survival (6.2 vs 6.9 months) and overall survival (17.5 vs 18.3 months).[246] Cisplatin combination therapy was superior mainly in the subgroup of patients who had not been exposed to it and the authors concluded that is still the key drug for patients who had not received any platinum agents.[247]

Despite the success of GOG 204 trial, only one-third of patients will respond to treatment and median overall survival did not exceed 12 months and concurrent chemotherapy and radiation have led to possibly more resistance to cisplatin-based regimens.

Antiangiogenic therapy
Angiogenesis plays a major role in cancer invasion, metastasis and progression.[248] VEGF has been identified as a poor prognostic factor in cervical cancer and has been a focus of targeted antiangiogenic therapy.[249] Bevacizumab, a humanized, monoclonal antibody that specifically targets VEGF-A is the most widely studied and most commonly used antiangiogenic therapy in patients with cervical cancer. Based on two phase II studies,[250,251] GOG conducted a phase III trial combining bevacizumab with cytotoxic therapy (cisplatin plus paclitaxel vs paclitaxel plus topotecan).[252]

There was no difference in outcomes noted between the chemotherapy regimens. However, when compared with chemotherapy alone, the addition of bevacizumab significantly improved OS (17 months vs 13.3 months), PFS (8.2 months vs 5.9 months), and RR (48% vs 36%) without a significant deterioration in health-related quality of life.[253] Major treatment-related toxicities included fistula (3%), thromboembolism (8%), and easily managed hypertension (25%).[253] The CECILIA trial evaluated the addition of bevacizumab with carboplatin and paclitaxel in a single-arm phase II study and among 150 patients. The objective response rate was 61% (95% CI: 52–69%), median progression-free survival was 10.9 (10.1–13.7) months and median overall survival was 25 months (20.9–30.4) months.[254] These results are comparable to GOG 240 and toxicity rates were also in line with GOG 0240, however, due to the results of JCOG0505, the authors state that for patients with good renal function, cisplatin-based regimen should still be the preferred treatment.[254] In 2014, the US Food and Drug Administration (FDA) approved bevacizumab in combination with chemotherapy for patients with metastatic, persistent, or recurrent cervix cancer.

EGFR inhibitors
EGFR is overexpressed in the majority of newly diagnosed cervical cancers is an adverse prognostic factor for survival and also predicts poor response to cytotoxic agents and radiation therapy.[255] Although EGFR seems a promising target, several phase II studies investigating either EGFR tyrosine kinase inhibitors (erlotinib[256] and gefitinib[257]) monotherapy or cetuximab (an anti-EGFR monoclonal antibody) as monotherapy[258] or in combination with cisplatin[259] have shown only limited activity. Finally, pazopanib (an oral agent targeting VEGFR) and lapatinib (dual inhibitor of EGFR and Her2/neu tyrosine kinases) have been studied in a phase II study with arms that included monotherapy of each drug and an arm that had a combination of the two drugs.[260] The arm with the combination of the two drugs was closed early due to futility Lapatinib monotherapy had lower OS than pazopanib (39.1 weeks vs 50.7 weeks) but the authors concluded that both drugs were well tolerated with modest activity in patient with recurrent or advanced cervical cancer.[260]

Poly ADP-ribose polymerase inhibitors
Poly ADP-ribose polymerase (PARP) is an enzyme utilized by tumor cells to repair errors in DNA replication in the setting of high mutational burden. PARP inhibitors are a class of drugs aimed at blocking DNA repair mechanisms in tumor cells.[261] In cervical cancer cells, PARP is found at higher levels compared to normal cells presenting a potential target for therapy.[262] Two trials[229,263] have shown some promise of the use of PARP inhibitors in combination with cytotoxic therapy but the patients who seem to benefit most were patients with low levels of PARP-1 on immunohistochemistry staining. This finding provides the possibility of PARP-1 as a potential biomarker, a marker that would identify patients who may benefit from this therapy.[263]

Immune checkpoint inhibitors
Over the past several years, there has been an increased focus on understanding the role of the immune system in the recognition and control of cancer progression. Intrinsic signaling via immune checkpoint receptors leads to suppression of antitumor immunity and contributes to tumor progression. Two different pathways are explicitly targeted with monoclonal antibody therapy to block the immunosuppression signaling.[264] Antiprogramed cell death (PD-1) and anticytotoxic T lymphocyte-associated antigen 4 (CTLA-4) are two targets for therapy being studied in multiple cancers including cervical cancer. In cervical cancer cells, it has been demonstrated that there is an upregulation of PD-1 and PD-L1, and possibly why utilization of this class of immunotherapy may work in patients with cervical cancer.[265]

Keynote 158 is a multi-cohort phase II basket trial that evaluated the safety and efficacy of pembrolizumab, a humanized monoclonal antibody that interacts with PD-1, preventing interaction with its ligands and resultant T cell exhaustion. In the cervical cancer subgroup of 98 patients, the overall response rate was 12.2% with three complete and nine partial responses. All 12 responses were in patients with PD-L1 positive tumors for an overall response rate of 14.6%. On the bases of these results, the FDA granted approval of pembrolizumab in the treatment of recurrent or metastatic cervical cancer patients with disease progression during or after chemotherapy treatment and who have at least 1% of PD-L1 positive staining cells on immunohistochemical detection.[266]

Similarly, nivolumab, another PD-1 inhibitor, has shown significant activity in advanced cervical cancer. In one study, monotherapy with nivolumab led to a 26% overall response rate.[267] Based on this result and the results from the KEYNOTE study, PD-1 inhibitors (pembrolizumab, nivolumab, cemiplimab) as well as PD-L1 inhibitors (atezolizumab, avelumab, durvalumab) are being evaluated in several ongoing trials (Table 9).[266,268–283] Presently, there is limited outcome data on immune checkpoint therapy in cervical cancer, however, the current trials that are presently ongoing hopefully will provide answers.

Therapeutic vaccines, antibody–drug conjugates and tumor-infiltrating lymphocyte (TiL) therapies
A variety of strategies have been used to try to enhance the innate immune response to the target and eliminate tumor cells. One of these strategies is to use therapeutic live vaccines targeting HPV using bacterial vectors. The first vaccine to be used in studies was axilimogene filolisbac (ADXS11-011 or AXAL), which is a *Listeria monocytogenes*-derived, live attenuated vaccine that secretes HPV-16 E7 protein. A phase II study included 110 patients with recurrent or persistent cervical cancer treated with the vaccine, with and without cisplatin. The study demonstrated an overall disease control rate of 43% and a 36% rate of 12-month survival.[284] The GOG also did a phase II study using AXAL in 50 patients with an OS of 12 months and 30% of the patients experienced stable disease and one patient had a complete response up to 18.5 months and was still disease free at 40.6 months.[285] Another study phase I/II has just completed accrual and results are pending.[286] Additional studies using alternating vaccine strategies are underway and one study is combining vaccine with pembrolizumab.[287]

Antibody–drug conjugates (ADCs) are targeted therapies where an antibody is linked to an active anticancer agent with the antibody targeting a specific cancer cell surface antigen, delivering the drug to the tumor cells, and avoiding nonmalignant cells.[288] Tisotumab vedoitin is an ADC that targets Tissue Factor which is highly expressed in many malignancies including cervical cancer. A phase I/II study investigated the safety and efficacy of tisotumab in recurrent, advanced, and metastatic cancer in different tumor sites including 34 patients with cervical cancer. The cervical cancer patients had a 26.5% ORR representing the second-highest response rate behind only bladder cancer.[289] Given the results of this study, two-phase II studies are assessing tisotumab in the treatment of cervical cancer. A phase II study has completed accrual using this ADC as monotherapy and results are

Table 9 Summary of immune checkpoint inhibitors studied in the treatment of cervical cancer.[a]

Drug	Additional therapy	Mechanism of action	Trial	Potential toxicities
Pembrolizumab	(Monotherapy) Carbo/cisplatin Concurrent Chemo-RT	Anti-PD1	KEYNOTE-158[266] MK-3475-826/KEYNOTE-826[268] NCT02635360[269]	Immune-related Side effects: Hypophysitis, Hepatitis, pneu- Monitis, Endocrine-related Side effects: hypo/hyperthyroidism T1DM
Nivolumab	(Monotherapy) Ipilimumab (Monotherapy)		CHECKMATE358[270] CHECKMATE358[271] NCT02257528[272]	
Cemiplimab	(Monotherapy)		REGN2810[273]	
Atezolizumab	Cisplatin/Paclitaxel/Bevacizumab Concurrent ChemoRT (Monotherapy)	Anti-PDL1	NCT03556839[274] NCT03612791[275] NRG-GY017[276]	
Avelumab	Valproic acid Axitinib		NCT03357757[277] NCT03826589[278]	
Durvalumab	Cisplatin/Carboplatin Tremelimumab + SBRT		CALLA[279] NCT0345233[280]	
Ipilimumab	Concurrent chemotherapy GITR receptor	Anti-CTLA-4	NCT01711515[281] NCT03126110[282]	

Abbreviations: CTLA-4, cytotoxic T-lymphocyte-associated antigen-4; GITR, glucocorticoid-induced TNFR family related; NCT, National Clinical Trials; PD1, programmed death-1; PDL1, programmed death ligand-1; SBRT, stereotactic body radiation therapy; TIDM, type-1 diabetes melitus.
[a]Source: Cohen et al.[283]

pending.[290] Another study is ongoing that combines tisotumab with carboplatin, bevacizumab, or pembrolizumab in recurrent and stage IVB cervical cancer.[291] Another phase 3 study is ongoing that is a randomized, open-label study of tisotumab versus investigator's choice chemotherapy in second or third line recurrent or metastatic cancer.[292]

Through emerging technologies, tumor-infiltrating lymphocytes (TILs) have been harvested from solid tumors and activated and expanded *ex vivo*.[293] An open-label phase II clinical trial has investigated LN-145, a TIL therapy developed to target cervical cancer. The trial treated 27 patients with advanced cervical cancer with at least one of prior chemotherapy. The preliminary results were presented at ASCO 2019, showing an ORR of 44% including one complete response.[294] In February 2019, the US FDA granted fast track designation to LN-145 for the treatment of patients with recurrent, metastatic, or persistent cervical who have progressed on or after prior therapy.

Summary

Cervical cancer incidence is decreasing with better screening and vaccine prophylaxis. In the past decade, we have seen advancement in technology that has led to better surgical techniques, image-guided radiation therapy, and better understanding of the molecular pathogenesis and aberrant signaling pathways in cervical cancers which has led to better patient outcomes. We are treating with less surgery thereby improving the quality of life. With image-guided radiation therapy, we are not only improving survival but again improving the quality of life of the patients by decreasing both acute and long-term toxicities. However, the biggest advances have been the new insights into the molecular pathogenesis, signaling pathways, and immunobiology of cervical cancer, leading to additional agents with activity against the disease. For the first time since 1999, we have multiple promising agents in clinical trials for patients with locally advanced or recurrent cervical cancer. However, key to success will be the translation of success seen in the developed countries to success in areas of the world where advanced-stage invasive cervical cancer is most common both in the reduction of the incidence of cervical cancer as well as the mortality from cervical cancer. The key to success worldwide will be the translation of success seen in the developed countries to success in other geographic areas where advanced-stage invasive cervical cancer is most common.

Key references

The complete reference list can be found on Vital Source version of this title, see inside front cover.

1. Arbyn M, Weiderpass E, Bruni L, et al. Estimates of incidence and mortality of cervical cancer in 2018: a worldwide analysis. *Lancet Glob Health*. 2020;**8**(2):e191–e203.
2. Siegel RL, Miller KD, Jemal A. Cancer statistics, 2019. *CA Cancer J Clin*. 2019;**69**(1):7–34.
56. Curry SJ, Krist AH, Owens DK, et al. Screening for cervical cancer: US preventive services task force recommendation statement. *JAMA*. 2018;**320**(7):674–686.
58. Kitchener HC, Almonte M, Gilham C, et al. ARTISTIC: a randomised trial of human papillomavirus (HPV) testing in primary cervical screening. *Health Technol Assess*. 2009;**13**(51):1–150, iii-iv.
63. Sawaya GF, Smith-McCune K, Kuppermann M. Cervical cancer screening: more choices in 2019. *JAMA*. 2019;**321**(20):2018–2019.
69. The FUTURE II Study Group. Quadrivalent vaccine against human papillomavirus to prevent high-grade cervical lesions. *N Engl J Med*. 2007;**356**(19):1915–1927.
70. Paavonen J, Jenkins D, Bosch FX, et al. HPV PATRICIA study group. Efficacy of a prophylactic adjuvanted bivalent L1 virus-like-particle vaccine against infection with human papillomavirus types 16 and 18 in young women: an interim analysis of a phase III double-blind, randomised controlled trial. *Lancet*. 2007;**369**(9580):2161–2170.
72. Kreimer AR, Herrero R, Sampson JN, et al. Evidence for single-dose protection by the bivalent HPV vaccine-Review of the Costa Rica HPV vaccine trial and future research studies. *Vaccine*. 2018;**36**(32 Pt A):4774–4782.
73. Lei J, Ploner A, Elfström KM, et al. HPV vaccination and the risk of invasive cervical cancer. *N Engl J Med*. 2020;**383**(14):1340–1348.
85. Bhatla N, Berek JS, Cuello Fredes M, et al. *Revised FIGO Staging for Carcinoma of the Cervix Uteri*. Paper presented at International Journal of Gynecology and Obstetrics; 14–19 October 2018, 2018; Rio de Janeiro, Brazil.
92. Gold MA, Tian C, Whitney CW, et al. Surgical versus radiographic determination of para-aortic lymph node metastases before chemoradiation for locally advanced cervical carcinoma: a Gynecologic Oncology Group Study. *Cancer-Am Cancer Soc*. 2008;**112**(9):1954–1963.
102. Peters WA 3rd, Liu PY, Barrett RJ 2nd, et al. Cisplatin, 5-fluorouracil plus radiation therapy are superior to radiation therapy as adjunctive therapy in high-risk, early-stage carcinoma of the cervix after radical hysterectomy and pelvic lymphadenectomy. Report of a phase III intergroup study. *Gynecol Oncol*. 1999;**72**(3):443–527.

107. Roman LD, Felix JC, Muderspach LI, et al. Influence of quantity of lymph-vascular space invasion on the risk of nodal metastases in women with early-stage squamous cancer of the cervix. *Gynecol Oncol.* 1998;**68**(3):220–225.
108. Eifel PJ, Burke TW, Delclos L, et al. Early stage I adenocarcinoma of the uterine cervix: treatment results in patients with tumors less than or equal to 4 cm in diameter. *Gynecol Oncol.* 1991;**41**(3):199–205.
138. Lécuru F, Mathevet P, Querleu D, et al. Bilateral negative sentinel nodes accurately predict absence of lymph node metastasis in early cervical cancer: results of the SENTICOL study. *J Clin Oncol.* 2011;**29**(13):1686–1691.
148. Ramirez PT, Frumovitz M, Pareja R, et al. Minimally invasive versus abdominal radical hysterectomy for cervical cancer. *N Engl J Med.* 2018;**379**(20):1895–1904.
149. Nitecki R, Ramirez PT, Frumovitz M, et al. Survival after minimally invasive vs open radical hysterectomy for early-stage cervical cancer: a systematic review and meta-analysis. *JAMA Oncol.* 2020;**6**(7):1019–1027.
158. Yeung AR, Pugh SL, Klopp AH, et al. Improvement in patient-reported outcomes with intensity-modulated radiotherapy (RT) compared with standard RT: a report from the NRG oncology RTOG 1203 study. *J Clin Oncol.* 2020;**38**(15):1685–1692.
163. Han K, Milosevic M, Fyles A, et al. Trends in the utilization of brachytherapy in cervical cancer in the United States. *Int J Radiat Oncol Biol Phys.* 2013;**87**(1):111–119.
164. Gill BS, Lin JF, Krivak TC, et al. National Cancer Data Base analysis of radiation therapy consolidation modality for cervical cancer: the impact of new technological advancements. *Int J Radiat Oncol Biol Phys.* 2014;**90**(5):1083–1090.
173. Keys HM, Bundy BN, Stehman FB, et al. Cisplatin, radiation, and adjuvant hysterectomy compared with radiation and adjuvant hysterectomy for bulky stage IB cervical carcinoma. *N Engl J Med.* 1999;**340**(15):1154–1161.
175. Rose PG, Bundy BN, Watkins EB, et al. Concurrent cisplatin-based radiotherapy and chemotherapy for locally advanced cervical cancer. *N Engl J Med.* 1999;**340**(15):1144–1153.
176. Whitney CW, Sause W, Bundy BN, et al. Randomized comparison of fluorouracil plus cisplatin versus hydroxyurea as an adjunct to radiation therapy in stage IIB-IVA carcinoma of the cervix with negative para-aortic lymph nodes: a Gynecologic Oncology Group and Southwest Oncology Group study. *J Clin Oncol.* 1999;**17**(5):1339–1348.
187. Thomakos N, Trachana S-P, Davidovic-Grigoraki M, Rodolakis A. Less radical surgery for early-stage cervical cancer: to what extent do we justify it?—our belief. *Taiwan J Obstet Gynecol.* 2016;**55**(4):495–498.
189. Rotman M, Sedlis A, Piedmonte MR, et al. A phase III randomized trial of postoperative pelvic irradiation in stage IB cervical carcinoma with poor prognostic features: follow-up of a gynecologic oncology group study. *Int J Radiat Oncol Biol Phys.* 2006;**65**(1):169–176.
193. Gupta S, Maheshwari A, Parab P, et al. Neoadjuvant chemotherapy followed by radical surgery versus concomitant chemotherapy and radiotherapy in patients with stage IB2, IIA, or IIB squamous cervical cancer: a randomized controlled trial. *J Clin Oncol.* 2018;**36**(16):1548–1555.
195. Chemotherapy for Cervical Cancer Meta-analysis Collaboration (CCMAC). Reducing uncertainties about the effects of chemoradiotherapy for cervical cancer: individual patient data meta-analysis. *Cochrane Database Syst Rev.* 2010;**2010**(1):Cd008285.
196. Shrivastava S, Mahantshetty U, Engineer R, et al. Cisplatin chemoradiotherapy vs radiotherapy in FIGO stage IIIB squamous cell carcinoma of the uterine cervix: a randomized clinical trial. *JAMA Oncol.* 2018;**4**(4):506–513.
200. Green JA, Kirwan JM, Tierney JF, et al. Survival and recurrence after concomitant chemotherapy and radiotherapy for cancer of the uterine cervix: a systematic review and meta-analysis. *Lancet.* 2001;**358**(9284):781–786.
209. Kunos CA, Radivoyevitch T, Waggoner S, et al. Radiochemotherapy plus 3-aminopyridine-2-carboxaldehyde thiosemicarbazone (3-AP, NSC #663249) in advanced-stage cervical and vaginal cancers. *Gynecol Oncol.* 2013;**130**(1):75–80.
222. Coleman RL, Keeney ED, Freedman RS, et al. Radical hysterectomy for recurrent carcinoma of the uterine cervix after radiotherapy. *Gynecol Oncol.* 1994;**55**(1):29–35.
228. Bonomi P, Blessing JA, Stehman FB, et al. Randomized trial of three cisplatin dose schedules in squamous-cell carcinoma of the cervix: a Gynecologic Oncology Group study. *J Clin Oncol.* 1985;**3**(8):1079–1085.
237. Monk BJ, Sill MW, McMeekin DS, et al. Phase III trial of four cisplatin-containing doublet combinations in stage IVB, recurrent, or persistent cervical carcinoma: a Gynecologic Oncology Group study. *J Clin Oncol.* 2009;**27**(28):4649–4655.
244. Dueñas-Gonzalez A, Lopez-Graniel C, Gonzalez A, et al. A phase II study of gemcitabine and cisplatin combination as induction chemotherapy for untreated locally advanced cervical carcinoma. *Ann Oncol.* 2001;**12**(4):541–547.
246. Kitagawa R, Katsumata N, Shibata T, et al. Paclitaxel plus carboplatin versus paclitaxel plus cisplatin in metastatic or recurrent cervical cancer: the open-label randomized phase III trial JCOG0505. *J Clin Oncol.* 2015;**33**(19):2129–2135.
247. Moore DH, Tian C, Monk BJ, et al. Prognostic factors for response to cisplatin-based chemotherapy in advanced cervical carcinoma: a Gynecologic Oncology Group Study. *Gynecol Oncol.* 2010;**116**(1):44–49.
248. Zhao Y, Adjei AA. Targeting angiogenesis in cancer therapy: moving beyond vascular endothelial growth factor. *Oncologist.* 2015;**20**(6):660–673.
252. Tewari KS, Sill MW, Long HJ 3rd, et al. Improved survival with bevacizumab in advanced cervical cancer. *N Engl J Med.* 2014;**370**(8):734–743.
254. Redondo A, Colombo N, McCormack M, et al. Primary results from CECILIA, a global single-arm phase II study evaluating bevacizumab, carboplatin and paclitaxel for advanced cervical cancer. *Gynecol Oncol.* 2020;**159**(1):142–149.
260. Monk BJ, Mas Lopez L, Zarba JJ, et al. Phase II, open-label study of pazopanib or lapatinib monotherapy compared with pazopanib plus lapatinib combination therapy in patients with advanced and recurrent cervical cancer. *J Clin Oncol.* 2010;**28**(22):3562–3569.
261. Lord CJ, Ashworth A. PARP inhibitors: synthetic lethality in the clinic. *Science.* 2017;**355**(6330):1152–1158.
266. Chung HC, Ros W, Delord JP, et al. Efficacy and safety of pembrolizumab in previously treated advanced cervical cancer: results from the phase II KEYNOTE-158 study. *J Clin Oncol.* 2019;**37**(17):1470–1478.
267. Hollebecque A, Meyer T, Moore KN, et al. An open-label, multicohort, phase I/II study of nivolumab in patients with virus-associated tumors (CheckMate 358): efficacy and safety in recurrent or metastatic (R/M) cervical, vaginal, and vulvar cancers. *J Clin Oncol.* 2017;**35**(15_suppl):5504.
268. U.S. National Library of Medicine. *Efficacy and Safety Study of First-Line Treatment with Pembrolizumab (MK-3475) Plus Chemotherapy Versus Placebo plus Chemotherapy in Women with Persistent, Recurrent, or Metastatic Cervical Cancer (MK-3475-826/KEYNOTE-826),* 2021; https://ClinicalTrials.gov/show/NCT03635567.
270. Naumann RW, Hollebecque A, Meyer T, et al. Safety and efficacy of nivolumab monotherapy in recurrent or metastatic cervical, vaginal, or vulvar carcinoma: results from the phase I/II CheckMate 358 trial. *J Clin Oncol.* 2019;**37**(31):2825–2834.
283. Cohen AC, Roane BM, Leath CA 3rd., Novel therapeutics for recurrent cervical cancer: moving towards personalized therapy. *Drugs.* 2020;**80**(3):217–227.
284. Basu P, Mehta A, Jain M, et al. A randomized phase 2 study of ADXS11-001 Listeria monocytogenes-Listeriolysin O immunotherapy with or without cisplatin in treatment of advanced cervical cancer. *Int J Gynecol Cancer.* 2018;**28**(4):764–772.
289. de Bono JS, Concin N, Hong DS, et al. Tisotumab vedotin in patients with advanced or metastatic solid tumours (InnovaTV 201): a first-in-human, multicentre, phase 1-2 trial. *Lancet Oncol.* 2019;**20**(3):383–393.
292. U.S. National Library of Medicine. *A Randomized, Open-Label, Phase 3 Trial of Tisotumab Vedotin vs Investigator's Choice Chemotherapy in Second- or Third-Line Recurrent or Metastatic Cervical Cancer,* 2021; https://clinicaltrials.gov/ct2/show/NCT04697628.
294. Jazaeri AA, Zsiros E, Amaria RN, et al. Safety and efficacy of adoptive cell transfer using autologous tumor infiltrating lymphocytes (LN-145) for treatment of recurrent, metastatic, or persistent cervical carcinoma. *J Clin Oncol.* 2019;**37**(15_suppl):2538–2538.

100 Endometrial cancer

Shannon N. Westin, MD, MPH ■ Karen H. Lu, MD ■ Jamal Rahaman, MD

Overview

Endometrial carcinoma is the most frequent gynecologic cancer in the United States with over 65,000 new cases diagnosed per year. Over 80% have the classic estrogen-dependent endometrioid histology with a favorable prognosis. Nonendometrioid histology types, including uterine serous carcinomas (USC), carcinosarcomas, and clear cell carcinomas, have a different molecular profile associated with more virulent disease and diminished survival. The Cancer Genome Atlas (TCGA) has defined four molecular subtypes of endometrial cancer, based on somatic mutations, copy number alterations, and microsatellite instability status. Over 75% of patients present with irregular or post-menopausal bleeding. Surgical staging includes a hysterectomy, bilateral salpingo-oophorectomy, with or without pelvic and para-aortic lymph node sampling done via a laparotomy, laparoscopy, or robotic surgery. Surgery, where possible, constitutes the definitive primary treatment for most patients with endometrial carcinoma. Primary radiation therapy and primary hormonal therapy are alternatives for inoperable patients. Adjuvant therapy for stage I disease is determined by age, depth of myometrial invasion, lymph-vascular space invasion, and tumor grade. For patients with advanced and recurrent disease radiation therapy, chemotherapy, and hormonal therapy are utilized. The combination of paclitaxel and carboplatin is the most effective and tolerable chemotherapy combination and currently serves as the backbone for a number of investigational strategies. Immune check-point inhibitors are FDA approved for the treatment of metastatic endometrial cancer, including pembrolizumab alone for microsatellite instability-high (MSI-H) cancers and pembrolizumab and lenvatinib for microsatellite stable (MSS) disease. The growing understanding of the molecular aberrations common in endometrial cancer has led to exploration of a number of therapies, targeting angiogenesis and the PI3K/AKT, HER2, RAS/RAF, and DNA damage repair pathways.

Epidemiology

In 2020, 65,620 new cases of uterine corpus cancer will be diagnosed in the United States and 12,590 women will die from this disease.[1] After declining between the mid-1980s and 1990s, the incidence rates for endometrial cancer increased by about 1.3% per year from 2007 to 2017.[1] The majority of patients are diagnosed at an early stage (75%) which yields 5-year survival rates of approximately 80% overall. However, outcomes for advanced-stage disease are poor, with 5-year survival rates of approximately 10%.[1]

While Black women have a lower incidence of endometrial carcinoma than White women, their mortality is higher.[2] Studies demonstrate that Black women are diagnosed with less favorable histologies, more advanced stage disease, and more poorly differentiated tumors than White women. Outcomes may also relate to access to optimal care. For more than two decades, studies have documented that Black women are treated differently from White women before and after surgery.[2] Recent studies that control for prognostic factors such as histology and stage still reveal worse outcomes for Black women with endometrial cancer.[3]

Risk factors

Risk factors for endometrial cancer include obesity, diabetes, nulliparity, history of colon and/or breast carcinoma, ovulatory failure, increased endogenous estrogen exposure, and exposure to exogenous oral estrogens.[4] Peripheral aromatization of estrogen precursors in body fat results in a higher level of circulating estrogen explaining, in part, the risk from obesity. Ultimately, excess weight and elevated hormone levels are the most important factors increasing risk for endometrial cancer. Lifestyle factors such as diet and physical activity contribute directly to these risks.[5]

Pathologic conditions that increase levels of endogenous estrogen or prompt exogenous estrogen supplementation increase endometrial cancer risk.[6] Gusberg and Kardon reviewed the endometrial histology from 115 patients with theca-granulosa cell ovarian tumors and found that 21% developed endometrial carcinoma and 43% had precancerous hyperplasia.[6] Others have not found the same incidence of adenocarcinoma but have identified a high incidence of atypical hyperplasias.[7,8] Patients with polycystic ovary syndrome usually do not ovulate and, thus, are exposed to endogenous unopposed estrogen production. When endometrial carcinoma occurs in women younger than 45 years of age, it is often in patients with polycystic ovary syndrome[9,10] and is most frequently surrounded by atypical hyperplasia histologically. Finally, patients who are treated for ovarian dysgenesis by oophorectomy and unopposed estrogen replacement may develop endometrial carcinoma in the residual uterus.[11] This association of continuous unopposed exposure to endogenous estrogens or exogenous oral estrogens and endometrial carcinoma has been widely reported.[12–20]

The Centers for Disease Control and Prevention reported that oral contraceptive use for at least 12 months diminished the risk of endometrial cancer by 50% compared with the risk for women who had never used oral contraception. Nulliparous women seemed to benefit most and the protection lasted for a decade following the discontinuation of oral contraceptive use.[21] In the Royal College of General Practitioners' Oral Contraception study of over 46,000 women, the risk of endometrial cancer was reduced by approximately 34% among women who ever used contraception compared to those who never used contraception.[22]

For more than 20 years, tamoxifen has been used to treat breast cancer, following the observation that it causes regression of metastatic tumor, diminishes the incidence of cancer in the contralateral breast, delays time to recurrence, and improves survival in subsets of patients.[23] Clinically, tamoxifen diminishes

---

Holland-Frei Cancer Medicine, Tenth Edition. Edited by Robert C. Bast, John C. Byrd, Carlo M. Croce, Ernest Hawk, Fadlo R. Khuri, Raphael E. Pollock, Apostolia M. Tsimberidou, Christopher G. Willett, and Cheryl L. Willman.
© 2023 John Wiley & Sons, Inc. Published 2023 by John Wiley & Sons, Inc.

serum cholesterol, increases sex hormone-binding globulin,[24] preserves bone density in the lumbar spine,[25] thickens the vaginal epithelium in some patients,[25,26] and is associated with the enlargement of uterine fibroids, the growth of endometrial polyps, and the development of endometrial neoplastic change. These are all estrogen-like functions. Paradoxically, the same drug is associated with features of estrogen deprivation, including vaginal atrophy, onset of vasomotor symptoms, and development of clinical dyspareunia.

The action of tamoxifen is organ specific and several investigators have described an increase in the incidence of endometrial cancers among patients with breast cancer who were treated with tamoxifen.[27-32] Two randomized control trials have clearly described the risk of endometrial cancer observed with tamoxifen treatment. The National Surgical Adjuvant Breast and Bowel Project (NSABP) described observations on 3863 patients prospectively studied.[28] In the B-14 protocol, 2843 patients with node-negative, ER-positive breast cancer received either tamoxifen (20 mg/d) or placebo. An additional 1020 patients taking tamoxifen were registered in this project. The relative risk calculated for the tamoxifen-treated group compared with the placebo group was 7.5, with an annual hazard rate of 0.2 per 1000 for the placebo group and 1.6 per 1000 for the randomized tamoxifen-treated group. In the Breast Cancer Prevention Trial (P-1) of the NSABP, 13,388 women were randomly assigned to receive placebo (6707) or 20 mg/d of tamoxifen (6681) for 5 years.[33] The rate of endometrial carcinoma was increased in the tamoxifen group (risk ratio = 2.53); this increase occurred primarily in women aged 50 years or older.

Neither ultrasound surveillance nor routine endometrial biopsy has proven effective in detecting endometrial cancer in women taking tamoxifen. A prospective longitudinal study in Canada of 304 women with breast cancer receiving tamoxifen found that routine surveillance with ultrasonography was not useful in asymptomatic patients.[34] Barakat and colleagues evaluated 159 tamoxifen-treated patients by serial office endometrial biopsies obtained at the start of tamoxifen therapy and at 6-month intervals for 2 years, followed by three additional annual biopsies.[35] Although the procedure was feasible, significant pathology requiring hysterectomy was observed in only three patients, and the authors concluded that the utility of routine endometrial biopsy for screening in tamoxifen-treated women is limited.[36] Prompt evaluation of any vaginal bleeding is, however, mandated and clinicians should not be reluctant to obtain endometrial biopsies or vaginal ultrasound in patients with multiple risk factors.

In addition to lifestyle factors and estrogen exposure, women with the hereditary cancer syndrome, Lynch syndrome, also have an increased risk of endometrial cancer. This autosomal dominant syndrome is caused by a germline defect in a DNA mismatch repair gene such as *MLH1, MSH2, MSH6,* or *PMS2.* Lynch syndrome confers increased risks of endometrial, colon, ovarian, and a number of other rare malignancies including, renal, liver, brain, and urinary tract.[37,38] Overall risk of cancer depends on the specific mutation. Lifetime risk of developing cancer ranges from 15% to 66%, 15% to 68%, and 1% to 20% for endometrial, colon, and ovarian cancer, respectively.[37,38] Screening for endometrial cancer is recommended for women with Lynch syndrome beginning at age 35. Endometrial biopsy is obtained annually until the patient has completed childbearing.[39] At that point, hysterectomy and bilateral salpingo-oophorectomy should be offered to reduce the risk of both endometrial and ovarian cancer in this patient population.[40] The NCCN guidelines and other oncology organizations recommend assessment of mismatch repair protein expression by immunohistochemistry for all women with endometrial cancer, regardless of age or risk factors. This testing can be utilized for Lynch syndrome screening as well as determination of eligibility for immunotherapy treatment (discussed below).

Pathology

Endometrial hyperplasia

There are a clear pattern of precursor abnormalities within the endometrium that occur prior to endometrial cancer. These range from a mild arrangement of densely crowded glands with eosinophilic cytoplasm through the spectrum of more disordered arrangements, characterized by intraluminal tufting, and an increase in mitosis, pseudopalisading, and bizarre nuclear morphology.[41] Hertig and Sommers similarly studied preinvasive changes in the endometrium and described three intensities of abnormality, which they called "adenomatous hyperplasia," "atypical hyperplasia," and "carcinoma *in situ.*"[42] Kurman and colleagues followed 170 patients with endometrial hyperplasia for a minimum of 1 year with a mean follow-up time of 13.4 years.[43] Only 1.6% of patients without cytologic atypia progressed to cancer compared with 23% of those with atypical cytology. Architectural abnormalities were not prognostically important. Table 2 presents the details of Kurman and colleagues' classification and observations. Their classification of simple or complex hyperplasia, with or without atypia, is accepted for describing these lesions.

Endometrioid adenocarcinoma

Endometrioid adenocarcinoma is the most common of the endometrial cancer histologies. It is characterized by the disappearance of stroma between abnormal glands that have infoldings of their linings into the lumens, disordered nuclear chromatin distribution, nuclear enlargement, and a variable degree of mitosis, necrosis, and hemorrhage. This classic variety accounts for approximately 80% of adenocarcinomas.

Uterine serous carcinoma

Described by Hendrickson and colleagues in 1982, uterine serous carcinoma (USC) comprises approximately 5% of endometrial carcinomas and is characterized by expansive papillary architecture with a fibrovascular matrix, marked cytologic atypia, bizarre nuclei, and widespread nuclear pleomorphism (Figure 1).[44,45] The features are suggestive of serous carcinoma of the ovary. The lesion is highly virulent, usually found with deep myometrial penetration at the time of diagnosis, often extrauterine in location in patients with clinical early-stage disease, and almost always incurable when the disease has spread beyond the uterus.[45-48]

Clear cell carcinoma

Kurman and Scully described clear cell cancers in detail.[49] Histologically, although there are a variety of patterns, a presentation of polygonal or flattened cells with clear cytoplasm accounts for more than half of the cells. This group constitutes approximately 5% of endometrial carcinomas and occurs more frequently in older women. The 5-year overall survival rate is approximately 40%,[50] but this may be a result of the older age of the patients and the fact that clear cell carcinomas are generally found in patients with higher stages of cancer. Further, clear cell tumors are often associated with serous tumors, conferring a worse prognosis.[51]

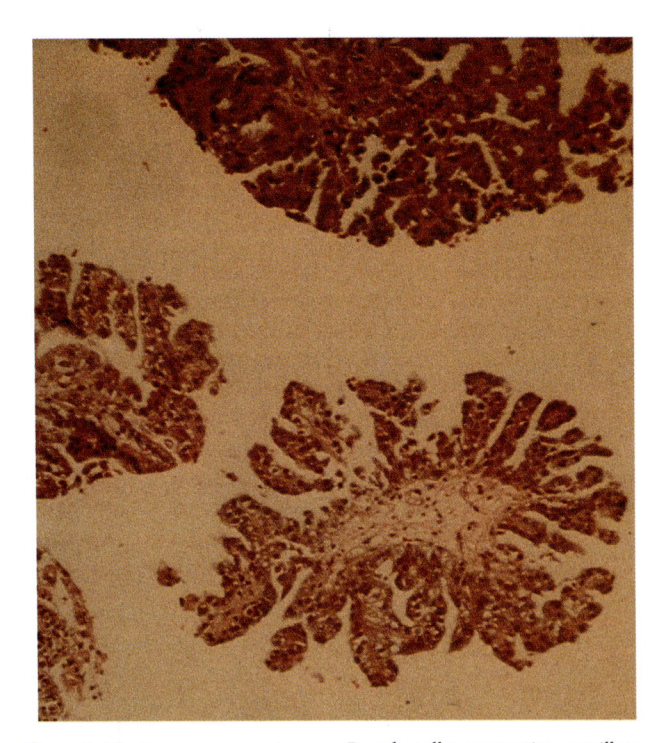

Figure 1 Uterine serous carcinoma. Broad stalks supporting papillary fronds, appearing like papillary ovarian carcinoma. Courtesy of Diane Deligdisch, MD, Mount Sinai School of Medicine. A four-color version of the figure is available on the CD-ROM) Correlation of the Federation Internationale de Gynecologie d'Obstetrique (FIGO), Unio Internationale Contre Cancrum (UICC), and American Joint Committee on Cancer (AJCC) nomenclatures.

Carcinosarcoma

Carcinosarcomas, also known as malignant mixed Müllerian tumors (MMMTs), contain two distinct cell types.[52] The malignant epithelial component may be made up of any of the histologic subtypes described above (endometrioid, serous, clear cell). The malignant mesenchymal component can either be homologous (containing uterine histotypes such as endometrial stromal sarcoma or leiomyosarcoma) or heterologous (containing nonuterine histotypes such as chondrosarcoma or rhabdomyosarcoma). Overall, carcinosarcomas have a very poor prognosis, and, in some studies, have worse outcomes than nonendometrioid or high-grade endometrioid tumors.[52]

Genomic alterations

The Cancer Genome Atlas (TCGA) provided a comprehensive mapping of DNA, RNA, and protein alterations in endometrioid and serous endometrial cancers.[53] In the decades leading up to TCGA, individual genes and proteins had been implicated in the pathogenesis of endometrial cancer. Based on these molecular alterations, as well as clinical features, endometrial cancers have been classically divided into endometrioid and nonendometrioid categories (Table 1). Endometrioid tumors demonstrate high estrogen and progesterone receptor positivity and aberrations in the PI3K pathway. Nonendometrioid tumors include serous, clear cell, and carcinosarcoma histologies and are characterized by high mutational rates in TP53.

The PI3K pathway is the most common dysregulated pathway in endometrial cancer, with mutations seen in multiple key members. Loss of PTEN (phosphate and tensin homolog deleted on chromosome 10) occurs in approximately 75–85% of tumors of the endometrioid histology,[54] and results in unopposed activation

Table 1 Clinical and molecular features of endometrial carcinoma.

Features	Endometrioid	Nonendometrioid
Clinical		
Risk factors	Unopposed estrogen	Age
Race	White > black	White = black
Degree of differentiation	Well differentiated	Poorly differentiated
Prognosis	Favorable	Unfavorable
Molecular		
K-ras overexpression	Yes	Yes
HER2/neu overexpression	No	Yes
TP53 overexpression	No	Yes
PTEN mutations	Yes	No
Microsatellite instability	Yes	Rare

of the PI3K pathway. Mutations account for the majority of PTEN loss and may occur early in endometrial carcinogenesis. However, other mechanisms including gene methylation and destabilization of the protein may also contribute to PTEN loss. Mutations have also been found in other components of the PI3K pathway, including PIK3CA, PIK3R1, and AKT.[55] A key downstream effector of the PI3K pathway is mTOR, which stimulates protein synthesis and entry into the G1 phase of the cell cycle.

There are a number of other alterations which are quite common in endometrial cancer. The Ras/Raf/MEK/ERK pathway is also frequently dysregulated and KRAS mutations occur in approximately 18–20% of endometrioid endometrial cancers. Mutations in the FGFR2 receptor tyrosine kinase occur in approximately 12% of endometrioid endometrial cancers and do not co-occur with tumors that have KRAS mutations. Among early-stage endometrioid endometrial cancer patients, KRAS mutations are associated with a more favorable prognosis while FGFR2 mutations are associated with a worse prognosis.[56] ARID1A has been shown to be mutated in approximately 25% of low-grade and 44% of high-grade endometrioid cancers.[57] The WNT pathway is another important dysregulated pathway in endometrioid endometrial cancer, with β-catenin, or CTNNB1, mutations occurring in approximately 10–28% of cases and conferring worse prognosis in early-stage disease.[58,59]

Microsatellite instability (MSI) occurs in approximately 35% of endometrioid endometrial cancers and <5% of nonendometrioid cell types.[56,60,61] The MSI phenotype primarily results from somatic silencing of MLH1 through promoter methylation. In a minority of cases, MSI results from germline mutations in the Lynch syndrome genes, including MLH1, MSH2, MSH6, or PMS2. In the past, MSI was only checked in patients deemed to be potentially at risk of Lynch syndrome based on family history. Given our growing understanding of this molecular abnormality and the potential implications for therapy, all patients with endometrial cancer should have this evaluation.

TP53 mutations occur in the majority of serous cancers and carcinosarcomas. In addition to mutations, stabilization of the protein can also lead to p53 overexpression. Similar to high-grade serous ovarian cancer, TP53 mutations occur early in the pathogenesis of uterine serous cancers. Other alterations that have been reported in uterine serous cancers include mutations in PPP2R1A and FBXW7, amplification and overexpression of ERBB2 (Her2/neu), and overexpression of cyclin E.[62–67]

Rather than through a single gene approach, TCGA performed a large scale, integrated genomic analysis of both endometrioid and serous endometrial cancers.[53] Four molecular subtypes of endometrial cancer were defined, based on somatic mutations, copy number alterations, and MSI status. These four groups are (1) POLE ultramutated, (2) hypermutated/microsatellite unstable,

(3) copy number low/microsatellite stable, and (4) copy number high (serous-like). The first group, called *POLE* "ultramutated" tumors, includes the clinically most favorable tumors with endometrioid histology. POLE refers to DNA polymerase epsilon, which is involved in DNA replication and harbors numerous hotspot mutations in tumors in this category. There are few copy number abnormalities in tumors of the POLE subtype, but a very high number of mutations. Mutations in *PTEN*, *PIK3R1*, *PIK3CA*, and *KRAS* are common. The second group, called MSI "hypermutated" tumors, includes endometrioid tumors with MSI, few copy number abnormalities, and mutation rates lower than the "ultramutated" *POLE* group but higher than the copy number low/MSS group. Mutations in *KRAS* and *PTEN* are frequent. The third group is the copy number low/MSS group which has *PTEN* and *PIK3CA* mutations, as well as frequent β-catenin mutations. The fourth group is the copy number high (serous-like) tumors with extensive copy number abnormalities. In addition to most of the serous tumors, approximately one-quarter of the patients with grade 3 endometrioid fall in this category. Interesting work is ongoing best utilize these classifications to direct clinical care.

Diagnosis

The median age for patients with adenocarcinoma of the endometrium is 61 years, with the highest prevalence during the sixth decade.[4,68] Only 5% develop adenocarcinomas before the age of 40 years, and many of these women have the genetic syndromes previously discussed. Eighty percent of patients are postmenopausal. Irregular or postmenopausal bleeding is the presenting symptom in at least 75% of patients, and at the time of diagnosis, the majority of patients have disease confined to the uterus. Thus, it is obvious that irregular bleeding is a critical symptom, and by explaining it histologically, one has an opportunity to identify endometrial cancer when it is highly curable by relatively uncomplicated therapy.[68]

Endometrial biopsy or fractional dilation and curettage of the uterus, with careful sampling of both the endometrial cavity and the endocervical canal, are essential for the diagnosis of endometrial cancer. Hysteroscopy, either by direct observation or with video-camera amplification, allows direct assessment of the topography of the endometrial cavity with the possibility for more selective sampling and the assurance of not missing any occult lesions.[69,70]

Imaging

Noninvasive radiographic imaging techniques, such as magnetic resonance imaging[71] and ultrasonography,[72] are not cost-effective for screening. For diagnosis and documenting recurrence, these techniques as well as CT scan and PET scan can achieve an accuracy rate above 80%.[73–80] Enthusiasm for preoperative imaging in low-grade tumors is tempered by the lack of cost-effectiveness and reproducibility.[81]

Laboratory evaluation and biomarker testing

Measurement of cancer antigen 125 (CA125) in the blood may be useful to anticipate and detect extrauterine disease.[82] Use of serum HE4 has been explored in endometrial cancer for both detection and monitoring response to treatment; however, this is still in early stages of exploration and has not yet been utilized broadly.[83] As noted above, all patients with endometrial cancer are suggested to undergo testing for mismatch repair protein expression. Further, biomarkers including HER2 expression/amplification and MSI can be utilized to direct therapy as discussed below.

Table 2 Comparison of follow-up of 170 patients with simple and complex hyperplasia and simple and complex atypical hyperplasia.[a]

	No. of patients	Regressed n (%)	Persisted n (%)	Progressed to carcinoma n (%)
Simple hyperplasia	93	74 (80)	18 (19)	1 (1)
Complex hyperplasia	29	23 (80)	5 (17)	1 (3)
Simple atypical hyperplasia	13	9 (69)	3 (23)	1 (8)
Complex atypical hyperplasia	35	20 (57)	5 (14)	10 (29)

[a]Source: Adapted from Kurman et al.[43]

Staging

Historically, endometrial cancer staging was clinical, based on physical examination, noninvasive radiographic testing, and measurement of the depth of the uterine cavity. In 1988, the International Federation of Gynecology and Obstetrics (FIGO) introduced the requirement for surgical staging of patients with endometrial carcinoma following the GOG 33 study that demonstrated that 9.6% of 843 patients in clinical stage I had lymph node metastasis on comprehensive surgical staging.[84–87]

In 2009, FIGO updated the surgical staging classification for Endometrial cancers as indicated in Table 2.[88] In addition in 2009, uterine carcinosarcomas continue to be staged using the epithelial endometrial cancer system and new specific Staging Classifications were developed for leiomyosarcomas, endometrial stromal sarcomas, and uterine adensarcomas (Table 3).

Comprehensive surgical staging includes performance of hysterectomy, bilateral salpingo-oophorectomy, with or without lymph node sampling. Controversy exists regarding the need for lymph node assessment (discussed below).

Prognostic factors

Several factors have been identified in large prospective surgical-pathologic staging studies by the GOG[84,87] that are predictive of extrauterine spread of disease at the time of initial diagnosis and with ultimate survival. Surgical stage and age are highly significant prognostic features that maintain their significance in each of the analyses performed in the various reports.

Histologic type

Whereas approximately 80% of endometrial cancers are classic endometrioid adenocarcinomas, the remainder constitutes a series of histologic types with a more unfavorable prognosis. These include serous, clear cell, carcinosarcoma, and undifferentiated cancers. These cell types confer an unfavorable prognosis, independent of other known prognostic factors.[89]

Tumor grade

Endometrial tumor grade is defined based on the percentage of tumor with a solid component (Table 4). Grade 1 is 5% or less solid, grade 2 is between 6% and 50% solid, and grade 3 has >50% solid. Within endometrioid adenocarcinomas, tumor grade is highly significant as an independent prognostic factor. Additionally, numerous studies have demonstrated that, in general, there is a greater tendency for the less differentiated tumors to be associated with other poor prognostic factors, including deep myometrial penetration, vascular space invasion, and increasing stage.[87,90,91] Salvesen and colleagues showed that morphometric

categories	FIGO[b] stages	Definition
Primary tumor (T)		
TX		Primary tumor cannot be assessed
T0		No evidence of primary tumor
Tis[c]		Carcinoma *in situ* (preinvasive carcinoma)
T1	I	Tumor confined to the corpus uteri
T1a	IA	Tumor limited to the endometrium or invades less than one-half of the myometrium
T1b	IB	Tumor invades one-half or more of the myometrium
T2	II	Tumor invades stromal connective tissue of the cervix but does not extend beyond the uterus[d]
T3a	IIIA	Tumor involves serosa and/or adnexa (direct extension or metastasis) ##
T3b	IIIB	Vaginal involvement (direct extension or metastasis) or parametrial involvement[e]
	IIIC	Metastasis to pelvic and/or para-aortic lymph nodes[e]
T4	IVA	Tumor invades bladder mucosa and/or bowel (bullous edema is not sufficient to classify a tumor as T4)
Regional lymph nodes (N)		
NX		Regional lymph nodes cannot be assessed
N0		No regional lymph node metastasis
N1	IIIC1	Regional lymph node metastasis to pelvic lymph nodes (positive pelvic nodes)
N2	IIIC2	Regional lymph node metastasis to para-aortic lymph nodes, with or without positive pelvic lymph nodes
Distant metastasis (M)		
M0		No distant metastasis
M1	IVB	Distant metastasis (includes metastasis to inguinal lymph nodes, intra-peritoneal disease, or lung, liver, or bone. It excludes metastasis to para-aortic lymph nodes, vagina, pelvic serosa, or adnexa)

[a]Source: Modified from Pecorelli[88] and Edge et al.[188]
[b]Either G1, G2, or G3.
[c]Note: FIGO no longer includes stage 0 (Tis).
[d]Endocervical glandular involvement only should be considered as stage I and no longer as stage II.
[e]Positive *cytology has to be* reported separately without changing the stage.

Table 4 Histopathology: degree of differentiation.

G1:	5% or less of a nonsquamous or nonmorular solid growth pattern
G2:	6–50% of a nonsquamous or nonmorular solid growth pattern
G3:	More than 50% of a nonsquamous or nonmorular solid growth pattern

nuclear grade was a stronger prognostic factor than subjective histologic grade.[92]

Myometrial invasion

The depth of myometrial invasion is an important independent prognostic factor for outcome in stage I disease. Deeper invasion is associated with higher probabilities of tumor recurrence and death.[87,90,93] Although increasing depth of invasion correlates with increasing grade of tumor, depth appears to be a more significant prognostic factor and predicts for the presence of extrauterine disease as detected at surgical staging procedures.[84] Regardless of grade, however, only 1% of patients with disease confined to the endometrium have extrauterine disease compared with patients with deep muscle invasion, for which the incidence of pelvic node invasion rises to 17% and para-aortic nodal involvement rises to 25%. DiSaia and colleagues found that patients with only endometrial involvement had an 8% recurrence rate compared with 12% if there was superficial or intermediate myometrial invasion versus 46% if there was involvement of the outer third of the myometrium.[93]

Lymphovascular space invasion

Vascular space invasion is a significant risk factor for recurrence, but it is not as important as the grade and depth of myometrial penetration. Approximately 15% of endometrial adenocarcinomas have capillary-like space invasion and are associated with a fivefold increase rate of positive pelvic (27%) and para-aortic lymph (19%) node involvement.[84,94]

Positive peritoneal cytology

Positive peritoneal cytology as the sole upstaging factor was dropped in the 2009 FIGO staging revisions as a stage-defining characteristic.[88] The presence of positive peritoneal cytology in washings is associated with an increased risk of relapse.[87] Approximately 15% of patients have positive peritoneal cytology,[87] and this is often related to other poor prognostic factors, such as high grade or deep myometrial penetration. Thus, it is not surprising that it is also associated with an increased risk of metastases to pelvic (25%) and paraaortic (19%) lymph nodes. Opinions and data in the literature conflict with respect to interpreting the independent prognostic significance of peritoneal cytology. Approximately 5% of patients with positive peritoneal cytology have no evidence of extrauterine disease,[84] but approximately one-third of patients with extrauterine disease do have positive cytology. In a review of the literature, Wethington categorized patients into groups based on low-risk uterine features (grade 1–2, <50% depth of invasion, no lymphovascular space invasion) with positive peritoneal cytology. In this group, positive cytology occurred in 11% of cases and had a recurrence rate of 4%. Patients with higher-risk features plus positive cytology had a 32% risk of recurrence.[95]

Race

When compared to White women, Black women have a higher incidence of unfavorable histology, advanced-stage disease, and poor differentiation. In fact, Black women have higher mortality rates than White women, even when controlling for poor prognostic factors.[3,96]

Hormone receptor status

The presence of cytoplasmic ER- and progesterone receptor (PR)-binding proteins has been quantitatively associated with better histologic differentiation,[97] favorable histologic subtype, and response to therapy.[98–100] Ligand binding to ER and PR was higher in well-differentiated lesions and was significantly lower in grade 3 lesions and the nonendometrioid carcinomas.[100] Clinically, reduced levels of ligand interaction with the ER, PR, or both in endometrial cancer samples significantly ($p < 0.01$) correlate with recurrence and death from disease.[99,100]

Treatment of primary disease

Surgery

The initial surgical staging procedure, outlined earlier (see Figure 2), is the standard therapeutic procedure as well. Minimally invasive techniques, including laparoscopy and robotic-assisted surgery, have been integrated into the management of endometrial cancer as standard of care.[101–111] A randomized controlled

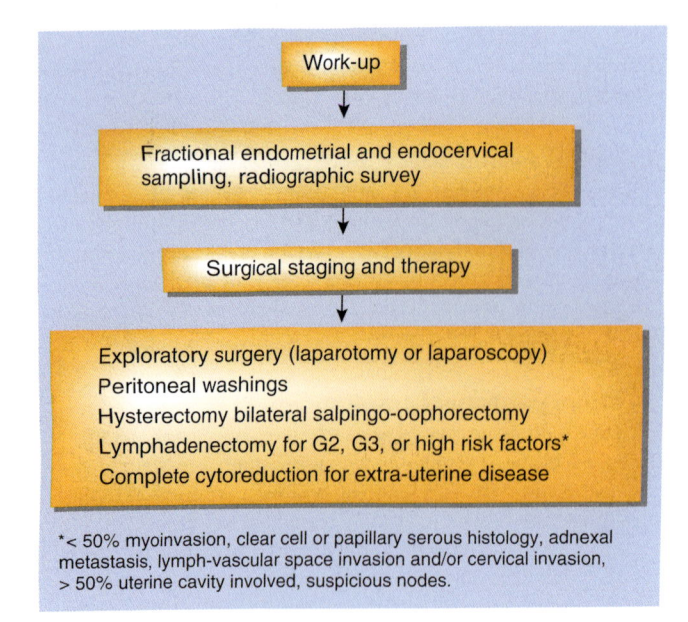

Figure 2 Surgical management of endometrial carcinoma.

Work-up → Fractional endometrial and endocervical sampling, radiographic survey → Surgical staging and therapy → Exploratory surgery (laparotomy or laparoscopy); Peritoneal washings; Hysterectomy bilateral salpingo-oophorectomy; Lymphadenectomy for G2, G3, or high risk factors*; Complete cytoreduction for extra-uterine disease

*< 50% myoinvasion, clear cell or papillary serous histology, adnexal metastasis, lymph-vascular space invasion and/or cervical invasion, > 50% uterine cavity involved, suspicious nodes.

trial revealed that use of laparoscopy compared to laparotomy in endometrial cancer did not negatively impact progression-free survival and led to less adverse events and shorter length of stay in the hospital.[101] Similarly, robotic surgery was found to have better operative outcomes, such as blood loss and complication rate, with a shorter length of stay after surgery when compared to laparotomy.[111]

Several randomized controlled trials have demonstrated that staging lymphadenectomy does not improve survival for women with endometrial cancer.[112,113] However, many clinicians use staging information to guide choice of adjuvant therapy and provide prognosis. Sentinel lymph node (SLN) mapping has been employed as a method to assess lymph node status while limiting postoperative complications. A number of prospective studies have been completed in high and low-risk stage I disease demonstrating that SLN mapping yields low false-negative rates when compared to full lymphadenectomy.[114–116]

There are occasions when, at the time of staging laparotomy, cervical or parametrial invasion is detected and a radical (Wertheim) hysterectomy is performed to achieve clearance of all disease. However, the addition of tailored external beam RT following surgery has largely reduced routine performance of such procedures.[117]

When there is disease outside the uterus and in the retroperitoneal nodes, there may be a potential benefit to surgical cytoreductive efforts. Several retrospective studies have demonstrated that complete resection of all disease is associated with improved survival.[118–121] However, there are no prospective studies confirming these observations.

Surgery for recurrent disease is generally confined to those patients who have symptoms of intestinal or urinary tract obstruction, isolated regional recurrence, or isolated lung metastases that have not responded to cytotoxic or hormonal therapy. For such patients, surgery may be useful to correct functional deficits or to excise isolated recurrences or resistant metastatic deposits.

Radiation therapy (RT)

Although surgery, where possible, constitutes the definitive primary treatment for most patients with endometrial carcinoma, many patients may require RT to prevent outcomes.

Definitive irradiation for inoperable patients

Modern surgical techniques and improved postoperative care have diminished the number of patients considered inoperable. Nevertheless, because endometrial cancer is frequently a disease of the elderly (over 65 years of age), who are often obese and sometimes diabetic, with other co-morbidities, surgery is not always possible. Several relatively large series have demonstrated pelvic RT as effective definitive management of endometrial cancer without initial surgery.[122–126]

The proportion surviving depends on tumor grade, just as for patients treated surgically; those with grade 1 tumors have better survival rates than do those with grade 3.[122] Significant numbers of patients die of causes unrelated to their primary carcinoma.[126] Inoperable patients who did not die from co-morbidities had a median 5-year survival rate that approached that of operable patients.[126]

Some patients with small uteri may be cured by intracavitary radiation only, but, usually, definitive management consists of both external beam and intracavitary irradiation because of more favorable radiation dosimetry. Further, a systematic meta-analysis demonstrated improved survival with combination therapy.[127] Complication rates are acceptable (usually less than 10%). After definitive irradiation, the pattern of failure, in contrast to that following surgery, consists mainly of central failure in the uterus. This observation is important for developing treatment strategies for patients with stage II disease. Removal of the uterus at some point in treatment provides better overall central control than that achieved by radiation alone. Three series indicate 5-year survival rates of approximately 50% for patients with stage II disease who received RT as definitive therapy.[117,122,128,129]

Adjuvant RT for stage I disease

The present recommendation to give postoperative RT in surgical stage I is dependent on prognosis as defined by the histologic features of the primary tumor within the endometrium. Extensive staging studies have identified that several of the aforementioned factors predict for the presence of clinically occult extrauterine disease.[87]

Although patients considered to be at high risk of recurrence (e.g., those with grade 2 or 3 disease with penetration of the outer 50% of the myometrium) have generally been treated with postoperative adjuvant RT, there is only one randomized trial addressing the benefit of adjuvant RT in surgically staged patients (GOG-99).[130] There are three randomized clinical trials in patients who had incomplete surgical staging (Alders,[90] PORTEC-1,[131] and PORTEC-2[132]).

The GOG-99 study stratified risk and validated pelvic radiation therapy for improved recurrence-free survival in the high intermediate risk (HIR) group. The HIR subgroup of patients was defined (as an increased recurrent rate of 25% at 5 years based on GOG 33) as those with (1) moderately to poorly differentiated tumor, the presence of lymphovascular invasion, and outer third myometrial invasion; (2) age 50 years or greater with any two of the risk factors listed above; or (3) age of at least 70 years with any risk factor listed above. The treatment difference was particularly evident among the HIR subgroup (2-year cumulative incidence of recurrence in NAT vs RT: 26% vs 6%; RH = 0.42). Overall, radiation had a substantial impact on pelvic and vaginal recurrences (18 in NAT and 3 in RT)[130] but did not achieve a significant difference in overall survival. In general, full pelvic radiotherapy is not utilized in this population. Instead, patients with high intermediate-risk disease are prioritized for vault irradiation as discussed in the next section.

Vault irradiation
On a theoretical basis, the patient who undergoes thorough staging might be at low risk of a pelvic sidewall recurrence in the absence of lymph node metastasis. Other occult pelvis sidewall disease not found at surgery, such as in the lymphatic channels in the parametrium or in parametrial lymph nodes, occurs infrequently and is an unlikely source of recurrence. The major site for possible recurrence within the pelvis for these patients would be the vaginal vault, which is amenable to brachytherapy with a lower morbidity.[133,134] PORTEC-2 evaluated this hypothesis in unstaged patients with HIR features by the PORTEC definition (where intermediate-risk factors were outer-half invasion, grade 3, or greater than 60 years of age, but excluded deeply invasive high-grade tumors, and where patients were deemed HIR with two of the three factors). At a median follow-up of 45 months, the estimated 5-year vaginal recurrence rates were 1.8% for brachytherapy alone and 1.6% for external irradiation. The nodal failure rate was significantly different at 3.8% for the brachytherapy-alone arm and 0.5% for external beam irradiation. Distant metastases, disease-free survival, and OS were similar in both arms.[132] Based on these results, as well as results from PORTEC-1 and GOG99, use of vaginal vault irradiation is prioritized for patients at high intermediate risk of recurrence. This modality provides the same reduction in risk of recurrence with lower overall toxicity.

Stage III
The 2009 FIGO surgical staging for endometrial cancer includes patients with metastases to pelvic and/or para-aortic lymph nodes as stage IIIC. The current staging classification covers a broad spectrum of prognostic groups that have diverse outcomes after standard surgery with or without adjuvant pelvic irradiation. Unfortunately, many of the published series include patients with microscopic extension to the adnexa (stage IIIA), those with malignant ascites (stage IIIA), and those with gross pelvic sidewall disease (stage IIIA or IIIC) without distinction, resulting in widely variable survival data.

Treatment recommendations at this time for patients with stage III disease must be made on an individual basis. Those in whom appropriate surgical staging has been completed without evidence of disease beyond the ovaries should be considered for chemotherapy with or without adjuvant postoperative pelvic irradiation based on two large randomized control trials.[135,136]

The primary endpoint of GOG 258, a randomized phase III trial was to determine if treatment with cisplatin and volume-directed radiation followed by carboplatin and paclitaxel for four cycles (C-RT, experimental arm) improved recurrence-free survival (RFS) when compared to carboplatin and paclitaxel for 6 cycles (CT, control arm) in patients with stages III–IVA (<2 cm residual disease) or FIGO 2009 stage I/II serous or clear cell endometrial cancer.[135] There were 201 (58%) > grade 3 toxicity events in the C-RT arm and 227 (63%) in the CT arm. Treatment hazard ratio for RFS was 0.9 (C-RT vs CT; CI 0.74–1.10). C-RT reduced the incidence of vaginal (3% vs 7%, HR = 0.36, CI 0.16–0.82), pelvic, and paraaortic recurrences (10% vs 21%, HR = 0.43, CI 02.8–0.66) compared to CT, but distant recurrences were more common with C-RT versus CT (28% vs 21%, HR 1.36, CI 1–1.86). Thus, although C-RT reduced the rate of local recurrence compared to CT, the combined modality regimen did not increase RFS in optimally debulked, stage III/IVA endometrial cancer.[135]

The randomized PORTEC-3 intergroup trial was initiated to investigate benefit of adjuvant chemotherapy during and after radiotherapy (CTRT) versus pelvic radiotherapy (RT) alone for women with high-risk endometrial cancer.[136] High risk included stage I grade 3 with deep myometrial invasion and/or LVSI; stage II or III; or serous/clear cell histology. Patients were randomly allocated (1 : 1) to RT or CTRT (two cycles of concurrent cisplatin week 1 and 4 of RT, followed by four cycles of carboplatin and paclitaxel. The co-primary endpoints were overall survival (OS) and failure-free survival (FFS). Grade 2 or worse adverse events were more common in the C-RT group (38%) versus the RT group (23%) ($p = 0.002$). At a median follow-up of 72.6 months, 5-year OS for CTRT versus RT was 81.4% versus 76.1%; adjusted HR 0.70 (95% CI 0.51–0.97, $p = 0.034$). Five-year FFS was 76.5% (CTRT) versus 69.1% (RT), overall HR 0.70 (0.52–0.94, $p = 0.016$). In the post hoc analysis of survival outcomes, patients with stage III and serous cancers or both had the greatest benefit. Thus, adjuvant chemotherapy given during and after pelvic radiotherapy showed significantly improved overall survival and failure-free survival compared to radiotherapy alone. This treatment schedule should be discussed and recommended, especially for women with stage III or serous cancers, or both, as part of shared decision-making between doctors and patients.[136,137]

The decision between chemotherapy alone versus CTRT remains quite controversial. Patients with nodal involvement certainly benefit from chemotherapy and may be treated with CTRT in order to reduce the risk of local recurrence and potentially improve FFS (Figure 3). Part of the decision-making for each patient will involve a thorough discussion of risks and benefits of these regimens. In general, rates of grade 3 toxicity are similar between CTRT and adjuvant chemotherapy, with chemotherapy demonstrating higher levels of myelosuppression and CTRT causing more gastrointestinal toxicity such as diarrhea and abdominal pain.[135,136]

Adjuvant chemotherapy for high-risk early-stage disease
Systemic therapy is a standard of care for stage IV endometrial cancer. Appropriate regimens and data are discussed in the section on recurrent disease.

With regard to chemotherapy in high-risk early-stage disease, Stringer et al.[138] studied 31 patients with high-risk stage I endometrial cancer and 2 patients with occult stage II disease. Postoperatively, the patients were treated with cisplatin, 50 mg/m^2, doxorubicin, 50 mg/m^2, and cyclophosphamide, 500 mg/m^2, (CAP) every 4 weeks for six cycles. The 2-year progression-free interval rate was 79%, and the 2-year survival was 83%. The median survival time for patients was not reached at 45 months. These results were considered superior to those of historical controls from the same institution. However, the GOG randomized patients with high-risk clinical stage I and stage II disease to postoperative whole-pelvis irradiation with or without doxorubicin and found no difference in PFI and OS.[139]

The Japanese GOG was designed to address the relative efficacy of CAP chemotherapy versus WPRT in stages IC to III. Although there was no difference in PFS or OS in the entire cohort—a subgroup analysis of 120 high intermediate-risk patients reported improved PFR and OS.[140] GOG 249 is a phase III trial that examined vaginal cuff brachytherapy followed by three cycles of paclitaxel/carboplatin chemotherapy versus external beam RT in patients with high-risk uterine confined endometrial carcinoma. Ultimately, there was no significant difference in survival

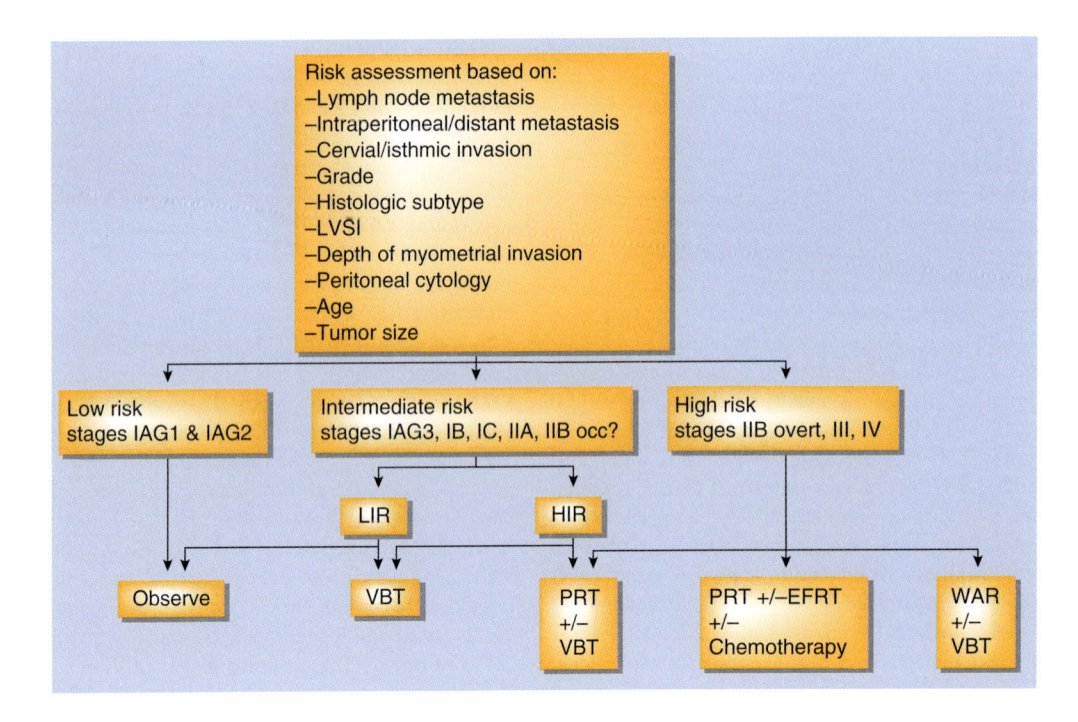

Figure 3 Postoperative management of endometrial carcinoma. EFRT, extended field radiation therapy; PRT, pelvic radiation therapy; VBT, vaginal brachytherapy; WAR, whole abdominopelvic radiotherapy; LIR, low intermediate risk; HIR, high intermediate risk based on Gynecologic Oncology Group 99: age <50, 50–70; >70, LVSI, lymph-vascular space invasion, outer third invasion, grade 2 or 3 (see text).

outcomes between the groups and worse toxicity in the cuff and chemotherapy group.[141]

In general, early-stage uterine serous cancers are treated with chemotherapy (paclitaxel/carboplatin) due to their poor prognosis and high likelihood of recurrence. The majority of data supporting this are retrospective in nature. In a study of 74 patients with stage I USC, Kelly et al. have demonstrated that all patients with residual disease (including disease confined to the endometrium) have improved PRI and OS with adjuvant platinum-based chemotherapy. There were no vaginal recurrences in those receiving vaginal brachytherapy.[45,142] Because clear cell carcinoma behaves like UPSC, despite the absence of data, they are treated in a similar fashion with paclitaxel and carboplatin chemotherapy and vaginal brachytherapy.[45,51]

Treatment of recurrent disease

Radiotherapy
Patients who develop isolated vaginal recurrences without previous radiation can expect a salvage rate of 80% with radiotherapy.[143] Those who develop a component of extra pelvic recurrence will require systemic therapy.

In the patient who has had initial adjuvant postoperative pelvic irradiation, there may rarely be a role for interstitial therapy at relapse if there is isolated central pelvic failure. For some systemic therapy may be applicable. For patients with other sites of disease or bony, cerebral, or nodal metastases, short courses of palliative irradiation may be useful in relieving the symptoms of disease. Similarly, palliative irradiation may be used for the uncommon patient (approximately 3% of those at presentation) who has stage IV disease.

Surgery
Surgery can be considered in specific cases of recurrent endometrial cancer. Isolated vagina recurrence after radiation can be definitively treated with pelvic exenteration (removal of all pelvic organs including bladder, rectum, vagina). Patients should be carefully chosen based on disease location, treatment-free interval, and performance status. In a large retrospective study of patients treated with exenteration, 5-year recurrence-free survival was 45% and overall survival was 55%.[144] These data are in line with other small retrospective studies that included this patient population.[145–147]

Support for secondary surgical cytoreduction in recurrent endometrial cancer has also been evaluated in a number of retrospective studies. Barlin and colleagues performed a meta-analysis of 672 patients in 14 studies that underwent cytoreduction in advanced or recurrent endometrial cancer and found that achieving a no gross residual disease resection was associated with overall survival benefit.[121]

Cytotoxic chemotherapy
If one selects only drugs that have achieved at least a 20% response rate in studies including at least 20 patients, the list of active agents in endometrial cancer is small (Table 6). The GOG studied single-agent doxorubicin at a dose rate of 60 mg/m^2 IV every 3 weeks and reported a 37% response rate in 43 patients.[148] Although the most frequent adverse effect was on the hematopoietic system, cardiac toxicity occurred in 12%, and there was one cardiotoxic death in a patient who had received more than 500 mg/m^2 of drug. This study was important because it clearly established the value of doxorubicin as a single agent in the chemotherapy of endometrial cancer. Studies by GOG and The Eastern Cooperative Oncology Group demonstrated no benefit from adding cyclophosphamide (Table 5).[149,150]

Table 5 Single-agent cytotoxic chemotherapy for endometrial cancer.[a]

Agent	References	N	Prior treatment	No CR + PR	(%)
Paclitaxel	151	28	No	4 + 6	36
Paclitaxel	152	19	Yes	2 + 5	37
Cisplatin	189, 190	75	No	3 + 18	28
Carboplatin	191–193	76	No	5 + 18	28
Doxorubicin	148, 153, 194	280	No	31 + 49	29
Epirubicin	195	27	No	2 + 5	26
Fluorouracil	196	34	NS	7	21
HMM	197	30	No	10	33
Docetaxel	198	35	No	3 + 4	21
Topotecan	199, 200	42	No	3 + 5	20

Note: Reported series with at least 20 patients with a response rate of at least 20%.
Abbreviations: HMM, Hexamethylmelamine; CR, complete response; PR, partial response; NS, not stated.
[a]Source: Modified from Muss[201] and Thigpen et al.[194]

Paclitaxel is an active drug in recurrent endometrial adenocarcinoma. Among 28 evaluable patients in a single-agent study of paclitaxel in recurrent endometrial cancer, four complete responses and six partial responses were observed, for an overall response rate of 35.7%.[151] Similarly, Lissoni and colleagues evaluated paclitaxel in 19 patients with advanced endometrial adenocarcinoma previously treated with cisplatin, doxorubicin, and cyclophosphamide.[152] Two complete responses and five partial responses were achieved, for an overall response rate of 37%.

Our best information on combination chemotherapy comes from the randomized phase III trials listed in Table 6. The randomized trials that have included hormonal therapy are listed in Table 7. The European Organisation for Research and Treatment of Cancer (EORTC) study reported by Aapro and colleagues, a survival advantage was demonstrated with a response rate of 43% for the doxorubicin and cisplatin combination versus 17% for single-agent doxorubicin ($p < 0.001$).[153] The GOG found no difference when doxorubicin and cisplatin were administered in a circadian fashion compared with a standard fashion.[154] The GOG also conducted a phase III study of doxorubicin plus cisplatin versus doxorubicin plus 24-hour paclitaxel in primary stage III or IV or recurrent endometrial carcinoma. This study found no difference in response rate, progression-free survival, or overall survival.[155]

The next phase III prospective randomized GOG study (Protocol 177) compared standard doxorubicin (60 mg/m^2) and cisplatin (50 mg/m^2), that is, AP against TAP with paclitaxel (Taxol 160 mg/m^2/3 h), doxorubicin (45 mg/m^2), and cisplatin (50 mg/m^2).[156] Two hundred and sixty-six patients were randomized, and the results indicated that TAP produced a significant improvement in response rate (57% vs 34%; $p < 0.01$), progression-free survival (median 8.3 vs 5.3 months; $p < 0.01$) and overall survival (median 15.3 vs 12.3 months; $p = 0.037$). Neurologic toxicity was worse for those receiving TAP, with 12% grade 3, and 27% grade 2 peripheral neuropathy.

The GOG followed up with GOG Protocol 209 which randomly assigned patients with advanced (stage IVB) or recurrent disease to either TAP or paclitaxel and carboplatin (TC). This phase III trial demonstrated similar oncologic outcomes in regards to PFS and OS, but the toxicity and tolerability profile favored TC.[157] This established the TC regimen as standard of care for upfront advanced stage or recurrent endometrial cancer. Doxorubicin is now utilized as a second-line agent as noted above.

Hormone therapy

Progestins

Endometrial cancer is driven by estrogen, thus, exploration of progesterone, which has an anti-estrogenic effect in the endometrium is rationale. The optimum dose for progestational treatment has not been determined and the doses employed in the most recent GOG studies were based on dose-seeking studies by Kohorn and Thigpen.[158,159] There is no evidence that lower doses are not equally effective, and there is no advantage for the parenteral route,[160] therefore, selecting lower doses in special circumstances may be permissible in order to avoid complications.

In summary, the following generalizations can be made concerning progestational therapy in the advanced and recurrent setting: (1) the response rate ranges from 10% to 30%, probably relating to the receptor level in the tumor; (2) well-differentiated cancers respond best; (3) the PR level diminishes sharply as the grade of the tumor increases; (4) clinical responses may not occur before 7 to 12 weeks of therapy; (5) two-thirds of patients will not respond; (6) there is no published evidence that progestational agents employed in an adjuvant mode offer any benefit; (7) appropriate oral doses based on GOG studies are 160 mg/d of megestrol or 200 mg/d of MPA, however, lower doses can be individualized.

Progestins can also be utilized to avoid hysterectomy in women with early-stage endometrial cancer. Ramirez and colleagues,

Table 6 Randomized trials of combination chemotherapy regimens for endometrial cancer.

Author	Year	Regimen	Number evaluable	RR (%)	Median PFS (months)	Median overall survival (months)
Thigpen et al.[150]	1994	A	132	22	3.2	6.7
		AC	144	30	3.9	7.3
Thigpen et al.[194]	2004	A	150	25	3.8	9.2
		AP	131	42[a]	5.7[a]	9.0
Aapro et al.[153]	2003	A	87	17	7.0	7.0
		AP	90	43[a]	8.0	9.0[a]
Gallion et al.[154]	2003	AP standard	169	46	6.5	11.2
		AP circadian	173	49	5.9	13.2
Fleming et al.[155]	2004	AP	157	40	7.2	12.6
		AT	160	43	6.0	13.6
Fleming et al.[156]	2004	AP	129	34	5.3	12.3
		TAP	134	57[a]	8.3[a]	15.3[a]

Abbreviations: PFS, Progression-free survival; RR, response rate = complete response + partial response; C, cyclophosphamide; A, doxorubicin (Adriamycin); P, cisplatin; F, 5-fluorouracil; T, paclitaxel.
[a]Significant difference.

Table 7 Randomized trials of combination chemotherapy + hormonal therapy for endometrial cancer.

Author	Year	Regimen	No evaluable	RR (%)
Horton et al.[202]	1982	CA + MA	55	27
		CAF + MA	56	16
Cohen et al.[203]	1984	F-Mel + MA	126	38
		CAF + MA	131	36
Ayoub et al.[204]	1988	CAF	20	15
		CAF + MPA/TAM	23	43[a]
Cornelison et al.[205]	1995	APE + MA	50	54
		F-Mel + MPA	50	48

Abbreviations: RR, response rate = complete response + partial response; C, cyclophosphamide; A, doxorubicin (Adriamycin); P, cisplatin; F, 5-fluorouracil; Mel, melphalan; MA, megestrol acetate; MPA, medroxyprogesterone acetate; TAM, tamoxifen.
[a]Significant difference.

in reviewing the literature, found that the majority of patients reported with well-differentiated endometrial adenocarcinoma who undergo conservative treatment with a progestational agent respond to treatment (62 of 81 = 76%). When an initial response is not achieved or when disease recurs after an initial response (15 of 62 = 24%), carcinoma extending beyond the uterus is rare.[161] In addition, several clinical trials have demonstrated that the levonorgestrel intrauterine device has acceptable levels of efficacy and toxicity in patients who are not ideal surgical candidates due to desire for future fertility or poor medical condition.[162,163]

Tamoxifen
Hormonal therapy by agents other than progestogens has been studied by many researchers. Extrapolating from the experience with breast cancer, investigators employed tamoxifen in doses of 20–40 mg daily for patients with advanced or recurrent endometrial carcinoma. In a review of eight published studies, Moore and colleagues described an overall response rate of 22%.[164] As one might predict, there is a wide spectrum of reported responses, ranging from 0% to 53%.[165] Not unlike the progestin experience, it would seem that tamoxifen is more likely to be effective in patients with low-grade tumors, receptor positivity, and either no previous hormone therapy or a previous response to progestin therapy.

Because progestins ultimately down-regulate PRs, and because tamoxifen induces these receptors in target tissues, the notion of the combined administration of these hormones has been examined by the GOG with two different strategies. In Whitney and colleagues' report, tamoxifen citrate 40 mg/d combined with alternating weekly cycles of MPA 200 mg/d in 58 patients with recurrent or measurable advanced endometrial carcinoma resulted in a 33% response rate (10.3% complete response and 23.4% partial response), with a median progression-free interval of 3 months and a median overall survival of 13 months.[166] In the Fiorica study, alternating 3-week courses of MA (160 mg/d) and tamoxifen citrate (40 mg/d) in 56 patients with recurrent or measurable advanced endometrial carcinoma produced a 27% response rate (21.4% complete response and 5.4% partial response), with a median progression-free interval of 2.7 months and a median overall survival of 14.0 months.[167] It is important to note that these agents are very well tolerated due to low risk of toxicity, however, an increased risk of thrombosis may be observed.

Other hormones
Gonadotropin-releasing hormone analogs have been tested in small phase II trials of patients with recurrent endometrial carcinoma, with response rates varying from 0% to 35%.[168–170]

Aromatase inhibitors have been tested in a limited fashion. The GOG phase II trial had a 9% response rate (2 partial responses of 23) with anastrozole,[171–173] whereas the Canadian National Cancer Institute study reported a 9.4% response rate (2 partial responses of 28) with letrozole.[174] These agents can be considered as second-line agents but we have seen improved response and clinical benefit when these agents are combined with other targeted therapies, discussed below.

Targeted therapy
Due to low response rates achieved by chemotherapy and the wealth of molecular aberrations found in endometrial cancer, a number of biologic therapies have been evaluated. Several anti-angiogenics have been explored, including bevacizumab, which have yielded a response rate of 13.5% and an overall survival of 10.5 months.[175] Subsequent studies of the addition of bevacizumab to chemotherapy in advanced stage and recurrent endometrial cancer did not yield a progression-free survival benefit.[176] The high rate of HER2 over-expression and amplification in uterine serous tumors led to exploration of HER2 targeted agents in this disease. In a randomized phase II trial with 61 patients, the addition of trastuzumab to carboplatin/paclitaxel increased PFS and OS in women with advanced/recurrent HER2/Neu-positive USC, with the greatest benefit seen for the treatment of stages III to IV disease.[177] Thus, testing for HER2 and inclusion of trastuzumab is indicated for women with uterine serous disease that is chemo-naïve. Use of other HER2-targeted agents in the recurrent setting is under exploration for this histology type.

As noted above, members of the PI3K/AKT pathway are frequently aberrant in endometrial cancer. Two trials of the mTOR inhibitor, temsirolimus, in endometrial cancer have demonstrated encouraging single-agent activity.[178,179] A phase II trial of the mTOR inhibitor everolimus combined with an aromatase inhibitor letrozole demonstrated a 32% response rate ($n = 35$; nine complete responses and two partial responses) in patients with recurrent endometrial cancer, leading to a subsequent randomized trial comparing this combination to dual hormonal therapy with medroxyprogesterone acetate and tamoxifen.[179,180] The combination of everolimus yielded improved PFS when compared to the hormonal regimen.

Immunotherapy
As immune therapy has expanded in the oncology world, endometrial cancer has been a key disease site for exploration due to high mutational burden. Pembrolizumab, a programmed death-1 (PD-1) inhibitor yielded impressive response rates in cancers with mismatch repair deficiency (MMRd) at different organ sites.[181] This led to an approval in any MMRd tumor, regardless of primary site. A number of other PD-1 and PD-L1 inhibitors have been studied in endometrial cancer, yielding consistent results and evidence of activity in MMRd tumors.[182–185] Conversely, in mismatch repair proficient (MMRp) tumors, activity of single-agent checkpoint inhibition has been rather low.[182–185] Thus, the combination of lenvatinib, a multi-target tyrosine kinase inhibitor with anti-angiogenic effects, was explored in a cohort of women with MMRp endometrial cancer. The impressive response rate of 38%, which included endometrioid, serous, and clear cell histotypes, yielded FDA approval of the combination in 2019. Impressively, duration of response is high at 21.9 months, but toxicity is quite high as well with 67% of patients experience grade 3 or above adverse events. Use of dose reductions and interruptions is critical

to manage issues such as fatigue, diarrhea, and hypertension.[186,187] The bottom line for patients with endometrial cancer is that all women should be tested for mismatch repair proteins and MSI to assist with the treatment decision between single-agent checkpoint inhibition versus the combination of pembrolizumab and lenvatinib.

The future

Efforts must continue to expand information about molecular characteristics to better define patient susceptibilities and therapeutic possibilities. Randomized studies understanding the role of targeted agents and immunotherapy in both early and advanced-stage disease will provide critical information to define a new standard of care. In addition, prioritization of rational combination strategies to improve success of targeted therapy and immune therapy is essential in this disease. Novel targets and agents including HER2, WEE1, PARP1, and MEK inhibitors have potential to change practice, both alone as well as part of doublet and triplet regimens. Certainly, with a cure rate in the United States of approximately 80%, it will be essential that patients with poor prognostic features or recurrent or metastatic disease be entered into collaborative trials to maximize the opportunities for improving survival.

Key references

The complete reference list can be found on Vital Source version of this title, see inside front cover.

1. Siegel RL, Miller KD, Jemal A. Cancer statistics, 2020. *CA Cancer J Clin.* 2020;**70**:7–30.
3. Doll KM, Snyder CR, Ford CL. Endometrial cancer disparities: a race-conscious critique of the literature. *Am J Obstet Gynecol.* 2018;**218**:474–482 e2.
4. Morice P, Leary A, Creutzberg C, et al. Endometrial cancer. *Lancet.* 2016;**387**:1094–1108.
5. Kaaks R, Lukanova A, Kurzer MS. Obesity, endogenous hormones, and endometrial cancer risk: a synthetic review. *Cancer Epidemiol Biomarkers Prev.* 2002;**11**:1531–1543.
13. Brinton LA, Hoover RN. Estrogen replacement therapy and endometrial cancer risk: unresolved issues. The Endometrial Cancer Collaborative Group. *Obstet Gynecol.* 1993;**81**:265–271.
22. Iversen L, Sivasubramaniam S, Lee AJ, et al. Lifetime cancer risk and combined oral contraceptives: the Royal College of General Practitioners' Oral Contraception Study. *Am J Obstet Gynecol.* 2017;**216**:580 e1–e9.
28. Fisher B, Costantino JP, Redmond CK, et al. Endometrial cancer in tamoxifen-treated breast cancer patients: findings from the National Surgical Adjuvant Breast and Bowel Project (NSABP) B-14. *J Natl Cancer Inst.* 1994;**86**:527–537.
32. Barakat RR, Wong G, Curtin JP, et al. Tamoxifen use in breast cancer patients who subsequently develop corpus cancer is not associated with a higher incidence of adverse histologic features. *Gynecol Oncol.* 1994;**55**:164–168.
36. Runowicz CD, Costantino MT, Kavanah M, et al. National surgical adjuvant breast and bowel project breast cancer prevention trial summary analysis of transvaginal sonography and endometrial biopsy in detecting endometrial pathology. *J Clin Oncol.* 1999;**358a**:18.
37. Hampel H, Stephens JA, Pukkala E, et al. Cancer risk in hereditary nonpolyposis colorectal cancer syndrome: later age of onset. *Gastroenterology.* 2005;**129**:415–421.
40. Schmeler KM, Lynch HT, Chen LM, et al. Prophylactic surgery to reduce the risk of gynecologic cancers in the Lynch syndrome. *N Engl J Med.* 2006;**354**:261–269.
43. Kurman RJ, Kaminski PF, Norris HJ. The behavior of endometrial hyperplasia. A long-term study of "untreated" hyperplasia in 170 patients. *Cancer.* 1985;**56**:403–412.
45. Boruta DM 2nd, Gehrig PA, Fader AN, Olawaiye AB. Management of women with uterine papillary serous cancer: a Society of Gynecologic Oncology (SGO) review. *Gynecol Oncol.* 2009;**115**:142–153.
51. Olawaiye AB, Boruta DM 2nd, Management of women with clear cell endometrial cancer: a Society of Gynecologic Oncology (SGO) review. *Gynecol Oncol.* 2009;**113**:277–283.
52. McCluggage WG. Malignant biphasic uterine tumours: carcinosarcomas or metaplastic carcinomas? *J Clin Pathol.* 2002;**55**:321–325.
53. Cancer Genome Atlas Research, Kandoth C, Schultz N, et al. Integrated genomic characterization of endometrial carcinoma. *Nature.* 2013;**497**:67–73.
55. Cheung LWT, Hennessy BT, Li J, et al. High frequency of PIK3R1 and PIK3R2 mutations in endometrial cancer elucidates a novel mechanism for regulation of PTEN protein stability. *Cancer Discov.* 2011;**1**:170–185.
60. Basil JB, Goodfellow PJ, Rader JS, et al. Clinical significance of microsatellite instability in endometrial carcinoma. *Cancer.* 2000;**89**:1758–1764.
68. Group SGOCPECW, Burke WM, Orr J, et al. Endometrial cancer: a review and current management strategies: part I. *Gynecol Oncol.* 2014;**134**:385–392.
78. Antonsen SL, Jensen LN, Loft A, et al. MRI, PET/CT and ultrasound in the preoperative staging of endometrial cancer — a multicenter prospective comparative study. *Gynecol Oncol.* 2013;**128**:300–308.
84. Creasman WT, Morrow CP, Bundy BN, et al. Surgical pathologic spread patterns of endometrial cancer. A gynecologic oncology group study. *Cancer.* 1987;**60**:2035–2041.
88. Pecorelli S. Revised FIGO staging for carcinoma of the vulva, cervix, and endometrium. *Int J Gynaecol Obstet.* 2009;**105**:103–104.
92. Salvesen HB, Iversen OE, Akslen LA. Prognostic impact of morphometric nuclear grade of endometrial carcinoma. *Cancer.* 1998;**83**:956–964.
101. Walker JL, Piedmonte MR, Spirtos NM, et al. Recurrence and survival after random assignment to laparoscopy versus laparotomy for comprehensive surgical staging of uterine cancer: gynecologic oncology group LAP2 study. *J Clin Oncol.* 2012;**30**:695–700.
111. Ind T, Laios A, Hacking M, Nobbenhuis M. A comparison of operative outcomes between standard and robotic laparoscopic surgery for endometrial cancer: A systematic review and meta-analysis. *Int J Med Robot Comput Assist Surg: MRCAS.* 2017:13.
112. ASTEC Study Group, Kitchener H, Swart AM, et al. Efficacy of systematic pelvic lymphadenectomy in endometrial cancer (MRC ASTEC trial): a randomised study. *Lancet.* 2009;**373**:125–136.
113. Benedetti Panici P, Basile S, Maneschi F, et al. Systematic pelvic lymphadenectomy vs. no lymphadenectomy in early-stage endometrial carcinoma: randomized clinical trial. *J Natl Cancer Inst.* 2008;**100**:1707–1716.
114. Darai E, Dubernard G, Bats AS, et al. Sentinel node biopsy for the management of early stage endometrial cancer: long-term results of the SENTI-ENDO study. *Gynecol Oncol.* 2015;**136**:54–59.
115. Soliman PT, Westin SN, Dioun S, et al. A prospective validation study of sentinel lymph node mapping for high-risk endometrial cancer. *Gynecol Oncol.* 2017;**146**:234–239.
116. Rossi EC, Kowalski LD, Scalici J, et al. A comparison of sentinel lymph node biopsy to lymphadenectomy for endometrial cancer staging (FIRES trial): a multicentre, prospective, cohort study. *Lancet Oncol.* 2017;**18**:384–392.
121. Barlin JN, Puri I, Bristow RE. Cytoreductive surgery for advanced or recurrent endometrial cancer: a meta-analysis. *Gynecol Oncol.* 2010;**118**:14–18.
127. Dutta SW, Trifiletti DM, Grover S, et al. Management of elderly patients with early-stage medically inoperable endometrial cancer: systematic review and National Cancer Database analysis. *Brachytherapy.* 2017;**16**:526–533.
130. Keys HM, Roberts JA, Brunetto VL, et al. A phase III trial of surgery with or without adjunctive external pelvic radiation therapy in intermediate risk endometrial adenocarcinoma: a Gynecologic Oncology Group study. *Gynecol Oncol.* 2004;**92**:744–751.
131. Creutzberg CL, van Putten WL, Koper PC, et al. Surgery and postoperative radiotherapy versus surgery alone for patients with stage-1 endometrial carcinoma: multicentre randomised trial. PORTEC Study Group. Post Operative Radiation Therapy in Endometrial Carcinoma. *Lancet.* 2000;**355**:1404–1411.
132. Nout RA, Smit VT, Putter H, et al. Vaginal brachytherapy versus pelvic external beam radiotherapy for patients with endometrial cancer of high-intermediate risk (PORTEC-2): an open-label, non-inferiority, randomised trial. *Lancet.* 2010;**375**:816–823.
135. Matei D, Filiaci V, Randall ME, et al. Adjuvant Chemotherapy plus Radiation for Locally Advanced Endometrial Cancer. *N Engl J Med.* 2019;**380**:2317–2326.
136. de Boer SM, Powell ME, Mileshkin L, et al. Adjuvant chemoradiotherapy versus radiotherapy alone for women with high-risk endometrial cancer (PORTEC-3): final results of an international, open-label, multicentre, randomised, phase 3 trial. *Lancet Oncol.* 2018;**19**:295–309.
137. de Boer SM, Powell ME, Mileshkin L, et al. Adjuvant chemoradiotherapy versus radiotherapy alone in women with high-risk endometrial cancer (PORTEC-3): patterns of recurrence and post-hoc survival analysis of a randomised phase 3 trial. *Lancet Oncol.* 2019;**20**:1273–1285.
141. Randall ME, Filiaci V, McMeekin DS, et al. Phase III trial: adjuvant pelvic radiation therapy versus vaginal brachytherapy plus paclitaxel/carboplatin in high-intermediate and high-risk early stage endometrial cancer. *J Clin Oncol.* 2019;**37**:1810–1818.
144. Westin SN, Rallapalli V, Fellman B, et al. Overall survival after pelvic exenteration for gynecologic malignancy. *Gynecol Oncol.* 2014;**134**:546–551.
153. van Wijk FH, Aapro MS, Bolis G, et al. Doxorubicin versus doxorubicin and cisplatin in endometrial carcinoma: definitive results of a randomised

154. Gallion HH, Brunetto VL, Cibull M, et al. Randomized phase III trial of standard timed doxorubicin plus cisplatin versus circadian timed doxorubicin plus cisplatin in stage III and IV or recurrent endometrial carcinoma: a Gynecologic Oncology Group Study. *J Clin Oncol*. 2003;**21**:3808–3813.
155. Fleming GF, Filiaci VL, Bentley RC, et al. Phase III randomized trial of doxorubicin + cisplatin versus doxorubicin + 24-h paclitaxel + filgrastim in endometrial carcinoma: a Gynecologic Oncology Group study. *Ann Oncol*. 2004;**15**:1173–1178.
156. Fleming GF, Brunetto VL, Cella D, et al. Phase III trial of doxorubicin plus cisplatin with or without paclitaxel plus filgrastim in advanced endometrial carcinoma: a Gynecologic Oncology Group Study. *J Clin Oncol*. 2004;**22**:2159–2166.
157. Miller DS, Filiaci VL, Mannel RS, et al. Carboplatin and Paclitaxel for Advanced Endometrial Cancer: Final Overall Survival and Adverse Event Analysis of a Phase III Trial (NRG Oncology/GOG0209). *J Clin Oncol*. 2020:JCO2001076.
159. Thigpen JT, Brady MF, Alvarez RD, et al. Oral medroxyprogesterone acetate in the treatment of advanced or recurrent endometrial carcinoma: a dose-response study by the Gynecologic Oncology Group. *J Clin Oncol*. 1999;**17**:1736–1744.
162. Westin SN, Fellman B, Sun CC, et al. Prospective phase II trial of levonorgestrel intrauterine device: nonsurgical approach for complex atypical hyperplasia and early-stage endometrial cancer. *Am J Obstet Gynecol*. 2020.
163. Minig L, Franchi D, Boveri S, et al. Progestin intrauterine device and GnRH analogue for uterus-sparing treatment of endometrial precancers and well-differentiated early endometrial carcinoma in young women. *Ann Oncol*. 2011;**22**:643–649.
166. Whitney CW, Brunetto VL, Zaino RJ, et al. Phase II study of medroxyprogesterone acetate plus tamoxifen in advanced endometrial carcinoma: a Gynecologic Oncology Group study. *Gynecol Oncol*. 2004;**92**:4–9.
167. Fiorica JV, Brunetto VL, Hanjani P, et al. Phase II trial of alternating courses of megestrol acetate and tamoxifen in advanced endometrial carcinoma: a Gynecologic Oncology Group study. *Gynecol Oncol*. 2004;**92**:10–14.
175. Aghajanian C, Sill MW, Darcy KM, et al. Phase II trial of bevacizumab in recurrent or persistent endometrial cancer: a Gynecologic Oncology Group study. *J Clin Oncol*. 2011;**29**:2259–2265.
177. Fader AN, Roque DM, Siegel E, et al. Randomized phase II trial of carboplatin-paclitaxel compared with carboplatin-paclitaxel-trastuzumab in advanced (stage III-IV) or recurrent uterine serous carcinomas that overexpress Her2/Neu (NCT01367002): updated overall survival analysis. *Clin Cancer Res*. 2020;**26**: 3928–3935.
178. Oza AM, Elit L, Tsao MS, et al. Phase II study of temsirolimus in women with recurrent or metastatic endometrial cancer: a trial of the NCIC clinical trials group. *J Clin Oncol*. 2011;**29**:3278–3285.
179. Fleming GF, Filiaci VL, Marzullo B, et al. Temsirolimus with or without megestrol acetate and tamoxifen for endometrial cancer: a gynecologic oncology group study. *Gynecol Oncol*. 2014;**132**:585–592.
180. Slomovitz BM, Jiang Y, Yates MS, et al. Phase II study of everolimus and letrozole in patients with recurrent endometrial carcinoma. *J Clin Oncol*. 2015;**33**: 930–936.
181. Le DT, Durham JN, Smith KN, et al. Mismatch repair deficiency predicts response of solid tumors to PD-1 blockade. *Science*. 2017;**357**:409–413.
182. Marabelle A, Le DT, Ascierto PA, et al. Efficacy of pembrolizumab in patients with noncolorectal high microsatellite instability/mismatch repair-deficient cancer: results from the phase II KEYNOTE-158 study. *J Clin Oncol*. 2020;**38**:1–10.
186. Makker V, Rasco D, Vogelzang NJ, et al. Lenvatinib plus pembrolizumab in patients with advanced endometrial cancer: an interim analysis of a multicentre, open-label, single-arm, phase 2 trial. *Lancet Oncol*. 2019;**20**:711–718.

101 Epithelial ovarian, fallopian tube, and peritoneal cancer

Jonathan S. Berek, MD, MMS ■ Malte Renz, MD, PhD ■ Michael L. Friedlander, MD, PhD ■ Robert C. Bast Jr., MD

Overview

Most epithelial ovarian, fallopian tube, and peritoneal cancers initially present in advanced-stage and respond to surgery and platinum-based chemotherapy. However, in the majority of these women, the disease eventually recurs and cannot be cured. Ovarian cancer has the highest fatality-to-case ratio of all gynecologic cancers.[1,2] The lifetime risk for ovarian cancer in the general population is 1 in 75; the prevalence in the postmenopausal population in the United States 1 in 2500. Germline mutations of *BRCA1* and *BRCA2* are associated with 10–15% of ovarian cancers and increase the risk of ovarian cancer dramatically. Factors that contribute to persistent ovulation increase the risk in women with sporadic disease, whereas oral contraceptives decrease its risk. While epithelial ovarian cancers were thought to arise from the ovarian surface epithelium or the lining of inclusion cysts beneath the ovarian surface, it has been recognized that many high-grade serous "ovarian" carcinomas and peritoneal cancers arise in the fimbriae of the fallopian tube.[3–10] Epithelial ovarian cancers can exhibit serous, endometrioid, mucinous or clear cell histotypes. Low-grade type I ovarian cancers grow slowly, can evolve from tumors of low malignant potential, bear predominantly *Ras* mutations, express wild type *TP53*, and respond less frequently to platinum- and taxane-based therapy. High-grade type II ovarian cancers grow rapidly, arise from precursors with *TP53* mutations, are driven by DNA copy number changes, present in late stage (III–IV) and frequently respond to platinum-based combination chemotherapy. Due to a lack of specific symptoms or effective screening, more than 70% of ovarian cancers are diagnosed in advanced stage (III–IV). Primary treatment of epithelial ovarian cancer involves cytoreductive surgery and six cycles of carboplatin and paclitaxel. Maintenance therapy has been established in primary and secondary treatment with targeted agents such as PARP-inhibitors and bevacizumab depending on for example, *BRCA* mutational status. Recurrent disease with few exceptions cannot be cured with currently available agents, but survival can be prolonged with combinations of cytotoxic agents including retreatment with paclitaxel and carboplatin. Palliative agents include liposomal doxorubicin, gemcitabine, topotecan, bevacizumab, and etoposide. New therapy for low-grade cancers involves MEK inhibitors, whereas trials of immunotherapy are underway in patients with high-grade epithelial ovarian cancers.

Epidemiology and etiology

Incidence, prevalence and mortality

In 2019, more than 22,500 new cases of ovarian cancer were diagnosed in the United States and almost 14,000 deaths registered.[2] Ovarian cancer prevalence is highest in women 55–64 years of age (median age 63), mortality is highest in women 65–74 years of age (median age 70).[2] Thus, ovarian, fallopian tube, and peritoneal cancers are predominantly diseases of postmenopausal women, with only 10–15% of all cases diagnosed in premenopause[1,2] and less than 1% in women younger than 30 years of age. The prevalence of ovarian cancer among postmenopausal women in the United States is 40 per 100,000 or 1 in 2500. The lifetime risk for a woman to develop ovarian cancer is approximately 1 in 75 (1.3%), compared to 1 in 8 for breast cancer. Based on surveillance, epidemiology, and end results (SEERs) data, both incidence and mortality of ovarian cancer have decreased over the years. The incidence decreased by 38% from 16 in 1976 to 10 per 100,000 women per year in 2016; mortality decreased by 32% from 10 to 6.8 over the same time span. In parallel, the 5-year survival for all stages increased from 33.6% in 1975 to 47.6% in 2009 to 2015.[2]

The incidence of ovarian cancer varies between ethnicities and different geographic locations. The incidence of epithelial ovarian cancer in the United States is about 1.5 times greater in Caucasians than Blacks. The incidence of epithelial ovarian cancer in Western countries, including the United States and the United Kingdom, is three to seven times greater than in Japan. Japanese immigrants to the United States, however, exhibit a significant increase in the incidence of ovarian cancer approaching that of white women from the United States.[10]

Etiology

In the past, most epithelial ovarian cancers were thought to arise from a single layer of epithelial cells covering the ovarian surface or lining so-called inclusion cysts located immediately underneath the ovarian surface. However, there is increasing molecular and genetic evidence that a majority of the high-grade serous ovarian cancers which form more than half of epithelial ovarian cancers are derived from the fimbriae of the fallopian tube.[5–9] Serous tubal intraepithelial carcinoma (STIC) appears to be the precursor of high-grade serous ovarian cancer.[11] Some high-grade serous ovarian cancers may be derived from developmental remnants of the secondary Müllerian system.[12] Regardless of origin, it is current belief that high-grade serous cancers of the ovary, fallopian tube carcinomas, and peritoneal carcinomas should be regarded as a single disease entity and managed with a common approach. Therefore, ovarian, fallopian tube and peritoneal carcinomas are included in the same Fédération Internationale de Gynécologie et d'Obstretique (FIGO) staging system.[4]

The causes of ovarian cancer are poorly understood. Prior reproductive history and number of ovulatory cycles are associated with the disease: low parity, infertility, early menarche and late menopause increase the risk.[13,14] Fertility-enhancing drugs, such as clomiphene citrate and gonadotropins used for ovulation induction were thought to increase the risk of ovarian cancer (ROCA), but the data have not consistently distinguished the influence of infertility per se from the use of fertility stimulating

Holland-Frei Cancer Medicine, Tenth Edition. Edited by Robert C. Bast, John C. Byrd, Carlo M. Croce, Ernest Hawk, Fadlo R. Khuri, Raphael E. Pollock, Apostolia M. Tsimberidou, Christopher G. Willett, and Cheryl L. Willman.
© 2023 John Wiley & Sons, Inc. Published 2023 by John Wiley & Sons, Inc.

agents.[15–18] A pooled analysis of eight case-control studies found an association of fertility stimulating drugs with serous borderline tumors, but not with invasive ovarian cancers.[18] Although many case-control and cohort studies failed to link hormone replacement therapy to an increased ROCA,[19] a large cohort study reopened controversy regarding this issue.[20] Women who had received estrogen replacement therapy only for more than 10 years without progestin were at increased risk of developing ovarian cancer. By 20 years, the relative risk was 3.2-fold. This is supported by a recent meta-analysis. Among women last recorded as current users, risk was increased even with <5 years of use (RR 1.43, CI = 1.31–1.56). The authors concluded that the increased risk may be causal and that women who use hormone therapy for 5 years from around age 50 years have about one extra ovarian cancer per 1000 users.[21] Case-control studies have pointed to an association of white race, high-fat diet and galactose consumption with a higher incidence of the disease.[22] Cigarette smoking has been linked to mucinous ovarian cancers, but not to the more common serous carcinomas.[23]

Prevention

Having at least one child reduces the relative ROCA by 30–40%. The use of oral contraceptives for 5 or more years reduces the risk by 50%.[24] Women who have had two children and used oral contraceptives for 5 or more years have a 70% reduction in risk. To date, oral contraceptive medication is the only documented method of chemoprevention for ovarian cancer. When counseling patients regarding birth control options, this important benefit of oral contraceptive use should be emphasized. This is also important for women with a strong family history of ovarian cancer, even in the absence of *BRCA1* or *BRCA2* (breast cancer gene 1 or 2) mutation.[25] Surgical prevention, that is, prophylactic salpingo-oophorectomy is important, but its use depends critically on identifying women at sufficient risk.

Genetic predisposition

Hereditary ovarian cancer

The ROCA is significantly higher than that of the general population in women with a family history of breast or ovarian cancer as well as in families with Lynch syndrome.[26–45] A strong hereditary component contributes to the development of the ovarian cancer in approximately 8–13% of cases. The vast majority are caused by germline mutations in *BRCA1* and *BRCA2*. Only a smaller fraction of about 3% is caused by germline mutations in other components of the homologous recombination (HR) pathway and the DNA mismatch repair system such as RAD51, BRIP1, PALB2.[46]

BRCA1 and *BRCA2*

Most hereditary ovarian cancer results from mutations in the *BRCA1* gene, located on chromosome 17, with a smaller fraction of familial ovarian cancers associated with mutations in *BRCA2*, located on chromosome 13. Both genes are involved in DNA double-strand break repair through HR. *BRCA1*-associated ovarian cancers generally occur in women approximately 10 years earlier than those with nonhereditary tumors.[33,38] There is no significant family history in about 44% of mutation-positive women, which underscores the importance of mutation testing in all women with high-grade nonmucinous ovarian cancer as reflected in current guidelines.[47]

There is a higher carrier rate of *BRCA1* and *BRCA2* mutations in women of Ashkenazi Jewish descent, in Icelandic women, and in some other ethnic groups.[32,33] There are three specific founder mutations that are carried by the Ashkenazi population: *185delAG* and *5382insC* on *BRCA1*, and *6174delT* on *BRCA2*. The carrier rate of at least one of these mutations for a patient of Ashkenazi Jewish descent is 1 in 40 or 2.5%, while it is 1 in 300 to 800 in the general population. The increased risk is a result of the *founder effect* – that is, a higher prevalence of a mutation is found within a specific population group that was geographically or culturally isolated in the past where one or more of their ancestors carried the mutant gene.

A combined analysis of 22 studies unselected for family history has found that women who have a *BRCA1* germ line mutation have a lifetime ROCA of 39% (18–54%), and the risk has been calculated to be 11% (10–27%) in women with a *BRCA2* mutation, dependent upon the study population. Women with a *BRCA1* or *BRCA2* mutation have a risk of breast cancer as high as 65% and 45%, respectively.[37,41] The breast cancers typically occur at a young age and may be bilateral. There is a higher incidence of triple-negative (ER-, PR-, HER2-) breast cancers in women with *BRCA1* mutations. Genetic risk modifiers, for example, on 4q32.2 and 17q21.31, may explain the variable risks inferred by *BCRA* mutations that have been reported.[48]

Lynch syndrome

There are other less common genetic causes of ovarian cancer. Lynch syndrome, formerly known as *hereditary nonpolyposis colorectal cancer (HNPCC) syndrome*, confers increased risk for colorectal cancer and a wide range of other malignancies (e.g., endometrial, ovarian, and gastric cancer) as a result of a germ line mismatch repair (MMR) genetic mutation. The mutations that have been associated with this syndrome are *MLH1*, *MSH2*, *MSH6*, *PMS2*, and *EpCAM*. The risk of endometrial cancer equals or exceeds that of colorectal cancer in women with Lynch Syndrome. The diagnosis of gynecologic cancer precedes that of colorectal cancer in over half the cases, making gynecologic cancer a "sentinel cancer" for Lynch syndrome. The lifetime ROCA in women with Lynch Syndrome has been estimated at approximately 6–12%. The mean age at diagnosis is 42.7–49.5 years. There is a higher risk of endometrioid and clear cell subtypes. The majority of cases are diagnosed in stage I or II.[45]

The management of women at high risk for ovarian cancer

The management of a woman with a strong family history of epithelial ovarian cancer must be individualized and will depend on her age, reproductive plans, and the estimated level of risk. A thorough pedigree analysis is important. A geneticist should evaluate the family pedigree for at least three generations. Decisions about management are best made after careful study of the pedigree and, whenever possible, verification of the histologic diagnosis of the family members' ovarian cancer as well as the age of onset and other tumors in the family.

Data suggest that the use of oral contraceptives is associated with an up to 50% lower ROCA in women who have a *BRCA1* or *BRCA2* mutation.[49–53] The data on the effect of oral contraceptives on breast cancer risk among *BRCA* mutations carriers is conflicting, but overall oral contraceptives do not appear to increase breast cancer risk.[52,53] Tubal ligation may also decrease the ROCA in patients with a *BRCA1* but not *BRCA2* mutation, but the protective effect is not nearly as strong as risk-reducing bilateral salpingo-oophorectomy.[51,54,55]

The value of prophylactic risk-reducing bilateral salpingo-oophorectomy in these patients has been well documented.[56–61] Occult ovarian/fallopian tube cancers detected at the time of risk-reducing bilateral salpingo-oophorectomy have been reported in many studies with wide variability in reported prevalence ranging from 2.3% to 23%. The performance of a prophylactic salpingo-oophorectomy reduces the risk of BRCA-related gynecologic cancer by 96%.[6] There remains a small risk of subsequently developing a peritoneal carcinoma. The risk of developing peritoneal carcinoma was 0.8% and 1%, respectively in two series.[57,58] As discussed above, many so-called "ovarian" cancers arise from the fallopian tube and it is essential that women having prophylactic surgery have their fallopian tubes removed as well and that these are carefully assessed by the pathologist as it is easy to miss small cancers or precursor lesions, particularly in the fimbrial end of the fallopian tube.[6] Prophylactic salpingo-oophorectomy in premenopausal women also reduced the risk of developing subsequent breast cancer by 50–80%.[57,58]

The survival of women who have a *BRCA1* or *BRCA2* mutation and develop ovarian cancer is longer than that for those who do not have a mutation. In one study, the median survival for mutation carriers was 53.4 months compared with 37.8 months for those with sporadic ovarian cancer from the same institution.[62] These findings have been confirmed in a population-based study from Israel in which Chetrit et al. reported that among Ashkenazi women with ovarian cancer those with *BRCA1* and *BRCA2* mutations had an improved long-term survival (38% vs 24% at 5 years). This may result from intrinsic growth properties or from a better response to chemotherapy.[63,64]

Box 1 Recommendations

All women with a nonmucinous high-grade epithelial ovarian, fallopian tube, or peritoneal cancer should be offered testing for *BRCA*1 to *BRCA*2 mutations or multigene panel testing. The recommendations for management of women at high risk for ovarian cancers are summarized below.

1. Women who wish to preserve their reproductive capability or delay prophylactic surgery should undergo periodic screening by transvaginal ultrasonography and CA125 every 6 months, although the efficacy of this approach has not been established.
2. Oral contraceptives should be recommended to young women before a planned family. Tamoxifen may reduce risk of breast cancer.
3. Women who do not wish to maintain their fertility or completed childbearing should undergo prophylactic bilateral salpingo-oophorectomy.
4. Annual mammographic and magnetic resonance imaging (MRI) breast screening should be performed commencing at age 30 years, or younger if there are family members with documented very early-onset breast cancer. Risk-reducing bilateral mastectomy should be discussed as it reduces the risks of breast cancer by >95%.
5. Women with a documented Lynch syndrome should be counseled about prophylactic hysterectomy and oophorectomy after childbearing, in view of the risk of both endometrial and ovarian cancer. Although there are no definitive studies to support screening, endometrial sampling and transvaginal ultrasound of the ovaries may be considered from ages 30 to 35. Colonoscopy is recommended every 1–2 years starting from age 20 to 25 or 10 years younger than the youngest person diagnosed in the family.[65,66]

Molecular, cellular, and clinical biology

Like most epithelial cancers, ovarian cancer is a clonal disease.[67] Despite origin from a single cell, ovarian cancers are markedly heterogeneous at a molecular and cellular level, but also related to the tumor microenvironment. A number of genetic abnormalities are observed in ovarian cancers, including loss of tumor suppressor genes, activation of oncogenes and epigenetic dysregulation. The tumor cancer genome atlas (TCGA) has sequenced the whole genome from more than 400 high-grade serous ovarian cancers and found mainly *TP53* (tumor protein p53) (98%) and *BRCA1-2* (15–20%) mutated, while only a few other genes were mutated in more than 1% (*NF1* (neurofibromatosis 1), *RB1* (retinoblastoma 1), *CSMD3* (CUB and Sushi Multiple Domains 3), and *CDK12* (cyclin dependent kinase 12)).[68] At a cellular level, the fraction of proliferating cells can vary from 1% to 90%.[69] The tumor microenvironment, specifically the tumor infiltrating T-lymphocytes, varies between metastatic sites and may determine which site progresses and which shrinks.[70,71] Ovarian cancers vary in histotype, exhibiting the serous, endometriod, mucinous and clear cell variants described below, related at least in part to the aberrant expression of *HOX* (homeobox) genes associated with normal gynecologic development.[72]

Biologically and clinically, there is a major distinction between low-grade (type I) and high-grade (type II) epithelial ovarian cancers.[11,73] Low-grade serous carcinomas (LGSCs) (comprising <10% of ovarian epithelial malignancies) are thought to develop from borderline tumors, and characterized by activating Ras-MAPK pathway mutations, including oncogenic RAS (rat sarcoma virus) (>50%), BRAF (B rapidly activated fibrosarcoma) (14%), *PIK3CA* (phosphatidyl 3-kinase catalytic domain) (30%), and *PTEN* (phosphatase and tensin homolog) (10%) mutations, and expression of the insulin-like growth factor receptor (IGFR) which responds to IGF produced by the tumor stroma. High-grade serous cancers (comprising 60% of all ovarian epithelial malignancies) develop from histologically normal ovarian and fallopian tube epithelial cells, present in late stage (III–IV) and depend upon amplification of multiple oncogenes and functional loss of tumor suppressor genes. Whereas *TP53* is rarely mutated in low-grade type I cancers, it is mutated in nearly all high-grade serous type II cancers. When germ line and somatic mutations of *BRCA1* and *2* are associated with epithelial ovarian cancer, the cancers are generally high grade. Defects in HR including *BRCA* and mutations other than in *BRCA*, so-called BRCAness, are associated with up to half of high-grade cancers,[68,74] but few, if any, low-grade cancers, possibly accounting for the fact that high-grade cancers are more sensitive to platinum-based chemotherapy than low-grade cancers. Current strategies exploit this deficiency using PARP inhibitors in the presence of *BRCA1-2* and BRCA-like mutations. The PI3 kinase pathway is a potential target in both type I and type II cancers.[75]

Clear cell ovarian cancers have mutations of *ARID1A* (AT-rich interaction domain 1A) (49%),[76] a chromatin processing enzyme and *PP2R1A* (6%), a phosphatase. Endometriod ovarian cancers also show mutations of *ARID1A* (30%).

Ascites formation results from increased leakage of proteinaceous fluid from capillaries under the influence of vascular endothelial growth factor (VEGF) produced by ovarian cancers and from inhibition of fluid outflow through diaphragmatic lymphatics that have been blocked by metastatic disease.[77] Immunobiological studies suggest that the peritoneal cavity may function as an immunoprivileged site, with elevated levels of immune suppressive molecules and growth factors. Angiogenesis in ovarian cancer has been shown to depend upon multiple factors

Table 1 Epithelial ovarian tumors.

Histologic type	Cellular type
I. Serous	Endosalpingeal
A. Benign	
B. Borderline	
C. Malignant	
II. Mucinous	Endocervical
A. Benign	
B. Borderline	
C. Malignant	
III. Endometrioid	Endometrial
A. Benign	
B. Borderline	
C. Malignant	
IV. Clear cell "mesonephroid"	Müllerian
A. Benign	
B. Borderline	
C. Malignant	
V. Brenner	Transitional
A. Benign	
B. Borderline ("proliferating")	
C. Malignant	
VI. Mixed epithelial	Mixed
A. Benign	
B. Borderline	
C. Malignant	
VII. Undifferentiated	
Anaplastic	
VIII. Unclassified	
Mesothelioma	
Other	

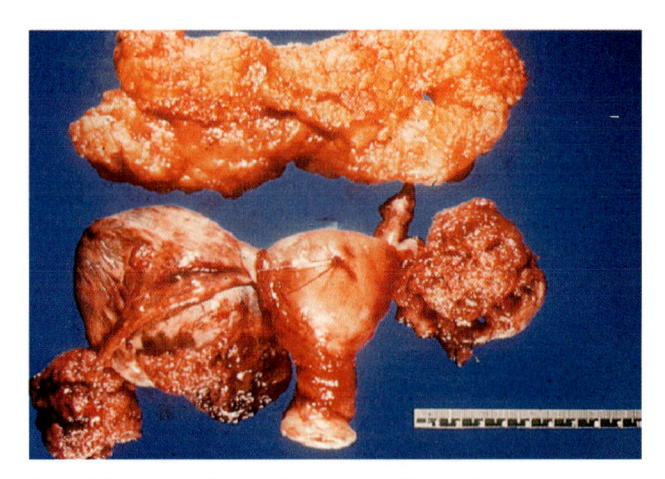

Figure 1 Serous cystadenocarcinoma gross with omentum.

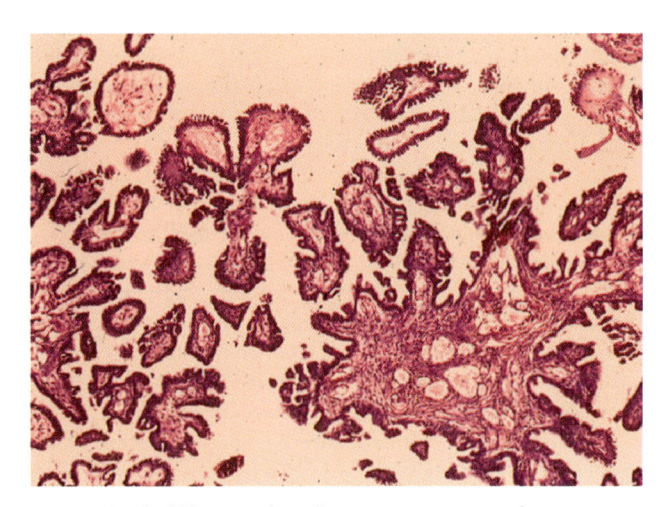

Figure 2 Poorly differentiated papillary serous carcinoma of ovary.

including VEGF and IL-8. Autophagy and tumor dormancy are regulated by ARHI, an imprinted tumor suppressor gene, that can be downregulated in low- and high-grade ovarian cancers.[78,79]

Upregulation and aberrant glycosylation of extracellular mucins have provided markers for monitoring disease. MUC-1 is a mucin expressed by more than 80% of ovarian cancers.[80] In transformed cells, aberrant glycosylation exposes peptide determinants recognized by murine monoclonal antibodies that have been used for serotherapy. CA125 is also a mucin (MUC-16) associated with cells that line the coelomic cavity during embryonic development. CA125 is shed from 80% of epithelial ovarian cancers and can be measured using the murine monoclonal antibody OC125.[81,82] The precise function of the glycoprotein is unknown,[83–85] but knockout of murine MUC-16 does not affect development or fertility.[86] In cancer cells, CA125 expression is upregulated transcriptionally and 80% of the CA125 is cleaved and shed. Interaction of CA125 with mesothelin at the peritoneal surface is likely the first point of contact for ovarian cancer cells metastasizing within the peritoneal cavity.

Classification and pathology

Primary ovarian cancers are classified according to the structures of the ovary from which they are derived.[87] As noted above, most have thought to be derived from the epithelial cells that cover the ovarian surface or that line inclusion cysts, although, as described above, this concept has recently been challenged by recognition that many high-grade serous cancers arise from the fimbriae of fallopian tubes. These cells are ultimately derived from the coelomic epithelium of mesodermal origin and share cytologic markers with mesothelium.

Epithelial malignancies account for 85–90% of ovarian cancers. A majority of epithelial lesions are seen in patients who are 40 years of age or older. Under the age of 40 years, epithelial malignancies are uncommon, and most malignancies seen in women under the age of 30 years are of germ cell origin. The histologic types of the epithelial tumors are listed in Table 1. The majority of lesions, about 75%, is of the serous type, followed by the mucinous, endometrioid, clear cell, mixed, Brenner, and undifferentiated histologies.[88]

Invasive histotypes

Serous carcinomas may have a complex admixture of cystic and solid areas with extensive papillations, or they may contain a predominantly solid mass with areas of necrosis and hemorrhage (Figure 1). The poorly differentiated tumors may have some areas with a papillary pattern, but other portions may be indistinguishable from the other histologic patterns described below (Figure 2). Stage I or II lesions are most frequently unilateral, with about 10–20% involving both ovaries. Conversely, about 50–70% of stage III serous carcinomas are bilateral.[88]

Epithelial malignancies that coat the surface of the ovary and peritoneum are referred to as peritoneal carcinomas.[89] The cells of the peritoneum have the ability to recapitulate any of the histologic patterns seen in ovarian cancers, although serous carcinomas occur most frequently and the other histologic types are rarely seen. Recognition of peritoneal carcinomas explains the occurrence of ovarian cancer after oophorectomy.[90] Also, peritoneal cancers can involve the surface of the ovaries without ovarian enlargement. Thus, ovaries can be innocent bystanders in a process originating in the peritoneal cavity. Therapeutically, peritoneal

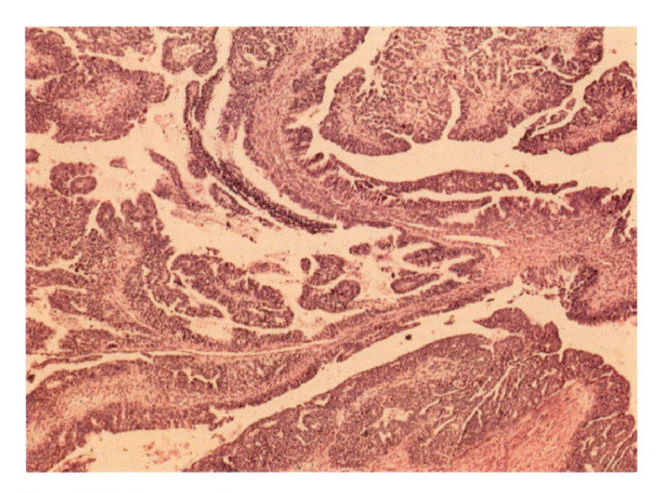

Figure 3 Mucinous carcinoma.

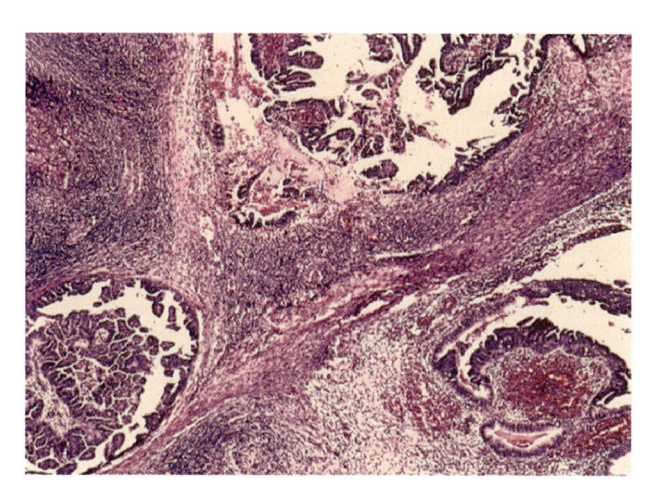

Figure 5 Borderline papillary serous tumor.

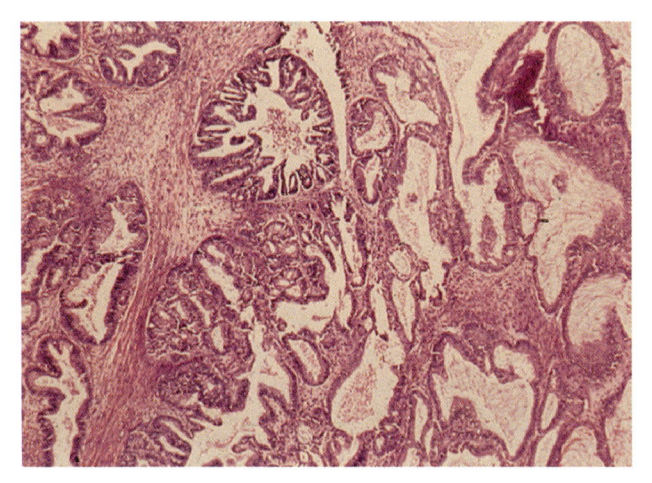

Figure 4 Endometrioid carcinoma.

malignancy should be treated as one would manage an epithelial ovarian cancer.

Mucinous tumors tend to be large, with many masses over 20 cm in diameter (Figure 3). The histologic pattern resembles uterine endocervical glands. The lesions frequently contain areas of hemorrhage, necrosis, and various quantities of mucin. These tumors are bilateral in 10–20% of cases. Occasionally, mucin is secreted into the peritoneal cavity and produces a condition known as pseudomyxoma or myxoma peritonei. A mucocele of the appendix may also be seen in conjunction with this tumor.

Endometrioid carcinomas of the ovary resemble typical carcinomas of the endometrium. These tumors may be seen with synchronous endometrial carcinoma, and when they are, both lesions may be of low-stage. Rarely, endometrioid carcinomas may arise in conjunction with pelvic endometriosis, resulting from malignant transformation of a benign process (Figure 4). Like endometrial cancers, endometrioid ovarian cancers are associated with inactivating mutations of *PTEN* and consequent activation of PI3 kinase signaling. Bilaterality is seen in 10–15% of stage I and II disease and in about 30% of stage III.

Ovarian clear cell carcinomas have abundant intracellular glycogen that is removed during histopathologic processing. About one-fourth of clear cell tumors are associated with endometriosis. Clear cell tumors are only rarely bilateral.[88]

Brenner tumors are uncommon, representing less than 1% of all epithelial malignancies. Mixed epithelial tumors may contain small areas of Brenner tumor histology, which have a histologic pattern similar to that of transitional cell. Malignant Brenner tumors are unilateral.[88]

Low-grade serous carcinomas (LGSC)
LGSC are a rare clinically and molecularly distinct subtype accounting for 5% of all epithelial ovarian cancers. Compared to high-grade serous carcinoma (HGSC), women with LGSC are diagnosed at younger average age of 47. LGSC share genetic alterations with serous borderline tumors and if borderline tumors recur they may present as LGSC, suggesting a pathway of progression from borderline tumor to low-grade carcinoma. However, LGSC can also arise de novo.

Borderline tumors
Borderline tumors, or low malignant potential tumors, need to be differentiated from invasive cancers. Borderline tumors tend to be confined to the ovary at the time of diagnosis, and occur in younger, premenopausal women (Figure 5). In women under the age of 40 years, about 60–70% of non-benign ovarian neoplasms are borderline, whereas in women over 40 years, only 10% are borderline.[88,91] Histologic criteria for borderline tumors include (1) the presence of epithelial cell proliferation with a "piling up" of cells, so-called pseudostratification; (2) cytologic atypia, but with rare mitoses; and (3) no evidence of stromal invasion. Borderline tumors of the ovary may be associated with peritoneal implants, which represent either dissemination or the multifocal evolution of the disease. Borderline tumors exist for all histological subtypes (Table 1). If invasive implants are found in serous borderline tumors, these are considered and treated as LGSCs.

Patterns of spread
Ovarian epithelial tumors spread primarily by direct exfoliation and implantation of cells throughout the peritoneal cavity (transcoelomic), but also metastasize via lymphatic and hematogenous routes.[88,92]

Exfoliated ovarian cancer cells spread directly to the pelvic and abdominal peritoneal surfaces, and tend to follow the path of circulation of peritoneal fluid from the right pericolic gutter cephalad to the right hemidiaphragm. At primary surgery, the parietal and visceral peritoneum can be studded with dozens to hundreds of metastatic nodules. Intestinal mesenteries can become involved by peritoneal metastases. Adhesions form between loops of small intestine producing mechanical obstruction, even though involvement of the lumen of the intestine by direct extension is uncommon. The intestinal dysfunction can also result from involvement by tumor of the myenteric plexus, the autonomic innervation of the intestine that is found in the mesentery. This condition has been referred to as "carcinomatous ileus." Large pelvic masses can also compress the rectum producing colonic obstruction.

Spread via the lymphatics is common in epithelial ovarian cancer. Apparent stage I and II tumors have retroperitoneal lymphatic dissemination in about 5–10% in most series, whereas lymphatic dissemination in stage III has been reported to be as high as 42–78% in carefully explored patients.[93] Most of these lymph nodes are not enlarged, but are microscopically positive for malignant cells. Spread through the retroperitoneal and diaphragmatic lymphatics can result in metastasis to the supraclavicular lymph nodes. Hematogenous metastasis of ovarian cancer to liver or lung paren chyma is uncommon at diagnosis and often a late finding in the disease. In advanced recurrent disease, parenchymal metastases are seen more frequently in lung, liver and even brain.

Clinical symptoms

Some patients with ovarian cancers confined to the ovary are asymptomatic, but the majority will have nonspecific symptoms. In one survey of 1725 women with ovarian cancer, 95% recalled symptoms prior to diagnosis, including 89% with stage I/II disease and 97% with stage III/IV disease.[94] 70% had abdominal or GI symptoms, 58% pain, 34% urinary symptoms, and 26% pelvic discomfort. At least some of these symptoms could have reflected pressure on the pelvic viscera from the enlarging ovary. Goff et al. have developed an ovarian cancer symptom index and reported that symptoms associated with ovarian cancer were pelvic/abdominal pain, urinary frequency/urgency, increased abdominal size or bloating and difficulty eating or feeing full when they were present for less than 1 year and occurred >12 days a month. The index had a sensitivity of 56.7% for early ovarian cancer and 79.5% for advanced-stage disease.[95] Interestingly, a population-based study from Australia found that there did not appear to be a significant difference in the duration of symptoms or the nature of symptoms in patients with early as opposed to advanced-stage ovarian cancer.[96]

Metastatic ovarian cancer is rarely asymptomatic. In addition to GI and urinary symptoms, ascites formation can produce an increase in abdominal girth. Pleural effusions may lead to dyspnea. Acute symptoms of adnexal rupture or torsion are uncommon. Vaginal bleeding is also uncommon in postmenopausal women, although premenopausal patients may present with irregular or heavy menses. Detection of an adnexal mass by pelvic examination can permit the early diagnosis of ovarian cancer. Since malignancy is rare and the majority of palpable adnexal masses are benign, an enlarged ovary discovered on pelvic examination is not likely to be an ovarian malignancy. In premenopausal women, ovarian cancer is uncommon and represents less than 7% of all adnexal masses.[88] Even in postmenopausal women, 70–80% of adnexal tumors are benign. In some patients who complain primarily of abdominal symptoms, however, a pelvic examination frequently is omitted and the tumor missed. Signs of advanced disease include abdominal distention and a fluid wave consistent with ascites. These signs are nonspecific and can be associated with many conditions arising in the abdominal cavity, especially malignancies of other primary sites or carcinomatosis from metastatic tumors of the GI tract or breast.

Diagnosis

The diagnosis of ovarian cancer requires histologic examination of a resected ovary. The primary workup for an adnexal mass includes history, physical exam and imaging studies. Transvaginal ultrasound is usually used for the initial workup, CT imaging to rule out metastases. Transvaginal ultrasound has better resolution than transabdominal ultrasonography for adnexal neoplasms. Doppler color-flow imaging may enhance the specificity of ultrasonography.

In pre- and postmenopausal women, simple cysts of up to 10 cm can be observed with repeat ultrasound. Those masses that regress in size can be managed with continued observation, whereas those that increase in size and complexity should be evaluated surgically. Ultrasonographic signs of malignancy include areas of complexity, such as irregular borders, multiple echogenic patterns within the mass, solid areas, and dense, multiple irregular septae. Bilateral tumors are more likely to be malignant, although the individual characteristics of the lesions are of greater significance. If a pelvic mass is suspicious and the most likely diagnosis is ovarian cancer, surgery should not be unnecessarily delayed.

Specific biomarkers and algorithms can aid in distinguishing malignant from benign pelvic masses. Ultrasound, CA125 and menopausal status have been combined to create a risk of malignancy index (RMI) that achieved a sensitivity of 71–88% and specificity of 74–97% for predicting the presence of ovarian cancers in women with pelvic masses.[97] An OVA1 panel including CA125, apolipoprotein A1, transthyretin, transferrin, and B2-microglobulin combined with imaging and menopausal status provides 92% sensitivity at 42% specificity in post-menopausal women and 85% sensitivity at 45% specificity for pre-menopausal women.[98] Similar sensitivity and higher specificity have been attained with a risk of ovarian malignancy algorithm (ROMA) calculated from CA125 and HE4 (human epididymis protein 4) values combined with menopausal status alone, without imaging.[99] In an initial trial of patients referred to academic centers the sensitivity for predicting a malignant pelvic mass was 93%, specificity 75% and negative predictive value 94%. In a subsequent community-based trial, a sensitivity of 94%, specificity of 75% and negative predictive value of 99% were attained.[100] The ROMA has been shown superior to the RMI.[101] A second generation OVERA panel test includes CA125, apolipoprotein A1, transferrin, follicle stimulating hormone, and HE4 producing a sensitivity of 91%, specificity of 69%, and negative predictive value of 97%.[102] Both the OVERA and the ROMA panels have been approved for use by the US FDA. Utilization of these panels could assure that women with suspicious adnexal masses are referred to gynecologic oncologists and receive optimal surgery. At present <50% of women in the United States with ovarian cancer have their initial operation with a gynecologic oncologist trained to perform optimal cytoreductive surgery.

The preoperative workup should exclude other primary cancers metastatic to the ovary. Colonoscopy and upper gastrointestinal endoscopy are indicated in women with GI symptoms. Mammography should be performed to exclude primary breast cancer. In patients with irregular menses or postmenopausal bleeding, an endometrial biopsy and endocervical curettage should be performed to exclude primary endometrial or endocervical pathology.

The differential diagnosis of an adnexal mass includes a variety of functional changes of the ovary, benign neoplasms of the reproductive tract, and inflammatory lesions of these organs. A hydrosalpinx, endometriosis, and pedunculated uterine leiomyomata can simulate an ovarian neoplasm. Non-gynecologic diseases, such as inflammatory processes of the colon and rectum, must be excluded.

Screening

The literature does not support screening for ovarian cancer in the general population.[103] Pelvic examination, transvaginal ultrasound and CA125 have been evaluated as screening tools in asymptomatic women.

Although some clinicians perceive that pelvic examination is a useful screening tool,[104] there is no evidence to confirm that.[105] The prostate, lung, colorectal and ovarian (PLCO) screening trial initially included bimanual examination, but this screening component was discontinued after 5 years because no case of ovarian cancer was detected by bimanual examination alone.[106,107]

Transvaginal ultrasonography has been reported to have up to 95% sensitivity for the detection of early-stage ovarian cancer but might result in up to 15 unnecessary laparotomies for every ovarian cancer detected, Doppler ultrasound may be a useful adjunct.[97,108–113]

CA125 is elevated in 50–60% of patients with stage I[114] and can rise 10–60 months prior to diagnosis with an average estimated lead time of 1.9 years prior to diagnosis of disease in all stages.[115] Therefore, CA125 screening might permit earlier diagnosis of ovarian cancer. In the PLCO screening trial, which included annual CA125 and transvaginal ultrasound, the stage distribution, however, was the same for the screening and control group (77% vs 78% stage III and IV).[106] Neither single values of CA125 and transvaginal ultrasonography exhibit adequate sensitivity or specificity for cost-effective early detection. Furthermore, a recent update of the trial with median 15-year follow-up confirmed no reduction in ovarian cancer mortality with screening.[116]

Data suggest that the specificity of CA125 is improved when followed over time.[117–119] Elevated CA125 levels in women without ovarian cancer remain static or decrease with time, whereas levels associated with ovarian malignancy tend to rise. This finding has been incorporated into an algorithm that uses age, rate of change of CA125 and absolute levels of CA125 to calculate an individual's ROCA. Patients with a rising CA125 underwent transvaginal sonography and, if abnormal, underwent surgery in two trials. The normal risk ovarian cancer screening study (NROSS) performed 24 operations in postmenopausal women to detect 15 cancers of which 13 (67%) were in stage I–II, rather than the 20–25% expected. The positive predictive value of the two-stage strategy was 62%, far better than the 10%, thought to be the least acceptable value, so that CA125 over time was sufficiently specific.[120,121] The UK Collaborative Trial of Ovarian Cancer Screening (UKCTOCS) assessed multimodal screening which included ROCA and transvaginal ultrasound versus transvaginal ultrasound alone versus no screening in a trial of 200,000 postmenopausal women, powered to detect a reduction in mortality. Preliminary results suggested that multimodal screening was more effective but at a median follow-up of 11 years there was no significant difference in mortality overall. A 20% mortality reduction was observed with multimodal screening, if prevalent cases were not included, but longer-term follow-up is needed to confirm this observation.[122] Currently, efforts are underway to create more sensitive panels of biomarker proteins (HE4, CA72.4), autoantibodies (anti-TP53), DNA mutations, copy number abnormalities and methylation, miRNAs, and metabolites, as well as more sensitive and specific imaging techniques.[121]

Current recommendations for screening women at high risk

Although transvaginal ultrasound and CA125-screening have been advocated for women at increased genetic ROCA, the efficacy of surveillance to reduce mortality or detect cancers at an earlier stage is unproven. The NCCN guidelines for screening in this population are vague and indicate that screening may be considered at clinician's discretion starting at age 30–35.

The findings of two prospective studies of annual transvaginal ultrasound and CA125 screening in 888 BRCA1 and BRCA2 mutation carriers in the Netherlands and 279 mutation carriers in the United Kingdom are not encouraging and suggest a very limited benefit of screening in high-risk women.[123,124] The UK Familial Ovarian Cancer Study (UKFOCCS) using ROCA every 3 months combined with transvaginal ultrasonography showed a possible shift to early-stage disease in the screened population.[125] Demonstration of a reduction in mortality would require a randomized controlled study that is ethically challenging to perform. Women in the high-risk population who request screening should be counseled about the current lack of evidence for the efficacy for either CA125 or for sonography as well as the associated false-positive rates. Many will still opt for screening despite the risks and limitations.

Treatment of early-stage epithelial cancer

Staging surgery

Ovarian, fallopian tube and peritoneal malignancies are staged according to the 2014 FIGO system (Table 2). A preoperative evaluation should exclude the presence of extraperitoneal metastases. In patients whose exploratory laparotomy does not reveal any macroscopic evidence of disease by inspection and palpation of the entire intra-abdominal space, a careful search for microscopic spread must be undertaken. This includes peritoneal washings, inspection and biopsies of peritoneal surfaces including the undersurface of the diaphragm, hysterectomy and bilateralteral salpingo-oophorectomy, infracolic omentectomy, and pelvic and para-aortic lymph node dissection. In an earlier series in which patients did not undergo careful surgical staging, the overall 5-year survival for patients with apparent stage I epithelial ovarian cancer was only about 60%. Survival rates of 90–100% have been reported for properly staged patients with stage IA or IB disease.[4] Metastases in clinically apparent stage I or II epithelial ovarian cancer are common. About 30% of patients whose ovarian epithelial cancers appear to be confined to the pelvis have occult metastatic disease in the upper abdomen or in the retroperitoneal lymph nodes.[126] Histologic grade was a significant predictor of occult metastasis, that is, 16% of patients with grade 1 lesions were upstaged, compared to 34% with grade 2 and 46% with grade 3 disease. Although accounting for only 15% to 20% of all cases after comprehensive staging, approximately one-third to one-half of all cured patients are derived from stage I.

A common situation is the apparently benign adherence of the tumor to adjacent structures in the absence of metastatic implants or obvious direct tumor extension. There is a considerable body of evidence that such benign adherence, when it is dense, is associated with a relapse risk equivalent to stage II, and that these patients should not be included in stage I, but rather in stage II.[127–130]

Management of invasive early-stage low-risk disease (stages IA and IB, low-grade)

Patients who have undergone a thorough staging laparotomy without evidence of spread beyond the ovary and have low-grade histology, do not need adjuvant chemotherapy. In fact, uterus and contralateral ovary can be preserved in women with stage IA lesions

Table 2 Figo staging of ovarian, fallopian tube, and peritoneal cancer (2014).

Stage	TNM
Stage I: Tumor confined to ovaries or fallopian tube(s)	T1-N0-M0
IA: Tumor limited to 1 ovary (capsule intact) or fallopian tube; no tumor on ovarian or fallopian tube surface; no malignant cells in the ascites or peritoneal washings	T1a-N0-M0
IB: Tumor limited to both ovaries (capsules intact) or fallopian tubes; no tumor on ovarian or fallopian tube surface; no malignant cells in the ascites or peritoneal washings	T1b-N0-M0
IC: Tumor limited to 1 or both ovaries or fallopian tubes, with any of the following:	
IC1: Surgical spill	T1c1-N0-M0
IC2: Capsule ruptured before surgery or tumor on ovarian or fallopian tube surface	T1c2-N0-M0
IC3: Malignant cells in the ascites or peritoneal washings	T1c3-N0-M0
Stage II: Tumor involves 1 or both ovaries or fallopian tubes with pelvic extension (below pelvic brim) or primary peritoneal cancer	T2-N0-M0
IIA: Extension and/or implants on uterus and/or fallopian tubes and/or ovaries	T2a-N0-M0
IIB: Extension to other pelvic intraperitoneal tissues	T2b-N0-M0
Stage III: Tumor involves 1 or both ovaries or fallopian tubes, or primary peritoneal cancer, with cytologically or histologically confirmed spread to the peritoneum outside the pelvis and/or metastasis to the retroperitoneal lymph nodes	T1/T2-N1-M0
IIIA1: Positive retroperitoneal lymph nodes only (cytologically or histologically proven):	
IIIA1(i) Metastasis up to 10 mm in greatest dimension	
IIIA1(ii) Metastasis more than 10 mm in greatest dimension	
IIIA2: Microscopic extrapelvic (above the pelvic brim) peritoneal involvement with or without positive retroperitoneal lymph nodes	T3a2-N0/N1-M0
IIIB: Macroscopic peritoneal metastasis beyond the pelvis up to 2 cm in greatest dimension, with or without metastasis to the retroperitoneal lymph nodes	T3b-N0/N1-M0
IIIC: Macroscopic peritoneal metastasis beyond the pelvis more than 2 cm in greatest dimension, with or without metastasis to the retroperitoneal lymph nodes (includes extension of tumor to capsule of liver and spleen without parenchymal involvement of either organ)	T3c-N0/N1-M0
Stage IV: Distant metastasis excluding peritoneal metastases	
Stage IVA: Pleural effusion with positive cytology	
Stage IVB: Parenchymal metastases and metastases to extra-abdominal organs (including inguinal lymph nodes and lymph nodes outside of the abdominal cavity)	Any T, any N, M1

who wish to preserve fertility. These women should be followed carefully with periodic pelvic examinations and CA125 levels. Generally, the other ovary and uterus are removed at the completion of childbearing. In a report by Guthrie et al., patients with early-stage epithelial ovarian cancer were studied. No patients with properly documented stage I, grade 1 cancer died of their disease and no adjuvant chemotherapy was needed.[131]

Management of invasive early-stage high-risk disease (stage IA and IB, high-grade and clear cell, stage IC and stage II)

The International Collaborative Ovarian Neoplasm Trial 1 (ICON1) and Adjuvant Chemotherapy Trial in Ovarian Neoplasia (ACTION)[130,132] randomized women with early-stage high-grade disease to platinum-based adjuvant chemotherapy versus observation. Both trials combined showed that progression-free survival and overall survival were significantly improved with chemotherapy (76% vs 65% and 82% vs 74%, respectively).[133] These results must be interpreted with caution, because most of the patients did not undergo thorough surgical staging, but the findings suggest that platinum-based chemotherapy should be given to patients who have not been optimally staged. GOG 157 compared three cycles of carboplatin and paclitaxel with six cycles patients with early-stage high-risk ovarian cancer.[129] The recurrence rate for six cycles was lower, but the difference did not reach statistical significance. While the authors concluded that three cycles of adjuvant carboplatin and paclitaxel was a reasonable option for women with high-risk early-stage ovarian cancer, particularly in women with non-serous cancers, patients with high-grade serous cancers had a statistically significant lower recurrence rate with six cycles of chemotherapy.

Management of early-stage borderline tumors

The principal treatment for borderline ovarian tumors is surgical resection of the primary tumor. There is no evidence that subsequent chemotherapy or radiation therapy improve survival. 10-year overall survival for stage I disease is 98% and all-stage 10-year survival is 87%. After performing a frozen section and determining that the histology is borderline, premenopausal patients who desire preservation of ovarian function may be managed with a fertility-sparing operation, that is, unilateral salpingo-oophorectomy. However, for staging purposes an omentectomy and peritoneal biopsies should be taken which may upstage a borderline tumor in up to 30% of cases. In patients in whom an ovarian cystectomy has been performed, a borderline tumor is documented in the permanent pathology and no residual disease is seen on CT imaging, no additional surgery is warranted.

Management of early-stage mucinous carcinoma

Mucinous carcinomas of the ovary are rare. More frequent are metastases from the GI tract to the ovary.[134] Mucinous cancers are often diagnosed at an early stage. 5-year survival for early stage is 80–90%. Fertility-sparing surgery for early stage is possible. Staging surgery includes peritoneal washings, peritoneal biopsies, omentectomy, and appendectomy. Based on retrospective data, lymph node metastases in clinically confined stage I disease is rare and lymphadenectomy should be omitted.[135,136]

Prognosis

Tumor stage, grade and size of metastatic disease after resection correlate best with outcome.[137] Among patients with low-stage disease, tumor grade correlates with prognosis, that is, patients with stage I high-grade lesions have a higher risk of recurrence and shorter survival than those with low-grade.[69] In patients with advanced-stage disease, the size of residual disease after surgery correlates most clearly with survival.[127] Complete removal of all

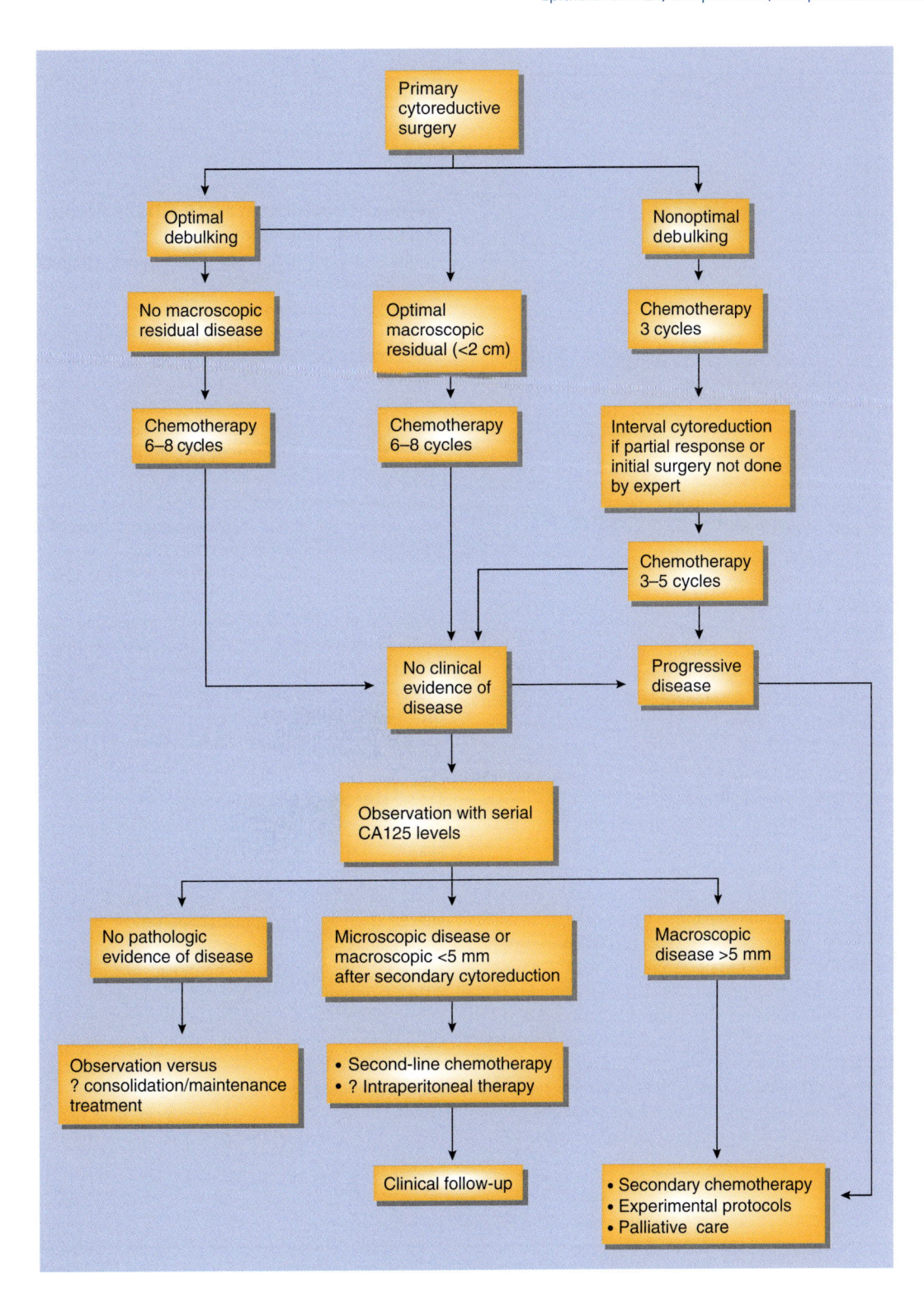

Figure 6 Treatment scheme for patients with advanced-stage ovarian cancer. Perform in a research setting where treatment will be based on outcome. Source: From Berek and Hacker.[24]

visible tumor has the best prognosis. The rapidity with which disease regresses during chemotherapy also correlates with survival. A short apparent half-life of the serum tumor marker CA125 correlated with improved survival in more than a dozen studies.[128] Normalization of CA125 by the third course of chemotherapy has been associated with a favorable prognosis. The presence of malignant ascites has been shown to also adversely impact on prognosis.

Treatment of advanced-stage epithelial cancer

Cytoreductive surgery

The principal goal of cytoreductive surgery is to remove all of the primary cancer and, if possible, its metastases (Figure 6). The operation usually includes the performance of a total abdominal

Table 3 Nomenclature for patient status-residual ovarian cancer.

Residual disease		Status
None	Pathologic	Complete remission
Microscopic disease	Only	Microscopic
Macroscopic disease	<5 mm	Minimal residual
Macroscopic disease	<1–2 cm	Optimal residual
Macroscopic residual disease	>1–2 cm	Suboptimal
Macroscopic disease	>2–3 cm	Bulky residual

Nomenclature for status of patient based on the extent of residual ovarian cancer prior to treatment.

hysterectomy and bilateral salpingo-oophorectomy, a complete omentectomy, and resection of metastatic lesions on the peritoneal surfaces or from the intestines. In addition, the pelvic tumor may directly involve the rectosigmoid colon, the terminal ileum, and the cecum. Based on recent data from the randomized lymphadenectomy in ovarian neoplasm (LION) trial, the removal of clinically negative lymph nodes during cytoreductive surgery, however, does not increase the progression-free survival and should not be undertaken.[138]

The rationale for cytoreductive surgery includes (1) potential physiologic benefits from excising the tumor, (2) improved tumor perfusion and increased growth fraction, that may increase the likelihood of response to chemotherapy or radiation therapy, and (3) enhanced immunologic competence of the patient.[139,140]

If resection of all metastases is not feasible, the goal is to reduce the tumor burden to an optimal status. The definition of "optimal" was initially proposed by Griffiths, who found that the survival of patients whose metastatic disease was resected to less than 1.5 cm in maximum dimension was significantly longer than the survival of those whose residual lesions were larger than 1.5 cm.[141] The optimal category of patients had a higher subsequent response rate to chemotherapy and longer disease-progression-free interval. Subsequently, Hacker et al.[142] showed that patients whose largest residual lesions were less than 5 mm survived much longer than those with larger nonresectable tumor deposits. The median survival of patients in this category was 40 months, compared with 18 months for patients whose disease was greater than 1.5 cm (Figure 6). The greatest benefit is observed in patients with no gross residual disease (R0) (Table 3).[143,144] In a meta-analysis of 81 studies of women who had undergone cytoreductive surgery, Bristow et al. documented that the greater the percentage of tumor reduction, the longer the survival. Each 10% increase in maximal cytoreduction was associated with a 5.5% increase in median survival time.[145]

Retrospective analysis suggests that these cytoreductive operations are feasible in 70–90% of patients when performed by gynecologic oncologists.[142,145–151] Major morbidity is in the range of 5% and operative mortality is 1%. Intestinal resection in these patients does not appear to increase the overall morbidity of the operation.

Adjuvant chemotherapy with platinum compounds and taxanes

Combination platinum- and taxane-based chemotherapy is the standard primary treatment for advanced epithelial ovarian cancer.[152–175] Combination chemotherapy has been shown to be superior to single-agent therapy (Table 4).[152,160] Cisplatin was introduced in the 1970s. Initially, it was combined with cyclophosphamide. In the 1990s, paclitaxel was incorporated into the combination treatment. Subsequent trials showed same efficacy but less toxicity of carboplatin compared to cisplatin.[174,175]

Docetaxel has a different toxicity profile compared to paclitaxel and its efficacy appeared to be equivalent in the SCOT-ROC trial.[168] Docetaxel is not commonly used but it is a reasonable substitute for paclitaxel in patients at greater risk of neuropathy or who have experienced a significant allergic reaction.

A five-arm study, GOG-182/ICON5 compared the standard combination of carboplatin and paclitaxel with these drugs in combination with gemcitabine, topotecan, or liposomal doxorubicin, respectively.[176] With over 4000 women, this was the largest randomized trial ever carried out in advanced ovarian cancer. There was no difference between any of the arms in progression-free or overall survival. The authors concluded that carboplatin and paclitaxel should remain the standard of care.

Dose-dense chemotherapy

There is preclinical and clinical evidence to suggest that dose-dense chemotherapy with paclitaxel given weekly and carboplatin given weekly or every 3 weeks may be more active than the same treatments given every 3 weeks. This may be due to anti-angiogenic effects, decreased repopulation of cancer cells between cycles, and reduced acquisition of drug resistance.[177,178] A phase III study by the Japanese Gynecologic Oncology Group (JGOG 3016) randomized women with stage II–IV ovarian cancer to receive either weekly paclitaxel (80 mg/m^2) in combination with three-weekly carboplatin (AUC 6) or three-weekly dosing of both drugs (carboplatin AUC 6 and paclitaxel 180 mg/m^2).[179] After a median follow-up of 29 months, a median PFS of 17.2 versus 28 months was reported (3-weekly vs dose-dense). Long-term follow up showed a difference in progression-free and overall

Table 4 Combination chemotherapy for advanced epithelial ovarian cancer: recommended regimens.

Drugs	Dose	Administration (h)	Interval	Number of treatments
Standard regimens				
Carboplatin	AUC = 5–6	3	Every 3 wk	6–8 cycles
Paclitaxel	175 mg/m^2			
Carboplatin	AUC = 5–6	3	Every 3 wk	Six cycles
Paclitaxel	80 mg/m^2		Every week	18 wk
Carboplatin	AUC = 5	3	Every week	Six cycles
Docetaxel	75 mg/m^2		Every 3 wk	
Cisplatin	75 mg/m^2	3	Every 3 wk	Six cycles
Paclitaxel	135 mg/m^2	24		
Carboplatin (single agent)[a]	AUC = 5	3	Every 3 wk	Six cycles, as tolerated

AUC, are under the curve dose by Calver formula.
[a] In patients who are elderly, frail or poor performance status.

survival of 17.5 versus 28.2 months and 62.2 versus 100.5 months, respectively.[180] The improvements in progression-free and overall survival exceeded any benefits previously seen in ovarian cancer. It is unclear whether these benefits relate to pharmacogenomic or pharmacodynamic differences in the Japanese population. This and other studies have suggested that Asian patients with ovarian cancer have a significantly better survival than Caucasian patients.[181] A GOG Phase III study of patients with advanced-stage ovarian cancer (Protocol 218) revealed that the overall survival was significantly higher in Asian patients when adjusted for age, stage, residual disease, performance status, and histology.[182]

The results of JGOG 3016 have not been confirmed in a predominantly Caucasian population. The Italian trial MITO-7 investigated weekly carboplatin (AUC 2) plus weekly paclitaxel (60 mg/m^2) compared with 3-weekly carboplatin (AUC 6) and paclitaxel (175 mg/m^2). The weekly regimen did not significantly improve progression-free survival (18.8 vs 16.5 months), but was associated with better quality of life and fewer toxic effects.[183] In the GOG 262 trial, patients were randomized to 3-weekly carboplatin and paclitaxel versus weekly paclitaxel and 3-weekly carboplatin.[184] Bevacizumab treatment was optional in both arms; and 84% of the patients received bevacizumab. No difference in progression-free survival was noted. ICON8 provided additional evidence that dose-dense therapy is not superior to 3-weekly regimens in Caucasian patients.[185] Carboplatin and paclitaxel every 3 weeks remain the standard of care.

Intraperitoneal chemotherapy

As ovarian cancer spreads over peritoneal surfaces, investigators have evaluated intraperitoneal (IP) chemotherapy to achieve high local drug concentrations. There have been several randomized trials on IP chemotherapy. Despite positive results in a number of trials, the role of IP chemotherapy remains contentious.

The first large randomized trial was performed by the Southwest Oncology Group (SWOG) and the GOG and compared IP cisplatin to IV cisplatin (100 mg/m^2), each given with cyclophosphamide (600 mg/m^2).[186] The IP cisplatin arm had a significantly longer overall median survival than the IV arm, 49 months versus 41 months. In the patients with the least residual disease (<0.5 cm maximum residual), who were expected to derive the most benefit, however, there was no statistically significant difference in median survival.

In the follow-up GOG 114 trial, a standard regimen of IV cisplatin (75 mg/m^2) and IV paclitaxel (135 mg/m^2 over 24 h) was compared to a dose-intense regimen that was initiated by giving moderately high-dose carboplatin (AUC = 9) for two induction cycles followed by IP cisplatin 100 mg/m^2 and IV paclitaxel (135 mg/m^2 over 24 h).[187] The dose-intense arm showed statistically significant improved progression-free survival (27.6 vs 22.5 months, but no difference in overall survival (52.9 vs 47.6 months).

The subsequent randomized GOG 172 study[188] compared IP cisplatin and paclitaxel with IV cisplatin and paclitaxel. The median PFS was 23.8 months in the IP arm versus 18.3 months in the IV arm ($p = 0.05$). The median overall survival was 65.6 months in the IP group and 49.7 months in the IV group ($p = 0.03$). However, only 42% of patients received the assigned six cycles of IP therapy with the remainder switching to IV therapy. The reasons for discontinuing were primarily for catheter-related problems, but there were also significantly more side effects in the IP group including severe fatigue, abdominal pain, hematological toxicity, nausea and vomiting, metabolic and neurotoxicity. The results of this and the previous studies led to an NCI Clinical Announcement recommending that women with optimally cytoreduced stage III ovarian cancer be considered for IP chemotherapy.

Simultaneously, a *Cochrane Review* and a separate meta-analysis concluded that IP chemotherapy was associated with better outcomes.[189,190] The meta-analysis included six randomized trials with a total of 1716 ovarian cancer patients. The pooled HR for PFS of IP cisplatin as compared to IV treatment regimens was 0.792 (CI = 0.688 – 0.912), and the pooled HR for OS 0.799 (CI: 0.702 – 0.910). Similar conclusions were reached in the Cochrane Review stating that IP chemotherapy is associated with increased progression-free and overall survival in patients with optimally debulked stage III advanced ovarian cancer. The authors, however, also commented on the potential for catheter-related complications and increased toxicity with IP therapy.

Long-term follow up of GOG 114 and 172 showed a significantly decreased risk of death associated with IP chemotherapy.[191] However, a long-term follow-up on patients of GOG 104, 114, and 172 showed no difference in proportion of recurrence-free patients for IP versus IV chemotherapy.[192]

The recently reported results of GOG 252 questioned the role of IP chemotherapy. Patients were randomized to weekly paclitaxel (80 mg/m^2) and 3-weekly carboplatin (AUC 6) versus weekly paclitaxel and 3-weekly IP carboplatin (AUC 6) versus 3-weekly paclitaxel and 3-weekly cisplatin as well as 3-weekly paclitaxel. In contrast to previous IP trials, all patients received bevacizumab. There was no difference in progression-free survival between the three groups; specifically, there was no difference in the subgroup with stage II or III and residual disease of ≤1 cm.[193]

Hyperthermic intraperitoneal chemotherapy (HIPEC) has mainly been used for the treatment of peritoneal metastases of appendiceal carcinoma, colorectal cancer and peritoneal mesothelioma.[194] There has been some recent data of the use of HIPEC in ovarian cancer. A Dutch phase III trial randomized patients with stage III ovarian cancer after neoadjuvant chemotherapy (NACT) to HIPEC at the time of interval debulking surgery versus surgery alone. Both groups were treated with subsequent adjuvant chemotherapy. Median PFS 10.7 versus 14.2 and median OS 33.9 versus 45.7 months improved with HIPEC.[195] In this trial, HIPEC was not compared to IP chemotherapy. Potential surgical side effects, including significant adhesion formation after HIPEC—some centers perform a routine cholecystectomy and appendectomy at the time of surgery to minimize the risk for a potential reoperation—support the need for further studies.

Neoadjuvant chemotherapy

Several investigators have suggested that NACT followed by interval cytoreduction might be appropriate in women whose performance status was poor.[196–199] In 2010, Vergote et al. reported the results of a randomized EORTC-NCIC (National Cancer Institute of Canada) study of primary debulking surgery (PDS) versus three cycles of neo-adjuvant chemotherapy followed by interval debulking.[200] All the patients had extensive stage IIIC or IV disease. Just over 60% had metastatic lesions larger than 10 cm in diameter, and 74.5% larger than 5 cm. Patients were randomly assigned either to PDS followed by at least six courses of platinum-based chemotherapy or to three courses of neoadjuvant platinum-based chemotherapy followed by interval debulking surgery in all patients with a response or stable disease, followed by at least three further courses of platinum-based chemotherapy. The median PFS in both groups was 12 months. The median overall survival was similar with 29 versus 30 months (primary-surgery vs

NACT). There was lower postoperative morbidity and mortality in the NACT group.

Complete tumor resection was the strongest independent predictor of overall survival in both groups. The results of this study have been widely debated.[201-204] du Bois et al. noted that the patients recruited to this study had a poorer performance status than those in most upfront randomized trials, and that the complete resection rates varied considerably from country to country and were low.[201] In the PDS group, only about 20% of patients were completely cytoreduced to no residual disease, lower than expected in experienced centers. The median OS was only 30 months, considerably less than the 60+ months expected with optimal cytoreduction followed by chemotherapy, suggesting that the study included a poor performance status cohort of patients with very advanced disease.

The Chemotherapy or Upfront Surgery (CHORUS) trial[205] randomized patients to NACT followed by interval debulking and then three additional cycles or primary debulking surgery followed by six cycles of platinum-based chemotherapy. The optimal debulking rate was only 16% in the PDS group, compared to 40% following NACT. The median duration of surgery was only 120 minutes in both groups, which does not appear long enough for aggressive debulking surgery. There was a 5.6% postoperative mortality rate in the PDS group, which is much higher than expected and may reflect patient selection. The median PFS was 12 months in both groups, and the median overall survival was similar with 22.6 versus 24.1 months (PDS vs NACT).

Two national trials are ongoing. Preliminary results of the Italian SCORPION trial show no difference in PFS for NACT and PDS.[206] Results of a JGOG trial are pending. A recent, pooled analysis of EORTEC 55971 and CHORUS shows a similar median overall survival (27.6 vs 26.9) but a better overall survival for stage IV disease (24.3 vs 21.2 months for NACT vs PDS).[207]

There remain divergent views regarding the place of NACT. A survey of SGO members found the 82% felt there was not enough evidence to justify the use of NACT.[208] In contrast, 70% of ESGO members felt there was sufficient evidence to recommend NACT. NACT appears indicated in patients who are medically unfit for upfront surgery or who have a high risk of surgical morbidity and mortality, including those with large pleural effusions, parenchymal liver and lung metastases. However, PDS should be considered standard of care for most patients.[209]

Laparoscopic scoring algorithms have been developed to triage patients to immediate or delayed debulking after three cycles of chemotherapy. Complete (R0) cytoreduction was achieved in 88% of patients with primary surgery and in 74% of patients receiving NACT, compared to 25% and 60% of patients treated prior to implementation of the laparoscopic algorithm.[210] Patients triaged to primary surgery had better PFS than did patuents receiving NACT (21.4 vs 12.9 months). In each group, patuents achieving complete cytoreduction (R0) had longer PFS than those with visible residual disease of <1 cm (R1).

Maintenance with chemotherapy and targeted therapies

Almost 80% of women with advanced ovarian cancer will relapse within 3 years following first-line chemotherapy. In view of this, several trials of maintenance therapy have been conducted to prolong PFS and possibly improve overall survival with chemotherapy and targeted therapies using bevacizumab and PARP-inhibitors.

Historically, trials on chemotherapy maintenance with paclitaxel[211,212] and topotecan[213] have been performed. Prior to the advent of PARP-inhibitors and bevacizumab, a Cochrane meta-analysis on maintenance chemotherapy concluded that there was no evidence that maintenance chemotherapy was more effective than observation alone.[214]

Bevacizumab

Inhibition of angiogenesis with drugs such as bevacizumab, a VEGF-A ligand monoclonal antibody, has demonstrated activity and benefit in women with recurrent ovarian cancer. Two large Phase III studies, (GOG 218 and ICON 7) have investigated the role of bevacizumab in the first-line setting. The GOG 218 trial randomized patients with stage III and macroscopic residual disease as well as stage IV ovarian cancer to (1) six cycles of carboplatin and paclitaxel plus placebo for cycle 2 through 22 (control group), (2) six cycles of carboplatin and paclitaxel in combination with bevacizumab (15 mg/kg) for cycles 2 through 6, followed by placebo (initiation group) and (3) six cycles of carboplatin and paclitaxel with bevacizumab for cycles 2 through 22 (throughout group).[215] The median PFS was 10.3 versus 11.2 versus 14.1 months in control versus initiation versus throughout group. There was no difference in median overall survival. However, in an exploratory subgroup analysis the median overall survival for stage IV disease was 32.6 versus 42.8 months (control vs throughout).[216]

The ICON7 trial included patients with early-stage high-risk disease (stage I or IIA clear cell or grade 3) and advanced stage IIB–IV and randomized to six cycles of chemotherapy or six cycles of chemotherapy plus bevacizumab (7.5 mg/kg), followed by 12 cycles of maintenance bevacizumab. Restricted mean progression-free survival was statistically different with 22.4 versus 24.1 months (control vs bevacizumab). An exploratory analysis of predefined subgroups showed a significant improvement in survival of 28.8 versus 36.6 months in the high-risk subgroups (defined as suboptimally debulked stage III and stage IV).[217] This was confirmed in the final survival data analysis, which showed that there was a 4-month improvement in median survival from 35 to 39 months in the high-risk subgroup.[218] Bevacizumab was associated with increased toxicity, including bleeding (mainly grade 1 mucocutaneous bleeding), ≥ grade 2 hypertension (18% vs 2%), grade ≥ 3 thromboembolic events (7% vs 3%), and gastrointestinal perforations (occurring in 10 vs 3 patients).

In contrast to the GOG 218 study, ICON7 included patients with advanced-stage cancer with no visible residual disease, as well as patients with high-risk early-stage disease. In the ICON7 study, a lower dose of bevacizumab was used (7.5 vs 15 mg/kg in GOG 218) for a shorter maintenance period (12 cycles, vs 16 cycles). In both studies, PFS curves converged a few months after bevacizumab was discontinued, suggesting that antiangiogenic treatment may delay, but not prevent, disease progression. There are no good biologic markers to identify which patients most likely benefit from bevacizumab in the first-line setting. The optimal dose is unclear.

PARP-inhibitors

The concept of synthetic lethality is deceptively simple and explains the selective and targeted effect of PARP-inhibitors in cells with dysfunction in the HR pathway. Loss of function of *BRCA 1* or *2* results in increased sensitivity to inhibition of PARP1 due to accumulation of unrepaired single-strand DNA breaks in proliferating cells which results in collapse of replication forks and consequently to double-strand DNA breaks (DSBs).[219,220] These DSBs are not repaired in *BRCA 1* or *2* tumor cells, which are deficient in HR and this leads to genetic instability and cell death. The initial Phase I trial reported a clinical benefit rate (CBR) of 63% in women with *BRCA* mutations and recurrent ovarian cancer treated with olaparib.[221] This led to the enrollment of an expanded cohort of patients with BRCA1 or 2 mutations which confirmed activity in a heavily pretreated group of patients with recurrent ovarian cancer with a CBR of 46%.[222] There was a correlation between response to olaparib and platinum sensitivity; platinum-sensitive patients had a 69% CBR compared with 46% and 23% in platinum-resistant and -refractory patients, respectively. Although the most mature data for PARP-inhibitor use is in recurrent ovarian cancer (see below), there is recent data to support their use as maintenance therapy in the first line setting.

In the SOLO1 trial, patients with stage III and IV high-grade serous and endometrioid ovarian cancer, a germline or somatic BRCA1 or 2 mutation and at least partial response to adjuvant platinum-based chemotherapy were randomized to olaparib maintenance or placebo. A 70% risk reduction for progression of disease or death was seen for olaparib (HR 0.3) with a median PFS not reached versus 13.8 months with placebo. Twice as many patients were progression free after 3 years, 60.4% versus 26.9%, which is unprecedented.[223]

The PRIMA trial enrolled patients similar to those in SOLO1, stage III and IV high-grade serous and endometrioid ovarian cancer with response to adjuvant chemotherapy, but regardless of BRCA status and with visible residual disease for stage III after surgery. Patients were randomized to niraparib or placebo. In the overall population, the median PFS was 8.2 versus 13.8 months (control vs niraparib). In the homologous recombination deficient (HRD) subgroup as determined with the Myriad myChoice test, the median PFS was 10.9 versus 22.1 months. In the HR proficient subgroup, the difference was smaller but still statistically significant (5.4 vs 8.1 months). This suggests that PARP inhibitors may have mechanisms other than those involved in DNA repair.

The VELIA trial randomized patients with advanced-stage ovarian cancer to (1) chemotherapy (control), (2) veliparib with chemotherapy, and (3) veliparib with chemotherapy followed by veliparib maintenance.[224] There was significant benefit from adding veliparib to chemotherapy and maintenance. In the BRCA mutation group, the median PFS was 22 versus 34.7 months; in the HRD group, 20.5 versus 31.9 months; and in the intention-to-treat population 17.3 versus 23.5 months. The results of the HR proficient patients were not reported.

In the PAOLA trial patients regardless of BRCA status with at least a partial response to previous therapy were randomized to bevacizumab or bevacizumab plus olaparib maintenance therapy.[225] The median PFS for the intention-to-treat population was 16.6 versus 22.1 months (without vs with olaparib), in the BRCA-mutated group 21.7 versus 37.2 months, in the HRD group excluding BRCA 16.6 versus 28.1 months. However, in the HRD-negative or unknown group the median PFS showed no difference (16 vs 16.9 months). The PAOLA design did not include olaparib monotherapy, making it difficult to ascertain the contribution of bevacizumab.

Taken together, it appears that maintenance therapy with PARP inhibitors provides the greatest impact on cancers with BRCA mutations, followed by cancers with HRDs, but with some modest benefit in cancers without biomarkers. The FDA has approved olaparib for front-line maintenance therapy in patients with BRCA-associated ovarian cancer and niraparib for all patients regardless of biomarker status.[226]

All PARP-inhibitors are associated with mainly low-grade side effects, such as nausea, fatigue and myelosuppression (anemia can be caused by all, neutropenia and thrombocytopenia mainly by niraparib) which can mostly be managed with dose reductions.

Management of advanced-stage borderline tumors

For advanced stage borderline tumors or for recurrent borderline tumors, the treatment is debulking surgery. If invasive implants are identified, the NCCN recommends to treat these tumors subsequently as LGSCs.

Management of advanced-stage low-grade serous cancer ovarian cancer

LGSCs have a low response rate to platinum-based chemotherapy. Available data is mainly derived from retrospective studies. In the neoadjuvant setting, platinum-based chemotherapy was reported to have only 4% objective response rate.[227] In the adjuvant setting, reported response rates were still low with up to 23%.[228] Most patients with advanced-stage LGSCs are treated with platinum-based chemotherapy. The majority will relapse, however, with a relatively long overall survival of 82 months.[229] Women who received hormonal maintenance treatment with for example, aromatase inhibitors following upfront surgery and chemotherapy have shown longer PFS than women who have been followed with observation alone.[230]

LGSCs show mutations in the MAP kinase pathway, particularly in KRAS (kirsten ras oncogene), BRAF, and NRAS. Preliminary results report improved objective response rates of 26.2% versus 6.2% and improved PFS with 13.0 versus 7.2 months in recurrent LGSC using the MEK-inhibitor trametinib compared to standard chemotherapy.[231]

Management of advanced stage mucinous ovarian cancers

Advanced-stage mucinous carcinomas are commonly chemoresistant, but usually treated with adjuvant platinum- and taxane-based chemotherapy or with a gastrointestinal cancer regimen such as 5-FU/leucovorin/oxaliplatin or capecitabine/oxaliplatin with or without bevacizumab. A planned randomized phase II trial comparing these regimens was closed due to slow accrual[134] and the optimal treatment approach is unknown.

Treatment assessment

Many patients who have undergone optimal cytoreductive surgery and subsequent chemotherapy for epithelial ovarian cancer will have no evidence of disease at the completion of treatment. Second-look operations, previously routine are no longer performed because there was no benefit associated with surgery,[232–234] although with novel PARP inhibitor maintenance and immunotherapy, this could be reexamined.

Follow-up examinations

The optimal frequency of follow-up examinations is unknown, but in those patients, who are in clinical remission it is reasonable to perform a pelvic examination and obtain a CA125 every 3 months for 2–3 years. Elevated CA125 levels are useful in predicting the presence of disease, but normal levels are an insensitive determinant of the absence of disease.[235] The Gynecologic Cancer Inter Group (GCIG) developed a standard definition for CA125 progression, which is now widely used in clinical trials. Patients with elevated CA125 pretreatment and normalization of CA125 must show evidence of CA125 greater than or equal to 2× the upper normal limit on two occasions at least 1 week apart or patients with elevated CA125 pretreatment, which never normalizes must show evidence of CA125 greater than or equal to 2× the nadir value on two occasions at least 1 week apart.

A UK-trial randomized patients to early treatment of relapse based on CA125 versus delaying treatment until the development of symptoms. CA125 rose 4.5 months prior to the development of symptoms, but no survival benefit was seen from early treatment.[236] Several flaws in design and execution question the validity of this study.[237]

A rising CA125 and or symptoms may prompt CT imaging. Combined [18]Fluorodeoxyglucose (FDG)-PET/CT may be more valuable to detect recurrent ovarian cancer and this technique may be useful for the selection of patients with late recurrent disease who may benefit from secondary cytoreductive surgery.[238]

Treatment of recurrent epithelial cancer

The majority of women who relapse will be offered further chemotherapy with the likelihood of benefit related in part to the initial response and the duration of response. The goals of treatment include improved control of disease-related symptoms, maintaining or improving quality of life, delaying time to progression, and possibly prolonging survival, particularly in women with platinum-sensitive recurrences.

Many active chemotherapy agents (platinum, paclitaxel, topotecan, liposomal doxorubicin, docetaxel, gemcitabine, and etoposide) as well as targeted agents (bevacizumab, cediranib, PARP-inhibitors) are available and the choice of treatment is based on many factors including likelihood of benefit, symptoms, *BRCA* status, histological subtype, potential toxicity and patient convenience.[239,240]

Women who relapse greater than 6 months after primary chemotherapy are classified as "platinum-sensitive" and usually receive further platinum-based chemotherapy with response rates ranging from 27% to 65% and a median survival of 18–24 months.[241,242] Patients who relapse within 6 months of completing first-line chemotherapy are classified as "platinum-resistant" and have a median survival of 6–9 months and a 10–30% likelihood of responding to chemotherapy. Patients who progress while on treatment are classified as "platinum-refractory." It is uncommon for high-grade serous ovarian cancers to be platinum-refractory and most cases involve other histological types such as clear cell cancers. Objective response rates to chemotherapy in patients with platinum-refractory ovarian cancer are typically less than 10%.

Platinum-sensitive disease

Secondary cytoreduction
Secondary cytoreduction is defined as the attempt to resect recurrent disease following first-line chemotherapy. While patients with platinum-resistant or -refractory disease are not suitable candidates, patients with long disease-free interval, localized recurrence and absence of ascites in whom all macroscopic disease could be resected are the best candidates. The DESKTOP III trial randomized patients with recurrent platinum-sensitive ovarian cancer and a positive AGO score, that is, ECOG status 0, ascites <500 mL, complete resection at initial surgery, to either chemotherapy or surgery followed by chemotherapy. The difference in median PFS, 14 versus 18.4 months, and median OS 46.2 versus 60.7 months) were statistically significant (without vs with secondary surgery and complete cytoreduction). Patients with surgery and incomplete resection did worse (median OS 28.8 months).[243] Results of the GOG 213 trial, however, showed no statistically significant difference in PFS with 18.9 versus 16.2 months and overall survival with 50.6 versus 64.7 months (with vs without secondary cytoreduction).[244] In the view of these two trials, secondary cytoreduction can be considered a safe option for carefully selected patients.

Chemotherapy

In general, randomized trials have shown that response rates, median PFS, and overall survival rates are superior for platinum-based combination chemotherapy compared to single-agent platinum chemotherapy. The use of platinum plus paclitaxel chemotherapy versus single-agent platinum has been tested in two randomized phase III trials[245] and a randomized phase II study.[246] In a report of the ICON4 and AGO-OVAR-2.2 trials,[245] women with platinum-sensitive ovarian cancer were randomized to platinum-based chemotherapy or paclitaxel plus platinum-based chemotherapy. Combining the trials for analysis, there was a significant survival advantage for the paclitaxel-containing therapy (HR = 0.82). There was a 5-month improvement in median survival (29 vs 24 months) and a 3-month prolongation in median PFS (13 vs 10 months). The toxicities were comparable, except for a significantly higher incidence of neurologic toxicity and alopecia in the paclitaxel group, whereas myelosuppression was significantly greater in non–paclitaxel-containing regimens.

Two randomized trials have compared carboplatin alone to carboplatin and gemcitabine or carboplatin and liposomal doxorubicin.[247,248] There was a higher response rate with the combination therapy and a longer PFS, but the studies were not powered to analyze overall survival. In the GCIG study comparing carboplatin and gemcitabine with carboplatin alone, the response rate was 47.2% for the combination and 30.9% for carboplatin, with the PFSs being 8.6 and 5.8 months, respectively. A SWOG study of carboplatin versus carboplatin and liposomal doxorubicin was closed early because of poor accrual, but with 61 patients recruited, the response rate was 67% for the combination and 32% for carboplatin. The PFS was 12 months versus 8 months; the overall survival 26 versus 18 months. A phase II study from France confirmed the high response rate of 67% with carboplatin and liposomal doxorubicin in patients with platinum-sensitive recurrent ovarian cancer.[249]

A large GCIG study (CALYPSO) comparing carboplatin and liposomal doxorubicin (CD) with carboplatin and paclitaxel (CP) recruited almost 1000 patients. The PFS for the CD arm was statistically superior to the CP arm (HR, 0.82); median PFS 11.3 versus 9.4 months. More frequent grade ≥ 2 alopecia (83.6% vs 7%), hypersensitivity reactions (18.8% vs 5.6%), and sensory neuropathy (26.9% vs 4.9%) were observed in the CP arm; more hand–foot syndrome (grade 2 to 3, 12% vs 2.2%), nausea (35.2% vs 24.2%), and mucositis (grade 2 to 3, 13.9% vs 7%) in the CD arm. This trial demonstrated superiority in PFS and better therapeutic index of carboplatin and liposomal doxorubicin compared to carboplatin and paclitaxel, and this regimen is now widely used.[250]

Some researchers have hypothesized that treating patients with non-platinum drugs to prolong the platinum-free interval will allow the tumor to again become more platinum-sensitive over time.[251] However, there are no data to support the hypothesis that the interposition of a non-platinum agents will result in an increase in platinum-sensitivity because of a longer interval since the last platinum treatment.

Targeted therapies

Bevacizumab combined with chemotherapy for recurrent platinum-sensitive ovarian cancer has been approved on the basis of two phase-III trials, OCEANS and GOG 213. OCEANS investigated the role of bevacizumab combined with carboplatin plus gemcitabine. Bevacizumab or placebo was continued until disease progression. The median PFS was 12.4 months in the bevacizumab arm compared to 8.4 months in the placebo arm. There was no difference in overall survival.[252,253] For the addition of bevacizumab to chemotherapy, GOG 213 showed a statistically not significant difference in overall survival of 5 months (42.6 vs 37.3 months) and a statistically significant increase in median PFS of 3.4 months (13.8 vs 10.4 months).[254] A recently published phase-III trial reported an increased PFS for carboplatin plus doxorubicin and bevacizumab compared to carboplatin plus gemcitabine and bevacizumab (13.3 vs 11.6 months).[255]

The PARP-inhibitors olaparib, niraparib, rucaparib have been approved for maintenance treatment of recurrent ovarian cancer or treatment of recurrent ovarian cancer after at least ≥2 prior lines. Study 19 was the first study to demomstrate benefit of olaparib maintenance (400 mg twice daily) in recurrent ovarian cancer following response to platinum-based chemotherapy.[256] Median PFS improved to 8 months compared to placebo (5 months). A separate analysis of Study 19 showed that *gBRCA* mutated patients had the greatest benefit (PFS 11 vs 4 months).[257] These results were confirmed in the SOLO2 trial; in *gBRCA* mutated patients with recurrent platinum-sensitive ovarian cancer the median PFS with olaparib (300 mg twice daily) was 19.2 versus 5.5 months[258] and median OS improved by 15 months (52.4 vs 37.4 months).[259]

Similarly, the NOVA trial randomized women with recurrent platinum-sensitive ovarian cancer to maintenance treatment with niraparib (300 mg daily) versus placebo. However, the NOVA trial enrolled also patients without *BRCA* mutations and stratified by *gBRCA* mutation, HRD and HR proficiency.[260] The study found statistically significant improvement of the median PFS in all subgroups, the *gBRCA* group 5.5 versus 21 months, HRD and *BRCAwt* 11 versus 20.9 months, and even HRD-negative 3.8 versus 6.9 months.

In ARIEL 3, patients with recurrent platinum-sensitive ovarian cancer and at least partial response were randomized to rucaparib (600 mg twice daily) versus placebo and stratified by HR status.[261] The median PFS in the intention-to-treat population was 5.4 versus 10.8 months, in the HRD group as assessed by loss of heterozygosity (LOH) 5.4 versus 13.6 months, and in the *BRCA* mutated group 5.4 versus 16.6 months.

Platinum-resistant disease

All randomized trials of combination versus single-agent chemotherapy in platinum-resistant/refractory ovarian cancer have failed to show superiority of combination chemotherapy over single-agent treatment. There are a variety of potentially active single agents, the most frequently used being paclitaxel, docetaxel, topotecan, liposomal doxorubicin, gemcitabine, ifosfamide, trabectedin, oral etoposide, tamoxifen, and bevacizumab as single-agent or in addition to chemotherapy.[262–267]

Patients with platinum-resistant ovarian cancer were randomized to gemcitabine or liposomal doxorubicin. Median PFSs were 3.6 versus 3.1 months, median overall survival 12.7 versus 13.5 months, and overall response rates 6.1% versus 8.3%, respectively. In the subset of patients with measurable disease, overall response rates were 9.2% versus 11.7. The liposomal doxorubicin group experienced significantly more hand–foot syndrome and mucositis, the gemcitabine group more constipation, nausea and vomiting, fatigue, and neutropenia.[268]

These findings are similar to the results of a large randomized phase III trial comparing patupilone to liposomal doxorubicin in patients with platinum-refractory/resistant ovarian cancer.[269] There was no difference in patient outcomes between the two treatments. The median PFS was 3.7 months in both arms, and the overall survival was 13.2 months in the patupilone arm and 12.7 months in the liposomal doxorubicin arm. The results highlight the poor prognosis of these patients and underscore the importance of symptom benefit and quality-of-life considerations.

Single-agent paclitaxel has shown objective responses in 20–30% of patients in phase II trials of women with platinum-resistant ovarian cancer.[270–273] The main toxicities have been asthenia and peripheral neuropathy. Weekly paclitaxel is more active than three-weekly dosing and is also associated with less toxicity.

Docetaxel also has some activity in patients with platinum-resistant disease.[274,275] The GOG studied 60 women with platinum-resistant ovarian or primary peritoneal cancer.[276] Although there was a 22% objective response rate, the median response duration was only 2.5 months, and therapy was complicated by severe neutropenia in three-quarters of the patients.

Topotecan is an active second-line treatment for patients with platinum-sensitive and platinum-resistant disease.[277–279] Topotecan at 1.5 mg/m^2 daily for 5 days, showed response rates of 19% and 13% in patients with platinum-sensitive and platinum-resistant disease.[277] The predominant toxicity of topotecan is hematologic, especially neutropenia. With the 5-day dosing schedule, 70–80% of patients have severe neutropenia, 25% febrile neutropenia.[277,280] In some studies, regimens of 5 days produce better response rates than regimens of shorter duration, but in others, reducing the dose to 1 mg/m^2/d for 3 days is associated with similar response rates but lower toxicity.[281,282] Topotecan at 2 mg/m^2/d for 3 days every 21 days showed a 32% response rate.[282] Continuous infusion topotecan (0.4 mg/m^2/d for 14–21 days) had a 27–35% objective response rate in platinum-refractory patients.[283,284] Weekly topotecan administered at a dose of 4 mg/m^2/wk for 3 weeks with a week off every month produced a response rate similar to the 5-day regimen with considerably less toxicity.[285] Therefore, this is considered the regimen of choice for this agent.

Liposomal doxorubicin (Doxil in the United States and Caelyx in Europe) has activity in platinum- and taxane-refractory disease. Its predominant severe toxicity is the hand–foot syndrome, also known as palmar–plantar erythrodysesthesia or acral erythema, which is observed in 20% of patients who receive 50 mg/m^2 every 4 weeks.[286–288] Liposomal doxorubicin does not cause neurologic toxicity or alopecia. It is administered every 4 weeks, which makes it convenient, and it is relatively well tolerated at the lower dose of 40 mg/m^2, which is widely used. In a study of 89 patients with platinum-refractory disease, liposomal doxorubicin (50 mg/m^2 every 3 weeks) produced a response in 17%.[288] In another study, an objective response rate of 26% was reported, although there were no responses in women who progressed during first-line therapy.[286]

Another study on patients with platinum-resistant or platinum-refractory disease compared liposomal doxorubicin (50 mg/m^2 every 4 weeks) with topotecan (1.5 mg/m^2/d for 5 days every 3 weeks). The two treatments had a similar overall response rate (20% vs 17%), time to progression (22 vs 20 weeks), and median overall survival (66 vs 56 weeks). The myelotoxicity was significantly lower in the liposomal doxorubicin–treated patients.[287] Comparing liposomal doxorubicin with single-agent paclitaxel, a different study showed overall response rates of 18% and 22% for liposomal doxorubicin and paclitaxel, respectively, and median PFS 5.4 versus 6 weeks.[289]

Gemcitabine is a nucleoside analogue of cytidine and has been reported to have response rates of 10–20% in patients who have platinum-resistant disease and 6% in those with platinum-refractory disease. Principal toxicities are myelosuppression and gastrointestinal side effects.[265,290]

Similarly, the most common toxicities with oral etoposide are myelosuppression, nausea and vomiting. Grade 4 neutropenia is observed in approximately one-fourth of patients, and 10–15% have severe nausea and vomiting. An initial study of intravenous etoposide reported an objective response rate of only 8%,[262] however, oral etoposide given for a prolonged period (50 mg/m^2 daily for 21 days every 4 weeks) had a 27–32% response rate in platinum-resistant disease.[264]

Targeted therapies

Bevacizumab
In the AURELIA trial, women with recurrent platinum-resistant ovarian cancer were randomized to standard of care, that is, weekly topotecan, weekly paclitaxel, or monthly liposomal doxorubicin versus these agents combined with bevacizumab (10 mg/kg every 2 weeks, or 15 mg/kg every 3 weeks).[291] Women in the experimental arm had a longer PFS with 6.7 versus 3.4 months and a higher overall response rate with 30.9% versus 12.6%. An exploratory subgroup analysis noted a remarkable increase in overall survival for weekly paclitaxel plus bevacizumab from 13.4 to 22.4 months (with and without bevacizumab).[292] The findings in the AURELIA trial changed the standard of care.

PARP-inhibitors

Although the best data for the use of PARP-inhibitors is in recurrent platinum-sensitive ovarian cancer, there is also some data, for example, in Study 42[293] and QUADRA study,[294] on the effectiveness of PARP-inhibitors in heavily pretreated ovarian cancer including platinum-resistant and -refractory ovarian cancer.

Immunotherapy

The results of immune checkpoint inhibitors in melanoma and in lung cancer stimulated trials in ovarian cancer. Hamanishi et al. presented a phase II study using nivolumab, an anti-PD-1 antibody, which showed an objective response rate of 15% in heavily pretreated platinum-resistant patients.[295] KEYNOTE-100 evaluated pembrolizumab, another anti-PD-1 antibody, in patients with recurrent ovarian cancer after multiple prior lines of treatment. The overall response rate was 8%, with a CPS (combined positive score, quantifying the number of PD-L1 positive cells) over 10 the objective response rate was 10%.[296] Similarly, the response rate with avelumab, an anti-PD-L1 antibody, was 10% in recurrent ovarian cancer.[297] The lower efficacy in ovarian cancer may be related to the unique immune environment in the abdominal cavity, where immune cells are shielded from environmental antigens. Ovarian cancer may particularly benefit from combination therapies. The phase I/II TOPACIO trial using niraparib and pembrolizumab in recurrent platinum-resistant ovarian cancer showed a response rate of 18%.[298] The combination of the CTLA-4 antibody ipilimumab with nivolumab, an anti-PD-1 antibody, induction followed by nivolumab maintenance had an objective response rate of 31.4% as preliminary results show.[299] Therapeutic cancer vaccines and cell-based vaccines with for example, dendritic cells as well as adoptive cell therapy using tumor-infiltrating lymphocytes (TILs), engineered T cell receptors and engineered T-cell chimeric antigen receptors (CARs) are being developed against several targets, including mesothelin and NY-ESO.[300]

Hormonal therapy

Tamoxifen,[301–304] aromatase inhibitors and GNRH-agonists[305] have been used either alone or in combination with cytotoxic chemotherapy in patients with advanced disease. A Cochrane review concluded that there is some data for tamoxifen use from observational studies but no (reliable) data from randomized studies.[306,307] The aromatase inhibitors, anastrozole[308] and letrozole,[309] provided some durable clinical benefit in patients with ER-positive recurrent platinum-resistant disease and may delay symptomatic progression. The greatest value of aromatase inhibitors may be in low-grade ER-positive cancers.

Palliative radiotherapy

Radiotherapy as a palliative modality even in chemoresistant ovarian cancer may be very useful if the sole dominant symptomatic problem for the patient is localized to an isolated site. For example, a fixed pelvic mass eroding the vaginal mucosa causing bleeding, may occur without obvious disseminated symptomatic peritoneal disease. Localized masses in lymph nodes or bony or brain metastases may benefit from palliative irradiation as would painful hepatomegaly from hepatic capsular distention.[310] For single or multiple brain metastases, cyberknife or palliative whole brain irradiation can be applied.

Future directions

A number of approaches to more effective detection and management of ovarian cancer are being pursued aggressively.[311] An effective strategy for early detection of ovarian cancer could reduce mortality by more than 20%. While this goal has not yet been achieved, two stage strategies hold promise in that algorithms measuring the rise of CA125 over time combined with transvaginal ultrasonography have proven adequately specific for effective screening in a postmenopausal population. The challenge is to develop panels of blood biomarkers with adequate sensitivity and lead time, as well as more sensitive imaging techniques. Heterogeneity has been documented at a molecular level between and within ovarian cancers of different histotypes, providing novel targets for therapy. Distinctive metabolic changes can also be targeted, including dependence on fatty acids, aberrant glycolysis, overexpression of SIK2 and dependence on arginine.[311] The tumor microenvironment can affect response to anti-angiogenic and immunotherapy and components of the microenvironment can be modified to enhance the effects of treatment. This could prove particularly important for optimizing the activity of bevacizumab and check point inhibitors. Treatment of ovarian cancer with targeted therapy upregulates signaling pathways and induces autophagy, producing "adaptive resistance." Measurement of changes in signaling during treatment can aid in choosing appropriate combinations of targeted agents to overcome resistance to individual drugs. PARP inhibitors are being combined with PI3K inhibitors, MEK inhibitors, ATR inhibitors and CHK1 inhibitors to overcome PARP inhibitor resistance. These advances promise further improvement in patient outcomes over the next years.

Key references

The complete reference list can be found on Vital Source version of this title, see inside front cover.

11 Kurman RJ, Shih Ie M. Pathogenesis of ovarian cancer: lessons from morphology and molecular biology and their clinical implications. *Int J Gynecol Pathol.* 2008;**27**(2):151–160.

16. Rossing MA, Daling JR, Weiss NS, et al. Ovarian tumors in a cohort of infertile women. *N Engl J Med*. 1994;**331**(12):771–776.
21. Collaborative Group On Epidemiological Studies Of Ovarian Cancer, Beral V, Gaitskell K, et al. Menopausal hormone use and ovarian cancer risk: individual participant meta-analysis of 52 epidemiological studies. *Lancet*. 2015;**385**(9980): 1835–1842.
32. Struewing JP, Hartge P, Wacholder S, et al. The risk of cancer associated with specific mutations of BRCA1 and BRCA2 among Ashkenazi Jews. *N Engl J Med*. 1997;**336**(20):1401–1408.
35. Ponder B. Genetic testing for cancer risk. *Science*. 1997;**278**(5340):1050–1054.
37. King MC, Marks JH, Mandell JB, et al. Breast and ovarian cancer risks due to inherited mutations in BRCA1 and BRCA2. *Science*. 2003;**302**(5645):643–646.
43. Lynch HT, Krush AJ. Cancer family "G" revisited: 1895–1970. *Cancer*. 1971;**27**(6):1505–1511.
49. Narod SA, Risch H, Moslehi R, et al. Oral contraceptives and the risk of hereditary ovarian cancer. Hereditary ovarian cancer clinical study group. *N Engl J Med*. 1998;**339**(7):424–428.
50. Modan B, Hartge P, Hirsh-Yechezkel G, et al. Parity, oral contraceptives, and the risk of ovarian cancer among carriers and noncarriers of a BRCA1 or BRCA2 mutation. *N Engl J Med*. 2001;**345**(4):235–240.
57. Schrag D, Kuntz KM, Garber JE, et al. Decision analysis--effects of prophylactic mastectomy and oophorectomy on life expectancy among women with BRCA1 or BRCA2 mutations. *N Engl J Med*. 1997;**336**(20):1465–1471.
59. Rebbeck TR, Lynch HT, Neuhausen SL, et al. Prophylactic oophorectomy in carriers of BRCA1 or BRCA2 mutations. *N Engl J Med*. 2002;**346**(21):1616–1622.
66. Schmeler KM, Lynch HT, Chen LM, et al. Prophylactic surgery to reduce the risk of gynecologic cancers in the Lynch syndrome. *N Engl J Med*. 2006;**354**(3):261–269.
68. Cancer Genome Atlas Research Network. Integrated genomic analyses of ovarian carcinoma. *Nature*. 2011;**474**(7353):609–615.
70. Jimenez-Sanchez A, Memon D, Pourpe S, et al. Heterogeneous tumor-immune microenvironments among differentially growing metastases in an ovarian cancer patient. *Cell*. 2017;**170**(5):927–938 e20.
71. Zhang AW, McPherson A, Milne K, et al. Interfaces of malignant and immunologic clonal dynamics in ovarian cancer. *Cell*. 2018;**173**(7):1755–1769 e22.
76. Wiegand KC, Shah SP, Al-Agha OM, et al. ARID1A mutations in endometriosis-associated ovarian carcinomas. *N Engl J Med*. 2010;**363**(16):1532–1543.
82. Bast RC Jr, Klug TL, John ES, et al. A radioimmunoassay using a monoclonal antibody to monitor the course of epithelial ovarian cancer. *N Engl J Med*. 1983;**309**(15):883–887.
119. Rosenthal AN, Fraser L, Philpott S, et al. Final results of 4-monthly screening in the UK Familial Ovarian Cancer Screening Study (UKFOCSS Phase 2). *J Clin Oncol*. 2013;**31**(15_suppl):5507.
122. Jacobs IJ, Menon U, Ryan A, et al. Ovarian cancer screening and mortality in the UK Collaborative Trial of Ovarian Cancer Screening (UKCTOCS): a randomised controlled trial. *Lancet*. 2016;**387**(10022):945–956.
133. Trimbos JB, Parmar M, Vergote I, et al. International Collaborative Ovarian Neoplasm trial 1 and Adjuvant ChemoTherapy In Ovarian Neoplasm trial: two parallel randomized phase III trials of adjuvant chemotherapy in patients with early-stage ovarian carcinoma. *J Natl Cancer Inst*. 2003;**95**(2):105–112.
138. Harter P, Sehouli J, Lorusso D, et al. A randomized trial of lymphadenectomy in patients with advanced ovarian neoplasms. *N Engl J Med*. 2019;**380**(9):822–832.
141. Griffiths CT. Surgical resection of tumor bulk in the primary treatment of ovarian carcinoma. *Natl Cancer Inst Monogr*. 1975;**42**:101–104.
142. Hacker NF, Berek JS, Lagasse LD, et al. Primary cytoreductive surgery for epithelial ovarian cancer. *Obstet Gynecol*. 1983;**61**(4):413–420.
145. Bristow RE, Tomacruz RS, Armstrong DK, et al. Survival effect of maximal cytoreductive surgery for advanced ovarian carcinoma during the platinum era: a meta-analysis. *J Clin Oncol*. 2002;**20**(5):1248–1259.
171. International Collaborative Ovarian Neoplasm Group. Paclitaxel plus carboplatin versus standard chemotherapy with either single-agent carboplatin or cyclophosphamide, doxorubicin, and cisplatin in women with ovarian cancer: the ICON3 randomised trial. *Lancet*. 2002;**360**(9332):505–515.
179. Katsumata N, Yasuda M, Takahashi F, et al. Dose-dense paclitaxel once a week in combination with carboplatin every 3 weeks for advanced ovarian cancer: a phase 3, open-label, randomised controlled trial. *Lancet*. 2009;**374**(9698): 1331–1338.
183. Pignata S, Scambia G, Katsaros D, et al. Carboplatin plus paclitaxel once a week versus every 3 weeks in patients with advanced ovarian cancer (MITO-7): a randomised, multicentre, open-label, phase 3 trial. *Lancet Oncol*. 2014;**15**(4): 396–405.
185. Clamp AR, James EC, McNeish IA, et al. Weekly dose-dense chemotherapy in first-line epithelial ovarian, fallopian tube, or primary peritoneal carcinoma treatment (ICON8): primary progression free survival analysis results from a GCIG phase 3 randomised controlled trial. *Lancet*. 2019;**394**(10214):2084–2095.
186. Alberts DS, Liu PY, Hannigan EV, et al. Intraperitoneal cisplatin plus intravenous cyclophosphamide versus intravenous cisplatin plus intravenous cyclophosphamide for stage III ovarian cancer. *N Engl J Med*. 1996;**335**(26): 1950–1955.
188. Armstrong DK, Bundy B, Wenzel L, et al. Intraperitoneal cisplatin and paclitaxel in ovarian cancer. *N Engl J Med*. 2006;**354**(1):34–43.
195. van Driel WJ, Koole SN, Sikorska K, et al. Hyperthermic intraperitoneal chemotherapy in ovarian cancer. *N Engl J Med*. 2018;**378**(3):230–240.
200. Vergote I, Trope CG, Amant F, et al. Neoadjuvant chemotherapy or primary surgery in stage IIIC or IV ovarian cancer. *N Engl J Med*. 2010;**363**(10):943–953.
205. Kehoe S, Hook J, Nankivell M, et al. Primary chemotherapy versus primary surgery for newly diagnosed advanced ovarian cancer (CHORUS): an open-label, randomised, controlled, non-inferiority trial. *Lancet*. 2015; **386**(9990):249–257.
217. Perren TJ, Swart AM, Pfisterer J, et al. A phase 3 trial of bevacizumab in ovarian cancer. *N Engl J Med*. 2011;**365**(26):2484–2496.
220. Farmer H, McCabe N, Lord CJ, et al. Targeting the DNA repair defect in BRCA mutant cells as a therapeutic strategy. *Nature*. 2005;**434**(7035):917–921.
221. Fong PC, Boss DS, Yap TA, et al. Inhibition of poly(ADP-ribose) polymerase in tumors from BRCA mutation carriers. *N Engl J Med*. 2009;**361**(2):123–134.
223. Moore K, Colombo N, Scambia G, et al. Maintenance olaparib in patients with newly diagnosed advanced ovarian cancer. *N Engl J Med*. 2018;**379**(26): 2495–2505.
230. Gershenson DM, Bodurka DC, Coleman RL, et al. Hormonal maintenance therapy for women with low-grade serous cancer of the ovary or peritoneum. *J Clin Oncol*. 2017;**35**(10):1103–1111.
236. Rustin GJ, van der Burg ME, Griffin CL, et al. Early versus delayed treatment of relapsed ovarian cancer (MRC OV05/EORTC 55955): a randomised trial. *Lancet*. 2010;**376**(9747):1155–1163.
243. Bois AD, Sehouli J, Vergote I, et al. Randomized phase III study to evaluate the impact of secondary cytoreductive surgery in recurrent ovarian cancer: final analysis of AGO DESKTOP III/ENGOT-ov20. *J Clin Oncol*. 2020; **38**(15_suppl):6000.
244. Coleman RL, Spirtos NM, Enserro D, et al. Secondary surgical cytoreduction for recurrent ovarian cancer. *N Engl J Med*. 2019;**381**(20):1929–1939.
245. Parmar MK, Ledermann JA, Colombo N, et al. Paclitaxel plus platinum-based chemotherapy versus conventional platinum-based chemotherapy in women with relapsed ovarian cancer: the ICON4/AGO-OVAR-2.2 trial. *Lancet*. 2003;**361**(9375):2099–2106.
247. Pfisterer J, Plante M, Vergote I, et al. Gemcitabine plus carboplatin compared with carboplatin in patients with platinum-sensitive recurrent ovarian cancer: an intergroup trial of the AGO-OVAR, the NCIC CTG, and the EORTC GCG. *J Clin Oncol*. 2006;**24**(29):4699–4707.
252. Aghajanian C, Blank SV, Goff BA, et al. OCEANS: a randomized, double-blind, placebo-controlled phase III trial of chemotherapy with or without bevacizumab in patients with platinum-sensitive recurrent epithelial ovarian, primary peritoneal, or fallopian tube cancer. *J Clin Oncol*. 2012;**30**(17):2039–2045.
256. Ledermann J, Harter P, Gourley C, et al. Olaparib maintenance therapy in platinum-sensitive relapsed ovarian cancer. *N Engl J Med*. 2012;**366**(15): 1382–1392.
260. Mirza MR, Monk BJ, Herrstedt J, et al. Niraparib maintenance therapy in platinum-sensitive, recurrent ovarian cancer. *N Engl J Med*. 2016;**375**(22): 2154–2164.
261. Coleman RL, Oza AM, Lorusso D, et al. Rucaparib maintenance treatment for recurrent ovarian carcinoma after response to platinum therapy (ARIEL3): a randomised, double-blind, placebo-controlled, phase 3 trial. *Lancet*. 2017;**390**(10106):1949–1961.
291. Pujade-Lauraine E, Hilpert F, Weber B, et al. *Bevacizumab combined with chemotherapy for platinum-resistant recurrent ovarian cancer: The AURELIA open-label randomized phase III trial*. *J Clin Oncol*. 2014;**32**(13):1302–1308.
294. Moore KN, Secord AA, Geller MA, et al. *Niraparib monotherapy for late-line treatment of ovarian cancer (QUADRA): a multicentre, open-label, single-arm, phase 2 trial*. *Lancet Oncol*. 2019.
295. Hamanishi J, Mandai M, Ikeda T, et al. *Safety and Antitumor Activity of Anti-PD-1 Antibody, Nivolumab, in Patients With Platinum-Resistant Ovarian Cancer*. *J Clin Oncol*. 2015;**33**(34):4015–4022.
308. Kok PS, Beale P, O'Connell RL, et al. PARAGON (ANZGOG-0903): a phase 2 study of anastrozole in asymptomatic patients with estrogen and progesterone receptor-positive recurrent ovarian cancer and CA125 progression. *J Gynecol Oncol*. 2019;**30**(5):e86.

102 Nonepithelial ovarian malignancies

Jonathan S. Berek, MD, MMS ■ Malte Renz, MD, PhD ■ Michael L. Friedlander, MD, PhD ■ Robert C. Bast, Jr., MD

Overview

Compared with epithelial ovarian cancers, nonepithelial ovarian tumors are uncommon, constituting <10% of all ovarian malignancies. They include germ cell malignancies, sex cord-stromal tumors, and a variety of extremely rare ovarian cancers, including sarcomas and lipoid cell tumors. Although there are many similarities in presentation, evaluation, and management of the patients, these tumors also have unique features that require special approaches to management.[1-5] Germ cell malignancies are derived from primordial germ cells of the ovary and can be distinguished by histotype and expression of the biomarkers α-fetoprotein (AFP) and/or human chorionic gonadotropin (hCG). They include dysgerminomas (AFP− hCG−), embryonal carcinomas (AFP+ hCG+), immature teratomas (AFP− hCG−), endodermal sinus (yolk sac) tumors (AFP+ hCG−), and ovarian choriocarcinomas (AFP− hCG+). Germ cell tumors occur in premenarchal girls and young women, grow rapidly, and can present with a symptomatic pelvic mass. As preservation of fertility is almost always an important priority, unilateral salpingo-oophorectomy should be performed often followed by adjuvant platinum-based therapy. Of note, dysgerminomas can be bilateral in 10-15% and are associated with gonadal dysgenesis in 5% of cases. Metastatic germ cell cancers are very sensitive to chemotherapy and the long-term survival rate is high, even in advanced stages. At some institutions, young patients with stage IA germ cell tumors are followed carefully after resection with excellent outcomes and chemotherapy given only if there is recurrence with excellent outcomes. Sex cord-stromal tumors include granulosa-stromal tumors, juvenile granulosa tumors, and Sertoli–Leydig cell tumors. Granulosa-stromal tumors can occur at all ages and produce estrogen resulting in pseudo-precocious puberty in a small fraction of girls, amenorrhea in premenopausal women, and endometrial hyperplasia in postmenopausal adults. Granulosa-stromal tumors are indolent and often confined to one ovary where surgery can cure stage I disease in more than 75% of cases. Adjuvant chemotherapy is generally not given after complete resection. Late recurrence has, however, been observed. Persistent or recurrent disease has responded to platinum-based and hormonal therapy, including progestational agents, GnRH agonists, and aromatase inhibitors. Inhibin B has been a useful biomarker. Sertoli–Leydig cell tumors generally present in the third or fourth decade, produce androgens, and induce virilization in more than 70% of patients. As many Sertoli–Leydig cell tumors are in early-stage and rarely bilateral, unilateral salpingo-oophorectomy is often performed with 70–90% 5-year survival.

Germ cell malignancies

Germ cell tumors are derived from the primordial germ cells of the ovary and occur with only about one-tenth the incidence of malignant germ cell tumors of the testis. Although they can arise in extragonadal sites such as the mediastinum and retroperitoneum, the majority of germ cell tumors arise in the gonad from undifferentiated germ cells. The site variation of these cancers is explained by the embryonic migration of germ cells from the caudal part of the yolk sac to the dorsal mesentery before their incorporation into the sex cords of the developing gonads.[1,2]

Germ cell tumors are curable.[6-9] The management of patients with ovarian germ cell tumors has largely been extrapolated from the much greater experience of treating males with the more common testicular germ cell tumors. There have been many randomized trials for testicular germ cell tumors, which have provided a strong evidence base for treatment decisions.[10,11] The outcome of patients with testicular germ cell tumors is better in experienced centers, and it is reasonable to suggest the same will be true for the less common ovarian counterparts. The cure rate is high, and attention is now being directed at reducing toxicity without compromising survival. Several factors have been associated with a higher risk of recurrence in ovarian germ cell tumors, including age >45, advanced stage, high human chorionic gonadotropin (hCG), and/or α-fetoprotein (AFP), yolk sac/endodermal sinus histology. A risk stratification initially established in males with metastatic germ cell cancers[12] has also been shown to be prognostic in females. The estimated 3-year progression-free survival (PFS) for the good-, intermediate-, and poor-risk patients were 88%, 78%, and 31%, respectively. The poor-risk group included nondysgerminomatous tumors with either nonpulmonary metastases or with AFP of >10,000 ng/mL, hCG > 50,000 mIU/mL, lactate dehydrogenase (LDH) > 10× upper limit of normal. This group of patients may benefit from more intensive chemotherapy.[13]

Histology and biomarkers

A histologic classification of ovarian germ cell tumors is presented in Table 1.[1,14,15] Both AFP and hCG are secreted by some germ cell malignancies. An elevated AFP and hCG can be clinically useful in the differential diagnosis of patients with a pelvic mass, and in monitoring patients after surgery. Placental alkaline phosphatase (PLAP) and LDH are elevated in up to 95% of patients with dysgerminomas, and serial monitoring of serum LDH levels may be useful for monitoring the disease. PLAP is more useful as immunohistochemical marker. The classification of germ cell tumors is based on both, histologic features and expression of tumor biomarkers (Figure 1).[17,18] In this scheme, embryonal carcinoma, which is composed of undifferentiated cells that synthesize both hCG and AFP, is the progenitor of several other germ cell tumors.[17] More differentiated germ cell tumors—such as the endodermal sinus tumor (EST), which secretes AFP, and choriocarcinoma, which secretes hCG—are derived from extraembryonic tissues; immature teratomas are derived from embryonic cells and do not secrete hCG, but may be associated with an elevated AFP. Elevated hCG levels are seen in 5% of dysgerminomas and the level is typically less than 100 International Units. AFP is never elevated in pure dysgerminomas.[1]

Table 1 Histologic typing of ovarian germ cell tumors.[a]

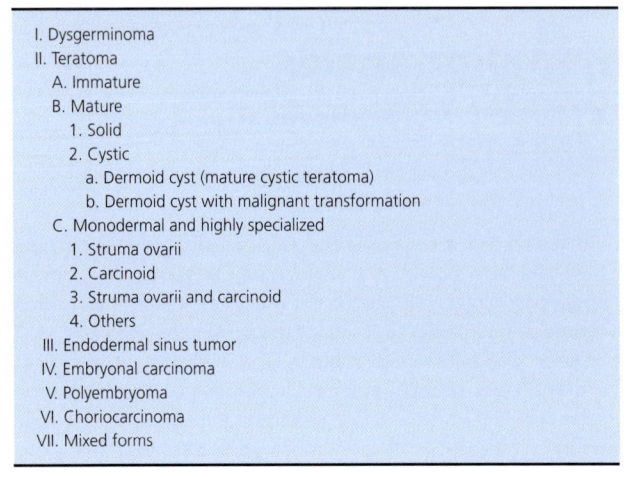

I. Dysgerminoma
II. Teratoma
   A. Immature
   B. Mature
      1. Solid
      2. Cystic
         a. Dermoid cyst (mature cystic teratoma)
         b. Dermoid cyst with malignant transformation
   C. Monodermal and highly specialized
      1. Struma ovarii
      2. Carcinoid
      3. Struma ovarii and carcinoid
      4. Others
III. Endodermal sinus tumor
IV. Embryonal carcinoma
V. Polyembryoma
VI. Choriocarcinoma
VII. Mixed forms

[a] Source: Adapted from Scully et al.[1]

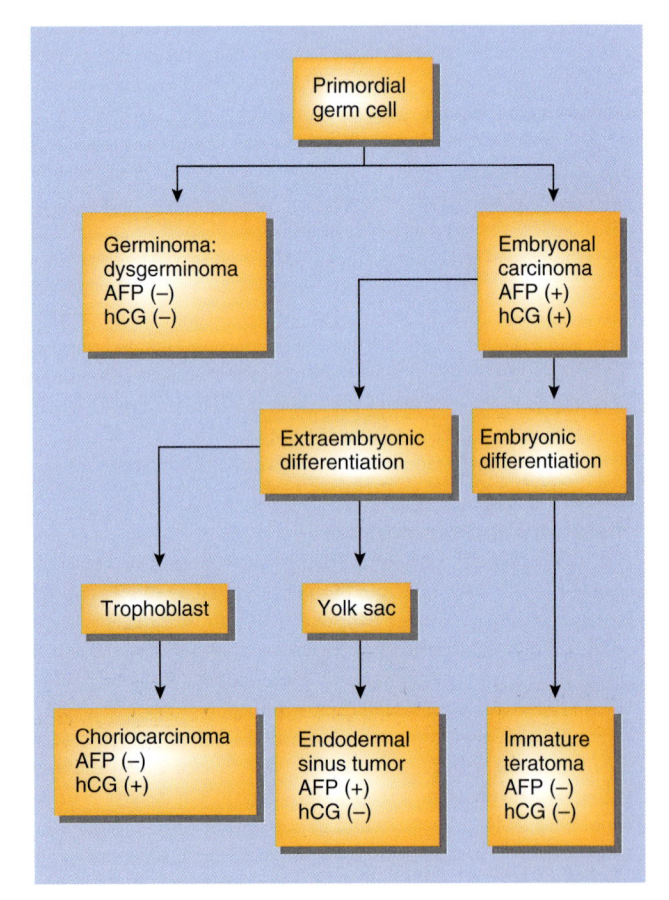

Figure 1 Relationship between examples of pure malignant germ cell tumors and their secreted substances. Abbreviations: AFP, α-fetoprotein; hCG, human chorionic gonadotropin. Source: Berek and Hacker.[16]

Epidemiology

Although 20–25% of all benign and malignant ovarian neoplasms are of germ cell origin, they account for only about 5% of all malignant ovarian neoplasms. In Asian and Black societies, where epithelial ovarian cancers are much less common, they may account for as many as 15% of ovarian cancers. In the first two decades of life, almost 70% of ovarian tumors are of germ cell origin, and one-third of these are malignant. Germ cell tumors account for two-thirds of the ovarian malignancies in this age group. Germ cell cancers also are seen in the third decade but become quite rare thereafter.[1,2,19,20]

Symptoms and signs

In contrast to the relatively slow-growing epithelial ovarian tumors, germ cell malignancies grow rapidly and often are characterized by pelvic pain related to capsular distention, hemorrhage, or necrosis. The rapidly enlarging pelvic mass may produce pressure symptoms on bladder or rectum. Menstrual irregularities may occur in menarchal patients. Some young patients may misinterpret the symptoms as those of pregnancy, and this can lead to a delay in diagnosis. Acute symptoms associated with torsion or rupture can develop. These symptoms may be confused with acute appendicitis. In more advanced cases, ascites may develop, and the patient may present with abdominal distention.[3]

In patients with a palpable adnexal mass, the evaluation can proceed as outlined above for epithelial cancers. Some patients with germ cell tumors will be premenarchal. If the lesions are principally solid, or a combination of solid and cystic on an ultrasonographic evaluation, a neoplasm is probable and a malignancy is possible. The remainder of the physical examination should search for signs of ascites, pleural effusion, and organomegaly.

Diagnosis

Adnexal masses measuring 2 cm or more in premenarchal girls, or cystic masses of 8–10 cm, or complex masses in premenopausal patients will usually require surgical exploration. In young patients, preoperative blood tests should include serum hCG, AFP, LDH, and CA125 levels, a complete blood count, and liver function tests. A radiograph of the chest is important because germ cell tumors can metastasize to lungs or mediastinum. A karyotype should ideally be obtained preoperatively on all premenarchal girls because of the propensity of these tumors to arise in dysgenetic gonads, but this may not be practical.[3] A preoperative computed tomographic (CT) scan or magnetic resonance imaging (MRI) may document the presence and extent of retroperitoneal lymphadenopathy or liver metastases, but unless there is very extensive metastatic disease, is unlikely to influence the decision to operate on the patient initially. If postmenarchal patients have predominantly cystic lesions up to 8–10 cm in diameter, they may undergo observation or a trial of hormonal suppression for two cycles.[21]

Dysgerminomas

Dysgerminomas are the most common malignant germ cell tumor, accounting for approximately 30–40% of all ovarian cancers of germ cell origin[2,18] (Figure 2). They represent only 1–3% of all ovarian cancers but represent as many one-third of ovarian cancers in patients younger than 20 years of age. Seventy-five percent of dysgerminomas occur between the ages of 10 and 30 years, 5% occur before the age of 10 years and they rarely occur after age 50.[1,5] They typically occur in young women and 20–30% of ovarian malignancies associated with pregnancy are dysgerminomas.

Association with abnormal ovaries

Approximately 5% of dysgerminomas occur in phenotypic females with abnormal gonads.[1,22] Dysgerminomas can be associated with patients who have pure gonadal dysgenesis (46XY, bilateral streak gonads), mixed gonadal dysgenesis (45X/46XY, unilateral

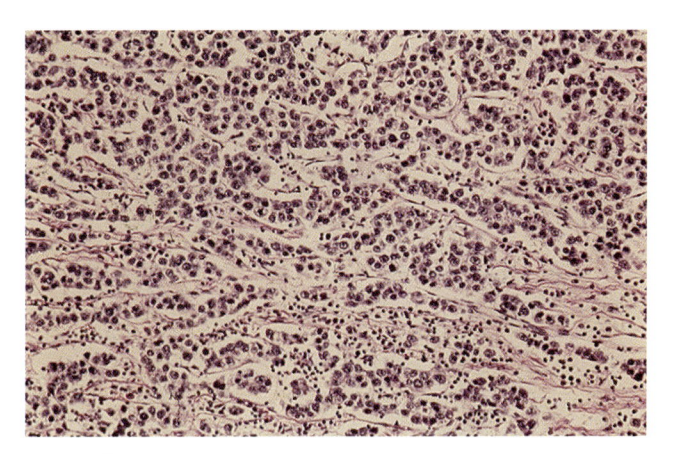

Figure 2 Dysgerminoma.

streak gonad, contralateral testis), and androgen insensitivity syndrome (46XY, testicular feminization). Therefore, in premenarchal patients with a pelvic mass, the karyotype should be determined, particularly if a dysgerminoma is considered as the likely diagnosis.

In most patients with gonadal dysgenesis, dysgerminomas arise in a gonadoblastoma, which is a benign ovarian tumor composed of germ cells and sex-cord stroma. If gonadoblastomas are left *in situ* in patients with gonadal dysgenesis, more than 50% will subsequently develop ovarian malignancies.[23]

Approximately 65% of dysgerminomas are stage I at diagnosis.[1,3,4,24–28] 85–90% of stage I tumors are confined to one ovary, while 10–15% are bilateral. All other germ cell tumors are rarely bilateral. In patients whose contralateral ovary has been preserved, a dysgerminoma can develop in 5–10% over the next 2 years. This figure includes patients who have not received systemic chemotherapy, as well as patients with gonadal dysgenesis.

Pattern of spread
In the 25% of patients who present with metastatic disease, the tumor most commonly spreads via the lymphatics, particularly to the higher para-aortic nodes.[26] They can also spread hematogenously, or by direct extension through the capsule of the ovary with exfoliation and dissemination of cells throughout the peritoneal surfaces. Metastases to the contralateral ovary may be present when there is no other evidence of spread. An uncommon site of metastatic disease is bone, and when metastasis to this site occurs, the metastases are seen typically in the lower vertebrae. Metastases to the lungs, liver, and brain are rare and seen mostly in patients with long-standing or recurrent disease. Metastasis to mediastinum and supraclavicular lymph nodes is also usually a late manifestation of disease.[24,25]

Treatment
The treatment of patients with early dysgerminoma is surgical, including resection of the primary lesion and limited surgical staging. Chemotherapy is administered to patients with metastatic disease. Because the disease principally affects young women, special consideration must be given to the preservation of fertility.[26,29] A comparison of outcomes based on treatment at the Norwegian Radium Hospital clearly demonstrates the superiority of chemotherapy over radiation. Survival was better and morbidity lower in the group treated with chemotherapy.[29]

Surgery
The minimum operation for ovarian dysgerminoma is unilateral oophorectomy.[8,27] If fertility preservation is desired, as usually is the case, the contralateral ovary, fallopian tube, and uterus should be left *in situ* even in the presence of metastatic disease, because of the sensitivity of the tumor to chemotherapy.[30] If fertility preservation is not required, it may be appropriate to perform a total abdominal hysterectomy and bilateral salpingo-oophorectomy in patients with advanced disease, although this will be appropriate in only a minority of patients.[4] In patients whose karyotype contains a Y chromosome, both ovaries should be removed, although the uterus may be left *in situ* for possible future embryo transfer. Cytoreductive surgery is of unproven value, but bulky disease that can be readily resected (e.g., an omental cake) should be removed at the initial operation. It is important not to undertake surgery that is potentially morbid and may delay the initiation of chemotherapy.

In patients in whom the dysgerminoma appears on inspection to be confined to the ovary, a careful staging operation should be undertaken to determine the presence of an occult metastatic disease. These tumors often metastasize to the para-aortic nodes around the renal vessels. Peritoneal washings should be taken for cytology, and a thorough exploration made of all peritoneal surfaces and retroperitoneal lymph nodes, with biopsy or resection of any noted abnormalities.[31] The contralateral ovary should be carefully inspected because dysgerminoma is the only germ cell tumor that tends to be bilateral, and not all of the bilateral lesions have obvious ovarian enlargement. Therefore, careful inspection and palpation of the contralateral ovary and excisional biopsy of any suspicious lesion are desirable.[4,8,27,28] If a small contralateral tumor is found, it may be possible to resect it and preserve some normal ovary.

Many patients with a dysgerminoma will have a tumor that is apparently confined to one ovary and will be referred after unilateral salpingo-oophorectomy without surgical staging. The options for such patients are (1) repeat laparotomy or laparoscopy for surgical staging, (2) regular pelvic and abdominal CT or MRI scans, or (3) adjuvant chemotherapy.[26] Because most dysgerminomas are confined to the ovary at presentation and are rapidly growing tumors, the author's preference is to offer regular and close surveillance to such patients.[32,33]

Radiation
Dysgerminomas are sensitive to radiation therapy; doses of 2500–3500 cGy may be curative. However, as (1) these tumors are very sensitive to platinum-based chemotherapy, and (2) infertility and secondary malignancies are important late effects of radiation therapy, radiation is no longer used as primary treatment. Radiation can be selectively used to treat recurrent disease.[4,28,29]

Chemotherapy
Chemotherapy is the adjuvant treatment of choice.[8,34–41] The obvious advantages are fertility preservation in most patients and reduced risk of secondary malignancies compared with radiation.[42–45] The most frequently used chemotherapeutic regimen is BEP (bleomycin, etoposide, and cisplatin) (Table 2). In the past, VBP (vinblastine, bleomycin, and cisplatin) and VAC (vincristine, actinomycin, and cyclophosphamide) were commonly used but are now rarely prescribed.[8,34–38]

The Gynecologic Oncology Group (GOG) studied three cycles of etoposide plus carboplatin (EC): Etoposide (120 mg/m^2 intravenously on days 1, 2, and 3 every 4 weeks) and carboplatin (400 mg/m^2 intravenously on day 1 every 4 weeks) in 39 patients with completely resected ovarian dysgerminoma, stages IB, IC, II, or III. The results were excellent, and GOG reported a sustained disease-free remission rate of 100%.[46]

Table 2 Combination chemotherapy for germ cell tumors of the ovary.

Regimens and drugs	Dosage and schedule[a]
BEP:	
Bleomycin	30 U[b] weekly to a maximum of 12 wk
	15 U[b]/m² /wk × 5; then on day 1 of course 4
Etoposide	100 mg/m² /d × 5 d every 3 wk
Cisplatin	20 mg/m² /d × 5 d, or 100 mg/m² /d × 1 d every 3 wk

[a] All doses given intravenously.
[b] 1 U = 1 mg.

For patients with advanced, incompletely resected germ cell tumors, the GOG studied cisplatin-based chemotherapy on two consecutive protocols. In the first study, patients received four cycles of VBP, that is, vinblastine (12 mg/m² every 3 weeks), bleomycin (20 unit/m² intravenously every week for 12 weeks), and cisplatin (20 mg/m²/day intravenously for 5 days every 3 weeks). Patients with persistent or progressive disease at second-look laparotomy were treated with six cycles of VAC.[35] In the second trial, patients received three cycles of BEP initially, followed by consolidation with VAC, which was later discontinued in patients with dysgerminomas. VAC does not appear to improve the outcome following the BEP regimen and is no longer used.[37] A total of 20 evaluable patients with stages III and IV dysgerminoma were treated in these two protocols, and 19 were alive and free of disease after 6–68 months (median = 26 months). Fourteen of these patients had a second-look laparotomy, and all findings were negative. In a series from MD Anderson Hospital, 26 patients with pure ovarian dysgerminomas received BEP chemotherapy, 54% of the patients had stage IIIC or IV disease, and 25 of 26 patients (96%) remained continuously disease free following three to six cycles of therapy.[36]

These results indicate that patients with advanced-stage, incompletely resected dysgerminoma have an excellent prognosis when treated with cisplatin-based combination chemotherapy. The optimal regimen is three to four cycles of BEP based on the data from testicular cancer with the number of cycles depending on the extent of disease and the presence of visceral metastases.[47–49] If bleomycin is contraindicated or omitted because of lung toxicity,[50] consideration should be given to four cycles of cisplatin and etoposide rather than three cycles of BEP.

There is no need to perform a second-look laparotomy in patients with dysgerminomas[51–53] as the vast majority of these patients will only have necrotic tissue and nonviable tumor. In general, these patients should be closely monitored with scans and tumor markers. A positron emission tomography (PET–CT) scan should be considered in patients who have bulky residual masses larger than 3 cm more than 4 weeks after chemotherapy. A positive PET–CT scan appears to be a sensitive predictor of residual seminoma in males in these circumstances,[54] with residual disease evident in 30–50% of patients. If the PET–CT is positive or if there is a suggestion of progressive disease on scans, ideally there should be histologic confirmation of residual disease before embarking on salvage therapy.[55]

Recurrent disease

Although recurrences are uncommon, 75% will occur within the first year after initial treatment, with the most common sites being the peritoneal cavity and the retroperitoneal lymph nodes.[1,2] These patients should be treated with either chemotherapy or radiation, depending on the location of disease and the primary treatment. Patients with recurrent disease who have had no therapy other than surgery should be treated with chemotherapy. If previous chemotherapy with BEP has been given, an alternative regimen such as TIP (paclitaxel, ifosfamide, and cisplatin), a commonly used salvage regimen in testicular germ cell tumors,[56] may be tried.

These treatment decisions should be made in a multidisciplinary setting with the input of physicians experienced in the management of patients with germ cell tumors. Consideration may be given to the use of high-dose chemotherapy with peripheral stem cell support in selected patients.[57] A number of high-dose regimens have been used in Phase II studies, and the choice depends on the previous chemotherapy, time to recurrence, and residual toxicity from the previous therapy.[58–60] It is unclear whether high-dose chemotherapy is superior to conventional-dose chemotherapy as first-line salvage therapy for patients with relapsed disease. The only randomized trial, conducted by the European Group for Blood and Marrow Transplantation (EBMT)-IT-94, did not demonstrate superiority for three cycles of VIP (vinblastine-ifosfamide-cisplatin) followed by high-dose chemotherapy compared with four cycles of conventional-dose chemotherapy.[58] An international randomized trial (TIGER) plans to randomize 390 patients with recurrent germ cell tumors to four cycles of conventional-dose cisplatin-based chemotherapy with TIP, compared with two cycles of paclitaxel-ifosfamide followed by three cycles of high-dose carboplatin and etoposide with autologous stem-cell support (paclitaxel, ifosfamide for cycles 1 and 2, carboplatin, etoposide for cycles 3, 4, 5 [TICE]).[59]

Radiation therapy may be considered in selected patients with dysgerminomas and localized recurrence, but this has the major disadvantage of causing loss of fertility if pelvic and abdominal radiation is required, and may also compromise the ability to deliver further chemotherapy if unsuccessful.[29]

Pregnancy

Because dysgerminomas tend to occur in young patients, they may coexist with pregnancy. When a stage IA cancer is found, the tumor can be removed intact and the pregnancy continued. In patients with more advanced disease, continuation of the pregnancy will depend on gestational age. In general, chemotherapy can be given in the second and third trimesters in the same dosages as given for the nonpregnant patient without apparent detriment to the fetus.[43,61] However, relatively few patients have been treated with BEP during pregnancy and some fetal malformations and complications have been reported, underscoring the importance of ensuring that only patients who definitely require chemotherapy during pregnancy should be treated.[62]

Prognosis

In patients with stage IA dysgerminoma, unilateral oophorectomy alone results in a 5-year disease-free survival rate of greater than 95%.[4,28] The features that have been associated with a higher tendency to recurrence include tumors larger than 10–15 cm in diameter, age younger than 20 years, and microscopic features that include numerous mitoses, anaplasia, and a medullary pattern.[1,18]

Kumar et al. abstracted data on malignant ovarian germ cell tumors from the Surveillance, Epidemiology, and End Results (SEER) program from 1988 through 2004.[63] There was a total of 1296 patients with dysgerminomas, immature teratomas, or mixed germ cell tumors, 613 (47.3%) of whom had lymphadenectomies. Lymph node metastases were present in 28% of dysgerminomas, 8% of immature teratomas, and 16% of mixed germ cell tumors ($p < 0.05$). The 5-year survival for patients with negative nodes was 95.7% compared to 82.8% for patients with positive nodes

($p < 0.001$). The same group updated the results recently and reported on 1083 patients with ovarian germ cell tumors who had surgery and who were believed to have disease clinically confined to the ovary.[64] This included 590 (54.5%) who had no lymphadenectomy and 493 (45.5%) who had a lymphadenectomy. Of the latter, 52 (10.5%) were upstaged to Fédération Internationale de Gynécologie et d'Obstétrique (FIGO) stage III due to nodal metastases. The 5-year survival was 96.9% for patients who did not have a lymphadenectomy, 97.7% for those who did, and 93.4% for patients who were found to have stage III disease after lymphadenectomy. These survivals were not statistically different, and underscore the excellent prognosis for patients with dysgerminomas.

Immature teratoma

Immature teratomas typically contain immature neuroepithelium and may be pure immature teratomas or occur in combination with other germ cell tumors as mixed germ cell tumors. The pure immature teratoma accounts for fewer than 1% of all ovarian cancers, but it is the second most common germ cell malignancy and represents 10–20% of all ovarian malignancies seen in women younger than 20 years of age.[1] Approximately 50% of pure immature teratomas of the ovary occur between the ages of 10 and 20 years, and they rarely occur in postmenopausal women.

Semi-quantification of the amount of neuroepithelium correlates with survival in ovarian immature teratomas and is the basis for the grading of these tumors.[65–67] Those with less than one lower-power field of immature neuroepithelium on the slide with the greatest amount of immature neuroepithelium (grade 1) have a survival of at least 95%, whereas greater amounts of immature neuroepithelium (grades 2 and 3) appear to have a lower overall survival (approximately 85%).[67] This may not apply to immature teratomas of the ovary in children, because they appear to have a very good outcome with surgery alone, regardless of the degree of immaturity. These findings are from an era when not all patients would have received platinum-based chemotherapy.[68,69]

Some pathologists have recommended a two-tiered grading system, suggesting that immature teratomas be categorized as either low grade or high grade because of the significant inter- and intra-observer difficulty with a three-grade system above,[66] which is the authors' current practice.

Immature ovarian teratomas may be associated with gliomatosis peritonei, which has a favorable prognosis if composed of completely mature tissues. Recent reports have suggested that these glial "implants" are not tumor derived, but represent teratoma-induced metaplasia of pluripotential Müllerian stem cells in the peritoneum.[68,70,71] SRY-box 2 (SOX2) is universally expressed in gliomatosis peritonei.[72]

Malignant transformation of a mature teratoma is a rare event. Squamous cell carcinoma is the most frequent subtype of malignancy, but adenocarcinomas, primary melanomas, and carcinoids may also rarely occur (see below).[73] The risk is reported to be between 0.5% and 2% of teratomas, and usually occurs in postmenopausal patients.

Diagnosis

The preoperative evaluation and differential diagnosis are the same as for patients with other germ cell tumors. Some of these tumors will contain calcifications similar to mature teratomas, and this can be detected by a radiograph of the abdomen or by ultrasonography. Rarely, they are associated with the production of steroid hormones and can be accompanied by sexual pseudoprecocity.[5] AFP may be elevated in some patients with a pure immature teratoma but hCG is not elevated.

Surgery

In a premenopausal patient where the tumor appears confined to a single ovary, unilateral oophorectomy, and limited surgical staging should be performed. In the rare postmenopausal patient with an immature teratoma, a total abdominal hysterectomy and bilateral salpingo-oophorectomy may be performed. Contralateral involvement is rare, and routine resection or wedge biopsy of the contralateral ovary is unnecessary.[2] Any suspicious lesions on the peritoneal surfaces should be sampled and submitted for histologic evaluation. The most frequent site of dissemination is the peritoneum and, much less commonly, the retroperitoneal lymph nodes. Hematogenous metastases to organ parenchyma such as the lungs, liver, or brain are uncommon. When present, they are usually seen in patients with late or recurrent disease and most often in tumors that are high grade.[5]

It is unclear whether debulking of metastases improves the response to combination chemotherapy.[74,75] Cure ultimately depends on the ability to deliver chemotherapy promptly. Any surgical resection that may be potentially morbid and therefore delay chemotherapy should be resisted, although surgical resection of any residual disease should be considered at the completion of chemotherapy.

Chemotherapy

In the pediatric patient, surveillance is considered standard by pediatric oncologists,[76] while in the adult patient, postoperative chemotherapy has been widely used for high-grade stage IA and stage II–IV pure immature teratomas.[77] Although this has been questioned even in the adult patient, as excellent results have been also reported with close surveillance and treating only patients who have a recurrence.[26,29,35,36,38,69,78–89] Chemotherapy for nondysgerminomatous germ cell tumors is discussed below.

Surgery for residual disease

Surgery should be considered in patients with metastatic immature teratomas who have residual disease at the completion of chemotherapy because they may have residual mature teratoma and are at risk of growing teratoma syndrome, a rare complication of immature teratomas.[90–94] Furthermore, cancers can arise at a later date in residual mature teratoma, and it is important to resect any residual mass and exclude persistent disease, as further chemotherapy may be indicated.

The principles of surgery are based on the much larger experience of surgery in males with residual masses following chemotherapy for germ cell tumors with a component of immature teratoma.[95] Mathew et al. reported their experience of laparotomy in assessing postchemotherapy residual masses in ovarian germ cell tumors.[96] Sixty-eight patients completed combination chemotherapy with cisplatin regimens, of whom 35 had radiologic evidence of residual masses. Twenty-nine of these 35 patients underwent laparotomy, and 10 patients (34.5%) had viable tumor, including seven cases (24.2%) of immature teratoma. Nineteen patients (65.5) had no evidence of malignancy, including three (10.3%) cases showing mature teratoma, and 16 (55.2%) showing necrosis or fibrosis only. None of the patients with a dysgerminoma or embryonal carcinoma and a radiologic residual mass of less than 5 cm had viable tumor present, whereas all patients with primary tumors containing a component of teratoma had residual tumor, strengthening the case for surgery in patients with metastatic immature teratoma and any residual mass.[96,97]

Prognosis

The most important prognostic feature of the immature teratoma is the grade and stage of the lesion.[1,5,66] Overall, the 5-year survival rate for patients with all stages of pure immature teratomas is 70–80%, and it is 90–95% for patients with surgical stage I tumors.[66,78]

The degree or grade of immaturity generally predicts the metastatic potential and prognosis. The 5-year survival rates have been reported to be 82%, 62%, and 30% for patients with grades 1, 2, and 3, respectively[66] but many of these patients were treated in an era before optimal chemotherapy was available, and these figures do not match current experience and more recently published data.[83] For example, Lai et al.[98] reported on the long-term outcome of 84 patients with ovarian germ cell tumors, including 29 immature teratomas, and the 5-year survival was 97.4%.

Occasionally, these tumors are associated with mature or low-grade glial elements that have implanted throughout the peritoneum. Such patients have a favorable long-term survival.[5] Mature glial elements can grow and mimic malignant disease and may need to be resected to relieve pressure on surrounding structures.

Endodermal sinus tumor

ESTs have also been referred to as yolk sac carcinomas because they are derived from the primitive yolk sac.[1] They are the third most frequent malignant germ cell tumor of the ovary. ESTs have a median age of 18 years at diagnosis.[1–3,99] Approximately one-third of the patients are premenarchal at presentation. Abdominal or pelvic pain occurs in approximately 75% of patients, whereas an asymptomatic pelvic mass is documented in 10% of patients. Most ESTs secrete AFP and rarely may also elaborate detectable α-1-antitrypsin (AAT). There is a good correlation between the extent of disease and the level of AFP, although discordance also has been observed. The serum level of AFP is useful in monitoring the patient's response to treatment, as well as in follow-up.[99–103]

Treatment

The treatment of an EST consists of surgical exploration, unilateral salpingo-oophorectomy, a frozen section for diagnosis, and limited surgical staging. A hysterectomy and contralateral salpingo-oophorectomy should not be done.[5,101,102] Conservative surgery and adjuvant chemotherapy allow fertility preservation as with other germ cell tumors.[8] In patients with metastatic disease, all gross disease should be resected if possible. At surgery, the tumors tend to be solid and large, ranging in size from 7 to 28 cm (median 15 cm) in the GOG series. Bilaterality is not seen in EST, and the other ovary is involved with metastatic disease only when there are other metastases in the peritoneal cavity. Most patients have early-stage disease: 71% stage I, 6% stage II, and 23% stage III.[102] All patients with ESTs should be treated with chemotherapy shortly after recovering from surgery. Prior to the routine use of combination chemotherapy, the 2-year survival rate was approximately 25%. After the introduction of the VAC regimen, the survival rate improved to 60–70%, which highlights the chemosensitivity of the majority of these tumors.[86,104] All patients should be treated with a cisplatin-based regimen such as BEP, which is considered the standard of care. The chance of cure now approaches 100% for patients with early-stage disease and is at least 75% for patients with more advanced-stage disease.[102]

Rare ovarian germ cell tumors

Embryonal carcinoma

Embryonal carcinoma of the ovary is an extremely rare tumor that is distinguished from choriocarcinoma of the ovary by the absence of syncytiotrophoblastic and cytotrophoblastic cells. The patients are very young, their ages ranging between 4 and 28 years (median 14 years) in two series.[105] Older patients have been reported.[106] Embryonal carcinomas may secrete estrogens, with the patient exhibiting symptoms and signs of precocious pseudopuberty or irregular bleeding.[1] The presentation is otherwise similar to that of EST. The primary lesions tend to be large, and approximately two-thirds are confined to one ovary at the time of presentation. These lesions frequently secrete AFP and hCG, which are useful for following the response to subsequent therapy.[107] The treatment of embryonal carcinomas is the same as that for ESTs.[67,108]

Choriocarcinoma of the ovary

Pure nongestational choriocarcinoma of the ovary is an extremely rare tumor. Histologically, it has the same appearance as gestational choriocarcinoma metastatic to the ovaries.[109] The majority of patients with this cancer are younger than 20 years. The presence of hCG can be useful in monitoring the patient's response to treatment. In the presence of high hCG levels, isosexual precocity has been seen, occurring in approximately 50% of patients whose tumors appear before menarche.[110,111]

There are only a few limited reports on the use of chemotherapy for these nongestational choriocarcinomas, but complete responses have been reported to the MAC regimen (methotrexate, actinomycin D, and cyclophosphamide) as described for gestational trophoblastic disease.[109] These tumors are so rare that no good data are available, but the options also include the BEP or cisplatin, vincristine (or oncovine), methotrexate, bleomycin, actinomycin, cyclophosphamide, etoposide (POMB-ACE) regimens. The prognosis for ovarian choriocarcinomas has been poor. The majority of patients have metastases to organ parenchyma of example lung, liver brain at the time of initial diagnosis, and they should be managed as high-risk germ cell tumors.

Polyembryoma

Polyembryoma of the ovary is another extremely rare tumor, which is composed of "embryoid bodies." This tumor replicates the structures of early embryonic differentiation (i.e., the three somatic layers: endoderm, mesoderm, and ectoderm).[1,18] They occur in very young, premenarchal girls with signs of pseudopuberty, and AFP and hCG levels are elevated. Women with polyembryomas confined to one ovary may be followed with serial tumor markers and imaging to avoid cytotoxic chemotherapy. In patients who require chemotherapy, the BEP regimen is appropriate.[112]

Mixed germ cell tumor

Mixed germ cell malignancies of the ovary contain two or more elements of the tumors described above. In one series, the most common component of a mixed germ cell tumor was dysgerminoma, which occurred in 80%, followed by EST in 70%, immature teratoma in 53%, choriocarcinoma in 20%, and embryonal carcinoma in 16%. The most frequent combination was dysgerminoma and EST. The mixed germ cell tumors may secrete either AFP or hCG—or both or neither—depending on the components.

These tumors should be managed with combination chemotherapy, preferably BEP. The serum marker, if positive initially, may become negative during chemotherapy, but this may reflect regression of only a particular component of the mixed lesion. Therefore, a second-look laparotomy may be indicated if there is residual disease following chemotherapy, particularly if there was an immature teratomatous component in the original tumor.[113]

The most important prognostic features are the size of the primary tumor and the relative percentage of its most malignant component. In stage IA lesions smaller than 10 cm, survival is 100%. Tumors composed of less than one-third EST, choriocarcinoma, or grade 3 immature teratoma also have an excellent prognosis, but it is possibly less favorable when these components comprise the majority of the tumor.

Chemotherapy for nondysgerminomatous ovarian germ cell tumors

The most frequently used combination chemotherapeutic regimen in the past was VAC,[86,104] but a GOG study reported a relapse-free survival rate in patients with incompletely resected disease of only 75%.[86] The approach over the last 30 years has been to incorporate cisplatin into the primary treatment of these tumors, and most of the experience has been with the VBP in the past and BEP more recently.

The GOG prospectively evaluated three courses of BEP therapy in patients with completely resected stage I, II, and III ovarian germ cell tumors. Overall, the toxicity was acceptable, and 91 of 93 patients (97.8%) with nondysgerminomatous tumors were clinically free of disease.[38] Some patients can progress rapidly postoperatively, and, in general, treatment should be initiated as soon as possible after surgery, preferably within 7–10 days, in those patients who require chemotherapy.

The switch from VBP to BEP has been prompted by the experience in patients with testicular cancer, where the replacement of vinblastine with etoposide has been associated with a better therapeutic index (i.e., equivalent efficacy and lower morbidity), with less neurologic and gastrointestinal (GI) toxicity, and improved outcomes. Furthermore, the use of bleomycin appears to be important in this group of patients. In a randomized study of three cycles of etoposide plus cisplatin with or without bleomycin (EP vs. BEP) in 171 patients with germ cell tumors of the testes, the BEP regimen had a relapse-free survival rate of 86% compared with 69% for the EP regimen ($p = 0.01$).[47]

Cisplatin is superior to carboplatin in metastatic germ cell tumors of the testis. Two hundred sixty-five patients with good-prognosis germ cell tumors of the testes were entered into a study of four cycles of EP versus four cycles of EC. There were four relapses with EP versus 16 with the EC regimen.[49]

A German group randomized patients to (1) a BEP regimen of three cycles at standard doses given days 1–5 versus (2) a carboplatin, etoposide, and bleomycin (CEB) regimen of carboplatin (target area under the curve (AUC) of 5 on day 1), etoposide 120 mg/m² on days 1–3, and bleomycin 30 mg on days 1, 8, and 15.[114] Four cycles of CEB were given, with the omission of bleomycin in the fourth cycle so that the cumulative doses of etoposide and bleomycin in the two treatment arms were comparable. Fifty-four patients were entered on the trial; 29 were treated with BEP and 25 with CEB chemotherapy. More patients treated with CEB relapsed after therapy (32% vs. 13%). Four patients (16%) treated with CEB died of disease progression in contrast to one patient (3%) after BEP therapy. The trial was terminated early after an interim analysis. The inferiority of carboplatin was confirmed in a larger randomized trial reported by Horwich et al. in males with nonseminomatous germ cell tumors.[115]

In view of these results, BEP is the preferred treatment regimen for women with ovarian germ cell tumors. The 3-day schedule has been found to be equivalent to a 5-day schedule for BEP chemotherapy.[116] A cycle of BEP consists of etoposide 500 mg/m², administered at either 100 mg/m² days 1 through 5 or 165 mg/m² days 1 through 3, cisplatin 100 mg/m², administered at either 20 mg/m² days 1 through 5 or 50 mg/m² days 1 and 2. Bleomycin 30 U is administered on days 1, 8, and 15 during cycles 1 through 3. Growth factor support is often required due to the risk of febrile neutropenia.

The optimal number of treatment cycles has not been established in ovarian germ cell tumors, but it is reasonable to extrapolate from the much larger experience in testicular germ cell tumors where three cycles of BEP is considered optimal for patients with low-risk tumors and four cycles for patients with intermediate to high-risk tumors.[116,117] In patients for whom bleomycin is omitted or discontinued because of toxicity, four cycles of cisplatin and etoposide are recommended. An alternative approach is to use VIP (etoposide, ifosfamide, and cisplatin) in patients with more advanced disease in whom bleomycin is contraindicated. Four cycles of VIP are equivalent to four cycles of BEP, but it is more myelotoxic and requires growth-factor support.[10,11] These patients should only be treated by clinicians experienced in the management of germ cell tumors as the outcomes of patients in inexperienced hands are compromised.

Neoadjuvant chemotherapy followed by fertility-sparing surgery may also be a reasonable option for patients with advanced ovarian germ cell tumors not suitable for optimal cytoreduction, as shown in a study of 21 patients from India.[118]

Over 40 years ago, the group from Charing Cross Hospital London developed the POMB-ACE (cisplatin, vincristine, methotrexate, bleomycin, actinomycin D, cyclophosphamide, etoposide) regimen for high-risk germ cell tumors of any histological type.[119,120] Results appear to be superior to BEP in patients with poor prognosis but have not been confirmed in randomized trials. This protocol introduces seven drugs into the initial treatment with the intention to reduce development of drug resistance which may be particularly relevant in patients with large-volume disease. The authors have used the POMB-ACE regimen as primary treatment for select patients with liver or brain metastases. The regimen is only moderately myelosuppressive, so the intervals between each course can be kept to a maximum of 14 days (usually 9–11), thereby minimizing the time for tumor regrowth. When bleomycin is given by a 48-h infusion, pulmonary toxicity is reduced. With a maximum of 9 years of follow-up, the Charing Cross group has seen no severe long-term side effects in patients treated with POMB-ACE. Children have developed normally, menstruation has been physiologic, and several completed normal pregnancies have been reported (Table 3).

There are a number of groups investigating different regimens to treat patients with testicular germ cell tumors who fall into the intermediate or high-risk group; the studied regimens include accelerated BEP every 2 weeks.[121]

Table 3 POMB/ACE chemotherapy for germ cell tumors of the ovary.

POMB	
Day 1	Vincristine 1 mg/m² IV; methotrexate 300 mg/m² as a 12-h infusion
Day 2	Bleomycin 15 mg[a] by 24-h infusion, folinic acid rescue started 24 h after the start of methotrexate in a dose of 15 mg[a] every 12 h for four doses
Day 3	Bleomycin 15 mg[a] by 24-h infusion
Day 4	Cisplatin 120 mg/m² as a 12-h infusion, given together with hydration and 3 mg magnesium sulfate supplementation
ACE	
Days 1–5	Etoposide (VP16) 100 mg/m², days 1–5
Days 3–5	Actinomycin D 0.5 mg IV, days 3–5
Day 5	Cyclophosphamide 500 mg/m² IV, day 5
OMB	
Day 1	Vincristine 1 mg/m² IV; methotrexate 300 mg/m² as a 12-h infusion
Day 2	Bleomycin 15 mg[a] by 24-h infusion; folinic acid rescue started at 24-h
Day 3	Bleomycin 15 mg[a] by 24-h infusion

The sequence of treatment schedules is two courses of POMB followed by ACE. POMB is then alternated with ACE until patients are in biochemical remission as measured by hCG and AFP, PLAP, and LDH. The usual number of courses of POMB is three to five. Following biochemical remission, patients alternate ACE with OMB until remission has been maintained for approximately 12 wk. The interval between courses of treatment is kept to the minimum (usually 9–11 d). If delays are caused by myelosuppression after courses of ACE, the first 2 d of etoposide are omitted from subsequent courses of ACE.
[a] 1 U = 1 mg.

Surveillance for stage I ovarian germ cell tumors

Surveillance is a common approach to the management of young men with apparent stage I testicular germ cell tumors. There is a large body of evidence to support this approach, as well as guidelines on what constitutes appropriate surveillance.[10,11] Although as many as 20–30% of patients will relapse, almost all will be cured with salvage chemotherapy with BEP, and the potential adverse effects of chemotherapy can be avoided in most patients.

Although this is a very common approach in young men, it has not been widely adopted in females with ovarian germ cell tumors. However, some data are now available to support surveillance in selected patients whose disease is confined to the ovary. Cushing et al. reported a study of 44 pediatric patients with completely resected ovarian immature teratomas who were followed for recurrence of disease with imaging and serum tumor markers.[122] Thirty-one patients (70.5%) had pure ovarian immature teratomas with a tumor grade of 1 ($n = 17$), 2 ($n = 12$), or 3 ($n = 2$). Thirteen patients (29.5%) had an ovarian immature teratoma plus microscopic foci of yolk sac tumor. The 4-year event-free and overall survival for the ovarian immature teratoma group and for the ovarian immature teratoma plus yolk sac tumor group was 97.7% (95% confidence interval, 84.9–99.7%) and 100%, respectively. The only yolk sac tumor relapse occurred in a child with ovarian immature teratoma and yolk sac tumor who was then treated and salvaged with chemotherapy.

The Charing Cross Group initially reported a prospective study of 24 patients with stage IA ovarian germ cell tumors who were also enrolled in a surveillance program. The group consisted of nine patients (37.5%) with dysgerminoma, nine (37.5%) with pure immature teratoma, and six (25%) with ESTs (with or without immature teratoma). Treatment consisted of surgical resection without adjuvant chemotherapy, followed by surveillance with clinical, serologic, and radiologic review. A second-look operation was performed, and all but one patient were alive and in remission after a median follow-up of 6.8 years. The 5-year overall survival was 95%, and the 5-year disease-free survival was 68%. Eight patients required chemotherapy for recurrent disease or a second primary germ cell tumor. This included three patients with a grade II immature teratoma, three patients with a dysgerminoma, and two patients with dysgerminoma who developed a contralateral dysgerminoma 4.5 and 5.2 years after their first tumor. All but one, who died of a pulmonary embolus, was successfully salvaged with chemotherapy.[123]

The same group updated its experience and reported on the safety of the ongoing surveillance program of all stage IA female germ cell tumors.[32] Thirty-seven patients (median age 26, range 14–48 years) with stage I disease underwent surgery and staging followed by intense surveillance, which included regular tumor markers and imaging. The median follow-up was 6 years. Relapse rates for stage IA nondysgerminomatous tumors and dysgerminomas were 8 of 22 (36%) and 2 of 9 (22%), respectively. In addition, one patient with mature teratoma and glial implants also relapsed. Ten of these 11 patients (91%) were successfully cured with platinum-based chemotherapy. Only one patient died from chemo-resistant disease. All relapses occurred within 13 months of initial surgery. The overall disease-specific survival of malignant ovarian germ cell tumors was 94%.

More than 50% of patients who underwent fertility-sparing surgery went on to have successful pregnancies. They concluded that surveillance of all stage IA ovarian germ cell tumors was safe and feasible and that the outcome was comparable with testicular tumors. They questioned the need for potentially toxic adjuvant chemotherapy in all patients with nondysgerminomas who have greater than 90% chance of being salvaged with chemotherapy if they relapse.

These results are supported by more recent studies. Park et al. reported of 31 young women with stage I tumors. The 10-year disease-free survival was 77%, but the 10-year overall survival was 97% with all but one of seven relapsed patients successfully salvaged with chemotherapy and surgery.[124] In a study by Marina et al., 44 pediatric patients with immature teratoma of the ovary, including 13 patients with immature teratoma mixed with another germ cell tumor, were treated with surgery alone. Only one patient with a mixed germ cell tumor relapsed and was salvaged with surgery and chemotherapy.[69]

This strategy is appealing and supported by a larger pediatric literature, but there is much less experience in adults. It deserves further study, but this will require international collaboration. If a surveillance program is to be instigated, it is essential that the protocols used by the Charing Cross group are closely adhered to and that patients understand that the data for adults are limited.

The surveillance policy is very strict and includes a CT scan of chest, abdomen, and pelvis after surgery, if not done preoperatively. At 12 weeks following surgery, a repeat MRI/CT of the abdomen and pelvis or a second-look laparoscopy should be performed if there has been inadequate initial staging. If all of these are negative, MRI/CT imaging should be repeated at 12 months. Patients are reviewed monthly in year one, every 2 months in year two, every 3 months in year three, and so on until year five, after which they are seen every 6 months for another 5 years. A pelvic ultrasound and chest X-ray should be done on alternate visits. Tumor markers including AFP, hCG, CA125, and LDH measurements should be done every 2 weeks for 6 months, and then monthly for 6 months, every other month in year two, every third month in year three, and so on until year five when they are repeated every 6 months for 5 years.[32,123] This surveillance program is more intense than the ones in males reflecting the lack of large prospective surveillance studies in women.[125]

Late effects of treatment of malignant germ cell tumors of the ovary

The toxicity of BEP chemotherapy has been well documented in men and includes significant pulmonary toxicity in 5% of patients, with fatal lung toxicity in 1%; acute myeloid leukemia or myelodysplastic syndrome in 0.2–1% of patients; neuropathy in 20–30%; Raynaud phenomenon in 20%; tinnitus in 24%; and high-tone hearing loss in as many as 70% of patients. In addition, late effects occur on gonadal function, there is an increased risk of hypertension and cardiovascular disease, and some degree of renal impairment in 30% of patients.[126,127] These side effects underscore the importance of limiting BEP to three cycles for low-risk and to four cycles for high-risk patients, and emphasize the need for these patients to be referred to major referral centers.[97,128] There is increased interest in substituting carboplatin for cisplatin in patients with dysgerminomas because of reduced acute and late toxicity. The Malignant Germ Cell International Consortium (MaGIC) is considering a trial of carboplatin-based chemotherapy for dysgerminomas.

Gonadal function

An important cause of infertility in patients with ovarian germ cell tumors is unnecessary bilateral salpingo-oophorectomy and hysterectomy. Although temporary ovarian dysfunction or failure is common with platinum-based chemotherapy, most women will resume normal ovarian function, and childbearing is usually preserved.[8,42–45,129] In one representative series of 47 patients treated with combination chemotherapy for germ cell malignancies, 91.5% of patients resumed normal menstrual function, and there were 14 healthy live births and no birth defects.[8] Factors such as older age at initiation of chemotherapy, greater cumulative drug dose, and longer duration of therapy all have adverse effects on future gonadal function.[44,97,128,130,131]

A large study of reproductive and sexual function after platinum-based chemotherapy in ovarian germ cell tumor survivors was reported by the GOG in 2007 and included 132 survivors. Only 71 (53.8%) had fertility-sparing surgery; of these, 87.3% had regular menstrual periods. Twenty-four survivors had 37 offspring after cancer treatment.[132]

Secondary malignancies

An important cause of late morbidity and mortality in patients receiving chemotherapy for germ cell tumors is the development of secondary tumors. Etoposide, in particular, has been implicated in the development of treatment-related leukemias.

The chance of developing treatment-related leukemia following etoposide is dose related. The incidence of leukemia is approximately 0.4–0.5% (representing a 30-fold increased likelihood) in patients receiving a cumulative etoposide dose of less than 2000 mg/m^2 compared with as much as 5% (representing a 336-fold increased likelihood) in those receiving more than 2000 mg/m^2.[133,134] In a typical three- or four-cycle course of BEP, patients receive a cumulative etoposide dose of 1500 or 2000 mg/m^2, respectively.

Despite the risk of secondary leukemia, risk–benefit analyses have concluded that etoposide-containing chemotherapy regimens are beneficial in advanced germ cell tumors; one case of treatment-induced leukemia would be expected for every 20 additionally cured patients who receive BEP as compared with PVB (cisplatin, vinblastine, and bleomycin). The risk–benefit balance for patients with low-risk disease, or for high-dose etoposide in the salvage setting, is less clear.[133]

Table 4 Sex cord-stromal tumors.[a]

A. Granulosa-stromal cell tumors
　1. Granulosa cell tumor
　2. Tumors in the thecoma-fibroma group
　　a. Thecoma
　　b. Fibroma
　　c. Unclassified
B. Androblastomas: Sertoli–Leydig cell tumors
　1. Well differentiated
　　a. Sertoli cell tumor
　　b. Sertoli–Leydig cell tumor
　　c. Leydig cell tumor; hilus cell tumor
　2. Moderately differentiated
　3. Poorly differentiated (sarcomatoid)
　4. With heterologous elements
C. Gynandroblastoma
D. Unclassified

[a]Source: Adapted from Scully et al.[1]

Sex cord-stromal tumors

Sex cord-stromal tumors of the ovary account for approximately 5–8% of all ovarian malignancies.[1–3,135–140] They are derived from the sex cords and the ovarian stroma or mesenchyme and are usually composed of various combinations of elements, including the "female" cells (i.e., granulosa and theca cells) and "male" cells (i.e., Sertoli and Leydig cells), as well as morphologically indifferent cells. A classification of this group of tumors is presented in Table 4.[14,15,141]

Granulosa-stromal cell tumors

Granulosa-stromal cell tumors include granulosa cell tumors (GCT), thecomas, and fibromas. The granulosa cell tumor is a low-grade malignancy. Thecomas and fibromas are benign but rarely may have morphologic features of malignancy and then may be referred to as fibrosarcomas.[1,142]

GCT, which may secrete estrogen, are seen in women of all ages, and are classified as either adult or juvenile GCT (Figure 3). Five percent of cases are found in prepubertal girls; the others are distributed throughout the reproductive and postmenopausal years.[138,139,143] They are bilateral in only 2% of patients.

Of the rare prepubertal lesions, 75% are associated with sexual pseudoprecocity because of the estrogen secretion. In the reproductive age group, most patients have menstrual irregularities or secondary amenorrhea. In postmenopausal women, abnormal uterine bleeding is frequently the presenting symptom. Endometrial cancer occurs in association with GCT in at least 5% of cases, and 25–50% are associated with endometrial hyperplasia. Rarely, GCT may produce androgens and cause virilization.[1,138–140,143]

The other symptoms and signs of GCT are nonspecific and the same as most ovarian malignancies. Ascites is present in approximately 10% of cases, and rarely a pleural effusion. Granulosa tumors tend to be hemorrhagic; occasionally they rupture and produce hemoperitoneum.[138,139]

GCT are usually stage I at diagnosis but may recur 5–30 years after initial diagnosis.[137,144] The tumors may also spread hematogenously, and metastases can develop in the lungs, liver, and brain years later. Malignant thecomas are extremely rare, and their presentation, management, and outcome are similar to those of the GCT.[142,145]

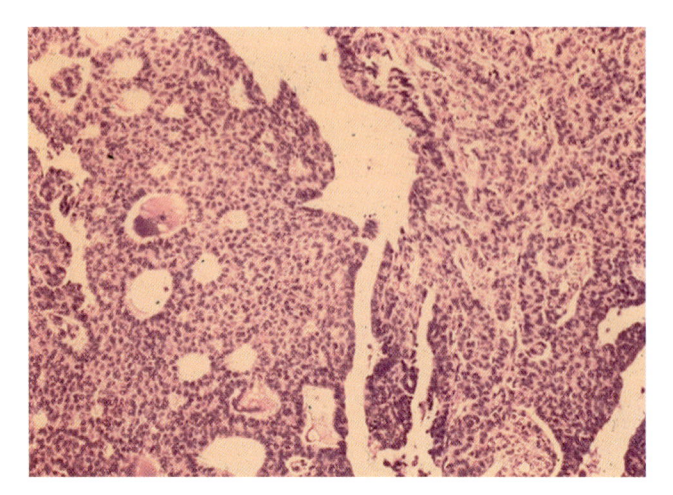

Figure 3 Granulosa cell tumor.

A somatic missense point mutation in the gene encoding the forkhead box protein L2 (*FOXL2*) has been found to be present in all adult-type GCT of the ovary. *FOXL2 402 CG* leads to a change of function and is believed to be a driver mutation for adult GCT. There is an effort to see if it can be targeted.[146-148]

Diagnosis

Inhibin is secreted by GCT and is a useful tumor marker for diagnosis and surveillance.[149-152] It is a polypeptide hormone secreted primarily by granulosa cells and an inhibitor of pituitary follicle-stimulating hormone (FSH) secretion. Inhibin decreases to nondetectable levels after menopause. However, certain ovarian cancers (mucinous epithelial ovarian carcinomas and GCT) produce inhibin, which may predate clinical recurrence.[153,154] An elevated serum inhibin level in a premenopausal woman presenting with amenorrhea and infertility is suggestive of a granulosa cell tumor.

There are now specific immunoassays to distinguish the inhibin subunits, inhibin A and B. Inhibin B is the predominant form of inhibin secreted by GCT and has been reported to reflect disease status more accurately than inhibin A. Measurement of serum inhibin B concentrations rather than total inhibin or inhibin A may be better for the follow-up of GCT.[155]

Anti-müllerian hormone (AMH), also called Müllerian inhibitory substance (MIS), is produced by granulosa cells, and is emerging as a potential marker for these tumors.[152,156-158] An elevated AMH level appears to have high specificity. The test is commercially available, and its role in the management of GCT is being investigated. A study included 123 patients with GCT and found that AMH is a useful marker for primary and recurrent disease with a sensitivity of 92% and specificity of 81%. Combing AMH and inhibin B was shown to improve detection of recurrent disease.[159] An elevated estradiol level is not a sensitive marker of this disease.[156]

The histologic diagnosis can be facilitated by staining for markers of ovarian GCT (e.g., inhibin, CD99, and AMH). Antibodies against inhibin appear to be the most useful, but they are not specific.[146] In one report, positive staining for inhibin was present in 94% of GCT and in 10–20% of ovarian endometrioid tumors and metastatic carcinomas to the ovary.[152] The latter demonstrated significantly weaker staining. Molecular testing for a mutation in FOXL2 is available to help with the diagnosis if it is in doubt.[147,148,160]

Treatment

The treatment of GCT depends on the age of the patient and the extent of disease. For most patients, surgery alone is sufficient primary therapy, with radiation and chemotherapy reserved for the treatment of recurrent or metastatic disease.[138,139,143,145,161,162]

Surgery

Because GCT are bilateral in only 2% of patients, a unilateral salpingo-oophorectomy is the appropriate therapy for stage IA tumors in children or in women of reproductive age. At the time of laparotomy, if a granulosa cell tumor is identified by frozen section, then a limited staging operation is performed, including an assessment of the contralateral ovary.[163,164] As with germ cell malignancies, staging is limited to washings, omental biopsy, careful palpation of the peritoneal surfaces and retroperitoneal nodes, and biopsy of any suspicious lesions. If the opposite ovary appears enlarged, it should be biopsied. If there is metastatic disease, an effort should be made to resect all disease because these tumors are typically slow growing and do not respond well to chemotherapy. In perimenopausal and postmenopausal women for whom ovarian preservation is not important, a hysterectomy and bilateral salpingo-oophorectomy should be performed. In premenopausal patients in whom the uterus is left *in situ*, a dilation and curettage of the uterus should be performed because of the possibility of a coexistent adenocarcinoma of the endometrium.[138]

Radiation

There is no evidence to support the use of adjuvant radiation therapy for GCT, although pelvic radiation may help to palliate isolated pelvic recurrences.[138,154] Radiation can induce clinical responses and occasional long-term remission in patients with persistent or recurrent GCT, particularly if the disease is surgically cytoreduced.[165] In one review of 34 patients treated at one center for more than 40 years, 14 (41.2%) were treated with measurable disease. Three (21%) were alive without progression for 10–21 years following treatment.[166]

Chemotherapy

There is no evidence that adjuvant chemotherapy in patients with stage I disease will prevent recurrence or improve survival.[167]

Patients with metastatic GCT have been treated with a variety of different antineoplastic drugs over the years. There has been no one consistently effective regimen, although complete responses have been reported anecdotally in patients treated with the single agents cyclophosphamide and melphalan, as well as the combinations VAC, PAC (cisplatin, doxorubicin, cyclophosphamide), PVB, and BEP.[5,168-178] More recently, carboplatin and paclitaxel (TC)[154] as well as bevacizumab[179] have shown benefit.

The rarity of these tumors has made it impossible to conduct well-designed randomized studies for patients with stages II–IV disease. In retrospective series, postoperative chemotherapy has been associated with a prolonged progression-free interval in women with stage III or IV disease, but an overall survival benefit has not been shown.[176] Despite the absence of data supporting a survival benefit, some experts recommend postoperative chemotherapy for women with completely resected stage II–IV disease, because of the high risk of disease progression and the potential for long-term survival after platinum-based chemotherapy.[154,169,175,180-182] Acceptable options include BEP, EP, PAC, and TC.

For patients with suboptimally cytoreduced disease, combinations of BEP have produced overall response rates of

58–83%.[154,172,175] In one study, 14 of 38 patients (37%) with advanced disease undergoing second-look laparotomy following four courses of BEP had negative findings.[175] With a median follow-up of 3 years, 11 of 16 patients (69%) with primary advanced disease and 21 of 41 patients (51%) with recurrent disease were progression free. This regimen was associated with severe toxicity and two bleomycin-related deaths. Carboplatin and etoposide,[173] PVB,[138,171,174] and PAC[168,170] have also been reported to have relatively high response rates. TC are reported to have a response rate of 60%[183–185] and are more commonly used today because of better tolerability, particularly in older patients. Ongoing clinical trials compare TC and BEP (NCT02429687 and NCT01042522).

Recurrent disease

The median time to relapse is approximately 4–6 years after initial diagnosis.[136,137] There is no standard approach to the management of relapsed disease. A common site of recurrence is the pelvis, although the upper abdomen may also be involved. Further surgery can be effective if the tumor is localized, but diffuse intra-abdominal disease is difficult to treat. Chemotherapy or radiation may be useful in selected patients.

Approximately 30% of these tumors are estrogen-receptor-positive and 100% are progesterone receptor-positive on immunostaining.[186] The pooled response rate with a range of hormonal therapies is >70% based on less than 100 patients in case reports and small retrospective studies.[187] The use of hormonal agents such as progestins, gonadotropin-releasing hormone (GnRH) agonists, and aromatase inhibitors has been suggested.[188,189]

GnRH agonists have been reported to have a 50% response rate in 13 patients from small clinical series and case reports,[190–192] whereas four of five patients (80%) were reported to respond to a progestational agent.[193] Freeman reported two patients with recurrent adult GCT who had received multiple treatment modalities, including chemotherapy, and had previously progressed on leuprolide. Both patients were treated with anastrozole, an aromatase inhibitor. Inhibin B levels normalized, as did clinical findings. Both were maintained on treatment for 14 and 18 months, respectively.[194] The numbers are too small to draw any conclusions, and it is likely that there has been significant publication bias, with more reports of responses to treatment.[195]

Preliminary results of the Phase II PARAGON trial of the use of anastrozole in patients with GCT showed a response rate of only 10% but many showed stable disease and 60% were progression free at 6 months.[196]

The role of bevacizumab combined with chemotherapy has been investigated in the ALIENOR trial. Sixty patients with recurrent sex cord-stromal tumors (predominantly GCT) after platinum-based chemotherapy were randomized to weekly paclitaxel with or without bevacizumab. The addition of bevacizumab increased the response rate from 25% to 44%; however, 6-month PFS and median PFS were unchanged with 70% and 15 months, respectively.[197]

Prognosis

The prognosis for granulosa cell tumor of the ovary depends on the surgical stage of disease.[137,139,154,198–201] Most GCT are indolent and confined to one ovary at diagnosis; the cure rate for stage I disease is 75–92%.[139,178,201] However, late recurrences are not uncommon.[136,137,139] In one report of 37 women with stage I disease, survival rates at 5, 10, and 20 years were 94%, 82%, and 62%, respectively. The survival rates for stages II–IV at 5 and 10 years were 55% and 34%, respectively.[154]

In adult tumors, cellular atypia, mitotic rate, and the absence of Call-Exner bodies are the only significant pathologic predictors of early recurrence. Neither an abnormal tumor karyotype nor p53 overexpression appears to be prognostic.[202] The DNA ploidy of the tumors has been correlated with survival. Holland et al. reported DNA aneuploidy in 13 of 37 patients (35%) with primary GCT.[203] The presence of residual disease was found to be the most important predictor of PFS, but DNA ploidy was an independent prognostic factor. Patients with no residual disease and DNA diploid tumors had a 10-year PFS of 96%.

Juvenile granulosa cell tumors

Juvenile GCT of the ovary are rare and make up less than 5% of ovarian tumors in childhood and adolescence.[173] Approximately 90% are diagnosed in stage I and have a favorable prognosis. The juvenile subtype behaves less aggressively than the adult type. Advanced-stage tumors have been successfully treated with platinum-based combination chemotherapy (e.g., BEP).[154]

Sertoli–Leydig cell tumors

Sertoli–Leydig tumors occur most frequently in the third and fourth decades, with 75% of the lesions seen in women younger than 40 years. They account for less than 0.2% of ovarian cancers. Sertoli–Leydig cell tumors are most frequently low-grade malignancies, although poorly differentiated tumors may behave more aggressively.

The tumors typically produce androgens, and clinical virilization is noted in 70–85% of patients.[204,205] Signs of virilization include oligomenorrhea followed by amenorrhea, breast atrophy, acne, hirsutism, clitoromegaly, a deepening voice, and a receding hairline. Measurement of plasma androgens may reveal elevated testosterone and androstenedione, with normal or slightly elevated dehydroepiandrosterone sulfate.[1] Rarely, the Sertoli–Leydig tumor can be associated with manifestations of estrogenization (i.e., isosexual precocity, irregular, or postmenopausal bleeding).[205]

Treatment

Because these low-grade tumors are bilateral in less than 1% of cases, the usual treatment is unilateral salpingo-oophorectomy and evaluation of the contralateral ovary in patients who are in their reproductive years.[205] In older patients, hysterectomy and bilateral salpingo-oophorectomy are appropriate.

There are limited data regarding the utility of chemotherapy in patients with persistent disease, but responses in patients with measurable disease have been reported with cisplatin in combination with doxorubicin or ifosfamide or both[205] as well as the regimens mentioned above for GCT. Because of their rarity, most series have included them with GCT.[169] Pelvic radiation can also be used for recurrent pelvic tumor but with limited responses.

Prognosis

The 5-year survival rate is 70–90%, and recurrences thereafter are uncommon.[1,2,205] The majority of fatalities occur with poorly differentiated lesions.

Uncommon ovarian cancers

There are several varieties of malignant ovarian tumors, which together constitute only 0.1% of ovarian malignancies. These lesions include lipoid (or lipid) cell tumors, primary ovarian sarcomas, and small-cell ovarian carcinomas.

Lipoid cell tumors

Lipoid cell tumors are thought to arise in adrenal cortical rests that reside in the vicinity of the ovary. More than 100 cases have been reported, and bilaterality has been noted in only a few.[1] Most are associated with virilization and occasionally with obesity, hypertension, and glucose intolerance, reflecting glucocorticoid secretion. Rare cases of estrogen secretion and isosexual precocity have been reported.

The majority of these have a benign or low-grade behavior, but approximately 20% develop metastatic lesions in the peritoneal cavity, or rarely at distant sites. The primary treatment is surgical, and there are no data regarding radiation or chemotherapy for this disease.

Carcinosarcomas

Malignant mixed mesodermal sarcomas of the ovary, or ovarian carcinosarcomas, are rare and account for <2% of ovarian cancers. They are diagnosed mainly in postmenopausal women.[206–211]

The current theory is that both the epithelial and sarcomatous component are monoclonal in origin and derived from pluripotent stem cells which undergo divergent differentiation.[212] Genomic analysis suggests that mutations in chromatin remodeling genes result in loss of genetic programing control in progenitor cells which leads to carcinosarcoma.[213] Carcinosarcomas are classified as homologous and heterologous based on the presence of a stromal component containing mesenchymal tissue. They are biologically aggressive, and their presentation and management are similar to that of other high-grade epithelial ovarian malignancies.

Most patients are treated with cytoreductive surgery and postoperative platinum-based chemotherapy. A Cochrane review of chemotherapy in combination with surgery for ovarian carcinosarcomas found no evidence to inform decisions about neoadjuvant or adjuvant chemotherapy.[214] Most of the available data is based on retrospective analyses.[215–217]

Silasi et al. reported their experience with 22 patients, all but two of whom presented with advanced-stage disease.[218] The median survival was 46 months for 18 optimally debulked (<1 cm) patients and 27 months for four suboptimally debulked (>1 cm) patients. After optimal cytoreduction, six patients were treated with cisplatin and ifosfamide; they had a median PFS of 13 months and a median survival of 51 months. TC were administered to four patients following optimal cytoreduction; their median PFS was 6 months, and median survival 38 months. The difference in survival between the cisplatin and ifosfamide group and the TC group was not statistically significant. First-line cisplatin/ifosfamide or carboplatin/paclitaxel can achieve survival rates comparable to those observed in epithelial ovarian cancer.

Leiser et al. reported the experience with platinum and paclitaxel in 30 patients with carcinosarcomas of the ovary.[219] Twelve patients (40%) had a complete response, seven (23%) a partial response, two (7%) stable disease, and nine (30%) progression of disease. The median time to progression for responders was 12 months; the median overall survival was 43 months. The 3- and 5-year survival rates were 53% and 30%, respectively. Brackman et al. described in 30 patients who received carboplatin/paclitaxel a median PFS of 17 months superior to an ifosfamide/paclitaxel regimen.[220]

Small-cell carcinomas of hypercalcemic type (SCCOHT)

This rare tumor occurs at an average age of 24 years (range 2–46 years).[221] The tumors are all bilateral. Approximately two-thirds of the tumors are accompanied by paraneoplastic hypercalcemia. This tumor accounts for one-half of all of the cases of hypercalcemia associated with ovarian tumors. Approximately 50% of the tumors have spread beyond the ovaries at the time of diagnosis.[222,223] They are associated with a very poor prognosis with only 33% survival in patients with stage I disease and much worse with advanced-stage disease.

Witkowski et al. recently identified germline or somatic mutation of *SMARCA4* in almost all patients tested. *SMARCA4* encodes BRG1 a central adenosine triphosphate hydrolase (ATPase) in chromatin remodeling complexes. The majority of tumors lost BRG1 expression on immunohistochemistry.[224,225] Given morphologic and molecular similarities it has been suggested to reclassify small-cell carcinomas of hypercalcemic type (SCCOHT) as malignant rhabdoid tumor of the ovary.[226] The differential diagnosis is difficult and requires expert review.

Management consists of surgery followed by platinum-based chemotherapy and/or high-dose chemotherapy with stem cell support. Radiation therapy may be considered in selected patients. In addition to the primary treatment of the disease, control of the hypercalcemia may require aggressive hydration, loop diuretics, calcitonin, and the use of bisphosphonates.

In a collaborative Gynecologic Cancer Intergroup study, data were collected for 17 patients treated in Australia, Canada, and Europe.[222] The median follow-up was 13 months for all patients and 35.5 months for surviving patients. Ten patients (58.8%) had FIGO stage I tumors, six (35.3%) stage III, and in one patient, stage was unknown. All underwent surgical resection and adjuvant platinum-based chemotherapy. Seven received adjuvant pelvic, whole-abdominal, or extended-field radiation. The median survival for stage I tumors was not reached, whereas it was 6 months for stage III tumors. For the 10 patients with stage I tumors, six also received adjuvant radiotherapy, with five alive and disease-free; four received no adjuvant radiotherapy, with one alive and disease-free. Of the seven patients with stage III or unknown tumor stage, all but one have died. The only long-term survivor was treated with platinum-based chemotherapy (BEP) followed by para-aortic and pelvic radiotherapy. Recurrences were most frequent in the pelvis and the abdomen. Patients receiving salvage treatment with chemotherapy and radiotherapy did poorly.

The optimal management is not known, and a variety of regimens has been used; including multimodal treatment with surgical resection, chemotherapy with carboplatin/paclitaxel or cisplatin/etoposide, plus involved-field radiation. Pautier et al. reported of a four-drug regimen followed by high-dose chemotherapy. Eight of 27 patients progressed on treatment. The 1- and 3-year overall survival were 58% and 49%, respectively.[223] High-dose chemotherapy with stem cell support has been advocated.[227] It has been suggested to alternate ifosfamide/carboplatin/etoposide with vincristine/doxorubicin/cyclophosphamide, a regimen used in patients with malignant rhabdoid tumors, given the close similarities with SCCOHT.[228]

Targeted agents such as tazemetostat, an EZH2 methyltransferase inhibitor, and ponatinib, a multi-targeted tyrosine kinase inhibitor, show activity in SCCOHT.[229,230] In addition, there have been recent case reports of responses to immunotherapy with PD-1/PD-L1 inhibitors.[231] Several approaches are being explored preclinically.[232]

Metastatic tumors

Approximately 5–6% of ovarian tumors are metastatic from other organs, most frequently from the female genital tract, the breast, or the GI tract.[233–250] The metastases may occur from direct extension of another pelvic neoplasm, by hematogenous spread, by lymphatic spread, or from transcoelomic dissemination, with surface implantation of tumors that spread in the peritoneal cavity.

Gynecologic primary

Nonovarian cancers of the genital tract can spread by direct extension or metastasize to the ovaries.[1] Under some circumstances, it is difficult to know whether the tumor originates in the fallopian tube or in the ovary when both are involved, especially because many high-grade serous carcinomas that were thought to be primary ovarian malignancies are now believed to actually arise in the fallopian tube, as discussed in the previous chapter.[251] Cervical cancer spreads to the ovary only in rare cases (<1%), and most of these are at an advanced clinical stage or are adenocarcinomas. Although adenocarcinoma of the endometrium can spread and implant directly onto the surface of the ovaries in as many as 5% of cases, two synchronous primary tumors probably occur with greater frequency. In these cases, an endometrioid carcinoma of the ovary is usually associated with the adenocarcinoma of the endometrium.[252]

Nongynecologic primary

The frequency of metastatic breast carcinoma to the ovaries varies according to the method of determination, but is relatively common, particularly in patients with estrogen receptor-positive metastatic breast cancer. In autopsy data of women who die of metastatic breast cancer, the ovaries are involved in 24% of cases, and 80% of the involvement is bilateral.[234–238,245,246] Similarly, when ovaries are removed as treatment for metastatic breast cancer in premenopausal women, approximately 20–30% of patients have evidence of ovarian metastases, 60% bilaterally. The involvement of ovaries in early-stage breast cancer is considerably lower, but precise figures are not available. In almost all cases, ovarian involvement is occult, but in some patients, a pelvic mass is discovered after other metastatic disease becomes apparent.

Krukenberg[1] tumor

Krukenberg tumors account for 30–40% of metastatic cancers to the ovaries and are characterized by mucin-filled, signet-ring cells in the ovarian stroma.[233,239] The primary tumor is most frequently the stomach, but less common primaries include the colon, breast, or biliary tract. Rarely, the cervix or the bladder may be the primary site. Krukenberg tumors can account for approximately 2% of ovarian cancers, and they are usually bilateral. The tumors are usually not discovered until the primary disease is advanced, and therefore most patients die of their disease within a year. In some cases, a primary tumor is never found.

Other gastrointestinal tumors

In other cases of metastasis from the GI tract to the ovary, the tumor does not have the classic histologic appearance of a Krukenberg tumor; most of these are from the colon and, less commonly, the small intestine. One to 2% of women with intestinal carcinomas will develop metastases to the ovaries during the course of their disease.[236,240,241,247–249] Before exploration for an adnexal tumor in a woman more than 40 years of age, a colonoscopy or gastroscopy should be performed to exclude a primary GI carcinoma with metastases to the ovaries if there are any GI symptoms.

Metastatic colon cancer can mimic a mucinous cystadenocarcinoma of the ovary histologically, and the histologic distinction between the two can be difficult.[240–244] Tumors that arise in the appendix may also be associated with ovarian metastasis and have frequently been confused with primary ovarian malignancies, especially when associated with pseudomyxoma peritonei.[240,244] When the ovaries are involved with metastasis, a bilateral salpingo-oophorectomy should be performed at the time of surgery for colon cancer.[247,250]

Melanoma

Rare cases of malignant melanoma metastatic to the ovaries have been reported,[253] and must be distinguished from the rare case of a melanoma arising in an ovarian teratoma.[254] In cases of metastatic disease, the melanomas are usually widely disseminated. Removal would be warranted for palliation of abdominal or pelvic pain, bleeding, or torsion.

Carcinoid

Metastatic carcinoid tumors represent fewer than 2% of metastatic lesions to the ovaries.[255] Conversely, only some 2% of primary carcinoids have evidence of ovarian metastasis, and only 40% of these patients have the carcinoid syndrome at the time of discovery of the metastatic carcinoid.[256] In perimenopausal and postmenopausal women explored for an intestinal carcinoid, it is reasonable to remove the ovaries to prevent subsequent ovarian metastasis. Furthermore, the discovery of an ovarian carcinoid should prompt a careful search for a primary intestinal lesion.

Primary ovarian carcinoid has four variants: insular, trabecular, mucinous, and mixed. About 30% of patients have symptoms of carcinoid syndrome, particularly with the insular type. In contrast to intestinal carcinoids, ovarian carcinoids cause carcinoid syndrome in the absence of metastatic disease, since the venous drainage bypasses the portal venous system. Bilaterality, peritoneal disease, absence of a teratomatous component suggest carcinoid tumor metastatic to the ovary. Immunostain with CDX2 may help define carcinoids of GI origin.[257–259]

Lymphoma and leukemia

Lymphomas and leukemia can involve the ovary. When they do, the involvement is usually bilateral.[260–263] Approximately 5% of patients with Hodgkin disease will have lymphomatous involvement of the ovaries, but this occurs typically with advanced-stage disease. With Burkitt lymphoma, ovarian involvement is very common. Other types of lymphoma involve the ovaries much less frequently, and leukemic infiltration of the ovaries is uncommon.

Sometimes the ovaries can be the only apparent sites of involvement of the abdominal or pelvic viscera with a lymphoma—in this circumstance, a careful surgical exploration may be necessary. An intraoperative consultation with a hematologist–oncologist should be obtained to determine the need for such procedures if frozen section of a solid ovarian mass reveals a lymphoma. In general, most lymphomas no longer require extensive surgical staging, although enlarged lymph nodes should generally be biopsied. In some cases of Hodgkin disease, a more extensive evaluation may be necessary. Treatment involves that of the lymphoma or leukemia in general. Removal of a large ovarian mass may improve patient comfort and facilitate a response to subsequent radiation or chemotherapy.[262]

---

[1] Friedrich Ernst Krukenberg (1871–1946): German Physician.

Key references

The complete reference list can be found on Vital Source version of this title, see inside front cover.

15. Kurman RJ, Carcangiu ML, Herrington CS, Young RH. *WHO Classification of Tumours of Female Reproductive Organs*, Vol. VI, 4th ed. WHO/ IARC Classification of Tumours. Lyon, France: IARC Press; 2014.
19. Gershenson DM. Management of ovarian germ cell tumors. *J Clin Oncol*. 2007;**25**(20):2938–2943.
30. Sessa C, Schneider DT, Planchamp F, et al. ESGO-SIOPE guidelines for the management of adolescents and young adults with non-epithelial ovarian cancers. *Lancet Oncol*. 2020;**21**(7):e360–e368.
33. Mangili G, Sigismondi C, Lorusso D, et al. Is surgical restaging indicated in apparent stage IA pure ovarian dysgerminoma? The MITO group retrospective experience. *Gynecol Oncol*. 2011;**121**(2):280–284.
34. Williams SD, Birch R, Einhorn LH, et al. Treatment of disseminated germ-cell tumors with cisplatin, bleomycin, and either vinblastine or etoposide. *N Engl J Med*. 1987;**316**(23):1435–1440.
35. Williams SD, Blessing JA, Moore DH, et al. Cisplatin, vinblastine, and bleomycin in advanced and recurrent ovarian germ-cell tumors. A trial of the Gynecologic Oncology Group. *Ann Intern Med*. 1989;**111**(1):22–27.
36. Gershenson DM, Morris M, Cangir A, et al. Treatment of malignant germ cell tumors of the ovary with bleomycin, etoposide, and cisplatin. *J Clin Oncol*. 1990;**8**(4):715–720.
37. Williams SD, Blessing JA, Hatch KD, et al. Chemotherapy of advanced dysgerminoma: trials of the Gynecologic Oncology Group. *J Clin Oncol*. 1991;**9**(11):1950–1955.
38. Williams S, Blessing JA, Liao SY, et al. Adjuvant therapy of ovarian germ cell tumors with cisplatin, etoposide, and bleomycin: a trial of the Gynecologic Oncology Group. *J Clin Oncol*. 1994;**12**(4):701–706.
43. Gershenson DM. Menstrual and reproductive function after treatment with combination chemotherapy for malignant ovarian germ cell tumors. *J Clin Oncol*. 1988;**6**(2):270–275.
46. Williams SD, Kauderer J, Burnett AF, et al. Adjuvant therapy of completely resected dysgerminoma with carboplatin and etoposide: a trial of the Gynecologic Oncology Group. *Gynecol Oncol*. 2004;**95**(3):496–499.
47. Loehrer PJ Sr, Johnson D, Elson P, et al. Importance of bleomycin in favorable-prognosis disseminated germ cell tumors: an Eastern Cooperative Oncology Group trial. *J Clin Oncol*. 1995;**13**(2):470–476.
49. Bajorin DF, Sarosdy MF, Pfister DG, et al. Randomized trial of etoposide and cisplatin versus etoposide and carboplatin in patients with good-risk germ cell tumors: a multiinstitutional study. *J Clin Oncol*. 1993;**11**(4):598–606.
52. Williams SD, Blessing JA, DiSaia PJ, et al. Second-look laparotomy in ovarian germ cell tumors: the gynecologic oncology group experience. *Gynecol Oncol*. 1994;**52**(3):287–291.
57. Einhorn LH, Williams SD, Chamness A, et al. High-dose chemotherapy and stem-cell rescue for metastatic germ-cell tumors. *N Engl J Med*. 2007;**357**(4):340–348.
63. Kumar S, Shah JP, Bryant CS, et al. The prevalence and prognostic impact of lymph node metastasis in malignant germ cell tumors of the ovary. *Gynecol Oncol*. 2008;**110**(2):125–132.
79. Culine S, Kattan J, Lhomme C, et al. A phase II study of high-dose cisplatin, vinblastine, bleomycin, and etoposide (PVeBV regimen) in malignant nondysgerminomatous germ-cell tumors of the ovary. *Gynecol Oncol*. 1994;**54**(1):47–53.
83. Mangili G, Scarfone G, Gadducci A, et al. Is adjuvant chemotherapy indicated in stage I pure immature ovarian teratoma (IT)? A multicentre Italian trial in ovarian cancer (MITO-9). *Gynecol Oncol*. 2010;**119**(1):48–52.
86. Slayton RE, Park RC, Silverberg SG, et al. Vincristine, dactinomycin, and cyclophosphamide in the treatment of malignant germ cell tumors of the ovary. A Gynecologic Oncology Group Study (a final report). *Cancer*. 1985;**56**(2):243–248.
125. Ray-Coquard I, Morice P, Lorusso D, et al. Non-epithelial ovarian cancer: ESMO Clinical Practice Guidelines for diagnosis, treatment and follow-up. *Ann Oncol*. 2018;**29**(Suppl 4):iv1–iv18.
133. Kollmannsberger C, Beyer J, Droz JP, et al. Secondary leukemia following high cumulative doses of etoposide in patients treated for advanced germ cell tumors. *J Clin Oncol*. 1998;**16**(10):3386–3391.
147. Shah SP, Kobel M, Senz J, et al. Mutation of FOXL2 in granulosa-cell tumors of the ovary. *N Engl J Med*. 2009;**360**(26):2719–2729.
149. Lappohn RE, Burger HG, Bouma J, et al. Inhibin as a marker for granulosa-cell tumors. *N Engl J Med*. 1989;**321**(12):790–793.
154. Schumer ST, Cannistra SA. Granulosa cell tumor of the ovary. *J Clin Oncol*. 2003;**21**(6):1180–1189.
157. Chang HL, Pahlavan N, Halpern EF, et al. Serum Mullerian inhibiting substance/anti-Mullerian hormone levels in patients with adult granulosa cell tumors directly correlate with aggregate tumor mass as determined by pathology or radiology. *Gynecol Oncol*. 2009;**114**(1):57–60.
163. Abu-Rustum NR, Restivo A, Ivy J, et al. Retroperitoneal nodal metastasis in primary and recurrent granulosa cell tumors of the ovary. *Gynecol Oncol*. 2006;**103**(1):31–34.
164. Brown J, Sood AK, Deavers MT, et al. Patterns of metastasis in sex cord-stromal tumors of the ovary: can routine staging lymphadenectomy be omitted? *Gynecol Oncol*. 2009;**113**(1):86–90.
167. Mangili G, Ottolina J, Cormio G, et al. Adjuvant chemotherapy does not improve disease-free survival in FIGO stage IC ovarian granulosa cell tumors: the MITO-9 study. *Gynecol Oncol*. 2016;**143**(2):276–280.
175. Homesley HD, Bundy BN, Hurteau JA, et al. Bleomycin, etoposide, and cisplatin combination therapy of ovarian granulosa cell tumors and other stromal malignancies: a Gynecologic Oncology Group study. *Gynecol Oncol*. 1999;**72**(2):131–137.
187. van Meurs HS, van Lonkhuijzen LR, Limpens J, et al. Hormone therapy in ovarian granulosa cell tumors: a systematic review. *Gynecol Oncol*. 2014;**134**(1):196–205.
196. Banerjee SN, Tang M, O'Connell R, et al. PARAGON: a phase 2 study of anastrozole (An) in patients with estrogen receptor(ER) and / progesterone receptor (PR) positive recurrent/metastatic granulosa cell tumors/sex-cord stromal tumors (GCT) of the ovary. *J Clin Oncol*. 2018;**36**(15_suppl):5524.
197. Ray-Coquard IL, Harter P, Lorusso D, et al. Effect of weekly paclitaxel With or without bevacizumab on progression-free rate among patients with relapsed ovarian sex cord-stromal tumors: the ALIENOR/ENGOT-ov7 randomized clinical trial. *JAMA Oncol*. 2020;**6**(12):1923–1930.
222. Harrison ML, Hoskins P, du Bois A, et al. Small cell of the ovary, hypercalcemic type—analysis of combined experience and recommendation for management. A GCIG study. *Gynecol Oncol*. 2006;**100**(2):233–238.
223. Pautier P, Ribrag V, Duvillard P, et al. Results of a prospective dose-intensive regimen in 27 patients with small cell carcinoma of the ovary of the hypercalcemic type. *Ann Oncol*. 2007;**18**(12):1985–1989.
225. Jelinic P, Mueller JJ, Olvera N, et al. Recurrent SMARCA4 mutations in small cell carcinoma of the ovary. *Nat Genet*. 2014;**46**(5):424–426.
231. Jelinic P, Ricca J, Van Oudenhove E, et al. Immune-active microenvironment in small cell carcinoma of the ovary, hypercalcemic type: rationale for immune checkpoint blockade. *J Natl Cancer Inst*. 2018;**110**(7):787–790.
232. Tischkowitz M, Huang S, Banerjee S, et al. Small-cell carcinoma of the ovary, hypercalcemic type-genetics, new treatment targets, and current management guidelines. *Clin Cancer Res*. 2020;**26**(15):3908–3917.
243. Lee KR, Young RH. The distinction between primary and metastatic mucinous carcinomas of the ovary: gross and histologic findings in 50 cases. *Am J Surg Pathol*. 2003;**27**(3):281–292.
253. Young RH, Scully RE. Malignant melanoma metastatic to the ovary. A clinicopathologic analysis of 20 cases. *Am J Surg Pathol*. 1991;**15**(9):849–860.

103 Molar pregnancy and gestational trophoblastic neoplasia

Neil S. Horowitz, MD ■ Donald P. Goldstein, MD ■ Ross S. Berkowitz, MD

Overview

Molar pregnancy and gestational trophoblastic neoplasia (GTN) comprise a group of interrelated diseases that includes complete hydatidiform mole (CHM) and partial hydatidiform mole (PHM), invasive mole, choriocarcinoma (CCA), placental site trophoblastic tumor (PSTT), and epithelioid trophoblastic tumor (ETT). Molar pregnancy and GTN produce a distinct tumor marker, human chorionic gonadotropin (hCG), which can be used for diagnosis, monitoring the effects of therapy, and follow-up to detect relapse. Complete and partial moles are noninvasive, localized tumors that develop as a result of an aberrant fertilization event that leads to a proliferative process. The other trophoblastic tumors which as a group are referred to as GTN represent malignant disease because of their local invasion and metastases. GTN most commonly develops from a molar pregnancy but can arise *de novo* after any gestation. Although these tumors are rare, it is important for medical oncologists to understand their natural history and management because of their life-threatening potential in reproductive-age females and their high degree of curability with preservation of reproductive function if treated early and appropriately.[1,2] Despite the advances made in the management of GTN over the past six decades, patients with protracted delays in diagnosis, particularly after nonmolar pregnancies, still present with extensive tumor burdens and are at substantial risk for treatment failure and death.

Incidence

The reported incidence of molar pregnancy and GTN varies substantially in different regions of the world.[3] The incidence of complete and partial molar pregnancy in North America and Europe is approximately 1:1250 and 1:650, respectively, while the incidence in Asian countries is 3–10 times greater.[4,5] Variations in the incidence rates of molar pregnancy throughout the world may result from differences between reporting hospital-based versus population-based data.

The incidence of GTN is also difficult to establish with certainty because accurate epidemiologic data is not available in most countries. Approximately 50% of GTN cases arise from molar pregnancy, 25% from miscarriages or tubal pregnancies, and 25% from term or preterm pregnancy.[6] GTN which develops after a nonmolar pregnancy is usually due to CCA, whereas metastatic PSTT and ETT occur rarely. The incidence of GTN following a nonmolar pregnancy in Europe and North America is estimated at 2–7 per 100,000 pregnancies, whereas in Southeast Asia and Japan the incidence is higher at 50–200 per 100,000 pregnancies, respectively.[7,8]

Risk factors

The two main risk factors for molar pregnancy and GTN are extremes of maternal age (especially over 35 and under 16) and a history of previous mole.[9–13] Gockley et al. reported that compared to average age women, women younger than 16, older than 40, and older than 45 have an increased risk of complete mole of 25.6, 1.9, and 15, respectively.[11] Ova from younger and older women may be more susceptible to abnormal fertilizations. Most cases of molar disease and GTN occur in women under 35 because of the greater number of pregnancies in this age group. The risk for PHM has not been associated with maternal age.

Histopathologic classification of GTN

Hydatidiform mole may be categorized as either complete or partial based on gross morphology, histopathology, and karyotype.[14,15] CHM is characterized by hydropic villi with trophoblastic hyperplasia. Embryonic or fetal tissues are not identifiable. Partial moles are characterized by the presence of two populations of chorionic villi, some appearing normal and some exhibiting focal swelling and focal trophoblastic hyperplasia. Fetal and embryonic tissues are commonly present. Locally invasive or metastatic GTN that develops after either a complete or partial mole can have the histologic features of either molar tissue or CCA.

CCA does not contain chorionic villi but is composed of sheets of both anaplastic cyto- and syncytiotrophoblasts. Although CCA is most commonly preceded by a CHM, it may develop after any gestation. After a nonmolar pregnancy, persistent GTN usually has the histologic pattern of CCA, but rarely can be present as PSTT or ETT. CCA is a highly vascular tumor that disseminates hematogenously, commonly metastasizing to the lungs. Distant sites such as the brain, liver, kidney, gastrointestinal tract, and spleen are usually late manifestations of the disease in patients where there has been delayed diagnosis.

PSTT and ETT are uncommon variants of CCA, which are composed almost entirely of mononuclear intermediate trophoblast and do not contain chorionic villi.[16,17] Both PSTT and ETT tend to infiltrate the myometrium and, in contrast to CCA, metastases are a late manifestation of the disease. These tumors display a wide clinical spectrum and when metastatic can be difficult to control even with surgery and chemotherapy. They are characterized by low hCG levels so a large tumor burden may be present before the disease is diagnosed.

Clinical presentation and diagnosis

Postmolar GTN

Complete moles develop uterine invasion or metastasis in about 15% and 4% of patients, respectively.[18] Approximately 1–4% of patients with PHM develop persistent tumor, which is generally nonmetastatic.[19] After molar evacuation, all patients must be monitored for development of postmolar GTN, defined as those patients who develop persistently elevated hCG levels, require chemotherapy and/or excisional surgery, or have evidence of metastases.[20] According to the International Federation of Gynecology and Obstetrics (FIGO) criteria, the presence of postmolar GTN should be diagnosed if the following is present: (1) serum hCG values that plateau (decline of <10% for at least 4 values over 3 weeks), (2) serum hCG levels rise (increase more than 10% over 2 consecutive weeks), or (3) histologic diagnosis of CCA.[21]

Patients on rare occasion present with a false positive elevation in their serum hCG concentration due to a number of factors other than GTN. The differential diagnosis of an elevated hCG value includes (1) pregnancy, (2) germ cell tumor of the ovary or other site, (3) nontrophoblastic gonadotropin-producing tumor (e.g., hepatoma), or (4) phantom hCG caused by heterophilic antibody.[22] Postmenopausal women have also been reported to have detectable low hCG levels of pituitary origin, which can be suppressed by hormone replacement therapy.[23]

Nonmetastatic GTN

Locally invasive GTN also occurs infrequently after nonmolar pregnancies.[18] These patients may present with persistently elevated hCG levels, irregular vaginal bleeding, uterine subinvolution, or asymmetric uterine enlargement. Theca lutein ovarian cysts are rare in the absence of high levels of hCG (>100,000 mIU/mL). The trophoblastic tumor may erode into uterine vessels, causing vaginal hemorrhage, or may perforate through the myometrium, producing intra-abdominal bleeding. Bulky necrotic tumors in the endometrial cavity may also serve as a nidus for sepsis, causing pelvic pain and purulent discharge.

Metastatic GTN

Metastases develop in approximately 4% of patients after complete mole and infrequently after other gestations.[18] When metastases occur, the pathology is usually CCA because this tumor has a propensity for early vascular invasion and dissemination. The presenting signs and symptoms in these patients depend on the sites of metastasis: hemoptysis from lung lesions, acute neurologic deficits from intracranial hemorrhage, etc.

The most common site of metastasis is the lung. Eighty percent of patients with metastatic GTN have pulmonary involvement on chest radiographs or computed tomography (CT). Because respiratory symptoms and radiographic findings may be striking, the patient may be thought to have a primary pulmonary process. Pulmonary hypertension can develop as a result of pulmonary arterial occlusion by trophoblastic emboli. The development of early respiratory failure requiring intubation is associated with a dismal outcome.[24] Gynecologic symptoms may be minimal or absent even when the patient has extensive metastases. *The diagnosis of GTN should be considered in any woman in the reproductive age group with unexplained pulmonary or systemic symptoms.*

Vaginal metastases are present in 30% of patients with metastatic GTN. Because these lesions are highly vascular, they may hemorrhage if biopsied so this should be avoided.[18]

Hepatic and cerebral metastases occur in approximately 10% of patients with metastatic GTN. Hepatic and cerebral lesions invariably have the histologic pattern of CCA, and usually follow a nonmolar pregnancy. These patients characteristically have protracted delays in diagnosis, extensive tumor burdens, and high risk of mortality. Virtually all patients with hepatic and cerebral metastases have concurrent pulmonary or vaginal involvement.[25,26]

Staging and risk assessment

An anatomic staging system for GTN was adopted by the FIGO in 1982[21]:

Stage I: Lesion confined to uterus.
Stage II: Lesion outside uterus but confined to vagina and pelvis.
Stage III: Lung metastases with or without evidence of uterine or pelvic disease.
Stage IV: Distant metastatic sites such as the brain, liver, kidney, gastrointestinal tract, spleen, etc.

In addition to anatomic staging, the World Health Organization (WHO) has adopted a prognostic scoring system (Table 1) that reliably predicts the risk of drug resistance to single-agent chemotherapy and assists in selecting the appropriate chemotherapy.[21,27] Prognostic scores less than 7 are associated with a low risk of resistance to single-agent chemotherapy. When the prognostic score is 7 or greater, the patient is considered to be

Table 1 Scoring system for gestational trophoblastic tumors based on prognostic factors.[a]

	Score[b]			
	0	1	2	4
Age (years)	<39	>39	—	—
Antecedent pregnancy	Mole	Abortion	Term	—
Interval[c]	<4	4–6	7–12	—
hCG (IU/L)	$<10^3$	$10^3–10^4$	$10^4–10^5$	—
Largest tumor, including uterine tumor	—	3–5 cm	>5 cm	—
Site of metastases	—	Spleen, kidney	Gastrointestinal tract, liver	Brain
Number of metastases identified	—	1–3	4–8	>8
Prior chemotherapy	—	—	Single drug	2 or more drug

[a]Source: Data from Ngan et al.[1]
[b]The total score for a patient is obtained by adding the individual scores for each prognostic factor. Total score: ≤6, low-risk; >7, high-risk; ≥12, ultra-high-risk.
[c]Interval is the time (months) between end of antecedent pregnancy and start of chemotherapy.

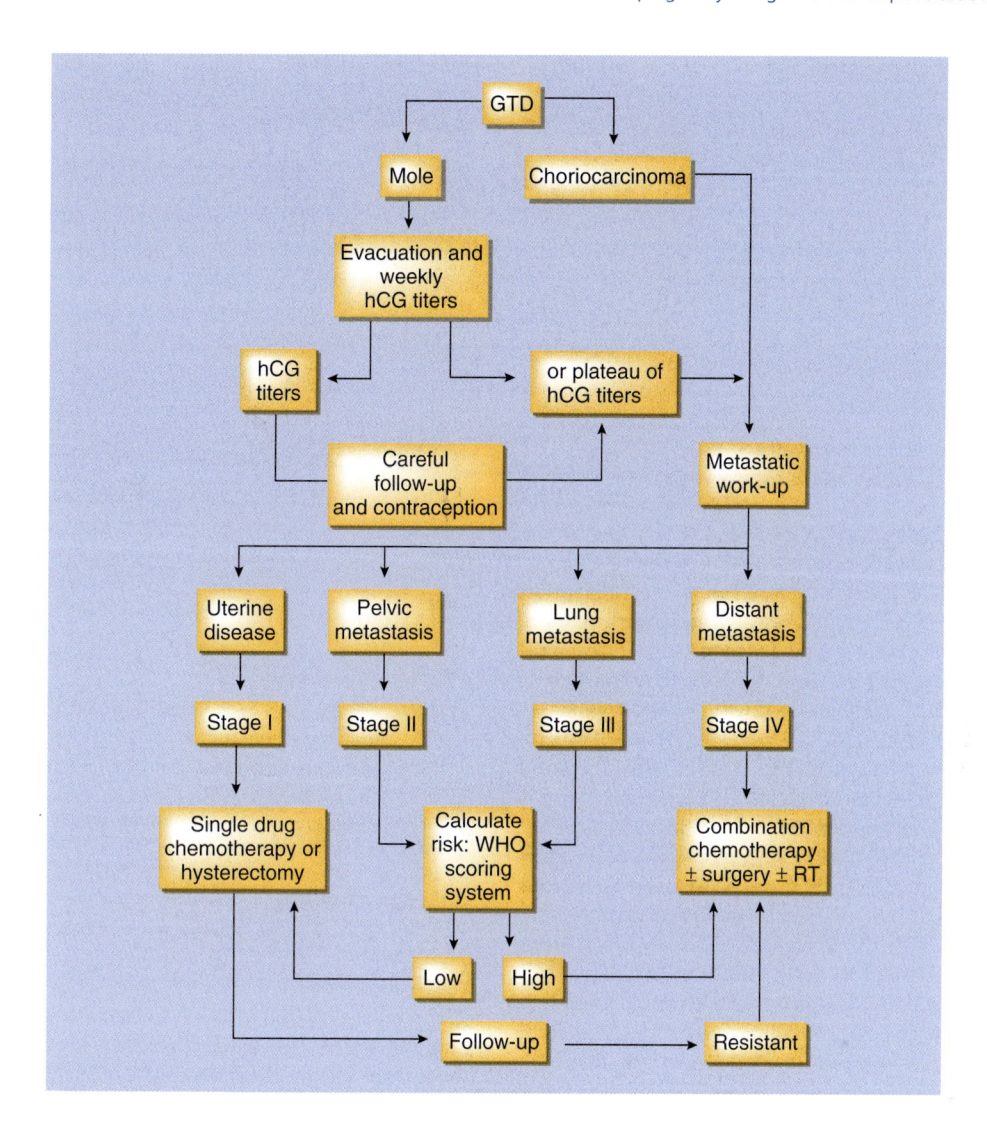

Figure 1 Algorithm for the management of gestational trophoblastic disease.

at high risk of developing drug resistance to single-agent therapy and requires intensive combination chemotherapy. A separate category of ultra high-risk, WHO score ≥12, represents a group of women at risk for early death and poor outcome. Patients with stage I GTN usually have a low-risk score, and those with stage IV disease generally have a high-risk score. Therefore, the distinction between low and high risk mainly applies to patients with stages II and III disease. The FIGO stage is designated by a Roman numeral and is followed by the modified WHO Prognostic Score designated by an Arabic number separated by a colon (e.g., II:6).

Data from Charing Cross Hospital indicate that only 30% of low-risk patients with a WHO Prognostic Score of 5–6 can be cured with monotherapy which suggests that a multidrug regimen should be considered initially. These patients characteristically present with pretreatment hCG levels >100,000 mIU/ml and ultrasound evidence of a large tumor burden.[28]

clinician in selecting the appropriate treatment (Figure 1). The physical examination should always include a vaginal speculum examination to detect implants, which can hemorrhage. Radiographic evaluation should include a pelvic ultrasound to look for evidence of retained trophoblastic tissue in the uterine cavity, myometrial invasion, and to evaluate the pelvis for local spread. Chest imaging is also required, as the lungs are the most common site of metastases. Although chest CT scans are more sensitive than a chest X-ray, they are not included in staging and risk score calculation, since detection of occult pulmonary metastases does not affect outcome. Pulmonary metastases can be detected by chest CT in up to 40% of patients with a negative chest X-ray.[29] In the absence of pulmonary and vaginal metastases, involvement of distant organs such as the brain and liver are rare. As long as the clinical picture is compatible with GTN, metastases need not be biopsied because of their vascularity and the risk of hemorrhage.

Management of GTN

Pretreatment evaluation and staging of GTN
Patients with GTN must undergo a thorough evaluation in order to determine their stage and risk status, which will guide the

Management of low-risk GTN

Primary therapy of low-risk GTN
Low-risk GTN includes patients with both stage I (nonmetastatic) and stages II and III (metastatic) GTN whose prognostic score is

Table 2 Single-agent regimen.

Methotrexate treatments
MTX-FA
MTX 1.0 mg/kg IM on days 1, 3, 5, and 7
FA 0.1 mg/kg IM or po on days 2, 4, 6, and 8
5-day MTX
MTX 0.4 mg/kg/day IV or IM daily for 5 days
Pulse MTX
MTX 50 mg/m^2 IM weekly
Actinomycin D treatments
5-day Act-D
Act-D 12 µg/kg/day IV for 5 days
Pulse Act-D
Act-D 1.25 mg/m^2 IV every 2 weeks

Abbreviations: FA, folinic acid; IM, intramuscular; IV, intravenous. Maximum dose of Act-D 2 mg.

Table 3 EMACO regimen.

Time	Treatment
Day	Etoposide 100 mg/m^2 by IV infusion in 200 mL of saline over 30 min
	Act-D 0.5 mg IV push
	MTX 100 mg/m^2 IV push
	MTX 200 mg/m^2 by IV infusion over 12 h
Day 2	Etoposide 100 mg/m^2 by IV infusion in 200 mL of saline over 30 min
	Act-D 0.5 mg IV push
	FA 15 mg IM or po every 12 h for four doses beginning 24 h after starting MTX
Day 8	Cyclophosphamide 600 mg/m^2 IV in saline Oncovin (vincristine) 1.0 mg/m^2 IV push

Abbreviations: Act-D, actinomycin D; FA, folinic acid; IM, intramuscular; IV, intravenous; MTX, methotrexate; po, per os (by mouth).

less than 7. In patients with stage I GTN, the selection of primary therapy is based on the patient's desire to preserve fertility. If the patient has completed her childbearing, hysterectomy should be considered.[30,31] At the time of surgery, we recommend the administration of one course of adjuvant single-agent chemotherapy, either methotrexate (MTX) or actinomycin D (ACTD) for treatment of occult metastases.

Single-agent chemotherapy with sequential MTX/ACTD is the preferred treatment in patients with stage I GTN who desire to retain fertility, as well as in patients with low-risk metastatic GTN. MTX with folinic acid (MTX-FA) **is** the preferred single-agent regimen at the New England Trophoblastic Disease Center (NETDC).[32] MTX-FA-induced complete remission in 147 (90.2%) of 163 patients with stage I GTN and in 15 (68.2%) of 22 patients with low-risk stages II and III GTN. ACTD is used as primary therapy in those patients with preexisting hepatic dysfunction, who develop hepatic toxicity to MTX, or sequentially in those patients who prove resistant to MTX.[21]

Single-agent chemotherapy with either MTX or ACTD has achieved excellent and comparable remission rates in both nonmetastatic (80–90%) and low-risk metastatic (60–70%) GTN.[2,18,21] Several protocols using MTX and ACTD have been used effectively in the treatment of GTN, but until recently, there has been no prospective randomized study comparing all of these regimens (Tables 2).[21] Single-agent chemotherapy should be administered at a fixed time interval. A decline in the hCG level less than a one log indicates that the patient's tumor is relatively resistant to that drug, and an alternative agent is substituted.

Salvage therapy of low-risk GTN

Patients with low-risk GTN who develop resistance to sequential single-agent chemotherapy can usually achieve remission with combination chemotherapy consisting of MTX, ACTD, cyclophosphamide, etoposide, and Oncovin^R (EMA/CO) (Table 3).[33] While there was an initial concern that etoposide was associated with an increased risk of secondary tumors, more recent data indicate that in general the relative risk for secondary tumors is not increased.[34] If the disease is resistant to both single-agent and combination chemotherapy, hysterectomy or local resection (if the patient wants to preserve fertility) may be considered. Ultrasonography, MRI scan, pelvic arteriography, and/or PET scan may aid in identifying the site of resistant uterine tumor when local resection is planned. After achieving nondetectable hCG levels, the administration of three additional courses of the last effective agent reduces the risk of relapse in patients with low-risk disease.[35]

Management of high-risk GTN, stages II and III

Primary therapy

Women with FIGO stages II and III and a WHO score of 7 or higher are at high risk for developing chemotherapy resistance and disease recurrence and should be treated with primary combination chemotherapy with EMACO which is associated with complete remissions in 76–86% of patients.[36–38]

Salvage therapy

Patients with disease resistant to EMACO may be treated by modifying that regimen by substituting cisplatin and etoposide (EMA/EP) on day 8, or using paclitaxel–etoposide alternating with paclitaxel-cisplatin (TE-TP).[39,40] Combination chemotherapy is administered at 2- to 3-week intervals, toxicity permitting, until the patient attains **three** consecutive weekly undetectable hCG levels, after which at least three additional courses of chemotherapy should be administered to reduce the risk of relapse.

Management of stage IV GTN

Patients with stage IV disease include patients who are at the highest risk of developing rapidly progressive disease and chemoresistance. The use of primary combination chemotherapy in conjunction with the selective use of radiation and surgical treatment has resulted in significantly improved survival. At the NETDC, before 1975 only 30% of patients with stage IV disease survived. After 1975, when the concept of early intensive multi-agent treatment was introduced, complete sustained remissions were achieved in 80% of patients.

Patients with stage IV GTN are generally managed with primary combination chemotherapy with EMA/CO. Patients with a risk score ≥12 are regarded as at ultra-high-risk and are treated with EMA-EP (1). When CNS metastases are present, the MTX dosage in the infusion is increased to 1 g/m^2 and urine is alkalinized.[37] Patients who develop resistance to EMA/CO should then be treated with EMA/EP (Table 4). A number of other salvage regimens have been reported to achieve remission in small series of patients. Second-line therapy with etoposide in combination with cisplatin, and bleomycin (BEP) or vinblastine in combination with cisplatin and bleomycin (PVB) have also been shown to be effective in patients with resistant GTN.[41]

Table 4 EMAEP regimen[a].

Time	Treatment
Day 1	Etoposide 100 mg/m² by IV infusion in 200 mL of saline over 30 min
	Act-D 0.5 mg IV push
	MTX 100 mg/m² IV push
	MTX 1000 mg/m² by IV infusion over 12 h
Day 2	Etoposide 100 mg/m² by IV infusion in 200 mL of saline over 30 min
	Act-D 0.5 mg IV push
	FA 30 mg IM or po every 12 h for six doses beginning 32 h after starting MTX
Day 8	Cisplatin 60 mg/m² IV with prehydration etoposide 100 mg/m² by IV infusion in 200 mL of saline over 30 min

Abbreviations: Act-D, actinomycin D; FA, folinic acid; IM, intramuscular; IV, intravenous; MTX, methotrexate; po, per os (by mouth).
[a]Source: From Newlands et al.[39]

The potential role of autologous bone marrow transplantation or stem cell rescue in GTN has yet to be well defined. Among 32 patients treated with high dose chemotherapy with autologous stem cell transplant, 7 achieved complete remission and 6 attained remission with additional treatment for a 41% complete remission rate.[42]

Despite the efficacy of well-recognized regimens, research continues to identify new agents effective in treating resistant disease. Wan et al.[43] demonstrated the efficacy of floxuridine (FUDR)-containing regimens which induced remission in all 21 patients with drug-resistant disease. Matsui et al.[44] reported that 5FU in combination with ACTD-induced remission in 9 of 11 (82%) of patients when used as salvage therapy.

Because GTN is at least a partial allograft, immunotherapy has been considered as a potentially important treatment. GTN is known to strongly express programmed cell death ligand 1 (PD-L1). Investigators administered pembrolizumab (a monoclonal antibody that acts as an immune checkpoint inhibitor against PD-L1) and 3 of 4 patients with drug-resistant GTN attained a complete remission.[45] Additionally, immunotherapy has been used successfully for women with single-agent chemotherapy-resistant GTN. In a recent phase II trial, avelumab cured approximately 50% of these women with minimal toxicity.[46]

Role of surgery

Surgery is performed either to treat complications or excise sites of resistant tumor.[47] Hysterectomy may be necessary to control uterine hemorrhage or sepsis or to reduce the tumor burden and thereby limit the need for chemotherapy. Bleeding from vaginal metastases may be managed by packing, wide local excision, or arteriographic embolization of the hypogastric arteries.[48] Thoracotomy may be performed to excise persistent viable tumor despite intensive chemotherapy.[49] However, fibrotic nodules may persist indefinitely on chest roentgenograms after complete gonadotropin remission is attained.[50] An extensive metastatic survey should be undertaken to exclude other sites of persistent tumor. A PET scan may be useful to identify occult sites of viable tumor.[51] Hepatic resection may be required to manage bleeding metastases although embolization has also been utilized in this setting.[26] Craniotomy may be necessary to provide acute decompression or to control bleeding, in addition to its role in the primary resection of solitary metastatic disease.[25]

Role of radiation therapy

When cranial metastases are identified stereotactic irradiation and systemic chemotherapy are promptly instituted at the NETDC to reduce the risk of cerebral hemorrhage. Yordan and colleagues[52] reported that deaths as a result of cerebral involvement occurred in 11 (44%) of 25 patients treated with chemotherapy alone but in none of 18 patients treated with brain irradiation and chemotherapy. Excellent results have also been achieved in selected cases with local resection, particularly when the metastasis is solitary and located peripherally.[25,53,54]

Newlands et al.[53] have documented excellent remission rates in patients with brain involvement who were treated with chemotherapy alone. Intensive combination chemotherapy including high dose intravenous and intrathecal MTX-induced sustained remission in 30 (86%) of 35 patients with cerebral lesions. The patients with superficial solitary brain metastases underwent craniotomy at the start of therapy.

Craniotomy may also be necessary to provide acute decompression or to control bleeding. Craniotomy should be performed to manage life-threatening complications thereby providing an opportunity to control the disease with chemotherapy. Infrequently, cerebral metastases may be resectable when they become resistant to chemotherapy. Athanassiou et al.[54] reported that four of five patients undergoing craniotomy for acute intracranial complications were ultimately cured. Fortunately, most patients with cerebral metastases who achieve remission have no residual neurological deficit unless a bleed has occurred.

However, we have observed rare cases of significant dementia and progressive memory loss in patients who received whole-brain irradiation. Although the controversy regarding the optimal treatment protocol for cerebral metastases has not been resolved, Neubauer et al.[55] have reported that multimodal therapy including chemotherapy, surgical resection, and radiation therapy (whole brain or stereotactic) has improved overall survival from 46% to 64%.

Management of PSTT and ETT

Patients with PSTT and ETT require special consideration because of the unique nature of their disease. We believe the primary therapy of all patients with nonmetastatic PSTT and ETT should be hysterectomy without adjunctive chemotherapy because this variant of CCA is relatively resistant to chemotherapy.[16,17,56–60] If deep myometrial involvement is present it is our policy to also perform a pelvic lymphadenectomy. Unlike CCA, these tumors tend to remain localized in the uterus for long periods of time before metastasizing. Once metastases occur, both PSTT and ETT have a high mortality rate. Kingdon et al.[59] in their review of deaths from GTN found that 30% of those dying from GTN had PSTT histology. In the absence of demonstrable metastases, no further treatment is required.

Although universally accepted guidelines on how to manage PSTT and ETT are not available because of their rarity, given their aggressive clinical behavior, the use of multimodal therapy with surgery and chemotherapy has improved survival. The use of EMA/EP has been shown to be curative in patients with metastases.[57] Papadopoulos et al.[60] reported that a long interval from the antecedent pregnancy to clinical presentation was the most important prognostic factor. Whereas all 27 patients survived when the interval was less than four years, all 7 patients died when the interval exceeded 4 years. Although not applicable to the majority of patients, fertility-sparing surgery has also been employed successfully.[61]

Results of therapy

Stage I GTN
Between July 1965 and December 2016, 646 patients with stage I GTN were treated at the NETDC and all attained remission. 493 out of 600 patients (82%) who were treated with primary single-agent chemotherapy achieved remission with sequential MTX/ACTD. All 37 patients managed with primary hysterectomy and adjuvant single-agent chemotherapy achieved remission with no further treatment. Seven patients with high-risk scores achieved remission with primary combination chemotherapy and 2 were treated with D and C. The remaining 107 patients resistant to primary treatment were treated successfully with either combination chemotherapy or surgical intervention.

Stages II and III GTN
Complete remission was achieved at the NETDC in all 37 patients with stage II GTN, and in 229 out of 232 (98%) patients with stage III GTN. Single-agent chemotherapy-induced remission in 16 (76%) of 21 patients with low-risk stage II disease, and in 114 (73%) of 154 patients with low-risk stage III disease. All patients with disease resistant to single-agent chemotherapy attained remission with combination chemotherapy. There were three deaths in the high-risk stage III group.

Stage IV GTN
Prior to 1975, only 6 of 20 patients (30%) with stage IV GTN achieved remission at the NETDC. However, after 1975, 25 of 33 patients (77.5%) with stage IV disease attained remission. This dramatic improvement in survival resulted from the use of intensive multimodal therapy early in the course of treatment. While brain irradiation is commonly employed in the United States for cerebral metastases, excellent remission rates have been reported in patients with cerebral metastases who were treated with chemotherapy alone.[53] Alifrangis et al. reported that the use of induction chemotherapy with low-dose etoposide and cisplatin resulted in improved survival in patients with ultra-high-risk GTN and large tumor volumes.[62]

Patients with high-risk GTN should particularly be considered for referral to a GTN Reference Center. Among 2186 Brazilian patients with GTN from 10 GTN Reference Centers, 84 (4.7%) died from their disease. Adjusting for the WHO-FIGO score, the relative risk of death from low-risk and high-risk GTN was 12.2 and 28.3, respectively when initial treatment was initiated outside of a GTN Reference Center. GTN is an uncommon but highly curable disease and the outcome is improved by experienced management.[63]

hCG follow-up and relapse
All patients with stages I-IV GTN are followed with weekly hCG values until undetectable for three consecutive weeks, and then monthly until undetectable for 12 months.[64,65] All patients must be encouraged to use effective contraception during the entire interval of monitoring. Relapse rates at the NETDC are as follows: stage I, 2.9%; stage II, 8.3%; stage III, 4.2%; and stage IV, 9.1%. The mean time to recurrence from the last nondetectable hCG level was 6 months, and this did not differ among the 4 stages.[64]

When relapse occurs, the patient should be reevaluated, and appropriate therapy begun with a new regimen not previously utilized in this patient.

Quiescent GTN
A rare cause of persistent (at least 3 months) low-level hCG is quiescent GTN (range 0.5–200 mIU/mL) that most commonly follows a molar pregnancy. Quiescent GTN is thought to be due to the presence of highly differentiated, noninvasive syncytiotrophoblast cells. This condition is characterized by the following: (1) foci of disease are not readily identifiable clinically and (2) hCG level is unresponsive to chemotherapy, presumably because the growth cycle of these cells is comparable to normal cells. Patients with quiescent GTN should not be treated with chemotherapy, but close follow-up is indicated because 6–10% will eventually develop active GTN requiring treatment. The presence of low levels of hyperglycosylated hCG indicates the presence of quiescent GTN. Increasing levels of hyperglycosylated hCG indicate the development of active GTN that requires treatment.[22]

Subsequent pregnancies
Patients with complete and partial mole can anticipate normal reproduction in the future.[66] However, these patients are at increased risk of developing molar pregnancy in later conceptions. Patients treated for GTN with chemotherapy can also expect normal reproduction in the future.[66] Importantly, the frequency of later major and minor congenital malformations is not increased. Data from the NETDC and 10 other centers have been reported concerning the outcome of 3191 pregnancies after chemotherapy.[66] These subsequent pregnancies resulted in 2342 (73.4%) live births, 89 (4.7%) premature deliveries, 40 (1.3%) stillbirths, and 457 (14.3%) spontaneous abortions. Although the frequency of stillbirths appears to be somewhat increased, congenital malformations were noted in only 46 (1.6%) infants, which is consistent with the general population.

Because the risk of a repeat molar pregnancy is increased 10-fold, an obstetrical ultrasound should be obtained in the late first trimester of subsequent pregnancies to confirm normal fetal development.[66] Additionally, an hCG test should be performed 6 weeks after completion of any subsequent pregnancy to rule out occult GTN. Later products of conception should also be evaluated by a pathologist following any spontaneous miscarriage or therapeutic abortion.

Key references
The complete reference list can be found on Vital Source version of this title, see inside front cover.

1. Ngan HYS, Seckl M, Berkowitz RS, et al. Update on the diagnosis and management of gestational trophoblastic disease. *Int J Gynecol Obstet.* 2018;**2**:79–85.
12. Elias KM, Goldstein DP, Berkowitz RS. Complete hydatitdform mole in women older than age 50. *J Reprod Med.* 2010;**55**:208–212.
18. Berkowitz RS, Goldstein DP. Chorionic tumors. *N Engl J Med.* 1996;**335**:1740–1748.
21. Elias KM, Berkowitz RS, Horowitz NS. State-of-the-art work up and initial management of newly diagnosed gestational trophoblastic disease. *JNCCN.* 2019;**17**:1396–1401.
24. Bakri YN, Berkowitz RS, Khan J, et al. Pulmonary metastases of gestational trophoblastic tumor: risk factors for early respiratory failure. *J Reprod Med.* 1994;**39**:175–178.
26. Ahamed E, Short D, North B, et al. Survival of women with gestational trophoblastic neoplasia and liver metastases: Is it improving? *J Reprod Med.* 2012;**57**:262–269.
28. McGrath S, Short D, Harvey R, et al. The management and outcome of women with post-hydatidiform mole 'low-risk' gestational trophoblastic neoplasia, but hCG levels in excess of 100,000 IU/L. *Br J Cancer.* 2010;**102**:810–814.
30. Clark RM, Nevadunsky NS, Ghosh S, et al. The evolving role of hysterectomy in gestational trophoblastic neoplasia at the New England Trophoblastic Disease Center. *J Reprod Med.* 2010;**55**:194–198.

32. Maesta I, Nitecki R, Horowitz NS, et al. Effectiveness and toxicity of first-line methotrexate chemotherapy in low-risk post-molar gestational trophoblastic neoplasia: The New England Trophoblastic Disease Center experience. *Gynecol Oncol.* 2018;**148**(1):161–167.
34. Savage P, Cooke R, O'Nions J, et al. Effects of single-agent and combination chemotherapy for gestational trophoblastic tumors on risks of second malignancy and early menopause. *J Clin Oncol.* 2015;**33**:472–478.
41. Lurain JR, Schink JC. Importance of salvage therapy in the management of high-risk gestational trophoblastic neoplasia. *J Reprod Med.* 2012;**57**:219–224.
51. Dhillon T, Palmieri C, Sebire NJ, et al. Value of whole body 18 FDG-PET to identify the active site of gestational trophoblastic neoplasia. *J Reprod Med.* 2006;**51**:879–883.
53. Newlands ES, Holden I, Seckl MJ, et al. Management of brain metastases in patients with high risk gestational trophoblastic tumor. *J Reprod Med.* 2002;**47**:465.
55. Neubauer NL, Latif N, Kalakota K, et al. Brain metastasis in gestational trophoblastic disease: an update. *J Reprod Med.* 2012;**57**:288–292.
59. Kingdon SJ, Coleman RE, Ellis L, Hancock BW. Deaths from gestational trophoblastic neoplasia. Any lessons to be learned? *J Reprod Med.* 2012;**57**:293–296.
62. Alifrangis C, Agarwal R, Short D, et al. EMA/CO for high-risk gestational trophoblastic neoplasia: good outcome with induction low-dose etoposide-cisplatin and genetic analysis. *J Clin Oncol.* 2013;**31**:280–286.

104 Gynecologic sarcomas

Jamal Rahaman, MD ■ Carmel J. Cohen, MD

Overview

Sarcomas are extremely rare and account for less than 1.5% of gynecologic cancers. Carcinosarcoma and leiomyosarcoma each account for 35–40% of uterine sarcomas, with endometrial stromal sarcoma (ESS) accounting for 10–15% and other sarcomas including adenosarcomas comprising 5–10 %. Uterine carcinosarcoma should be classified as a metaplastic carcinoma of the uterus. Most adenosarcomas and ESSs have good prognosis and respond to hormonal therapy. Undifferentiated endometrial sarcoma (UES) and adenosarcomas with sarcomatous overgrowth are rare and have poor prognosis and require chemotherapy. ESS are histologically and clinically distinct from UES and each have distinct gene rearrangements. More than 50% of stage I leiomyosarcomas and carcinosarcomas patients will recur. Chemotherapy is required for advanced or recurrent disease. In leiomyosarcomas, the active drugs are doxorubicin, ifosfamide, gemcitabine, and docetaxel. For uterine carcinosarcomas, the drugs of choice are ifosfamide, cisplatin/carboplatin, and paclitaxel. Adjuvant radiation therapy may provide locoregional control in select cases of uterine carcinosarcomas. Hormonal therapy, including progestational agents, GnRH analogs, and aromatase inhibitors, has a role in the treatment of advanced or recurrent low-grade ESSs and adenosarcomas.

Historical perspective

Sarcomas (including mesenchymal and mixed epithelial–mesenchymal malignancies) of the vulva, vagina, cervix, uterus, and ovaries account for less than 1.5% of the cancers of these organs. Classification of these cancers was a taxonomic dilemma until Ober, in 1959,[1] proposed a classification which Kempson and Bari[2] revised in 1970, and the World Health Organization[3] and the College of American Pathologist[4] reclassified in 2003 (see Table 1). Uterine carcinosarcomas are not classified as a uterine sarcoma any longer, and should be classified as a metaplastic carcinoma of the uterus[5,6] but will be discussed in this article. The principles of etiology, histopathology, molecular and genetic alterations, and multidisciplinary management concepts overlap with the other soft tissue sarcomas and will be explored in greater detail in this article.

Incidence and epidemiology

The most common site for sarcoma in the female pelvis is the uterus comprising only 4–9% of uterine cancers, with an annual incidence rate of less than 20 per million females.[7,8] Overall incidence for Blacks is twice that of Whites, but there were no differences in survival for women receiving similar therapy.[7,8] Risk of carcinosarcoma increases sharply with age. Incidence rate per million women per year is 8.2 for carcinosarcomas, 6.4 for leiomyosarcomas (LMSs), 1.8 for endometrial stromal sarcomas (ESSs), and 0.7 for unclassified sarcomas.[7,8] Authors have reported that carcinosarcoma and LMS each account for 35–40% of uterine sarcomas, ESS accounting for 10–15%, and other sarcomas comprising 5%.[8]

Risk factors

Epidemiologic risk factors for uterine sarcoma are undefined except for radiation exposure[9–12] and previous tamoxifen use.[13,14]

Pathology

The uterus is the most common site of gynecologic sarcomas arising from the endometrium only (ESS), the myometrium only (LMS), or contributions from both (carcinosarcomas).[1,15] The homologous tumors include carcinoma plus a sarcoma indigenous to the uterus, while the heterologous tumors include a sarcoma resembling tissue from some extrauterine source (bone, cartilage, striated muscle). Müllerian adenosarcomas are mixed Müllerian tumors composed of malignant stroma and benign epithelium.[3,16,17]

Endometrial stromal lesions

Endometrial stromal nodules (ESN) are rare. They are characterized by a well-defined noninfiltrating border without evidence of myometrial or vascular invasion. Two-thirds are found as isolated lesions within the myometrium with no apparent connection to the endometrium.[3]

ESS is low-grade with metastatic potential. Like ESN, they are composed of uniform cells that mimic proliferative endometrium. However, they exhibit myometrial and/or vascular invasion.[3] Histologically, they are characterized by densely uniform stromal cells with minimal cellular pleomorphism, mild nuclear atypia, and rare mitotic figures. Of note, an isolated finding of increased mitotic figures does not confer an adverse prognosis in an otherwise typical low-grade ESS.[18]

The diagnosis of ESS may be complicated by variant morphologic features (see Table 1).[3] In tumors with focal smooth muscle differentiation, the tumor is categorized as ESS if the smooth muscle component involves <30% of the total tumor volume. Tumors composed of a larger smooth muscle component are designated as mixed endometrial stromal and smooth muscle tumors.[3,19]

Undifferentiated endometrial sarcoma (UES—previously referred to as high-grade ESSs) is characterized by marked cytologic atypia, nuclear pleomorphism, high mitotic activity, and extensive invasion. In addition, UES usually show destructive myometrial invasion.[3]

Holland-Frei Cancer Medicine, Tenth Edition. Edited by Robert C. Bast, John C. Byrd, Carlo M. Croce, Ernest Hawk, Fadlo R. Khuri, Raphael E. Pollock, Apostolia M. Tsimberidou, Christopher G. Willett, and Cheryl L. Willman.
© 2023 John Wiley & Sons, Inc. Published 2023 by John Wiley & Sons, Inc.

Table 1 Classification of uterine sarcomas.[a]

Histologic type (select all that apply)
Leiomyosarcoma
Low-grade endometrial stromal sarcoma
Low-grade endometrial stromal sarcoma with:
- Smooth muscle differentiation
- Sex cord elements
- Glandular elements

Other (specify): _____
High-grade endometrial stromal sarcoma
Undifferentiated uterine/endometrial sarcoma
Adenosarcoma
Adenosarcoma with:
- Rhabdomyoblastic differentiation
- Cartilaginous differentiation
- Osseous differentiation
- Other heterologous element (specify): _____

Adenosarcoma with sarcomatous overgrowth
Other (specify): _____

College of American Pathologist Classification of Uterine Sarcomas. Low-grade endometrial sarcoma is distinguished from benign endometrial stromal nodule by infiltration into the surrounding myometrium and/or lymphovascular invasion. Minor marginal irregularity in the form of tongues <3 mm (up to 3) is allowable for an endometrial stromal nodule. This protocol does not apply to endometrial stromal nodule
[a]Source: Modified from Tavassoli and coworker[3] and Otis et al.[4]

Molecular and genetic alterations

The following molecular features are characteristic of ESS and are also found in ESN: The majority are immunoreactive for the ER and PR. They are typically immunohistochemically positive for CD10 and negative for desmin and h-caldesmon and loss of heterozygosity of PTEN, and deregulation of the Wnt signaling pathway.[5,20,21]

UES shows increased staining for proliferation markers (Ki67, p16, and p53) and does not generally exhibit immunoreactivity against ER, PR, desmin, or smooth muscle antigen (SMA).[5] UES also expresses the receptor tyrosine kinase CD117 (c-KIT),[22] cyclin D1,[23] and human epidermal growth factor receptor 2 (HER2 or ERBB2), which are not typically found in ESS.[5]

Mutations, translocations, amplifications, deletions

Gene rearrangements have been described and validated in patients with ESSs with at least 75% having a gene rearrangement.[24,25] The t(7;17) translocation resulting in the JAZF1-SUZ12 gene fusion is the most common translocation found in approximately 35% to 50% of ESSs.[25] Other noted gene fusions are JAZF1-PHF1, EPC1-PHF1, JAZF1 only, and PHF1 only.[24–28]

UESs lack these JAFZ1-based rearrangements but instead appear to frequently harbor the YWHAE-FAM22A/B genetic fusion[29–32] which may be specific to these tumors since this rearrangement was not detected in 827 other cases representing 55 tumor types.[30]

Patterns of spread

Uterine sarcomas are spread by lymphatic, hematogenous, local extension, and peritoneal dissemination.[33–41]

Rose and colleagues[33] studied the autopsy findings of 73 patients with uterine sarcoma, including 43 patients with carcinosarcoma, 19 with LMS, 9 with ESS, and 2 with endolymphatic stromal myosis. The peritoneal cavity and omentum were the most frequently involved sites (59%), followed by lung (52%), pelvic (41%) and para-aortic (38%) lymph nodes, and liver parenchyma (34%). Of note, the presence of lung metastasis was often a sole metastatic site.

Lymph node metastasis in adult soft-tissue sarcomas is <3%, with some variation among histologic subtypes.[42] The risk of lymph metastasis in LMS overall was approximately 6.4% in a series of 357 patients.[43] However, the rate of occult lymph node metastasis in clinically normal nodes and disease clinically confined to the uterus was only 3.5% among 57 surgically staged patients with LMS.[38] Carcinosarcomas have a higher rate of both overall (25%)[44] and occult (18%)[38] lymph node metastasis. The rate of overall and occult lymph node metastasis in ESS is 16% and 6%, respectively.[45] Deep myometrial invasion and extensive lymph–vascular space invasion (LVSI) further increase the risk of occult metastasis.[35,46] The rate of lymph node metastasis in adenosarcomas is approximately 3%.[47]

Clinical profile

Uterine endometrial stromal tumors

Patients with endometrial stromal tumors are commonly perimenopausal with irregular vaginal bleeding. The tumor tissue may protrude through the cervical os and may grow large without penetrating through the uterine wall. The diagnosis is usually made by endometrial sampling.[19,48,49]

LMS

LMS commonly occurs during the fourth and fifth decades of life, with a peak incidence at 45 years, after which there is a gradual decline in incidence until the eighth decade. The lesion is frequently associated with benign leiomyomas, although among leiomyomas, sarcoma is found less than 1% of the time.[50,51] There is debate over whether the lesion "develops" from a benign leiomyoma or occurs independently. Ferenczy and colleagues were unable to demonstrate a developmental relationship,[52] whereas Spiro and Koss[53] found intermediate changes in leiomyomas and proposed malignant transformation. Often LMSs are discovered by chance at the time of myomectomy or hysterectomy.[50,54,55]

Carcinosarcoma

The incidence of carcinosarcoma increases at 50 years and plateaus after age 75 years. Vaginal bleeding, heavy discharge, and abdominal pain is characteristic. Endometrial sampling is more often diagnostic than in LMS because LMS invades the endometrial cavity infrequently.

Tumor biomarkers

Goto et al. reported that serum lactate dehydrogenase (LDH) was elevated in a small series of LMS and was useful in combination with dynamic MRI. The positive predictive value was 91% using the combined assessment compared to 39% for LDH alone and 71% for MRI alone.[56]

Huang et al. reported that preoperative CA125 elevation was a marker of extrauterine disease and deep myometrial invasion in patients with uterine CS. Postoperative CA125 elevation was an independent prognostic factor for poor survival.[57]

Imaging studies

ESS has a nonspecific appearance on ultrasound.[58] The characteristic pattern of ESS consists of worm-like tumor projections along the vessels or ligaments, which are best visualized on MRI with diffuse weighted imaging.[59] There are few studies describing the characteristic appearance of UES.[60]

Kurjak and colleagues evaluated the role of transvaginal color Doppler ultrasonography in differentiating uterine sarcomas from leiomyomas.[61] Computed tomography will identify extrauterine spread, and magnetic resonance imaging can assess the depth of myometrial invasion. Imaging studies are performed preoperatively to characterize the uterine mass and evaluate lymph node involvement and other metastases but cannot reliably differentiate between a uterine sarcoma and other uterine findings. There are few data suggesting the best choice of imaging.[60,62,63] The FDG-PET showed a better detection rate than the abdominal CT scan for extra pelvic metastatic lesions.[64–67]

Diagnosis

Of patients with uterine sarcomas, 75–95% present with abnormal vaginal bleeding.[68,69] Pelvic pain, discharge, and aborting tissue occur frequently. Endometrial biopsy may confirm carcinosarcoma in the majority of cases[70]; however, LMS and ESS are missed in at least 40% and 20% of cases, respectively.[19,37,71,72]

TNM and FIGO staging classification

Uterine sarcomas require surgical staging. The International Federation of Gynecology and Obstetrics (FIGO) did not have a sarcoma-specific system until recently and the endometrial staging criteria were applied until 2009. FIGO devised a uterine sarcoma-specific staging system in 2009 for LMS, EES, and UES and another specific for adenosarcoma (see Tables 2 and 3).

Carcinosarcomas are to be staged using the 2009 revised FIGO Staging for endometrial carcinomas (see *Endometrial cancer*).

Prognostic factors and prognosis

Prognostic factors differ for the three major types of uterine sarcomas. Major and colleagues reported the GOG clinicopathologic study of clinical stages I and II uterine sarcoma, which included 59 patients with LMS and 301 patients with carcinosarcoma.[38] Of the 453 patients eligible for analysis, 430 underwent complete surgical staging that included lymphadenectomy. The median survival was 62.6 months for homologous carcinosarcoma, 22.7 months for heterologous carcinosarcoma, and 20.6 months for LMS. The overall recurrence rate for homologous carcinosarcoma was 56%.

In patients with LMS, lymph vascular space involvement and involvement of the cervix and isthmus were common, whereas lymph node metastases, adnexal metastases, and positive peritoneal cytology were infrequent findings. The only surgicopathologic finding that correlated with progression-free interval was the mitotic index.[2,38,40,73] Whereas there were no treatment failures among the three women who had less than 10 mitoses per 10 high-power fields, 61% of women with 10–20 mitoses per 10 high-power fields and 79% of women with greater than 20 mitoses per 10 high-power fields developed recurrences.

Table 2 STAGING—leiomyosarcoma, endometrial stromal sarcoma, and undifferentiated uterine sarcoma.[a]

TNM categories	FIGO stages	Definition
Primary tumor (T)		
TX		Primary tumor cannot be assessed
T0		No evidence of primary tumor
T1	I	Tumor is limited to the uterus
T1a	IA	Tumor is 5 cm or less (≤5 cm) in greatest dimension
T1b	IB	Tumor is greater than 5 cm (>5 cm) in greatest dimension
T2	II	Tumor extends beyond the uterus but is within the pelvis (tumor extends to extrauterine pelvic tissue)
T2a	IIA	Tumor involves the adnexa
T2b	IIB	Tumor involves other pelvis tissue
T3	III	Tumor invades abdominal tissues (not just protruding into the abdomen)
T3a	IIIA	Tumor invades abdominal tissues at one site
T3b	IIIB	Tumor invades abdominal tissues at more than one site
T4	IVA	Tumor invades bladder mucosa and/or rectum
Regional lymph nodes (N)		
NX		Regional lymph nodes cannot be assessed
N0		No regional lymph node metastasis
N1	IIIC	Regional lymph node metastasis to pelvic lymph nodes
Distant metastasis (M)		
M0		No distant metastasis
M1	IVB	Distant metastasis (excluding adnexa, pelvic and abdominal tissues) Specify site(s), if known:

[a]Source: Modified from Otis et al.[4] and D'Angelo and Prat.[5]

Table 3 STAGING—uterine adenosarcoma.[a]

TNM Categories	FIGO Stages	Definition
Primary tumor (T)		
TX		Primary tumor cannot be assessed
T0		No evidence of primary tumor
T1	I	Tumor limited to the uterus
T1a	IA	Tumor is limited to the endometrium/endocervix without myometrial invasion
T1b	IB	Tumor invades less than or equal to 50% (≤50%) total myometrial thickness
T1c	IC	Tumor invades greater than 50% (>50%) total myometrial thickness
T2	II	Tumor extends beyond the uterus but is within the pelvis (tumor extends to extrauterine pelvic tissue)
T2a	IIA	Tumor involves the adnexa
T2b	IIB	Tumor involves other pelvis tissue
T3	III	Tumor invades abdominal tissues (not just protruding into the abdomen)
T3a	IIIA	Tumor invades abdominal tissues at one site
T3b	IIIB	Tumor invades abdominal tissues at more than one site
T4	IVA	Tumor invades bladder mucosa and/or rectum
Regional lymph nodes (N)		
NX		Regional lymph nodes cannot be assessed
N0		No regional lymph node metastasis
N1	IIIC	Regional lymph node metastasis to pelvic lymph nodes
Distant metastasis (M)		
M0		No distant metastasis
M1	IVB	Distant metastasis (excluding adnexa, pelvic and abdominal tissues) Specify site(s), if known:

[a]Source: Modified from Otis et al.[4] and D'Angelo and Prat.[5]

In contrast to patients with LMS, surgicopathologic factors of carcinosarcoma that related to progression-free interval included adnexal spread, lymph node metastasis, histologic cell type (heterologous versus homologous), and the grade of sarcoma. Of note, patients with carcinosarcoma had high rates of nodal and adnexal metastases and positive peritoneal cytology. Pelvic nodes were involved twice as often as aortic nodes (15% vs 7.8%), and both nodal groups were involved in 5% of the patients.[38]

Morcellation

In patients undergoing laparoscopic hysterectomy for a presumed uterine sarcoma, power morcellation should not be attempted. Wright used a large insurance database to identify 36,470 women undergoing minimally invasive hysterectomy with power morcellation performed to demonstrate that the prevalence of uterine cancers was 27 per 10,000 (99 cases).[74] In addition in this cohort, 26 cases of other gynecologic malignancies were found (a prevalence of 7/10,000), 39 uterine neoplasms of uncertain malignant potential (11/10,000), and 368 cases of endometrial hyperplasia (101/10,000).[74]

LMS

Morcellation of a uterine leiomyosarcoma is associated with a worsened outcome.[51,75] Park et al. reported a series in which the 5-year disease-free survival was 40% in women who underwent tumor morcellation and were subsequently diagnosed with leiomyosarcoma, compared to 65% in those with leiomyosarcoma who had not undergone morcellation ($p = 0.04$).[76] Similarly, the 5-year OS was 46% after morcellation compared to 73% in those not morcellated ($p = 0.04$).[76]

ESS

In one study, tumor morcellation in women with ESS was associated with a lower 5-year disease-free survival (DFS) compared with those who did not have a morcellation (55% vs 84%, respectively, odds ratio 4.03, 95% CI 1.06–15.3).[77] However, no significant impact on overall survival (OS) was reported.

Surgical treatment

The initial therapy for sarcomas of the gynecologic tract is surgical except for embryonal rhabdomyosarcomas. Patients with uterine sarcoma require total abdominal hysterectomy and careful staging including pelvic and para-aortic lymph node sampling. In patients with carcinosarcoma limited to the uterus by pathologic staging, the cytologic presence of malignant cells in the peritoneal washings is a poor prognostic factor. Minimal invasive laparoscopic or robotic surgery may be appropriate in selected cases with early-stage disease provided no power morcellation is used and it appears that patterns of recurrence and survival were not impacted by surgical approach.[78]

The ovaries could be retained in premenopausal patients with LMS because this does not appear to affect prognosis.[15,72,79–81] However, a bilateral salpingo-oophorectomy should be performed in all other patients, including those with low-grade ESS,[82,83] because these tumors may be hormone dependent or responsive and have a propensity for extension into the parametria, broad ligament, and adnexal structures.

For carcinosarcoma, a high percentage of patients with clinical stages I or II disease is upstaged at the time of laparotomy;[84,85] thus all patients should undergo a lymphadenectomy. In addition, lymphadenectomy may be associated with an improvement in overall survival.[86,87] Surgical cytoreduction to no gross visible disease is a reasonable option in selected advanced stage carcinosarcoma patients.[88]

There is a paucity of data regarding the role of lymph node sampling in patients with LMS[79] and ESS, but it appears that almost all patients with these sarcomas who have lymph node metastases also have evidence of intraperitoneal disease spread.[50]

Unlike other gynecologic malignancies, there is a role for thoracotomy or video-assisted thoracoscopy in patients with uterine sarcoma metastatic to the lung. Levenback and colleagues reviewed 45 patients whose pulmonary metastases from uterine sarcoma were resected at Memorial Sloan-Kettering Cancer Center, the majority of which were LMS (84%).[89] The mean survival of patients with unilateral disease (39 months) was significantly greater than that of patients with bilateral disease (27 months). Recurrent or metastatic low-grade ESS may also be amenable to surgical excision of pelvic disease or pulmonary metastases.

Postsurgical therapy for gynecologic sarcomas

Although complete surgical removal is the ideal initial therapy for patients with sarcoma of the gynecologic tract, there is no randomized study proving that surgical cytoreduction influences overall survival for patients with advanced or recurrent disease. Similarly, the therapeutic benefit of lymphadenectomy has not been proven but is rational. For patients with sarcoma of the uterus or ovary, no formal trial has evaluated the role of lymphadenectomy in addition to hysterectomy and bilateral salpingo-oophorectomy.

For patients with uterine sarcoma, there is no definitive evidence from prospective trials that adjuvant therapy of any type leads to overall improvement in survival. To review the currently understood role of radiotherapy and chemotherapy in sarcomas, LMS is separated from the remaining homologous and heterologous carcinosarcomas because the patterns of relapse for the former are somewhat different from those of the latter group.

Radiation oncology

Radiation therapy for LMS

In contrast to other sarcomas, patients with LMS confined to the uterus appear to have a dominant pattern of failure outside the pelvis and abdominal cavity (65%) with a minority of patients with a first recurrence confined to the abdomen and or pelvis (28%).[90–92] Thus, in LMS, although the rate of failure in the pelvis is not insubstantial, little is to be potentially gained by delivering pelvic irradiation as a postoperative adjuvant treatment insofar as two-thirds of patients have some component of distant disease at first recurrence. Radiation treatment is reserved for isolated pelvic relapse only.

Radiation therapy for carcinosarcoma

Historically, pre- or postoperative pelvic irradiation has been used as an adjunct to surgery for carcinosarcoma. Many retrospective reviews illustrate this common use.[68,85,93–99] In several reports for carcinosarcoma, the pelvic recurrence rate was 56%, whereas the distant metastasis rate was 45%. This represents a higher risk of pelvic recurrence than that seen in patients with LMS.[68,93–95,99] It also demonstrates that surgery alone, even for disease apparently confined to the uterus, is inadequate for control of disease in the pelvis. Some but not all studies have shown benefit from postoperative irradiation,[100–102] especially in local control.[68,97,101,103–107] Rates of distant metastases in series of patients treated with or without adjuvant pelvic irradiation are similar, in the order of 35–45%.[68,94,97]

There has been only one randomized clinical trial evaluating the role of adjuvant pelvic radiotherapy in stages I and II Uterine Sarcomas. The EORTC enrolled 224 patients (103 LMS, 91 carcinosarcoma, and 28ESS) from 1998 to 2001 and demonstrated an improved local control rate for patients with carcinosarcoma (24% recurrence in RT vs 47% in observation) but no survival benefit. There was no improvement in local control for LMS (20% local recurrence in RT vs 24% in observation group).[107]

The morbidity associated with pelvic recurrence in uterine sarcomas may be substantial; therefore, it is reasonable to offer adjuvant pelvic irradiation to patients with carcinosarcoma to improve locoregional control rates. The doses of radiation have not been standardized; however, it is probable that doses should be at least 50 Gy, fractionated over 5 weeks.

The GOG[108] also conducted a phase III study of whole-abdomen irradiation (WAI) versus three cycles of cisplatin–ifosfamide and mesna (CIM) in 206 eligible patients with optimally debulked stages I–IV carcinosarcoma. Although there was no significant advantage the observed difference favored the use of chemotherapy. The adjusted recurrence rate was 21% lower for CIM patients and the adjusted death rate was 29% lower. Moreover, there was a significant increase in late adverse events in the WAI patients.[109]

Primary pelvic irradiation has been employed rarely in patients with sarcoma deemed inoperable. Literature reports suggest that in approximately half or two-thirds of patients, pelvic disease could be controlled with standard fractionated irradiation; a small proportion of patients are cured with such treatment.[68,93–95]

Finally, radiation may be useful as a palliative measure for recurrent or uncontrolled pelvic tumor causing pain or bleeding.

Chemotherapy

Two characteristics of uterine sarcomas increase the likelihood that systemic therapy will be required: a recurrence rate of at least 50% even in stage I disease and a tendency to recur at distant sites. Nevertheless, the amount of meaningful data on the use of systemic therapy is limited by the low incidence of these lesions. Studies by the GOG first identified the differential sensitivity of carcinosarcoma and LMS to drug therapy.[110] Because these two cell types respond differently to chemotherapy, they are discussed separately.

Single-agent therapy

Several drugs have been studied in advanced or recurrent carcinosarcoma and/or LMS (Tables 3 and 4), including cisplatin,[114–117] ifosfamide,[111–113] doxorubicin,[110,118] liposomal doxorubicin,[119] etoposide,[120–122] mitoxantrone,[123] paclitaxel,[124,125] topotecan,[126] gemcitabine,[127] Trimetrexate,[130] and docetaxel.[129,131]

Carcinosarcoma

Ifosfamide is the most active single agent in the treatment of advanced or recurrent carcinosarcoma of the uterus with a 32.2% overall response rate in chemo-naïve patients.[111] Paclitaxel[125] and cisplatin[114] are the two other very active single agents with overall response rates of 18.2% and 18%, respectively.

Leiomyosarcoma

Of the single agents that have been tested in patients with LMS (Table 4), the most active are doxorubicin,[110] gemcitabine,[127] ifosfamide,[112] and trabectedin[128] with response rates of 25%, 20.5%, 17.2%, and 10%, respectively. Trabectedin was recently approved for advanced LMS after progression on an anthracycline-based treatment. The most active and commonly employed single-agent chemotherapy for first line or recurrence remains doxorubicin at a dose of 60–75 mg/m^2.[132] Randomized clinical trials have demonstrated no improvement when doxorubicin is combined with cyclophosphamide,[133] trabectedin,[134] or olaratumab[135,136] and

Table 4 Single-agent activity in uterine sarcomas.

Drug	Prior chemotherapy	Schedule	Response, n (%)			
			CS	LMS	ESS	References
Ifosfamide	No	1.5 g/m²/d + mesna, 0.3 g/m²/d, d 1–5 q 4 weeks	9/28 (32)	6/35 (17)	7/21 (33)	111–113
Cisplatin	No	50 mg/m² q 3 weeks	12/63 (19)	1/33 (3)		114
	Yes	50 mg/m² q 3 weeks	5/28 (18)	1/19 (5)		115, 116
	No	75–100 mg/m² q 3 weeks	5/12 (42)			117
Doxorubicin	No	60 mg/m² q 3 weeks	4/41 (10)	7/28 (25)		110
	No	50–90 mg/m² q 3 weeks	0/9 (0)			118
Liposomal doxorubicin	No	50 mg/m² q 4 weeks		5/32 (16)		119
Etoposide	Yes	100 mg/m²/d, d 1–3 q 4 weeks	2/31 (6)	3/28 (11)		120
	Yes	50 mg/m², d 1–21 q 4 weeks		2/29 (7)		121
	No	100 mg/m²/d, d 1–3 q 3 weeks		0/28 (0)		122
Mitoxantrone	Yes	12 mg/m² q 3 weeks	0/17 (0)	0/12 (0)		123
Paclitaxel	No	175 mg/m² q 3 weeks		3/34 (9)		124
Paclitaxel	Yes	170 mg/m² q 3 weeks	8/44 (18.)			125
Topotecan	No	1.5 mg/m²/d, d 1–5 q 3 weeks		3/36 (8)		126
Gemcitabine	Yes	1000 mg/m² d 1, 8, 15 q 4 weeks		9/44 (20.5)		127
Trabectedin	No	1.5 mg/m² q 3 weeks		2/20 (10)		128
Docetaxel	No	100 mg/m² q 3 weeks		0/16 (0)		129

Abbreviations: ESS, endometrial stromal sarcoma; LMS, leiomyosarcoma; CS, carcinosarcoma.

no difference when compared to the combination of gemcitabine and docetaxel.[132]

Endometrial stromal sarcoma
There are few data in the gynecologic literature regarding the use of chemotherapy for ESS.[37,71,137] Ifosfamide[78,113] had an overall response rate of 33.3% in 21 women with metastatic ESS. Tanner reported on 13 patients with high-grade undifferentiated uterine sarcoma who received first-line chemotherapy for measurable disease, with the overall response rate of 62% using gemcitabine/docetaxel (6 of 8) and doxorubicin in (2 of 5).[138]

For metastatic YWHAE-rearranged HG-ESS, prolonged disease control following diagnosis was seen, with notable responses (33% complete response) to anthracycline-based therapy suggesting a role for appropriate molecular testing of uterine mesenchymal malignancies to define chemo-sensitivity.[139]

Combination chemotherapy

Leiomyosarcoma
The most active combination is Gemcitabine 900 mg/m^2 intravenously on days 1 and 8 plus docetaxel 100 mg/m^2 intravenously on day 8, with granulocyte colony-stimulating factor subcutaneously on days 9–15. The GOG conducted two phase II studies with this regimen with gemcitabine at a fixed dose rate of 10 mg/m^2/min as first-line and second-line therapy for metastatic LMS. As initial therapy for metastatic uterine leiomyosarcoma, this combination achieved a 36% response rate among 42 patients and an additional 26% with stable disease.[140] This doublet achieved a 27% response rate in the second-line study among the 48 patients with an additional 50% with stable disease (median duration 5.4 months).[141]

The other highly active combination is Adriamycin and ifosfamide. The GOG[142] reported a 30% response rate in 33 patients treated as first line with conventional doses of ifosfamide. Levyraz and colleagues[143] achieved a 49% response rate in 37 patients treated with a dose-intensive regimen with ifosfamide, 10 g/m^2 as a continuous infusion over 5 days, plus doxorubicin intravenously, 25 mg/m^2/day for 3 days.

Carcinosarcoma
In uterine carcinosarcoma, three randomized clinical trials have defined the best combination chemotherapy regimens. GOG-0108 evaluated the combination of ifosfamide-mesna with or without cisplatin as first-line therapy in patients with advanced, persistent, or recurrent uterine CS. The combination regimen demonstrated a significantly improved overall response rate (54%) when compared to the single-agent regimen (36%) but no survival advantage.

In the GOG-0161, there was a 31% decrease in the adjusted hazard of death and a 29% decrease in the adjusted hazard of progression in those patients receiving paclitaxel-ifosfamide /mesna-growth factor relative to ifosfamide alone for uterine CS.[144] Thus paclitaxel /ifosfamide became the standard arm for future GOG studies testing combination chemotherapy for uterine CS.

The GOG phase II trial (GOG-0232B) formally tested the efficacy of paclitaxel and carboplatin (T/C) in 55 patients with advanced uterine CS. The proportions of patients with confirmed complete and partial responses were 13% and 41%, respectively, resulting in a total overall response rate of 54% with a median progression-free survival of 7.0 months and median survival was 14.4 months.[145]

Thus, the GOG 261 phase III trial for uterine CS was designed as a noninferiority trial to test the efficacy of T/C compared to paclitaxel/ifosfamide in 637 women with stages I–IV carcinosarcoma or recurrent chemotherapy-naïve disease. The trial presented at ASCO 2019 confirmed paclitaxel and carboplatin to be noninferior with regards to overall survival (OS 37 vs 29 months) and resulted in a longer PFS (16 vs 12 months: HR = 0.73). Therefore, T/C has emerged as the best chemotherapy regimen for carcinosarcoma.[146]

Adjuvant chemotherapy for limited disease

Leiomyosarcoma
The role of adjuvant chemotherapy following complete resection of early-stage uterine leiomyosarcoma is still under investigation. The only randomized trial (GOG Protocol 20) of adjuvant chemotherapy in early-stage uterine sarcomas to date assigned patients to either doxorubicin 60 mg/m^2 every 3 weeks for eight cycles or no further therapy. There were only 48 patients in the LMS subset and with these small numbers it was underpowered to assess a significant difference in recurrence or survival.[147]

The Sarcoma Alliance for Research through Collaboration conducted a phase II, multicenter study (SARC 005) of four cycles of adjuvant fixed-dose-rate gemcitabine docetaxel followed by 4 cycles of doxorubicin in 47 patients with uterus-limited leiomyosarcoma.[148] Although 78% of the patients remained progression-free at 2 years, this dropped to 50% at the 3-year follow-up.[148] A phase III multicenter randomized trial (GOG 277) comparing gemcitabine and docetaxel followed by doxorubicin to the current standard approach of observation was closed after slow accrual of only 38 patients. Unfortunately, there were the same number of recurrences in both arms, no difference in PFS and OS was worse in the chemotherapy arm. These data suggest observation as a reasonable option for this population and are supported by a large retrospective study in the California-Colorado population-based health plan.[149,150]

Carcinosarcoma
The GOG also reported a study (GOG Protocol 117) of adjuvant ifosfamide, mesna, and cisplatin in 65 patients with completely resected stage I or II carcinosarcoma of the uterus in which no postoperative radiotherapy was allowed. Progression-free survival and overall survival rates, respectively, were 69% and 82% at 24 months and 54% and 52% at 84 months. The overall 5-year survival rate was 62%.[108] Since more than half of the recurrences involved the pelvis, the study suggested that a combined sequential approach with chemotherapy and radiotherapy might be beneficial for this group of patients and there is limited phase II data demonstrating feasibility.[151] Based on GOG261 T/C chemotherapy is now employed.

Hormone and biologic therapy
Receptors for estrogen and progesterone are identified in patients with uterine sarcoma.[43,44,48,152] Sutton and colleagues studied 43 patients with various uterine sarcomas and found estrogen receptors in 55.5% of the tumors and progesterone receptors in 55.8%.[152] The presence of receptors was not influenced by stage or grade, but levels were much higher and more prevalent in patients with ESS of low grade, and this group of tumors frequently

responds to progestational hormone treatment.[48,49,137,153–155] The cessation of estrogen replacement therapy and tamoxifen is also advised.[48,156] Recent use of aromatase inhibitors[66,157] and gonadotropin-releasing hormone analogs[158] has been described in ESS, with dramatic and prolonged responses.[48,156,159]

Pazopanib (800 mg once daily) an oral multikinase inhibitor was approved in 2012 for the treatment of metastatic soft tissue sarcoma after progression on an anthracycline-based treatment based on a phase III study of 372 patients with an improvement in PFS of 5 versus 2 months compared to placebo.[160]

The addition of bevacizumab to fixed-dose rate gemcitabine–docetaxel failed to improve overall response rate, PFS, or OS in a GOG0250 phase III trial of 102 chemo-naïve patients with metastatic uterine leiomyosarcoma.

Müllerian adenosarcomas

The term "Müllerian adenosarcoma" was coined in 1974 for a distinctive uterine tumor characterized by a malignant, usually low-grade, stromal component, and a generally benign, but occasionally atypical, glandular epithelial component.[16] Most adenosarcomas arise in the endometrium and, rarely, in the endocervix, lower uterine segment, and myometrium.[17,161,162] In a Gynecologic Oncology Group study in 1993, adenosarcomas accounted for 7% of uterine sarcomas.[38] Uterine adenosarcoma occurs in all age groups but is most common in women after the menopause. In the largest reported series, the peak incidence was in the eighth decade with 38% occurring in patients aged below 50 years.[161] The most common presenting symptom is abnormal vaginal bleeding but some patients present with pelvic pain, an abdominal mass, or vaginal discharge.

Grossly, the majority are solitary polypoid masses with a spongy appearance secondary to the presence of small cysts.[17,161] Minimal histologic criteria were described by Clement and Scully in a review of 100 cases of adenosarcoma published in 1990.[161] They include at least one of the following: two or more stromal mitoses per 10 HPF, marked stromal hypercellularity, and significant stromal cell atypia. A minority of cases have "sarcomatous overgrowth," when more than 25% of the tumor is composed of pure sarcoma. In these cases, the sarcoma is typically high-grade and the lesions are aggressive.[17,163] Most adenosarcomas without stromal overgrowth express estrogen and progesterone receptors in the sarcomatous component and this may be used for therapeutic purposes. However, hormonal receptors are negative in adenosarcomas with stromal overgrowth.[17,164,165] Besides stromal overgrowth, the only other histopathological feature associated with decreased survival is myometrial invasion.[17,47,161,163,165]

Müllerian adenosarcomas have been described in extrauterine sites including the ovary and areas of endometriosis in the vagina, rectovaginal-septum, gastrointestinal tract, urinary bladder, pouch of Douglas, peritoneum, and liver.[17,162,165–167] Ovarian adenosarcomas are much more likely to exhibit malignant behavior than their uterine counterparts, probably due to the lack of an anatomic barrier to peritoneal dissemination.[17,167]

Nonuterine gynecologic sarcomas

The vulva

Fewer than 700 patients with vulvar sarcoma have been described in the literature. LMS,[168] rhabdomyosarcoma, and fibrosarcoma are the most frequently diagnosed vulvar tumors.[169] The clinical behavior of these tumors is related to their grade, mitotic count, histology, and stage.[169,170] For the lowest-grade tumors, wide local excision should suffice. However, for the more aggressive histologic patterns, radical vulvectomy with lymphadenectomy followed by cytotoxic chemotherapy should be considered, although the role of adjuvant chemotherapy has not been studied in these tumors.[170] For vulvar epithelioid sarcomas, there may be a role for consolidation radiation therapy.[171,172]

The vagina

Sarcomas represent 3% of primary vaginal cancers.[173] Leiomyosarcomas are the most common vaginal sarcoma in adults and present most commonly with vaginal bleeding in a patient above the age of 40. Although vaginal sarcomas are highly virulent, Peters et al.[174] has reported on survivors among those treated by hysterectomy, oophorectomy, and vaginectomy.[174]

Embryonal rhabdomyosarcomas, formerly termed sarcoma botryoides, occur most frequently in children and have a typical grape cluster-like appearance. The disease was once uniformly fatal, provoking radical extirpative surgery that resulted in exenteration for young girls. Pediatric embryonal RMS of the vagina is best approached with induction multiagent-combination therapy, such as VAC (Vincristine, Actinomycin D, and Cyclophosphamide) followed by local resection with or without brachytherapy, with radical surgery being reserved for those with persistent or recurrent disease.[175–177]

The ovary

Most types of sarcomas described in the vagina, vulva, or uterus have been found in the ovary as well.[178,179] Ovarian carcinosarcomas are rare and aggressive tumors, associated with a poor prognosis, and account for only 1–4% of all ovarian cancer.[180,181] The mainstay of treatment remains maximal cytoreductive surgical effort for metastatic disease followed by platinum-based chemotherapy usually T/C.[182,183] Survival is better for patients with early-stage disease and those whose tumors have homologous stromal elements.[180,184]

The fallopian tube

The fallopian tube is the least frequent site of primary sarcomas in the gynecologic tract. The most common histologic type is carcinosarcoma[185–189] with treatment identical to ovarian carcinosarcomas with maximal cytoreduction for metastatic disease followed by platinum-based chemotherapy usually T/C.[184,185]

Key references

The complete reference list can be found on Vital Source version of this title, see inside front cover.

2   Kempson RL, Bari W. Uterine sarcomas. Classification, diagnosis, and prognosis. *Hum Pathol.* 1970;**1**(3):331–349.

3   Tavassoli FA, Devilee P. *Tumors of the Uterine Corpus. World Health Organization Classification of Tumours Pathology and genetics of Tumours of the Breast and Female Genital Organs.* Lyons, France: IARC Press; 2003:217–258.

4   Otis COAC, Nucci MR, McCluggage WG. Protocol for the Examination of Specimens From Patients With Sarcoma of the Uterus. College of American Pathologists; 2013 [cited 01/04/2015]. Available from: https://webapps.cap.org/apps/docs/committees/cancer/cancer_protocols/2013/UterineSarcomaProtocol_3000.pdf

5   D'Angelo E, Prat J. Uterine sarcomas: a review. *Gynecol Oncol.* 2010;**116**(1):131–139. Epub 2009/10/27.

6. Somarelli JA, Boss MK, Epstein JI, et al. Carcinosarcomas: tumors in transition? *Histol Histopathol*. 2015;30(6):673–687. Epub 2015/01/15.
8. Brooks SE, Zhan M, Cote T, Baquet CR. Surveillance, epidemiology, and end results analysis of 2677 cases of uterine sarcoma 1989–1999. *Gynecol Oncol*. 2004;93(1):204–208. Epub 2004/03/30.
16. Clement PB, Scully RE. Mullerian adenosarcoma of the uterus. A clinicopathologic analysis of ten cases of a distinctive type of mullerian mixed tumor. *Cancer*. 1974;34(4):1138–1149. Epub 1974/10/01.
17. McCluggage WG. Mullerian adenosarcoma of the female genital tract. *Adv Anat Pathol*. 2010;17(2):122–129. Epub 2010/02/25.
18. Feng W, Malpica A, Robboy SJ, et al. Prognostic value of the diagnostic criteria distinguishing endometrial stromal sarcoma, low grade from undifferentiated endometrial sarcoma, 2 entities within the invasive endometrial stromal neoplasia family. *Int J Gynecol Pathol*. 2013;32(3):299–306. Epub 2013/04/03.
24. Chiang S, Ali R, Melnyk N, et al. Frequency of known gene rearrangements in endometrial stromal tumors. *Am J Surg Pathol*. 2011;35(9):1364–1372. Epub 2011/08/13.
32. Ried T, Gaiser T. A recurrent fusion gene in high-grade endometrial stromal sarcoma: a new tool for diagnosis and therapy? *Genome Med*. 2012;4(3):20. Epub 2012/03/21.
33. Rose PG, Piver MS, Tsukada Y, Lau T. Patterns of metastasis in uterine sarcoma. An autopsy study. *Cancer*. 1989;63(5):935–938.
38. Major FJ, Blessing JA, Silverberg SG, et al. Prognostic factors in early-stage uterine sarcoma. A gynecologic oncology group study. *Cancer*. 1993;71(4 Suppl):1702–1709.
47. Arend R, Bagaria M, Lewin SN, et al. Long-term outcome and natural history of uterine adenosarcomas. *Gynecol Oncol*. 2010;119(2):305–308. Epub 2010/08/07.
48. Amant F, Floquet A, Friedlander M, et al. Gynecologic Cancer InterGroup (GCIG) consensus review for endometrial stromal sarcoma. *Int J Gynecol Cancer*. 2014;24(9 Suppl 3):S67–S72. Epub 2014/07/18.
49. Rauh-Hain JA, del Carmen MG. Endometrial stromal sarcoma: a systematic review. *Obstetr Gynecol*. 2013;122(3):676–683. Epub 2013/08/08.
50. Leibsohn S, d'Ablaing G, Mishell DR Jr, Schlaerth JB. Leiomyosarcoma in a series of hysterectomies performed for presumed uterine leiomyomas. *Am J Obstet Gynecol*. 1990;162(4):968–974, discussion 74-6.
56. Goto A, Takeuchi S, Sugimura K, Maruo T. Usefulness of Gd-DTPA contrast-enhanced dynamic MRI and serum determination of LDH and its isozymes in the differential diagnosis of leiomyosarcoma from degenerated leiomyoma of the uterus. *Int J Gynecol Cancer*. 2002;12(4):354–361. Epub 2002/07/30.
73. Gadducci A, Cosio S, Romanini A, Genazzani AR. The management of patients with uterine sarcoma: a debated clinical challenge. *Crit Rev Oncol/Hematol*. 2008;65(2):129–142. Epub 2007/08/21.
74. Wright JD, Tergas AI, Burke WM, et al. Uterine pathology in women undergoing minimally invasive hysterectomy using morcellation. *JAMA*. 2014;312(12):1253–1255. Epub 2014/07/23.
76. Park JY, Park SK, Kim DY, et al. The impact of tumor morcellation during surgery on the prognosis of patients with apparently early uterine leiomyosarcoma. *Gynecol Oncol*. 2011;122(2):255–259. Epub 2011/05/14.
77. Park JY, Kim DY, Kim JH, et al. The impact of tumor morcellation during surgery on the outcomes of patients with apparently early low-grade endometrial stromal sarcoma of the uterus. *Ann Surg Oncol*. 2011;18(12):3453–3461. Epub 2011/05/05.
78. Fader AN, Java J, Tenney M, et al. Impact of histology and surgical approach on survival among women with early-stage, high-grade uterine cancer: An NRG Oncology/Gynecologic Oncology Group ancillary analysis. *Gynecol Oncol*. 2016;143(3):460–465. Epub 2016/10/17.
79. Seagle BL, Sobecki-Rausch J, Strohl AE, et al. Prognosis and treatment of uterine leiomyosarcoma: a national cancer database study. *Gynecol Oncol*. 2017;145(1):61–70. Epub 2017/03/21.
80. Aaro LA, Symmonds RE, Dockerty MB. Sarcoma of the uterus. A clinical and pathologic study of 177 cases. *Am J Obstet Gynecol*. 1966;94(1):101–109.
81. Garg G, Shah JP, Liu JR, et al. Validation of tumor size as staging variable in the revised International Federation of Gynecology and Obstetrics stage I leiomyosarcoma: a population-based study. *Int J Gynecol Cancer*. 2010;20(7):1201–1206. Epub 2010/10/14.
85. Silverberg SG, Major FJ, Blessing JA, et al. Carcinosarcoma (malignant mixed mesodermal tumor) of the uterus. A gynecologic oncology group pathologic study of 203 cases. *Int J Gynecol Pathol*. 1990;9(1):1–19.
107. Reed NS, Mangioni C, Malmstrom H, et al. Phase III randomised study to evaluate the role of adjuvant pelvic radiotherapy in the treatment of uterine sarcomas stages I and II: an European organisation for research and treatment of cancer gynaecological cancer group study (protocol 55874). *Eur J Cancer*. 2008;44(6):808–818. Epub 2008/04/02.
109. Wolfson AH, Brady MF, Rocereto T, et al. A gynecologic oncology group randomized phase III trial of whole abdominal irradiation (WAI) vs. cisplatin-ifosfamide and mesna (CIM) as post-surgical therapy in stage I-IV carcinosarcoma (CS) of the uterus. *Gynecol Oncol*. 2007;107(2):177–185.
110. Omura GA, Major FJ, Blessing JA, et al. A randomized study of adriamycin with and without dimethyl triazenoimidazole carboxamide in advanced uterine sarcomas. *Cancer*. 1983;52(4):626–632.
128. Monk BJ, Blessing JA, Street DG, et al. A phase II evaluation of trabectedin in the treatment of advanced, persistent, or recurrent uterine leiomyosarcoma: a gynecologic oncology group study. *Gynecol Oncol*. 2012;124(1):48–52. Epub 2011/10/15.
132. Seddon B, Strauss SJ, Whelan J, et al. Gemcitabine and docetaxel versus doxorubicin as first-line treatment in previously untreated advanced unresectable or metastatic soft-tissue sarcomas (GeDDiS): a randomised controlled phase 3 trial. *Lancet Oncol*. 2017;18(10):1397–1410. Epub 2017/09/09.
134. Martin-Broto J, Pousa AL, de Las Penas R, et al. Randomized phase II study of trabectedin and doxorubicin compared with doxorubicin alone as first-line treatment in patients with advanced soft tissue sarcomas: a Spanish group for research on sarcoma study. *J Clin Oncol*. 2016;34(19):2294–2302. Epub 2016/05/18.
135. Tap WD, Wagner AJ, Schoffski P, et al. Effect of doxorubicin plus olaratumab vs doxorubicin plus placebo on survival in patients with advanced soft tissue sarcomas: the ANNOUNCE randomized clinical trial. *JAMA*. 2020;323(13):1266–1276. Epub 2020/04/08.
136. Moroncini G, Maccaroni E, Fiordoliva I, et al. Developments in the management of advanced soft-tissue sarcoma - olaratumab in context. *OncoTargets Therapy*. 2018;11:833–842. Epub 2018/03/03.
138. Tanner EJ, Garg K, Leitao MM Jr, et al. High grade undifferentiated uterine sarcoma: surgery, treatment, and survival outcomes. *Gynecol Oncol*. 2012;127(1):27–31. Epub 2012/07/04.
140. Hensley ML, Blessing JA, Mannel R, Rose PG. Fixed-dose rate gemcitabine plus docetaxel as first-line therapy for metastatic uterine leiomyosarcoma: a gynecologic oncology group phase II trial. *Gynecol Oncol*. 2008;109(3):329–334. Epub 2008/06/07.
141. Hensley ML, Blessing JA, Degeest K, et al. Fixed-dose rate gemcitabine plus docetaxel as second-line therapy for metastatic uterine leiomyosarcoma: a Gynecologic Oncology Group phase II study. *Gynecol Oncol*. 2008;109(3):323–328. Epub 2008/04/09.
143. Leyvraz S, Zweifel M, Jundt G, et al. Long-term results of a multicenter SAKK trial on high-dose ifosfamide and doxorubicin in advanced or metastatic gynecologic sarcomas. *Ann Oncol: Off J Eur Soc Med Oncol*. 2006;17(4):646–651. Epub 2006/02/28.
144. Homesley HD, Filiaci V, Markman M, et al. Phase III trial of ifosfamide with or without paclitaxel in advanced uterine carcinosarcoma: a gynecologic oncology group study. *J Clin Oncol*. 2007;25(5):526–531.
145. Powell MA, Filiaci VL, Rose PG, et al. Phase II evaluation of paclitaxel and carboplatin in the treatment of carcinosarcoma of the uterus: a gynecologic oncology group study. *J Clin Oncol*. 2010;28(16):2727–2731. Epub 2010/04/28.
146. Powell M, Filiaci V, Hensley M. A randomized phase 3 trial of paclitaxel (P) plus carboplatin (C) versus paclitaxel plus ifosfamide (I) in chemotherapy-naive patients with stage I-IV, persistent or recurrent carcinsarcoma of the uterus or ovary: an NRG oncology trial. *J Clin Oncol*. 2019;37S:5500.
147. Omura GA, Blessing JA, Major F, et al. A randomized clinical trial of adjuvant adriamycin in uterine sarcomas: a gynecologic oncology group study. *J Clin Oncol*. 1985;3(9):1240–1245.
148. Hensley ML, Wathen JK, Maki RG, et al. Adjuvant therapy for high-grade, uterus-limited leiomyosarcoma: results of a phase 2 trial (SARC 005). *Cancer*. 2013;119(8):1555–1561. Epub 2013/01/22.
149. Littell RD, Tucker LY, Raine-Bennett T, et al. Adjuvant gemcitabine-docetaxel chemotherapy for stage I uterine leiomyosarcoma: Trends and survival outcomes. *Gynecol Oncol*. 2017;147(1):11–17. Epub 2017/07/28.
150. Hensley ML. Difficult choices in stage I uterine leiomyosarcoma — it's okay to "stand there". *Gynecol Oncol*. 2017;147(1):1–2. Epub 2017/09/20.
154. Cheng X, Yang G, Schmeler KM, et al. Recurrence patterns and prognosis of endometrial stromal sarcoma and the potential of tyrosine kinase-inhibiting therapy. *Gynecol Oncol*. 2011;121(2):323–327. Epub 2011/02/01.
161. Clement PB, Scully RE. Mullerian adenosarcoma of the uterus: a clinicopathologic analysis of 100 cases with a review of the literature. *Hum Pathol*. 1990;21(4):363–381. Epub 1990/04/01.
167. Eichhorn JH, Young RH, Clement PB, Scully RE. Mesodermal (mullerian) adenosarcoma of the ovary: a clinicopathologic analysis of 40 cases and a review of the literature. *Am J Surg Pathol*. 2002;26(10):1243–1258. Epub 2002/10/03.
170. Curtin JP, Saigo P, Slucher B, et al. Soft-tissue sarcoma of the vagina and vulva: a clinicopathologic study. *Obstetr Gynecol*. 1995;86(2):269–272. Epub 1995/08/01.
175. Raney RB Jr, Gehan EA, Hays DM, et al. Primary chemotherapy with or without radiation therapy and/or surgery for children with localized sarcoma of the bladder, prostate, vagina, uterus, and cervix. A comparison of the results in Intergroup Rhabdomyosarcoma Studies I and II. *Cancer*. 1990;66(10):2072–2081. Epub 1990/11/15.

176 Andrassy RJ, Wiener ES, Raney RB, et al. Progress in the surgical management of vaginal rhabdomyosarcoma: a 25-year review from the Intergroup Rhabdomyosarcoma Study Group. *J Pediatr Surg*. 1999;**34**(5):731–734; discussion 4-5. Epub 1999/06/08.

178 Oliva E, Egger JF, Young RH. Primary endometrioid stromal sarcoma of the ovary: a clinicopathologic study of 27 cases with morphologic and behavioral features similar to those of uterine low-grade endometrial stromal sarcoma. *Am J Surg Pathol*. 2014;**38**(3):305–315. Epub 2014/02/15.

179 Lan C, Huang X, Lin S, et al. Endometrial stromal sarcoma arising from endometriosis: a clinicopathological study and literature review. *Gynecol Obstet Invest*. 2012;**74**(4):288–297. Epub 2012/09/19.

180 del Carmen MG, Birrer M, Schorge JO. Carcinosarcoma of the ovary: a review of the literature. *Gynecol Oncol*. 2012;**125**(1):271–277. Epub 2011/12/14.

181 Rauh-Hain JA, Gonzalez R, Bregar AJ, et al. Patterns of care, predictors and outcomes of chemotherapy for ovarian carcinosarcoma: a National Cancer Database analysis. *Gynecol Oncol*. 2016;**142**(1):38–43. Epub 2016/04/25.

182 Kanis MJ, Kolev V, Getrajdman J, et al. Carcinosarcoma of the ovary: a single institution experience and review of the literature. *Eur J Gynaecol Oncol*. 2016;**37**(1):75–79. Epub 2016/04/07.

183 Boussios S, Karathanasi A, Zakynthinakis-Kyriakou N, et al. Ovarian carcinosarcoma: current developments and future perspectives. *Crit Rev Oncol/Hematol*. 2019:134, 46–155. Epub 2019/02/18.

184 Rauh-Hain JA, Birrer M, Del Carmen MG. Carcinosarcoma of the ovary, fallopian tube, and peritoneum: prognostic factors and treatment modalities. *Gynecol Oncol*. 2016;(2):142, 248–154. Epub 2016/06/21.

185 Yokoyama Y, Yokota M, Futagami M, Mizunuma H. Carcinosarcoma of the fallopian tube: report of four cases and review of literature. *Asia Pac J Clin Oncol*. 2012;**8**(3):303–311. Epub 2012/08/18.

105 Neoplasms of the breast

Debu Tripathy, MD ■ Sukh Makhnoon, PhD, MS ■ Banu Arun, MD ■ Aysegul Sahin, MD ■ Nicole M. Kettner, PhD ■ Senthil Damodaran, MD, PhD ■ Khandan Keyomarsi, PhD ■ Wei Yang, MBBS, FRCR, MD ■ Kelly K. Hunt, MD ■ Mark Clemens, MD ■ Wendy A. Woodward, MD ■ Melissa P. Mitchell, MD ■ Rachel Layman, MD ■ Evthokia A. Hobbs, MD ■ Bora Lim, MD ■ Megan Dupuis, MD ■ Rashmi Murthy, MD ■ Omar Alhalabi, MD ■ Nuhad Ibrahim, MD ■ Ishwaria M. Subbiah, MD, MS ■ Carlos Barcenas, MD

> **Overview**
>
> Breast cancer is the most common cancer among women in the United States and growing in incidence worldwide, while mortality due to breast cancer is slowly decreasing. The last two decades have witnessed many changes in the diagnostic landscape both in terms of imaging studies and laboratory tests, most notably next-generation sequencing both on tumor and blood. Our understanding of breast oncogenesis, tumor heterogeneity, and metastasis has deepened. Segmental mastectomy and sentinel lymph node (SLN) biopsy have been used in the majority of cases coupled with radiation therapy. In cases managed with mastectomy, radiation of one to three positive nodes has been utilized more often. Gene expression profiling has been used to identify women with hormone receptor-positive (HR+) breast cancer who would benefit from adjuvant chemotherapy. Targeted therapy has been developed for HR+, HER2 amplified, and triple-negative breast cancer. Immune checkpoint inhibitors have improved the management of triple-negative disease. poly(adenosine diphosphate [ADP]–ribose) (PARP) inhibitors have improved outcomes for breast cancer patients with BRCA1/2 mutations. Combinations of targeted therapies and hormonal therapies have proved effective for adjuvant therapy and in recurrent disease.

Epidemiology, etiology, and risk factors

Prevalence

In industrialized countries, breast cancer is the most prevalent malignancy in women and accounts for 31% of all women's cancers in the United States.[1] In 2022, an estimated 287,850 new cases of breast cancer were diagnosed among US women, and 43,250 women died from the disease.[1] The lifetime risk for a woman developing breast cancer is 1 in 8 (13%).[2] A higher risk is found in women with a strong family history or known genetic mutations. While less than one percent of breast cancers occur in men, approximately 2710 men were diagnosed with breast cancer in 2022.[1]

Some 2.2 million cases of breast cancer were diagnosed in 2020 worldwide, accounting for 25% of all cancer cases in women.[3] Approximately half are diagnosed in developed countries. In less developed regions, the cumulative breast cancer risk to age 74 is 3.3% compared to 8% in more developed areas. These differences in incidence are likely to relate both to differences in risk factors and to availability of early detection methods.[4] The incidence of breast cancer has been increasing in Asia, South America, and Africa, possibly because of changes in lifestyle, including reproductive patterns, diet, obesity, and physical activity.[4] Some 61% of breast cancers are diagnosed when breast cancer is localized to the breast, 32% when it has spread to regional nodes, and only 6% when it has already metastasized. Five-year survival rates correlate with the extent of spread at diagnosis with 98.6% alive when cancer is limited to the breast, 84.9% alive when tumor is found in regional lymph nodes, and only 26% when diagnosed with distant metastases.

Over the most recent 5-year period with available data (2012–2016), breast cancer incidence rate increased slightly by 0.3% per year, largely due to rising rates of local stage and hormone receptor-positive (HR+) disease. Rates vary significantly by race and ethnicity, as described in Table 1. However, rates between White and African American women in the United States are now converging (see below).

The mortality rate from breast cancer in the United States slowly increased by 0.4% from 1975 to 1990, then decreased by 34% from 1990 to 2010.[2] This decrease has been attributed to improvements in treatment as well as early detection,[5] with the largest decrease in women below 50 years of age. Mortality rates vary by race and ethnicity with African American women experiencing a 40% higher death rate than White women (28.4 vs 20.3 deaths per 100,000) despite a lower incidence rate (126.7 vs 130.8). This black–white disparity has been attributed to variations in biologic subtype, later stage of disease at diagnosis, and poorer survival by stage, driven in large part by differences in socioeconomic status. Despite this difference, overall death rates declined 40% from their peak in 2017, resulting in 375,900 breast cancer total deaths averted.

Risk factors

The risk of developing breast cancer depends on several factors, particularly female gender and increasing age. Germline mutations in BRCA1, BRCA2, and other DNA repair genes markedly increase the lifetime risk of developing breast and several other cancers and increase the risk of cancer occurring at younger ages. Several lifestyle factors have a more modest impact on risk, and the impact of altering modifiable factors on an individual's risk of developing breast cancer is largely unknown.[6] The risk factors associated with the development of breast cancer are indicated in Figure 1.

Gender

The incidence of age-adjusted breast cancer is more than 100-fold higher in White women than in White men in the United States, but about 70-fold higher in Black women than Black men. Male breast

Table 1 Female breast cancer incidence (2012–2016) and mortality (2013–2017) by race/ethnicity in the United States.[a]

	Non-Hispanic White	Non-Hispanic Black	Hispanic-Latino	American Indian/Alaskan Native	Asian/Pacific Islander
Incidence rates (per 100,000)	130.8	126.7	93.7	94.7	93.2
Mortality rates (per 100,000)	20.3	28.4	14.0	14.6	11.5

[a]Source: Siegel 2019.[3] Reproduced with permission of Wiley.

cancer represents less than 1% of all cancers in men and about 1% of all breast cancers. Lifetime risk of breast cancer for men is about 1 in 833 and germline mutations in *BRCA1* and *BRCA2* are the best-understood risk factors, with a range of lifetime risk of just over 1% (*BRCA1*) to almost 7% (*BRCA2*).

Age
At diagnosis, the median age of women with breast cancer in the United States is 62, and a majority of cases are diagnosed in women between the ages of 60 and 69. In other parts of the world, where life expectancy is shorter, the median age of development of breast cancer is 10–15 years younger. Age-related mortality rates increase with age and are highest at 80 years or older.

Socioeconomic status
Women with higher socioeconomic status have higher breast cancer incidence, which may be explained by reproductive factors (e.g., age at first childbirth), mammography screening, use of HRT, and lifestyle factors such as diet and alcohol consumption.[7] However, mortality is higher in women of lower socioeconomic status, correlating with observed differences including higher stage at diagnosis, more aggressive tumor biology, comorbidity, and reduced access to care.

Ethnicity and race
The incidence and mortality rates of breast cancer vary considerably by ethnicity and race, as outlined in Table 1. In the United States, the incidence of breast cancer is highest in Whites, followed closely by Blacks and are lowest in Asian/Pacific Islanders. Studies of migrant populations showed that when people living in low-risk geographic areas move to high-risk areas (e.g., a move from Asia to the United States), their incidence of breast cancer increases, approaching the rates of the host population within one to two generations, suggesting an important role of lifestyle in the determination of risk, even within ethnic and racial groups.[8]

Breast density
Breast density is a common and significant risk factor for breast cancer across ethnicities and is inversely associated with age and body mass index (BMI).[9–12] Numerous state laws require reporting of breast density information to women at the time of screening mammography.[12] The highest quartile of breast density appears to have a significantly elevated risk, with a 4.5- to 5-fold higher risk than those with the least dense breast tissue. The impact of breast density is modified by individual risk factors, as measured by the Breast Cancer Surveillance Consortium (BCSC) 5-year risk model, where women at moderate or high risk for breast cancer using this model and extremely high density had the highest risk for interval cancer.[13]

Benign breast disease (BBD)
Most forms of BBD appear to be unrelated to an increased breast cancer risk, and the majority of women with lumpy breasts and most of those with BBD do not have a significantly increased risk of breast cancer. However, a number of studies, including a recent meta-analysis, suggest that the presence (or history) of BBD, particularly in those with a previous biopsy for benign disease, is associated with an increase in breast cancer risk.[14] This association is generally limited to biopsy-proven lesions with histologic atypia or proliferation (atypical ductal or lobular hyperplasia) (Table 2).[16]

Family history and genetic mutations
Family history and germline mutations are significant risk factors for breast cancer and are discussed in depth in **Chapter 32**, Genetic predispositions to cancer and risk models.

Exogenous hormones
The large Women's Health Initiative provided definitive evidence of the risks associated with postmenopausal hormone replacement therapy (HRT) with combined estrogen and progesterone. In this study, 16,608 postmenopausal, otherwise healthy, women were randomly assigned to conjugated estrogen plus medroxyprogesterone acetate (MPA) or placebo.[17] The combined estrogen and progesterone arm was stopped early because health risks (excess breast cancer risk, adverse cardiovascular effects) exceeded health benefits (reduction in colorectal cancer and hip fractures) among women on hormonal replacement. Although risk decreased right after stopping HRT, the overall increased risk persisted during long-term follow-up. The Million Women Study and the HERS II study reached similar conclusions.[18–20] The attributable risk of breast cancer in women in their 50s, the group most likely to take HRT for menopausal symptoms, is very low (three cases per 1000 women for 5 years of combined conjugated estrogen MPA use). The United States Preventive Services Task Force (USPSTF) concluded that the harmful effects of combined estrogen and progestin exceed the prevention of chronic disease effects in most women. Although short-term use of HRT might be beneficial for the control of vasomotor symptoms related to menopause, long-term use is not indicated.

The use of oral contraceptives has long been associated with a slightly increased risk of breast cancer. A recent large study of a US health care delivery system in women between the ages of 20 and 49 years has found an increased risk in recent users taking high-dose estrogen preparations, but not in those taking low-dose estrogen contraceptives.[21] Risk does not appear to be sustained after cessation of use.

Exercise and obesity
Lack of physical activity is a risk factor for postmenopausal breast cancer and a relative reduction in breast cancer risk is observed in active women.[22,23] Little or no benefit from exercise is, however, observed in obese women ($\geq 30 \, \text{kg/m}^2$). Regular strenuous exercise decreased breast cancer risk by 25% when compared to that of less active women.[24] Even 1.25–2.5 h per week of brisk walking was associated with an 18% relative decrease in breast cancer risk compared with sedentary women.[24]

The effect of physical activity is stronger in specific population subgroups and for certain types of physical activity. Stronger

Major increase

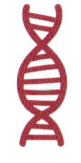

Mutations in *BRCA1* or *BRCA2* (45–87%), *PTEN* (up to 50%), *TP53* (up to 93%), *STK11* (up to 45%), *CDH1* (39–52%)
Percentages are lifetime breast cancer risks

Increasing age
(majority of cases in US diagnosed between 55 and 64 years)

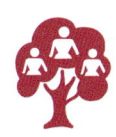

Living in developed countries

Family history of breast or ovarian cancer in first-degree relatives *(early age of diagnosis related to higher risk)*

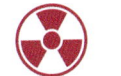

Atypical hyperplasia, LCIS before the age of 45

Exposure to ionizing radiation

Moderate increase

Prior diagnosis of breast cancer

Early menarche
(3–4% increased risk annually) [SM2]

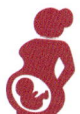

Late menopause
(3–4% increased risk annually) [SM2]

Nulliparity or delayed first full-term pregnancy
(above age 30)

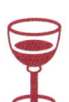

High socioeconomic and educational status
(related to lifestyle factors)

Alcohol intake *(risk increases with higher daily consumption)*

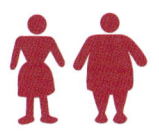

Atypical hyperplasia, LCIS over the age of 45

Obesity
(postmenopausal women only)

High breast density
(those with highest quartile of breast density have 4.5- to 5-fold higher risk than those with least dense breast tissue)

Diagnosis of soft-tissue sarcoma in son or daughter

Prior diagnosis of uterine, ovarian, or colon cancer

Modest increase

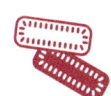

Benign breast disease with hyperplasia
(no atypia)

Oral contraceptives
(for longer than 10 years)

Postmenopausal estrogen replacement therapy

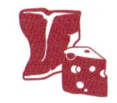

Questionable increase
(no evidence to support)

High-fat diet

Complex fibroadenoma

Interrupted first pregnancy

No effect

Breast reduction

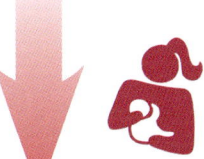

Decreased risk

Full-term pregnancy before age 20

Multiple pregnancies
(each birth decreased risk ratio by 7%)

Breastfeeding *(each year of breastfeeding reduced risk ratio by an additional [SM3] 3.4% over multiple pregnancies)*

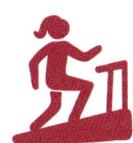

Ovariectomy before age 45

Regular exercise, particularly during adolescence and early adulthood

Risk of disease rises as number of factors increases

Figure 1 Risk factors associated with the development of breast cancer.

Table 2 Relative risk[a] of invasive breast carcinoma based on histologic examination of breast tissue without carcinoma.[b]

No increased risk (no proliferative disease)
Adenosis
Apocrine change
Duct ectasia
Mild epithelial hyperplasia of usual type
Slightly increased risk (1.5–2 times) (proliferative disease without atypia)
Hyperplasia of usual type, moderate, or florid
Papilloma (probably)
Sclerosing adenosis
Moderately increased risk (4–5 times) (atypical hyperplasia or borderline lesion)
Atypical ductal hyperplasia
Atypical lobular hyperplasia
High risk (8–10 times) (carcinoma in situ)[c]
Lobular carcinoma *in situ*—both breasts
Ductal carcinoma *in situ* (non-comedo)—unilateral, local

---

[a] Women in each category are compared with women matched for age who have had no breast biopsies for the risk of invasive breast cancer during the ensuing 10–20 years. These risks are not lifetime risks.
[b] Source: Dupont and Page.[15]
[c] Only smaller examples of non-comedo ductal carcinoma have consistently been assessed as risk indicators after biopsy only.

decreases in risk are observed for recreational activity, lifetime or later life activity, vigorous activity, among postmenopausal women, women with normal BMI, those with HR− tumors, and non-white racial groups. A high BMI (>25 kg/m^2), particularly when associated with weight gain after menopause and abdominal obesity, has been clearly associated with an increased risk of postmenopausal breast cancer.[6,25–27] The relative risk for postmenopausal women is about 1.5 for those with a BMI > 25 and 2 for those who are obese (BMI > 30). In the WHI trials, obesity was also associated with an increased risk of HR+ breast cancer and more advanced disease at diagnosis.[28] The data in premenopausal women are more complicated, without a clear relationship between weight and risk of breast cancer.[29]

Higher physical activity and reduced BMI have been associated with lower relative levels of estradiol and estrone as well as serum insulin levels, which may in part explain the impact of exercise on breast cancer risk.[30–32] The ACS has published guidelines on exercise and nutrition to reduce cancer risk.[33] Adherence to these guidelines has been associated with a lower risk of breast cancer.[34]

Metformin and diabetes mellitus

A higher risk of breast cancer has been associated with diabetes mellitus in some, but, not all studies.[28,35–37] Breast cancer patients who have diabetes do have a worse outcome.[38] In the WHI, the use of metformin in diabetic women reduced the risk of breast cancer. Metformin is known to increase insulin sensitivity and reduce hyperinsulinemia, and hyperinsulinemia has been associated with carcinogenesis and proliferation in preclinical models.[39] In addition, signaling through expression of the insulin-like growth factor receptor is related to both proliferation and therapeutic resistance in breast cancer, and metformin may inhibit downstream signaling through the mammalian target of rapamycin (mTOR).[40–43] However, a large placebo-controlled trial of adjuvant metformin showed no benefit in progression-free survival.[44]

Alcohol

Alcohol is considered to be causally related to breast cancer risk, with a 7–10% increase in risk for each 10 g (~1 drink) of alcohol consumed daily by adult women.[29,45–47] Alcohol is thought to be involved in breast tumorigenesis though increasing sex hormone levels, enhancing breast epithelial cell responsiveness to sex hormones, and epigenetic regulation of gene expression in the breast. When compared with women who never drink, those who were reported to consume more than seven drinks per week had almost a twofold increased risk of invasive lobular cancer, but there was no difference in the risk of invasive ductal cancer, even when both subtypes were HR+.

Radiation exposure

Exposure to ionizing radiation is a known risk factor for breast cancer. Atomic bomb survivors and patients treated in the past with irradiation for postpartum mastitis, acne, hirsutism, or arthritic conditions and repeated fluoroscopic chest radiography used to monitor tuberculosis have an increased incidence of breast cancer, even after low or moderate radiation doses.[48,49] Survivors of Hodgkin's disease who received radiation therapy to the chest in adolescence or at a young age, particularly when the radiation was combined with chemotherapy, have a marked increase in breast cancer risk.[50] The latency period between radiation exposure and development of breast cancer is long, with a median of 30 years although this time is shorter in those treated with both radiation and chemotherapy. The risk of developing breast cancer as a result of common diagnostic radiologic procedures is minimal, and radiology technicians do not have an increased incidence of breast cancer.[51] Recent evidence has suggested that therapeutic radiation administered to treat primary breast cancer modestly increases (~30%) the risk of developing contralateral breast cancer more than 5 years after treatment.[52]

Bisphosphonates

The use of adjuvant bisphosphonates, the most commonly prescribed and effective class of drugs for osteoporosis treatment, has been associated with a reduced risk of invasive breast cancer. Any use of bisphosphonates postdiagnosis was associated with a 35% decreased risk for second breast cancer, and a 50% reduction in recurrence risk when used within 3 years after diagnosis. When used for at least one year, the risk of dying from breast cancer was reduced by 60%.[53]

Dietary factors

A diet high in animal fat and low in fruits and vegetables has been associated with a higher risk of breast cancer. However, this is closely related to additional factors such as exercise and body fat. A primary prevention trial was conducted in more than 48,000 postmenopausal women without a history of breast cancer.[54] One study arm had low total fat intake (20% of energy) and consumption of five to six servings of vegetables, fruits, and grains daily. With eight years of follow-up, there was no reduction in invasive breast cancer risk, but a trend toward decreased risk was found among the most adherent participants.

Breast cancer risk assessment models

Several prediction models can be used to estimate a woman's risk of breast cancer (Table 3). Generally, models are designed for two types of populations: (1) high-risk women and (2) low-risk women. These models also differ in the type of risk factors they incorporate but may include age, age at first live birth, age at menarche, information on affected relatives, BMI, menopause, and HRT use. The genetic factors used by the models also differ, with some assuming one risk locus (e.g., the Claus model),[61] two loci (e.g., IBIS and BRCAPRO), or multiple loci including a polygenic component (e.g., BOADICEA model.[58–60] The utility of these models is to

Table 3 Breast cancer risk assessment models.

Target population	Model examples	Model parameters
Low-risk women without genetic mutation or strong family history of Breast and Ovarian Cancer	Gail model, which is the basis for the Breast Cancer Risk Assessment Tool [BCRAT],[55] and the Colditz and Rosner model I[56]	Limited family history information required (e.g., number of first degree relatives with breast cancer)
High-risk women with personal or family history of Breast and Ovarian cancer	Tyrer-Cuzick or the International Breast Cancer Intervention Study [IBIS] model and the BRCAPRO model,[57] Breast and Ovarian Analysis of Disease Incidence and Carrier Estimation Algorithm [BOADICEA] model[58–60]	Detailed personal and family history required (e.g., ages at onset of cancer, carrier status of specific BC susceptibility alleles)

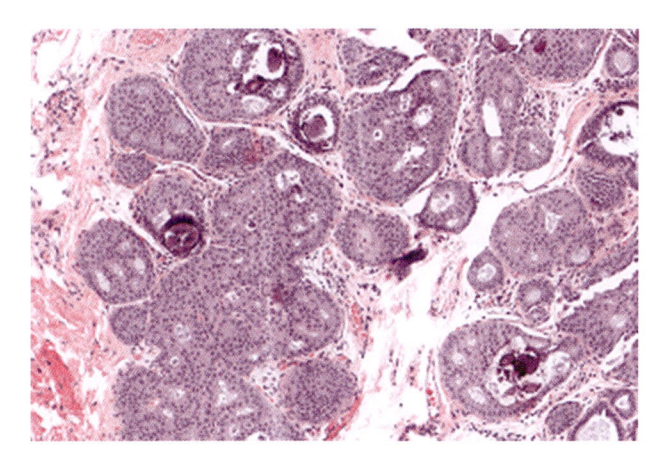

Figure 2 Ductal carcinoma *in situ*.

Breast cancer screening

The topic of breast cancer screening and early detection is reviewed in detail in **Chapter 36** and is also considered below in the section titled "Diagnosis". As with other cancers, the use of screening can improve mortality and morbidity in screened individuals but, can also lead to "overdiagnosis" of low risk or preinvasive cancers that would not impact on mortality and introduce short and long-term complications due to cancer therapy itself. Risk-adapted processes for screening that utilize some of the risk models outlined in this article are being tested in a prospective manner.

Pathology

In situ carcinomas

Ductal carcinoma in situ (DCIS)
Ductal carcinoma *in situ* (DCIS) (Figure 2) is a neoplastic epithelial cell proliferation confined to the mammary ductal-lobular system without stromal invasion and is considered a nonobligatory precursor of invasive breast cancer. DCIS is a heterogeneous lesion in terms of presentation, morphologic features, biomarker expression, and clinical behavior. In most cases, DCIS is a unicentric lesion; true multicentric disease is unusual. There are many morphologic variants of DCIS, including different architectural patterns and nuclear grades. A large fraction of DCIS lesions contain more than one morphologic variant. The College of American Pathologists recommends that a DCIS diagnosis should include a description of nuclear grade, architectural pattern, and the presence and type of necrosis. Grading DCIS is currently based on cytologic atypia. Three grades are identifiable: low (grade 1), intermediate (grade 2), and high (grade 3). Compared to low- and intermediate-grade DCIS, high-grade DCIS is more likely to recur and progress into invasive carcinoma. Low- and intermediate-grade DCIS usually expresses estrogen receptor (ER) and progesterone receptor (PR) strongly, while high-grade DCIS can be negative for ER/PR and positive for human epidermal receptor 2 (HER2) overexpression. Common architectural patterns of DCIS include solid, cribriform, papillary, and micropapillary. Although some patterns may be associated with nuclear grade, the growth patterns are not directly associated with progression to invasive carcinoma. DCIS is usually associated with microcalcifications, which is the most common initial finding on mammography. Necrosis can be extensive (comedo) or focal (individual cell necrosis). Comedonecrosis within a solid pattern is commonly seen in high-grade DCIS, but it can also be identified in intermediate-grade DCIS with other growth patterns.

Usually, the diagnosis of DCIS is straightforward. However, it may occasionally be difficult to distinguish DCIS from non-malignant intraductal proliferations. This is particularly true

guide clinicians in decisions regarding the age of initiation and periodicity of surveillance, need for genetic testing, and need to discuss additional risk-reducing interventions. These models have limited discriminatory power (i.e., ability to discriminate between cancer affected and unaffected individuals) ranging between 0.56 and 0.63.[62] In the United States, the Gail Risk Assessment model, BRCAPRO, and the Claus model are the most frequently used models to predict a woman's risk of breast cancer.[63] The models are highly dependent on the age of the person: a very low short-term risk for a young woman may be accompanied by a high lifetime risk.[64] BRCAPRO is demonstrated to be increasingly universal due to its population-adjustable prevalence and penetrance guides and has been shown to perform equally well in Hispanics as well as non-Hispanic populations.[65]

More recently, newer models have emerged that include breast density, exposures, family history, and single nucleotide polymorphisms such as the BCSC model which has been validated in over 1 million women.[66]

The Gail Risk Assessment model is the most commonly used statistical model for estimating the risk of developing breast cancer in women undergoing annual screening. In a landmark 1989 paper, Gail and colleagues used data from 5998 predominantly White women to develop the Gail model to identify women who might benefit from chemoprevention. This is an unconditional logistic regression model based on risk factors including age, age at menarche, age at first live birth, number of first-degree relatives with breast cancer (mother, sisters, or daughters only), number of breast biopsies, and breast pathology exhibiting atypical hyperplasia. Since then, the reference Gail model has been modified,[67–72] validated,[71–75] and studied in other populations in subsequent research. The Gail model is applicable to the largest number of women and is currently used widely for clinical decision-making for individual patients.

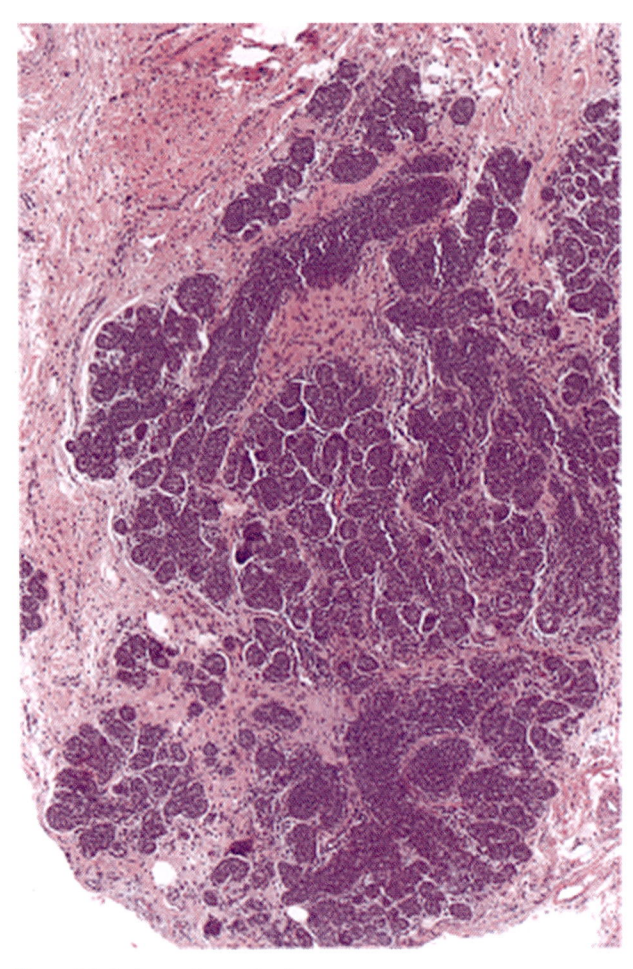

Figure 3 Lobular carcinoma *in situ*.

for small, low-grade DCIS with cribriform and micropapillary patterns without comedonecrosis. In distinguishing these lesions from atypical ductal hyperplasia, both qualitative and quantitative criteria are used. At the other end of the spectrum, it may be difficult to separate extensive pure DCIS from DCIS with stromal invasion due to extension of DCIS into lobular units and distortion of involved ducts by areas of periductal fibrosis and inflammation. Immunohistochemical (IHC) staining for myoepithelial markers can be used to identify areas of invasion.

Lobular carcinoma in situ (LCIS)
Lobular carcinoma *in situ* (LCIS) (Figure 3) still uses the term "carcinoma" *in situ*, but it is currently considered a high-risk lesion rather than a precursor lesion of invasive breast cancer. The eighth editions of the UICC TNM classification and AJCC cancer staging system recommend not staging LCIS as *in situ* carcinoma (pTis).[76] In addition to classic LCIS, there are specific morphologic subtypes of LCIS, including pleomorphic, apocrine, and florid LCIS. These LCIS variants can have a high nuclear grade with comedonecrosis and may mimic DCIS. Compared with classic LCIS, a higher chance of identifying invasive carcinoma is associated with these variants of LCIS. Thus, in clinical practice, these lesions are managed more like DCIS.

Special types of in situ carcinomas
Three specific carcinomas of the breast—Paget disease, encapsulated papillary carcinoma, and solid papillary carcinoma without invasive carcinoma—are classified as *in situ* carcinomas (pTis).[77,78]

Paget disease of the breast (Figure 4) is defined as intraepidermal proliferation of neoplastic epithelial cells in the nipple-areolar area without dermal invasion. It is usually associated with underlying DCIS or invasive breast carcinoma. Paget cells are typically positive for HER2 and low-molecular-weight cytokeratins (such as CK7) and negative for S100, which can be used to distinguish two skin tumors with similar morphology: melanoma *in situ* and squamous carcinoma *in situ*.

Encapsulated (intracystic) papillary carcinoma (Figure 5) and *solid papillary carcinoma* are two specific noninvasive papillary carcinomas of the breast. The two papillary carcinomas have low to intermediate nuclear grade with classic or delicate papillary architecture histologically and are typically positive for hormone receptors (HRs) ER/PR. Occasionally, the two papillary carcinomas may have a stromal invasion, but lack of peripheral myoepithelial cells cannot be used to differentiate *in situ* from invasive carcinoma in these two specific papillary carcinomas. In addition, these papillary carcinomas may be associated with other special- or nonspecial-type invasive breast carcinomas. In the absence of invasive carcinoma, the two papillary carcinomas have excellent prognosis after adequate local resection.

Invasive breast carcinoma

Invasive breast carcinoma encompasses a heterogeneous group of malignant epithelial neoplasms and is characterized by stromal invasion of malignant cells. Stromal invasion incites a pronounced stromal fibroblastic proliferation called desmoplastic response, which creates a palpable mass. A broad spectrum of histologic features can be seen, and invasive breast cancer is classified based on morphologic features into two general categories: (1) No special type and (2) special types.[77]

Nottingham histologic score is recommended to grade all invasive breast carcinomas, which provides a general histologic appearance of invasive breast carcinoma and has been shown to be a reliable prognosis indicator. The Nottingham grading system semi-qualitatively evaluates three morphologic characteristics (scored 1–3 for each factor)—tubule and gland formation, nuclear pleomorphism, and mitosis count—and then produces a total score (3–9) to grade the carcinoma as follows: grade 1 (well differentiated, with score 3–5), grade 2 (moderately differentiated, with score 6–7), and grade 3 (poorly differentiated, with score 8–9).

Invasive breast cancer of no special type (IBC-NST)
This is the most common histologic subtype (70–80%) of invasive breast carcinoma; invasive breast cancer of no special type (IBC-NST) refers to a large spectrum of invasive carcinomas that lack specific histologic patterns. Commonly, it is called invasive ductal carcinoma (IDC) (Figure 6), which is not indicative of ductal origin. The great majority of breast cancers originate from terminal ductal lobular units. Grossly, IDC usually presents as an ill-defined, firm mass, which may be accompanied by central scar, necrosis, or satellite lesion. Histologically, IDC shows considerable variation in architectural pattern; the tumor cells can be arranged in well-formed glands, trabeculae, solid, or even extensively infiltrative-like invasive lobular carcinoma (ILC) on a background of variable stromal reaction and lymphocytic infiltration. Cytologically, the tumor cells can range from monotonous low-grade to pleomorphic high-grade nuclear atypia, and show some special morphologic features such as oncocytic, clear cell, and signet-ring cell differentiation. Notably, carcinomas with medullary features (syncytial architecture, pushing board, prominent tumor-infiltrating lymphocyte (TIL) infiltrate, and high

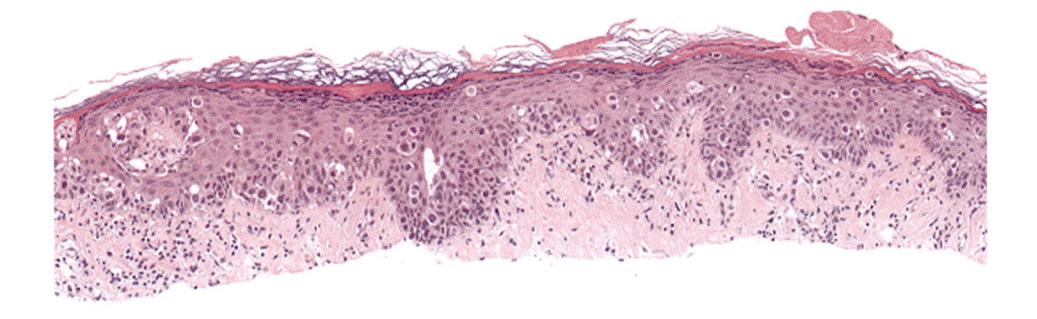

Figure 4 Paget disease.

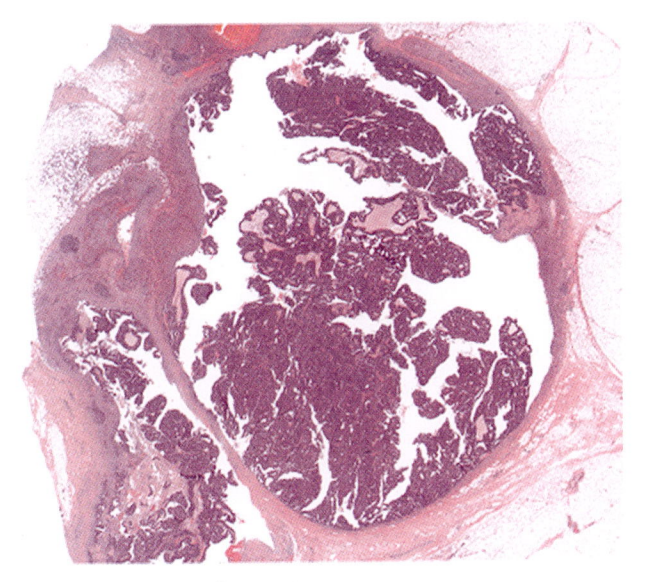

Figure 5 Intracystic papillary carcinoma.

nuclear grade with brisk mitosis), previously considered as one of the special types of invasive carcinoma, is currently interpreted as IBC-NST with medullary pattern, according to the fifth edition of the WHO classification of breast tumors, as this kind of tumor has histologic features and clinical significance correlated with those of basal-like breast carcinoma with abundant TILs. In addition, several rare breast carcinomas with characteristic morphologic patterns, including carcinoma with osteoclast-like stromal giant cells, carcinoma with pleomorphic features, and carcinoma with choriocarcinomatous features, are considered special variants of IDC. IDC may coexist with other special types of invasive carcinoma, such as mixed ductal and lobular carcinoma or mixed ductal and mucinous carcinoma; it is recommended to report the percentage and histologic grade of each type of carcinoma. The expression of breast biomarkers (ER/PR and HER2) is closely related to the differentiation of the carcinoma. Nottingham histologic grade 1 IDC is almost always ER/PR positive and HER2 negative, while Nottingham histologic grade 3 IDC is ER/PR negative in >one-half of cases and HER2 positive in >1/3 of cases. The prognosis of IDC is profoundly influenced by multiple clinicopathologic factors, including Nottingham histologic grade, pathologic and clinical stage, lymph node and distant metastasis, molecular subtype, and response to chemotherapy.

Special types of invasive breast carcinoma

These types include a number of invasive carcinomas with specific and predominant histologic patterns, including ILC, tubular

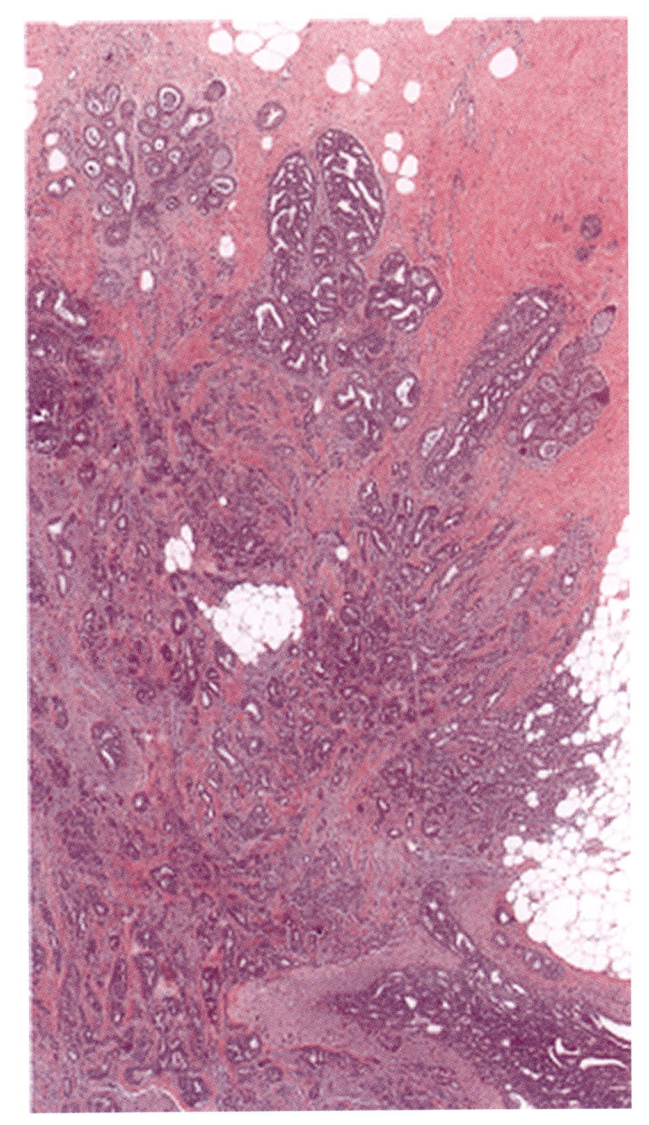

Figure 6 Invasive ductal carcinoma.

carcinoma, cribriform carcinoma, mucinous carcinoma, invasive micropapillary carcinoma, carcinoma with apocrine differentiation, metaplastic carcinoma, and other rare types. Recognizing and reporting these specific morphologies has considerable significance as they may be associated with prognosis or have specific clinical characteristics.

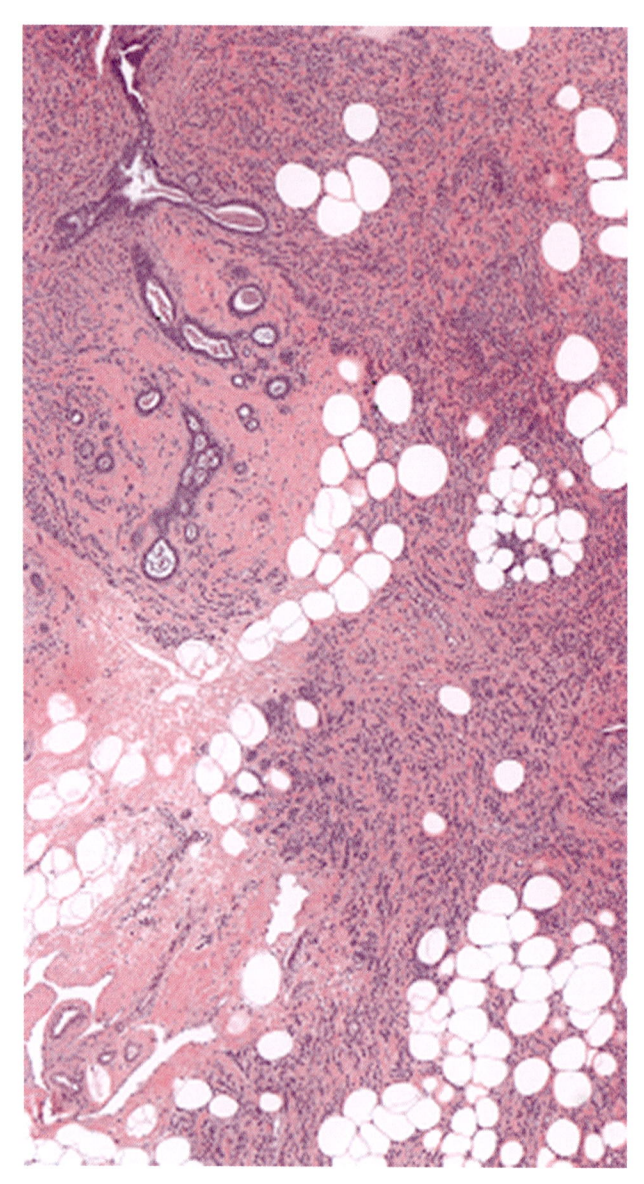

Figure 7 Invasive lobular carcinoma.

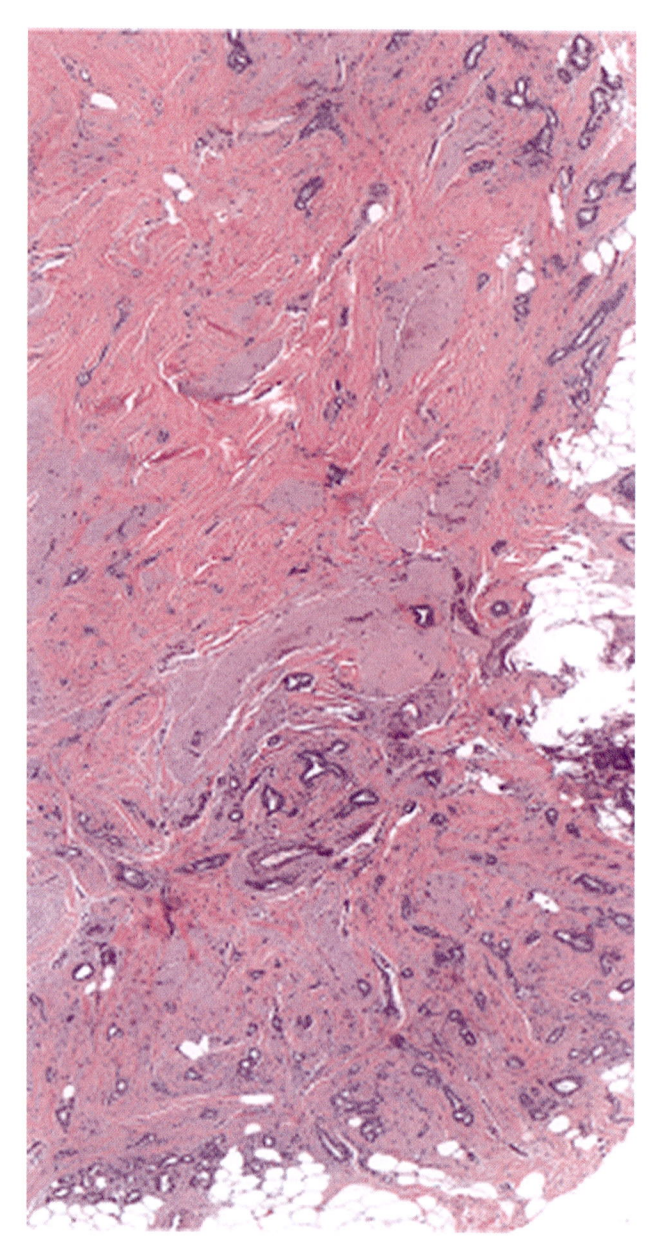

Figure 8 Tubular carcinoma.

1. *Invasive lobular carcinoma (ILC)* (Figure 7) is the second most common type (5–15%) of invasive breast carcinoma. Classic ILC is composed of discohesive tumor cells infiltrating the stroma in a single linear pattern; the neoplastic cells are relatively uniform and round, with inconspicuous nucleoli and a thin rim of cytoplasm. Although intracytoplasmic vacuoles and mucin (signet-ring cell features) can be seen in all types of breast carcinoma, they are more frequently seen in ILC. Uncommon variant ILCs refer to carcinoma cells arranged in solid, alveolar, and tubulobular patterns. Different from IDC, lobular carcinoma cells lack membranous expression of E-cadherin due to genetic alteration involving the *CDH1* gene. Classic ILC is usually well to moderately differentiated (Nottingham histologic grade 1 or 2), ER/PR positive, and HER2 negative, but most pleomorphic ILC is poorly differentiated (Nottingham histologic grade 3) and can be ER/PR negative and HER2 positive. ILC has been reported to have high rates of multicentricity, bilaterality, development of contralateral carcinoma, and metastasis, including peritoneal involvement. In addition, ILC does not respond well to neoadjuvant systemic therapy and has a much lower rate of pathologic complete response (pCR) than IDC.
2. *Tubular carcinoma* (Figure 8) and *cribriform carcinoma* are two well-differentiated carcinomas (Nottingham histologic grade 1) with predominantly (>90%) tubular and cribriform architectures, respectively. They are uncommon breast carcinomas, account for 1–5% of all invasive breast carcinomas. These two special-type carcinomas have similar molecular profiles—strongly/diffusely positive ER/PR and negative HER2—and excellent long-term outcome.
3. *Mucinous carcinoma* (Figure 9), characterized by clusters of malignant epithelial cells floating in a pool of extracellular mucin, represents 1–2% of all invasive breast carcinomas. Typically, mucinous carcinoma is well to moderately differentiated (Nottingham histologic grade 1–2) with strongly/diffusely positive ER/PR and negative HER2; rarely, mucinous carcinoma can have high nuclear grade and positive HER2 overexpression.

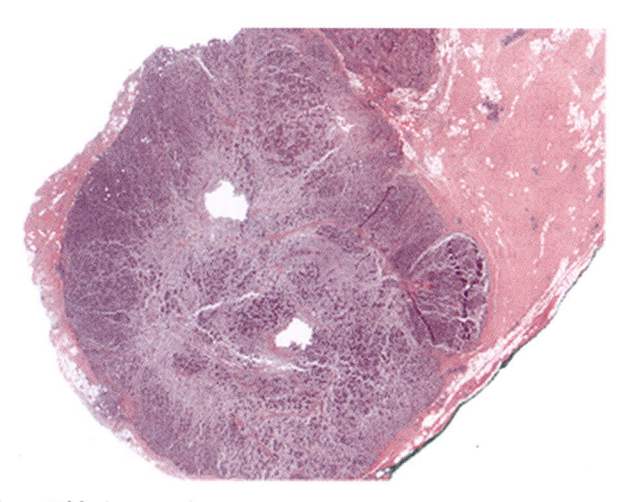

Figure 9 Mucinous carcinoma.

Pure mucinous carcinoma has excellent 5- and 10-year survival rates and low rates of recurrence.

4. *Invasive micropapillary carcinoma* (Figure 10) is a clinically aggressive variant of invasive breast carcinoma with a high risk of lymphovascular invasion and lymph node metastasis and thus a relatively worse prognosis. Like micropapillary carcinoma in other organs, the tumor cells are arranged in small solid or morular-like clusters with surrounding clear space and no obvious fibrovascular core. Invasive micropapillary carcinoma is typically moderately to poorly differentiated (Nottingham histologic grade 2–3) and ER/PR positive. HER2 overexpression/amplification is observed in approximately 30% of these special-type carcinomas; the tumor cells have a typical U-shaped basolateral staining pattern of HER2, which is recommended to be graded as equivocal HER2 overexpression (2+) and reflexed to *in situ* hybridization (ISH) by the fifth edition of WHO classification of breast tumors. There is morphological overlap among some micropapillary carcinomas and mucinous carcinomas, especially the hypercellular variant of mucinous carcinoma. To diagnose pure mucinous carcinoma or invasive micropapillary carcinoma, the mucinous component or micropapillary component is required to be >90% of the entire invasive carcinoma.

5. *Carcinoma with apocrine differentiation* (Figure 11) is invasive carcinoma with predominant apocrine features—large tumor cells with abundant eosinophilic granular cytoplasm, large vesicular nuclei, and prominent nucleoli—constituting about 1% of breast carcinomas. Most invasive apocrine carcinomas are moderately to poorly differentiated (Nottingham histologic grade 2–3), with a characteristic molecular profile of positive androgen receptor (AR) and negative ER/PR. Positive HER2 is reported in 30–60% of apocrine carcinomas.

6. *Metaplastic carcinoma* (Figure 12) refers to a heterogeneous group of invasive breast carcinomas with squamous, spindle cell, and/or mesenchymal differentiation and accounts for <1% of all invasive breast carcinomas. Although most metaplastic carcinomas are triple-negative (negative ER/PR and HER2) with rare lymph node metastasis, their prognosis largely depends on the metaplastic elements. Low-grade adenosquamous carcinoma and fibromatosis-like carcinoma are two types of metaplastic carcinoma with favorable prognosis, but metaplastic carcinomas with high-grade spindle cell component, squamous cell component, or heterologous mesenchymal element (such as chondroid or osseous differentiation) are associated with worse prognosis, as these metaplastic components do not respond to chemotherapy. With another coexisting type of invasive breast carcinoma or DCIS, diagnosis of metaplastic carcinoma is not challenging in the presence of the abovementioned heterologous elements/differentiation, but without the background of *in situ* or invasive breast carcinoma, cautious differentiation is essential. Pure squamous cell carcinoma is a diagnosis of exclusion of metastasis from other organs; with the morphology of spindle cell carcinoma, and/or mesenchymal elements such as chondrosarcoma or osteosarcoma, primary sarcoma of the breast must be ruled out, although it is extremely rare in the breast. In addition, an IHC panel for cytokeratin, especially high-molecular-weight cytokeratin, is typically used to prove the epithelial origin of metaplastic components; at least one positive cytokeratin is required to diagnose metaplastic carcinoma of the breast.

7. *Adenoid cystic carcinoma (AdCC)* (Figure 13) and *secretory carcinoma* (Figure 14) are two rare, salivary gland-type breast carcinomas that are triple-negative. Like AdCC of the salivary gland, most AdCCs of the breast harbor a characteristic *MYB-NFIB* fusion gene and are composed of malignant epithelial and myoepithelial cells arranged in cribriform (classic type) and/or solid (solid type) patterns morphologically. Classic-type AdCC is usually low to intermediate grade and contains pale-bluish-grey material and pink basement substance in the lumen of cribriform architecture; negative ER/PR is critical to differentiate this histotype from invasive cribriform carcinoma. Solid-type AdCC is typically composed of high-grade basaloid tumor cells in solid nests with surrounding myxoid stroma; strong/diffuse expression of MYB is helpful to differentiate from other carcinomas with similar morphology, such as basaloid triple-negative ductal carcinoma and small-cell neuroendocrine carcinoma. AdCC of the breast generally has an excellent prognosis, especially the classic-type AdCC; the solid-type AdCC may show aggressive behaviors, such as metastasis to lymph nodes, lungs, and bones. Secretory carcinoma is usually a low-grade invasive carcinoma with a characteristic *ETV6-NTRK* fusion gene, which is composed of neoplastic cells with eosinophilic or vacuolated cytoplasm and mild to moderate nuclear atypia in a microcytic or tubular growth pattern; pink secretion can be seen in the intracytoplasmic and extracellular microcysts, which are positive for PAS and mucicarmine. Secretory carcinoma has an excellent prognosis, even in patients with axillary lymph node metastasis.

Malignant nonepithelial neoplasms

Mesenchymal tumors

A number of malignant mesenchymal neoplasms, including liposarcoma, leiomyosarcoma, angiosarcoma, or even extra-skeletal chondrosarcoma and osteosarcoma, have been reported to primarily occur in the breast, although they are extremely rare. Excluding metaplastic carcinoma with mesenchymal differentiation and malignant phyllodes tumor with mesenchymal elements is always the first step when a sarcomatous neoplasm is identified in the breast tissue, especially in the limited biopsy sample.

As radiation therapy of the chest wall is a standard treatment for breast carcinoma after segmental mastectomy, there is an increased risk of angiosarcoma in patients who received radiation therapy, with an incidence of up to 1%. Postradiation

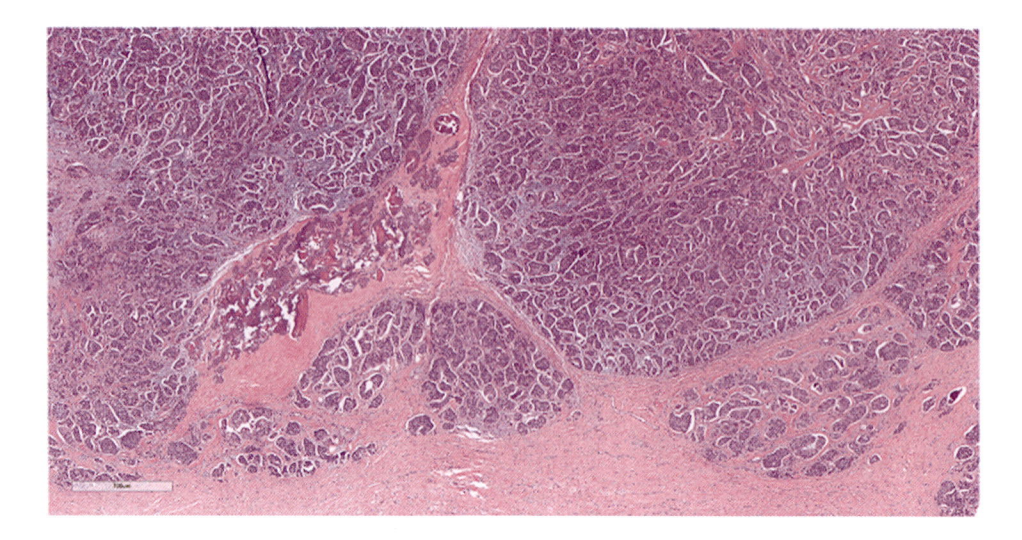

Figure 10 Invasive micropapillary carcinoma.

angiosarcoma usually arises in the radiation area a median of 6 years after radiation; rarely, it can occur 1–2 years after radiation. Unlike primary angiosarcoma, which usually occurs in the deep breast parenchyma, postradiation angiosarcoma usually involves the dermis diffusely or multifocally with variable infiltration into the subcutaneous tissue and deeper breast parenchyma. In addition, *MYC* amplification is a molecular characteristic of radiation-induced angiosarcoma but not primary angiosarcoma. Postradiation angiosarcoma, whether well-differentiated with well-formed vessels or poorly differentiated with solid growth histologically, is associated with high risk of local recurrence and distant metastasis and poor survival time.

Hematopoietic tumors
Primary lymphoma occurring in the breast is a rare malignancy, accounting for <0.5% of all breast malignancies. Diffuse large B-cell lymphoma, MALT lymphoma, and follicular lymphoma are the most common lymphomas, accounting for >90% of lymphomas in the breast, although any type of lymphoma can occur in the breast.

Breast implant-associated anaplastic large cell lymphoma (BIA-ALCL) is a rare and special type of T-cell lymphoma that occurs in the fibrous capsule surrounding breast implants; the *risk of developing BIA-ALCL ranges from about 1 in 1000 to 1 in 30,000 for people with textured breast implants*. Anaplastic tumor cells can infiltrate breast tissue, which may mimic poorly differentiated carcinoma morphologically. BIA-ALCL has a favorable prognosis, especially after complete excision of the capsule and implant.

Fibroepithelial tumors
Phyllodes tumor is a biphasic neoplasia including epithelial and stromal components with characteristic intracanalicular architecture—leaf-like stromal fronds capped by epithelial lining—which accounts for <1% of all breast neoplasia. Phyllodes tumors can be classified as benign, borderline, and malignant. Stromal overgrowth, defined as the absence of epithelial elements in one low-power microscopic field, is the most significant feature of malignant phyllodes tumor; other malignant features include stromal hypercellularity, marked cytologic atypia, brisk mitotic activity, infiltrative tumor border, and heterologous elements of mesenchymal malignancy that should be differentiated from metaplastic carcinoma.

Biomarkers of clinical value
ER and PR, the most critical HRs in the breast, play an important role in breast development, differentiation, and tumorigenesis. ER and PR are nuclear receptors mostly expressed in the luminal cells. Most invasive breast carcinomas, including the majority of well- to moderately differentiated and some poorly differentiated carcinomas, express ER and PR. It is not common to see cases with positive PR and negative ER, as PR expression is regulated by ER. Expression of ER and PR is detected by IHC staining. According to the current ASCO/CAP guidelines, breast cancer samples with ER or PR expression in >10% of tumor nuclei should be interpreted as ER or PR positive, 1–10% as low positive, and <1% as negative.[79]

HER2, a member of the HER family is a tyrosine kinase growth factor receptor. Amplification and overexpression of *HER2* can activate its downstream targets, including the PI3K-AKT and MAPK signaling pathways, and thus initiate tumor development and growth. As recommended by the updated 2018 ASCO/CAP guidelines, accurate HER2 status designation (positive or negative) is based on combined interpretation of HER2 expression by IHC staining and *HER2* amplification by ISH.[80] HER2 expression by IHC staining is graded into three levels: IHC negative (0 and 1+), IHC equivalent (2+), and IHC positive (3+). Equivocal (2+) IHC prompts ordering an ISH test.

Ki-67 is a widely used marker of cell proliferation in breast carcinomas, but it is not universally accepted or officially recommended due to lack of reproducibility and consensus for cutoff values. The Ki-67 index generally correlates with other clinicopathologic characteristics such as tumor grade and molecular status. High Ki-67 is more commonly seen in high-grade, HER2-positive, and triple-negative breast cancers. Breast carcinomas with high Ki-67 usually respond well to chemotherapy. A threshold of 14% has been proposed to determine Luminal A-like (<14%) or Luminal B-like type (>14%) breast carcinomas with positive ER and negative HER2.

PD-L1 is a ligand for the PD-1 immune checkpoint receptor on T lymphocytes. Monoclonal antibodies that bind to PD-1 or to PDL1, disrupting the PD-1/PD-L1 interaction and enhancing antitumor immunity have been approved and are widely used to treat multiple cancer types, including melanoma, non-small-cell lung carcinoma, renal cell, urothelial, and breast cancers. PD-L1 can be overexpressed on the cancer cells and normal immune cells in the tumor microenvironment (TME). In breast carcinoma,

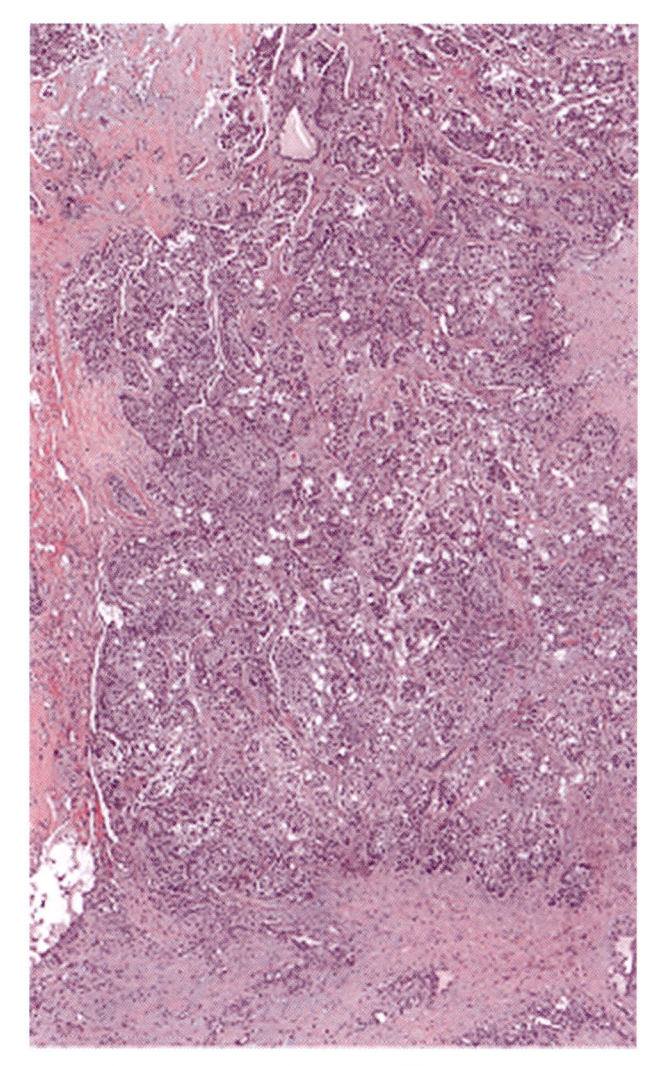

Figure 11 Invasive carcinoma with apocrine differentiation.

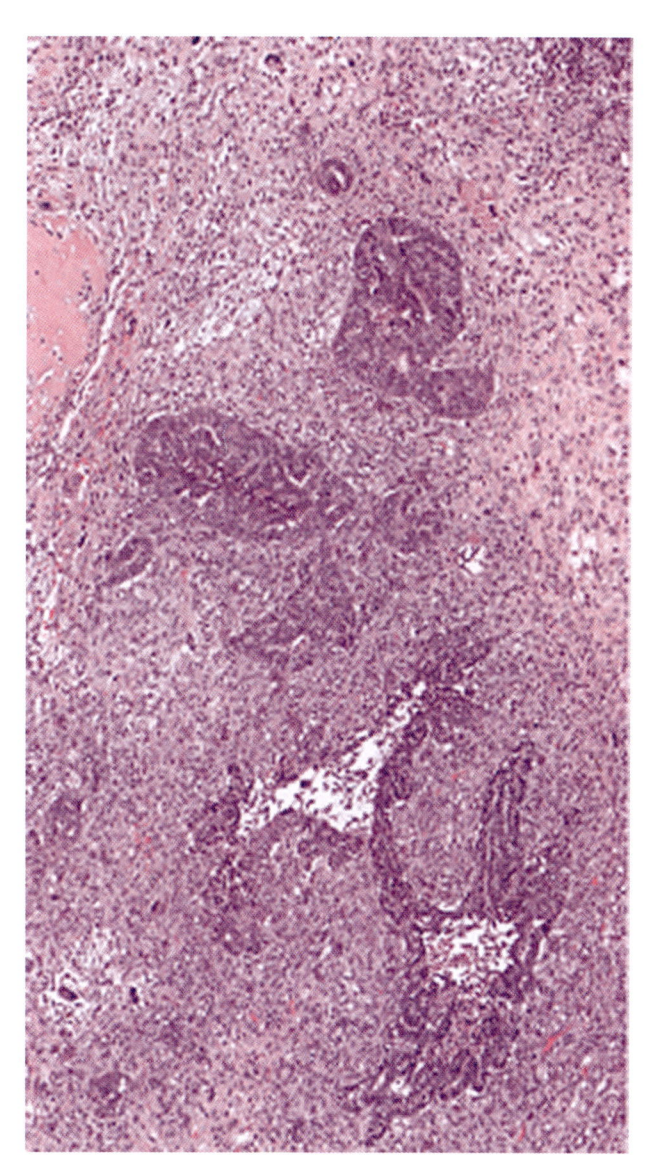

Figure 12 Metaplastic carcinoma.

PD-L1 expression is relatively higher in the triple-negative and HER2-positive groups than in the luminal groups. Response to immune checkpoint inhibitory antibodies has correlated with elevated PD-L1 levels. The use of specific assays for PD-L1 scoring to qualify the use of checkpoint inhibitors is reviewed in the section on TNBC treatment.

Molecular classification

A widely accepted classification of breast cancers was proposed by Perou et al., in 2000.[81] Hierarchical cluster analysis of gene expression by cDNA microarray identified four major intrinsic subtypes of invasive breast cancer: *luminal A-like*, with the highest expression of ER and ER-related genes, negative HER2, and low Ki-67, responding well to endocrine therapy (ET); *luminal B-like*, with ER expression, low PR, and high K-67, responding better to chemotherapy, but with a poorer prognosis than luminal A-like; *HER2-enriched*, with amplification and high expression of the HER2 gene, although about 50% of HER2-overexpressing breast cancers express ER as well and are classified luminal B type; and *basal-like* that express genes associated with basal myoepithelial cells that surround breast ducts, including CK5/6 and CK14, where about 70% are triple-negative and fail to express ER, PR, or HER2, associated with the poorest prognosis.

Additional genomic biomarkers that aid in personalizing therapy

Advances in tumor genome sequencing have enabled the identification of actionable mutations and have increasingly defined treatment selection in solid tumor patients including breast cancers (Table 4). Typically, paired germline DNA testing is typically not utilized for clinical tumor testing in order to minimize cost and turnaround time. Nevertheless, it is important to recognize that incidental germline alterations can be uncovered with tumor-only sequencing and this could have significant implications for patients and their families.

BRCA1/2 mutations

Approximately, 5–10% of breast cancers are associated with germline alterations in *BRCA1* and *BRCA2*. Inhibition of poly(adenosine diphosphate [ADP]–ribose) polymerase (PARP) offers a synthetic lethal therapeutic strategy in cells with loss-of-function *BRCA1* or *BRCA2*. Currently, two PARP inhibitors, olaparib, and talazoparib are approved in patients with germline *BRCA* mutations and HER2-negative locally advanced or metastatic breast cancer (MBC) based on improvement in

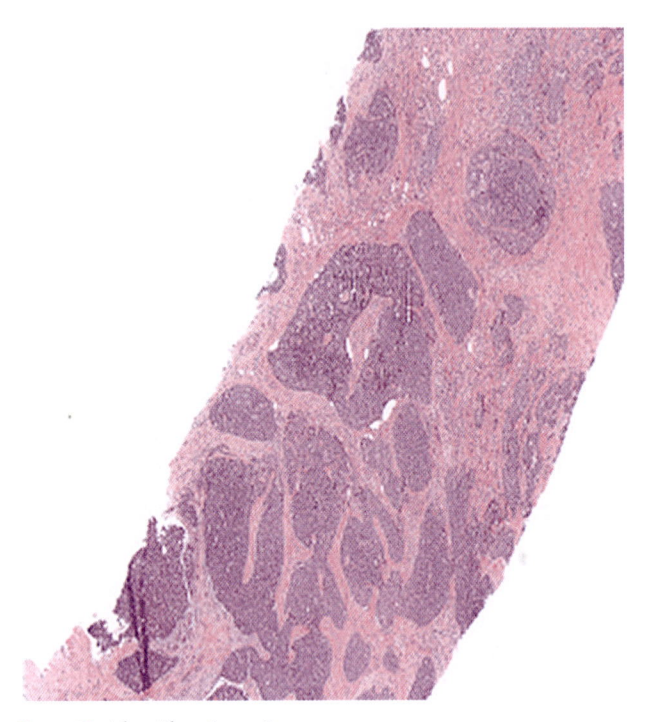

Figure 13 Adenoid cystic carcinoma.

Table 4 Actionable genomic alterations.

Gene	Alteration	Agents
BRCA1/2	Mutation	Olaparib
		Talazoparib
ERRB2	Amplification	Trastuzumab
		Pertuzumab
		Ado-Trastuzumab-emtansine (TDM-1)
		Fam-trastuzumab-deruxtecan-nxki
		Lapatinib
		Neratinib, DS-8201a
		Tucatinib
PIK3CA	Mutation	Alpelisib
NTRK1/2/3	Fusion	Entrectinib
		Larotrectinib

progression-free survival (PFS) compared to physician's choice of chemotherapy.[82,83]

The *phosphatidylinositide-3-kinase (PI3K)/Akt/mammalian target of rapamycin (mTOR)* pathway is an integral pathway in mediating tumor survival cells and alterations involving this pathway have been observed in multiple tumors including breast, colon, and bladder cancers.[84,85] Mutations in the p110 catalytic α-subunit are observed in about 35–40% of HR-positive breast cancers, primarily in exons 9 and 20. The BOLERO2 study evaluated the use of everolimus, an mTOR inhibitor, in combination with exemestane in HR-positive advanced breast cancer.[86] Though, PFS benefit was observed independent of *PIK3CA* mutational status, data suggested that patients with mutations in exon 9 were likely to benefit with the addition of everolimus.[87] The BELLE-3 study, evaluated buparlisib, a pan-PI3K inhibitor in combination with fulvestrant, a selective estrogen receptor downregulator (SERD), in HR-positive MBC who had progressed on prior endocrine therapy.[88] Although improvement in PFS was noted in patients with *PIK3CA* mutations, significant grade 3/4 toxicities were observed with the addition of buparlisib. Taselisib, a β-sparing PI3K inhibitor, was evaluated in combination with fulvestrant in the phase-3 SANDPIPER study.[89] While the combination showed a statistically significant improvement in PFS (7.4 months vs 5.4 months with fulvestrant alone) (HR 0.70; $p = 0.0037$) in *PIK3CA* mutant patients, it was associated with significant toxicity leading to frequent discontinuations.

The SOLAR-I, phase-3 study evaluated an α isoform-selective PI3K inhibitor, alpelisib, and fulvestrant to fulvestrant alone in patients with HR-positive, HER2-negative MBC, who had progressed on prior endocrine therapy.[90] PFS was 11 months with combination compared to 5.7 months with fulvestrant alone (HR 0.65; $p < 0.001$) in patients with PIK3CA mutations, leading to FDA approval of alpelisib in HR-positive MBC with *PIK3CA* alterations in tumor tissue or in circulating tumor DNA (ctDNA). Significant on-target toxicities, with hyperglycemia and diarrhea, were, however, observed in patients treated with alpelisib. While the study primarily enrolled patients who were CDK4/6 naïve, the combination also showed clinical activity in a small group of patients who received prior CDD4/6 inhibitors and thus alpelisib

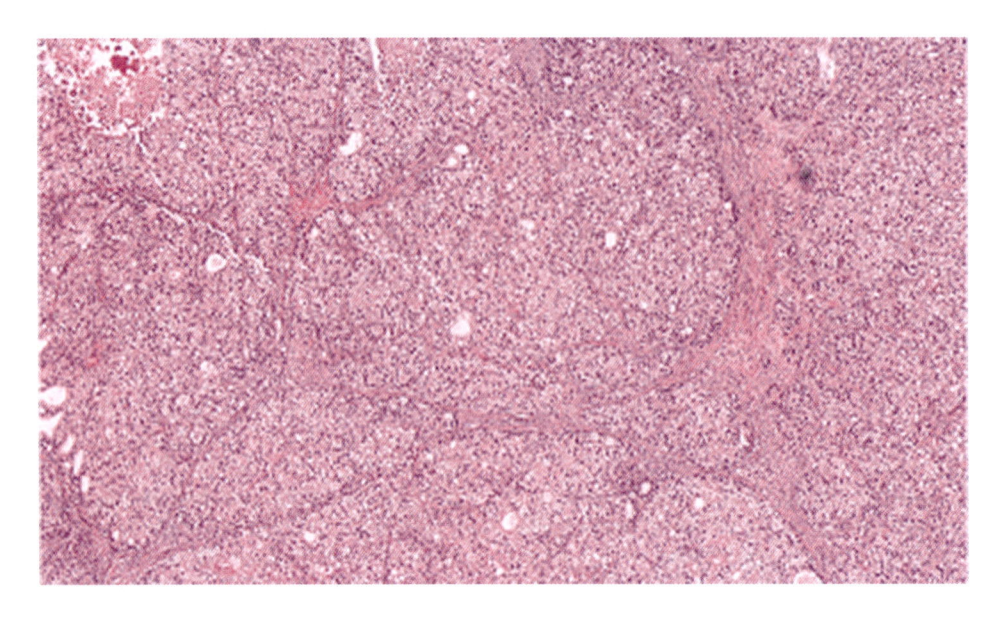

Figure 14 Secretory carcinoma.

is currently being evaluated in this setting (NCT03056755). In addition to mutations in helical and kinase domains, deletions in C2 domain, that relieve the inhibitory effect of p85 subunit on p110 α have also been shown to mediate sensitivity to PI3K inhibition.[91]

In the FAKTION study, which evaluated the combination of fulvestrant with capivasertib, an ATP-competitive pan-AKT inhibitor, median PFS was significantly longer in patients who received capivasertib combination than in those who received fulvestrant alone (PFS 10.3 vs 4.8 months, HR 0.58; $p = 0.0044$).[92] However, PIK3CA mutations or PTEN loss by immunohistochemistry did not predict for clinical activity of capivasertib. Capivasertib was also evaluated in combination with paclitaxel as first-line therapy for metastatic TNBC. The addition of capivasertib resulted in a significant improvement in PFS and OS in patients with PIK3CA/AKT1/PTEN-altered tumors.[93] In addition to PIK3CA, mutations in some of the other pathway genes such as AKT, PIK3R1, PTEN, and TSC1 are also considered to be clinically actionable.[94,95]

Acquired mutations in ESR1 are common in MBC patients exposed to estrogen deprivation with aromatase inhibitors (AIs) limiting clinical activity.[96-99] ESR1 mutations are infrequent in primary breast cancers, suggesting clonal selection with exposure.[100,101] In the BOLERO-2 study, ESR1 mutations (D538G and Y537S) were identified in nearly 30% of patients and associated with inferior OS. However, compared to WT (32 months), Y537S ESR1 mutations (20 months) were associated with worse OS compared to D538G (26 months) suggesting differences in the ESR1 variants.[102] Currently, the most effective therapy for patients harboring ESR1 mutations is unclear; though data have suggested that these mutations may exhibit greater sensitivity to fulvestrant.[103] In the SOFEA trial, which compared the activity of fulvestrant plus anastrozole or placebo versus exemestane alone, ESR1 mutations were observed in nearly 40% of HR-positive MBC patients and those with mutations had improved PFS with fulvestrant compared with exemestane ($p = 0.02$) while no PFS difference was observed in WT ESR1.[104] However, Y537S ESR1 is selected with fulvestrant exposure, suggesting that this variant mediates resistance.[105,106] ESR1 targeting is an important unmet clinical need and multiple clinical trials evaluating novel SERDs (e.g., elacestrant, LSZ102, and ZN-C5) as well as selective ER modulators (e.g., lasofoxifene) are currently in progress.

Amplification of FGFR1 and FGFR2
Deregulation of FGFR signaling due to gene amplification, mutation, or fusion has been reported in multiple tumor types including breast, bladder, and cholangiocarcinoma.[107] In breast cancers, amplifications in FGFR1 and FGFR2 are commonly observed with mutations and rearrangements seen infrequently.[108] Amplification of FGFR1 has been shown to be associated with resistance to endocrine therapy and associated with early relapse and poor survival in patients with HR-positive breast cancers.[109] Alterations in FGFR1/2 have also been observed in ctDNA in approximately 40% of patients post-CDK4/6 progression, suggesting aberrant FGFR signaling promotes resistance to CDK4/6 inhibitors.[110] Also, patients with FGFR1 amplification exhibited a shorter PFS (11 months) compared to patients with WT FGFR1 (25 months) ($p = 0.075$) with the addition of ribociclib to letrozole in HR-positive MBC in the MONALEESA-2 study.[110] Clinical trials with single-agent FGFR inhibitors have shown limited activity suggesting that combination with endocrine therapy or other rational targeted agents may be clinically more meaningful and clinical trials to this end are in progress.[111]

NTRK1/2/3 fusion
Oncogenic fusions involving neurotrophic tyrosine receptor kinase NTRK1/2/3 leading to constitutive TRKA kinase activity have been reported in lung, breast, papillary thyroid, and salivary gland tumors.[112-114] Currently two TRK inhibitors, larotrectinib and entrectinib, have been approved by the FDA for treatment of any solid tumor patients with NTRK fusions that are metastatic or inoperable.[115,116] While NTRK fusions are uncommon in breast cancers, ETV6-NTRK3 are typically seen in secretory breast cancers and are eligible candidates for matching inhibitors.

Breast cancer biology
Breast cancer is highly heterogeneous and is classified into different subtypes based on numerous features such as histopathology, grade, stage, and HR status. Historically, breast cancer has been classified based on immunostaining for the HRs such as ER, PR, and HER2.[117] Further classification with clinical implications have been defined through differential gene expression, which are commonly separated into luminal-like (HR-positive), HER2-enriched, and basal-like (HR-negative and HER2-negative or triple-negative).[118] This molecular classification revealed that there are at least two distinct cell types, luminal and basal epithelial cells, present in breast tumors suggesting that breast cancer initiation is a result of the dysregulation of normal mammary gland development processes and pathways.

The mature mammary gland is organized into two main epithelial compartments, the inner luminal compartment, and the outer basal or myoepithelial compartment. The majority of human breast cancer, which is HR-positive comprising 70% of all breast cancer patients, is thought to arise mainly in the luminal epithelial compartment. The luminal cell compartment is comprised of two cell lineages hormone sensing (ERα-positive) and secretory cells (ERα-negative) that have been identified to arise from unipotent luminal progenitor cells.[119] Mammary luminal progenitors can display a remarkable degree of plasticity dependent on molecular signals to control commitment to a specific cell type. A master regulator of luminal cell fate is GATA-3, which is necessary for the maintenance of the differentiated luminal epithelium in the adult mammary gland.[120] ERα not only is positively regulated by GATA3, but it can also stimulate GATA3 transcription, in a positive feedback loop. GATA-3 expression has implications in luminal subtypes of breast cancer, with high expression indicative of better overall survival (OS) in ERα-positive tumors[121] due to improved response to hormonal therapy, the mainstay treatment for HR-positive tumors.[122] GATA3 is not expressed in basal cells that do not contain HRs. Mammary cell balance is maintained via complex paracrine signaling between the cellular compartments.

The basal cell layer, which secretes the components of a basement membrane, is required to polarize the luminal epithelial cell layer and promote luminal cell survival.[123] Basal cells depend on WNT and receptor activator of nuclear factor kappa-B ligand (RANKL) paracrine signals from the luminal layer to proliferate and maintain the putative mammary stem cell population.[124] Thus, basal cells are considered to be less differentiated than luminal cells and correlate with the feature of basal-like breast cancers. Certain breast cancer models have supported the idea that normal mammary stem cells are the target for transformation. For instance, hyperactivation of the WNT pathway in mice results in an expanded stem cell population in preneoplastic mammary glands, and the development of heterogeneous tumors.[125,126] These initiating events in the distinct

Table 5 Overview of genetic engineered mouse models by breast cancer subtype.

Subtype(s)	Promoter	Targeted gene	Effect on expression	Time to tumor development	References
Luminal	MMTV	Cyclin D1	Overexpression	20–23 mo	128
Luminal	MMTV	Cyclin D1 (T286A)	Constitutive activation	16–20 mo	128
Luminal	MMTV	PIK3CA (H1047R)	Activating mutation	5–16 mo	129
Luminal	MMTV	AIB1	Overexpression	12–25 mo	130
Luminal	MMTV	ESPL1	Overexpression	10–12 mo	131
Luminal	MMTV	AKT (Myc)	Myristoylated Overexpression		132
Luminal	N/A	Stat1	Knockout	18–26 mo	133
HER2	MMTV	neu/ErbB2	Overexpression	5–10 mo	134
Basal	MMTV	Cyclin E	Overexpression	10–18 mo	135
Basal	MMTV	BRCA1; p53	Loss of function	6–8 mo	136
Basal	N/A	p53	Knockout	11–12 mo	137
Basal	MMTV	Wnt1	Overexpression	8–10 mo	138
Luminal and Basal	MMTV	PyMT	Overexpression	2–3 mo	139
Luminal and Basal	MMTV	c-Myc	Overexpression	10–15 mo	140

cell types of the mammary gland are an example of the genetic complexity of breast cancer.

To understand breast cancer initiation and progression, *in vivo* mouse models have become an important tool. Genetically engineered mice (GEM) have been developed that overexpress an oncogene, silence a tumor suppressor, or include a mutation found in human breast cancer. The majority of breast cancer GEMs use a mammary-specific promoter that limits the genetic alteration of interest to the mammary gland. The most extensively used promoter is from the mouse mammary tumor virus (MMTV), identified in the 1930s. MMTV restricts expression to mammary epithelial cells in the luminal and basal compartments.[127] Many transgenic mouse models of breast cancer have been generated and this article only provides a brief review of some of the models due to their high clinical relevance based on subtype and current therapeutic targets (Table 5).

A GEM model that is been widely used is the expression of the polyoma virus middle T oncoprotein (PyMT) under the control of MMTV. MMTV-PyMT mice (Table 1) display mammary hyperplasia as early as 4 weeks of age and develop carcinomas at 14 weeks.[139] Depending on the stage of tumor progression, tumors are more luminal-like (ER-positive) at early stages but become more basal-like (ER-negative) at late stages. PyMT is not expressed in human breast cancer; however, it has been a model to study breast tumorigenesis due to the induction of several signal transduction pathways that are altered in human breast cancer, such as c-myc, errb2 (HER2), PIK3CA, and cyclin D1.[141]

Luminal-like breast cancers have several genes that have been identified as drivers of oncogenesis. Cyclin D1 overexpression has been observed in 40–50% of human breast cancers, mainly in luminal cases. MMTV-CyclinD1 and MMTV-CyclinD1^{T286A} (constitutively activated) mouse models develop ER-positive (luminal-like) tumors (Table 5).[128,142] Even though tumor development occurs in the MMTV-Cyclin D1, it takes almost 1 year, indicative of a long latency suggesting that other additional changes are necessary for oncogenesis. Targeted therapies have been developed to overcome cyclin D1 overexpression by inhibiting CDK4/6 activity that is needed to promote cell proliferation. A mutation in phosphatidylinositol 3-kinase (PIK3CA) that is commonly found in ~30% of luminal breast cancers was generated in mice with a conditional knock-in of the activating mutation (H1047R) detected in human cases. This model referred to as MMTV-Cre; PIK3CA(H1047R) produces ductal hyperplasia and the formation of ER-positive breast cancers (Table 5).[143] Targeted therapies have now been developed against PIK3CA that can effectively inhibit the proliferation of those luminal cells that have an activating or gain of function mutations in PIK3CA. ErbB2 (HER2/neu) genomic amplifications have been reported in about 20–30% of breast cancers. MMTV-ErbB2 (MMTV-Neu) mice were developed and characterized (Table 5).[134] The tumors developed in these murine models are both histologically and genetically similar to the human cases. Targeted therapy directly blocking the HER2 pathway is currently used as a standard of care either as a single agent or in combination therapy for HER2-positive breast cancers. Cyclin E (cytoplasmic) overexpression has been observed as a marker of aggressive disease. Overexpression of cyclin E on the MMTV promoter led to abnormal development of the mammary epithelium that progresses to basal-like mammary carcinomas[135] (Table 5) Cyclin E and TP53 also cooperate to induce mammary cancers with a shorter latency than that observed with cyclin E overexpression alone.[135]

Some breast cancers arise from germline mutation in the human tumor suppressor genes TP53 or BReast CAncer genes 1 and 2 (BRCA1 and 2). Carriers of germline BRCA1 mutations frequently have a basal-like phenotype. Different mouse models with BRCA1 dysfunction have the basal phenotype. For example, MMTV-BRCA1 deletion combined with aberrant p53 expression leads to mammary tumor formation (Table 5).[136] Two additional mouse models of BRCA1 tumorigenesis have been studied to determine the cell of origins. Luminal-derived *Blg-Cre; BRCA1$^{f/f}$; p53$^{+/-}$* tumors resemble those found in human BRCA1 patients, whereas the basally derived *K14-Cre BRCA1$^{f/f}$ p53$^{+/-}$* tumors do not.[144] Another study, however, found that luminal progenitors from BRCA1 patients have a basal-like expression profile, suggesting that the progenitors from these patients or transgenic mouse models may not have fully differentiated (Table 5).[145] Thus, when modeling the tumorigenic process of breast cancer, multiple GEMs need to be considered since there is not one model that can perfectly recapitulate the tumorigenic state for any subtype as it occurs in patients.

These mutations are often compensated during development, skewing the cellular state in a way which may or may not be representative of human oncogenesis. Most of these models use only the most aggressive drivers of tumorigenesis. While GEM models have been invaluable in understanding how particular oncogenes promote oncogenesis, oncogenes expressed in a transgenic mouse

Table 6 Overview of establishment of patient-derived xenograft models.

References	# of patients	Patient subtype	# PDX established	PDX subtype	Host mouse model
140, 147, 148	44	Luminal (10) HER2 (3) Basal (29) Not reported (2)	51	Luminal (7) HER2 (6) Basal (37) Not reported (1)	SCID/Bg and NSG
149, 150	27	Luminal (9) HER2 (4) Basal (14)	29	Luminal (10) HER2 (4) Basal (15)	NSG
151, 152	15	Luminal (5) HER2 (2) Basal (8)	18	Luminal (8) HER2 (2) Basal (8)	NSG
153, 154	64	Luminal (36) HER2 (3) Basal (25)	29	Luminal (9) HER2 (1) Basal (19)	Nude
155	24	Luminal (18) HER2 (0) Basal (6)	10	Luminal (8) HER2 (0) Basal (2)	NSG

do not necessarily behave as they would when introduced *de novo* in mature human breast tissue.[146] Furthermore, paracrine signaling is critical to homeostasis in most tissues, and the expression of an oncogene from every cell in a tissue compartment may radically change the TME. Techniques such as single-cell RNA-sequencing and mass cytometry (CyTOF) are revealing this heterogeneity and furthering our understanding of signaling between compartments.

Patient-derived xenografts (PDXs) provide an alternative model. PDXs maintain the heterogeneity of the human breast cancer since the tumor tissue is biopsied from a patient and placed subcutaneously into immunocompromised mice to prevent rejection. Characteristics of several PDX models are summarized in Table 6. Establishing PDX models, particularly those that are HR-positive, has proven difficult. Since immunocompromised mice must be utilized for PDX to avoid rejection, PDXs do not permit the study of the immune response in tumor prevention, promotion, and therapy. PDX models have, however, furthered the development of targeted therapies.

Recent advancements in 3D *ex vivo* culturing of patient tumor biopsies as "organoids" that maintain disease heterogeneity.[156] Organoid culture technology can also preserve complex progenitor and differentiated cell types and mammary stem cell populations.[157] Organoid models are being used to test for targeted therapeutics, which can be done in a higher-throughput fashion.[158] Further development and characterization of organoid culture techniques will help accelerate therapeutic advancements.

Diagnosis

Current mammographic screening guidelines

The American College of Radiology (ACR) recommends annual mammographic screening beginning at age 40 for women at average risk.[159] This is based on maximizing proven benefits which include reduction in breast cancer mortality in women who participate in regular screening.[159] Meta-analyses have shown a net benefit to mammographic screening for women 39–49 years of age at study entry across seven randomized controlled trials demonstrating a 15% reduction in mortality.[160] For women aged 50–74 years at study entry, a 22% reduction in mortality from screening was observed.[160] Observational studies report the impact of screening mammography in clinical practice. In a Pan-Canadian analysis of observational data, a 44% reduction in mortality was observed from screening at age 40–49.[160] The identification of early-stage breast cancer is balanced by the diagnosis of indolent or very slow-growing cancers that may represent overdiagnosis and overtreatment.[161] Reasonable estimates show the overdiagnosis rate with screening mammography to be between 1% and 10%.[162] Until science can reliably discriminate breast cancers that will not cause harm or metastasize from those that will, this level of deemed excess diagnosis is likely to persist.[162] In spite of limitations, mammography remains the single most effective screening test that reduces breast cancer mortality and is the only breast cancer screening test that is supported by the USPSTF and the American Cancer Society.[163,164]

Women with specific predisposition for breasts including African American women and women of Ashkenazi Jewish descent should undergo formal risk evaluation at age 30. Establishing an elevated risk will allow women to benefit from annual high-risk screening at an earlier age.[165] Depending on individual patient risk factors, appropriate supplemental screening tests can be personalized to the needs of each patient.

Advances in screening mammography

Two key changes have improved screening mammography performance in recent decades.[166] The first is the transition from screen-film to digital mammography beginning in 2000, and the second is the expansion of training programs to enhance interpretive skills for radiologists who interpret screening mammograms.[166] Digital mammography has been shown to improve the diagnostic accuracy in certain subgroups of women, including women 49 years of age or younger, and women with dense breast tissue.[167–169] An update to performance benchmarks for modern screening digital mammography in the US community practice showed the cancer detection rate (CDR) to be 5.1 per 1000 screening examinations.[166]

Digital breast tomosynthesis (DBT) has gained wide acceptance into clinical practice in the past decade and has demonstrated improvement of radiologist reader performance by lowering recall rates while increasing sensitivity.[170–172] With DBT, an X-ray source emits multiple low-dose X-rays as it moves in an arc over the compressed breast.[173,174] The resulting projection images are reconstructed to produce thin-slice cross-sectional images of the breast.[175] Thin slices reduce false-positive findings and recall rates related to overlapping breast tissue for women with both dense

Table 7 Incremental cancer detection rates of selected imaging modalities.[a,177]

Modality	Incremental cancer detection rate (per 1000)
Digital breast tomosynthesis	1.6
Supplemental screening with ultrasound	2.8
Supplemental screening with contrast-enhanced breast MRI	10
Supplemental screening with molecular breast imaging	8.8

[a]Source: Adapted from Berg and Leung[160]; Lehman et al.[166]; Marinovich et al.[173]

and nondense breast tissue.[174–176] A meta-analysis of 17 studies reported a 2.2% absolute decrease in recall rate, and a pooled incremental CDR of 1.6/1000 (Table 7) by addressing the "masking" of breast cancer by overlapping breast tissue.[173,174]

The largest performance improvements with DBT have been demonstrated in women less than 50 years of age, and in women with high breast density.[176,178–181] Thus, younger women who tend to have dense tissue and higher-risk women who begin screening at an earlier age, are expected to benefit from DBT.[165]

Screening women at high risk

Although BRCA mutation carriers are susceptible to radiation, the low radiation dose from screening mammography does not demonstrably increase their breast cancer risk.[182] BRCA1 carriers receive less benefit from mammography before age 40, while a significant proportion of cancer is found only on mammography in BRCA2 carriers.[183] Mammography also remains important for the early detection of cancer in women treated at a young age with chest radiation therapy. By age 40–45 years, 13–20% of these women will develop breast cancer.[184–190] If a woman has received chest radiation between the ages of 10 and 30, she should begin screening mammography 8 years after the radiation therapy but not before age 25.[191]

Contrast-enhanced mammography (CEM)
An emerging modality in breast imaging is contrast-enhanced mammography (CEM), which combines digital mammography with the administration of intravenous contrast material.[192] Breast cancer can be identified not only by its density and morphology but also by neovascularity associated with the malignancy.[192–194] CEM has been shown to have comparable sensitivity to breast MRI for the detection of cancer, but with a shorter acquisition time and cost.[192] Early data suggests that CEM may provide a low-cost and more accessible alternative to MRI in the evaluation of disease extent.[195] CEM has primarily been evaluated in the diagnostic setting with higher sensitivity, specificity, and accuracy compared to digital mammography.[196] A limited number of studies have evaluated the potential of CEM as a screening test and further evaluation is warranted to investigate this emerging technology in the context of breast cancer screening and diagnosis.[197,198]

Supplemental screening with ultrasound
Dense fibro-glandular tissue obscures breast cancers and reduces the effectiveness of mammographic screening and is also an independent risk factor for the development of breast cancer.[199–201] As of February 2019, Federal law requires mammography facilities to include breast density information in reports sent to patients and their physicians. The law specifies there must be standard reporting language that includes at a minimum, how breast density may mask cancer on a mammogram, a qualitative assessment of breast density by the interpreting radiologist, and a reminder to individuals with dense breast tissue to speak with their provider if they have questions. Research has shown that women in states with laws requiring specific recommendations for supplemental screening had higher rates of receiving ultrasound studies and higher cancer detection after implementation of the law.[202] The same study found no changes in states that only required notifications regarding breast density.[202]

Supplemental screening breast ultrasound performed in addition to screening mammography of women with dense breasts has been shown to reduce the interval cancer detection rate (IDCR) to that of women with nondense breasts at 1-year follow-up.[203] The ICDR of supplemental screening ultrasound ranges from 0.5 to 12 additional cancers/1000 women.[204] Supplemental screening ultrasound has been reported to increase the detection of small node-negative invasive cancers thus supporting the rationale that it may offer a mortality reduction benefit.[204] ACRIN 6666, a multi-institutional trial of screening ultrasound for women with dense breast tissue and intermediate/high risk for breast cancer, showed increased CDR of 4.2/1000 women in year 1 of screening.[205] The sensitivity of screening increased from 50% with digital mammography alone to 77.5% for digital mammography combined with ultrasound.[205] Follow-up at year 3 of supplemental screening ultrasound showed a sustained incremental CDR of 3.7/1000 women in the incident second- and third-year screening rounds.[206]

A multicenter Italian study, the ASTOUND trial, compared the sensitivity of DBT and supplemental ultrasound.[207] In women with dense breasts and negative findings on 2D screening mammograms, DBT showed ICDR of 2.8/1000 in comparison to physician performed hand-held ultrasound that showed ICDR of 4.9/1000 women screening.[207]

Supplemental screening with breast MRI
In high-risk populations, dynamic contrast-enhanced breast MRI screening detects more breast cancer than either mammography or ultrasound.[189,208–216] For high-risk women with ≥20–25% lifetime risk of developing breast cancer, supplemental screening with dynamic contrast-enhanced breast MRI is recommended annually beginning between ages 25 and 30.[165,217] In one study of BRCA mutation carriers and women of 20% or higher lifetime risk for breast cancer, MRI sensitivity for detecting breast cancer was 90%, compared to 37.5% for mammography and 37% for ultrasound.[213]

High-risk patients include women who are carriers of pathogenic mutations (BRCA1/BRCA2 or other disease-causing mutation), untested women with a first degree relative BRCA carrier, women who have been risk-assessed by various models due to strong family history, and women with a personal history of chest radiation therapy before age 30.[165,207] In this latter group of women, screening MRI is recommended to begin 8 years after completion of chest radiation but not earlier than age 25.[165] For BRCA gene mutation carriers, MRI is recommended beginning at age 25, in addition to annual mammography at and beyond age 30.[165] In high-risk patients, excluding those with previous history of breast cancer, the ICDR averages 10/1000 screening MR examinations.[160]

For intermediate-risk women with 15–25% lifetime risk of developing breast cancer, breast MRI may be considered as a supplement to mammography to screen women.[207] Annual screening MRI may be beneficial for women with a personal history of breast cancer and dense breasts and for women diagnosed with breast cancer

Table 8 Definitions of TNM categories

Category	Definitions
Tis	*In situ* (ductal not lobular) should specify separately if Paget's disease
T1	≤2 cm (invasive component)
T1mic	≤1 mm
T1a	>1 mm and ≤5 mm
T1b	>5 mm and ≤10 mm
T1c	>10 mm and ≤2 cm
T2	>2 cm and ≤5 cm
T3	>5 cm
T4	Any size with extension to chest wall/skin as described below
T4a	Extension to chest wall with adherence
T4b	Extension to skin with ulceration, satellitosis, edema, and/or redness (not meeting T4d criteria)
T4c	Both T4a and T4b apply
T4d	Inflammatory breast cancer (peau d'orange edema, redness, clinically rapid onset)
cN0	No palpable or imaging-apparent adenopathy
cN1a	Ipsilateral axillary level 1 or 2 nodes
cN2b	No axillary node, but ipsilateral internal mammary (IM) nodes present
cN3a	Ipsilateral infraclavicular (axillary level 3) node(s)
cN3b	Ipsilateral and internal mammary and axillary nodes
cN3c	Ipsilateral supraclavicular node
pN0	Histologically negative axillary nodes
pN0[i+]/pN0[mol+]	Isolated tumor cells only, ≤0.2 mm/molecularly + (by RT-PCR*)
pN1	Involvement of 1–3 axillary nodes (>0.2 mm)
pN1mic	Micrometastases only to axillary nodes (>0.2 and ≤2 mm)
pN1a	Involvement of 1–3 axillary nodes, at least one >2 mm
pN1b	Involvement of IM node >0.2 mm
pN1c	Both pN1a and pN1b apply
pN2	Refers to either pN2a or pN2b
pN2a	Involvement of 4–9 nodes, at least one >2 mm
pN2b	Involvement of IM node(s) clinically without axillary nodes
pN3	Refers to either pN3a, pN3b, or pN3c
pN3a	Involvement of 10+ nodes, at least one >2 mm, or infraclavicular (axillary level 3) node(s)
pN3b	pN1a or pN2a with cN2b or pN2a with pN1b
pN3c	Involvement of ipsilateral supraclavicular node(s)
For all pN categories, suffix (sn) is used if regional node metastasis identified only by sentinel node, or suffix (f) if by fine needle aspirate or core biopsy	
cM0	No tissue-based, clinical, or radiographic distant metastases (beyond breast and ipsilateral regional nodes). Imaging not required
cM0[i+]	cM0, but circulating or bone marrow tumor cells or tissue deposits ≤0.2 mm
cM1	Distant metastases noted by physical exam or imaging
pM1	Histologically demonstrated distant metastases >0.2 mm

IM, internal mammary; RT-PCR, reverse transcriptase–polymerase chain reaction.

under the age of 50.[165,207] Mammography has been shown to be less sensitive in women with a personal history of breast cancer.[218]

Staging with breast MRI

Dynamic contrast-enhanced breast MRI is the imaging examination of choice to estimate disease extent and guide appropriate treatment.[219] Breast MRI is particularly sensitive in identifying multifocal, multicentric, and contralateral disease.[220,221] For patients with newly diagnosed breast malignancy, dynamic contrast-enhanced breast MRI can detect occult malignancy in the contralateral breast in up to 5% of patients.[220,222–226] This may reduce the incidence of metachronous contralateral cancer.[227]

A few retrospective studies have evaluated the use of MBI for the evaluation of disease extent. One study described the detection of additional ipsilateral foci in 6% of patients, and contralateral foci in 5%.[228] MBI may serve as an alternative for patients who cannot undergo MRI due to renal insufficiency, claustrophobia, weight/body habitus limitations, or an MRI-incompatible implanted device.[229]

CEM has also been used to demonstrate disease extent, particularly in patients with contraindications to MRI.[192] Studies have demonstrated comparable sensitivity and performance of CEM and MRI for evaluating disease extent in patients with newly diagnosed breast cancer.[219,230]

Staging

The most recent eighth edition of the American Joint Committee on Cancer (AJCC) staging of breast cancer enacted a fundamental change to supplement anatomic staging with prognostic indices including tumor grade, hormone, and HER2 receptor status and gene profiling to not only refine prognosis but also the interaction with standard therapies including those that are guided by these indices.[231] The anatomic component still follows the TNM categories for tumor size, regional nodal involvement, and distant disease beyond the breast and regional nodes, respectively (Table 8). The timing in relationship to presentation and treatment is indicated by a prefix for each TNM category with "c" indicating the best clinical estimation by physical exam and/or imaging, "p" indicating pathological assessment, "y" indicating posttherapy (systemic or radiation), "r" indicating recurrent disease before any treatment, and "a" for autopsy incidental finding with no prior diagnosis. Prefixes "y" and "r" precede "c" and "p" as applicable. The TNM components are summarized in Table 8, noting that T stage definitions are the same for clinical and pathological even though ascertained differently and refer to the greatest dimension and largest tumor in the case of multifocal disease, while nodal stage definitions use different criteria. The "x" designation after T, N, or M indicates data are missing to designate a category. The TNM classification has been used to develop an anatomic staging system (Table 9).

Table 9 AJCC anatomic breast cancer staging chart.

Stage	TNM
Stage 0	Tis, N0, M0
Stage IA	T1, N0, M0
Stage IB	T0, N1mi, M0
	T1, N1mi, M0
Stage IIA	T0, N1, M0
	T1, N1, M0
	T2, N0, M0
Stage IIB	T2, N1, M0
	T3, N0, M0
Stage IIIA	T0, N2, M0
	T1, N2, M0
	T2, N2, M0
	T3, N1, M0
	T3, N2, M0
Stage IIIB	T4, N0, M0
	T4, N1, M0
	T4, N2, M0
Stage IIIC	Any T, N3, M0
Stage IV	Any T, Any N, M1

Prognostic indices are added to anatomic staging to yield prognostic stage groups, including grading of invasive cancers using Nottingham combined grade, or Nottingham modification of the Scarff, Bloom, Richardson (SBR) grading system that incorporates tubular formation, each on a 1–3 scale for the degree of tubular/ductal formation, nuclear grade and mitotic index for a cumulative score of 3–5 (low), 6–7 (intermediate), and 7–8 (high).[232] Estrogen, progesterone, and HER2 receptor status based on ASCO/CAP criteria as described in the Pathology section of this article is also gathered and entered into AJCC eighth edition staging as this provides additional prognostic factors that are also predictive of treatment effect, resulting in more prognostic precision in the context of standard of care therapy receptor subtype-based therapy, as evidenced by two independent validation of this staging system showing better performance that anatomic staging alone.[233] For in situ carcinomas, nuclear grade and ER/PR status should be included. Finally, the staging system also calls for gene profiling results to complete the prognostic stage grouping as these assays provide prognostic and even predictive (response to chemotherapy) information for HR+ cases such that the totality of staging best approaches a real-world outcome prediction.[234]

Surgery

The locoregional management of breast cancer has changed markedly over the last few decades. As a result, radical mastectomy is rarely utilized in the surgical management of breast cancer patients. A series of randomized controlled clinical trials comparing radical mastectomy to breast-conserving surgery (BCS) led to a National Institutes of Health (NIH) consensus statement in 1990 recommending that breast-conserving therapy be the preferred loco-regional treatment for women with stage I–II breast cancer, because it provides equivalent survival outcomes compared with total mastectomy while, at the same time, preserving the breast.[235]

It is widely appreciated that at diagnosis breast cancer may have spread through lymphatic and hematogenous routes. Treatment should therefore be designed to address both loco-regional and systemic diseases. Since breast cancer is a heterogeneous disease, the treatment plan must be crafted around patient and tumor characteristics.[15,236] Molecular profiling has demonstrated that biologic properties in addition to tumor size and nodal status can distinguish different subtypes of breast cancer with different outcomes and vulnerabilities, helping to tailor treatment accordingly.

Historically, patients were classified as low risk based on the lack of nodal metastasis and high risk based on the presence of nodal metastasis. This classification based on anatomic features alone (TNM staging system) does not adequately address the biologic behavior of many breast cancers and was the impetus for the modification of the staging system to include both anatomic and biologic features that more adequately reflect the high risk of developing metastases. Traditionally, excisional biopsy was performed for the diagnosis of both palpable and nonpalpable breast lesions. This two-stage approach of biopsy followed by definitive surgery increased the volume of tissue excised in patients undergoing breast-conserving operations and also led to delays in the initiation of adjuvant therapy.[237] Core needle biopsy is now considered the standard, so that the surgeon has a definite diagnosis of invasive or noninvasive disease, facilitating planning with a multidisciplinary team and making an informed decision between upfront surgery and neoadjuvant systemic therapy.

If a definitive diagnosis cannot be made based on core biopsy, excisional biopsy should be performed with the intent of complete excision with negative margins. If invasive cancer is identified at final pathology, axillary staging can be performed at a second procedure. Most breast cancer operations, excisional biopsies, BCS, and even mastectomy are performed as outpatient procedures or require only brief hospitalization with low rates of surgical complications.

Neoadjuvant systemic therapy

When systemic therapy is indicated based on the characteristics of the primary tumor, treatment in the neoadjuvant (preoperative) setting should be considered. Neoadjuvant systemic therapy increases breast conservation rates and decreases the incidence of positive lymph nodes found at the time of surgery.[238] Similar results have been reported in patients receiving chemotherapy and HER2-targeted therapy for HER2-positive disease (CALGB 40601) and for patients with HR-positive tumors receiving neoadjuvant endocrine therapy (ACOSOG Z1031). Neoadjuvant chemotherapy allows many patients with large breast tumors to have clinically meaningful tumor reduction that facilitates breast conservation. Response rates vary, however, with different breast cancer subtypes. In the ISPY-1 trial, concordance between tumor size on MRI and surgical pathology was higher in well-defined tumors, particularly those with a triple-negative phenotype, and was lower in HR-positive tumors.[239] In the ACOSOG Z1071 trial, 50% of patients with triple-negative disease achieved a pCR in the axilla and those with HER2+ disease had a nodal pCR in almost 70% of cases. Response to chemotherapy is an important prognostic indicator and residual disease is an indication for adjuvant chemotherapy in certain subtypes (triple-negative and HER2+ disease). Sequencing of surgery following chemotherapy can also facilitate reconstruction since any postoperative complications would be less likely to delay adjuvant therapy while providing the patient more time to consider surgical options and to adjust to the diagnosis.

Breast-conserving therapy

Breast conservation has been studied as an alternative to mastectomy for more than four decades. After initial success was reported from single institutions, a number of phase III clinical trials were initiated, which compared outcomes of patients treated with breast conservation to those treated with mastectomy.[240–242] The NSABP B-06[243] trial was initiated in 1976 and enrolled 1843 women. Patients with T1 or T2, N0, or N1, M0 tumors less than or equal to 4 cm were randomly assigned to one of three treatment groups: (1) modified radical mastectomy; (2) segmental mastectomy and axillary dissection; or (3) segmental mastectomy and axillary dissection, followed by radiation therapy. At 20 years of follow-up, this trial demonstrated that breast-conservation therapy (BCT) provided survival equivalent to mastectomy.

The goal of breast conservation is to remove the tumor with a margin of normal tissue while preserving the contour of the breast and symmetry with the contralateral breast. Positive margins increase the risk of ipsilateral breast tumor recurrence (IBTR) which can lead to an increased risk of distant metastasis. While phase III trials have demonstrated that BCS with whole-breast irradiation results in equivalent survival outcomes compared with mastectomy, the optimal margin width for a negative margin has been debated. The Society of Surgical Oncology (SSO) and the American Society for Radiation Oncology (ASTRO) developed a multidisciplinary consensus panel to review available data on margin width in patients with stage I–II breast cancer undergoing BCS with whole-breast irradiation.[244] They performed a systematic review of 33 studies including 28,162 patients and used a meta-analysis of margin width and IBTR to develop consensus. The median prevalence for IBTR was 5.3% at a median follow-up of 79.2 months. Positive margins, defined as ink on invasive carcinoma or DCIS, were associated with a twofold increase in the risk of IBTR compared with negative margins. This increased risk was not mitigated by favorable tumor biology, use of endocrine therapy in HR+ disease, or use of a radiation boost. Close margins did not significantly increase the recurrence risk and therefore the panel concluded that more widely negative margins than "no ink on tumor" were not necessary. This was also true in younger patients, unfavorable biologic subtypes, lobular cancers, and those with an extensive intraductal component. These guidelines, published in 2014, have been widely adopted in clinical practice resulting in a reduction in re-operative surgery for re-excision of margins or completion mastectomy. After breast conservation, 90% of IBTR, in the first decade after diagnosis, are in the same quadrant and histologically similar to the primary cancer. Longer follow-up studies have demonstrated an ongoing risk for developing new cancers in the breast after 10 years, often occurring in other quadrants. These tumors in the treated breast may be of different histologic types with differing biomarker profiles and are best classified as new primary tumors with a better prognosis compared with true recurrences.[245] Some patients are not candidates for breast conservation as they are at high risk for radiation complications. Specific examples include those previously treated with radiation, women who are pregnant, and patients with certain connective tissue diseases. For women early in the course of their pregnancy, radiation scatters from irradiation of the intact breast can reach lethal and teratogenic dose levels.[246] Collagen vascular diseases, such as systemic scleroderma, polymyositis, dermatomyositis, lupus erythematosus, and mixed connective tissue disorders have been associated with significant risks, including breast fibrosis and pain, chest wall necrosis, and brachial plexopathy.[247]

Technical considerations

In order to achieve optimal cosmetic outcomes, incisions should be planned based on the extent of tumor in the breast, the location of the tumor, and plans for reshaping the breast to restore the contour and symmetry. The extent of parenchymal resection depends on tumor size although larger resections may be performed when the oncologic procedure is performed in the setting of breast reduction surgery. Oncoplastic surgical techniques are now commonly performed on the index breast at the time of tumor resection, with or without a contralateral symmetry procedure, in order to achieve optimal cosmesis and prevent the need for a second surgical procedure. Oncoplastic surgery can range from local tissue rearrangement to mastopexy or reduction depending on the tumor size, the parenchymal defect, the degree of ptosis, and whether resection of skin is planned to achieve negative margins. If there is significant volume loss due to parenchymal or skin resection, local flaps can be performed to fill the defect and restore the contour of the breast. A breast reduction procedure can be utilized in patients with a large breast size who have larger tumors or when there is multifocal or multicentric disease. Reducing the degree of ptosis in women with larger breasts can also facilitate the delivery of radiation therapy and reduce skin toxicity.

Careful planning of incision placement facilitates the removal of the tumor without the need for extensive tunneling through the breast. Periareolar incisions can be used for tumors located in any quadrant of the breast but can increase the difficulty of resection depending on the distance from the nipple. When oncoplastic surgery is performed at the same procedure, it is important to leave clips in the tumor resection cavity for postoperative radiation treatment planning and to facilitate re-excision should the final margins be positive. When a mastopexy or reduction mammoplasty is being performed, the same incisions can be utilized for resection and reconstruction. In instances where lumpectomy cannot be carried out because of the inability to obtain tumor-free margins, mastectomy incisions can be modified to accommodate the lumpectomy incision.

Skin removal is generally not required in BCS unless there is direct tumor extension or concern about achieving a negative margin. Removal of skin can lead to displacement of the nipple–areolar complex and asymmetry with the contralateral breast. Skin edges should not be undermined when the excision is being performed, as this can lead to thin flaps with poor perfusion.

Tumor removal and examination of specimen margins

The tumor resection should be performed with the intent of achieving a margin of normal tissue in all directions around the lesion. Nonpalpable lesions or those with extensive microcalcifications require preoperative localization with wires or nonwire guided techniques (radioactive seeds, magnetic seeds, etc.). A specimen radiograph should be performed on the resected specimen to document removal of the target lesion and removal of the localizing device and any biopsy clips. While it is typical to use sutures marking the lateral (long stitch) and superior (short stitch) margins, recent studies have shown that three points of orientation (clip anterior or ink posterior)[248] improves the accuracy of margin orientation. At our institution, we also obtain a second specimen radiograph after the specimen has been inked and sectioned. This improves the chance of identifying positive margins that can be re-excised at the same surgery reducing the need for a second operative procedure to achieve negative margins (Figure 15).

Radiographic and pathologic assessment intraoperatively can be helpful to assess the need for additional resection; however, definitive margin assessment is better done with permanent sections in a detailed manner. If one or more margins are found to be involved microscopically following BCS, a multidisciplinary discussion should be the next step to determine if re-excision is recommended.[249] In some circumstances of microscopically

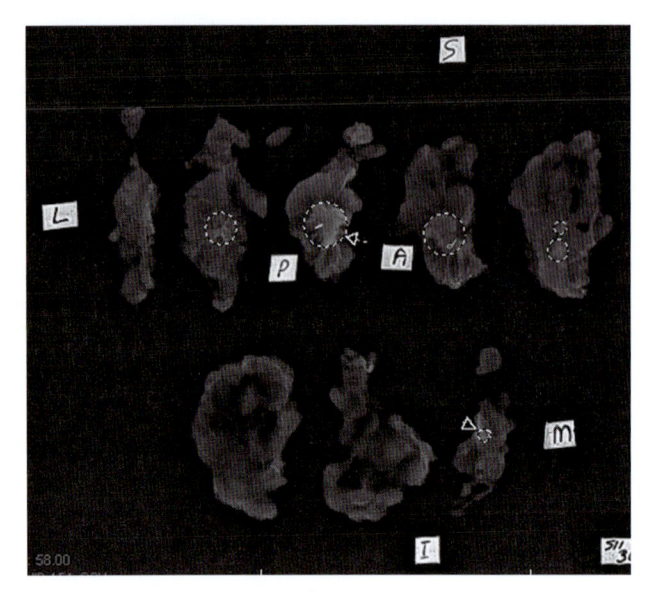

Figure 15 Sectioned specimen radiograph.

positive margins, when it is clear that gross tumor has not been transected, it may be appropriate to proceed with radiation and systemic therapy. Some studies have shown that recurrence rates are the same for focally positive margins as for true negative ones.[250] Many pathologists infer margin involvement by subjective designations as tumor "very close" to a margin. It is preferred that the pathologist measure the distance from the tumor to the inked margin to include in the final pathology report. This is also part of the synoptic reporting template required by the College of American Pathologists (CAP) for reporting on breast resection specimens. Multiple wires or seeds can be placed in the breast to bracket large areas of calcifications or multifocal lesions. Specimen radiograph can confirm the presence of the lesion(s) as well as the location relative to the margins. Nonpalpable lesions can also be localized using ultrasound in radiology preoperatively or intraoperatively by the radiologist or surgeon who has been trained to use ultrasound and is skilled in interventional ultrasound techniques.

Mastectomy

Patients who undergo mastectomy for early-stage breast cancer are considered for immediate breast reconstruction unless they have significant medical comorbidities that would increase their risk for perioperative complications. Patients with advanced disease who require comprehensive chest wall and nodal irradiation are usually considered for delayed reconstruction. Cosmetic considerations are important, regardless of whether the patient chooses reconstruction or prefers to go flat. It is important to try to leave a flat surface on the chest wall so that wearing a prosthesis is possible and comfortable. Avoiding excess skin in the lateral chest wall and axilla can be accomplished through techniques such as V-Y advancement flap or other plastic surgery techniques to avoid excess skin and lateral fullness. Immediate reconstruction has been shown to be safe,[251] when appropriate multidisciplinary planning is used. When mastectomy is preferred or required, the patient should be educated about reconstructive options, both immediate and delayed. Complications after reconstruction are common and should be fully discussed with the patient by both the oncologic and reconstructive surgeons. It is important to discuss expectations regarding cosmetic outcomes and that multiple surgical procedures may be required to optimize the reconstructive outcome. When immediate breast reconstruction is performed, this can increase the length of surgery and postoperative recovery and requires patient and caregiver education for optimal outcomes.

For women who are ambivalent about reconstruction, delayed reconstruction may be optimal. However, cosmetic outcomes are better when reconstruction is performed immediately, since more skin can be preserved and scars can be minimized and tailored to the type of reconstruction that has been chosen. It may be difficult to make decisions about reconstruction within a short interval, and women who are deciding should be reassured that an extra week or two to consider their options and make good decisions will not impact their survival outcome.

Two basic types of reconstruction can be offered: implant-based reconstruction and autologous tissue reconstruction. Implants can be placed directly or following use of tissue expanders (TEs). Expanders are the most commonly used form of reconstruction and can be placed under the pectoralis muscle or on top of the muscle with an overlay of acellular dermal matrix. The pocket is gradually expanded until it is larger than the desired breast size. Then the expander is exchanged for a permanent implant and the breast shape is contoured. The entire process can take several months. An alternative technique, used in conjunction with skin-sparing mastectomy (SSM) or nipple-sparing mastectomy (NSM), is the direct placement of permanent implants. The majority of implants used for reconstruction are saline. Silicone implants had been pulled off the market because of a concern that they increased the risk for developing autoimmune disease; however, several large studies have failed to show a definitive connection, and as a result, silicone implants are once again an option for reconstruction.[252]

Decisions about the type of reconstruction depend largely on patient preference, although treatment considerations can also play an important role. If radiation is anticipated, most reconstructive surgeons prefer to delay autologous tissue reconstruction since radiation can cause shrinkage of the flap and lead to fat necrosis. While flaps can tolerate radiation, there have been several published reports detailing significant deleterious effects on the flap from radiation. There could be a difference in toxicities between pedicled flaps versus free flaps, and the higher doses of radiation (up to 6500 cGy including the boost) utilized in patients with more advanced disease resulting in higher complication rates. More recently, some institutions are utilizing neoadjuvant radiation therapy followed by immediate reconstruction with free flaps or implant-based reconstruction. Evaluation of outcomes including complication rates, local–regional control, and cosmetic outcomes will help to determine whether this approach is favored over adjuvant postoperative radiation therapy.

Another technique for mastectomy is the total SSM or NSM, which has been increasingly utilized for prophylactic and therapeutic mastectomy.[253,254] This technique removes all of the breast tissue, including the tissue behind the nipple and areola, but preserves the overlying dermis. There have been numerous single institution and multicenter reports that show the technique is reliable and that various incisions can be used to achieve excellent results. Although follow-up is limited, early results show that the local recurrence rate is extremely low (<2%). Systematic reviews have shown that the total skin-sparing technique does not result in a higher local recurrence risk. The key is the complete resection of the mammary gland with the removal of the ductal tissue behind the nipple. This technique can be combined with any reconstructive technique including direct to implant reconstruction. There have been some reports of increased rates of skin and nipple necrosis with direct to implant reconstruction with complete filling of the TE. The plan for reconstruction is largely dependent on the perfusion of the skin flaps following mastectomy. The NSM is technically more challenging in order to assure removal of the entire mammary gland but definitely offers superior cosmetic results. Relative contraindications include those with extensive DCIS, tumors within 2 cm of the nipple areolar complex, and those with significant ptosis.

Axillary lymph node dissection

Axillary lymph node dissection (ALND) has historically been utilized for axillary staging in patients with clinically negative nodes and for regional control in those with axillary lymph node metastasis.

ALND is performed through an incision below the axillary hairline and typically includes level 1 and level 2 nodes, with level 3 dissection reserved for patients with advanced nodal disease. The boundaries of the axillary dissection include the latissimus dorsi muscle laterally, the axillary vein superiorly, and the pectoralis minor muscle medially. Removal of the pectoralis minor muscle is not required to access the level 2 nodes which lie posterior to the pectoralis minor. The nerves to the serratus anterior (long thoracic) and latissimus dorsi (thoracodorsal) muscles should be identified and preserved. There are several branches of the intercostal brachial nerves that course through the axilla that can be preserved as well. The axillary vein should be visualized and followed under the pectoralis minor muscle to the medial border. The average number of nodes removed in a level 1 and 2 ALND is about 15–20.

Sentinel lymph node dissection

The management of the axilla has changed significantly since the introduction of sentinel node dissection. This procedure limits the extent of surgery in the axilla and, for patients with negative axillary lymph nodes, precludes the need for formal ALND. The concept of sentinel node dissection is that there is a node or nodes that drain from a specific anatomic region of the breast and identification and removal of these sentinel node(s) permits the pathologist to perform a more detailed assessment that would not be feasible with the entire contents of an ALND. The detection of micrometastases is significantly increased by combining light microscopy, immunohistochemistry, and even more sensitive molecular techniques. The identification of occult metastasis in the sentinel nodes is more frequent using more sensitive techniques although most studies suggest that isolated tumor cells should not be used in clinical decision-making regarding chemotherapy, radiation therapy, or more extensive axillary surgery. Several large cooperative group studies have examined the role of sentinel node biopsy, including the National Surgical Adjuvant Breast and Bowel Project (NSABP) and the American College of Surgeons Oncology Group (ACOSOG). The ACOSOG Z0010 trial enrolled patients with clinically negative lymph nodes and subjected H&E negative sentinel nodes to immunohistochemistry for cytokeratin. Isolated tumor cells and small metastatic deposits identified on central review did not impact prognosis or local–regional control. The NSABP B-32 trial randomized 5611 women with negative SLNs to either sentinel lymph node dissection (SLND) alone or SLND followed by ALND. Women with positive SLNs proceeded to complete ALND. This study is the largest randomized trial of SLN biopsy versus ALND with 232 participating surgeons from 80 different centers. Local–regional control and survival were not different between patients undergoing ALND versus SLN surgery alone.[255] On average, three SLNs were removed per patient; the SLN identification rate was 97.2% and improved with surgeon experience. There were 26% of patients with a positive SLN. In 61.5% with a positive SLN, the additional axillary nodes were negative (38.5% had additional positive nodes). The false-negative rate (axillary lymph node involvement when the SLN was negative) was 9.7%, which did not change with the experience of the surgeon. The false-negative rate (FNR) was significantly affected by the type of biopsy used for diagnosis, 8.0% in those with FNA or core biopsy, 14.3% with incisional biopsy, and 15.2% after excisional biopsy. The number of SLNs identified was also important with a lower FNR in those with 2 or more SLNs removed. Nomograms have been developed that predict the likelihood of a positive SLN based on clinical and pathologic factors of the primary tumor.

The technique of SLN dissection was first performed with vital blue dyes but later included a combination of blue dye with radiotracer materials which increased identification rates and reduced FNRs. The ACOSOG Z0011 trial was designed to assess whether the addition of ALND versus SLND alone improved survival outcomes in patients with one or two positive SLN undergoing BCS and whole breast irradiation. There was no difference in local–regional recurrence or survival between the two groups, but the rates of lymphedema were lower after SLND (<7%) compared with ALND (17–25%).[256]

The use of SLND for axillary staging following neoadjuvant chemotherapy[257] has been debated as the initial reports showed lower identification rates and higher false-negative rates, especially in patients with initial node-positive disease at diagnosis. The benefits of using SLND after neoadjuvant therapy are that the patient is spared an additional operation before starting chemotherapy—they may avoid ALND as tumor positive nodes may respond to chemotherapy—and that the information about the presence of tumor in the nodes after chemotherapy is beneficial in determining prognosis and determining the need for adjuvant systemic and radiation therapy.[258] Intraoperative detection of SLN metastases is beneficial as it enables the surgeon to proceed to a full axillary dissection if necessary, thereby avoiding a second procedure. There have been several prospective trials evaluating the FNR of SLND following chemotherapy in patients with initial node-positive disease including ACOSOG Z1071, SENTINA, and SN FNAC. The trials all demonstrated FNRs in the 12–14% range. The FNR was decreased in all three trials with dual tracer mapping (blue dye with radioactive tracer), removal of three or more SLNs, and use of immunohistochemistry for cytokeratin to detect occult metastases.

More recently, the technique of targeted axillary dissection (TAD) has been described to increase the accuracy of axillary staging following neoadjuvant chemotherapy.[259] TAD relies on clip placement at the time of initial lymph node biopsy and SLND with localization of the clipped axillary node at the time of surgery. Localization of the clipped node prior to surgery (wire or non-wire guided localization) is necessary as the clipped node is not identified as a sentinel node in 25% of cases. TAD is currently being examined as an alternative to ALND in selected patients with initial node-positive disease and a favorable response to systemic therapy. There are two important ongoing clinical trials evaluating local–regional management of patients with the initial node-positive disease following neoadjuvant chemotherapy. The Alliance A011202 trial randomizes patients with positive SLNs to ALND plus postoperative radiation versus radiation alone. The NSABP B-51 trial randomizes patients with a pCR in the axilla to regional nodal irradiation (RNI) versus no radiation.

As these data mature, the role of sentinel node dissection and axillary dissection will need to be clarified in the setting of pCR after neoadjuvant therapy. The increasing use of SLND after neoadjuvant chemotherapy in women regardless of nodal status

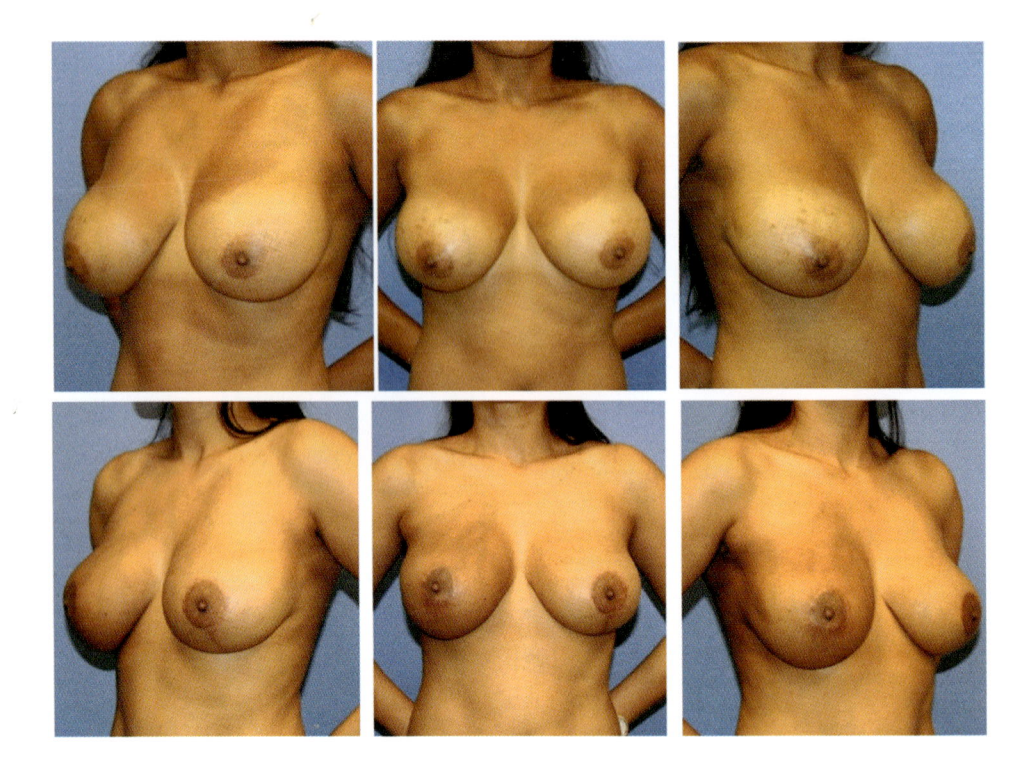

Figure 16 A 42-year-old female with a 2 cm invasive ductal carcinoma of the right breast. She was treated with a lumpectomy and an immediate bilateral circumareolar mastopexy. Bottom photos are 2 years postoperatively.

pretreatment is an example of modifying the extent of surgical treatment based on response to therapy. The need for ALND has also been questioned in older women with ER-positive disease who are planned for adjuvant endocrine therapy. In this setting, the status of the axillary nodes would not likely alter the decision about the administration of adjuvant therapy. In almost all cases with a clinically negative axilla, however, SLND is a standard part of staging and surgical management and can be successfully performed in most women with very low morbidity. In the setting of positive SLNs, a level 1 and 2 ALND is considered standard management for patients who fall outside of the Z0011 criteria.

Reconstructive surgery

Reconstruction in the setting of breast-conservation therapy

The goal of BCT is to remove the tumor with negative margins while preserving the contour and shape of the breast. Increasingly, oncoplastic surgeries are performed as a joint procedure between breast surgery and plastic surgery to achieve optimal cosmesis. In a series of 9861 patients treated at the MD Anderson Cancer Center, combining oncoplastic reconstruction with BCT compared to BCT alone lowered the rate of seroma formation (13.4% vs 18%; $p = 0.002$) and positive or close margins (5.8% vs 8.3%; $p = 0.04$)[260] while not compromising OS or recurrence-free survival.[261] Oncoplastic surgery is useful and several studies have confirmed long-term outcomes and patient satisfaction (Figure 16). In order to achieve the best cosmetic results, incisions should be planned based on the extent of tumor in the breast, the location of the tumor, and the original shape of the breast. Traditionally, BCT was reserved for early-stage disease; however, oncoplastic techniques have expanded the indications to larger tumors and multifocal disease in select patients.[240,241] The extent of tissue resection depends on the tumor size and breast size.

Plastic surgery techniques can be used to improve symmetry, both with and without surgery on the contralateral breast. Once the breast tissue is removed, care is taken to not rotate any tissue away from the ablation cavity. Breast surgeons will place a number of medium-sized clips to demarcate the ablation cavity edges, and these ideally should be collapsed upon themselves so that the cavity appears as a small contained area of clips on postoperative imaging to facilitate disease surveillance and focus the delivery of radiation therapy (Figure 17). Smaller defects are amendable to reconstruction with local tissue rearrangement. The technique proceeds by undermining the breast tissue at the level of the fascia which provides the opportunity to arrange the closure of the breast tissue in a medial to lateral direction, thereby avoiding the displacement of the nipple either superiorly or inferiorly. Mastopexy or reduction can be performed on the contralateral breast to improve symmetry based upon the patient's goals of reconstruction. Mastopexy techniques include Benelli (donut), circumareolar, circumvertical, and Wise patterns. If there is a significant degree of ptosis in the breast, a partial mastectomy can be accomplished by performing a breast reduction, thereby combining a cosmetic enhancement with the oncologic procedure of removing the breast tissue. In a breast reduction procedure, more than half of the breast tissue can be removed; thus, this technique can be used for larger tumors or when there is extensive *in situ* disease in a single quadrant.

Incisions do not necessarily need to be placed directly over the tumor in order to perform a satisfactory lumpectomy. For example, tunneling from either a periareolar incision or inframammary fold incision will lessen the stigmata of breast scars (Figure 18). If there is concern that a mastectomy may eventually be necessary, the incision should be made with some thought as to what type of incision would be made if a mastectomy were required such as a radial incision medial or lateral of the nipple. In instances where lumpectomy cannot be carried out because of the inability to obtain tumor-free margins, mastectomy incisions can be modified

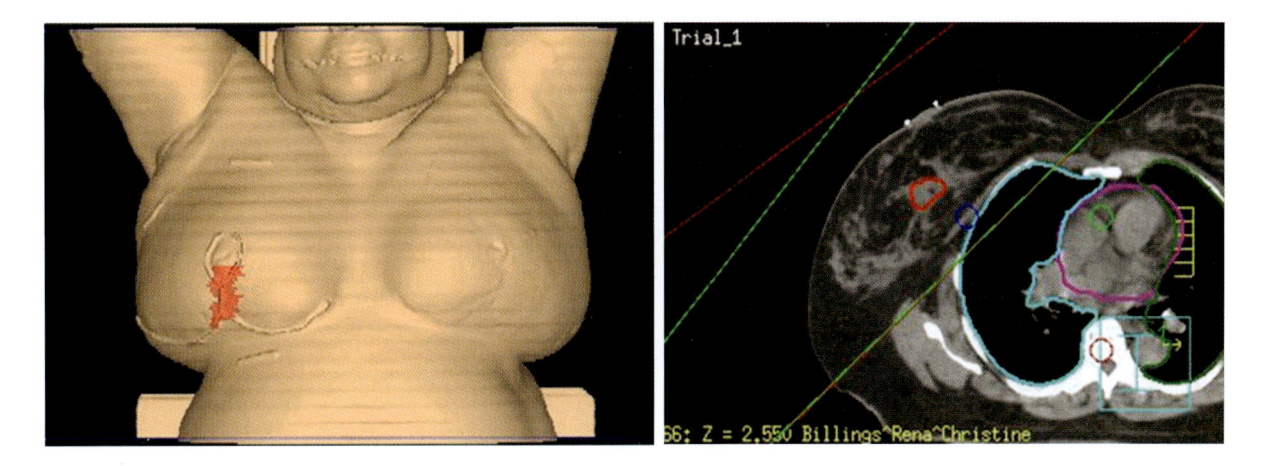

Figure 17 *Collapsing of the ablation cavity.* Once the breast tissue is resected, care is taken to not rotate any tissue away from the ablation cavity. Postoperative imaging is shown following oncoplastic breast reduction with a Wise pattern of tissue reduction (a). Breast surgeons place a number of medium-sized clips to demarcate the ablation cavity edges, and these ideally should be collapsed upon themselves so that the cavity appears as a small contained area l of clips on postoperative imaging to facilitate disease surveillance and focus radiation delivery (b).

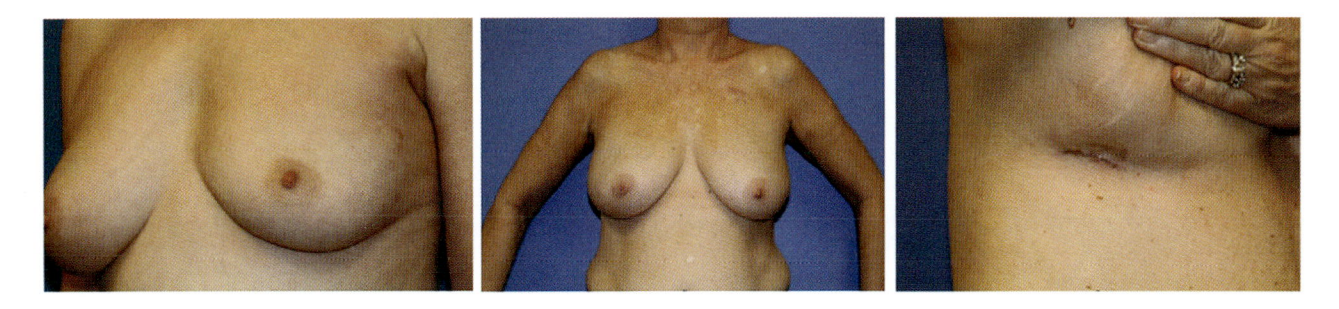

Figure 18 The appearance of postoperative scars can be minimized by placing incisions either in the skin along the areola transition or within the inframammary fold. This requires tunneling to the lumpectomy site. A periareolar incision is demonstrated in panel a and an inframammary fold incision is demonstrated in panels b and c.

to accommodate the lumpectomy incision. Skin removal is not required for lumpectomy. If a prior biopsy was performed, skin encompassing the biopsy scar can be removed when lumpectomy is done, but it is not essential.

Postmastectomy breast reconstruction
Prior to a mastectomy, patients should undergo consultation with plastic and reconstructive surgery to have an extensive discussion of their options, and the risks and benefits of possible procedures. The Women's Health and Cancer Rights Act of 1998 requires health plans that offer breast cancer coverage to also provide for breast reconstruction and prostheses. Despite this, less than half of all women requiring a mastectomy are currently offered breast reconstruction surgery.[242] The 2016 Breast Cancer Patient Education Act requires the Secretary of Health and Human Services to plan and implement an education campaign to inform breast cancer patients about the availability and coverage of breast reconstruction and other available alternatives postmastectomy. The disbursement of educational materials during the discussion of mastectomy is important to inform women of their right to breast reconstruction under federal law and provide women with information about when breast reconstruction or prostheses may be appropriate within their recovery plan. Patients who undergo mastectomy can opt for reconstruction or not, and any procedure should be agreed upon through shared decision-making. Aesthetic considerations are important, regardless of the diagnosis of breast cancer.

Immediate reconstruction has been shown to be safe, even in the setting of locally advanced disease and should be offered to patients with all stages of disease, when appropriate multimodal therapy is used (Figure 19). Therefore, any woman considering mastectomy should also be told about options for reconstruction, both immediate and delayed. Complications after reconstruction are common and should be expected by both the surgeon and patient. The most common complications include infection (9–16%), explantation (5–9%), seroma (6–11%), and hematoma (1%) with an overall complication rate of 24–38%.[262] Expectations about outcomes should be appropriately set, and women should be prepared for the possibility of multiple surgical procedures to optimize the reconstructive outcome.

For women who are ambivalent about reconstruction, delayed reconstruction may be optimal. However, cosmetic outcomes are better when reconstruction is performed immediately, the breast "footprint" can be preserved, and scars can be minimized and tailored to the type of reconstruction that has been chosen.

Implants can be placed as expanders or permanent implants. Expanders are the most commonly used form of immediate reconstruction. They are placed most commonly on top of the pectoralis muscle (prepectoral) and the skin envelope is gradually expanded until is it larger than the desired breast size. Expanders are most

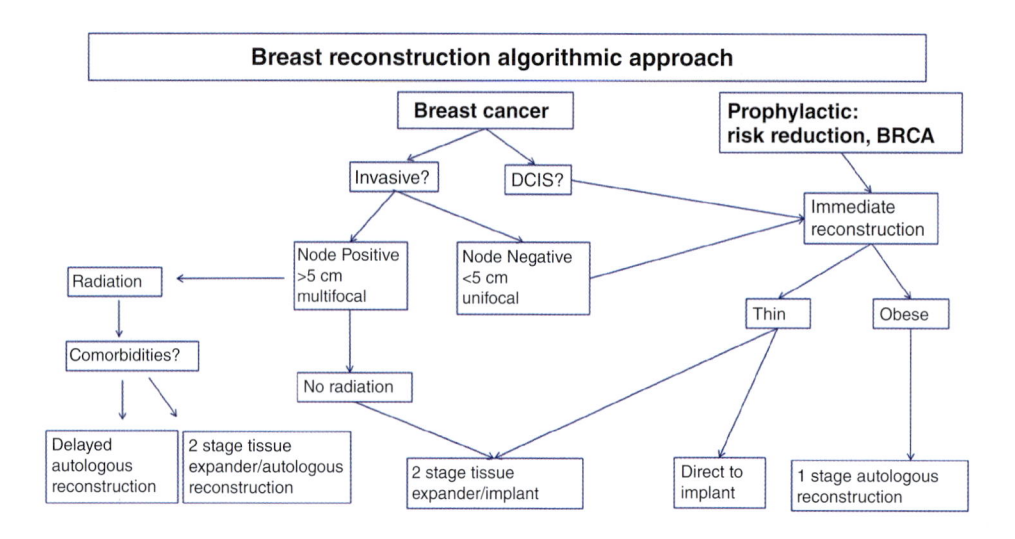

Figure 19 Postmastectomy breast reconstruction algorithm.

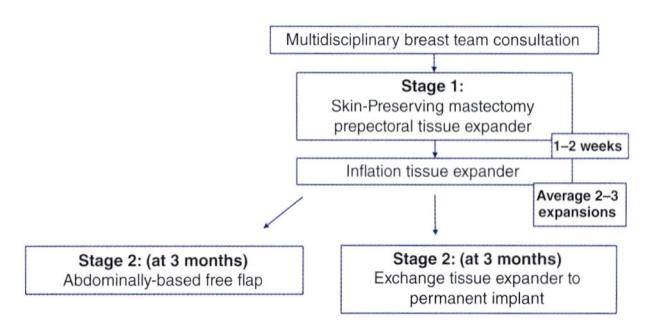

Figure 20 Two-stage breast reconstruction with tissue expander placement followed by implant exchange or conversion to autologous reconstruction.

commonly air filled at the time of surgery to reduce pressure on mastectomy skin flaps which is then exchanged to saline 1–2 weeks postoperatively. Then the expander is exchanged for a permanent implant and the breast shape is contoured. The entire process can take 2–3 months. (Figure 20). An alternative technique, used in conjunction with NSM, is the immediate placement of permanent implants. Modern generation silicone implants are solid highly cohesive silicone used to decrease the spread of contents in the event of a rupture. Implants and TEs are most commonly smooth surface as rough or textured surface implants have been found to be associated with the occurrence of an uncommon malignancy, breast implant-associated anaplastic large cell lymphoma (BIA-ALCL). This association led to a 2019 FDA Class I device recall of Allergan corporation textured surface implants and TEs, which were the most commonly placed devices worldwide at the time.[263] Importantly, this disease is most commonly treated with surgical resection alone, is highly curative in the majority of patients, and there are no recommendations for prophylactic explantation in patients with existing devices. Consequently, the majority of implants and expanders placed worldwide are now smooth surface.

Autologous tissue reconstruction most commonly employs abdominal-based tissue. Flaps include the deep inferior epigastric artery perforator (DIEP) flap, muscle-sparing transverse rectus abdominis muscle (msTRAM) flap, and the superficial inferior epigastric artery (SIEA) flap. Pedicled TRAM flaps and full muscle TRAM flaps have increasingly fallen out of favor due to concerns of donor site morbidity. Secondary autologous options include the posterior artery perforator (PAP) flap and the pedicled latissimus dorsi flap in combination with an implant.

Decisions about the type of reconstruction depend largely on patient preference, although treatment considerations can also play an important role. If radiation is anticipated, complications are less if autologous tissue is used to reconstruct the breast following radiation therapy. Radiation causes significant deleterious effects on DIEP and TRAM flaps and therefore autologous reconstruction is generally delayed until after the delivery of radiation therapy.

There are growing trends in breast surgery toward NSM. This technique removes all breast tissue, excluding the tissue of the areola, nipple, and the overlying dermis. This technique can be combined with any reconstructive technique including the use of permanent implants. The immediate expansion of the skin is dependent upon the preserved vascularity of the skin flaps. Flap thickness is not as important as the preservation of intercostal perforators coming off the internal mammary vessels. Flaps may be thick or thin, but it is the intact arborization of the vascular tree that is essential for mastectomy skin flap survival (Figure 21). The opportunity to use NSM is particularly important when considering prophylactic mastectomy for women at highest risk and may enable them to feel comfortable about the cosmetic result to undergo the surgery.

Managing lymphedema following axillary dissection
Lymphedema of the arm is characterized by regional swelling because of the accumulation of protein-rich fluid within body tissues, leading to disfigurement and decreased mobility and function. Lymphedema rates after SLND are reported to be <7% compared with 17–25% with ALND.[256] In one study over 1400 patients with a positive SNLB were randomized to receive either axillary dissection or axillary irradiation, and at 6 years there was no statistical difference in axillary recurrence. The rate of upper extremity lymphedema was significantly higher for patients who underwent dissection.[243,264] It affects approximately 21% of breast cancer survivors with variable incidence depending on the type of surgery. In addition to decreased functionality, patients experience paresthesia, pain, and psychologic distress, resulting in a reduced quality of life (QOL). Early physiotherapy, including manual lymph drainage, massage of scar tissue, and shoulder exercises, starting within days of surgery results in a lower incidence of lymphedema. Treatment options for lymphedema include physical therapy to

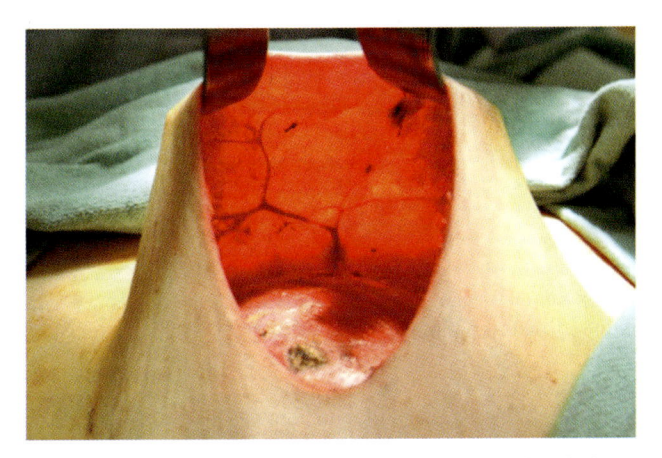

Figure 21 Perforator-sparing mastectomy. Mastectomy skin flap thickness is not as important as the preservation of intercostal perforators coming off of the internal mammary vessels. Flaps may be thick or thin, depending on body habitus, but it is the intact arborization of the vascular tree that is essential for mastectomy skin flap survival.

optimize range of motion, progressive resistance training with compression garments, weight loss, and properly fitted compression garments. Operative therapies include lymphovenous bypass and lymph node transfer.[265] The lymphovenous bypass procedure involves identification of obstructed lymphatic vessels and targeted bypass of these into neighboring venules. The vascularized lymph node transplant procedure involves microvascular anastomosis of functional lymph nodes into an extremity, either to an anatomical (orthotopic) or nonanatomical (heterotopic) location, to restore physiologic lymphatic function. Observational case-control and cohort studies support the efficacy of lymphovenous bypass and vascularized lymph node transplantation for lymphedema in reduction of limb volume and episodes of cellulitis.[266] Increasingly, select patients undergoing axillary dissection are offered prophylactic lymphovenous bypass at the time of initial surgery.

Integrating postmastectomy radiation therapy (PMRT) with breast reconstruction

Two trends on a collision course over the last decade have been the expanding indications for postmastectomy radiation therapy (PMRT), particularly in younger patients, versus the increasing use of elective mastectomy combined with reconstruction in this population. While breast reconstruction, both implant- and tissue flap-based, poses certain challenges for the treating radiation oncologist, it should never be considered a contraindication to PMRT. While plastic surgery practice patterns are highly variable, there are certain common principles that have developed over time. In general, immediate reconstruction (in a patient requiring PMRT) is best accomplished with a TE/implant-based technique. This is the most popular modality as it consolidates surgical procedures and allows full-tissue expansion through the months long course of adjuvant chemotherapy and or radiation therapy. TEs are most commonly placed in a prepectoral position with an acellular dermal matrix wrap for soft tissue support. The TE may be swapped for the permanent implant before PMRT or left in place through the course of PMRT, allowing its deflation to improve radiation dosimetry.[267,268] Alternatively, autologous flap techniques are the procedures of choice for delayed reconstruction, where vascularized tissue is brought into the irradiated field for improved wound healing and cosmetic results. Increasingly, patients are receiving neoadjuvant radiation therapy which allows for the immediate reconstruction of a mastectomy patient with autologous tissue.

Radiation therapy

For more than 100 years, radiation has had a vital function in the effective treatment of breast cancer. Radiation therapy is a component of care for the majority of breast cancer patients at some point during the course of their disease. At present, radiation therapy is undergoing a technological renaissance, creating challenges and controversies in the balance of evidence-based medicine and personalized, highly technical care. The hope is that advancing technology can bring cost-effective efficient radiotherapy solutions to nations with limited resources and limited access to radiotherapy.

Role of radiation in breast-conserving surgery (BCS) for ductal carcinoma *in situ* (DCIS)

Before the advent of screening, DCIS comprised about 3% of breast cancers detected. DCIS now accounts for approximately 20–25% of screen-detected breast cancers. Long-term combined follow-up of the NSABP B-17 and B-24 trials shows that an *invasive* recurrence after surgery only for DCIS increases the risk of breast cancer-related death and that radiation reduces this risk of invasive recurrence by more than half (19.4% vs 8.9%).[269–271] As such, NCCN guidelines recommend whole breast radiation after BCS for standard risk DCIS.[272]

An ongoing therapeutic question related to the treatment of "low-risk" DCIS is the role of omitting radiotherapy after BCS. Risk factors for in-breast recurrence that influence the decision to omit whole breast radiation include age >50, small tumor size, low grade, lack of clinical symptoms, and wide margin width. In 1998, the Radiation Therapy Oncology Group (RTOG) initiated a trial for selected women with low-/intermediate-grade DCIS ≤ 2.5 cm in the highest extent with ≥3-mm margins.[273] Unfortunately, the study was ended in 2006 due to poor accrual; however, in the 636 patients enrolled, radiation reduced the local failure rate from 11.4% to 2.8% at 12 years ($p = 0.0001$).[274] The clinical impact of this small absolute benefit is up for discussion, and patients must be counseled regarding the trade-offs of toxicity and inconvenience of adjuvant radiation versus the higher risk of a (possibly invasive) recurrence and need for subsequent salvage therapy. An emerging clinical tool to counsel patients and tailor adjuvant recommendations for DCIS may be genomic sequencing. In a tissue analysis of over 300 patients treated on the ECOG 5194 trial, the 21-gene Oncotype DX assay (see section on adjuvant therapy) was used to assign a score according to the risk of invasive recurrence and was found to be predictive for recurrence, independent of clinical factors.[275] An alternative immunohistochemistry-based test PreludeDX estimated DCIS risk in a multisite study of 474 patients.[276] It remains to be seen whether biology-based strategies provide cost-effective utility over the currently used clinical selection factors, such as age, tumor grade, tumor size, and margin width.

Among DCIS patients, breast cancer-specific mortality is associated with age at diagnosis, ethnicity, and DCIS characteristics such as ER status, grade, size (>5 cm), and comedonecrosis. Despite their significance in a multivariable analysis, high-risk characteristics, such as ER-negativity and high grade, often overlap. Only a small minority of patients will have one or more of these high-risk characteristics. Young women (<40 years of age) who present with symptomatic DCIS, such as a palpable mass or nipple discharge, comprise about 5% of the DCIS population and represent a different disease than the average DCIS. In addition, African American women and patients with hormone-receptor negative DCIS are at higher risk of breast cancer-specific mortality and should continue to be treated according to the current standards. In total, these groups probably constitute about 20% of the population of DCIS patients.

Role of radiation for early-stage invasive disease

Defining the role of radiation in BCT has been the focus of numerous randomized prospective clinical trials conducted over the past 30 years.[277,278] Together, these trials have demonstrated that radiation after breast-conserving surgery significantly improves local control, minimizes the risk of subsequent distant metastases, and decreases breast cancer death rates.

The NSABP B-06 trial was one of the first randomized studies to evaluate the benefit of radiation after lumpectomy. This trial showed that for patients treated with BCS, WBRT offered significant clinical benefits. After 20 years, the recurrence rates in the breast were 40% and 14% for those treated with lumpectomy only and lumpectomy plus WBRT, respectively. The almost two-thirds reduction in the risk of recurrence (ROR) was very similar to reductions observed in other similarly designed trials.[279] The data from NSABP B-06 and 16 other randomized prospective clinical trials assessing the role of radiation for patients with invasive disease treated with breast conservation have been analyzed by the Early Breast Cancer Trialists Collaborative Group (EBCTCG). In this large meta-analysis, the individual patient data from 10,801 women were studied. Breast irradiation after lumpectomy reduced the 10-year rate of any recurrence from 31% to 16% for patients with negative lymph nodes and from 64% to 43% for patients with positive lymph nodes. More importantly, radiation use significantly decreased the 15-year risk of dying from breast cancer. For patients with negative lymph nodes, breast cancer mortality decreased from 20% to 17% and for patients with positive lymph nodes, it decreased from 51% to 43%.[280]

Use of a "boost" after WBRT

A strategy to reduce local recurrence after WBRT even further is dose escalation via an additional boost of radiation to the tissue at the highest risk in the postoperative tumor bed. The first randomized trial investigating the impact of a 1000-cGy lumpectomy bed boost following 5000-cGy WBRT was performed in Lyons, France. The use of a boost led to a small but statistically significant reduction in the rates of local recurrence at 5 years (3.6% vs 4.5%; $p = 0.04$).[281] Subsequently, the EORTC completed a much larger trial that randomized over 5000 patients to 5000-cGy WBRT with or without an additional tumor bed boost of 1600 cGy. This trial again demonstrated a reduced breast recurrence rate in patients treated with a boost (10.2% vs 6.2% at 10 years; $p < 0.001$).[282] In a subset analysis, this benefit was noted across all age groups but was most pronounced in younger women. Given the now well-understood association of local recurrence risk and receptor subtype of breast cancer, it is reasonable to personalize the use of a boost, with consideration of omission in postmenopausal women with low grade, strongly ER+ early breast cancers. There is also data to support the omission of a radiation boost in patients with HER2-positive disease who have an exceptional response to neoadjuvant systemic therapy.[283]

Omission of radiation for selected patients

Although the data are conclusive that radiation is beneficial for the majority of patients treated with breast-conserving surgery, identifying subsets of patients who do well with surgery only remains an area of active study. Initial trials for the omission of radiation used tumor size to stratify patients with low-risk disease and were unable to show that surgery alone was an acceptable option. A trial conducted in Milan, Italy, randomized patients who underwent quadrantectomy and axillary clearance for tumors ≤2.5 cm to undergo WBRT versus no further therapy. The 10-year results showed that radiation reduced the breast recurrence rate from 24% to 6% ($p < 0.001$).[284] For patients with even smaller primary tumors (stage I), randomized trials in Sweden and Finland showed that radiation reduced the 5-year breast recurrence rate from 18% to 2% ($p < 0.0001$) and from 14.1% to 6.2% ($p = 0.029$), respectively.[285,286]

There has been a question about the need for radiation in the setting of improving systemic therapy. Data from early trials have also indicated that the use of systemic treatment (either chemotherapy or tamoxifen) does not negate the benefit of breast radiation. In the aforementioned NSABP B-06 trial, chemotherapy was used in patients with lymph node-positive disease, and the 20-year breast recurrence rate for these patients was decreased from 44% to 9% when radiation was used.[279] A trial from Scotland that required systemic treatment for all of the 589 enrolled patients yielded a 6-year breast recurrence rate of 6% in the surgery, systemic therapy, and radiation arm versus 25% in patients randomized to forego radiation.[287]

Four more modern trials conducted among very low-risk subgroups of patients diagnosed in the mammographic era have further refined the selection criteria.[288–291] In all four of these studies, radiation achieved a statistically significant reduction in breast recurrence rate, although the absolute benefit for some subcategories of patients treated with surgery only was relatively small. The NSABP B-21 trial enrolled patients with node-negative breast cancers whose primary tumors measured ≤1.0 cm. All patients underwent lumpectomy and ALND and were randomized to tamoxifen only, radiation only, or tamoxifen plus radiation.[288] The 8-year risk of IBTR was 16.5% with tamoxifen alone, 9.3% with radiation alone, and 2.8% with the combination. A Canadian trial had very similar eligibility criteria and results with 5-year local relapse rates of 7.7% for tamoxifen alone and 0.6% when combined with radiation.[289] Finally, two trials recently tested the omission of radiation for older women with the early-stage, biologically favorable disease. Long-term results of the CALGB study of stage I ER+ tumors showed that for patients over the age of 70, the 10-year recurrence rates were 10% vs 2% in the tamoxifen only vs tamoxifen plus radiation arms, respectively.[290] Furthermore, there were no differences in the rates of salvage mastectomy, distant metastases, or OS between the two groups. The Scottish PRIME II trial enrolled over 1300 patients with early-stage disease of age ≥65 and found 5-year local recurrence rates of 4% versus 1% for those on tamoxifen only vs tamoxifen plus radiation ($p = 0.0002$), respectively.[291] As the overall benefit from radiation is small in older patients with biologically favorable diseases, this is one cohort for which the addition of radiation should be based on the patients' life expectancy and personal preferences.

Outside of patients over the age of 70 with HR-positive disease, radiation remains standard after BCS. However, future guidelines may incorporate tumor biology into clinical decision-making for adjuvant radiation for younger patients. In a trial of lumpectomy +/− radiation in Toronto-British Columbia, for patients over 60 with luminal A tumors, the 10-year ipsilateral breast recurrence was only 1.3% with lumpectomy alone.[292] Several ongoing trials are prospectively assessing the omission of radiation in patients with favorable tumor biology (ER+, T1N0) as young as 50 years

Table 10 Outcomes for selected randomized clinical trials comparing conventionally fractionated radiotherapy (CFRT) to hypofractionated radiotherapy (HFRT).

Trial	Median follow-up (years)	N	Dose (cGy)	# fractions	IBTR[a] (%)	LRR[a] (%)	DFS[a] (%)	OS[a] (%)	Cosmesis[a] (% good or excellent)	Acute toxicity[a] (% ≥grade 3)
Canada[293]	10	612	5000	25	6.7	—	—	84	71.3	3.0
		622	4250	16	6.2	—	—	85	69.8	3.0
Royal Marsden[294]	10	470	5000	25	12	—	—	—	71	—
		466	4290	13	9.6	—	—	—	74	—
		474	3900	13	15	—	—	—	58[b]	—
START A[295,296]	9	749	5000	25	6.7	7.4	77	80	—	0.3
		750	4160	13	5.6	6.3	77	82	—	0.0
		737	3900	13	8.1	8.8	76	80	—	0.0
START B[296,297]	10	1105	5000	25	5.2	5.5	78	81	—	1.2
		1110	4050	15	3.8	4.3	82[c]	84[c]	—	0.3
MDACC[298]	3	149	5000	25	1	1	99	100	78.2	0.9
		137	4256	16	1	1	99	100	73.2	0

Abbreviations: N, number of patients; FRAC, fractions; IBTR, in-breast tumor recurrence; LRR, locoregional recurrence; DFS, disease-free survival; OS, overall survival.
[a]All statistical p values are nonsignificant in the comparison of CFRT to HFRT, unless otherwise specified.
[b]Measure found to be statistically inferior to CFRT ($p < 0.05$).
[c]Measure found to be statistically superior to CFRT ($p < 0.05$).

old using existing gene assays that are predictive of recurrence. This includes the IDEA trial (NCT02400190), which enrolled postmenopausal patients with low Oncotype Dx recurrence score (RS) (<18), the PRECISION trial (NCT02653755), enrolling women with low PAM50 ROR score, and the EXPERT trial (NCT02889874), randomizing use of radiation in women with a low PAM50 ROR score.

Whole breast radiation dose for early-stage breast cancer
Historically, all breast cancer treatment entailed 25–28 treatments of 180–200 cGy per day to the breast or chest wall with or without the inclusion of lymphatic regions at risk (total dose 4500–5040 cGy). This protracted course is known as conventionally fractionated radiation therapy (CFRT). This treatment was typically followed by five to eight supplemental treatments of 180–200 cGy per day to the tumor bed region (the aforementioned boost) for an additional 1000–1600 cGy. In the first decade of the 2000s, data matured from randomized trials in postlumpectomy patients comparing hypo-fractionated courses of 15–16 fractions of whole breast radiation to 25 fractions, which led to the 15–16 fractions replacing the 25 regimen for most postlumpectomy patients.[293–299] It is anticipated based on new data comparing 15 fractions to 5, this shortened course of 15–16 fractions of hypo-fractionated radiation therapy (HFRT) will be replaced by 5.[300,301]

Some patients treated with lumpectomy for breast cancer fail to receive recommended radiation due to difficulties with access to care. Furthermore, a number of patients who are excellent candidates for BCT elect to be treated with mastectomy to avoid radiation.[302,303] A major factor that contributes to both of these scenarios concerns the inconvenience and expense associated with 5–7 weeks of CFRT. This schedule is particularly burdensome for patients who have significant home or work responsibilities, patients in rural areas who need to travel for access to the nearest radiation facility, and patients who rely on public transportation. In addition, worldwide, there are too few radiation oncologists, facilities, and equipment to offer this type of treatment schedule to all patients with breast cancer who will benefit from radiation. For these reasons, strategies were developed to shorten the radiation treatment schedule and lessen the burdens of time and out-of-pocket expense. With 15–16 fractions of HFRT, the amount of radiation delivered per treatment is increased to decrease the overall treatment course by about one-half. As the amount of radiation per fraction increases, the total dose delivered is commensurately adjusted downward to provide radiobiologic equivalence to CFRT dosing. Results of large randomized trials of HFRT are shown in Table 10.

In 1986, a clinical trial was initiated at the Royal Marsden Hospital, which included approximately 1500 patients randomized to receive CFRT versus one of two HFRT schedules, 3900–4290 cGy in 13 fractions over 5 weeks.[294] The results were promising and led to the establishment of the UK Standardisation of Breast Radiotherapy (START) Trialists' Group, which developed two randomized trials comparing CFRT and HFRT for approximately 4500 women with early-stage breast cancer. In the HFRT arms of the START A trial,[295] patients received either 4160 or 3900 cGy in 13 fractions over 5 weeks, and in START B,[297] patients received a dose of 4050 cGy in 15 fractions over 3 weeks. Long-term follow-up at 10 years in the START trials showed that HFRT is a safe and effective treatment for early-stage breast cancer, equivalent in every way to CFRT.[295–297] During the same period of time, Whelan and colleagues initiated a randomized trial evaluating HFRT (4256 cGy in 16 fractions) in more than 1000 patients with early-stage node-negative breast cancer. After 10 years of follow-up, patients in both arms were noted to have equivalent cosmetic outcomes and recurrence and survival rates.[293,304] Based on the results of these randomized trials, hypofractionation is now the recommended treatment of choice for any early breast cancer patient treated with lumpectomy, who is receiving radiation to the breast +/− the low axilla.[299]

A second strategy, called accelerated partial breast irradiation (APBI), shortens the total treatment time to only 1–2 weeks by both increasing fraction size and minimizing the volume of breast tissue being irradiated. The rationale is that 80% of patients who undergo lumpectomy for small primary tumors have no residual disease after lumpectomy or disease that is within 2 cm of the index cancer.[305] Early studies of interstitial or intracavitary brachytherapy as a method to deliver the radiation dose led to large randomized studies using widely available linear accelerator-based three-dimensional (3D) conformal external beam technology or intensity-modulated external radiotherapy techniques.[306–311] During interstitial or intracavitary brachytherapy, patients have catheters implanted around (multicatheter technique) or directly into (balloon catheter technique) the lumpectomy cavity. Subsequently, high-dose-rate radioactive seeds are temporarily placed within the catheters in two sessions per day for 5 days. 3D conformal external beam APBI and IMRT use sophisticated external beam planning to replicate the favorable dosimetry of brachytherapy with a noninvasive technique.[309]

NSABP and RTOG sponsored a phase III trial (NSABP B-39/RTOG 0413) of over 4000 patients with stage 0, I, or II breast cancer randomized to undergo CFRT or APBI (brachytherapy or 3D conformal external beam).[310] In the same timeframe, investigators in Canada, New Zealand, and Australia conducted a similar study called the RAPID trial, of 2135 women randomized to CFRT or APBI (all 3D conformal external beam).[311] The primary endpoint of noninferiority was met in the RAPID trial and 8-year in-breast tumor recurrence rates were 3% versus 2.8% in the APBI vs. CFRT arms. In NSABP B-39/RTOG 0413, the statistical requirements for noninferiority were not met, although there was no statistically significant difference in the low breast tumor recurrence rates between the arms at 10.2 years (4% vs 3% APBI vs CFRT). While no significant differences in cosmesis or toxicity between arms emerged in the NSABP B-39/RTOG 0413 study, the RAPID trial found APBI was associated with a higher percentage of patient- and physician-reported fair or poor cosmesis compared to CFRT. This led RAPID investigators to conclude this regimen would not become the standard of care in these regions. Notable differences are seen between these trials, with the inclusion of higher-risk patients, including node-positive patients, and the use of brachytherapy-based APBI on the NSABP B-39/RTOG 0413 trial. In the RAPID trial, the whole breast arm allowed hypo-fractionated 3-week radiation. Together, these trials provide strong evidence that the APBI regimen of 38.5 Gy given in twice-daily fractions over 5 days offers equivalent tumor control outcomes for women well represented in these trials, largely postmenopausal women with invasive or noninvasive breast cancer which is small, node-negative, and HR+. The potential for increased toxicity, especially identified in the RAPID study, may be acceptable to patients for whom convenience is a higher priority. Alternatively, 10-year results from a 5-day external beam APBI regimen delivered using IMRT once every other day instead of daily also demonstrate noninferiority and no cosmetic or toxicity difference.[312] These data offer another safe APBI option in terms of tumor efficacy that may strike a better balance for toxicity.

Treatment recommendations will continue to change, as data emerge on faster and more convenient treatment regimens. In the UK FAST-forward trial, early-stage breast cancer patients were randomized to conventional whole breast radiation of 40.05 Gy in 15 fractions delivered over 3 weeks versus whole breast radiation with 26 Gy in five fractions delivered once daily for 5 days.[300] The 5-year rates of tumor recurrence were 2.1% and 1.4%, respectively. The study met its endpoint for noninferiority and there were no significant differences in long-term toxicity between the two groups. While longer-term data are desirable, the low absolute rates of toxicity and recurrence make it unlikely this will be deemed unsafe. Patients over 50 with HR-positive early-stage breast cancer were well represented in this trial and are a population for whom to routinely consider this treatment option, and it is difficult to rationalize twice daily APBI regimens when the whole breast can be treated safely in five fractions.

Radiation as a substitute for radical axillary surgery in early-stage node-positive patients
In the era of mammographically detected disease, systemic therapy, and the use of SLN surgery, there has been an enormous interest in reducing the use of axillary dissection for not only node-negative patients but also low-volume node-positive patients. The interest in eliminating radical axillary surgery is particularly important for patients in whom radiation is planned, as the risk of lymphedema and its impact on QOL are higher when these modalities are combined. The ACOSOG Z0011 trial showed that for patients undergoing BCS with WBRT for early-stage disease with one to two positive nodes, the addition of axillary dissection to SLNB did not improve disease-free or OS at 10 years.[313] The EORTC 10981-22023 (AMAROS) trial analyzed a similar patient population, including patients with more than two positive nodes (5%) and patients who had undergone mastectomy (18%).[314] Over 1400 patients with a positive SLN were randomized to receive either axillary dissection or axillary irradiation, and at 10 years there was no statistical difference in axillary recurrence, 0.93% versus 1.82% (HR 1.71; $p = 0.37$).[315] Although the trial was underpowered because of the low overall number of events, the rate of upper extremity lymphedema was significantly higher for patients who underwent dissection. These two trials taken together have had a broad, practice-changing effect on the locoregional treatment of early-stage node-positive patients, directing therapy away from radical surgery. Given that axillary recurrences are rare events, typically occurring within 2 years[279,316] longer-term follow-up of these two trials is unlikely to alter their significant impact on clinical practice. It should be noted that in patients for whom SLN biopsy is positive and axillary nodal surgery omitted, radiation should be directed to the entire level I and II axilla. In patients with larger tumors, large nodal disease burden, or patients with positive nodes after chemotherapy, radiation should not be a substitute for a completion axillary dissection.

Role of radiation after mastectomy for locally advanced disease

A strong rationale exists for combining the beneficial effects of radiation and mastectomy for selected women with locally advanced breast cancer, in whom areas of subclinical disease extend beyond the operative field. The initial studies that investigated radiation after mastectomy began in the 1950s and represented some of the first controlled clinical trials in oncology history. After five decades of study, controversies still remain regarding the selection criteria and value of PMRT. This relates to two factors: the late-term morbidity of early radiation techniques and the addition of systemic therapy as a routine component of care. In general, however, as PMRT techniques have improved and systemic therapies decrease the competing risk of distant metastases, improvements in locoregional control gained by radiation have had a consequential positive effect on survival.

There have been several meta-analyses conducted to quantify the value and risk of PMRT, the most comprehensive and important being the work of the EBCTCG. This group was able to obtain the raw data from every randomized prospective trial of PMRT, including nearly 10,000 randomized to radiation versus observation following mastectomy and axillary clearance. For node-positive patients, PMRT reduced the 10-year risk of locoregional recurrence threefold (26 vs 8%), which led to an 8% absolute decrease in breast cancer mortality (66% vs 58%) at 20 years. For patients with node-negative disease, the locoregional benefit was smaller (3–1.6%) and not associated with a significant difference in survival.[317] Overall, data from the EBCTCG meta-analysis suggested that a long-term survival benefit was only manifested in the trials where there was a ≥10% improvement in 5-year locoregional control.[318] As such, there is a clear indication that the role of PMRT in the eradication of persistent postsurgical microscopic disease is to prevent the development of a subsequent local source for distant metastasis, which eventually can lead to death.

The three PMRT randomized trials that most heavily influenced the EBCTCG meta-analysis all involved relatively modern radiation techniques and the judicious use of systemic therapy. The Danish Breast Cancer Cooperative Group (DBCCG) 82b trial, randomized 1708 premenopausal women with stage II or III breast cancer to mastectomy and CMF-based chemotherapy with or without PMRT.[319] The majority of patients had one to three positive lymph nodes; however, the median number of axillary lymph nodes resected was only seven, fewer than generally recovered from a formal level I/II axillary dissection. Patients randomized to PMRT had an improved OS rate at 10 years (54% vs 45%; $p < 0.001$), likely a consequence of decreased locoregional recurrence (9% vs 32%; $p < 0.001$). Investigators in Vancouver, British Columbia, conducted a similar, albeit smaller trial in which 318 premenopausal women with lymph node-positive disease were randomized to receive mastectomy and CMF with or without PMRT.[320] The results were nearly identical, with PMRT providing a 10% absolute benefit in long-term OS (20-year rates: 47% vs 37%; $p = 0.03$) and an even higher benefit in locoregional control (87% vs 61%; $p < 0.0001$).

Finally, the DBCCG 82c trial randomized 1300 postmenopausal patients to mastectomy and tamoxifen with or without PMRT.[321] The stage of disease and extent of axillary surgery were similar to the 82b trial. The magnitude of benefits in OS and local control was similar to the two previous studies in terms of 10-year OS (45% vs 36%; $p = 0.03$) and locoregional control (92% vs 65%; $p < 0.001$). At almost 20 years of follow-up, updates of the DBCCG 82b and 82c combined data show continued benefits of PMRT for both locoregional control (86% vs 51%; $p < 0.0001$) and distant metastasis-free survival (47% vs 36%; $p < 0.0001$).[322]

While the extent of the radiation field has been debated for many years, recent studies have confirmed the benefit of radiation to the regional nodes in relatively early-stage patients. The National Cancer Institute of Canada MA.20 trial randomly assigned high-risk lumpectomy-treated patients to whole breast radiation +/− RNI.[323] This trial demonstrated that regional nodal radiation significantly improved 10-year locoregional recurrence-free survival (hazard ratio, 0.59; $p = 0.009$; absolute improvement of 3%), disease-free survival (DFS) (HR, 0.76; $p = 0.01$; absolute improvement of 5%), and distant DFS (HR, 0.76; $p = 0.03$; absolute improvement of 4%). The EORTC 22922 trial of high-risk lumpectomy and mastectomy patients similarly showed that RNI significantly improved DFS (HR, 0.89; $p = 0.04$; absolute improvement of 3%), distant DFS (HR, 0.86; $p = 0.02$; absolute improvement of 3%), and breast cancer-specific mortality (HR, 0.82; $p = 0.02$; absolute improvement of 1.9%).[324] Importantly, both of these trials in early-stage patients demonstrate systemic benefits from RNI in spite of relatively small local benefits, adding more complexity to the EBCTCG findings discussed above suggesting distant benefit is solely a fraction of local benefit. Although these trials were predominantly postlumpectomy patients, the benefit of RNI may be extrapolated to PMRT decisions discussed further below.

Current indications for postmastectomy radiation

The American Society of Clinical Oncology (ASCO) consensus guidelines for PMRT, published almost 20 years ago, recommended treatment for patients with stage III disease (defined by T3 with involved lymph nodes, T4 primaries, or four or more involved lymph nodes) after mastectomy, standard axillary dissection, and chemotherapy, due to the magnitude of survival benefit for these locally advanced patients.[325] However, the landmark publication left the role of PMRT for patients with stage II disease, with one to three positive nodes, unsettled and hence controversial. The reason for this is that although most of the patients in the Danish and British Columbia trials had one to three positive lymph nodes, the benefit of PMRT for this subset has been challenged by surgeons who point to the inadequate clearance of the axilla in the standard arm of the larger Danish trial. Indeed, the long-term locoregional recurrence rate for these patients in the Danish trials, who were treated without PMRT, was 41% versus 21% in patients who underwent a more complete axillary clearance in similar trials.[322] It is important to note that inadequate axillary surgery may have led to an underestimation of the true number of positive lymph nodes and that many of these patients would likely have had four or more lymph nodes if subject to more extensive surgery.

The findings and critiques of the Danish and Canadian Studies heavily influenced the ASCO consensus guidelines for PMRT (published in 2001), which in turn have guided clinical practice patterns for over a decade. A meta-analysis by the EBCTCG published in 2014 has sought to clarify the utility of PMRT for the most controversial patients, those with small primary tumors and one to three positive nodes.[317] Data from 22 randomized trials including over 3700 patients treated with PMRT after axillary dissection to at least level II were analyzed for differences in 10-year locoregional recurrence and 20-year survival. For patients with one to three positive nodes in whom systemic therapy was followed ($n = 1133$), PMRT significantly reduced locoregional recurrence by more than three-quarters (20% vs 4%; $p < 0.0001$) and improved breast cancer-specific mortality by approximately 8% (50% vs 42%; $p = 0.01$). The magnitude of benefit in this controversial subgroup was nearly the same as that for patients with four or more positive nodes for both locoregional recurrence (32% vs 13%; $p < 0.00001$) and breast cancer mortality (80% vs 70%; $p = 0.04$).

While these studies of PMRT indicate a benefit for all node-positive and locally advanced patients, our increasing understanding of biologic subtypes has led to a dramatic change in the staging system incorporating grade and receptor status to re-classify patients, including those with node-positive disease. Taking into account the EORTC 22922 and MA-20 studies showing benefits in early-stage patients, including high-risk node-negative, and the trend toward SLN surgery identifying node-positive patients that would have previously been considered node-negative, it is critical to consider all contemporary risk stratifiers in PMRT decision making. In addition to the number of positive nodes, the size of nodal metastases and other adverse pathologic features such as the receptor subtype, presence of LVSI, grade, tumor size, RS, if available, and age should be used to guide clinical decision-making. A retrospective analysis of the Oncotype Dx RS in patients treated on NSABP B-28, SWOG 8814, and ECOG 2197 showed that the RS correlated with local recurrence in node-positive patients treated with mastectomy.[326–328] An ongoing randomized trial tailoring radiotherapy use in N1 patients with Oncotype Dx scores ≤18 will provide prospective data on whether this assay can be utilized for routine clinical decision making on the use of radiotherapy.[329]

Integrating PMRT with breast reconstruction

As noted previously, the indications for PMRT have been expanded, particularly in younger patients, and we are seeing more patients pursue mastectomy combined with reconstruction.[267,330,331] We have usually preferred a TE for patients undergoing mastectomy who require PMRT.[268] This allows full-tissue expansion during the course of adjuvant chemotherapy. The TE may be left in place through the course of PMRT, and its deflation can improve radiation dosimetry.[332] Importantly, as prepectoral placement of the TE becomes more popular, consideration must be given to the potential breast target deep to the expander and fields adjusted accordingly. Consultation between the plastic surgeon and radiation oncologist is important to determine when a prepectoral TE overly compromises the radiation plan. Similarly, care must be taken to remove air from TEs prior to radiotherapy planning when air-filled devices are used to ensure there is adequate tissue or water for dose build-up and to reduce heterogeneity. Autologous flap techniques are the procedures of choice for delayed reconstruction, where vascularized tissue is brought into the irradiated field for improved wound healing and cosmetic results.[333] As breast reconstruction after mastectomy proves vital to many patients in terms of QOL posttreatment, the choice for PMRT in patients with low-risk disease can incorporate cosmesis goals into patient decision-making. However, it is important that high-risk patients, such as those who are very young, or have high-risk features such as unfavorable tumor biology, not change their oncologic therapy for fear of consequences that are cosmetic and rectifiable.

Breast conservation after neoadjuvant chemotherapy
One of the reasons to investigate sequencing chemotherapy before surgery was to determine whether breast conservation could be offered to selected patients with larger primary tumors needing mastectomy at diagnosis. The NSABP and EORTC independently conducted clinical trials that compared neoadjuvant chemotherapy with adjuvant chemotherapy for patients with stage II or III breast cancer. Although both trials found that breast conservation rates were higher in the neoadjuvant chemotherapy arms,[334–336] the NSABP study showed that this increase was largely due to a near tripling of breast conservation use for patients with T3 disease postchemotherapy (22% vs 8%).[337]

For patients with large initial primaries, resection must be directed at the postchemotherapy tumor bed rather than the initial volume of disease. However, some breast cancers do not shrink concentrically to a solitary nidus in response to neoadjuvant chemotherapy, but rather break up into nests of residual disease over the initially involved volume.[338] In such cases, surgery directed at the residual core may identify more microscopic disease around the tumor bed site, which may be associated with higher rates of breast cancer recurrence.

In the NSABP B-18 trial, the overall rate of breast cancer recurrence did not statistically differ in the patients treated with neoadjuvant chemotherapy compared with those treated with adjuvant chemotherapy (16-year rates of 13% vs 10%, respectively).[336] However, breast cancer recurrence rates were higher in patients with large primary tumors in whom a response to neoadjuvant chemotherapy permitted a BCS. In this subset of patients treated with neoadjuvant chemotherapy, the breast recurrence rate at 8 years was 16%, more than twice the rate in patients with smaller tumors who were treated with breast-conserving surgery first. Other multicenter series have also shown relatively higher breast cancer recurrence rates in patients who receive neoadjuvant chemotherapy.[339]

By contrast, single-institution studies with careful selection criteria and a high degree of multidisciplinary coordination have reported excellent rates of local control. Investigators at MD Anderson published the results of one of the largest studies investigating breast conservation after neoadjuvant chemotherapy.[340] In this study, 340 carefully selected patients who had a favorable response to chemotherapy were treated with breast-conserving surgery and radiation. Despite the fact that 72% of patients in the study had clinical stage IIB or III disease, the 5- and 10-year breast cancer recurrence rates were only 5% and 10%, respectively.

Four tumor-related factors were associated with breast cancer recurrence and locoregional recurrence: clinical N2 or N3 disease, lymphovascular space invasion, a multifocal pattern of residual disease, and residual disease larger than 2 cm in diameter. These investigators developed a prognostic index from these factors and found that for patients with a score of 0 or 1, breast conservation will offer similar excellent outcome as mastectomy and radiation. However, mastectomy and radiation were associated with a lower risk of locoregional recurrence in patients with three or more adverse factors.[341]

PMRT after neoadjuvant chemotherapy
Over the past three decades, the use of neoadjuvant chemotherapy has significantly increased. This strategy was first adopted for patients with unresectable or marginally resectable disease. Subsequently, this approach became frequent in patients with large, resectable, or node-positive breast cancers at diagnosis. Neoadjuvant chemotherapy ensures there is an *in situ* indication of the efficacy of the first-line systemic therapy and provides resulting prognostic information obtained from the assessment of pathologic response. Importantly, among patients with HER2 over-expressing or triple-negative breast cancer (TNBC), the presence of residual disease is an indicator for adjuvant therapies.[342,343]

Neoadjuvant chemotherapy changes the extent of disease in 80–90% of cases, and this may hold implications for locoregional recurrence. Therefore, both the pretreatment clinical stage and the extent of pathologically defined residual disease need to be considered when assessing the risk of locoregional recurrence in patients treated with neoadjuvant chemotherapy and mastectomy. In one analysis of patients treated with neoadjuvant chemotherapy, mastectomy, and no radiation, a multivariate analysis of locoregional recurrence predictors revealed that both pre- and posttreatment factors were independent predictors.[344] One large retrospective study of PMRT after neoadjuvant chemotherapy compared outcomes of 542 patients who received radiation following neoadjuvant chemotherapy and mastectomy with 134 patients who were treated with neoadjuvant chemotherapy and mastectomy only.[345] Despite the fact that the PMRT cohort had more extensive disease than those treated without radiation, irradiated patients had a significantly lower isolated locoregional recurrence rate at 10 years (8% vs 22%; $p = 0.001$). In the subgroup of patients with clinical T4 tumors, clinical-stage IIIB/C disease, and in those with four or more positive lymph nodes after chemotherapy, the absolute improvement in locoregional recurrence risk was approximately 30–40%. The use of radiation in these same subgroups was associated with an approximately 15–20% improvement in overall and cause-specific survival. In a subsequent analysis that focused only on patients who achieved a pCR, the locoregional recurrence rate for them with clinical stage III disease was improved with radiation therapy (33% vs 7%; $p = 0.04$).[346]

Patients enrolled on the NSABP B-18 and NSABP B-27 trials who received neoadjuvant chemotherapy and mastectomy were not allowed to receive PMRT.[347] In this study of 1947 mastectomy patients, patients who were pathologically node-positive had a greater than 12% risk of locoregional recurrence at 10 years. Based on this data, radiation is recommended for any patient with pathologically positive nodal disease following neoadjuvant chemotherapy. The utility of PMRT in patients who achieve a pCR in the nodes is currently under investigation in the NSABP B-51/RTOG 1304 trial.[348]

On the basis of the available data, it is reasonable to recommend PMRT for all patients with clinical stage III disease at initial presentation. It is also reasonable to infer that patients with clinical stage I or II disease who have any positive lymph nodes after chemotherapy should receive radiation. De-escalation of local therapy in this population is currently being investigated on the Alliance A011202 trial that randomizes patients who remain node-positive after chemotherapy to axillary dissection versus level I/II axillary radiation with sentinel node biopsy. All patients receive comprehensive PMRT to the breast or chest wall and other draining lymphatics.[348]

Systemic therapy

Early-stage hormone receptor (HR) positive/HER2-negative breast cancer

HR-positive breast cancer is the largest receptor subtype of breast cancer, likely a manifestation of other cancers that are driven by pathways responsible for proliferation and survival of the normal cell of origin. Approximately 65–70% of breast cancer are positive for either ER and/or PR and nonamplified for the human epithelial receptor 2 (HER2), hereafter defined as HR+ and HER2-negative (HER2−). As with other subtypes, receptor determination at initial diagnosis and recurrence/progression is important for treatment decision-making. HR status is defined by IHC positivity of either ER or PR-positivity (as defined in the section titled "Pathology and biomarkers"), although recent updates have suggested that responsiveness to endocrine therapy is primarily seen at ER or PR levels of 10% or more.

Endocrine therapy for early-stage HR+ breast cancer

Systemic adjuvant treatment with ET is recommended for most HR+ early-stage breast cancers. Approved agents include tamoxifen and AIs.

Tamoxifen is a selective estrogen receptor modulator (SERM), which competitively inhibits estrogen from binding ER with resultant antagonist and agonist effects depending on the target tissue. The differential effects may be due to variable interactions with coactivator and corepressor proteins involved in ER-mediated gene regulation. Adjuvant tamoxifen efficacy is backed by substantial long-term clinical trial data (see Table 11). A 2011 EBCTCG meta-analysis demonstrated that 5 years of tamoxifen significantly improved outcomes,[350] with reduction of annual breast cancer recurrence by almost 40% and death by 31%, independent of age, chemotherapy, LN, and menopausal status. Unfortunately, the ROR persists over time, with over half of recurrences and two-thirds of deaths occurring >5 years after diagnosis. Therefore, two large phase III clinical trials, ATLAS and aTTom, evaluated the efficacy of an additional 5 years of tamoxifen after the completion of 5 years of treatment.[362,363] In ATLAS, patients with ER+ disease randomized to extended therapy had significant benefit 15 years postdiagnosis with decreased breast cancer recurrence and improved mortality; benefits were primarily observed >10 years postdiagnosis.[362,364]

Tamoxifen is associated with notable side effects and adverse events. Hot flashes are the most commonly reported side effect, occurring in approximately 80% of patients. Tamoxifen's agonist activity on uterine tissue increases the risk of endometrial cancer by approximately 2.4-fold (primarily in women >50 years), but without worsened mortality. Venous thromboembolic events are increased by two- to threefold. A greater absolute risk in these side effects is seen with 10 compared to 5 years of therapy Additional side effects include vaginal discharge, sexual dysfunction, menstrual irregularities, and cataracts.

Aromatase inhibitors decrease circulating estrogen by blocking aromatase, which converts androgens to estrogen in peripheral tissues. Since ovarian-secreted estrogen persists, AIs are only effective in postmenopausal women. The nonsteroidal agents, anastrozole, and letrozole, reversibly bind aromatase, while the steroidal AI exemestane binds irreversibly. Common side effects include accelerated bone loss, increased fracture risk, arthralgias, joint stiffness, bone pain, hot flashes, and sexual dysfunction.

Adjuvant endocrine therapy for postmenopausal women
AIs are generally preferred over tamoxifen in postmenopausal women with HR+ ESBC given superior efficacy demonstrated in several pivotal phase III trials. AI monotherapy improves multiple outcomes, including DFS, compared to tamoxifen.[351,352,365] Furthermore, several schedules of sequenced therapy of tamoxifen and AI have been evaluated with results favoring the addition of AI compared to 5 years of tamoxifen alone[366,367] (Table 11).

The rate of distant recurrence is generally 1–2% per year following 5 years of adjuvant ET.[368] Therefore, multiple clinical trials have investigated the efficacy of extended AI therapy beyond 5 years. While outcomes such as DFS[369,370] have varied Table 12, longer follow-up is required to fully capture the impact. The 2018 ASCO guidelines recommend extending adjuvant AI therapy to 10 years for node-positive HR+ early-stage breast cancer and consideration of extended therapy in higher-risk node-negative patients.[379]

Adjuvant endocrine therapy for premenopausal women
Addition of ovarian suppression to endocrine therapy. Tamoxifen has historically been the standard adjuvant endocrine therapy for premenopausal women with HR+ early-stage breast cancer. More recently, the role of pharmacologic ovarian suppression (OvS) and AI therapy in premenopausal women have been evaluated. The ABCSG-12 trial did not reveal DFS benefit with AI compared to tamoxifen, both combined with a 3-year course of goserelin,[359,360] though the addition of zoledronic acid was advantageous.

In contrast, combined analysis of the SOFT and TEXT studies demonstrated superior DFS for AI therapy over tamoxifen.[361] However, direct comparison of the TEXT/SOFT and ABCSG-12 study results is problematic given differences in trial design and study therapy. The TEXT trial compared the use of adjuvant tamoxifen or exemestane plus OvS over a 5-year period.[361] The SOFT trial had three arms: OvS plus tamoxifen, OvS plus exemestane, and tamoxifen only for 5 years.[361] The original plans for TEXT and SOFT were to compare DFS between treatment groups within each trial separately, but because of fewer than anticipated DFS events, trial amendments allowed for a combined analysis of the TEXT and SOFT arms comparing OvS plus tamoxifen or exemestane. The 8-year DFS rate was 86.8% for exemestane with OvS compared to 82.8% for tamoxifen with OvS ($p < 0.001$).[361] The majority of patients had HER2-negative breast cancer (86.0%), in whom the absolute DFS benefit was 5.4% with exemestane (HR 0.70; 95% CI, 0.60–0.83) (see Table 11).

Further analysis of SOFT and TEXT data showed that ROR based on several prognostic factors correlates with the degree of therapeutic benefit according to subpopulation treatment effect pattern plot (STEPP) analysis. Escalated therapy resulted in absolute benefit in breast cancer-free interval and freedom from distant recurrence of up to 15% in the highest risk patients.[380,381] Improved outcomes were most evident in patients who received chemotherapy, a population with higher risk factors, and patients who were

Table 11 Adjuvant endocrine therapy in early-stage breast cancer for 5 years.

Trial	Study treatment (n)	Patient population	Breast cancer events	Breast cancer recurrence	Time to distant recurrence	DFS/EFS	Breast cancer mortality	OS/all-cause mortality	Median follow-up
Tamoxifen monotherapy									
NATO[349]	TAM × 5 yr (564) vs PBO (567)	Any nodal, menopausal, ER status	RR 0.64 p = 0.0001					RR 0.71 p = 0.0062	5.5 yr
EBCTCG meta-analysis[350]	TAM × 5 yr vs PBO (10,645 overall)	ER+ patients		RR 0.61 p < 0.00001 at 15 yr			RR 0.70 p < 0.00001 at 15 yr		13 yr
Aromatase inhibitor monotherapy									
ATAC[351]	ANA × 5 yr (3125) vs TAM (3116) × 5 yr	Postmenopause			HR 0.87	DFS HR 0.91 p = 0.04		HR 0.97 p = 0.6	10 yr
BIG 1-98[352,353]	LET × 5 yr (2463) vs TAM × 5 yr (2459)	Postmenopause			p = 0.03 HR 0.86	DFS HR 0.86 p = 0.007		HR 0.87 p = 0.048	8.7 yr
		HR+			p = 0.047 HR 0.85	HR 0.91 p = 0.08		HR 0.89 p = 0.087	12.6 yr
		ITT			p = 0.057				
AI sequential therapy									
IES[354,355]	TAM 2–3 yr, complete 5 yr with EXE (2362) vs TAM × 5 yr (2380)	Postmenopause				DFS HR 0.76 p = 0.0001		HR 0.85 p = 0.08	4.6 yr
		ER+/unknown						HR 0.89 p = 0.08	10 yr
ABCSG-8/ARNO 95[356]	TAM × 2 yr, ANA × 3 yr (1618) vs TAM × 5 yr (1606)	Postmenopause				HR 0.81 p < 0.001			2.3 yr
		HR+				EFS HR 0.60 p = 0.0009			
ITA[357]	TAM × 2–3 yr, complete 5 yr with ANA (223) vs TAM × 5 yr (225)	Postmenopause ER+ Node-positive				EFS HR 0.71 p = 0.03		HR 0.79 p = 0.3	10.7 yr
TEAM[358]	EXE × 5 yr (3075) vs TAM × 2.5 yr, complete 5 yr with EXE (3045)	Postmenopause HR+		HR 0.88 p = 0.03		DFS HR 0.96 p = 0.39		HR 0.98 p = 0.74	9.8 yr
Ovarian suppression									
ABCSG-12[359,360]	ANA/goserelin × 3 yr (903) vs TAM/goserelin × 3 yr (900)	Premenopause				DFS HR 1.13 p = 0.335		HR 1.63 p = 0.030	7.9 yr
SOFT[361]	EXE/OvS[a] × 5 yr (1014) vs TAM/OvS[a] × 5 yr (1015) vs TAM × 5 yr (1018)	Premenopause HR+				DFS EXE + OvS vs TAM HR 0.65 TAM + OvS vs. TAM HR 0.76 p = 0.009		EXE + OvS vs TAM HR 0.85 TAM + OvS vs. TAM HR 0.67 p = 0.014	8 yr
TEXT/SOFT[361]	EXE/OvS[a] × 5 yr (2346) vs TAM/OvS[a] × 5 yr (2344)	Premenopause HR+				DFS HR 0.77 p < 0.001		HR 0.98 p = 0.84	9 yr

Abbreviations: EBSC, early-stage breast cancer; n, number of patients; DFS, disease-free survival; EFS, event-free survival; OS: overall survival; RR, relative risk; HR, hazard ratio; HR+ hormone-receptor-positive; ER+, estrogen-receptor-positive; ITT, intention to treat; TAM, tamoxifen; PBO, placebo; ANA, anastrazole; LET, letrozole; EXE, exemestane; OvS, ovarian suppression; GOS, goserelin.

[a] OvS achieved chemically, surgically, or by irradiation.

Table 12 Extended adjuvant endocrine therapy in early-stage breast cancer.

Trial	Study treatment (n)	Patient population	Breast cancer recurrence	DFS/RFS	Breast cancer mortality	OS/all-cause mortality	Median follow-up
Tamoxifen monotherapy							
ATLAS[362]	TAM x 5 more yr; 10 yr total. (3428 ER+ patients) vs stop TAM; 5 yr total (3418 ER+ patients)	Any nodal, menopausal status	RR 0.84 $p=0.002$		RR 0.71 $p=0.01$	639 vs 722 deaths $p=0.01$	Analysis at 15 yr postdiagnosis (10 yr post-ATLAS entry)
aTTom[363]	TAM x 10 yr (3468) vs TAM x 5 yr (3485)	Completed TAM x 5 yr ER+/untested	16.7% vs. 19.3% $p=0.003$		392 deaths vs 443 deaths $p=0.05$	849 deaths vs 910 deaths $p=0.1$	9 yr
Aromatase inhibitor ≤5 yr							
MA.17[371,372]	LET x 5 yr (2575) vs PBO (2582)	Postmenopause HR+		DFS HR 0.57 $p=0.00008$ HR 0.68 $p=0.0001$		HR 0.76 $p=0.25$ HR 0.98 $p=0.853$	2.4 yr 4 yr[a]
B-33[373]	EXE x 5 yr (783) vs PBO (779)	Postmenopause HR+		DFS RR 0.68 $p=0.07$ RFS RR 0.44 $p=0.004$			2.5 yr
ABCSG-6a[374]	ANA x 3 yr (386) vs PBO (466)	Completed TAM x 5 yr Postmenopause HR+	HR 0.62 $p=0.031$				5.2 yr
Aromatase inhibitor >5 yr							
MA.17R[369]	LET x 5 yr (959) vs PBO (959)	Completed TAM x 5 yr Postmenopause HR+	HR 0.66 $p=0.01$			HR 0.97 $p=0.83$	6.3 yr
B-42[370]	LET x 5 yr (1983) vs PBO (1983)	Completed AI x 5 yr Postmenopause HR+		DFS HR 0.85 $p=0.048$			6.9 yr
DATA[375]	ANA x 6 yr (931) vs ANA x 3 yr (929)	Completed 5 yr of ET, which included AI Postmenopause HR+		DFS HR 0.79 $p=0.066$		HR 0.91 $p=0.6$	4.2 yr
IDEAL[376]	LET x 5 yr (915) vs LET x 2.5 yr (909)	Completed 2–3 yr TAM Postmenopause HR+		DFS HR 0.92 $p=0.49$		HR 1.04 $p=0.79$	6.6 yr
SOLE[377]	LET intermittent x 5 yr (2425) vs LET continuous x 5 yr (2426)	Completed 5 yr of ET, which included AI Postmenopause HR+		DFS HR 1.08 $p=0.31$			5 yr
ABCSG-16[378]	ANA x 5yr vs ANA x 2yr	Completed 4–6 yr of ET Postmenopause HR+ Completed 5yr of ET		DFS HR 0.997 $p=0.982$			106.2 mo

Abbreviations: DFS, disease-free survival; RFS, relapse-free survival; OS, overall survival; ESBC, early-stage breast cancer; RR, relative risk; HR, hazard ratio; HR+, hormone-receptor-positive; ER+, estrogen-receptor-positive; TAM, tamoxifen; PBO, placebo; ANA, anastrazole; LET, letrozole; EXE, exemestane.
[a]Intention to treat analysis includes patients on placebo who crossed over to letrozole after unblinding.

persistently premenopausal following chemotherapy particularly benefitted.[380,381] Given the additional toxicities associated with AI therapy and OvS, clinical features and risk factors for an individual patient should be considered when making adjuvant ET decisions. Tamoxifen alone is appropriate adjuvant ET for lower-risk patients.

Adjuvant chemotherapy for HR+/HER2− early-stage breast cancer

Multigene assays
Several multigene assays, including Oncotype DX, MammaPrint (MP), and the Breast Cancer Index, are commercially available to aid in risk assessment and choice of adjuvant therapy.

Oncotype DX is prognostic for HR+ early-stage breast cancer and is predictive for adjuvant chemotherapy benefit.[382] The multigene assay quantifies the expression of 21 genes (16 cancer-related genes and 5 housekeeping for normalization) from a single formalin-fixed paraffin-embedded breast cancer tissue sample. The prospective TAILORx trial randomized >6000 patients with node-negative, HR+/HER2− ESBC with intermediate RS 11–25 to adjuvant endocrine or chemo-endocrine therapy.[383] Patients with RS<11 received only ET and patients with RS>25 received chemo-endocrine therapy. Based on available data, adjuvant chemotherapy is not beneficial for RS<15 but does benefit patients with RS>25. For RS 16–25, no benefit is seen for women >50 years old, though women ≤50 years old derived some benefit, postulated to be possibly or partially due to the ovarian suppressive effect of chemotherapy.

Predictive tools for node-positive patients have been less fully validated and data is largely retrospective. However, the prospective MINDACT study assessed the role of the 70-gene MammaPrint (MP) assay in predicting benefit for patients with early-stage breast cancer and 0–3 positive nodes who had discordant clinical risk (per Adjuvant! online and other available tables) and genomic risk by MP.[384] In the group of patients of interest with high clinical but low genomic risk, there was a slightly lower rate of distant metastases at 5 years if adjuvant chemotherapy was used; however, the study was underpowered to assess statistical significance.[384] Accordingly, MP should be reserved for patients with high-clinical risk. The prospective RxPONDER trial evaluated Oncotype DX in pN1a HR+/HER2− early-stage breast cancer with 1–3 nodes involved and randomized patients to endocrine therapy or chemotherapy followed by endocrine therapy and showed no benefit in postmenopausal women but did benefit premenopausal women with regard to invasive recurrence and distant metastases.[385]

Adjuvant drug regimens
Commonly used adjuvant chemotherapy regimens include (1) an anthracycline-based regimen with or without paclitaxel or (2) a combination of docetaxel plus cyclophosphamide (TC). In the TAILORx trial, 36% of the patients received an anthracycline-containing regimen and 56% received TC.[383] Other regimens, such as CMF, which were historically much more common, are used less now.

Neoadjuvant therapy
Preoperative neoadjuvant chemotherapy for early-stage breast cancer has been well-studied (described in more detail in the sections on HER2+ and TNBC), demonstrating that administration in the pre- compared to postoperative settings has no impact on DFS or OS while allowing more conservative surgery.[239,337] Pathologic response to preoperative therapy is prognostic. pCR predicts relapse-free survival and is often used as a surrogate marker of long-term treatment benefit.[336] However, compared to other sub-types, HR+ breast cancers, especially lower-grade tumors, attain much lower pCR rates with standard chemotherapy.[386] As chemotherapy regimens do not include ET, pCR may not reflect long-term outcomes.

Neoadjuvant endocrine therapy has also been studied in HR+ early-stage breast cancer patients with evidence that neoadjuvant AI therapy in postmenopausal women has similar efficacy as neoadjuvant chemotherapy but with less toxicity.[387] Neoadjuvant AI is superior to tamoxifen in terms of breast conservation rates.[388–390] Parameters other than pCR, such as markers of proliferation, have been assessed in HR+ disease. Ongoing trials are assessing the role of Ki-67 suppression during treatment as a marker for treatment efficacy.[391,392] The preoperative endocrine prognostic index (PEPI) score, which is composed of the pathological tumor stage, nodal involvement, ER expression, and Ki67 percent expression (%) following surgery has been validated prospectively although its use in clinical decision-making has not been formally tested.

Targeted therapies in the adjuvant/neoadjuvant settings

Adjuvant therapy with biological treatments that are known to improve outcomes when added to endocrine therapy are ongoing or awaiting follow-up. The SWOG 1207 trial is comparing either tamoxifen or AI therapy to placebo or the mTOR inhibitor everolimus for 1 year. Three large trials have assessed AI therapy with palbociclib or abemaciclib compared to placebo for 2 years, or 3 years of ribociclib vs. placebo for 3 years. The palbociclib trial (PALLAS) recently failed to show benefit at interim analysis and trial was terminated.[393] On the other hand, the monarchE trial testing abemaciclib in high-risk patients found a 25% relative reduction in invasive DFS.[394]

Endocrine therapy combined with targeted agents is also being explored in the neoadjuvant setting. The ALTERNATE Trial compared anastrozole to fulvestrant to a combination of the two for 6 months in patients with stage II–III ER+HER2− breast cancer.[395] Neither fulvestrant nor fulvestrant plus anastrozole improved upon anastrozole with regard to the fraction of patients who achieved a PEPI score of 0 (pT1–2, pN0, Ki 67 <2.7) or a pCR at the surgery. Data are not yet available regarding the breast cancer-free interval. Neoadjuvant trials of different designs combining AIs with cyclin-dependent kinase (CDK) 4/6 inhibitor have demonstrated much greater decreases in Ki67-based proliferation indices compared to AI alone but still very low pCR rates. Interestingly, activation of markers of immunity has been seen, providing some support to further examine CDK 4/6 and immune targeted therapy combinations in the advanced setting.

Metastatic ER+/HER2− breast cancer

As the goals of MBC treatment are life-prolongation and palliation, patients with HR+/HER2− MBC should initially be treated with endocrine-based therapy unless rapid disease regression is urgently indicated.[394] Chemotherapy should be reserved for the management of visceral crisis or when patients develop irreversible resistance to endocrine-based therapies. A meta-analysis of older trials comparing chemotherapy alone to endocrine therapy alone as initial treatment for advanced breast cancer found that while response to chemotherapy was more rapid, there was no difference in OS.[396]

Endocrine-based therapies for HR+/HER2− metastatic breast cancer

Most endocrine-based therapies for HR+ MBC utilize an AI, SERD, or tamoxifen. As AIs and SERDs are approved for postmenopausal women, premenopausal women may receive tamoxifen or undergo OvS or bilateral oophorectomy to achieve postmenopausal levels of circulating estrogen, permitting the use of treatments approved for postmenopausal patients.[395] Additional ETs, including ethinyl estradiol and megestrol acetate, have been employed in special circumstances, though their use has declined with the advent of novel targeted therapies.

When choosing endocrine therapy for HR+/HER2− MBC, it is important to consider in what context metastatic disease presented: de novo, early-stage which progressed to metastatic disease, or early-stage which relapsed as metastatic disease. In most cases, the development of MBC suggests an element of endocrine resistance. Primary endocrine resistance denotes relapsed disease during the first 2 years of adjuvant ET or progressive disease within 6 months of initiating treatment with frontline endocrine therapy for metastatic disease.[397] Secondary endocrine resistance conveys relapsed disease ≥2 years after adjuvant ET initiation, relapse within 1 year of completing adjuvant endocrine therapy, or progressive disease ≥6 months after starting endocrine therapy for metastatic disease.

The SERD, fulvestrant, is effective as monotherapy in HR+ metastatic disease.[398–400] The CONFIRM trial established the approved dosing regimen of 500 mg every 28 days (with an additional 500 mg on day 14 of the first month).[401,402] Additionally, fulvestrant combined with anastrozole in the S0226 study demonstrated a nearly 8-month OS benefit compared to anastrozole alone as frontline therapy.[403] By contrast, the FACT and SoFEA trials did not demonstrate benefit with the combination of AI and fulvestrant therapy in the metastatic setting.[404,405] However, there were differences in trial designs and patient populations. Most patients in S0226 did not receive prior adjuvant endocrine therapy,[406] while approximately 70% of patients in FACT had adjuvant endocrine therapy. In addition, the SoFEA study required relapse or progression on a prior nonsteroidal AI. As patients in FACT and SoFEA were more heavily pretreated, they likely had a higher risk of not responding to combination endocrine therapy (see Table 3).[402]

Combination of endocrine-based therapy and targeted drugs for ER+HER2− metastatic breast cancer

Nearly all patients with MBC will develop resistance to endocrine therapy. To improve outcomes and to delay the onset of endocrine resistance targeted therapy has been combined with endocrine therapy.

Endocrine therapy and CDK 4/6 inhibitors

Cyclin proteins interact with CDKs to regulate cell cycle progression. Cyclin D1, frequently overexpressed in HR+ breast cancer, interacts with CDK4 and CDK6, which inactivate the tumor suppressor protein Rb.[407] Inhibitors of CDK4/6 synergize with endocrine therapy to produce cell growth arrest and apoptosis in HR+ breast models.[408] Three CDK4/6 inhibitors (palbociclib, ribociclib, and abemaciclib) have been approved by the US FDA for the treatment of HR+/HER2− MBC in combination with an AI or fulvestrant.

Randomized phase III studies with each of the three CDK4/6 combined with an AI reveal substantial efficacy in the frontline setting,[409–414] with most trials showing approximately 10- to 12-month improvement in PFS, or roughly a doubling of PFS, when compared to AI monotherapy. Similarly, fulvestrant was evaluated in combination with CDK4/6 inhibitors in patients who had recent AI therapy, also demonstrating improved PFS of about two-fold.[415–417] OS was significantly improved with ribociclib and abemaciclib,[418,419] but the statistical significance has not yet been reached with palbociclib.[420] Given differences in trial enrollment criteria and sample size, efficacy comparisons between the different CDK4/6 inhibitors are fraught with biases and the drugs have not been compared directly in the same trial. The decision of whether to pair a CDK4/6i with an AI or fulvestrant is based on provider/patient choice with consideration of prior therapies (see Table 13).

Most studies included postmenopausal women, although some included pre- or peri-menopausal patients. A randomized phase III study exclusively in premenopausal women revealed that the addition of ribociclib to a nonsteroidal AI or tamoxifen following pharmacologic OvS with goserelin improved PFS and OS.[421,427] Finally, abemaciclib monotherapy has produced an ORR of nearly 20% in a single-arm phase II study of women with HR+ MBC that had been heavily pretreated with prior endocrine therapy and chemotherapy.[423]

CDK4/6 inhibitors have important toxicities to monitor, including neutropenia, mild anemia, and mild fatigue. Ribociclib is associated with QTc prolongation, requiring EKG monitoring. Consequently, ribociclib is typically not coadministered with tamoxifen, which can also prolong the QTc interval. Abemaciclib is associated with GI toxicities, particularly diarrhea, which can be quite significant in some patients.

Endocrine therapy and PI3K/Akt/mTOR pathway inhibitors

The PI3K/Akt/mTOR pathway is involved in cellular proliferation, metabolism, and survival. In breast cancer, hyperactivation of this pathway has been identified as a resistance mechanism to endocrine therapy.[86,406,425] For example, downstream targets of mTOR can mediate ligand-independent activation of the ER.[423] Inhibitors of this pathway are now utilized in the treatment of HR+ MBC, though they have not been compared directly to CDK4/6is in large clinical trials (see Table 13).

Randomized studies have established that the addition of the oral mTOR inhibitor, everolimus, to an AI, tamoxifen, or fulvestrant results in improved progression-free survival but have not shown survival benefits.[422,423,426] Notable side effects of everolimus include stomatitis, fatigue, and hyperglycemia, though the incidence of grade 3/4 events was <10% for each of these in the BOLERO-2 trial.

PI3K inhibitor treatment is an option for patients with activating PIK3CA somatic mutations. Activating mutations of PIK3CA (which encodes the catalytic p110α subunit of PI3K) are present in 30–40% of HR+/HER2− invasive ductal breast cancer samples and lead to increased activity of the PI3K/Akt/mTOR pathway.[90,406] The PI3K inhibitor, alpelisib, in combination with fulvestrant improved PFS in patients with PIK3CA mutated HR+/HER2− MBC who had disease recurrence or progression with prior AI treatment.[426] Despite its efficacy, alpelisib has significant side effects, most notably hyperglycemia, diarrhea, and potentially severe rash. Grade 3 hyperglycemia is common; accordingly, alpelisib use is strongly discouraged in patients with type 1 or poorly controlled type 2 diabetes mellitus.

Table 13 Endocrine and targeted therapies for HR+/HER2− advanced breast cancer/metastatic breast cancer.

Trial	Study treatment (n)	Patient population	Time to progression	PFS	OS/all-cause mortality	Median follow-up
Fulvestrant monotherapy						
Osborne et al.[397]	FUL 250 mg (206) vs ANA (194)	Postmenopause HR-sensitive or HR+ PD/Recurrent after ET	HR 0.92 $p = 0.43$			16.8 mo
EFECT[398]	FUL 250 mg (351) vs EXE (342)	Postmenopause HR+ PD or recurrent after NSAI	HR 0.963 $p = 0.65$			13 mo
FALCON[399]	FUL 500 mg (230) vs ANA (232)	Postmenopause HR+ No prior ET		HR 0.797 $p = 0.049$		25 mo
CONFIRM[400,401]	FUL 500 mg (362) vs FUL 250 mg (374)	Postmenopause ER+ Prior ET—adj/MBC setting		HR 0.80 $p = 0.006$	HR 0.81 $p = 0.02$	
Fulvestrant + AI						
FACT[404]	ANA + FUL (258) vs ANA (256)	Postmenopause or premenopause on OvS HR+ No prior therapy for MBC	HR 0.99 $p = 0.91$		HR = 1.0 $p = 1.00$	8.9 mo
SoFEA[405]	ANA + FUL (243) vs FUL (231) vs EXE (249)	Postmenopause HR+ Relapsed/progressed on NSAI		ANA+FUL vs FUL HR = 1.00 $p = 0.98$ FUL vs EXE HR = 0.95 $p = 0.56$	ANA+FUL vs FUL HR = 0.95 $p = 0.61$ FUL vs EXE HR = 1.05 $p = 0.68$	37.9 mo
S0226[402]	ANA + FUL (349) vs ANA (345)	Postmenopause HR+ No prior therapy for MBC		HR 0.81 $p = 0.007$	HR 0.82 $p = 0.03$	7 yr
Endocrine therapy + CDKi						
PALOMA-2[408,411]	PAL + LET (444) vs LET (222)	Postmenopause ER+ No prior therapy for ABC		HR 0.63 $p < 0.0001$		38 mo
MONALEESA-2[410,412]	RIB + LET (334) vs LET (334)	Postmenopause HR+ No prior therapy for ABC		HR 0.568 $p < 9.6 \times 10^{-8}$		26.4 mo
MONARCH-3[409,413]	ABE + NSAI (328) vs NSAI (165)	Postmenopause HR+ No prior therapy for ABC		HR 0.54 $p = 0.000001$		26.7 mo
PALOMA-3[414,417]	PAL + FUL (347) vs FUL (174)	Any menopausal status. OvS if pre/perimenopausal HR+ Relapsed or PD on prior ET		HR 0.42 $p < 0.001$	HR 0.81 $p = 0.09$	44.8 mo
MONALEESA-3[415,417]	RIB + FUL (484) vs FUL (242)	Postmenopause HR+ Firstline or following prior therapy		HR 0.59 $p < 0.001$	HR 0.72 $p = 0.0046$	39.4 mo
MONARCH-2[416,418]	ABE + FUL (446) vs FUL (223)	Any menopausal status. OvS if pre/perimenopausal HR+ PD on prior ET (neoadjuvant, adjuvant, or first-line MBC setting)		HR 0.55 $p < 0.001$	HR 0.76 $p = 0.01$	47.7 mo
MONALEESA-7[420,421]	RIB + ET (TAM or NSAI) + OvS with GOS (335) vs ET (TAM or NSAI) + OvS with GOS (337)	Pre/peri-menopause HR+ 0–1 line of chemotherapy and no prior ET or CDKi for ABC		HR 0.55 $p < 0.0001$	HR 0.71 $p = 0.0097$	34.6 mo
PI3K/Akt/mTOR pathway						
TAMRAD[422]	TAM + EVR (54) vs TAM (57)	Postmenopause HR+ PD on AI in adjuvant or metastatic setting	HR 0.54 $p = 0.002$			23.7 mo
BOLERO-2[423,424]	EVR + EXE (485) vs EXE (239)	Postmenopause ER+ Recurrence or PD on NSAI		HR 0.45 $p < 0.0001$		18 mo

Table 13 (continued)

Trial	Study treatment (n)	Patient population	Time to progression	PFS	OS/all-cause mortality	Median follow-up
PrE0102[425]	EVR + FUL (66) vs FUL (65)	Postmenopause ER+ Recurrence or PD on AI		HR 0.61 $p=0.02$		19.3 months
SOLAR-1[426]	ALP + FUL (169 PIK3CA-mutated; 284 total) vs FUL (172 PIK3CA-mutated; 288 total)	Postmenopause HR+ Recurrence or PD on NSAI Analysis of PIK3CA-mutated group		HR 0.65 $p<0.001$		20 months
FAKTION[90]	CAP + FUL (69) vs FUL (71)	Postmenopause ER+ Relapsed/progressed on AI No prior exposure to fulvestrant or PI3K/AKT inhibitor		HR 0.56 $p=0.0044$		4.9 months

Abbreviations: PFS, progression-free survival; OS, overall survival; PD, progressive disease; HR, hazard ratio; HR+, hormone-receptor-positive; ER+, estrogen-receptor-positive; Adj, adjuvant; MBC, metastatic breast cancer; ABC, advanced breast cancer; ET, endocrine therapy; NSAI, nonsteroidal AI (ANA or LET); FUL, fulvestrant; ANA, anastrozole; LET, letrozole; EXE, exemestane; PAL, palbociclib; RIB, ribociclib; ABE, abemaciclib; EVR, everolimus; ALP, alpelisib; CAP, capivasertib; OvS, ovarian suppression; GOS, goserelin.

A novel means of targeting the PI3K/AKT pathway in patients independent of *PIK3CA* mutation status has recently emerged with the AKT inhibitor capivasertib.[92] In the randomized phase II FAKTION study, the addition of capivasertib to fulvestrant improved PFS compared to fulvestrant alone.[90] Notable toxicities observed with capivasertib were hypertension, rash, and diarrhea.

Ductal carcinoma *in situ*
Endocrine therapy can be considered in patients with DCIS to reduce the ROR in the ipsilateral breast and development of contralateral breast cancer[428,429] but does not improve OS.[92,428,430] Benefit is primarily evident with HR+ DCIS.[92,428] Both tamoxifen[92,431] and anastrozole for postmenopausal women[428,432] have demonstrated efficacy (see Table 14).

Management of HER2-positive breast cancer
Fifteen to 20% of breast cancers have amplified *HER2* DNA and overexpress HER2 protein, of which approximately 2/3 are also HR+. The *HER2* oncogene encodes a transmembrane glycoprotein receptor with intracellular tyrosine kinase activity. The HER2 receptor is a member of the human epithelial (ErbB) family of receptors, which are involved in the activation of signal transduction pathways that regulate the growth and differentiation of normal and malignant breast epithelial cells. HER2 overexpression is prognostic and predictive of response to specific chemotherapies and HER2-directed therapies.

HER2 testing has become increasingly complex, as testing modalities have become more sensitive. Here, we recommend following the 2018 ASCO/CAP guidelines for defining HER2+ samples using a combination of IHC and FISH (refer to section titled "Pathology").

HER2-directed therapies for early-stage breast cancer
The landscape of HER2-targeted therapies has broadened considerably in the past 20 years, and current treatments fall into three broad categories: HER2-targeted antibodies, tyrosine kinase inhibitors (TKIs), and antibody–drug conjugates (ADCs). In the vast majority of the trials presented here, disease-free survival (DFS) or pathologic CR (pCR) are used as surrogates for overall survival (OS) when evaluating these agents. A recent meta-analysis of DFS and OS in HER2+ trials[433] found that the correlation coefficient of DFS and OS is 0.90, suggesting that DFS remains an appropriate surrogate marker for OS. pCR is an accepted surrogate for DFS and OS by the FDA.[434] This has motivated further study and yielded standard-of-care neoadjuvant approaches for HER2+ disease.

The first antibody to be approved in early-stage HER2+ breast cancer was trastuzumab, a humanized monoclonal antibody that prevents HER2 homodimerization and subsequent downstream signaling and may also have an immunotherapeutic component. A series of landmark studies (and their subsequent analyses) demonstrating that trastuzumab plus chemotherapy in the adjuvant setting increases OS and PFS have been summarized in Table 15. Collectively, these trials and their subsequent updates have demonstrated a reduction in the 3-year recurrence risk of approximately 50%, although longer-term follow-up and a recent patient-level meta-analysis show these reductions to be in the range of 34% with a reduction In the odds of mortality of 33%. This supports the use of trastuzumab as part of adjuvant therapy for all patients with HER2-positive disease with the possible exception of T1aN0 tumors and T1bN0 tumors that are of low/intermediate grade and HR-positive. For stage 1 breast cancer, the de-escalated APT regiment of weekly paclitaxel x 12 with concurrent trastuzumab that is given for 1 year with a 7-year DFS of 93% and accepted as a standard of care (Figure 22).

The question of optimal duration of adjuvant trastuzumab therapy was first addressed in the HERA trial (as summarized in Table 15), which demonstrated no significant benefit of extending treatment for more than 1 year. A series of trials have shown that shorter courses of trastuzumab are not equivalent in efficacy to 1 year, and thus 52 weeks of treatment remains the standard. This is further supported by a recent meta-analysis which demonstrates better DFS and OS with a 52-week course of treatment.[435] The PERSEPHONE trial has shown noninferiority of 6-month adjuvant trastuzumab compared to 12-month treatment highlighting that there may be potential to further de-escalate therapy, but long-term follow-up is still awaited from this trial. Trastuzumab can cause cardiomyopathy, usually subclinical, which may require holding or stopping trastuzumab, such that monitoring of cardiac ejection fraction is necessary. Infusion reactions, cutaneous,

Table 14 Randomized trials of systemic therapy for DCIS.

	Study treatment[a] (n)	Patient population	Breast cancer events	Ipsilateral breast cancer	Contralateral breast cancer	Invasive breast cancer	Noninvasive breast cancer	Median follow-up
NSABP B-24[92]	Tamoxifen (899) vs Placebo (899)	DCIS[b] – BCS[c] + RT[d]	HR[e] 0.63 $p=0.009$	HR 0.70 $p=0.04$	HR 0.48 $p=0.01$	HR 0.57 $p=.004$	HR 0.69 $p=0.08$	5 yr
UK/ANZ[430]	Tamoxifen (794) vs none (782)[f]	DCIS – BCS +/– RT	HR 0.71 $p=0.002$	HR 0.78 $p=0.04$	HR 0.44 $p=0.005$	HR 0.81 $p=0.2$	HR 0.67 $p=0.008$	12.7 yr
NSABP B-35[428]	Anastrazole (1552) vs Tamoxifen (1552)	HR+[g] DCIS – BCS + RT Postmenopause	HR 0.73 $p=0.0234$	HR 0.83 $p=0.34$	HR 0.64 $p=0.0322$	HR 0.62 $p=0.0123$	HR 0.88 $p=0.52$	9.0 yr
IBIS-II[431]	Anastrozole (160) vs Placebo (166)[h]	ER+[i] DCIS – ipsilateral mastectomy Postmenopause	HR 0.44 95% CI[j] 0.17–1.15	—	—	—	—	5 yr

[a] All treatments given for 5 years.
[b] DCIS, ductal carcinoma in situ.
[c] BCS, breast-conserving surgery.
[d] RT, radiation therapy.
[e] HR, hazard ratio.
[f] 2 × 2 factorial randomization: radiation vs none; tamoxifen vs none.
[g] HR+, hormone receptor-positive.
[h] DCIS is a subset of study population including women at increased breast cancer risk. 3864 total patients enrolled.
[i] ER+, estrogen receptor+.
[j] CI, confidence interval.

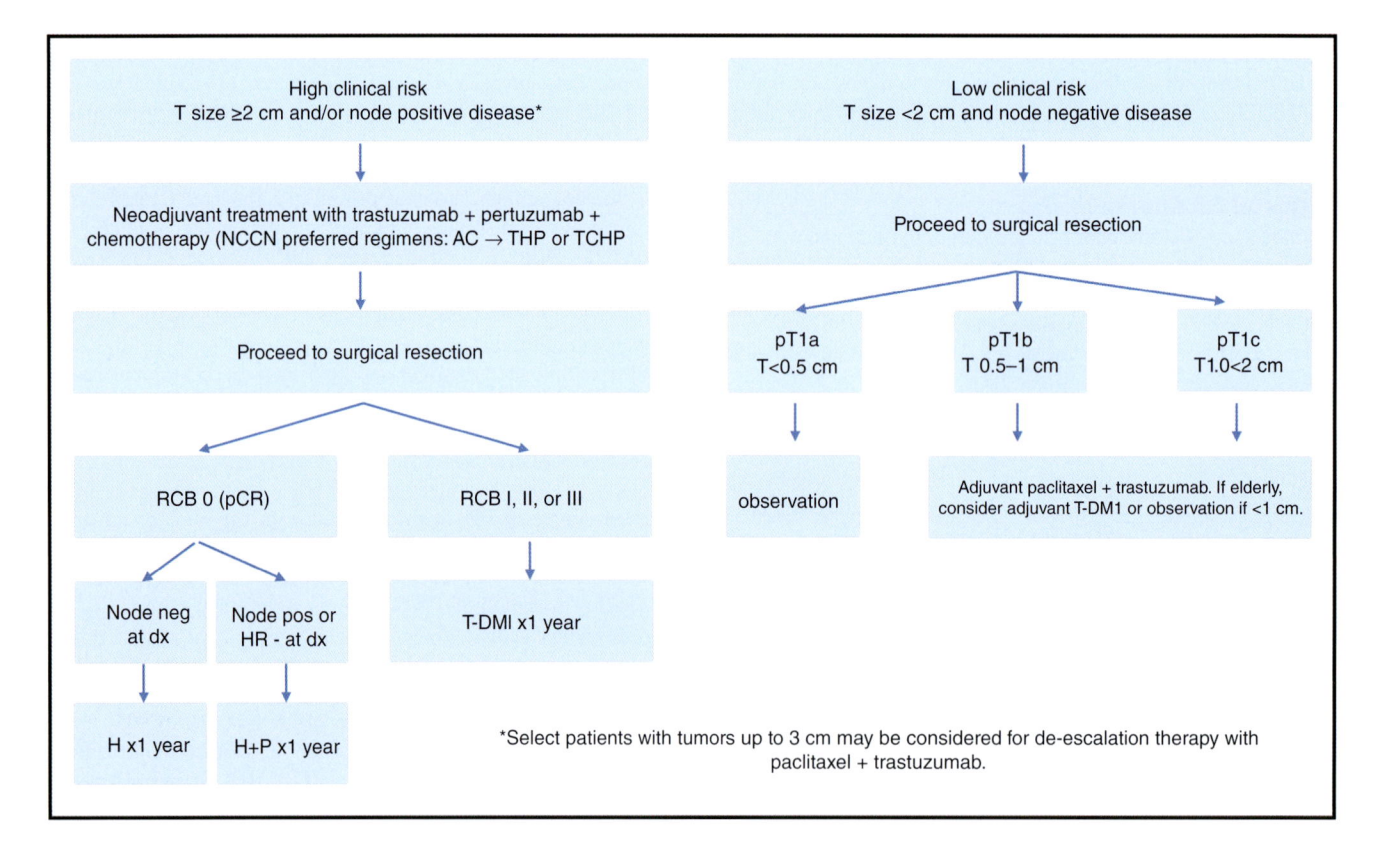

Figure 22 Clinical pathway for HER2+ breast cancer.

gastrointestinal, and rare, but serious interstitial lung disease has been observed. The use of anthracycline-free regimens that include taxane and platinum therapy is preferred as less cardiotoxicity is observed. The addition of the pertuzumab, a humanized monoclonal antibody, which prevents HER2 heterodimerization with HER3 to trastuzumab-based adjuvant regimen yields a small improvement in DFS primarily seen in node-positive cases.

Trastuzumab with chemotherapy has also been extensively studied in the neoadjuvant setting, and the pivotal trials show high rates of pCR (30–55%).

Neoadjuvant therapy allows for downstaging tumors for possible breast-conserving therapy, but also to evaluate the biology of the disease. The second antibody approved for use in HER2+ early-stage breast cancer is pertuzumab, a humanized

Table 15 Adjuvant trastuzumab studies.

Study	Primary completion date	Trial design	Primary endpoint	Secondary endpoint	Results
NSABP-B31	2005	Phase III, randomized, open-label study. Enrolled 2130 participants and randomized to AC-T or AC-T-H, followed by H meant for 40 weeks	DFS, cardiotoxicity	OS, long-term cardiotoxicity	NSABP and N9831 were combined for all interim analyses due to similarities in design. Significantly longer DFS in H-containing arms, with an absolute difference in DFS of 12% at 3 yr. H-containing arms had 53% risk reduction in distant recurrence and reduction in mortality by 1/3
NCCTG N9831	2005	Phase III, randomized, open-label study. Enrolled 3506 participants and randomized to AC-T or AC-T-H, followed by H maint for 40 weeks, or AC-T followed by H maint for 52 weeks	DFS	OS	
NSABP-B31 and N9831 final OS analysis	2014	Eight-year interim analysis completed after definitive number of events for OS (710) reached in 2012	As above	As above	Chemo—H had a 37% relative improvement in OS and an increase in 10-year OS rate from 75.2% to 84%. DFS had a relative improvement of 40% and 10-yr DFS rate increased from 62.2% to 73.7%
NSABP-B31 and N9831 analysis of late relapses	2019	Analysis of relapse rates in patients on both trials, analysis broken down by HR+ vs HR− disease	As above	N/A	Patients with HR+ disease had lower cumulative hazard for RFS in first 5 years but no difference in years 5–10 trastuzumab yielded benefits in HR− and HR−+ groups
HERA	2005	Multicenter randomized trial of 5081, node-positive or node-negative, HER2-positive patients who received either 1 or 2 years of adjuvant trastuzumab after receiving at least four cycles of adjuvant or neoadjuvant chemotherapy	DES	OS, safety, site of first DFS event, time to distant recurrence	Initial report only discussed results of control arm vs 1 year H. Treatment with H resulted in absolute benefit in DFS of 8.4% and the unadjusted HR was 0.54
PACS-04	2009	Randomized, phase III trial with 528 HER2+ ESBC patients randomized to receive H or observation following completion of adjuvant chemotherapy	DFS	Safety, EFS, OS	After a 47-mo median follow-up, H administered sequentially after adjuvant chemotherapy is not associated with a statistically significant increase in DFS
BCIRG006	2011	Randomized phase III trial with 3222 women, randomized to one of three arms: AC–Taxotere, AC–TH, or TCH	DFS	OS, safety	At median 2 years follow-up, women who received H had significant improvement in DFS, with 51% reduction in relapse risk in the AC-TH arm and 39% in the TCH arm
BCIRG006 QOL update	2013	Patients on BCIRG006 were evaluated with a survey tool at baseline, midway, at the end of chemo, and at 6, 12, and 24 months to assess QOL measures	QOL measures – side effects, physical functioning, and global health scores	N/A	HRQL outcomes favored TCH over AC–TH or AC–T regimens, PF
APT	2015, 2019	Uncontrolled, single group, investigator initiated study of 410 women with small (<3 cm), node-negative HER2+ disease	IDFS, death from any cause		Among women with primarily stage I HER2+ breast cancer, taxol +H is associated with a DFS of 93% and a 7-year OS of 95%
HERA 11 year update	2017	Final analysis of the ITT population described above after 11 years	As above	As above	Significant DFS and OS benefits were seen in the groups that received H compared to no H. There was no additional benefit of 2 years of H compared to 1 year

Abbreviations: AC-T, doxorubicin, cyclophosphamide, and paclitaxel; AC-TH, doxorubicin, cyclophosphamide, paclitaxel, and trastuzumab; DFS, disease-free survival; H, trastuzumab; HR, hormone receptor; HRQOL, health-related quality of life; IDFS, invasive disease-free survival; ITT, intention to treat. OS, overall survival; QOL, quality of life; RFS, relapse-free survival; TCH, docetaxel, carboplatin, and trastuzumab.

monoclonal antibody which prevents HER2 heterodimerization with HER3 and induced higher pCR rates when added to standard trastuzumab and chemotherapy. The current NCCN guidelines reflect the recommendation to add pertuzumab to trastuzumab and chemotherapy in the neoadjuvant setting when the patient has ≥T2 or ≥N1 disease and to continue trastuzumab and pertuzumab in the adjuvant setting in patients who achieve a pCR and are clinically node-positive. In patients who are clinically node-negative and achieve a pCR, adjuvant trastuzumab alone may be considered.

Patients with residual disease after neoadjuvant therapy remain at high risk for recurrence.[386] The ADC ado-trastuzumab emtansine (T-DM1) is approved as adjuvant therapy for patients with the residual disease based on the trial results from KATHERINE study which showed a 50% reduction in the risk of disease recurrence or death favoring treatment with adjuvant TDM1 compared to trastuzumab (95% CI 0.39–0.64; $p < 0.001$). Trials are ongoing to use pathological responses to neoadjuvant therapy to de-escalate by removing more toxic chemotherapy components or escalate therapy with newer HER-2 targeted therapies.

Multidisciplinary input is critical for all newly diagnosed patients with breast cancer but is particularly important for HER2+ disease, where neoadjuvant therapy is the preferred approach for patients with tumors >2–3 cm if nodes are—negative or if any nodes are positive. Conversely, surgery may be preferable for patients with clinical T1N0 disease for definitive staging as they may qualify for de-escalated medical therapy.

Neratinib, which targets HER2, HER4, and EGFR, has been evaluated in the adjuvant setting in the ExteNET study wherein patients received neratinib or placebo after completion of a year of adjuvant trastuzumab therapy. Patients did have an improved DFS in comparison to placebo (90.2% vs 97.7%; HR 0.73; $p = 0.0083$), but this was at the expense of grade 3 diarrhea. Additionally, there are no data regarding the benefit of neratinib following adjuvant TDM1 in patients who did not achieve pCR. Neratinib is FDA approved in the extended adjuvant setting, given for 1 year following completion of maintenance HER2 antibody therapy, with the largest benefits seen in ER+ cases, within a year of completing adjuvant trastuzumab and in higher-risk cases. Specific strategies can mitigate the high incidence of Grade 3/4 diarrhea seen especially in the first 2 months of therapy.

HER2-directed therapies for metastatic breast cancer

Trastuzumab was the first anti-HER2 therapy to be approved for use in the metastatic setting by the FDA in 1998 based on the pivotal phase III trial by Slamon et al.[436] comparing either doxorubicin plus cyclophosphamide or paclitaxel with or without trastuzumab until disease progression. The combination of trastuzumab plus anthracyclines leads to high rates of cardiotoxicity and these agents should not be combined in the metastatic setting. The addition of platinum agents also adds toxicity without improving outcomes.

Similar to the neoadjuvant and adjuvant settings, the treatment options for HER2+ MBC have broadened well beyond trastuzumab. Pertuzumab, described above under adjuvant treatment, received approval in the MBC setting following the unprecedented results of the CLEOPATRA study. This trial randomized HER2+ MBC patients to trastuzumab/docetaxel/placebo or trastuzumab/docetaxel/pertuzumab in the first-line setting. The addition of pertuzumab led to a 6.3-month improvement in PFS and a 15.7-month improvement in OS, without significant increases in cardiotoxicity. This regimen is now considered the standard first-line therapy for HER2+ MBC in patients who are treatment-naïve or >1-year postcompletion of adjuvant trastuzumab. Studies that used less toxic paclitaxel or nab-paclitaxel instead of docetaxel (albeit with higher incidence of neuropathy) have shown equivalent outcome with response and PFS but were not powered for survival. Currently, the regimen studied in CLEOPATRA remains an NCCN category 1 recommendation for first-line therapy in HER2+ MBC. For patients who may not be candidates for chemotherapy for metastatic HR+ and HER2+ breast cancer, the ALTERNATIVE and PERTAIN trials evaluated the efficacy of dual-HER2 blockade plus endocrine therapy using lapatinib + trastuzumab + anastrozole (ALTERNATIVE) or pertuzumab + trastuzumab + anastrozole (PERTAIN). Both trials demonstrated PFS benefits in the dual-HER2 blockade arms compared to single-agent blockade, suggesting that the degree of HER2 inhibition plays a role in efficacy in HR+ patients, similar to what has been demonstrated in the HR-negative population. However, direct comparisons with chemotherapy-containing regimens have not been performed. Following progression on first-line therapy, the ADC T-DM1 has been typically favored in the second line based on the results of the EMILIA trial which demonstrated superior PFS and OS with T-DM1 when compared to lapatinib and capecitabine. There is also notable activity of TDM1 in more heavily pretreated patients based on the THR3SA trial. More recently, the newer generation antibody–drug conjugate (ADC) trastuzumab deruxtecan, which also uses trastuzumab linked to deruxtecan, a synthetic analog of camptothecin and potent topoisomerase I inhibitor that showed significant activity in a phase II trial of heavily pretreated patient with metastatic HER2+ breast cancer, was compared to T-DM1 in the second line in a pivotal phase III trial and showed a remarkable improvement in PFS (HR0.23), although at the time of this article writing had not yet been approved in this setting.

Following progression after the CLEOPATRA regimen, T-DM1 has been typically favored in the second line based on the results of the EMILIA trial, which demonstrated superior PFS and OS with T-DM1 when compared to lapatinib and capecitabine. There is also notable activity of TDM1 in more heavily pretreated patients based on the THRESA trial.

Newer agents targeting HER2 in the second/third line and beyond

In late 2019, the HER2 treatment landscape expanded to include several more options with newer HER2-targeting drugs. In the randomized NALA trial, neratinib, a potent HER1 (EGFR) and HER2 kinase inhibitor was studied in combination with capecitabine compared to lapatinib plus capecitabine. There was a small but statistically significant improvement in PFS favoring the neratinib + capecitabine arm, with a toxicity profile included significant diarrhea, even with mandated antidiarrheal prophylaxis. This can be explained by the fact that neratinib is a potent pan-HER inhibitor, including the EGFR which has wide expression in gastrointestinal mucosal tissue. Another TKI recently developed includes tucatinib, which has high specificity for HER2 relative to EGFR and hence is expected to have a more tolerable safety profile. This agent was recently evaluated in the phase III HER2 CLIMB trial, which compared trastuzumab + capecitabine + tucatinib versus trastuzumab + capecitabine + placebo in a heavily pretreated population previously exposed to at least 3 HER2-targeted agents (trastuzumab, pertuzumab, and TDM1). Further, the trial participants included patients with brain metastasis (BM) that were either already subject to local therapy or had minimal symptoms with no treatment. When compared to placebo, the tucatinib combination group significantly increased 1-year PFS, median duration of

PFS, OS at 2 years, and median OS (HR 0.66). Remarkably, in pts with CNS disease, median PFS at 1 year was 24.9% in the tucatinib-containing arm versus 0% in the placebo arm. In addition, the regimen was well tolerated, and only 12.9% of patients experienced grade 3 diarrhea in the tucatinib arm compared to 9% in the control arm. In patients with a history of locally treated CNS disease as well as untreated CNS disease, PFS (HR 0.32 and 0.36, respectively) and OS (HR 0.58 and 0.49, respectively) were also significantly improved. Taken together, these data suggest that among the TKIs, tucatinib will be the putative first choice in the heavily pretreated setting or in patients with CNS disease.

The phase III clinical trial SOPHIA has recently compared the novel agent margetuximab plus chemotherapy when compared to trastuzumab plus chemotherapy. Margetuximab is an Fc-engineered anti-HER2 monoclonal antibody that targets the same epitope as trastuzumab and exerts similar antiproliferative effects but has a higher affinity for CD16A on Fc receptors D compared to trastuzumab, enhancing both innate and adaptive immunity. The first prospective analysis demonstrates an increase in PFS and a trend toward improvement in OS with margetuximab + chemotherapy compared to trastuzumab + chemotherapy (one of several agents based on physician's choice).

The appropriate treatment in the third line for patients without CNS disease remains unclear. Given the success of the ADC T-DM1 in the metastatic setting, the novel and more optimized ADC trastuzumab-deruxtecan, consisting of trastuzumab linked to a synthetic topoisomerase I inhibitor has been developed and tested. In the DESTINY-Breast01 phase II trial, heavily pretreated patients (including with prior T-DM1) received trastuzumab-deruxtecan, yielding a 60.9% response rate, a median response duration of 14.8 months, and median PFS of 16.4 months. Treatment was well tolerated, but the safety profile was notable for deaths related to interstitial lung disease/pneumonitis in approximately 2% of patients, requiring special monitoring and treatment. The composite results suggest that either a tucatinib-based regimen or trastuzumab dertuxtecan could be appropriate third-line options for patients with HER2+ MBC, and the appropriate agent should be chosen based on patient factors such as sites of disease, prior therapies received, and toxicity profile. However, given the result of randomized DESTINY-Breast03 trial showing a dramatic superiority in the activity of trastuzumab deruxtecan over that of T-DM1, is likely this agent will be approved in the second line.

Patients with metastatic HER2+ breast cancer may have up to a 50% likelihood of developing CNS metastasis. With the observation that some patients receiving systemic HER2-targeted therapies do have responses in the CNS, there have been trials testing HER2-targeted therapies in situations where local treatment options are not feasible. In addition to earlier described CNS activity seem with tucatinib, capecitabine, and trastuzumab, responses have also been seen with capecitabine in combination with both lapatinib and neratinib. For patients who are able to receive local therapy with surgery and/or radiation for new or progressive CNS metastases, continuation of the same HER2-targeted therapy is recommended in the absence of systemic (extra CNS) progression.

Management of triple-negative breast cancer

TNBC accounts for 10–15% of all breast cancers and lacks clinically significant expression of ER, PR, and HER2 as defined by the American Society of Clinical Oncology (ASCO) and College of American Pathologists (CAP). As a group, TNBC is heterogeneous and is associated with aggressive clinical features such as high recurrence and mortality rate, younger age onset, and African Americans/Hispanic ethnicity.[437,438] Therapeutically, both early- and late-stage TNBC harbor clinical challenges that have given the lack of effective therapeutic targets.[439,440]

Molecular characterization of TNBC

Recently, molecularly-defined TNBC subtypes have been identified with subgroup-specific biomarkers that serve as potential therapeutic targets (Table 16).[441,442] Additionally, several important driver mutations have been identified in TNBC, such as somatic mutations of P53 (60–70%), PIK3CA (9–10%) as the most common mutations, followed by PTEN and RB1 (8%).[443,444] Copy number alterations in tumor suppressors and oncogenes occur at lower frequency (~5%) and most commonly in RB1, PTEN, and EGFR, and fusion events are infrequent. The basal-like subtype is uniquely enriched in P53 mutations/functional loss (84%), cell cycle pathway aberrations, high expression of AKT3, MYC amplification, and BRCA1/2 inactivation. These molecular subgroups dissect the characteristics of TNBC with the aim to discover novel targets. However, to date, TNBC is still treated as if they were a single entity as such efforts to identify molecular aberrations have not yet been translated into the development of novel therapies as part of standard care.

Management of early-stage TNBC

The mainstay of treatment for early-stage TNBC is combination cytotoxic chemotherapy, which was largely established from early trials that included all subtypes of breast cancer. Multiple-drug regimens have been refined over the years since the early 1970s after the Milan Study, which established the cyclophosphamide, methotrexate, and 5-fluorouracil (CMF) regimen that significantly reduced treatment failure in all subgroups of patients.[445] Subsequent regimens containing anthracyclines and later taxanes were later clearly defined in a large number of prospective trials were conducted to determine optimal combinations as well as treatment frequency and length and has become the standard adjuvant chemotherapy regimen.

The NSABP B-15 compared a course of anthracycline and cyclophosphamide (AC) given every 3 weeks for four cycles compared to the CMF regimen given every 4 weeks for six cycles and no significant difference in DFS or OS was observed.[446] Thus, the AC regimen was preferred over the CMF regimen given its shorter treatment duration. Several clinical trials later established the sequential administration of anthracycline and taxane in early stage, including the NSABP B-30, Eastern Cooperative Oncology Group (ECOG) 1199, GEICAM 9906, CALGB 9344/INT1048, and NSABP B-38.[447-451] A majority of these pivotal adjuvant chemotherapy trials failed to specify outcomes for the TNBC subgroup; however, the available retrospective analyses of tumor subtypes clearly demonstrate significant benefits with anthracycline and taxane-based regimens. The comprehensive Early Breast Cancer Trialists' Collaborative Group (EBCTCG) meta-analyses, which included many of these trials, demonstrated a significant improvement in OS and DFS with combination chemotherapy in TNBC.[452] In summary, sequential dose-dense AC and taxane is the standard of care for adjuvant therapy in early-stage TNBC.

Historically, adjuvant chemotherapy was the standard of care for early-stage disease; however, The National Surgical Adjuvant Breast and Bowel Project (NSABP) studies B-18 and B-27, established that neoadjuvant therapy provides equivalent long-term outcomes to adjuvant therapy, and is now neoadjuvant chemotherapy is the preferred option.[336] Neoadjuvant therapy offers several advantages over adjuvant therapy with primary goal of down-staging tumor size for the conversion of an inoperable tumor to operable

Table 16 Molecularly defined TNBC subtype based on newly refined four subtypes.

Molecular subtype	Common mutations	Summary of pathway aberrations	Characteristics
Androgen receptor positive	PIK3CA, CDH1, PTEN, RB1	Steroid hormone biosynthesis Androgen/estrogen metabolism AR FOXA1 GATA3	More common in older postmenopausal women. Lobular histology with apocrine differentiation similar to luminal HR+ tumors. Associated with lower-grade, however, more frequent LN involvement at time of diagnosis and higher incidence of bone metastases. Low pCR rates to neoadjuvant chemotherapy
Mesenchymal	PTEN, RB1, TP53, PK3CA, TP53	EMT Proliferation-associated genes IGF/mTOR WNT ALK TGFb	Have metaplastic and/or medullary histological presentation with increased lymphocytic infiltration. Higher expression of proliferation-associated genes, stem cell-like, mesenchymal genes and low expression of epithelial and intercellular tight-junction genes. Shares similar features with basal-like subtypes. Clinical significance is under investigation
Basal like 1	BRCA1, BRCA2, TP53, CTNND1, STAT4, UTX, TOP2B, CAMK1, MAPK13, MDC1, PTEN, RB1, SMAD4, CDKN2A	DNA damage response Cell proliferation/cell cycle regulation ATR/BRCA	BL1/2 make up 70% of TNBC and are exclusively ductal histology and tend to be high-grade. BL1 has higher pCR rates compared to BL2 (41% vs 18%) and other subtypes
Basal like 2	BRCA1, RB1, TP53, CDKN2A, UTX	DNA damage response Cell proliferation/cell cycle Growth factor signaling EGF NGF MET WNT/b-catenin IGF1R	Similar characteristics to BL1 but with enrichments in growth factor signaling and myoepithelial markers

and improving rates of breast-conservation surgery. Additionally, response to neoadjuvant therapy can serve as a surrogate endpoint for the prediction of long-term clinical benefit and allow for early regulatory approval of treatments while waiting for long-term endpoints to result. Approximately 30% of TNBCs treated with neoadjuvant chemotherapy achieve a pCR, defined as eradication of tumor from both breast and lymph nodes.[386,453] In the CTNeoBC pooled analysis, those who achieve a pCR have improved long-term outcomes with event-free survival HR of 0.24 (95% CI 0.18–0.33) compared to those who do not achieve a pCR. Lastly, neoadjuvant chemotherapy serves as an invaluable research tool to compare effectiveness of standard of care and novel therapies and facilitates the study of biological factors that influence treatment sensitivity and resistance as well as what changes the treatment may exert on the primary tumor or TME.

De-escalating chemotherapy

Patients with T1a/bN0 (tumor size ≤ 1 cm and node-negative) have a good prognosis and the optimal regimen has not been well defined. There have been no randomized trials of chemotherapy versus no chemotherapy; however, in retrospective studies, the 5-year DFS is 90–95% with or without the use of chemotherapy.[454–456] The largest retrospective study from the NCCN database showed a slight trend toward improvement of chemotherapy in T1a/bN0 patients. With the lack of prospective data, treatment decisions remain controversial; however, it is generally accepted to consider observation for T1aN0 and chemotherapy for T1bN0 TNBC. Additional risk factors such as the absence/presence of lymphovascular invasion, other aggressive features and age should be considered when omitting chemotherapy for this population.

The pivotal joint analysis of the anthracyclines in early breast cancer (ABC) trials included three prospective noninferiority trials aimed to address whether anthracyclines can be omitted from early-stage HER2-negative breast cancer.[457] The individual trial designs compared docetaxel plus cyclophosphamide (TC) for six cycles compared against several anthracycline and taxane-based regimens. A preplanned subgroup analysis of TNBC patients showed a benefit with the addition of anthracycline to taxane with a HR for invasive DFS of 1.42 (95% CI, 1.04–1.94). In an exploratory analysis, TNBC with node-positive disease derived the most benefit. Therefore, TC regimen may be saved only for lower-risk node-negative TNBC or in those with underlying cardiac co-morbidities.

Immunotherapy with chemotherapy

Several trials have explored the addition of anti-PD-1 or anti-PD-L1 checkpoint inhibitors with varying results (Table 17) In the I-SPY2 trial, subset analysis of TNBC patients demonstrated that the addition of pembrolizumab to standard NACT dramatically improved pCR rates from 22% to 60%.[458] However, this was not observed in the phase II trial GeparNuevo trial, which examined the addition of durvalumab to nab-paclitaxel followed by epirubicin and cyclophosphamide (EC), nor the phase III NeoTRIP trial with the addition of atezolizumab to neoadjuvant paclitaxel and carboplatin.[459,460]

The Keynote-522 trial, randomized patients with stage II/III TNBC to receive neoadjuvant chemotherapy using paclitaxel and carboplatinum followed by AC with placebo or pembrolizumab followed by postoperative pembrolizumab or placebo for about 6 months followed by EC with or without pembrolizumab, followed by adjuvant pembrolizumab for up to nine cycles. In the first interim analysis, there was an improvement in pCR of 64.8% versus 51.2% and an improvement in disease progression, defined as local or distance recurrence, second primary tumor, or death.[461] Addition of pembrolizumab showed a better event-free survival (HR 0.63), leading to FDA approval in this setting.[461]

Additional treatment after neoadjuvant therapy

Patients who have residual disease after completing neoadjuvant chemotherapy carry a high ROR. For these patients, in the post-neoadjuvant chemotherapy setting, the CREATE-X (JBCRG-04)

Table 17 Immunotherapy-based studies (both ongoing and completed) in early-/late-stage of TNBC.

Early-stage						
Study	Phase	Population	N	Treatment	pCR	
I-SPY2	II	TNBC	29	Pembrolizumab +/− AC-T	22% −> 60%	Bayesian design, probability superior to control 99.6%
GeparNuevo	II	TNBC	174	Durvalumab +/− nab-paclitaxel -> EC	44.2% −> 53.4%	p = 0.287
NeoTRIP	III	TNBC	280	Atezolizumab +/− nab-paclitaxel + Cb	40.8% −> 43.5%	p = 0.066
Keynote-522	III	TNBC	602	Pembrolizumab +/− TCb -> AC	51.2% −> 64.8%	p < 0.001
Metastatic						
Study	Phase	Population	N	Regimen	PD-L1 threshold	ORR
Emens et al.	Ia	TNBC, first line or pretreated	21	Atezolizumab	Unselected	24%
Schmid et al.	Ia	TNBC, first line or pretreated	115	Atezolizumab	Unselected	10%
Adams et al.	Ib/II	TNBC, first line or pretreated	32	Atezolizumab + Nab-paclitaxel	Unselected	42%
IMpassion130	III	TNBC, first line	452	Atezolizumab + Nab-paclitaxel Nab-paclitaxel	Unselected	56% 45.9%
KEYNOTE-012	Ib	TNBC, pretreated	32	Pembrolizumab	PD-L1 positive (≥1% in tumor cells or stroma)	18.5%
ENHANCE-1	Ib/II	TNBC, first line or pretreated	39	Pembrolizumab + Eribulin	Unselected	33.3%
KEYNOTE-086	II	TNBC, Cohort A pretreated; Cohort B, first line	84	Pembrolizumab	PD-L1 positive (≥1% in tumor cells or stroma)	Cohort A: 5% Cohort B: 23%
KEYNOTE-119	III	TNBC, pretreated	622	Pembrolizumab	Unselected	TMB ≥ 10: 14.3% TMB < 10: 12.7%
JAVELIN	Ib	Unselected, pretreated	168	Avelumab	Unseleted	5.4%

trial randomized patients with HER2-negative breast cancer who did not achieve pCR after anthracycline and taxane containing therapy to either capecitabine 2500 mg/m^2/day in divided doses on days 1–14 every 3 weeks versus placebo for six to eight cycles. In a preplanned subgroup analysis among the patients with TNBC, the 5-year DFS improved from 56.1% to 69.8% and OS improved from 70.3% to 78.8% with the addition of capecitabine.[343] The GEICAM/2003-11_CIBOMA/2004-01 trial also examined the use of adjuvant capecitabine in TNBC with either lymph node-positive or node-negative with tumors ≥1 cm, however, was unable to show an improvement in DFS.[462] A meta-analysis of eight randomized controlled trials demonstrated there was an improved OS benefit in TNBC.[463] Thus, adjuvant capecitabine has become a standard of care. In these trials, 2500 mg/m^2/day dosing led to significant palmar–plantar erythrodysesthesia (hand and foot syndrome), and it is reasonable to start with 2000 mg/m^2/day and to adjust the dose based on tolerance. The role of capecitabine in patients who receive immunotherapy (pembrolizumab) remains unclear.

Management of metastatic TNBC

Chemotherapy for advanced TNBC
In the metastatic setting, sequential single-agent cytotoxic chemotherapy remains the most common treatment, unless patients are symptomatic or in visceral crisis warranting urgent cytoreduction. The selection of chemotherapy agents is guided by prior chemotherapy, toxicities, underlying co-morbidities, and patient preference. Anthracyclines and taxanes are amongst the most active agents in TNBC, but they form the backbone of NACT. As a result, they have limited roles in the metastatic setting, particularly if disease recurrence occurs <12 months after NACT. Additionally, there is a cumulative risk of cardiotoxicity with additional anthracycline exposure and neuropathy with taxanes, thus re-challenging requires caution. Pegylated liposomal doxorubicin is an enhanced form of doxorubicin that is encapsulated in liposomes to minimize cardiotoxicity and adverse effects with less alopecia and nausea, while maintaining treatment efficacy. Several phase III studies comparing pegylated liposomal doxorubicin to doxorubicin demonstrated similar efficacy.[464–466] Eribulin, a novel synthetic inhibitor of tubulin polymerization. In a pooled analysis of eribulin in the phase III trials EMBRACE and Study 103, demonstrated a survival benefit compared to the physician's choice of chemotherapy, and those with TNBC appear to have the most benefit compared to other subtypes.[467] Other approved chemotherapies for the treatment of metastatic TNBC include capecitabine, ixabepilone, gemcitabine, and vinorelbine with similar efficacy with response rates of 10–30% in second line and beyond.[468]

TNBC in the context of germline BRCA1/2 mutations
Poly ADP-ribose polymerase (PARP) represents a family of proteins that are involved in the repair of DNA single-strand breaks and mutations in *BRCA1/2* selectively renders tumor cells to PARP inhibition and can induce synthetic lethality.[469] Currently, two PARP inhibitors, olaparib and talazoparib, are approved

for use in MBC with gBRCA-mt based on the results of two phase III trials, OlympiAD[82] and EMBRACA.[83] In these studies, PARP inhibitors led to improvement in median PFS by roughly 3 months compared to physician's choice of chemotherapy in heavily pretreated patients with HER2-negative breast cancer. Disappointingly, despite impressive response rates of ~60%, resistance often emerges. Therefore, significant investigations are underway on how to optimize these agents with novel combinations. Several ongoing trials test these combinations using PARP inhibitor and either chemotherapy or other novel agents ClinicalTrials.gov (accessed on 14 May 2020).

Immunotherapy for metastatic disease

Prior to the emergence of immunotherapy as a treatment in cancer, TILs were recognized as an important prognostic marker in early-stage TNBC.[470–472] These data suggest that antigens in breast cancer may be immunogenic, and immune modulation could be an important strategy. However, unlike "immunogenic tumors," the success of currently available immune-modulating therapies in TNBC remains controversial. The optimal treatment strategy for individual patients might be eventually overcome with improved understanding of immuno-biology, emerging biomarkers, and the development of new therapeutic targets beyond PD-1, PD-L1, and CTLA-4.[473]

A series of trials with single-agent anti-PD-1 or anti-PD-L1 inhibitor demonstrated poor response rates, particularly when given after several lines of chemotherapy: pembrolizumab (KEYNOTE-012, KEYNOTE-086, and KEYNOTE-119), atezolizumab, and avelumab (JAVELIN Solid Tumor Study).[474–478] Despite these initial negative trials, subsequent data led to the approval of combinations with chemotherapy and a shift in the current stand of TNBC care. The phase III IMpassion130 trial demonstrated improved outcomes when atezolizumab was combined with nab-paclitaxel as the first line in those with PD-L1 positivity defined by the Ventana SP142 IHC assay ($\geq$1% on immune cells).[479,480] There was no difference in PFS or OS in the intention-to-treat population, which included patients with PD-L1 negative disease. In the exploratory analysis, there was a benefit in PFS and OS in patients with PD-L1 positive disease, which led to approval of the combination. Atezolizumab approval was voluntarily withdrawn when a confirmatory study IMpassion131 reported negative results.[479,480] Since that time, pembrolizumab was approved in combination with one of several chemotherapy agents for PD-L1+ tumors using a different antibody assay (DAKO 22C3)[481] showing a combined pathological score (CPS) of $\geq$10.

Key studies are summarized in Table 17. Lower response rates with immunotherapy in the advanced stage after multiple lines of treatment, maybe in part because compared to primary tumor, metastatic sites have lower level of TILs and PD-L1 expression possibly due to immune exhaustion, yet the exact biology requires further studies.

Newly emerging-targeted therapies

With new understanding of the molecular characteristics of TNBC, multiple therapies show future potential and are under investigation with a limited list of agents in Table 18. Of significant interest is targeting the phosphoinositide 3-kinase (PI3K) pathway. Although PIK3CA mutations are most prevalent in luminal A HR+ breast cancer, mutations and amplifications are frequent in every major component of this pathway in TNBC including upstream activators of PI3K such as epidermal growth factor receptor (EGFR) and downstream regulators such as AKT, mTOR, and PTEN. Current investigational agents include pan- or isoform-specific PI3K inhibitors, or dual inhibitors of AKT and mTOR.

Additional efforts are underway to exploit the DDR pathway beyond the limited scope of PARP inhibitors in patients with gBRCA1/2-mt breast cancer. This includes combination of PARP or other novel DDR inhibitors such as ATR and CHEK1/2 inhibitors with other therapies that can induce an "HRD" phenotype or immunotherapy as preclinical studies suggest DDR agents lead to immune activation through cGAS-STING pathway.[482,483]

The serine/threonine CDK protein family regulates the cell cycle and overexpression of CDK4/6 or loss of cell cycle negative regulators result in uncontrolled cell proliferation. The basal-like subgroup of TNBC has derangements in several cell cycle checkpoints, offering a novel targeting strategy that needs to be explored.

Additionally, ADCs are emerging as potential therapeutics in TNBC. Sacituzumab govitecan-hziy (SC) against the Trop-2 antigen and using that active irinotecan metabolite (SN-38) as a payload was recently granted accelerated approval by the FDA for use beyond second-line therapy in metastatic TNBC on the basis of a phase I/II study that demonstrated an ORR of 33.3% and median duration of response of 7.7 months.[484] The randomized ASCENT Trial comparing SC to several chemotherapy agents of physician choice in this population showed a dramatic improvement in PFS and OS (HR 0.48), leading to final FDA approval.[485] Various other targets that have shown efficacy include anti-HER2 with trastuzumab deruxtecan in TNBC with low HER2 expression,[486] and the TROP-2-targeting ADC datopotamab deruxtecan.[487]

Cross talk between pathways via common downstream effectors, and interchangeable signaling makes targeting individual pathway challenging. Ras is a GTPase that has downstream effects on proliferation and cell regulation. Despite a small fraction of Ras mutations in breast cancer (only about 2%), this pathway harbors several potential opportunities for therapeutic targeting.[488] For example, Ras can be activated by estrogen, IGF, and EGF ligands, while IGF and EGF RTK pathways showed their aberration in basal-like TNBC.[489] Recently, Mittal et al.[490] reported a cross-talk between Ras/MAPK pathway and the Notch pathway that can be suppressed by combinatorial therapy in preclinical experiments in aggressive breast cancer. Therefore, additional exploration of this pathway is warranted.

TNBC is enriched for mutations in TP53. Despite past attempts to re-activate normal p53 function or inhibit the mutant p53, new drugs are being developed and tested in this space.[491–493] Given the participation of p53 in the induction of apoptosis in response to DNA damage, targeting apoptosis is an attractive pathway in TNBC. Many inhibitors of antiapoptotic effectors have been developed, such as inhibitors of Bcl-2 family and IAP family, however, without too much success in translation to date in TNBC.

Management of inflammatory breast cancer (IBC)

The current American Joint Committee on Cancer (AJCC) defines inflammatory breast cancer (IBC) as a separate "clinicopathological entity" with the erythema and edema occupying at least one-third of the breast, that can extend to the whole breast and across to the contralateral breast involving mediastinum, upper extremities, and neck area.[494] The term inflammatory in the context of IBC refers to the inflamed appearance of the breast skin, which is attributed to tumor emboli physically clogging diffuse lymphatic networks through the breast and breast skin causing redness and swelling. It does not denote a frank inflammatory infiltrate. Indeed, pathologically, IBC tumor foci resemble other aggressive non-IBC

Table 18 Emerging therapeutics ion TNBC.

Pathway	Investigational drug	Molecular target/mechanism of action
PIK3CA/AKT/mTOR	Alpelisib (BYL719)	PI3Kα inhibitor
	Buparlisib (BKM120)	Pan-class 1 PI3K inhibitor
	Copanlisib (BAY-90-6946)	PI3Kα/d inhibitor
	Capivasertib (AZD5363), Ipatasertib (GDC-0068), MK2206	AKT inhibitor
	AZD2014	mTOR inhibitor
	Sapanisertib (TAK-228)	TORC1/2 inhibitor
	Dactolisib (BEZ-235), Gedatolisib (PKI-587)	Dual PI3K/mTOR inhibitor
DNA damage repair	Talazoparib, Olaparib, Veliparib, Niraparib, Rucaparib	PARP inhibitor
	Prexasertib (LY606368)	CHEK1/2 inhibitor
	ZEN003694	BET bromodomain inhibitor
	Berzosertib (VX-970)	ATR kinase inhibitor
Androgen	CR1447, Enobosarm (GTx-024)	Androgen receptor modulator
	Enzalutamide (MDV-3100)	Androgen receptor antagonist
	Bicalutamide	GnRH analogue
	Orteronel (TAK-700)	Nonsteroidal CYP17A1 inhibitor
Growth factor receptor	Trastuzumab deruxtecan	HER2 antibody–drug conjugate
	Cetuximab, Panitumumab	EGFR mAb
	Dacomitinib (PF-00299804)	EGFR inhibitor
	Cediranib Maleate, Tivozanib (AV-951)	VEGFR1-3 inhibitor
	Apatinib (YN968D1)	VEGFR2 inhibitor
	Tanibirumab (TTAC-0001)	VEGFR2 mAb
	Onartuzumab (PRO-143966)	c-MET mAb
Ras	Binimetinib (ARRY-162), Cobimetinib (GDC-0973), Trametinib (GSK2141795), GSK1120212	MEK inhibitor
	Selumetinib (AZD6244), OTS167PO	MELK inhibitor
Cell cycle	Palbociclib (PD-0332991), Ribociclib (LEE-001), Abemaciclib (LY2835219), Trilaciclib (G1T28)	CDK4/6 inhibitor
	Dinaciclib (SCH-727964)	CDK1/5 inhibitor
Epigenetic modulators	Entinostat (MS-275), Panobinostat (LBH589)	HDAC inhibitor
	ASTX727	HDAC and cytidine deaminase inhibitor
	Azacitidine	DNMT inhibitor
Immune cell	Cabiralizumab (FFA008)	CSF-1R mAb
	Pexidartinib (PLX3397)	CSF-1R, KIT inhibitor
	Reparixin (DF1681Y)	CXCR1/2 inhibitor
	Sarilumab	IL-6R mAb
	PF 04518600	OX40 agonist
	Balixafortide (POL6326)	CXCR4 inhibitor
	M7824	Bifunctional mAB TGFb trap linked to anti-PD-L1
	Leramilimab (LAG525)	LAG-3 mAb
	Utomilumab (PF-05082566)	CD137 mAb
	Oleclumab (MDI9447)	CD73 mAb
	Daclizumab (BEZ-235)	CD25 mAb
	Bempegaldesleukin (NKTR-214)	Pegylated IL-2
Stem cell-like	Sonidegib (LDE225), Vismodegib (GDC-0449)	Smoothened receptor inhibitor
	RO492907	Gamma secretase inhibitor
Apoptosis	LCL161	SMAC mimetic
Others	Sacituzumab govitecan-hziy (IMMU-132), SKB264	Trop-2 antibody–drug conjugate
	Mirvetuximab soravtansine (IMGN853)	Folate receptor alpha antibody–drug conjugate
	PMD-026	RSK2 inhibitor
	PF-06647020	PTK7 antibody–drug conjugate
	Onalespib (AT13387)	Hsp90
	Trebananib (AMG386), LC06, MEDI13617	ANG-Tie2
	Ladiratuzumab vedotin (SGNLIV1A)	LIV1A antibody–drug conjugate

breast cancers. Clinically, changes of overlying skin and nipple of the affected breast (erythema, edema, and *peau d'orange* affecting a large area of the breast) along with the pathological confirmation of invasive breast carcinoma are integral to the diagnosis of IBC. These symptoms often appear abruptly and must be described as having occurred within a 6-month time frame, which is an important distinguishing feature form non-IBC.[495] While a skin punch biopsy may be informative if the diagnosis of invasive cancer is elusive, it is not required. Typical presentation of IBC is depicted in Figure 23; however, it is important to recognize there is significant heterogeneity in IBC presentation. Diffuse skin change without explicit erythema should not preclude a diagnosis of IBC. Pretreatment photographs are critical to ensuring all affected skin is ultimately addressed by locoregional therapy.

While tri-modality therapy is critical in the treatment of IBC, the adaptation of multimodality therapy ranged from 58.4% to 73.4% annually in IBC patients who were diagnosed between 1998 and 2010 who had local resection. For this study, patients without all three modality treatments were associated with a lower 5- and 10-year OS.[496] Based on the analysis of 107 patients with stage III IBC, only 25.8% received treatment concordant with NCCN guidelines.[497] From the same analysis, IBC patients receiving guideline-based treatment survived longer with a statistically significant difference. The same trends were observed between 2003 guidelines and 2013 guidelines. Among 10,197 patients with nonmetastatic IBC from 1998 to 2010 analyzed by SEER data, the rate of utilization of full trimodality fluctuated between 58.4% and 73.4%. Both 5 years and 10 years survival of patients who had trimodality therapy in this study, showed to be highest amongst all subgroups with different treatments.

The cornerstone of IBC management is trimodally therapy incorporating the standard of care targeted therapies based on

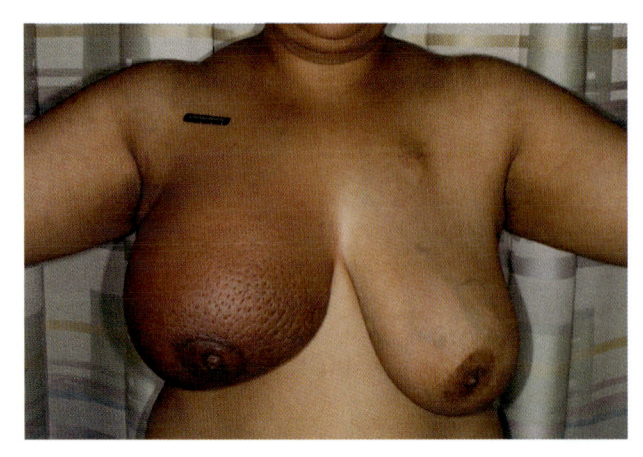

Figure 23 *Classic clinical presentation of IBC*: global breast swelling, diffuse skin change, and nipple inversion. The patient first noted a small area of red patch, which soon spread within 4 weeks period of time. Biopsy confirmed invasive ductal carcinoma.

subtype. In IBC, the incidence of the HR-positive subtype is relatively lower than in non-IBC, and both HER2 positive and TNBC are higher than in non-IBC—40% HER2 positive, and 30% TNBC.[498] In some studies, HR-positive IBC does not have a better prognostic outcome compared to other subtypes.[499] Histological type of lobular versus ductal did not affect survival.[500] It is important to review the bilateral nodal basins as contralateral nodes in the absence of contralateral breast disease is common and may be addressed with aggressive loco-regional therapy. N3 regional nodes are common in IBC and in all cases cross section neck imaging prechemotherapy is helpful for radiotherapy planning.

All patients with stage III IBC undergo neoadjuvant induction systemic therapy first before local therapies are delivered, using subtype-based therapeutics, and strongly encouraged to enroll into IBC specific targeted clinical trials to optimize this systemic response. Patients who achieve pCR have significantly improved outcomes compared to patients who did not.[501] Historical collection of patient IBC data showed that the pCR rate in stage III IBC was about 15.2%; HR-positive/HER2-negative, HR-negative/HER2-positive, triple-negative were 7.3%, 30.6%, 18.6%, respectively. Unlike non-IBC HR-positive breast cancer, the pCR in HR-positive IBC also was able to predict the long-term survival.[400] In previous analysis of 68 stage III IBC patients with 10 years follow-up, the 5 years and 10 years OS rate were 44% and 32%, respectively.[502]

Mastectomy and ALND remain the standard surgical procedure for all IBC patients. The surgical goal is the complete removal of the breast and all initially involved breast skin to pathologically negative margins. Removal of all involved areas in the skin is strongly recommended, as the remnant cells within the skin can further manifest as a recurrence of disease.[503] Patients with developing disease progression are offered additional systemic therapeutic options before surgical approach can be optimized, and yet these patients should also be closely monitored to not lose the window of operability when this control is desired. Local progression or recurrence in IBC is very morbid and difficult to control. While advances in the treatment of non-IBC have gradually focused more on breast-conserving operation with sentinel node biopsy, more extensive surgery in the form of mastectomy with axillary node dissection is still the optimal method of surgery in patients with IBC.[504] Skin sparing approaches including placement of a TE are discouraged to avoid leaving disease behind. Sentinel node mapping is not recommended for IBC patients, as it has not proved to be accurate in this population,[505] and axillary node dissection is recommended.

Immediate reconstruction further compromises planning and monitoring of frequent local recurrence. Contralateral mastectomy should be delayed until reconstruction of ipsilateral breast and can be planned with the management of lymphedema.

Consistent with current NCCN Guidelines for breast cancer,[506] radiation therapy, after chemotherapy and surgery is a major and necessary treatment modality. Postmastectomy radiation including the chest wall, un-dissected high axilla (level III), supraclavicular, and internal mammary lymph nodes is the standard of care.[507] Medical photography at diagnosis can ensure all affected skin areas are covered with radiation. It is important to treat the field with large radiation coverage in patients with IBC, given the involvement of skin and dermal lymphatic system at presentation. This often involves crossing the midline to provide adequate margin on the medial scar. Contralateral nodal basins should always be imaged prior to beginning systemic therapy, and consideration should be given to bilateral therapy in selected cases where metastases are limited to the contralateral regional nodes or breast. Additionally, postoperative changes to blood flow and lymphatic drainage can allow progression to the contralateral breast, lymph node areas, or the skin of the upper abdomen. Anecdotally, many treatment failures are seen at the most medial aspect of the surgical scar or within the contralateral skin and lymph nodes. Inadequate coverage of this area can promote progression and recurrence in these areas.[508,509] Dose escalation in IBC can prevent local recurrence, more so than non-IBC patient. Twice daily treatment, as well as radio-sensitizer combinations with radiation, may help to lower the local failure rate in young patients and women with inadequate response to therapy. Boost targets are dependent on sites of initially involved gross disease.

Finally, receptor subtype-based adjuvant therapies should be offered to IBC patients where indicated. About 33% of IBC patients have stage IV disease at diagnosis.[510–512] A topic of debate in IBC management is the role of local therapy for de novo stage IV patients. The indisputable benefit of local therapy in IBC is the control of local disease. While this may not contribute to OS, this benefit alone is felt to be warranted for many patients to avoid the morbidity of local failure and progression in IBC.[513] Given this, patients with stage IV IBC are still encouraged to see all tri-modality physicians and get appropriate plan of local therapy if they can defer systemically therapy safely for the window required and are expected to live long enough to benefit from local control.[514]

Management of brain metastases in breast cancer

Breast cancer (BC) is the second leading solid tumor that metastasizes to the brain,[515] with a cumulative incidence of 25%[516] and a prevalence of up to 36% in autopsy series.[517] It may present at any stage of the disease: the reported 5-year cumulative incidence of BM from BC is 3.1% in stage I, 3.6% in stage II, 8.6% in stage III, and reaches 12.6% in stage IV patients.[518] BM is considered a late event in the progression of breast cancer occurring at a median of 32 months from the initial cancer diagnosis, frequently (90%) with extracranial metastases.[519] However, BM can be an early event occurring with a median of 12.8 months in patients without an extracranial disease (10%).[520] Historically, BC patients with BMs had a median OS of less than 6 months;[520] however, with recent advances in locoregional and systemic management, the average median OS has increased to about 14 months, in general, and up to

17.1 months in HER2 positive patients receiving anti-HER2 therapy, in particular.[521,522] Up to 50% of all patients with HER2+ BC may develop BM during their disease course with notable continuous risk over time.[523] This problem is likely to only worsen over time as the development of more novel drugs potentially control systemic disease more effectively.

The predictive factors of recurrence with BMs in patients with treated locoregional BC, include positive HER-2 status, nodal involvement, negative HR status, larger primary tumor, higher grade, African American race, and younger age.[524,525] In patients with metastatic disease, the predictive factors for subsequent BM include younger age, higher grade, higher number of metastatic sites, lung involvement, shorter DFS, and negative hormone status.[319,526,527]

Comparison of biomarker expressions of paired primary and brain metastatic tumors showed that HER-2 expression was highly concordant between the primary and the metastatic brain lesion, however, changes in the ER and PR status occurred in a substantial proportion of patients.[528] Comparison of the tumor profiles of BM with those of primary tumors (lung, breast, and melanoma) and extracranial metastasis[529] showed that TOP2A expression was increased in BM from all three cancers, as well as, BM overexpressed multiple proteins clustering around functions critical to DNA synthesis and repair and implicated in chemotherapy resistance, including RPM1, TS, ERCC1, and TOPO1. Brain metastatic lesions, therefore, may particularly benefit from therapeutic targeting of enzymes associated with DNA synthesis, replication, or repair. Many attempts are under way, as well, to identify a genomic profile that may predict primary tumor genes with predilection to BM.

Current clinical practice guidelines recommend brain imaging for breast cancer patients with neurologic symptoms or signs.[530] Management of BM involves a multidisciplinary approach including medical oncology, radiation oncology, neurosurgery, and neuro-oncology (specially if leptomeningeal carcinomatosis [LMC] is suspected). Management will depend on the size, number, and location/distribution of the lesion(s), in addition to the clinical symptoms/signs, comorbidities, performance status, and overall prognosis. Favorable prognostic features include Karnofsky Performance Score (KPS) 70 or higher, age <65 years, <3 BM lesions, controlled primary tumor, and controlled or absent extracranial metastases.[531]

Treatment options include surgery, stereotactic radiosurgery (SRS), WBRT, or any combination henceforth: SRS added to S,[532] WBRT added to S,[533] or WBRT added to SRS,[534,535] resulting in better disease control. To guide the appropriate clinical decision-making and outcomes, three prognostic indices were developed. The recursive partitioning analysis (RPA)[536,537] was built on KPS >70 or ≤ 70, age older or younger than 65 years, control of the primary tumor, and presence/absence of extracranial metastasis. The Score for Radiosurgery (SIR)[538] included in addition to age, KPS and status of the systemic disease, the number of the lesions and the largest lesion volume. The Basic Score Index for Brain Metastasis (BSBM)[539] integrated KPS, control of the primary tumor and the extracranial disease. Evaluation of many of the variables is subjective and may result in the inaccuracy of assessment. Therefore, more objectively measured variables were needed.

A fourth index was developed,[540,541] the graded prognostic assessment (GPA) index, a prognostic index, based on age, KPS, number of CNS metastases, and whether extracranial metastasis is present or not. It was shown to be as prognostic as RPA, but its application is less subjective. The GPA index was further developed to include the genetic subtypes of the breast cancer, in addition to the KPS and age.[542] The modified-breast GPA included, in addition, a fourth variable, the number of brain metastatic lesions.[543]

In lesions that are ≤ 4 in number and < 4 cm in diameter, local progression is similar when comparing SRS to surgical resection.[544] Patient selection for surgery may be aided using the RPA index.[330,331] SRS is usually the preferred approach. The addition of WBRT, however, postoperatively, post-SRS, or SRS postoperatively, results in improved time to progression.[327–329] If the BM is >4 cm in diameter, surgery is preferred. Postoperative SRS or WBRT may decrease the risk of local progression. WBRT, when used postmetastatectomy or SRS, may result in additional lower incidence of further secondary BMs, but with an increased risk of cognitive impairment.[545] In the event of a second BM, SRS should be considered if possible, and to reserve WBRT if not previously utilized, to scenarios where additional SRS is not possible.[546,547] Finally, if surgical or SRS options are ruled out, WBRT remains the treatment of choice.

If there were >4 lesions, the indication for SRS, versus WBRT, may vary with the number (and size) of lesions in the brain. In a prospective, multicenter, single-arm, observational study of SRS alone for 1–10 brain metastases (10% were BC patients), no difference in OS between patients with 5–10 and 2–4 metastases.[548] A definitive prospective randomized trial to compare SRS alone vs WBRT in patients with >5 is underway.[549] In cases where SRS is not available or indicated and the patient is symptomatic, WBRT remains the standard of care. Furthermore, in patients with brain metastases from HER2-positive disease, systemic therapy can be considered as an adjunct or maintenance therapy. It should not be used as an alternative to local therapy unless the last is not a valid option.

Neurocognitive impairment following WBRT may represent a significant deterioration of the patient's QOL. The use of memantine and hippocampal shielding during radiation therapy are recommended.[550,551] On the other hand, and in addition to the well-documented side effects associated with craniotomy,[552] tumor cell spillage secondary to the piecemeal tumor resection, may result in the development of leptomeningeal seeding and LMC, especially in tumors close to the cerebrospinal fluid pathway.[553]

Systemic therapy for brain metastases

The effectiveness of a systemic agent on intracranial metastasis may depend on its ability to penetrate the blood–brain (or blood–tumor) barrier,[554] and its possible modification or interaction with the tumor's microenvironment. There is no confirmed activity of a systemic agent against HER2 negative BM. On the other hand, patients with HER2-positive tumors with BM, treated with either lapatinib plus capecitabine or lapatinib alone, the overall response rate (RR) was 29%, and 21%, respectively.[555] Other anti-HER2 agents such as trastuzumab,[556,557] pertuzumab,[558] trastuzumab-emtansine (T-DM1),[559,560] neratinib,[561] or tucatinib[562] show clinically meaningful intracranial activity. In patients with extracranial metastasis and treated BMs, change of systemic therapy is recommended only with extracranial disease progression; with intracranial progression; however, the option would be further locoregional management, as tolerated, including clinical trials. On the other hand, patients with treated BM but no evidence of extracranial metastasis, continuation of active surveillance is suggested for the HER negative patients, and the initiation of anti-HER2 agent may be considered for the HER positive patients.

Leptomeningeal disease
The prognosis of patients with LMC remains guarded, with a one-year survival rate of 13% and a median OS of 3–4 months.[563,564] The OS may differ, however, according to different biologic subtypes, with a median of 4.4 months in HER2+ BC patients, and 3.7 and 2.2 months in HR+/HER2− BC, and TNBC patients, respectively.[352] Radiation therapy (e.g., WBRT, SRS, and craniospinal irradiation) is often recommended for patients with nodular symptomatic spinal or cerebral LMC.[565] However, intra-CSF (intrathecal or intraventricular) therapy with methotrexate, cytarabine, liposomal cytarabine, or Thiotepa are used with comparable OS and, trastuzumab, is used with encouraging outcomes for HER 2 positive tumors, thus representing the standard of care therapy options for HER2 negative and HER2 positive LMC, respectively.[566,567] Multiple ongoing clinical trials are in progress.

Quality of life

Recognizing the interplay between symptoms
The clinical approach to comprehensive symptom management hinges on the broader recognition of the whole-person impact of breast cancer from diagnosis through the patient's cancer journey. The recognition of the interplay between these symptoms forms the cornerstone of delivering patient-centered care. In clinical practice, the most perceptible symptoms are often physical manifestations of suffering such as pain, nausea, or shortness of breath. However, management of physical symptoms is inextricably intertwined with the patient's social, financial, functional, and psychosocial domains of well-being among others.

Toxicities and healthcare-related quality of life outcomes of systemic therapy
Rapid advances for breast cancer over the past decade have brought entirely new classes of systemic therapy such as CDK4/6 inhibitors in addition to adding newer agents to established classes such as anti-HER-2 therapies.[568,569] The variability in the toxicity profiles among these different classes calls for comprehensive symptom management in conjunction with the delivery of the cancer-directed treatment.[570,571] The early integration of a subspecialty supportive/palliative care team serves to provide this multidisciplinary symptom care in collaboration with the primary oncology services.[572,573] Resources for symptom-specific management include guiding documents from the National Comprehensive Cancer Network (NCCN) and American Society of Clinical Oncology (ASCO).[574–576] The NCCN Clinical Practice Guidelines for supportive care during cancer therapy provide consensus statements and management approaches to adult cancer pain, anti-emesis, cancer-associated fatigue, distress management, Palliative Care, smoking cessation, and survivorship.[577]

Integration of patient-reported outcomes into breast cancer care
The recognition of the individual symptoms as well as their interplay highlights the role of systematic comprehensive symptom management through the integration of patient-reported outcomes (PROs). Deploying PRO measures mitigate the variability in definitions of QOL as well as approaches to symptom assessment. Commonly studied measures of symptom burden provide a validated approach to assessing different domains of a person's well-being.

A recent study of industry-sponsored clinical trials for patients with MBC characterized PRO utilization as endpoints.[570] Of the 38 trials that included a PRO endpoint, the more commonly used questionnaires were the Functional Assessment of Cancer Therapy—Breast (FACT-B, $n = 18$, 47%) as well as the European Organization for Research and Treatment of Cancer Quality of Life Questionnaire—Core 30 (EORTC QLQ-C30, $n = 14$, 37%), the EuroQol 5-Dimensions (EQ-5D, $n = 8$, 21%), and the EORTC QLQ—Breast Cancer Module (EORTC QLQ-BR23, $n = 5$, 13.2%). Most broad PRO questionnaires cover domains of treatment-related, physical and emotional symptoms and functioning and provide valuable insight in patient perception of symptoms at a specific stage of illness or on a particular therapy. The overall characterization of patient performance on a specific therapy is an amalgam of clinician-reported findings, imaging laboratory, and other objective measures of disease, in combination with the patient's own report of symptom evolution over the course of treatment. Integration of holistic symptom management and systematic measure of patient performance in both real-world settings and in cancer clinical trials not only provide valuable information but also serve as crucial components of patient-centered cancer care.

Survivorship
The estimated number of breast cancer survivors in the United States as of January 2019 is over 3.8 million, representing over 40% of all female cancer survivors, and this number is expected to grow to about 5 million in the next decade.[578] Breast cancer survivors are at risk for developing recurrence of disease,[579] or a new primary cancer including a second breast primary cancer, which can occur even several decades after the initial diagnosis. The multidisciplinary treatment of non-MBC includes a highly strategized combination of surgery, radiation therapy, chemotherapy, biotherapy, and endocrine therapy, which has been proven to be very effective but can also lead to long-term or late side effects including physical, psychological, and socioeconomic consequences such as financial hardship.[580,581] Breast cancer patients usually complete their local management and systemic therapy within the first year after diagnosis, and many may continue adjuvant endocrine therapy for 5–10 years. An important goal in the care of breast cancer survivors is to return to their baseline or to an improved health status after the completion of treatment.

Guidelines
The American Cancer Society (ACS) in collaboration with the American Society of Clinical Oncology (ASCO) has serially published updated guidelines for the follow-up and management of breast cancer survivors.[582] These guidelines have consistently recommended a periodic history and physical exam with an annual breast surveillance imaging if indicated, and they also specifically recommend against routine blood work including tumor markers, and other surveillance body imaging.[583] Although early detection of a new primary breast cancer or of local–regional recurrence may have an OS benefit, it has never been proven that the early detection of recurrent distant metastatic disease provides any benefit to OS.[584,585] Additionally, routine body imaging surveillance can generate false-positive findings that can trigger unnecessary invasive tests, increased costs, unnecessary medical procedures, and increased anxiety for the patient.[586] We do recommend

ordering corresponding tests to workup specific symptoms or signs, or abnormal lab values, and we advocate a low threshold to order such tests in high-risk patients.

Models of survivorship care

Several models of care delivery for cancer survivors have been proposed, including ones where the primary oncologists or oncology-trained advanced clinical practitioners deliver such care, versus models where the survivorship care is delivered by community primary care physicians or by primary advanced practitioners.[587–591] All models have pros and cons and no specific model has shown to improve outcomes such as QOL, stress, comorbidities, or survival.[592] An oncology practice should adopt a model that will deliver the highest quality of cancer survivorship care provided their available resources seeking cost-effectiveness. At our institution, which is a tertiary comprehensive cancer center, we adopted a model where the survivorship care is mainly provided by breast medical oncology trained advanced clinical practitioners in specialized clinics who have immediate access to the primary breast medical oncologist as needed. We created specific institutional guidelines for the management of breast cancer survivors, which closely follow the ACS/ASCO guidelines.[593] We are sensitive to the fact that our survivorship care model may not be suited for the general community oncology practice in the United States or the world.

Clinical surveillance visit

During each routine surveillance visit, breast cancer survivors should be screened for symptoms and signs of local and distant recurrence of disease, and also for long-term and late side effects from the treatment received. A thorough review of systems should include screening for pain, headaches, weight changes, fatigue, organ-specific symptoms, neuropathy, depression, anxiety, insomnia, cognitive dysfunction, menopausal symptoms, and sexual-related problems including infertility.[594] A complete physical examination should focus on bilateral breasts, nipple–areolar complexes (or reconstructed breasts), chest wall, and bilateral nodal basins searching for suspicious skin changes, abnormal nodules, lumps, masses, or lymphadenopathy. It is common for breast cancer survivors to have benign posttreatment findings, such as skin hyperpigmentation, fat necrosis, cysts, reactive lymph nodes, postsurgical seromas, keloid scars, among others. Survivors should also be assessed for lymphedema, signs of heart failure, hepatomegaly, lower extremity deep venous thrombosis, neurological deficits, and screened for osteoporosis and for other primary cancers. We also recommend a routine gynecological and pelvic examination usually performed by the patient's gynecologist, family practice physician, or advanced clinical practitioner.[595,596]

Genetic counseling

The guidelines which recommend screening and testing for hereditary breast and ovarian cancer syndrome have evolved over time and the cancer family history of a breast cancer survivor can also change over time. We therefore recommend routinely screening for changes in the family history of cancer and consulting a genetic counselor for those breast cancer survivors who have not been tested yet but meet current criteria for genetic testing.[597]

Surveillance imaging

Annual breast surveillance imaging is the only routine imaging test recommended by national guidelines for breast cancer survivors.[586,593,598] At our institution we schedule the first posttreatment diagnostic mammogram for patients who underwent BCS at 6 months after completing radiation therapy. Annual diagnostic mammograms are performed thereafter for the first 5 years since diagnosis and then switched to annual screening mammography with tomosynthesis. The use of breast ultrasound as an adjunct to mammography in patients with dense breast tissue is an area of controversy considering the limited data of its potential benefits in reducing breast cancer-specific mortality and potential harms from false-positive biopsies.[599,600] Although very sensitive, a breast MRI is also not recommended for routine surveillance purposes in all breast cancer survivors due to low specificity and increased the risk of overdiagnosis, but it is justified for patients who are at high risk (>20%) of developing a new primary breast cancer.[593,601–603]

Management of endocrine therapy-induced side effects

For hot flashes, a regular exercise program and behavioral interventions such as relaxation-based methods or acupuncture are recommended.[604] If patients require medications, selective serotonin or serotonin–norepinephrine reuptake inhibitors avoiding strong CYP2D6 inhibitors among patients who are taking tamoxifen can be tried, while gabapentin and pregabalin are also treatment options. The use of estrogen systemic therapy or herbal products therapies that contain phytoestrogens are not recommended for prolonged use.[605] For vaginal dryness nonhormonal lubricants and moisturizers are advised; however, for extreme urogenital atrophy, there are some data to support the use of topical estrogen for 6–12 weeks to help rebuild the vaginal mucosa.[593,606] For the management of AI-associated musculoskeletal pain a regular exercise program is recommended initially, and a short course or intermittent use of nonsteroidal anti-inflammatory agents can be recommended. If needed, one can offer a 2- to 8-week holiday[607] and explore alternate endocrine therapy options, such as a different AI or tamoxifen. A randomized control trial showed that duloxetine was superior to placebo in improving AI-associated arthralgias, but also had more toxicities.[608]

Bone health

We recommend calcium and vitamin D supplementation coupled with weight-bearing and muscle-strengthening exercises, and to avoid tobacco products and to limit alcohol intake. We obtain a baseline bone mineral density (DEXA) scan and a vitamin D 25-OH level and if normal we reinforce universal recommendations and repeat tests in 2 years. If the vitamin D level is insufficient, we recommend a higher dose of supplementation and rechecking a level in 8–12 weeks. If the DEXA scan shows osteopenia we consider treatment with a bisphosphonate or denosumab and repeating the DEXA scan in 1 year to assess bone density changes. If the DEXA scan shows osteoporosis we recommend treatment with a bisphosphonate or denosumab with close monitoring of potential side effects of these medications.[609,610]

Screening for primary cancer sites and lifestyle modifications

Breast cancer survivors who are free of cancer should undergo age-appropriate screening for other primary cancers, such as cervical screening, colonoscopy, skin and lung cancer screening. A healthy lifestyle, consisting of routine physical activity,[611] a healthy balanced diet, a healthy body weight,[612,613] limited alcohol intake,[594,614] and a tobacco-free lifestyle should be advised for all survivors.

Other important aspects

Additional information is available in the general section on cancer survivorship. It is best practice to routinely assess and refer breast cancer survivors as indicated for lymphedema,[615] cardiac toxicity,[616] chronic fatigue,[617] chemotherapy-induced neuropathy,[618] cognitive dysfunction,[619] anxiety,[620] depression, insomnia,[621] sexual health,[622,623] fertility issues,[624,625] and financial hardship.[597,598]

Acknowledgments

The authors gratefully acknowledge the previous contributors to this article including Hope S. Rugo, MD, Melanie Majure, MD, Anthony Dragun, MD, Merideth Buxton, PhD, and Laura Esserman, MD, MBA.

Key references

The complete reference list can be found on Vital Source version of this title, see inside front cover.

1. Siegel RL, Miller KD, Fuchs HE, et al. Cancer statistics, 2022. *CA Cancer J Clin.* 2022;**72**:7–33.
3. Bray F, Ferlay J, Soerjomataram I, et al. Global cancer statistics 2018: GLOBOCAN estimates of incidence and mortality worldwide for 36 cancers in 185 countries. *CA Cancer J Clin.* 2018;**6**:394–424.
5. Berry DA, Cronin KA, Plevritis SK, et al. Effect of screening and adjuvant therapy on mortality from breast cancer. *NEJM.* 2005;**353**:1784–1792.
13. Sprague BL, Gangnon RE, Burt V, et al. Prevalence of mammographically dense breasts in the United States. *J Natl Cancer Inst.* 2014;**106**:dju255.
54. Prentice RL, Caan B, Chlebowski RT, et al. Low-fat dietary pattern and risk of invasive breast cancer: the Women's Health Initiative Randomized Controlled Dietary Modification Trial. *JAMA.* 2006;**295**:629–642.
62. Anothaisintawee T, Teerawattananon Y, Wiratkapun C, et al. Risk prediction models of breast cancer: a systematic review of model performances. *Breast Cancer Res Treat.* 2012;**133**:1–10.
64. Tyrer J, Duffy SW, Cuzick J. A breast cancer prediction model incorporating familial and personal risk factors. *Stat Med.* 2004;**23**:1111–1130.
66. Vachon CM, Pankratz VS, Scott CG, et al. The contributions of breast density and common genetic variation to breast cancer risk. *J Natl Cancer Inst.* 2015;**107**:dju397.
79. Allisson KH, Hammond MEH, Dowsett M, et al. Estrogen and progesterone receptor testing in breast cancer: ASCO/CAP Guideline Update. *J Clin Oncol.* 2020;**38**:1346–1366.
80. Wolff AC, Hammond MEH, Allison KH, et al. Human epidermal growth factor receptor 2 testing in breast cancer: American Society of Clinical Oncology/College of American Pathologists Clinical Practice Guideline Focused Update. *Arch Pathol Lab Med.* 2018;**142**:1364–1382.
82. Robson M, Im SA, Senkus E, et al. Olaparib for metastatic breast cancer in patients with a germline BRCA mutation. *N Engl J Med.* 2017;**377**:523–533.
83. Litton JK, Rugo HS, Ettl J, et al. Talazoparib in patients with advanced breast cancer and a germline BRCA mutation. *N Engl J Med.* 2018;**379**:753–763.
86. Baselga J, Campone M, Piccart M, et al. Everolimus in postmenopausal hormone-receptor-positive advanced breast cancer. *N Engl J Med.* 2012;**366**:520–529.
264. Giuliano AE, Hunt KK, Ballman KV, et al. Axillary dissection vs no axillary dissection in women with invasive breast cancer and sentinel node metastasis: a randomized clinical trial. *JAMA.* 2011;**305**:569–575.
270. Narod SA, Iqbal J, Giannakeas V, et al. Breast cancer mortality after a diagnosis of ductal carcinoma in situ. *JAMA Oncol.* 2015;**1**:888–896.
277. Veronesi U, Cascinelli N, Mariani L, et al. Twenty-year follow-up of a randomized study comparing breast-conserving surgery with radical mastectomy for early breast cancer. *N Engl J Med.* 2002;**347**:1227–1232.
279. Fisher B, Anderson S, Bryant J, et al. Twenty-year follow-up of a randomized trial comparing total mastectomy, lumpectomy, and lumpectomy plus irradiation for the treatment of invasive breast cancer. *N Engl J Med.* 2002;**347**:1233–1241.
280. Early Breast Cancer Trialists' Collaborative Group (EBCTCG), Darby S, McGale P, et al. Effect of radiotherapy after breast-conserving surgery on 10-year recurrence and 15-year breast cancer death: meta-analysis of individual patient data for 10,801 women in 17 randomized trials. *Lancet.* 2011;**378**:1707–1716.
282. Bartelink H, Horiot JC, Poortmans PM, et al. Impact of a higher radiation dose on local control and survival in breast-conserving therapy of early breast cancer: 10-year results of the randomized boost versus no boost EORTC 22881-10882 trial. *J Clin Oncol.* 2007;**25**:3259–3265.
342. von Minckwitz G, Huang CS, Mano MS, et al. Trastuzumab emtansine for residual invasive HER2-positive breast cancer. *N Engl J Med.* 2019;**380**:617–628.
343. Masuda N, Lee SJ, Ohtani S, et al. Adjuvant capecitabine for breast cancer after preoperative chemotherapy. *N Engl J Med.* 2017;**376**:2147–2159.
350. Early Breast Cancer Trialists' Collaborative Group, Davies C, Godwin J, et al. Relevance of breast cancer hormone receptors and other factors to the efficacy of adjuvant tamoxifen: patient-level meta-analysis of randomised trials. *Lancet.* 2011;**378**:771–784.
351. Cuzick J, Sestak I, Baum M, et al. Effect of anastrozole and tamoxifen as adjuvant treatment for early-stage breast cancer: 10-year analysis of the ATAC trial. *Lancet Oncol.* 2010;**11**:1135–1141.
362. Davies C, Pan H, Godwin J, et al. Long-term effects of continuing adjuvant tamoxifen to 10 years versus stopping at 5 years after diagnosis of oestrogen receptor-positive breast cancer: ATLAS, a randomised trial. *Lancet.* 2013;**381**:805–816.
367. Coombes RC, Hall E, Gibson LJ, et al. A randomized trial of exemestane after two to three years of tamoxifen therapy in postmenopausal women with primary breast cancer. *N Engl J Med.* 2004;**350**:1081–1092.
369. Goss PE, Ingle JN, Pritchard KI, et al. Extending aromatase-inhibitor adjuvant therapy to 10 years. *N Engl J Med.* 2016;**375**:209–219.
370. Mamounas EP, Bandos H, Lembersky BC, et al. Use of letrozole after aromatase inhibitor-based therapy in postmenopausal breast cancer (NRG Oncology/NSABP B-42): a randomised, double-blind, placebo-controlled, phase 3 trial. *Lancet Oncol.* 2019;**20**:88–99.
382. Paik S, Shak S, Tang G, et al. A multigene assay to predict recurrence of tamoxifen-treated, node-negative breast cancer. *N Engl J Med.* 2004;**351**:2817–2826.
383. Sparano JA, Gray RJ, Makower DF, et al. Adjuvant chemotherapy guided by a 21-gene expression assay in breast cancer. *N Engl J Med.* 2018;**379**:111–121.
384. Cardoso F, van't Veer LJ, Bogaerts J, et al. 70-gene signature as an aid to treatment decisions in early-stage breast cancer. *N Engl J Med.* 2016;**375**:717–729.
386. Cortazar P, Zhang L, Untch M, et al. Pathological complete response and long-term clinical benefit in breast cancer: the CTNeoBC pooled analysis. *Lancet.* 2014;**384**:164–172.
394. Rugo HS, Rumble RB, Macrae E, et al. Endocrine therapy for hormone receptor-positive metastatic breast cancer: American society of clinical oncology guideline. *J Clin Oncol.* 2016;**34**:3069–3103.
409. Finn RS, Martin M, Rugo HS, et al. Palbociclib and letrozole in advanced breast cancer. *N Engl J Med.* 2016;**375**:1925–1936.
411. Hortobagyi GN, Stemmer SM, Burris HA, et al. Ribociclib as first-line therapy for HR-positive, advanced breast cancer. *N Engl J Med.* 2016;**375**:1738–1748.
419. Sledge GW Jr, Toi M, Neven P, et al. The effect of abemaciclib plus fulvestrant on overall survival in hormone receptor-positive, ERBB2-negative breast cancer that progressed on endocrine therapy-MONARCH 2: a randomized clinical trial. *JAMA Oncol.* 2020;**6**:116–124.
421. Im SA, Lu YS, Bardia A, et al. Overall survival with ribociclib plus endocrine therapy in breast cancer. *N Engl J Med.* 2019;**381**:307–316.
424. Yardley DA, Noguchi S, Pritchard KI, et al. Everolimus plus exemestane in postmenopausal patients with HR(+) breast cancer: BOLERO-2 final progression-free survival analysis. *Adv Ther.* 2013;**30**:870–884.
427. Tripathy D, Im SA, Colleoni M, et al. Ribociclib plus endocrine therapy for premenopausal women with hormone-receptor-positive, advanced breast cancer (MONALEESA-7): a randomised phase 3 trial. *Lancet Oncol.* 2018;**19**:904–915.
428. Fisher B, Dignam J, Wolmark N, et al. Tamoxifen in treatment of intraductal breast cancer: National Surgical Adjuvant Breast and Bowel Project B-24 randomised controlled trial. *Lancet.* 1999;**353**:1993–2000.
429. Margolese RG, Cecchini RS, Julian TB, et al. Anastrozole versus tamoxifen in postmenopausal women with ductal carcinoma in situ undergoing lumpectomy plus radiotherapy (NSABP B-35): a randomised, double-blind, phase 3 clinical trial. *Lancet.* 2016;**387**:849–856.
433. Saad ED, Squifflet P, Burzykowski T, et al. Disease-free survival as a surrogate for overall survival in patients with HER2-positive, early breast cancer in trials of adjuvant trastuzumab for up to 1 year: a systematic review and meta-analysis. *Lancet Oncol.* 2019;**20**:361–370.
434. Prowell TM, Pazdur R. Pathological complete response and accelerated drug approval in early breast cancer. *N Engl J Med.* 2012;**366**:2438–2441.
435. Inno A, Barni S, Ghidini A, et al. One year versus a shorter duration of adjuvant trastuzumab for HER2-positive early breast cancer: a systematic review and meta-analysis. *Breast Cancer Res Treat.* 2019;**173**:247–254.
443. Koboldt DC, Fulton R, McLellan M, et al. Comprehensive molecular portraits of human breast tumours. *Nature.* 2012;**490**:61–70.

448 Sparano JA, Zhao F, Martino S, et al. Long-term follow-up of the E1199 phase III trial evaluating the role of taxane and schedule in operable breast cancer. *J Clin Oncol*. 2015;**33**:2353–2360.

457 Blum JL, Flynn PJ, Yothers G, et al. Anthracyclines in early breast cancer: the ABC trials-USOR 06-090, NSABP B-46-I/USOR 07132, and NSABP B-49 (NRG Oncology). *J Clin Oncol*. 2017;**35**:2647–2655.

461 Schmid P, Cortes J, Pusztai L, et al. Pembrolizumab for early triple-negative breast cancer. *N Engl J Med*. 2020;**382**:810–821.

479 Schmid P, Rugo HS, Adams S, et al. Atezolizumab plus nab-paclitaxel as first-line treatment for unresectable, locally advanced or metastatic triple-negative breast cancer (IMpassion130): updated efficacy results from a randomised, double-blind, placebo-controlled, phase 3 trial. *Lancet Oncol*. 2020;**21**:44–59.

480 Schmid P, Adams S, Rugo HS, et al. Atezolizumab and nab-paclitaxel in advanced triple-negative breast cancer. *N Engl J Med*. 2018;**379**:2108–2121.

481 Cortes J, Cescon DW, Rugo HS, et al. Pembrolizumab plus chemotherapy versus placebo plus chemotherapy for previously untreated locally recurrent inoperable or metastatic triple-negative breast cancer (KEYNOTE-355): a randomised, placebo-controlled, double-blind, phase 3 clinical trial. *Lancet*. 2020;**396**:1817–1828.

485 Bardia A, Hurvitz SA, Tolaney SM, et al. Sacituzumab govitecan in metastatic triple-negative breast cancer. *N Engl J Med*. 2021;**384**:1529–1541.

495 Dawood S, Merajver SD, Viens P, et al. International expert panel on inflammatory breast cancer: consensus statement for standardized diagnosis and treatment. *Ann Oncol*. 2011;**22**:515–523.

499 Masuda H, Brewer TM, Liu DD, et al. Long-term treatment efficacy in primary inflammatory breast cancer by hormonal receptor- and HER2-defined subtypes. *Ann Oncol*. 2014;**25**:384–391.

509 Woodward WA. Postmastectomy radiation therapy for inflammatory breast cancer: is more better? *Int J Radiat Oncol Biol Phys*. 2014;**89**:1004–1005.

533 Patchel RA, Tibbs PA, Walsh JW, et al. A randomized trial of surgery in the treatment of single metastasis to brain. *NEJM*. 1990;**322**:494–500.

543 Subbiah IM, Lei X, Weinberg JS, et al. Validation and development of a modified breast cancer graded prognostic assessment as a tool for survival in patients with breast cancer and brain metastasis. *JCO*. 2015;**33**:2239–2245.

558 Swain SM, Baselga J, Miles D, et al. Incidence of central nervous system metastasis in patients with HER-2 positive metastatic breast cancer treated with pertuzumab, trastuzumab and docetaxel: results from the randomized phase III study CLEOPATRA. *Ann Oncol*. 2014;**25**:1116–1121.

562 Murthy RK, Loi S, Okines A, et al. Tucatinib, trastuzumab, and capecitabine for HER2-positive metastatic breast cancer. *N Engl J Med*. 2019;**382**:597–609.

106 Malignant melanoma

Michael J. Carr, MD, MS ▪ Justin M. Ko, MD, MBA ▪ Susan M. Swetter, MD ▪ Scott E. Woodman, MD, PhD ▪ Vernon K. Sondak, MD ▪ Kim A. Margolin, MD ▪ Jonathan S. Zager, MD

> **Overview**
>
> Melanoma comprises a wide variety of malignant cell types arising from the skin, the mucous membranes, and the pigmented cells of the eye. While these tumors are all classified as melanoma and share a common molecular biology of pigmentation and biological resemblance to cells of neural crest origin, important distinctions in other molecular characteristics and patterns of exposure to ultraviolet light as a carcinogen determine their clinical natural history, including the response to therapeutic interventions. While the majority of melanomas are diagnosed at an early stage and curable with minimal surgery, melanoma has the potential for early and widespread dissemination via lymphatic and hematogenous routes. Surgery remains the mainstay of therapy for primary, regional, and many cases of single- or oligo-metastatic disease, but systemic therapies have dramatically improved the prognosis for metastatic melanoma, particularly immunotherapies that enhance existing cellular immunity. The rapid discovery of new molecular targets, immunotherapy combinations, and understanding of the mechanisms of therapeutic resistance is likely to lead to even greater improvements in the prognosis for patients with melanoma in the near future.

Dermatologic principles in melanoma

Epidemiology and etiology

Melanoma incidence and mortality rates continue to rise worldwide, driven by increased ultraviolet (UV) light exposure (both natural and artificial sources) and differences in prognosis according to age and sex. Incidence has more than doubled among non-Hispanic whites over the past 30 years, faster than that of nearly all cancers. Western states with increased ultraviolet radiation (UVR) have a greater incidence than those with lower UVR. From 2010 to 2014, US incidence rates decreased slightly in younger men and women but continued to rise significantly in women 45 years and older and men 55 years and older.[1]

The increase in melanoma incidence has been attributed to factors including increased intermittent UVR exposure in fair-skinned populations, higher rates of skin biopsies and screening resulting in the detection of thinner, biologically indolent lesions, and potential changes in the histologic interpretation of early evolving lesions from atypical melanocytic hyperplasia or severe dysplasia to melanoma *in situ*, which is a nonobligate precursor to invasive melanoma.[2,3] However, continued increases in the incidence rates of thicker tumors, including steep rises among individuals of lower socioeconomic status, points to a true increase in potentially fatal cases and lack of screening as a critical factor accounting for melanoma incidence trends.[4] Recent favorable trends in melanoma mortality are a result of more efficacious immune and targeted therapies for patients with advanced disease; mortality rates dropped by 6.2% per year between 2013 and 2016, with an even larger decline (8.3% per year) in men 50 years and older since 2014.

Risk factors

Environmental factors
The risk of developing melanoma is related to both intermittent and chronic UVR exposure from UV-A and UV-B light. Melanomas associated with intermittent UVR tend to occur in areas with less cumulative sun damage (i.e., trunk, proximal extremities) and in patients with higher nevus count, as opposed to those in chronically sun-exposed sites (i.e., head/neck, forearms), which tend to occur in patients with lower nevus counts.[5,6] Age of onset also tends to differ between melanomas related to intermittent vs chronic UVR,[7] around 55 years for those developing on intermittently-exposed sites, which likely reflects a period of vulnerability to UVR early in life and a latency to full melanomagenesis that may be triggered by ongoing UVR and other host factors.[8] Conversely, melanomas on chronically exposed sites tend to occur in older age individuals. Signature DNA mutations induced by UV are found commonly in driver mutations identified in melanoma[9] but not as often as in nonmelanoma skin cancers that are more directly related to chronic sun exposure, so alternate sources of mutagenesis are likely. Nevertheless, a randomized study in Australia showed that consistent daily application of both UVA- and UVB-filtering broad-spectrum sunscreen (compared with discretionary or nonuse) resulted in a decreased incidence of melanoma.[10] Indoor tanning is now proven to be a major contributor to the increased incidence of cutaneous melanoma among young women, with greater melanoma risk proportional to increasing years, hours, and sessions of indoor tanning.[11,12] Alarmingly, 76% of melanomas in light-skinned participants were attributed to tanning bed use at young ages. A strong association of tanning bed use with recreational drugs,[13] suggesting a common genetically mediated addiction, is consistent with animal studies showing sunlight-seeking behaviors mediated by opioid-related substances through endorphin receptors.[14]

Host factors
Although the process by which normal melanocytes transform into melanoma cells is not entirely understood, it is believed to involve progressive genetic mutations that alter cell proliferation, differentiation, and death and impact cellular susceptibility to the carcinogenic effects of UVR. Melanoma is mainly a disease of individuals of lighter skin complexion, particularly those with red hair,

who burn easily or have a history of severe sunburn, or who are unable to tan.[15] Non-Hispanic whites with an increased number of nevi are also at increased risk for developing melanoma.[16] The risk of cutaneous melanoma in the presence of increased numbers of common/typical nevi, large nevi, and/or clinically atypical nevi (CAN) on the body was confirmed in a pooled analysis of melanocytic nevus phenotype, even at different latitudes.[17] Both prior personal history and family history are important risk factors for the development of melanoma. Solid-organ transplant recipients are at increased risk of developing melanoma compared to the general population, with more aggressive melanoma behavior related to transplant-associated immunosuppression.[18,19]

Genetic predisposition and familial melanoma
The majority of melanomas appear to be sporadic, with only 5–10% of cases attributable to an identified familial predisposition. Familial melanoma is characterized by an increased risk of developing melanoma, a higher incidence of multiple primary melanomas, and typically an earlier age at onset.[20] Specific genetic alterations have been implicated in the pathogenesis of familial melanoma. Mutations at the CDKN2A locus on chromosome 9p21, which codes for the tumor suppressor p16 and p14/ARF, account for about one-third of familial cases. Additional melanoma risk occurs in CDKN2A mutation carriers who express variants of the melanocortin receptor gene MC1R, which is associated with red hair, fair skin, and freckling. As mutations of either of these genes are present in only a subset of familial melanoma kindreds, other melanoma susceptibility genes likely exist. Formal recommendations for p16 mutation testing have been proposed in patients with a personal or family history of three or more invasive melanomas or cancer events, defined as two invasive melanomas and one pancreatic cancer in the patient or family members, or vice versa, which conveys a >20% risk of carriage.[21] However, owing to the low frequency of mutations even among high-risk individuals and the lack of implications for dermatologic surveillance, genetic testing other than for research purposes is generally not recommended.

Atypical mole syndrome/phenotype
The presence of numerous CAN, histologically termed dysplastic nevi, is the most important clinical risk factor for melanoma. Compared with the general population, patients with CAN have a 2- to 15-fold elevated risk of developing melanoma, and risk increases with the number of CAN and/or personal or family history of melanoma.[22] An atypical mole phenotype is characterized by numerous (>50–100) common nevi along with multiple (generally >5), large (>6–8 mm) nevi with color variegation, border irregularity, and asymmetric shape. Melanomas seldom arise in association with preexisting atypical nevi, and over 70% of melanomas in patients with any type of melanocytic nevus (common, atypical, or congenital) are believed to develop de novo, although CAN with severe histologic dysplasia may more often be true melanoma precursors.[23] Melanomas associated with atypical/dysplastic nevi are generally thin superficial spreading type, possibly due to increased skin surveillance in affected individuals.

Congenital melanocytic nevi
Congenital melanocytic nevi (CMN) are evident in 1–6% of neonates and uncommonly transform into melanoma.[24] Patients with congenital nevi >20 cm in diameter in an adult, >6 cm on the body of an infant, or >9 cm on the head of an infant have a less than 5% lifetime risk of developing a melanoma[25–28] with about half arising during the first few years of life.[29] The risk of melanoma arising within small-sized (<1.5 cm) and medium-sized CMN is low and virtually nonexistent before puberty.[30] Management of CMN hinges on many variables including ease of monitoring and potential psychosocial benefits and harms of surgical procedures.

Melanoma risk assessment
Several risk assessment tools have been used to target individuals at high risk for developing melanoma. One risk assessment tool was derived from a large case-control study of 718 non-Hispanic white patients and 945 controls that involved inspection of the back for suspicious moles and asked two questions about complexion and history of sun exposure.[31] Mild freckling and light complexion were demonstrated as risk factors for both men and women. In addition, >17 small moles and ≥2 large moles in men or ≥12 small moles on the backs of women were also significant risk factors. These data led to the Melanoma Risk Assessment Tool, which is available from the National Cancer Institute (http://www.cancer.gov/melanomarisktool/) and calculates absolute risk of melanoma over the next 5 years up to age 70. A more recent risk assessment tool was developed using data from Australia and Sweden and incorporates self-assessed hair color, nevus density, first-degree family history of melanoma, previous nonmelanoma skin cancer, and lifetime sunbed use to calculate melanoma risk.[32]

Prognostic factors
A number of clinical factors affect patient prognosis including age, gender, and anatomic location of the primary tumor. In general, men, older age individuals, and those with melanoma on the head and neck tend to fare worse. A population-based study in France during 2004–2008 showed that male patients had thicker and more frequently ulcerated tumors. Older patients had thicker and more advanced melanomas, with more frequent head and neck location.[33] While newer concepts in the taxonomy of melanoma suggest distinct molecular, genetic, anatomic, and UV-exposure-linked characteristics, growth kinetics of certain histological subtypes also appear to play a role in prognosis. The rapidly growing nodular subtype of melanoma tends to elude early detection based on clinical characteristics alone. Nodular melanoma (NM) comprises <15% of subtyped melanoma cases in the United States and Australia, but accounts for a disproportionate number of thicker tumors (>2 mm) and melanoma deaths compared with other histologic subtypes.[34]

Clinical presentation

Cutaneous melanoma can occur anywhere but is most common on the lower extremities and back in women and on the trunk in men. From a clinical standpoint, a new or changing mole or skin lesion is the most common warning sign for melanoma. The so-called "ABCDEs" of early diagnosis pioneered by Sigel et al.[35] are an easy mnemonic to improve recognition of the classic early signs of melanoma (Table 1). To simplify further, Weinstock[36] succinctly focused the message by emphasizing that the most important warning sign is a new or changing skin lesion. The "ugly duckling" warning sign refers to a pigmented or clinically amelanotic lesion that looks different from the rest, which may be of value to identify melanomas that lack the classic ABCD criteria (e.g., nodular, amelanotic, or desmoplastic subtypes).[37,38]

Table 1 ABCDEs: clinical features of melanoma.

A	Asymmetry—the two halves of the lesion do not match each other
B	Border irregularity—may appear ragged, notched, or scalloped
C	Color variation—color is not uniform or lesion may be many colors displaying shades of tan, brown, or black. White, reddish, or blue-gray discoloration is of particular concern
D	Diameter—usually >6 mm (roughly the diameter of a pencil eraser) although melanomas may be smaller in size; any growth in a nevus warrants an evaluation
E	Evolving lesion—changes in size or color; critical for nodular or amelanotic melanoma, which may not exhibit the ABCD criteria above

As histologic features of a primary melanoma are critical for melanoma staging and prognostication, proper initial biopsy of a suspicious lesion is paramount. An excisional/complete biopsy with narrow clinical margins (1–3 mm) of normal-appearing skin around the pigmented lesion is preferred when possible to provide accurate diagnosis and histologic microstaging; complete biopsy may be performed via elliptical or punch excision versus saucerization shave removal. An important exception to this rule is the lentigo maligna (LM) subtype of melanoma *in situ*, in which the risk of misdiagnosis is high if small or partial biopsy specimens are taken. The best diagnostic biopsy technique, in this case, is often a broad shave biopsy that extends into at least the papillary dermis, provides the opportunity to exclude microinvasive melanoma, and allows for optimal histopathologic interpretation of the tumor.

Pathologic features

Dermal invasion confers metastatic potential, although the greatest risk occurs in the setting of a vertical growth (tumorigenic) phase.[39] With the exception of NM, the growth patterns of the other clinicopathologic subtypes are characterized by a preceding *in situ* (radial growth) phase that lacks the biologic potential to metastasize and may last from months to years before dermal invasion (vertical growth) occurs. Immunohistochemical staining for lineage [S-100, human melanoma black 45 (HMB-45), melan-A/Mart-1] or proliferation markers (Ki67) may be helpful in some cases for histologic differentiation from melanoma simulators such as melanocytic nevi, Spitz nevi, cellular blue nevus, clear cell sarcoma, or malignant peripheral nerve sheath tumor.[40] A study of melanoma biomarker expression in melanocytic tumor progression examined differential expression of melanoma biomarkers between nevi, primary melanoma, and metastases.[41] Approaches combining Ki67/MART-1 (Melan-A) and HMB-45/MITF immunostains have been used for melanoma diagnosis, along with newer immunostains such as nuclear transcription factor (SOX10) and melanoma associated antigen (PReferentially expressed Antigen in Melanoma [PRAME]).[42]

A pathology report for melanoma should include tumor thickness (Breslow depth) and presence of ulceration, dermal mitotic rate (measured as number per mm^2), microsatellites, and lymphovascular invasion. Anatomic level of invasion (Clark's level) has less prognostic significance and is no longer used in pathology reporting.

Atypical melanocytic lesions in children and adolescents, in particular, may be difficult to distinguish from true melanoma, including atypical Spitz tumors and Spitz tumors of uncertain malignant potential. As such, molecular techniques such as comparative genomic hybridization (CGH) and fluorescence *in situ* hybridization (FISH) have been utilized to assist in the determination of malignant versus benign lesions.[43–46] Gene expression profiling remains controversial in the diagnosis of challenging atypical melanocytic neoplasms,[47–50] but integration of next-generation sequencing with cytomorphology has also been shown to improve biologic and prognostic classification of atypical Spitz/spitzoid neoplasms.[51]

Clinicopathologic subtypes

The four major classical histogenetic subtypes of primary cutaneous melanoma are based on histopathologic findings, anatomic site, and degree of sun damage. These include superficial spreading melanoma, NM, lentigo maligna melanoma (LMM), and acral lentiginous melanoma. In addition, there are other rarer variants (<5% of melanomas), which include (1) desmoplastic/neurotropic melanoma, (2) mucosal melanoma, (3) blue nevus-like melanoma, and (4) melanoma arising in a giant/large congenital nevus (Figure 1).[50]

Superficial spreading melanoma
Superficial spreading melanoma accounts for nearly 70% of cutaneous melanoma, commonly displays the ABCDE signs, and is the most common subtype in individuals aged 30–50 years, as well as those with atypical/dysplastic nevi. It is most common on the trunk in men and women and on the legs in women.

Nodular melanoma
NM is the next most common melanoma subtype and occurs in 15–30% of patients, most commonly on the legs and trunk in men and women. It typically presents as a dark brown-to-black papule or dome-shaped nodule with rapid growth over weeks to month but may be amelanotic, which may ulcerate and bleed with minor trauma. This subtype is responsible for most thick melanomas at diagnosis.[52]

Lentigo maligna melanoma
LMM incidence is rising in the United States.[53] It is typically located on chronically sun-damaged skin (CSD) (head, neck, and arms) of fair-skinned older individuals (average age 65 years), slowly growing over years to decades. The *in situ* precursor lesion termed LM is typically a longstanding large >1–3 cm flat (macular) lesion, demonstrating pigmentation ranging from dark brown to black, although white or hypopigmented areas are common within LM. Dermal invasion denoting progression to LMM is characterized by the development of raised brown-black nodules within the *in situ* lesion.

Acral melanoma
Acral melanoma is the least-common subtype of melanoma in white persons (2–8% of melanoma cases), although the most-common subtype of melanoma in darker-complexioned individuals (i.e., African American, Asian, and Hispanic persons), representing 29–72% of melanoma cases in these populations. Acral lentiginous melanoma occurs on the palms, soles, or beneath the nail plate (subungual melanoma), which may manifest as diffuse nail discoloration or a longitudinal pigmented band (melanonychia striata) within the finger or toenail. Pigment spread to the proximal or lateral nail folds is termed the Hutchinson sign, which is a hallmark for subungual melanoma. Because of the atypical locations of occurrence, there may be a delay in diagnosis associated with advanced presentation.[54,55]

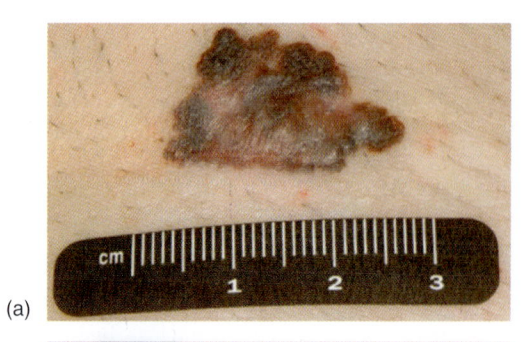

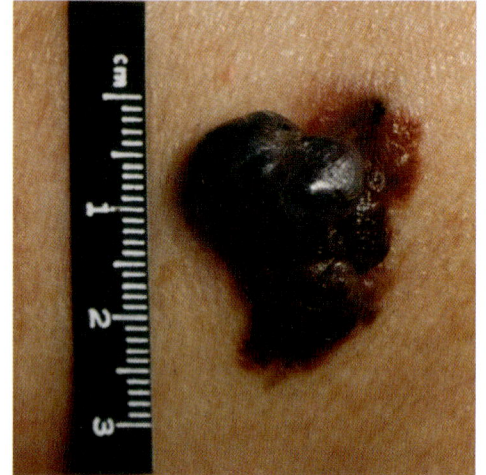

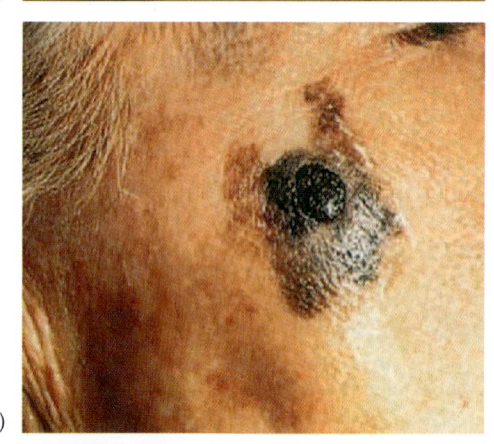

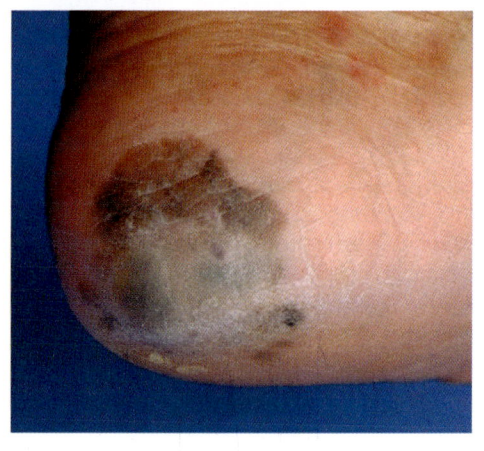

Figure 1 (a) Superficial spreading melanoma. Note the irregular borders, a variegation in color, and size >6 mm. (b) Nodular melanoma. (c) LMM with a nodular area of accelerated growth. (d) Acral lentiginous melanoma of heel. Source: Courtesy of Jeffrey E. Gershenwald, MD.

Less-common subtypes

Desmoplastic melanoma is a less common but important melanoma subtype, given its predilection for older age individuals, clinical features similar to nonmelanoma (keratinocytic) skin cancer, and potential indication for adjuvant radiation therapy following wide excision (depending on tumor thickness, perineural invasion, and margin status). Amelanotic melanoma (<5% of melanomas) can occur with any subtype and often mimics basal cell or squamous cell carcinoma, dermatofibroma, or a ruptured hair follicle. It occurs most commonly in the setting of the nodular or desmoplastic subtype or melanoma metastasis to the skin, presumably because of the inability of these poorly differentiated cancer cells to synthesize melanin pigment.

Genetics and molecular pathology

Significant complexity exists in the clinical and histopathological presentation, cells of origin, causative relationship to UVR, age of onset, somatic mutations, and germline genetic predisposition. Melanoma is not a homogeneous disease but instead is composed of biologically distinct subtypes, the phenotype of which is driven by underlying genetic alterations.[56]

Recognitiong of a a key growth factor pathway in melanoma resulted in development of groundbreaking therapies targeting the RAS–RAF–MAPK–ERK (mitogen-associated protein kinase, MAPK) signaling cascade. A unique mutation at position 1799 of the gene for the serine–threonine kinase BRAF in the MAPK pathway—occurring in about half of cutaneous melanomas—results in a substitution of glutamine (about 75–80% of cases) or lysine for valine (most of the remaining cases) at position 600 which confers constitutive activity, resulting in hyperproliferation and resistance to apoptosis among cells driven by this oncogenic mutation.[57] The biology of melanoma in cells dependent on a BRAF mutation is also impacted by coexisting mutations or other alterations of gene expression in linked pathways, particularly the phosphatase and tensin homolog (PTEN)/AKT/PI3K/mTOR pathway that is critical in the control of metabolic sensors and the cancer/microenvironment nutrient balance. Activating mutations of NRAS, as well as less-common oncogenes such as c-kit (covered in greater detail below), result in downstream activation of both of these pathways.

Most BRAF-mutated melanomas arise in intermittently sun-exposed skin, while melanomas from chronically sun-exposed areas have a lower incidence of BRAF mutations and occasionally carry a mutation or amplification of c-Kit[58,59] a receptor tyrosine kinase that may be altered in about 15–20% of acral and mucosal melanomas.[60-62] Activation of c-Kit results in the stimulation of both the MAPK and PI3K–AKT pathways, producing both proliferative and survival advantages.[61]

The observation that BRAF mutations noted in benign melanocytic nevi typically arising by early adolescence occurred with the same frequency as in non-CSD melanoma led to the proposition that patients with acquired nevi and non-CSD melanomas may have a particular susceptibility for developing BRAF-mutated melanocytic neoplasms at relatively low doses of UV radiation.[62] This concept was supported in subsequent studies that demonstrated a germline polymorphism in the melanocortin receptor 1 (MC1R) to significantly contribute to this susceptibility. More specifically, polymorphisms of MC1R were shown to strongly increase the risk for non-CSD melanomas with BRAF mutation.[63]

None of the oncogenes or tumor suppressor genes identified in melanoma are thought to be solely responsible for melanoma pathogenesis, and some appear to be mutually exclusive due to overlapping downstream functions. For instance, activating NRAS mutations, occurring in 15–20% of melanomas from any site (with the exception of uveal), cause enhanced signaling through cell-surface growth factor receptors with downstream stimulation of Raf and Raf-dependent kinases. Activating mutations of NRAS practically never occur in the same cells as BRAF v600 mutations.[64] The loss of the p16 tumor suppressor and other alterations of the cyclin-dependent kinases (CDKs) are relatively frequent somatic alterations in melanoma, and there is significant overlap with BRAF mutation.[65] PTEN alterations, most commonly loss-of-function mutations and less often genetic deletion, have been described in a fraction of melanomas and appear to coincide with BRAF mutation, rendering these cells more resistant to targeted therapy but providing the potential for the development of regimen that also target the cellular pathways downstream from the suppressive effects of PTEN, particularly the PI3K/AKT/mTOR pathway.[66]

Surgical management of melanoma

Management of primary cutaneous melanoma

Surgery remains the mainstay of treatment for primary cutaneous melanoma. Primary melanoma is treated by wide excision with a defined margin of adjacent normal-appearing skin. The margin of resection is dependent on the Breslow depth of the tumor and the site of the primary. Margin widths are measured from the biopsy scar or residual pigment at the time of surgery; it is not expected to equate to a histopathologic measurement on the resection specimen. A histologically negative margin, however, is always the goal in excising the primary tumor. Current recommendations for width of the excision in invasive melanoma (Table 2) are supported by randomized trials, summarized in Table 3.[67–71] For melanoma in situ, the recommended margin is 0.5–1 cm. For invasive melanomas ≤1 mm in depth, 1 cm margins are recommended and are associated with low rates of local recurrence. For melanomas between 1 and 2 mm, 1–2 cm margins are recommended, taking into consideration cosmetic or functional outcome. For melanomas >2 mm, 2 cm margins are recommended, whenever feasible. A meta-analysis found that margins >2 cm are unnecessary even for thick primaries, and margins should not be <1 cm for any invasive melanoma.[72] A Phase 3, multicenter, international randomized study (MelmarT, NCT02385214) is currently underway to evaluate the use of 1 cm versus 2 cm margins for excision of lesions ≥1 mm thick, with the endpoints of comparing rates of local recurrence and melanoma-specific survival.

Management of the regional lymph nodes

The role of sentinel lymph node biopsy

The presence of occult tumor deposits within clinically negative lymph nodes is a key predictor of outcome in clinical stage I and II melanoma,[73,74] and evidence suggests even tiny nodal micrometastases have clinical relevance.[75,76] Melanoma micrometastases in the regional lymph nodes cannot reliably be detected by any imaging modality, including PET–CT[77,78] or ultrasonography.[79,80] Sentinel lymph node biopsy (SLNB) can identify micrometastases with low morbidity. In 2018, an evidence-based assessment of the indications for SLNB in melanoma was issued jointly by ASCO and the Society of Surgical Oncology (SSO) (Table 3).[81]

Table 2 Recommended margins of wide excision for cutaneous melanoma based on primary tumor thickness and location.[a]

Breslow thickness	Primary site	Recommended excision margin (cm)
Melanoma in situ	Anywhere on the skin	0.5–1
0.01–1.00 (mm)	Anywhere on the skin	1
1.01–2.00 (mm)	Head/neck, distal extremity[b]	1
	Trunk or proximal extremity[c]	2
>2.00 (mm)	Head/neck, distal extremity[b]	1
	Trunk or proximal extremity	2

[a]Source: Adapted from Sondak and Gibney.[67]
[b]Subungual primary tumors may require distal digital amputation.
[c]If a skin graft would be required to reconstruct the excision defect, it is acceptable to take a 1 cm excision margin.
Local anatomic constraints and specific patient factors may justify minor deviations from the standard margin recommendations.

Table 3 Summary of ASCO-SSO recommendations for sentinel lymph node biopsy in melanoma.[a]

- SLNB is recommended for patients with cutaneous melanomas with Breslow thickness of >1–4 mm at any anatomic site
- SLNB may be recommended for staging purposes and to facilitate regional disease control for patients with melanomas that are >4 mm in Breslow thickness
- There is insufficient evidence to support routine SLNB for patients with T1a melanomas (nonulcerated lesions <0.8 mm in Breslow thickness). SLNB may be considered for T1b patients (0.8–1.0 mm Breslow thickness or <0.8 mm with ulceration), after thorough discussion of benefits and risks of harm with the patient.
- Either completion lymph node dissection or careful observation may be recommended for all patients with a positive SLNB, with due consideration of clinicopathological factors and patient autonomy.

SLNB, sentinel lymph node biopsy.
[a]Source: Adapted from Wong et al.[68]

The panel found that the strongest evidence supported SLNB for patients with intermediate-thickness melanomas, based on results from the prospective randomized Multicenter Selective Lymphadenectomy Trial I (MSLT-1).[73,74] Key ASCO–SSO SLNB recommendations are summarized in Table 3. The results of MSLT-1 (Table 4) and retrospective institutional series also support SLNB for patients with clinically node-negative thick melanomas (>4 mm).[82–85] Controversy remains regarding the use of sentinel node biopsy in patients with thin melanomas (<1 mm), which were not adequately assessed in the MSLT-1 study nor included in the prospective but nonrandomized Sunbelt Melanoma Trial.[86]

The majority of newly diagnosed cutaneous melanomas are ≤1 mm in thickness, with a low overall risk of nodal metastasis or death from melanoma.[87] Sentinel node biopsy for all patients with T1 melanomas is not associated with favorable cost-effectiveness or risk-benefit advantages and is therefore not routinely recommended.[88] ASCO–SSO recommends that SLNB for thin melanoma be considered in selected cases with high-risk features (Table 5).[81,89–96]

On the basis of the large retrospectively collected registry data, the current AJCC Cancer Staging Manual Eighth Edition (AJCC 8) defines the T-category thresholds at 1, 2, and 4 mm melanoma thickness. T1 subcategories are defined as T1a, nonulcerated melanoma <0.8 mm in thickness, and T1b, ulcerated

Table 4 Summary of selected final results of the Multicenter Selective Lymphadenectomy Trial 1 (MSLT-1).[a]

	Result	Comment
Feasibility	At least one sentinel node was identified in 99.5% of patients undergoing SLNB	SLNB highly feasible in a worldwide experience
Yield and false-negative rate	The sentinel node was positive in 19% of patients with melanomas ≥1.2 mm: 16% for melanomas 1.2–3.5 mm and 33% for melanomas >3.5 mm	SLNB is an effective staging procedure with an acceptable false-negative rate
Prognostic significance	A positive sentinel node was associated with ~2.5-fold increases in disease recurrence and death from melanoma for melanomas 1.2–3.5 mm; 10-year melanoma-specific survival was 85% for patients with a negative sentinel node versus 62% for patients with a positive sentinel node	Sentinel node status is the strongest known prognostic indicator in clinically node-negative intermediate-thickness melanoma
Survival impact of SLNB	There was a nonsignificant 3% increase in 10-year melanoma-specific survival for intermediate-thickness melanoma patients randomized to SLNB versus observation	SLNB does not significantly affect survival for all patients subjected to the procedure
Relapse-free survival impact	Patients randomized to SLNB had a statistically significant improvement in relapse-free survival compared to observation	SLNB significantly reduces melanoma recurrence for intermediate and thick melanomas, mostly by decreasing subsequent nodal relapse
Impact on node-positive patients	Patients with intermediate-thickness melanoma and positive nodes who were randomized to SLNB (with completion lymphadenectomy) had statistically significantly improved distant metastasis-free survival and melanoma-specific survival compared to observation arm patients who failed clinically in the regional nodal basin; there were no significant differences for patients with thick melanomas and positive nodes between the SLNB and observation arms	Early treatment of intermediate-thickness node-positive melanoma by radical lymphadenectomy improves outcomes significantly; patients with thick node-positive melanomas may be at such high risk of distant disease that timing of lymphadenectomy loses importance

SLNB, sentinel lymph node biopsy.
[a]Source: Adapted from Sondak and Gibney[67] Original data from Morton.

Table 5 High-risk features for selecting T1 melanomas for sentinel lymph node biopsy.

High-risk criterion	Impact on likelihood of finding a positive node	Comment
Thickness 0.76–0.99 (mm)	In a registry series of 1250 patients with melanomas ≤1 mm selected by a wide variety of criteria to undergo SLNB, metastases were detected in 6.3% of 891 melanomas ≥0.76 mm but in only 2.5% of 359 melanomas ≤0.75 mm. No metastases were detected in sentinel nodes from patients with melanomas <0.5 mm.[89] In a large contemporary single-institution experience from a center where SLNB was routinely offered to patients with melanoma ≥0.76 mm without requiring any other high-risk feature to be present, 8.4% of patients had a positive sentinel node[82]	Most patients with thin melanomas and a positive sentinel node are found in this upper end of the thickness spectrum; very few unselected patients with melanomas <0.76 mm are at sufficient risk of nodal metastasis to justify SLNB
Ulceration	18.3% of patients in a registry series[89] and 23.5% of patients in a single-institution series[90] who had ulcerated melanomas ≤1 mm had a positive sentinel node	Relatively rare finding in melanomas ≤1 mm (present in <10% of cases) but perhaps the highest risk factor for sentinel node positivity in thin melanoma. Presence of ulceration upstages the tumor from a to b in all T subcategories in the AJCC 8 staging system[91]
Mitotic count	Mitotic count ≥1/mm^2 was not predictive of nodal metastases in a registry series[89] but was predictive in a single-institution series.[90] In a multicenter observational study of 4249 patients with melanomas ≤1 mm, those with melanoma <0.8 mm had SLN positivity rate of 3.4% which rose to 20% with ≥2/mm^2. In 0.8–1.0 mm melanoma the overall SLN positivity rate was 8%, which fell to 3.6% with mitotic rate of 0/mm^2 [92]	Although no longer included in T subcategory criteria, mitotic activity has been associated with increased risk of SLN metastasis[91]
Patient age	In a National Cancer Database study of 8772 patients with melanomas 0.5–1.0 mm, rate of SLN positivity decreased consistently with increasing age[93]	Younger patients have a higher risk of positive sentinel nodes across all tumor thickness categories as well as more years at risk for nodal recurrence
Clark level	Clark level was a significant predictor of sentinel node status in a registry series[89] but not in a single-institution series[90]	Clark level IV melanomas are more likely to be thicker (≥0.76–1.00 mm) where most nodal metastases are encountered. The value of SLNB for Clark IV melanomas <0.76 mm has not been demonstrated

SLNB, sentinel lymph node biopsy.

melanoma <0.8 mm in thickness or any melanoma 0.8–1.0 mm in thickness.[89] SLNB seems well justified for many patients with melanomas 0.8–1.00 mm, but not for the majority of patients with melanomas <0.8 mm in thickness. Consideration should be given for SLNB in T1a melanoma with high mitotic rate (>2/mm^2) or T1b melanoma without mitoses or low mitotic rate. In addition, patient age, preference, and comorbidities need to be considered in the decision regarding SNLB. A few other clinical situations pertaining to the use of SLNB deserve mention. Desmoplastic melanomas, in general, appear to have a lower risk of nodal metastases, and some authors advocate abandoning SLNB in this histologic type. However, the risk of nodal metastases has been shown to be high enough to justify routine consideration of SLNB in all patients with desmoplastic melanomas ≥1 mm in thickness.[97-99] Pediatric melanoma patients have a higher incidence of nodal metastases, yet an apparent better overall prognosis compared to adults, and the role of SLNB in these patients remains controversial, especially for the so-called atypical melanocytic proliferations of childhood.[100–103]

Lymphadenectomy for node-positive disease
The MSLT-1 trial showed that outcomes for patients with intermediate-thickness melanoma and a positive SNLB undergoing completion lymphadenectomy (CLND) were superior to those for patients whose melanoma recurred in the nodal basin, but by the nature of the trial, the contribution of the CLND over and above removal of the sentinel node could not be assessed, and nonsentinel nodes were only found to have tumor involvement in a minority of cases[73,74] The morbidity of lymphadenectomy, especially severe lymphedema, has been shown to be less for CLND after a positive SLNB than for therapeutic lymphadenectomy in patients whose disease recurs.[104,105]

The second Multicenter Selective Lymphadenectomy Trial (MSLT-2) evaluated the benefit of CLND for patients with SLNB positive disease, comparing ultrasound surveillance of the lymph node basin to immediate CLND for sentinel node-positive patients. There was an increase in regional disease control in patients randomized to undergo CLND; the prognostic value of identifying nonsentinel-node metastasis is most important for decisions regarding adjuvant systemic therapy, which is now superior to the therapies that were available during the time period in which the MSLT-2 was conducted. However, given that limitation, the primary endpoint of melanoma-specific survival was not improved with CLND. Additionally, postoperative lymphedema was significantly higher in the CLND group, and CLND was associated with a higher morbidity and risk of infection, particularly in the inguinal area.[106] The MSLT-2 study was limited in adaptation into clinical practice by exclusion of sentinel node-positive patients with extranodal extension, microsatellitosis, and/or >3 positive sentinel lymph nodes. A propensity-score matched comparison of nodal surveillance versus CLND in patients with these high-risk factors found similar relapse-free survival (RFS) and melanoma specific survival (MSS), suggesting that ultrasound surveillance of the lymph node basin is also appropriate in these patients.[107]

NCCN guidelines, strongly supported by decades of clinical experience, call for routine performance of a therapeutic lymphadenectomy in all melanoma patients with clinically (palpable on examination or considered likely to be involved with melanoma on radiographic assessment) positive nodes and no radiographic evidence of distant metastases. However, the routine use of CLND after a positive SLNB is no longer the preferred treatment.[108] Recommendations made by the ASCO/SSO guidelines are considered standard of care, based on consideration of clinicopathologic factors, include CLND or preferably close surveillance with nodal bed ultrasound every 4 months for the first 3 years, every 6 months for another 2 years, and then yearly out to 10 years after positive SLNB.[81]

Management of in-transit and locoregional recurrent melanoma
Wide excision remains the first-line treatment for biopsy-proven local, satellite, or in-transit recurrence when a limited number of lesions can be resected without adverse functional or cosmetic outcomes and in the absence of distant disease. Therefore, radiographic staging with full-body PET/CT and brain MRI should be performed before curative-intent excision of the recurrent tumor.

Intra-arterial regional perfusion therapies
Hyperthermic isolated limb perfusion (HILP) and isolated limb infusion (ILI) are methods of treating unresectable locally recurrent or in-transit metastatic melanoma limited to an extremity and without distant metastasis. The extremity is isolated from systemic circulation through vascular occlusion, enabling the intra-arterial injection of high-dose chemotherapy with limited systemic exposure. HILP is performed by exposing the major vessels of the extremity through direct dissection and circulating chemotherapy via a cardiopulmonary bypass machine, which allows increased temperature and an oxygenated perfusate.[109,110] Response rates in the range of 80–90% with complete response (CR) rates as high as 60–70% have been reported.[110–114]

Melphalan is the most common cytotoxic agent used in the United States, while melphalan plus tumor necrosis factor-alpha (TNF-α) is often used in Europe. The value of TNF-α has not been clearly demonstrated, as a large multicenter randomized trial found no statistically significant differences in either overall or CR rates or survival, and the addition of TNF-α was associated with significantly higher regional toxicity. Significant morbidity may occur, the most common being lymphedema, which has been reported to occur in 12–36% of patients. Severe regional toxicities including compartment syndrome in up to 5% of cases as well as limb loss in up to 3.3% of cases have been described.[110]

ILI is the less-invasive counterpart to HILP and is a manually circulated low-flow infusion conducted in a mildly hyperthermic, acidotic, and hypoxic environment. Catheters are percutaneously placed into the artery and vein of the uninvolved limb and advanced into the vessels of the involved limb proximal to the extent of disease, avoiding the need for open surgical cannulation with its attendant morbidity.[114] Regional CR rates after ILI are in the range of 23–44% with partial response (PR) rates in the range of 27–56%.[115] Although the two techniques have not been prospectively compared in a head-to-head manner in a clinical trial setting, a retrospective comparison found a significantly higher overall response rate for HILP (53% vs 80%, $p < 0.001$), yet no difference in median overall survival (OS) (46 vs 40 months, $p = 0.31$). However, burden of disease (BOD) was higher for the ILI group (high BOD 58% vs 44%, $p = 0.04$), notable as lower BOD has been associated with improved rates of response.[116–119] ILI can be readily repeated if necessary and appears to have less regional toxicities than HILP (erythema and edema of the skin are among the most common side effects with tissue loss seen <1% of the time), virtually no systemic toxicities, and is well tolerated in octo- and nonagenarians.[119,120]

Intralesional and topical therapies
Intralesional therapy in melanoma has several advantages over regional or systemic therapy. Local drug administration allows for delivery of an increased concentration of the agent and reduced regional and systemic exposure, potentially increasing efficacy and lowering toxicity. Moreover, alterations in the tumor microenvironment can be immunogenic and induce local immune responses that result in the bystander effect, where uninjected distant lesions exhibit a response.

Bacille Calmette–Guèrin (BCG) was one of the first intralesional therapies used for in-transit metastases, based on the regression of injected metastases and occasional regression of uninjected lesions, suggesting the achievement of a substantial local antitumor immune response that could result in systemic immunity against distant metastases. Other immunomodulatory agents, including Interleukin-2 (IL-2) and alpha-interferon (IFN-α), and

Rose Bengal, a xanthine dye otherwise used for imaging purposes, have also demonstrated activity against injected lesions, but durable control and antitumor activity against distant metastases are rarely achieved, and there is no uniform practice for dose, schedule, or potential combination with other therapies.

PV-10 is a 10% solution of Rose Bengal, shown to preferentially enter melanoma cell lysosomes, resulting in tumor cell death secondary to the release of proteases.[121,122] Responses have been reported in patients refractory to previous systemic ipilimumab, anti-PD1, and vemurafenib, with evidence of bystander effects in uninjected lesions.[123] A Phase 1b/2 study of 23 patients with stage III and IV melanoma treated with PV-10 in combination with immune checkpoint inhibitor pembrolizumab found a 77% CR in injected lesions with overall CR in 9% and overall PR in 57%.[124] Two expansion cohorts have been opened to patients refractory to prior checkpoint inhibition and patients with in-transit or satellite disease (NCT02557321).

Talimogene laherparepvec (TVEC) is a genetically modified oncolytic herpesvirus incorporating the coding sequence for human granulocyte-macrophage colony-stimulating factor (GM-CSF). Oncolytic viruses are designed to selectively replicate in tumors, thereby infecting and destroying cancer cells, inducing immune responses that target the cancer cell. Expression of the GM-CSF gene in tumor cells results in the recruitment and activation of antigen-presenting cells and immune effectors that mediate potent antitumor T cell cytotoxicity. Tumor destruction in this fashion may also induce T cells capable of circulating and exerting antitumor effects in nearby and distant uninjected metastases. The Phase III OPTiM study included 436 patients randomized in a 2:1 manner to intralesional TVEC or subcutaneous GM-CSF alone, respectively. There was a 26.4% objective response rate for TVEC compared to a 5.7% for GM-CSF ($p < 0.001$). There was a statistically significant increase in the primary endpoint of durable response rate (DRR), defined as a partial or CR lasting for 6 months or more. DRR was 16.3% for TVEC and 2.1% for GM-CSF ($p < 0.001$). TVEC also showed a borderline OS benefit over GM-CSF. While this study had shortcomings, such as the use of an inactive control and the potential impact of prior and postprotocol therapy on the study outcomes,[125] TVEC became the first intratumoral oncolytic virotherapy to win FDA approval and set the stage for several newer strategies under investigation. This viral-mediated immune gene therapy was also evaluated in combination with immune checkpoint blockers based on the promising data seen in combination with CTLA-4 blockade (ipilimumab), and an in-depth analysis of immunologic correlates of TVEC in combination with PD-1 blockade (pembrolizumab), showing that responders had increased intratumoral CD8+ T cells, elevated PD-L1, and IFN-γ gene expression after TVEC treatment.[126] The definitive Phase III study to test the benefit of adding TVEC injections to systemic pembrolizumab (NCT02263508) failed to show an advantage for patients randomized to the combination over pembrolizumab alone.[127] Other oncolytic tumor viruses currently under investigation include the RP-1 virus, a herpesvirus expressing a fusogenic glycoprotein and GM-CSF, in combination with nivolumab for melanoma and other malignancies (NCT03767348), and the Coxsackie virus Cavatak plus pembrolizumab in patients with advanced melanoma (NCT02565992).

Several other approaches to intratumoral immunomodulatory therapy of melanoma have been taken using cytokines or Toll-like receptor (TLR) agonists in combination with immune checkpoint blockade.[127] IMO2125 and CMP-001 are TLR 9 agonists given by intratumoral injection, and tavokinogene telseplasmid is a plasmid-encoded interleukin-12 gene administered by electroporation into the tumor mass. Each of these agents has shown promising activity and a favorable safety profile in Phase I and II studies and is entering Phase III trials to test the benefit of adding intratumoral immunomodulatory therapy to a backbone of immune checkpoint blockade in metastatic melanoma.

Imiquimod and diphencyprone (DPCP) are topically applied agents that have been used for patients with multiple small cutaneous metastases. Imiquimod, a TLR 7/8 agonist immunomodulator, stimulates antigen-presenting cells and has mainly been used to control melanoma *in situ*/LM. Topical application of imiquimod, with or without additional agents such as topical 5-fluorouracil, resulted in regression of up to 90% of treated superficial lesions.[128] DPCP is a contact sensitizer that induces hypersensitivity; in a cohort of 50 patients treated with DPCP, 23 patients (46%) achieved a CR and an additional 19 patients (38%) showed a PR. The side effect profile of DPCP is tolerable, with skin reactions such as blistering and irritation being the most common side effects.[129] Topical agents produce transient benefits without inducing sufficient systemic antitumor immunity to control distant metastatic disease, and their use will likely be eclipsed by the intratumoral agents summarized above as well as by the systemic therapies discussed in detail later in this article. Topical immunomodulators may remain valuable for the management of noninvasive disease and avoidance of surgery, such as extensive melanoma *in situ*/LM.[129,130]

Systemic therapy

Treatment of in-transit or regional disease with immune checkpoint inhibitors and targeted therapies as first-line therapy has been based on evidence from multicenter, randomized trials for advanced melanoma. However, the percentage of patients with disease limited to in-transit lesions or nodal disease in these studies is difficult to assess and at best a small portion of the total cohort. While demonstrating improved OS in advanced melanoma, severe adverse events and development of resistance should be considered on an individual basis. Although failure of regional therapies does not preclude subsequent use of systemic agents, current NCCN guidelines list systemic therapy as preferred treatment for recurrent, in-transit, or satellite unresectable disease.

Radiation therapy

In patients with in-transit or regional recurrence, radiation may offer a benefit. Treatment protocols are not well defined, but the potential for symptom control makes radiation an option for selected patients with unresectable locoregional melanoma[131,132] and is now under active investigation as an immunomodulator, detailed later in this chapter. The principles of palliative radiotherapy for melanoma are similar to those used for other malignancies, although the relative radioresistance of melanoma has led to many attempts to improve its therapeutic index by alternative fractionation schemes, particularly hypofractionated treatment with large fraction sizes.

Surgical metastasectomy for stage IV melanoma

Patients with isolated, resectable distant metastatic melanoma are candidates for surgical management aimed at removing all known sites of metastatic disease. Identifying which patients will benefit from metastasectomy requires good clinical judgment and a thorough preoperative staging that includes PET–CT of the body and

MRI of the brain to rule out occult sites of metastasis.[133] While the main purpose of metastasectomy is to achieve a surgical NED status, followed if appropriate by systemic adjuvant therapy (discussed in detail below), a small fraction of patients may be candidates for palliative metastasectomy for symptom management.

Response to systemic therapy must be considered when evaluating patients for metastasectomy, to confirm no development of additional metastatic disease will develop in the near future. The Southwest Oncology Group conducted trial S9430, a prospective, nonrandomized evaluation of surgery for patients with stage IV melanoma, enrolled patients as soon as the determination of potential resectability was made, allowing the investigators to estimate resectability rate and define relapse-free and OS after complete resection. Among the 77 study patients, 3 had no evidence of melanoma in the resected specimen (the suspected metastatic deposit was either a second primary malignancy or a benign finding) and 2 patients had only stage III disease. An additional 8 patients were not able to have all disease resected, leaving 64 patients (88.9%) in total resected to a disease-free state. After a median follow-up of 5 years, all but 6 (9.4%) had recurred, with a median RFS of approximately 5 months. Median OS was 21 months with an estimated 12-month survival of 75% and 4-year survival of 31%.[134] Analysis from the MSLT-1 trial also found survival benefit in 161 patients who underwent resection for distant recurrence with versus without systemic therapy, noting that over half of patients with distant recurrence were eligible for metastasectomy.[135] Improved OS was shown in patients with disease stabilized by systemic therapy and undergoing hepatic resection for melanoma compared to systemic therapy alone (median 5-year OS 8 vs 25 months, respectively, $p < 0.001$).[136] Undergoing surgery while receiving BRAF targeted therapy has been shown to be safe, with a trend toward improved OS with both a longer duration of systemic treatment and for patients who underwent elective surgery.[137] Similar findings have been reported with more recently developed immunotherapies and targeted therapies.[138,139]

The role of adjuvant therapy for resected, high-risk melanoma

Interferon and chemotherapy

Immunotherapy has been the adjuvant treatment approach evaluated most extensively in melanoma, starting with injections of BCG in the 1970s[140] and continuing with high-dose IFN-α in the 1980s and 1990s. While BCG and early vaccine preparations produced from melanoma cells did not show meaningful adjuvant activity, the 1-year high-dose IFN-α regimen, consisting of a 1-month intravenous induction phase at 20 million units of IFN-α2b/m2 of body surface area given 5 days per week for 4 weeks, followed by an 11-month subcutaneous maintenance phase at 10 million units/m² subcutaneously three times a week showed improved RFS in three randomized trials using different comparators (observation or a vaccine containing GM-CSF and multiple melanoma peptides).[141,142] However, the impact on OS was minimal, and the toxicities of high-dose IFN-α (flu-like symptoms, fatigue, anorexia, and a variety of organ toxicities) were intolerable for most patients. The subsequent Phase III Sunbelt Melanoma study, investigating both the value of high-dose IFN-α as well as molecular staging of the sentinel lymph node, showed no RFS or OS benefit for this agent.[143]

Polyethylene glycol-conjugated (pegylated) IFN-α was developed to extend the half-life of IFN-α and potentially reduce its toxicities. This derivative of IFN-α, which was also used for both chronic myelogenous leukemia and chronic hepatitis C prior to the emergence of superior drugs, was approved in the United States as an alternative adjuvant treatment for stage III melanoma in 2011, based on the results of a single randomized trial that demonstrated a statistically significant improvement in RFS, in keeping with trials of standard IFN-α, but did not show an OS benefit.[144] In subset analysis, however, patients with sentinel node-positive melanoma and an ulcerated primary showed a significant survival benefit (41% improvement) when treated with pegylated IFN-α.[145,146] Although some other IFN-α trials have seen a similar benefit in this subset,[147] IFN-α has been relegated to a very low level of recommendation in view of the far superior results from adjuvant immune checkpoint blockade, the low fraction of ulcerated melanomas, and rapid improvements in therapeutic agents that have emerged from a growing understanding and incorporation of immunobiology and molecular biology into regimen design.

Cytotoxic chemotherapy has also not demonstrated high activity and tolerability in the adjuvant therapy of melanoma, although a single randomized study in patients with mucosal melanoma was positive for RFS and OS.[148] Cisplatin appears to be the most active cytotoxic agent, but randomized trials in advanced melanoma as well as in the adjuvant setting failed to demonstrate the superiority of multidrug regimens, including all cytotoxic agents or combinations with immunomodulatory drugs or even the early, nonspecific kinase inhibitor sorafenib.[149,150]

Adjuvant immune checkpoint blockade

The investigation of ipilimumab in the adjuvant setting for high-risk melanoma began soon after the discovery that immune checkpoint blockade, first in the form of CTLA-4 blocking antibodies and later with the advent of PD-1 blockade, could lead to prolonged remissions in a fraction of patients with advanced melanoma. The toxicities of CTLA-4 blockade mirrored the preclinical experience, consisting predominantly of a wide spectrum of immune-related inflammatory effects that generally reversed with immunosuppressive agents such as glucocorticoids. A randomized 950-patient trial in patients with resected stage III cutaneous melanoma compared ipilimumab at 10 mg/kg (a dose higher than that approved for use in the treatment of unresectable metastatic melanoma, discussed below) to placebo, on a schedule of every 3 weeks × 4 infusions followed by the same dose every 12 weeks to complete 3 years of adjuvant therapy. The results of this study included significantly improved RFS and OS with hazard ratios of approximately 0.7 for the ipilimumab arm.[151] Unfortunately, the toxicity of the regimen was unexpectedly severe, consisting of immune-related adverse events (irAEs) of grade 3–4 severity in nearly half of the patients. In order to better understand the dose-toxicity relationship for ipilimumab, a randomized trial was then conducted to evaluate ipilimumab at 10 and 3 mg/kg, and compare ipilimumab to high-dose IFN-α. The results suggested noninferiority for the 3 mg/kg dose of ipilimumab in the adjuvant setting and a substantial reduction in irAEs, establishing this dose, similar to that used in advanced melanoma, as the recommended dose for adjuvant therapy.[152]

The safety and tolerability of anti-PD1 antibodies for advanced melanoma were demonstrated at about the same time that ipilimumab emerged as the gold standard for melanoma adjuvant therapy, and the results of two large Phase III adjuvant studies for high-risk melanoma demonstrated the superiority of PD-1 blockade over CTLA-4 blockade. In the 906-patient Checkmate

238 study, there was a significantly longer recurrence-free survival (hazard ratio 0.65) and lower rate of grade 3 or 4 adverse events with nivolumab compared to ipilimumab in resected stage IIIB, IIIC, or IV melanoma.[153] The 1000-patient Keynote-054 study comparing adjuvant pembrolizumab to placebo for resected Stage III melanoma patients showed that pembrolizumab was far superior to placebo for RFS with a hazard ratio of 0.56, which was similar across a variety of subgroups such as patients with tumors expressing PD-L1 or BRAF v600 mutations. This study was unique in featuring a required crossover to pembrolizumab at the time of relapse for patients initially randomized to placebo, and it is believed that the lack of OS benefit for adjuvant pembrolizumab is due to the comparable benefits of PD-1-directed immune checkpoint blockade given in the adjuvant setting (to all patients) or at the time of relapse (only for the subset of patients who relapse).[154] This observation also has implications for the design of a newer approach for locally advanced melanoma, which is neoadjuvant immunotherapy (and targeted therapy), further detailed below. The Checkmate 238 study of adjuvant ipilimumab versus nivolumab similarly lacks an OS benefit despite a strong RFS benefit for nivolumab, since the majority of patients who relapse after adjuvant treatment on this study would be candidates for off-study PD-1 blockade or even combination CTLA-4 plus PD-1 blockade.

Two studies have assessed the value of ipilimumab plus nivolumab in unique adjuvant settings: The Immuned study from the German Dermatologic Oncology Cooperative Group was a randomized 167-patient Phase II trial for patients with no evidence of residual disease after resection or curative-intent radiation of single-site or oligometastatic melanoma. Patients received adjuvant ipilimumab plus nivolumab, nivolumab, or placebo. Despite the randomized Phase II trial design, the differences between cohorts were sufficiently large to report direct comparisons, which showed a hazard ratio of 0.23 for RFS between combination checkpoint blockade and placebo and a hazard ratio of 0.56 for RFS between adjuvant nivolumab and placebo.[155] There are many caveats with this approach and the study details, so a general recommendation to use double immune checkpoint blockade adjuvantly in this infrequent and challenging patient population could not be made until more data and particularly more insight into patient selection and toxicity management were generated by additional trials. The second study introducing ipilimumab plus nivolumab in the adjuvant study was a comparison with standard nivolumab alone in the Checkmate 915 trial, a very large >1900 patient trial for melanoma patients with resected stage IIIB, IIIC, or IIID melanoma or stage IV single-or oligometastatic disease. Patients were randomized to standard regimens of both immune checkpoint blocking antibodies versus nivolumab alone and, in the first report (unpublished; released by sponsor BMS online in October, 2020 http://businesswire.com/), the data showed no advantage for the combination of CTLA-4 plus PD-1 blockade over PD-1 blockade alone. Clearly, there is a need to improve the results of adjuvant therapy for all stages of melanoma at substantial risk of relapse, but the contradictory results of these two adjuvant trials highlight the gaps in current knowledge of optimal therapy and patient selection.

Adjuvant targeted therapy

As detailed earlier in this article, the molecular drivers of melanoma are complex and heterogeneous but tend to converge on the MAP kinase pathways; likewise, mechanisms of resistance to MAPK-directed therapies predominantly involve reactivation of this pathway. To date, the druggability of melanoma with molecularly targeted agents has been limited to inhibitors of the constitutively activated v600-mutant BRAF and the resulting upregulated MEK (usually wild-type) downstream of BRAF. This driver pathway is present in about half of cutaneous melanomas, and while it does not impact substantially the response to immunotherapy or the overall prognosis (although it confers a slightly higher incidence of eventual brain metastasis), it is required for the response to pathway-directed therapy. There are now three combinations of BRAF plus MEK inhibitors that have been approved in advanced melanoma on the basis of Phase III trials against single-agent BRAF inhibitors. COMBI-d and COMBI-v demonstrated the superiority of dabrafenib (BRAF inhibitor) plus trametinib (MEK inhibitor) over single-agent dabrafenib or vemurafenib (BRAF inhibitor), respectively.[156] The 870-patient COMBI-AD trial was designed to test this combination in the adjuvant setting and compared the active regimen against placebo, since immune checkpoint blockade had not become standard adjuvant therapy at the time COMBI-AD was opened. The combination was highly active, with a hazard ratio for RFS of 0.47. Although direct comparisons could not be made, the targeted regimen was also associated with lower rates of grade 3–4 adverse events than the immunotherapies available at that time, consisting of interferon or ipilimumab. With this result, the dabrafenib/trametinib combination was approved by the FDA for patients with resected stage III melanoma.[157]

Adjuvant radiation to the resected nodal basin

Criteria for identifying patients at high risk of regional recurrence in the resected nodal basin after radical lymphadenectomy include multiple (≥4) or matted tumor-involved lymph nodes, the presence of extranodal extension of tumor in at least one node, large size (≥3 cm) of any one lymph node, location on the head or neck, extensive neurotropism, and pure desmoplastic histologic subtype. In the prospective Trans-Tasman trial, 217 eligible patients possessing at least one of these criteria were randomized to observation or postoperative nodal basin irradiation after lymphadenectomy. After a median follow-up of 40 months, nodal basin relapse occurred in 34 of 108 patients (31.5%) in the observation arm, confirming the high risk of regional recurrence in these patients. Nodal basin relapse was significantly reduced in the adjuvant radiotherapy group compared with the observation group, but no differences were noted for RFS when all sites of relapse were included or for OS.[158] This confirmed the ability of postoperative radiation to significantly decrease recurrence within the nodal basin in patients at high risk of such recurrence, and radiation should be considered for selected high-risk cases. Ongoing studies of the interaction of adjuvant locoregional radiotherapy with systemic immune checkpoint blockade as well as newer approaches to locoregionally advanced disease, most importantly neoadjuvant therapy (see below) will add important insight regarding the value of postoperative radiotherapy for high-risk melanoma.

Surveillance for high-risk melanoma patients

A variety of algorithms have been proposed regarding the frequency and nature of the follow-up evaluation of melanoma patients after surgical treatment.[159,160] One study evaluating the results of follow-up after surgery in stage III melanoma patients themselves found that half of all recurrences were detected by patients as opposed to medical professionals or more intense or frequent imaging follow-up. While most proposed follow-up algorithms involve more frequent follow-up in the initial years after surgery, the conditional probability of recurrence of stage I and II melanoma is actually fairly constant over the first decade

Table 6 Summary of NCCN follow-up guidelines for patients with completely resected melanoma, staged according to the AJCC eighth edition.

Stage	Physical examination	Imaging
Stage IA–IIA	Every 6–12 months × 3 years with annual follow-up beyond 3 years as clinically indicated	No imaging needed unless clinically indicated
Stage IIB–IIC	Every 3–6 months × 2 years, then every 3–12 months for an additional 3 years with annual follow-up beyond 5 years as clinically indicated[a]	Cross-sectional body imaging considered for higher-risk patients: CT and/or PET/CT, to screen for recurrent disease every 3–12 months. Consider brain MRI annually[b]
Stage III–IV	Every 3–6 months × 2 years, then every 3–12 months for an additional 3 years with annual follow-up beyond 5 years as clinically indicated[c]	Cross-sectional body imaging should be considered for higher-risk patients: CT and/or PET/CT, to screen for recurrent disease every 3–12 months. Consider brain MRI annually[b]

These guidelines have not been prospectively validated and hence should only be considered as recommendations.
CT, computed tomography; CXR, chest X-ray; PET/CT, positron emission tomography/computed tomography.
[a]Consider more frequent and longer follow-up in high-risk stage II patients with thick and/or ulcerated primary tumors.
[b]Ultrasonography can be considered to evaluate regional nodal basins.
[c]Consider more frequent and longer follow-up in high-risk stage IIIB/C patients.

after surgery.[161] The MELanoma Follow-up (MELFO) study, a multicenter, prospective, randomized clinical trial, compared the conventional Dutch Melanoma guideline of the time to a reduced stage-adjusted follow-up schedule in patients with stage IB–IIC SLNB staged melanoma. Where prior convention had all patients return to clinic every 3 months for the 1st year, 4 months for the 2nd year, 6 months years 3–5, and annually thereafter until year 10, the experimental schedule reduced the frequency to annually for stage IB patients, every 6 months for the first 2 years and then annually for stage IIA patients, and every 4 months for the first 2 years, 6 months for the 3rd year, and annually thereafter for stage IIC patients. Results over 3 years of the study noted no difference in detection of recurrences and secondary primary melanomas, healthcare cost reduction, and no differences in patient-reported outcome measures.[162] The current NCCN guidelines reflect the results of this study but also stress the importance of tailoring follow-up to the individual[108] (Table 6).

Education is key and should be focused on both the patient and family as well as the primary care physicians, dermatologists, and surgeons alike. Patients should be willing to return to the melanoma center for evaluation of suspected recurrence, because properly diagnosing recurrence (e.g., documenting nodal recurrence by needle aspiration cytology instead of open biopsy) is important to successful treatment.

Uveal melanoma and rare melanomas of the eye

Uveal melanoma (UM) is the most common primary intraocular cancer of the eye in adults and represents 5% of all melanomas. The term UM is used for melanomas that arise within the uveal tract (i.e., iris, ciliary body, or choroid), while the broader term ocular melanoma includes such sites as conjunctiva and eyelid, which behave like cutaneous melanoma. UMs are further designated as anterior (iris) or posterior (ciliary body and/or choroid) chamber tumors. Anterior chamber UM is rarer (<10% of UMs) and tends not to metastasize, whereas approximately half of the patients diagnosed with posterior chamber UM will develop metastases.

Local therapy for UM employs radioactive plaque, proton therapy, or enucleation of the primary UM tumor. In a randomized study comparing ^{128}I plaque brachytherapy with enucleation, 85% of patients receiving radiation retained their eye, and 37% had visual acuity better than 20/200 in the irradiated eye 5 years after therapy. No survival difference was seen between the radioactive plaque and enucleation groups.[163] Thus, a radiotherapeutic approach has become the strategy of choice for primary UM treatment, with enucleation reserved for the remaining <10% of cases in which radiotherapy is not possible (e.g., bulky disease, technically difficult tumor location, patient preference). Because most patients do not undergo enucleation, fine-needle aspiration techniques are now often used to obtain the pathologic and molecular diagnostic information that is critical to prognosis.

Unlike cutaneous melanoma, UM infrequently metastasizes to lymph nodes or brain. UM metastases are hematogenous, because the uveal tract does not appear to contain clear lymphatic channels with draining lymph nodes. The liver is ultimately involved in 95% of metastatic UM cases and is the sole site of metastatic UM in approximately 50% of patients. The most common other sites of metastatic UM are lung (24%), bone (16%), and skin (11%). The clinical course of patients with UM is highly dependent on disease progression in the liver. The median survival after diagnosis of patients with liver metastases is approximately 4–6 months with a 1-year survival of approximately 10–15%. Patients with metastases limited to extrahepatic sites have a median survival of approximately 19–28 months with a 1-year survival of approximately 76%. Thus, hepatic versus extrahepatic-only disease may represent distinct biological entities.[164]

Approximately 90% of UM harbor activating, mutually exclusive, recurrent mutations in the g-protein alpha q (*GNAQ*) or 11 (*GNA11*) subunit genes. Nearly all *GNAQ/11* gene mutations localize to a hotspot in exon 5 (Q209), although a small number localize to exon 4 (R183). *GNAQ/11* gene mutations are early tumorigenic events that are insufficient to initiate metastatic disease, but some of the downstream pathways in UM resulting from additional molecular aberrations, such as protein kinase C and others, may be targetable with investigational agents in development.[165] Additional recurrent missense mutations in *SF3B1* (altering the R625 amino acid position in most cases) or *EIF1AX* (exons 1 or 2) genes occur in equal proportion in approximately 40% of UM tumors and are essentially mutually exclusive with each other. Truncating and nontruncating mutations are observed in the nuclear ubiquitin carboxy-terminal hydrolase *BAP1* gene located on chromosome 3p21.1. Genetic aberrations in *BAP1* tend to co-occur with monosomy 3, resulting in the loss of heterozygosity of BAP1. Both *BAP1* gene mutations and monosomy 3 tend not to co-occur with *SF3B1* or *EIF1AX* gene mutations, and the former are associated with a high risk of developing metastatic UM.[166] Consistent with *BAP1* mutations leading to loss of tumor suppression, there have been multiple reports of germline *BAP1* mutations within families that result in a high incidence of UM.[167] Another recurrent chromosomal aberration observed in UM is 8q copy number gain (often with 8p loss), which tends to accompany monosomy 3 and is associated with a shorter time to relapse. Conversely, 6p copy number gain (often with 6q loss) is usually present in tumors that lack monosomy 3 or 8q copy number gain and is associated with a low risk of metastasis. Less frequent chromosomal aberrations, such as 1p and/or 16q loss, have also been described. With the exception of BAP1, the identification of specific genes that correlate functionally with these chromosomal aberrations is less clear.[168]

Multiple anatomic, histologic, and molecular features within primary tumors are associated with poor prognosis: (1) location in ciliary body (poorer) > choroid ≫ iris (rarely metastasize); (2) greater tumor size; (3) extrascleral invasion; (4) epithelioid > spindle cell histology; (5) higher mitotic rate; (6) presence of monosomy 3 ± chr 8q gain; and (7) class 2 ≫ class 1b ≫ class 1a gene expression profile (a 15-gene expression profile that accurately predicts outcome and does not require chromosomal analysis). However, the strongest risk factors for metastasis are copy number profile (e.g., presence of monosomy 3/chr 8q gain) and/or a class 1b/2 gene expression profile.[169,170]

Metastatic UM has proven essentially recalcitrant to traditional chemo- and immunotherapeutic approaches. Given the current inability to therapeutically target the aforementioned molecular aberrations characteristic of UM, there has been a major focus on targeting the effector molecules associated with these genetic alterations. The most successful systemic approach to date has been to target the MEK–MAPK pathway that is clearly activated by GNAQ/11 mutations. A Phase II randomized clinical trial showed that treatment of metastatic UM patients with single-agent selumetinib (a small-molecule MEK inhibitor) resulted in tumor regression in 50% and RECIST responses in 15% of cases. A significant difference in median progression-free survival following treatment with selumetinib (15.9 weeks) compared to dacarbazine (7 weeks) was shown, although without an improvement in OS.[171]

Immunotherapies with high activity against metastatic cutaneous melanoma, such as combined CTLA-4 and PD-1 blockade, have a low response rate against metastatic UM. One study of intratumoral immune/inflammatory cell infiltrates and gene expression patterns in metastatic UM showed a positive association between inflammatory and immune gene signatures and tumor response to these agents,[172] suggesting that UM may be amenable to immunomodulatory therapy, especially with novel agents under development.

Targetable effectors of mutant BAP1/monosomy 3 are still under investigation. Retrospective analyses of metastatic UM patients from multiple centers treated with ipilimumab suggest that long-term tumor response was observed in a subset (~5%), as well as prolonged stable disease (SD) in a slightly larger subset of advanced disease patients.[173] More recently, therapy of metastatic UM with antibodies blocking PD-1 or PD-L1 was reported from a multi-institution retrospective series and also showed very low activity,[174] further evidence that the successful therapy of this melanoma variant requires strategies that focus on its unique molecular biology and targets in its immune tumor microenvironment. For example, the bispecific immunomodulator IMCgp100, composed of an agonistic, T cell-activating anti-CD3 domain linked to an HLA-A0201-restricted T cell receptor for an immunogenic epitope from the melanoma differentiation (median 22 months) antigen gp100, has been reported to show a survival advantage over physician's choice therapy of either single immune checkpoint blockade or dacarbazine (median 16 months) in a randomized study for patients with metastatic UM.[175]

For patients with liver-only or -dominant metastatic UM, multiple therapies specifically directed at the liver have been explored: isolated or percutaneous hepatic perfusion (PHP) of chemotherapy, transarterial chemoembolization (TACE), radioembolization or cryoembolization, or selective internal radiation therapy (SIRT). Liver-directed therapy studies tend to have low patient numbers, but when taken in aggregate, suggest relatively high tumor response, prolonged time-to-progression, and/or survival in the target population. Nine studies (totaling 209 patients) using TACE (mostly cisplatin-based) reveal a 2% CR, 24% PR, and 33% SD rate when taken in aggregate. One retrospective comparison of liver-directed therapies in 30 patients showed improved PFS in patients treated with PHP versus TACE or radioembolization. Other studies of PHP have reported response rates of up to 83%, with median hepatic PFS of 11 months and median OS of 27 months.[176–179]

There may be a role for resection of metastatic UM if there is a relatively stable and safely resectable solitary lesion(s). In a study in which 61 patients had resection in addition to chemotherapy, a 22-month median OS was observed among patients who could undergo resection with curative intent compared to 10 months among those who could not. Variations in patient referral and selection criteria are important factors in all of these outcomes, which must be validated by performing well-controlled prospective randomized trials.

With one of the most predictive sets of molecular markers of metastatic risk, the identification of clear genetic drivers within primary UM tumors, and a wide spectrum of clinically relevant approaches (molecular inhibitors, immunotherapies, radiation, and surgery) now available, there is tremendous excitement that truly effective therapies for UM in both the adjuvant and advanced settings are within practical reach.

Melanoma of the conjunctival surface of the eye is rare and may complicate primary acquired melanosis. Reports demonstrating the presence of typical activating BRAF mutations in 29% and NRAS mutations in 18% of a cohort of 78 conjunctival melanomas provide further evidence of the close relationship of melanomas in this site to cutaneous melanomas, with case reports of clinical responses to vemurafenib that corroborate the importance of BRAF as an oncogenic driver in conjunctival melanoma.[180,181]

Biology and therapy of advanced melanoma

The diagnosis of metastatic melanoma may be triggered by new symptoms or signs in a patient with a history of melanoma (about half of the presentations) or a new but asymptomatic finding on radiographic surveillance scans, based on guidelines and practice that take into account the initial stage, time-dependent risk of relapse, and likelihood that intervention will change the natural history of the disease. Skin and soft tissue are more common sites of initial metastatic disease than visceral sites, and a minority of patients have widespread metastatic disease secondary to hematogenous spread, such as is common with mucosal melanomas.

Uncommonly, advanced melanoma may present as a solitary or multiple metastases—even in the central nervous system—without a known history or evidence of a concurrent new primary melanoma. It has been postulated that immune-mediated control or regression of a missed primary controlled by a local immune response explains this phenomenon, which also has a slightly more favorable prognosis than matched cases with a known primary.[182] Melanoma spreads widely and spares few organs or sites, with a particular affinity for the brain, where it is often the immediate or major contributing cause of death due to bleeding and edema. Other sites of melanoma metastasis that are rare for other cancers include the small and large intestine and even the heart. Characteristics of primary melanoma that pose increased propensity to specific sites of metastasis are under investigation. For example, the CCL25 and CCR9 chemokine: chemokine receptor interaction has been reported in intestinal metastases,[183] and increased activity of the AKT and PI3K pathways downstream from suppression mediated by PTEN is associated with a higher rate of eventual metastasis to the brain.[184] Many other molecular alterations, notably the expression of a variant CD44v6 molecule, a receptor for hyaluronic acid that is highly expressed by brain,[185] have been reported to impact the risk and/or the biological behavior of established brain metastases.[186] Driver oncogenes that are targetable by approved therapies may also be associated with an increased risk of brain metastases, including BRAF v600 mutations, and NRAS mutations have also been reported to confer an increased incidence of brain metastases.[187]

Molecularly targeted therapy for advanced melanoma

Metastatic or stage IV melanoma is now divided into four substages based on the survival curves used in the AJCC version 8 staging system. Stage M1a is metastatic disease limited to skin and soft tissue; M1b adds lung metastasis with/without skin/soft tissue involvement; M1c adds metastasis in any visceral organ; and M1d is used when brain metastasis is present, with/without any other site. Substages of M1 disease are also defined by the serum lactate dehydrogenase (LDH) as (1) (above the institutional upper limit of normal) or (0) (LDH within normal limits). It remains to be seen whether rapid advances in molecular-based prognostication will supersede the traditional size, site, and ulceration-based staging criteria in future staging systems.

Melanoma, together with lung cancer, has the highest frequency of mutations per cell among all human malignancies, which is largely attributable to frequent C → T transitions resulting from solar UV exposure.[7] A few mutations result in driver oncogenes (such as activating BRAF v600E/K mutations or NRAS mutations at G12, G13, or Q61) and/or important passenger alterations that collaborate to varying degrees in oncogenesis (such as PTEN loss of function, which occurs in at least 20–30% of melanomas, often in association with BRAF mutations, and many others such as TP53 and p16INK4a and p14ARF).[7] Simultaneous mutation of BRAF and NRAS is rarely found in primary melanomas untreated with BRAF inhibitors. The importance of the PTEN pathway, which exerts a suppressive effect on the downstream mediators (PI3K/AKT and mTOR) of a wide variety of proliferative, metabolic, and antiapoptotic functions is illustrated by a large number of mechanisms for pathway activation, including hypermethylation of the PTEN promoter and rare mutations of AKT or PI3 kinase isoforms.[188]

The molecular drivers currently targetable by therapeutic agents approved for melanoma are limited to BRAF-activating mutations, tested by gene sequencing[189] for the mutations encoding BRAF v600E or one of the less-common activating mutations at residue 600 of the BRAF serine–threonine kinase. BRAF v600E has a change from valine to glutamic acid (V → E) and accounts for approximately 75% of cases, while the next most common is valine to lysine (V → K) in about 17%. Other amino acid substitutions account for the small number of remaining cases.[190] Tumors carrying V600K are associated with more advanced age, chronic sun damage, and a somewhat less favorable outcome even with BRAF inhibition.[191] There are many assays available for next-generation genomic sequencing that detect additional alterations with therapeutic implications, for example, activating c-kit mutations in about 20% of mucosal and 15% of acral melanomas with occasional responsiveness to imatinib or dasatinib[192,193] and NRAS mutations, which have shown modest responsiveness to MEK and CDK 4/6 inhibitors. These assays are also valuable for discovery of new mechanisms of resistance, especially when performed sequentially on biopsies before and during therapy. Also of interest is the observation of BRAF gene fusions with several other molecular species that provide unique targets for several agents already in testing.[194]

Disease regression occurs in the majority of patients treated with single-agent BRAF or MEK inhibitors (Table 7) and can be improved with the combination of inhibitors, which have shown survival benefit over single-agent BRAF inhibition.[200–203] As BRAF inhibitors may lead to paradoxical activation of MAPK signaling from upstream pathways that also activate MEK, these effects are less prominent during combined therapy; furthermore, the secondary low-grade cutaneous proliferations (keratoacanthoma and squamous cancers) attributed to mutant HRAS activation upstream of MEK[204] are also reduced during combination therapy. Such combinations also yield higher response rates and additional disease regression, as shown on the waterfall plots of maximum regression in individual subjects that sentence is redundant with essentially same statement earlier in paragraph. Toxicities of single-agent therapy with either BRAF or MEK inhibitors are generally tolerable but may require dose reduction, brief drug holiday, or a switch in agent(s). Further management guidelines will undoubtedly emerge with more experience, particularly since the regulatory approval of these agents has led to their more widespread use.

Acquired resistance to single MAPK inhibitors occurs after a median of 6 months and somewhat later (median 8–11 months) with combined MAPK inhibitors (Table 7), although a fraction of patients may enjoy prolonged control.[195] The mechanisms of resistance as well as protection against resistance are becoming evident from the many clinical trials that provide tissue for analysis before therapy and during therapy or at the time of progression. Reactivation of MEK signaling occurs in most cases of acquired resistance to MAPK inhibition, via alterations in BRAF (gene amplification or truncation mutations); secondary mutations in NRAS with the downstream consequence of increased CRAF heterodimerization with blocked mutant BRAF to reactivate downstream signaling; rare MEK mutations or related (COT1) activation; and several receptor kinase alterations (Figure 2) that also activate the PI3K/AKT pathway.[196,197]

Adaptive resistance is an earlier-onset form of therapy resistance, involving shifts in metabolic or receptor tyrosine kinase signaling that confer growth advantage or resistance to apoptosis and may also be targetable with small-molecule inhibitors or antibodies but have been less extensively studied than acquired mechanisms.[198] Therapeutic trials to delay or prevent the emergence of resistance will be critical, as established resistance is difficult to overcome with any form of targeted therapy. For example, the activity of combination MEK plus BRAF inhibitor after BRAF inhibition fails is modest (only 15% response, PFS <4 months[199]), and current efforts are focused on preventing or delaying resistance by improving front-line therapy and molecular typing. The use of intermittent dosing, based on strong preclinical data and clinical anecdotes,[205] was tested in a Phase III trial randomizing patients who were candidates for first-line MAPK inhibition to receive dabrafenib plus trametinib in the standard doses and schedule of daily, continuous administration versus an

Table 7 Antitumor activity and toxicities of molecularly targeted agents.

DRUG (references)	Vemurafenib[195]	Vemurafenib[196]	Dabrafenib[197]	Trametinib[198]	Encorafenib[199]	Dab/Tram[197]	Dab/Tram[196]	Vem/Cobi[a,195]	Enco/Bini[199]
Patient number	239	352	212	214	194	211	352	254	192
Objective response (%)	45	51	51	22	52	67	64	68	63
CR (%)	4	8	9	2	5	10	13	10	16
Progression-free survival (median, mo)	6.2	7.3	8.8	4.8	9.6	9.3	11.4	9.9	15
TOXICITIES[b]									
All grade 3 (%)	49	57	34	Grade 3 or 4	65	32	48	49	51
All grade 4 (%)	9	1.4	3	8	1	3	1	13	7
Fever	22	21	28	—	29	51	53	26	35
Fatigue	31	—	35	26	48	35	—	32	55
Headache	—	—	29	—	52	30	—	—	42
Nausea or emesis	24	15	26	18	74	30	29	10	79
Chills	—	8	16	—	—	30	31	—	—
Arthralgia	40	51	27	—	84	24	24	32	59
Diarrhea	28	38	14	43	26	24	32	17	69
Rash	35	43	22	57 (acneiform 19)	41	23	22	17	27
Hypertension	—	—	14	15	11	22	—	—	21
Peripheral edema	—	—	5	26	—	14	—	—	—
Increased transaminase	18	—	5	—	30	11	—	18	50
Photosensitivity	15	22	—	—	7	—	4	28	8
Hyperkeratosis	29	25	32	—	73	9	4	10	27
Keratoacanthoma	20	KA or SCC	21	—	12	—	KA or SCC	1	4
Squamous cancer	11	18	9	—	—	—	1	3	—
Alopecia	—	26	26	17	107	—	—	2	26
Hand-foot syndrome	—	25	27	—	98	5	4	—	13
Decreased LVEF	—	—	2	—	—	4	8	—	—

[a]Thirty percent of patients had asymptomatic grade 1–2 creatinine phosphokinase elevation.
[b]Reversible transient drug-induced retinopathy, rarely reported.

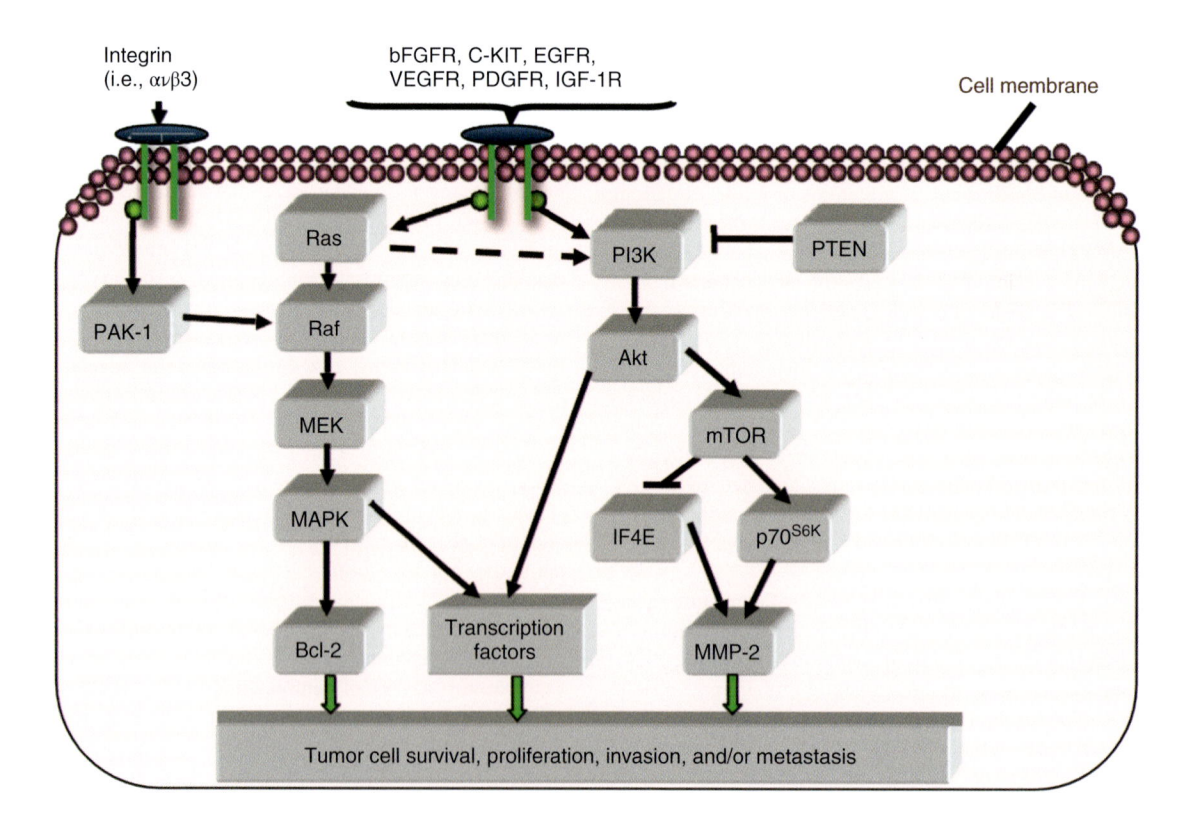

Figure 2 Multiple molecular pathways, such as the RAF/MEK/MAPK and PI3K/AKT pathways, have been found to support melanoma proliferation and survival. Understanding these pathways will enable the development of targeted therapies for melanoma.

8-week lead-in on therapy followed by 3 weeks off and 5 weeks on, every 8 weeks until progression or toxicity. This study failed to demonstrate a benefit with intermittent dosing, and it is unlikely that testing this hypothesis using one of the other two pairs of approved MAPK inhibitors would show different outcomes.[206] It is more likely that other molecularly designed strategies designed to overcome or forestall the onset of resistance to MAPK inhibition, including combinations with immunotherapy, detailed below, will fill this need.

The choice between immunotherapy and targeted agents for the first-line therapy of patients whose melanoma carries a BRAF activating mutation remains unclear, as the kinetics of benefit early during therapy are so different. MAPK inhibitors work quickly and relieve symptoms within days to weeks, while immunotherapy responses, especially when only a single agent is used, may require weeks to months for definitive and maximum benefit to be confirmed. This feature is particularly true for single-agent CTLA-4 blockade, which has shown several patterns of response, including both delayed responses after objective progression as well as the appearance of new lesions before an overall objective response at all sites of metastatic disease.[205] Until the completion of planned drug-sequencing trials (see below) to answer this question, it had generally been recommended that patients with a BRAF-mutated advanced melanoma and rapidly growing, symptomatic, or very high tumor burden disease be treated first with combination MAPK inhibitorss. This critical question was tested in a large U.S. cooperative group trial (NCT02224781) led by the Eastern Cooperative Onology Group with the collaboration of the American College of Radiology Imaging Network and the other U.S. cooperative oncology groups (SWOG and the Alliance). Patients with advanced melanoma carrying an activating BRAF mutation were randomized to initial therapy with dabrafenib plus trametinib versus ipilimumab plus nivolumab. Upon progression, patients who meet eligibility criteria are crossed over to the opposite treatment. The trial results have recently been reported[207] and demonstrated a significant benefit in 2-year survival for immunotherapy over targeted agents. Among the still unresolved questions include whether and how to continue targeted agents in patients requiring palliative radiotherapy (which can interact to enhance skin and liver toxicities) or surgery for single sites of symptomatic progression during disease control in other sites.

Additional molecular targets are likely to be identified in the near future; for example, the FDA approved the NTRK inhibitor larotrectinib for adult and pediatric solid tumors with activating alterations of the NTRK gene, irrespective of tumor histology. As it has become more common practice to perform whole genome sequencing of tumors rather than targeted sequencing of a prespecified number of mutations, patients with rare somatic alterations of targetable oncogenes will more commonly be identified and provided access to potentially effective drugs.[208]

Immunotherapy for advanced melanoma

Ipilimumab is a fully human antibody to CTLA-4, a molecule that provides an immune checkpoint on activated effector T cells by engaging with the ligand B7.1 on tumors or on dendritic cells and removing it from the activating receptor CD28. In the presence of anti-CTLA-4, activation is restored, and a preexisting but ineffective immune response against tumors is enhanced. CTLA-4 blockade also promotes homing of effector T cells to tumor and elimination of Treg cells.[209,210] Additional mechanisms for CTLA-4 blockade have been reported, including the expansion of type 1 CD4 cells (associated with antitumor response) and stimulation of exhausted-like CD8 cells to enhance their antitumor cytotoxicity.[211] When used at the approved dose of 3 mg/kg × 4 doses at 3-week intervals, ipilimumab provides objective response in 10–15% of advanced melanoma patients, with less than partial regressions or disease stabilization in another 10–15%. The survival appears to plateau after 2.5 years at about 20%, so these patients may be cured by a durable and effective immune response.[212]

The patterns of response to CTLA-4 blockade may be atypical and delayed, making it more difficult to know when to switch a patient to second-line therapy upon the appearance of progression, which should always be confirmed by either clinical evidence of increased tumor burden or by radiologic evidence of unequivocal progression, ruling out pseudoprogression, defined as radiologic or clinically increased tumor measurements or a new lesion without clinical deterioration; a subsequent tumor assessment must show reversal of this increase in order to designate pseudoprogression. While the original observations of durable remissions in a fraction of advanced melanoma patients represented a true breakthrough in the immunotherapy of cancer, the advent of antibodies that block the PD-L1/PD-1 interaction (see below and Table 8, Refs 216–219, elevated this breakthrough to new heights that have since found a therapeutic niche in almost all adult solid tumors and some hematologic malignancies. As with ipilimumab, the elucidation of fine mechanisms for the activity of PD-1 blockade—in

Table 8 Activity and toxicities of selected CTLA-4 and PD-1 blocking antibodies from Phase III trials for advanced melanoma.

Drug (references)	Nivolumab[213]		Pembrolizumab[a,214]		Ipilimumab[215]		Ipilimumab[215]		Ipi/Nivo[215]		Nivolumab[215]		Pembrolizumab[b,224]	
Patient number	206		277		256		315		314		316		178	
ORR (%)	40		33		12		19		58		44		38	
Overall survival	1-yr 79%		1-yr 74%		1-yr 58%		NR		NR		NR		NR	
Toxicity (%),[c] grades	All	3–4	All	3–4	All	3–4	All	3–4	All	3–4	All	3–4	All	3–4
Fatigue	20	0	21	0	15	1	28	1	35	4	34	1	21	1
Colitis/diarrhea	16	1	17	2.5	23	3	33	6	44	9	19	2	8	0
Dermatitis/pruritus/rash	17	0.5	15	0	25	1	35	2	40	5	26	0.6	21	0
Hypophysitis/other endocrinopathy[c]	NR	NR	0.4	0.4	1	2	4	0	15	0.3	9	0	5	0
Hepatitis	NR	NR	1	1	1	0.4	4	0.6	18	8	4	1	NR	NR
Pneumonitis	NR	NR	0.4	0	0	0	NR	NR	NR	NR	NR	NR	NR	NR
Nephropathy	NR	NR	0	0	0.4	0.4	NR	NR	NR	NR	NR	NR	NR	NR
Fever	NR	NR	NR	NR	NR	NR	7	0.3	18	0.6	6	0	NR	NR
Arthralgia	6	0	9	6	5	0.8	6	1	10	0.3	8	0	7	1
Nausea	16	0	10	0	9	0.4	16	0.6	26	2	13	0.6	4	0

[a]Pembrolizumab 10 mg/kg every 3 weeks.
[b]Pembrolizumab 2 mg/kg every 2 weeks.
[c]NR, not reported.

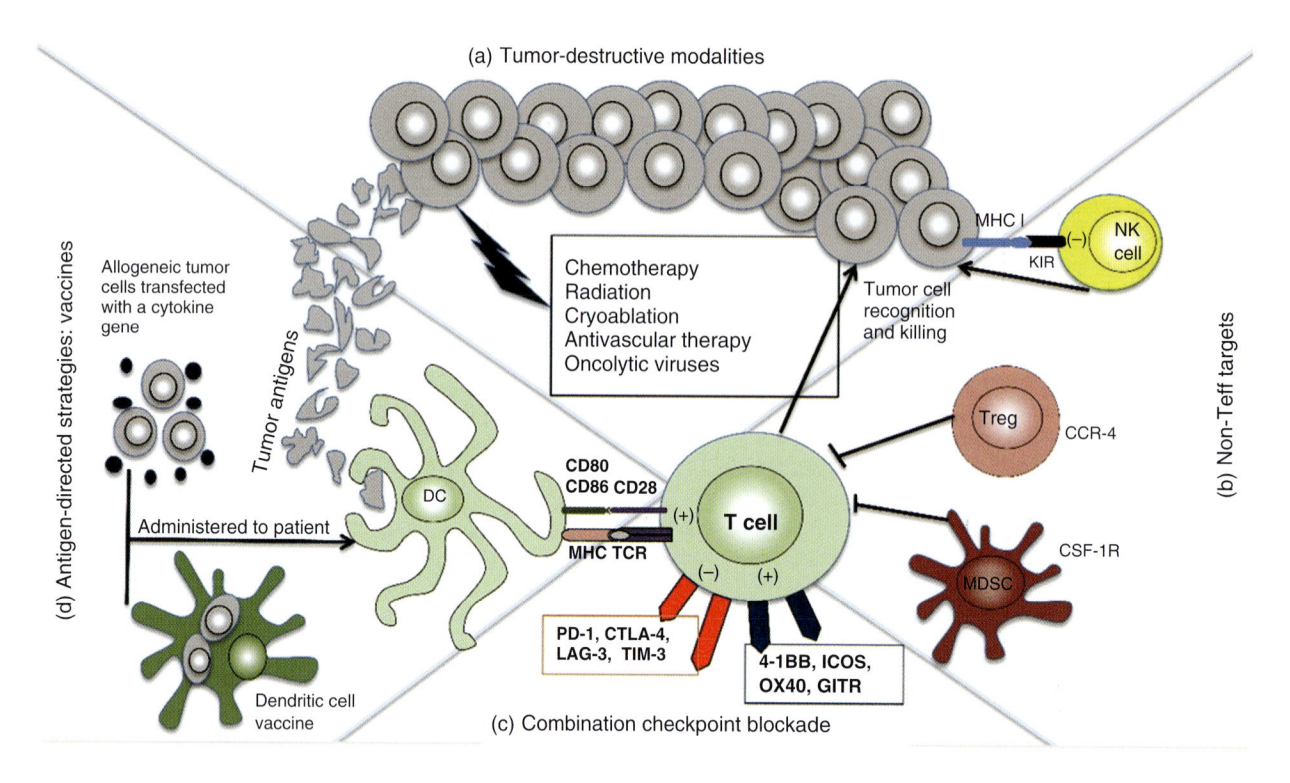

Figure 3 Combination strategies with cytotoxic T-lymphocyte-associated antigen 4 (CTLA-4) blockade—(a) conventional and novel therapies may efficiently destroy tumor and liberate tumor-associated antigens (TAAs), thereby enhancing antigen presentation and tumor-specific adaptive immunity; (b) novel-targeted agents may inhibit the suppressive effects of regulatory T cells (Treg) and myeloid-derived suppressor cells (MDSCs) or enhance innate immunity via natural killer (NK) cell-killer immunoglobulin-like receptor (KIR) activity; (c) immune checkpoints and costimulatory receptors can be targeted in combination with CTLA-4 to enhance T-cell function; (d) adaptive immunity to known TAAs can be enhanced via vaccine strategies employing peptides, whole proteins, whole cells, DNA, or virus-based vectors. CSF-1R, colony-stimulating factor 1 receptor; DC, dendritic cell; GITR, glucocorticoid-induced tumor necrosis factor receptor (TNF) receptor-related protein; ICOS, inducible T-cell costimulator; LAG-3, lymphocyte activation gene 3; MHC, major histocompatibility complex; PD-1, programmed cell death 1; TCR, T-cell receptor; Teff, effector T cell; TIM-3, T-cell immunoglobulin and mucin-containing domain 3. Source: Funt et al.[220] Reproduced with permissions of UBM Medica.

this case, stimulation of the exhausted-like subset of antitumor CD8 cells—has provided insights that inform the design of new trials across the spectrum of malignancies. Among the remaining questions regarding the use of immune checkpoint blockade are the optimal dosing, duration of therapy, and sequencing with other agents and modalities such as surgery and radiotherapy, as well as the potential for new agents with complementary or synergistic mechanisms in the therapy of melanoma and other malignancies (Figure 3). For example, the addition of GM-CSF (daily for 2 of every 3 weeks) to a 10 mg/kg dose of ipilimumab, given every 3 weeks × 4 and then every 12 weeks, was shown in a randomized Phase II study to both enhance survival and reduce ipilimumab's toxicities,[221] an intriguing result that has been followed by a trial of GM-CSF added to combined CTLA-4 and PD-1-directed immune checkpoint blockade (NCT02339571) that is in progress. Although the BRAF mutation has been associated with a higher likelihood of relapse and slightly more aggressive metastatic disease,[222] it does not appear to impact the activity of ipilimumab in melanoma.[223]

Hypofractionated or other schemes of radiation may also overcome resistance to ipilimumab and other immunomodulatory therapies via multiple mechanisms that include enhanced antigen and MHC expression, reduction of suppressive cells and molecules, and induction of inflammatory substances that promote dendritic cell function, which in turn enhances tumor antigen-specific responses, and many clinical trials have been initiated to study these effects in melanoma and other tumors.[213,214,224] Important interactions among these modalities are shown in Figure 3. While there is abundant proof of these principles in animal models, the human experience to date for beneficial interactions between radiotherapy and immunotherapy has been limited and disappointing.

Ipilimumab's toxicities are immune-based and include pruritus, rash, fatigue, and diarrhea (about 1/3 to half of patients), while colitis requiring intervention is less common (7–10%) but can cause bleeding and even bowel perforation (<1%). Hypophysitis may result in adrenal, thyroid, and reproductive hormone insufficiency requiring replacement hormone therapy and sometimes a brief course of therapeutic glucocorticosteroid for local inflammation, especially if vision is compromised by compression of the optic chiasm by the inflamed pituitary. Immune-related hepatitis and rare cases of other organ involvement such as neuropathy have been reported. The first line of therapy for most irAEs is generally a course of therapeutic glucocorticoids followed, if necessary, by anti-tumor necrosis factor antibody (for rare cases of steroid-resistant hepatitis, mycophenolate mofetil is preferred over TNF blockade).[215] While an association between autoimmune reactions and tumor regression has been reported for CTLA-4 antibody therapy,[225] and the generation during therapy of a higher circulating lymphocyte count has also correlated with therapeutic benefit, these associations are imperfect and do not provide insight into pretreatment biomarkers that can be used to foresee the likelihood of either benefit or toxicity. However, one report details the presence in pretreatment melanoma biopsies of common exomic mutation sequences creating immunogenic MHC class I-binding tumor neoepitopes from the tumors of patients who benefited from CTLA-4 blockade.[220] This report, along with others that demonstrate benefit associated with antigen-specific immune responses to melanoma in patients benefiting from ipilimumab,[226] lends support to the concept that immune checkpoint inhibition exploits existing antitumor immune responses, which in many cases are now believed to be tumor-specific mutations, presumably derived from the damage induced by carcinogens of known importance in tumorigenesis.[227] Thus, combinations with other immunomodulators that provide costimulation, reduce negative signaling in the tumor microenvironment, or enhance the functions of antigen-presenting cells are under investigation.

Insights from further study of pre- and posttreatment tumor and circulating cells and their gene expression and patterns of activation may also lead to better selection criteria for initial therapy in individual patients. PD-1 has two important ligands, PD-L1 (expressed on a wide variety of cells and variably inducible in tumors, generally by cytokines produced by infiltrating lymphocytes) and PD-L2 (predominantly expressed on hematopoietic cells). Ligand engagement of PD-1 triggers negative signaling in effector T cells, rendering them unresponsive to further antigen stimulation and eventually apoptotic, a cascade that, in the case of tumor expressing PD-L1, may be one mechanism of tumor resistance to immune control. This may be of particular importance in adaptive resistance, a term used to describe the induction of PD-L1 on tumor cells by γ-interferon produced by infiltrating CD8 lymphocytes, which may set the stage for effective immunotherapy by PD-1 or PD-L1 blocking antibodies.[228,229] Such antibodies, fully human or extensively humanized, have been studied in patients with advanced melanoma and several other malignancies, and the results of these studies, which showed objective responses in about 25–30% of patients previously treated with ipilimumab and, if BRAF mutant, with a BRAF inhibitor, led to the approvals of pembrolizumab and nivolumab in late 2014 for advanced pretreated melanoma. However, the randomized trial that demonstrated a dramatic progression-free and OS benefit of nivolumab over dacarbazine (HR for death 0.42, 1-year survival 73% vs 42%) in the first randomized study for patients with untreated BRAF wild-type melanoma[217] (Figure 4) quickly led to the routine use of these antibodies in the first-line setting, even for patients with BRAF mutant melanoma.

The toxicity data for PD-1 blocking antibodies have demonstrated the expected superior therapeutic ratio over single-agent ipilimumab, which has lower benefit and higher immune-related side effects (Table 8). Most toxicities affect the same tissues targeted by ipilimumab's immune-related adverse effects but appear to be less frequent and severe; unique toxicities such as pneumonitis, nephritis, and neuritis have been reported in occasional patients on PD-1 axis blockade, and rare case reports describe other unusual events likely to represent loss of immune tolerance resulting from this form of checkpoint blockade. However, also shown in Table 8, while the combination of CTLA-4 and PD-1 blockade has shown higher response rates and progression-free survival over single-agent ipilimumab (further detailed below), the toxicities of the combination are much more frequent, of higher grade, and include events not reported previously for either agent alone.

Combination therapy with concurrent ipilimumab and nivolumab showed particularly dramatic antitumor effects in initial Phase I and II trials that were confirmed in a 945-patient Phase III study comparing the combination with each of the single agents in untreated advanced melanoma. This landmark study, published in 2015 with the most recent followup report in 2021,[230] demonstrated the highest-ever objective response rate, progression-free and OS reported as of that time but also highlighted the substantial toxicities and management challenges—essentially all immune-related, as detailed above—of combined immune checkpoint blockade. While there has been substantial uptake of this combination in standard practice, many clinicians feel safer using single-agent PD-1 blockade for advanced melanoma, where response rates around 30–40% have been achieved at the cost of minimal immune-related toxicity. For analogous reasons, the combination of CTLA-4 and PD-1 blockade has rarely been used for the control arm of subsequent randomized trials, which have nearly all used single-agent PD-1 blockade as the control. This permits a clean comparison of activity and a reasonable, if indirect, comparison of the toxicities to those of combined checkpoint blockade. While several retrospective, unplanned subgroup analyses that emerged from the Phase III trial of combined immune checkpoint blockade versus single-agents suggested that patients with BRAF mutant melanomas and those with PD-L1-negative tumors benefited from the combination over nivolumab alone, the trial was not powered to compare double immune checkpoint versus nivolumab, and the subsets (outcomes by PD-L1 expression and by BRAF status) were considered hypothesis-generating rather than practice-defining.

Sequential or simultaneous administration of molecularly targeted and immunotherapeutic agents

The initial data from retrospective series had strongly supported the likelihood that patients with BRAF-mutated melanoma who started with single targeted therapy (the first such drug to be approved was the BRAF inhibitor vemurafenib) and then received ipilimumab at the time of progression had more unfavorable outcomes than patients who started with immunotherapy and crossed over to targeted therapy at the time of treatment failure.[231,232] While this outcome may have resulted from a true treatment-sequence effect, it may also reflect the bias resulting from the treatment of patients with more aggressive disease to targeted therapy first and patients with less aggressive tumor to immunotherapy first. The Phase III prospective, randomized study of initial targeted therapy versus immunotherapy followed by crossover at progression and detailed in the earlier section on molecularly-targeted therapy, answered the question definitively for patients who are good candidates for combined immune checkpoint blockade and who don't "require" the almost-immediate therapeutic effects resulting from initial treatment with targeted agents. However, important questions remain for the next generation of trials: is immunotherapy also the best first-line therapy when the patient is not a candidate for both CTLA-4 and PD-1 blockade but should be treated with the safer single-agent PD-1 antibody? Will newer immune checkpoint antibodies that combine well for antitumor activity and improved safety supplant the current regimen of ipilimumab and nivolumab? Can a sufficiently improved therapeutic index of those two antibodies in combination be achieved by using the so-called "flipped dose" regimen that features a lower dose of ipilimumab during induction but maintains the nivolumab dose throughout?[233]

Concurrent therapy with MAPK inhibitors and CTLA-4 blockade was attempted early on, since both vemurafenib and ipilimumab were FDA-approved in 2011. While initial combination therapy with vemurafenib and ipilimumab proved excessively hepatotoxic,[234] many other combinations of molecularly targeted therapy with immunotherapy are under investigation, based in part on promising data supporting the importance of BRAF muta-

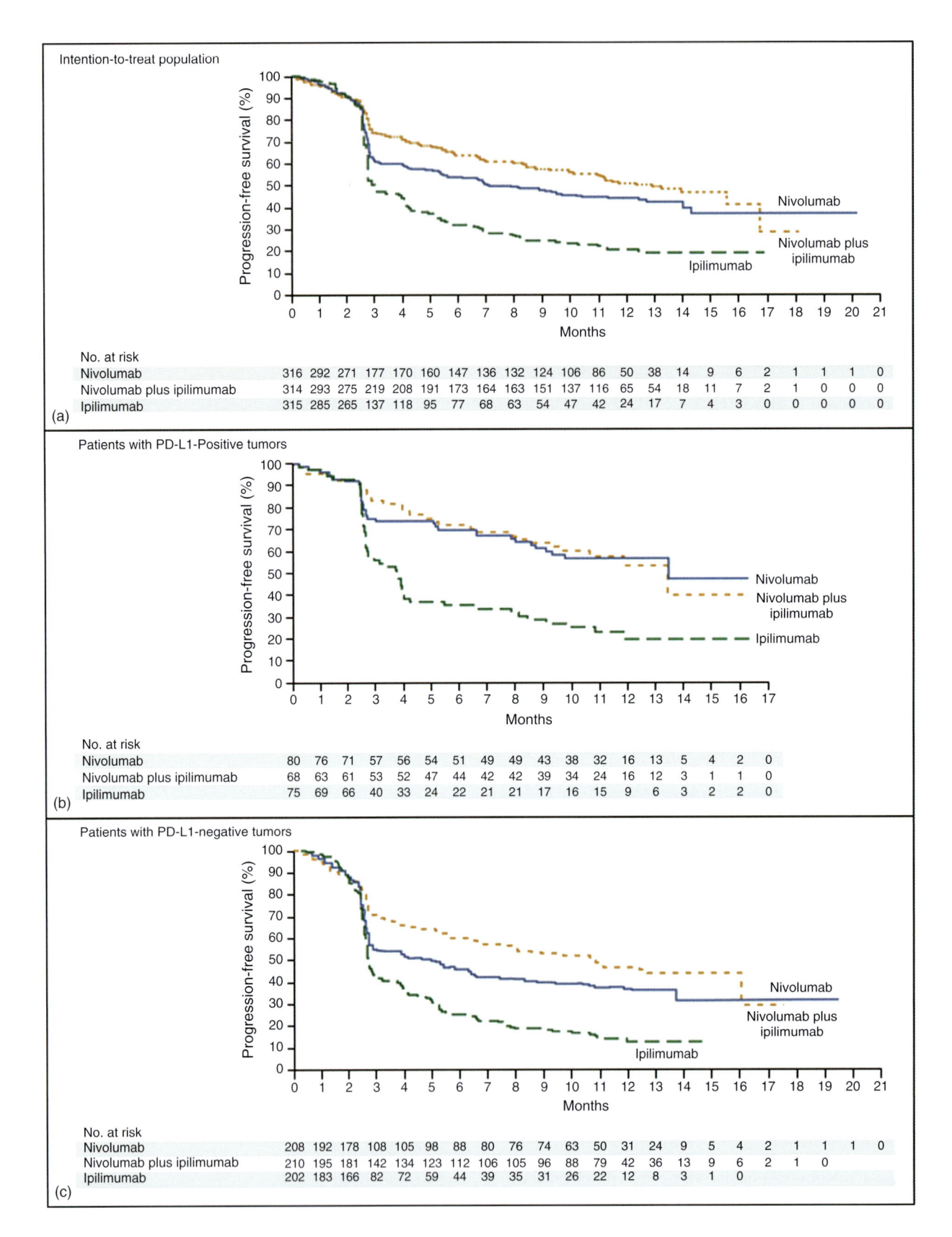

Figure 4 PFS, nivolumab plus ipilimumab versus either single agent. (a) Kaplan–Meier curves for progression-free survival in the intention-to-treat population. The median progression-free survival was 6.9 months (95% CI, 4.3–9.5) in the nivolumab group, 11.5 months (95% CI, 8.9–16.7) in the nivolumab-plus-ipilimumab group, and 2.9 months (95% CI, 2.8–3.4) in the ipilimumab group. Significantly longer PFS was observed for nivolumab plus ipilimumab than for ipilimumab (hazard ratio for death or disease progression, 0.42; 99.5% CI, 0.31–0.57; $P < 0.001$) and for nivolumab versus ipilimumab (hazard ratio, 0.57; 99.5% CI, 0.43–0.76; $P < 0.001$). (b) PFS for patients with PD-L1-positive tumors, and (c) PFS for patients with PD-L1-negative tumors. Source: Larkin et al.[215] Reproduced with permission of the New England Journal of Medicine.

tion in resistance to immunotherapy and, conversely, BRAF (and MEK) inhibition in promoting immune response.[235]

While the majority of studies for PD-1/PD-L1 axis blockade in melanoma have used the human or humanized PD-1 antibodies nivolumab or pembrolizumab, respectively, the PD-L1 antibody atezolizumab was used in a novel combination with the MAPK-targeted agents vemurafenib and cobimetinib for advanced melanoma. The 514-patient Phase III Imspire 150 trial showed that atezolizumab, when added to vemurafenib plus cobimetinib for patients with advanced, BRAF v600 mutant melanoma, significantly improved the median progression-free survival from 11 to 15 months. The objective response rate and OS were similar between the groups, but the duration of response was also significantly longer for the triplet (median 21 vs 13 months).[236] Two other studies that were conducted in a similar time-frame failed to show improvements of this magnitude when PD-1 blockade was added to double MAP kinase inhibition but trended in the same direction,[237,238] and the FDA approved the combination of atezolizumab plus vemurafenib and cobimetinib for BRAF mutant advanced melanoma in mid-2020. Of note is that the toxicities of this combination are essentially additive, with a high rate of grade 3 and 4 adverse events; while many of these toxicities were asymptomatic and most resolved with dose reduction of the MAP kinase inhibitors, if judged attributable to those agents, their management can be challenging to the treating oncologist and dangerous for the patient. Importantly, none of the trials to date has used PD-1 blockade as the control and tested the addition of targeted therapy. Another strategy of importance for which final results are anticipated soon is that of the Secombit trial, which evaluates the strategy of crossing over from initial targeted therapy to immunotherapy, before disease progression, since waiting for disease progression appears to be associated with loss of activity for the subsequent line of therapy especially if the first line of treatment is MAP kinase inhibition. (NCT02631447).

Many reports have already described patient and tumor factors associated with benefit from immune checkpoint blockade in melanoma and other tumor types, including the expression of PD-L1 on tumor and/or stromal cells, the presence of a brisk CD8 lymphocyte infiltrate within the tumor, a high tumor mutational burden (TMB), and molecular correlates of a favorable immune response, including patterns of gene expression[239] and oligoclonality of T-cell receptors among the tumor-infiltrating CD8 cell. However, much additional work is needed to clearly define biomarkers of benefit and toxicity and to further elucidate mechanisms of action and of resistance to both classes of agents.

Since cutaneous melanoma tends to have a high PD-L1 expression and a high TMB, these two factors do not perform as well in identifying melanoma patients likely to benefit from immune checkpoint blockade as well as they do for other malignancies like lung and bladder cancers. The mechanisms of innate resistance to therapy may be distinct for melanoma and thus require melanoma-specific strategies to overcome them. Other factors that help to identify patients with favorable outcomes are only available once the patient has undergone a period of treatment, such as the well-known association of irAEs with clinical benefit. Truly predictive factors that can be assessed prior to therapy and have a high positive and negative predictive value are the holy grail of immunotherapy for melanoma and many other malignancies and remain under active investigation and lively discussions.

Many new approaches to enhancing immunotherapy with checkpoint antibodies include engineering to add or enhance selected functions, for example by altering the Fc portion of the antibody or adding a cleavable moiety that depends on tumor-associated proteases to localize the signal. Other checkpoint blocking antibodies and related immunomodulatory agents also hold promise in melanoma, including agonistic antibodies that costimulate T cells through ligands associated with activation (agonistic anti-CD137, anti-OX40, anti-CD40, anti-CD27) and dendritic cells (TLR ligands and tumor vaccine antigens bound to dendritic cell-targeting antibodies). Recent reports have demonstrated high antitumor activity and modest toxicities with combinations of antibodies against the immune checkpoint LAG 3 on T lymphocytes (ligand on tumor is MHC class II) with PD-1 blocking antibodies.[240,241] Altering gene expression with epigenetic modulators like selected histone deacetylase or heat shock protein inhibitors, interrupting signaling by receptors associated with tumor angiogenesis and immunosuppression, and blocking upregulated cell-cycle pathways in selected melanomas may also hold promise—more likely in rational combinations than as single agents.

Other strategies—less specific to melanoma and under investigation for immunotherapy of other malignancies—include manipulation of the gut (or other) microbiome, metabolomics of tumor and immune cells, and immune tumor microenvironment. include the inhibition of other immunosuppressive signals in the tumor microenvironment, such as indoleamine dioxygenase or signaling receptors on suppressive tumor-associated macrophages.

Cytokine therapy of melanoma

IL-2 is an immunomodulatory, type I cytokine with pleiotropic effects on immune effectors that has activity against melanoma when given at high pharmacologic doses. Most data show a 15–25% rate of objective response and an RFS plateau of 20%.[207] To date, clinical criteria for safety and the availability of an expert team to administer high-dose IL-2 and the associated supportive care are used to select patients for this form of treatment; although many dose and schedule alterations and the addition of a variety of toxicity modulators have been studied, no modification of the original regimen has improved its unfavorable therapeutic index. The toxicities of high-dose IL-2 result from a generalized capillary leak syndrome mediated by small-molecule vasoactive mediators such as nitric oxide and a reversible systemic inflammatory response syndrome with multiorgan dysfunction that may also be attributed to the effects of IL-2-induced inflammatory mediators such as tumor necrosis factor and interferon-γ.[242] Studies are now underway to identify immunologic or genetic predictors of benefit, for example the Cytokine Working Group's "Melanoma Select" trial of high-dose IL-2. The results of that study will potentially complement those under investigation for selection of other immunotherapies (detailed below) as single agents or, more likely, in combination or carefully sequenced strategies. Other trials test the activity of regimens that combine or sequence IL-2 with immune checkpoint blockers as well as the potential role for newer cytokines such as engineered IL-2 molecules and other gamma-c cytokines (those which, like IL-2, signal on target cells through the common receptor gamma chain), particularly IL-15, which also promotes NK cell expansion and cytotoxicity.[243] The predominant goal of these newer-generation cytokines is to stimulate cytotoxic T cells without also enhancing regulatory T cells or other counterregulatory effects that would dampen the desired antitumor immune response as well as to reduce the toxicities of high-dose IL-2. However, high-dose IL-2 remains an essential component of the complex regimens used for tumor-infiltrating lymphocyte (TIL) therapy of melanoma, detailed at the end of this chapter.

Neoadjuvant therapy of melanoma

The last several years have ushered in a growing level of interest and important data for the use of systemic therapy, predominantly immune checkpoint blockade, prior to surgery in patients with resectable, locally advanced melanoma. Largely the work of investigators at the Netherlands Cancer Institute (NKI), remarkably high clinical objective response rates between 65% and 75% for regimens with concurrent ipilimumab and nivolumab, including even higher rates of pathologic complete and near-complete remissions in the 75–80% range, have been reported.[244] This discordant rate of clinical versus pathologic responses favoring the latter suggests that clinical residual masses overestimate the rate of incomplete responses to immunotherapy, a phenomenon that requires further investigation aimed at reconciling clinical, radiologic, pathologic and immunomolecular data to optimize patient assessment and ultimately their management. The NKI studies used ipilimumab and nivolumab, investigating the optimal regimen based on therapeutic index and pathologic findings. Smaller, non-randomized studies using single-agent PD-1 blockade have shown somewhat inferior outcomes,[245,246] as expected from the activity of these agents in metastatic disease, and caution is advised regarding the use of less-active single agents, since tumor progression during the treatment window may result in loss of the opportunity for curative-intent resection. The results of a just-completed cooperative group trial, S1801 (NCT03698019), are expected to provide more definitive answers to this question for single-agent PD-1 blockade but will also need to be supplemented by results from studies of newer agents such as Opdualag.

In the case of neoadjuvant therapy with MAPK inhibitors, the response rate is very high regardless of whether they are used in a neoadjuvant approach or for advanced disease, and their adjuvant activity has also been proven with randomized trials, as detailed earlier in this article. However, their role in cytoreduction prior to surgery remains unproven by large, randomized trials. The next few years will see these questions answered in the form of Phase III studies to directly compare neoadjuvant to adjuvant therapies and to study correlates of outcome that should also define which patients benefit most from each approach. This is also a fine testing ground for new agents in multi-drug regimens, as illustrated by the Phase Ib DONIMI study (NCT04133948) that adds the histone deacetylase inhibitor domatinostat to nivolumab and ipilimumab.

Cytotoxic agents and combinations with immunotherapy for advanced melanoma

Until the advent of high-dose IL-2, therapy for metastatic melanoma was of very limited benefit, with low rates of objective response to single-agent cytotoxic therapies and limited response durations for both IL-2 and cytotoxic agents or combinations. The standard and only FDA-approved drug was dacarbazine, with response rates in the 10–12% range, and an oral equivalent of this drug, temozolomide (technically approved only for primary brain malignancies), has often been used with similar outcomes but better tolerance.[247] Although expectations were high for temozolomide as treatment for patients with brain metastases due to its central nervous system penetration and its widespread use in primary brain tumors, the low activity of dacarbazine and temozolomide in melanoma tempered enthusiasm, and it is now used predominantly for patients who have failed or cannot tolerate the other agents detailed above (and with very low expectations for its antitumor activity). Alternative multiagent regimens have been more toxic and without proven benefit despite reports of higher response rates, particularly to biochemotherapy combinations with at least 3 cytotoxic agents and 2 immunotherapies, usually IL-2 and IFN-α.[248] Nanoparticle-albumin-bound paclitaxel or unmodified paclitaxel as a single agent or in combination with carboplatin are cytotoxic regimens with modest activity against melanoma but have not demonstrated survival benefit in prospective trials.[249]

Melanoma metastatic to the brain

Melanoma has the highest propensity of any adult solid tumor to spread hematogenously to the brain, and due to its vascular nature and its high growth rate in many cases, it poses serious threats to the survival and well-being of patients. Resection may be required for diagnosis and is often necessary for immediate relief of the complications of edema, bleeding, and rapidly progressive neurologic deficits. The impact of whole-brain radiation given in standard or alternative dose and fractionation schedules has been minimal and cannot be distinguished from the benefits of simply treating patients with glucocorticosteroids.[250] Stereotactic radiotherapies have the most favorable outcomes despite the lack of randomized, controlled comparisons, the maximum size and number of lesions amenable to treatment varying by center and type of modality (gamma-knife or cyberknife).[251] Whole-brain radiotherapy is of limited palliative benefit and may be offered to patients with numerous lesions or failure of prior therapy, including systemic agents, which are increasingly showing activity against melanoma brain metastases (molecularly targeted agents and immunotherapy).

Several studies have tested the activity of BRAF inhibitors alone[252,253] or in combination with MEK inhibitors[254,255] and shown a modest response rate and duration which in each case was lower than reported for these drugs in patients with metastatic BRAF mutant melanoma without brain metastases. Whether the lower activity in the brain is due to molecular biologic differences of melanoma brain metastases[256] or a sign of a more aggressive melanoma with greater intrinsic resistance to therapy[257] has not been elucidated. However, the use of targeted therapy alone for management of brain metastases from BRAF mutant melanoma is not routinely recommended[258] unless the lesions are too numerous to treat with stereotactic radiosurgery (SRS), which can be given in combination with systemic therapy.

In the case of immune checkpoint blocking antibodies, despite the presumed lack of ability to cross an intact blood–brain barrier (see below), their level of activity against melanoma brain metastases is in the same range reported for metastases outside of the central nervous system, probably due to several factors, including the loss of blood–brain barrier integrity resulting from tumor growth and inflammation as well as peripherally activated lymphocytes that gain access and migrate to the melanoma metastases in the CNS.[259]

Immunotherapy in patients with melanoma metastatic to the brain has evolved from the use of single-agent ipilimumab to PD-1 blockade and then the combination of CTLA-4 and PD-1 blockade, analogous to the evolution of these therapies for systemic therapy in patients without brain involvement. Ipilimumab demonstrated, in a 51-patient trial for patients without neurologic symptoms or steroid requirement, activity in the brain comparable to its extracranial activity in these patients and its activity in patients without brain metastases.[260] Subsequent studies with single-agent pembrolizumab also showed modest activity against brain metastases with response rates in the 25% range,[261] but the low level of activity and ease of its combination with brain radiation have led to more common use of PD-1 blockade plus SRS outside of clinical trials. The combination of ipilimumab and nivolumab was used successfully in 101 neurologically asymptomatic and steroid-free patients, who achieved a remarkably high response rate of 58% (with long durability) in the brain with similar outcomes in extracranial sites and globally.[262] A small cohort of patients with neurologic symptoms or steroid requirements had a lower response rate of 22%.[263] Others have published smaller series showing the same results.[264] This combination is now recommended for patients with small-volume brain metastases who are good candidates for dual immune checkpoint blockade, do not require steroids for symptoms or edema, and have no immediate need for surgical or radiotherapeutic intervention.

Further understanding of the process of brain metastasis to guide their prevention, as well as optimal selection of therapy, will depend on factors that include the molecular characteristics of the primary site as well as changes occurring as melanoma cells experience other metastatic niches before the brain. Investigation of earlier-stage disease has provided limited and heterogeneous insights, but reports suggesting the importance of the PTEN/AKT/PI3 kinase pathway either intrinsically or via signals from nearby astrocytes and other studies of the molecular and immunobiology of brain metastasis in melanoma and other malignancies are providing insights with likely near-term therapeutic implications.[265]

Tumor-infiltrating lymphocyte (TIL) therapy in melanoma

The ability to isolate, expand, and infuse large numbers of autologous tumor-derived cytotoxic T lymphocytes, usually obtained from dissected fragments of excised tumor and expansion of predominantly CD8 lymphocytes in IL-2-containing medium into patients with advanced melanoma, has been under investigation for several decades. Recently, improvements in all aspects of this technology have led to its commercialization and testing in multicenter studies outside of the U.S. National Cancer Institute and a few other specialty centers. Investigations remain ongoing to better define the antigens, effector cell characteristics, and growth conditions associated with maximum yield and highest objective response rates with durability and persistence of the activated effector cells. These regimens require acquisition of a tumor fragment, lymphodepleting chemotherapy, and postinfusion high-dose IL-2 and are now associated with an OR rate in the range of 35–40% in patients who have failed to achieve durable disease control with immune checkpoint blockade and, if applicable, targeted agents.[266,267] It is expected that this modality will be approved by the FDA within the next year and then become more widely available, while at the same time clinical trials will continue to optimize the technique for patient selection, efficacy, and safety.

Observations regarding the immunobiology of TIL cells in melanoma are consistent with the findings detailed earlier for effective melanoma immunotherapy with PD-1 checkpoint blockade, including the presence of multiple immune checkpoints (PD-1, LAG3, TIM3) and costimulatory molecules (4-1BB, ICOS) on CD8 effector T cells and oligoclonality of T-cell receptor beta gene sequences on CD8 cells with antigen specificity for tumor-specific mutations.[266,268] Further, there are several new engineered IL-2 molecules designed to improve the activity and enhance the safety of this therapy, and the use of these cytokines may also improve the TIL regimen for melanoma.

The advent of multiple new targeted agents and immune checkpoint inhibitors will provide ample opportunities to study the role of TIL cell therapies both for patients who fail to achieve durable benefit from the former agents and as part of multicomponent strategies for optimal therapy of advanced melanoma. While advanced melanoma will continue to be a lethal disease for a fraction of patients, the rapid emergence of highly active molecularly targeted therapies and immunotherapies with mechanisms of action and resistance that are more successfully probed and manipulated promise to counter the threat of this constellation of diseases and to continue to lead the way in new therapeutic discoveries.

Summary

Melanoma is rising in incidence and mortality in a pattern reflecting exposure to UV light (both natural and artificial) and other carcinogens that have not been fully elucidated. Familial risk factors include rare mutations of cyclin kinase genes and more common polymorphisms of genes such as the melanocortin receptor that control pigmentation of the skin and hair. Other risk factors include large numbers of moles or atypical nevi. Among the clinicopathologic subtypes, NM has the most unfavorable prognosis owing to more rapid growth, the absence of an initial noninvasive radial growth phase, and a propensity to be nonpigmented, resulting in thicker tumors at diagnosis. Surgical excision guidelines include the need for adequate margins around the primary site to reduce the probability of local relapse; sentinel node biopsies guided by lymphoscintigraphic and lymphatic-tracking dyes at the time of wide local excision; and CLND for patients with one or more involved sentinel nodes. Imaging guidelines are often tailored to the calculated risk of relapse based on Breslow thickness, ulceration, mitotic rate, and number and size of nodal metastases. Metastasis occurs via predominantly hematogenous spread for uveal and mucosal melanoma and some cutaneous melanomas, while lymphatic spread is also common with cutaneous melanomas. Surgical management of metastatic melanoma depends on the number and location of metastases but can be associated with prolonged survival. Metastatic melanoma is divided by prognosis into skin/soft tissue only, lung, and visceral metastasis and/or elevation of serum LDH. Metastasis to the brain is more common in melanoma than any other malignancy and carries the most unfavorable prognosis, although improvements have resulted from SRS and new molecularly targeted as well as immunotherapies have shown activity against brain metastases. Melanoma is an immunogenic tumor that has been successfully treated with ex vivo expanded TILs and antibodies that block the CTLA-4 and PD-1/PD-L1 immune checkpoints. Combinations with radiation therapy have also shown promise through multiple modulations of suppressive factors in the tumor immune microenvironment. Molecularly targeted agents, particularly those that inhibit sequential steps in the mitogen-activated protein kinase pathway in melanomas carrying an oncogenic activating mutation of BRAF, have also improved survival, and new agents to prevent or overcome resistance as well as to target other molecular drivers are under investigation. The challenge of brain metastases, likely originating from cells with molecular features predisposing them to traffic to and thrive in the brain, is still an important cause of melanoma death despite some responsiveness to targeted and immunotherapies and remains under intense investigation.

A. Appendix

See Table A1.

Table A1 Summary of major randomized trials evaluating width of excision for primary cutaneous melanoma.

Author	Number of patients	Breslow thickness (mm)	Margins widths evaluated (cm)	Recurrence rates (local or regional)	Overall or disease-specific survival
Veronesi[67]	612	<2	1 versus 3	Locoregional recurrence 4.6% versus 2.3% at 55 months (p = NS)	No difference in overall survival or disease-specific survival at 55 months
Cohn-Cedermark[69]	989	>0.8–2.0	2 versus 5	Recurrence-free survival 71% versus 70% at 10 years (p = NS)	Overall survival 79% versus 76% at 10 years (p = NS)
Balch[70]	468	1–4	2 versus 4	Local recurrence 2.1% versus 2.6% at 10 years (p = NS)	Overall survival 70% versus 77% at 10 years (p = NS)
Thomas[71]	900	2	1 versus 3	Local recurrence 37% versus 31% at 3 years (p = 0.05)	No difference in overall survival and disease-specific survival at 3 years

NS, not significant.

Key references

The complete reference list can be found on Vital Source version of this title, see inside front cover.

1 Purdue MP, Freeman LE, Anderson WF, et al. Recent trends in incidence of cutaneous melanoma among US Caucasian young adults. *J Invest Dermatol.* 2008;**128**:2905–2908.
2 Welch HG, Woloshin S, Schwartz LM. Skin biopsy rates and incidence of melanoma: population based ecological study. *BMJ.* 2005;**331**:481.
3 Swerlick RA, Chen S. The melanoma epidemic: more apparent than real? *Mayo Clin Proc.* 1997;**72**:559–564.
4 Berk-Krauss J, Stein JA, Weber J, et al. New Systematic Therapies and Trends in Cutaneous Melanoma Deaths Among US Whites, 1986–2016. *Am J Public Health.* 2020;**110**:731–733.
5 Beral V, Robinson N. The relationship of malignant melanoma, basal and squamous skin cancers to indoor and outdoor work. *Br J Cancer.* 1981;**44**:886–891.
6 Vagero D, Ringback G, Kiviranta H. Melanoma and other tumors of the skin among office, other indoor and outdoor workers in Sweden 1961-79. *Br J Cancer.* 1986;**53**:507–512.
7 Whiteman DC, Bray CA, Siskind V, et al. A comparison of the anatomic distribution of cutaneous melanoma in two populations with different levels of sunlight: the west of Scotland and Queensland, Australia 1982-2001. *Cancer Causes Control.* 2007;**18**:485–491.
8 Whiteman DC, Whiteman CA, Green AC. Childhood sun exposure as a risk factor for melanoma: a systematic review of epidemiologic studies. *Cancer Causes Control.* 2001;**12**:69–82.
9 Hodis E, Watson IR, Kryukov GV, et al. A landscape of driver mutations in melanoma. *Cell.* 2012;**150**:251–263.
10 Green AC, Williams GM, Logan V, Strutton GM. Reduced melanoma after regular sunscreen use: randomized trial follow-up. *J Clin Oncol.* 2011;**29**:257–263.
11 Lazovich D, Vogel RI, Berwick M, et al. Indoor tanning and risk of melanoma: a case-control study in a highly exposed population. *Cancer Epidemiol Biomark Prev.* 2010;**19**:1557–1568.
12 Cust AE, Armstrong BK, Goumas C, et al. Sunbed use during adolescence and early adulthood is associated with increased risk of early-onset melanoma. *Int J Cancer.* 2011;**128**:2425–2435.
13 Mosher CE, Danoff-Burg S. Addiction to indoor tanning: relation to anxiety, depression, and substance use. *Arch Dermatol.* 2010;**146**:412–417.
14 Fell GL, Robinson KC, Mao J, et al. Skin β-endorphin mediates addiction to UV light. *Cell.* 2014;**157**:1527–1534.
15 Olsen CM, Carroll HJ, Whiteman DC. Estimating the attributable fraction for melanoma: a meta-analysis of pigmentary characteristics and freckling. *Int J Cancer.* 2010;**127**:2430–2445.
16 MacKie RM, Freudenberger T, Aitchison TC. Personal risk-factor chart for cutaneous melanoma. *Lancet.* 1989;**2**:487–490.
17 Chang YM, Newton-Bishop JA, Bishop DT, et al. A pooled analysis of melanocytic nevus phenotype and the risk of cutaneous melanoma at different latitudes. *Int J Cancer.* 2009;**124**:420–428.
18 Manson JE, Rexrode KM, Garland FC, et al. The case for a comprehensive national campaign to prevent melanoma and associated mortality. *Epidemiology.* 2000;**11**:728–734.
19 Robbins HA, Clarke CA, Arron ST, et al. Melanoma Risk and Survival among Organ Transplant Recipients. *J Invest Dermatol.* 2015;**135**:2657–2665.
20 Florell SR, Boucher KM, Garibotti G, et al. Population-based analysis of prognostic factors and survival in familial melanoma. *J Clin Oncol.* 2005;**23**:168–177.
21 Goldstein AM. Familial melanoma, pancreatic cancer and germline CDKN2A mutations. *Hum Mutat.* 2004;**23**:630.
22 Leachman SA, Carucci J, Kohlmann W, et al. Selection criteria for genetic assessment of patients with familial melanoma. *J Am Acad Dermatol.* 2009;**61**:677.
23 Choi JN, Hanlon A, Leffell D. Melanoma and nevi: detection and diagnosis. *Curr Probl Cancer.* 2011;**35**:138–161.
24 Betti R, Santambrogio R, Cerri A, et al. Observational study on the mitotic rate and other prognostic factors in cutaneous primary melanoma arising from naevi and from melanoma de novo. *J Eur Acad Dermatol Venereol.* 2014;**28**:1738–1741.
25 Price HN, Schaffer JV. Congenital melanocytic nevi-when to worry and how to treat: facts and controversies. *Clin Dermatol.* 2010;**28**:293–302.
26 Swerdlow AJ, English JS, Qiao Z. The risk of melanoma in patients with congenital nevi: a cohort study. *J Am Acad Dermatol.* 1995;**32**:595–599.
27 Berg P, Lindelöf B. Congenital melanocytic naevi and cutaneous melanoma. *Melanoma Res.* 2003;**13**:441–445.
28 Zaal LH, Mooi WJ, Klip H, van der Horst CM. Risk of malignant transformation of congenital melanocytic nevi: a retrospective nationwide study from The Netherlands. *Plast Reconstr Surg.* 2005;**116**:1902–1909.
29 Bett BJ. Large or multiple congenital melanocytic nevi: occurrence of cutaneous melanoma in 1008 persons. *J Am Acad Dermatol.* 2006;**54**:767–777.
30 Egan CL, Oliveria SA, Elenitsas R, et al. Cutaneous melanoma risk and phenotypic changes in large congenital nevi: a follow-up study of 46 patients. *J Am Acad Dermatol.* 1998;**39**:923–932.
31 Tannous ZS, Mihm MC, Sober AJ, Duncan LM. Congenital melanocytic nevi: clinical and histopathologic features, risk of melanoma, and clinical management. *J Am Acad Dermatol.* 2005;**52**:197–203.
32 Fears TR, Guerry D, Pfeiffer RM, et al. Identifying individuals at high risk of melanoma: a practical predictor of absolute risk. *J Clin Oncol.* 2006;**24**:3590–3596.
33 Barbe C, Hibon E, Vitry F, et al. Clinical and pathological characteristics of melanoma: a population-based study in a French regional population. *J Eur Acad Dermatol Venereol.* 2012;**26**:159–164.
34 Ankeny JS, Labadie B, Luke J, et al. Review of diagnostic, prognostic, and predictive biomarkers in melanoma. *Clin Exp Metastasis.* 2018;**35**(5):487–493.
35 Sigel DS, Friedman RJ, Kopf AW, et al. ABCDE—an evolving concept in the early detection of melanoma. *Arch Dermatol.* 2005;**141**:1032–1034.
36 Weinstock MA. ABCD, ABCDE, and ABCCCDEEEEFNU. *Arch Dermatol.* 2006;**142**:528a.
37 Grob JJ, Bonerandi JJ. The 'ugly duckling' sign: identification of the common characteristics of nevi in an individual as a basis for melanoma screening. *Arch Dermatol.* 1998;**134**:103–104.
38 Gachon J, Beaulieu P, Sei JF, et al. First prospective study of the recognition process of melanoma in dermatological practice. *Arch Dermatol.* 2005;**141**:434–438.
39 Guerry DT, Synnestvedt M, Elder DE, Schultz D. Lessons from tumor progression: the invasive radial growth phase of melanoma is common, incapable of metastasis, and indolent. *J Invest Dermatol.* 1993;**100**:342S–345S.
40 Ohsie SJ, Sarantopoulos GP, Cochran AJ, Binder SW. Immunohistochemical characteristics of melanoma. *J Cutan Pathol.* 2008;**35**:433–444.
81 Wong SL, Faries MB, Kennedy EB, et al. Sentinel lymph node biopsy and management of regional lymph nodes in melanoma: American Society of Clinical Oncology and Society of Surgical Oncology Clinical Practice Guideline Update. *J Clin Oncol.* 2018;**36**:399–413.
89 Gershenwald JE, Scolyer RA, Hess KR. Melanoma staging: evidence-based changes in the American Joint Committee on Cancer eighth edition cancer staging manual. *CA Cancer J Clin.* 2017;**67**(6):472–492.

90. Tejera-Vaquerizo A, Ribero S, Puig S, et al. Survival analysis and sentinel lymph node status in thin cutaneous melanoma: a multicenter observational study. *Cancer Med*. 2019;**8**:4235–4244.
91. Sinnamon AJ, Neuwirth MG, Yalamanchi P, et al. Association between patient age and lymph node positivity in thin melanoma. *JAMA Dermatol*. 2017;**153**(9):866–873.
92. Amin MB, Greene FL, Edge SB, et al. The eighth edition AJCC cancer staging manual: continuing to build a bridge from a population-based to a more "personalized" approach to cancer staging. *CA Cancer J Clin*. 2017;**67**(2):93–99.
93. Bartlett EK, Gimotty PA, Sinnamon AJ. Clark level risk stratifies patients with mitogenic thin melanomas for sentinel lymph node biopsy. *Ann Surg Oncol*. 2014;**21**(2):643–649.
96. Tejera-Vaquerizo A, Pérez-Cabello G, Marínez-Leborans L, et al. Is mitotic rate still useful in the management of patients with thin melanoma? *J Eur Acad Dermatol Venereol*. 2017;**31**(12):2025–2029.
117. Carr MJ, Sun J, Kroon HM, et al. Oncologic outcomes after isolated limb infusion for advanced melanoma: an international comparison of the procedure and outcomes between the United States and Australia. *Ann Surg Oncol*. 2020;**27**(13):5107–5118. doi: 10.1245/s10434-020-09051-y.
118. Miura JT, Kroon HM, Beasley GM, et al. Long-term oncologic outcomes after isolated limb infusion for locoregionally metastatic melanoma: an International Multicenter Analysis. *Ann Surg Oncol*. 2019;**26**:2486–2494.
120. Teras J, Kroon HM, Miura JT, et al. International multi-center experience of isolated limb infusion for in-transit melanoma metastases in octogenarian and nonagenarian patients. *Ann Surg Oncol*. 2020;**27**:1420–1429.
122. Mousavi H, Zhang X, Gillespie S, et al. Rose Bengal induces dual modes of cell death in melanoma cells and has clinical activity against melanoma. *Melanoma Res*. 2006;**16**:S8.
124. Agarwala SS, Ross MI, Zager JS, et al. Phase 1b study of PV-10 and anti-PD-1 in advanced cutaneous melanoma. *J Clin Oncol*. 2019;**37**(15_suppl):9559.
126. Ribas A, Dummer R, Puzanov I, et al. Oncolytic virotherapy promotes intratumoral T cell infiltration and improves anti-PD-1 immunotherapy. *Cell*. 2018;**174**(4):1031–1032.
128. Tio D, van der Woude J, Prinsen CAC, et al. A systematic review on the role of imiquimod in lentigo maligna and lentigo maligna melanoma: need for standardization of treatment schedule and outcome measures. *J Eur Acad Dermatol Venereol*. 2017;**31**(4):616–624.
129. Damian DL, Saw RP, Thompson JF. Topical immunotherapy with diphencyprone for in transit and cutaneously metastatic melanoma. *J Surg Oncol*. 2014;**109**:308–313.
131. Keilholz L, Altendorf-Hofmann A, et al. Palliative radiotherapy for recurrent and metastatic malignant melanoma. Prognostic factors for tumor response and long-term outcome: a 20-year experience. *Int J Radiat Oncol Biol Phys*. 1999;**44**:607–618.
135. Howard JH, Thompson JF, Mozzillo N, et al. Metastasectomy for distant metastatic melanoma: analysis of data from the first Multicenter Selective Lymphadenectomy Trial (MSLT-I). *Ann Surg Oncol*. 2012;**19**(8):2547–2555.
136. Faries MB, Leung A, Morton DL, et al. A 20-year experience of hepatic resection for melanoma: is there an expanding role? *J Am Coll Surg*. 2014;**219**(1):62–68.
137. He M, Lovell J, Ng BL, et al. Post-operative survival following metastasectomy for patients receiving BRAF inhibitor therapy is associated with duration of pre-operative treatment and elective indication. *J Surg Oncol*. 2015;**111**(8):980–984.
238. Dummer R, Lebbé C, Atkinson V, et al. Combined PD-1, BRAF and MEK inhibition in advanced BRAF-mutant melanoma: safety run-in and biomarker cohorts of COMBI-I. *Nat Med*. 2020;**26**:1557–1563.

107 Other skin cancers

Stacy L. McMurray, MD ■ William G. Stebbins, MD ■ Eric A. Millican, MD ■ Victor A. Neel, MD, PhD

Overview

Nonmelanoma skin cancer (NMSC) includes squamous cell carcinoma (SCC), basal cell carcinoma (BCC), Merkel cell carcinoma (MCC), and other premalignant and malignant tumor types. The incidence of NMSC has increased significantly in recent years. These cancers are diverse in their clinical presentation, biology, and capacity to metastasize. Our understanding of the molecular biology of NMSC has grown considerably in recent years, leading to the development of new treatment options. In addition to malignant NMSC, this article will discuss several benign skin tumors that arise due to underlying internal malignancies.

Introduction

The skin is a heterogeneous organ, consisting of elements of ectodermal, endodermal, and mesodermal origin. This diverse group of tissues gives rise to a wide variety of benign and malignant tumors. Many of these tumors are rare and will not be discussed in this article. Table 1 lists the more common premalignant and malignant tumors, which we discuss in detail. These are tumors relevant to the oncologist because they have the capacity to metastasize and cause significant morbidity and mortality. We also briefly mention several tumor syndromes that may present with unusual benign skin tumors that, if recognized, should prompt the clinician to conduct a detailed search for an internal malignancy. Melanoma, Kaposi sarcoma, the malignant histiocytoses, and the cutaneous lymphomas are discussed elsewhere in this book.

The incidence of nonmelanoma skin cancer (NMSC), which includes squamous cell carcinoma (SCC) and basal cell carcinoma (BCC), is increasing (Table 2). In the United States, approximately 480,000 persons were diagnosed with NMSC in 1983,[4] over 1 million in 2008,[5] and an estimated 5.4 million new lesions in 2012.[1] The ratio of BCC to SCC among Caucasians in the United States, Australia, and the United Kingdom is about 4:1.[4,6,7] Together, these two tumors account for approximately 90% of all skin cancers. In recent years, the role of the sun in the causation of these common skin tumors has received much attention.[8]

Ultraviolet radiation in the pathogenesis of skin cancers

In the past several decades, research on the relationship between the sun and skin cancer has escalated principally because of fear of the consequences of increased ultraviolet B (UVB) radiation on the earth's surface as a result of ozone depletion in the stratosphere. There is now general consensus over the role of sunlight in the etiology of NMSC.[9,10] Chuang et al.[11] reported a 45-fold increase in NMSC in the Japanese population in Kauai, Hawaii, as compared with the Japanese population in Japan. Another study showed the incidence of SCC, but not BCC, in a group of Caucasian fishermen in Maryland correlated directly with the amount of sun exposure.[12] A population-based study on nearly 12,000 patients also demonstrated the close correlation between chronic cumulative sun exposure and SCC.[13] Geographically, the incidence of skin cancer in Caucasians increases toward the equator, further supporting the role of sunlight in carcinogenesis.

UVB imprints a unique signature on the DNA it damages. Cellular attempts to repair this damage can lead to CC>TT mutations or C→T transitions. UVA can also induce these mutations, though likely indirectly through the creation of reactive oxygen species.[14,15] In the precursors of SCC (known as actinic keratoses), inactivating mutations of the tumor suppressor p53 harbor these UV-induced errors.[16] Because p53 is involved in the transcriptional regulation of DNA repair genes, cell-cycle control genes, and the induction of cell death, damage to this important regulator by UV irradiation is one mechanism that allows for the overgrowth of damaged cells.

In addition to natural sun exposure, indoor tanning is increasingly recognized as carcinogenic. According to a meta-analysis, patients who reported ever using a tanning bed had a 67% increased risk of developing SCC and a 29% increased risk of BCC.[17] Two independent case-control studies also found a greater than 60% increase in the risk of early-onset (younger than age 50) BCC.[18,19] Overall, more than 419,000 cases of skin cancer in the United States are attributable to indoor tanning annually.[20] These and other similar findings led the International Agency for Research on Cancer to classify UV tanning devices as Group 1 carcinogens.[21] More recently, the US FDA reclassified tanning devices as class II (moderate-to-high risk) devices, and several states have passed legislation limiting their use among minor children. UVB (280–320 nm) and UVA (320–400 nm) also have direct and indirect effects on the cutaneous immune system, lowering cell-mediated immunity, and inducing T-suppressor cell production.[22] Loss of local immunity is thought to be another factor influencing carcinogenesis.

Tumors arising from the epidermis

Actinic keratosis

Definition
Actinic keratosis (AK), also known as solar keratosis, is a very common lesion occurring in susceptible persons as a result of prolonged and repeated solar exposures. Ultraviolet radiation results in damage to the keratinocytes and produces single or multiple, discrete scaly macules or thin papules. These premalignant lesions may, in time, progress to SCCs.

Holland-Frei Cancer Medicine, Tenth Edition. Edited by Robert C. Bast, John C. Byrd, Carlo M. Croce, Ernest Hawk, Fadlo R. Khuri, Raphael E. Pollock, Apostolia M. Tsimberidou, Christopher G. Willett, and Cheryl L. Willman.
© 2023 John Wiley & Sons, Inc. Published 2023 by John Wiley & Sons, Inc.

Table 1 Common premalignant and malignant neoplasms of the skin.

	Premalignant	Malignant
Epidermis	Keratoacanthoma Actinic keratosis Arsenical keratosis HPV-induced premalignant papules (epidermodysplasia verruciformis, Bowenoid papulosis) Mucosal leukoplakia	Basal cell carcinoma Merkel cell carcinoma Squamous cell carcinoma
Dermal		Dermatofibrosarcoma protuberans Atypical fibroxanthoma/pleomorphic dermal sarcoma Angiosarcoma
Appendageal	Nevus sebaceous	Sebaceous carcinoma Extramammary Paget disease

Benign cutaneous tumors associated with cancer syndromes
   Trichilemmomas → Cowden disease (breast/visceral tumors)
   Sebaceous tumors → Muir–Torre syndrome (GI/GU tumors)
   Mucosal neuromas → MEN3 (thyroid carcinoma/pheochromocytoma)		

Abbreviations: GI, gastrointestinal; GU, genitourinary; HPV, human papillomavirus; MEN, multiple endocrine neoplasia.

Table 2 Nonmelanoma skin cancer statistics.

	BCC and SCC	Merkel cell carcinoma
Magnitude of the problem (yearly)	>5.4 million new lesions in 3.3 million people[1]	2488 new cases[2]
Severity of the problem (yearly)	Approximately 8800 deaths from SCC[3] Disfigurement Disability	700 deaths Incidence increasing

Epidemiology

AK predominantly affects sun-exposed areas of fair-skinned people. The incidence in elderly whites may approach 100% in some populations.[4] AK may appear at a much younger age (under 30 years) in individuals with an outdoor occupation (e.g., farmers, ranchers, and sailors) or an outdoor lifestyle. The lesions are more common in transplant recipients[23] and albinos.[24] It is rare in darker-skinned individuals.

Clinical features

The onset of AK is typically insidious and therefore often passes unnoticed for some time. The characteristic lesion is rough and gritty to palpation, similar to the feel of coarse sandpaper. Lesions are usually skin-colored or yellow-brown, often with a reddish tinge, and round-to-ovular in shape, often less than 1 cm in diameter. They may be macules or papules, as in the hypertrophic variety of AK (Figure 1). There may be single or multiple scattered discrete lesions, typically limited to sun-exposed areas. A pigmented variant, named spreading pigmented AK, is a brown, slowly growing, slightly scaly lesion that tends to appear on the face and may be larger than 1.5 cm in diameter, making it difficult to distinguish from lentigo maligna.

Diagnosis

The diagnosis of AK is usually based on clinical examination alone. The hypertrophic variant may sometimes be confused with early SCC. Suchniak et al.[25] demonstrated histologically the presence of *in situ* or invasive SCCs in 50% of lesions diagnosed clinically as hypertrophic AK.

Treatment

Macular AK is most easily treated with cryotherapy.[26] Brief applications of liquid nitrogen with a cotton-tipped swab or cryo gun will suffice in the majority of cases. Retreatment may be necessary for more resistant lesions. It is not necessary to freeze to

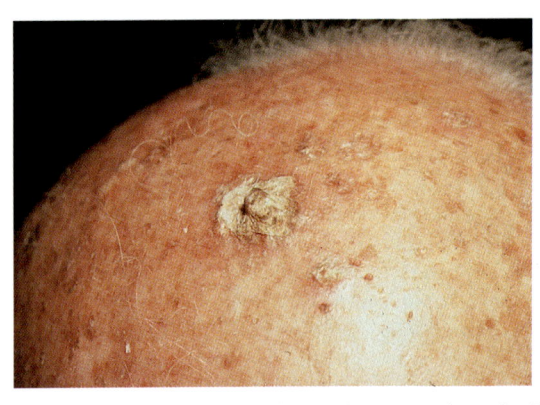

Figure 1 Actinic keratosis. Multiple discrete lesions on the scalp. These lesions are "gritty" to palpation. The largest lesion in the center of the picture represents the hypertrophic variant. This must be differentiated from a squamous cell carcinoma *in situ*.

the point of blistering. Electrodessication and curettage (ED&C) of the lesions is equally effective but carries a slightly greater risk of scarring and dyspigmentation. Hypertrophic lesions are best evaluated by biopsy to rule out invasive SCC.

Where large areas of skin are involved, topical 5-fluorouracil may be applied twice a day to the affected areas for up to 4 weeks as a field treatment. This results in a brisk reaction in the treated areas, ranging from redness, soreness, and weeping to shallow ulcerations and crusting (Figure 2), which gradually subsides after discontinuation of the cytotoxic cream. Newer formulations containing 0.5% 5-fluorouracil used once daily for 4 weeks may cause less skin irritation.[27]

Multiple additional topical approaches are available. 5% imiquimod cream has been used twice weekly for 16 weeks for nonhypertrophic, AK of the face/scalp in immunocompetent individuals. Side effects include erythema, pruritus and/or burning, and hypopigmentation at the treatment site. Imiquimod acts via upregulation of inflammatory cytokines primarily through

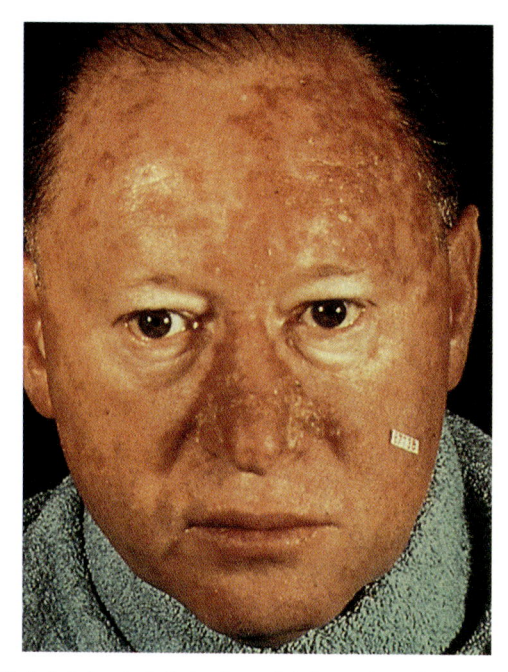

Figure 2 Actinic keratosis. Extensive actinic keratosis on the face. Note that the right half has been used as control and the left half of the forehead and the nose were treated with 5% 5-fluorouracil cream for 14 days.

stimulation of toll-like receptor 7 (TLR7). Topical 3% diclofenac gel has been reported to be efficacious for AK when used twice daily for 60–90 days.[28] Studies have demonstrated that topical 5-fluorouracil and imiquimod produce superior clearance rates when compared to topical 3% diclofenac gel.[29,30] 5% 5-fluorouracil cream has also demonstrated efficacy when combined 1:1 with 0.005% calcipotriene cream applied twice daily for 4 days.[31] Side effects are similar to 5-fluorouracil alone, but combination therapy can produce brisk responses that peak 4–5 days after completion of treatment.

Lastly, photodynamic therapy (PDT) utilizes a topically applied photosensitizer, aminolevulinic acid, which is preferentially absorbed by the premalignant cells and photoactivated upon exposure to blue or red light. PDT results in clearance of up to 90% of AK in patients with extensive AK of the face and scalp.[32] Stinging of the treated skin may occur during light exposure. A sunburn-like reaction follows therapy.

Course and prognosis
The lesions of AK may resolve spontaneously, but generally, they persist if left untreated. There is modest lifetime risk (<10%) of an individual AK transforming into SCC. Marks et al.[33] reported that 60% of SCCs arise from preexisting solar keratoses.

Keratoacanthoma

Definition
Keratoacanthoma (KA) is a common, rapidly growing low-grade tumor that may involute spontaneously, even if untreated. It is believed to originate from the hair follicles.

Epidemiology
Few studies have been done on the incidence of KA.[34] Chuang et al.[35] reported an incidence rate of 103.6 per 100,000 based on the small population in Kauai, Hawaii. It is most common between the ages of 60–65 and is rare in persons younger than age 20.

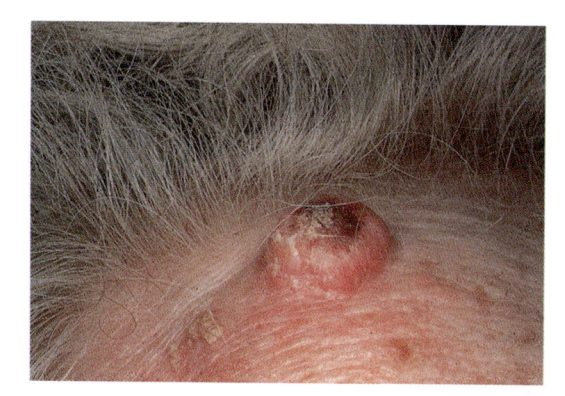

Figure 3 Keratoacanthoma. A pink, dome-shaped lesion with a central core of keratin. This rapidly growing lesion is located on the mid-forehead. Source: Courtesy of P.L. McCarthy, MD.

In contrast to SCC and BCC, there is no increase in frequency in old age. It is uncommon in black or Japanese patients and is approximately 2–3 times more common in males. The majority of patients have a solitary lesion.

Sun exposure and exposure to chemical carcinogens such as tar are thought to be etiologic factors, and the possibility of a viral etiology is still debated. The presence of HPV has been demonstrated by DNA hybridization and polymerase chain reaction (PCR) studies.[36] The possibility of a genetic defect has also been proposed because these tumors are more common in patients with Muir–Torre syndrome (MTS) than in the general population.

Clinical features
Keratoacanthomas characteristically arise on hair-bearing skin. The most common areas of involvement are the central parts of the face: cheeks, nose, ears, lips, eyelids, and forehead, as well as the dorsa of the hands, wrists, and forearms. The trunk and scalp are uncommon sites. Typically, the lesion presents as a solitary, rapidly growing, firm, dome-shaped, skin-colored to slightly pink lesion with a central keratin plug (Figure 3). The evolving lesion typically grows rapidly for 2–4 weeks to a size of up to 2 cm in diameter. The mature lesion involutes spontaneously after a few months, leaving a scar. The complete cycle of growth to spontaneous resolution takes 4–6 months.[37] Multiple or recurrent lesions may occur, particularly in cases associated with tar exposure. Multiple lesions associated with defects in cell-mediated immunity and with multiple internal malignant neoplasms and sebaceous adenomas, as part of MTS, have been noted. There is no evidence that the solitary type KA is associated with internal malignancy.

Diagnosis
The main differential diagnosis is to distinguish KA from SCC. The rapid evolution and spontaneous involution, the characteristic dome shape with a central plug of keratin, and the relatively young age of the patient are all clues to the diagnosis. In most cases, evaluation of the base of the lesion is essential to exclude an invasive SCC.

Treatment
Keratoacanthomas may resolve spontaneously. Surgical excision of the lesion will produce better cosmetic results and provide tissue for histopathologic diagnosis. Intralesional (IL) therapy with various agents has also been studied with some success. Cure rates with intralesional therapy approach 98% for 5-FU, 91% for methotrexate (MTX), 100% for bleomycin, 100% for IFN alpha (α)-2, 83%

for IFN α-2a, and 100% for IFN α-2b.[38] Intradermal triamcinolone has also been used successfully as a therapy for treatment of solitary and multiple reactive KA.[39–42] Radiotherapy[43] has been used to treat lesions that cannot be distinguished from SCCs, as well as the so-called giant aggressive keratoacanthomas.[44,45] The dosage used, 4000–6000 cGy, is the same as the tumoricidal dosage used for SCCs. A biopsy of the lesion to rule out SCC prior to treatment may be prudent.

Course and prognosis
Keratoacanthoma is a low-grade tumor that carries a very good prognosis. Reports of malignant transformation or metastasizing lesions are probably misdiagnosed SCCs.

Squamous cell carcinoma

Definition
SCC is a malignant tumor arising from epidermal or appendageal keratinocytes or from squamous mucosal epithelium. There is often a history of damage by exogenous agents acting as carcinogens, such as sunlight, ionizing radiation, local irritants, or arsenic. The tumor cells have a tendency toward keratin formation. Variants include Bowen disease, an *in situ* SCC; verrucous carcinoma, a low-grade SCC with a clinicopathologically distinct warty appearance; Buschke–Loewenstein tumor, the subset of verrucous carcinoma found on the genitals; oral florid papillomatosis, which involves the oral cavity; and epithelioma cuniculatum which involves the plantar surface.

Epidemiology
The incidence of cutaneous SCC varies greatly for different parts of the world, different ethnic backgrounds, and different life habits and occupations. The incidence was reported as 41.4 cases per 100,000 in 1983,[4] and is increasing.[5] Over the past 3 decades, SCC incidence has increased over 200% in the United States, and more than 1 million cases are diagnosed annually.[1,3]

As previously mentioned, mutations in the p53 tumor-suppressor gene have been found in a number of SCC.[46] Phototherapy patients who received broadband UVB or psoralen plus ultraviolet A (PUVA) for the treatment of skin diseases, such as psoriasis or mycosis fungoides (cutaneous T-cell lymphoma), are also at increased risk.[47,48] The incidence of SCC is much higher in immunosuppressed patients, and these patients should be followed closely. Many dermatology departments now have dedicated clinics for immunosuppressed and transplant patients.[49] Depending on the dose of immunosuppressive drugs and previous sun exposure, transplant patients have up to a 65-fold increased risk of developing SCC.[50] The SCC to BCC ratio also reverses from 0.25 to 1 in the general population to 1.5–3 to 1 in transplant patients. Tumors in such patients tend to behave more aggressively.[47,51]

Verrucous carcinoma of the skin is a rare tumor, with more than 100 reported cases.[52] Approximately 80–90% of patients are male, with a mean age of 52–60 years. The Buschke–Loewenstein tumor is a verrucous carcinoma of the anogenital mucosa. Penile Buschke–Loewenstein tumor is the most common, with an incidence between 5% and 24% of all penile cancers. Vaginal, cervical, perianal, and perirectal Buschke–Loewenstein tumors are less common than penile ones. The etiology of these tumors is linked to HPV, particularly to HPV serotypes 6 and 11.[52]

The incidence of Bowen disease has not been extensively investigated. The incidence has been reported as 14 per 100,000 population in Rochester, Minnesota,[53] and 142 per 100,000 population in Kauai, Hawaii.[54]

Progress has been made in the identification of heritable risk factors in NMSC.[55] Polymorphisms of the melanocortin-1 receptor, which are linked to an increased risk of melanoma, segregate with patients at an elevated risk for both SCC and BCC.

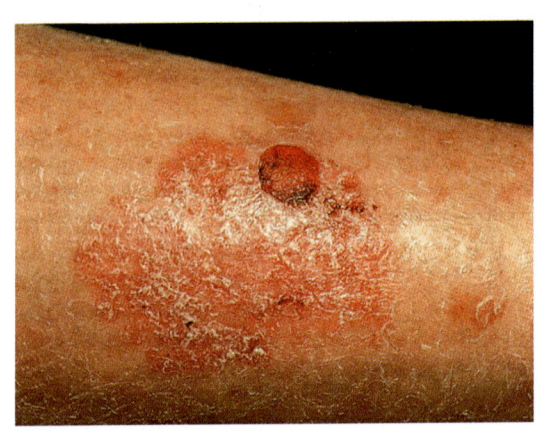

Figure 4 Squamous cell carcinoma (SCC) arising in SCC *in situ*. A nodule of invasive SCC on the lower leg arising within the well-demarcated, erythematous scaly plaque of SCC *in situ*.

Clinical features
SCC often arises in skin that is damaged or has been subjected to chronic irritation. Thus, the skin adjacent to the carcinoma may show evidence of solar damage, such as AK, wrinkling, dryness, telangiectasias, and irregular pigmentation. Alternatively, there may be features of radiodermatitis from previous radiation therapy,[56] a sinus tract associated with an underlying osteomyelitis, or scarring from a burn ("Marjolin ulcer").[57] Chronic venous ulcers of the lower extremities are also associated with increased risks of developing SCC.[58] Chronic ulcers that show features of proliferation beyond the expected granulation process should raise the suspicion of malignant transformation.

SCC usually evolves faster than BCC but not as rapidly as KA. The earliest lesion, the intraepidermal SCC or carcinoma *in situ*, typically appears as a scaly, erythematous plaque on sun-exposed areas, often with a sharply demarcated but irregular outline (Figure 4). Bowen disease is clinically identical to SCC *in situ*. Bowen disease on the glans penis is also known as erythroplasia of Queyrat.

Invasive SCC (Figure 5) almost always arises from a preexisting premalignant lesion or an *in situ* carcinoma, although *de novo* SCC has been reported.[59] The lesion is typically an erythematous, indurated papule, plaque, or nodule, which may be polygonal, oval, round, or verrucous in shape (Figures 6 and 7). The tumor tends to increase both in elevation and diameter with time. A hallmark of SCC is its firmness on palpation. The late lesion is often eroded, crusted, and ulcerated with an indurated margin. The ulcer is often covered with a purulent exudate and bleeds easily (Figure 7). Early ulceration is often a marker for anaplastic lesions. Regional lymphadenopathy may be present either as a response to infection of the ulcer or from metastases. The latter tend to be rubbery and more irregular and may be fixed to adjacent tissues.

Verrucous carcinoma of the skin is most commonly found on the soles of men.[52] Typically, it presents as a slowly enlarging cauliflower-like mass. It is locally aggressive and may grow to a significant size. The ball of the foot is involved in more than 50% of cases. Other locations include the face, buttocks, oral cavity,

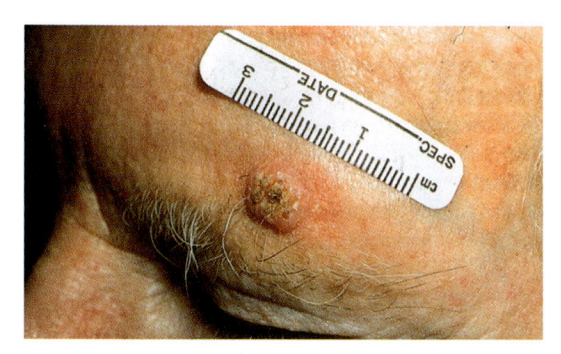

Figure 5 Invasive squamous cell carcinoma. Erythematous, hyperkeratotic nodule on the forehead resembling a keratoacanthoma (see Figure 3). An incisional or excisional biopsy is necessary to distinguish the two lesions.

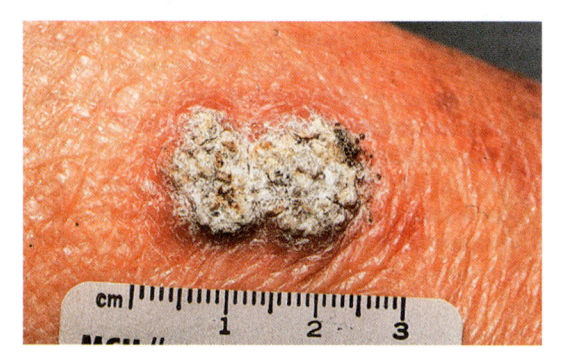

Figure 6 Invasive squamous cell carcinoma. A hyperkeratotic, crusty plaque on the forearm. Note the evidence of sun damage in the surrounding skin: wrinkling, bruising, and a lackluster appearance.

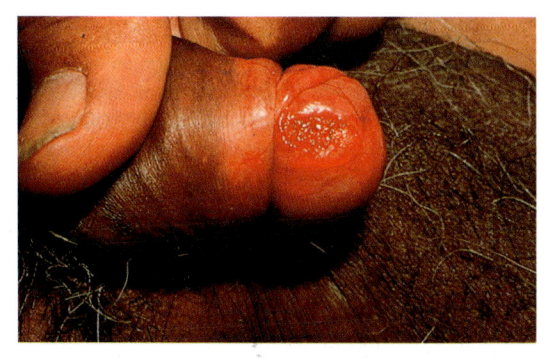

Figure 7 Invasive squamous cell carcinoma. An ulcerated lesion on the glans penis with an indurated margin. The ulcer typically bleeds easily.

trunk, and extremities. The bulk of the tumor is soft and may be foul-smelling. If left untreated, the tumor will eventually penetrate the underlying soft tissue and bone. However, metastasis is rare.

The Buschke–Loewenstein tumor most commonly affects the penile glans and prepuce of uncircumcised males, presenting as a cauliflower-like, fungating, foul-smelling tumor on the coronal sulcus. In women, it may present on the vagina, cervix, or vulva. The Buschke–Loewenstein tumor tends to infiltrate deeply, causing destruction of underlying tissues.

SCC of the lip may arise from an area of leukoplakia or actinic cheilitis, and almost always occurs on the lower lip. This tumor is typically much more aggressive than those on glabrous skin and has a higher rate of metastasis.

Carcinomas arising in longstanding radiation dermatitis tend to be histologically anaplastic and extremely aggressive, with a high rate of metastasis.[60]

Treatment

The choice of treatment modality depends on the degree of differentiation of the tumor and the presence or absence of metastasis. The size, shape, location of the tumor, and the predisposing factors should also be considered. In the case of a localized, well-differentiated tumor with no evidence of metastasis, the goal should be complete eradication of the lesion. In the presence of lymph node metastases or unresectable tumors, palliative treatment may be considered. The variety of modalities available for consideration include ED&C, excisional surgery, Mohs surgery, cryosurgery, electrosurgery, and radiation therapy.[43,61–63]

Electrodessication and curettage

ED&C is an option for SCC *in situ*, particularly on the trunk. The primary drawback is the lack of histologic confirmation of clear tumor margins, but in properly chosen patients the recurrence rate is similar to excisional surgery.[64] Invasive SCC and tumors with high-risk features have a higher risk of recurrence, however, and the preferred treatment for these tumors would allow for proper margin assessment. The larger, circular scar left from the ED&C procedure is also a deterrent for some patients.

Excisional surgery

Surgical excision with primary closure or repair with skin graft or flap is the treatment of choice for relatively small lesions with distinct borders. There should be an adequate margin of clearance of 3–5 mm to minimize the risk of recurrence. Brodland and Zitelli[65] reported that margins of 4 mm were required to achieve a 95% tumor clearance rate. For invasive or large tumors (>2 cm in diameter), or tumors on high-risk areas such as the scalp, ears, nose, eyelids, or lips, Mohs micrographic surgery (MMS) is the preferred modality.

Prophylactic lymph node dissection is not recommended because of the relatively low rate of metastasis. Sentinel lymph node biopsy is an emerging approach for high-risk tumors, though the specific indications remain undefined.[66] Tumors that have metastasized to regional lymph nodes are best treated with excision, lymph node dissection, and chemoradiation.

Mohs surgery

MMS is a technique wherein a single physician excises the tumor and performs a histologic examination of 100% of the surgical margin. This technique has the lowest local recurrence rate of all treatment modalities while also allowing maximum conservation of surrounding healthy tissue, allowing for an optimal cosmetic result.[65] It is the treatment of choice for tumors on cosmetically or functionally sensitive areas, as well as for recurrent tumors. It is also indicated for immunocompromised patients, tumors in previously irradiated skin, or tumors with high-risk features including poor differentiation, Breslow depth ≥2 mm, diameter ≥2 cm, or perineural invasion. Appropriate use criteria for Mohs surgery have been published.[65,67]

Cryosurgery

Treatment of SCC by freezing with liquid nitrogen is best restricted to the carcinoma *in situ* on low-risk areas that are not cosmetically sensitive. This modality has the advantage of simplicity with a high cure rate when employed in the proper situation.[62,68]

Radiation therapy

Radiation therapy is an option for patients who cannot tolerate other more invasive treatment modalities. The treatment schedule is determined by the treatment modality, size, depth, and location of the tumor and the particular time-dose-fractionation schedule used. A fractionated dose provides the best cure rate and the lowest risk of adverse events, but fractionation schedules vary from 5 to 30 fractions.[43] Most radiation for skin cancers in the United States is delivered using electron beam or superficial X-ray therapies with a dose between 4000 and 6000 cGy. The reported 5-year control rates for these approaches are 89% and 68% for primary and recurrent SCC, respectively.[69] While reasonable, these are significantly below the 5-year cure rates for excisions or MMS. More recently, high-dose-rate electronic brachytherapy has become a popular treatment approach with high clearance rates and good cosmesis, but long-term data are lacking.[70,71] Postoperative radiation therapy may be considered as an adjuvant treatment for certain high-risk tumors including those with perineural invasion or other high-risk features (see AJCC and BWH high-risk features below). However, adjuvant radiation has not been shown to improve outcomes when compared to surgical monotherapy in all cases, and further studies are needed to define the subset of cutaneous SCC that benefits most from adjuvant radiation.[72]

Patient and tumor site selection are critical for all radiation therapy. Good cosmetic results can be obtained for carefully selected small lesions of the nose, lip, eyelid, and canthus, though these may deteriorate with time. Lesions on the dorsum of the hand and those over bony and cartilaginous structures should not be treated with radiation due to the risk of radiation necrosis. Lesions in younger patients should be approached with caution given the risk of tumors arising secondary to the treatment. Tumors that do arise in areas of chronic radiation dermatitis should not be treated with further radiation.

Systemic therapy
The use of oral acitretin has decreased the incidence of SCC when given as a chemopreventive agent. The benefit from such long-term use must be weighed against the toxicity, which includes hypertriglyceridemia, arthralgias, mucocutaneous xerosis, and alopecia. In organ transplant recipients, where the risk of developing skin cancer and risk of death from SCC is increased, chronic use of retinoids may be justified.[73]

Immunotherapy offers a relatively novel treatment option for patients with advanced disease. Cemiplimab and pembrolizumab are anti-programmed cell death protein 1 (PD-1) antibodies that inhibit the immune checkpoint blockade. These PD-1 inhibitors have been recently approved for the treatment unresectable locally advanced or metastatic cutaneous SCC that cannot be cured with radiation. Common side effects include fatigue, rash, diarrhea and other immune-mediated reactions.

Course and prognosis
The risk factors correlated with local recurrence and metastasis include treatment modality, prior treatment, location, size, depth, histologic differentiation, histologic evidence of perineural involvement, precipitating factors other than ultraviolet light, and host immunosuppression. SCC in skin carries an overall metastatic rate of 3–6%.[74] Those arising from sun-damaged skin typically have a low risk for metastasis whereas those arising from chronic osteomyelitic sinus tracts, irradiated areas, and burn scars have a much higher metastatic rate (31%, 20%, and 18%, respectively). Carcinoma on the lower lip, although mostly sun induced, has a metastatic incidence of about 15%. Tumor arising in areas such as the glans penis (see Figure 7), the vulva, and the oral mucosa also have a high rate of metastasis. Disease-specific mortality from cSCC in the United States is approximately 1.5%.[3]

The 8th edition of the American Joint Committee on Cancer (AJCC 8) staging system for head and neck cutaneous SCC was released in 2017.[75] Staging factors include size in greatest dimension (e.g., >2 cm but less than 4 cm is stage T2) and number of high-risk features: deep invasion (defined as invasion beyond the subcutaneous fat or >6 mm), perineural invasion (defined as tumor cells invading the perineural space of nerves lying deeper than the dermis or measuring ≥0.1 mm in caliber, or clinical or radiographic involvement of named nerves), and minor bone invasion.[75] Studies demonstrate improved ability of AJCC 8 to stratify tumors with a significant risk of disease-related poor outcomes when compared to AJCC 7.[76] However, alternative staging systems, such as the Brigham and Women's Hospital (BWH) staging system, may more accurately stratify high-risk tumors into different prognostic groups.[77,78] The BWH system stages tumors based on the number of high-risk factors including tumor diameter ≥ 2 cm, poorly differentiated histology, perineural invasion ≥0.1 mm, and tumor invasion beyond fat, excluding bone invasion, which automatically upgrades tumors to stage T3. A cohort study by Ruiz et al.[79] found that the bulk of poor outcomes (i.e., metastases, deaths) occurred in high tumor classes for both staging systems, AJCC 8 (T3/T4) and BWH (T2b/T3). The BWH staging system was found to have a higher specificity (93%) and positive predictive value (30%) for identifying cases at risk for metastasis or death. Specifically, statistical analysis showed superiority of BWH for predicting nodal metastasis and disease-specific death, but there was no statistical difference between staging systems for local recurrence or overall survival.[79]

With proper treatment, the overall 5-year remission rate is 90%, including SCC of the lip.[74] Frankel et al.[80] recommended follow-ups at least every 3 months for a year after treatment of SCC, and semiannually thereafter for up to 4 years.

Basal cell carcinoma

Definition
BCC is a malignant tumor that very rarely metastasizes. It is composed of cells that arise from the epidermis and the appendages which resemble the basal layer of the epidermis and is associated with a characteristic stroma. It tends to grow slowly and invade locally over many years. Eventually, it can ulcerate, hence its archaic name "rodent ulcer."

Epidemiology
BCCs account for more than 75% of NMSC diagnosed in the United States each year.[81,82] Incidence varies from 422 per 100,000 general population in Kauai, Hawaii,[34] to 146 per 100,000 in Rochester, Minnesota.[83] BCC is the most common form of skin cancer in whites[4] and is rare in darkly pigmented people. It most frequently occurs in persons older than 40 years of age. The frequency is slightly higher in males. Other risk factors include geographic locations with high solar intensity, exposures to inorganic trivalent arsenic, ionizing radiation, and immunosuppression. Phototherapy patients receiving UVB or PUVA for treatment of certain dermatoses, such as psoriasis or mycosis fungoides, are also at increased risk.[47] Recent studies suggest a correlation between BCCs and exposures to sunlight in early life and intense intermittent (recreational) sun exposures.[84,85] This is contrary to the previous belief that BCCs result from cumulative lifetime sunlight exposures. Genetic studies show that loss-of-function mutations in the tumor-suppressor gene Patched, or gain-of-function mutations in the Smoothened gene, lead to the formation of sporadic basal cell tumors.[86,87] Germline mutations in these genes lead to Gorlin syndrome or basal cell nevus syndrome.

Clinical features

BCC is characteristically slow growing over months to years. It is usually asymptomatic unless ulceration occurs, and then there is bleeding. It most frequently occurs on sun-exposed areas such as the face and upper trunk and is not seen on the palms and soles.

Early lesions are round-to-oval papules or nodules, firm to palpation, often with an umbilicated center that may be ulcerated. The color is pink to red and often has a translucent or pearly quality (Figure 8). If left untreated, the lesion enlarges slowly and is destructive to neighboring structures by direct invasion. Longstanding lesions are ulcerated as a rule (Figure 9). The surrounding skin often shows telangiectasias and other evidence of solar damage, such as AK, atrophy, wrinkling, dryness, and irregular pigmentation. Some BCCs are pigmented and may exhibit a bluish hue.[88] These may be confused with malignant melanoma (Figure 10). Superficial-type BCC usually presents on the trunk as an irregular, atrophic pink plaque with a slightly raised border and can be mistaken for psoriasis or dermatophytic infection (Figure 11). Infiltrative-type BCCs can be difficult to detect. They are often ivory-white and may resemble morphea and are therefore called morpheaform BCCs. This type of lesion usually occurs on the face and has a more aggressive behavior.[89]

Treatment

The choice of therapy depends on the type and size of the lesion, the location, the general condition of the patient, the cosmetic considerations, and, not least, the experience and skill of the operator.[81] Morpheaform BCCs usually have indistinct borders clinically and may result in underestimation of the extent of the tumor. Lesions situated in the nasolabial crease, around the eye, and behind the ear also tend to undermine deeply and extend far beyond the clinical border (Figure 12). Lesions that ulcerate early tend to be more aggressive. Knowledge of the behavior of the different clinical and pathologic types of BCC is essential in determining the choice of therapy. Treatment of BCCs should be aimed at a cure in the first instance. Under-treatment will result in recurrence and deep invasion.

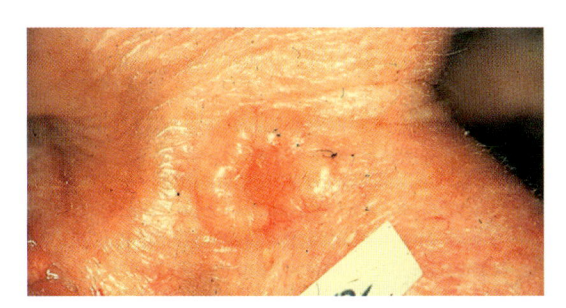

Figure 8 Basal cell carcinoma. A pearly nodule with an umbilicated, ulcerated center and telangiectasia.

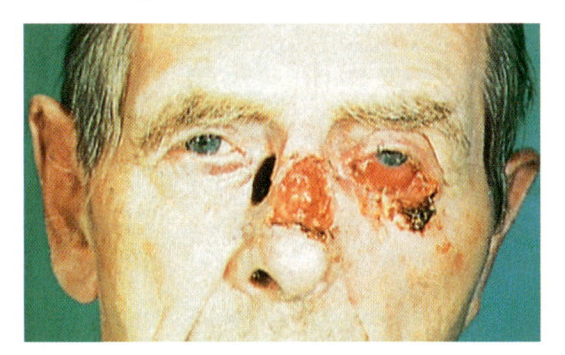

Figure 9 Basal cell carcinoma. Note the erosive nature of such a long-standing lesion.

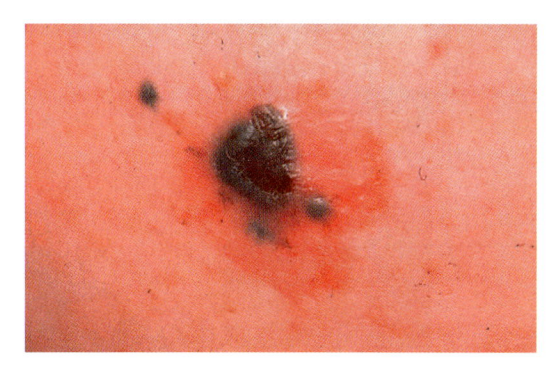

Figure 10 Pigmented basal cell carcinoma. A pink, irregular plaque with dark blue to black pigmentation at the center that mimics a superficial spreading melanoma. The shiny quality is one clue to the diagnosis.

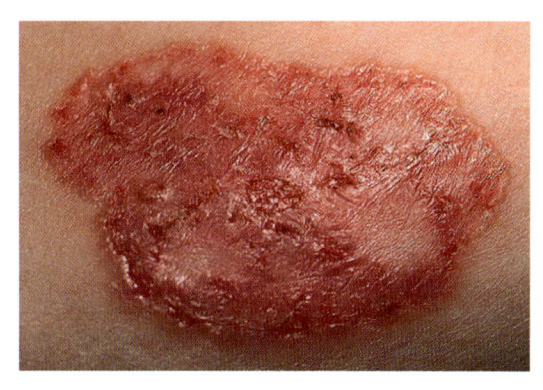

Figure 11 Superficial basal cell carcinoma. A large, 5-cm lesion on the abdomen. The pearly, string-like border is the clue to the clinical diagnosis.

Electrodesiccation and curettage

ED&C can be a reasonable option for small (<1 cm) tumors in low-risk areas that lack high aggressive histologic features. In carefully selected patients, the recurrence rate is similar to excision, but in less appropriate lesions the recurrence rate can exceed 20%.[90] Primary drawbacks include the lack of histologic confirmation of clearance and the appearance of a round, hypopigmented scar.

Surgical excision

Surgical excision of the tumor with 4 mm margins followed by primary closure produces good cosmetic results and allows the surgical margins to be examined by the pathologist to confirm adequate margins.[91] Tumor present at the lateral excision margins will result in marginal recurrences, which tend to present early and may be re-excised with relative ease. Inadequate deep margins result in recurrences which tend to present late, together with invasion of deep structures. For lesions without aggressive histologic features on the trunk or extremity, the recurrence rate is less than 5%.[91]

Mohs surgery

MMS offers the lowest recurrence rate of all treatment options while allowing maximum conservation of healthy surrounding tissue (see Figure 12). According to the appropriate use criteria published in 2012, Mohs surgery is indicated for tumors with aggressive histologic features including morpheaform, infiltrative,

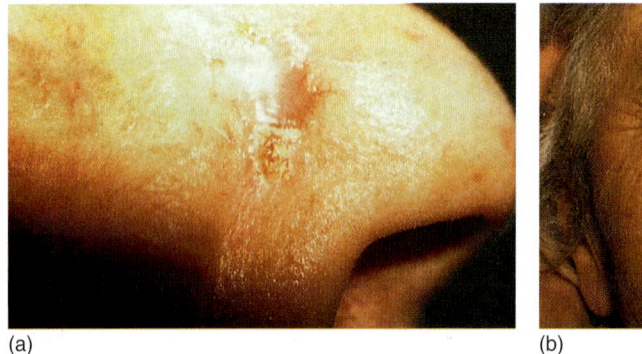

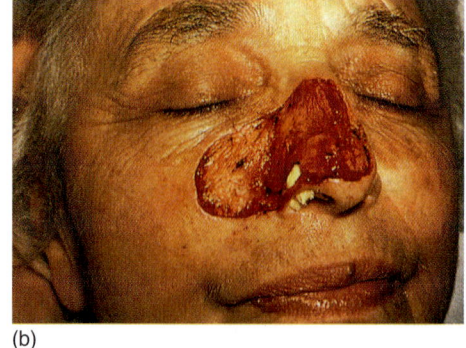

Figure 12 (a) Basal cell carcinoma. The lesion is quite limited clinically. (b) Same patient after treatment with Mohs surgery, illustrating the cryptic extension far beyond the clinically evident border.

metatypical, and micronodular patterns. It is also indicated for nearly all recurrent tumors, lesions on the head, neck, genitals, pretibial legs, hands, and feet as well as nodular tumors >2 cm on the trunk.[67] Advantages include complete margin assessment of the tumor and maximal tissue preservation. Disadvantages include cost and, in some areas, limited availability of trained Mohs surgeons.[92]

Radiation therapy

Treatment with ionizing radiation is an option in selected patient populations, in particular, elderly or fragile patients who cannot tolerate invasive procedures. Electron beam and superficial X-ray therapies yield 5-year control rates of 95% and 86% in primary and recurrent BCCs, respectively.[69] Electron beam brachytherapy has been used with early success in BCC, but large studies and 5-year data are lacking.[70] Lesions >5 cm have higher recurrence rates than smaller tumors.[93] The treatment schedule is chosen according to the type, location, size, and depth of the tumor, the total dose of radiation, and the number of fractions that will be given. Atrophy, necrosis, and scarring may be kept to a minimum when the total dose, typically in the range of 4000–6000 cGy, is divided into several smaller fractions over several weeks. Hypo-fractionated schedules with five to eight treatments have been suggested, particularly with high-dose-rate brachytherapy, to minimize patient inconvenience. However, these may have more adverse events and poorer cosmesis compared to traditional 20–30 fraction regimens.[94]

Chemotherapy

Topical applications of 5% 5-fluorouracil cream to the tumor twice a day for several weeks is best suited only for small, superficial tumors in elderly patients who cannot tolerate other more aggressive forms of treatment. The rate of recurrence, however, is considerably higher. Intralesional 5-fluorouracil has also been tried in nodular lesions.[95,96] Five percent imiquimod cream five times per week for 6 weeks has been shown to be effective therapy for the majority of biopsy-proven superficial BCCs in immunocompetent individuals on the trunk and extremities. Lesions >2.0 cm or lesions located on the head, neck, hands, and feet are excluded in the FDA indications.

Two systemic medications have been FDA approved for metastatic or "locally advanced" BCC, vismodegib, and sonidegib. These agents act via inhibition of the transmembrane protein smoothened, blocking the hedgehog signaling cascade. In the pivotal phase 2, nonrandomized trial for vismodegib, 30% of patients with metastatic disease and 43% of patients with locally advanced (inoperable) disease showed at least a partial response. The median response duration was 7.6 months.[97] Adverse events are almost universal and often lead to discontinuation of the drug, including muscle spasms, dysgeusia, alopecia, diarrhea, and amenorrhea[98] Alternative dosing schedules have demonstrated efficacy with reduced side effect profiles.[99–101]

Course and prognosis

BCCs are slow growing as a rule. However, if left untreated, they may reach a large size, with consequent extensive tissue destruction. In a comprehensive review of recurrence rates for primary BCCs, the results are highly comparable for the various treatment modalities.[92] Most studies reported a 95% or higher cure rate.[90,102] A lower 5-year recurrence rate has been reported with Mohs surgery than with other commonly used modalities. Metastasis, although rare, may occur, particularly in large or recurrent lesions.[103] In such cases, the prognosis is usually poor, with a 1-year survival rate of less than 20%, and a 5-year survival rate of approximately 10%. In general, the 5-year occurrence rate of new BCCs developing in patients with a previous BCC may be as high as 45%.[104]

Merkel cell carcinoma

Definition

The Merkel cell was first described by Merkel in 1875. It is a nondendritic, nonkeratinocytic epithelial clear cell normally found in the epidermis and dermis of mammals and humans. Merkel cell carcinoma (MCC) was first described by Toker in 1972 and is thought to arise from the cutaneous Merkel cell. It is a high-grade malignant tumor, with a high rate of local recurrence and metastasis. Mortality of approximately 33% at 3 years exceeds that seen in cutaneous melanoma.

Epidemiology

MCC is a relatively uncommon neoplasm. Data from SEER show a 95% increase from 2000 to 2013 (0.7 cases/100,000 person-years) in the number of MCC, corresponding to 2488 cases yearly.[2] This is thought to be due to the aging population as well as partially due to improved diagnostic accuracy with the advent of targeted immunostains such as cytokeratin 20 (CK20). The incidence increases exponentially with age, and 90% of patients are older than 50 years. There is a slight male predominance. Higher rates of MCC are seen in patients with HIV, hematologic malignancy, as well as those on immunosuppressive agents for solid organ transplantation or autoimmune disease. A polyoma virus has been identified in 80% of MCC tumors.[105]

Clinical features
The most common sites of involvement are head and neck (49%), extremities (38%), with the lower extremities more frequently involved than the upper extremities, and trunk (13%), mainly lower back and buttocks. The lesions present as papules or nodules, pink to red to violet, often with overlying telangiectasia. Typically, the tumors are <2 cm in size. MCC can be suspected based on the mnemonic AEIOU (asymptomatic/lack of tenderness, expanding rapidly, immune suppression, older than 50 years, UV-exposed site on a person with fair skin).[106] CK20 immunostaining (perinuclear dot pattern) has greatly assisted diagnosis of MCC.

Treatment
Wide local excision is the standard treatment modality.[107] Alternatively, local excision with margin control by frozen-section histology (Mohs surgery) may be of value.[108] Studies have shown that sentinel lymph node biopsy (SLNB) is predictive of nodal involvement and should be considered in all patients without clinically detectable nodes.[109] Postoperative adjuvant radiation therapy to the primary tumor bed remains controversial in patients with established clear surgical margins. However, it has been shown to improve local and regional control in patients with subtotal resection and microscopically positive margins.[110] Radiation is strongly recommended in patients with bulky regional disease and multiple metastatic lymph nodes and may also be beneficial for local recurrences or local control after node dissection.[111] Chemotherapy regimens have not been shown to extend life.

The advent of checkpoint inhibitors has resulted in major developments in the treatment of advanced MCC. Avelumab, an anti-programmed cell death ligand 1 (PD L1) antibody, is approved as first or second-line treatment of metastatic MCC. Pembrolizumab, an anti PD-1 antibody, has also been approved to treat locally advanced or metastatic Merkel cell carcinoma.

Course and prognosis
MCC 5-year overall survival (OS) ranges from 50.6% for patients with local disease to 13.5% for patients with distant metastases.[112] Outcome is based on primary tumor size and stage of disease. In 2017, the AJCC updated staging criteria to include lymph node pathology and distant metastasis, as well as overall tumor diameter.[75] Immunosuppressed patients have a higher mortality than immunocompetent patients.[113]

Tumors arising from the dermis

Dermatofibrosarcoma protuberans

Definition
Dermatofibrosarcoma protuberans (DFSP) is a locally malignant, slow-growing tumor originating in the dermis. The tumor cells resemble fibroblasts with various degrees of atypia.

Epidemiology
DFSP is an uncommon tumor that typically presents during early to mid-adult life, and rarely in children. Males are affected four times more often than females. It may be more common in black patients than in Caucasians. Associations with arsenic exposure, burn or surgical scars, acanthosis nigricans, and rapid growth during pregnancy have been reported.

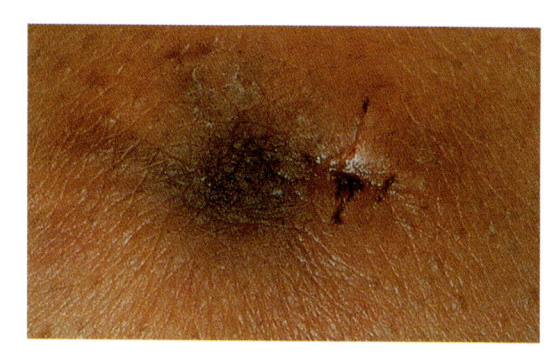

Figure 13 Dermatofibrosarcoma protuberans on the back of the neck. Firm papule resembling a dermatofibroma. Source: Courtesy of R.A. Johnson, MD.

Clinical features
DFSP is most commonly located on the trunk and proximal extremities. It typically presents as a solitary, slow-growing nodule with multiple palpable surface irregularities.[114] The early lesion may resemble a dermatofibroma, keloid scar, or SCC (see Figure 13). The lesion is firm to palpation and varies from skin-colored to reddish to yellow. The center may be ulcerated. The tumor can achieve an enormous size with multiple satellite nodules, if untreated. The characteristic irregular surface on a firm, plaque-like base may suggest the diagnosis. A biopsy will provide confirmation. The average size at the time of surgery is approximately 5 cm.

DFSP harbor chromosomal translocations that fuse the collagen type I alpha gene with the gene for platelet-derived growth factor B (COL1A1-PDGFB).[115] The presence of this specific t(17;22) translocation permits the diagnosis of DFSP in equivocal cases.

Treatment
DFSP has a high recurrence rate after conventional surgical excision, with a range of 30–50%.[116] Lateral surgical margins of at least 3 cm excised through the deep fascia are the current recommendation for conventional excision. In one large series, this yielded a recurrence rate of approximately 10%. Because of the potential for deforming surgical defects, MMS with microscopic control of the excision margins is the treatment of choice. This allows the subclinical margins to be mapped at the time of surgery, and, consequently, the surgical margins more precisely determined. Prophylactic lymph node dissection is not recommended because of the low initial risk of metastasis. Targeted therapy with the receptor tyrosine kinase inhibitor imatinib has been used with success in treating multiple recurrent and metastatic cases of DFSP.[117]

Course and prognosis
In a review of 136 cases of DFSP treated with Mohs surgery, a local recurrence rate of 6.6% was determined, although smaller studies have shown fewer recurrences.[118] The experience of the Mohs surgeon is critical in preventing tumor recurrence. Historically, late recurrences are frequent, thus long-term follow-up is recommended.

Cutaneous angiosarcoma

Definition
Angiosarcoma (AS) is an aggressive malignancy of endothelial cells, arising in the setting of chronic lymphedema, chronic radiation dermatitis, or on the face and scalp of the elderly patients.

Epidemiology
Cutaneous AS (cAS) affects elderly men more often than women. Sun does not appear to be an important factor because the tumor often appears under cover of hair.[119] cAS developing in areas of chronic lymphedema (so-called Stewart–Treves syndrome) is an infrequent complication of mastectomy, axillary node dissection for melanoma, lymphedema secondary to filarial infection, and chronic idiopathic lymphedema. Unfortunately, up to 0.5% of women undergoing mastectomy and lymph node dissection develop cAS within 1–30 years. Radiation-associated cAS (RAAS) is a rare iatrogenic complication of radiation that develops in or near the irradiated site. The incubation period may be up to 40 years in some cases.

Clinical features
In all three presentations, the clinical features can be similar. Purpuric macules, papules, and nodules develop and tend to enlarge quickly. Ulceration can occur in advanced lesions. On the face, facial edema can be the presenting sign. In all cases, the lesions extend beyond the clinical borders.

There is heterogeneity in the genomic alteration of cAS with mutations enriched in the mitosis-activated kinase (MAPK) pathway.

Treatment
Treatment for cAS is not promising. One problem is that by the time a diagnosis is made the tumors have spread several centimeters beyond the clinically appreciated borders. AS of the face and scalp is rarely less than 10 cm in diameter at presentation. Surgical resection with or without radiotherapy is the mainstay of treatment.[120] In a study of 24 patients with AS of the face and scalp, local control was obtained in 57%. However, of those patients, 47% developed distant metastases.[121] Treatment with a taxane (e.g., paclitaxel) has been shown to be effective for maintenance therapy in patients following surgical resection and postoperative radiation.[122] In surgically unresectable tumors or metastatic disease, paclitaxel may be considered as first-line therapy.[123] Other treatments that may be considered as second-line for cAS include the microtubule targeting agent eribulin mesylate, the histone deacetylase inhibitor trabectedin, the vascular endothelial growth factor (VEGF) receptor inhibitor bevacizumab, the multityrosine kinase inhibitor pazopanib, and propranolol.[124]

Course and prognosis
Survival at 5 years is approximately 12%.[119]

Tumors arising from appendages

Sebaceous carcinoma

Definition
Sebaceous carcinoma is an uncommon but potentially aggressive malignant adnexal neoplasm that arises from the sebaceous glands of the eyelid. Extraocular sebaceous carcinoma is rare and has an indeterminant origin.

Epidemiology
Sebaceous carcinoma is an uncommon cutaneous malignancy that represents less than 1% of skin cancers.[125,126] Advanced age and immunosuppression are established risk factors for sebaceous carcinoma. Historical data have suggested a slight female predominance and an increased incidence in Asian patients.[127–130] However, more recent studies contradict these findings.[131]

Clinical features
Misdiagnosis of sebaceous carcinoma is frequent. The tumor usually appears as a painless, skin-colored papule, or nodule on the upper or lower eyelid where it is easily dismissed as a chalazion or chronic blepharitis. Ulceration is often the feature that stimulates clinical suspicion and biopsy. Focal loss of eyelashes and a yellowish hue are other diagnostic clues. Sebaceous tumors are frequently associated with the MTS, as described later in this article. Individuals with extraocular sebaceous carcinoma may be selected for genetic testing based on calculated Mayo MTS risk score. Screening for MTS is not recommended for periocular sebaceous carcinoma.[132]

Treatment
Treatment of sebaceous carcinoma is primarily surgical. Recent consensus guidelines recommend MMS or complete circumferential peripheral and deep margin assessment (CCPDMA), followed by WLE as first-line treatment.[132] For extraocular sebaceous carcinoma, primary radiotherapy, and staging by SLNB or nodal dissection are not recommended, although adjuvant radiation to the nodal basin may be considered to assist with regional control. For periocular sebaceous carcinoma, CCPDMA or MMS are the treatments of choice.[133–135] Topical mitomycin or cryotherapy may be considered for conjunctival involvement after surgical intervention. For periocular tumors stage T2c or higher by the AJCC 8, consideration of SLNB is recommended.[132]

Course and prognosis
Extent of disease at the time of diagnosis remains the most significant predictor of reduced survival.[136] While periorbital sebaceous carcinoma has been associated historically with a poor prognosis, a recent review of the literature found significantly lower rates of cancer-specific mortality (3–6.7%).[137] Overall, factors associated with poor outcomes include location on the eyelid, previously irradiated sites, and poor histopathological differentiation. The impact of perineural involvement and immunosuppression is less clear.[132]

Extramammary paget disease

Definition
Extramammary Paget disease (EMPD) is a neoplasm of apocrine glands that clinically resembles Paget disease of the breast but occurs in areas rich in apocrine glands, including the perineum and axilla.

Epidemiology
More frequent in women and Caucasians, EMPD arises after the fifth decade.

Clinical features
EMPD is a scaly, sharply demarcated plaque, most commonly found in the vulva. Because itching and burning are common symptoms, it is often mistaken for intertrigo or flexural eczema, and the diagnosis is delayed. Progressive enlargement of the plaque in the face of topical steroid or antifungal medications is a diagnostic clue.

Treatment

Evaluation to identify the presence of underlying malignancy is crucial. MMS is the treatment of choice for primary EMPD. A recent study found a 12.2% recurrence rate with MMS compared to a recurrence rate of 36% with WLE, with a nearly 40% reduction in estimated 5-year recurrence-free survival rates.[138] Lymph node dissection should be considered in patients with invasion of the reticular dermis or invasion to subcutaneous tissue, even in patients without clinical or pathological lymph node metastasis.[139]

Imiquimod 5% cream offers a potential viable alternative to surgery. While response rates are high, complete response rates vary and recurrence is common. Patients should be monitored for recurrence even when complete response is confirmed histopathologically.[140] Systemic side effects to imiquimod are common and may limit treatment.

Other treatments that have been studied include radiotherapy and photodynamic therapy. However, evidence is limited to small case series and case reports with significant recurrence rates. Ablative carbon dioxide laser treatment is palliative, as recurrence rates are very high. There is no clear chemotherapeutic established for EMPD.

Course and prognosis

When EMPD is associated with an adenocarcinoma, the prognosis is poor. However, even primary EMPD can eventually ulcerate and become locally invasive and spread to lymph nodes, with depth of invasion >1 mm being an important prognostic factor. Regardless of the treatment modality, long-term recurrence is common and close surveillance is key.

Benign cutaneous tumors associated with cancer syndromes

Trichilemmoma (in Cowden disease)

Definition

Trichilemmoma is a tumor that exhibits features of outer root sheath differentiation of hair. In Cowden disease, multiple trichilemmomas are associated with multiple hamartomatous neoplasms of ectodermal, mesodermal, and endodermal origin, the most important include fibrocystic disease and carcinoma of the breast, adenoma and follicular adenocarcinoma of the thyroid, gastrointestinal polyps, and lipomas.[141]

Epidemiology

Cowden disease is a rare autosomal dominant condition with variable expressivity. It is part of a group of genetic disorders linked to phosphatase and tensin homolog (PTEN) germline mutations collectively referred to as the PTEN hamartoma tumor syndromes (PHTS).

Clinical features

In Cowden disease, trichilemmomas present as small lichenoid, skin-colored to yellow-tan papules with a smooth surface. They are concentrated on the face, especially around the orifices and the ears. Similar papules may appear on the extremities, including palmoplantar surfaces, and the oral cavity, particularly on the gingiva and the tongue (Figures 14 and 15). The presentation of these papules may herald an associated internal malignancy, particularly breast, thyroid, and endometrium or a benign overgrowth of a variety of tissues (e.g., skin, colon, thyroid, etc.).[142] Broad variability exists in clinical presentation, even within families with the same mutation.

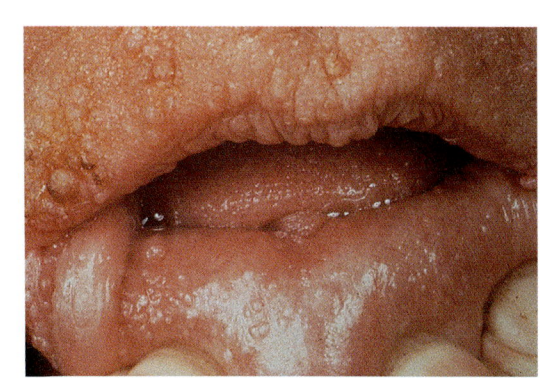

Figure 14 Cowden disease. Multiple trichilemmomas on the upper lip. Similar papules are present on the mucosal surface of the lower lip.

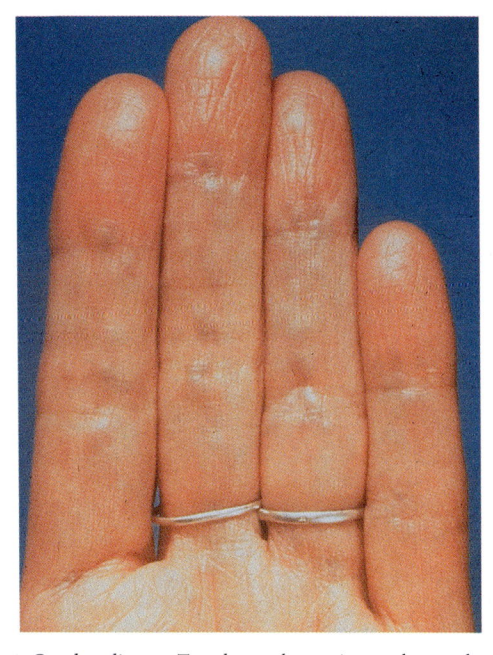

Figure 15 Cowden disease. Translucent keratotic papules on the palmar surface. Source: Courtesy of R.A. Johnson, MD.

Genetics

Germline mutations in the protein tyrosine phosphatase PTEN have been linked to multiple families with Cowden disease.[143] However, recent evidence suggests that only 30–35% of patients meeting clinical diagnostic criteria for Cowden syndrome have a detectable PTEN mutation.[142]

Treatment

Therapies are directed toward achieving good cosmetic appearance and treatment of the various associated benign and malignant tumors, as indicated. Consensus diagnostic criteria were revised in 2013 and the National Comprehensive Cancer Network (NCCN) has established guidelines for appropriate testing and management, including screening guidelines for underlying malignancies.[144]

Sebaceous adenoma (in Muir–Torre syndrome)

Definition
Sebaceous adenoma is a rare, benign tumor consisting of incompletely differentiated sebaceous lobules within the dermis. In MTS, multiple sebaceous adenomas, carcinomas, and keratoacanthomas are associated with multiple visceral malignant neoplasms, most commonly carcinoma of the colon and carcinoma of the ampulla of Vater. These sebaceous tumors are rare enough that the presence of a single lesion in an otherwise healthy patient warrants an investigation for internal neoplasms.

Epidemiology
Solitary sebaceous adenoma is a rare tumor that occurs in elderly patients with a slight male predilection. The multiple type, associated with MTS, is familial, with more than 50% of reported patients having an immediate family member with a history of internal cancer, most frequently of the colon.[145]

Clinical features
Sebaceous adenoma typically appears as a firm, flesh-colored to waxy-yellow papule or pedunculated lesion, usually less than 1 cm in size. The surface may be smooth or verrucous. Older lesions may be plaque-like or ulcerated. It is usually located on the face or scalp and is usually slow growing.

Genetics
Germline mutations in the DNA mismatch repair genes MSH2 (most common), MLH1, MSH6, and PMS2 have been identified in a majority of cases.[146] Mismatch repair gene immunohistochemistry (IHC) of sebaceous neoplasms is imperative as part of the workup of patients with suspected MTS. Loss of IHC staining of combinations of certain gene products (e.g., MLH1 and MSH6; or MSH2, MLH1, and MSH6) have shown a positive predictive value of 100% for MTS.[146]

Treatment
The treatment of choice is surgical excision, including MMS. Radiation therapy may be used as an adjuvant or palliative treatment option but not as sole treatment due to higher rates of recurrence and morality.

Multiple mucosal neuromas (multiple endocrine neoplasia 3, MEN3)

Definition
Mucosal neuromas present as small, discrete and coalescing, painless nodules, usually involving the lips, and sometimes studding the margins of the tongue. The association of multiple mucosal neuromas, medullary thyroid carcinoma, and pheochromocytoma has been established as a familial syndrome.

Epidemiology
Discrete mucosal neuromas are common and often result from direct trauma, as in the typical bite neuroma. More than 150 cases of multiple neuromas associated with endocrine tumors have been described in the literature.[147] The prevalence of MEN3 (formerly MEN2B) approximates 0.2 per 100,000.[148]

Clinical features
In MEN3, diffusely enlarged lips are an early cutaneous feature. Diffuse and symmetric fleshy papules and nodules occur on the tongue by the end of first decade. Any mucosal surface may be involved. Musculoskeletal deformities, including a Marfanoid habitus, joint laxity, bowing of the extremities, and kyphoscoliosis are common. Medullary thyroid carcinoma is often the initial presentation, and pheochromocytomas develop in about half of patients. These tumors produce calcitonin and can stimulate parathyroid hyperplasia.

Genetics
In all cases studied to date, mutation in the protooncogene RET, a receptor tyrosine kinase, has been uncovered.[149]

Course and prognosis
Medullary thyroid carcinoma is often the cause of death. Routine screening for this tumor with ultrasonography and by measuring serum calcitonin levels is useful, but current recommendations suggest prophylactic thyroidectomy in cases where a RET mutation is documented.[150]

Metastatic tumors to the skin

Cutaneous metastases of internal cancers are uncommon. In a report of 7316 nonmelanoma cancer patients,[151] only 1% of patients had cutaneous metastases at the time of diagnosis. In a study of 2298 patients reported as having died of visceral carcinoma, only 2.7% had evidence of cutaneous metastases.[152] In a more recent retrospective study of 4020 patients with metastatic carcinomas and melanoma, 10% had cutaneous metastases. In general, the incidence of the various cancers metastatic to the skin correlates well with the incidence of the particular primary tumor.[153]

The spectrum of metastatic tumors differs slightly between the two sexes.[153] In one study, the most common primary sources of metastatic carcinoma to the skin in males were malignant melanoma (32%), lung (12%), large intestine (11%), carcinoma of the oral cavity (9%) and larynx (5.5%), and kidney (5%). In females, breast is by far the most common source (70%), followed by melanoma (12%), and ovary (3%), and large intestine, lung, and oral cavity, each accounting for 1.3–2.3% of the cases.[153] In females, the incidence of lung carcinoma has increased dramatically in recent years, resulting in a corresponding rise in the incidence of cutaneous metastatic lung carcinoma deposits. Other carcinomas that metastasize to the skin include thyroid, pancreas, liver, gallbladder, urinary bladder, endometrium, prostate, and testis. However, these are quite rare.

Typically, metastatic cancer presents as multiple, firm, nonulcerated nodules. When solitary, they may be misdiagnosed as primary skin tumors. Inflammatory skin metastases mimicking cellulitis may occur in 10% of metastases from breast cancer. The most common sites for skin metastases are chest and abdomen, followed by head and neck; metastasis to the extremities is rare. Metastases in the scalp can be associated with alopecia ("alopecia neoplastica"). Dissemination may be via the bloodstream or via the lymphatics. Carcinomas of the breast and of the oral cavity tend to spread through the lymphatics, whereas others tend to spread hematogenously. Lymphatic dissemination may explain the observation that skin metastases tend to be close to the site of the primary tumor: chest in lung carcinoma, abdominal wall in gastrointestinal tumors, and lower back in renal cell carcinoma.

The prognosis for patients with cutaneous metastases is generally poor. In Lookingbill and colleagues,[153] the average time from diagnosis of skin metastases to death for the various primary tumors varies from 1 to 34 months. The variability in prognosis may be the result of advances in cancer therapy during the past decades. Some patients with metastatic melanoma to skin as the sole site of metastasis may have prolonged disease-free survival.

Key references

The complete reference list can be found on Vital Source version of this title, see inside front cover.

2. Paulson KG, Park SY, Vandeven NA, et al. Merkel cell carcinoma: current US incidence and projected increases based on changing demographics. *J Am Acad Dermatol*. 2018;**78**(3):457–463 e2.
11. Chuang TY, Reizner GT, Elpern DJ, et al. Nonmelanoma skin cancer in Japanese ethnic Hawaiians in Kauai, Hawaii: an incidence report. *J Am Acad Dermatol*. 1995;**33**(3):422–426.
12. Vitasa BC, Taylor HR, Strickland PT, et al. Association of nonmelanoma skin cancer and actinic keratosis with cumulative solar ultraviolet exposure in Maryland watermen. *Cancer*. 1990;**65**(12):2811–2817.
13. Franceschi S, Levi F, Randimbison L, La Vecchia C. Site distribution of different types of skin cancer: new aetiological clues. *Int J Cancer*. 1996;**67**(1):24–28.
17. Wehner MR, Shive ML, Chren MM, et al. Indoor tanning and non-melanoma skin cancer: systematic review and meta-analysis. *BMJ*. 2012;**345**:e5909.
18. Ferrucci LM, Cartmel B, Molinaro AM, et al. Indoor tanning and risk of early-onset basal cell carcinoma. *J Am Acad Dermatol*. 2012;**67**(4):552–562.
19. Karagas MR, Zens MS, Li Z, et al. Early-onset basal cell carcinoma and indoor tanning: a population-based study. *Pediatrics*. 2014;**134**(1):e4–e12.
25. Suchniak JM, Baer S, Goldberg LH. High rate of malignant transformation in hyperkeratotic actinic keratoses. *J Am Acad Dermatol*. 1997;**37**(3 Pt 1):392–394.
33. Marks R, Rennie G, Selwood TS. Malignant transformation of solar keratoses to squamous cell carcinoma. *Lancet*. 1988;**1**(8589):795–797.
38. Chitwood K, Etzkorn J, Cohen G. Topical and intralesional treatment of nonmelanoma skin cancer: efficacy and cost comparisons. *Dermatol Surg*. 2013;**39**(9):1306–1316.
60. Maalej M, Frikha H, Kochbati L, et al. Radio-induced malignancies of the scalp about 98 patients with 150 lesions and literature review. *Cancer Radiother*. 2004;**8**(2):81–87.
64. Lansbury L, Bath-Hextall F, Perkins W, et al. Interventions for non-metastatic squamous cell carcinoma of the skin: systematic review and pooled analysis of observational studies. *BMJ*. 2013;**347**:f6153.
65. Brodland DG, Zitelli JA. Surgical margins for excision of primary cutaneous squamous cell carcinoma. *J Am Acad Dermatol*. 1992;**27**(2 Pt 1):241–248.
66. Heppt MV, Steeb T, Berking C, Nast A. Comparison of guidelines for the management of patients with high-risk and advanced cutaneous squamous cell carcinoma – a systematic review. *J Eur Acad Dermatol Venereol*. 2019;**33**(Suppl 8):25–32.
69. Locke J, Karimpour S, Young G, et al. Radiotherapy for epithelial skin cancer. *Int J Radiat Oncol Biol Phys*. 2001;**51**(3):748–755.
72. Ruiz ES, Koyfman SA, Que SKT, et al. Evaluation of the utility of localized adjuvant radiation for node-negative primary cutaneous squamous cell carcinoma with clear histologic margins. *J Am Acad Dermatol*. 2020;**82**(2):420–429.
76. Karia PS, Morgan FC, Califano JA, Schmults CD. Comparison of tumor classifications for cutaneous squamous cell carcinoma of the head and neck in the 7th vs 8th edition of the AJCC cancer staging manual. *JAMA Dermatol*. 2018;**154**(2):175–181.
79. Ruiz ES, Karia PS, Besaw R, Schmults CD. Performance of the American Joint Committee on Cancer Staging Manual, 8th Edition vs the Brigham and Women's Hospital Tumor Classification System for Cutaneous Squamous Cell Carcinoma. *JAMA Dermatol*. 2019;**155**(7):819–825.
80. Frankel DH, Hanusa BH, Zitelli JA. New primary nonmelanoma skin cancer in patients with a history of squamous cell carcinoma of the skin. Implications and recommendations for follow-up. *J Am Acad Dermatol*. 1992;**26**(5 Pt 1):720–726.
90. Silverman MK, Kopf AW, Grin CM, et al. Recurrence rates of treated basal cell carcinomas. Part 2: Curettage-electrodesiccation. *J Dermatol Surg Oncol*. 1991;**17**(9):720–726.
91. Silverman MK, Kopf AW, Bart RS, et al. Recurrence rates of treated basal cell carcinomas. Part 3: Surgical excision. *J Dermatol Surg Oncol*. 1992;**18**(6):471–476.
92. Rowe DE, Carroll RJ, Day CL. Mohs surgery is the treatment of choice for recurrent (previously treated) basal cell carcinoma. *J Dermatol Surg Oncol*. 1989;**15**(4):424–431.
93. Wilder RB, Kittelson JM, Shimm DS. Basal cell carcinoma treated with radiation therapy. *Cancer*. 1991;**68**(10):2134–2137.
94. Gauden R, Pracy M, Avery AM, et al. HDR brachytherapy for superficial non-melanoma skin cancers. *J Med Imaging Radiation Oncol*. 2013;**57**(2):212–217.
97. Sekulic A, Migden MR, Oro AE, et al. Efficacy and safety of vismodegib in advanced basal-cell carcinoma. *N Engl J Med*. 2012;**366**(23):2171–2179.
105. Feng H, Shuda M, Chang Y, Moore PS. Clonal integration of a polyomavirus in human Merkel cell carcinoma. *Science*. 2008;**319**(5866):1096–1100.
110. Harrington C, Kwan W. Radiotherapy and conservative surgery in the locoregional management of merkel cell carcinoma: the british columbia cancer agency experience. *Ann Surg Oncol*. 2016;**23**(2):573–578.
112. Harms KL, Healy MA, Nghiem P, et al. Analysis of prognostic factors from 9387 merkel cell carcinoma cases forms the basis for the new 8th edition AJCC staging system. *Ann Surg Oncol*. 2016;**23**(11):3564–3571.
118. Snow SN, Gordon EM, Larson PO, et al. Dermatofibrosarcoma protuberans: a report on 29 patients treated by Mohs micrographic surgery with long-term follow-up and review of the literature. *Cancer*. 2004;**101**(1):28–38.
121. Sasaki R, Soejima T, Kishi K, et al. Angiosarcoma treated with radiotherapy: impact of tumor type and size on outcome. *Int J Radiat Oncol Biol Phys*. 2002;**52**(4):1032–1040.
132. Owen JL, Kibbi N, Worley B, et al. Sebaceous carcinoma: evidence-based clinical practice guidelines. *Lancet Oncol*. 2019;**20**(12):e699–e714.
137. Kyllo RL, Brady KL, Hurst EA. Sebaceous carcinoma: review of the literature. *Dermatol Surg*. 2015;**41**(1):1–15.
138. Kim SJ, Thompson AK, Zubair AS, et al. Surgical treatment and outcomes of patients with extramammary paget disease: a cohort study. *Dermatol Surg*. 2017;**43**(5):708–714.
146. John AM, Schwartz RA. Muir-Torre syndrome (MTS): an update and approach to diagnosis and management. *J Am Acad Dermatol*. 2016;**74**(3):558–566.
148. Znaczko A, Donnelly DE, Morrison PJ. Epidemiology, clinical features, and genetics of multiple endocrine neoplasia type 2B in a complete population. *Oncologist*. 2014;**19**(12):1284–1286.

108 Bone tumors

Timothy A. Damron, MD, FACS

> **Overview**
>
> As a group, bone tumors are uncommon lesions arising from a wide array of cells, affecting all ages of patients, and involving any bone in the body. Benign bone lesions are quite common and range from inactive to active and aggressive tumors. Treatment of inactive bone lesions is most often observation. Active benign bone lesions are frequently treated surgically by curettage. Benign aggressive tumors often require extended intralesional curettage with adjuncts. Among malignant bone lesions, the most common bone malignancy is metastatic carcinoma, and the most common primary bone malignancy is myeloma. The focus on bone involvement in these tumors is fixation of pathologic fractures and prediction of impending fractures. Primary bone sarcomas are rare tumors with characteristic clinical, radiographic, and pathologic features. Treatment of bone sarcomas most often requires wide surgical resection with or without chemotherapy and/or radiotherapy. Although often numerous specialties may contribute to their evaluation and care, orthopedic oncology is the only subspecialty focused specifically on all aspects of bone tumors.

Introduction

As a group, bone tumors are uncommon lesions arising from a wide array of cells, affecting all ages of patients, and involving any bone in the body. They include benign lesions, primary bone sarcomas, metastatic carcinomas to bone, myeloma, and lymphoma. The benign bone lesions may behave in an inactive, active, or aggressive fashion. Despite the broad spectrum of bone tumors, each individual entity has a distinct clinical and radiographic presentation, with a predilection for specific locations, which lends itself to narrowing the differential diagnosis and selecting appropriate management.

Bone sarcomas account for less than 0.2% of all cancers.[1] During 2014, approximately 3020 new cases of primary bone sarcomas were diagnosed and approximately 1460 deaths occurred. The three most common bone sarcomas are osteosarcoma (45%), chondrosarcoma (36%), and Ewing sarcoma (18%).[2] In pediatric patients, the most common bone sarcomas are osteosarcoma and Ewing sarcoma in order of diminishing numbers. In adults, the most common bone sarcoma is chondrosarcoma. However, the most common primary malignancy of bone is myeloma, and the most common cancer that involves bone is metastatic carcinoma. Malignancies of bone as a group are only the tip of the iceberg, as the vast majority of bone lesions are benign.

The pathologic classification of bone tumors continues to evolve. To a large extent, classification continues to be according to the cell of origin or tissue type. Primary bone tumors may derive from cartilage cells—chondrocytes (enchondromas, periosteal chondromas, chondroblastomas, chondromyxoid fibromas, chondrosarcomas), bone cells—osteoblasts and osteocytes (osteoma, osteoid osteoma, osteoblastoma, osteosarcoma), and vascular cells (hemangioma and angiosarcoma), among others, but for some tumors, the cell of origin is unknown. The most widely accepted pathologic classification system to date is that of the World Health Organization, and their terminology is used to a large degree in this article, although some tumors, such as benign fibrous tumors, are grouped differently.[3] The WHO Classification of bone tumors has been updated since the last publication of this text.

The introductory sections of this chapter deal with the pretreatment phase (evaluation, staging, and biopsy), the middle sections with surgical treatment (surgical margins through reconstructive options), radiation therapy and medical management, and the final sections with the specific benign and malignant bone tumors as well as congenital syndromes related to bone tumors.

Evaluation

Crucial information about bone lesions is derived from the history, physical examination, and radiographic features. The goal of evaluation of any bone lesion is to arrive at a narrow differential diagnosis which will guide subsequent action. In some cases, a specific diagnosis may be determined, and, depending upon the diagnosis, a specific action will be taken. Although the examples that follow in parentheses are by no means exhaustive, specific actions may include observation (e.g., nonossifying fibroma, enchondroma), biopsy confirmation (e.g., aneurysmal bone cyst, chondroblastoma, giant cell tumor, osteosarcoma, Ewing sarcoma, metastatic carcinoma among many others), irrigation/debridement (e.g., osteomyelitis), aspiration/injection (e.g., unicameral bone cyst), radiofrequency ablation (e.g., osteoid osteoma and some bone metastases), curettage and grafting or cementation, sometimes with surgical adjuvants (e.g., chondroblastoma, osteoblastoma, giant cell tumor of bone, aneurysmal bone cyst, chondromyxoid fibroma), simple excision (e.g., osteochondroma, periosteal chondroma), preoperative embolization (e.g., aneurysmal bone cyst, metastatic renal carcinoma), radiotherapy (Ewing sarcoma, metastatic carcinoma, myeloma, lymphoma), preoperative chemotherapy (osteosarcoma, Ewing sarcoma), bone modifying agents such as bisphosphonates (metastatic carcinoma, myeloma, lymphoma), pathologic fracture fixation (e.g., metastatic carcinoma, benign aggressive bone lesions), or prophylactic stabilization (e.g., established metastatic carcinoma, myeloma). In other cases, the lesion may only be categorized according to a general category of biologic behavior: latent, active, or aggressive. Latent bone tumors may be observed. Active lesions often require biopsy and curettage with or without grafting. Aggressive bone tumors almost always require biopsy confirmation prior to treatment and include both benign aggressive lesions (e.g., chondroblastoma, osteoblastoma, giant cell tumor of bone, aneurysmal bone cyst, chondromyxoid fibroma) and malignancies (e.g., primary bone sarcomas, metastatic carcinoma, myeloma, lymphoma).

Holland-Frei Cancer Medicine, Tenth Edition. Edited by Robert C. Bast, John C. Byrd, Carlo M. Croce, Ernest Hawk, Fadlo R. Khuri, Raphael E. Pollock, Apostolia M. Tsimberidou, Christopher G. Willett, and Cheryl L. Willman.
© 2023 John Wiley & Sons, Inc. Published 2023 by John Wiley & Sons, Inc.

Important historical features are the patient's age and the means by which the lesion was discovered. Age divisions are particularly helpful when the patient is less than 5 years old, where metastatic neuroblastoma has its peak occurrence, Langerhans cell histiocytosis is relatively more common and sarcomas are rare, and when the patient is older than 40, where the differential diagnosis, in order of decreasing frequency, includes metastatic carcinoma, myeloma, lymphoma, and primary bone sarcomas such as chondrosarcoma, secondary osteosarcoma, malignant fibrous histiocytoma of bone, and fibrosarcoma. Some of the most common lesions in the skeletal maturity to 40 age group are giant cell tumor of bone, enchondromas, enostoses, and lymphoma (although bone lymphomas may occur at practically any age). In the age group from 5 to skeletal maturity, many benign tumors may occur, but the most common malignancies are osteosarcoma, Ewing sarcoma, and bone lymphoma.

The means of discovery of a bone lesion are variable but can generally be grouped into one of three presentations: (1) incidental discovery, (2) pain, and (3) pathologic fracture. Bone lesions discovered incidentally during evaluation for other reasons are usually latent lesions that require nothing further than observation. In adult patients, the most common lesions discovered incidentally are enostoses (bone islands) and enchondromas; in pediatric patients, nonossifying fibromas (or fibrous cortical defects if limited to the cortex) are by far the most common lesion. Other lesions that may be discovered incidentally, although not uniformly, include bone cysts (unicameral and aneurysmal), fibrous dysplasia, infection, and Langerhans cell histiocytosis. Painless bony masses are usually osteochondromas, but other surface bone lesions may present in this fashion. The broadest category is the painful bone lesion, and this includes a wide variety of active and aggressive bone lesions. They can generally be divided into pediatric and adult groupings, as the differential diagnosis differs. In children, some of the more common painful nonmalignant lesions are chondroblastoma, aneurysmal bone cysts, fibrous dysplasia, Langerhans cell histiocytosis, and infection. Most pediatric malignancies will present with pain, and those include osteosarcoma, Ewing sarcoma, lymphoma, and metastatic neuroblastoma. In adults, painful bone lesions include both benign aggressive (fibrous dysplasia, osteomyelitis, Langerhans cell histiocytosis, osteoblastoma, giant cell tumor of bone, aneurysmal bone cyst, and chondromyxoid fibroma) and malignancy (metastatic carcinoma, myeloma, lymphoma, and the adult bone sarcomas, including chondrosarcoma, Paget's osteosarcoma, postradiation osteosarcoma, and undifferentiated pleomorphic sarcoma of bone, among others). Pathologic fractures may be divided into those preceded by pain, which are usually associated with active or aggressive bone tumors, and those not preceded by pain, which are more commonly latent lesions. Pathologic fractures preceded by pain should usually be biopsied, whereas those not preceded by pain may often be observed at least until the fracture heals, although exceptions exist.

Plain radiographs are standard for the radiologic evaluation of any bone tumor. These should be evaluated for location (epiphyseal, metaphyseal, diaphyseal, surface, or intracortical), lesional border characteristics (Type 1: geographic, Type 2: motheaten, or Type 3: permeative), bone response to the lesion (periosteal reaction), and matrix mineralization pattern (cartilaginous, osseous, ground glass) when present (Tables 1 and 2). Classification of the Type 1 border can be broken down into three specific subtypes.[5] Type 1A is characterized by a thick, sclerotic margin and usually represents a benign lesion. Type 1B is still well defined but lacks the thick, sclerotic margin, as these lesions potentially have a slightly faster growth pattern and in unusual cases may actually represent low-grade malignancies. Type 1C begins to blend with the motheaten pattern, representing a more aggressive pattern, including cortical destruction. Type 1C is characteristic of giant cell tumor of bone or lymphoma.[5] Hyaline cartilage tumors are one exception to the general rule that benign lesions usually have a sclerotic rim, as most benign enchondromas lack a 1A border. Putting these radiographic features together with the clinical features will often yield a narrow differential diagnosis.

Table 1 Classification of bone tumors by 4th edition of WHO classification on bone and soft tissue tumours.[a]

Chondrogenic tumors
Osteochondroma
Chondromas: enchondroma, periosteal chondroma
Chondromyxoid fibroma
Osteochondromyxoma
Subungual exostosis and bizarre parosteal osteochondromatous proliferation
Synovial chondromatosis
Chondroblastoma
Chondrosarcoma (grades I–III) including primary and secondary variants and periosteal chondrosarcoma
Dedifferentiated chondrosarcoma
Mesenchymal chondrosarcoma
Clear cell chondrosarcoma
Osteogenic tumors
Osteoma
Osteoid osteoma
Osteoblastoma
Low-grade central osteosarcoma
Conventional osteosarcoma
Telangiectatic osteosarcoma
Small-cell osteosarcoma
Parosteal osteosarcoma
Periosteal osteosarcoma
High-grade surface osteosarcoma
Fibrogenic tumors
Desmoplastic fibroma of bone
Fibrosarcoma of bone
Fibrohistiocytic tumors
Nonossifying fibroma and benign fibrous histiocytoma of bone
Ewing sarcoma
Hematopoietic neoplasms
Plasma cell myeloma
Solitary plasmacytoma of bone
Primary non-Hodgkin lymphoma of bone
Osteoclastic giant cell-rich tumors
Giant cell lesion of the small bones
Giant cell tumor of bone
Notochordal tumors
Benign notochordal cell tumor
Chordoma
Vascular tumors
Haemangioma
Epithelioid haemangioma
Epithelioid haemangioendothelioma
Angiosarcoma
Myogenic, lipogenic, and epithelial tumors
Leiomyosarcoma
Lipoma
Liposarcoma
Adamantinoma
Tumors of undefined neoplastic nature
Aneurysmal bone cyst
Simple bone cyst
Fibrous dysplasia
Osteofibrous dysplasia
Langerhans cell histiocytosis
Erdheim–Chester disease
Chondromesenchymal hamartoma
Rosai–Dorfman disease

[a]Source: Fletcher et al.[3]

Table 2 Classic examples of bone tumors fitting specific patterns of lesional borders, bone response, and lesional matrix on plain radiographs.[a]

Radiographic category	Type	Classic examples[b]	
Lesional border	Geographic (well-defined)	1A	Nonossifying fibroma Unicameral bone cyst
		1B	Aneurysmal bone cyst Chondroblastoma
		1C	Giant cell tumor Lymphoma
	Motheaten (blurred)	Metastatic carcinoma Myeloma Lymphoma Osteomyelitis	
	Permeative (poorly-defined)	Osteosarcoma Ewing sarcoma Metastatic carcinoma Lymphoma	
Bone response	Marginal sclerosis	Nonossifying fibroma Fibrous dysplasia	
	Cortical thickening	Osteoid osteoma Osteomyelitis	
	Laminar periosteal response	Stress fracture	
	Endosteal expansion and scalloping	Low- to intermediate-grade chondrosarcoma	
	Periosteal rimming	Aneurysmal bone cyst Giant cell tumor of bone	
	Codman's triangle Cumulus cloud reaction	Osteosarcoma	
	Onion-skinning periosteal response	Ewing sarcoma	
Lesional matrix	Punctate rings and arcs	Hyaline cartilage tumors (enchondromas/chondrosarcomas)	
	Ground glass appearance	Fibrous dysplasia	
	Osteoblastic	Osteoid osteoma Osteoblastoma Osteosarcoma Metastatic carcinoma (prostate, breast) Lymphoma	

[a]Source: Damron.[4]
[b]None of the radiographic findings here are specific, and there is considerable overlap; hence, those lesions listed may be considered classic but by no means the only ones that may present with such findings.

Bone scans help to determine whether the lesion shows uptake of the Tc[99] radionuclide, indicating an active or aggressive lesion, and whether the lesion is solitary or only one of numerous lesions. Myeloma deposits in bone serve as an exception to the rule, often being cold on bone scan. Some aggressive lesions, such as renal carcinoma metastases, may not be hot on bone scan if tumor destruction outpaces the bone's ability to form bone in response.

Positron emission tomography (PET) has come to play an increasing role in evaluation and staging of bone lesions.[6] On average, PET avidity is greater for malignant bone tumors than for benign bone tumors. However, 18F-FDG PET avidity has been shown to be nonspecific for malignancy, and many benign tumors, ranging from nonossifying fibroma to osteoid osteomas, also show this finding, albeit with greater variability. PET scans have come to play an increasing role in staging for malignant bone tumors, but they are less sensitive than routine chest CT for pulmonary metastases.[6]

Magnetic resonance imaging (MRI) of bone tumors is indicated when the diagnosis is not evident from the plain radiographs and for determining the local extent of bone sarcomas. Specific bone tumors that may be strongly suspected on MRI include simple bone cysts (rim enhancement of a fluid-filled lesion) and aneurysmal bone cysts (septations separating multiple loculated areas filled with blood, as indicated by fluid-fluid levels). Perilesional edema is common surrounding bone sarcomas and other bone malignancies but may also be seen in certain benign conditions, including osteomyelitis, osteoid osteoma, chondroblastoma, Langerhans cell histiocytosis, and chondromyxoid fibroma. Computerized tomography (CT) is indicated to find the radiolucent nidus of an osteoid osteoma within the surrounding reactive bone, to assess for endosteal scalloping in a cartilage tumor to distinguish enchondroma from chondrosarcoma, to find the pattern of lesional mineralization when it is unclear, and to supplement MRI in difficult anatomic locations such as the spine, sacrum, pelvis, and scapula.

Staging

Staging of bone sarcomas requires assessment of both the primary site and distant disease. For assessment of the primary site, radiographs and MRI of the entire involved bone should be obtained in order to check for other "skip" lesions. The two most common sites of metastases from bone sarcomas are lung followed by bone. Hence, the most crucial staging studies to obtain are chest radiograph and CT to evaluate the lungs as well as a total body bone scan or PET scan to evaluate the rest of the skeleton.

Traditionally, the staging system most commonly used for musculoskeletal sarcomas was that originally described by Doctor William Enneking and adopted by the Musculoskeletal Tumor Society (MSTS) (Table 3). Variables incorporated into the MSTS surgical staging system include the presence or absence of metastases, grade (high or low), and local extent of the tumor (intraosseous or with extension into the soft tissues). The typical chondrosarcoma is low-grade and intra-compartmental (confined to the bone), so it is usually stage IA. The conventional high-grade osteosarcoma usually extends into the soft tissue, and since 80% present without evidence of distant metastases, the typical stage is IIB. Evidence of metastases equates to a stage III in this system.

The current most widely accepted staging system for bone sarcomas is that of the American Joint Commission on Cancer (AJCC)[8–10] (Tables 4–6). This system has the most well-documented prognostic significance (Figure 1). For extremity tumors, variables incorporated into the AJCC system include presence or absence of metastases (with multiple/discontinuous bone tumors separated from distant metastases), grade (grade 1 versus grade 2 or 3), and size (8 cm or smaller vs larger than 8 cm). This system is similar to the MSTS system in separating Stage I from II or III based on grade, but the A–B designation is based upon size here. For osteosarcoma and Ewing sarcoma, Stage IIB patients have higher rates of metastases than Stage IIA patients. Patients with "skip lesions" (discontinuous lesions in the same bone) are designated as Stage III. Distant metastases in this system are Stage IV, but since

Table 3 Musculoskeletal tumor society staging system.[a,1]

Stage	Grade	Local extent	Metastases
I	Low	A – Intracompartmental B – Extracompartmental	None
II	High	A – Intracompartmental B – Extracompartmental	
III	Any	Any	Present

[a]Source: Adapted from Enneking et al.[7]

Table 4 American Joint Commission on cancer staging system for bone sarcomas: T–N–M definitions (8th edition).[a]

Definition of primary tumor (T)		Definition of regional lymph node (N)		Definition of distant metastasis (M)		Histologic grade (G)	
T	T Criteria	N	N Criteria	M	M Criteria	G	G Definition
TX	Primary tumor cannot be assessed	NX	Regional lymph node cannot be assessed	M0	No distant metastasis	GX	Grade cannot be assessed
T0	No evidence of primary tumor	N0	No regional lymph node metastasis	M1	Distant metastasis	G1	Well-differentiated, low grade
T1	Tumor ≤ 8 cm in greatest dimension	N1	Regional lymph node metastasis	M1a	Lung	G2	Moderately differentiated, high grade
T2	Tumor > 8 cm in greatest dimension			M1b	Bone or other distant sites	G3	Poorly differentiated, high grade
T3	Discontinuous tumors in the primary bone site						

[a]Source: Amin et al.[9] and Tanaka and Ozaki.[10]

Table 5 American Joint Commission on cancer staging system for bone sarcomas for appendicular skeleton, trunk, skull, and facial bones (8th edition).[a]

Stage	Primary tumor (T)	Regional lymph node (N)	Distant metastasis (M)	Histologic grade (G)
IA	T1	N0	M0	G1 or GX
IB	T2 or T3	N0	M0	G1 or GX
IIA	T1	N0	M0	G2 or G3
IIB	T2	N0	M0	G2 or G3
III	T3	N0	M0	G2 or G3
IVA	Any T	N0	M1a	Any G
IVB	Any T	N1	Any M	Any G
	Any T	Any N	M1b	Any G

[a]Source: Amin et al.[9] and Tanaka and Ozaki.[10]

metastases to sites other than the lung (such as bone) carry a worse prognosis than lung metastases patients alone, a separate designation is reserved for those two groups (IVA and IVB). Hence, for a less than 8 cm low-grade chondrosarcoma, the typical staging would be Stage IA. For a larger than 8 cm high-grade osteosarcoma without skip lesions or metastases, the typical staging is Stage IIB. There were no changes in the AJCC staging between the 2002 and 2012 versions, but as of January 2018, the 8th edition of the AJCC bone sarcoma staging was published with changes compared to earlier versions.[11]

Biopsy

Biopsy of bone tumors is indicated when a specific benign diagnosis cannot be determined based on radiographic evaluation alone. When the clinico-radiographic diagnosis of a latent lesion such as nonossifying fibroma, unicameral bone cyst, osteochondroma, or enchondroma can be made, biopsy is generally unnecessary. Some active lesions, such as fibrous dysplasia and intraosseous lipoma do not always require biopsy if the diagnosis can be established radiographically. For most other active and all aggressive lesions, biopsy should be done to determine or confirm the diagnosis. Suspected high-grade sarcomas should be biopsied prior to initiating treatment neoadjuvant.

Careful consideration must be given when the diagnosis of metastatic carcinoma or myeloma is suspected, because the treatment of these disseminated cancers of bone differs dramatically from that of a primary bone tumor. Hence, even for patients with a history of a known carcinoma with predilection to bone (breast, prostate, lung, renal, thyroid), the first bone metastases should generally be established by biopsy unless the clinical situation represents a terminal state (known wide metastases to other sites). The diagnosis of myeloma will usually be suggested by monoclonal gammopathy but should be confirmed by bone biopsy prior to any orthopedic procedure if the diagnosis has yet to be proven. When dealing with suspected metastatic disease or myeloma requiring a biopsy, reamings are not the best way to submit a biopsy specimen, because once the intramedullary canal to and through the lesion has been breached, all associated bone and soft tissue have been potentially contaminated with tumor. If the pathology shows sarcoma, rather than metastatic disease or myeloma, unnecessary contamination of previously uninvolved tissue will have already occurred.

There are four general biopsy techniques applicable to bone tumors: (1) fine needle biopsy, (2) core needle biopsy, (3) incisional open biopsy, and (4) excisional biopsy. Fine needle aspiration (FNA) biopsy provides only cells for cytology and is usually done by interventional radiologists. An FNA is useful in two general clinical situations where bone tumors are involved: (1) when the diagnosis of a bone lesion is strongly suspected (metastatic carcinoma, recurrent sarcoma) and (2) for difficult to access lesions (spine, pelvis, scapula). Core needle biopsies allow for interpretation of the tissue architecture in addition to the cytological detail. For bone lesions, core biopsies may be done in the same situations as FNA and for bone lesions with soft-tissue extension. Percutaneous needle biopsy has been shown to be safe, efficacious, and cost-effective in some patient groups.[12] However, a nondiagnostic needle biopsy should be viewed with caution.[13] Incisional open biopsy has traditionally been the workhorse biopsy tool for bone lesions, as it provides more tissue for histological interpretation. There are numerous pitfalls to open biopsy which must be considered, and for most incisional biopsies, the surgeon who will be doing the definitive surgery, no matter what the final diagnosis, is the person who should do the open biopsy.[14,15] Excisional biopsy, where the entire lesion is excised without a preceding incisional biopsy, is usually reserved for bone tumors such as osteochondromas, where the radiographic features establish the diagnosis, the morbidity of excision is small, and the surface location of the lesion lends itself to excision.

Surgical margins

Surgical margins depend upon the type of excision done, and the appropriate type of excision varies according to bone tumor type.

Table 6 American Joint Commission on cancer staging system for bone sarcomas for pelvic bones (8th edition).[a]

Pelvis T Criteria							
T	TX–T1 Criteria	T	T2 Criteria	T	T3 Criteria	T	T4 Definition
TX	Primary tumor cannot be assessed	T2	Tumor confined to 1 pelvic segment with extraosseous extension or 2 segments without extraosseous extension	T3	Tumor spanning 2 pelvic segments with extraosseous extension	T4	Tumor spanning 3 pelvic segments or crossing the sacroiliac joint
T0	No evidence of primary tumor	T2a	Tumor ≤ 8 cm in greatest dimension	T3a	Tumor ≤ 8 cm in greatest dimension	T4a	Tumor involves sacroiliac joint and extends medial to sacral neuroforamen
T1	Tumor confined to 1 pelvic segment with no extraosseous extension	T2b	Tumor > 8 cm in greatest dimension	T3b	Tumor > 8 cm in greatest dimension	T4b	Tumor encasement of external iliac vessels or presence of gross tumor thrombus in major pelvic vessels
T1a	Tumor ≤ 8 cm in greatest dimension						
T1b	Tumor > 8 cm in greatest dimension						

[a]Source: Amin et al.[9] and Tanaka and Ozaki.[10]

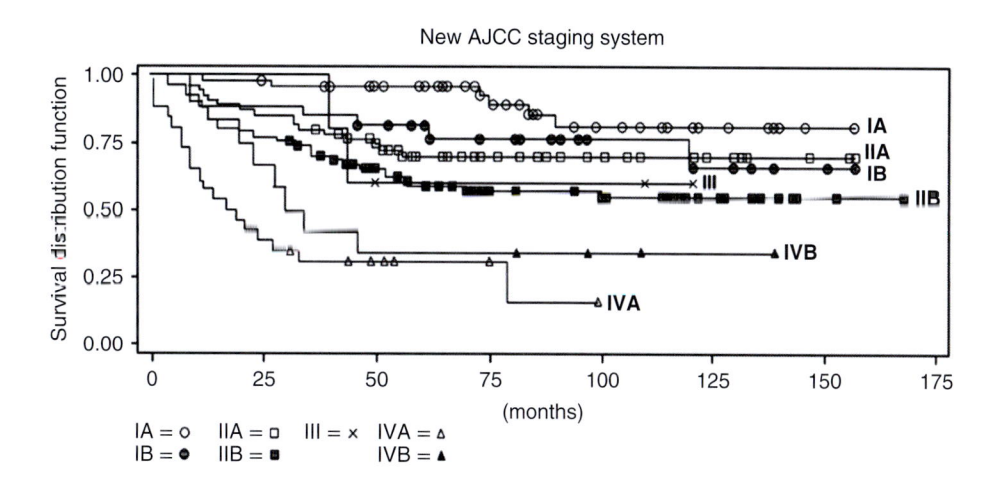

Figure 1 Survival according to staging by the new American Joint Commission on Cancer staging system for bone sarcomas. Source: Based on American Cancer Society.[1]

There are four types of excisions: (1) intralesional, (2) marginal, (3) wide, and (4) radical.[16] For most benign bone lesions, an intralesional excision by way of a curettage is appropriate. When necessary, metastatic bone lesions undergoing surgery for stabilization may be treated by debulking curettage. For aggressive benign lesions (chondroblastoma, osteoblastoma, giant cell tumor of bone, aneurysmal bone cyst, and chondromyxoid fibroma), an extended intralesional curettage is usually indicated. This differs from a simple curettage in that it utilizes mechanical (high-speed burr, pulsatile lavage) and adjunctive (phenol, laser, liquid nitrogen, argon beam coagulation) techniques to extend the margin into normal bone. Bone cement is also considered by some to serve as a local adjunct due to its exothermic effects. Recent trends suggest that most extremity low-grade (grade 1) chondrosarcomas may also be treated in this way. Marginal en bloc excision (through the pseudocapsule surrounding the tumor, is appropriate for osteochondromas, but wide resection (excision with a cuff of normal tissue) is indicated for most bone sarcomas being treated operatively.

Limb salvage versus amputation

Two issues must be considered in making the decision regarding limb salvage versus amputation: oncologic safety and function. First and foremost, in order for a patient to be a candidate for limb salvage, the oncologic procedure should not lower the expected survival beyond that which could be achieved with an amputation. This question has been addressed prospectively, and—in properly selected patients—survival is no less with limb-sparing surgery when compared to amputation.[17,18] However, this decision still needs to be made carefully for each patient. Oncologic safety considers two variables: response to chemotherapy (when applicable) and surgical margin. The poorer the response to chemotherapy, the greater the likelihood of local recurrence for any given margin achieved intra-operatively. Hence, for a poor response to chemotherapy (tumor progression), limb salvage surgery is a relatively strong contraindication. A wide surgical margin is the goal of bone sarcoma surgery, and it can almost always be achieved with the appropriately planned level of amputation but not always with limb-sparing surgery. If vital structures (major vessels and nerves) are encased by the soft-tissue extent of the sarcoma, necessitating their resection along with the tumor, limb salvage is contraindicated and amputation is preferable.

As with oncologic safety, if limb salvage is to be done, the expected function of the planned reconstruction should be at least equivalent to that of a comparable level amputation. In the lower extremity, function with a below-knee amputation is generally thought to be better than a distal tibia reconstruction, so a distal tibial location is a relative indication for amputation. In the upper extremity, it is preferable to be able to preserve 2 of the 3 major nerves (radial, ulnar, median) for limb salvage. Patients who undergo limb salvage report higher outcome measures when compared to those who undergo amputation.[19] Tumor encasement of more than one major upper extremity nerve and/or the axillary or brachial vessels is an indication for amputation.

Operative management of metastatic carcinoma, myeloma, lymphoma

There are four settings that potentially require operative management for patients with bone lesions from metastatic carcinoma, myeloma, and lymphoma: (1) biopsy to establish diagnosis, (2) prophylactic stabilization of impending pathologic fracture, (3) operative fixation of pathologic fracture, and (4) en bloc resection of isolated lesions. Biopsy issues have been previously discussed but cannot be emphasized enough: the diagnosis should be established before embarking upon an operative treatment plan. Prediction of impending fracture risk is evolving. Currently, fractures are predicted based upon clinical and radiographic criteria. A rating system devised by Mirels has been devised based upon four variables (Tables 7 and 8).[20] The Mirels system is valid across experience levels, but it still has a low specificity of approximately 33%.[21] A CT-based biomechanical structural rigidity analysis improves specificity but is not widely available.[22,23] Axial cortical involvement greater than 30 mm and circumferential involvement greater than 50% (or 45 mm and 30%) are also better predictors of fracture compared to Mirels.[24–26] Finite element analysis, although promising, remains under study.[27–29] Similarly, work is underway on the use of FDG-PET and machine learning in this setting.[30–32]

Table 7 Mirels scoring system for predicting risk of pathologic fracture in metastatic disease.[a]

	1 Point	2 Points	3 Points
Site	Upper extremity	Lower extremity	Peritrochanteric
Size	<1/3	1/3–2/3	>2/3
Nature	Blastic	Mixed	Lytic
Pain	Mild	Moderate	Functional

[a] Source: Mirels.[20]

Table 8 Mirels definitions, fracture risk, and treatment recommendations based upon point totals.[a]

Definition	Points	Fracture risk	Recommendation
Nonimpending	≤7	<10%	Observe
Borderline	8	15%	Consider fixation
Impending fracture	9	33%	Prophylactic fixation
Impending fracture	≥10	>50%	Prophylactic fixation

[a] Source: Mirels.[20]

When pathologic fractures occur in the setting of disseminated malignancies, they usually warrant operative fixation in order to improve function since these patients have limited life expectancy. Exceptions include moribund immediately preterminal patients, those who cannot tolerate operative intervention, and fractures that are usually managed by nonoperative means. In order for the patient to benefit from the procedure, life expectancy should be longer than the expected time required to recover from any proposed procedure. Tools for life expectancy both for extremity and spine tumors due to disseminated malignancies have become increasingly sophisticated and accessible.[33,34]

The principles of operative fixation for fractures in this clinical situation differ from those of standard fracture fixation. Since later lesions may develop elsewhere in the bone, intramedullary nail fixation, as opposed to plate/screw fixation, is preferred in the long bones in order to protect the remainder of the bone. Immediate stability is the goal in order to avoid prolonged recovery that diminishes patient function, so bone cement is much more commonly used to supplement fixation in this situation. Although ideally the entire long bone should be protected, recent evidence suggests that not only is this unnecessary in some situations, but it also carries the additional morbidity of pulmonary embolic events.[35,36] However, all identified lesions should be protected.[37] Fracture healing in the setting of metastatic carcinoma and myeloma may be prolonged, so fixation should be planned assuming there will be no fracture healing. Postoperative radiotherapy has been shown to improve function, slow local tumor progression, and reduce reoperation rates.[38,39]

Reconstructive alternatives

Benign bone tumors

The defects created after curettage of benign bone tumors can be filled with autologous bone graft, allograft bone, synthetic filler material, or bone cement.[4] Bone cement is usually reserved for defects created after extended intralesional curettage of giant cell tumors of bone. Bone cement provides immediate stability that allows full weight-bearing, solidifies with an exothermic reaction that extends the margin, and provides a clear radiographic border to facilitate diagnosis of local recurrence. In cases where large lesions have been curetted, prophylactic stabilization with pins or plates/screws may be used to minimize the chance of fracture.

Primary bone sarcomas

Following resection of bone sarcomas, numerous alternatives are available to reconstruct the large bone and associated soft-tissue deficits that result. Selection of the appropriate reconstruction in each instance requires consideration of the patient age and expectations, prognosis, adjuvant treatments, type of resection, and anatomic site. In general, reconstructive techniques include endoprostheses, structural allografts, allograft-prosthetic composites, and vascularized bone grafts. Over time, the use of endoprosthetic and allograft-prosthetic composite reconstructions following resections that include a joint has increased, while the indications for structural allografts in the United States have continued to decline. Apart from allograft-prosthetic composite reconstructions, the main role for structural allografts has been for intercalary reconstructions (when the joints above and below the diaphyseal segment can be preserved). The most frequent type of resection for sarcomas is intra-articular (removal of the bone up to and including the joint surface), requiring reconstruction of the joint surface, usually with a joint replacement. When the tumor invades the joint, an extra-articular resection (removal of both sides of the joint) is indicated, and this is often better reconstructed with a joint fusion using intervening allograft bone.

Patient age is a major consideration, since skeletally immature patients may develop limb length discrepancy unless the reconstruction accommodates the loss of growth on the operative side. For patients less than 8 years old, the potential limb length discrepancy is so profound that standard means of reconstruction are generally contra-indicated. In these difficult situations, amputation, rotationplasty, or vascularized fibula grafting with open growth plates are viable alternatives.[40–47] Rotationplasty in the lower extremity after resection of a tumor around the knee involves fixing the foot and ankle in a position rotated 180° from normal so that the heel points forward and the ankle is situated at the level of and functions as the patient's knee. In this situation, the patient is able to function as a below-knee amputee rather than having to settle for a higher above knee amputation. In patients older than 8 years old, expandable endoprosthetic reconstructions are available.[48–52] In recent years, the availability of such growing prostheses with a noninvasive mechanism has increased their attraction.[51] However, the complication rates have proven to be high, and their durability once the patient reaches skeletal maturity has been less than optimal.[53]

Upper extremity

For reconstructions following bone sarcoma resection about the shoulder, function is most dependent on whether the deltoid muscle may be preserved during resection of the tumor.[54–56] If a tumor of the proximal humerus extends into the deltoid, and the deltoid has to be removed to achieve a wide margin, function of the shoulder will be poor regardless of the reconstruction. When the deltoid can be preserved, consideration is often given to using an allograft-prosthetic composite reconstruction.[57] In this way, the patient's remaining rotator cuff tendons can be repaired to the allograft tendons, and there is potential for improved function. If an osteoarticular allograft reconstruction is chosen, there is an increased risk of nonunion of the allograft-host junction, fracture, and subchondral collapse. The scapula and all portions of the humerus may be reconstructed with an endoprosthesis. The distal upper extremity is an unusual site for bone sarcomas.

Lower extremity

Following limb-preserving bone sarcoma resection of the pelvis (internal hemipelvectomy), no reconstruction is needed when the hip joint is able to be preserved (e.g., anterior pubic/ischial rami and supra-acetabular iliac resections), and some surgeons do not reconstruct even following resection of the acetabular portion of the pelvis. The numerous reconstructive alternatives for the acetabulum and hip joint following internal hemipelvectomy are fraught with complications.[58,59] For the proximal femur, reconstruction is often done with either an endoprosthetic hemiarthroplasty (replacing the femoral head side but without a cup in the pelvis) or an allograft-prosthetic composite.[60–62] The latter reconstruction allows attachment of the patient's hip abductors to the allograft tendon, which may improve stability and gait.

Most reconstructions of the distal femur utilize a distal femoral replacement endoprosthetic total knee reconstruction. Because of the attachment of the extensor mechanism through the patellar tendon to the tibial tuberosity, resection of the proximal tibia necessitates consideration of extensor mechanism reconstruction. Here, the primary alternatives are endoprosthetic proximal tibial total knee reconstruction or allograft-prosthetic composite reconstruction. For both reconstructions, the medial head of the gastrocnemius muscle is often used both to cover the allograft and/or prosthesis and to reconstruct the extensor mechanism. With an allograft-prosthetic composite reconstruction of the proximal tibia, the patient's remaining patellar tendon may be sutured to the allograft tendon, further augmenting the extensor mechanism reconstruction.

Complications

Complications after resections and reconstructions for bone sarcomas are numerous and frequent. Infection is a concern with all reconstructions, particularly considering the large dead space created following these procedures, the prolonged wound healing while receiving adjuvant treatments, and the prevalence of chemotherapy-induced neutropenia. However, certain complications are associated with specific anatomic sites and types of reconstructions. The proximal tibia is an anatomic site particularly prone to infection and wound breakdown given the paucity of soft-tissue coverage. For endoprosthetic reconstructions of the shoulder and hip, joint instability and frank dislocation are relatively common complications with hemiarthroplasties, although reverse total shoulder arthroplasties are being used more frequently and may improve function over conventional arthroplasty.[63,64] All endoprosthetic reconstructions are prone to loosening, but prosthetic survival is acceptable (proximal femur: 90%, distal femur: 60%, proximal tibia: 50%).[65] Exciting new developments in alternative compliant means of fixation other than those commonly used with joint arthroplasties have been reported and warrant continued close follow-up.[66] Reports of their use around the knee show 80% ten-year survivorship.[67] Allografts, particularly when used alone, are prone to nonunion at the allograft-host junction and to fracture.

Radiotherapy for bone tumors

Radiotherapy plays a limited role in the treatment of primary tumors of bone, but it is a mainstay of local treatment for bone lesions resulting from metastatic carcinoma, myeloma, and lymphoma.[39] Radiotherapy should generally be avoided in the treatment of benign bone tumors, but low dose radiotherapy has been advocated in recalcitrant symptomatic spine cases of Langerhans cell histiocytosis.[68] For bone sarcomas, radiotherapy may be considered for the treatment of Ewing sarcoma, but it is not part of standard treatment for osteosarcoma or chondrosarcoma.

Potential complications of bone irradiation include postradiation sarcoma, spontaneous and fragility fracture, osteonecrosis, and—in pediatric patients—growth arrest or angular deformities. Postradiation sarcomas (most commonly osteosarcoma) typically occur at a minimum of 3 years following the radiation exposure and after mean doses of 50 Gy, although the risk may be as low as <1%.[64,69] Risk factors for postradiation fracture include periosteal stripping, neoadjuvant chemotherapy, femoral location, higher dose irradiation, and circumferential irradiation.[70] Following radiation of the femur for metastatic disease, the rate of fracture is >10% and most common in the proximal femur and within 3 months of treatment regardless of the risk of fracture based on Mirels scoring.[71] Fractures occurring in this setting more than 3 months after treatment have been attributed to radiation-induced bone fragility.[71] Postradiation fractures are gaining increasing attention because of their difficulty in management, prolonged healing times, and high nonunion rates (45–67%), and the frequent need for surgical treatment, multiple operations, radical bone resection/reconstruction, and/or amputation.[70]

Medical management of bone tumors

The roles for medical management of bone tumors continue to expand. As a rule, high-grade bone sarcomas warrant chemotherapy to address systemic microscopic disease. Chemotherapy for bone sarcomas is usually initiated prior to (neoadjuvant chemotherapy) and completed after local surgical or radiation treatment. Hence, the treatment of both conventional high-grade osteosarcoma and Ewing sarcoma begins with neoadjuvant chemotherapy. There is no established role for chemotherapy in the treatment of low-grade chondrosarcoma. Unfortunately, there have been no major advances in the medical oncology management of bone sarcomas over the last several decades.

Use of bisphosphonates to inhibit osteoclast-mediated bone destruction has become standard of care for myeloma and many metastatic carcinomas, including breast, prostate, and lung.[72] Bisphosphonates drugs have also been used for specific benign bone lesions, including for pain relief in symptomatic fibrous dysplasia, but their efficacy is variable. Giant cell tumor of bone has also been treated with TNF-alpha inhibitors with some success, but the specific role for their use remains unclear.[73,74] Of concern with bisphosphonates and Denosumab are osteonecrosis of the jaw and atypical subtrochanteric proximal femur fractures.[72,75,76]

Specific benign bone tumors

Cartilage tumors

Cartilage tumors can be divided into those that derive from mature hyaline cartilage (chondromas and osteochondromas) versus those that derive from immature cartilage (chondroblastoma and chondromyxoid fibroma).

Chondromas

The World Health Organization classification lists enchondromas and periosteal chondromas under the general heading of "chondromas."[3] Enchondromas are the intramedullary variety of these benign hyaline cartilage tumors and periosteal chondromas are the variety that reside on the bone surface. Enchondromatosis (multiple enchondromas/Ollier's disease and Maffucci's syndrome) is discussed under the "Congenital syndromes" section. The latter represents multiple enchondromas combined with hemangiomas.

Enchondromas are relatively common among primary bone tumors, representing up to 17% overall. They likely represent residual rests of hyaline growth plate cartilage left behind during skeletal immaturity. Most of these lesions are asymptomatic and incidentally noted on imaging studies done for other causes of pain.[77] Enchondromas represent the most common bone lesion seen in the small bones of the hands and feet. In the long bones, they are most commonly located in the femur (where they are frequently picked up on X-rays of patients with hip or knee pain) and the humerus (where they are picked up during radiologic evaluation of patients with common causes of shoulder pain). Solitary enchondromas of the flat bones are rare, and the possibility of chondrosarcoma needs to be considered when a cartilage lesion occurs there. Because the radiographic characteristics of hyaline cartilage are fairly typical, the primary challenge is distinguishing enchondromas from chondrosarcomas.

The natural history of enchondromas is that they become more calcified over time. Hence, mature lesions in adults almost always display a characteristic punctate pattern of calcified arcs and rings which is so distinctive as to often allow the diagnosis to be confirmed radiographically without biopsy (Figure 2). They can be associated with some endosteal scalloping. However, when they have periosteal reaction, expansion of the surrounding bone, more extensive cortical destruction, or soft-tissue extension, they have to be considered chondrosarcomas. MRI characteristics of enchondromas are a lobular pattern of organization which is dark on T1-weighted (T1W) images and bright on T2-weighted (T2W) images. Increased uptake on bone scan is typical of enchondromas and should not be considered to be a sign of malignancy; it is likely due to ongoing remodeling of the surrounding bone.

Under the microscope, enchondromas are comprised of benign, sparsely cellular hyaline cartilage, but the degree of cellularity and atypia is variable. In certain locations, such as the fingers and other small bones, the histologic features often appear more aggressive despite their benign behavior. Differentiation of benign enchondromas from low-grade (grade 1) chondrosarcomas by pathologists, radiologists, and clinicians remains problematic.[78–80]

The vast majority of enchondromas, especially when they present as asymptomatic lesions with typical radiological findings, can simply be observed to ensure that they do not progress.[81] This approach has been shown to be cost-effective and safe.[81] However, when either the radiographic features or associated pain cast doubt on the diagnosis, the lesion may require a complete curettage and complete histological review to differentiate from chondrosarcoma. Cartilage lesions rarely recur after curettage.

Periosteal chondromas, by contrast, are distinctly unusual benign hyaline cartilage lesions. They more commonly present as a bump on a digit or as a low-grade painful lesion elsewhere. Radiographically, the usually show a typical "saucerization" of the underlying cortex of this surface lesion. They need to be distinguished from periosteal chondrosarcoma. Smaller lesions (less than 7 cm) are usually chondromas. Depending upon the location, periosteal chondromas may be removed by curettage or en bloc excision.

Chondroblastoma

This immature cartilage-derived tumor is an uncommon benign process that typically presents with joint pain, is difficult to diagnosis, and occurs in the epiphysis of the long bones.[82] The vast majority of cases occur in skeletally immature patients, and their presentation with joint pain (due to their location at the end of long bones), mimicking symptoms of far more common processes, and their initially subtle radiographic findings may lead to a prolonged course prior to diagnosis. Although they may occur in numerous bones, their most common locations are the proximal humerus, distal femur, and proximal tibia.

Radiograph appearance can be subtle, since its immature cartilage usually does not cause the calcification seen so characteristically with hyaline cartilage lesions. Furthermore, the subtle epiphyseal round radiolucency of chondroblastoma is not usually surrounded by a very obvious sclerotic rim. Easier to recognize on MRI, chondroblastoma is dark on T1W and bright on T2W images and shows extensive perilesional edema. Bone scans are hot at the site of the lesion.

Chondroblastoma histology shows a preponderance of rounded cells with distinct folded "coffee-bean" nuclei arranged in a pseudolobulated "cobblestone" pattern of organization. Giant cells and chondroid matrix may also be seen.

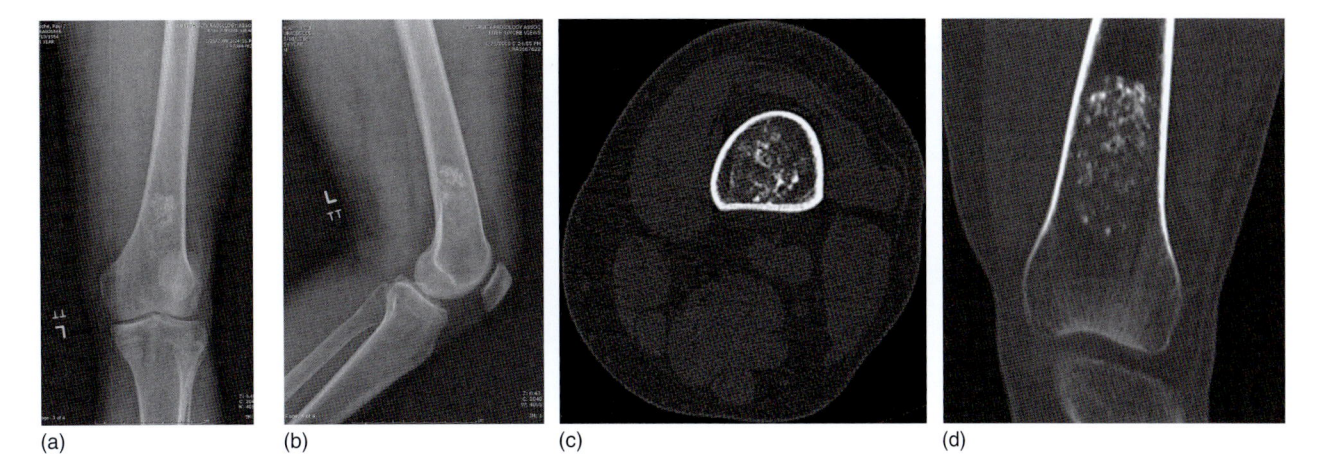

Figure 2 Enchondroma. Anteroposterior (a) and lateral (b) distal femur radiographs as well as axial (c) and coronal (d). CT scans show the characteristic punctate arcs and rings of hyaline cartilage without prominent endosteal scalloping or cortical destruction to suggest features of chondrosarcoma.

Treatment of chondroblastoma must take into account the fact that while is usually behaves only as an active lesion, it may also behave in an aggressive fashion. An extended intralesional curettage with burring remains the classic treatment of choice, but more recently radiofrequency ablation has been employed in selected lesions with considerable success.[83,84] When RFA is used for large lesions beneath weight-bearing articular surfaces the risk of collapse must be considered.[83] Chondroblastoma is also one of two benign bone lesions (along with giant cell tumor) that carry the potential to develop pulmonary metastases, so initial screening and subsequent surveillance of the lungs should be considered.

Chondromyxoid fibroma

Like chondroblastoma, chondromyxoid fibroma is a benign tumor of immature cartilage.[85] Unique from chondroblastoma, however, is the metaphyseal eccentric location in long bones, often immediately adjacent to the growth plate. It is a rare tumor, representing less than 1% of bone tumors. The most common long bone involved is the tibia. One-third of these tumors occur in flat bones. Chondromyxoid fibromas usually present with pain.

Radiographic features of chondromyxoid fibroma include its eccentric metaphyseal location, lytic lobulated, soap-bubble appearance usually without matrix mineralization, and associated cortical thinning. In some cases, the appearance may be of an aggressive tumor, with cortical breakthrough and even soft-tissue extension (Figure 3). Under the microscope, the tumor is arranged in lobules which are more cellular around the periphery than the sparsely cellular myxoid center. The characteristic cells are "stellate" in shape.

Treatment is typically by curettage and grafting. Local recurrence rates range from 15% to 25%. Chondromyxoid fibromas do not metastasize.

Osteochondroma

The most common tumor of bone, osteochondroma, is an exophytic growth of physical cartilage away from the growth plate and joint but paralleling the temporal course of long bone growth.[86] As the cartilage grows, it leaves behind either a sessile or pedunculated bony prominence. These tumors form and grow during the period of skeletal immaturity, cease growing at or around the time of skeletal maturity, and remain throughout a patient's life unless excised. They may present as a painless mass or with pain. Pain is usually from irritation of the overlying soft tissues or bursitis but may also result from fracture of the stalk or malignant degeneration. Malignant degeneration is rare in solitary osteochondromas, but it occurs somewhat more commonly in patients with the hereditary form, multiple hereditary exostoses (see section titled "Congenital syndromess").[87]

Osteochondromas may be diagnosed radiographically with confidence. They are an exophytic metaphyseal projection characterized by continuity of the cortical and underlying medullary bone. When they have a stalk, the cap of the osteochondroma is directed away from the nearest joint. MRI is sometimes used to assess the thickness of the cartilage cap, which may be up to 3 cm in children. In adults, however, the cap should be less than 1.5 cm; thicker caps should cause suspicion for chondrosarcoma arising from the underlying osteochondroma. Under the microscope, osteochondromas have a benign hyaline cartilage cap overlying normal trabecular bone.

Treatment of osteochondromas is based on symptoms and clinical presentation. When they are asymptomatic, they may be observed. When they are painful in children, they may be excised, but the older the child and the farther away from the growth plate, the lower the risk of recurrence. In adults, any symptomatic or enlarging osteochondroma should be investigated further with an MRI to make sure that it has not developed into a chondrosarcoma.[86]

Fibrous tumors

These three lesions are grouped together based on their histologic similarity in giving the light microscopic appearance of being comprised of fibrous tissue. In the latest WHO classification system for bone lesions, however, fibrous dysplasia and osteofibrous dysplasia are listed together under "Tumors of Undefined Neoplastic Nature." Nonossifying fibromas" are classified as "Fibrohistiocytic Tumors" under the current WHO outline of bone tumors.[3]

Fibrous dysplasia

The etiology of fibrous dysplasia has been identified to be a mutation of the GNAS gene, creating a developmental anomaly of bone formation. It is a relatively common bone process which has its onset in children but may also be diagnosed in adults. The spectrum of clinical presentation is broad and depends upon age, number of lesions, and site(s) of involvement. Patients may present with incidental lesions, painful lesions, or pathologic fracture. Monostotic (solitary) fibrous dysplasia is most commonly located

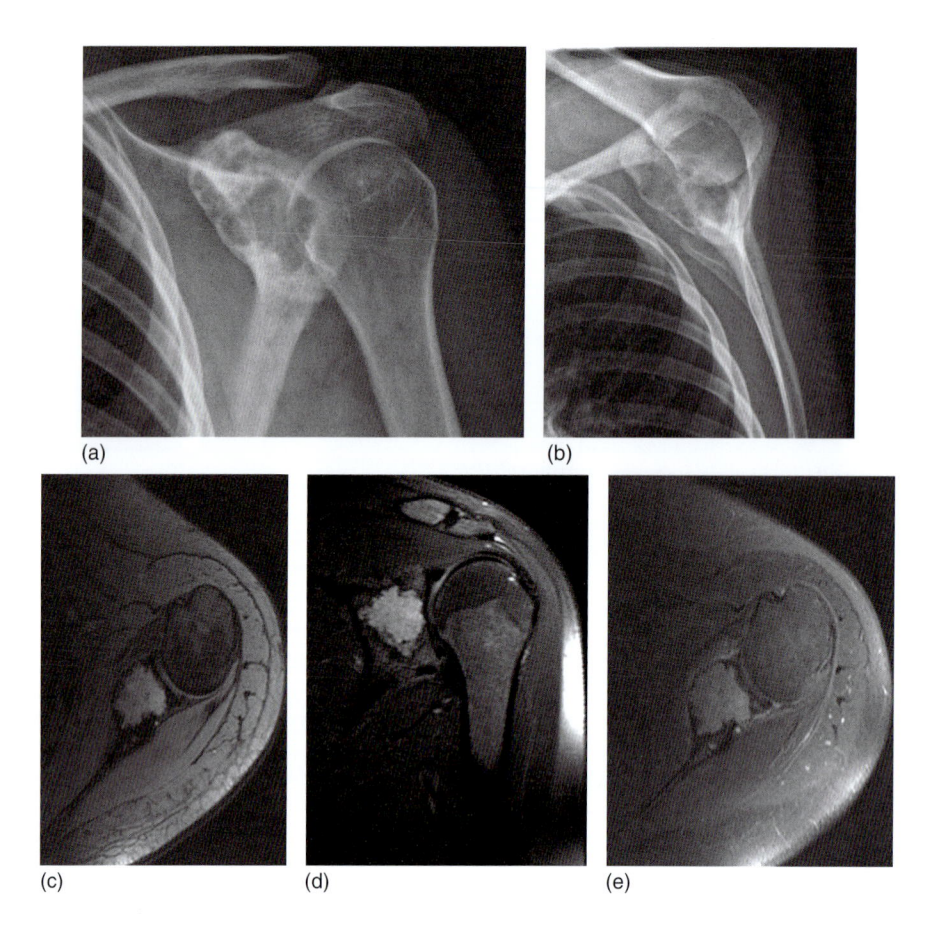

Figure 3 Chondromyxoid fibroma. Anteroposterior shoulder (a) and scapular-Y (b) radiographs, T2-weighted axial (c) and coronal (d), and proton-density axial (e) MRI images show the features of a chondromyxoid fibroma, in this case involving a flat bone, the scapula. Note the cortical thinning and focal cortical destruction that characterizes aggressive behavior and may lead to confusion with chondrosarcoma.

in the skull, followed by the femur, tibia, and ribs. Polyostotic lesions (less common than the monostotic form) most often involve the femur, pelvis, and tibia. The polyostotic form may also present as McCune–Albright syndrome (see section titled "Congenital syndromes") or Mazabraud's syndrome (associated intramuscular myxomas).[88]

Radiographically, lesions of fibrous dysplasia usually present as geographic lytic lesions. In long bones, they are frequently described as "long lesions in long bones." They affect any portion of the bone (epiphysis, metaphysis, or diaphysis) and have a characteristic "ground glass" appearance of the matrix. In the proximal femur, extensive involvement may lead to a "shepherd's crook" deformity. Uptake on Tc99 bone scan is usually intense. Under the microscope, immature woven bone classically described as taking the form of "Chinese characters" lacks the osteoblastic rimming seen with osteofibrous dysplasia and is surrounded by bland appearing fibroblasts.

Orthopedic treatment is based upon age, location, and symptoms. When the radiographic appearance is classic, symptomatic lesions may be observed. For some symptomatic lesions, curettage and grafting may be done, but structural bone graft is usually preferred, as particulate graft materials are usually resorbed. Prophylactic stabilization is often considered in the proximal femur, where the disorganized trabecular bone of fibrous dysplasia predisposes to stress fracture and remodeling. For symptomatic patients with polyostotic fibrous dysplasia, bisphosphonates have been used with some success.[89,90] If associated FGF-23-mediated hypophosphatemia is identified, referral to a metabolic bone specialist with experience in phosphate wasting disorders is suggested.[88]

Nonossifying fibroma and fibrous cortical defect

Nonossifying fibromas and fibrous cortical defects are variants of a spectrum of developmental abnormalities of skeletally immature bone.[91] Fibrous cortical defects are smaller and generally confined to the cortex while nonossifying fibromas are larger, extending into the medullary canal. They are so common as to almost be considered variants of normal. Fully 1/3 of children seen in the emergency room for knee injuries will show evidence of one or more of these lesions. They are almost always an incidental, asymptomatic finding. In the rare instance where they are discovered after a fracture has occurred through one, the characteristic history is the absence of pain leading to the time of fracture. This absence of pain underscores their latent nature without active features. The metaphysis of long bones is affected most frequently, particularly around the knee.

These lesions may be diagnosed with confidence on plain x-rays in nearly all cases. Their characteristic features are an at least partially intra-cortical, eccentric metaphyseal position, a soap-bubble lytic geographic appearance, and a thin rim of sclerotic bone around the periphery of the lesion. MRI, when necessary, shows a low signal center on both T1W and T2W sequences that is also characteristic. Perilesional edema is absent in the absence of fracture. Rarely, biopsy is needed to establish the diagnosis, and in those instances, the histopathology features a storiform, whirling background of fibroblasts with scattered giant cells.

Treatment of the vast majority of fibrous cortical defects and nonossifying fibromas should be observation alone. The unusual associated pathologic fracture should be treated according to the location and type of fracture, combining curettage and grafting of the lesion when operative management is indicated.

Osteofibrous dysplasia

In the past, osteofibrous dysplasia has been referred to as ossifying fibroma and Campanacci's disease.[91] It is unique among fibrous tumors in its location (anterior tibial shaft almost exclusively) and histology (bone islands surrounded by osteoblastic rimming and separated by a bland fibrous background). It is almost exclusively a tumor of children, and most cases occur in patients less than 8 years old. Its restricted sites of occurrence within bones that have a relatively superficial location (tibia, fibula, ulna, radius) is distinctive, as is the fact that it may be bilateral and multifocal within a single bone. It should be distinguished from adamantinoma, a bone sarcoma that also occurs most frequently in the anterior aspect of the tibia. Clinical presentation of osteofibrous dysplasia is variable, with some patients noticing a painless lump over the tibia, others presenting with episodic pain from associated stress fractures, and rare patients developing progressive tibial bowing.

Radiographically, osteofibrous dysplasia presents most commonly in the tibia within the middle or proximal third in an eccentric anterior position with a lytic, soap-bubble, or saw-toothed appearance. In older patients, there is radiographic overlap with adamantinoma, from which it must be distinguished. Unlike in adamantinoma, soft-tissue extension is not seen on MRI in osteofibrous dysplasia. As an active lesion, osteofibrous dysplasia shows increased uptake on bone scan. Under the microscope, osteofibrous dysplasia must be distinguished from both fibrous dysplasia and adamantinoma. While both osteofibrous dysplasia and fibrous dysplasia have woven bone islands within a sea of benign fibrous tissue, only osteofibrous dysplasia has osteoblastic rimming around those islands. The distinction from adamantinoma is that osteofibrous dysplasia does not show islands of epithelioid cells seen in the more aggressive condition. Although the two lesions are related in some aspects, there is no good evidence to suggest that osteofibrous dysplasia progresses to adamantinoma.[92]

Treatment of osteofibrous dysplasia varies according to age, symptoms, and radiographic appearance. Prior to closure of the growth plate, an asymptomatic and radiographically classic lesion may be observed. If stress fractures occur, bracing should be considered. When the radiographic features are atypical, biopsy should be undertaken to establish the diagnosis. Surgical excision with or without grafting is only indicated for progressive deformity or in symptomatic patients after skeletal maturity. Some authors have suggested that due to the high incidence of recurrence after curettage and grafting, an extra-periosteal resection should be performed in all cases.[93]

Giant cell tumors

Giant cell tumor of bone is a relatively common (5–10% of all bone tumors) benign tumor of bone characterized by its distinct histology and behavior.[94] In the current WHO classification system, it is classified as with "Osteoclastic Giant Cell Rich Tumours." It is one of the few benign bone tumors (along with chondroblastoma, osteoblastoma, aneurysmal bone cyst, and chondromyxoid fibroma) that have the potential to behave in an aggressive fashion. In addition, along with chondroblastoma, it is unique in its potential to create pulmonary metastases despite its benign designation. Because giant cell tumor typically behaves in an active or aggressive fashion, it presents clinically with pain, swelling, limited range of motion at the associated joint, and sometimes with pathologic fracture. It is a tumor of adulthood, peaking in young adults aged 20 to 40, and it is very unusual in skeletally immature patients. The most common locations are around the knee (distal femur and proximal tibia), wrist (distal radius), sacrum, and shoulder (proximal humerus).

Radiologically, giant cell tumor has its epicenter within the metaphysis of the long bones but almost always extends to involve the epiphysis, creating an eccentric radiolucency typically with geographic type 1C borders that abuts the subchondral bone of the adjacent joint. In skeletally immature patients, however, the lesion is usually metaphyseal. It is purely lytic without matrix mineralization, and it may show radiographic signs of aggressive behavior complete with cortical destruction and an associated soft-tissue extension. Although histologically, the predominant feature is the multi-nucleated giant cell, it is the background stromal cell with identical nuclear features which is the true neoplastic cell.

Local treatment of giant cell tumor depends upon location. In expendable locations, such as the proximal fibula or distal ulna, en bloc excision is appropriate. For most sites, however, the conventional recommended treatment is extended intralesional curettage and either grafting or cementing of the defect. Extended curettage involves mechanical removal (curettes) combined with a high-speed burr and additional means of extending the margin (e.g., phenol, liquid nitrogen, argon beam). The local recurrence rate for intralesional curettage of giant cell tumor varies from 30% to 47% after simple curettage but is less than 25% with extended curettage. An integral part of the care of patients with giant cell tumor is assessment for potential pulmonary metastases and extended follow-up for early diagnosis of local recurrence. Recurrences have been described up to 20 years later.[94] For "unresectable" giant cell tumors, options include radiotherapy, embolization, or denosumab. Denosumab is a Rank-ligand inhibitor which inhibits the ability of the background stromal cells in giant cell tumor from coalescing to form giant cells.[95] Although early results have been promising, questions remain regarding its role in long-term use and complications that may be associated with such application.[74,96]

Hemangioma of bone

The most common benign bone tumor of the spine, hemangioma of bone is a proliferation of blood vessels that may rarely be seen in other locations. The vast majority of hemangiomas of bone, particularly in the spine, are asymptomatic incidental findings, and the true source of any presenting symptoms should be sought apart from this tumor. Rarely, they may cause expansion of the bone or pathologic fracture. In the spine, these problems may cause neurologic compromise.

In the spine, the radiographic characteristics of hemangioma of bone are so typical that in the majority of cases, no biopsy is needed for confirmation. Radiographs show "jailbar" vertical striations. Axial CT and MRI scans show a "polka-dot" pattern. On T2-weighted MRI images, hemangiomas show high signal; after contrast administration, these lesions enhance markedly. When radiographic features are atypical, biopsy will usually show variably sized benign blood vessels, but numerous histologic subtypes have been described. In nonspinal sites, appearances are variable, and biopsy is often needed.

Since most hemangiomas are asymptomatic, management in the majority should simply be observation. For the rare truly symptomatic, "atypical" or "aggressive" lesion, consideration may be given to excision, radiotherapy, embolization, and sclerosing therapy.[97,98] Interventional radiologists are playing an increasing role in the treatment of symptomatic intraosseous hemangiomas.[98]

Osteogenic tumors

Enostosis

Enostosis, or bone island, is a localized region of dense lamellar bone within cancellous bone of the medullary canal.[99] Enostoses are uniformly benign latent lesions that are incidental asymptomatic findings during radiographic evaluation of other problems. They are most concerning when they occur in adults as part of the autosomal dominant condition osteopoikilosis, where they present as multiple lesions and must be distinguished from osteoblastic metastatic disease.

On plain radiographs and CT scans, enostoses are densely sclerotic areas within medullary bone that are distinguished by the lack of a central nidus (as seen in osteoid osteoma), presence of radiating spicules emanating from the periphery of the lesion, and absence of uptake on bone scan (except in giant enostoses) (Figure 4). Recently, CT attenuation values have shown high sensitivity and specificity in distinguishing bone islands from sclerotic metastases.[100,101] They usually do not require biopsy, but under the microscope, the histology is that of mature lamellar bone.

No treatment is necessary for classic bone islands. Once the diagnosis is established radiographically, nothing more that observation is warranted.

Osteoid osteoma

A benign bone-forming condition that typically presents with a unique and distinctive pain pattern, osteoid osteoma is most common in adolescents and young adults.[102] The pain pattern is that of pain that is worse at night and relieved (in 70% of patients) dramatically and completely over a very short time course (20–30 min) with nonsteroidal anti-inflammatory drugs (NSAIDs). Relief with NSAIDs is theorized to be due to the beneficial effect these agents have on lowering the elevated prostaglandin levels known to be present within the nidus of osteoid osteoma. Osteoid osteomas occur with greatest frequency in the femur and tibia, but they are also one of the three most common tumors of the posterior elements of the spine (along with osteoblastoma and aneurysmal bone cyst). In the spine, they may cause painful scoliosis, where they are located in the concavity of the curve. In juxta-articular locations, they may cause an arthropathy, with associated effusion and synovitis.

The characteristic radiographic finding in an osteoid osteoma is the radiolucent nidus, which is less than 2 cm in diameter and usually surrounded by dense sclerotic reactive bone. The lesion is usually intracortical, appearing eccentrically in the bone, so the reactive bone may extend both into the medullary canal and also cause expansion of the bone externally. The reactive bone may be so dense that the nidus is only evident on CT or MRI evaluation. On MRI, the extensive perilesional edema associated with osteoid osteoma is characteristic. Osteoid osteomas are always intensely hot on bone scan. Histologically, the nidus of an osteoid osteoma is characterized by irregularly arranged seams of variably mineralized osteoid surrounded by both osteoblasts and osteoclasts within a highly vascular fibrous stroma.

Treatment of osteoid osteoma has evolved considerably over time. The mainstay of operative treatment currently is percutaneous techniques including radiofrequency ablation (RFA) and microwave ablation (MWA).[103,104] Success of first-time RFA or MWA in eliminating symptoms is 90–100% in both pediatric and adult populations.[103–105] When percutaneous techniques are not feasible (spinal lesions close to nerve roots, juxta-articular, or difficult to access sites), surgical excision of the nidus will eliminate the symptoms. However, the nidus is sometimes difficult to localize intra-operatively, and numerous techniques have been described. The third option is medical management with NSAIDs, but the mean duration of treatment needed before the lesion ceases to cause symptoms is 2.5 years.

Osteoblastoma

Osteoblastoma shares a great deal of similarity with osteoid osteoma, and to a large degree, the primary distinguishing feature of osteoblastoma is the larger size of its nidus.[102] Similarities include their peak occurrence in adolescent and young adult patients, predilection for the posterior elements of the spine, and their underlying histology. Differences include the absence of the typical pain pattern of osteoid osteoma, the potential for aggressive behavior, and a nidus of larger than 2 cm in osteoblastoma. In addition, a much higher proportion of osteoblastomas (up to 70%) are located in the spine, making the long bones an unusual site.

Radiological features are similar to osteoid osteoma but with a larger nidus that typically shows some faint calcifications. The microscopic appearance overlaps considerably with that of osteoid osteoma, showing irregularly arranged seams of variably mineralized osteoid surrounded by both osteoblasts and osteoclasts within a highly vascular fibrous stroma.

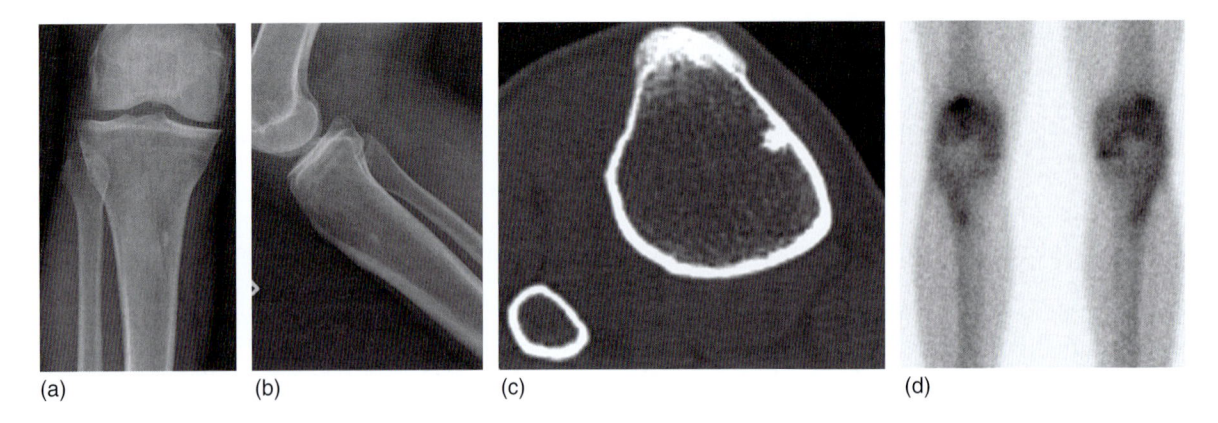

Figure 4 Enostosis (bone island). Anteroposterior (a) and lateral (b) radiographs of the knee show an incidental small radiodense bone lesion. Axial CT (c) shows the characteristic radiating spicules that extend from the periphery of the sclerotic bone island and interdigitate with the surrounding bone trabeculae. As in this case (d), there is usually absence of uptake on bone scan.

Because of its larger size and potential for more aggressive behavior than osteoid osteoma, treatment of osteoblastoma has classically involved excision, usually by extended intralesional curettage.[106] Recurrence rates range from 10% to 30%. However, more recently, percutaneous interventional ablative techniques such as RFA have been employed with success in small series, particularly in the spine.[107] Radiation should be reserved for recurrent lesions in difficult locations such as the spine.

Cysts and other tumors

Aneurysmal bone cyst

Aneurysmal bone cyst may occur as a primary or a secondary lesion.[108] Primary aneurysmal bone cysts are neoplastic proliferations characterized by gene rearrangements involving the oncogene USP6 and the promoter CDH11.[109,110] Secondary aneurysmal bone cysts occur in association with other primary bone lesions and do not carry the same chromosomal abnormalities.[110] Along with chondroblastoma, osteoblastoma, giant cell tumor, and chondromyxoid fibroma, aneurysmal bone cyst is one of the few benign bone tumors that have the potential to behave in an aggressive manner. Peak age range is from 1 to 20 years. They typically present with pain and sometimes with swelling and/or pathologic fracture. Anatomic distribution is predominately within the long bones, with the femur and tibia being the most common, but aneurysmal bone cyst is also one of the three most common tumors of the posterior elements of the spine (along with osteoid osteoma and osteoblastoma).

Radiographically, the classic appearance of an aneurysmal bone cyst is that of an eccentric, osteolytic, aneurysmal like "blown-out cortex" surrounded only by an "eggshell thin rim" of reactive bone. However, these features are not present in all cases, and the plain films may show an appearance that overlaps with other benign conditions such as simple bone cyst, nonossifying fibroma, and fibrous dysplasia (Figure 5). In those cases, MRI of aneurysmal bone cyst will often show septations separating loculated regions filled with blood, manifest as fluid–fluid levels. The radiographic presence of these characteristic findings, however, is not pathognomonic, and underlying primary lesions should be sought. Biopsy is indicated to establish the diagnosis and to distinguish from telangiectatic osteosarcoma, which has an overlapping radiographic appearance. The microscopic appearance of aneurysmal bone cyst is that of blood-filled lakes separated by bland fibroblastic septa with evidence of hemosiderin deposition and scattered giant cells.

Because of its potential for aggressive local behavior and its highly vascular tissue, treatment of aneurysmal bone cyst is challenging, and the natural history is sometimes difficult to predict.[111] In most cases, an initial thorough curettage is preferred in order to allow complete histologic examination that may reveal other underlying primary lesions and to distinguish from telangiectatic osteosarcoma. Before curettage, consideration should be given to preoperative embolization, particularly for central lesions that do not lend themselves to intra-operative tourniquet control of bleeding. Intraoperative bleeding may be life-threatening. Some authors have suggested embolization or aspiration/injection as definitive treatments, but these options do not allow complete histologic review.[112] Local recurrences do not always progress in an aggressive fashion, so these may sometimes be observed closely. Low-dose irradiation should be reserved for incompletely excised, aggressive, recurrent lesions in difficult to access locations such as the spine.

Simple bone cyst

In contrast to aneurysmal bone cyst, simple (or unicameral) bone cyst is usually an inactive lesiona and at worst an active lesion. Without a prior fracture, it is a single cavity within bone filled with serous or serosanguinous fluid. Most simple bone cysts are diagnosed during childhood and are located in the proximal humerus, proximal femur, or calcaneus. In young adults, they are more common in the calcaneus and ilium. Simple bone cysts are usually asymptomatic until fracture, and many present with pathologic fracture following minimal trauma.

Radiographically, simple bone cysts are usually centrally located within the metaphysis or metadiaphysis of a long bone, are purely radiolucent in the absence of prior fracture, lack prominent marginal sclerosis, thin and sometimes slightly expand the surrounding cortex, and may rarely demonstrate the pathognomonic "fallen fragment sign" after fracture. The fallen fragment (or leaf) sign is a thin wafer of cortical bone that is situated at the caudad aspect of the bone cyst because it passed through the fluid in the cyst to reach that position. MRI of simple bone cyst shows homogenous fluid signal within the lesion, dark on T1W and bright on T2W sequences. Peripheral rim enhancement without any central enhancement is the norm. In some cases after fracture

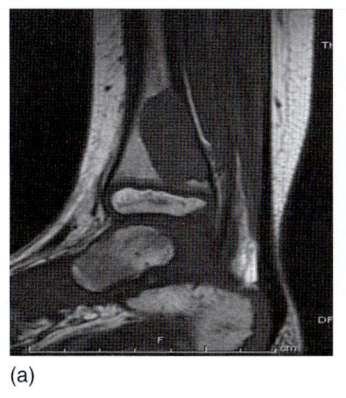

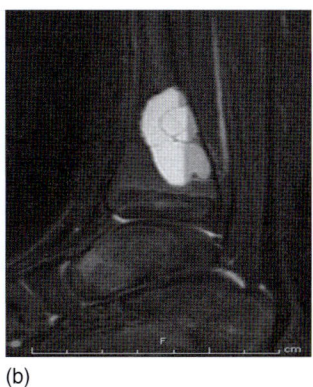

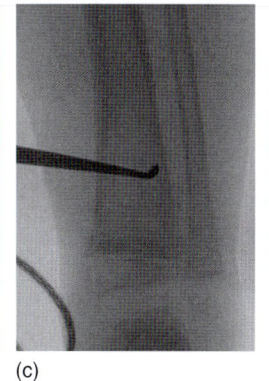

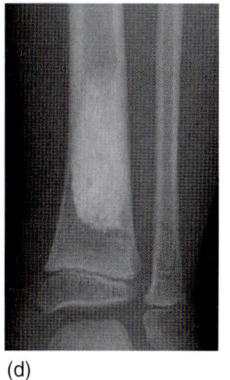

Figure 5 Aneurysmal bone cyst. Magnetic resonance images of this radiolucent bone lesion that presented with pain in a 4-year-old show fluid signal characteristics on T1-weighted sagittal images (a), but the septations and fluid-fluid levels characteristic of aneurysmal bone cyst are best seen in this case on the T2-weighted sagittal images (b). Intraoperative fluoroscopic images (c) show that this lesion does not show aggressive features seen with many aneurysmal bone cysts (ballooned out cortex). This lesion was curetted completely and filled with synthetic graft material (d).

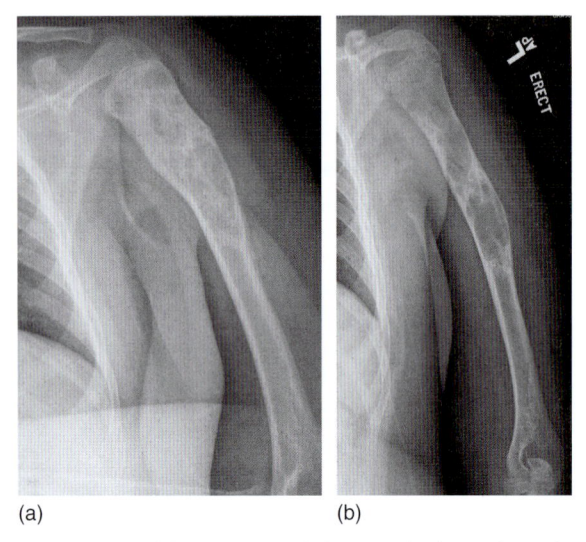

Figure 6 Unicameral bone cyst (simple bone cyst). Plain radiographs of the left humerus of a 9-year old (a) who has incurred two prior fractures with minimal trauma through this lytic geographic proximal humeral bone lesion abutting the proximal humeral growth plate. At this point, there is evidence of healing within the cyst, which occurs in approximately 1/7th of simple bone cysts after fracture. However, 2 years later (b), the cyst shows signs of recurrence, with increased radiolucency in the mid-diaphysis. Note that the proximal humeral growth plate has grown away from the bone cyst. These lesions are only active during skeletal immaturity.

blood products mixed with the serous fluid may produce a single low fluid–fluid level, but the lack of septations and numerous fluid–fluid levels should distinguish a simple bone cyst. When aspirated, clear serous fluid is obtained unless there has been a fracture, in which case, the fluid can be bloody. After curettage, histologic findings reveal only a bland fibrous membrane with scattered histiocytes.

Treatment of simple bone cysts depends upon location, age, and presentation. In the proximal humerus, pathologic fractures should be allowed to heal first. Approximately one of seven simple bone cysts will heal after fracture (Figure 6). If the cyst does not heal with fracture healing, then definitive treatment options usually employ some form of aspiration and injection. Various agents have been used in the injection, including methylprednisolone, demineralized bone matrix, bone marrow, and combinations of agents. In the only level I study comparing bone marrow with steroid injection, the steroid was superior to bone marrow alone in radiographic evidence of healing.[113] In the proximal femur, the risk of fracture through unicameral bone cysts is higher and the consequences potentially more devastating, so consideration should be given to open curettage and grafting here in order to prevent fracture. The addition of proximal femoral hardware lessens the risk of additional surgery and speeds return to normal activities.[114] When a proximal femoral simple bone cyst has caused a pathologic fracture, open reduction and internal fixation of the fracture should be accompanied by curettage and grafting. In some locations, such as the calcaneus and ilium, observation may be elected if the cyst is asymptomatic, since pathologic fractures in these sites are very unusual. Regardless of the means of treatment, approximately 60% respond with progressive healing of the lesion. Partial healing may occur in another 30%, but 10% persist or recur. The natural history of simple bone cyst must always be borne in mind, as those in the typical locations resolve after skeletal maturity. Hence, the closer the patient is to skeletal maturity, the less aggressive the approach should be.

Langerhans cell histiocytosis

Langerhans cell histiocytes, the cells of origin of this disease entity, are a component of the reticuloendothelial system involved in phagocytizing foreign debris and originating in the bone marrow.[68] The group of disease entities encompassed by Langerhans cell histiocytosis classically includes solitary eosinophilic granuloma, Hand–Christian–Schuller disease (may include classic triad of multifocal bone lesions, exophthalmos, and diabetes insipidus), and Litterer-Siwe disease (disseminated, often fatal form). The younger the patients at clinical presentation, the more likely they are to have disseminated disease, with most disseminated disease patients being less than 2 years, and most patients with eosinophilic granuloma being between 5 and 20 years of age. Current classifications of LCH include involvement of "nonrisk" organs, including bone, skin, and lymph node, "risk" organs (liver, spleen, lung, and bone marrow), and "CNS risk" areas (orbit, mastoid, and temporal skull), the latter due to the risk for development of diabetes insipidus, other endocrine abnormalities, and brain lesions. Isolated nonrisk involvement is generally considered a benign disease.[115] Solitary eosinophilic granuloma is more common in flat bones such as the skull, pelvis, ribs, and vertebral bodies; in the long bones, it occurs as a diaphyseal or metaphyseal lesion. In multifocal disease, the skull and jawbones, as well as bones of the hands and feet, are more commonly involved.

Clinical presentation varies depending upon the stage of the disease. Patients with solitary or isolated multifocal bone disease often present with pain localized to the site of involvement or a limp with involvement in the lower extremity, but the bone lesions may also be asymptomatic and discovered as incidental findings. Systemic manifestations of this disease spectrum may include diabetes insipidus, exophthalmos, fevers, infections, hepatosplenomegaly, lymphadenopathy, papular rash, among others.

Radiological presentation is variable, and hence bone lesions in Langerhans cell histiocytosis are "great mimickers" (along with osteomyelitis), often simulating more aggressive processes including sarcomas (Figure 7). They typically show a lytic appearance with permeative margination and soft-tissue extension, and they are often mistaken for Ewing sarcoma. In the spine, they create a "vertebra plana" appearance, with profound flattening of the vertebral body. On MRI, these lesions will also show considerable perilesional edema. Bone scan has a 30% false-negative rate, so a skeletal survey should always be performed in patients with any form of Langerhans cell histiocytosis. Because of the overlap in clinical presentation with other entities, including Ewing sarcoma and lymphoma, biopsy is indicated in order to establish the diagnosis. Under the microscope, the characteristic Langerhans histiocyte (large, basophilic, coffee-bean shaped nucleus) predominates, often accompanied by numerous eosinophils.

Treatment of biopsy-proven Langerhans cell histiocytosis depends upon the stage and the symptoms, location, size, and number of bone lesions. Systemic involvement involving "risk" organs warrants consideration of chemotherapy. Low-dose radiotherapy is sometimes employed for vertebral lesions at risk for collapse. Surgical treatment for isolated bone involvement may involve curettage alone, curettage and grafting, prophylactic stabilization, and corticosteroid aspiration/injection. Patients with solitary eosinophilic granuloma generally do well with little treatment, and in some cases, the bone lesions resolve after biopsy alone. Patients with systemic disease have prognosis inversely proportional to age at presentation and extent of involvement.

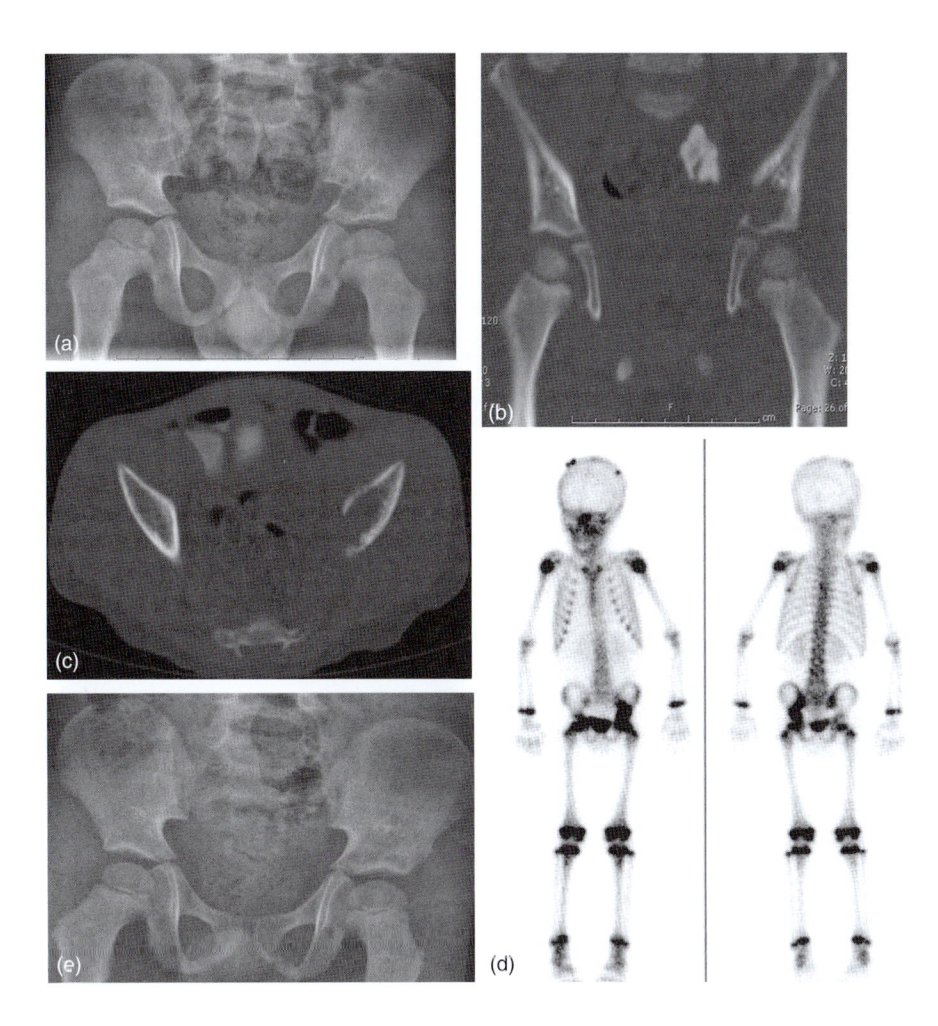

Figure 7 Langerhans cell histiocytosis (eosinophilic granuloma). This anteroposterior pelvis radiograph (a) of a 4-year-old boy shows a left supra-acetabular lytic bone lesion with motheaten borders. Cortical destruction seen on coronal (b) and axial (c) CT scans cause concern for metastatic neuroblastoma or Ewing's sarcoma, but biopsy showed sheets of Langerhans cells interspersed with eosinophils. Bone scan (d) showed increased uptake in this lesion, and a skeletal survey was done to exclude other lesions that might not show up on bone scan. In this case, there was only a solitary lesion and no visceral involvement. One year after biopsy and curettage, the lesion is less apparent on radiograph (e), and the patient remains asymptomatic.

Primary bone sarcomas

Adamantinoma

An epithelial neoplasm, adamantinoma is a rare primary bone sarcoma of low grade that is thought to be derived from ectopic rests of epithelial cells.[116] It represents approximately 0.4% of all bone tumors. Older children and young adults are most commonly affected, and 95% affect the tibia, particularly the anterior aspect, or both the tibia and fibula. The most common presentation is of progressive pain and swelling localized to the middle third of the lower leg.

Radiographically, adamantinoma is an eccentric destructive lytic process that usually destroys the anterior cortex of the mid-tibia and leads to an associated soft-tissue mass. The medullary border usually has a rim of sclerotic reactive bone surrounding the radiolucent areas. On MRI, the lesion is dark on T1W and bright on T2W sequences with soft-tissue extension commonly and sometimes multifocal disease. Under the microscope, it shows a biphasic arrangement with epithelial groups of cells often forming glandular structures and surrounded by a background of fibrous tissue.

Treatment of adamantinoma is surgical and involves achieving a wide surgical resection of all involved bone and soft tissue with a margin of uninvolved tissue. Although cure is achieved in 85% of cases, long-term follow-up is necessary, as these tumors may recur or metastasize over 15 years later.[117]

Chondrosarcoma

Chondrosarcomas derive from chondrocytes, the cartilage cells that are crucial to bone growth and development.[118-121] Among bone tumors, they are relatively common, representing the second most common bone sarcoma after osteosarcoma. The vast majority of chondrosarcomas are low-grade tumors arising in adults in a wide variety of anatomic sites. The most common locations are the pelvis, followed by the femur, ribs, humerus, scapula, and tibia. Chondrosarcomas are often painful, and this symptom often leads to their discovery. Because of the prevalence of cartilage neoplasms of bone and the overlap in clinical, radiographic, and even histologic appearance between benign and malignant, one of the most difficult challenges is the differentiation of enchondromas from chondrosarcomas.

Chondrosarcomas may be classified in other ways than grade. Specific histologic subtypes (clear cell, dedifferentiated, and mesenchymal) other than conventional low-grade chondrosarcoma are discussed individually below. Conventional low-grade chondrosarcomas may arise *de novo* as "primary chondrosarcomas" or in association with preexisting benign cartilage lesions

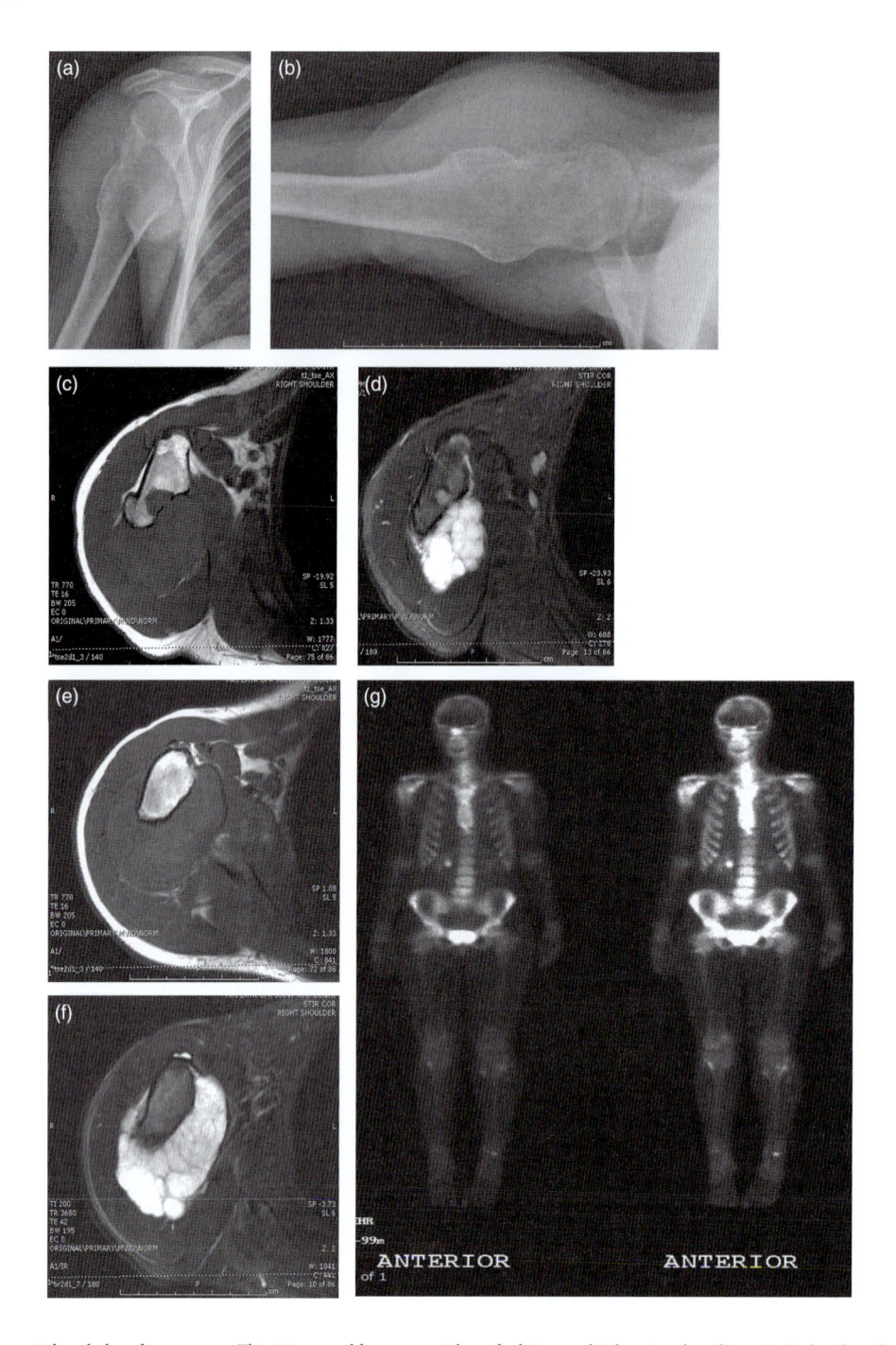

Figure 8 Secondary peripheral chondrosarcoma. This 26-year-old woman with underlying multiple osteochondromatosis developed pain and swelling in her right shoulder. Anteroposterior (a) and axillary lateral (b) right shoulder radiographs show numerous osteochondromas arising from the proximal humeral metaphysis but also a large soft tissue shadow associated with the bone. In addition, particularly on the lateral view, there is cortical irregularity. Magnetic resonance axial T1-weighted (c, e) and T2-weighted (d, f) images show that there is a cartilage cap measuring more than 2 cm thick, indicative of a chondrosarcoma arising from the underlying osteochondroma and extending into the underlying bone as well. Uptake is noted in the right proximal humerus on bone scan. This patient underwent proximal humeral resection and prosthetic reconstruction.

(enchondromas and osteochondromas) as "secondary chondrosarcomas" (Figure 8). Further, chondrosarcomas that arise within the medullary bone are "central" whereas those arising on the surface of the bone (periosteal/juxtacortical chondrosarcoma or secondary chondrosarcoma arising within a preexisting osteochondroma) are "peripheral."

On plain radiographs, conventional chondrosarcomas usually show the same sort of hyaline cartilage mineralization in the forms of arcs and rings that typify enchondromas. However, a number of features that accompany this mineralization pattern point towards a malignant diagnosis. These include cortical destruction with soft-tissue extension, progressive enlargement over time, cortical expansion and >50% endosteal scalloping, enlarging regions of radiolucency, and periosteal reaction. MRI may be more sensitive at showing soft-tissue extension and perilesional edema, but the pattern of being dark on T1W images and bright on T2W images holds true for both benign and malignant cartilage tumors. CT scan is often best at delineating the degree of scalloping and cortical destruction. Bone scans usually show increased uptake in any hyaline cartilage tumor, so they do not play a major role in distinguishing benign from malignant cartilage tumors. The classic histologic distinction between enchondromas and chondrosarcomas is the presence of "encasement" (hyaline cartilage lobules isolated and surrounded by rimming reactive bone) in enchondromas compared to "permeation" (cartilage tumor permeating around preexisting bone trabecular) in chondrosarcomas. In addition, increased cellularity, cytologic atypia, and binucleation favor chondrosarcoma. The anatomic site has to be considered as well. The histologic appearance of enchondromas arising in the hand or in the setting of Ollier's disease may have a malignant histologic appearance but nonetheless have a benign course. Overall, the histologic distinction between benign and low-grade malignant cartilage tumors is fraught with difficulty, and this process should always consider the clinical presentation and radiographic features.[78–80] In many hyaline cartilage tumors, a firm diagnosis may be established based largely on clinical and radiographic grounds.

Because of the large amount of matrix and relatively low cellularity, current treatment is usually restricted to surgical means. There is no standard role for either radiotherapy or chemotherapy in most low-grade chondrosarcomas. In recent years, there has been a shift to performing extended intralesional curettage with local adjuvants (phenol, liquid nitrogen, or laser) followed by bone grafting or cementation for grade I intramedullary chondrosarcomas rather than the classic treatment recommendation, which was to perform a wide resection of the tumor.[122–124] However, this less aggressive approach has been limited to chondrosarcomas without soft-tissue extension and generally does not apply to grade II or grade III chondrosarcomas. Prognosis for chondrosarcoma is closely related to grade (Table 9). As with other predominantly low-grade tumors, long-term follow-up is recommended.

New work has explored the role of systemic treatment and/or radiotherapy for high-grade chondrosarcomas. For select high-risk chondrosarcomas in difficult locations or with positive margins after resection, a National Cancer Database study suggests there may be a role for high-dose radiotherapy.[126] Some limited survival benefit has been shown with standard chemotherapy agents and antiangiogenics for inoperable or metastatic chondrosarcomas.[127,128]

Clear cell chondrosarcoma
Similar to conventional chondrosarcoma in being a low-grade sarcoma, clear cell chondrosarcoma has a distinctive location (the epiphysis of long bones) and histology (large cells with abundant clear cytoplasm in a cartilage matrix). The most common locations of this rare tumor are the proximal epiphysis of the femur, tibia, or humerus. Peak ages are 20 to 40 years. Pain is the usual presenting symptom.

Given its epiphyseal location, clear cell chondrosarcoma should be considered in the differential diagnosis of chondroblastoma but in older patients (since most chondroblastomas are in skeletally immature patients). On plain radiographs, clear cell chondrosarcoma is seen as a radiolucent lesion that extends to subchondral bone and can have an appearance very similar to that of giant cell tumor of bone. The large clear cells are distinctive under the microscope and the permeative pattern belies its malignant behavior.

Wide en bloc resection is the standard of care for clear cell chondrosarcoma. Prognosis is very good with appropriate treatment. Overall recurrence rate is approximately 15%.

Dedifferentiated chondrosarcoma
Among chondrosarcomas, dedifferentiated chondrosarcoma is the most aggressive and carries the worst prognosis. By definition, it consists of a conventional low-grade chondrosarcoma adjacent to a region of high-grade sarcoma, often osteosarcoma. The most common locations are the femur, pelvis, humerus, ribs, and scapula. Radiographically, a lytic region developing within an otherwise typical chondrosarcoma may signify a dedifferentiated chondrosarcoma. Treatment for chondrosarcoma should be directed at the high-grade component, but the role for chemotherapy remains to be established, and prognosis is uniformly poor, with a 10–15% 5-year survival rate.[118,129,130] A recent report showed a survival advantage with ifosfamide-based chemotherapy compared to standard nonifosfamide chemotherapy when combined with surgery in one series.[129]

Mesenchymal chondrosarcoma
The rarest of all chondrosarcomas of bone, mesenchymal chondrosarcoma is a highly aggressive chondrosarcoma which predominately affects teenagers and young adults. The most common locations are in the axial skeleton, and the tumor is usually eccentric. Under the microscope, mesenchymal chondrosarcomas show nodules of cellular chondroid tissue surrounding vascular spaces. As with most chondrosarcomas, surgery is the mainstay of treatment, although recent reports continue to explore the potential benefits of chemotherapy.[119] Prognosis has been reported as ranging from <30% to 52% 5-year survival.[2]

Chordoma

Chordoma is a low-grade malignancy arising from vestigial notochordal remnants that exist in the midline of the spine. Following the distribution of those remnants, chordoma is a midline tumor involving the sacrococcygeal, spheno-occipital, and other mobile spine regions. Chordoma predominately involves adults, and in the adults, the sacrum is the most common location. It is very rare in African-Americans. In younger patients, the skull is the most common location. It accounts for only 3–4% of all primary bone tumors. Clinical presentation is dependent upon location, although pain is usually a presenting symptom. In the sacrum, bowel, bladder, or sexual symptoms may be present. In the skull, cranial nerve deficits may be present. In the mobile spine, back or leg pain predominates.

Radiographs of chordoma may be difficult to interpret as the findings of lytic destruction are often subtle in these anatomically complex sites. Only CT or MRI will show the extensive anterior soft-tissue mass that usually accompanies the bone destruction in chordoma. Under the microscope, chordoma is composed of nests or cords of physaliferous cells, distinctive large cells with bubbly vacuolated cytoplasm.

Treatment of chordoma involves wide surgical resection when possible, but irradiation improves the disease-free interval in patients with marginal or contaminated margins.[131] Overall survival has been associated with >65 Gy and advanced techniques.[132]

Table 9 Chondrosarcoma survival, metastatic potential, and local recurrence rates according to grade.[a]

Type	5-Year survival (%)	Metastatic potential (%)	Recurrence rate
Grade I	90	0	Low
Grade II	81	10–15	Intermediate
Grade III	29	>50	High

[a]Modified from Randall and Hunt.[125]

Chemotherapy does not play a role in this low-grade malignancy. Local recurrence is common (up to 70%), and overall survival drops from 75–85% at 5 years to 40–50% at 10 years.

Ewing sarcoma

Overall, Ewing sarcoma is the third most common bone sarcoma after osteosarcoma and chondrosarcoma.[2] In patients 5–30 years old (the peak ages for Ewings), Ewings is second only to osteosarcoma. Thought to be derived from primitive mesenchymal cells, Ewing sarcoma is a poorly differentiated malignant small round blue cell tumor closely related to other tumors within the Ewing family of tumors.[133] The Ewing family of tumors includes Ewing sarcoma, PNET/primitive neuroectodermal tumor, and Askin's tumor, all of which have translocations involving the EWS gene on chromosome 22. The most common locations are the femur and pelvis, but vertebral body and rib involvement are also relatively common. Presenting symptoms usually include both pain and swelling, but in approximately 20%, the symptoms may be accompanied by fever and malaise. In 10%, pathologic fractures are present at diagnosis. Increased ESR is common, and some patients may also have anemia and leukocytosis.

Radiographically, Ewing sarcoma has a varied presentation depending upon the location. Within the long bones, it has a predilection of diaphyseal involvement, and onion-skinning periosteal reaction (numerous layers of reactive new bone a few millimeters apart formed as the periosteum is lifted off by the expanding tumor and repetitively forms reactive bone) is frequent, accompanied by permeative poorly defined borders, cortical destruction, and usually an associated soft-tissue mass. The radiographic pattern is almost always lytic. Under the microscope, Ewing sarcoma is a prototypical small round blue cell tumor and is difficult to distinguish from other such entities (such as lymphoma and metastatic neuroblastoma) without special studies. Immunohistochemistry is positive for CD-99 (the MIC2 protein) in 95% of cases. The most definitive test is demonstration of the t(11;22)(q24;q12) or similar translocation (t(21;22)) by fluorescent in situ hybridization (FISH). Resulting fusion proteins that result from these translocations are EWS-FLI1 and EWS-ERG.

Treatment of Ewing sarcoma involves neoadjuvant multi-agent chemotherapy for systemic disease and either wide surgical resection or irradiation for local disease.[133] The standard chemotherapeutic approach in Ewing sarcoma is alternating cycles of vincristine–doxorubicin–cyclophosphamide (VDC) and ifosfamide–etoposide (IE), with improved event-free survival using 2 week instead of 3-week cycles.[134] It has been the chemotherapy that has led to the greatest improvement in survival. The latest trend is for increased surgical resection in sites that previously would have received radiotherapy, but historically Ewing sarcoma has been considered a radiosensitive tumor. Radiotherapy is still utilized for unresectable central locations (some pelvic tumors, sacrum, spine, cranium), for metastatic disease, and as a surgical adjuvant if margins of resection are close or microscopically positive. Surgical resection has evolved from being used initially only for expendable bones (iliac wing, rib, fibula, proximal radius, distal ulna) to now being used more frequently for most reconstructable anatomic sites (femur, tibia, humerus). The pelvis remains a controversial site for local treatment of Ewing sarcoma, where surgery has been used with increasing frequency and acceptable results.[135] However, there have been no randomized studies comparing radiotherapy to surgical resection in Ewings patients, and retrospective studies suffer from selection bias, as radiotherapy has traditionally been used for the worst centrally located tumors. Currently, some trials have suggested that the

Table 10 Osteosarcoma variants according to grade.

Low grade	Intermediate grade	High grade
Low-grade intra-medullary Parosteal	Periosteal	Conventional High-grade surface Secondary Pagetoid Postradiation Small cell

prognosis is as good as 65–70% 5-year survival, but based on minimum 5-year follow-up for 3225 Ewing's sarcomas collected in the National Cancer Database, 5-year survival was only 50.6% for Ewing sarcoma.[2]

Osteosarcoma

The most common bone sarcoma, osteosarcoma comprises a somewhat heterogeneous group of sarcomas that are predominately high grade but with three low to intermediate-grade variants (Table 10). The common thread is that they are felt to be derived from the osteoblast cell line and are bone-forming sarcomas.[136,137] Ninety percent of osteosarcomas are conventional high-grade. The three most common histologic subtypes are osteoblastic, chondroblastic, and fibroblastic, but there are multiple clinical and radiographic subtypes. Classically, the age distribution has been described as bimodal, but the peak age is during the second and third decades of life; cases in older adults usually occur in the setting of Paget's disease (Pagetoid osteosarcoma) or following irradiation (postradiation osteosarcoma). Clinical presentation almost always involves progressively worsening pain and may involve associated swelling. The most common locations reflect the most active areas of growth in skeletally immature patients ... the distal femur followed by the proximal tibia and proximal humerus. Overall, there is a 1.5:1 male to female ratio.

Radiographically, osteosarcomas, in general, are bone-forming, relatively poorly defined metaphyseal tumors that frequently have associated soft-tissue extension accompanied by cumulus cloud-type bone formation (Figure 9). Some histologic subtypes, especially the fibroblastic and telangiectatic osteosarcomas, form radiolucent tumors without the classic bone formation. Telangiectatic osteosarcoma, due to its blood-filled lakes, can closely resemble a benign aneurysmal bone cyst (ABC) on imaging studies, so this tumor should always be considered in the differential diagnosis of an apparent ABC. On MRI, the typical osteosarcoma is dark on T1W and bright but heterogeneous on T2W sequences, usually shows soft-tissue extension, and may show skip lesions within the medullary canal. They show increased uptake on bone scan. Under the microscope, there is some variation, particularly between the low and high-grade variants, but the key element is malignant osteoid production. Osteoid production in typical high-grade variants is seen as pink, lace-like osteoid being produced by pleomorphic cells, but in the low-grade variants, osteoid takes the form of broad osteoid seams with a more monotonous population of background cells. The most common histologic subtype is osteoblastic, followed by chondroblastic, fibroblastic, and—rarely—telangiectatic.

Treatment depends upon grade and extent of the tumor. For all high-grade variants, neoadjuvant multidrug chemotherapy is key, and this involves adriamycin, ifosfamide, cisplatin, and methotrexate.[138] The advantage of neoadjuvant chemotherapy is that it allows determination of percent tumor necrosis after resection and often reduces the size of the soft-tissue extension of the tumor, facilitating surgical resection. Tumor necrosis

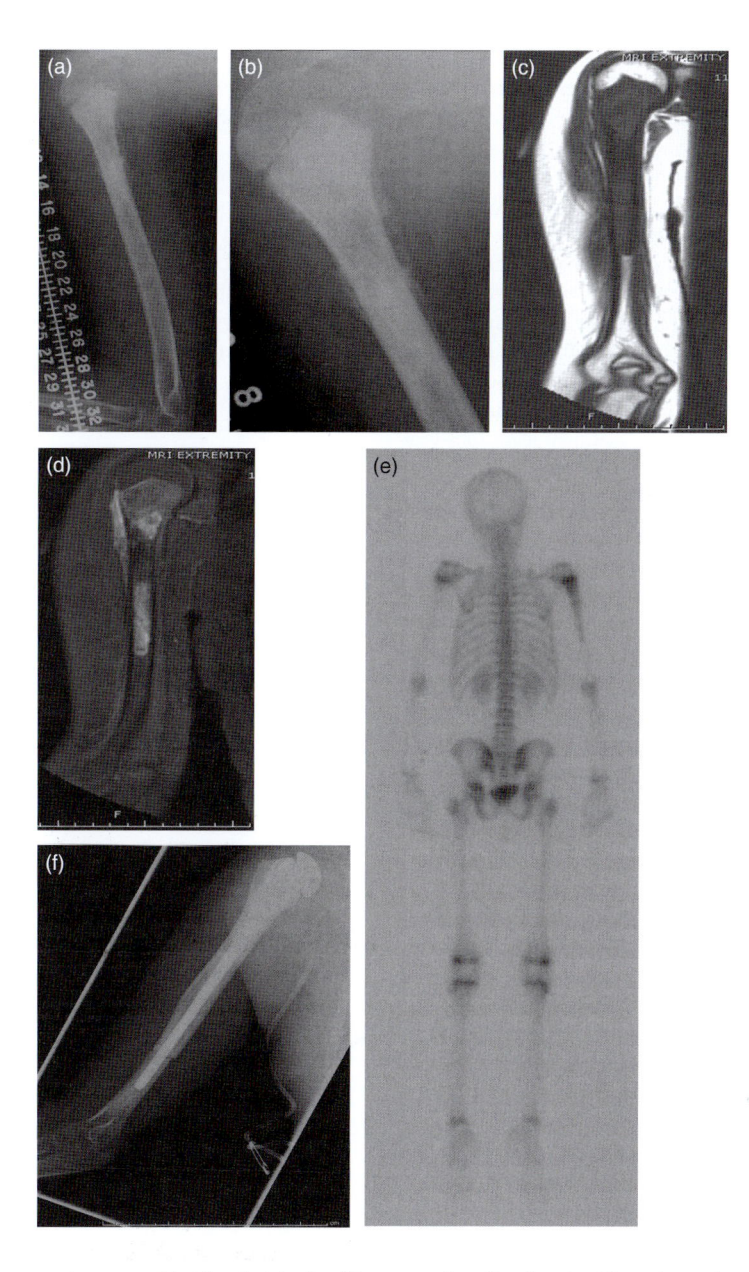

Figure 9 Conventional osteosarcoma. A 13-year-old girl with right shoulder pain and swelling has shoulder radiographs (a, b) showing a radiodense proximal humeral metaphyseal lesion with permeative borders and Codman triangle periosteal reaction and soft-tissue extension. Coronal T1-weighted (c) and T2-weighted (d) MRI images show the soft-tissue extension and extent of the tumor within the medullary canal. Bone scan (e) shows increased uptake in the proximal humerus. In a young patient, these features are nearly diagnostic of osteosarcoma, and a biopsy confirmed the diagnosis of high-grade osteosarcoma. After neoadjuvant chemotherapy, the patient underwent wide resection and proximal humeral allograft-prosthetic reconstruction (f).

>95% is strongly predictive of disease-free and overall survival. Drug resistance is sometimes seen due to the p-glycoprotein membrane-bound pump (coded for by the MDR-1 gene), which pumps the chemotherapeutic agents out of the cell. Local disease is addressed by wide surgical resection. There is no role for radiotherapy in standard treatment of osteosarcoma. For low-grade central and parosteal osteosarcoma (the low-grade variants), treatment only involves wide surgical resection; neither chemotherapy nor radiotherapy play a role.

Features unique to the various clinicopathologic subtypes will be presented below.

Conventional osteosarcoma

As the classic osteosarcoma, conventional high-grade osteosarcoma has the typical radiographic appearance of a metaphyseal tumor most common in the distal femur, proximal tibia, and proximal humerus. It usually demonstrates a cloud-like bone formation with permeative borders on plain radiographs and often has cortical breakthrough with an associated soft-tissue extension bordered by Codman's triangles (reactive bone formed by the bordering periosteum as it is lifted away from the bone surface by the expanding tumor) (Figure 9).

Histologically, osteosarcoma is comprised of pleomorphic cells with frequent mitoses forming lace-like pink osteoid. Conventional osteosarcoma may show a predominance of bone formation (osteoblastic), chondroid matrix (chondroblastic), fibrous background (fibroblastic), or blood-filled pools (telangiectatic). Differentiation of chondroblastic osteosarcoma from chondrosarcoma and fibroblastic osteosarcoma from fibrosarcoma is based upon the presence of malignant osteoid.

Prognosis for osteosarcoma has improved considerably due primarily to the use of multi-agent chemotherapy but has not improved much recently. Clinical trials involving patients with nonmetastatic disease report actuarial 5-year survival rates of 75–80%. For all comers, including all ages and those with metastatic disease, data from the National Cancer Database of the American College of Surgeons suggests a less optimistic outlook.[2] Based upon 8104 osteosarcomas cases with a minimum 5-year follow-up from 1985 to 1998, the relative 5-year survival rate for high grade was 52.6%. For osteosarcoma patients younger than 30 years, the relative 5-year survival rate was 60%; for those aged 30 to 49 years, it was 50% and for those aged 50 years or older it was 30%. For the approximately 20% of patients with osteosarcoma that present with metastases, aggressive treatment leads to 5-year survival in 30–40%, but for patients who develop metastases after treatment, 5-year survival is only 15–20%.

High-grade surface

Although the other two surface osteosarcomas (parosteal and periosteal) are low or intermediate grade, respectively, this surface variant is defined by its more aggressive radiographic and histologic appearance and clinical behavior. Otherwise, the clinical presentation, demographic features, pathology, and treatment are identical to those of conventional high-grade osteosarcoma.

Low-grade intramedullary

Along with parosteal osteosarcoma, low-grade central intramedullary osteosarcoma is the only other low-grade osteosarcoma. In contrast to the two other low to intermediate-grade osteosarcomas (parosteal and periosteal, respectively), this one is not a surface tumor; conversely, this is the only intramedullary low-grade osteosarcoma. A rare tumor, it represents only 1–2% of all osteosarcomas. Clinical presentation usually involves pain. The typical patient is slightly older than classic osteosarcoma, often being in the third decade of life.

Radiographically, the well-demarcated radiodensity that characterizes low-grade intramedullary osteosarcoma is often confused with fibrous dysplasia (Figure 10). Under the microscope, the appearance is distinctly different from high-grade conventional osteosarcoma. Like parosteal osteosarcoma, low-grade central osteosarcoma is comprised of broad bands of osteoid separated by a hypocellular fibroblastic stroma with minimal atypia and rare mitoses.

As for both of the low-grade osteosarcomas, low-grade intramedullary osteosarcoma is treated by wide surgical resection alone without chemotherapy or radiotherapy. Overall prognosis is quite good, with local recurrences in only approximately 5% following appropriate surgery and a 90% 5-year survival rate that drops slightly to 85% at 10 years. In rare cases, dedifferentiation may occur by way of an adjacent high-grade sarcomatous component.

Parosteal

The low-grade surface osteosarcoma, parosteal osteosarcoma is a distinct clinical, radiographic and pathologic entity that accounts for 5% of osteosarcomas. Similar to its intramedullary counterpart, the peak age is in the third decade of life. Females are affected more commonly than males (M:F 1:2). Parosteal osteosarcoma has a strong predilection for the posterior aspect of the distal femur (80% of cases); the proximal tibia and proximal humerus are other relatively common locations. It usually presents as a painless posterior distal thigh mass that may decrease knee range of motion.

Radiographically, parosteal osteosarcoma usually shows a lobulated, fairly densely ossified knob-like mass that has the appearance of being "stuck on" the underlying bony cortex. In unusual cases, the tumor may encircle the bone, and the underlying cortex may show reactive changes. Under the microscope, parosteal osteosarcoma looks like low-grade central osteosarcoma, with a sparsely cellular fibroblastic stroma between broad bands of osteoid.

Treatment for parosteal osteosarcoma involves wide surgical resection alone; there is no established role for chemotherapy or radiotherapy. In rare instances, dedifferentiated areas may arise. Overall prognosis is 86% 5-year survival.[2]

Periosteal

Another surface tumor, periosteal osteosarcoma accounts for only 1–2% of osteosarcomas. Clinical presentation and peak age are the

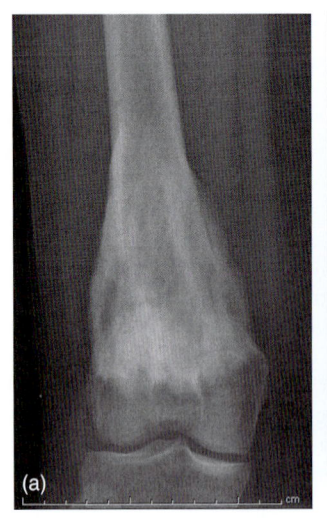

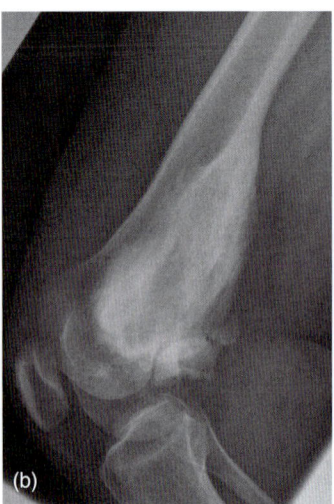

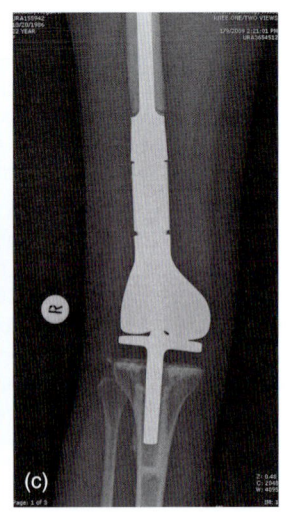

Figure 10 Low-grade central osteosarcoma. This 26-year-old woman was diagnosed with low-grade central osteosarcoma after a prolonged course with pain and swelling over several years. Plain anteroposterior (a) and lateral (b) radiographs show a sclerotic predominately intramedullary lesion of the distal femoral metaphysis. Biopsy showed streaming osteoid separated by a relatively bland fibrous background. Following wide surgical resection, the distal femur was reconstructed with a distal femoral replacement total knee arthroplasty (c).

same as for conventional osteosarcoma, but it has a predilection for the tibial diaphysis and the femoral diaphysis. Radiographically, in addition to its diaphyseal surface predilection, periosteal osteosarcoma is characterized by mineralization, which may present as a sunburst periosteal reaction or patchy calcification reflecting its often chondroblastic histology. Under the microscope, periosteal osteosarcoma is similar to conventional osteosarcoma except for being intermediate grade and usually having a chondroblastic pattern. Treatment usually employs conventional neoadjuvant chemotherapy followed by wide surgical resection. Prognosis is intermediate between parosteal and conventional osteosarcoma.

Secondary

Secondary osteosarcomas have a peak age in older patients, have the worst prognosis of all osteosarcomas, and arise within the setting of a predisposing condition, either Paget's disease of bone or previous irradiation. Osteosarcoma arising as the high-grade component of a dedifferentiated chondrosarcoma is discussed in the chondrosarcoma section.

Pagetoid

Sarcomatous degeneration within Paget's disease occurs in a small percentage (1–15%) of patients with this metabolic bone condition characterized by rapid bone turnover. Peak age is in 55 to 85 years old. Clinical presentation is usually heralded by a change in the patient's baseline pain and/or a new soft-tissue mass or swelling. Due to the prevalence of Paget's disease in flat bones, Paget's osteosarcoma has a predilection for the scapula, pelvis, and ribs. Radiographic presentation is usually of an aggressive osteoblastic or osteolytic area arising within Pagetoid bone. Treatment involves chemotherapy—if the patient can tolerate it—and wide surgical resection. The benefits of chemotherapy in this group remain unproven. Prognosis is poor, with 5-year survival 5–18%.[2]

Postradiation

The criteria for defining postradiation sarcoma is that the sarcoma arises within a previously irradiated area without a preexisting sarcoma of the same histologic type and that a latent period of at least 3–4 years has elapsed since the initial radiotherapy and the development of the sarcoma. Postradiation osteosarcoma arises within previously irradiated bone and represents 70% of postradiation bone sarcomas. Other pathologies include malignant fibrous histiocytoma and fibrosarcoma. Clinical presentation is that of swelling and pain arising within the previously irradiated region. Radiographically, postradiation sarcomas of bone appear as an aggressive lesion within the previously irradiated field. Under the microscope, they may show the histology of high-grade conventional osteosarcoma, malignant fibrous histiocytoma, or fibrosarcoma. Treatment is by surgical resection and adjuvant chemotherapy when the patient can tolerate it, although the benefits of chemotherapy in this group are unproven.[139] Prognosis is extremely poor, ranging from 5% to 30% 5-year survival.

Small cell

Other than their histologic appearance, small-cell osteosarcomas resemble high-grade conventional osteosarcomas. Under the microscope, the only feature that distinguishes this tumor—comprised predominantly of small round blue cells with indistinct cytoplasm—from Ewing sarcoma is the presence of osteoid, which is sometimes difficult to identify on biopsy. Treatment and prognosis are as for conventional osteosarcoma.

Vascular sarcomas

There are two major subtypes of vascular sarcomas in the current WHO classification which may involve bone: epithelioid hemangioendothelioma and angiosarcoma.[140–142] Hemangiopericytoma, which has previously been included in this category, has been reclassified as a solid fibrous tumor in the latest WHO schema.[3] These tumors represent a spectrum of disease, with hemangioendothelioma at the less aggressive end of the spectrum and angiosarcoma at the aggressive end. These are rare tumors, as a group representing less than 1% of bone sarcomas. Clinically, they have a broad age range but are most common in middle-aged and older adults. As with most bone sarcomas, presenting symptoms include pain and swelling. Rarely, pathologic fracture may occur, more commonly with angiosarcoma. One-third of patients with vascular sarcomas will have multifocal disease, either "skipping joints" in a single limb or involving disseminated sites throughout the body. Any bone may be affected, but long bones predominate.

Radiographically, these tumors are typically lytic and destructive, but a combination of osteolysis and sclerosis may be seen. Soft-tissue extension is not usually seen in these tumors. Under the microscope, each tumor has a characteristic appearance with some evidence of rudimentary vascular channels.

Treatment of vascular sarcomas may involve wide surgical resection or radiotherapy. Epithelioid hemangioendothelioma is a particularly radiosensitive tumor and may be treated primarily with radiotherapy. The role of chemotherapy for this group of tumors is not well established. For extensive or multifocal disease, radiotherapy has efficacy.

Metastatic disease to bone

The most common malignancy to affect bone is metastatic carcinoma. It is far more common than bone sarcoma or myeloma. The most common "osteophilic" primary tumors to affect bone arise from primaries of the breast, prostate, lung, kidney, and thyroid. Patients with breast and prostate cancer have usually had their primary cancer treated and then develop delayed metastatic disease to bone. Patients with metastatic lung carcinoma more commonly present with metastatic bone disease as the presenting symptom of their lung cancer. Patients with kidney and thyroid cancer may present with either concurrent or delayed metastatic disease. For a primary carcinoma metastatic to bone in a patient with no history of cancer, the most common sources are lung and kidney primaries. Metastatic carcinoma to bone most commonly involves patients older than 40 years. In patients less than 5, metastatic neuroblastoma predominates, and in older pediatric patients, rhabdomyosarcoma is the most common primary source. Presenting symptoms may involve pain, swelling, or pathologic fracture, but in some cases, the bone lesions are asymptomatic and are discovered on routine staging studies. In the spine, neurologic symptoms and even paraplegia may be seen. The most common sites are the spine, proximal femur, pelvis, ribs, sternum, proximal humerus, and skull. Metastases distal to the elbow and knee are unusual, and when they are present, the most common source is lung carcinoma.

Evaluation of bone lesions suspected of being due to metastatic disease involves a comprehensive physical examination, laboratory parameters, and a radiographic evaluation of common sites of primary disease. Since myeloma is often in the differential diagnosis of metastatic carcinoma in adults, serum and urine protein electrophoresis is often requested. Lactate dehydrogenase may be elevated in lymphoma, although it is nonspecific. Prostate-specific

Table 11 Examples of immunohistochemistry markers for evaluation of metastatic disease to bone.

Immunohistochemistry marker	Primary tumor source
Prostate-specific antigen (PSA)	Prostate carcinoma
Thyroid transcription factor (TTF-1)	Lung carcinoma
Leukocyte common antigen (LCA)	Lymphoma

antigen is usually elevated in prostate cancer. Renal cell carcinoma may cause hematuria. Standard radiographs of any involved bone, a total skeleton bone scan, and CT's of the chest, abdomen, and pelvis comprise the classic radiographic evaluation. Increasingly, PET-CTs are being utilized in this setting.

Radiographically, metastatic carcinoma may have a myriad of appearances. Some tumors, such as prostate metastases, are typically osteoblastic. Breast cancer metastases usually show a combination of osteolysis and sclerosis. Metastases from lung, kidney, and thyroid cancer are usually purely osteolytic. Bone scans usually show increased uptake at multiple sites, but solitary metastatic lesions are not uncommon, and certain very aggressive bone metastases, such as those from renal or thyroid carcinoma, may not show increased uptake. Pathology often falls into a general descriptive category, such as adenocarcinoma, squamous cell carcinoma, or poorly-differentiated carcinoma. In these cases, immunohistochemistry markers are of greater importance in identifying the source (Table 11). Some tumors have specific histopathology patterns, such as clear cell carcinoma of the kidney, well-differentiated follicular carcinoma of the thyroid, and metastatic pigmented malignant melanoma of the skin.

Treatment of metastases can be viewed as systemic and local. Systemic treatment is directed both at the primary tumor (discussed in other chapters throughout the text) and at the mediator of bone destruction, the osteoclast. Bisphosphonates have become widely accepted in the setting of metastatic bone disease to inhibit the osteoclastic bone destruction. Operative management of metastatic carcinoma, myeloma, lymphoma has been discussed in a previous section. Once bone metastases are diagnosed, prognosis is poor, but survival varies according to the underlying primary tumor (Table 12).

Myeloma

Myeloma represents the most common primary bone malignancy. As it is covered elsewhere in this text, only the details related to bone will be presented here. Myeloma predominately affects adults aged 50 to 80 and has a propensity to affect blacks greater than Caucasians by a ratio of 2:1. Clinical presentation may involve pain, pathologic bone fracture, bone marrow failure (manifesting as fatigue and weakness from anemia, bruising and bleeding from thrombocytopenia, recurrent infections from neutropenia), renal failure, or hypercalcemia. A solitary plasmacytoma in the bone does not clinch the diagnosis of myeloma. Diagnostic criteria for myeloma include at least 10% plasma cells in the bone marrow, monoclonal protein in the serum (monoclonal gammopathy on serum protein electrophoresis) or urine (Bence-Jones proteins on urine protein electrophoresis), and end-organ failure (hypercalcemia, renal insufficiency, anemia, or bone lesions).

Radiographic manifestations of myeloma include single or multiple "punched-out" small lytic lesions sometimes coalescing into much larger lesions. Since 80% of myeloma bone lesions do not show increased uptake on bone scan, a skeletal survey should be considered to search for other lesions during the initial evaluation. Under the microscope, myeloma is comprised of sheets of plasma cells with large round, clockface, eccentric nuclei, and perinuclear clearing.

Bone lesions from myeloma are very sensitive to radiotherapy but for large lesions or those with pathologic fracture, surgical fixation is warranted. For surgical management of myeloma bone manifestations, please refer to the earlier section.

Bone lymphoma

Primary lymphoma of bone was first described as "reticulum cell sarcoma" and is comprised of malignant lymphoid infiltrate within bone in the absence of concurrent lymph node or visceral involvement. Just about any age may be affected, and the most common locations are the femur, ilium, and ribs. Clinical presentation may include pain, an associated soft-tissue mass, or pathologic fracture. Unlike diffuse lymphoma, these patients rarely have systemic symptoms.

Radiographically, lymphoma may be diaphyseal or metaphyseal and typically has a permeative, poorly defined border on plain films. Many cases are osteolytic, but in some cases, a sclerotic appearance may simulate osteosarcoma. Under the microscope, primary lymphoma of bone is a small round blue cell tumor which requires immunohistochemistry in order to distinguish it from Ewing sarcoma. Ninety percent of primary bone lymphomas are large B-cell type. Immunohistochemical markers for B-cells include CD19 and CD20.

Treatment of primary bone lymphoma requires a multidisciplinary approach. Chemotherapy is the primary treatment modality, with surgery reserved for biopsy, fracture fixation, and prophylactic fixation of impending fractures. Chemotherapy often involves CHOP (cyclophosphamide, doxorubicin, vincristine, and prednisone) and rituximab (monoclonal antibody against CD20). Although local radiotherapy is often employed in addition to chemotherapy, recent reports are beginning to question its benefits to overall survival, particularly in light of its adverse effects on bone fragility and fracture healing.

Table 12 Common primary tumors metastatic to bone: frequency of bone involvement and survival after metastases.[a]

Primary tumor	Percentage of patients that develop metastatic disease (%)	Fraction of patients with mets who have bone involvement clinically (%)	Median survival after diagnosis of mets (months)	Mean 5 year survival (%)
Breast carcinoma	65–75		24	20
Prostate carcinoma	65–75	30–40	40	25
Lung carcinoma	30–40	20–40	<6	<5
Renal carcinoma	20–25	15–25	6	10
Thyroid carcinoma	60	20–40	48	40

[a]Source: Data from Coleman[143] and Table from Damron.[144]

Congenital syndromes
A number of congenital syndromes either involve bone lesions, predispose to development of bone malignancies, or both. Some of these syndromes are covered in this section.

Enchondromatosis
Enchondromatosis may involve simply multiple enchondromas (Ollier disease) or the combination of multiple enchondromas with multiple soft-tissue hemangiomas (Maffucci syndrome). Both syndromes occur sporadically. Neither has a known cause. They are uncommon and are typically diagnosed in childhood. Radiographically, the enchondromas individually are not different than those of solitary disease. The most important distinguishing feature of these two syndromes is the risk of developing malignancy.

Ollier disease
Multiple enchondromatosis carries up to a 20–30% risk of developing one or more chondrosarcomas. Hence, these patients should be followed on an annual basis for surveillance. The most common locations for chondrosarcomas in Ollier disease are the pelvis, proximal femur, and proximal humerus.

Maffucci syndrome
Patients with Maffucci syndrome are also at risk of developing chondrosarcomas, but they are at increased risk of developing numerous other types of malignancies as well. In fact, the risk of malignancy in Maffucci patients approaches 100%. Common primaries include acute lymphocytic leukemia, astrocytoma, and gastrointestinal malignancies. Vigilant surveillance is essential for early diagnosis of these tumors.

Familial adenomatous polyposis
The early onset of multiple colorectal polyps characterizes this autosomal dominant condition caused by a mutation in the adenomatous polyposis coli (APC) gene. The only bone lesion associated with familial adenomatous polyposis (and the related Gardner syndrome) is osteoma. These lesions do not require specific treatment nor do they predispose to bone malignancy. The only malignancy associated with this familial adenomatous polyposis is colon cancer.

Polyostotic fibrous dysplasia, McCune–Albright syndrome, and Mazabraud's syndrome While most fibrous dysplasia lesions occur in a single location (monostotic), some involve multiple bones (polyostotic fibrous dysplasia). In addition, polyostotic fibrous dysplasia may be accompanied in 30–50% of cases by extraskeletal manifestations of disease, including distinctive pigmented cutaneous markings with a "coast-of-Maine" irregular border in a distribution respecting the midline of the body, Gonadotropin-independent sex steroid production causing precocious puberty, recurrent ovarian cysts in girls or autonomous testosterone production in boys and men, thyroid lesions, growth hormone excess, or neonatal hypercortisolism, a syndrome named McCune–Albright (or Albright's syndrome).[88] However, the diagnosis of McCune–Albright disease may also be made based upon presence of two extraskeletal manifestations of the GNAS gene aberration.[88] Rarely, fibrous dysplasia may occur in the setting of soft tissue myxomas (Mazabraud's syndrome). The common etiologic thread for these conditions is the presence of activating mutations of the GNAS1 gene. Usually, these patients are diagnosed in childhood or adolescence either with manifestations of their underlying bone disease (pain, limp, swelling, angular deformity, limb-length discrepancy, or craniofacial abnormalities), the characteristic skin lesions, precocious puberty, or one of aforementioned extraskeletal manifestations.

Radiographically and histologically, the individual fibrous dysplasia lesions are the same as those described previously for solitary fibrous dysplasia. Treatment should address any associated condition (particularly the FGF-23-associated hypophosphatemia and associated endocrinopathies) as well as the bone manifestations. Since polyostotic fibrous dysplasia is more often associated with progressive deformity, particularly in the proximal femur, more aggressive prophylactic treatment—including both surgical intervention and bisphosphonate therapy—should be considered. Malignancy in these conditions is rare and usually preceded by radiotherapy.

Multiple osteochondromatosis
An autosomal dominant condition attributable to mutation of either the EXT1 or EXT2 gene, multiple osteochondromatosis (multiple hereditary exostoses) is rare compared to the solitary occurrence of osteochondromas, the most common benign bone tumors.[87] The underlying pathology is related to absent or abnormal heparin sulfate due to the EXT1 and EXT2 gene alterations, resulting in abnormal growth plate cartilage function through downstream mediators believed to include Indian hedgehog, fibroblastic growth factors, bone morphogenic proteins, Wnt signaling pathway, and parathyroid related protein.[87] The condition is usually diagnosed in early childhood between ages 2 and 10. Typical manifestations include "knobby" protuberances near joints, short stature, shortened limbs, coax valga, genu valgum, radial head dislocation, and pain. Radiologic features consist of multiple osteochondromas, each of which has the characteristic features of a solitary osteochondroma. As for solitary osteochondromas, excision is only recommended for symptomatic tumors. Risk of malignant degeneration has been estimated at between 3% and 10% and typically involves a low-grade chondrosarcoma (Figure 11).

Osteopoikilosis and related syndromes
Osteopoikilosis is the presence of multiple bone islands (enostoses). Its main importance is in distinguishing it from osteosclerotic metastases such as those from prostate cancer, and the use of CT attenuation values has become a valuable tool in this regard.[100,101] Buschke–Ollendorff syndrome (also known as dermatofibrosis lenticularis disseminata, dermato-osteopoikilosis, and familial cutaneous collagenoma) is an autosomal recessive disease resulting from mutations in the LEMD3 gene and characterized by painless cutaneous connective tissue nevi (elastomas, collagenomas, or fibromas) combined with osteopoikilosis and sometimes other noncutaneous manifestations.

Gardner syndrome
Gardner syndrome, an autosomal dominant genetic condition related to mutations in the APC gene, is characterized by multiple colorectal polyps and numerous types of both benign and malignant tumors. From an orthopedic perspective, the syndrome may be associated with osteomas of bone as well as fibromas, lipomas, and desmoid tumors of the soft tissue. Close monitoring of these patients for development of colon cancer is pertinent due to their high risk. However, numerous other cancers, including those of visceral and endocrine origin occur at increased frequency in these patients.

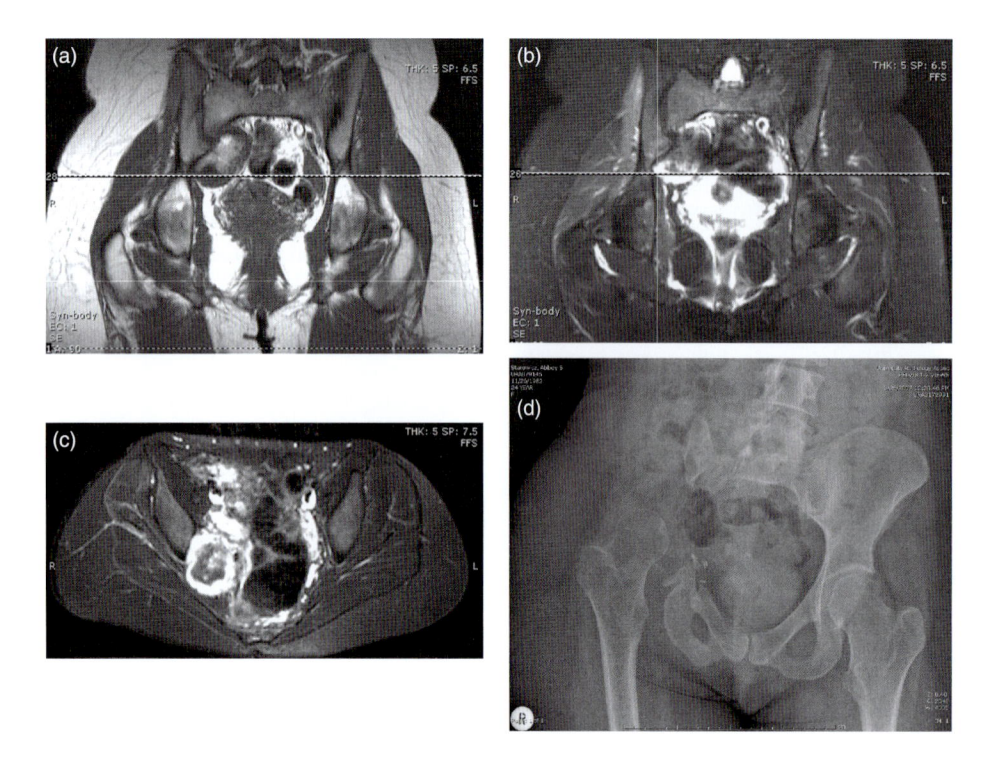

Figure 11 Secondary chondrosarcoma in osteochondromatosis. A 23-year-old woman with known multiple hereditary exostoses developed pelvic pain. Radiographs were not revealing, but MRI images (a–c) revealed a mass arising from a small osteochondroma on the inner table of the pelvis beginning at the level of the sacroiliac joint and extending to the sciatic notch. Biopsy confirmed low-grade chondrosarcoma. The patient underwent internal hemipelvectomy without reconstruction (d). The pelvis is a common location for development of chondrosarcomas in osteochondromatosis, and regular screening in these patients is advisable.

Retinoblastoma syndrome

Patients with a germline mutation of the RB1 gene are predisposed to develop not only retinoblastoma but also—via a "second hit" somatic mutation—other malignancies, the most common of which is osteosarcoma. Hence, this syndrome has also been referred to as "retinoblastoma/osteogenic sarcoma syndrome." Patients with retinoblastoma are usually diagnosed before age 3, and the potential for osteosarcoma peaks in the adolescent age range. Radiographic presentation, histology, and treatment of the osteosarcoma are the same as for conventional high-grade osteosarcoma, discussed previously.

Rothmund–Thomson syndrome

This rare syndrome is important in the context of bone tumors because of its predisposition for development of osteosarcoma. An autosomal recessive genetically transmitted syndrome attributable to mutation in the RECQL4 helicase gene on chromosome 8, Rothmund–Thomson syndrome is usually diagnosed within the first 6 months of life based on a characteristic sun-sensitive erythematous rash that eventually leaves a hyper- and hypo-pigmented poikiloderma. Genetic testing confirms the disorder in a substantial number of cases, but related conditions such as Werner syndrome and Bloom syndrome should be excluded. Other orthopedic associated manifestations include osteoporosis, clavicular hypoplasia, syndactyly, patellar aplasia, genu valgum, and benign osseous lesions. There is no specific treatment for Rothmund–Thomson syndrome. High vigilance should be maintained to diagnosis musculoskeletal malignancies such as osteosarcoma.

Werner syndrome

A syndrome related to Rothmund–Thomson syndrome by gene homology and clinical overlap, Werner syndrome (adult progeria) is another autosomal recessive disorder and is caused by mutation in the WRN gene on chromosome 8. The resultant RecQ helicase deficiency predisposes to development of a wide variety of malignancies, including osteosarcoma, although soft-tissue sarcomas, thyroid cancer, and melanomas are much more common. Diagnosis is not usually made until adulthood due to manifestations of premature aging (scleroderma, premature graying and alopecia, nonsenile cataracts, calcific valvular deposits, atherosclerosis, diabetes, and hypogonadism) confirmed by genetic testing and elevation of urinary hyaluronic acid level. Orthopedic associated conditions include osteoporosis, muscle wasting, calcific deposits, and pes planus. For patients with an established diagnosis of Werner syndrome, vigilance should be maintained for the early diagnosis of malignancy.

Key references

The complete reference list can be found on Vital Source version of this title, see inside front cover.

1. American Cancer Society. *American Cancer Society: Cancer Facts and Figures 2014*. Atlanta: American Cancer Society; 2014. http://www.cancer.org/acs/groups/content/@research/documents/webcontent/acspc-042151.pdf (accessed 13 July 2021).
2. Damron TA, Ward WG, Stewart A. Osteosarcoma, chondrosarcoma, and Ewing's sarcoma: National Cancer Data Base Report. *Clin Orthop Relat Res.* 2007;**459**:40–47.
3. CDM F, Bridge JA, Hogendoorn P, Mertens F (eds). *WHO Classification of Tumours of Soft Tissue and Bone*, 4th ed. WHO Press; 2013.

4. Kelly C. Chapter 4.2. Benign tumors of bone. In: Damron TA, ed. *Orthopaedic Essentials: Oncology and Basic Science*. Lippincott, Williams, and Wilkins; 2008:54–60.
5. Davies AM, Sundaram M, James SJ (eds). *Imaging of Bone Tumors and Tumor-Like Lesions: Techniques and Applications*. Springer Science & Business Media; 2009.
7. Enneking WF, Spanier SS, Goodman MA. A system for the surgical staging of musculoskeletal sarcoma. *Clin Orthop Relat Res*. 1980;**153**:106–120.
8. Heck RK Jr, Peabody TD, Simon MA. Staging of primary malignancies of bone. *CA Cancer J Clin*. 2006;**56**:366–375.
9. Amin MB, Edge SB, Greene FL, et al. (eds). *AJCC Cancer Staging Manual*, 8th ed. Switzerland: Springer; 2017.
10. Tanaka K, Ozaki T. New TNM classification (AJCC eighth edition) of bone and soft tissue sarcomas: JCOG Bone and Soft Tissue Tumor Study Group. *Jpn J Clin Oncol*. 2019;**49**(2):103–107. doi: 10.1093/jjco/hyy157.
11. AJCC. Bone sarcoma. In: *AJCC Cancer Staging Manual*, 7th ed. New York, NY: Springer:2010.
14. Mankin HJ, Lange TA, Spanier SS. The hazards of biopsy in patients with malignant primary bone and soft tissue tumors. *J Bone Joint Surg Am*. 1982;**64**:1121–1127.
15. Mankin HJ, Mankin CJ, Simon MA. The hazards of the biopsy, revisited. Members of the musculoskeletal tumor society. *J Bone Joint Surg Am*. 1996;**78**:656–663.
16. Wolf RE, Enneking WF. The staging and surgery of musculoskeletal neoplasms. *Orthop Clin North Am*. 1996;**27**(3):473–481.
19. Wilke B, Cooper A, Scarborough M, et al. Comparison of limb salvage versus amputation for nonmetastatic sarcomas using patient-reported outcomes measurement information system outcomes. *J Am Acad Orthop Surg*. 2019;**27**(8):e381–e389. doi: 10.5435/JAAOS-D-17-00758.
20. Mirels H. Metastatic disease in long bones. *Clin Orthop*. 1989:256–264.

109 Soft tissue sarcomas

Katherine A. Thornton, MD ■ Elizabeth H. Baldini, MD, MPH, FASTRO ■ Robert G. Maki, MD, PhD, FACP, FASCO ■ Brian O'Sullivan, MD ■ Yan Leyfman, MD ■ Chandrajit P. Raut, MD, MSc, FACS

Overview

The management of soft tissue sarcomas is driven by the anatomic site as well as the histologic subtype of the primary disease. In this chapter, we focus on the importance of a multidisciplinary approach to this diverse group of over 75 different tumor types.

We will discuss in this chapter the etiology, clinical presentation, staging, histopathologic classification and prognostic factors for patients with soft tissue sarcoma. Surgery remains paramount to achieving cure for the vast majority of sarcomas. We will discuss how adjunctive therapies, like radiation and chemotherapy can improve overall outcome, as well as highlight the limitations and unanswered questions, both with respect to local recurrence and distant metastases. Where appropriate, we attempt to link specific histologies or molecular changes to the therapeutic approach to disease. We hope to draw attention to the fact that in a field that has traditionally had stagnation in the development of new therapeutic strategies, there has been a renaissance of new molecularly and mechanistically targeted therapies helping to improve outcomes for soft tissue sarcoma patients.

Sarcomas of nonosseous tissues, known traditionally as soft tissue sarcomas (STS), comprise a group of rare malignancies that exhibit tremendous diversity of anatomic site, specific genetic alterations, and histopathologic characteristics. These tumors share a common embryologic origin, arising primarily from mesodermal tissues. The notable exceptions are (1) sarcomas of the neural tissues (such as malignant peripheral nerve sheath tumors [MPNST]) and possibly the Ewing sarcoma/primitive neuroectodermal tumor (PNET) family of tumors, which are believed to arise from ectodermal tissues and (2) angiosarcomas, which are derived from endoderm. Despite the fact that the somatic nonosseous tissues account for as much as 75% of total body weight, primary neoplasms of these connective tissues are comparatively rare, accounting for <1% of adult malignancies and 15% of pediatric malignancies. About 13,460 people receive a diagnosis of STS in the United States each year, with approximately 5,350 deaths annually.[1] An understanding of these cancers is important because patients' outcomes will be compromised if initial management is not thoughtfully planned and judiciously executed. Furthermore, biologic insights about sarcomas are providing new strategies for the detection, treatment, and prevention of more common malignancies.

This article reviews current concepts in the diagnosis, staging, and multidisciplinary management of patients with sarcomas of nonosseous tissues. The evolving and expanding contributions of molecular biology and basic scientific principles underlying the varied differentiation and clinical behavior of these tumors will also be reviewed. Although histopathologic aspects of sarcomas are increasingly important in categorizing these tumors, the anatomic site of primary disease remains an important variable on which treatment and outcome may depend. Extremity soft tissue sarcomas (ESTS), retroperitoneal sarcomas (RPS), gastrointestinal stromal tumors (GIST), and dermatofibrosarcoma protuberans (DFSP) are addressed separately in the article. Sarcomas at other anatomic sites are not discussed because of their rarity. Throughout the article, the emphasis is on identifying what is known from definitive data and what requires additional research.

Etiology

Most sarcomas are believed to arise spontaneously.[2] The conceptual frameworks that address the neoplastic transformation of mesenchymal stem cells are in rapid evolution owing to new insights from the molecular analysis of sarcomatous and normal tissues from STS patients and family members. Genetics and environmental factors each appear to play a role in the neoplastic transformation of soft tissues into sarcomas.[3]

Sarcomas can arise in persons with certain genetic predispositions to cancer development. One such autosomal dominant genetic predisposition, Li–Fraumeni syndrome, has been characterized at the molecular level as a germline mutation of the *TP53* gene, which acts as a faulty tumor suppressor.[4,5]

Other genetic disorders are also associated with an increased risk of developing specific sarcomas. The best-studied example of this is the predilection of patients with neurofibromatoses to develop MPNSTs (also referred to as neurofibrosarcomas or malignant schwannomas).[6,7] Type 1 neurofibromatosis (von Recklinghausen disease) is an autosomal dominant disease that can disrupt the function of the *NF1* gene, located on chromosome 17q11.2. The endogenous function of the *NF1* gene product, neurofibromin, remains incompletely understood, but it appears to act as a tumor suppressor via stimulation of guanosine triphosphatase activity. Common mutations in *NF1* include truncations, with loss of function leading to uncontrolled signaling through *ras* pathways, which impact therapeutic options.[8,9] *NF1* loss appears to be a fundamental process that facilitates the development of MPNSTs over time in patients with neurofibromatosis. Patients with type 1 neurofibromatosis have up to a 10% cumulative lifetime risk of developing sarcoma (usually MPNST); it is unclear why the risk is not greater, given the protean effects of *ras* activation; other factors such as inactivation of epigenetic regulators in the PRC2 complex may contribute to the neoplastic phenotype.[10–12]

Survivors of childhood retinoblastoma have also been noted to have an increased risk of sarcoma development.[13,14] These data provide another model of a dysfunctional or deleted tumor suppressor genetic element (in this case, the product of the *Rb* gene on chromosome 13q14). The risk of STS in retinoblastoma patients and their families is accompanied by the risk of developing several other types of neoplasms, including osteosarcomas, breast cancer, and lung cancer. No reasons have been convincingly posited for the development of one type of malignancy over another in patients with *Rb* mutations, and this remains an important question to be addressed by future research on mechanisms of neoplastic transformation.

Gardner syndrome represents an important genetic connection between dysfunctional regulation of epithelial and mesenchymal cells. Gardner syndrome represents a subset of familial adenomatous polyposis disorders of the bowel (usually the colon); patients with the syndrome also have extracolonic abnormalities such as epidermoid cysts and osteomas. The molecular lesion has been identified as a defect within the *APC* (adenomatous polyposis coli) gene on chromosome 5q21. Patients with Gardner syndrome are at much increased risk of developing mesenteric and intraperitoneal desmoid tumors.[15,16] Desmoid tumors are mesenchymal cells proliferating in a pattern of aggressive fibromatosis, characterized by bland cells that—although histologically benign—act in a malignant fashion with uncontrolled proliferation and infiltration of vital structures; spontaneous desmoid tumors more commonly demonstrate mutations in the beta-catenin gene, *CTNNB1*, which is in the same signaling pathway as *APC*.[17,18] It remains poorly understood why some patients with Gardner syndrome develop desmoid tumors whereas others do not, and the lifetime risk of developing desmoid tumors has been estimated at approximately 10–20%, representing a nearly 1000 times greater risk than that of the general population.

Certain environmental exposures have also been associated with the development of sarcomas. One of the most important is ionizing radiation. Radiation-associated sarcoma is most often a late effect of radiotherapy (RT) given to treat another condition (often a prior malignancy). Sarcomas have been noted as a late effect of RT for breast cancer, Hodgkin lymphoma, non-Hodgkin lymphomas, various childhood malignancies, and other tumor types.[19] The radiation dose appears to be correlated with the later development of sarcoma, with a very low risk in patients who received less than 10 Gy. The molecular mechanisms may be complex, since it has been noted clinically that sarcomas appear at the margins of prior RT fields. This suggests that the mutagenic effect may be maximal at the edges of prior RT where scatter radiation leads to a dose sufficient to induce mutations but insufficient to kill the mutated cells. Traditionally, radiation-associated sarcomas were thought to arise with a median of ~9 years following RT, although RT-associated sarcomas are observed earlier in some patients. MPNSTs, angiosarcomas, osteosarcomas, and undifferentiated pleomorphic sarcomas (UPS), angiosarcoma, MPNST and osteosarcomas comprise the majority of radiation-associated sarcomas. Clinical outcomes are worse in patients with radiation-associated sarcomas compared to histology matched controls. Radiation-associated sarcomas should be approached as new primary disease and treated appropriately to optimize the patient's outcomes.

Certain chemical exposures have also been weakly linked to sarcomagenesis, although chemical-induced development of sarcomas in animal models is one of the more reliable models of studying neoplastic transformation in the laboratory. Hepatic angiosarcomas are associated with exposure to several classes of chemicals, such as polyvinyl chloride and arsenic compounds.[20] The relationship between exposure and development of sarcoma is more tenuous for other compounds, including dioxins (such as Agent Orange and other phenoxyacetic acid-based herbicides) and chlorophenols used in wood preservatives.[21]

Chronic irritation or inflammation of tissues is a controversial potential cause of sarcomas. Certainly, there is an increased sarcoma risk in the lymphedematous arms of women who have undergone radical mastectomy (the Stewart–Treves syndrome), often with the additional complicating variable of prior RT.[22,23] Limited data, typically case reports only, suggest that other sources of chronic tissue irritation and inflammation might be associated with sarcomagenesis.[24] Although a history of trauma is not infrequently elicited from patients with STSs, the impact of such trauma on sarcoma development is dubious.

Severe and chronic immunosuppression following solid organ transplantation represents yet another risk factor for the development of sarcomas. Sarcomas represent a disproportionate percentage of tumors (10%) in patients following solid organ transplantation, with Kaposi sarcoma comprising the majority of these.[25,26]

Screening

Given the rarity of sarcomas in the general population, no general screening is indicated beyond routine health care surveillance. However, it is important for physicians to be aware of the predisposing genetic tendencies and environmental exposures that might increase patients' risk of sarcoma development. A complete family history should reveal clues about genetic predispositions, including a family history of polyposis, neurofibromatosis, retinoblastoma, any cancer at a young age in first-degree relatives, or sarcomas. Genetic counseling is appropriate to discuss issues relating to these predispositions, in particular given the finding of Li–Fraumeni in families that lack the canonical *TP53* mutations.[27] In patients at increased risk of sarcoma, a more detailed clinical evaluation might be required at a lower threshold of intervention than one might use in general practice. Rapidly growing masses, especially symptomatic ones, in patients with neurofibromatosis should be considered for biopsy and surgical removal to rule out the potential of sarcomatous transformation of a neurofibroma. Similarly, any superficial or deep abnormalities of skin or soft tissues in patients with a history of prior RT should be evaluated very thoroughly.

Clinical presentation, classification, and diagnosis

Sites of origin

Sarcomas of nonosseous tissues have been noted to arise at virtually all anatomic sites. The anatomic sites and site-specific histologic subtypes of more than 5113 sarcomas treated at a single referral institution are outlined in Figure 1. Approximately one-third to one-half of all sarcomas of nonosseous tissues occur in the lower extremities, where the most common histopathologic subtypes have traditionally been noted to include liposarcomas as well as UPS, formerly termed "malignant fibrous histiocytoma." With improved pathologic tools to categorize sarcomas (e.g., immunohistochemistry and genomic analysis), it is increasingly recognized that UPS may have some features in common with poorly differentiated liposarcomas or leiomyosarcomas, as well as other histologic subtypes.[28] RPS comprise 15–20% of all STSs, with well-differentiated/dedifferentiated liposarcoma and leiomyosarcoma being the predominant histologic subtypes. Visceral sarcomas including GIST account for an additional 24%, and head and neck sarcomas comprise approximately 4% of sarcomas.

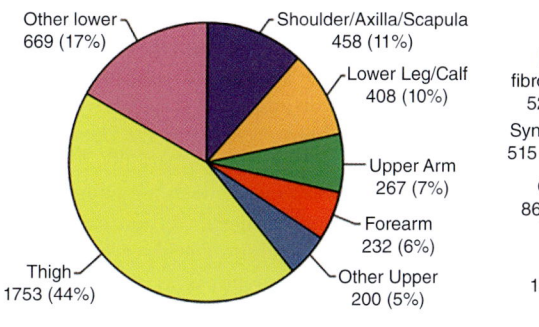

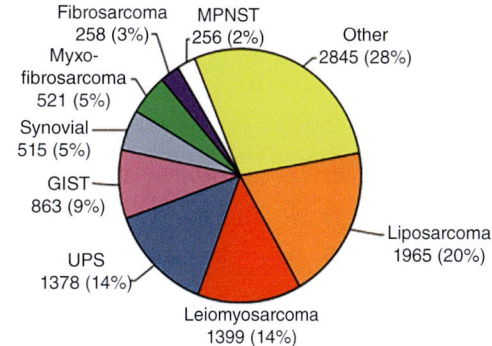

Figure 1 Anatomic distribution and site-specific histologic subtypes of 5113 consecutive STSs seen at the University of Texas MD Anderson Cancer Center Sarcoma Center (MDACC Sarcoma Database, June 1996 to June 2005).

Clinical presentation

The majority of patients with non-osseous sarcomas present with a painless mass, although pain is noted at presentation in up to one-third of cases.[29] Delay in diagnosis of sarcomas is common, with the most common incorrect diagnosis for extremity and trunk lesions being hematoma or "lipoma." Late diagnosis of RPS is extremely common, since tumors in this area can grow to massive size before causing any symptoms (such as abdominal distention or psoas irritation with back or groin discomfort) or functional compromise such as hydronephrosis from ureteric obstruction.

Physical examination should include an assessment of the size and mobility of the mass. Its relationship to the fascia (superficial vs deep) and nearby neurovascular and bony structures should be noted. A site-specific neurovascular examination and assessment of regional lymph nodes should also be performed. Sarcomas rarely metastasize to lymph nodes, with those that do being limited to a few specific histopathologic subtypes. Presence of true nodal metastases should prompt the clinician to investigate whether the diagnosis of sarcoma is accurate.

Histopathologic classification

Methods of classification

In broad terms, sarcomas can be classified as neoplasms arising in bone versus those arising from the nonosseous or peri-osseous soft tissues. Sarcomas of nonosseous tissues can be further grouped into those that arise from the viscera (e.g., gastrointestinal or gynecologic organs) and those that originate in nonvisceral soft tissues such as muscle, tendon, adipose tissue, pleura, synovium, and other connective tissues.

The most universally applied classification scheme for STS is based on histogenesis, as outlined in the recently updated WHO sarcoma classification system.[30] This classification system is reproducible between pathologists for the better differentiated tumors. However, as the degree of histologic differentiation declines, the determination of cellular origin becomes increasingly difficult. For example, pathologists may vary in their criteria to consider a tumor a UPS versus a poorly differentiated leiomyosarcoma; the use of specific DNA tests and ready availability of an increasing battery of immunohistochemical markers has improved consistency in diagnosis. Nonetheless, the lack of familiarity with sarcomas in general leads to misdiagnosis in over 20% of outside cases reviewed at reference centers.[31]

Previously, difficulties in establishing the specific cellular origin of STS were viewed as having limited clinical importance because clinical investigators did not have sufficient data to tie the histologic subtype directly to biologic behavior or to specific therapeutic interventions. Important exceptions to this generalization include epithelioid sarcoma, clear cell sarcoma, angiosarcoma, and embryonal rhabdomyosarcoma (ERMS), all of which have a greater risk of regional lymph node metastasis.[32,33] In a single-institution study, the overall rate of nodal metastasis at the time of presentation was only 2.7%; however, the rate was much higher for specific histologic subtypes: angiosarcoma (13%), ERMS (14%), and epithelioid sarcoma (17%), though the data were based on limited numbers.[32] While the impact of sentinel lymph node biopsy or lymphadenectomy on prognosis is still uncertain, additional treatment strategies may be considered for these histologies. For the remaining histologic subtypes, biologic behavior appears to be determined more by histologic grade than by histologic subtype. However, as the fundamental biologic and molecular understanding of the mechanisms of malignant transformation in sarcomas has increased and as understanding of individual histologic outcomes has improved, detailed categorization is proving to have important clinical ramifications. The tools required to categorize or subclassify sarcomas at the molecular level are now increasingly available for many sarcoma subtypes (Table 1). Clinical trials now generally take histologic and molecular characteristics into account in a more sophisticated manner than in the past three decades of research when markers were not so readily available.

Histologic grade

Biologic aggressiveness can often be predicted based on histologic grade.[34] The spectrum of grades varies among specific histologic subtypes. In careful comparative multivariate analyses, histologic grade has been the most important prognostic factor in assessing the risk of distant metastasis and tumor-related death.[34,35] Several grading systems have been proposed, but there is no consensus regarding the specific morphologic criteria that should be employed in the grading of STS.

Two of the most commonly employed grading systems, both first published in 1984, are the US National Cancer Institute (NCI) system developed by Costa and colleagues[28,29,36] and the system developed by the Federation Nationale des Centres de Lutte Contre le Cancer (FNCLCC) Sarcoma Group. The NCI system is based on the tumor's histologic subtype, location, and amount of tumor necrosis, but cellularity, nuclear pleomorphism, and mitosis count are also to be considered in certain situations. The FNCLCC system employs a score generated by the evaluation of three parameters: tumor differentiation, mitotic rate, and amount of tumor necrosis.

Table 1 Selected cytogenetic aberrations in nonosseous sarcomas.

Histologic subtype	Cytogenetic finding	Genes
Myxoid liposarcoma	t(12;16)	FUS-DDIT3
Well-differentiated liposarcoma	Rings and giant markers	Amplified 12q13-15
		HMG1C
		CDK4
		MDM2
Lipoma (minimal atypia)	12q abnormalities	Amplified 12q13-15
Lipoma	12q14-15 abnormalities	
	6p abnormalities	
Synovial sarcoma	t(X;18)	SS18-SSX1, SSX2, or SSX4
Ewing's family/PNET	t(11;22) and others	EWSR1-FLI1 and others
Rhabdomyosarcoma	t(2;13) or t(1;13)	PAX3(or 7)-FOXO1 (alveolar)
Clear cell sarcoma	t(12;22)	EWSR1-ATF1
Extraskeletal myxoid chondrosarcomas	t(9;22)	EWSR1-NR4A3
	t(9;17)	TAF15-NR4A3
Dermatofibrosarcoma protuberans	t(17;22)	COL1A1-PDGFB
Endometrial stromal sarcoma (low grade)	t(7;17)	JAZF1-SUZ12
Desmoplastic small round-cell tumor	t(11;22)	EWSR1-WT1
Alveolar sarcoma of soft parts	t(X;17)	ASPSCR1-TFE3

Abbreviation: PNET, primitive neuroectodermal tumors.

In a retrospective comparison of these two grading systems, in a population of 410 adult patients with nonmetastatic STS, univariate and multivariate analyses suggested that the FNCLCC system has a slightly better ability to predict distant metastasis and tumor-related death.[37] Significant discrepancies in assigned grade were observed in one-third of cases. An increased number of grade 3 tumors, reduced number of grade 2 tumors, and better correlation with overall and metastasis-free survival were observed in favor of the FNCLCC system. The FNCLCC system is the best presently available grading system and is employed as part of the AJCC (American Joint Committee on Cancer)/UICC STS staging system, with the caveat that several new diagnostic categories have been identified since 1984 whose histological grades are undefined by FNCLCC criteria.

In discussing grade, it is important to note well-described characteristics of sarcomas. First, there is often substantial intratumoral heterogeneity within individual sarcomas. Therefore, diagnoses based on very limited amounts of tumor may be inaccurate (e.g., diagnoses based only on fine-needle aspiration (FNA) biopsy specimens). This is particularly true for such histopathologic subtypes as de-differentiated liposarcomas, where one area of the tumor might have a relatively low-to-intermediate grade appearance and another area within the same tumor might have high-grade components more evident. Any discussion of the clinical relevance of grading must take into account this variability inherent in the diagnostic process, which will add to the clinical variability in outcomes among patients with any given grade of sarcomas.

Second, the grade of tumors may evolve over time. This process is best described in the evolution of de-differentiated liposarcoma arising in conjunction with well-differentiated liposarcoma in the same patient. Additional examples include the round cell liposarcoma growing from what was previously myxoid liposarcoma, and fibrosarcomatous degeneration that will occasionally accompany multiply recurrent DFSPs.

Imaging

Optimal imaging of the primary tumor is dependent on the anatomic site. For soft tissue masses of the extremities, trunk, and occasionally head and neck, magnetic resonance imaging (MRI) generally has been regarded as the imaging modality of choice (Figures 2 and 3) because MRI enhances the contrast between tumor and muscle and between tumor and adjacent blood vessels and provides multiplanar definition of the lesion.[38] A study by the Radiation Diagnostic Oncology Group that compared MRI and computed tomography (CT) in patients with malignant bone ($n = 183$) and soft tissue ($n = 133$) tumors demonstrated no specific advantage of MRI over CT, however.[39] That said, although it may be true that the diagnostic evaluation is equally served by both modalities, surgery and RT planning may require additional information provided by the multiplanar capability of MRI and the ability to perform MRI/CT image fusion.[40,41] For pelvic lesions or evaluation of specific fixed organs, such as rectum or liver, the multiplanar capability of MRI may provide superior single-modality imaging (Figure 3), whereas in the retroperitoneum and abdomen, CT usually provides satisfactory anatomic definition of the lesion. Occasionally, MRI with gradient sequence imaging can better delineate the relationship of a tumor to midline vascular structures, particularly the inferior vena cava and aorta (Figure 4). More invasive studies such as angiography or cavography are rarely used in evaluation of STS.

Cost-effective imaging to exclude the possibility of distant metastatic disease is dependent on the size, grade, and anatomic location of the primary tumor. In general, patients with low- and intermediate-grade tumors or high-grade tumors 5 cm or less in diameter require only a chest radiograph for satisfactory staging of the chest. This directly reflects the comparatively low risk of presentation with pulmonary metastases in these patients.[42,43] However, patients with high-grade tumors larger than 5 cm (T2) should undergo more thorough staging of the chest by CT owing to the increased risk of presentation with established metastatic disease in this group.[43,44] Patients with RPS and intra-abdominal visceral sarcomas should undergo imaging of the liver to exclude the possibility of synchronous hepatic metastases; the liver is a more common site of first metastasis from these lesions. CT is usually adequate in these patients to assess the liver, although the increased sensitivity of MRI of the liver may be valuable if any questionable findings are noted on initial CT.

Positron emission tomography (PET) scans may be used selectively to look for extent of disease, particularly when evaluating an ambiguous lesion that could represent a potential metastasis noted on other imaging. However, PET scans are not routinely utilized in staging work-up of STS.

Biopsy

Biopsy of the primary tumor is essential for most patients presenting with soft tissue masses. In general, any soft tissue mass in an adult that is enlarging (even if asymptomatic), is larger than 5 cm, or persists beyond 4–6 weeks should be biopsied. The preferred biopsy approach is generally the least invasive technique required to allow a definitive histologic diagnosis and assessment of grade. In most centers, core-needle biopsy provides sufficient tissue for diagnosis and results in substantial cost savings compared with open surgical biopsy.[45,46] When core-needle biopsy yields insufficient tissue for diagnosis, incisional biopsy is considered to yield optimal amounts of tissue to assess histopathology over a larger area of tumor volume, given the known heterogeneity of sarcomas, as well as to provide sufficient material for detailed molecular and

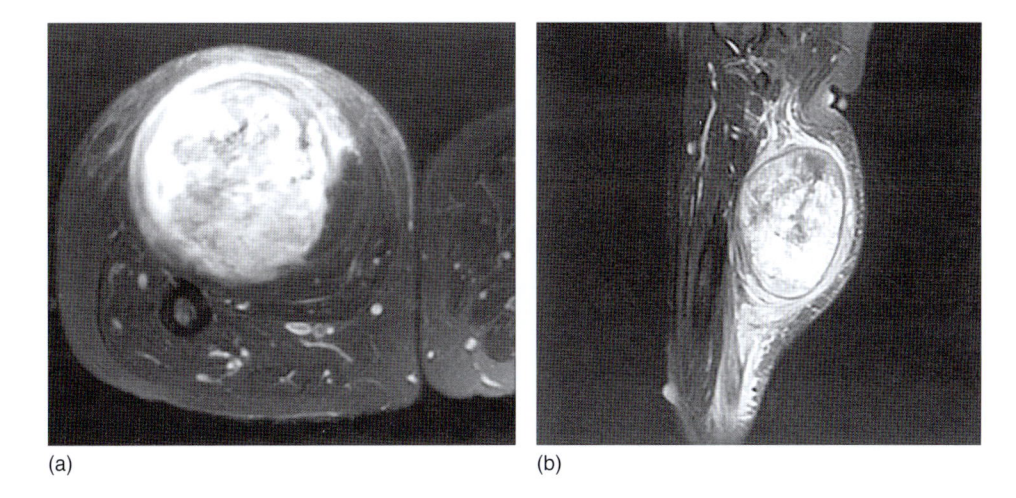

Figure 2 (a) Weighted T2-fat-saturated magnetic resonance image of a TNM T2b high-grade sarcoma in the posterior thigh compartment of a 55-year-old woman. Note the containment by the superficial fascia overlying the posterior thigh muscles, where there is a "strip" of peritumoral edema. Anteriorly, the lesion can be seen to be separate from the femur, but the edge of the tumor is less clearly defined than its superficial component, presumably because of muscle infiltration. (b) Sagittal MRI of the same patient. The main lesion manifests a well-defined border. However, a clear zone of peritumoral edema is evident tracking proximally toward the head of the femur, seen at the top of the figure. Inferiorly, the edema seems to be even more pronounced as evidenced by the triangular signal enhancement pointing inferiorly. Whether the zone of edema harbors microscopic disease is uncertain, and this uncertainty can complicate accurate treatment planning (see text).

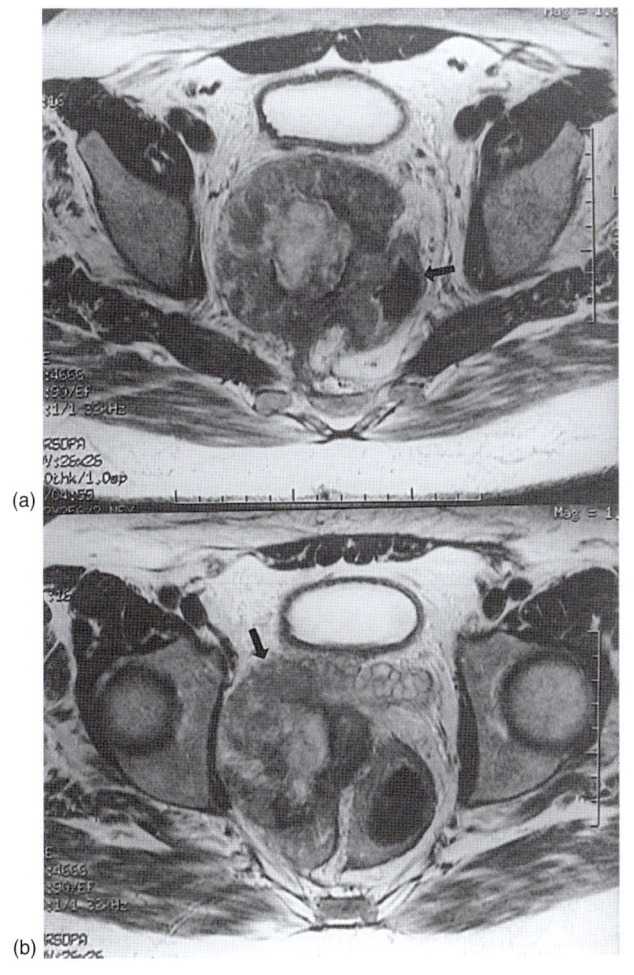

Figure 3 A 57-year-old man with T2 pelvic leiomyosarcoma. (a) Axial T2-weighted fast-spin echo MRI reveals a heterogeneous mass involving the rectum (*arrow,* air in rectal lumen). (b) Note that the mas abuts right seminal vesicle (*arrow*).

cytogenetic assays. Direct palpation can be used to guide needle biopsy of most superficial lesions, but less accessible sarcomas often require imaging-guided biopsy for safe percutaneous sampling of the most radiographically suspicious area(s) of the mass. Tumor recurrences within the needle track after percutaneous biopsy are exceedingly rare but have been reported, leading some physicians to advocate tattooing the biopsy site for subsequent excision. FNA generally does not provide sufficient material for initial diagnosis but can be used to confirm recurrence or metastatic disease. Exceptions to this idea exist; endoscopic ultrasound-guided FNA for visceral sarcomas such as GISTs may provide enough tissue for diagnosis while minimizing risk of tumor rupture; in this scenario, it is not feasible to assess mitotic rate. The need for sufficient tissue to conduct more specific molecular testing is a final major rationale for use of core needle biopsy over FNA. Another major limitation of FNA (compared to core-needle biopsy) is that there is no semblance of preserved tissue architecture to evaluate characteristics such as degree of tissue necrosis.

Small (<5 cm) superficial lesions on an extremity where the morbidity of excisional biopsy is minimal (i.e., remote from joints, tendons, and neurovascular structures that would compromise the surgical margin) are easily biopsied by excisional biopsy with microscopic assessment of surgical margins. For extremity lesions, incisions used for excisional biopsies should be oriented longitudinally along the length of the limb. T2 lesions, T1 lesions located beneath the investing fascia of the extremity, or superficial T1 lesions situated in proximity to joints, tendons, or neurovascular structures are best biopsied by percutaneous core-needle biopsy.

Staging and prognostic factors

Staging

The relative rarity of STS, the anatomic heterogeneity of these lesions, and the presence of more than 50 recognized histologic subtypes of variable grades have made it difficult to establish a

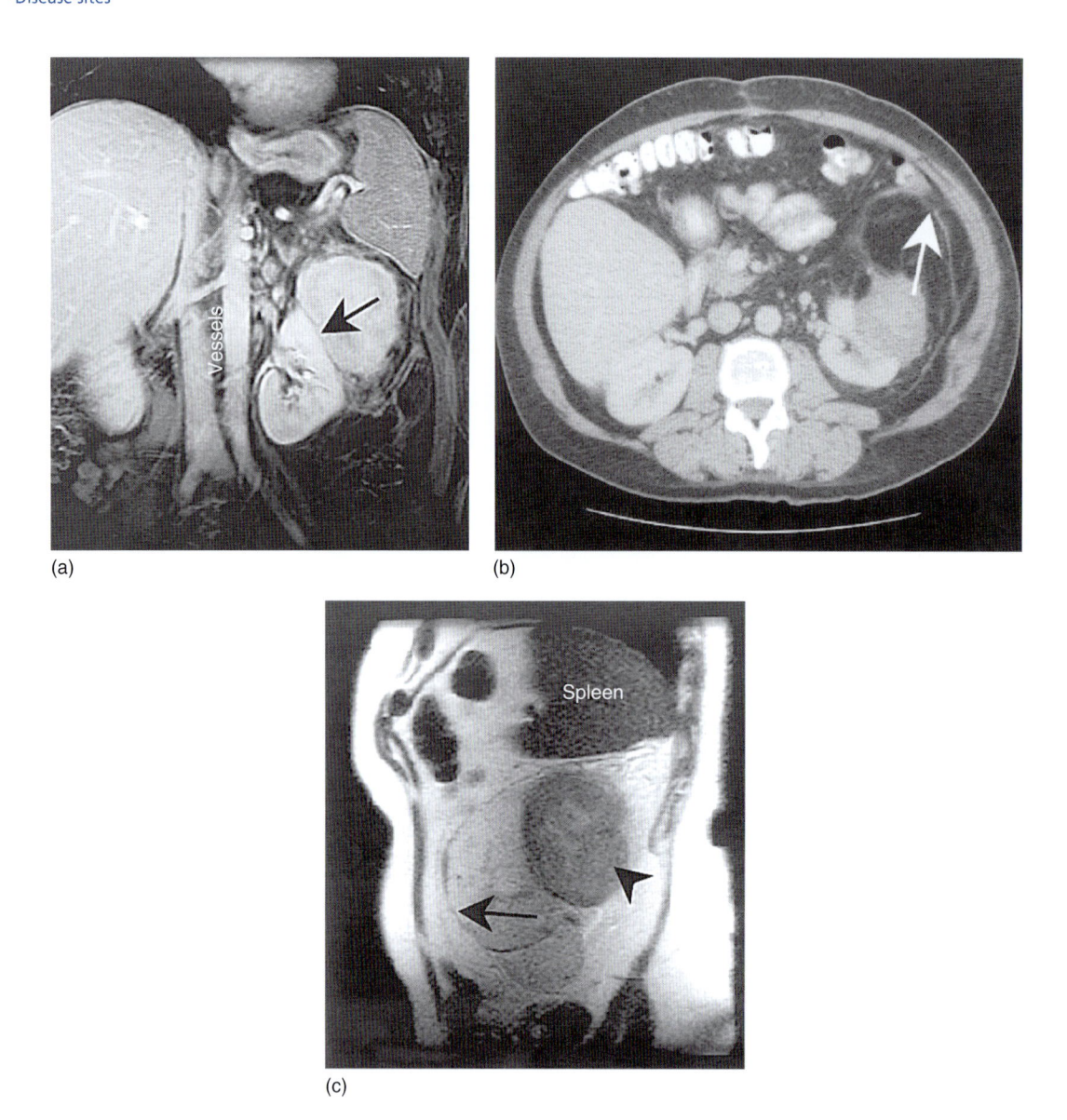

Figure 4 (a) Coronal fat-saturated gadolinium-enhanced MRI showing a solid liposarcoma, 8.3 × 6.6 cm, adjacent to and compressing the upper pole of the left kidney. The mass lies below the spleen and is separate from the kidney (line of demarcation, *arrow*) but is part of a larger fatty tumor. The midline vessels are well visualized. (b) CT image of the same lesion. The mass can be seen adjacent to the kidney, as before. An additional mass of fatty attenuation with gray areas of edema, inflammation, or increased cellularity can be seen bounded by a rim anteriorly (*arrow*). This mass has the appearance of abnormal fat, which must be considered in treatment planning. Note the displacement of bowel containing contrast. (c) Sagittal MR image of the same case but without gadolinium. The potential advantage of MR imaging in separating the anterior edge of the retroperitoneal sarcoma (*long arrow*) from the normal fat anteriorly is seen. The more solid component can also be seen (*arrowhead*) inferior to the spleen. In addition, these images can be exported digitally to a three-dimensional RT treatment planning workstation or CT simulator workstation where the MR images can be fused to the CT planning slices. This can provide more accurate demonstration of tumor in selected cases for contouring the gross tumor volume and clinical target volume than may be possible with CT images alone. This is particularly helpful in situations where CT does not show tumor as well as MRI.

functional system that can accurately stage all forms of this disease. The staging system (eighth edition) of the AJCC and the Union for International Cancer Control is the most widely employed staging system for STS (Table 2).[47] The system is designed to optimally stage extremity tumors but is also applicable to torso, head and neck, and retroperitoneal lesions; a separate staging system is provided for GIST.

A major limitation of the present staging system is that it does not take into account the anatomic site of STS. Anatomic site, however, has been recognized as an important determinant of outcome.[48,49] Therefore, although site is not a specific component of any present staging system, outcome data should be reported on a site-specific basis, when feasible. Furthermore, the staging system also fails to include histology, a critical prognostic factor.

Conventional prognostic factors

A thorough understanding of the clinicopathologic factors known to impact outcome is essential in formulating a treatment plan for the patient with STS. Several multivariate analyses of prognostic factors for patients with localized sarcoma have been reported.[50–52] However, with few exceptions, most studies have analyzed fewer than 300 patients.

Studies have established the clinical profile of what is now accepted as the high-risk patient with ESTS: the patient with a

Table 2 American Joint Committee on Cancer Staging System for STSs.[a]

T1	Tumor 5 cm or less in greatest dimension			
T2	Tumor more than 5 cm or less than or equal to 10 cm in greatest dimension			
T3	Tumor greater than 10 cm and less than or equal to 15 cm in greatest dimension			
T4	Tumor greater than 15 cm in greatest dimension			
N0	No regional lymph node metastasis or unknown lymph node status			
N1	Regional lymph node metastasis			
M0	No distant metastasis			
M1	Distant metastasis			
Stage IA	T1	N0	M0	G1
Stage IB	T2, T3, T4	N0	M0	G1
Stage II	T1	N0	M0	G2–3
Stage IIIA	T2	N0	M0	G2–3
Stage IIIB	T3, T4	N0	M0	G2–3
Stage IV	Any T	N1	M0	Any G
	Any T	Any N	M1	Any G

[a]Source: From Cates. American Joint Committee on Cancer AJCC cancer staging manual. 8th ed. Journal of the National Comprehensive Cancer Network Volume 16; Issue 2, February 2018.

large (≥5 cm), high-grade, deep lesion. In addition, unappreciated prognostic significance includes specific histologic subtypes, for example MPNST, and the increased risk of adverse outcome associated with a microscopically positive surgical margin or presentation with locally recurrent disease. The type of microscopically positive surgical margins also appears important. Patients with low-grade liposarcomas have a relatively low risk of local recurrence (LR), as do those patients in whom the positive margin is planned before surgery to preserve critical structures and RT can sterilize the small amount of residual disease. However, patients with two categories of positive margin remain at relatively higher risk of LR. These include patients who underwent "unplanned" excision and still have positive margins on re-excision and those with unanticipated positive margins after primary resection.[53] An "unplanned excision" is defined as an excisional biopsy or resection carried out without adequate preoperative staging or consideration of the need to remove normal tissue around the tumor.

Unlike for other solid tumors, the adverse prognostic factors for LR of a STS are distinct from those that predict distant metastasis and tumor-related death.[50] In other words, patients with a constellation of adverse prognostic factors for LR are not necessarily at increased risk of distant metastasis or tumor-related death. Therefore, staging systems that are designed to stratify patients for risk of distant metastasis and tumor-related death will not necessarily stratify patients for risk of LR.

Kattan et al.[49] from the Memorial Sloan-Kettering Cancer Center (MSKCC) have utilized a database of over 2000 prospectively followed adult patients with STS to predict the probability of sarcoma-specific death by 12 years. The results have been used to construct and internally validate a nomogram to predict sarcoma-specific death; this and similar nomograms have been validated in a variety of clinical situations, for example retroperitoneal sarcoma, or for disease-specific contexts, for example liposarcoma, for individual patients.[54–57] These tools may be used for patient counseling, follow-up scheduling, and clinical trial eligibility determination.

Potential molecular prognostic factors

Specific molecular parameters evaluated for prognostic significance in STS have included TP53 mutation, MDM2 amplification, Ki-67 status, and altered expression of the *RB* gene product in high-grade sarcomas. Histologic grade, but not SS18-SSX fusion type, appears to be an important prognostic factor in patients with synovial sarcoma.[58] Complete discussion of the extensive literature on molecular prognostic factors in sarcoma is beyond the scope of this article. Readers are referred to more detailed reviews.[59,60]

As an example of the difficulty of using even the most commonly recognized markers as prognostic factors, one need look no further than Ki-67, an antigen expressed throughout the majority of the cell cycle. Ki-67 is used as a measure of the fraction of cells undergoing division. Preliminary reports of series of heterogeneous sarcomas in adults suggested Ki-67 nuclear staining correlated with histologic grade but was not an independent prognostic factor when histologic grade was taken into account.[61] Conversely, additional studies in larger numbers of patients indicated Ki-67 status was an independent prognostic factor for clinical outcomes.[62] It is only with the development of consensus guidelines regarding the nature of Ki67 immunohistochemistry and its interpretation that we can expect to see more careful accurate assessment of this biomarker in sarcoma outcomes.[63] It is also with the inconsistencies in the Ki-67 data that one can extrapolate the difficulty of using increasingly available genetic markers for outcome determination. Although specific protein, DNA and RNA parameters have been identified as having independent prognostic significance, there is presently no consensus on how these prognostic factors should be used in clinical practice.

Demicco et al.[64] published a clinicopathological study evaluating one particular tumor sub-type, solitary fibrous tumor. Based on review of over 100 patients, they developed a three-tiered model to help prognosticate the risk of distant metastasis. Scores were assigned based upon age, tumor size, and mitotic figures, with total scores tabulated to determine the risk of aggressive disease.

Treatment of localized primary disease of the extremities

Surgery

General issues
Surgical resection remains the cornerstone of therapy for localized primary STS. The discussion that follows focuses on STSs in the limbs, the most common site of origin, but the principles are equally applicable to sarcomas of other primary anatomic sites.

With the development of limb-sparing techniques in the 1970s and 1980s, there was a marked decline in the rate of amputation as the primary therapy for ESTS. Today, the widespread application of multimodality treatment strategies means that the vast majority of patients with localized STS of the extremities undergo limb-sparing, usually function-sparing treatment; fewer than 10% of patients presently undergo amputation.[65–67] In selected patients, limb-sparing can be approached with surgery alone.

Amputation
Most surgeons consider definite major vascular, bony, or nerve involvement by STS as relative indications for amputation. Complex *en bloc* bone, vascular, and nerve resections with interposition grafting can be undertaken, but the associated morbidity is high. Therefore, for a few patients with critical involvement of major bony or neurovascular structures, for example in the foot, amputation remains the only surgical option but offers the prospect of prompt rehabilitation with excellent local control and survival rates. Other indications for amputation include tumor fungating through the skin or associated with a pathologic fracture with lack of reasonable salvage option.

Table 3 Phase 3 trials of adjuvant radiotherapy for localized extremity and trunk sarcoma stratified by grade.

Histologic grade	First author/institution	Treatment group	Radiation dose (Gy)	No of patients	No. local failure (%)	LRFS (%)	OS (%)
High grade	Pisters/MSKCC[70]	Surgery + BRT	42–45	56	5 (9)	89	27
		Surgery	—	63	19 (30)	66	67
	Yang/NCI[69]	Surgery + EBRT	45 + 18 (boost)	47	0 (0)	100	75
		Surgery	—	44	9 (20)	78	74
Low grade	Pisters/MSKCC[70]	Surgery + BRT	42–45	22	8 (36)	73	96
		Surgery	—	23	6 (26)	73	95
	Yang/NCI[69]	Surgery + EBRT	45 + 18 (boost)	26	1 (4)	96	NR
		Surgery	—	24	8 (33)	63	NR

Abbreviations: BRT, brachytherapy; LRFS, local recurrence-free survival; MSKCC, Memorial Sloan-Kettering Cancer Center; NCI, National Cancer Institute; NR, not reported; OS, overall survival; EBRT, external-beam radiotherapy.

Combined-modality limb-sparing treatment

Currently, at least 90% of patients with localized extremity sarcomas can undergo limb-sparing procedures. The use of limb-sparing multimodality treatment approaches for extremity sarcoma stems from a phase 3 trial from the NCI published in 1982, in which patients with extremity sarcomas amenable to limb-sparing surgery were randomly assigned to receive amputation or limb-sparing surgery with postoperative RT.[68] The arms of this trial included postoperative chemotherapy with doxorubicin, cyclophosphamide, and methotrexate. With over 9 years of follow-up, this study established that for patients for whom limb-sparing surgery is an option, limb-sparing surgery combined with postoperative RT and chemotherapy yielded disease-related survival rates comparable to those for amputation while simultaneously preserving a functional extremity.

Satisfactory local resection involves resection of the primary tumor via a longitudinally oriented incision with a margin of normal tissue. Dissection along the tumor pseudocapsule (enucleation) is associated with LR rates in 1/3 to 2/3 of patients. In contrast, wide local excision with a margin of normal tissue around the lesion is associated with LR rates in the range of 10–31%, as noted in the control arms (surgery alone) of randomized trials evaluating postoperative RT and in single-institution reports.[50]

In the modern era, a discussion of limb-preserving approaches must be linked to a discussion of the role of adjuvant therapies, most commonly RT. Several randomized controlled trials have addressed issues surrounding the use of adjuvant therapy and collectively have established important milestones in the evolution of the local management of STS. With a single exception, these trials have focused on extremity lesions and the themes of surgery and adjuvant RT.

Yang et al.[69] randomized 91 patients with high-grade extremity lesions following limb-sparing surgery to receive adjuvant chemotherapy alone or concurrent chemotherapy and RT. An additional 50 patients with low-grade tumors were to receive adjuvant RT or no further treatment following limb-sparing surgery. The local control rate for those who received RT was 99% compared with 70% in the no-RT group ($p = 0.0001$). The results were similar for high- and low-grade tumors (Table 3).

Adjuvant RT was also evaluated in a randomized trial of 126 cases treated between 1982 and 1987 (Table 3).[70] Brachytherapy (BRT) was administered postoperatively, via an iridium-192 implant that delivered 42–45 Gy over 4–6 days. At 5 years, the local control rate for high-grade tumors was 91% with BRT compared with 70% in surgery-alone controls ($p = 0.04$). Of note, no improvement in local control with BRT was evident for the low-grade tumors (the local control rate was 74% with surgery alone and 64% with BRT). The full explanation for grade-specific differences in local control with BRT remains unresolved, although one suggestion implicates the relatively long cell cycle of low-grade tumors: low-grade tumor cells may not enter the radiosensitive phases of the cell cycle during the relatively short BRT time. The finding may also be spurious and perhaps related to small numbers, (45 low-grade tumors, 27% of study population). Additional discussion of the pros and cons of BRT compared to external beam radiotherapy (EBRT) is included in the section titled "Methods of radiotherapy delivery" later.

Satisfactory surgical margins to omit radiotherapy

There are no randomized data to define what constitutes a satisfactory gross resection margin for a sarcoma. In general, every effort should be made to achieve a wide margin (2 cm is often an arbitrary choice) around the tumor mass, except in the immediate vicinity of functionally important neurovascular structures, where, in the absence of frank neoplastic involvement, dissection is performed in the immediate perineural or perivascular tissue planes. Technical details of the surgical approach to extremity sarcomas are beyond the scope of this article but are reviewed elsewhere.[71] The principle remains that adequate clearance of potential tumor-bearing tissues can be achieved if there is sufficient distance between the surgical margin and the edge of any grossly evident tumor (e.g., at least 2 cm for the closest margin), or where an intact barrier to tumor spread is excised *en bloc* with the tumor. In such cases, there is little evidence that RT is required even when potential adverse prognostic factors, such as large high-grade tumors are present. The exception is cases of "unplanned" excision where significant contamination of surrounding tissues may have taken place and the precise extent of the tumor is essentially unknown. Depending on histology, margins of less than 2 cm are reasonable when an appropriate biological barrier (such as muscle fascia) constitutes that margin. Histologies with infiltrative borders, such as myxofibrosarcoma may require wider resection margins. On the other hand, tumors with good prognoses, such as well-differentiated liposarcoma/atypical lipomatous tumor, may be managed by a more limited, marginal resection.

Management of regional lymph nodes

Given the low (2–3%) prevalence of lymph node metastasis in adults with sarcomas, there is no role for routine regional lymph node dissection in most patients.[32] However, patients with angiosarcoma, ERMS/ARMS (alveolar rhabdomyosarcoma), and epithelioid sarcoma have an increased incidence of lymph node metastasis and should be carefully examined for lymphadenopathy on examination and imaging. Sentinel lymph node biopsy is also reasonable to consider for these select histologies.[72] Inclusion of clinically negative lymph node regions electively in adjuvant RT fields is not recommended.

For patients with STS, lymph node metastasis has been regarded as a particularly adverse finding conferring similar risk to distant metastasis in TNM (tumor-nodes-metastasis) stage classification. Nevertheless, therapeutic lymph node dissection results in a 34% actuarial survival rate, and thus in the rare patient with regional nodal involvement who has no evidence of extranodal disease, therapeutic lymphadenectomy, and/or lymph node basin radiation should be considered.[32] Although formerly classified as being prognostically as adverse as distant metastasis in the TNM staging classification, isolated lymph node metastasis (as opposed to synchronous distant metastasis), if treated intensively, appear to have a prognosis similar to patients with Stage III tumors (i.e., those with high-grade, deep lesions and lesions larger than 5 cm). The impact of isolated nodal disease was adjusted in the AJCC/UICC staging system by moving N1 disease alone into the Stage III Group.[47] The validity of including N1 disease into Stage III was questioned in a follow-up manuscript, in which survival for N1 patients more closely parallels survival with Stage IV than node-negative AJCC Stage III disease.[73]

Radiotherapy

Rationale for combining radiotherapy with surgery

The use of RT in combination with surgery for STS is supported by two-phase three clinical trials and is based on two premises: microscopic nests of tumor cells can be destroyed by RT, and less radical surgery can be performed when surgery and RT are combined.[50,69] Although the traditional belief was that STSs were resistant to RT, radiosensitivity assays performed on sarcoma cell lines grown in vitro have confirmed that the radiosensitivity of sarcomas is similar to that of other malignancies; this confirmation supports the first premise.[74,75] The second premise stresses the philosophy of preservation of form (including cosmesis where possible) and functions as a goal for many patients with extremity, truncal, breast, and head and neck sarcomas.[76–78] Similar principles govern the frequent use of RT for sarcomas at nonextremity problematic sites such as RPS, high-risk sarcomas of the head and neck with skull base invasion, or spinal canal invasion by paravertebral lesions. While the efficacy of RT has been confirmed through prospective randomized clinical trials for extremity sarcomas, it has not been confirmed for other sites.

Visceral sarcomas are not ordinarily managed with RT, in part because of the mobile nature of these structures within the pelvic, abdominal, or thoracic compartments. After resection of visceral sarcomas, accurate identification of the field at risk of residual disease is particularly problematic. Contaminated loops of bowel or mesentery may relocate remotely within the abdominal cavity after surgery, and pleural contamination and mediastinal shift may occur following intrathoracic resections. Fixed tumors in the pelvis or tumors attached to internal truncal walls may occasionally be suited to preoperative or postoperative RT. Typically, however, the vast size of the radiation fields needed to cover entire body cavities, coupled with the limited RT doses that can be safely administered to the organs within the cavities, and the overwhelming risk of distant rather than LR, confines adjuvant RT for visceral sarcomas to the investigational setting. A phase III randomized study of preoperative RT plus surgery versus surgery alone failed to demonstrate a benefit for RPS. In an exploratory analysis, there may be a sub-type-specific advantage for well-differentiated liposarcomas.[79] Further discussion is included in the section titled "Retroperitoneal sarcomas."

Essential elements in the treatment planning of external beam radiotherapy

Accurate tumor localization is the first essential element for RT planning. Radiation planning is primarily CT-based for dosimetric reasons, but MRI imaging can provide complementary information about tumor extent and can be assimilated in the computer planning workstation through image fusion technology.[40,41] Further essential information is obtained from the pathology and operative reports, discussion with the surgeon, and metallic clips placed at the time of surgery may also help define the tumor bed.

It is usually helpful to secure the targeted area to minimize set-up variations and eliminate movement during treatment. Simple maneuvers such as comfortable limb positioning or fashioning of customized thermoplastic molds for immobilization will facilitate reliable and consistent treatment setups. RT of superficial tissues, including the scar following definitive resection, with appropriate application of tissue-like bolus material should be considered, but with the recognition that fibrosis, atrophy, and telangiectasias may result. Traditionally, dose uniformity within irregular volumes was optimized using 3D conformal radiation (3D-CRT) with beam segmentation, compensators, or wedge filters. However, 3D-CRT has now largely been replaced by the use of intensity-modulated radiotherapy (IMRT) including volumetric modulated arc therapy (VMAT). These more modern technologies enable delivery of more conformal dose distributions, and consequently, improved normal tissue sparing. IMRT is the preferred technique for most STS.[80] Whenever possible, the entire limb circumference, whole joints, or pressure areas (e.g., elbow or heel) should not be treated with what is considered to be a full RT dose, as this may adversely affect limb function, cause distal edema, pain, and stiffness.

It is also prudent to assess baseline function before initiating RT. This is especially important with paired organs, such as eyes or kidneys, if the functional ablation of one organ by RT is expected. Radiation ablation (and subsequent nephrectomy) of the ipsilateral kidney is a frequent occurrence in RPS. Some large right-sided RPS may infiltrate the liver capsule or be "hooded" by the liver, making delivery of adequate RT doses to tumor with appropriate sparing of normal liver surrounding the tumor extremely difficult. This area may be particularly appropriate for IMRT techniques because of the exquisite conformality that is possible with this approach which permits sufficient liver and other normal tissue to be excluded from the irradiated volume.[81,82] Fortunately, although the tolerance of the entire liver to radiation is low, part of the liver may be safely treated to much higher doses. In these instances, if a subsequent liver resection is needed because of tumor infiltration or adherence to the capsule, detailed consultation between the surgical and radiation oncology teams is needed to ensure that an adequate volume of nonirradiated liver remains *in situ*.

Dose fractionation issues

Total radiation doses administered postoperatively for sarcoma depend on involvement of the surgical margin.[69,83,84] Typical total doses are 60–66 Gy in the setting of negative resection margins and 66 Gy for positive margins, respectively. When RT is given preoperatively, the total dose used in most institutions is 50 Gy in 2 Gy daily fractions administered over 5 weeks.[84,85] However, data regarding radiation dose–response are very limited and based on underpowered retrospective studies. Based on current data, higher doses of RT are probably indicated in the postoperative setting (compared with preoperative RT), but the search for an alternative lower dose postoperative schedule seems desirable. There is an ongoing randomized trial in Canada evaluating postoperative

RT doses of 50 Gy versus 66 Gy for STS resected with negative margins.

The fraction size used in conventional fractionation schemes is usually 1.8 or 2 Gy.[84,86] Several altered fractionation schemes have been described including hyperfractionated, hypofractionated, and accelerated schedules.[87–90] A preoperative hypofractionated RT schedule of 5 Gy delivered for five consecutive days for extremity and trunk wall STS was evaluated in a series of 272 patients. The 3-year LR rate of 19% is higher than reported rates for many contemporary series.[91] Longer follow-up of this novel strategy is warranted.

Radiation dose and target volumes

Guidelines on how to address the technical design of the radiation volumes have been published and should be reviewed for additional detail regarding this topic.[92]

Many STS respect barriers to tumor spread in the axial plane of the extremity, such as bones, interosseous membranes, or major fascial planes. Consequently, ESTS tend to spread preferentially in the longitudinal direction of muscles. Therefore, the margins of the RT volume must be wide in the cephalocaudal direction. Bone, interosseous membranes, and fascial planes are considered barriers to tumor spread in the axial direction, and, therefore radial radiation margins are typically smaller than those in the cephalocaudal direction. For nonextremity lesions, the preferred direction of spread is also along the direction of the involved musculature, but care must be taken to ensure that the fascial planes are appropriately recognized and encompassed in the radiation target volume. For subcutaneous STS, the area of potential spread is similar in longitudinal and radial dimensions.

The basic elements in RT planning are to first define a gross tumor volume (GTV) and then place a margin around it to encompass tissues at risk of harboring microscopic residual disease (clinical target volume [CTV]) (Figure 5).[86] Generally, RT is phased so that an initial volume (CTV1) around the risk zone is treated to doses that are capable of sterilizing microscopic amounts of tumor cells (e.g., 50–50.4 Gy in 1.8 or 2.0 Gy fractions). If delivering RT postoperatively it is then customary to have at least one field reduction to permit additional dose to a reduced volume surrounding the highest risk zone (CTV2). This dose is usually 10–16 Gy for negative margins and 16 Gy for microscopic positive margins but can be higher if there is gross residual disease.[94] In the postoperative setting, for CTV1, the surgical bed is expanded with a 1.5 cm radial margin and a 4 cm cranio-caudal margin to encompass microscopic disease in the surrounding tissues; CTV2 encompasses the original sarcoma localization with a 1.5 cm radial

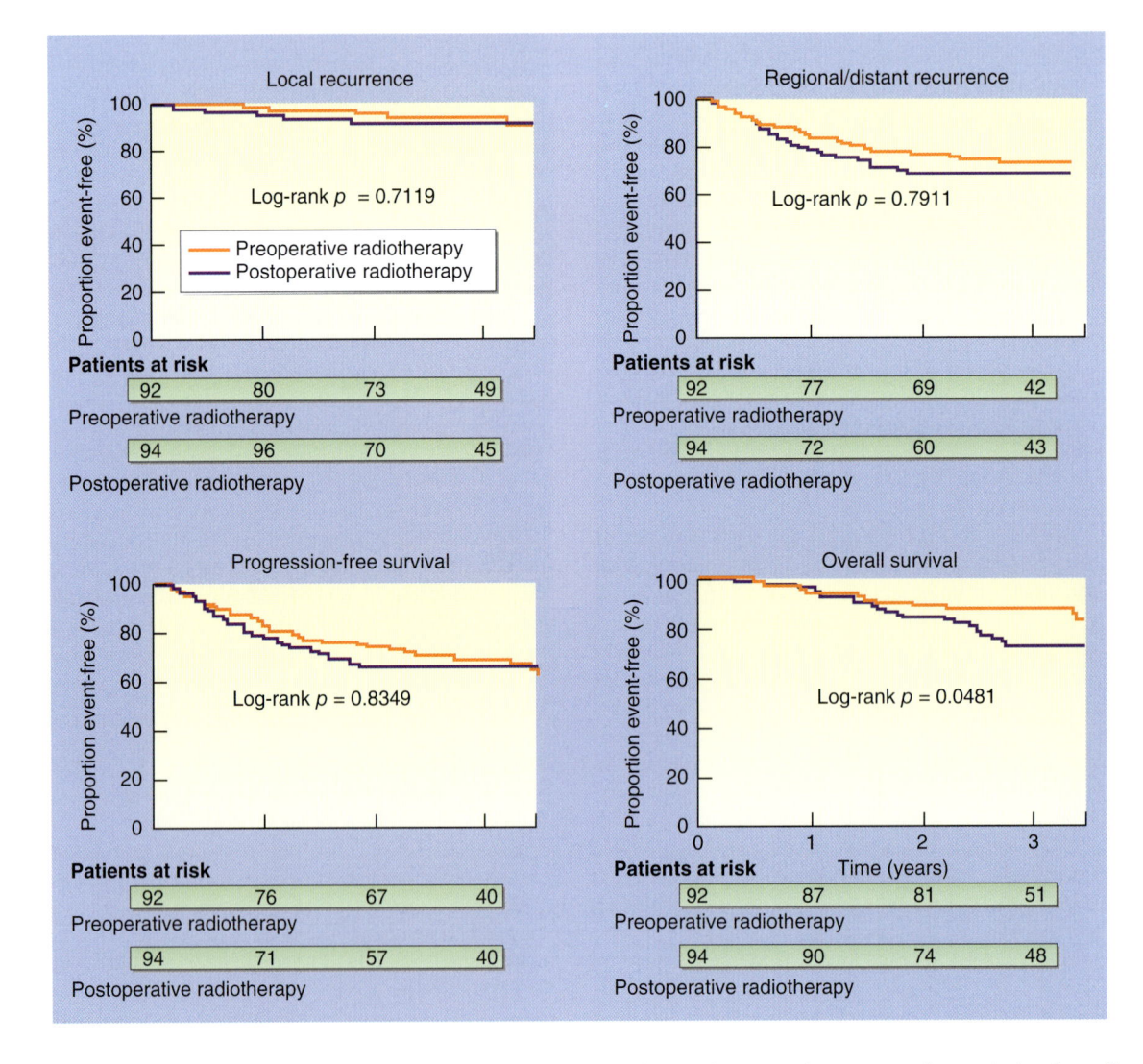

Figure 5 Kaplan–Meier plots for probability of local recurrence, metastasis (local and regional recurrence), progression-free survival, and overall survival in the Canadian Sarcoma Group randomized trial of the NCI of Canada Clinical Trials Group comparing preoperative and postoperative radiotherapy.[93]

margin and a 2 cm cranio-caudal margin. In preoperative RT, the GTV is treated to a dose of 50 Gy in 25 fractions over 5 weeks with surgery following 4–6 weeks later. In general, the CTV encompasses the GTV with a 4 cm cranio-caudal and a 1.5–2.0 cm radial margin for microscopic disease coverage. If feasible, the CTV should also include peritumoral edema since it may harbor tumor cells at some distance from the GTV.[87] Following preoperative RT, a postoperative "boost" had traditionally been delivered for cases of margin-positive disease at surgery in order to decrease the chance of LR. However, the efficacy of a boost dose in this setting has been questioned given the lack of demonstrated benefit in two retrospective reviews.[95,96] These results suggest that a benefit from a delayed postoperative boost following preoperative RT and surgery with positive margins is at best debatable, and the increased risk and challenges of managing later RT morbidity (e.g., radiation-induced fractures) resulting from the higher radiation doses involved should be considered when contemplating this approach.

The defined external beam volumes for ESTS reflect those of the prospective Canadian Sarcoma Group randomized clinical trial discussed later.[93] However, the United Kingdom postoperative phase III randomized "VORTEX" trial (NCT NCT00423618) compared a standard volume 5-cm longitudinal margin from GTV to a reduced volume 2-cm margin for 216 patients. Preliminary results showed no statistically significant differences for local recurrence-free survival (LRFS) nor late radiation toxicity.[97] The RTOG-0630 trial (NCT NCT00589121) defined slightly smaller preoperative RT volumes (longitudinal 3 cm) and demonstrated acceptable local control. However, these results are less easily interpreted due to the trial's nonrandomized nature.[98] In any event, the appropriate size of RT volume margins on tumor is not appreciably smaller than the 4-cm longitudinal margin noted above and further outcome reports will be needed before target volumes can reliably be reduced in the interest of normal tissue protection.

Local control rates reported for ESTS using combinations of surgery and RT are excellent (approximately 90%). With further study, we may learn it is appropriate to reduce RT treatment volumes. For example, improvements in surgical technique may lessen the degree of intraoperative tumor dissemination, and irradiation of all surgically handled tissues, scars, and drain sites may be unnecessary. This seems particularly relevant for major centers where surgery is performed by teams with extensive experience in sarcoma management.

Sequencing of radiotherapy and surgery

The two most common sequencing methods of EBRT delivery are preoperatively or postoperatively. There are several advantages for preoperative RT. Preoperative RT is delivered to an undisturbed and potentially better oxygenated tumor site, which may be one reason why lower preoperative radiation doses do not appear to compromise local control.[99] Nielsen et al.[100] repeated RT planning in patients who had undergone preoperative RT and surgery and observed that the field size and number of joints irradiated in preoperative RT were significantly less than if the treatment had been administered postoperatively. Another advantage of preoperative RT is that it promotes collaboration between the surgical and radiation oncologists and facilitates the formulation of a coordinated management plan prior to any treatment.

The Canadian Sarcoma Group SR2 clinical trial represents the only prospective randomized comparison of preoperative versus postoperative RT.[93] Local control was similar between arms. As was anticipated, the trial showed that preoperative RT results in an increased rate of temporary acute wound complications (WC). On the other hand, as also anticipated, the trial showed that postoperative delivery is associated with increased permanent limb fibrosis, edema, joint stiffness, and bone fractures.

Long-term follow-up of patients treated in the Canadian Sarcoma Group NCIC trial (SR2) showed that, of 129 patients evaluable for late toxicity, 48% in the postoperative group compared to 32% in the preoperative group had grade 2 or greater fibrosis ($p = 0.07$).[101] Edema was more frequently seen in the postoperative group (23% vs 16%), as was joint stiffness (23% vs 18%). Patients with these complications had lower function scores (all p-values < 0.01) on the Toronto Extremity Salvage Score and the Musculoskeletal Tumor Society Rating Scale. Field size predicted greater rates of fibrosis ($p = 0.002$) and joint stiffness ($p = 0.006$), and marginally predicted edema ($p = 0.06$). Acute wound healing complications were twice as common with preoperative compared to postoperative RT. The increased risk was almost entirely confined to the lower extremity (43% associated with preoperative vs 21% with postoperative timing; $p = 0.01$). Of interest, additional reports, including ones from Dana-Farber/Brigham and Women's Hospital and the University of Texas M.D. Anderson Cancer Center, using the same criteria for classifying WCs as were used in the Canadian NCI trial, found almost identical results.[65,102]

The influence of time interval between preoperative EBRT and surgery on the development of WC in extremity sarcoma has also been studied. While the interval had little influence, the data still suggested that the optimal interval to reduce potential WC was 4 or 5 weeks between RT and surgery.[66]

In the initial report of the SR2 trial with 3.3 years median follow-up, an improvement in overall survival (OS) ($p = 0.048$) in the preoperative RT arm was noted and partially explained by increased deaths in the postoperative RT unrelated to sarcoma.[93] The local failure rate was identical in the two arms (7%). However, updated results were recently presented and the preliminary survival difference had dissipated.[101] The 5-year results for preoperative versus postoperative, respectively, were, local control: 93% versus 92%; metastatic relapse-free: 67% versus 69%; recurrence-free survival: 58% versus 59%; OS: 73% versus 67% ($p = 0.48$); cause-specific survival: 78% versus 73% ($p = 0.64$). Cox modeling showed only resection margins as significant for local control. Tumor size and grade were the only significant factors for metastatic-relapse, OS, and cause-specific survival. Grade was the only consistent predictor of recurrence-free survival.

The sequencing of surgery and RT for ESTS should be decided after multidisciplinary evaluation. Preoperative RT is typically preferred to postoperative RT, but decisions should be individualized taking into account tumor location, tumor size, RT volumes needed, comorbidities, and risks.

Methods of radiotherapy delivery

In general terms, the most accepted methods of delivering RT include EBRT and BRT. The former also includes the controversy about its sequencing (pre- vs postoperative) discussed earlier and can be delivered using 3D-CRT or IMRT as mentioned earlier. No randomized trials directly comparing EBRT and BRT have been undertaken, but both forms of RT have been compared with surgery alone. There also have been no randomized trials addressing IMRT.

Intensity-modulated radiotherapy

Target coverage and protection of normal tissues from high-dose areas appear to be superior for IMRT compared to traditional 3D-CRT in ESTS.[103] A recent retrospective review spanning noncoincident treatment time periods compared surgery combined with either IMRT ($n = 165$) or conventional EBRT ($n = 154$). Allowing for known limitations associated with studies involving treatments deployed over different eras, IMRT showed significantly reduced LR for primary ESTS (7.6% LR for IMRT vs 15.1% LR for conventional RT; $p = 0.02$).[104]

Two recently completed prospective phase II trials (from Princess Margaret (PMH) (NCT00188175) and the Radiation Therapy Oncology Group (RTOG 0630: NCT00589121)) investigated if preoperative image-guided radiotherapy (IGRT) using conformal RT/IMRT could reduce RT-related morbidities.[93,98] The characteristics of the PMH and RTOG 0630 trials differed in several ways, including the exclusion of upper extremity lesions in the PMH trial, the use of a boost dose following preoperative RT in RTOG 0630, the potential to use chemotherapy in the RTOG trial, and some aspects of the choice of target coverage mentioned below. The two trials also differed regarding their primary endpoints.

The PMH trial showed reduced WC rates (31%) in lower extremity compared to the 43% risk in the previous Canadian Sarcoma Group NCIC SR2 trial that used 3D-CRT.[93] The need for tissue transfer, RT chronic morbidities, and subsequent secondary operations for WCs were reduced while maintaining good limb function and local control (93%). The RTOG-0630 trial reported a significant reduction of late toxicities in comparison to the NCIC-SR2 trial (11% vs 37% in SR2), which is very similar to the IGRT PMH trial. Importantly, both the PMH and RTOG-0630 trials defined the CTV differently (longitudinal margin of 3-cm from the gross tumor for high-grade lesions and 2-cm for low-grade lesions vs 4-cm longitudinal margins in the PMH trial). Potentially, the reduction in CTV margins of this degree could explain the improvement in limb function for the RTOG trial. An alternative possibility is the reduction in normal tissues receiving the target dose due to IMRT explains the improved toxicity profile for the PMH and RTOG trials compared to the SR2 trial which employed 3D-CRT. Perhaps the greatest advantage to IMRT in addition to the possibility of improving local control is the ability to spare bone toxicity and reduce late fracture risk by achieving bone avoidance. This point is often overlooked in the discussion of combined modality treatments of extremity sarcoma. A study addressed evidence-based dose volume bone avoidance objectives for IMRT planning in 230 patients (176 lower and 54 upper extremity) with a median follow-up of 41.2 months.[105] The overall risk of fracture was 2% (4/230 patients), which compares favorably to a previously reported incidence of 6%, and suggests that efforts to achieve bone avoidance are appropriate.

Brachytherapy

BRT has some putative advantages over external beam, including a shorter overall treatment time (4–6 days vs 5–6.5 weeks) and quicker initiation of RT after surgery (compared to postoperative RT) while clonogenic numbers are theoretically at a minimum. Because of its brevity, BRT is also more easily integrated into protocols that include systemic chemotherapy than is EBRT, with its protracted courses. The irradiated volume is also smaller with BRT, which may confer functional advantages. The use of BRT with surgery in previously irradiated tissues is another situation to achieve limb salvage.[106,107] As noted earlier, no apparent benefit for BRT over surgical excision alone is evident with low-grade lesions, and external beam appears more effective for these tumors (Table 3).[69,70,108] BRT also permits radiation volumes to be mapped according to intraoperative findings. The American Brachytherapy Society Guidelines differ from those for EBRT and also advise that BRT as a sole treatment modality is contraindicated in the following situations: (1) the CTV cannot be adequately encompassed by the implant geometry, (2) the proximity of critical anatomy, such as neurovascular structures, is anticipated to interfere with meaningful dose administration, (3) the surgical resection margins are positive, and (4) there is skin involved by tumor.[109,110]

In addition, BRT was compared retrospectively to IMRT in 134 high-grade ESTS where both cohorts had similar adverse features.[111] The 5-year local control rate was 92% for IMRT compared to 81% for BRT ($p = 0.04$). However, there is no randomized controlled trial comparing IMRT and BRT.

Most published BRT studies, including those mentioned above, used low dose rate (LDR) techniques. High-dose-rate (HDR) BRT has potential logistic advantages including lower radiation staff exposure, outpatient delivery, and optimized dose distributions by varying dwell times. However, infection and wound healing complications may occur and caution is recommended with this approach.[112] As yet, no large series evaluating HDR BRT for STS is available nor has it been directly compared to LDR.

Additional approaches to RT delivery

In addition to EBRT (3D-CRT, IMRT) and BRT, several other approaches for RT delivery exist. These include particle beam RT (electrons, protons, pions, or neutrons), intraoperative radiotherapy (IORT) using external beam or BRT techniques, and combinations of other modalities (e.g., hyperthermia) with RT. IORT has been used most often in the management of RPS and will be discussed later. Some reports also describe IORT for extremity sarcomas.[113,114] Formal clinical trials have not compared the relative merits of these approaches, and their use may be governed as much by their availability at a given center as by any special advantage they may confer. In the case of proton beam RT, its ability to achieve accurate targeting provides an advantage when tumors lie in proximity to critical structures.[115,116] In general, however, although reports on the use of many of these approaches exist, the problems of selection bias need to be considered in interpreting small series in which treatments were not randomly assigned.[117,118]

Systemic therapy

Systemic agents, including both traditional cytotoxic chemotherapy drugs as well as newer small molecule oral kinase inhibitors (SMOKIs), are used widely in the metastatic setting for patients with STSs. The use of chemotherapy in the adjuvant setting remains somewhat controversial. This section will review the use of chemotherapy in the adjuvant and metastatic settings. A brief discussion of chemotherapy combined with radiation therapy is also included in this section.

Adjuvant systemic therapy following primary surgical resection

Although local or local-regional recurrence is a problem for a small subset of patients following primary therapy, the primary driver of disease-related mortality is development of metastatic disease. As such, the question as to whether systemic chemotherapy can be a driver in improvement in OS has been a long-standing question in sarcoma multidisciplinary care.

Certainly for Ewing sarcoma/PNET, rhabdomyosarcoma, and osteogenic sarcoma, adjuvant or neoadjuvant chemotherapy have a long-standing, well-established role, with proven benefit on OS in randomized study with significant benefit in most cases.[119–122] However, for more common STSs such as leiomyosarcoma, liposarcoma, and high-grade undifferentiated pleomorphic sarcoma, the benefit of chemotherapy is questionable.[123]

There have been over a dozen studies of anthracycline-based adjuvant chemotherapy for STSs that date back nearly as long as the initial development of doxorubicin.[124,125]

The Italian Sarcoma Study Group (ISSG) examined patients with primary or recurrent resected STS of the extremity or limb girdle treated or not treated with radiation.[126,127] A total of 104 patients were randomized to receive ifosfamide (1800 mg/m^2/day for five consecutive days with mesna) and epirubicin (60 mg/m^2 on two consecutive days) versus no chemotherapy, with filgrastim support. Interim analysis led to early termination of the trial because the study had reached its primary endpoint of improved distant metastasis-free survival (DFS). At a median follow-up of 36 months, OS in the chemotherapy arm was 72%, compared with 55% for the control arm ($p = 0.002$). However, with longer-term follow-up, the OS difference showed only a trend toward statistical significance in an intention-to-treat analysis.[126] This study is the strongest single study in the literature supporting the use of adjuvant chemotherapy for STS.

Conversely, no survival benefit was observed in an European Organization for Research and Treatment of Cancer (EORTC) phase III study of adjuvant chemotherapy versus observation (doxorubicin 75 mg/m^2, ifosfamide 5 g/m^2 per cycle for five cycles, with filgrastim support).[128] A total of 351 patients were accrued between 1995 and 2003, and 130 (80%) of the 163 patients receiving chemotherapy completed all five cycles. OS was not statistically different between arms (hazard ratio (HR) 0.94 [95% confidence interval (CI) 0.68–1.31] for the treatment arm, $p = 0.72$), and relapse-free survival was also not statistically different (HR 0.91, CI 0.67–1.22, $p = 0.51$). The 5 year OS rate was 67% for the treatment arm and 68% for the control group. The major differences between this study and the ISSG study were a lower dose of ifosfamide and use of epirubicin in the ISSG trial, but it is unclear based on data from metastatic disease of the relevance of these differences.

In 2008, Ghert and colleagues[129] published a follow-up to their 1997 Sarcoma Meta-analysis Collaboration paper and included 18 studies encompassing sarcomas of all anatomic sites. In this analysis, 93 potential studies were considered, and 18 ultimately selected, constituting 1953 patients with STSs of extremity and nonextremity. Pathology review was not centralized.

Study data from the 18 trials were combined without examining individual patient data. Combining all data, LR risk, distant recurrence risk, overall recurrence risk, and OS were superior with chemotherapy. For OS, the relative risk of death was 0.77 with chemotherapy (95% CI 0.64–0.93), $p = 0.01$, and relative recurrence risk was 0.67 (95% CI 0.56–0.82), $p = 0.0001$. The absolute risk reduction of any recurrence was 10% and absolute risk reduction for OS was 6%. However, as pointed out in a commentary on the prior meta-analysis,[130] these data have to be interpreted with caution. For example, (1) individual patient data were not reviewed and interrogated, (2) in an older analysis, 18% of patients did not have histology available for review, recognizing the error rate in pathology review at expert centers, (3) ineligibility rates were high, and (4) the largest individual trial was not included (published after the meta-analysis publication) (Table 4).

Most recently, the STBSG (Soft Tissue and Bone Sarcoma Group)–EORTC pooled analysis of two 2 prospective, randomized phase III studies evaluating adjuvant chemotherapy in over 800 patients with localized high-grade STS was published. Ultimately, although chemotherapy was an independent favorable prognostic factor for recurrent free survival, there was no improvement in OS. The authors concluded, that based on this data, adjuvant chemotherapy should remain investigational and not a routine

Table 4 Relative risks and 95% confidence intervals for clinical outcomes with adjuvant chemotherapy (2008 meta-analysis).[a]

	Doxorubicin	Doxorubicin-ifosfamide	Combined
Local RFI	0.75 (0.56–1.01)	0.66 (0.39–1.12)	0.73 (0.56–0.94)
Distant RFI	0.69 (0.56–0.86)	0.61 (0.41–0.92)	0.67 (0.56–0.82)
Overall RFS	0.69 (0.56–0.86)	0.61 (0.41–0.92)	0.67 (0.56–0.82)
Overall survival	0.84 (0.68–1.03)	0.56 (0.36–0.85)	0.77 (0.64–0.93)

[a]Source: Pervaiz et al.[129]

standard of care, and chemotherapy cannot be used to salvage inadequate initial surgery.[131]

Preoperative (neoadjuvant) chemotherapy

Preoperative chemotherapy has a theoretic advantage over postoperative treatment. First, preoperative chemotherapy provides an *in vivo* test of chemotherapy sensitivity. Patients whose tumors show objective evidence of response are potentially a subset of patients that may benefit from further postoperative systemic treatment. In contrast, it is assumed that the population of nonresponding patients will derive minimal or no benefit from further chemotherapy and can therefore be spared its toxicity. Conversely, it is conceivable that the patients whose tumors respond to chemotherapy may be those destined to do well irrespective of any systemic treatment.

A second potential advantage of neoadjuvant treatment is that chemotherapy-induced cytoreduction may permit a less radical and consequently less morbid surgical resection than would have been required initially. In patients with large STS of the extremities, cytoreduction may reduce the morbidity of limb-sparing surgical procedures and possibly even allow patients who might otherwise have required an amputation to undergo limb-sparing surgery.

Investigators from the MD Anderson Cancer Center reported long-term results with doxorubicin-based preoperative chemotherapy for AJCC Stages IIC and III (formerly AJCC Stage IIIB) ESTS.[132] In a series of 76 patients treated with doxorubicin-based preoperative chemotherapy, radiologic response rates included: complete response, 9%; partial response, 19%; minor response, 13%; stable disease, 30%; and disease progression, 30%. The overall objective major response rate (complete plus partial responses) was 27%. At a median follow-up of 85 months, 5-year actuarial rates of LRFS, DMFS, DFS, and OS were 83, 52, 46, and 59%, respectively. The event-free outcomes reported from MD Anderson are similar to those observed with chemotherapy in the phase 3 postoperative chemotherapy trials. Furthermore, comparison of responding patients (complete and partial responses) and nonresponding patients did not reveal any significant differences in event-free outcome. Conversely, only 1/29 patients in a smaller study from Memorial Sloan-Kettering demonstrated WHO defined tumor-shrinking after two cycles of doxorubicin-based therapy.[133]

Ifosfamide-containing combinations also have been used in the preoperative setting. Selected patients treated with aggressive ifosfamide-based regimens have had major responses, and preliminary results suggest that response rates may be higher than in historic controls treated with non-ifosfamide-containing regimens.[134] However, as noted above, the randomized phase 2 neoadjuvant study of doxorubicin and ifosfamide chemotherapy showed no benefit for the treatment arm, although the study was not specifically designed to determine a survival advantage.[135]

The Italian Sarcoma Group recently published the results of ISG-STS 1001, an international, open-label, randomized, controlled, phase 3 multicenter trial examining histology tailored neoadjuvant chemotherapy versus standard chemotherapy in patients with high-risk STS. 287 patients were randomized to either receive ifosfamide and epirubicin versus a histology tailored regimen. High-grade myxoid liposarcomas received trabectedin, leiomyosarcoma receive gemcitabine and dacarbazine (DTIC), synovial sarcoma received high-dose ifosfamide, MPNST received ifosfamide and etoposide and undifferentiated pleomorphic sarcoma received gemcitabine and docetaxel, all based on previously reported studies supporting these regimens for those specific sub-types of sarcoma. Ultimately, the study did not see any benefit of tailoring chemotherapy based on any particular histologic subtype over utilizing a standard chemotherapy regimen.[136] If neoadjuvant chemotherapy is to be given, 3 cycles of ifosfamide and an anthracycline represent a reasonable standard f care.

Regional administration of chemotherapy

In an effort to try to improve upon outcomes in regional control and long-term disease-free survival, various groups have explored alternative chemotherapy administration techniques. Isolated limb perfusion (ILP) and isolated limb infusion (ILI), more commonly utilized in melanoma, have been explored in extremity sarcomas with varying success. It is more commonly used outside of the United States. Neuwirth et al.[137] recently performed a contemporary systematic review and meta-analysis of ILP for extremity sarcoma. Nineteen studies were identified that met the inclusion criteria of >10 patients and adequate outcome data with a total of 1288 patients. About 88% of patients had ILP as compared to ILI. The most common regimens utilized included melphalan with tumor necrosis factor-alpha (TNF-α), melphalan and actinomycin, and "other." The overall limb salvage rate was 73.8% and median time to local in-field progression ranged from 4 to 28 months.

Hyperthermic intraperitoneal chemotherapy (HIPEC) has been explored in diseases like desmoplastic small round cell tumor, where peritoneal disease is common and in limited studies may suggest a longer disease-free survival compared to historical controls. Given the rarity of the sub-type, prospective studies are difficult to perform.[138]

Combined preoperative chemotherapy and RT

As with combinations with hyperthermia, the primary putative advantage of preoperative chemotherapy with radiation is the potential to reduce tumor size and allow for a less morbid surgical procedure.

Concurrent chemotherapy and radiation have been employed extensively by Eilber and colleagues[139,140] at UCLA and have been modified and examined by other groups. The first chemotherapy–radiation treatment protocol typically involved intra-arterial doxorubicin with high dose per fraction RT (35 Gy of external beam radiation delivered in 10 daily fractions, which was reduced to 17.5 Gy in five daily fractions to minimize local toxicity). Although the intra-arterial route delivers chemotherapy more directly to the tumor, it is more complex, expensive, and prone to complications than intravenous chemotherapy.[141] Indeed, a prospective randomized trial comparing preoperative intra-arterial doxorubicin with intravenous doxorubicin, both followed by 28 Gy of radiation delivered over 8 days and then surgical resection, showed no differences in LR or survival.[140]

Ifosfamide and cyclophosphamide have been routinely combined with radiation therapy as part of the definitive therapy for Ewing sarcoma and rhabdomyosarcoma in an attempt to continue systemic therapy at the same time as maximizing local control.[119] This is a feasible approach; however, skin toxicity from the combination was greater in one study than that seen with radiation alone.[142]

An alternative sequential chemotherapy and radiation strategy in patients with localized, high-grade, large (>8 cm) ESTSs has been examined.[143–145] This treatment protocol involved three courses of doxorubicin, ifosfamide, mesna, and DTIC (mesna, adriamycin, ifosfamide, and dacarbazine (MAID)) with two 22-Gy courses of radiation (11 fractions each) for a total preoperative radiation dose of 44 Gy. This was followed by surgical resection with assessment of surgical margins. An additional 16-Gy (eight fraction) boost was delivered for microscopically positive surgical margins. The outcomes of 48 patients treated with this regimen were compared with those of matched historical controls and were superior to that of the historical controls.[143] The 5-year actuarial local control, freedom from distant metastasis, DFS, and OS rate were 92% versus 86% ($p=0.1155$), 75% versus 44% ($p=0.0016$), 70% versus 42% ($p=0.0002$), and 87% versus 58% ($p=0.0003$) for the MAID and control groups, respectively. Febrile neutropenia was a complication in 25% of patients. Wound healing complications were substantial and occurred in 14 (29%) patients receiving the chemotherapy/radiation sequential therapy. One patient who received chemotherapy developed late fatal myelodysplasia. Given the favorable results of this study in comparison to historical controls for high-risk ESTS, the RTOG conducted a multi-institutional trial, modifying the chemotherapy in an attempt to address the local toxicity issue. The report of the trial suggested combined-modality treatment can be delivered successfully in a multi-institutional setting albeit with some toxicity. Efficacy results are consistent with previous single-institution results.[144,145] The question remains whether this approach in high-risk, ESTS, confers any OS benefit and as such, should be considered in the setting of a clinical trial.

Pisters et al.[132] examined concurrent doxorubicin and irradiation in the neoadjuvant setting in 27 patients with ESTS. Preoperative external beam radiation was administered in 25 fractions of 2 Gy each. Doxorubicin was administered in escalating doses with a bolus followed by 4-day continuous infusion weekly. Radiographic restaging was performed 4–7 weeks after chemoradiation. Patients with localized disease underwent surgical resection. The maximum tolerated dose of continuous infusion doxorubicin combined with standard preoperative radiation was 17.5 mg/m^2/week; 7 of 23 (30%) patients had grade 3 dermatologic toxicity at this dose level. Macroscopically complete resection (R0 or R1) was performed in all 26 patients who underwent surgery. For 22 patients who were treated with doxorubicin at the maximum tolerated dose and subsequent surgery, 11 patients (50%) had 90% or greater tumor necrosis, including two patients who had complete pathologic responses. This approach appears valid with other radiation-sensitizing agents as well, such as gemcitabine.[146] Further studies of combination therapy are also discussed later in the section titled "Retroperitoneal sarcomas."

"Pediatric" sarcomas and adjuvant therapy

The standard of care for Ewing sarcoma, osteosarcoma, and rhabdomyosarcoma involves chemotherapy, typically both neoadjuvant and adjuvant.

Neoadjuvant chemotherapy followed by definitive resection and then adjuvant chemotherapy is the standard of care for the initial treatment of osteogenic sarcoma.[121] In the era before systemic therapy, cure rates for osteosarcoma, even in the setting of amputation for primary disease, were only on the order of 15%. With chemotherapy, the survival rate improved significantly to

65–70%. Regimens typically follow a backbone of cisplatin and doxorubicin, with methotrexate employed in most pediatric and some adult patients. The benefit for methotrexate as part of adjuvant treatment was called into question in a 1997 paper in which the combination of doxorubicin and cisplatin alone was shown equivalent to the more complicated regimen containing high-dose methotrexate.[147] However, the methotrexate component of neoadjuvant therapy has been observed to be important in a variety of studies and remains an integral part of combination therapy for osteosarcoma.[148]

Rhabdomyosarcoma is the most common STS in children and is comprised of a high-grade malignant neoplasm with cells having the propensity for myogenic differentiation. ARMS and ERMS are the two main sub-types of rhabdomyosarcoma.[149] The mainstay of treatment for both subtypes typically involves an induction course of multi-agent chemotherapy, followed by combination chemotherapy ± radiation, followed by the completion of chemotherapy depending on the stage and risk grouping of the tumor. The standard of care is in the United States is typically a combination of vincristine, dactinomycin, and cyclophosphamide.[119] Whereas, in Europe, the standard is typically ifosfamide, vincristine, and actinomycin D (known as IVA).[119] The addition of doxorubicin to the vincristine, dactinomycin, and cyclophosphamide regimen did not appear to improve OS and is omitted in the treatment of pediatric rhabdomyosarcoma.[150] Children with this diagnosis appear to fare better than adults with the same diagnosis stage for stage in most studies, as well as in everyday practice.[151,152]

For patients with Ewing sarcoma, in distinction from rhabdomyosarcoma, the addition of additional agents (ifosfamide and etoposide) to an existing backbone of vincristine, doxorubicin, and cyclophosphamide chemotherapy improved outcome for localized disease, with a 2-week schedule superior to a 3-week schedule of treatment.[122] Due to the limited number of adult patients in the dose-compressed trial, decisions to adhere to a shorter more intense regimen should be made on a case-by-case basis. As with rhabdomyosarcoma, children with Ewing sarcoma fare better than adults with the same diagnosis.[153–155]

Treatment of locally advanced disease

Hyperthermic isolated limb perfusion, isolated limb infusion, and regional hyperthermia

Hyperthermic isolated limb perfusion (HILP), an investigational technique in the United States (although approved by regulatory agencies in other parts of the world), has received considerable attention in the treatment of locally advanced, unresectable sarcomas of nonosseous tissues. ILP involves local perfusion of high-dose chemotherapy (most commonly melphalan) and when available TNF-α under hyperthermic conditions. An oxygenated circuit is established by local arterial and venous cannulation on a bypass pump. Systemic circulation is minimized by placement of a tourniquet proximally.

ILP has been evaluated in two settings: (1) attempted limb preservation in cases of locally advanced extremity lesions surgically amenable only to amputation and (2) function extremity preservation for the short survival duration anticipated in cases of locally advanced extremity lesions with synchronous pulmonary metastases (Stage IV disease).

A multicenter phase 2 trial evaluated a series of 55 patients with radiologically unresectable ESTS using HILP with high-dose TNF-α and melphalan and interferon-α in some patients.[156] A major tumor response was seen and limb salvaged in over 80% of patients. Regional toxicity was limited, and systemic toxicity was minimal to moderate. There were no treatment-related deaths. Despite the high rate of complete responses (15–30%) and limb sparing (>80%) achieved by ILP, no randomized trials have compared ILP to aggressive limb-sparing resection with RT for STS. Therefore, ILP should be considered as a potential treatment, when other options are limited or not available, in appropriately selected patients. Eligible patients should be referred to centers where this therapy is available.

ILI has been evaluated in ESTS in a more limited fashion, and parallels work done with intra-arterial chemotherapy. Like IPL, ILI relies on circulating high-dose chemotherapy in an isolated extremity. Unlike ILP, ILI is conducted through percutaneously placed catheters and is performed under hypoxic conditions. Similar to ILP, ILI has not been directly compared to aggressive limb-sparing resection with EBRT in a randomized trial. However, patients under consideration for ILP and ILI are often not candidates for surgery with EBRT at first evaluation, and therefore ILP and ILI may be considered as potential therapies in appropriately selected patients.

Treatment of metastatic disease

Clinical problem of metastases

The development of metastatic disease in STS often relegates the goal of treatment from one of cure to one of control. The role of the multidisciplinary sarcoma team in the management of patients with metastatic sarcoma is to recognize opportunities in which multimodality care might still improve important outcomes such as survival or quality of life. Both surgery and systemic chemotherapy can play an important role in improving these outcomes in select patients. Overall, it is important to recognize that chemotherapy is usually given with the palliative aim of prolonging life and improving quality of life.

The most common site of metastasis in STS of the extremities is the lungs. Indeed, the lungs are the only site of metastasis in approximately 80% of patients with metastases from primary extremity and trunk STS.[59] Primary GIST metastasize to liver and peritoneum, while other visceral sarcomas can metastasize to lungs or demonstrate local regional recurrences in the body cavity in which they arose. Extrapulmonary metastases are uncommon forms of first metastasis from extremity sarcomas and usually occur as a late manifestation of widely disseminated disease. The median survival after development of distant metastases is approximately 12 months,[157] though more contemporary data suggest median survival may presently be 15–18 months for unselected patients who receive cytotoxic chemotherapy. The optimal treatment of patients with metastatic STS requires an understanding of the natural history of the disease and individualized selection of treatment options based on patient factors, disease factors, and limitations imposed by prior treatment.

The approach to patients with advanced or metastatic sarcoma has evolved over time. Studies of "sarcomas" without stratification by histology or molecular features are generally akin to undertaking studies of "cancer" without further qualification. Mesenchymal-derived diseases lumped under the heading of "sarcoma" are quite diverse in their responses to various treatments, and studies need to take that heterogeneity into account. To generate studies of sufficient size and power, large-scale collaborations on a national and international level are required. With international and cross-institutional collaborations, it is hoped that further research will rapidly translate research findings into the novel therapeutics that are so desperately required by patients with sarcomas.

Resection of metastatic disease

Many investigators have reported their experience with pulmonary metastasectomy for metastatic STS in adults.[157,158] Three-year survival rates following thoracotomy for pulmonary metastasectomy range from 23% to 54%.

It remains difficult to predict which patients with pulmonary metastases will benefit from pulmonary resection. A number of clinical criteria have been evaluated by univariate analysis in this regard, including the disease-free interval, number of metastatic nodules, and tumor doubling time. Multivariate analyses from both the NCI and Roswell Park Cancer Institute confirm that a short disease-free interval and incomplete pulmonary resection are adverse prognostic factors for survival for patients with pulmonary metastases.[158–161] A multivariate analysis from MD Anderson suggested that, in addition, the presence of more than three metastatic pulmonary nodules on preoperative chest CT is an adverse prognostic sign. The most important prognostic factor impacting survival appears to be the ability to completely resect all disease. In the review of postmetastasectomy outcomes in one series, the median survival among patients who were able to undergo complete resection of metastases was 20 months as compared with 10 months among patients who did not have complete resection.[157] In summary, the ability to achieve complete resection and the number of pulmonary nodules present appear to best define the postoperative prognosis for these patients.

Unfortunately, metastasectomy benefits only a fraction of patients who develop pulmonary metastases. This is best illustrated by data from MSKCC, where patients who presented with primary extremity sarcoma were followed for the subsequent development and treatment of pulmonary metastases.[162] Of an initial group of 716 patients, 148 patients (21%) developed pulmonary metastases. Isolated pulmonary metastases occurred in 135 (91%) of these 148 patients. Of the 135 patients with pulmonary-only metastases, 78 (58%) were considered to have operable disease, and 65 (83%) of those taken to thoracotomy were able to undergo complete resection of all of their pulmonary metastatic disease. Thus, 44% of all patients with pulmonary metastases were able to undergo complete metastasectomy. The median survival from the time of complete resection was 19 months, and the 3-year survival rate was 23%. All patients who did not undergo thoracotomy died within 3 years. For the entire cohort of 135 patients developing pulmonary-only metastases, the 3-year survival rate was only 11%.

Several series of repeat pulmonary metastasectomy also have been published. In a series of 43 patients thus treated at the NCI, 72% of patients could be rendered free of disease at the second thoracotomy, with a median survival duration from the time of second thoracotomy of 25 months.[163]

The disappointing overall results of treatment of metastatic disease underscore the importance of careful patient selection for resection of pulmonary metastases. The following criteria are generally agreed upon: (1) the primary tumor is controlled or is controllable, (2) there is no extrathoracic disease, (3) the patient is a medical candidate for thoracotomy and pulmonary resection, and (4) complete resection of all macroscopic disease appears possible. With careful patient selection, the morbidity of thoracotomy (or repeated thoracotomies) can be limited to the subset of patients who are most likely to benefit from this aggressive treatment approach.

Chemotherapy for metastatic disease

Natural history of metastases

A good place to begin a discussion of chemotherapy for unresectable metastatic sarcoma is the expected course of the disease. The EORTC contributed greatly to define the expected course of unresectable metastatic sarcoma by publishing its large series of more than 2000 patients with advanced sarcomas of soft tissues to describe prognostic features and the response to anthracycline-based chemotherapy in an era before GIST was recognized as a unique entity.[164] In this study reviewing more than 20 years of experience, the median OS was approximately 1 year. Subsets of patients had longer median survival; such patients were typically those who were younger, had a better performance status, had low-grade sarcoma, had no liver metastases, and had developed metastatic disease following a longer interval from initial diagnosis. Importantly, this study concluded that the variables predicting improved survival were actually different from variables predicting objective response to chemotherapy (the latter variables including such items as high-grade tumor and liposarcoma subtype). Thus, one interpretation that is reasonable is that the most important predictors of survival with metastatic sarcoma are variables dependent on the tumor biology itself, as well as certain patient factors such as age and comorbid disease.

Individualized therapy

The approach to patients with advanced or metastatic sarcomas is evolving as are new therapeutics, and in this context, the use of therapies directed at specific histologies or DNA alterations is evolving, as are the entirely orthogonal approaches involving immunotherapy. It is increasingly recognized that clinical trials must be stratified rationally for data of value to be derived. To generate studies of sufficient size and power, large-scale collaborations on a national and international level will be required.

Anthracyclines and ifosfamide

With the caveat that specific sarcomas demonstrate differential sensitivity to different chemotherapy agents, doxorubicin and ifosfamide remain the most active agents for metastatic sarcoma, with response evaluation criteria in solid tumors (RECIST) response rates in the 10–20% range for each drug.[165] Depending on the ratio of sensitive versus less sensitive subtypes of STSs in past studies, the response rate can be significantly higher. For example, synovial sarcoma and myxoid/round-cell liposarcomas are relatively sensitive to ifosfamide (as well as doxorubicin), while GIST, alveolar soft part sarcoma, and extraskeletal myxoid chondrosarcoma appear to be largely resistant to both agents.

It is important to recognize that response rates *per se* increasingly are being criticized as poor surrogates of clinical benefit. Objective response rates based on imaging may underestimate the antitumor efficacy of chemotherapy. Conversely, simply shrinking a tumor and achieving a nondurable response may not be worth the toxicities of aggressive multiagent chemotherapy. Thus, from both standpoints, RECIST-defined responses may not be an ideal indicator of antitumor efficacy in sarcoma management in general, with GIST a case in point.[166,167] Increasing attention in the field of sarcoma drug development is thus being paid to other important indicators of clinical outcomes, such as progression-free survival duration and OS rate.

Some drugs may slow disease progression and prolong survival even if objective response rates are low, although the clinical data to support those claims must be generated with rigor and careful attention to consistency of follow-up. Nonetheless, despite observations that clinical benefit might be underestimated by RECIST, it remains the yardstick by which radiologic responses are measured.

Dose–response relationships

The sensitivity of sarcomas to chemotherapy was first convincingly demonstrated with doxorubicin in the early to mid-1970s.[124] Subsequent studies of doxorubicin in sarcomas have widely been viewed as supporting a dose–response relationship, with doses of 50 mg/m^2/cycle or less associated with less antitumor activity than doses of 60 mg/m^2/cycle or higher. Although a dose–response relationship is evident, it is important to recognize that other variables may affect antitumor efficacy, such as histopathologic subtype of sarcoma, as noted above. Nonetheless, since a dose threshold for optimal activity has been documented with doxorubicin in another chemotherapy-sensitive solid tumor, specifically breast cancer, it seems reasonable to conclude that doxorubicin is best used at doses above 60 mg/m^2/cycle. Also analogous to breast cancer, improved response rates above 75 mg/m^2/cycle dose range are difficult to demonstrate.

A wide variety of dose- and schedule-ranging studies have been performed with ifosfamide. It is clear that antitumor response is improved by higher doses of ifosfamide.[133,168] This point has been made most convincingly by the responses to high-dose ifosfamide (>10,000 mg/m^2/cycle) in patients who had previously failed to respond to the same drug at lower doses (i.e., <6000 mg/m^2/cycle). However, given the toxicities of this drug at higher doses, high-dose ifosfamide is best reserved for a subset of patients with disease that is expected to be chemotherapy sensitive to achieve meaningful responses (e.g., prior to planned surgical extirpation of metastases).

Single-agent versus combination chemotherapy

A continuing controversy is whether the optimal approach to patients with advanced sarcomas is combination chemotherapy regimens or sequential single agents. One of the best prospective randomized trials of combination chemotherapy for advanced disease came from a US intergroup study in which ifosfamide was or was not given to previously untreated patients with metastatic or advanced STS receiving doxorubicin plus DTIC. This study demonstrated no survival advantage for the group receiving ifosfamide in combination with doxorubicin plus DTIC, although this group had a statistically significant increase in objective response rate.[169,170] The role of combination chemotherapy is further called into question for broad use given the statistically significant increase in toxicities when ifosfamide was added. Thus, despite the increased anticancer activity as evidenced by the small but significant improvement in response rates, no survival benefit was obtained by adding a third drug.

In a similar fashion, the addition of higher dose ifosfamide (10 g/m^2 per cycle) to doxorubicin (75 mg/m^2 per cycle) was associated with a statistically significantly higher RECIST response rate (26% vs 14%), median progression-free survival rate (7.4 vs 4.6 months), greater toxicity burden, but no OS advantage.[171] It was not clear from these data if sequential use of the two agents would yield similar outcomes to combination treatment. The survival data in particular serve as a touchstone by which we determine success for therapy in metastatic sarcomas. The data from these two randomized trials support the use of combination chemotherapy for patients with symptomatic disease who are in need of a response; by the same token, it is not unreasonable to use single agents sequentially to minimize patient toxicity for less symptomatic or asymptomatic patients who remain in need of therapy.

Doxorubicin

Recently, the ANNOUNCE study was presented at the 2018 American Society of Clinical Oncology (ASCO) plenary session. This was a large phase III multicenter, international trial of doxorubicin plus placebo versus doxorubicin plus olaratumab, a fully human immunoglobin G class 1 monoclonal antibody targeting platelet derived growth factor receptor (PDGFR)-α. The combination demonstrated superior progression free survival (PFS) and OS (26.5 months vs 14.7 months; stratified HR = 0.46; 95%CI, 0.3–0.71) compared with doxorubicin and placebo among 129 patients in the phase 2 study. This ultimately led to an accelerated approval by the United States Food and Drug Administration (FDA), with the phase 3 to act as confirmation. The phase 3 study failed to meet the primary endpoint of prolonged OS, with median OS of 20.4 months in the olaratumab arm and 19.7 months in the placebo arm. This led to withdrawal of olaratumab from commercial use. Although this study was disappointing with regards to its primary goals, it did reveal that patients are living longer than earlier OS data had suggested. This is likely multifactorial in nature, with better surgical outcomes, more second and third-line systemic therapeutics available, and better supportive care, like growth factor support, possibly contributing to the result.[172,173]

Strategies to improve the therapeutic index of chemotherapy

Encapsulated anthracyclines

Another strategy to increase the therapeutic index of anthracyclines is to encapsulate the drug within a liposomal vehicle. At least three liposomal preparations of anthracyclines have been tested, and all have shown some efficacy against sarcomas. Pegylated liposomal doxorubicin (Doxil/Caelyx) is a small liposome with polyethylene glycol anchored within the lipid bilayer, acting as a hydrophilic coating to preserve the circulating half-life of the liposome and prevent degradation within the reticuloendothelial system. This preparation, given at a dose less than that of unencapsulated doxorubicin, is typically better tolerated than doxorubicin, with substantially less myelotoxicity, cardiac toxicity, and alopecia at the cost of hand-foot syndrome and idiosyncratic reactions to the first dose of therapy; while its dose is lower, its long half-life in the circulation (30–70 h), leads to an increased area under the curve for 50 mg/m^2 that is 300 times that of doxorubicin itself. In a randomized phase 2 study, pegylated liposomal doxorubicin demonstrated similar activity to normal doxorubicin (9% vs 10% response rate in the era before GIST was recognized as a separate type of sarcoma); formal noninferiority or equivalence was not determined, but pegylated liposomal doxorubicin was significantly less toxic than doxorubicin.[174]

Beyond anthracyclines and ifosfamide

It is recognized that DTIC has minor activity in STS, and studies have demonstrated that leiomyosarcoma and to a lesser degree solitary fibrous tumor are two diagnoses in which DTIC and its orally absorbed relative temozolomide have greatest activity.[175–177] Gemcitabine and docetaxel as a combination was first demonstrated to have activity in uterine leiomyosarcoma, after relatively disappointing phase II trials of gemcitabine as a single agent, suggesting true synergy between the two agents.[178,179] A randomized study of gemcitabine and docetaxel showed the combination was superior to gemcitabine alone with respect to both PFS and OS in a group of unselected sarcomas.[180] Notably, responses were most common in UPS and pleomorphic liposarcoma, more than leiomyosarcoma. A randomized study demonstrated the superiority in PFS and OS of gemcitabine and DTIC over DTIC alone.[181] Thus either the gemcitabine-docetaxel or gemcitabine-DTIC combinations are good options after failure of doxorubicin and–or ifosfamide. Indeed, the perception of toxicity of gemcitabine-based therapy versus doxorubicin-based therapy has led to its acceptance in first line in metastatic sarcoma patients in the U.S.[174] Given the data supporting gemcitabine and docetaxel as a possible first-line regimen in leiomyosarcoma and pleomorphic high-grade sarcoma, Seddon et al.[182] performed the GeDDiS trial, a randomized phase 3 trial performed in 24 UK hospitals and one Swiss group. Patients were randomized to receive doxorubicin 75 mg/m^2 on day 1 of a 21-day cycle versus gemcitabine 675 mg/m^2 on days 1 and 8 and docetaxel 75 mg/m^2 on day 8 every 3 weeks. The proportion of patients alive and progression free at 24 weeks did not differ between those who received doxorubicin versus those who received gemcitabine and docetaxel (46.3% vs 46.4%). Toxicity was greater in the combination chemotherapy arm and thus, doxorubicin was felt to remain the standard first-line treatment for most patients with advanced STS soft tissue sarcoma.

Newer agents

Sarcomas represent a fertile ground for the field of drug development. Doxorubicin was first recognized as an effective agent against sarcomas and subsequently was developed into one of the most widely used anticancer agents ever discovered. The efficacy of imatinib in a chemotherapy-resistant diagnosis like GIST provided a proof of principle that has since been borne out in other solid tumors with EGFR inhibitors, BRAF inhibitors, and the like. Although investigators are always seeking out the "next imatinib" with a more targeted approach to cancer therapy, the results are typically less promising.

Trabectidin (ET-743, ecteinascidin)

Trabectedin is a marine-derived drug from the marine tunicate *Ecteinascidia turbinata*. It covalently binds to the minor groove of the DNA and blocks the cell cycle in late S and G2, and affects the transcription in part by prevention of binding of transcription factor NF-Y, thus decreasing expression of a variety of genes, including multidrug resistance genes. After initial promising results in phase 1 studies, multiple phase 2 trials were performed, the most successful of which (a randomized phase II study of two schedules of drug) led to the drug's approval in Europe for refractory STS.[183,184] A follow-up randomized study showed greater activity of trabectedin than DTIC.[185]

The randomized phase 3 study of trabectedin in patients with metastatic leiomyosarcoma and liposarcoma was performed by Demetri et al.[186] Patients were randomized in a 2 : 1 ratio to receive trabectedin or DTIC intravenously every 3 weeks. The primary endpoint was OS. A total of 518 patients were enrolled and randomly assigned to receive trabectedin or DTIC. Trabectedin resulted in 45% reduction in the risk of disease progression or death compared to DTIC (median PFS for trabectedin vs DTIC 4.2 vs 1.5 months, HR 0.87; $p < 0.001$). This helped support the eventual approval of trabectedin in the US.

Eribulin In a similar manner, the microtubule targeted agent eribulin demonstrated activity in a phase II study,[187] which led to the conduct of a study similar to that of the trabectedin trial above, in which eribulin was tested against DTIC in a phase III trial in leiomyosarcoma and liposarcoma. It was ultimately approved by the FDA in 2016 for the treatment of patients with unresectable or metastatic liposarcoma who have received a prior anthracycline-based regimen. Estimated median OS was 13.5 months in the eribulin arm and 11.3 months in the DTIC arm.[188]

Pazopanib Beyond cytotoxics, the most important result to date involves the TKI pazopanib. After the demonstration of activity in a phase II trial,[189] a phase III study termed pazopanib for metastatic soft-tissue sarcoma (PALETTE) was conducted, involving 369 patients with STS progressing after standard therapy. With a 2 : 1 randomization for pazopanib 800 mg versus placebo, the pazopanib arm demonstrated statistically superior PFS. Median PFS in the placebo arm was 1.6 months and 4.6 months in the pazopanib arm, with a corresponding HR of 0.35 ($p < 0.001$) as assessed by independent radiology review. Median OS at final analysis was 10.7 month in the placebo arm versus 12.6 month in the pazopanib arm, HR = 0.87, $p = 0.26$.[190] These data were sufficient to obtain broad international approval for pazopanib for metastatic STS who have received prior therapy.[190]

Diagnosis specific agents Increasingly, the molecular characteristics of specific sarcomas will dictate therapeutic options. Based on tumor DNA alterations (gene loss, translocation, or mutation), mTOR inhibitors such as sirolimus have activity in perivascular epithelial cell tumors (PEComas),[191] imatinib, and other inhibitors of PDGFR and CSF1 receptor have activity in GIST, DFSP,[192] and tenosynovial giant cell tumor.[193,194] Crizotinib, the ALK inhibitor, is active in *ALK* translocation positive inflammatory myofibroblastic tumor (IMT).

Highlighting the current trend toward more histology-driven studies, the FDA recently granted accelerated approval to tazemetostat, an EZH2 inhibitor, for adult patients and pediatric patients aged 16 years and older with metastatic or locally advanced epithelioid sarcoma not eligible for complete resection. Efficacy was investigated in a single-arm cohort of a multi-center international trial in patients with epithelioid sarcoma. Patients were required to have INI1 loss. The overall response rate (ORR) was 15% with 1.6% achieving a complete response and 13% having partial response, with 67% of those patients having sustainable responses lasting 6 months or longer. A confirmatory phase III study is ongoing.[195]

Additionally, two recent FDA approvals for the rare histologic subtypes of PEComa and tenosynovial giant cell tumor (TGCT) include nab-rapamycin and pexidartinib respectively, providing more evidence that as we parse soft-tissue sarcomas down to specific sub-types, more focused clinical trials may lead to improved results.[196]

Management of local recurrence

If an isolated LR is identified, the treatment goals are the same as for patients with primary tumors, namely, optimal local control while maintaining as much function and cosmesis as possible.[107] Early identification of local relapse may improve the chance of successful salvage therapy, and, like newly diagnosed patients, these patients are probably best managed in specialized multidisciplinary sarcoma centers. The initial evaluation must include a full review of previous therapy because this will have a bearing on the therapeutic options available. Therefore, all prior surgery and pathology reports should be examined, as should reports on previous chemotherapy and previous RT, especially volume treated, dose, and energy of radiation.

Staging should be performed in the same way as for newly presenting patients. The areas adjacent to the original lesion and potentially contaminated by previous surgical interventions should be scrutinized carefully. Both these areas and tissues adjacent to the recurrent tumor, containing potential tumor extensions, should be considered at risk and candidates for resection and/or inclusion in radiation fields.

Several distinct groupings are evident under the rubric of "locally recurrent" disease: (1) cases in which prior treatment did not include RT, (2) cases treated with RT in the past, (3) cases in which distant metastases are also present, and (4) cases in which it is difficult to distinguish between recurrence and secondary tumors induced by RT. Although the therapeutic options available are more limited in recurrent disease and the challenge posed by these cases are much more formidable, a proportion of these patients can be cured. Clinical experience is needed to determine which therapeutic options are appropriate in a given case of recurrent disease.

Gastrointestinal stromal tumors

No discussion of sarcomas would be complete without noting the remarkable advances made with one particular sarcoma subtype, GIST, which has changed the way people think about solid tumors. With the recognition of KIT as a good marker for GIST to distinguish it from other sarcomas and the recognition of *KIT* and *PDGFRA* activating mutations responsible for the constitutive activation of *KIT*,[197] clinical studies followed rapidly, and have been done in parallel to studies investigating the biology of GIST.

Surgical principles for management of primary GIST differ than those for other sarcomas and visceral adenocarcinomas. In general, resection requires a minimal margin of normal tissue, not the wide margins of other sarcomas or visceral adenocarcinomas. Unlike gastric cancer, GISTs do not generally metastasize to local-regional lymph nodes (except in some GISTs arising in the pediatric population), rendering lymph node dissection unnecessary in the vast majority of patients. Thus, gastric GISTs can often be removed by simple wedge resections, and large gastric resections are only rarely required, generally due to anatomic constraints. Similarly, GISTs arising in the small intestine, colon, or rectum may be resected with minimal margins. Furthermore, patients with GIST undergoing a macroscopically complete resection but with positive microscopic margins are not at increased risk for LR compared to those resected with negative margins.[198]

After the recognition of *in vivo* efficacy of imatinib in a GIST cell line,[199] treatment of metastatic disease has rapidly advanced from treating a single patient to phase 1, 2, and 3 studies for patients with metastatic disease.[199–202] The results have been remarkably consistent. Imatinib is at least 10-fold more active than any agent ever examined for treatment of GIST (formerly called GI leiomyosarcoma). The response rate to imatinib is approximately 50%, 30–35% with stable disease, and ~15% with overt progression on therapy. US phase 3 data indicate that 400 and 800 mg yield equivalent time-to-progression curves, but the European/Australian phase 3 study indicates that time to progression is improved with the higher dose (800 mg daily) arm.[200] Remarkably, patient kinase genotype determined relative sensitivity to therapy (Figure 6).[203] Patients with *KIT* exon 11 mutation had an 80–90% response rate, while patients with *KIT* exon 9 mutation had less sensitivity. Patients with no mutation in *KIT* or *PDGFRA* had a much lower response rate, but still higher than that observed for any other chemotherapy drugs. For the time being, for patients with Exon 11 and Exon 9 mutations, imatinib remains the first-line standard of care for metastatic GIST. A dosage of 400 mg daily is a reasonable starting point for most patients, with some data suggesting 800 mg for GISTs with the presence of exon 9 mutation.[204]

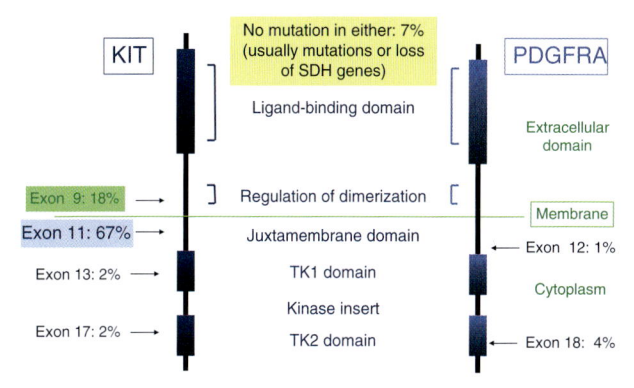

Figure 6 Mutation status of gastrointestinal stromal tumors and location on the KIT or PDGFRA protein.[203]

The median time to progression for patients with metastatic GIST on imatinib is approximately 2 years. Patients with progression on a lower dose of imatinib can respond further with dose increases. The phase 1 study of imatinib indicated that the maximum tolerated dosage is 800 mg daily (400 mg by mouth bid). Patients with progression of disease have had unusual patterns of progression, so-called "tumor within a tumor," which represents clone(s) with second resistant *KIT* mutations.[156] In some cases, tumor regrowth in an apparently necrotic tumor is observed, and in others, only one metastatic deposit is seen to progress instead of the multiplicity of lesions seen in many patients with advanced GIST. As a result, some patients have been treated with carefully planned operations to remove problematic individual sites of metastatic disease.

The rationale for consideration of metastasis surgery for patients with responding or stable metastatic disease on imatinib is based on the observations that: (1) pathologic complete response to imatinib is very rare (<5%) and many (perhaps most) patients will eventually develop secondary resistance to imatinib owing chiefly to development of secondary resistance mutations. Reports from high-volume centers demonstrate that carefully selected patients treated by imatinib and subsequent metastectomy appear to have very favorable progression-free survival rates. Whether this is due to case selection or bona fide clinical benefit related to surgery is unclear.[156,205] Randomized controlled trials of the impact of metastectomy in patients with stable or responding disease were planned in the United States, Europe, and China. Poor accrual led to the closure of the European and Chinese trials, and the American trial was never started.

The utility of imatinib in metastatic GIST spawned new tyrosine kinase inhibitors (TKIs), with subsequent regulatory approval. Sunitinib is active in imatinib-resistant GIST and is associated with both significantly improved progression-free survival and OS in comparison to placebo.[203] With the demonstration of activity of sorafenib in GIST,[206,207] regorafenib (a fluorinated form of sorafenib) was found active in phase III trial of drug against placebo; in this phase 3 "efficacy and safety of regorafenib for advanced gastrointestinal stromal tumors after failure of imatinib and sunitinib: an international, multicenter, prospective, randomized, placebo-controlled phase 3 trial (GRID)" study, the patients on placebo were crossed over more rapidly to drug than the study involving sunitinib, perhaps accounting for the lack of OS benefit seen in the GRID study.[208] After failure of other agents, some form of TKI appears to be beneficial; including the use of imatinib which was superior to placebo in late-stage patients in a randomized trial.[209] Most recently, in January 2020, the FDA approved avapritinib for adults with unresectable or metastatic GIST harboring a platelet-derived growth factor receptor alpha exon 18 mutation, including the D842V mutation. The D842V mutation is universally unresponsive to imatinib, and this was an example of an approval in a very small, niche population of patients with a rare disease. The drug has been associated with serious but less common side effects including cerebrovascular bleeding and cognitive effects.[210,211] Following shortly thereafter was the approval of ripretinib in advanced GIST patients who have received prior treatment with three or more kinase inhibitors.[212]

Given the remarkable activity of imatinib in the metastatic setting, it is not surprising that imatinib has been tested in the adjuvant setting as well. Data for studies of 0 versus 1 year of imatinib, 0 versus 2 years of imatinib, and 1 versus 3 years of imatinib have all consistently demonstrated the benefit of the longer course of therapy. Adjuvant imatinib was initially approved in the United States by virtue of the ACOSOG Z9001 study, in which 1 year of imatinib (400 mg/daily) was compared to placebo following complete resection of GISTs greater than 3 cm in size. This study was halted to further accrual after accruing 762 patients when a planned interim analysis for the primary endpoint demonstrated superior progression-free survival in the imatinib arm (97% vs 83% in the placebo arm).[213] A randomized trial comparing one versus 3 years of adjuvant imatinib subsequently demonstrated not only an improvement in recurrence-free survival but also demonstrated improvement in OS favoring longer duration of adjuvant therapy.[214] Whether longer adjuvant treatment with imatinib for longer periods adds further benefit is uncertain and is the subject of a single-arm 5-year trial of imatinib. At this juncture, the best recommendation that can be made is that 3 years of adjuvant treatment be considered for patients with intermediate and high-risk resected primary GISTs. Some high risk patients may benefit from longer treatment.[215–217]

Retroperitoneal sarcomas

RPS comprise about 15% of STS. RPS typically present late and are frequently located in regions where the administration of optimal surgery and RT are difficult (e.g., adjacent to the small bowel, kidney, and liver). Consequently, the excellent local control rates achieved with combined-modality treatment of ESTSs are not seen in RPS.[35,52,218–221] For example, in a series of 102 RPS patients treated at PMH, complete excision was achieved in only 45, gross disease remained in 29, and only a biopsy was possible in 28.[221] The overall local-regional relapse-free rates were 28% and 9% at 5 and 10 years, respectively. RT did not improve survival but appeared to significantly lengthen the time to local-regional relapse, especially with higher doses. Complete tumor resection was the only significant prognostic variable for survival and local-regional and distant failure, similar to other series referenced above. RPS patients should be evaluated in a multidisciplinary clinic prior to treatment so that patients can benefit from the expertise and investigational approaches available in such centers.

Controversial reports from Europe explored extended surgery termed compartmental resection as a strategy to improve local control for patients with RPS.[222,223] These retrospective reports from France and Italy have suggested that local control may be enhanced by resecting adjacent involved viscera—primarily the kidney and colon. Interpretation of these reports is complicated by significant selection bias and, as outlined in an editorial that accompanied these papers,[224] no specific therapeutic recommendation could be made based on these data. At this time, there are no clinical trials demonstrating improved local control with more radical surgery that involves resection of adjacent uninvolved viscera.

Radiotherapy for RPS

RPS is rare and in fact represents a group of diseases comprised of several histologic sub-types with different biologic behaviors. Because of this rarity and heterogeneity, rigorous data testing the role of RT does not exist and surgery alone remains the standard of care. A prospective randomized trial compared an IORT boost (20 Gy) to the tumor bed followed by postoperative external beam (35–40 Gy) with conventional postoperative RT (50–55 Gy). In this study of 35 patients, the incidence of local-regional recurrence was lower in the experimental treatment arm, but no improvement in survival was demonstrated.[225] IORT was associated with a high rate of peripheral neuropathy and gastrointestinal complications were more common in the control group, in whom higher doses were delivered to the bowel. Since RT was included in both arms of the trial, the role of RT in addition to surgery cannot be assessed. There are several retrospective trials comparing pre- or postoperative RT to surgery alone for RPS. These studies all have potential selection biases and provide mixed results regarding the potential local control efficacy of adding RT to surgery.[226–232] There is only one completed randomized trial addressing the role of RT for RPS. The EORTC STRASS (a phase III randomized study of preoperative radiotherapy plus surgery versus surgery alone for patients with retroperitoneal sarcoma) trial compared 50.4 Gy preoperative RT followed by surgery to surgery alone for 266 patients with primary, localized RPS.[79] The primary endpoint was a composite endpoint of abdominal recurrence-free survival (ARFS). Median follow-up is relatively short at 43.1 months. There was no statistically significant benefit due to the addition of RT to surgery. On sub-group analysis, there was a suggestion of benefit for RT for low-grade liposarcoma. Given the limited data, it is not possible to endorse *routine* use of RT in addition to surgery for RPS. With further study, RPS sub-groups that benefit from RT may be identified.

(1) After multidisciplinary evaluation, acknowledgment of the lack of firm data to support a role for RT, and incorporation of patient preferences, it may be reasonable to consider RT in select cases to improve local control. If RT is going to be delivered, preoperative RT is preferred to postoperative RT for several reasons. Advantages for preoperative RT for RPS include: the tumor bulk often displaces small bowel from the high-dose RT region, resulting in a safer and less toxic treatment; (2) bowel is unlikely to be fixed by surgical adhesions as when RT is given postoperatively, enabling safe delivery of a higher dose to the true area at risk; (3) optimum knowledge of the gross tumor location is possible, permitting better radiation targeting; (4) the tumor is contained by an intact peritoneal covering, providing a physical barrier to immediate tumor dissemination; (5) the risk of intraperitoneal tumor dissemination at the time of surgery may be reduced by the biologic impact of preoperative RT; and (6) using traditional principles of sarcoma RT, the radiation dose believed to be biologically effective is lower in the preoperative setting. Although RT planning for RPS can be complex, studies have shown that preoperative RT can be delivered safely, without significant gastro-intestinal toxicity nor increased morbidity following resection.[233,234]

When preoperative RT is planned, it is imperative that the surgeon and radiation oncologist discuss the details of the resection especially with respect to whether the ipsilateral kidney will be resected and the extent of any liver resection planned.[235] In such situations it is important to document adequate function of the contralateral kidney and minimize RT dose to the remaining kidney and liver. At the time of simulation, evaluation of motion with a 4D-CT is recommended to define an internal gross tumor volume (iGTV) (which incorporates motion of the tumor). Typical volume expansions from GTV to CTV are 1.5 cm with editing at liver, kidney, bone, and retroperitoneal compartment and expansion 5 mm into bowel.[235] IMRT or VMAT is the favored technique.[236,237] The standard dose is 50 Gy in 2 Gy fractions over 5 weeks. Dose escalation to areas of expected positive margins (posterior abdominal wall, vertebral body, great vessels) has been reported in several studies.[238–241] Reported toxicity is acceptable and local control encouraging, but follow-up is short. Dose escalation has not been compared to conventional dose RT nor to surgery alone and thus is best delivered on a trial or at experienced institutions.

Postoperative RT is typically not recommended. Following surgery alone, surveillance is preferred with consideration of preoperative RT at the time of a localized recurrence. Postoperative RT might be considered in highly select situations such as cases at very high risk for recurrence where the target volume is well defined, can be treated safely, and in situations where future salvage surgery is not considered to be an option.

Chemoradiation approaches

Although chemotherapy alone has not been associated with obvious improvements in outcome of RPS, chemoradiation, as in other solid tumors, is a subject of interest as a treatment strategy for RPS. This is especially relevant in high-grade RPS, which have a more adverse prognosis than the more common low-grade lesions.

Pilot studies using concurrent preoperative chemotherapy and external beam radiation have been reported, often in patients with extremely large tumors, with acceptable toxicity and with achievement of local control in patients in whom a negative-margin resection was possible.[141,146] These reports demonstrate that chemoradiation approaches are feasible. Additional phase 2 studies will be necessary to clarify response rates and toxicity profiles and determine whether chemoradiation should be tested in phase 3 trials. As discussed earlier, the RTOG completed a phase 2 study of preoperative doxorubicin and ifosfamide followed by preoperative RT and then by surgical resection with an intra- or postoperative radiation boost in patients with intermediate- and high-grade RPS. This study demonstrated significant toxicities and event-free outcomes that were considered modest.[143,145]

Additional issues in STS management

Functional outcome and morbidity of treatment

The functional result of extremity sarcoma management has become an important component of outcome assessment. Assessing the functional result is difficult, as it requires methods that are valid and reproducible. Many centers have yet to become experienced in the development and use of these methods, and much of the literature contains significant heterogeneity in patient samples.

Thus far, the variables associated with poorer functional outcome include large tumor size, higher doses and larger volumes of radiation, nerve sacrifice, postoperative fracture, and wound-healing complications.[242,243] To evaluate and compare functional outcome, it is imperative that functional data be reported consistently. Three disease-specific scoring scales have been reported as useful in assessing functional outcome.[244] This area has been discussed in detail by Davis,[244] who observed that "function" has many meanings in the literature. The concepts of impairment, disability, and handicap following ESTS are likely misunderstood and certainly not used consistently. Davis noted that impairment is a disorder of structure or function whereas disability is a restriction or lack of ability to perform an activity. Handicap results from impairment and disability and prevents or restricts an individual from performing in a role that is normal for the individual. For sarcoma patients, impairments can be manifested as soft tissue fibrosis, loss of motion at a joint, and decreased muscle strength; disability can be manifested as limited mobility and difficulty performing routine self-care and activities of daily living; and handicap can be evident in limitation in family roles, social functioning, and the capacity for employment.

Impairments are the most frequently reported deficits following limb-preserving therapy for ESTS, and up to 50% of patients appear to experience significant impairments.[244] Disability occurs less frequently, although reports are contradictory. It seems likely that many sarcoma patients learn to accommodate their impairments. Handicap has received little attention in the literature. However, the limited data suggest that up to 50% of patients may experience changes in their employment and vocation status after treatment of ESTS. The continuing challenge in treating sarcomas is to define the therapeutic ratio for the patient with sarcoma of the extremity. Specifically, the aim of the multidisciplinary team will be to minimize the amount of treatment while maintaining or improving current standards of disease control to reduce treatment morbidity and enhance patient outcome.

Wound complications

Considerable variability in reporting wound-healing complications exists in the literature. WCs have been reported in up to 40% of patients undergoing extremity sarcoma surgery.[88,245–247] Differences in the definition of WCs probably account for some of the variability in reporting. The retrospective data suggest that factors associated with compromised wound healing include advanced patient age, poor nutritional status, lower extremity tumor location, large tumor size, and preoperative adjuvant treatment, especially RT.[245,246,248] Particularly high complication rates were noted with combination preoperative RT and hyperthermia.[117] Although many authors have reported an association of WCs with preoperative RT, reports of high rates of surgical complications without RT or chemotherapy also exist.[249] Most likely, these relate to the risk of major WCs associated with extensive tumor resection, particularly in the lower extremities. The use of vascularized tissue transfers to replace resected tissues and optimize wound closure may decrease the risks of major WCs and allow for more extensive limb-sparing surgical approaches.[242,248,250] As noted earlier, the SR2 trial results have confirmed the adverse effect of preoperative RT on wound healing in a prospective manner but did not resolve the contribution of tissue transfer for wound reconstruction as its use was determined on an individual basis at the surgeon's discretion.[93] Recently, enhanced recovery after surgery (ERAS) pathways have been developed for sarcomas. Preliminary, single-institution data suggest ERAS principles, including judicious management of perioperative fluids, minimizing long-acting narcotics, and early mobilization and diet advancement may reduce rates of postoperative WCs and shorten hospital length of stay.[251]

Molecularly and pathologically based sarcoma management

Management of sarcomas is increasingly being driven by the specific nature of the disease entity, most importantly the pathophysiologic subtype. The work of Pasteur and Koch was fundamental for the recognition and definition of pathogenic microbes; similarly, many laboratories today are identifying molecular changes that are redefining the field of sarcoma research. An example of this work is in the recognition of soft tissue Ewing sarcoma/PNET family of tumors as relatives of their bony primary counterparts by virtue of the same spectrum of translocations in each clinical setting. These tumors should be treated with curative intent using an aggressive multimodality approach that begins with multi-agent chemotherapy. If primary surgery has removed measurable disease, adjuvant chemotherapy is definitely indicated, with consideration of adjuvant RT. By adopting similar strategies for PNETs and Askin tumors as for conventional Ewing sarcomas, outcomes improved. The molecular similarities between tumors of this family have led to the current convention of considering them morphologic and clinicopathologic variants of the same underlying molecular disease process.[252,253]

Greater understanding of the biology of translocation gene products points to epigenetic events being important in sarcomagenesis and should impact on the efficacy of chemotherapy. Ewing sarcoma and synovial sarcoma are chemotherapy-responsive STS subtypes. While *TP53* could be posited as a reason that certain sarcomas are chemotherapy sensitive, *TP53* status is not the only factor dictating chemotherapy sensitivity as there are other *TP53* wild-type sarcomas that are far less sensitive to chemotherapy, for example extraskeletal myxoid chondrosarcoma and alveolar soft part sarcoma. Striking research on the epigenetic mSWI/SNF (BAF) complexes and their role in synovial sarcoma hopefully will shed light on some of the basic mechanistic aspects permitting synovial sarcoma survival, in order to better engender tumor cell death.[254,255]

As a final example, the multiple histopathologic subtypes of liposarcomas are becoming increasingly well researched and well understood, and mechanisms by which some forms acquire their characteristic DNA signature are beginning to become understood.[256] Myxoid and round-cell liposarcomas usually exhibit a characteristic chromosomal rearrangement t(12;16) (q13;p11) *FUS-DDIT3*. These liposarcomas tend to be relatively sensitive to chemotherapy, with trabectedin standing out as most active in this specific diagnosis. Trabectedin appears to inhibit the binding of the FUS-DDIT3 fusion protein to DNA, which then causes liposarcoma cell death or differentiation.[257,258] The rarer pleomorphic liposarcoma subtype has more in common with undifferentiated pleomorphic sarcoma than other liposarcomas. Finally, well-differentiated liposarcomas exhibit ring and giant marker chromosomes on cytogenetic analysis and these karyotypic abnormalities, often involving massive amplification of chromosome 12q, carry through in de-differentiated liposarcomas. Unraveling the ability of the CDK4 and MDM2 loci on 12q to amplify hundreds of times in well well-differentiated–dedifferentiated liposarcoma may provide insight on how better to attack these relatively chemotherapy insensitive sarcomas.[259-261]

Immunotherapy for STS

Engineered T cell therapy in NY-ESO-1-positive and MAGE/LAGE positive sarcomas such as synovial sarcoma and myxoid liposarcoma have been evaluated by Robbins et al.[262,263] and are currently being evaluated in several on-going clinical trials. One of the largest studies in sarcoma to date using pembrolizumab, an anti-PD-1 antibody failed to meet its primary endpoint of overall response. However, pembrolizumab showed encouraging activity in patients with undifferentiated pleomorphic sarcoma or dedifferentiated liposarcoma. Recent approval of pembrolizumab for tumors with tumor mutational burden (TMB) >10 in a tissue agnostic manner, may prove helpful to patients with radiation-associated sarcomas like postradiation angiosarcoma, or scalp angiosarcoma, that tend to have better sensitivity to immunotherapy approaches.[264]

Summary

It is clear that STS management has improved in the past 20 years. In fewer than three decades, the standard of care has shifted toward coordinated multimodality care in specialty centers, with increased rates of function-sparing surgery and better outcomes for patients. Judicious use of aggressive multimodality approaches shows promise to decrease relapse rates and improve survival rates. The genomic and immunological revolutions in cancer are furthering the fundamental understanding of these unusual diseases and providing novel approaches for diagnostic techniques, which will banish the vagaries and lack of consistency that have plagued this field of clinical investigation, and also will provide resources for selecting new targets for therapy. New therapeutic initiatives are attacking the basic mechanisms of sarcomatous transformation of cells in some subtypes of STS, and it is hoped that these initiatives will improve outcomes for patients with less morbidity than current treatments entail. Large collaborative studies should further this work.

Key references

The complete reference list can be found on Vital Source version of this title, see inside front cover.

3   Thomas DM, Ballinger ML. Etiologic, environmental and inherited risk factors in sarcomas. *J Surg Oncol*. 2015;**111**(5):490–495. doi: 10.1002/jso.23809.

6   Kolberg M, Holand M, Agesen TH, et al. Survival meta-analyses for >1800 malignant peripheral nerve sheath tumor patients with and without neurofibromatosis type 1. *Neuro Oncol*. 2013;**15**(2):135–147. doi: 10.1093/neuonc/nos287.

17 Couture J, Mitri A, Lagace R, et al. A germline mutation at the extreme 3' end of the APC gene results in a severe desmoid phenotype and is associated with overexpression of beta-catenin in the desmoid tumor. *Clin Genet*. 2000;**57**(3):205–212.

19 Gladdy RA, Qin LX, Moraco N, et al. Do radiation-associated soft tissue sarcomas have the same prognosis as sporadic soft tissue sarcomas? *J Clin Oncol*. 2010;**28**(12):2064–2069. doi: 10.1200/JCO.2009.25.1728.

22 Cozen W, Bernstein L, Wang F, et al. The risk of angiosarcoma following primary breast cancer. *Br J Cancer*. 1999;**81**(3):532–536. doi: 10.1038/sj.bjc.6690726.

31 Raut CP, George S, Hornick JL, et al. High rates of histopathologic discordance in sarcoma with implications for clinical care. *J Clin Oncol*. 2011;**29**(15_suppl):10065. doi: 10.1200/jco.2011.29.15_suppl.10065.

34 Brennan MF, Antonescu CR, Moraco N, Singer S. Lessons learned from the study of 10,000 patients with soft tissue sarcoma. *Ann Surg*. 2014;**260**(3):416–421; discussion 421–422. doi: 10.1097/SLA.0000000000000869.

43 von Mehren M, Randall RL, Benjamin RS, et al. Soft tissue sarcoma, Version 2.2018, NCCN Clinical Practice Guidelines in Oncology. *J Natil Compr Canc Netw*. 2018;**16**(5):536–563.

52 Gronchi A, Miceli R, Shurell E, et al. Outcome prediction in primary resected retroperitoneal soft tissue sarcoma: histology-specific overall survival and disease-free survival nomograms built on major sarcoma center data sets. *J Clin Oncol*. 2013;**31**(13):1649–1655. doi: 10.1200/JCO.2012.44.3747.

54 Cahlon O, Brennan MF, Jia X, et al. A postoperative nomogram for local recurrence risk in extremity soft tissue sarcomas after limb-sparing surgery without adjuvant radiation. *Ann Surg*. 2012;**255**(2):343–347. doi: 10.1097/SLA.0b013e3182367aa7.

55 Eilber FC, Kattan MW. Sarcoma nomogram: validation and a model to evaluate impact of therapy. *J Am Coll Surg*. 2007;**205**(4 Suppl):S90–S95. doi: 10.1016/j.jamcollsurg.2007.06.335.

57 Shuman AG, Brennan MF, Palmer FL, et al. Soft tissue sarcoma of the head & neck: nomogram validation and analysis of staging systems. *J Surg Oncol*. 2015;**111**(6):690–495. doi: 10.1002/jso.23868.

59 Brennan MF, Antonescu CR, Maki RG. *Management of Soft Tissue Sarcoma*. New York: Springer; 2013:380.

64 Demicco EG, Park MS, Araujo DM, et al. Solitary fibrous tumor: a clinicopathological study of 110 cases and proposed risk assessment model. *Mod Pathol*. 2012;**25**(9):1298–1306. doi: 10.1038/modpathol.2012.83.

66 Griffin A, Dickie C, Catton C, et al. The influence of time interval between preoperative radiation and surgical resection on the development of wound healing complications in extremity soft tissue sarcoma. *Ann Surg Oncol*. 2015;**22**:2824–2830.

68 Rosenberg SA, Tepper J, Glatstein E, et al. The treatment of soft-tissue sarcomas of the extremities: prospective randomized evaluations of (1) limb-sparing surgery plus radiation therapy compared with amputation and (2) the role of adjuvant chemotherapy. *Ann Surg*. 1982;**196**(3):305–315.

71 Karakousis CP. *Atlas of Operative Procedures in Surgical Oncology*. New York: Springer; 2015:397.

72 Andreou D, Boldt H, Werner M, et al. Sentinel node biopsy in soft tissue sarcoma subtypes with a high propensity for regional lymphatic spread--results of a large prospective trial. *Ann Oncol*. 2013;**24**(5):1400–1405. doi: 10.1093/annonc/mds650.

73 Maki RG, Moraco N, Antonescu CR, et al. Toward better soft tissue sarcoma staging: building on american joint committee on cancer staging systems versions 6 and 7. *Ann Surg Oncol*. 2013;**20**(11):3377–3383. doi: 10.1245/s10434-013-3052-0.

77 McGowan TS, Cummings BJ, O'Sullivan B, et al. An analysis of 78 breast sarcoma patients without distant metastases at presentation. *Int J Radiat Oncol Biol Phys*. 2000;**46**(2):383–390.

79 Bonvalot S, Gronchi A, Le Pechoux C, et al. Preoperative radiotherapy plus surgery versus surgery alone for patients with primary retroperitoneal sarcoma (EORTC-62092: STRASS): a multicentre, open-label, randomised, phase 3 trial. *Lancet Oncol*. 2020;**21**(10):1366–1377. doi: 10.1016/S1470-2045(20)30446-0.

80 Guadagnolo BA. IMRT should be considered a standard-of-care approach for radiation therapy for soft tissue sarcoma of the extremity. *Ann Surg Oncol*. 2019;**26**(5):1186–1187. doi: 10.1245/s10434-019-07192-3.

92 Haas RL, Delaney TF, O'Sullivan B, et al. Radiotherapy for management of extremity soft tissue sarcomas: why, when, and where? Review. *Int J Radiat Oncol Biol Phys*. 2012;**84**(3):572–580. doi: 10.1016/j.ijrobp.2012.01.062.

93 O'Sullivan B, Davis AM, Turcotte R, et al. Preoperative versus postoperative radiotherapy in soft-tissue sarcoma of the limbs: a randomised trial. *Lancet*. 2002;**359**(9325):2235–2241.

94 Salerno KE, Alektiar KM, Baldini EH, et al. Radiation therapy for treatment of soft tissue sarcoma in adults: executive summary of an ASTRO clinical practice guideline. *Pract Radiat Oncol*. 2021;**11**(5):339–351. doi: 10.1016/j.prro.2021.04.005.

95 Al Yami A, Griffin AM, Ferguson PC, et al. Positive surgical margins in soft tissue sarcoma treated with preoperative radiation: is a postoperative boost necessary? *Int J Radiat Oncol Biol Phys*. 2010;**77**(4):1191–1197. doi: 10.1016/j.ijrobp.2009.06.074.

98 Wang D, Zhang Q, Eisenberg B, et al. Significant reduction of late toxicities in patients with extremity sarcoma treated with image-guided radiation therapy to a reduced target volume: results of Radiation Therapy Oncology Group RTOG-0630 trial. *J Clin Oncol*. 2015;**33**:2231–2238. doi: 10.1200/JCO.2014.58.5828.

102 Baldini EH, Lapidus MR, Wang Q, et al. Predictors for major wound complications following preoperative radiotherapy and surgery for soft-tissue sarcoma of the extremities and trunk: importance of tumor proximity to skin surface. *Ann Surg Oncol*. 2013;**20**(5):1494–1499. doi: 10.1245/s10434-012-2797-1.

104 Folkert MR, Singer S, Brennan MF, et al. Comparison of local recurrence with conventional and intensity-modulated radiation therapy for primary soft-tissue sarcomas of the extremity. *J Clin Oncol*. 2014;**32**(29):3236–3241. doi: 10.1200/JCO.2013.53.9452.

109 Holloway CL, Delaney TF, Alektiar KM, et al. American Brachytherapy Society (ABS) consensus statement for sarcoma brachytherapy. Review. *Brachytherapy*. 2013;**12**(3):179–190. doi: 10.1016/j.brachy.2012.12.002.

111 Alektiar KM, Brennan MF, Singer S. Local control comparison of adjuvant brachytherapy to intensity-modulated radiotherapy in primary high-grade sarcoma of the extremity. Comparative Study. *Cancer*. 2011;**117**(14):3229–3234. doi: 10.1002/cncr.25882.

119 Crist WM, Anderson JR, Meza JL, et al. Intergroup rhabdomyosarcoma study-IV: results for patients with nonmetastatic disease. *J Clin Oncol*. 2001;**19**(12):3091–3102.

121 Whelan JS, Bielack SS, Marina N, et al. EURAMOS-1, an international randomised study for osteosarcoma: results from pre-randomisation treatment. *Ann Oncol*. 2015;**26**(2):407–414. doi: 10.1093/annonc/mdu526.

122 Womer RB, West DC, Krailo MD, et al. Randomized controlled trial of interval-compressed chemotherapy for the treatment of localized Ewing sarcoma: a report from the Children's Oncology Group. *J Clin Oncol*. 2012;**30**(33):4148–4154. doi: 10.1200/JCO.2011.41.5703.

123 Bramwell VH. Adjuvant chemotherapy for adult soft tissue sarcoma: is there a standard of care? *J Clin Oncol*. 2001;**19**(5):1235–1237.

128 Woll PJ, Reichardt P, Le Cesne A, et al. Adjuvant chemotherapy with doxorubicin, ifosfamide, and lenograstim for resected soft-tissue sarcoma (EORTC 62931): a multicentre randomised controlled trial. *Lancet Oncol*. 2012;**13**(10):1045–1054. doi: 10.1016/s1470-2045(12)70346-7.

129 Pervaiz N, Colterjohn N, Farrokhyar F, et al. A systematic meta-analysis of randomized controlled trials of adjuvant chemotherapy for localized resectable soft-tissue sarcoma. *Cancer*. 2008;**113**(3):573–581. doi: 10.1002/cncr.23592.

131 Le Cesne A, Ouali M, Leahy MG, et al. Doxorubicin-based adjuvant chemotherapy in soft tissue sarcoma: pooled analysis of two STBSG-EORTC phase III clinical trials. *Ann Oncol*. 2014;**25**(12):2425–2432. doi: 10.1093/annonc/mdu460.

136 Gronchi A, Ferrari S, Quagliuolo V, et al. Histotype-tailored neoadjuvant chemotherapy versus standard chemotherapy in patients with high-risk soft-tissue sarcomas (ISG-STS 1001): an international, open-label, randomised, controlled, phase 3, multicentre trial. *Lancet Oncol*. 2017;**18**(6):812–822. doi: 10.1016/S1470-2045(17)30334-0.

137 Neuwirth MG, Song Y, Sinnamon AJ, et al. Isolated Limb perfusion and infusion for extremity soft tissue sarcoma: a contemporary systematic review and meta-analysis. *Ann Surg Oncol*. 2017;**24**(13):3803–3810. doi: 10.1245/s10434-017-6109-7.

144 Kraybill WG, Harris J, Spiro IJ, et al. Long-term results of a phase 2 study of neoadjuvant chemotherapy and radiotherapy in the management of high-risk, high-grade, soft tissue sarcomas of the extremities and body wall: Radiation Therapy Oncology Group Trial 9514. *Cancer*. 2010;**116**(19):4613–4621. doi: 10.1002/cncr.25350.

145 Kraybill WG, Harris J, Spiro IJ, et al. Phase II study of neoadjuvant chemotherapy and radiation therapy in the management of high-risk, high-grade, soft tissue sarcomas of the extremities and body wall: Radiation Therapy Oncology Group Trial 9514. Clinical Trial, Phase II Multicenter Study Research Support, N.I.H., Extramural. *J Clin Oncol*. 2006;**24**(4):619–625. doi: 10.1200/JCO.2005.02.5577.

146 Pisters PW, Patel SR, Prieto VG, et al. Phase I trial of preoperative doxorubicin-based concurrent chemoradiation and surgical resection for localized extremity and body wall soft tissue sarcomas. *J Clin Oncol*. 2004;**22**(16):3375–3380. doi: 10.1200/JCO.2004.01.040.

151 Dumont SN, Araujo DM, Munsell MF, et al. Management and outcome of 239 adolescent and adult rhabdomyosarcoma patients. *Cancer Med*. 2013;**2**(4):553–563. doi: 10.1002/cam4.92.

156 Raut CP, Posner M, Desai J, et al. Surgical management of advanced gastrointestinal stromal tumors after treatment with targeted systemic therapy using kinase inhibitors. *J Clin Oncol*. 2006;**24**(15):2325–2331. doi: 10.1200/JCO.2005.05.3439.

164 Van Glabbeke M, van Oosterom AT, Oosterhuis JW, et al. Prognostic factors for the outcome of chemotherapy in advanced soft tissue sarcoma: an analysis of 2,185 patients treated with anthracycline-containing first-line regimens--a European Organization for Research and Treatment of Cancer Soft Tissue and Bone Sarcoma Group Study. *J Clin Oncol*. 1999;**17**(1):150–157.

171 Judson I, Verweij J, Gelderblom H, et al. Doxorubicin alone versus intensified doxorubicin plus ifosfamide for first-line treatment of advanced or metastatic soft-tissue sarcoma: a randomised controlled phase 3 trial. *Lancet Oncol*. 2014;**15**(4):415–423. doi: 10.1016/S1470-2045(14)70063-4.

172 Tap WD, Wagner AJ, Schoffski P, et al. Effect of doxorubicin plus olaratumab vs doxorubicin plus placebo on survival in patients with advanced soft tissue sarcomas: The ANNOUNCE randomized clinical trial. *JAMA*. 2020;**323**(13):1266–1276. doi: 10.1001/jama.2020.1707.

173 Tap WD, Jones RL, Van Tine BA, et al. Olaratumab and doxorubicin versus doxorubicin alone for treatment of soft-tissue sarcoma: an open-label phase 1b and randomised phase 2 trial. *Lancet*. 2016;**388**(10043):488–497. doi: 10.1016/S0140-6736(16)30587-6.

178 Hensley ML, Maki R, Venkatraman E, et al. Gemcitabine and docetaxel in patients with unresectable leiomyosarcoma: results of a phase II trial. *J Clin Oncol*. 2002;**20**(12):2824–2831.

180 Maki RG, Wathen JK, Patel SR, et al. Randomized phase II study of gemcitabine and docetaxel compared with gemcitabine alone in patients with metastatic soft tissue sarcomas: results of sarcoma alliance for research through collaboration study 002 [corrected]. *J Clin Oncol*. 2007;**25**(19):2755–2763. doi: 10.1200/JCO.2006.10.4117.

182 Seddon B, Strauss SJ, Whelan J, et al. Gemcitabine and docetaxel versus doxorubicin as first-line treatment in previously untreated advanced unresectable or

185 Demetri G, von Mehren M, Jones R. Efficacy and safety of trabectedin or dacarbazine for metastatic liposarcoma or leiomyosarcoma after failure of conventional chemotherapy: results of a phase III randomized multicener clinical trial. *J Clin Oncol*. 2016;**34**(8):786–793.

187 Schoffski P, Ray-Coquard IL, Cioffi A, et al. Activity of eribulin mesylate in patients with soft-tissue sarcoma: a phase 2 study in four independent histological subtypes. *Lancet Oncol*. 2011;**12**(11):1045–1052. doi: 10.1016/S1470-2045(11)70230-3.

191 Wagner AJ, Malinowska-Kolodziej I, Morgan JA, et al. Clinical activity of mTOR inhibition with sirolimus in malignant perivascular epithelioid cell tumors: targeting the pathogenic activation of mTORC1 in tumors. *J Clin Oncol*. 2010;**28**(5):835–840. doi: 10.1200/JCO.2009.25.2981.

194 Tap W, Gelderblom H, Palmerini E, et al. Pexidartinib versus placebo for advanced tenosynovial giant cell tumor (ENLIVEN): a randomized phase 3 trial. *The Lancet*. 2019;**394**(10197):478–487.

196 Wagner A, Ravi V, Riedel R, et al. Nab-Sirolimus for patients with malignant perivascular epitheliod cell tumors. *J Clin Oncol*. 2021;**39**(33):3660–3670.

metastatic soft-tissue sarcomas (GeDDiS): a randomised controlled phase 3 trial. *Lancet Oncol*. 2017;**18**(10):1397–1410. doi: 10.1016/S1470-2045(17)30622-8.

201 Demetri GD, von Mehren M, Blanke CD, et al. Efficacy and safety of imatinib mesylate in advanced gastrointestinal stromal tumors. *N Engl J Med*. 2002;**347**(7):472–480. doi: 10.1056/NEJMoa020461.

208 Demetri GD, Reichardt P, Kang YK, et al. Efficacy and safety of regorafenib for advanced gastrointestinal stromal tumours after failure of imatinib and sunitinib (GRID): an international, multicentre, randomised, placebo-controlled, phase 3 trial. *Lancet*. 2013;**381**(9863):295–302. doi: 10.1016/S0140-6736(12)61857-1.

210 George S, Jones RL, Bauer S, et al. Avapritinib in patients with advanced gastrointestinal stromal tumors following at least three prior lines of therapy. *Oncologist*. 2021;**26**(4):e639–e649. doi: 10.1002/onco.13674.

212 Blay JY, Serrano C, Heinrich MC, et al. Ripretinib in patients with advanced gastrointestinal stromal tumours (INVICTUS): a double-blind, randomised, placebo-controlled, phase 3 trial. *Lancet Oncol*. 2020;**21**(7):923–934. doi: 10.1016/S1470-2045(20)30168-6.

214 Joensuu H, Eriksson M, Sundby Hall K, et al. One vs three years of adjuvant imatinib for operable gastrointestinal stromal tumor: a randomized trial. *JAMA*. 2012;**307**(12):1265–1272. doi: 10.1001/jama.2012.347.

110 Myelodysplastic syndromes

Uma M. Borate, MD, MS

Overview

Primary, secondary, and familial myelodysplastic syndromes (MDS) became a reportable group of malignancies in 2001. Over the past 20 years, there have been tremendous strides in genetic and translational research, which has influenced the pathological diagnosis and classification, risk stratification scoring systems, and genomic characterization of MDS. In certain cases, this has led to more personalized therapy options such as Luspatercept in RARS patients with SF3B1 mutations. In this chapter, we discuss the history behind the various MDS prognostic risk stratification and classifications. We also examine our current understanding of MDS pathophysiology, the complexities with establishing an MDS diagnosis including the evolving diagnostic criteria, and the use of next-generation sequencing analyses. Then, we outline both the standard of care therapeutic options including hypomethylating agents, and their impact over the past decade, as well as multiple clinical trials and treatment options being investigated for MDS patients. Finally, we discuss what personalized treatments and possible preventative strategies we may expect to see – in the next decade – for MDS development in high-risk patient populations.

Myelodysplastic syndromes (MDSs), derived from a multipotent hematopoietic stem cell, are characterized clinically by a hyperproliferative bone marrow, ineffective hematopoiesis, and one or more peripheral cytopenias. These group of disorders became reportable as a group of malignancies in the Surveillance, Epidemiology, and End-Results Program in 2001.[1] These neoplasms are reported as either primary, secondary, or familial.[2] Primary MDS arise de novo while patients with a history of cancer treatment, environmental exposure, inherited genetic abnormalities (Fanconi anemia or paroxysmal nocturnal hemoglobinuria) are placed in the secondary MDS (sMDS) category.[3]

Estimates of the incidence of MDS range from a frequency equal to that of acute myeloid leukemia (AML), or approximately 14,000 new cases per year in the United States, to almost twice that of AML.[4-6] The incidence rate of sMDS—more specifically therapy-related MDS (t-MDS) which constitutes approximately 10–20% of all MDS cases—is estimated to increase by 2% annual as a result of increased use of chemotherapy, radiotherapy, and extended survival of patients with prior malignancies.[7-12] The Surveillance, Epidemiology, and End Results (SEER) database now tracks the disease, thus more accurate data will be available in the future. An estimate based on medical insurance claims indicated a total of 107,000 cases in the observation period from 2009 to 2011.[13] The consensus is that the incidence is increasing owing to a number of factors, including those described above, greater awareness, greater diagnostic precision, and the aging of the population. Ultimately, approximately 30% of patients with MDS progress to a leukemic state known as secondary AML.[14,15]

Classically, MDS and secondary AML have been classified as distinct entities. In recent years, the identification of clonal hematopoiesis (CH) in myeloid genes that are commonly mutated has been identified as a distinct entity known as clonal hematopoiesis of indeterminate potential (CHIP). There have been additional disease entities characterized in the CH spectrum such as idiopathic clonal cytopenia of undetermined significance (ICCUS), clonal cytopenia of unknown significance (CCUS), and age-related clonal hematopoiesis (ARCH). These will be discussed more in detail in the section titled "Clonal origin" of this chapter. This is an emerging area in the field of MDS where identification, close observation, and possibly early treatment of these entities may form part of the future strategy of the care of the MDS patient.[16,17]

Classification

The most recent classification of MDS released in 2016 incorporated molecular genetic features of these disorders due to novel methods of genetic analysis using next-generation sequencing (NGS). The 2016 WHO classification of MDS is as follows: (1) MDS with single lineage dysplasia (MDS-SLD), (2) MDS with ringed sideroblasts (MDS-RS), (3) MDS with multilineage dysplasia (MDS-MLD), (4) MDS with excess blasts (MDS-EB), (5) MDS with isolated deletion (5q), (6) MDS, unclassifiable (MDS-U), and (7) Refractory cytopenia of childhood (provisional).[18] Within MDS-RS are two more categories (a) MDS-RS-SLD and (b) MDS-RS-MLD while MDS-EB also has two subgroups (a) MDS-EB-1 and (b) MDS-EB-2 (Table 1).[18]

The heterogeneity of these disorders prompted specifically categorizing patients into prognostic risk groups to guide clinical decision-making. The International Prognostic Scoring System (IPSS) has been advanced based on the percentage of bone marrow blasts, cytogenetics, and degree of cytopenias.[19] The IPSS has predictive value for both survival and risk of transformation to acute leukemia. However, this prognostic scoring system did not consider sMDS or chronic myelomonocytic leukemia (CMML) patients and did not consider depth of cytopenias in these patient groups.

In 2002, the WHO created the World Health Organization Prognostic Scoring System (WPSS) which included a unique MDS subtype defined by del(5q).[20] The main advantage of WPSS, compared to IPSS, was its use for serial prognostication; an important characteristic given the pathophysiology of MDS. Similarly, to IPSS, limitations included the exclusion of sMDS or CMML patients.

The MD Anderson Risk Model Score for MDS (MDAS) was the next scoring system created based on the identification of several adverse factors that affected prognostication of MDS patients

---

Holland-Frei Cancer Medicine, Tenth Edition. Edited by Robert C. Bast, John C. Byrd, Carlo M. Croce, Ernest Hawk, Fadlo R. Khuri, Raphael E. Pollock, Apostolia M. Tsimberidou, Christopher G. Willett, and Cheryl L. Willman.
© 2023 John Wiley & Sons, Inc. Published 2023 by John Wiley & Sons, Inc.

Table 1 World Health Organization (WHO) 2016 classification.[a]

MDS with single lineage dysplasia (MDS-SLD)
MDS with ringed sideroblasts (MDS-RS)
With single lineage dysplasia (MDS-RS-SLD)
With multi-lineage dysplasia (MDS-RS-MLD)
MDS with multilineage dysplasia (MDS-MLD)
MDS with excess blasts (MDS-EB)
Type 1 (MDS-EB-1)
Type 2 (MDS-EB-2)
MDS with isolated del(5q)
Myelodysplastic syndrome, unclassifiable (MDS-U)
Refractory cytopenia of childhood (provisional)

[a]Source: Modified after Hong and He.[18]

including Eastern Cooperative Oncology Group (ECOG) performance status, age, platelet count, white blood cell (WBC) counts, hemoglobin count, bone marrow blast count, cytogenetics, and history of transfusions.[20] The MDAS included patients not included in IPSS and WPSS, could be used for serial prognostication, and included new factors to risk stratify patients into four groups.

Finally, The IPSS was revised (IPSS-R) and now separates patients into five subcategories with greater predictive value and utilizes peripheral blood count values in a more discriminatory manner. The cytogenetic subgroups have also been revised based on further risk assessment. These revisions were based on analyses of 7012 patients compared to 816 for the original IPSS. The IPSS-R is better able to segregate patients into risk categories and predict prognoses for, not only, newly diagnosed patients but also for patients at any time during their course of disease. The new cytogenetic classification defined 16 cytogenetic abnormalities that were grouped into 5 categories. These classifications have been validated and have become, along with the World Health Organization (WHO) classification,[4] the standard classifications (Tables 2–4). If cytogenetic data are not available, however, the predictive power of the IPSS models diminishes significantly.

A number of other relevant prognostic approaches—such as flow cytometry, cytogenetic analysis, and molecular analysis—are most likely to contribute to the formation of the next version of the IPSS-R and other MDS prognostic models that were discussed here; similarly, to the 2016 WHO Classification of MDS. In addition, the recent advancements in genetic analysis and technology have offered rapid and accurate genomic profile with whole-genome and NGS across various cancer types including MDS and AML.[21,22] Even though MDS and AML are molecularly heterogenous, these technologies have provided an opportunity to identify subgroups of individuals that reflect distinct paths in the evolution of MDS and AML.[22] It has been discovered that genes found in at least 5% of primary MDS patients have prognostic impact (Table 5).[20] Future prognostic models may incorporate NGS results for improved disease classification, prognostication, and prediction of therapy response.

Table 3 International prognostic scoring system – revised (IPSS) classification of MDS according to prognostic risk subgroups.[a]

International prognostic scoring system (IPSS)	Risk of transformation to acute myeloid leukemia (in 25% of patients) (yr)	Median survival (yr)
Very low	Not reached	8.8
Low	10.8	5.3
Intermediate-1	3.2	3.0
High	1.4	1.6
Very high	0.73	0.8

[a]Source: Modified after Vardiman et al.[4]

Table 4 World Health Organization (WHO) 2016 classification.[a]

MDS with single lineage dysplasia (MDS-SLD)
MDS with ringed sideroblasts (MDS-RS)
With single lineage dysplasia (MDS-RS-SLD)
With multilineage dysplasia (MDS-RS-MLD)
MDS with multilineage dysplasia (MDS-MLD)
MDS with excess blasts (MDS-EB)
Type 1 (MDS-EB-1)
Type 2 (MDS-EB-2)
MDS with isolated del(5q)
Myelodysplastic syndrome, unclassifiable (MDS-U)
Refractory cytopenia of childhood (provisional)

[a]Source: Modified from Vardiman et al.[4]

Table 5 Prognostic impact of recurrent (>5%) mutations in MDS.[a]

Function	Gene
Epigenetic/chromatin modifiers	TET2,[b] DNMT3A,[c] ASXL1,[c] EXH2[c]
Splicing	SF3B1,[b] SRSF2,[c] U2AF1,[c] ZRSR2[c]
Differentiaton	RUNX1[c]
DNA damage response/apoptosis	TP53,[c] BCOR[c]
Cohesion complex	STAG2[d]
Signaling	CBL[d]

[a]Source: Modified after Jonas and Greenberg.[20]
[b]Favorable prognostic impact.
[c]Negative prognostic impact.
[d]Neutral prognostic impact.

Table 2 IPSS score.[a]

Prognostic variable	Score value				
	0	0.5	1.0	1.5	2.0
Bone marrow blasts (%)	<5	5–10	—	11–20	21–29
Karyotype	Good	Interm	Poor	—	—
Cytopenias	0/1	2/3	—	—	—
Scores	Cytogenetics				
Low: 0	Good: normal				
Intermediate-1: 0.5–1.0	−y				
Intermediate-2: 1.5–2.0	del (5q)				
High: >2.5	del (20q)				
	Poor: chromosome 7 abnormalities				
	Complex ≥3 abnormalities				
	Intermediate: other				

[a]Source: Modified after Vardiman et al.[4]

Table 6 Research performed in the past 20 years investigating the probability of T-MDS development after prior malignancy/associated chemotherapy.[a]

Primary malignancy	Risk factors
Hodgkins lymphoma	Treatment with alkylating agents 14-yr cumulative probability was 2.8%
Breast cancer treated with mitoxantrone	1.8% incidence of t-MDS + 3.6% incidence of t-AML at 72 mo
Acute myeloid leukemia	6-yr cumulative probability: 13.5%. Peripheral blood HSCT
Ovarian cancer	Dose-dependent increased risk with carboplatin and cisplatin
HL and NHL autologous HSCT	5-yr cumulative survival: 4.6% for HL and 3% for NHL Higher risk with older age and exposure to total body irradiation
Testicular cancer	Dose-dependent radiation. Cumulative dose of cisplatin
HL and NHL autologous HSCT	Cumulative probability of MDS/AML 8.6% at 6 yr. Stem cell priming with etoposide (RR = 7.7)
Acute leukemia	Incidence was 0.88% Myelosuppressive chemotherapy and pegfilgrastim
Acute lymphoblastic leukemia	15-yr cumulative incidence was 0.3%Relapse of primary disease was associated with increased risk
Indolent lymphoma randomized to autologous HSCT versus IFN	5-yr risk for secondary hematologic neoplasia was 3.8% in patients with radiochemotherapy and autologous STC. In contrast, in the IFN-α arm, the 5-yr risk of hematologic neoplasia was 0%
NHL autologous HSCT	Median latency to develop t-MDS was 6 mo (range: 6–44 m). Slow collectors were found to be at fourfold higher risk of developing t-MDS/AML (RR = 4.0; 95% CI, 0.5–35.1) compared with rapid collectors
Ewing sarcoma	5-yr cumulative incidence of 2%Increasing exposure for cyclophosphamide from 9.6 to 17.6 g/m^2 and doxorubicin from 375 to 450 mg/m^2
Hodgkin's lymphoma	10-yr cumulative incidence ranged from 0.3% to 5.7%
US population-based cancer registries	t-AML risks increased after chemotherapy for NHL, declined for ovarian cancer, myeloma, and possibly lung cancer and were significantly heterogeneous for breast cancer and HL
Hodgkin's lymphoma	Median time from HL treatment to t-AML/MDS was 31 mo. Patients who received >4 cycles of escalated BEACOPP had a higher risk compared with BEACOPP (1.7% vs 0.7%)

[a]Source: Modified after Candelaria and Dueñas-Gonzalez.[32]

Etiology

Although the etiologic agent cannot be identified in the majority of patients with MDS, in some, exposure to ionizing radiation, chemicals, drugs, or other environmental agents can be implicated.

Radiation exposure has been clearly linked to the development of stem cell abnormalities,[23] as seen in the leukemias that developed in survivors of atomic bomb explosions were often preceded by a preleukemic state.[24] They also continued to exhibit an increased incidence of genetic instability seen as structural and numerical chromosomal abnormalities long after the initial exposure, which may contribute to the development of MDS and AML.[25] Chemical injury to the marrow is a well-established phenomenon, and an increased risk of leukemogenesis has been noted among workers exposed to petrochemicals, particularly benzene, and the rubber industry.[26–28] Many of the initial cases of benzene-induced leukemia were associated with a preleukemic syndrome.[29] Exposure of human cell lines to hydroquinone, a benzene metabolite, is associated with the development of abnormalities of chromosomes 5, 7, and 8 and may be responsible, in part, for the DNA damage associated with the chemical exposure.[30] In patients with or without ringed sideroblasts exposure to diesel oil fumes ($p < 0.01$), diesel oil liquids ($p < 0.01$), or ammonia ($p < 0.05$) was associated with the development of MDS.[31] A careful history of exposure to environmental and occupational hazards should be an integral part of the work-up of all patients with MDSs. Additional environmental factors may include the use of hair dye and cigarette smoking.[5]

In contrast to chemical exposure, both a history of chemotherapy and radiation therapy are associated with a subset of MDS named t-MDS. The incidence rate of t-MDS and leukemia is estimated to increase by 2% annually as a result of increased use of chemotherapy, radiotherapy, and extended survival of patients with prior malignancies.[7–12] In the past 20 years, it has been recognized that certain cancer types, and the chemotherapy agents used to treat those cancers, are more associated with increased risk of t-MDS compared to others such as alkylating agents, topoisomerase II inhibitors, and platinum compounds (Table 6).[32] Chemotherapy agents have also been linked to certain genetic mutations (i.e., balance rearrangements within mixed-lineage leukemia (MLL) gene, promyelocytic leukemia/retinoic acid receptor alpha (PML-RARA) fusion, balanced translocation between RUNX1 and CBFB genes (21q22 or 16q22) have been linked to topoisomerase II inhibitors).[33] On the other hand, alkylating agents have lower risks and other classes of agents, such as fluoropyrimidines, have no known association with t-MDS development.[34] Radiotherapy, unfortunately, has been associated with t-MDS development but the overall risk is unclear.[34–37]

With the introduction of new chemotherapeutic agents, increased neoadjuvant and adjuvant chemotherapy, and chemoimmunotherapy, there have been various reports of increased risk for t-MDS after solid tumor treatment as well as decreased risk of t-MDS development for immunotherapy.[34,38–41] For example, research performed using the SEER identified that t-MDS and AML risks were statistically significantly elevated after chemotherapy for 22 of 23 solid cancers (all except colon cancer).[34] On the other hand, a study examining chronic lymphocytic leukemia (CLL) chemoimmunotherapy found that rare incidences (1/1000) of secondary hematological malignancies and especially myeloid malignancies.[39] Most recently, in a safety meta-analysis, poly (ADP-ribose) polymerase (PARP) inhibitors (an agent used for ovarian cancer) were associated with a higher development of AML and t-MDS compared to placebo.[41]

Yet, exposure history is only a small component of the complex etiology of MDS and t-MDS. The physiology specific to stem cell hematopoiesis and CH, bone marrow microenvironment, and inflammatory pathways have also been found to play a role in recent years.

Pathobiology

Clonal origin

In recent years, the identification of CH in myeloid genes that are commonly mutated has been identified as a distinct entity known as CHIP. The development of NGS technology has permitted researchers to define CHIP and further categorize the pre-MDS conditions into the following CH spectrum: ICCUS, idiopathic dysplasia of unknown significance (IDUS), CCUS, and ARCH

Table 7 Major diagnostic features and criteria of Pre-MDS conditions as defined by WHO 2019.[a]

Pre-MDS	Major diagnostic features and criteria, does not meet MDS criteria
ICUS	Peripheral cytopenia(s), no MDS-related mutation found, no or only mild (<10%) dysplasia, blast cells <5%
CCUS	Peripheral cytopenia(s), one or more MDS-related mutations found, no or only mild (<10%) dysplasia, blast cells <5%
IDUS	No peripheral cytopenia(s), no MDS-related mutation found, dysplasia in ≥10% of neutrophilic, erythroid, and/or megakaryocytes found, blast cells <5%
CHIP	No peripheral cytopenia(s), one or more MDS-related mutations found, no or only mild (<10%) dysplasia, blast cells <5%

[a]Source: Modified after Valent[42]; Kwok et al.[43]

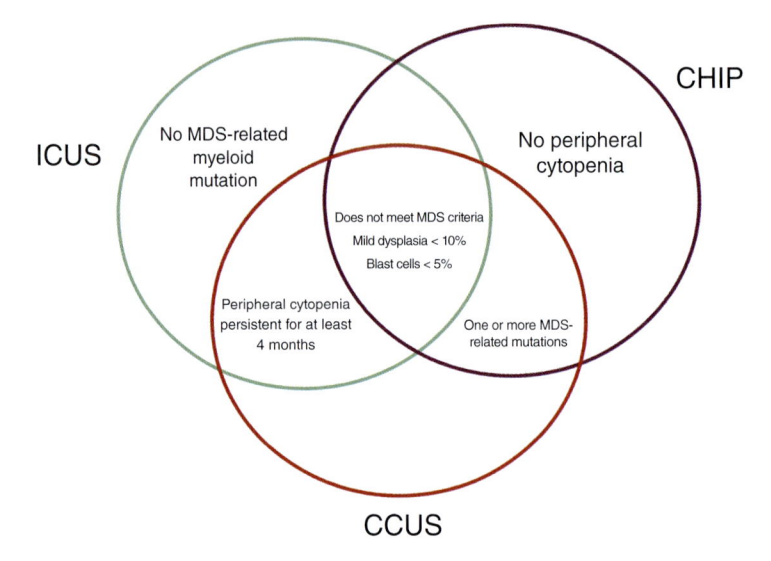

Figure 1 Venn diagram outlining the similarities and differences between pre-MDS syndromes such as clonal cytopenias of unknown significance, clonal hematopoiesis of indeterminate potential, idiopathic cytopenias of unknown significance. Source: From Valent;[42] Kwok et al.[43]

(Table 7).[40,42] In general, there has been limited research on the prevalence and therapeutic interventions for these disorders. It is hypothesized that CCUS, may have a higher prevalence than MDS.[43] Therefore, the following information is more specific to diagnostic criteria as there is little information on current therapeutic interventions, rate of MDS transformation, and risk stratification for certain CH conditions.[43]

All of these conditions are similar in that the patients who are diagnosed with these conditions may present with clinical manifestations or be diagnosed incidentally. These conditions are also all capable of progression to MDS or other hematological malignancies such as myeloid or lymphoid neoplasms or autoimmune conditions.[42] These pre-MDS conditions' diagnostic criteria are similar in that the minimal diagnostic criteria for MDS cannot be met (Figure 1). However, they are dissimilar in that some of these disorders are categorized by cytopenic states (ICCUS or CCUS) versus noncytopenic states (IDUS and CHIP).[42] Neither IDUS and ARCH have been defined by the WHO as a pre-MDS condition; however, they are used in clinical practice as a descriptor and are an entity of the Pre-MDS spectrum (Table 7).

More specifically, ICCUS is defined as a mild, moderate, or severely persistent cytopenia (>4 months) in one or more blood cell lineages (Figure 1). ICCUS is further classified into four variants depending on the cellular line that is affected (ie anemia, neutropenia, thrombocytopenia, or pan/bi-cytopenias). The subtyping of ICUS has been defined, however, its use in clinical practice is limited and there have been no studies that show that classification of ICUS has a prognostic impact. It is suspected, however, that patients with pan-cytopenias may have a higher rate of transformation than those with cytopenias specific to one cell line.[42] In contrast, IDUS is typically defined as dysplasia (>10%) in any cell line within the bone marrow but the absence of peripheral cytopenias or somatic mutations associated with MDS. History of autoimmune diseases or anti-neoplastic treatments is highly associated with bone marrow dysplasia. Before the diagnosis of IDUS, other conditions must be ruled out such as vitamin B12 deficiency, copper deficiency, or drug-induced bone marrow injury and dysplasia. Typically, this condition is provisional, and commonly after observation, it is diagnosed as another underlying disease, CHIP, or MDS.

In contrast, CHIP does *not* have a persistent cytopenia in any cell line and has *one or more* MDS-related mutation found using NGS (Figure 1). The variant allele frequency (VAF) of these mutations must be at least 2% to be considered significant. CCUS, on the other hand, has one or more MDS-related mutation is present but, in addition, one or more cytopenias in a peripheral cell line has been present for at least 4 months (Figure 1). Patients with CCUS are typically diagnosed with this disorder as peripheral cytopenias are found during routine screening examinations or in response to symptoms. In contrast, CHIP is found incidentally given the absence of peripheral cytopenias and accessibility of NGS technology. More specifically, the pathophysiology of CHIP stems from the theory of multihit and multiphase concept of cancer evolution.[44,45] It begins with a single somatic mutation in a blood cell that is commonly associated with the development of MDS, AML (Table 9). This somatic mutation favors survival of that cell, which allows it to expand and clone itself in order to survive. However, this is not yet a cancer. Many subclonal mutations must be acquired in order for this, initially benign clone, to transform into a myeloid malignancy.

Risk of transformation to myeloid malignancy has been mainly investigated in patients with CHIP given the ability to monitor the presence or absence of somatic mutations known to be associated with MDS, AML, or other hematological malignancies. CHIP has been stratified into different risk categories depending on the mutation detected. For most patients, three leukemic driver mutations are commonly identified (DMNT3A, TET2, ASXL1); DMNT3A has historically been accounted for >50% of all mutations identified in elderly patient cohorts.[17] For a person diagnosed with low-risk CHIP, the risk of transformation to a myeloid malignancy is approximately 0.5–1% annually. This risk of transformation increases if the patient has a history of hematological malignancy or radiation exposure and/or has a high-risk mutation. For patients with a TP53 mutation, risk of transformation increases by three to five fold annually.[40,46]

It is hypothesized that common mutations in CCUS and CHIP have both intrinsic and noncellular effects on the microenvironment of the bone marrow; making the survival of these clones favorable and leading to myeloid malignancy.[47] Studies have shown that loss of function in certain genes lead to distinct hyperinflammatory gene expression linked to increased inflammasome and cytokine signaling.[48] The use of anti-inflammatory agents to possibly slow the progression of CH and, as result, slow the progression to myeloid malignancy is an emerging area of scientific focus.

CH has also been linked to nonmalignant diseases specifically cardiovascular disease, diabetes mellitus type 2, and chronic obstructive pulmonary disease.[49–51] Definitive causation has not been linked for the latter two diseases; however, research within the past 10 years has found causal links between CHIP status and incidence of cardiovascular events.[50,51] Analysis has revealed that patients who are CHIP positive have double the risk of ischemic stroke and myocardial infarction, and those who harbor gene mutation associated with CHIP had poorer outcomes for postinfarction congestive heart failure.[49,50]

Bone marrow microenvironment

Histologic examination of bone marrow trephine biopsies has pointed to abnormalities of the microenvironment.[52] They noted the presence of clusters of immature precursor cells in the central intertrabecular region of the marrow, rather than along the endosteal surfaces. They cited this as evidence of abnormal localization of immature precursors (ALIP).[53] In a series of 40 patients, the presence of ALIP correlated significantly with shortened survival and was associated with an increased risk of transformation to AML. These findings were independent of the French-American-British classification (FAB) subtype and were detected even in patients with refractory anemia. However, care must be applied to differentiate true ALIP from pseudo-ALIP. In the latter case, the clusters of cells are either of erythroid or megakaryocytic origin and do not convey the same prognostic information compared with the former, where the immature cells are of myeloid origin. The determination of the immature precursor phenotype by immunohistochemical methods may be helpful in distinguishing pseudo- and true ALIP.[53] ALIP is not, however, specific to patients with MDS and, therefore, not helpful as a diagnostic tool.[53]

Recent data in a mouse model suggest that osteoblasts have a modulating influence on leukemic blasts in the bone marrow microenvironmental niche. Reduction in osteoblasts is associated with leukemic progression and shortened survival.[54] This opens a possibility of osteoblast number could be a drug target in modulating progression of MDS/AML.

Signal transduction

The disordered maturation seen in hematopoietic progenitor cells may be intrinsic or could be augmented by or derived from their interaction with accessory cells and other microenvironmental factors. Hematopoietic cell defects could reflect abnormalities in signal transduction in response to cytokines or other regulatory molecules that trigger proliferation and differentiation pathways. Hematopoietic cells from MDS patients display impaired responses to a number of cytokines and are unable to respond to external signals owing either to abnormalities in number or function of cytokine receptors or to dysfunctional postbinding signal transduction.[55]

Hematopoietic progenitors have impaired responses to cytokine stimulation with decreased CFU-GM, CFU-GEMM, and BFU-E colony number.[56] Purified blast cells from MDS patients proliferate but do not mature in response to granulocyte colony-stimulating factor (G-CSF) and granulocyte-macrophage colony-stimulating factor (GM-CSF). Purified populations of CD34+ cells from MDS patients also demonstrate impaired responses to G-CSF.[57] Defects in signal transduction appear to play a larger role in the aberrant response of hematopoietic progenitors to regulatory molecules. This pertains both to the cytokine signal transduction pathways and factors which regulate apoptosis.[58–60] Epigenetic changes resulting in transcriptional silencing are another potential mechanism affecting cytokine signaling. Evidence demonstrates aberrant hypermethylation of the suppressor of cytokine signaling-1 (SOCS-1) gene in 31% of MDS patients associated with increased activity of the JAK/STAT pathway.[61] Hypermethylation which occurs in other genes such as p15 may be explained in part by the overexpression of DNA methyltransferase 1 and 3A that has been identified in bone marrow of MDS patients.[62]

Cytogenetics

Chromosomal abnormalities, found in 30–70% of MDS patients, are similar to those seen in patients with AML and involve complete or partial deletions, most frequently involving chromosomes 5(−5,5q−), 7(−7,7q−), and 8(8+).[63] Certain karyotypic abnormalities that are associated with core-binding factor rearrangements, such as t(15;17) in acute promyelocytic leukemia (M3), t(8;21) in AML (M2), and inv 16 in AML (M4), have only rarely been identified in MDS.[55,63–65] Moreover, patients with these AML subtypes have good prognoses with potential for cure. Thus, they should be viewed as having AML and should be managed accordingly. Furthermore, abnormalities involving partial deletions of the long arm of chromosome 20 (20q−), seen frequently in MDS, particularly arginyl-TRNA synthetase 1 (RARS), polycythemia vera, and myeloproliferative syndromes, are usually not seen in patients with de novo AML.[63,66] Abnormalities are identified most frequently in patients with higher-risk. Although specific chromosomal abnormalities have been identified, unlike AML, no specific abnormality has been associated with any specific subcategory.[63]

Many studies have demonstrated that the presence of karyotypic abnormalities is an independent prognostic variable.[63,67] Furthermore, more complex abnormalities are associated with shortened survival compared with either single clonal abnormality or a normal karyotype.[68,69] Certain specific clonal subtypes have varying prognostic significance for both survival and the risk of leukemic transformation. Monosomy 7 or 5 and 7q are associated with shortened survival, while deletions of the long arms of chromosome 20 (20q−) and 5(5q-syndrome) and deletion of y as the sole abnormality are associated with longer survival.[63] In the IPSS, cytogenetic findings are an independent prognostic variable classifying

Table 8 Cytogenetics: revised cytogenetic IPSS-R groupings.[a]

Risk group	Cytogenetic groupings	Doublet	Complex	Median overall survival (mo)
Very low	Del 11q −Y	—	—	60.8
Low	Normal del (5q) del (12p) del (20q)	Including del(5q)	—	48.6
Intermediate	del 7q +8 i(17p) +19 Any other independent clones	Any other	—	26
High	Inv(3)/t(3q)/del(3q) −7	Including −7/del(7q)	3	15.8
Very high	—	—	>3	5.9

[a]Source: Modified after Valcárcel et al.[68]; Jacobs et al.[69]

patients according to 3 subgroups: good, intermediate, and poor risk.[19] Further review of additional databases demonstrated that cytogenetics was underweighted as a risk factor in the IPSS and suggested that poor-risk cytogenetics was just as poor a risk factor in patients as those with > 20% blasts (Table 8).[70] This led to a revision of the IPSS cytogenetics group. These groups were categorized into five prognostic subgroups including very good, good, intermediate, poor, and very poor and were incorporated into the revised IPSS (Table 8).[71]

Genetic instability as demonstrated by clonal evolution occurs in a substantial percentage of patients. Around 20–35% have been found to undergo clonal evolution during the course of the disease, independent of karyotypic status at the outset.[72] The significance of clonal evolution with respect to leukemic transformation and survival is contradictory.[72–75] In some studies, clonal evolution was associated with a poor prognosis without an increased risk of leukemic transformation.[74] In contrast, Glenn et al.[75] have demonstrated karyotypic changes in clinically stable patients. Assessment of the clonal architecture in the marrow of MDS patients demonstrates that there is a founding clone and multiple secondary clones with acquisition of additional mutations leading to clonal evolution.[5]

One particular abnormality involving a deletion of part of the long arm of chromosome 5 (5q−) deserves special note. As originally described, the del 5q-syndrome is associated with a refractory macrocytic anemia, a normal or increased platelet count, giant thrombocytes, dyserythropoiesis, hypo-lobulated megakaryocytes, female predominance, prolonged survival, and a low rate of leukemic transformation.[72,76–78] It is important to differentiate the del 5q-syndrome from instances where this deletion is found in combination with other chromosomal abnormalities or in association with FAB subtypes other than refractory anemia that have a more aggressive clinical course associated with shorter survival. Patients with del 5q have been identified to have a deficiency in RPS14 ribosomal RNA as the genetic defect responsible for the bone marrow failure in these patients (see section titled "Gene mutations and dysregulation").[79]

Patients with MDS secondary to exposure to mutagenic or carcinogenic agents have similar findings in terms of the types and significance of the chromosomal abnormalities.[80–82] Patients treated with epipodophyllotoxins (etoposide and teniposide) can develop specific translocations involving the breakpoint at 11q23.[83,84] This leads to transcription of a fusion protein involving the MLL gene.[85]

Gene mutations and dysregulation

Alterations in the control and expression of proto-oncogenes in the cellular genome, leading to abnormalities of cellular proliferation and differentiation, are thought to contribute to the molecular basis of neoplastic transformation.[86] Point mutations of the *ras* family of oncogenes have been identified in association with a number of human tumors, including lung, pancreatic, colorectal, and hematopoietic neoplasms.[87–89] Activated *ras* genes with specific point mutations involving codons 12, 13, and 61 have been identified in 20–30% of patients with AML and 9–48% of patients with MDS. These findings have suggested that activation of *ras* genes either may contribute to the development of MDS or, once established, to the process of transformation of the commonly affected stem cell. Ki-*ras* with H-*ras* are involved in only a few cases. CMML was the FAB subtype most frequently associated with a *ras* mutation. The abnormality was found in 40% of cases.[90]

Recently, a number of genes have been identified with recurrent somatic mutations in patients with MDS involving a number of different pathways including those involved in epigenetic regulation, RNA splicing, signal activation, and transcription factors (Table 9). Many of these mutations are oncogenic and there are patterns of association or mutual exclusions in some of these abnormalities. These mutations are not exclusive to MDS but are seen in the myeloid spectrum of disease including AML and myeloproliferative neoplasms (MPNs).[91,92] The data in some of these studies indicate that there are mutations that appear early in the process of MDS whereas others are later appearing mutations. The presence of some mutations have prognostic significance particularly EZH2, TP53, RUNX1, DNAMT3A, and ASLX1.[93] Some of these mutations may lead to an increased propensity to subclonal evolution and an increased number of mutations appears to be associated with poorer outcome and higher rate of transformation to AML. The functional dysregulation of some such as TET2 or IDH1 and IDH2 mutations result in abnormalities of the hydroxymethylation but the major impact on pathways of these abnormalities is unknown. These recurring mutations will provide insight into disease mechanisms, prognostic information, and offer potential for therapeutic targets.

Deletion of all or part of chromosome 5 in a substantial number of patients with either de novo or sMDS has led to the hypothesis of a tumor suppressor gene located within a short segment of the long arm in the so-called critical region at 5q21–5q34.[94] This region has been the focus of intensive study, and candidate genes either deleted or dysregulated have been identified, narrowing the region of interest.[95] The interferon regulatory factor-1 (IRF-1) is a DNA binding regulatory factor that regulates, in part, expression of interferon and interferon-inducible genes by binding to promoter regions. It functions as an activator, has antiproliferative and antioncogene activity, and can reverse a transformed phenotype.[96] The *IRF-1* gene has been mapped to the 5q31 region.[97] A loss of one or both IRF-l alleles in patients with MDS[192] or AML with a del 5q has been described.[98–100] *In vitro* studies have suggested that loss of the *IRF-1* gene is associated either with a transformed phenotype and/or with chemo- and radiation-induced apoptosis. Although these data suggest a potential role for the *IRF-1* gene, studies have not confirmed these observations. A recent study suggests a role for overexpression of IRF-1 leading to upregulation of Toll-like receptors resulting in an activated apoptotic pathway.[101] The lack of identification of a definitive tumor suppressor gene responsible for the disease has led to other approaches investigating the underlying

Table 9 Gene mutations in MDS.[a]

Pathway/function	Candidate gene	Chromosome	Frequency in MDS (%)	Putative functional significance
Chromatin modification	ASXL1 *612990	20q	11–15	Unknown
	EZH2*601573	7q	2–6	Decreased survival
DNA methylation	IDH1/IDH2*147700/*147650	2q/15q	4–11	Decreased survival
	DNMT3A*602769	2p	8	Decreased survival
	TET2*612839	4q	11–26	Unknown
Signaling	JAK2*147796	9p	2	Unknown
	N/KRAS*164790/*190070	1p/12p	3–6	Increased risk of progression to AML
	CBL*165360	11q	1	Unknown
	FLT3 ITD*136351	13q	0–2	Decreased survival
Transcription regulation	RUNX1*151385	21q	4–14	Decreased survival; more common in therapy-related MDS
Cell cycle	TP53*191170	17p	10–18	Decreased survival and increased risk of progression to AML
RNA splicing	SF3B1	—	14	Alternate protein splicing
	SRSF2	—	12	Alternate protein splicing
	U2AF1	—	7	Alternate protein splicing
	ZRSR2	—	3	Alternate protein splicing
Others	NPM1*164040	5q	2	Unknown
	SETBP1	18	—	Unknown

[a]Source: Modified after Abdel-Wahab and Figueroa[91]; Papaemmanuil et al.[92]; Bejar et al.[93]

mechanism. Ebert and colleagues used RNA-mediated interference (RNAi) to identify genes that might be involved. They identified a partial loss of function of the ribosomal subunit protein, *RSP14* gene, that was associated with a block in erythroid differentiation in progenitor cells from patients with the del 5q-. Using the RNAi *in vitro*, they were able to recapitulate the phenotype of cells from patients with del 5q-. Overexpression of the *RSP14* gene in cells from patients with del 5q-was able to rescue the phenotype and restore normal erythropoiesis, suggesting that this gene is causal for the del 5q-hematopoietic picture. The loss of function of the RSP14 results in reduction in processing of the 18s pre-rRNA levels. This is similar to the mechanism involved in the Diamond–Blackfan anemia, the congenital bone marrow failure state.[79]

Point mutations in the TP53 tumor suppressor gene have been reported in 8% of MDS cases.[102,103] In one series, patients with sMDS or therapy-related AML (tAML) were found to have a higher than expected prevalence of TP53 mutations in leukemic but not germline tissues. Accumulation of TP53 abnormalities with sequential follow-up was identified in patients as they transform to AML.[104] Microsatellite instability was identified and was consistent with a mutator phenotype, suggesting that these patients were at higher risk of developing t-MDS/AML.[105] Patients have been described with a 17p-syndrome characterized by dysgranulopoiesis with pseudo-Pelger–Huet hypolobulation and small vacuoles in neutrophils. In one series, 15 of 16 patients with this deletion had an associated deletion of TP53, suggesting a potential role for loss of a tumor suppressor gene as a contributing factor to the morphologic, cytogenetic, and molecular phenotype of this syndrome.[106] The expression of several other genes, including EVI-1, c-mpl, platelet derived growth factor (PDGF), MLL, and the colony stimulating factor (CSF)-1 receptor have recently been described to be dysregulated in some patients with MDS.[98,107–109] The EVI-1 gene, located on chromosome 3, has been shown to play a role in both myeloid and erythroid differentiation. Dysregulation of gene expression is associated with blocks in myeloid and erythroid maturation.[110,111]

The V617F JAK 2 mutation has been described in patients with the MPDs, polycythemia vera, myelofibrosis, and essential thrombocythemia. There is also a small subset of patients with MDS with the mutation. These patients usually have high platelet counts and may have sideroblastic anemia. Some have designated this small subset RARS-T (T = thrombocytosis).[112]

Clinical and laboratory features

The clinical and laboratory picture in patients with MDS is dominated by and derives from the defect involving a multipotent hematopoietic stem cell. Although the disease has occasionally been described in children and adolescents, it is primarily encountered in adults in their sixth decade or older.[113] In most reports, the median age is over 65, and there appears to be a male predominance. The clinical presentation is nonspecific. The symptoms relate primarily to the cytopenias, with those attributable to anemia being the most common. These include fatigue, weakness, pallor, dyspnea, angina pectoris, and cardiac failure. Other signs and symptoms encountered less frequently include easy bruising, ecchymosis, epistaxis, gingival bleeding, petechiae, and bacterial infections, particularly respiratory and dermal. Physical findings are nonspecific. Hepatic and/or splenic enlargement is reported in 10–40% of patients and is most commonly found in CMML. Lymphadenopathy and skin infiltration are uncommon.[114–118] Nontherapy-related MDS has been reported in association with other neoplasms, including lymphoproliferative and plasma cell disorders as well as carcinomas.[119]

The characteristic hematologic findings include peripheral blood cytopenias associated with dysmyelopoietic morphology and functional abnormalities involving one or more of the cell lines and are detailed in Table 10. The bone marrow is hypercellular in the majority and features the dysmyelopoietic morphology of part or all of the progenitors. Abnormalities involving erythrocyte enzymes, surface antigens, hemoglobin production, and iron metabolism have been described. Some of the changes in enzyme activity, such as pyruvate kinase, may affect red cell survival.[120,135] Impaired activity of A and H transferase and galactosyltransferase has resulted in changes in blood types.[121,122] Hemoglobin production is affected with increased fetal hemoglobin, aberrant globin chain synthesis, and disordered ferrokinetics.[123,124]

The myeloid series often reveals leukopenia with immature forms and increased numbers of large unstained cells (LUC). Neutropenia is more commonly found in patients with refractory anemia with excess blasts (RAEB) and RAEB-T than RA and RARS.[119] Leukocytosis most often accompanies CMML, and by definition, requires an absolute monocytosis ($>1 \times 10^9$/L) for diagnosis. Monocytosis may, however, also be present in the other MDS subtypes.[119] Cytoplasmic abnormalities result in cells with hypo- or defective granule formation, Auer rods, or abnormal azurophilic granules. Histocytochemical studies reveal cells with

Table 10 Morphologic and functional cellular abnormalities in myelodysplastic syndromes.[a]

Erythrocytes
Morphology
Anisocytosis
Poikilocytosis
Oval macrocytes
Microcytes
Basophilic stippling
Howell–Jolly bodies
Circulating nucleated red cells
Megaloblastoid maturation
Multinucleated precursors
Nuclear budding
Karryohexis
Defective hemoglobinization
Ringed sideroblasts
Increased stainable iron
Enzymes
Increased hexokinase
Decreased pyruvate kinase
Decreased 2,3 diphosphoglycerate mutase
Decreased phosphofructokinase
Increased adenosine deaminase
Increased pyruvate kinase
Decreases or loss of blood group antigens
Increased fetal hemoglobin
Aberrant globin chain synthesis
Disordered ferrokinetics
Leukocytes
Morphology
Pseudo–Pelger-huet cells
Abnormal chromatin clumping
Abnormal nuclear bridging
Monocytosis
Defective granule formation (hypogranulation)
Megaloblastoid maturation
Auer rods
Increased LAP
Decreased myeloperoxidase
Increased muramidase (CMML)
Loss of granule membrane glycoproteins
Inappropriate surface antigens
Lineage infidelity
Decreased adhesion
Defective chemotaxis
Deficient phagocytosis
Impaired bacteriocidal activity
Megakaryocytes
Morphology
Micromegakaryocytes
Hypolobulated nuclei
Large mononuclear forms
Circulating megakaryocyte fragments
Giant thrombocytes
Defective platelet aggregation
Deficiency in thromboxane A2
Bernard–Soulier-like defect
Immune deficiencies
Decreased T-cell IL-2 receptors
Decreased IL-2 production
Decreased NK activity
Decreased NK response to gamma interferon
Decreased response to mitogens
Decreased T4 cells
Immunoglobulin abnormalities
Autoantibodies
Autoimmune phenomenon
Impaired self-recognition

[a]Source: Modified after Tani et al.[120]; Dreyfus et al.[121]; Yoshida et al.[122]; Uchida et al.[123], Peters et al.[124]; Hokland et al.[125]; Felzmann et al.[126]; Lowe et al.[127]; Felman et al.[128]; Ohmori et al.[129]; Russell et al.[130]; Duetz et al.[131]; Porwit et al.[132]; Westers et al.[133]; Patnaik et al.[134]

increased or decreased levels of leukocyte alkaline phosphatase, decreased myeloperoxidase staining, and loss of granule membrane glycoproteins.[135] Surface antigen analysis has shown loss of lineage-specific antigens, with persistent or increased expression of inappropriate antigens and lineage infidelity.[125] In some instances, the abnormal persistence of antigens or an increased proportion of cells expressing those antigens was associated with an increased risk of leukemic transformation and shortened survival. Abnormal expression of an activated surface phenotype on monocytes has been demonstrated in patients within all FAB subtypes, while expression of activated surface antigens on granulocytes was almost exclusively seen in patients with excess blasts.[126] Impaired granulocyte function includes impaired respiratory burst, deficit in chemotaxis and superoxide release, as well as a defect in neutrophil stimulation signaling.[126,127] Nuclear and functional abnormalities are outlined in Table 10.[128,129]

Megakaryocytes can be decreased and their morphology is often bizarre (Table 10). Patients with RAEB and RAEB-T more commonly have thrombocytopenia, decreased megakaryocytes, and greater degrees of dysmegakaryopoiesis.[119] Megakaryocyte fragments and giant thrombocytes may circulate in the peripheral blood. Hemorrhagic symptoms in these patients may be due not only to thrombocytopenia but to functionally defective platelets as well. Dysfunction can result from defective platelet aggregation, deficiencies in thromboxane A2 activity, or the development of a Bernard–Soulier-type platelet defect. This latter defect has developed from a deficiency in the membrane glycoprotein GP Ib-IX complex.[130,136]

A small percentage of patients present with hypoplastic bone marrows and cytopenias that morphologically may be difficult to distinguish from aplastic anemia.[137] Cytogenetic analysis with or without interphase fluorescent *in situ* hybridization (FISH) may be helpful in establishing a diagnosis.

The relationship of MDS to abnormalities of the immune system is of particular interest given the broad range of abnormalities described. There is a decrease in the number of T-cell interleukin-2 (IL-2) receptors, as well as IL-2 production. The latter is due, in part, to a failure of immunoregulatory B cells.[138] NK cell activity and responsiveness to α-interferon are decreased, as is α-interferon production, while total numbers of NK cells are variable.[138,139] There are decreases in the number of T cells, responsiveness to mitogenic stimulation, the total number of cells, and the T4/T8 ratio.[125,140,141] The latter is due predominantly to a decrease in T4 cells.

Establishing a diagnosis

The diagnosis in most patients is readily established with standardized testing, which should include history and physical examination, complete blood count, and review of the peripheral blood smear. The findings of cytopenias in the absence of explanation from biochemical, vitamin deficiency, hemorrhage, toxin/drug, or infectious etiology should lead to a bone marrow aspirate and biopsy. Routine cytogenetic evaluation should be included as well. The diagnosis of MDS is based primarily on morphologic criteria demonstrating dysmorphic features in the peripheral blood and bone marrow precursors (Table 10). Although some of the classification systems include cytogenetic information (IPSS, IPSS-R, and WHO), they are based primarily on bone marrow and peripheral blood morphology. Analysis of the marrow population using flow cytometric analysis has become standard for the diagnosis and subtyping in patients with acute leukemia. It is more routinely being applied to establish a diagnosis of MDS as well (Table 10).[131–133,142] Abnormal populations and skewed antigen expression can be identified. However, comparative studies of bone marrow morphology and flow cytometry results have not been conducted, and thus one cannot be certain if used alone whether flow cytometry results can reliably establish a diagnosis and classification of MDS. Accurate classification according to FAB, IPSS, IPSS-R, or WHO criteria must be based, at least in part, on bone marrow morphology. Thus, flow cytometry should be viewed as a complementary examination but not sufficient to establish the diagnosis and classification. Cytogenetics is abnormal in up to 70% of patients, with abnormalities that are not diagnostic but may be suggestive of the diagnosis. Gene mutation analyses of genes commonly mutated in myeloid diseases, are becoming commercially available and can be used to support a diagnosis of MDS. However, gene mutations have been described in normal patients with no manifestation of a hematologic malignancy and whose significance is uncertain.[50] So gene mutations alone are insufficient to establish a diagnosis.

Diagnostic dilemmas

Some patients with MDS present with features also suggestive of an MPN, representing an "overlap syndrome."[134,143] In these patients, cytopenias may present simultaneously with elevated white or platelet counts. In some patients, an increased leukocyte count may be accompanied by monocytosis. Under current classification systems, some of these patients will be clearly defined as MPN, while others are still categorized as MDS, depending on the upper limit of WBC permitted in the classification system. Others may have myelofibrosis with or without marked splenomegaly and peripheral blood cytopenias, yet also have dysplastic features suggesting MDS.[144] These patients are more difficult to classify. Those with myelofibrosis with markedly enlarged spleens and a leukoerythroblastic peripheral smear are more likely classic myelofibrosis with myeloid metaplasia, while patients without significant splenomegaly and/or the peripheral leukoerythroblastic picture may be considered to have primary MDS with fibrosis. The presence of V617F Jak2 mutation would favor a diagnosis of an MPN over MDS except in patients with RARS-T.[112]

The hypoplastic MDS variant is often indistinguishable from aplastic anemia and may have many features in common.[145] Those patients with increased expression of HLA-DR 15 and the PNH phenotype (decreased expression of CD59), whether MDS or aplastic anemia, may respond to immunomodulatory treatments. Cytogenetic abnormalities, if present, involving chromosomes frequently abnormal in MDS, may suggest the diagnosis of MDS, but do not completely exclude aplastic anemia.[145] In these patients, therapeutic options may be the determinants in the orientation of the diagnosis in the absence of other criteria.

Finally, there are patients who present with severe pancytopenia and bone marrow findings that are nondiagnostic (i.e., minimal, if any, dysmorphic changes; no increase in myeloblasts) and without any cytogenetic abnormalities. Some of these patients may have MDS, and only with continued observation and testing will a diagnosis be unequivocally established. Gene mutations may also suggest MDS. Others may have been exposed to a bone marrow insult (toxin, infectious agent, etc.), which may never be identified, but which may permit eventual, complete, or partial marrow recovery; which takes months or years. In these latter individuals, in the absence of clear diagnostic evidence, patience, continued observation, and supportive care (SC) is usually the best approach pending a declarative diagnosis. One other consideration for these patients would be an immune-mediated injury to hematopoietic stem cells. The differential in these patients would include large granular lymphocytic (LGL) leukemia, where T-cell receptor and immunoglobulin gene rearrangement studies and T-cell subsets may be informative.[146,147]

Pathogenesis and relation to leukemic transformation

Initiation and promotion of an abnormality affecting a multipotent stem cell may be related to a variety of factors, including chemical insult, radiation, or infection, leading to modification of gene expression. Since most patients with MDS are in the sixth, seventh, or eighth decades, cell senescence may also play a role. Once established, the clonal lesion follows the multistep process of oncogenesis and results in the transformation to acute leukemia in up to 40% of patients. It is likely that multiple events occur and lead to evolution of the disease and ultimate emergence of a dominant clone of cells.[148] Based on the knowledge of a number of abnormalities that do occur, one may speculate on the possible interrelationship of these events that contribute to the pathogenesis. Mutations of the *ras* oncogene, either as an early or late event in the development of the disease, may be one of the steps in this process.[149–151] One model of *ras* mutation results in impaired growth and differentiation along with impaired response to erythropoietin and increased apoptosis, similar to the response of the *in vivo* phenotype.[152] Such mutations may serve to confer a growth advantage to the mutated cells, resulting in their progressive expansion.[153] As a late event, the selective growth advantage may be sufficient to trigger a leukemic transformation. However, when alteration of the *ras* gene occurs as an early event, it may be insufficient to trigger further progression and may require the concerted action of other factors such as those accompanying chromosomal abnormalities and the attendant gene dysregulation that occurs. The identification of many more somatic mutations involving differing pathways including those involved in epigenetic regulation, signaling, transcription factors, and RNA splicing suggests the pathogenesis is more complex. Models that will allow the study of the role of these mutations will be critical.[154]

The impaired response of hematopoietic progenitors suggests an underlying abnormality of signal transduction. Mutations of cytokine receptors can result in a signal that is muted or overexpressed. Mutations have been identified of the FLT3 and G-CSF receptor in association with transformation to AML in patients with MDS.[155] Most studies, however, have not identified abnormalities of cytokine receptors, suggesting a defect further downstream from the ligand-receptor interaction. The increase in apoptosis in the bone marrow with apparent dysregulation of tumor necrosis factor (TNF)-α and transforming growth factor (TGF)-β further suggest cytokine dysregulation. Hematopoietic progenitors with impaired cellular response to cytokine signals could behave as though deprived of obligate survival factors, and thus undergo accelerated apoptosis. This would be the predominant phenotype until further genetic or growth regulatory changes occurred that would trigger a proliferative advantage and transformation to AML. In patients with severe congenital neutropenia, evolution to an MDS or acute leukemia is usually accompanied by acquired mutations in the G-CSF receptor.[156] Point mutations of the G-CSF receptor gene cause truncation of the C-terminal cytoplasmic region of the receptor. Cells with this defect fail to undergo terminal maturation to granulocytes in response to the G-CSF.[157] In a mouse model, the equivalent G-CSF receptor mutation leads to expansion of the G-CSF receptor responsive progenitor population.[158] Treatment with G-CSF leads to neutrophilia, accompanied by increased activation of transcription factors and prolonged external cell surface expression owing to defective internalization. Further genetic mutations in the face of clonal expansion can contribute to leukemogenesis.

Karyotypic abnormalities have been described in up to 79% of patients with MDS and appear to be a later phenomenon.[72] This is suggested by the identification of karyotypic abnormalities in cells belonging to already established clones derived from a multipotent stem cell and by their greater frequency in patients with increased bone marrow blasts.[73,76,136] The association in some studies of complex karyotypic abnormalities with an increased risk of leukemic transformation further suggests that these anomalies confer a growth advantage to a clone, as well as reflecting underlying genetic instability.[63,66,68,69,71,73,74,118] This instability, manifest by clonal evolution with the subsequent acquisition of additional chromosomal abnormalities, has also been associated with disease progression, either to a more malignant subtype or frank AML.[63,66–69,71,73,118] Finally, most of the karyotypic abnormalities involve complete or partial deletions of chromosomes and suggest that gene loss may play a role in the pathogenesis.[68] The critical region on the long arm of chromosome 5, in the interstitial region q13–q34, contains genes encoding a number of important proteins, including GMCSF, IL-3, IL-4, IL-5, CSF-1, and the oncogene *cfms*, which codes for the CSF-1 receptor.[159–162] Changes in this critical region may result in the production of an abnormal gene product or a point mutation. Deletion or loss of chromosomal material may result in a cell hemizygous for a mutant allele, which can be expressed, or loss of a tumor suppressor gene. Several chromosomal regions that are commonly deleted in patients with MDS have been identified, including del 1q, del 5q, del 17p, and del 3p, and may contain tumor suppressor genes whose loss may contribute to the transformation process.[162]

Dysregulation of the cell cycle may occur and contribute to the leukemic transformation. The cyclin-dependent kinase inhibitor (CDKI) gene p15INK4B undergoes aberrant methylation of the CpG islands in up to 50% of patients with MDS studied in one series. Patients with high-risk MDS had the highest frequency of hypermethylation, compared to those with low-risk MDS. In addition, hypermethylation became more prominent as disease progressed.[163]

Treatment

For many years, the management of patients with MDS was challenging due to the lack of treatment options for various risk categories and clinical presentations. In the last few years, there has been an expanded interest in the treatment of MDS, with the identification of new effective therapeutic strategies and several novel agents in advanced phase studies.

Growth factors

Myeloid growth factors

The hematopoietic growth factors are regulatory glycoproteins that control the proliferation and differentiation of bone marrow stem cells.[164] Several phase I studies were initiated to investigate the use of these stimulating factors to determine whether increasing WBC counts improved symptoms and ineffective hematopoiesis in MDS patients. In a controlled study, patients were randomized to observation or treatment with rhGM-CSF.[165,166] Those treated had significant increases in neutrophils, eosinophils, monocytes, and lymphocytes, while the frequency of infections was decreased in comparison with those observed in the absence of this cytokine.

There were no differences in platelet count, hemoglobin, or transfusion requirements between the two groups. The risk of leukemic transformation appeared greatest for those patients with greater than 15% blasts in the bone marrow and may be a critical level with respect to leukemic transformation.[166]

Unfortunately, most clinical trials showed minimal efficacy in symptomatic improvement as well as increased risk for leukemic transformation in those who were given growth factors as monotherapy.[167–169] Current, the National Cancer Center Network (NCCN) does not recommend the routine use of these growth factors in the treatment regimens of MDS patients.[170] However, other clinical trials have investigated the tolerability and efficacy of growth factors in combination with erythropoiesis-stimulating agents and have found improved outcomes.[171]

Erythropoietin

Erythropoietin has also been studied in patients with MDS, with red cell responses being demonstrated in 20–25% of the patients tested.[172–174] Responses were confined to the erythroid lineage. A meta-analysis suggests that efficacy declines as bone marrow failure progresses.[172] Patients with lower serum erythropoietin levels and less transfusion need are more likely to respond. The observation that *in vitro* erythropoiesis improved in patients treated *in vivo* with G-CSF led to two clinical trials of erythropoietin and G-CSF in combination. The response rate ranged from 35% to 40% and appeared to enhance the activity of erythropoietin. Serum erythropoietin levels in these trials, as in others, are of predictive value with few responses in patients with levels above 500 U/L. In another report, the response-enhancing effect of G-CSF was not substantiated.[171,175] Effects of erythropoietin therapy on survival suggest that elimination of a transfusion requirement may be beneficial.[176]

Historically, patients that have low-risk MDS would commonly receive erythrocyte stimulating factors (ESAs) as needed for symptom relief related to severe anemia; such as cardiac or pulmonary manifestations.[177,178] Unfortunately, only about 20–50% of patients with low-risk MDS have been shown to respond to ESAs and further, response after chronic ESA use typically declines after 2 years with a peak duration of response from 13 to 18 months.[177,178] A S3B1 mutation has been associated with a higher rate of transfusion dependence (TD) as well as ineffective response to ESAs.[177,178]

Anti-tumor necrosis factor (anti-TNF) and the immunomodulatory imide drugs (IMiDs)

Lenalidomide, an analog without sedative or neuropathic side effects and with more potent *in vitro* anti-TNF and anti-VEGF effects, was tested in a phase II trial. Of the 148 patients with low and intermediate-1 disease with del 5q either isolated or combined with other cytogenetic abnormalities, 67% of patients became red cell transfusion independent.[179] The median duration of transfusion independence was 115 weeks.[179] These findings were confirmed in a second study confirming that 10 mg/d should be the initial dose. In a second study of low and intermediate-1 disease in patients without a deletion 5q, 26% of patients achieved transfusion independence for a median of 41 weeks.[180] Lenalidomide has been combined with azacitidine (AzaC) and produced an overall response rate (ORR) of 67%.[181] The combination was well tolerated but will require more testing to determine if it is better than either agent alone.

Luspatercept was approved for low-risk MDS as a second-line agent after patients' failed initial ESA agent therapy or had contraindications for an ESA agent.[182] This agent is a fusion protein that acts as a ligand trap against TGF-β; a ligand that is thought to play a role in myelosuppression and in inhibiting erythroid differentiation by induction of apoptosis and cell cycle arrest in erythroblasts.[182,183] The success of preclinical and early phase trials, the phase III (MEDALIST) randomized, double-blinded, controlled study was performed ($n = 153$).[184-187] Of those who received Luspatercept, more achieved red blood cell (RBC) transfusion independence for at least 8 weeks (37.9% vs 13.2%, $p = 0.0001$) and 12 weeks (28.1% vs 7.9%, $p = 0.0002$) compared to placebo, as well as improved neutrophil count (59% vs 17%).[184] The toxicity profile was minimal (31% vs 30% of those had a serious adverse event) and patients showed responses regardless of S3B1 status; leading to its FDA approval in 2020.[184] The phase 3 COMMANDS trial is currently investigating the use of Luspatercept as a first-line agent for patients with MDS (ClinicalTrials.Gov Identifier: NCT03682536).[182]

Iron chelation

For patients with lower-risk disease who are red cell transfusion-dependent accumulation of iron leading to iron overload and ultimate tissue damage from hemochromatosis is a long-term problem. Use of chelation is recommended for patients who have received ≥20–25 units of lifetime transfused RBC or a serum ferritin >1000–2000 ng/mL.[188] Use of deferasirox has been shown to reduce serum ferritin and labile plasma iron.[189] Some studies have suggested an impact on survival but there have been no randomized trials and other factors could be at play as well including patient selection bias. However, chelation should be part of the management strategy for lower-risk RBC transfusion-dependent patients. In patients with higher risk MDS, the role of chelation is undetermined. And, unless MDS patients achieve a hematological response to primary therapy, chelation therapy is not warranted.[188]

Hypomethylating agents

Epigenetic Combinations, Use of HMAs as MDS therapy in the Community, Novel agents in combination with HMA Agents The hypomethylating agent (HMA) AzaC has produced significant benefits (Table 11).[190,191] The promoter region of genes that are not expressed are often associated with hyper-methylated CpG islands. Aberrant acquired changes in methylation, or epigenetic events, affecting intergenic and intron regions as well, result in gene silencing and can have important effects on genes regulating the cell cycle and differentiation programs. A series of experiments by Christman, Acs, Taylor and Jones, and colleagues led to the development of a biochemical model that provided an explanation for the action of AzaC as an inducer of differentiation through its effects on DNA methylation.[192,193]

AzaC, once incorporated into DNA, covalently binds to DNA methyltransferase, the enzyme in mammalian cells responsible for methylation of newly synthesized DNA.

In 2002, the Cancer and Leukemia Group B (CALGB) conducted two—multiple phase—clinical trials comparing AzaC to SC in patients with MDS.[190,191] Patients who received the AzaC displayed statistically significant clinical responses (7% CR, 16% PR, 37% improved), delay in transformation or death, lower probability of transformation, longer median survival, and improved quality of life (QOL); specifically, decreased fatigue, dyspnea, and psychosocial distress as well as increased positive affect and physical functioning than those that received AzaC.[190,191] Patients who initially received SC then crossed over to investigational treatment after anywhere from 4 to 6 months demonstrated longer median survival compared to patients who continued on SC.[190,191] Significant differences persisted after controlling for RBC transfusions. Additional analyses demonstrated that AzaC results in transfusion independence in 45% of patients and is effective in producing responses in patients according to the WHO AML classification (blasts >20%) with a median survival of 19.3 months suggesting a potential benefit in this patient population.[194] Thus, AzaC is the only agent other than allogeneic bone marrow transplantation to alter the natural history of MDS. Furthermore, AzaC is not age restricted, as is marrow transplantation.

A second randomized phase III controlled trial named AZA-001 has confirmed and extended these observations demonstrating a significant survival advantage for patients treated with AzaC compared to a conventional care regimen (a physician-directed choice of either best SC, low-dose cytarabine, or induction chemotherapy with an anthracycline and cytarabine) with median OS for AzaC of 24.4 months compared to 15 months for the conventional care regimen (Figure 2).[195] Time to AML or death, and time to AML, was significantly delayed for patients in the AzaC treated group. Transfusion independence occurred in 45% of patients and there was a reduction by 33% in the infections requiring intravenous (IV) antibiotics in the AzaC treated patients. Time to initial response is slow requiring repetitive monthly cycles to see a response, with the median time to response of three cycles an observation seen consistently across all AzaC studies. Additional analyses suggest that maintenance therapy with AzaC is also beneficial.[196]

Another HMA decitabine, (2-deoxy-5-AzaC) has also been evaluated.[197,198] Although response criteria are different, decitabine, like AzaC, produces responses. In a randomized North American

Table 11 Randomized controlled trials in patients with MDS drug versus supportive care +/− placebo.[a]

Agent	Response to treatment	Quality of life	Frequency of transformation to AML	Time to progression	Time to AML or death	Survival at 24 mo
Cis-retinoic acid	NSSD	—	—	—	—	NSSD
Low-dose cytarabine	Cytarabine	—	NSSD	NSSD	NSSD	NSSD
G-CSF	G-CSF	—	NSSD	NSSD	SC[b]	SC[b]
GM-CSF	GM-CSF	—	NSSD	—	—	NSSD
Azacitidine	Azacitidine[c]	Azacitidine[d]	Azacitidine[c]	Azacitidine[e]	Azacitidine[f]	Azacitidine[g]
Decitabine	Decitabine	Decitabine	NSSD	NSSD	NSSD	NR

Abbreviations: NSSD, no statistically significant difference between agent tested and placebo or supportive care (SC); –, endpoint not assessed in trial; NR, not reported.
[a]Source: Modified after Vadhan-Raj et al.[165]; Hoelzer et al.[166]
[b]Differences are for patients with RAEB. For those with RAEB-T, there was NSSD between G-CSF and SC.
[c]$p < 0.001$.
[d]Fatigue ($p = 0.001$); physical functioning ($p = 0.002$); dyspnea ($p = 0.0014$); mental health index ($p = 0.0077$).
[e]$p < 0.0001$.
[f]$p = 0.004$.
[g]$p = 0.03$.

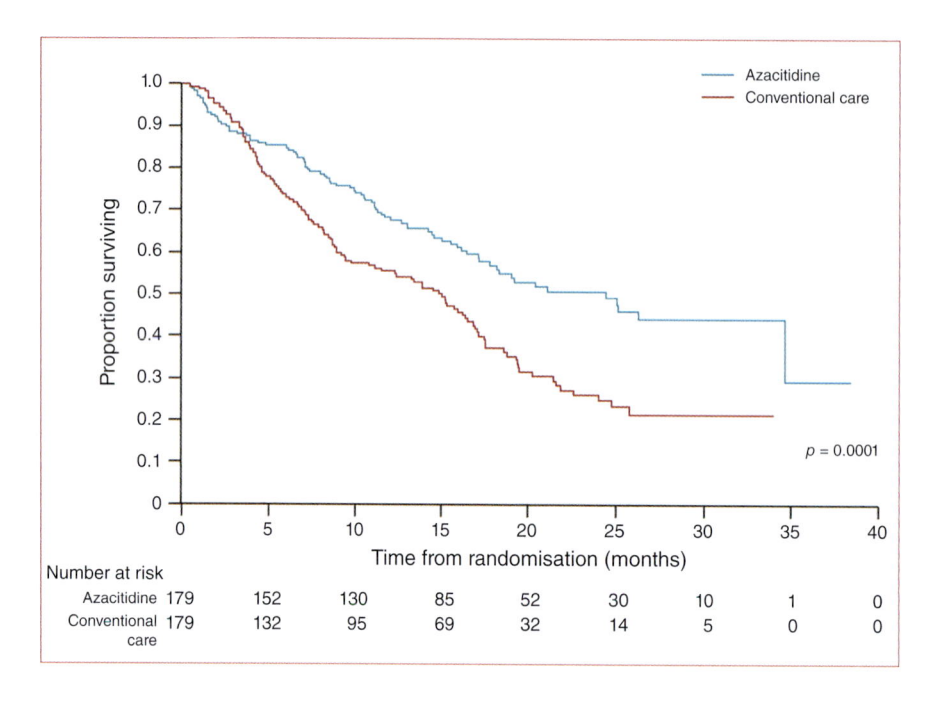

Figure 2 Time to transformation or death in patients treated with azacitidine compared to supportive care. Measured from time of study entry to first event, either transformation to AML or death, and estimated according to the method of Kaplan–Meier. Median time 21 versus 13 months, respectively ($p = 0.007$). Source: From Fenaux et al.[195]

randomized trial of decitabine compared to SC, decitabine was superior with a response rate of 17% CR+PR compared to 0% for SC. However, there was no difference in the second co-primary endpoint of time to AML or death between the two groups.[199] In a second randomized trial conducted in Europe by the EORTC of decitabine compared to SC in patients with intermediate-2 or high-risk disease, there was no difference in time to AML or death or survival between the two groups.[200] An alternative dosing regimen of 20 mg/m^2/day × 5 days every 4 weeks has yielded response rates that are comparable but maybe less myelosuppressive.[201,202] However, this was not a controlled trial and the effects on modifying disease outcome are uncertain.[203] In 2020, the FDA approved decitabine plus cedazuridine (Inqovi) tablets for the treatment of adults with intermediate- or high-risk MDS, including patients with CMML.[204] Inqovi is an orally administered fixed-dose combination of the HMA agent decitabine plus the cytidine deaminase inhibitor cedazuridine. Inqovi is the first and only orally administered HMA agent approved for the treatment of this patient population.[204] The FDA approval of decitabine plus cedazuridine was based on data from the phase 3 clinical trial ASCERTAIN, which compared the efficacy and safety of 5-day administration of oral decitabine plus cedazuridine versus IV decitabine, as well as on supporting data from phase 1 and phase 2 clinical trials.[204–207] Findings from these trials showed similar drug concentrations between the 2 treatments. In addition, approximately 50% of the patients who were previously dependent on transfusions no longer required transfusions during an 8-week period.[204–207]

Epigenetic combinations
Single-agent HMAs produce responses in half the patients treated but are not curative. Combination epigenetic therapy with HMAs and a variety of histone deacetylase inhibitors (HDACs) has been explored.[203] *In vitro* combinations of HMAs and HDACs are synergistic in re-expressing epigenetically silenced genes. The effect is sequence dependent with the HMA required to be administered before the HDAC to see the effect and this observation has led to a series of combination translational trials. AzaC has been combined with Entinostat, in a randomized trial comparing the single agent to the combination. There was no difference between the combination compared to AzaC monotherapy in response or overall survival. Analysis of the methylation differences between the two arms suggests that there was a negative interaction between the combinations compared to monotherapy with reduced hypomethylation in the patients treated with the combination.[208]

AzaC combined with vorinostat in phase I–II study demonstrates a response rate up to 75% with an increase in time to AML or death and overall survival in the cohort of azacitidine 75 mg/m^2/day 1–7 and vorinostat 200 mg twice daily (BID) day 3–9.[209] In contrast, a phase II/III study looking at AzaC in combination with vorinostat or lenalidomide which found that patients with higher-risk MDS who received combination had similar ORR compared to the those who received AzaC monotherapy but with increased toxicity.[210] The combination studies are associated with GI toxicity, nausea, and vomiting, and fatigue being described in many patients. This toxicity can be tolerated by some but may hinder longer-term tolerance among patients and may contribute to an inability to maintain patients on treatment to obtain the full effect.

Use of HMAs as MDS therapy in the community
Since their FDA approval in 2004 and 2006, AzaC and decitabine have been the gold standard for MDS treatment in high-risk and elderly patient populations, respectively.[211] Community-based and clinical trial research has found alternate dosing schedules shown to result in similar outcomes to those who receive HMA for seven consecutive days.[202,212] Further, retrospective studies and metanalyses of various databases—within the past decade—supports the effectiveness, practicality, and tolerability of both HMAs in a community setting. It was also found that patients treated with HMAs in community practice are more likely to achieve a response (either complete or partial) when treated with a greater number of consecutive cycles.[213,214]

Novel agents in combination with HMA agents

For patients with high-risk MDS or ineligible for stem cell transplant, pevonidostat—a small-molecular inhibitor responsible for degrading cullin-RING E3 ubiquitin ligases (CRLs) thereby decreasing tumor cell growth and survival—has been shown to be effective in recent clinical trials.[215–217] Most recently, a randomized phase II study showed combinatory therapy resulted in increases in overall survival (median 21.8 vs 19.0 months; $P = 0.334$), and event-free survival (median 21.0 vs 16.6 months; $P = 0.076$) compared to patients who received AzaC monotherapy.[218] Interestingly, the safety profile of combination therapy was also similar to AzaC monotherapy.[218] Current phase III clinical trials are currently recruiting (ClinialTrials.gov identifier: NCT03268954).

Eprenetapopt (APR-243, APR) has been developed for high-risk MDS patients with p53 mutations and has shown efficacy in several clinical trials.[219,220] Eprenetapopt is a methylated derivative of PRIMA-1—a molecule that induces apoptosis in tumor cells via the restoration of an originally mutant p53 – and has been shown to work synergistically with AzaC.[219] One phase I/II trial found combinatory therapy resulted in higher complete remission rates (73% vs 50%), complete molecular remission rates, and median overall survival (14.6 vs 7.5 months; $P = 0.0005$).[220] Consistent findings were identified in a phase II trial by the Groupe Francophone des Myélodysplasies.[221] A, phase III, multicenter, randomized study of this combinatory treatment was underway (ClinicalTrials.gov identifier: NCT03745716); however, the trial did not meet its primary endpoint as the complete response rate was 53% higher in the combination arm; but was not statistically significant.[222]

Signal inhibitors—multikinase inhibitors

Rigosertib is a RAS mimetic molecule with multikinase inhibitory activity. It is a broad inhibitor of the PI3 kinase/AKT pathway and has been tested alone and in combination in MDS. As a single-agent, rigosertib administered IV has shown improvement in peripheral blood counts and a reduction in marrow blast percentage in patients that were predominantly HMA failures.[223] In a randomized phase III study (ONTIME), patients were randomized to either rigosertib or best supportive care (BSC) (which could include low-dose cytarabine) with OS as the primary endpoint in patients who were HMA failures. The trend was in favor of rigosertib, 8.2 months versus 5.9 [$p = 0.33$, HR 0.87 (95% CI 0.67–1.14)]. Although the trial did not meet the primary endpoint there were several subgroups that demonstrated a survival benefit.[224] The drug was then tested in a new phase III study (INSPIRE trial) adapted to include high-risk MDS patients after failing HMA agent therapy; making the patient population more homogenous. However, this trial also failed to meet primary endpoints with the overall survival being 6.4 months in the treatment group versus 6.3 months ($p = 0.33$).[225] Retinoic acid and related compounds, highly effective inducers of differentiation *in vitro*, have been disappointing in their lack of efficacy in several clinical trials.[226–229]

Chemotherapy

Chemotherapeutic agents, alone and in combination, have been used to treat patients with MDS. These agents have been employed in a variety of regimens ranging from attenuated low-dose schedules to the more conventional antileukemic myelotoxic-type strategies. These have been employed to treat patients at all stages of disease. Antileukemic-type treatments have not substantially altered the outcome of the disease for most patients and have been associated with significant toxicity in many. In a retrospective analysis of chemotherapy induction compared to an HMA the trend suggested a benefit for the HMA.[230]

The combination of fludarabine, cytarabine, and filgrastim (FLAG) or without (FA) G-CSF has been tested in patients with MDS and de novo AML.[231] The two regimens yielded comparable complete response rates of 60% and 55%, respectively, with the response rate generally higher in the subgroups of MDS-EB. Overall, 27% of patients (MDS and AML) died during induction. The median projected survival was 29 weeks for FA and 39 weeks for FLAG. These differences were not statistically significant. In patients with deletion of chromosome 5 or 7, FLAG produced a response rate of 64% versus 36% for FA. However, the differences were attributed by the authors to factors other than an effect of treatment. Use of G-CSF was associated with a more rapid recovery of neutrophil count, but this did not translate into decreased rates of infection or infection-related mortality.[231] Overall, there were no differences in treatment outcomes for patients with MDS compared with AML.

In 2017, the combination of cytarabine and daunorubicin was approved by the FDA for secondary AML or AML with myelodysplastic-related changes. The agents are encapsulated in a liposome (Vyxeos, CPX -351).[232] This liposome was manufactured to deliver a fixed molar ratio of 5 : 1.[232] This novel therapy showed improvements of overall survival compared to the SC (the standard 7 + 3 model with anthracycline and cytarabine) for these secondary or tAML patients (9.56 vs 5.95 months, HR 0.69; 95% CI: 0.52–0.90, $p = 0.005$).[232,233] Unfortunately, this drug has not yet been approved for MDS. However, several clinical trials are investigating the use of Vyxeos in combination with various small molecular inhibitors or monoclonal antibodies for high-risk MDS patients as well as patients with relapsed/refractory MDS (Clinic Trial Reference Number: NCT03896269, NCT04493164, NCT04128748, NCT04915612).

In general, responses to treatment of patients with either MDS or AML following MDS are less favorable than treatment of de novo AML.[234,235] Age appears to influence the rate and duration of response, with younger patients achieving CR more frequently and remaining in remission longer compared with older patients.[236–238] Achievement of a CR in MDS is associated with improved survival in comparison to nonresponding patients, but the duration of the response is substantially shorter in comparison with patients with de novo AML who achieve response.[234,235] Treatment prior to the transformation to AML, and patients with shorter intervals between the diagnosis of MDS and leukemic transformation, is associated with higher response rates.[234,235] However, aggressive anti-leukemic type treatment is associated with high rates of morbidity and mortality, with up to 30% of the patients dying from drug-related complications.

Novel immunotherapy combinations

Magrolimab—an IgG4 anti-CD47 monoclonal antibody—has shown clinical promise in intermediate to high-risk MDS patients. Instead of targeting the adaptive immune system, the primary function of this antibody is to bind to CD47 proteins located on cancer cells.[239] Typically, these proteins evade macrophages by expressing these proteins. Human antibodies cause an "unmasking" of the originally hidden cancer cell; resulting in phagocytosis and destruction of said cancer cell.[239] Phase I/Ib clinical trials have investigated the use of magrolimab in combination with AzaC.[240] Researchers found a similar safety profile in combinatory therapy compared to monotherapy and patients who received combinatory therapy had a higher objective response (54% CR, 39% marrow CR, 7% hematological improvement) than the monotherapy cohort; some data indicating that combination therapy may be uniquely effective in patients harboring a TP53 mutation and extension cohorts are being investigated currently (ClinicalTrials.gov Identifier: NCT03248479).[240]

Similarly, Sabatolimab (MBG453) is an IgG4 anti-TIM-3 antibody.[241] TIM-3 is expressed on leukemic cells and blasts, but not hematopoietic stem cells, making it a favorite target while restoring immune function.[241,242] In a phase IB clinical trial, combination therapy (AzaC or decitabine) in high-risk or very high-risk newly diagnosed or relapsed/refractory MDS patients had an ORR of 62.9% with encouraging response rates both patient cohorts with high-risk MDS (ORR 50% [11/22]) and very high-risk MDS (ORR 84.6% [11/13]).[242] No patients with MDS had to discontinue treatment due to toxicity.[242] The STIMULUS clinical trial program – a multicenter group of phase II and phase III clinical trials investigating treatment-naive MDS patients – is now underway (ClinicalTrials.gov Identifier: NCT03946670 and NCT04266301).[243]

Bone marrow transplantation
Results of allogeneic and syngeneic bone marrow transplantation from a series of reports containing small numbers of MDS patients have suggested that 35–40% can achieve durable long-term disease-free remissions when treated with this modality.[244,245] This has been substantiated with the results from two larger single-institution series.[246,247] In one large series, 251 patients treated between 1981 and 1996 were evaluated.[244] Appelbaum and colleagues reported an estimated (Kaplan-Meier) 5-year disease-free survival (DFS) of 40%. Younger age, shorter duration of disease, female gender, and de novo MDS were predictors of better DFS. Patients under the age of 20 years had a 60% DFS rate, compared with 40% and 20% for those 20–50 years old or over the age of 50, respectively. Patients with low-risk MDS had a 55% DFS at 6 years compared with only 30% for those with high-risk MDS. This difference correlated with a higher rate of relapse among those with more advanced diseases. Among patients with low and intermediate-1 risk according to the IPSS score, there were almost no relapses. The 5-year DFS for those in the low and intermediate-1 groups was 60%, 36% for those in intermediate-2, and 28% for those in the high-risk group. Patients undergoing matched unrelated donor (MUD) marrow transplants fare less well. In an analysis of results from the National Marrow Donor Program, patients receiving MUD transplants during the first 4 years of registry data (1986–1990) had a disappointing DFS of only 18% at 2 years and 24% an overall survival at 2 years.[248] In one study, patients with primary MDS demonstrated a survival advantage over those with sMDS (56% vs 27%).[249]

The exact role and timing of bone marrow transplantation remain to be determined, as does the optimal conditioning regimen. A recent analysis of patients with low-risk disease, suggests that watchful waiting until evidence of disease progression increases life expectancy compared with immediate transplantation. For patients with high-risk diseases, transplantation shortly after diagnosis was associated with better life expectancy.[249] These data were recently updated for patients 60–70 years old and favors transplant for higher-risk patients with some gain in life expectancy whereas nontransplant approaches are favored for lower-risk patients.[250] For patients 40 years or younger with a compatible related donor, however, transplantation should be favored, since no other therapy thus far is curative. However, selection of transplant candidates for patients under the age of 50 remains problematic. There are some younger patients with low-risk MDS with a median survival greater than 15 years treated with SC alone.[251] Fewer patients over the age of 40 have been transplanted given the high risk of morbidity and mortality during conditioning and after transplant.

Because of the age of most MDS patients and the potential toxicity of fully ablative transplantation regimens, reduced-intensity conditioning hematopoietic stem cell transplantation (RIC HCT) has been developed as an alternative. These treatment strategies use conditioning regimens, often fludarabine-based, which are better tolerated and not intended to be fully ablative. They permit chimerism to be established with either sibling or volunteer unrelated matched donors. Recent publications have found the benefit of these regimens in patients who once were not candidates for this type of therapy. For example, a multicenter, biologic assignment clinical trial was performed in 50–75-year-old patients with primary MDS who underwent either RIC HCT or non-HCT therapy. There was a significant overall survival advantage in patients with high-risk MDS (Intermediate-2 and High IPSS risk) who received RIC HCT and had an HLA-matched donor.[252,253] More importantly, there were no significant differences between QOL for both arms; a general concern given the toxicity of higher dose ablative regimens.[252,253]

AzaC has been explored as both a bridge to transplant with administration prior to allogeneic transplant and also as a maintenance strategy post allogeneic transplant.[254,255] Treatment is well tolerated in both the pre- and posttransplant setting but randomized trials will be required to assess whether AzaC in either the pre or posttransplant setting positively impacts disease outcome.

For patients with a variant of MDS characterized by severe hypoplasia and pancytopenia, which may resemble severe aplastic anemia (hypoplastic MDS), administration of anti-thymocyte globulin produced responses in 11 of 25 patients treated (9 of 14 RA; 2 of 6 RAEB).[256] Responses were characterized predominantly by loss of transfusion requirement and 3 of 25 had normalization of their counts. There were no changes in the dysplastic features or in bone marrow cellularity. In the completed study, 61 patients were treated, with 21(34%) responding. Transfusion requirement was eliminated in 76% of responding patients or 25% overall.[257] The effect may be mediated, in part, through an immunosuppressive effect alleviating a T-cell suppression of hematopoietic progenitors.[258] Patients who are younger, have more cytopenias, shorter duration of red cell TD, and the presence of HLA-DRB1-15, appear more likely to respond.

Clinical management
The management of patients with MDS presents a series of difficult choices. For patients with RA or RARS, low- or intermediate-1-risk groups, who have better prognoses and in whom the disease is manifest predominantly as asymptomatic anemia, observation and SC should be the mainstay. For those who require red cell transfusions, which in and of itself is a negative prognostic variable, a trial of erythropoietin with or without GCSF appears reasonable.[259] Treatment with lenalidomide or AzaC in patients who fail an ESA or have severe leukopenia or thrombocytopenia are a consideration. Those patients with a karyotypic abnormality (other than the 5q-syndrome, very good risk cytogenetics) have a less favorable prognosis. Such patients warrant closer follow-up and are candidates for investigational studies, particularly if they manifest an increasing number of blasts in the bone marrow or develop significant neutropenia or thrombocytopenia. Patients with low-risk disease who fail therapy with erythropoietin with or without G-CSF for anemia or who have severe cytopenias in other lineages can be considered for treatment with AzaC, which

has demonstrated efficacy in low-risk disease with amelioration of symptoms. Single-agent lenalidomide or an HMA can lead to transfusion independence in between 25% (lenalidomide) and 50% (AzaC) of patients. For patients with lower-risk disease that is progressing, who fail lenalidomide or HMA and, who have a compatible donor, allogeneic bone marrow transplantation should be considered, since it is the only therapy that has so far achieved cures.[250,260]

Patients with higher-risk disease (intermediate-2-or high-risk; high risk and very high risk—IPSS-R) have a poorer prognosis and are candidates for treatment with an HMA. Those with RAEB 1 (5–10% blasts) without other poor prognostic features (i.e., abnormal karyotype, severe thrombocytopenia, or severe neutropenia) could be closely observed to determine the relative stability of the disease. Those with evidence of progression are candidates for immediate intervention.

Patients with higher risk of disease can benefit from treatment with AzaC which should be considered the standard first-line therapy for these patients. It has demonstrated significant benefits compared with SC, induces remission, decreases transfusion requirements, extends survival, and improves the QOL. This therapy may now represent the SC.[181,190,192,195,203,208,210,211,213,218,220,221,241,255,261] Alternatively, they can be treated as part of an investigational program. Stem cell transplantation is a consideration for those patients as a potentially curative strategy and should be considered early in the evaluation process after the diagnosis is established, if a donor is available, and dependent on the patient's age. However, the rate of relapse is high, and many centers will not consider these patients as candidates. Strategies aimed at inducing a remission prior to transplantation may be useful.[250,260,262]

For patients who have transformed to leukemia, aggressive antileukemic chemotherapy can be undertaken or an HMA is a consideration for older patients. The CR rate for antileukemic chemotherapy ranges between 30% and 60% but is associated with a high rate of treatment-related morbidity and mortality. Most patients relapse. The HMAs have been used in these patients and in may improve survival.[199] Patients with hypoplastic MDS, particularly if younger, may benefit from antithymocyte globulin with or without cyclosporine or other immunomodulatory effects. Patients who have either primary or secondary HMA failure have a poor prognosis and an investigational agent should be considered.[261]

Future directions

Progress in the prevention and therapy of MDS depends on a better understanding of the basic biochemical and molecular defects that contribute to the development of this syndrome. Identification of gene mutations affecting various pathways including the epigenetic landscape of MDS will help to individualize therapeutic decisions. Well-designed clinical trials using clearly defined biological end points are critical. Improvement in survival is the ultimate goal, but focusing on this singular end point disregards multiple aspects of the disease that are important from a patient's perspective including TD, hospitalization for infections, fatigue, and other QOL measures. QOL assessments have gained favor as useful tools in the measure of the effects of treatment. These assessments should be included routinely in phase II and III studies and help as a critical measure of therapeutic efficacy. Cost analysis is another useful gauge of treatment efficacy and such measurements should ideally be included in future phase III studies.

In a disease characterized by the development of a progressive uncoupling of cellular maturation and proliferation, induction differentiation is an attractive approach. This has proven to be a highly provocative strategy in the treatment of acute promyelocytic leukemia with trans-retinoic acid. AzaC, which may act in part as a biologic response modifier with effects on the epigenome and gene signaling, may be advantageously combined with other agents such as HDACs.[203] Drugs that interfere with or block abnormal signal transduction (e.g., tyrosine and multikinase inhibitors) may prove beneficial.[223] Tumor vaccines and the use of immunomodulatory strategies that can stimulate auto- or allogeneic T cells will be explored in the coming years with PD-1/PDL-1 checkpoint inhibitors.

Key references

The complete reference list can be found on Vital Source version of this title, see inside front cover.

4 Vardiman JW, Thiele J, Arber DA, et al. The 2008 revision of the World Health Organization (WHO) classification of myeloid neoplasms and acute leukemia: rationale and important changes. *Blood.* 2009;**114**(5):937–951.
6 Walter MJ, Shen D, Shao J, et al. Clonal diversity of recurrently mutated genes in myelodysplastic syndromes. *Leukemia.* 2013;**27**(6):1275–1282.
11 Steensma DP. Myelodysplastic syndromes current treatment algorithm 2018. *Blood Cancer J.* 2018;**8**(5):1–7.
13 Demakos EP, Silverman LR, Lawrence ME, et al. *Incidence and Treatment of Myelodysplastic Syndrome in the US: Treatment Approaches, Optimization of Care and the Need for Additional Therapeutic Agents.* Washington, DC: American Society of Hematology; 2014.
16 Gibson CJ, Steensma DP. New insights from studies of clonal hematopoiesis. *Clin Cancer Res.* 2018;**24**(19):4633–4642.
17 Steensma DP. Clinical consequences of clonal hematopoiesis of indeterminate potential. *Hematology.* 2018;**2018**(1):264–269.
18 Hong M, He G. The 2016 revision to the World Health Organization classification of myelodysplastic syndromes. *J Transl Int Med.* 2017;**5**(3):139–143.
19 Greenberg P, Cox C, LeBeau MM, et al. International scoring system for evaluating prognosis in myelodysplastic syndromes. *Blood.* 1997;**89**(6):2079–2088.
20 Jonas BA, Greenberg PL. MDS prognostic scoring systems–past, present, and future. *Best Pract Res Clin Haematol.* 2015;**28**(1):3–13.
21 Duncavage EJ, Schroeder MC, O'Laughlin M, et al. Genome sequencing as an alternative to cytogenetic analysis in myeloid cancers. *N Engl J Med.* 2021;**384**(10):924–935.
22 Papaemmanuil E, Gerstung M, Bullinger L, et al. Genomic classification and prognosis in acute myeloid leukemia. *N Engl J Med.* 2016;**374**(23):2209–2221.
23 Kantarjian HM, Keating MJ. Therapy-related leukemia and myelodysplastic syndrome. *Semin Oncol.* 1987;**14**(4):435–443.
29 Sobecks RM, Le Beau MM, Anastasi J, et al. Myelodysplasia and acute leukemia following high-dose chemotherapy and autologous bone marrow or peripheral blood stem cell transplantation. *Bone Marrow Transplant.* 1999;**23**(11):1161–1165.
30 Stone RM. Myelodysplastic syndrome after autologous transplantation for lymphoma: the price of progress. *Blood.* 1994;**83**(12):3437–3440.
34 Morton LM, Dores GM, Schonfeld SJ, et al. Association of chemotherapy for solid tumors with development of therapy-related myelodysplastic syndrome or acute myeloid leukemia in the modern era. *JAMA Oncol.* 2019;**5**(3):318–325.
35 McNerney ME, Godley LA, Le Beau MM. Therapy-related myeloid neoplasms: when genetics and environment collide. *Nat Rev Cancer.* 2017;**17**(9):513.
40 DeZern AE, Malcovati L, Ebert BL. CHIP, CCUS, and other acronyms: definition, implications, and impact on practice. *Am Soc Clin Oncol Educ Book.* 2019;**39**:400–410.
41 Morice PM, Leary A, Dolladille C, et al. Myelodysplastic syndrome and acute myeloid leukaemia in patients treated with PARP inhibitors: a safety meta-analysis of randomised controlled trials and a retrospective study of the WHO pharmacovigilance database. *Lancet Haematol.* 2021;**8**(2):e122–e134.
42 Valent P. ICUS, IDUS, CHIP and CCUS: diagnostic criteria, separation from MDS and clinical implications. *Pathobiology.* 2019;**86**(1):30–38.
43 Kwok B, Hall JM, Witte JS, et al. MDS-associated somatic mutations and clonal hematopoiesis are common in idiopathic cytopenias of undetermined significance. *Blood.* 2015;**126**(21):2355–2361.
45 Valent P, Orazi A, Steensma DP, et al. Proposed minimal diagnostic criteria for myelodysplastic syndromes (MDS) and potential pre-MDS conditions. *Oncotarget.* 2017;**8**(43):73483–73500.
46 Desai P, Mencia-Trinchant N, Savenkov O, et al. Somatic mutations precede acute myeloid leukemia years before diagnosis. *Nat Med.* 2018;**24**(7):1015–1023.

49. Jaiswal S, Ebert BL. Clonal hematopoiesis in human aging and disease. *Science*. 2019;**366**(6465):eaan4673.
50. Jaiswal S, Fontanillas P, Flannick J, et al. Age-related clonal hematopoiesis associated with adverse outcomes. *N Engl J Med*. 2014;**371**(26):2488–2498.
51. Zink F, Stacey SN, Norddahl GL, et al. Clonal hematopoiesis, with and without candidate driver mutations, is common in the elderly. *Blood*. 2017;**130**(6):742–752.
78. Teerenhovi L. Specificity of haematological indicators for '5q- syndrome' in patients with myelodysplastic syndromes. *Eur J Haematol*. 1987;**39**(4):326–330.
91. Abdel-Wahab O, Figueroa ME. Interpreting new molecular genetics in myelodysplastic syndromes. *Hematology Am Soc Hematol Educ Program*. 2012;**2012**:56–64.
92. Papaemmanuil E, Gerstung M, Malcovati L, et al. Clinical and biological implications of driver mutations in myelodysplastic syndromes. *Blood*. 2013;**122**(22):3616–3627; quiz 3699.
93. Bejar R, Stevenson K, Abdel-Wahab O, et al. Clinical effect of point mutations in myelodysplastic syndromes. *N Engl J Med*. 2011;**364**(26):2496–2506.
134. Patnaik MM, Lasho TL. Genomics of myelodysplastic syndrome/myeloproliferative neoplasm overlap syndromes. *Hematology Am Soc Hematol Educ Program*. 2020;**2020**(1):450–459.
143. Patnaik MM, Tefferi A. Myelodysplastic syndromes with ring sideroblasts (MDS-RS) and MDS/myeloproliferative neoplasm with RS and thrombocytosis (MDS/MPN-RS-T) – "2021 update on diagnosis, risk-stratification, and management". *Am J Hematol*. 2021;**96**(3):379–394.
177. Castelli R, Schiavon R, Rossi V, et al. Management of anemia in low-risk myelodysplastic syndromes treated with erythropoiesis-stimulating agents newer and older agents. *Med Oncol*. 2018;**35**(5):76.
187. Cappellini MD, Viprakasit V, Taher AT, et al. A phase 3 trial of luspatercept in patients with transfusion-dependent β-thalassemia. *N Engl J Med*. 2020;**382**(13):1219–1231.
190. Kornblith AB, Herndon JE 2nd, Silverman LR, et al. Impact of azacytidine on the quality of life of patients with myelodysplastic syndrome treated in a randomized phase III trial: a Cancer and Leukemia Group B study. *J Clin Oncol*. 2002;**20**(10):2441–2452.
191. Silverman LR, Demakos EP, Peterson BL, et al. Randomized controlled trial of azacitidine in patients with the myelodysplastic syndrome: a study of the cancer and leukemia group B. *J Clin Oncol*. 2002;**20**(10):2429–2440.
195. Fenaux P, Mufti GJ, Hellstrom-Lindberg E, et al. Efficacy of azacitidine compared with that of conventional care regimens in the treatment of higher-risk myelodysplastic syndromes: a randomised, open-label, phase III study. *Lancet Oncol*. 2009;**10**(3):223–232.
196. Silverman LR, Fenaux P, Mufti GJ, et al. Continued azacitidine therapy beyond time of first response improves quality of response in patients with higher-risk myelodysplastic syndromes. *Cancer*. 2011;**117**(12):2697–2702.
199. Kantarjian H, Issa JP, Rosenfeld CS, et al. Decitabine improves patient outcomes in myelodysplastic syndromes: results of a phase III randomized study. *Cancer*. 2006;**106**(8):1794–1803.
200. Lübbert M, Suciu S, Baila L, et al. Low-dose decitabine versus best supportive care in elderly patients with intermediate- or high-risk myelodysplastic syndrome (MDS) ineligible for intensive chemotherapy: final results of the randomized phase III study of the European Organisation for Research and Treatment of Cancer Leukemia Group and the German MDS Study Group. *J Clin Oncol*. 2011;**29**(15):1987–1996.
201. Kantarjian H, Oki Y, Garcia-Manero G, et al. Results of a randomized study of 3 schedules of low-dose decitabine in higher-risk myelodysplastic syndrome and chronic myelomonocytic leukemia. *Blood*. 2007;**109**(1):52–57.
207. Garcia-Manero G, McCloskey J, Griffiths EA, et al. Pharmacokinetic exposure equivalence and preliminary efficacy and safety from a randomized cross over phase 3 study (ASCERTAIN study) of an oral hypomethylating agent ASTX727 (cedazuridine/decitabine) compared to IV decitabine. *Blood*. 2019;**134**(Supplement_1):846–846.
208. Prebet T, Sun Z, Figueroa ME, et al. Prolonged administration of azacitidine with or without entinostat for myelodysplastic syndrome and acute myeloid leukemia with myelodysplasia-related changes: results of the US Leukemia Intergroup trial E1905. *J Clin Oncol*. 2014;**32**(12):1242–1248.
210. Sekeres MA, Othus M, List AF, et al. Randomized phase II study of azacitidine alone or in combination with lenalidomide or with vorinostat in higher-risk myelodysplastic syndromes and chronic myelomonocytic leukemia: North American Intergroup Study SWOG S1117. *J Clin Oncol*. 2017;**35**(24):2745–2753.
220. Sallman DA, DeZern AE, Garcia-Manero G, et al. Eprenetapopt (APR-246) and azacitidine in TP53-mutant myelodysplastic syndromes. *J Clin Oncol*. 2021;**39**(14):1584–1594.
221. Cluzeau T, Sebert M, Rahmé R, et al. Eprenetapopt plus azacitidine in TP53-mutated myelodysplastic syndromes and acute myeloid leukemia: a phase II study by the Groupe Francophone des Myélodysplasies (GFM). *J Clin Oncol*. 2021;**39**(14):1575–1583.
222. Aprea Therapeutics. *Aprea Therapeutics Announces Results of Primary Endpoint from Phase 3 Trial of Eprenetapopt in TP53 Mutant Myelodysplastic Syndromes (MDS)*. Aprea Therapeutics; 2020, https://ir.aprea.com/news-releases/news-release-details/aprea-therapeutics-announces-results-primary-endpoint-phase-3.
240. Sallman DA, Asch AS, Al Malki MM, et al. The first-in-class anti-CD47 antibody magrolimab (5F9) in combination with azacitidine is effective in MDS and AML patients: ongoing phase 1b results. *Blood*. 2019, Supplement_1;**134**:569–569.
242. Brunner AM, Esteve J, Porkka K, et al. Efficacy and safety of sabatolimab (MBG453) in combination with hypomethylating agents (HMAs) in patients with acute myeloid leukemia (AML) and high-risk myelodysplastic syndrome (HR-MDS): updated results from a phase 1b study. *Blood*. 2020;**136**(Supplement 1):1–2.
243. Zeidan A, Esteve J, Kim H-J, et al. AML-187: the STIMULUS clinical trial program: evaluating combination therapy with MBG453 in patients with higher-risk myelodysplastic syndrome (HR-MDS) or acute myeloid leukemia. *Clin Lymphoma Myeloma Leuk*. 2020;**20**:S188.
259. Malcovati L, Porta MG, Pascutto C, et al. Prognostic factors and life expectancy in myelodysplastic syndromes classified according to WHO criteria: a basis for clinical decision making. *J Clin Oncol*. 2005;**23**(30):7594–7603.
261. Prebet T, Gore SD, Esterni B, et al. Outcome of high-risk myelodysplastic syndrome after azacitidine treatment failure. *J Clin Oncol*. 2011;**29**(24):3322–3327.

111 Acute myeloid leukemia in adults: mast cell leukemia and other mast cell neoplasms

Richard M. Stone, MD ■ Charles A. Schiffer, MD ■ Daniel J. DeAngelo, MD/PhD

Overview

Acute myeloid leukemia (AML) is a heterogeneous disease characterized by unbridled proliferation of myeloid stem cells resulting in bone marrow failure and death without effective therapy. The median age of AML is approximately 70; predisposing factors include inherited mutations, exposure to industrial solvents, ionizing radiation, or certain chemotherapy given for other malignancies or conditions. The disease results from the accumulation of mutations in pathways that promote cellular proliferation or impairing differentiation. Prognosis is based on a combination of host and disease factors, especially diagnostic cytogenetics and genomics. In younger fit patients, therapy consists of myelosuppressive induction chemotherapy to minimize disease burden and allow restoration of normal hematopoiesis. Postremission chemotherapy with additional myelo-intense chemotherapy and/or allogeneic stem cell transplant is required to potentiate cure. In older and less fit patients (perhaps those with adverse prognosis) the current standard is repetitive cycles of a hypomethylating agent or low-dose cytarabine plus the BCL-2 inhibitor, venetoclax. The application of molecularly targeted therapies at both diagnosis and relapse may change the natural history of the disease, the management of which requires a comprehensive integration of disparate fields including social work, nutrition, pharmacy, blood bank, and medical oncology.

Acute myeloid leukemia (AML) is the most common variant of acute leukemia occurring in adults, with estimates of almost 20,000 new cases in 2021 with a 5 year survival of 29%.[1] The relatively poor outcome is attributed in part a 70 year median age of onset.[1,2] Decades of stagnation have given way to optimism based on advances in transfusion medicine, antifungals, increased use of safer allogeneic transplantation and notably FDA approvals of at least seven new agents in the past 4 years. A more sophisticated understanding of pathophysiology, particularly in the area of genomics,[3] and the ability to detect small numbers of leukemia cells in the posttherapy state has helped provide optimism for the achievement of greater strides in the near future.

AML can present either as a *de novo* leukemia without an apparent antecedent illness or as an evolution from marrow disorders such as myelodysplasia, myeloproliferative neoplasms, aplastic anemia, and Fanconi anemia, or after the administration of therapy for other types of cancers or nonmalignant disorders. AML presenting without prior marrow disease or antineoplastic therapy is termed *de novo*, whereas other types are considered secondary. Such terms may be less important predictors of response to therapy and long-term outcome than the mutational profile reflecting the biological heterogeneity of this condition.[4] The proper care of patients with AML is a multidisciplinary effort, benefiting from a team approach. Expertise in transfusion medicine, infectious disease, placement and care of indwelling catheters, nutrition, and antineoplastic drug pharmacology are required as well as the availability of sophisticated diagnostic laboratory facilities and psychosocial counseling for both patients and their families. Optimally, allogeneic stem cell transplant, now employed in patients up to age 75, should be available. These disciplines are described elsewhere in this book, but their critical importance in the care of the leukemia patient cannot be overestimated.

Pathogenesis and etiology

Pathophysiology

The pathophysiology of AML can be partially explained by the acquisition of genetic changes in hematopoietic stem cells that both promote self-renewal and impair normal hematopoietic differentiation, resulting in an accumulation of immature cells. Genetic changes in AML were first recognized by the identification of genes at cytogenetic breakpoints involved in balanced translocations. Many of these chromosomal abnormalities, for example, $t(8; 21)$, $t(15; 17)$, and inv (16), are associated with specific AML subtypes. The fusion proteins generated by the translocations generally result in disruption of transcription factors believed to be critical in myeloid differentiation.[5,6] Murine experiments indicate that transfection of mutated genes that primarily alter cell differentiation, such as RUNX1-RUX1T1 resulting from the $t(8;21)$ translocation, produce abnormal hematopoiesis but are not sufficient to generate frank AML.[7]

The genetic landscape of *de novo* AML has been recently characterized.[3,8] An average of five mutations are found in an individual patients' leukemia cells and "only" 30 mutations are recurrent (seen in more than 3% of patients). Of the 30 recurrent mutations, several are relatively common, including changes which lead to gain-of-function mutations such as those on the *FLT3* gene, encoding a trans membrane tyrosine kinase.[9] Blasts from about 25% of AML patients have length or internal tandem duplications (ITDs) mutations in which the protein is elongated in the juxtamembrane region by between three and greater than 100 amino acids. This type of mutation is associated with an adverse prognosis due to a high relapse rate. Both the ITD mutation and the less common tyrosine kinase domain point mutation (occurs in approximately 10%; usually D835Y) cause ligand-independent constitutive activation of the receptor. A second common mutation is a point mutation in the *NPM1* shuttle protein.[10] Mutations in the *RAS* guanine nucleotide-binding protein occur in about 20% of patients with AML and are associated with increased proliferation.[11] Mutations in the isocitrate dehydrogenase genes *IDH1* and *IDH2* occur in about 20% of patients with AML (approximately 10% for each case).[12] Enzymes encoded by IDH mutant genes generate the neomorphic production of 2-hydroxyglutarate (2HG) instead of the usual reaction product, alpha-ketoglutarate. 2 HG levels may correlate with disease activity and yield pro-leukemic epigenetic (posttranslational modification of the DNA) changes which phenocopy those seen with inactivating *TET2* mutations.[13] Mutations in transcriptional machinery and mutations in enzymes which affect epigenetics potentially leading to profound effects on gene expression, are common in AML.[8] *DNMT3A* mutations in occur in about 20% of patients with AML.[14] The presence of some of the mutations encoding so-called spliceosome complex enzymes (U2AF1, SF3B1, ZRSR2, SRSF2) or chromatin modifying enzymes (ASXL1, BCOR, EZH2, STAG2) are often associated with AML that has arisen from an MDS prodrome.[4] *TP53* mutations are often associated with complex karyotype.[15]

Not only are individual cases of AML heterogeneous, but the makeup of the disease can change over time, particularly in response to therapy. First, a precursor entity termed CHIP, clonal hematopoiesis of indeterminant potential, applies to patients who are found to have mutations in the marrow or blood but do not have hematological abnormalities. Such individuals develop MDS or AML at a slightly higher rate than expected, but the biggest clinical issue is a propensity to cardiovascular disease, suggesting disordered inflammation.[16,17] Those with MDS who tend to have mutations in epigenetic machinery-encoding genes may spontaneously acquire another "hit," for example a *FLT3* or *NRAS* mutation, and transition to leukemia.[14,18] This "clonal hematopoiesis" leads to the production of mature cells with the same mutations, so NGS analysis of the blood cells can be useful in cases where marrow is not obtained. Sub-clones may persist at clinical remission [see minimal or measurable residual disease (MRD) below] and clones may emerge with "progression" mutation that might have been present at undetectably small amounts at diagnosis. Thus, NGS panel testing should be carried out at relapse as well as diagnosis as it can lead to the ability to give an alternative targeted therapy.

The genetic complexity of AML is only one important feature of disordered molecular pathophysiology. The epigenetic profiles, mRNA, and micro RNA profiles in AML can differ widely in different cases and in suggest the importance of AML–immune system interactions.[19] Integration of the vast potential array of data from both bulk and single-cell analysis[20] including genomic lesions, epigenomic changes, and RNA[21] and microRNA expression patterns yield a daunting amount of information and will be the subject of intense research over the coming decade.

Exposure and risk

Although more acquired genetic lesions that lead to leukemia are being defined, DNA damage from a known cause accounts for only a small fraction of patients with AML. Leukemia occurs with increased frequency after nuclear bomb[22] or therapeutic radiation exposure,[23] after certain types of chemotherapy,[24,25] and with heavy and continuous occupational exposures to benzene or petrochemicals.[26] It is now recognized that there are two types of chemotherapy-related leukemias: (1) the classic alkylating agent-induced type in which the leukemia is usually preceded by a myelodysplastic prodrome and is characterized by clonal abnormalities, often with loss of chromosome 5 and/or 7[24] and (2) an epipodophyllotoxin/topoisomerase II inhibitor-associated type with a shorter (median 2-vs 5-year) incubation period, often with myelomonocytic or monocytic differentiation and abnormalities at the 11q23 region.[25] Recent studies challenge preconceived notions about the origin of therapy-related leukemia: (1) some patients who have been exposed to chemotherapy have genetic[4] or cytogenetic lesions[27] and clinical behavior indistinguishable from *de novo* AML; (2) preexisting TP53 mutant hematopoietic clones due to the "normal" stochastic accumulation of mutations may be selected for survival after genotoxic therapy and thus predispose to the development of AML.[28]

Familial AML

Patients with a germline predisposition to AML are being recognized with increasing frequency.[29] (Chart 110-1) (Table 1). Inherited conditions such as Fanconi's anemia, Schwachman-Diamond Syndrome, Dyskeratosis Congenita, Bloom's syndrome, and Ataxia telangiectasia predispose to the development of AML, sometimes at an age older than expected. A careful family cancer and bleeding (e.g., *RUNX1* mutations that also lead to a familial platelet defect) history should be obtained from all patients).[30]

Table 1 Selected Known Heritible syndromes that predispose to AML.[a]

Gene	Disorder	Hematologic phenotype	Other phenotype	Inheritance
ETV6	Thrombocytopenia-5	t-penia, bleeding, mecrocytosis	Possible: esophogeal dysmotility	AD
RUNX1	FPD/AML	Chronic t-penia, easy bruising/bleeding, and platelet aggregation defect	Eczema	AD
DDX41	Famila MDS/AML with mutated *DDX41*	Hypocellular marrow, myeloid dysplasia, erythroleukemia	Possible: autoimmune disorders	AD
CEBPα	Familial AML with CEBPα	None pre-AML	None	AD
GATA2	Familial MDS/AML with *GATA2* mutation	Mild cytopenias, chronic neutropenia, B-NK lymphopenia, monocytopenia	Warts, dyspnea, opportunistic infections	AD
TERC/TERT	Telomere syndrome with familial MDS/AML predisposition	Mild cytopenia macrocytosis, and cytopenia	Anogenital cancer, head and neck cancer, osteoporosis, pulmonary fibrosis, nail dystrophy	AD/AR
Multiple genes	Fanconi anemia	Cytopenia, macrocytosis, elevated HgbF		AR/X-linked
TP53	Li-Fraumeni syndrome	Therapy-related leukemia possible	Adrenocortical carcinoma, brain cancer, breast cancer, others	AD
BRCA1/BRCA2	Hereditary breast and ovarian cancer	Therapy-related leukemia possible	Breast cancer, pancreatic cancer	AD
MLH1, MSH2, others	Lynch syndrome	None pre-AML	Colorectal cancer, others	AD

Abbreviations: t-penia, Thrombocytopenia; AD, autoimmune dominant; AR, autosomal recessive.
[a]Modified from Churpek et al.[29]

Prognosis

As noted, AML is a heterogeneous disease genetically and biologically; thus, it is not surprising that a patient's prognosis at the time of diagnosis can vary widely from over a 90% cure rate in acute promyelocytic leukemia (APL) to virtually zero in those patients who have monosomal karyotype and/or a loss of functional TP53 protein in their malignant cells. A reasonably accurate prognosis can be derived from knowledge of host and disease factors. In addition to chronological age, co-morbid disease and frailty in the elderly are among those parameters that predict success with antileukemic therapy. A more sophisticated and comprehensive geriatric assessment (compared to, e.g., ECOG performance status) may accurately determine a patient's success with chemotherapy.[31] Older adults have an increased likelihood of co-morbid disease, a more limited stem cell reserve, as well as a decline in hepatic and renal function with age. Moreover, leukemias arising in older adults tend to be more biologically aggressive having an increased ratio of adverse chromosomal abnormalities to favorable abnormalities,[32] an increased likelihood of so-called myelodysplasia-related genetic abnormalities, and the increased likelihood of an antecedent clinical marrow stem cell disorder.

The sole reliance on chromosomal abnormalities to discern prognosis, and thus make therapeutic choices has yielded to an approach that integrates this data with diagnostic molecular findings.[33] Both the ELN and NCCN have promulgated such integrated prognostic algorithms, thus making critical the availability of cytogenetic and molecular findings as soon as possible after diagnosis. The ELN system requires information about the mutational state of the following genes: FLT3, NPM1, TP53, ASXL1, RUNX1, CEBPA, thus making the use of a multiple gene platform "Next-Generation Sequencing" more efficient than single-gene assays.[34]

About 15% have more favorable prognostic abnormalities (not including APL) that include core-binding factor translocations including t(8; 21) and inversion of chromosome 16. Such patients have a high complete remission (CR) rate and a relatively low relapse rate, although at least two-thirds are destined to relapse with an increased likelihood of an adverse outcome in those with an associated mutation in the KIT tyrosine kinase gene.[35] Those with bi-allelic CEPBPA mutations fare extremely well with standard chemotherapy.[36] Those with a normal karyotype and an NPM1 mutation without or with a low allelic ratio of FLT3-ITD also have favorable outcome.[33] Approximately 15% have unfavorable chromosomal abnormalities[33] consisting of those with complex karyotypes, generally greater than 3, although in some classifications 5 distinct chromosomal abnormalities or those with the so-called monosomal karyotype (2 monosomies or 1 monosomy plus one structural abnormality).[37] Patients in this adverse prognostic category taken together have a 15% likelihood of long-term disease-free survival, but those with monosomal karyotype are destined to fare even worse.[37] This is partially explained by high incidence of TP53 gene mutations in this subgroup, but ASXL1, RUNX1, or FLT3 ITD high allelic ratio mutations without NPM1 associated mutations are also considered adverse.[33] Other so-called adverse chromosomal abnormalities include 3q26, t(6;9), and 11q abnormalities except t(9;11). Some patients have well-characterized abnormalities such as trisomy 8; those with a high allelic ratio of FLT3 ITD with an NPM1 mutation are also in the intermediate category.[33]

Table 2 depicts a modification of the European leukemia net (ELN) classification scheme showing the frequency and general prognosis of those younger adults with various combinations of cytogenetic and genetic findings. It is expected that this list will change over time as other genetic abnormalities are introduced into the equation.

Table 2 2017 ELN risk stratification by genetics/cytogenetics.[a]

Risk category[b]	Genetic abnormality
Favorable	t(8;21)(q22;q22.1); RUNX1-RUNX1T1
	inv(16)(p13.1q22) or t(16;16)(p13.1;q22); CBFB-MYH11
	Mutated NPM1 without FLT3-ITD or with FLT3-ITD[low c]
	Biallelic mutated CEBPA
Intermediate	Mutated NPM1 and FLT3-ITD[high c]
	Wild-type NPM1 without FLT3-ITD or with FLT3-ITD[low c] (without adverse-risk genetic lesions)
	t(9;11)(p21.3;q23.3); MLLT3-KMT2A[d]
	Cytogenetic abnormalities not classified as favorable or adverse
Adverse	t(6;9)(p23;q34.1); DEK-NUP214
	t(v;11q23.3); KMT2A rearranged
	t(9;22)(q34.1;q11.2); BCR-ABL1
	inv(3)(q21.3q26.2) or t(3;3)(q21.3;q26.2); GATA2,MECOM(EVI1)
	−5 or del(5q); −7; −17/abn(17p)
	Complex karyotype,[e] monosomal karyotype[f]
	Wild-type NPM1 and FLT3-ITD[high c]
	Mutated RUNX1[g]
	Mutated ASXL1[g]
	Mutated TP53[h]

Frequencies, response rates, and outcome measures should be reported by risk category, and, if sufficient numbers are available, by specific genetic lesions indicated.
[a]Source: Modified from Dohner et al.[33]
[b]Prognostic impact of a marker is treatment-dependent and may change with new therapies.
[c]Low, low allelic ratio (<0.5); high, high allelic ratio (≥0.5); semiquantitative assessment of FLT3-ITD allelic ratio (using DNA fragment analysis) is determined as ratio of the area under the curve "FLT3-ITD" divided by area under the curve "FLT3-wild type"; recent studies indicate that AML with NPM1 mutation and FLT3-ITD low allelic ratio may also have a more favorable prognosis and patients should not routinely be assigned to allogeneic HCT.[38–41]
[d]The presence of t(9;11)(p21.3;q23.3) takes precedence over rare, concurrent adverse-risk gene mutations.
[e]Three or more unrelated chromosome abnormalities in the absence of 1 of the WHO-designated recurring translocations or inversions, that is, t(8;21), inv(16) or t(16;16), t(9;11), t(v;11)(v;q23.3), t(6;9), inv(3) or t(3;3); AML with BCR-ABL1.
[f]Defined by the presence of 1 single monosomy (excluding loss of X or Y) in association with at least 1 additional monosomy or structural chromosome abnormality (excluding core-binding factor AML).[42]
[g]These markers should not be used as an adverse prognostic marker if they co-occur with favorable-risk AML subtypes.
[h]TP53 mutations are significantly associated with AML with complex and monosomal karyotype.[37]

Presentation

Patients with AML generally present with symptoms related to complications of pancytopenia including combinations of weakness, easy fatigability, infections of variable severity, or hemorrhagic findings such as gingival bleeding, ecchymoses, epistaxis, or menorrhagia. Occasional patients present because of prominent extramedullary sites of leukemia usually related to either cutaneous or gingival infiltration by leukemia cells. Bone pain is infrequent in adults with AML, although some individuals describe sternal discomfort or tenderness, occasionally with aching in the long bones, particularly of the lower extremities. It is generally difficult to date the onset of AML precisely, at least in part because individuals have different symptomatic thresholds for choosing to seek medical attention. It is likely that most patients have had more subtle evidence of leukemia for weeks, to perhaps months, before diagnosis.

The findings on physical examination are variable and generally nonspecific. If fever is present an infectious site must be vigorously sought and treated, if necessary, empirically with broad-spectrum antibiotics. A sizable number of patients have fever related solely to the underlying leukemia, which abates with appropriate chemotherapy. Examination of the skin can reveal pallor, infiltrative lesions suggestive of leukemic involvement, cutaneous sites of infection, which may be either primary or embolic, or, most commonly, petechiae or ecchymoses related to thrombocytopenia and/or coagulopathy. Examination of the fundus reveals hemorrhages and/or exudates in the majority of patients (see the section titled "Ophthalmic complications"). The conjunctivae may be pale, according to the magnitude of the anemia. Careful examination of the oropharynx and teeth is important because of the occasional occurrence of leukemic involvement. Palpable adenopathy is uncommon in patients with AML, and significant lymph node enlargement is rare. Similarly, hepatomegaly and splenomegaly are uncommon and, if found, may suggest the possibility of ALL or chronic myeloid leukemia in blast crisis. None of these findings is diagnostic of acute leukemia, and the final diagnosis and categorization depends on appropriate evaluation of peripheral blood and bone marrow.

Most patients with AML present with anemia (median hemoglobin 8 gm/dL), thrombocytopenia (median platelet count 40,000–50,000/μL), and leukocytosis (median white blood cell (WBC) count 10,000–20,000/μL). The red blood cell morphology is usually relatively normal. Large, sometimes hypogranular, platelets can be seen, and functional defects can contribute to hemorrhagic manifestations. Most patients are neutropenic, and morphologic abnormalities (nuclear hyperlobulation, hypogranulation, Pelger–Huet anomaly) are often noted in the remaining neutrophils. Careful examination will detect blasts in most patients, although it can be difficult to distinguish among leukemia subtypes (or occasionally even to be confident of the diagnosis of acute leukemia) in patients with a low number of circulating blasts. In occasional patients, marked leukopenia at presentation (so-called aleukemic leukemia) may obscure the diagnosis until a marrow examination is performed.

Morphologic classification and clinical and laboratory correlates

Traditionally, the key to the diagnosis of AML was the delineation of the percentage of immature hematopoietic elements termed myeloblasts [distinguished from lymphoid blasts based on the presence of Auer rods, myeloperoxidase or nonspecific esterase (monocytoid) cytochemistry or immunophenotype] in the marrow aspirate and or peripheral blood while cell differential. A marrow biopsy is not absolutely required but can be helpful when immunohistochemical stains for CD34 or C117 are applied to help enumerate blasts and posttherapy to delineate cellularity. The diagnostic classification has evolved from solely morphologically based (FAB classification) to a revised WHO scheme which incorporate new findings from immunologic, cytogenetic, and molecular studies.

The diagnosis of AML requires that myeloblasts constitute 20% or more of bone marrow cells or circulating WBCs, generally evaluated on Wright or Wright–Giemsa stained smears. Auer rods are concretions of lysosomes that can be seen on Wright–Giemsa staining in a 50% of AML cases in younger adults. Cytochemical stains: myeloperoxidase (myeloid), nonspecific esterase (monocytoid), and PAS (periodic acid Schiff stains glycogen "blocks" in ALL, and more punctate staining in so-called acute erythroleukemia and acute megakaryoblastic leukemia) have largely been supplanted by immunophenotypic staining to assigned lineage. Key myeloid antigens are CD 11b, CD13, CD14, CD15, CD33, and CD117.[43] The predominant clone can change with time, especially given the selective pressure exerted by chemotherapy. Representative examples of different subtypes of AML are shown in Figures 1–10. The immunologic, cytogenetic, and (where they exist) clinical correlates of these morphologic subtypes are reviewed in Table 3.

2016 WHO classification

The most recent WHO classification incorporates features of the older FAB morphologic categories with the recognition of distinct entities associated with certain cytogenetic and molecularly detected mutations.[44] Some biologic and clinical implications of these categories are summarized herewith.

AML with recurrent genetic abnormalities

AML with $t(8;21)$ and $inv(16)$ are referred to as "core binding factor" (CBF) leukemias because of the molecular abnormalities in transcription produced by these translocations. The presence of these abnormalities is residual AML regardless of blast enumeration.[44] The patients with inv(16) (about 5% of *de novo* AML) have typical morphologic features of myelomonocytic leukemia with the presence of variable numbers of dysplastic eosinophils at various stages of maturation.

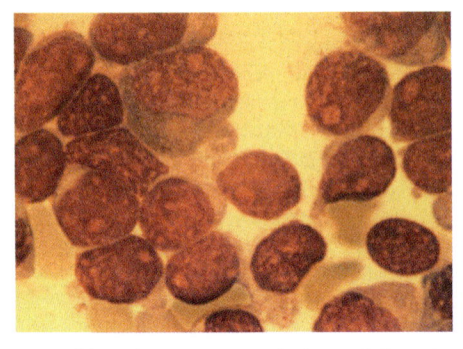

Figure 1 Marrow blasts from patients with this undifferentiated type of acute myelogenous leukemia can have variable amounts of agranular cytoplasm. Cells are peroxidase- and Sudan Black-negative Myeloid commitment of those blasts can be confirmed by immunophenotyping with antibodies against myeloid antigens and/or demonstration of ultrastructural peroxidase-positive granules using transmission electron microscopy.

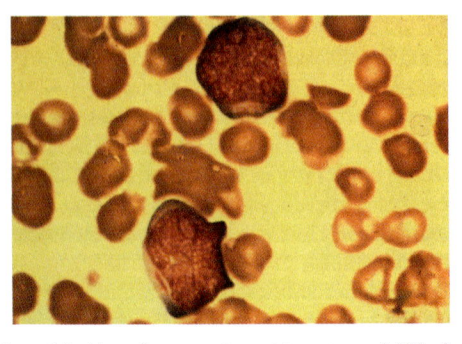

Figure 2 One of the blasts from a patient with acute myeloid leukemia contains a prominent Auer rod.

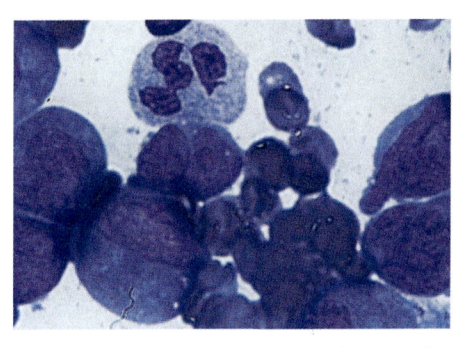

Figure 3 This AML is characterized by evidence of continued myeloid differentiation with myelocytes and more mature myeloid elements present.

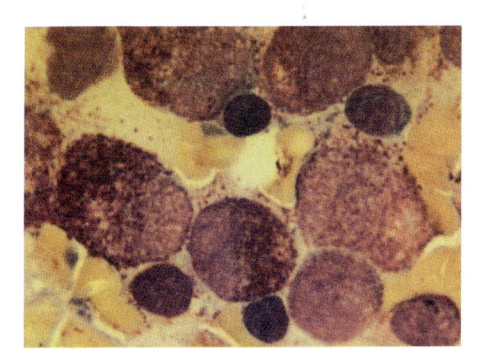

Figure 4 Promyelocytic leukemic cells usually have spherical nuclei with heavily granulated cytoplasm. Extracellular granules are often noted and blasts with multiple Auer rods (not shown) are common. This leukemia has typical 15;17 translocation and a characteristic clinical picture of disseminated intravascular coagulation.

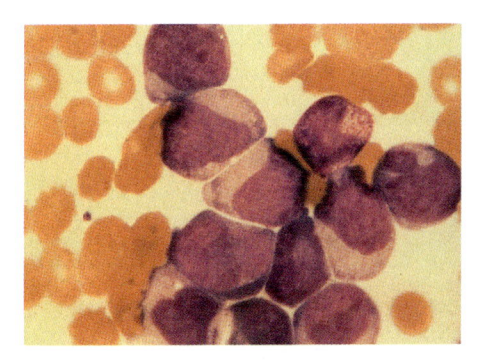

Figure 5 Myelomonocytic leukemia has blasts with both myeloid and monocytoid appearance.

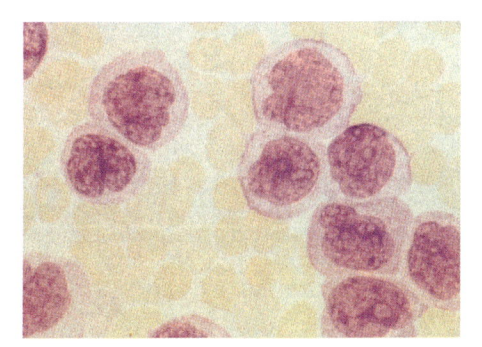

Figure 6 Monocytic leukemia. Prominent nuclei filled with nucleoli in some cells, light granulation, and large amounts of lightly basophilic cytoplasm give these cells the appearance of promonocytes.

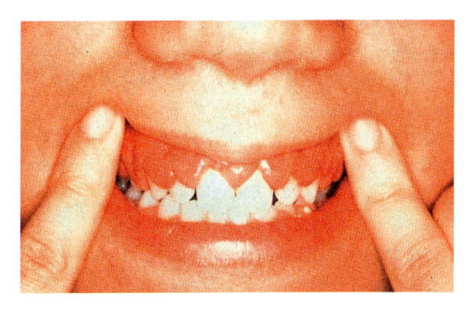

Figure 7 Gingival hypertrophy due to infiltration by leukemic cells in acute monocytic leukemia.

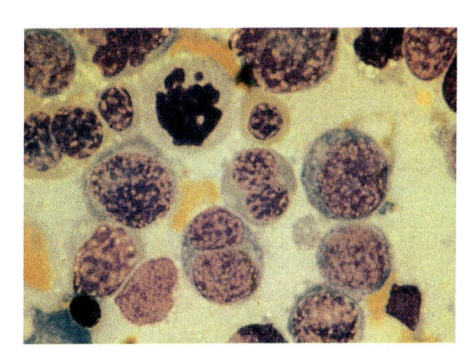

Figure 8 Erythroleukemia is characterized by the presence of bizarre megaloblastic and often multinucleated erythroid precursors. Karyorrhexis is seen in some cells. The somewhat arbitrary distinction between FAB M6 and myelodysplastic syndrome with excess blasts in transformation is made by quantification of the fraction of myeloid blasts.

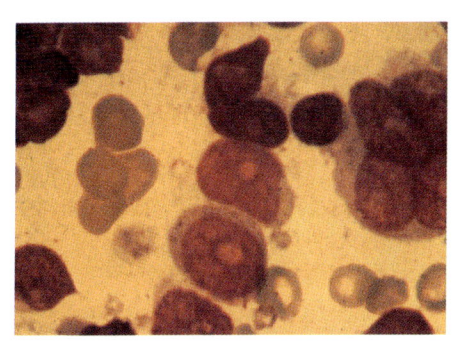

Figure 9 Megakaryocytic leukemia. Blasts in this category are often morphologically undifferentiated. The presence of multinucleated cells, dysplastic micromegakaryocytes, and cytoplasmic budding can be useful diagnostic clues. The diagnosis is confirmed by immunophenotyping or ultrastructural studies.

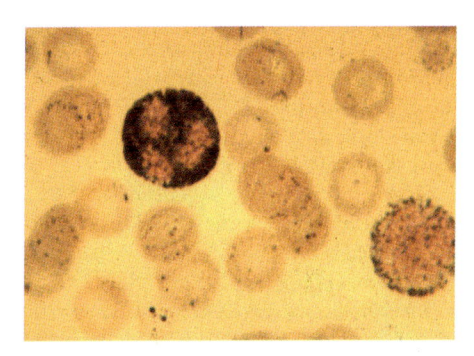

Figure 10 Typical granular staining with Sudan Black B of a blast and a neutrophil from a patient with acute myeloid leukemia.

Table 3 Recurring karyotypic and molecular abnormalities in AML.

Cytogenetic abnormality	FAB morphology	Affected genes	Median age	Approximate incidence in de novo AML	Prognostic effects	Comments
t(8;21)	M2	AML1/ETO	30 years	5–7%	Favorable	Auer rods usually present
t(15;17)	M3	PML-RARa	40	5–8%	Favorable-high cure rate with ATRA-based therapy	DIC
t(11;17)	Similar to M3	PLZF/RARa	?	<1%	Poor response to ATRA-based therapy	
abn 16q22	M4 with eosinophilia	CBFA/MYH11	35–40	5%	Favorable	High reinduction rate post relapse
abn11q23	M5	MLL + many partners	>50	3%	Poor except t(9;11)	Hyperleukocytosis, extra medullary disease
+8	Varied		>60	5–10%	Poor	Common in patients with secondary AML, prior MDS
del 5, del 7, 5q–, 7q–, or combinations	Varied; common in FABM6		>60	15–20%	Poor	
Inv 3	Abnormal megakaryocytes	Ribophorin/EVI1	?	<1%	Poor	Increased platelet count; other abnormalities common (del 5, del 7)
+13	Varied; sometimes undifferentiated		Probably >60	~1–2%	Poor	Higher frequency of hybrid features
t(6;9) (p2;q34)	M2/M4 with basophilia	DEK/CAN	?	<1%	Poor	Prominent basophilia
t(9;22)	Usually M1	BCR/ABL	Probably >50	~1%	Poor	Splenomegaly
t(1;22)	Often M7	MOZ/CBP	Infants	<1%	Poor	Organomegaly
t(8;16)	M4,5	KAT6A/CREBP	?	<1%	Poor	Erythrophagocytosis, often threap-related
Molecular abnormality						
Fms-related tyrosine kinase gene mutations	Varied—most common in CN-AML; can be found with (6;9); t(15;17)	Internal tandem repeat or point mutation of	?	~30% in CN-AML	Adverse	
Nucleophosmin (NPM1)—(5q35) mutation	Varied	Nucleophosmin (NPM1); often found with other mutations	?	~35% of AML, ~50% of CN-AML	Favorable DFS except when associated with mutation	
CEBPα gene	Varied	Mutation results in decreasing levels of CEBPα (CCAAT entamer binding protein)	?	~15% of CN-AML	Favorable when biallic with FLT3 ITD mutation	
Overexpression of BAALC (brain and acute leukemia cytoplasmic) protein	Varied	Overexpression of BAALC	?	Studied most extensively in CN-AML	Adverse—further studies needed	
Partial tandem duplication of MLL (mixed lineage leukemia) gene	Varied	Affects HOX gene function	?	~8% of CN-AML	Unclear—further studies needed	
IDH1, IDH2	Varied	Isocitrate dehydrogenase	?	IDH1 in 10%, IDH2 in 18%	Variable	Specific inhibitors in clinical trials
TET2	Varied (common in MDS)	DNA methylation	>60	15%	Adverse	Increased with older age
DNMT3A	Varied	DNA methylation	>60	20%	Adverse	Increased with older age
ASXL1	Varied	Epigenetic regulation	?	6%	Adverse	Associated with other mutations

Abbreviations: AML, acute myelogenous leukemia; ATRA, all trans retinoic acid; DIC, disseminated intravascular coagulation; FAB, French, American, and British; MDS, myelodysplastic syndrome.

The distinctive eosinophils usually represent only 5–10% of the cells in the marrow.[45] These cells generally contain large basophilic granules in addition to typical eosinophilic granules. This breakpoint involves a fusion between the CBF-β chain and the gene encoding the smooth muscle myosin heavy chain. The fusion protein thus generated may recruit nuclear corepressor activity (in the form of histone deacetylase), which prevents transcription of genes required for myeloid differentiation in a fashion analogous to the RUNX-1-RUNX1T1 fusion in t(8;21) M2 AML.[35]

The recurrent genetic abnormalities group also includes inv3(q21;q26.2), t(3;3)(q21;26.2) (the *MECOM* gene resides at 3q6, t(9;11)(p21l q23.3) [MLLT3-KMT2A} and t(1;22) (p13;q13) [RBM15-MLK1] usually found in infants (see M7 later) as well as t(6;9) (p23;q23)[DEK-NUP214].[44] The t(6;9) is very uncommon, may occur more frequently in younger patients, and can be found in association with a variety of AML morphologies, often with prominent basophilia.[46] *FLT3 ITD* mutations are found in approximately two-thirds of patients with t(6;9).[47]

Solely molecular genetic-based categories include AML with mutated *NPM1* and AML with biallelic mutations of *CEBPA* and provisional entities: AML with *BCR-ABL* and AML with mutated *RUNX1*.[44]

AML with MDS-related changes

The addition of this category reflects the recognition that a substantial fraction of AML, particularly in older patients, evolves from a prior myelodysplastic disorder. This group includes patients with a prior history of MDS (myelodysplastic syndrome), those with >50% dysplasia in at least two cell lines and patients with so-called "MDS cytogenetics" including, −5, −7, i(17)/t(17p), −13, del 11q, del (12p), del 9q and those with complex karyotypes, which may include these changes as well as the presence of marker chromosomes.[48,49] These leukemias seem to arise in a very early hematopoietic stem cell and tend to have low response rates with short durations of response. *TP53* mutations are often associated with complex karyotypes and auger for a very poor prognosis, especially if both alleles are deleted and/or nonfunctional.[50,51] However, patients in this category solely on the basis of morphological abnormalities may have a variety of oncogenic pathways based on mutational profile and thus may not have a uniformly poor prognosis.[4]

Therapy-related AML

This category includes patients whose AML followed treatment with chemotherapy and/or radiation therapy for other disorders. Morphology and karyotypes are often similar to those seen in MDS with the addition of a group of patients with abnormalities of 11q23 associated with prior treatment with topoisomerase II inhibitors and often with a short interval until the development of AML.[25] Therapy-related AML tends to be more resistant to chemotherapy, and allogeneic transplant should be considered in suitable patients who achieve remission. Of note is that occasional patients with therapy-related AML can have inv(16), t(8;21), and t(15;17) (APL) and can respond well to standard approaches for these subtypes, although perhaps not as well as those with these karyotypes with *de novo* disease.

Extramedullary AML (formerly termed myeloid sarcoma)

Occasionally patients will present for medical attention because of lesions identified to be comprised of myeloblasts by histochemical staining but without apparent bone marrow involvement. Masses can involve the skin, gastrointestinal tract, ovaries, central nervous system, and virtually every body organ. There is little systematic literature about the management of such patients although there is a high rate of eventual systemic relapse without treatment.[52] Most clinicians consider induction and consolidation treatment in medically fit patients after the diagnosis is established. Despite such "early" treatment, the recurrence rate is high; the role of stem cell transplant is unclear, but it is reasonable to consider transplantation to maintain the remission. Some of these patients have a t(8;21) chromosomal translocation, but in this setting, may not have the same favorable prognostic input as found in more typical t(8;21) AML.[53]

Distinct clinico-pathologic categories

Acute promyelocytic leukemia

APL is one of the most distinctive subtypes of AML with regard to morphologic, clinical, cytogenetic features, and response to differentiating agent therapies, such as all-trans-retinoic acid (ATRA) and arsenic.[54] In most patients, the morphologic diagnosis is straightforward, with the marrow being replaced by blasts that resemble unusually heavily granulated progranulocytes. The nuclei are round, with obvious nucleoli, and the cytoplasm is filled with multiple, large, and often coalesced azurophilic granules (Figure 4). Auer rods are usually seen, and multiple Auer rods (so-called faggot cells) are frequently noted. In a minority of patients, the blasts are hypogranular and granules sometimes can only be seen with electron microscopy.[55] This hypogranular variant often has cells with bilobed or lobulated nuclei, which can sometimes be confused with monocytic variants of AML. In contrast to the typical leukopenic presentation of APL, patients with the hypogranular variant tend to have higher white cell counts. In both types of APL, staining with either Sudan black B or myeloperoxidase is strongly positive. Class II HLA antigens (HLA DR), which are found on all hematopoietic precursors, are usually not detected on the surface of the malignant progranulocytes. The explanation for and biologic implications of this finding is not known. In contrast, CD33 is consistently strongly expressed.[56]

Patients with APL tend to be somewhat younger, with a median age of 30–40 years, although APL is seen in patients of all ages. APL accounts for approximately 10% of AML and may be more prevalent in Latinos[57] and obese people.[58] APL is almost uniformly characterized by hypofibrinogenemia, variable depletion of other coagulation factors, elevated levels of fibrin degradation products, and accelerated consumption of endogenous and transfused platelets. The granules contain potent procoagulants, and disseminated intravascular coagulation (DIC) is generally accelerated following lysis of blasts by chemotherapy,[59] often with increased bleeding, although the problem can be rapidly ameliorated with the use of ATRA.[60] In some patients, there is evidence that accelerated fibrinolysis may be the primary event triggering the coagulopathy.[61] APL is associated with the highest frequency of hemorrhagic morbidity and mortality, the latter usually related to intracranial hemorrhage, emphasizing the need to initiate ATRA at the first thought of APL.[38] Before DIC is controlled with ATRA, severe hypofibrinogenemia (<100 mg/dL) may require supplementation with cryoprecipitate, and thrombocytopenia should be managed with aggressive use of platelet transfusions.

Almost all patients with APL have a characteristic translocation involving chromosomes 15 and 17 [t(15;17) (q22;q12)],[39] which may be accompanied by additional cytogenetic abnormalities, such as trisomy 8.[40] RT-PCR can be used to detect the fusion transcript, is useful for assessing for minimal residual disease,[62] and permits the proper classification of the occasional patient with clinically and morphologically typical APL but with an apparently normal karyotype. The breakpoint on chromosome 17 is in an intron of the retinoic acid receptor alpha gene. A gene that has been termed *PML*, also with DNA-binding capability, is translocated from chromosome 15, resulting in the formation of a fusion protein that functions in a dominant fashion to block transcription of genes controlled by *RAR*-α, probably by recruiting nuclear corepressor activity. Retinoic acid treatment relieves the corepressor activity,[63,64] allowing transcription of genes involved in differentiation.[65] FLT3 *ITD* mutations can be detected in approximately a third of patients with APL, are associated with higher WBC counts and M3 variant morphology, but unlike the case for non-APL AML, does not seem to be associated with inferior outcome.[66,67] A group of patients with a leukemia similar in morphology to APL but with alternate translocations such as *t*(11;17)(q23;q21) have been described. Although *RAR*-α is rearranged, these patients fail to respond to ATRA. A novel zinc finger gene termed PZLF from chromosome 11 is translocated to the *RAR*-α, rather than the *PML* gene from chromosome 15, creating a fusion protein that does not allow the ATRA-mediated release of transcriptional corepressor activity.[68]

Myelomonocytic leukemia

Myelomonocytic leukemia is characterized morphologically by a mixture of myeloid and monocytic elements and represents about 15–20% of newly diagnosed patients with AML. The monocytic elements often resemble partially differentiated monocytes with lightly granulated, grayish cytoplasm and folded nuclei, which are frequently seen in the peripheral blood (Figure 5). Monocytic derivation can be confirmed by staining with nonspecific esterases such as α-naphthyl acetate or α-naphthyl butyrate. Other than a higher incidence of extra medullary leukemia, here is no distinct clinical picture associated with this variant.

Monocytic leukemia

Monocytic leukemia can exist with minimal or significant amounts of relatively mature monocytes: the latter (Figure 6) can sometimes be difficult to distinguish from chronic myelomonocytic leukemia (see **Chapter 110**).

Although seen in patients of all ages, monocytic leukemias are somewhat more common in older adults. Patients have higher blast counts at diagnosis, and problems with hyperleukocytosis are most common in this morphologic variant (see the section titled "Complications").[69] In addition, the incidence of extramedullary leukemia is highest in monocytic leukemia, particularly in those with evidence of morphologic differentiation.[70] For example, it is common for patients to present to the dentist with gingival hypertrophy, an example of which is seen in Figure 7. Skin infiltration is common both at diagnosis and relapse and frequently represents the initial site of recurrence, sometimes while the bone marrow is still morphologically normal. Other less common areas of extramedullary involvement include the gastrointestinal tract, conjunctivae, and the CNS. It is likely that extramedullary infiltration is related to active migration of the leukemic promonocytes to these sites.

Serum levels of lysozyme are elevated in most patients with AML but are generally much higher in patients with monocytic leukemia.[71] Lysozyme can affect renal tubular function, and severe, symptomatic hypokalemia can occur in patients with monocytic subtypes of leukemia. This problem generally resolves with cytoreduction but can also be additive to the hypokalemic side effects of vomiting and diarrhea.

A variety of cytogenetic abnormalities can be detected, although the most common findings involve abnormalities of chromosome 11 at band q23. This break point, at what has been termed the mixed-lineage leukemia (*MLL*) gene, can be involved in leukemias of myeloid or lymphoid origin as well as in leukemias following therapy with epipodophyllotoxins and other drugs directed at topoisomerase II.[72] The *MLL* gene, also called *KMT2A*, may partner with at least 16 different genes in balanced translocation.[73] *MLL* is homologous to a gene important in Drosophila development and includes DNA binding elements. The t(9;11) is a relatively common translocation involving the MLL gene, which may actually confer a better prognosis than formerly thought, with high initial CR rates.[74,75] There is an association between extensive erythrophagocytosis and the t(8;16)(p11;p13), a translocation involving the CBP class of translocation factors that are positive regulators of myeloid differentiation.[76]

Erythroleukemia

Erythroleukemia, often termed de Guglielmo syndrome in earlier literature, is the variant of AML in which morphologic abnormalities of erythropoiesis are most prominent.[77] Cases of pure erythroleukemia, in which the predominant malignant cell is clearly identified as a pronormoblast, are rare. Rather, this is a disease of the myeloid stem cell with marked dysplastic changes in all three hematopoietic lines. Along with the increase in myeloid-appearing blasts, there is persistence of morphologic abnormalities in the erythroid series with profound megablastosis, multinuclearity, karyorrhexis, increased numbers of mitoses, and staining with PAS, often in a block pattern (Figure 8). Increased iron stores are usually seen, often with ringed sideroblasts. These changes are morphologically identical to those seen in patients with myelodysplasia, and many observers feel that most cases of erythroleukemia are biologically similar, if not identical, to patients with refractory anemia with excess blasts. This contention is supported by the very poor response to therapy in both groups, the tendency for the disease to occur in patients of older age, and the presence of similar cytogenetic abnormalities (complex karyotypic abnormalities, loss of part, or all of chromosomes 5, and/or 7, and marker chromosomes).[77] Prior controversy as to how to quantify the myeloblasts in patients with >50% has been rectified by applying the term AEL (acute erythroleukemia) only to those with >20% blasts.

Megakaryocytic leukemia

Morphologic abnormalities of megakaryocytopoiesis, usually characterized by the presence of mono- or binucleated micromegakaryocytes, are common in many variants of AML and can be particularly prominent in patients with erythroleukemia or myelodysplasia. A minority of these patients have thrombocytosis and abnormalities of chromosome 3 [inv(3) (q21;q26)]. This cytogenetic abnormality is often found in association with other chromosomal deletions, with a variety of primary morphologies, and in patients with a prior background of MDS.[78] These patients have a poor response to initial treatment and low overall survival. Thrombocytosis is not unique to patients with the inv(3) karyotype but can also be present in other patients with AML at the time of diagnosis.[41] The gene at the chromosome 3q21 break point is associated with the activation of MECOM transcription factor.[79]

In some patients, there is obvious evidence of megakaryocytic dysplasia or multinucleated cells that strongly points toward principal involvement of the megakaryocyte (Figure 9). In others, however, the leukemia is undifferentiated morphologically, with variable amounts of generally agranular cytoplasm, and can sometimes be confused with relatively undifferentiated AML or even ALL. Sudan black B (Figure 10), myeloperoxidase, and α-naphthyl butyrate stains are negative, whereas PAS and acid phosphatase may be positive, usually in a diffuse, speckled pattern. Histochemical staining is nondiagnostic, however, and the definitive diagnosis depends on either the detection of platelet-specific peroxidase by ultrastructural techniques or, more commonly, by the demonstration of a variety of platelet antigens (usually glycoprotein IIb/IIIa [CD41] or von Willebrand's factor) on the surface of the blasts.[80] At times, the diagnosis can be quite difficult to confirm, particularly because there is increased marrow reticulin in most patients, rendering the marrow fibrotic and in-aspirable. Careful evaluation of peripheral blood blasts is necessary in such patients. It is likely that most patients with what has been termed acute myelosclerosis actually have acute megakaryocytic leukemia. Acute megakaryocytic leukemia should not be confused with the late stages of primary myelofibrosis, and, indeed, prominent splenomegaly is not a clinical feature. Although an uncommon variant of AML, most series suggest that this subtype is associated with a very poor prognosis. Prolonged aplasia is common following induction chemotherapy, and, because of the marrow fibrosis, it is often difficult to follow the results of therapy with repeated marrow aspirations. There have been relatively few cytogenetic evaluations of this variant, and except for the inv(3) and cases of t(1;22) (p13;q13) [RBM15/MKL1 gene fusion] found in infants,[81] no consistent abnormality has been identified.

Acute panmyelosis with myelofibrosis (APMF)
This very rare variant of AML is felt to derive from the hematopoietic stem cell: the marrow demonstrates a marked increase in reticulin fibers with evidence of morphologically abnormal trilineage hematopoiesis and a variable number of blasts with an immature myeloid immunophenotype.[82] Patients usually present with pancytopenia and constitutional symptoms. It can sometimes be difficult to distinguish acute panmyelosis with myelofibrosis (APMF) from acute megakaryocytic leukemia or myelodysplastic syndromes with myelofibrosis. APMF responds poorly to standard chemotherapy.

Mixed phenotypic leukemia
There are certain cases of acute leukemia that lack straightforward categorization because the cells may have features of both lymphoid and myeloid derivation. The WHO uses the term "mixed phenotype acute leukemias" (MPAL) to encompass these heterogenous group of neoplasms. MPALs are defined by immature cells which display cytochemical or immunophenotypic features of both myeloid and lymphoid lineage (biphenotypic) or there are two different populations of leukemia cells, one myeloid and one lymphoid (bilineal). The difference between bilineal and biphenotypic generally does not alter the diagnostic add or between daignostic or therapeutic therapeutic approach. Certain entities in which there is evidence of derivation from both lineages are not included as MPALs if there is a known recurrent genetic or lesion such as Philadelphia chromosome-positive leukemia, MLL rearranged leukemia, or those with AML-defining balanced translocation such as t(8;21). MPALs also exclude secondary leukemias, leukemias with FGFR1, mutations, and CML in blast crisis.[83]

The essential features of an MPAL are the specific expression of certain lineage-defining markers. Although the algorithm is more complex, simply put, CD3 expression is evidence of T-lymphoid derivation, and CD19 plus one or two other markers indicate B-lymphoid origin. Myeloid origin can be determined by a set of monocytic immunophenotypic markers or most commonly by myeloperoxidase expression. Terminal d-oxynucleotide transferase (TdT) is characteristically seen in ALL but since 25% of AML patients express TdT this is not considered to be a lineage defining abnormality. It is also important to point out that many AMLs may have lymphoid antigens detectable by flow cytometry but do not merit the criteria for biphenotypic leukemia. Such cases should be considered in the AML prognostic and therapeutic rubric. ALL-type regimens followed by allogeneic transplant are often used in MPAL patients.

Therapeutic considerations at diagnosis

Because of the rigorous nature of the chemotherapy, even the less aggressive type now routinely employed in older adults, required for the successful treatment of AML, particular attention should be paid to other medical problems that could complicate the patient's management. A history of congestive heart failure or other heart disease may preclude therapy with anthracyclines and mandates careful monitoring of the large amounts of intravenous fluids, including antibiotics, blood and platelet transfusions, hydration for nephrotoxic antimicrobial agents, and sometimes parenteral nutrition, given during the 3–4 weeks of chemotherapy-induced pancytopenia. Prior transfusion for other disorders or multiple previous pregnancies may presage difficulties with platelet transfusions or herald the occurrence of transfusion reactions after red blood cell or platelet administration. Careful appraisal for possible drug allergies is critical, since virtually every patient will require antibiotic therapy. A history of prior herpes simplex infections (or the presence of an elevated antibody titer) provides justification for prophylactic administration of acyclovir, although this is commonly used without any known risk factors.[84] Prophylactic antibacterial and antifungal agents are commonly but not universally employed. In premenopausal women, menses should be suppressed with a GNRH agonist or estrogens and/or progestational compounds until thrombocytopenia has resolved. Considerations of fertility preservation should be discussed with appropriate patients. Sperm-banking in males wishing to have a family should be considered, if time permits, although many patients are either oligo- or azoospermic at the time of diagnosis. GNRH antagonist therapy, by shutting down the pituitary-ovarian axis during chemotherapy, may preserve fertility in females with childbearing potential.[85]

After the diagnosis is established, the physician and staff must present the goals of therapy and the side effects of treatment to the patient and family. For almost all patients, this discussion can rightfully emphasize the potential benefits of treatment with regard to both the short- and long-term outcome. It is frequently appropriate and necessary to repeat this discussion and counsel later during the patient's course. In general, for younger patients, induction therapy followed by postremission treatment with intensive chemotherapy and/or allogeneic transplant is appropriate. For older (>60–65 years old), there may be merit to the standard, more aggressive approach, but hypomethylating agent-based therapy should be discussed. A guide to initial workup is presented in Table 4.

Table 4 Initial diagnostic evaluation.

History and physical examination—In addition to an overall comprehensive evaluation, emphasis should be placed on the following:
- Duration of symptoms
- Menstrual history
- Prior pregnancies, transfusions, history of transfusion reactions
- Drug allergies (antibiotics)
- Sites of infection: rectum, vagina, oropharynx, gingiva, skin
- Signs of hemorrhage
- Signs of extramedullary leukemia—skin, gingiva
- Dentition status

Bone marrow aspirate and biopsy
- Morphologic classification
- Cytochemistry
- Immunophenotyping
- Cytogenetics
- Terminal deoxynucleotidyl transferase
- Genomic studies

Blood chemistries
- Blood urea nitrogen, creatinine, electrolytes, uric acid
- Transaminases, alkaline phosphatase, bilirubin, lactate dehydrogenase, calcium, phosphorus

Coagulation studies
- Prothrombin time, activated partial thromboplastin time, fibrinogen, fibrin split products

Chest radiograph, electrocardiogram, left ventricular ejection fraction if clinically indicated
HLA typing (patient and family); lymphocytotoxic (anti-HLA) antibody screen
Herpes simplex and cytomegalovirus serology
Lumbar puncture (only if symptomatic)

Abbreviation: HLA, human leukocyte antigen.

Therapy-general

For most patients under age 65–75 years, the goal of therapy should be cure, often requiring an allogeneic stem cell transplant. Older adults and those with significant co-morbidities usually warrant treatment to improve blood counts and prolong life. The initial aim is to achieve CR, defined primarily on morphologic grounds and includes the development of a bone marrow containing less than 5% blast elements, absence of any signs of extramedullary leukemia, and return of normal neutrophil (>1500/μL) and platelet (>150,000/μL) counts. Other forms of response such as partial response (reduction of blast count by 50% to less than 25% with restoration of blood counts, and CRp (platelets not recovered), CRi (neutrophils not recovered), and CRh (plts recovered to >50 K and ANC to >0.5 K), MLFS (no recovery), are newer monikers referring to states wherein the blasts are reduced but blood count recovery is less complete than required for "full" CR. The "best" CR is "deep." The ability to quantify malignant blasts using flow cytometric or molecular genetics allows the delineation of the degree of AML burden reduction (MRD) beyond that possible using light microscopically based morphologic analysis. Thus, attainment of an MRD-negative remission, optimally without major toxicity, should become the optimal standard for initial therapy.[86,87]

Patients who fail to achieve a response after initial therapy (20–40% based on age and AML biology) fare poorly. Patients who fail to respond or who relapse after an initial remission may sometimes be "salvaged" with additional therapy followed by allogeneic stem cell transplantation if feasible based on a reduction in tumor burden and patient factors, Those who do respond well to initial therapy may thereafter receive ("postremission") additional cycles of the original therapy (generally the approach in older adults treated with hypomethylating agent/venetoclax), intensified cytarabine (consolidation), or stem cell transplantation (generally allogeneic). The factors involved in choosing amongst these options include patient age, co-morbidities, intrinsic AML responsiveness, and degree of leukemic burden reduction after initial therapy. Recent data suggest that low-dose therapy after the completion of postremission therapy, so-called maintenance therapy, may have an important role in prolonging survival in certain patients.[88]

What initial therapy should be given?

Before 2000, options were limited to intensive induction or no therapy. The use of lower dose therapy, with low-dose cytarabine or with decitabine or azacitidine (hypomethylating agents), provided a different choice for older adults. The addition of venetoclax to these agents has proven to be a significantly more effective, albeit somewhat more toxic, approach. The addition of targeted agents such as midostaurin in *FLT3* mutant patients and gemtuzumab in core binding factor AML has provided upgrades to standard induction, yet demand a rapid delineation of molecular and cytogenetic factors. First, it is critical to rule/out APL in which devastating CNS bleeding or thrombotic consequences may occur if the diagnosis is missed. ATRA 45 mg/m^2 twice daily, which can rapidly ameliorate the coagulopathy, should be started if APL is suspected. ATRA can be stopped if non-APL AML is definitively diagnosed without deleterious effect.

Our algorithm guiding the choice of initial therapy is shown in Table 5. After ruling out APL, the next task is to determine if the patient should receive an intensive induction therapy. Patients over age 75 should almost always receive repetitive cycles of HMA/Venetoclax, the details of which are described below. For younger patients, most should presumptively receive intensive initial or "induction" chemotherapy. However, patients who have particularly adverse biology, notably complex cytogenetics and or *TP53* mutations are also candidates to receive a nonintensive approach. However, except for patients with significant comorbidities based on the so-called Ferrara et al.[94] criteria (e.g., reduction in DLCO, CHF, renal failure), there are no prospective comparative data. supporting this approach. Nonetheless, many leukemia specialists feel that intensive chemotherapy is not indicated for those with particularly adverse biology. Another consideration to determine fitness for chemotherapy in older adults is the geriatric assessment tool,[95] which can provide more precise information than obtained from an ECOG performance status.

As noted above, rapidly determining the genetic and molecular profile of a patient who could receive intensive chemotherapy is critical in choosing amongst the various options. If rapid metaphase chromosome analysis is not possible, fluorescent *in situ* hybridization (FISH) can determine if there is an inv 16 or t(8; 21) (core binding factor [CBF] abnormality). Gemtuzumab ozogamicin (GO), an antibody–drug conjugate targets the CD 33[96] epitope frequently expressed on leukemic cells. GO was formerly approved in relapsed disease using higher doses[97] and then withdrawn due to lack of efficacy in a SWOG trial.[98] However, based on a meta-analysis looking at five intensive chemo+/−GO trials G.O.+3+7 was shown to be superior to 3+7 alone in AML,[89] with the greatest benefit in CBF disease. However, the specter

Table 5 General therapeutic algorithm.

Initial therapy
A. Fit: with t(8;21) or inv16 (CBF) 3 + 7 + G.O.[89]
B. Fit FLT3 ITD or FLT3 TKD mutation (≥5% allele burden) 3 + 7 + midostaurin.[90]
C. Fit: MRC (myelodysplastic-related changes, or treatment related (AML) CPX-51.[91]
D. Fit: TP53 mutation: azacitidine/venetoclax or clinical trial.[92]
E. Fit: no CBF, FLT3 mutation, MRC or p53 mutation: 3 + 7.[93]
F. Age 75 or unfit: azacitidine/venetoclax.[92]
Post-remission therapy
A. Fit: CBF or NPM1 mutant/FLT 3 WT high-dose cytarabine.[33]
B. Fit: allogeneic transplant.
C. Unfit: continue azacitidine/venetoclax.[92]
D. Fit: but no allogeneic transplant, age >55: oral azacytidine.[88]

Abbreviation: CBF, core binding factor.

of hepatotoxicity, apparently lessened by the fractionated dosing schedules generally employed in this after trial, does give pause to some clinicians. The dose of daunorubicin used with GO is 60 mg/m^2; 90 mg/m^2, superior to 45 mg/m^2 in a large randomized trial in all subtypes of AML,[93] must be used with caution if adding GO.

The CALGB 10603 trial randomized patients with FLT3 mutant (both ITD and TKD mutations, with a minimum allelic ratio of 5%) AML aged 18 – 59 to 3 + 7 (with 60 mg//2 daunorubicin) +placebo or midostaurin (50 mg bid days for 14 days starting the day after the completion of 3 + 7).[90] Midostaurin is a multi-kinase inhibitor with preclinical[99] and clinical[100] activity in mutant FLT3 AML. Patients who achieved CR received midostaurin or placebo with four cycles of high-dose cytarabine and a year of maintenance. The statistically significant overall survival benefit lead in the experimental arm,[90] lead to the approval of this regimen for any chemotherapy fit mutant FLT3 AML patient. Midostaurin should be used with caution if daunorubicin at 90 mg/m^2 is used. While midostaurin is currently the only FLT3 inhibitor approved to be used with intensive chemotherapy other more potent and specific agents are being tested against placebo (quizartinib) or midostaurin (gilteritinib, crenolanib) in this setting.

"Standard" 3 + 7 (3 days of anthracycline, usually daunorubicin at 60–90 mg/m^2/d) and 7 days of continuous infusion cytarabine 100–200 mg/m^2/d is still the mainstay of induction therapy in fit patients without myelodysplasia-vetted changes, CBF or FLT3 (or possibly TP53) mutant AML Approximately 1 week after standard induction therapy is completed (generally 2 weeks after the initiation of treatment), bone marrow aspirates and biopsies are done to evaluate the magnitude of cytoreduction. If the marrow is profoundly hypoplastic, one waits for count recovery. If the marrow is not hypoplastic and only leukemia cells are noted on the day 14 marrow, then a second course of therapy (either repeat 3 + 7 or 2 + 5) is generally. At times, particularly if the "day 14" marrow is hypocellular, it can be difficult to distinguish between residual leukemia cells and normal undifferentiated hematopoietic progenitors. In this instance, it is advisable to delay retreatment and perform another marrow aspirate in a few days. If there is no evidence of further maturation, then a second course of treatment is indicated. The presence of erythroid precursors, juvenile megakaryocytes, or increases in the peripheral blood platelet or neutrophil counts, serve as clues that normal regeneration is occurring and that a second course of treatment should be delayed. The second marrow is performed at day 21 in the 3 + 7 + midostaurin regimen. With standard regimens, approximately 30% of patients with AML require two courses of treatment to enter remission administered. If 90 mg/m^2 of daunorubicin is employed, the second course should be at 45 mg/m^2.[93] Approximately 30% of patients will require a second course of chemotherapy.

CPX-351 (liposomal encapsulated daunorubicin/cytarabine) is an emerging alternative to 3 + 7 currently approved in adults of any age with secondary AML defined as prior MDS (treated or not), prior antineoplastic therapy for another cancer or MDS-related marrow changes (significant dysplasia, or MDS-type chromosomal abnormalities). The drug releases cytarabine and daunorubicin in a fixed molar ratio of 5 : 1,[101] apparently optimal for AML cell killing and persists in the bone marrow compartment. These favorable properties may be the reason why a head-to-head trial of CPX 351 v 3 + 7 in secondary AML in patients aged 60–75 showed a superior overall survival in the experimental arm without added toxicity except for prolonged cytopenias.[91,102] Patients who received an alloSCT survived longer if they had been induced with CPX than with 3 + 7, presumptively because the newer drug elicited CRs a lower disease burden. However, the drug does not appear to overcome TP53 mutations (compared with 3 + 7)[103] and has not been definitely treated against 3 + 7 in a broader population nor against HMA/ven in any group.

Modifications to "3 + 7" (outside of addition of midostaurin in mutant FLT3 disease, adding GO, or increasing the daunorubicin dose as noted above) have been unsuccessful. Although idarubicin at 12 mg/m^2/d is seen as equivalent or slightly better than 45 mg/m^{2104} of daunorubicin, comparisons to higher daunorubicin doses are lacking. Alternative anthracyclines or other agents such as mitoxantrone, rubidazone, aclacinomycin, amsacrine, mitoxantrone, and doxorubicin have been used in several trials but are not clearly superior.[105,106] Etoposide has been added to 3 + 7 without clear-cut beneficial results.[107]

Because high-dose ara-C (HIDAC) is a beneficial postremission therapy (see below), several groups have tested the concept of using this approach during induction in younger patients. Studies have compared standard 7 and 3 to daunorubicin plus intermediate- or high-dose ara-C (2–3 g/m^2 for 8–12 doses).[107,108] These studies failed to show an improved CR rate for the recipients of HIDAC, although one study documented a more prolonged duration of CR (but no change in overall survival) in the patients randomized to HIDAC.[108] The addition of HIDAC to standard daunorubicin/ara-C during induction has also been studied. Although a small trial demonstrated an 87% remission rate in patients under 60 years old,[109] a cooperative group trial failed to confirm those positive results.[110] Results seem to be equivalent if HIDAC is used either as part of induction or only as postremission therapy.[111] The use of continuous infusion high-dose ara-C plus idarubicin has led to favorable results in nonrandomized phase 2 studies at MD Anderson Cancer Center,[112] but did was not superior to "3 + 7" in the context of a large phase III trial.[113]

The addition of other nucleoside analogs to 3 + 7 type chemotherapy holds promise. The Polish Acute Leukemia Study Group showed that the addition of cladribine to anthracycline/cytarabine was superior to 3 + 7[114]; however, the CR rate in the control group in these younger adults was lower than expected and these results need to be confirmed by additional studies. The FLAG-IDA regimen, while quite intensive and toxic, led to a high remission rate and favorable disease-free survival rate.[115] The addition of venetoclax to FLAG-IDA,[92] to standard "3 + 7,"[116] or to "2 + 5"[42] has shown promising results as has the so-called "G-CLAM" regimen (G-CSF, cladribine, cytarabine, mitoxantrone).[117]

Less intensive induction

Patients over age 75 fare poorly with standard 3 + 7. Less intensive approaches have been attempted to lessen toxicity while preserving efficacy in both the older group as well as in younger patients with significant co-morbidities or whose disease biology predicts for a poor outcome with standard intensive chemo. While cytarabine and HMA (hypomethylating agents, azacytidine and decitabine) have been the mainstay of these efforts, clofarabine has been tested, A phase 2 trial using 30 mg/m^2 of clofarabine for 5 days produced a 35% CR rate with a 10% rate of toxic death.[118] In part because of difficulties in defining a group of patients "unfit for intensive therapy" this trial did not result in FDA approval. (Clofarabine was not superior to "3 + 7" evaluated in a large ECOG-led phase III trial).[119]

The mainstays of lower intensity initial therapy are the HMA and low-dose cytarabine. Low-dose cytarabine, often used in Europe and Asia, seems to be somewhat better than hydroxyurea.[120] While both azacitidine and decitabine are approved in the US for MDS and frequently used in AML the lack of clear-cut survival benefit compared to intensive chemo in a defined patient population likely prevented US FDA approval. A trial compared decitabine (25% CR rate) to low-dose ara-C or supportive care but did not meet its primary endpoint of extending overall survival.[121] A comparison of azacitidine to conventional care regimens (doctor's prerandomization choice of supportive care, low-dose cytarabine or intensive induction) in older AML patients whose white counts were less than 15,000/μL again did not meet its primary endpoint but certainly suggested that azacitidine was a reasonable therapy although was not powered to detect a 3 + 7 versus, azacitidine difference.[122]

Anthracycline, decitabine, or low-dose cytarabine should rarely be used as single agents based on the results of the VIALE-A[123] and VIALE-C[124] trials. The VIALE-A trial compared azacitidine alone to azacitidine/venetoclax in adults age ≥ 75 or in younger patients with significant comorbidities not appropriate for chemotherapy. The overall response rate was 67% for the doublet versus 35%. The median overall survival in the control arm was 10 months compared to 15 months (HR 0.68, p-0.0004) with the dual therapy approach. Patients of all AML subtypes benefitted, although the survival benefit was more modest in the *TP53* mutants and impressively long in those with *IDH1* or *IDH2* mutant disease. *FLT3* mutant patients also responded to the combination therapy at a high rate. While a direct comparison of HMA/venetoclax to HMA/FLT3 inhibitor is not available, the results from the VIALE-A trial and the recent press release noting that gilteritinib/azacitidine was not better than azacytidine/venetoclax (Astellas.com/en/news/16296) suggest that the latter may be the best current option for the chemo unfit FLT3 mutant patient, at least until triplets such as azacitidine/venetoclax/FLT3 inhibitor[125] can be safely developed. Of note patients less than age 75 who went on the VIALE-A trial due to significant co-morbidities experienced a more modest benefit with the doublet therapy, likely owing to the major influence of comorbidities on outcome. The combination was more myelosuppressive than the single agent and dose adjustments were more frequent. Low-dose cytarabine +/− venetoclax was compared in the VIALE-C trial[124] in a similar patient population enrolled in VIALE-A, except that patients could have received treatment for prior MDS. The results showed a real but more modest survival benefit favoring the combined approach. It seems unlikely that patients ≥75 will receive 3 + 7 chemotherapy due to the results of the aforementioned studies which repeated venetoclax. Nonetheless, the role of venetoclax/low-dose chemotherapy combinations compared to intensive chemotherapy, such as 3 + 7 or CPX-351, especially in those with adverse prognosis (or in particularly responsive subsets such as IDH mutant AML), remains to be defined. Decitabine given for 10 days instead of the traditional 5[126,127] yields a high initial response rate, but the durability of these responses is questionable. Older adults under age approximately 75, who respond to initial therapy should be considered for a nonmyeloablative allogeneic transplant.[128] This is usually thought of only in people who elect or are given aggressive chemotherapy but may be nonetheless a consideration even in those who receive a less intensive chemotherapy.

Glasdegib is a smoothin/hedgehog inhibitor which inhibits a critical pathway involved in the survival of leukemic stem cells.[129] A prospective randomized trial in newly diagnosed AML patients unfit for chemotherapy demonstrated a superior overall survival for glasdegib plus low-dose cytarabine compared to low-dose cytarabine alone[130] and lead to FDA approval of the agent in this setting. However, the results in the control group were very poor and the experimental arm performed significantly worse than what was seen in the doublet arm of the VIALE-A trial, so this regimen is rarely used.

Postremission therapy

It is estimated that as many as 10^9 leukemia cells may still be present in patients in apparent morphologic CR; it is generally accepted that some form of therapy after CR is required to achieve long-term disease-free survival. Older trials that compared some post-CR treatment to none demonstrated a 100% relapse rate in the control arm.

One of the momentous decisions facing an AML patient in initial remission is whether to perform an allogenic transplant or use chemotherapy as the primary modality to achieve cure. Most patients now have a donor (matched sibling, matched unrelated, partially matched unrelated, haploidentical, or cord blood- in order of preference at most institutions). Allogeneic transplantation has become safer and more widely available; indeed, it is a consideration for most CR1 AML patients up to age 75. Umbilical cord blood may offer an alternative source of stem cells for those without matched siblings or unrelated donors. The incidence of graft-versus-host disease is much lower following cord blood transplants despite the fact that many of these transplants utilize mismatched donors. Engraftment can be delayed, however, and dosage considerations represent an issue for many adult recipients, although the use of double cord transplants has helped to address this problem.[131] Haploidentical transplantation from partially matched siblings, parents, or children is also now readily available thanks to the use of posttransplant cyclophosphamide, such that donors are now available for almost all recipients, with haplo donors generally preferred over cord blood.[132] Debate about matched unrelated "vs" haploidentical donors continues.[133]

Indeed alloSCT has become the mainstay of therapy for all those with any type of AML other than CBF patients and normal karyotype/*NPM1* mutant/*FLT3* WT patients. Moreover, patients who fail to clear MRD (measurement of fusion transcript for CBF or NPM1 by RT PCR after two chemo cycles) should be considered for alloSCT,[134] though the results with alloSCT are less than optimal if MRD is present.

For those not having an alloSCT in CR1, a high-dose ara-C consolidation program is probability best. Two important randomized trials have shown that HIDAC in the postremission setting is better than lower doses of the drug in younger patients. In an ECOG study, patients randomized to receive one course of very intensive postremission consolidation with a HIDAC-type regimen had a longer median duration of remission than patients receiving 2 years of lower-dose maintenance therapy.[135] The CALGB randomized 596 AML patients in CR to receive four courses of ara-C administered at three different dose levels [100 mg/m^2 by continuous IV infusion (CIV) for 5 days, 400 mg/m^2 CIV for 5 days, 3 g/m^2 IV for 3 h q12h on days 1, 3, and 5 (total 6 doses/course)].[136] There was no benefit from the higher-dose arms in patients >60 years of age with a median duration of CR of approximately 13 months and with only 10–12% long-term disease-free survival.[136] In addition, there was a substantial incidence of CNS neurotoxicity in the older patients, manifested primarily as cerebellar dysfunction. In contrast, patients younger than 60 years of age benefited substantially from the HIDAC regimen in terms of both relapse-free and overall survival.[136]

These studies strongly support the use of HIDAC-based consolidation programs in younger patients with AML. How many courses of such therapy are needed, the optimal dose and schedule of HIDAC, and whether the addition of other active agents will improve on these results are still unclear. It is likely that ara-C incorporated into DNA is maximal at 1–1.5 gm/m^2 per dose; a randomized study has shown identical overall survival when doses of 1.5 gm/m^2 were compared to the original CALGB doses of 3 gms/m^2.[137] Studies from the Medical Research Council in Britain which used multiple postremission courses using a variety of different drugs produced similar overall outcomes.[138,139] The CALGB data suggest that the benefit from HIDAC was most pronounced in patients with favorable cytogenetic findings [t(8; 21); and inv(16)][140] as well as those with RAS mutant disease; there was much less effect in patients with unfavorable karyotypes typically associated with drug resistance.[141]

High-dose cytarabine consolidation programs, carry up to a 5% mortality rate in CR so this risk must be carefully explained to the patient, although the use of myeloid growth factors after consolidation can appreciably shorten the duration of severe neutropenia and potentially make the administration of this therapy safer.[142] An alternative way to deliver high-dose chemotherapy in AML is autologous SCT.[143] Most studies have suggested that this approach is equivalent to chemotherapy but is now rarely performed in AML.

Allogeneic transplant "vs" high-dose cytarabine-based chemo in the CR1 patient

In the 1990s, several large prospective trials "genetically" assigned patients with histocompatible siblings to allogeneic BMT (usually only in those 45 years old or less) while randomizing the others to either autologous BMT or chemotherapy. Meta-analysis has suggested that in general, all patients with nonfavorable cytogenetics should fare slightly better with a stem cell transplantation approach.[144,145] The only subgroup in the intermediate prognosis group for whom this is not clear-cut are those with normal cytogenetics and an NPM1 mutation but without a FLT3 ITD mutation. Such patients do well with a chemotherapy-based approach; it would be reasonable to reserve stem cell transplantation for second remission for such patients as well as for those with favorable translocations. The recommendation for alloSCT in first remission takes into account the risk of mortality from graft "vs" host disease, as well as the potential for chronic GVHD, secondary tumors, and other late complications.[146]

Maintenance therapy

Maintenance therapy, or low-dose longer-term chemotherapy as successfully used in ALL, until recently, was not considered useful in AML. An older ECOG study demonstrated no benefit from the addition of 2 years of maintenance therapy following two courses of postremission treatment with DAT (daunorubicin, ara-C, thioguanine).[147] Studies from Germany reported by Buchner et al.[148,149] suggested a modest prolongation of CR duration when long-term maintenance therapy was administered after a single course of postremission DAT, although with a questionable effect on long-term survival. There was less effect of maintenance in later studies when more intensive postremission consolidation was used before the maintenance.[148,149] However, the recent QUASAR trial has altered the landscape and led to the approval of oral azacitidine. Patients age 55 and over who were treated with intensive remission therapy and who remained in remission after 0–3 cycles of post-remission chemotherapy (but were not undergoing alloSCT) courses were randomized to twelve 28 d courses of oral azacitidine or placebo in a blinded fashion. The patients receiving oral azacitidine experienced a clear prolongation in relapse-free and overall survival.[88] Oral azacytidine differs pharmacologically from IV or SC aza and should not be considered interchangeable.

Post-alloSCT maintenance is an important strategy to limit relapse after alloSCT. Post-alloSCT HMA trials have produced inconclusive results, but azacytidine/venetoclax needs to be tested regarding safety and efficacy in this setting. Patients with mutant FLT3 disease who undergo allogeneic transplant often receive sorafenib maintenance based on the results of the SORMAIN trial in which 80 patients were randomized to sorafenib or placebo; sorafenib demonstrated a survival benefit despite the small trial size.[150] A large trial comparing gilteritinib to maintenance in a similar population has completed accrual. Similarly, trials with IDH1 and IDH2 inhibitors in the relevant post-alloSCT context are ongoing.

Therapy of relapsed and refractory AML

There are a number of agents available that have clear-cut activity when used alone or in combination in patients with relapsed or refractory AML, including amsacrine, mitoxantrone, diaziquone, idarubicin, fludarabine, 2-chlorodeoxy-adenosine, etoposide, homoharringtonine, topotecan, carboplatin, and clofarabine. Because many patients are now receiving an alloSCT in CR1, a second transplant, or donor lymphocyte infusion can be considered to consolidate the response to salvage chemotherapy. There is considerable heterogeneity among relapsed patients, and a number of factors in addition to the specific drugs used to influence the outcome of treatment.[151,152] Some consistent trends are evident: (1) Response rates are uniformly low in patients with primary refractory leukemia, in those with short initial CR durations, or in those who relapsed while receiving postremission chemotherapy; (2) leukemias that evolved from a prior hematologic disorder, and patients with poor-risk cytogenetics are particularly resistant to further therapy; (3) patients in second and subsequent relapse have a poorer prognosis than patients in first relapse, and the durations of subsequent remissions tend to decrease progressively (4) Patients who progress on HMA/Venetoclax have a particularly dismal prognosis; (5) one of the most important prognosis for outcome after relapse is the duration of prior remission.[153]

The type and timing of therapy for relapsed patients should be individualized. Patients with other medical problems who have had poor responses to initial therapy have a small likelihood of sustained benefit from re-induction therapy and, indeed, may have their life shortened by intensive therapy. Some of these patients can be supported for many months, with maintenance of a reasonable quality of life, with a more conservative approach using red blood cell and platelet transfusions and oral hydroxyurea to control elevated WBC counts or symptoms such as bone pain. However, there is no potential for long-term benefit. Conversely, younger patients with longer initial responses may derive prolonged benefit from intensive re-induction therapy, if a remission or at least a good response can be followed by allogeneic stem cell transplant.

Recurrence of leukemia is often detected when the patient is asymptomatic, blood counts are normal, and there is modest marrow infiltration by blasts. Although it is logical to begin re-induction therapy at the earliest sign of relapse, when tumor burden is presumably the lowest, there are no data to demonstrate the validity of this approach except possibly as preparation for subsequent SCT. The drawback to early treatment is that re-induction therapy is often unsuccessful and may result in excessive early morbidity and premature patient death, but if long-term survival is the goal (e.g., an allogeneic stem cell transplant) there is no reason to delay.

There are essentially no comparative trials providing guidance about the choice of agents to be used. The initial decision is generally between reuse of drugs that have previously been effective in a given patient, compared with the use of new drugs, some of which may be investigational. If a patient has relapsed while receiving chemotherapy, it makes little sense to use these same agents for re-induction. The often-quoted guidance is to repeat the induction regimen if the disease-free interval is greater than 1 year; otherwise mitoxantrone/etoposide/cytarabine[154] or FLAG: IDA[155] are two of the most commonly used intensive "salvage regimes. For patients resistant or unable to receive an anthracycline, cytarabine/clofarabine[156] is a reasonable option. HMA/venetoclax is often used for relapsed patients who are not deemedable to withstand one of the aforementioned aggressive regimens[157] but its efficacy is limited in this setting. There is no proven benefit of postremission chemotherapy in patients achieving second or third remissions. The obvious downside to postremission chemotherapy is this setting is that one is potentially depriving patients of time when they would be asymptomatic and out of hospital by the administration of therapy of variable toxicity but no proven long-term efficacy.

Three so-called mutationally targeted agents have been approved for the treatment of subgroups of patients with relapsed AML. The potent and specific FLT3 inhibitor, gilteritinib, was shown to yield a response rate of over 50% in relapsed patients in an early phase trial.[158] The ADMIRAL trial was a prospective randomized trial in which patients with relapsed or refractory mutant FLT3 AML (either am ITD or TKD mutation) were randomized on a 2 to 1 basis to gilteritinib at 120 mg orally daily or doctor's choice chemotherapy (either standard salvage therapy or low-dose approaches).[159] The trial led to the approval of the drug in this setting, by demonstrating a higher response rate in gilteritinib-treated patients and meeting its primary endpoint of improvement of overall survival. Whether gilteritinib should be used alone or in combination with other agents remains to be determined.

IDH1 and *IDH2* mutations occur in approximately 9% and 12% of AML patients respectively. The mutant enzyme catalyzes a neo-morphic reaction product called 2 hydroxyglutarate which phenocopies a *TET2* mutation thereby causing pro-leukemic panic epigenetic changes.[160] Ivosidenib is an IDH1 inhibitor and enasidenib is an IDH 2 inhibitor. Both these drugs were tested in single-agent phase one trials in relapsed/refractory patients who had the respective IDH mutation.[161,162] In each case, the drug lead to approximately 15% to 20% CR rate and 30% to 35% overall response rate. This led to the approval of each agent in relapsed/refractory disease. Ivosidenib is also approved as a single agent upfront therapy in newly diagnosed patients but is rarely used because of the good results in this mutational setting with azacitidine/venetoclax. Just as the case with gilteritinib, is unclear if single-agent therapy alone is ideal; combination trials are underway. It is also important to note that the IDH inhibitors can give rise to a differentiation type syndrome[163] similar to that seen with retinoic acid in APL. Steroids should be used when patients develop pleural and pericardial effusions or other evidence of third spacing and or cytokine release while on these drugs.

Although SCT could be offered at the time of initial relapse, most will receive a salvage attempt and undergo transplant only when a second remission is achieved. Unfortunately, most patients do not achieve second remission, and some develop medical problems during re-induction therapy that preclude subsequent transplantation. Although allogeneic BMT can produce long-term survival in some patients with primary refractory or relapsed leukemia, such attempts are generally now considered inadvisable due to very high relapse rates. Though many patients under age 75 have an allogeneic transplant in CR1, many relapses today occur after such a procedure. Relapse after allogeneic SCT is ominous.[164] However, selected patients who relapse following BMT can derive benefit from donor lymphocyte infusions[165] or a second BMT[166] and, in general, can receive and tolerate further chemotherapy. Targeted therapies, such as sorafenib or gilteritinib in *FLT3 ITD* mutant AML,[167] or immune checkpoint inhibitors[168] hold promise for better results in the post-SCT relapse setting.

Therapy of acute promyelocytic leukemia (APL)

APL needs to be recognized and retinoic acid begun rapidly to avoid a hemorrhagic death. That APL is highly sensitive to anthracycline therapy, and that remission with chemotherapy in APL does not require bone marrow aplasia[56] were perhaps clues that so-called differentiation-based therapy n APL would be extremely useful. Indeed, almost all APL patients are now treated with ATRA in combination with arsenic trioxide with the expectation for a very high likelihood of cure.[54]

The differentiation paradigm was verified by dramatic responses in patients with APL reported from China with ATRA administered orally for 30–90 days.[169] CRs were seen in >80% of both relapsed and previously untreated individuals. Marrow aplasia did not occur and serial bone marrows demonstrated what appeared to be maturation of the abnormal, hypergranulated promyelocytes. DIC resolved promptly, with a profound reduction in the requirement for platelet transfusions following ATRA treatment. Although the hemorrhagic complications are decreased, approximately 20–30% of patients treated with ATRA alone develop significant side effects that can include fever, rapidly evolving pulmonary insufficiency, pericarditis, and pleurisy. This syndrome can occur independently of the leukocytosis frequently observed with

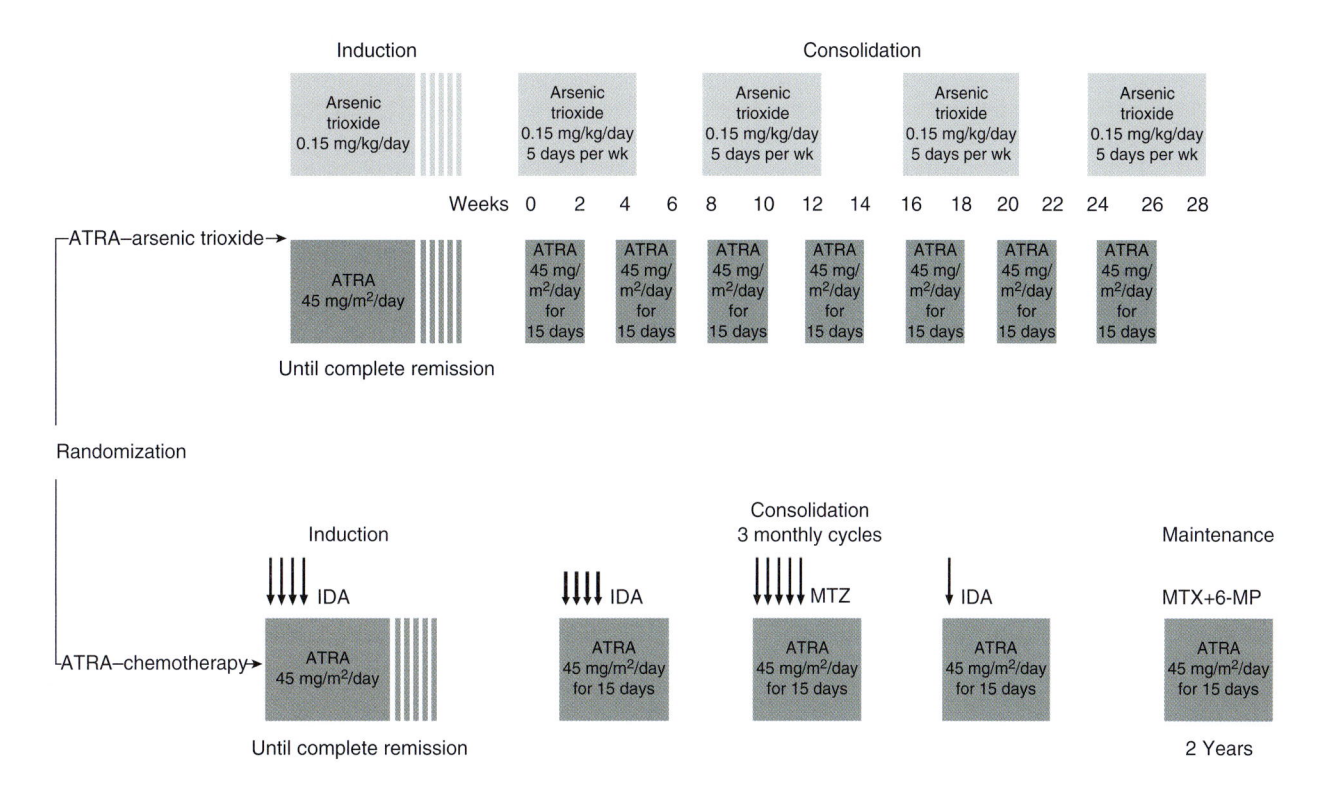

Figure 11 Treatment groups in the all-trans retinoic acid-chemotherapy group, the chemotherapy regimen was as follows: idarubicin (IDA) at a dose of 12 mg/m² of body surface area per day on days 2, 4, 6, and 8 of the induction phase. IDA at a dose of 5 mg/m²/d on days 1–4 of the first cycle of consolidation therapy; mitoxantrone (MTZ) at a dose of 10 mg/m²/d on days 1–5 of the second cycle of consolidation therapy; IDA at a dose of 12 mg/m²/d on day 1 of the third cycle of consolidation therapy; and intramuscular or oral methotrexate at a dose of 15 mg/m²/week and oral 6-mercaptopurine at a dose of 50 mg/m²/d, alternating with ATRA at a dose of 45 mg/m²/d for 15 days every 3 months for 2 years. The vertical lines in the induction therapy boxes indicate variability in the duration of remission induction therapy. The arrows indicate the approximate timing and doses of different chemotherapeutic agents. Source: Lo-Coco et al.[54] Reproduced with permission of NEJM.

ATRA therapy and can be fatal. Optimal management includes the prompt administration of corticosteroids at the first signs of the "ATRA" syndrome.[170]

Once the efficacy of ATRA in APL was recognized, several efforts were undertaken to determine the optimal way to use this agent. Trials conducted on both sides of the Atlantic showed that combinations of retinoic acid and anthracycline-based chemo are better than either agent alone both during induction and postremission therapy.[60,171] A risk score based on the platelet count and white count at diagnosis derived from results in these trials, notably from successive Spanish (PETHEMA) trials, indicated that those with the poorest long-term outcome, are those with white counts greater than 10,000/uL and those with the best long-term outcomes were those with white counts less than 10,000/uL and platelet counts greater than 40,000/uL at the time of diagnosis.[172]

The demonstration, again in China, that intravenous arsenic trioxide produces a high rate of CR even in patients with advanced, multiply relapsed disease,[173] spurred a major change in our approach to APL. Oral arsenic may someday replace IV arsenic leading to an oral therapy for this disease.[174] Arsenic trioxide initially became the standard therapy for relapsed APL[175] and can be used effectively as a single agent in newly diagnosed disease.[176] Using only ATRA and arsenic in patients not deemed to be candidates for anthracycline-based therapy, with GO added for patients with high WBC or insufficient response, the MD Anderson group demonstrated a leukemia-free survival rate as high as that seen in cooperative trials employing more standard therapy.[177] The North American Intergroup evaluated the addition of two courses of arsenic as consolidation therapy postremission and showed a survival benefit compared to the standard treatment without arsenic.[178] Patients with high-risk disease (WBC > 10 K) fared very well with this approach. Australian investigators also showed the value of a combined chemo/ATRA/arsenic approach.[179]

One of the most dramatic changes in the way we treat APL derived from a GIMEMA-led trial which compared a chemotherapy-free based approach (ATRA and arsenic trioxide given together as both induction and postremission therapy) to the aforementioned PETHEMA approach using anthracyclines and retinoic acid (Figure 11).[54] The trial was designed as a noninferiority effort and was restricted to patients under age 70 whose white counts were less than 10,000/uL at diagnosis. Patients assigned to the ATRA/arsenic arm had a 93% event free and 95% overall survival, which was statistically superior to the outcome in the patients assigned to the chemotherapy-containing arm. As such, the new standard of care for those with white counts less than 10,000/uL at diagnosis, is now the regimen of ATRA and arsenic as used in the GIMEMA trial. The standard of care for those patients whose white counts are greater than 10,000/uL has not yet emerged but it is reasonable to add idarubicin[179] or gemtuzumab to ATRA/arsenic.[180]

Other issues

Hematopoietic growth factors

Because myelosuppression-associated toxicity and mortality are high, particularly in older adults with AML, the development of hematopoietic growth factors (HGFs) held promise to ameliorate such side effects. Granulocyte-macrophage colony-stimulating factor (GM-CSF), granulocyte colony-stimulating factor (G-CSF), and interleukin (IL)-3 have been evaluated as well as the thrombopoietic factors, megakaryocyte growth and development factor (MGDF), IL-11, and the newer thrombopoietic agents (romiplostim and eltromopag). The use of these agents in AML lagged behind that in solid tumors because of the concern that pharmacologic doses would lead to blast proliferation and a poor clinical outcome. Although fears regarding this clinical problem have proven unfounded, the HGFs have not lived up to their promise for other reasons.

In aggregate, it would appear that the benefits of growth factors administered after the completion of induction therapy are modest at best.[181] In contrast, G-CSF following intensive consolidation therapy has appreciably shortened the duration of neutropenia,[142] and thrombopoietin, and other agents shorted duration of thrombocytopenia albeit without improvement in CR duration or survival.[182] Because of the potential for eliminating the need for hospitalization, the use of HGF can be recommended following consolidation therapy.

Minimal or measurable residual disease (MRD)

A number of techniques can detect residual leukemia cells in patients in morphologic CR, including (in approximate descending order of sensitivity) conventional cytogenetics, Southern blotting for known gene rearrangements, FISH, multiparameter flow cytometry, and RT-PCR.[183] Serial measurement of MRD is an important component of the management of APL, chronic myelogenous leukemia, and childhood ALL but is not sufficiently standardized to be used routinely in patients with AML.[184] Technical problems abound, including the requirement for a known and already clonal abnormality when applying molecular techniques and the potential for changes in antigen expression over time when using immunologic monitoring. There are few large prospective studies available. Although preliminary data are compatible with the logical premise that persistence of detectable disease presages eventual relapse, false-positive and false-negative rates may be appreciable and could result in incorrect decisions about further treatment. Serial monitoring is cumbersome, and it is hoped that future studies will determine specific time points after completion of therapy when detection of MRD is prognostically significant. It is also likely that different sampling strategies will be needed for different AML subtypes. The key clinical question is whether intervention with further therapy or allogeneic SCT will be of value if applied earlier, prior to gross relapse. There are no prospective data addressing this issue, but retrospective studies have shown much higher than expected relapse rates in allogeneic transplant recipients with detectable MRD. Because of the presence of residual disease, autologous collection and high-dose therapy may be predicted to be of less value in this circumstance.

Small molecules inhibitors and other novel approaches

A comprehensive discussion of all agents in development for AML is beyond the scope of this article; however, it is worth highlighting progress in mutationally targeted, leukemic stem cell niche, and immunologically targeted approaches.

Mutationally targeted therapies. Inhibition of the activated FLT3 transmembrane tyrosine kinase in patients with mutations has led to the approval of midostaurin with chemotherapy and gilteritinib as a single agent in relapsed disease. Quizartinib[185] (specific but only inhibits the *FLT3* ITD mutation subtype, resistance via outgrowth of mutant *FLT3* TKD clones) and crenolanib[186] are two additional FLT3 inhibitors in late-stage development for possible use with chemotherapy in upfront patients. Sorafenib is approved as a vascular endothelial growth factor receptor inhibitor in patients with advanced renal and hepatocellular carcinomas but has FLT3 inhibitory activity and data supports its use for post-alloSCT maintenance.

Given that a sizable minority of patients with favorable chromosome (so-called-CBF translocations) AML has either overexpression of c-KIT and/or mutations in the *KIT* tyrosine kinase, the *KIT* inhibitor dasatinib has been added to chemotherapy in this cytogenetic subset of patients with AML. Preliminary results are encouraging[187] and a randomized trial is ongoing. IDH inhibitors are approved in relapsed AML with the relevant mutations. MEK pathway inhibitors in patients with activating mutation of the RAS oncogene[188] are in early-stage development. TP53 mutations are generally loss of function and therefore harder to target but refolding agents are in development.[189] Both SYK kinase[190] and menin inhibitors[191] may be useful in NPM1 and MLL (on 11q23) rearranged AML. In each of these mutational subtypes, a pro-transcriptional complex involving menin leads to activation of genes in the pro-leukemic HOX9-ME1S1 program.[192,193]

In addition to these genomically based therapies, there are a host of other agents in development which take advantage of potential biologic differences between AML cells and normal stem cells. AML cells in the marrow niche have their survival promoted by factors elaborated by endothelial and other cells in the marrow stroma.[194] Drugs such as the CXCR4 inhibitor, plerixafor or the E-selectin inhibitor uproleselan, may disrupt the survival signals making AML cells more amenable to killing via cytotoxic agents.[195] Selinexor is a nuclear export protein inhibitor which works primarily by preventing expulsion of tumor suppressor genes from the nucleus of cancer cells, in general, and in AML cells in particular.[196] There are several antibodies and immunoconjugates targeting CD123[197] believed to be specifically expressed on leukemic stem cells, including a drug approved in blastic plasmacytoid dendritic cell neoplasm, tagraxofusp,[197] which is an IL3 molecule bound to diptheria toxin. The developmental pathway for any agent in AML is a bit daunting since one has to determine if single-agent utility in advanced patients and whether it should be added in chemotherapy in patients in earlier stages of the disease. In the latter case, given the relatively high initial response rate to chemotherapy in patients, large trials or trials with a novel design are needed.

A critical component of the therapeutic benefit associated with allogeneic SCT is related to the graft-versus leukemia effect. Although this is a complex, multifactorial set of events, further studies may enable the rational application of lymphokines to stimulate the appropriate cells in patients treated with chemotherapy alone. Efforts to harness the immune system in the non-alloSCT context have been difficult. Augmenting with autologous natural killer (NK) cells that may mediate GVL and/or with Interleukin 2 have been variably successful but many patients refused randomization or refused IL-2 if they were randomized to receive it.[198] A randomized trial showed that a combination of histamine plus IL-2 was beneficial in the late postremission setting,[199] but has been criticized because of the heterogeneity of the prerandomization chemotherapy. Immune checkpoint inhibitors have yet to show great promise in AML though the CTLA4 inhibitor ipilimumab has shown activity in post-alloSCT extra-medullary relapse.[168] Vaccine-based approaches using dendritic cell fusions to present leukemia-associated antigens,[200] bispecific antibodies capable of juxtaposing effector CD3 postive T cells to CD33 or CD123 positive AML cells, or chimeric antigen receptor T cells are alternative means to leverage immune cells against AML.[201]

Complications

Hyperleukocytosis

Leukemic blasts are considerably less deformable than mature myeloid cells and are "stickier" than lymphoblasts because of the expression of cell surface adhesion molecules. With increasing blast counts, usually at levels greater than 100,000/μL in the myeloid leukemias, blood flow in the microcirculation can be impeded by plugs of these more rigid cells. Local hypoxemia may be exacerbated by the high metabolic activity of the dividing blasts, with endothelial damage and hemorrhage. Red blood cell transfusions can potentially further increase the blood viscosity and make the situation worse and should be either withheld or administered slowly, until the WBC decreases. Coagulation abnormalities, including DIC, further increase the risk of local hemorrhage. Liberal use of platelet transfusions is recommended, particularly since the platelet count is frequently overestimated because of the presence of fragments of blasts on blood smears, which can be mistakenly counted as platelets by automated blood cell counters.[202]

Although pathologic evidence of leukostasis can be found in most organs in patients with extremely high blast cell counts, clinical symptomatology is usually related to CNS and pulmonary involvement.[203] Occasionally, dyspnea with worsening hypoxemia can occur following therapy and lysis of trapped leukemic cells. Spurious elevation of serum potassium can occur because of the release from WBCs during clotting, and it is sometimes necessary to measure potassium levels on heparinized plasma. Similarly, pO_2 can appear falsely decreased because of the enhanced metabolic activity of the WBCs, even when the specimen is appropriately placed on ice during transport to the laboratory. Pulse oximetry provides an accurate assessment of O_2 saturation in such circumstances. Hyperleukocytosis is more common in patients with myelomonocytic or monocytic leukemia, and it is possible that the clinical manifestations are exacerbated by the migration of leukemic promonocytes into tissue where further proliferation occurs.

The initial mortality rate for patients with AML and symptomatic hyperleukocytosis is high.[203] If patients survive the initial period, they tend to have somewhat lower remission rates and shorter CR durations. Symptomatic hyperleukocytosis in AML (and rarely in ALL) constitutes a medical emergency, and efforts should be made to lower the WBC count rapidly. In most patients, rapid cytoreduction can be achieved by chemotherapy, with either standard induction agents with high doses of hydroxyurea (30–40 mg/1 g) or a single 1 gm dose of cytarabine. Some centers also advocate low-dose cranial irradiation, including the retina, in order to prevent further proliferation of leukemic cells in CNS sites where drug delivery may theoretically be compromised. This treatment is well tolerated, although there are no comparative studies to determine whether the results are superior to chemotherapy alone.

In some patients, it is impossible to initiate chemotherapy immediately because of renal insufficiency, metabolic problems, delays in initiating allopurinol therapy so as to prevent hyperuricemia, or similar considerations. In such patients, emergency leukapheresis has been used to lower or stabilize the white count.[204] Although intensive leukapheresis, with procedure times often lasting many hours, can produce improvement of pulmonary and CNS symptomatology, there are theoretic and practical limitations to its benefits. It is difficult, for example, for leukapheresis to affect already established vascular plugs, particularly if vascular invasion has taken place. In such cases, chemotherapy is the primary modality, although theoretically, leukapheresis could decrease further accumulation of leukocytes at these sites. Furthermore, it is precisely the patient in whom leukostasis is most likely to occur, that is, the patient with high and rapidly rising blasts counts, in whom the technical limitations of leukapheresis are apparent, in that it is often difficult, even with highly efficient cell separators, to reduce the rising count. In such patients with a high proliferative thrust, cycle-specific chemotherapeutic agents are more likely to be most immediately effective. Leukapheresis is also of modest benefit to patients who develop pulmonary problems during cytotoxic treatment, since in some such patients the symptoms are related at least in part to a local inflammatory response following leukocyte lysis.

Central nervous system leukemia

Involvement of the CNS is considerably less common in patients with AML than in both adults and children with ALL. Most clinicians have the impression that the incidence has decreased even further in recent years, perhaps related to the use of higher doses of ara-C, which can penetrate into the CNS. The incidence of CNS leukemia has been less than 5% in large AML clinical trials in recent years.[205] Therefore, diagnostic lumbar punctures are not routinely indicated in the absence of CNS symptoms, and chemotherapy regimens do not include CNS prophylaxis. Symptoms are consequences of increased intracranial pressure and usually consist of a constant headache, sometimes associated with lethargy or other mental changes. Cranial nerve signs (most commonly cranial nerves III or VI) and, occasionally, peripheral nerve manifestations are secondary to nerve root involvement and can be accompanied by headaches or occur alone.[206]

The diagnosis is usually suspected clinically and/or by meningeal enhancement on MRI with gadolinium and confirmed by examination of cytocentrifuge preparations of cerebrospinal fluid (CSF) after lumbar puncture. Cell counts can vary from as few as 5/μL to >1000. Most patients have moderate elevations in CSF protein with a moderate decrease in glucose. Treatment consists of the administration of intrathecal chemotherapy, with the addition of cranial radiation (usually 2400 cGy), to patients who do not respond fully to chemotherapy or in whom cranial nerve involvement is present.[206] Either methotrexate (15 mg/dose when administered by lumbar puncture) or ara-C (50 mg/dose) can be used as initial therapy, with a crossover to the other agent in the event of refractoriness or relapse. A typical schedule includes treatment two to three times a week until the CSF has cleared, generally occurring after a few injections. Treatment is then given at weekly intervals for two more doses to be followed by monthly administration for a total of a year. An Ommaya reservoir to permit intraventricular drug administration is frequently needed either because of difficulties in performing repeated lumbar punctures or because of concern that in some individuals, the CSF flow does not deliver sufficient amounts of the drug from the lumbar space to the entire CNS.[207] Successful therapy with systemically administered agents that penetrate the CNS, such as high-dose methotrexate, or high-dose ara-C, may be used. Unfortunately, the relapse rate is high, either concomitantly with bone marrow relapse or independently, even after initial successful therapy.

It has been suggested that the incidence of CNS leukemia is higher in patients with myelomonocytic or monocytic leukemia and/or high circulating blast counts. This may no longer be the case using more contemporary treatment regimens, and prophylactic therapy is not indicated in such individuals. As noted, CNS involvement can occur in patients with APL with high white blood count.

Ophthalmic complications

Essentially every ocular structure can be involved in the leukemias, sometimes dominating the clinical picture in the prechemotherapy era. Leukemia cells can infiltrate the conjunctiva and lacrimal glands, producing obvious masses that may require treatment with radiation therapy. Involvement of the choroid and retina is most common, however. A prospective study of 53 newly diagnosed adults with AML documented retinal or optic nerve abnormalities in 64% of patients.[208] Hemorrhage and cotton-wool spots (a consequence of nerve fiber ischemia) were most frequent, and the occurrence of these findings was unrelated to patient age, FAB type, WBC count or hematocrit. Initial platelet counts were lower in patients with retinopathy. Ten patients had decreased visual acuity, including five with macular hemorrhages. It was felt that many of the cotton-wool spots were either a consequence of or exacerbated by ischemia due to anemia. Definite leukemic infiltrate of the retina could not be confirmed. All patients received aggressive chemotherapy and platelet transfusion support; no patient received cranial or ocular irradiation. All ocular findings resolved in patients achieving CR and there was no residual visual deficit in any patient. Infectious ocular problems were not noted and seem to be uncommon, perhaps because the prompt empiric use of antibacterial and antifungal antibiotics has decreased the possibility of hematogenous spread of infections to the eye.

Pregnancy

AML is occasionally diagnosed during pregnancy, either because of clinical manifestations or as an incidental finding during blood count checks. If detected during the first trimester, termination of pregnancy followed by treatment of the leukemia is advisable. The management of patients diagnosed later in pregnancy, such as late in the second trimester or during the third trimester, is more problematic. If the leukemia is relatively indolent, it is sometimes possible to manage patients conservatively with leukapheresis and/or transfusion with induction of labor and delivery of the fetus as soon as possible. There have also been many reports of patients treated with chemotherapy later in their pregnancy. The majority of these women have not aborted, and there have been no reports of leukemia occurring in the children or an increased incidence of abnormalities in the infants.[209]

Metabolic abnormalities

Patients receiving therapy for AML can experience a wide range of metabolic problems as a consequence such as vomiting, diarrhea, impaired nutrition, or renal dysfunction, potentially because of the leukemic process itself. Hyperuricemia, occasionally accompanied by urate nephropathy with renal insufficiency, is the most frequent metabolic accompaniment of AML. All patients should receive allopurinol, 300 mg/d or more, as soon as the diagnosis of acute leukemia is established, so that chemotherapy can be administered as soon as is medically appropriate. In most patients, urate nephropathy can be avoided or ameliorated with vigorous hydration and urinary alkalization with systemic or oral administration of sodium bicarbonate. Allopurinol can usually be discontinued within a day or two after chemotherapy is completed. In occasional patients with markedly elevated levels of uric acid, the use of recombinant urate oxidase, which can rapidly lower levels within a few hours, may be advisable.[210] A single dose is almost always sufficient with the decision about subsequent doses dependent on serial monitoring of uric acid.[211]

Tumor lysis syndrome occurs more frequently in patients with ALL, although some AML patients experience hyperphosphatemia, hypocalcemia, hyperkalemia, and renal insufficiency as a consequence of massive leukemic cell death. The inciting cause seems to be release of large amounts of phosphate from lysed blasts, which coprecipitates with calcium in the kidneys, leading to hypocalcemia and sometimes to oliguric renal failure. Hyperuricemia further contributes to this problem, which is usually self-limited and responds to judicious hydration.

Despite markedly hypercellular marrows, hypercalcemia is extremely unusual in patients with AML. Severe, occasionally symptomatic, hypokalemia is not infrequent, particularly in patients with monocytic leukemias. The mechanism appears to be renal potassium loss because of tubular damage induced by the high levels of lysozyme often noted in these patients. Aggressive replacement with parenteral potassium is required; the syndrome usually abates after cytoreduction by chemotherapy. Lastly, rare patients have been described in whom lactic acidosis has been a constant metabolic accompaniment of the leukemia both at the time of presentation and relapse.[212]

Summary

Dramatic advances in molecular genetics and increased understanding of leukemia biology have led to the development of small molecules, monoclonal antibodies, cytokines, and HGF with clinical utility. Further clarification of mechanisms of drug resistance with the possibility of enhancement of the effectiveness of currently available drugs and using MRD to guide therapy are exciting and achievable prospects. These strategies, along with improvements in alloSCT provide the hope that therapy for AML will be both more successful and less empiric in the future.

Mast cell leukemia and other mast cell neoplasms

Mast cell activation syndrome, in which mast cells degranulate, thereby producing severe symptoms such as flushing, wheezing, rash, and hypotension may or may not be associated with excessive numbers of mast cells, is generally not considered a neoplasm.[213] Mast cell excess may be reactive[214] (associated with other hematologic neoplasm or with allergic phenomena such as rhinitis) or clonal. Clonal proliferation range from purely cutaneous involvement (i.e., urticaria pigmentosa) to life-threatening aggressive diseases such as advanced systemic mastocytosis, including mast cell leukemia. Such clonal or neoplastic growth of (morphologically abnormal) mast cells are no longer considered under the myeloproliferative neoplasm rubric but rather as a separate category.[215]

Classification of neoplastic mast cell disease

Urticaria pigmentosa (cutaneous mastocytosis) is by far the most common manifestation of neoplastic mast cell proliferation.[216] The typical eruption of urticaria pigmentosa consists of multiple discrete hyperpigmented nodulopapular lesions and portends a benign clinical course, especially in children. Cutaneous symptoms may include the classic urticarial wheals that result from mast cell degranulation in response to mechanical insult (Darier's sign), pruritus, or episodic flushing. Cutaneous involvement may be a manifestation of the more aggressive disease (systemic mastocytosis [SM]) seen in adults.[217] SM can be associated with a second myeloid neoplasm which may be clonally related.[218] Systemic mastocytosis may present with a variety of constitutional and/or gastrointestinal symptoms, each of which can be attributed to excessive elaboration of mast cell mediators. Such symptoms, often associated with elevation of serum tryptase, which may also be present to a lesser degree in patients with urticaria pigmentosa, include rhinitis, asthma, nausea, vomiting, diarrhea, syncope, chest pain, bone pain, and rectal discomfort.[217] The bony skeleton, the gastrointestinal tract, and the spleen can also be sites of mast cell infiltration.

The diagnostic workup of suspected SM should include serum tryptase, marrow biopsy (include stains for tryptase CD25 by Immunohistochemistry and molecular testing for *KIT* D816V mutation). One should determine if criteria for systemic mastocytosis are met: (required major criterion of multi-focal dense infiltrates of mast cells (>15 mast cells in aggregates) in marrow or other extracutaneous organs and at least three of the following minor criteria: (1) >25% of the mast cells in the infiltrate are spindle shaped or have atypical morphology, or of all mast cells in marrow aspirate, 25% are immature or atypical; (2) activating point mutations at codon 816 of *KIT*; (3) mast cells express CD25; (4) serum tryptase persistently exceeds 20 mg/μL. Once a diagnosis of SM is made, patients can be subdivided into SM-AHN (if another myeloid neoplasm is identified); aggressive systemic mastocytosis (ASM) if there are "C" findings (marrow dysfunction; palpable liver, ascites, portal hypertension; skeletal involvement with osteolytic lesions; palpable splenomegaly with hyperplasia, or malabsorption due to gastrointestinal mast cell infiltration); indolent SM [ISM] if there are no "C" findings (ISM includes the subcategory of smoldering SM if there are two or more "B" findings (high mast cell marrow burden, dysplasia with proliferation not meeting criteria of associated neoplasm or enlarged liver or spleen without functional consequences); or mast cell leukemia if there are >20% of mast cells on the aspirate smear. The natural history of SM is similar or slightly worse than age-matched controls, but the ASM category is clearly more adverse. Models not solely based on SM subcategories may add useful information.[217]

While the diagnostic algorithm is complex, another detail includes the misinterpretation rather than undermeaning of an elevated tryptase in SM-AHN (since neoplasms such as MDS can be associated with elevated tryptase.[219]) Interestingly, the D816V *KIT* mutation, both pathophysiologically and therapeutically critical is not universally detected in the associated heme neoplasm in SM-AHN.[220] Particularly in patients with concomitant eosinophils, it is important to exclude the FIPIL1-PDGRA translocation, since such patients will benefit from low-dose imatinib.[221]

Treatment

Treatment of mast cell neoplasms is based on the disease subtype and clinical manifestations. Patients with cutaneous mastocytosis usually require no treatment. Systemic mast cell disease, however, has protean clinical manifestations. For example, those with hematological abnormalities may require supportive care, which could include transfusions or the empiric use of HGFs. Avoidance of mast cell stimulants such as anesthesia, alcohol, aspirin, and morphine may diminish flushing, pruritus, and diarrhea. Full "antimast cell degranulation" therapy should be employed. Such therapy may include H1 and H2 antihistamines, leukotriene antagonists, proton pump inhibitors, anti-IL-5 antibody, disodium chromoglycolate, or steroids which may offer palliative benefit.[217] Osteoperosis is often present, mandating the use of bisphonates.[217] If such measures fail to control symptoms, mast cell debulking may be required.

"Non-specific" mast cell debulking agents used in ASM have included interferon-alpha,[222] cladribine,[223] or allogeneic stem cell transplant.[224] Treatment may additionally need to be directed to the "other" hematological neoplasm in SM-AHN.

The ability to inhibit the activated KIT enzyme with small molecules has led to clinical benefit in the management of patients ASM (and possibly ISM). Midostaurin (100 mg/bid) is approved for the treatment of ASM based on a 75% overall response rate, but few CRs were noted).[225] Nausea, vomiting, diarrhea, and fatigue are common side effects and frequently lead to discontinuation. A novel potent D816V KIT inhibitor, avapritinib, was recently approved based on high activity in ASM, even in those with prior exposure to midostaurin.[226,227] Though there is a risk of thrombocytopenia and CNS hemorrhage, avapritinib holds significant promise as an agent capable of improving the quality of life in patients with potentially devastating SM.

Key references

The complete reference list can be found on Vital Source version of this title, see inside front cover.

2   Shallis RM, Wang R, Davidoff A, et al. Epidemiology of acute myeloid leukemia: recent progress and enduring challenges. *Blood Rev.* 2019;**36**:70–87.

3   Cancer Genome Atlas Research Network. Genomic and epigenomic landscapes of adults de novo acute myeloid leukemia. *N Engl J Med.* 2013;**368**:2059–2074.

4   Lindsley RC, Mar BG, Mazzola E, et al. Acute myeloid leukemia ontogeny is defined by distinct somatic mutations. *Blood.* 2015;**125**:1367–1376.

25 Pui C-H, Ribeiro RC, Hancock ML, et al. Acute myeloid leukemia in children treated with epipodophyllotoxins for acute lymphoblastic leukemia. *N Engl J Med.* 1991;**325**:1682–1687.

28 Wong TN, Ramsingh G, Young AL, et al. Role of TP53 mutations in the origin and evolution of therapy-related acute myeloid leukaemia. *Nature.* 2015;**518**:552–555.

29 Churpek JE, Pyrtel K, Kanchi K-L, et al. Genomic analysis of germ line and somatic variants in familial myelodysplasia/acute myeloid leukemia. *Blood.* 2015;**126**:2484–2490.

33 Dohner H, Estey E, Grimwade D, et al. Diagnosis and management of AML in adults: 2017 ELN recommendations from an international expert panel. *Blood.* 2017;**129**:424–447.

44 Arber DA, Orazi A, Hasserjian R, et al. The 2016 revision to the World Health Organization classification of myeloid neoplasms and acute leukemia. *Blood.* 2016;**127**:2391–2405.

54 Lo-Coco F, Avvisati G, Vignetti M, et al. Retinoic acid and arsenic trioxide for acute promyelocytic leukemia. *N Engl J Med.* 2013;**369**:111–121.

64 Grignani F, De Matteis S, Nervi C, et al. Fusion proteins of the retinoic acid receptor-alpha recruit histone deacetylase in promyelocytic leukaemia. *Nature.* 1998;**391**:815–818.

79 Birdwell C, Fiskus W, Kadia TM, et al. EVI1 dysregulation: impact on biology and therapy of myeloid malignancies. *Blood Cancer J.* 2021;**11**:64.

83 Wolach O, Stone RM. How I treat mixed phenotype acute leukemia. *Blood.* 2015;**125**:2477–2485. doi: 10.1182/blood-2014-10-551465.

86 Ngai LL, Kelder A, Janssen J, et al. MRD tailored therapy in AML: what we have learned so far. *Front Oncol.* 2020;**10**:603636.

87 Short NJ, Zhou S, Fu C, et al. Association of measurable residual disease with survival outcomes in patients with acute myeloid leukemia: a systematic review and meta-analysis. *JAMA Oncol.* 2020;**6**:1890–1899.

88 Wei AH, Dohner H, Pocock C, et al. Oral azacitidine maintenance therapy for acute myeloid leukemia in first remission. *N Engl J Med*. 2020;**383**:2526–2537.

89 Hills RK, Castaigne S, Appelbaum FR, et al. Addition of gemtuzumab ozogamicin to induction chemotherapy in adult patients with acute myeloid leukaemia: a meta-analysis of individual patient data from randomised controlled trials. *Lancet Oncol*. 2014;**15**:986–996.

90 Stone RM, Mandrekar SJ, Sanford BL, et al. Midostaurin plus chemotherapy for acute myeloid leukemia with a FLT3 mutation. *N Engl J Med*. 2017;**377**:454–464.

91 Lancet JE, Uy GL, Cortes JE, et al. CPX-351 (cytarabine and daunorubicin) liposome for injection versus conventional cytarabine plus daunorubicin in older patients with newly diagnosed secondary acute myeloid leukemia. *J Clin Oncol*. 2018;**36**:2684–2692.

92 DiNardo CD, Lachowiez CA, Takahashi K, et al. Venetoclax combined with FLAG-IDA induction and consolidation in newly diagnosed and relapsed or refractory acute myeloid leukemia. *J Clin Oncol*. 2021;**39**:2768–2778.

93 Fernandez HF, Sun Z, Yao X, et al. Anthracycline dose intensification in acute myeloid leukemia. *N Engl J Med*. 2009;**361**:1249–1259.

94 Ferrara F, Barosi G, Venditti A, et al. Consensus-based definition of unfitness to intensive and non-intensive chemotherapy in acute myeloid leukemia: a project of SIE, SIES and GITMO group on a new tool for therapy decision making. *Leukemia*. 2013;**27**:997–999.

95 Klepin HD, Geiger AM, Tooze JA, et al. Geriatric assessment predicts survival for older adults receiving induction chemotherapy for acute myelogenous leukemia. *Blood*. 2013;**121**:4287–4294.

102 Lancet JE, Uy GL, Newell LF, et al. CPX-351 versus 7+3 cytarabine and daunorubicin chemotherapy in older adults with newly diagnosed high-risk or secondary acute myeloid leukaemia: 5-year results of a randomised, open-label, multicentre, phase 3 trial. *Lancet Haematol*. 2021;**8**:e481–e491.

114 Holowiecki J, Grosicki S, Giebel S, et al. Cladribine, but not fludarabine, added to daunorubicin and cytarabine during induction prolongs survival of patients with acute myeloid leukemia: a multicenter, randomized phase III study. *J Clin Oncol*. 2012;**30**:2441–2448.

117 Halpern AB, Othus M, Huebner EM, et al. Phase 1/2 trial of GCLAM with dose-escalated mitoxantrone for newly diagnosed AML or other high-grade myeloid neoplasms. *Leukemia*. 2018;**32**:2352–2362.

120 Burnett AK, Milligan D, Prentice AG, et al. A comparison of low-dose cytarabine and hydroxyurea with or without all-trans retinoic acid for acute myeloid leukemia and high-risk myelodysplastic syndrome in patients not considered fit for intensive treatment. *Cancer*. 2007;**109**:1114–1124.

122 Dombret H, Seymour JF, Butrym A, et al. International phase 3 study of azacitidine vs conventional care regimens in older patients with newly diagnosed AML with >30% blasts. *Blood*. 2015;**126**:291–299.

123 DiNardo CD, Jonas BA, Pullarkat V, et al. Azacitidine and venetoclax in previously untreated acute myeloid leukemia. *N Engl J Med*. 2020;**383**:617–629.

124 Wei AH, Montesinos P, Ivanov V, et al. Venetoclax plus LDAC for newly diagnosed AML ineligible for intensive chemotherapy: a phase 3 randomized placebo-controlled trial. *Blood*. 2020;**135**:2137–2145.

128 Devine SM, Owzar K, Blum W, et al. Phase II study of allogeneic transplantation for older patients with acute myeloid leukemia in first complete remission using a reduced-intensity conditioning regimen: results from cancer and leukemia group B 100103 (Alliance for Clinical Trials in Oncology)/blood and marrow transplant clinical trial network 0502. *J Clin Oncol*. 2015;**33**:4167–4175.

132 Gooptu M, Romee R, St Martin A, et al. HLA-haploidentical vs matched unrelated donor transplants with posttransplant cyclophosphamide-based prophylaxis. *Blood*. 2021;**138**:273–282.

136 Mayer RJ, Davis RB, Schiffer CA, et al. Intensive postremission chemotherapy in adults with acute myeloid leukemia. Cancer and Leukemia Group B. *N Engl J Med*. 1994;**331**:896–903.

140 Bloomfield CD, Lawrence D, Byrd JC, et al. Frequency of prolonged remission duration after high-dose cytarabine intensification in acute myeloid leukemia varies by cytogenetic subtype. *Cancer Res*. 1998;**58**:4173–4179.

141 Neubauer A, Maharry K, Mrozek K, et al. Patients with acute myeloid leukemia and RAS mutations benefit most from postremission high-dose cytarabine: a Cancer and Leukemia Group B study. *J Clin Oncol*. 2008;**26**:4603–4609.

142 Heil G, Hoelzer D, Sanz MA, et al. A randomized, double-blind, placebo-controlled, phase III study of filgrastim in remission induction and consolidation therapy for adults with de novo acute myeloid leukemia. The International Acute Myeloid Leukemia Study Group. *Blood*. 1997;**90**:4710–4718.

144 Koreth J, Schlenk R, Kopecky KJ, et al. Allogeneic stem cell transplantation for acute myeloid leukemia in first complete remission: systematic review and meta-analysis of prospective clinical trials. *JAMA*. 2009;**301**:2349–2361.

145 Stelljes M, Krug U, Beelen DW, et al. Allogeneic transplantation versus chemotherapy as postremission therapy for acute myeloid leukemia: a prospective matched pairs analysis. *J Clin Oncol*. 2014;**32**:288–296.

150 Burchert A, Bug G, Fritz LV, et al. Sorafenib maintenance after allogeneic hematopoietic stem cell transplantation for acute myeloid leukemia with FLT3-internal tandem duplication mutation (SORMAIN). *J Clin Oncol*. 2020;**38**:2993–3002.

152 DeWolf S, Tallman MS. How I treat relapsed or refractory AML. *Blood*. 2020;**136**:1023–1032.

153 Breems DA, Van Putten WL, Huijgens PC, et al. Prognostic index for adult patients with acute myeloid leukemia in first relapse. *J Clin Oncol*. 2005;**23**:1969–1978.

154 Archimbaud E, Thomas X, Leblond V, et al. Timed sequential chemotherapy for previously treated patients with acute myeloid leukemia: long-term follow-up of the etoposide, mitoxantrone, and cytarabine-86 trial. *J Clin Oncol*. 1995;**13**:11–18.

155 Westhus J, Noppeney R, Duhrsen U, et al. FLAG salvage therapy combined with idarubicin in relapsed/refractory acute myeloid leukemia. *Leuk Lymphoma*. 2019;**60**:1014–1022.

156 Faderl S, Gandhi V, O'Brien S, et al. Results of a phase 1-2 study of clofarabine in combination with cytarabine (ara-C) in relapased and refractory acute leukemias. *Blood*. 2005;**105**:940–947.

157 Stahl M, Menghrajani K, Derkach A, et al. Clinical and molecular predictors of response and survival following venetoclax therapy in relapsed/refractory AML. *Blood Adv*. 2021;**5**:1552–1564.

159 Perl AE, Martinelli G, Cortes JE, et al. Gilteritinib or chemotherapy for relapsed or refractory FLT3-mutated AML. *N Engl J Med*. 2019;**381**:1728–1740.

160 Waitkus MS, Diplas BH, Yan H. Biological role and therapeutic potential of IDH mutations in cancer. *Cancer Cell*. 2018;**34**:186–195.

161 DiNardo CD, Stein EM, de Botton S, et al. Durable remissions with ivosidenib in IDH1-mutated relapsed or refractory AML. *N Engl J Med*. 2018;**378**:2386–2398.

162 Stein EM, DiNardo CD, Fathi AT, et al. Molecular remission and response patterns in patients with mutant-IDH2 acute myeloid leukemia treated with enasidenib. *Blood*. 2019;**133**:676–687.

163 Fathi AT, DiNardo CD, Kline I, et al. Differentiation syndrome associated with enasidenib, a selective inhibitor of mutant isocitrate dehydrogenase 2: analysis of a phase 1/2 study. *JAMA Oncol*. 2018;**4**:1106–1110.

164 Yanada M, Konuma T, Yamasaki S, et al. Relapse of acute myeloid leukemia after allogeneic hematopoietic cell transplantation: clinical features and outcomes. *Bone Marrow Transplant*. 2021;**56**:1126–1133.

166 Moukalled NM, Kharfan-Dabaja MA. What is the role of a second allogeneic hematopoietic cell transplant in relapsed acute myeloid leukemia? *Bone Marrow Transplant*. 2020;**55**:325–331.

168 Davids MS, Kim HT, Bachireddy P, et al. Ipilimumab for patients with relapse after allogeneic transplantation. *N Engl J Med*. 2016;**375**:143–153.

170 Sanz MA, Montesinos P. How we prevent and treat differentiation syndrome in patients with acute promyelocytic leukemia. *Blood*. 2014;**123**:2777–2782.

177 Ravandi F, Estey E, Jones D, et al. Effective treatment of acute promyelocytic leukemia with all-trans-retinoic acid, arsenic trioxide, and gemtuzumab ozogamicin. *J Clin Oncol*. 2009;**27**:504–510.

179 Iland HJ, Bradstock K, Supple SG, et al. All-trans-retinoic acid, idarubicin, and IV arsenic trioxide as initial therapy in acute promyelocytic leukemia (APML4). *Blood*. 2012;**120**:1570–1580.

184 Dillon R, Potter N, Freeman S, et al. How we use molecular minimal residual disease (MRD) testing in acute myeloid leukaemia (AML). *Br J Haematol*. 2021;**193**:231–244.

206 Bleyer WA, Poplack DG. Prophylaxis and treatment of leukemia in the central nervous system and other sanctuaries. *Semin Oncol*. 1985;**12**:131–148.

209 Milojkovic D, Apperley JF. How I treat leukemia during pregnancy. *Blood*. 2014;**123**:974–984.

217 Pardanani A. Systemic mastocytosis in adults: 2021 Update on diagnosis, risk stratification and management. *Am J Hematol*. 2021;**96**:508–525.

226 Gotlib J, Reiter A, Radia D, et al. Efficacy and safety of avapritinib in advanced systemic mastocytosis: interim analysis of the phase 2 PATHFINDER trial. *Nat Med*. 2021. doi: 10.1038/s41591-021-01539-8.

112 Chronic myeloid leukemia

Jorge Cortes, MD ■ Richard T. Silver, MD ■ Hagop Kantarjian, MD

Overview

Chronic myeloid leukemia (CML) was the first malignancy where a unique chromosomal abnormality, the Philadelphia chromosome (Ph), was directly linked to it. The unraveling of the molecular and physiologic consequences of this abnormality, with a fusion gene (BCR-ABL1) translating into a chimeric protein with increased tyrosine kinase activity, led to the development of specific tyrosine kinase inhibitors (TKIs). The use of such agents as initial therapy has resulted in a dramatic change in the natural history of CML where patients properly managed can have a normal life expectancy. Several treatment options are also available for patients who may not have optimal response to their initial therapy. Current research goals are to improve the safety, efficacy, and wide availability of TKIs and to achieve a response such that patients can eventually discontinue therapy. With these approaches and ongoing research, the goal of eradication of chronic myeloid leukemia is ever closer.

Chronic myeloid leukemia (CML) is a myeloproliferative neoplasm affecting a pluripotent progenitor and involving myeloid, erythroid, megakaryocytic, B, and sometimes T, lymphoid cells, but not marrow fibroblasts. It is characterized by the presence of a unique chromosomal abnormality, the Philadelphia chromosome (Ph).

Historical perspective

In 1960, a minute chromosome was identified in patients with CML, an abnormality later identified as a balanced translocation between chromosomes 9 and 22.[1,2] Later studies demonstrated this translocation resulted in the creation of a chimeric gene, BCR-ABL1 that, when transfected into mice, induced CML.[3] Translation of this chimeric gene results in a fusion protein with constitutive tyrosine kinase activity.[4] Interferon alfa was the first therapy to induce the disappearance of the Ph chromosome, establishing complete cytogenetic responses as the gold standard of response to therapy.[5] The knowledge of the activation of a tyrosine kinase led to the development of tyrosine kinase inhibitors (TKIs), initially imatinib[6] and later second and third-generation drugs that radically changed the natural history of the disease (Figure 1).[7] Today, patients diagnosed with CML, if properly managed have a life expectancy similar to that of the general population.

Incidence and epidemiology

CML accounts for 15% of all leukemias.[1,2] The median age of onset of CML is 55–65 years, and the incidence increases with age with a slight male preponderance (ratio 1.67 : 1).[8] It is estimated that 9110 new cases of CML will be diagnosed in the United States in 2021 with 1220 patients dying from their disease.[9] The incidence in the United States has remained constant at about 1.9 : 100,000. With modern therapy the annual mortality has decreased from 15–20% to 2% and the estimated median survival may exceed 20 years. Thus, the prevalence of CML in the United States in the next three decades may exceed 200,000 cases.[10]

Risk factors

In most patients with CML, a causative factor cannot be identified. Although ionizing radiation is leukemogenic, the most common leukemia following radiation is acute myeloid leukemia. CML has been reported following the atomic bombing in Japan, and in earlier studies in radiologists and in patients with ankylosing spondylitis treated with radiation therapy.[11,12] No other known risk factors have been recognized.

Pathology

CML typically follows a bi- or triphasic course with a chronic phase, followed by an accelerated phase, and a blast phase.[13] Leukocytosis is common, with white cell counts frequently $>100 \times 10^9$/L. Historically, the median survival for patients in chronic phase was 3–6 years, with an estimated annual risk of transformation to the blast phase of 5–10% in the first 2 years, and 15–20% subsequently. Accelerated-phase CML is characterized by increasing maturation arrest. Different criteria have been used to define accelerated phase. One common classification defines accelerated phase as the presence of any of the following: ≥15% blasts, ≥30% blasts plus promyelocytes, ≥20% basophils, platelets $<100 \times 10^9$/L unrelated to therapy, or cytogenetic clonal evolution.[14] Other criteria have been proposed, such as the World Health Organization (WHO) proposal, but all the main TKI trials have used the earlier standard classification. The median survival for patients in accelerated phase was 1–2 years[15] but has greatly improved with the use of TKI.[16] The blast phase is defined by the presence of ≥30% blasts (≥20% in the WHO classification) in the peripheral blood or bone marrow, or the presence of extramedullary disease with immature cells.[17] The blast phase can be classified according to the immunophenotype as myeloid, lymphoid, megakaryocytic, erythroblastic, undifferentiated, biphenotypic, or mixed lineage. Lymphoid blast phase occurs in 20–30% of patients, myeloid in 50%, and undifferentiated in 25%.[18] The median survival in blast phase is 3–6 months. Patients with lymphoid blast phase have a better prognosis, with a response rate of ≥90% and a median survival of >18 months with TKI combined with chemotherapy.[19]

Laboratory features in the chronic phase include leukocytosis with left maturation shift and frequently basophilia and

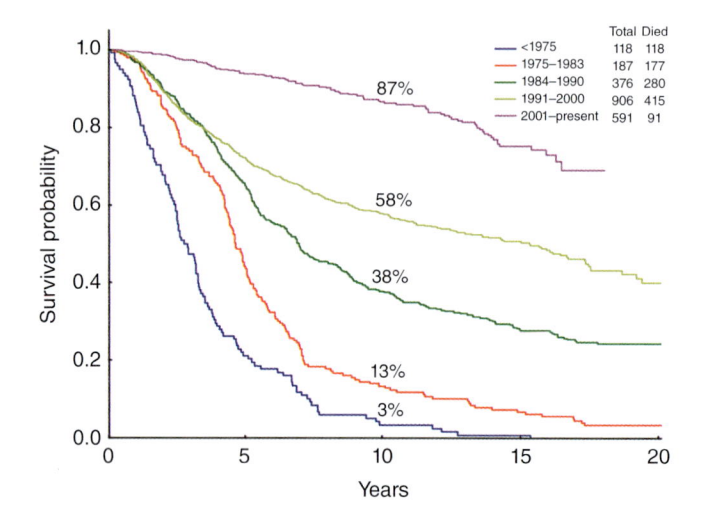

Figure 1 Survival of patients with newly diagnosed CML in chronic phase referred to MD Anderson Cancer Center ($N = 1148$; 1965–2010). Source: Kantarjian et al.[7]

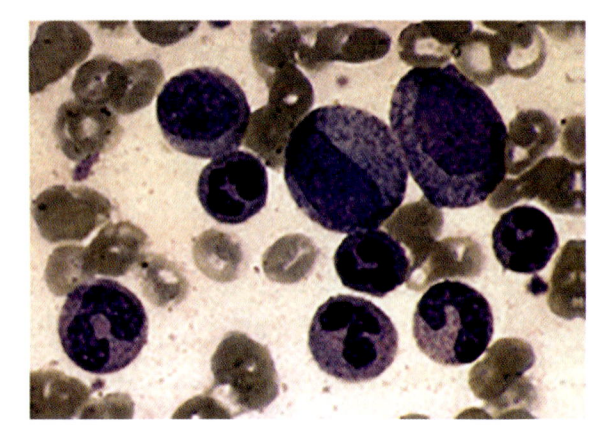

Figure 2 Chronic myeloid leukemia. Leukocytosis with myelocytes, metamyelocytes, band cells, and polymorphonuclear leukocytes are characteristics of the peripheral blood in the chronic phase of this disease.

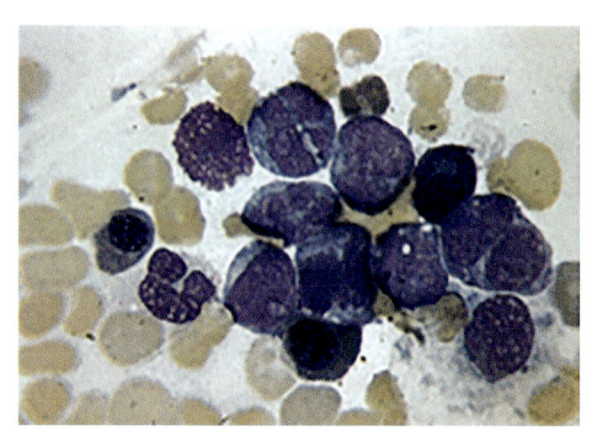

Figure 3 Chronic myeloid leukemia, myeloid blast crisis. The marrow aspiration shows predominance of blast forms, which have a myeloid appearance.

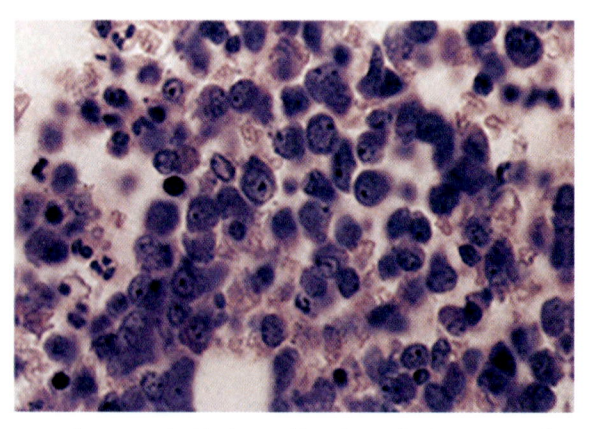

Figure 4 Chronic myeloid leukemia, blast phase. This bone marrow biopsy shows "blasts" with prominent nucleoli comprising about 75% of the marrow cells.

eosinophilia (Figure 2). Thrombocytosis is common but thrombotic phenomena are unusual. Some degree of anemia is common. There is a reduction in leukocyte alkaline phosphatase (LAP) activity and a marked elevation of serum B12 levels.

The bone marrow is hypercellular. In chronic phase, all stages of differentiation are present, but the myelocytes predominate, whereas myeloblasts and promyelocytes account for <10% of cells (Figures 3 and 4). Megakaryocytes may be increased, and there might be increased reticulin fibrosis, which may worsen with disease progression, but is reversed with TKIs.[20]

In the blast phase, lymphoid blasts contain terminal deoxynucleotidyl transferase (TdT). Lymphoblasts usually express CD10, CD19, and CD22 or other B-cell markers;[18] T-cell blast phase is uncommon. The myeloid blast phase may mimic acute myeloid leukemia. The myeloblasts stain with myeloperoxidase and express myeloid markers, including CD13, CD33, and CD117.

Occasionally, patients may present in lymphoid or myeloid blast phase without a recognized antecedent chronic phase. The differentiation between this presentation and Ph-positive acute lymphoblastic or myeloid leukemias may be impossible, but the distinction is semantic as the treatment and prognosis are the same. Megakaryoblastic, erythroblastic, and basophilic transformations are uncommon.

Prognostic classification

Prognosis in CML is variable. Risk classifications have been proposed to stratify patients and assist in treatment decisions. The Sokal model is most frequently used[21] and defines three risk groups: low (about 40–60% of all patients), intermediate (about 20–30%), and high risk (10–20%), with median survivals of 4.5, 3.5, and 2.5 years, respectively, with busulfan or hydroxyurea.

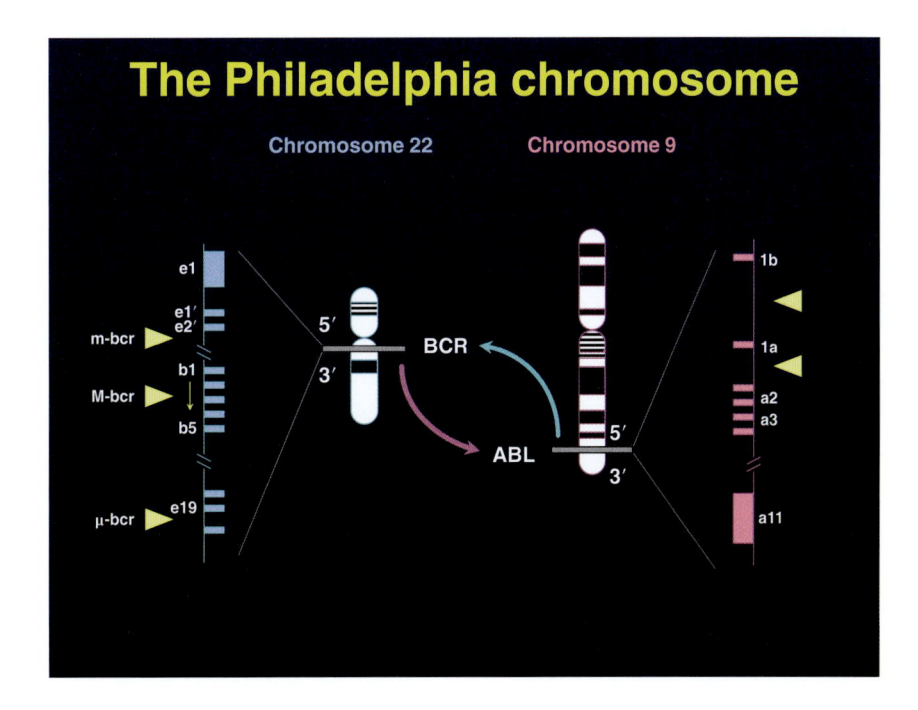

Figure 5 Schematic of 9.22 chromosome translocation.

The model still predicts response to therapy and progression-free survival (PFS) with imatinib therapy, although outcomes for all risk groups are significantly better than in the past. Other classifications have been proposed such as the Harford score (designed for interferon-treated patients),[22] the simpler European treatment and outcome study for CML (EUTOS) score (based only on percentage of basophils and size of spleen),[23] and the most recent EUTOS long-term survival score (ELTS), designed to estimate the risk of death from CML-related causes.[24] With TKI therapy, the significance of several prognostic factors (older age, marrow fibrosis, deletion of derivative 9q, complex Ph chromosome) has been reduced or eliminated.[25–28] Adolescents and young adults may have a worse outcome, arguably because of poor adherence to therapy.[29]

Pathogenesis

The primary biologic defect in CML is unregulated proliferation with discordant maturation, reduced apoptosis, and defective adherence to the bone marrow stroma.[30–32]

Cytogenetics

The hallmark of CML is the Ph chromosome. This results from a reciprocal translocation between chromosome 9 and chromosome 22, t(9;22)(q34.1;q11.21) that transposes the 3′ segment of the *ABL1* gene to the 5′ segment of the *BCR* gene.[2] This creates the chimeric *BCR-ABL1* oncogene (Figure 5).

The Ph chromosome is found in ~95% of patients with CML. It is also observed in 5% of children and 15–30% of adults with acute lymphoblastic leukemia and in 2% of patients with newly diagnosed acute myeloid leukemia.[33] Some patients have variant translocations, which may be simple (involving chromosome 22 and one additional chromosome other than chromosome 9) or complex (involving chromosomes 22, 9, and at least one other chromosome).[34] These patients historically had an inferior outcome, but with TKIs they have a similar prognosis to patients with the classic Ph chromosome.[28]

Progression of CML is frequently accompanied by additional cytogenetic abnormalities. The most common abnormalities include a second Ph chromosome, isochromosome 17, trisomy 8, trisomy 19, and deletion 20q.[35] The molecular consequences of these abnormalities are not known. Mutations or deletions of tumor suppressor genes such as *p16* and *TP53*, and methylation of *ABL1*, *BCR*, p15, and cadherin-13 may contribute to transformation.[36–40] Activation of Janus kinase 2 (JAK2)–signal transducer and activator of transcription (STAT) pathway might be responsible for the survival of the leukemic stem cell.[41,42] In blast phase, granulocyte-macrophage progenitors are the candidate stem cells and activation of β-catenin may enhance the self-renewal activity of these cells.[43]

After successful treatment with TKI, chromosomal abnormalities are found in the Ph-negative cells in 10–15% of patients, most frequently trisomy 8, monosomy 7 or 5, and deletion 20q.[44] These may regress spontaneously in some cases but in rare instances (<1%) may lead to development of a myelodysplastic syndrome or acute myeloid leukemia.[45–47]

Molecular biology

The chimeric oncogene, *BCR-ABL1*, codes for a Bcr-Abl oncoprotein that has constitutional tyrosine kinase activity.[42,48]

There is some heterogeneity in the breakpoints on chromosomes 9 and 22. On chromosome 9, breaks may occur in a region 200 kb or more in length, resulting in most of the c-*abl* gene being translocated.[42] The breakpoints within the *ABL* gene occurs either upstream of exon Ib, downstream of exon Ia, or more frequently, between exons Ib and Ia. Breakpoints in *BCR* occur most frequently in the major breakpoint cluster region that includes exons e12–e16 (formerly b1–b5), resulting in either e13a2 (b2a2) or e14b2 (b3a2) transcripts, both of them generating a 210-kDa

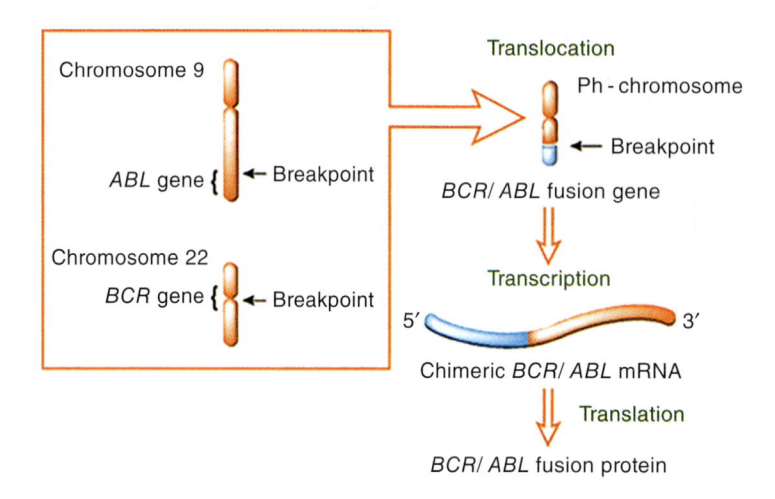

Figure 6 Summary of the cytogenetic and molecular effects of the Ph chromosome.

protein (p210[Bcr-Abl]). In few patients with CML (and most with Ph-positive acute lymphoblastic leukemia (ALL)) the breakpoint may occur in the minor breakpoint cluster region, resulting in an e1a2 fusion.[49] Less frequently, the breakpoint may occur in a different, more telomeric breakpoint region, μ-bcr, resulting in e19a2 fusion oncogene. Rarely, atypical fusion genes may be present (e.g., e13a3 or e14a3).

Transcription of the fusion *BCR-ABL1* oncogene results in a chimeric *BCR-ABL1* mRNA that is translated into fusion proteins p190[Bcr-Abl], p210[Bcr-Abl], and p230[Bcr-Abl], according to the breakpoint on *BCR* (Figure 6). In all instances, the fusion protein has unregulated constitutive tyrosine kinase activity that triggers intracellular signaling pathways such as *STAT, RAS, RAF, JUN* kinase, *MYC, AKT,* and *BCL-2*, which confer the malignant phenotype.[48] Mutations in other cancer-associated genes have been identified in a subset of patients with CML at the time of diagnosis, most frequently *ASXL1, RUNX1,* and *IKZF1*, and the methyltransferase *SETD1B*.[50] The presence of these mutations is associated with poor response to therapy and transformation to blast phase. Upon transformation, patients in blast phase frequently express these and other mutations as well as non-Ph-related fusions frequently with partners that are associated with other cancers.[50]

The clinical features, response to treatment, and prognosis are similar in patients with e13a2 and e14a2. Patients with Ph-positive ALL may express either p210[Bcr-Abl] (30–50%) or p190[Bcr-Abl] (50–70%). Rare patients with CML in chronic phase express e1a2 (p190[Bcr-Abl1]) and have a worse prognosis.[49,51] The p230[Bcr-Abl] is associated with a more indolent disease and a phenotype similar to chronic neutrophilic leukemia.

In approximately 5–10% of morphologically typical cases of CML, the Ph-chromosome cannot be identified. In one-third of these the *BCR-ABL1* rearrangement is present. These patients have similar characteristics, response to treatment, and prognosis as Ph-positive CML.[52] The other two-thirds lack the *BCR-ABL1* rearrangement, usually representing "atypical CML" in the WHO classification. Reverse transcriptase-polymerase chain reaction (RT-PCR) can detect the *BCR-ABL1* transcript with a sensitivity of 10^{-5}.[53] *BCR-ABL1* rearrangement has been identified in up to 25–30% of normal adults using RT-PCR approximately 3-log more sensitive (sensitivity $\sim 10^{-8}$) than the one used clinically.[54] This suggests that clonal disease requires escape from immune surveillance and/or a second oncogenic event to become clinically relevant.

A subset of patients treated with TKI develop resistance. Several mechanisms of resistance have been identified; the most common are mutations in the *BCR-ABL1* kinase domain (KD). More than 50 different mutations have been reported, and involve any of the domains in the BCR-ABL1 structure, including the P-loop (the area where adenosine triphosphate (ATP) binds), the activation loop, and the catalytic domain, as well as the amino acids where imatinib makes contact with Bcr-Abl1.[55] Different mutations vary in their sensitivity to different TKIs. Mutational analysis is useful in patients with resistance to a particular TKI to identify the TKI predicted to have clinical efficacy based on the half-maximal inhibitory concentration (IC_{50}) for particular agents. For example, F317L and V299L are insensitive to dasatinib, V299L is insensitive to bosutinib, and F359V and E255K/V are insensitive to nilotinib, while T315I is sensitive only to ponatinib.[56,57] Selecting a TKI with *in vitro* efficacy is associated with better probability of response and PFS for patients in chronic phase, but is much less predictive in the blast phase, likely because of the greater role of other molecular pathways (Table 1).

Diagnosis

Approximately 90% of patients are diagnosed in the chronic phase, which is usually asymptomatic.[13] When symptoms occur, they are usually due to splenomegaly (pain, abdominal fullness, early satiety) or hyper-proliferation (fatigue, night sweats, unexplained fever, gout, weight loss). Some patients may have signs of platelet dysfunction (e.g., ecchymoses or hemorrhage). Patients with very high white blood cells (WBC) may have signs of hyperviscosity (priapism, cerebrovascular accidents, tinnitus, confusion, retinal hemorrhage). Symptoms associated with advanced phase, particularly blast phase, include constitutional symptoms (night sweats, weight loss, fever, bone pain), anemia, infections, and/or bleeding.

When the diagnosis of CML is suspected, a bone marrow aspiration is mandatory. Although the diagnosis of CML can be made in peripheral blood, proper staging and recognition of all features of the disease can only be made with evaluation of the bone marrow and peripheral blood. The bone marrow aspiration should include: (1) cell differential for proper staging; (2) assessment of fibrosis and other bone marrow architectural features; and (3) cytogenetic analysis by G-banding to confirm the presence of the Ph chromosome and possibly additional chromosomal abnormalities;

Table 1 *In vitro* sensitivity of different BCR-ABL mutants to tyrosine kinase inhibitors.[a]

	IC$_{50}$-fold increase (WT = 1)			
	Imatinib	Bosutinib	Dasatinib	Nilotinib
WT	1	1	1	1
L248V	3.54	2.97	5.11	2.80
G250E	6.86	4.31	4.45	4.56
Q252H	1.39	0.31	3.05	2.64
Y253F	3.58	0.96	1.58	3.23
E255K	6.02	9.47	5.61	6.69
E255V	16.99	5.53	3.44	10.31
D276G	2.18	0.60	1.44	2.00
E279K	3.55	0.95	1.64	2.05
V299L	1.54	26.10	8.65	1.34
T315I	17.50	45.42	75.03	39.41
F317L	2.60	2.42	4.46	2.22
M351T	1.76	0.70	0.88	0.44
F359V	2.86	0.93	1.49	5.16
L384M	1.28	0.47	2.21	2.33
H396P	2.43	0.43	1.07	2.41
H396R	3.91	0.81	1.63	3.10
G398R	0.35	1.16	0.69	0.49
F486S	8.10	2.31	3.04	1.85

Abbreviations: Mutations can be classified as sensitive (IC$_{50}$-fold increase ≤2), resistant (between 2.01 and 10), or highly resistant (>10). T315I mutation.
[a]Source: Based on Shah et al.[58]

at least 20 metaphases are required for a proper interpretation of the karyotype and assessment of response. In addition, RT-PCR is recommended at the time of diagnosis. Although the number of *BCR-ABL1* transcripts has no bearing on the prognosis (and is not reliable at baseline when using *ABL1* as the control gene), it permits investigation of unusual transcripts (e.g., e19a2, e13a3, e14a3) not detected by standard PCR, although some laboratories may have multiplex PCR that may detect these rearrangements. Even then, these rearrangements cannot be quantified in the international scale. These should be suspected in a patient that has the Ph-chromosome but is PCR-negative.

While on treatment, a bone marrow aspiration with cytogenetic analysis may be performed every 6–12 months until a complete cytogenetic response is confirmed. Then a bone marrow is needed less frequently or perhaps not at all in most patients. Fluorescent *in situ* hybridization (FISH) can be used to assess a cytogenetic response, and it can be done in peripheral blood, but it does not provide information on the presence of additional chromosomal abnormalities whether in Ph-positive cells (i.e., clonal evolution) or in Ph-chromosome negative cells, unless specific probes are used for already identified abnormalities in a standard karyotype. A bone marrow should be done in all patients with unexplained changes in peripheral blood counts, or in those with loss of major molecular response (MMR) (and definitely if levels are close to 1% using the international scale). During treatment, patients should also be monitored with RT-PCR at 3, 6, and 12 months after the start of therapy and every 6 months after that once an MMR is confirmed. For patients with atypical transcripts, FISH is the most sensitive test available for monitoring response.

Assessment for mutations is unnecessary at the time of diagnosis in patients in chronic phase as mutations have not been found in this setting with the standard methodology. A search for mutations should be done when there is loss of complete cytogenetic response. Patients that do not meet the recommended response criteria at the given times as per the European Leukemia Net recommendations may have a mutation analysis performed, but mutations are more commonly found among patients with secondary resistance (i.e., loss of cytogenetic response) than those with primary resistance (i.e., not achieving optimal response).

Staging and prognostic factors

CML has three stages, chronic, accelerated, and blast phase. The features that define each phase are described above (section titled "Pathology"). For patients in the chronic phase, risk classifications have been proposed. These include the Sokal,[21] Hasford (Euro),[22] EUTOS,[23] and the ELTS[24] classifications. These classifications identify groups with low, intermediate, and high-risk (low and high only in the EUTOS) that predict outcome and are frequently used to identify patients who benefit the most of second-generation TKI therapy compared to imatinib. In the United States, only 10% or less of patients have a high-risk score at the time of diagnosis, whereas in other areas of the world these can represent up to one-third of all patients.

Treatment

Initial treatment for all patients with CML is with TKI. Imatinib mesylate, a selective Bcr-Abl1 TKI introduced in the 1990s, has changed the natural history of CML.[7] Patients in chronic phase at the time of diagnosis treated with TKI have a life expectancy that matches that of the general population.[59,60]

Imatinib mesylate

Imatinib is a potent inhibitor of Bcr-Abl1 and few other tyrosine kinases such as c-kit and platelet-derived growth factor receptor (PDGFR).[6,61] It was first used in CML after failure or intolerance to interferon-alpha.[62,63] Imatinib 400 mg orally daily, given to 454 patients, resulted in a complete cytogenetic response of 57%. The estimated 5-year survival rate was 76%.[62]

The efficacy of imatinib in previously untreated patients was demonstrated in a multicenter randomized trial comparing imatinib to the combination of interferon-alpha plus low-dose cytarabine (International Randomized Study of Interferon and STI571 (IRIS) trial).[64] With 10 years of follow-up, the cumulative rate of complete cytogenetic response with imatinib was 83%, resulting in an event-free survival (EFS) of 80%, transformation free-survival of 92%, and overall survival of 83%.[65] The 10-year probability of achieving MMR was 88%, and for MR4.5 70%.[66]

Second-generation tyrosine kinase inhibitors

Dasatinib, bosutinib, and nilotinib are second-generation TKI that are more potent than imatinib and have preclinical and clinical activity against most of the mutations associated with imatinib resistance.[67–69] They were first investigated and approved for treatment of patients who have experienced resistance or intolerance to imatinib. Subsequently, trials demonstrated that these second-generation TKIs produced high rates of cytogenetic and molecular responses which were achieved early.[70,71] Randomized trials compared to imatinib confirmed their benefit compared to imatinib, with higher rates of response, faster and deeper responses, and fewer transformations to accelerated and blast phase. There were no improvements in progression-free or overall survival with any of them compared to imatinib. All three are approved and considered standard for the initial treatment of patients with chronic phase CML.

In the randomized trial of dasatinib versus imatinib, the rate of confirmed complete cytogenetic response by 12 months was 77% with dasatinib versus 66% with imatinib, and the cumulative 5-year rates of MMR 76% versus 64%, and MR4.5 42% and 33%, respectively. At 3-months, 84% of patients treated with dasatinib achieved *BCR-ABL1/ABL1* transcript <10% compared to 64%

with imatinib. Transformation to accelerated and blast phase occurred in 5% and 7%, respectively.[72] The standard starting dose of dasatinib for patients with newly diagnosed CML in chronic phase is 100 mg once daily. Lower dose of dasatinib 50 mg daily were found to be equally effective to the historical experience with 100 mg daily in frontline chronic phase therapy with fewer adverse events.[73]

A similar randomized trial investigated two different dose schedules of nilotinib (300 mg twice daily and 400 mg twice daily) compared to imatinib. By 12 months the rate of complete cytogenetic response was 80% with nilotinib 300 mg twice daily and 78% with 400 mg twice daily, compared to 65% with imatinib. The 5-year rates of MMR were 77%, 77%, and 60%, respectively. The corresponding 5-year MR4.5 rates were 54%, 52%, and 31%. BCR-ABL1/ABL1 levels of <10% were achieved by 91% treated with nilotinib 300 mg twice daily, 89% with nilotinib 400 mg twice daily, and 67% with imatinib, and the 5-year rates of freedom from progression to accelerated or blast phase were 99%, 99%, and 95%, respectively. The 5-year estimated PFS were 97%, 98%, and 95%, and overall survival 94%, 96%, and 92%.[74] Nilotinib 300 mg twice daily is standard therapy for newly diagnosed CML in chronic phase.

In the randomized trial of bosutinib 400 mg orally daily compared to imatinib, with a follow-up of 12 months, the 12-month rate of MMR was 47% with bosutinib and 37% with imatinib, and corresponding rates of complete cytogenetic response were 77% and 66%. At 3 months, 75% and 57% had achieved transcript levels of ≤10%. Transformation to accelerated and blast phase was observed in 2.5% and 1.6%, respectively. By 12 months, 3.7% of bosutinib-treated patients had experienced an event compared to 6.4% of imatinib-treated patients.[75] Bosutinib is approved as frontline therapy at a dose of 400 mg daily.

Treatment algorithm

Achievement of a complete cytogenetic response is associated with near eradication of the risk of transformation to accelerated and blast phase, and a significant survival benefit, with a 10-year survival probability of 70–80% equivalent to that of the general population. Achieving MMR by 18 months increases the probability of EFS. The 7-year probability of EFS for patients that achieve MMR is 95% compared to 86% among those with complete cytogenetic response but no MMR. Deep molecular responses open the possibility of considering treatment discontinuation.

In addition to the depth of response, the time to response is important to improve long-term outcomes. The European Leukemia Net recommendations are thus based on the level of response at specific times (Table 2). Patients with BCR-ABL1/ABL1 transcripts <10% at 3 months from the start of therapy have significantly better probability of EFS (approximately 95%) compared to those with >10% transcripts (approximately 80%).[76–79] There is also a significant but smaller difference in overall survival. Patients with confirmed BCR-ABL1/ABL1 transcripts >10% at 3 months are considered to have failure to therapy by these recommendations. One study has investigated the benefit of changing therapy to dasatinib versus continuing imatinib for patients with BCR-ABL1/ABL1 transcripts >10% at 3 months. Although the rate of MMR at 12 months is higher with dasatinib compared to imatinib (29% vs. 13%), the long-term outcomes have not been described to show a possible benefit.[80] Therefore, the management of these patients remains controversial.

Both imatinib and second-generation TKIs are excellent options for frontline therapy. The choice depends on availability, disease features, the patient's goals and co-morbidities, among others.

Table 2 Suggested management of some common adverse events associated with TKIs.

Adverse events	Management
Nausea/vomiting	Take with food (except nilotinib)
	Antiemetics
Diarrhea	Loperamide
	Diphenoxylate atropine
Peripheral edema	Diuretics
Periorbital edema	Steroid-containing cream
Skin rash	Avoid sun exposure
	Topical steroids
	Systemic steroids (early intervention important)
Muscle cramps	Tonic water or quinine
	Electrolyte replacement as needed
	Calcium gluconate
Arthralgia, bone pain	Nonsteroidal anti-inflammatory agents
Elevated transaminases (uncommon)	Hold therapy and monitor closely
	Dose reduction upon resolution
Pleural effusion	Diuretics, corticosteroids
	Thoracentesis in refractory instances
Myelosuppression	
Anemia	Treatment interruption/dose reduction usually not indicated
	Consider erythropoietin or darbepoietin[a]
Neutropenia	Hold therapy if grade ≥ 3 (i.e., ANC < 1 × 10^9/L)
	Consider filgrastim if recurrent/persistent, or sepsis
Thrombocytopenia	Hold therapy if grade ≥ 3 (i.e., platelets <50 × 10^9/L)
	Consider eltrombopag[a]

[a]The use of erythropoietin, darbepoetin, filgrastim, and eltrombopag in this setting is not standard and should be considered investigational.

Patients with greater risk of arterio-occlusive disease have a lower risk of such events with imatinib; if a second-generation TKI is preferred, bosutinib may have the lowest risk of arterio-occlusive events among them. Patients whose primary goal is treatment-free remission (TFR) may have a better probability if treated with a second-generation TKI. For those with high-risk Sokal scores, second-generation TKIs may also be preferable. Patients who achieve an optimal therapy can continue therapy unchanged. Those that meet the definition of warning per the European LeukemiaNet (ELN) recommendations can continue therapy but adherence should be assessed, therapy optimized, and patients monitored rigorously every 3 months with treatment change considered if failure is identified. Once the definition of failure is met, treatment changes should be implemented.[81]

Patients who develop intolerance may also need a change of therapy. Despite the excellent overall tolerability of TKI, they all have adverse events that need monitoring and adequate management. With proper management,[82] that may include transient treatment interruptions, dose adjustments, medical management of adverse events, and supportive care, most patients can continue therapy an experience an adequate response. In general, patients should not be changed to a different TKI based on the first occurrence of an adverse event unless this is life threatening (e.g., Stevens–Johnson's, myocardial infarction, stroke, etc.). True intolerance to TKI occurs in only approximately 5% of all patients. Suggestions for the management of the most common adverse events are presented in Table 3.

Treatment options after failure of prior TKI

Several TKIs are available for the management of patients with resistance (as defined by the ELN[81]) or intolerance to prior TKI. These include dasatinib, bosutinib, nilotinib, and ponatinib. In addition, omacetaxine, a protein-synthesis inhibitor (not a TKI),

Table 3 Response criteria according to the European Leukemia Net.[a]

Time (mo)	Response		
	Failure	Warning	Optimal
Baseline	NA	High-risk ACA, high-risk ELTS score	NA
3	BCR-ABL1 > 10% if confirmed within 1–3 mo	BCR-ABL1 > 10%	BCR-ABL1 ≤ 10%
6	BCR-ABL1 > 10%	BCR-ABL1 1–10%	BCR-ABL1 ≤ 1%
12	BCR-ABL1 > 1%	BCR-ABL1 > 0.1–1%	BCR-ABL1 ≤ 0.1%
Any	BCR-ABL1 > 1%, resistance mutations, high-risk ACA	BCR-ABL1 > 0.1–1%, loss of ≤ 0.1% (MMR)[b]	BCR-ABL1 ≤ 0.1%

Abbreviations: CHR, complete hematologic response; Ph+, percentage of metaphases with presence of the Philadelphia chromosome (a minimum of 20 required for full assessment); CCyR, complete cytogenetic response; MMR, major molecular response; CCA/Ph+, clonal chromosomal abnormalities in cell with the Philadelphia chromosome.
[a]Source: Adapted from Hochhaus et al.[81]
[b]Loss of MMR (BCR-ABL1 > 0.1%) indicates failure after TFR.

is also approved for patients who have received at least two prior TKIs.

Among patients who have received imatinib as their only prior TKI and experienced resistance or intolerance, dasatinib, at a dose of 100 mg once daily induced a complete cytogenetic response in 44% of patients with resistance and 67% of those with intolerance. The 7-year cumulative rate of MMR was 46% overall, with PFS of 42% and overall survival of 65%.[58] Nilotinib, at the standard second-line dose of 400 mg twice daily, induced complete cytogenetic response in 41% of patients with resistance to imatinib and 51% of those with intolerance, for a 4-year PFS of 57% and overall survival of 78%.[83] Bosutinib has also been effective in this patient population, with a 5-year cumulative rate of complete cytogenetic response of 50%. The cumulative rate of transformation to accelerated or blast phase by 5 years was 5%, and the 5-year overall survival 84%.[84] None of these agents is active in patients with the T315I mutation.

Bosutinib and ponatinib have been investigated among patients who have received two or more TKIs. With bosutinib, 500 mg once daily, of the 4-year cumulative rate of major cytogenetic response was 40% among 112 patients who had received imatinib and were then resistant or intolerant to dasatinib, or resistant to nilotinib, with a corresponding rate of complete cytogenetic response of 32%. The 4-year estimates of transformation or death were 24%, and the 4-year overall survival 78%.[85] Ponatinib is a potent inhibitor of Abl1 tyrosine kinase activity as well as other kinases including c-kit, fms-like tyrosine kinase 3 (FLT3), and vascular endothelial gene receptor (VEGFR). It has potent inhibitory activity against unmutated BCR-ABL1 or in the presence of any of the KD mutations tested, including the gatekeeper mutation T315I.[86] With ponatinib 45 mg daily, among 267 patients of whom 93% had received at least two prior TKIs (60% had received at least 3), a major cytogenetic response was achieved in 60% (complete in 54%), MMR in 40%, and MR4.5 in 24%. Major cytogenetic response was sustained for 5 years in 82% and the 5-year overall survival was 73%. For patients with T315I, the response rates were 72%, 70%, 58%, and 38%, respectively, with similar durability of response and overall survival.[87] With omacetaxine, 18% of patients treated in chronic phase after resistance to at least two prior TKI achieved a major cytogenetic response, with a median overall survival of 40.3 months.[88] Responses can be seen regardless of mutation status, including patients with T315I.[89]

Stem cell transplantation

Allogeneic stem cell transplant (SCT) may be curative in 40–80% of patients who receive a transplant from an human leukocyte antigen (HLA)-identical sibling or an unrelated donor;[90] is currently used mostly after failure to multiple TKI or after transformation to blast phase. Despite its curative potential, late relapses may occur. Among patients who have been alive and in continuous complete remission for ≥5 years the cumulative incidence of relapse was 8% after sibling donor transplant and 2% after unrelated donor, with relapses documented as late as 18 years after transplant. Transplanted patients have a higher mortality than the general population until approximately 14 years after transplantation.[91] Previous exposure to TKI does not adversely affect the outcome after SCT although time from diagnosis to SCT remains an important prognostic factor for outcome after transplant.[92,93] Comparisons of series treated with TKI with registry data with allogeneic SCT have suggested that survival in chronic phase is superior with TKI than with SCT, equivalent for both options in accelerated phase, and superior with SCT in blast phase.[94]

Treatment-free remission

Elective treatment discontinuation has emerged as an important goal for many patients. Among patients with sustained deep molecular response who have discontinued therapy, approximately 50–60% have remained off therapy and in remission.[95] The minimum criteria required to consider this option is a deep molecular remission defined as MR4.5 sustained for at least 2 years with at least five determinations during that period. Upon discontinuation, patients should be monitored closely, typically monthly for the first 6 months when the highest risk of relapse occurs, then every 2 months for 6 months, then every 3 months for 1 year, then every 6 months probably indefinitely as late relapses may occur. Some variations of this monitoring schema exist but all emphasize frequent monitoring. Patients who lose MMR at any time, or with two assessments with loss of MR4 should resume therapy, usually with the same TKI as they were receiving at the time they stopped therapy.[96,97] Although most of the earlier data was generated with imatinib, recent studies with nilotinib or dasatinib have shown that similar results can be expected with other TKIs.[98,99] A greater duration of MR4.5 may decrease the probability of relapse to 10–15% and may be preferable in some patients.[100] Some studies have used laxer rules for discontinuation, such as defining deep molecular remission as MR4, or requiring a duration of only 1 year of deep molecular response. Although some patients may still have a successful discontinuation, the results appear inferior to those with the initial stricter (and currently standard) criteria.[101] Patient receiving a second-generation TKI after resistance or suboptimal response to a prior TKI have a lower probability of TFR of approximately 30%, whereas those receiving them after intolerance of a prior TKI seem to have similar results as those receiving it as frontline therapy.[102] Patients who have relapsed after a prior attempt who again meet criteria for discontinuation after resuming therapy also have about a 30% probability of successful discontinuation, but it might be advisable to have a more sustained and deeper response prior to a second attempt.[103]

Treatment recommendations in CML in 2020

The results with imatinib to date have been excellent and durable. Second-generation TKI (dasatinib, bosutinib, and nilotinib) offer earlier and deeper responses, and lower rate of transformation, with no difference in event-free or overall survival. The life expectancy of patients treated with TKI is similar to that of the general population, particularly for patients achieving a complete cytogenetic response or better. Based on this, TKIs are standard initial therapy for all patients with CML in chronic phase. Second-generation TKIs may be preferable for patients with high and possibly intermediate-risk scores, and for those interested in eventually considering treatment discontinuation. However, imatinib is likely to remain the treatment of choice for a large percentage (perhaps the majority) of patients throughout the world. It should be emphasized that imatinib is adequate treatment, and generic versions with adequate quality control offer similar benefits and lower costs.[104] The most important requirement to offer a patient the best possible long-term outcome is the proper management. This includes close follow-up to recognize and manage adverse events. All TKIs have adverse events associated with them, but most of these are manageable through transient treatment interruptions, dose adjustments, and/or medical interventions. Very few patients (around 5%) are truly intolerant to a given drug. Until ongoing studies[80] demonstrate a long-term benefit of early change in therapy, patients not having an early molecular response (i.e., those with *BCR-ABL1/ABL1* transcripts >10%) at 3 months may continue therapy unchanged but they need to be checked again at 6 months. A change of therapy is indicated when the criteria for failure are met (as defined by the European Leukemia Net).[81] In these instances, randomized trials have demonstrated that a change of therapy from imatinib to a second-generation TKI improves outcome compared to a dose increase of imatinib.[105] There is minimal data on the best approach for patients with resistance to a second-generation TKI used as frontline therapy.[106] A mutation analysis is always indicated when the criteria of failure are met, and a bone marrow aspiration is also needed to determine the cytogenetics and stage of the patient before change. If a mutation is identified, this can guide which TKI is predicted to induce a response (e.g., if F317L or V299L identified, consider nilotinib or ponatinib; if F359V, consider bosutinib, dasatinib, or ponatinib; for T315I, ponatinib, or omacetaxine).[107,108] If no mutation is identified, or there is a mutation for which there is no available information or no meaningful difference between the various TKI then other considerations may help in the decision of what drug to use, such as comorbidities that might expose the patient more to adverse events associated with one drug or another, the adverse event profile that might be more acceptable for a given patient, and the dose schedule that a patient might find more acceptable to optimize adherence. Patients resistant to second-generation TKI without a guiding mutation still respond very well to ponatinib. The Food and Drug Administration (FDA)-approved dose of ponatinib is 45 mg daily with a reduction to 15 mg once BCR-ABL1/ABL1 transcripts reach <=1%. Patients with resistance to at least two TKI can be considered for SCT. Allogeneic SCT may also be considered in other settings where long-term therapy might not be optimal or feasible (e.g., for cost considerations).

Patients with accelerated phase features at the time of diagnosis can be treated with a TKI, particularly dasatinib, bosutinib, or nilotinib, as their prognosis in this setting is nearly identical to that of patients in chronic phase.[109] SCT for these patients is not required unless not responding adequately. Patients who progress to accelerated phase while on treatment with TKI for chronic phase should receive a different TKI and considered for SCT.[110] Patients with blast phase CML should receive TKI, usually in combination with chemotherapy,[19,111-113] and SCT strongly considered. Although results for SCT in this setting are best with the least residual disease, once the patient achieves a hematologic complete remission or is back in chronic phase transplant should proceed, as further chemotherapy may cause co-morbidities that may make SCT impossible or of greater risk, and response may not improve further.

Adverse events

Patients with CML should be followed closely with attention to co-morbidities and possible side effects. Mild adverse events are common but generally manageable in most instances.[114,115] There is increased awareness of adverse events that will need continued assessment. These include arterio-occlusive events such as ischemic heart disease (including angina and myocardial infarction), cerebrovascular events (including transient ischemic attacks and strokes), and peripheral arterial occlusive disease, particularly with ponatinib, nilotinib, and dasatinib.[116,117] Attention should be paid to monitoring and managing risk factors such as hypertension (frequently caused or aggravated by ponatinib), diabetes (might be more difficult to control with nilotinib), hyperlipidemia (also associated with TKI therapy), and others. Recent analyses also suggest there might be impairment of renal function with TKI, particularly with imatinib and bosutinib.[118,119] Patients on dasatinib with respiratory symptoms should be evaluated for pleural effusion or pulmonary hypertension. Patients with recurrent abdominal pain should be evaluated for pancreatitis and for mesenteric occlusive disease. Although most adverse events occur early during the course of the disease, for some (such as pleural effusion or arterio-thrombotic events) the incidence is constant and a first event may occur after several years of treatment.

Conclusion

The outcome of patients with CML has improved significantly since the introduction of TKIs. A patient diagnosed with CML today may have a near-normal life expectancy provided the patient has access to proper therapy, monitoring, and management. Adequate management includes adequate dose optimization, proper management of adverse events, continued periodic monitoring of disease response, timely intervention when indicated, and continued support throughout the life of the patient. With this approach, transformation to advanced stages is uncommon and few patients will die of CML.

Summary

CML is characterized by the presence of the Ph. This results in the creation of the BCR-ABL1 fusion gene, which is in turn translated into a tyrosine kinase with constitutive kinase activity. The disease evolves in three stages: chronic, accelerated, and blast phase. Most patients are diagnosed in the chronic phase and are asymptomatic at the time of diagnosis. Treatment with TKIs has changed the natural history of the disease with a life expectancy which is similar to that of the general population. Imatinib was the first TKI to be used and is still standard and effective frontline therapy. Most patients achieve a complete cytogenetic response making transformation to accelerated and blast phase very rare. Higher doses of imatinib have been suggested to provide higher rates of response, including deeper molecular responses. Dasatinib, bosutinib, and nilotinib are also approved treatment options for frontline therapy and may improve the rates of complete cytogenetic, MMR, and deeper molecular response, with fewer instances of transformation to the accelerated and blast phase, but have not resulted in improved event-free or overall survival compared to imatinib in randomized trials. For patients who experience resistance or intolerance to one TKIs, alternative inhibitors can be used. In this setting, an alternative appropriate second-generation TKI and ponatinib are additional options. Overall, approximately 40% of patients with resistance or intolerance to initial therapy might achieve a complete cytogenetic response with a subsequent TKI. The most common mechanism of resistance is the emergence of mutations of the KD. Different mutations may have differing sensitivities to the various TKIs and the presence of such mutations, when present, may allow selection of the most appropriate therapy. Although generally well tolerated, TKIs may cause adverse events, some of them potentially serious, which require proper identification and management; this may include in some instances change of therapy. Allogeneic SCT remains a useful and potentially curative treatment modality for patients who have not experienced adequate response to various lines of therapy. With adequate access to treatment and proper management, patients diagnosed with CML should be able to have a normal life expectancy.

Key references

The complete reference list can be found on Vital Source version of this title, see inside front cover.

1. Nowell PC, Hungerford DA. A minute chromosome in human chronic granulocytic leukemia. *Science*. 1960;**132**:1497–1501.
6. Druker BJ, Tamura S, Buchdunger E, et al. Effects of a selective inhibitor of the Abl tyrosine kinase on the growth of Bcr-Abl positive cells. *Nat Med*. 1996;**2**(5):561–566.
9. Siegel RL, Miller KD, Jemal A. *American Cancer Society. Cancer Facts & Figures 2021*, Atlanta: American Cancer Society; 2021.
19. Strati P, Kantarjian H, Thomas D, et al. HCVAD plus imatinib or dasatinib in lymphoid blastic phase chronic myeloid leukemia. *Cancer*. 2014;**120**(3):373–380.
47. Kovitz C, Kantarjian H, Garcia-Manero G, et al. Myelodysplastic syndromes and acute leukemia developing after imatinib mesylate therapy for chronic myeloid leukemia. *Blood*. 2006;**108**(8):2811–2813.
48. Quintas-Cardama A, Cortes J. Molecular biology of bcr-abl1-positive chronic myeloid leukemia. *Blood*. 2009;**113**(8):1619–1630.
50. Branford S, Wang P, Yeung DT, et al. Integrative genomic analysis reveals cancer-associated mutations at diagnosis of CML in patients with high-risk disease. *Blood*. 2018;**132**(9):948–961.
53. Hughes T, Deininger M, Hochhaus A, et al. Monitoring CML patients responding to treatment with tyrosine kinase inhibitors: review and recommendations for harmonizing current methodology for detecting BCR-ABL transcripts and kinase domain mutations and for expressing results. *Blood*. 2006;**108**(1):28–37.
57. Branford S, Rudzki Z, Walsh S, et al. High frequency of point mutations clustered within the adenosine triphosphate-binding region of BCR/ABL in patients with chronic myeloid leukemia or Ph-positive acute lymphoblastic leukemia who develop imatinib (STI571) resistance. *Blood*. 2002;**99**(9):3472–3475.
58. Shah NP, Rousselot P, Schiffer C, et al. Dasatinib in imatinib-resistant or -intolerant chronic-phase, chronic myeloid leukemia patients: 7-year follow-up of study CA180-034. *Am J Hematol*. 2016;**91**(9):869–874.
60. Sasaki K, Strom SS, O'Brien S, et al. Relative survival in patients with chronic-phase chronic myeloid leukaemia in the tyrosine-kinase inhibitor era: analysis of patient data from six prospective clinical trials. *Lancet Haematol*. 2015;**2**(5):e186–e193.
62. Hochhaus A, Druker B, Sawyers C, et al. Favorable long-term follow-up results over 6 years for response, survival, and safety with imatinib mesylate therapy in chronic-phase chronic myeloid leukemia after failure of interferon-{alpha} treatment. *Blood*. 2008;**111**(3):1039–1043.
65. Hochhaus A, Larson RA, Guilhot F, et al. Long-term outcomes of imatinib treatment for chronic myeloid leukemia. *N Engl J Med*. 2017;**376**(10):917–927.
66. Hehlmann R, Lauseker M, Saussele S, et al. Assessment of imatinib as first-line treatment of chronic myeloid leukemia: 10-year survival results of the randomized CML study IV and impact of non-CML determinants. *Leukemia*. 2017;**31**(11):2398–2406.
72. Cortes JE, Saglio G, Kantarjian HM, et al. Final 5-year study results of DASISION: the dasatinib versus imatinib study in treatment-naive chronic myeloid leukemia patients trial. *J Clin Oncol*. 2016;**34**(20):2333–2340.
74. Hochhaus A, Saglio G, Hughes TP, et al. Long-term benefits and risks of frontline nilotinib vs imatinib for chronic myeloid leukemia in chronic phase: 5-year update of the randomized ENESTnd trial. *Leukemia*. 2016;**30**(5):1044–1054.
75. Cortes JE, Gambacorti-Passerini C, Deininger MW, et al. Bosutinib versus imatinib for newly diagnosed chronic myeloid leukemia: results from the eandomized BFORE trial. *J Clin Oncol*. 2018;**36**(3):231–237.
76. Jain P, Kantarjian H, Nazha A, et al. Early responses predict better outcomes in patients with newly diagnosed chronic myeloid leukemia: results with four tyrosine kinase inhibitor modalities. *Blood*. 2013;**121**(24):4867–4874.
80. Cortes JE, Jiang Q, Wang J, et al. Dasatinib vs. imatinib in patients with chronic myeloid leukemia in chronic phase (CML-CP) who have not achieved an optimal response to 3 months of imatinib therapy: the DASCERN randomized study. *Leukemia*. 2020;**34**:2064–2073.
81. Hochhaus A, Baccarani M, Silver RT, et al. European LeukemiaNet 2020 recommendations for treating chronic myeloid leukemia. *Leukemia*. 2020;**34**:966–984.
83. Giles FJ, le Coutre PD, Pinilla-Ibarz J, et al. Nilotinib in imatinib-resistant or imatinib-intolerant patients with chronic myeloid leukemia in chronic phase: 48-month follow-up results of a phase II study. *Leukemia*. 2013;**27**(1):107–112.
84. Gambacorti-Passerini C, Cortes JE, Lipton JH, et al. Safety and efficacy of second-line bosutinib for chronic phase chronic myeloid leukemia over a five-year period: final results of a phase I/II study. *Haematologica*. 2018;**103**(8):1298–1307.
85. Cortes JE, Khoury HJ, Kantarjian HM, et al. Long-term bosutinib for chronic phase chronic myeloid leukemia after failure of imatinib plus dasatinib and/or nilotinib. *Am J Hematol*. 2016;**91**(12):1206–1214.
87. Cortes JE, Kim DW, Pinilla-Ibarz J, et al. Ponatinib efficacy and safety in Philadelphia chromosome-positive leukemia: final 5-year results of the phase 2 PACE trial. *Blood*. 2018;**132**(4):393–404.
88. Cortes JE, Kantarjian HM, Rea D, et al. Final analysis of the efficacy and safety of omacetaxine mepesuccinate in patients with chronic- or accelerated-phase chronic myeloid leukemia: results with 24 months of follow-up. *Cancer*. 2015;**121**(10):1637–1644.
94. Nicolini FE, Basak GW, Kim DW, et al. Overall survival with ponatinib versus allogeneic stem cell transplantation in Philadelphia chromosome-positive leukemias with the T315I mutation. *Cancer*. 2017;**123**(15):2875–2880.
96. Hughes TP, Ross DM. Moving treatment-free remission into mainstream clinical practice in CML. *Blood*. 2016;**128**(1):17–23.
98. Ross DM, Masszi T, Gomez Casares MT, et al. Durable treatment-free remission in patients with chronic myeloid leukemia in chronic phase following frontline nilotinib: 96-week update of the ENESTfreedom study. *J Cancer Res Clin Oncol*. 2018;**144**(5):945–954.
99. Kimura S, Imagawa J, Murai K, et al. Treatment-free remission after first-line dasatinib discontinuation in patients with chronic myeloid leukaemia (first-line DADI trial): a single-arm, multicentre, phase 2 trial. *Lancet Haematol*. 2020;**7**(3):e218–e225.
101. Saussele S, Richter J, Guilhot J, et al. Discontinuation of tyrosine kinase inhibitor therapy in chronic myeloid leukaemia (EURO-SKI): a prespecified interim analysis of a prospective, multicentre, non-randomised, trial. *Lancet Oncol*. 2018;**19**(6):747–757.

102 Rea D, Nicolini FE, Tulliez M, et al. Discontinuation of dasatinib or nilotinib in chronic myeloid leukemia: interim analysis of the STOP 2G-TKI study. *Blood.* 2017;**129**(7):846–854.

104 Abou Dalle I, Kantarjian H, Burger J, et al. Efficacy and safety of generic imatinib after switching from original imatinib in patients treated for chronic myeloid leukemia in the United States. *Cancer Med.* 2019;**8**(15):6559–6565.

108 Redaelli S, Piazza R, Rostagno R, et al. Activity of bosutinib, dasatinib, and nilotinib against 18 imatinib-resistant BCR/ABL mutants. *J Clin Oncol.* 2009;**27**(3):469–471.

113 Jain P, Kantarjian HM, Ghorab A, et al. Prognostic factors and survival outcomes in patients with chronic myeloid leukemia in blast phase in the tyrosine kinase inhibitor era: cohort study of 477 patients. *Cancer.* 2017;**123**(22):4391–4402.

115 Rea D. Management of adverse events associated with tyrosine kinase inhibitors in chronic myeloid leukemia. *Ann Hematol.* 2015;**94**(Suppl 2):S149–S158.

116 Jain P, Kantarjian H, Boddu PC, et al. Analysis of cardiovascular and arteriothrombotic adverse events in chronic-phase CML patients after frontline TKIs. *Blood Adv.* 2019;**3**(6):851–861.

113 Acute lymphoblastic leukemia

Elias Jabbour, MD ■ Nitin Jain, MD ■ Hagop Kantarjian, MD ■ Susan O'Brien, MD

> **Overview**
>
> Acute lymphoblastic leukemia (ALL) is characterized by clonal proliferation of lymphoid progenitors. In the last decade, significant advances in understanding the disease pathogenesis, refining prognostic groups, and developing novel therapies that target specific subsets, have improved our treatment strategies and patient outcomes. Therapies targeting either specific transcripts (e.g., BCR-ABL1 tyrosine kinase inhibitors) or specific leukemic cell surface antigens (e.g., CD20, CD22, and CD19 monoclonal antibodies, chimeric antigen receptor T-cell therapies) produced major therapeutic breakthroughs. These novel therapies and combinations are transforming our strategies for adults with ALL and are resulting in significant improvements in survival. Many of these approaches focus on decreasing or eliminating the role of chemotherapy, with the goal of making these regimens more tolerable in older adults and decreasing the morbidity and mortality associated with myelosuppression-related infections and other complications of intensive chemotherapy.

Introduction

Acute lymphoblastic leukemia (ALL) is a heterogeneous disease. Identification of cytogenetic-molecular features in ALL has translated into more accurate classification of disease subtypes, institution of risk-adapted therapies, and identification of new drugs. Advances in ALL therapy over only a few decades have led to cures for most children with ALL. The adaptation of successful pediatric ALL treatment strategies into therapeutic algorithms for adult ALL patients has also resulted in significant improvements in outcome, although long-term disease-free survival (DFS) rates of around 40% in young adults are still inferior. Nonetheless, the ongoing molecular dissection of ALL subtypes, the refinements of multidrug chemotherapy in combination with the development of new and targeted drugs, comprehension of the kinetics of residual disease, and an increasing grasp of the impact of pharmacogenomic features and drug resistance are expected to contribute to further improvement in the prognosis for adults with ALL.

Epidemiology and etiology

ALL is predominantly a disease of children, and it constitutes about 80% of all childhood leukemias and 25% of all childhood cancers. It peaks between the ages of 2 and 5 years and is diagnosed at an incidence of 3.5–4/100,000.[1] In contrast, it makes up less than 1% of malignancies in adults. The age-adjusted overall incidence of ALL in the United States is about 1.7/100,000. In 2020, the American Cancer Society estimated that 6150 individuals would be diagnosed with ALL in the United States that year, and 1520 patients would succumb to the disease.[1]

ALL is more frequent among Caucasians. Geographic variations in its frequency have been described with higher rates among Hispanic populations in Spain and Latin America.[2] While there is a slightly higher incidence in males than in females among childhood ALL, the rate is more predominant in males among patients older than 20 years (1.3 : 1). A higher incidence of ALL has also been observed in industrialized and urban areas giving rise to speculation about socioeconomic factors in the etiology of ALL.[2]

In most cases, no etiology can be established. Among children, only a few cases (<5%) are associated with inherited, predisposing genetic disorders (e.g., Down's syndrome, Bloom's syndrome, ataxia-telangiectasia, Nijmegen breakage syndrome).[3] There is an extensive list of conflicting or isolated papers reporting an increased risk of childhood ALL based on parental occupation, maternal reproductive history, parental tobacco or alcohol use, maternal diet, prenatal vitamin use, exposure to pesticide or solvents, and exposure to the highest levels (>0.3 or 0.4 μT) of residential, power-line associated magnetic fields.[4] Studies have also focused on genetic variability in drug metabolism, DNA repair, and cell-cycle checkpoints that might interact with environmental, dietary, maternal, and other external factors to affect leukemogenesis. Genome-wide association studies have identified several genes (such as *ARID5B, IKZF1, CDKN2A, TP63, GATA3*) that are associated with an increased risk of developing ALL.[5–7]

The peak age for developing childhood ALL of 2–5 years, an association of ALL with industrialized and affluent societies, and the occasional clustering of childhood ALL cases (especially in new towns), have fueled two hypotheses: (1) population-mixing and (2) delayed infection.[8,9] The first hypothesis suggests that clusters of childhood cases result from exposure of susceptible (nonimmune) individuals to a common, fairly nonpathologic infection after mixing naïve hosts with carriers.[8] The second hypothesis is based on a two-hit model where susceptible individuals with a prenatally acquired preleukemic clone have had low or no exposure to common infections early in life because of their affluent hygienic environment.[9] Insulation from infection predisposes the immune system of these individuals to aberrant or pathological responses to common infections at an age commensurate with when they encounter pathogens with increased lymphoid proliferation. Indeed, retrospective studies of archived neonatal blood spots and monozygotic twin pairs have identified preleukemic clones, and support the notion that additional postnatal transforming events are needed for full leukemic transformation.[10–12]

A significantly higher rate of Philadelphia chromosome (Ph)-like ALL is observed in patients of Hispanic ethnicity. Genome-wide association studies in children and adolescent and young adults (AYAs) with ALL have identified inherited genetic variants in GATA3 that are associated with Ph-like ALL and show an increased frequency in Hispanics and individuals with Native American or indigenous genetic ancestry.[13]

Holland-Frei Cancer Medicine, Tenth Edition. Edited by Robert C. Bast, John C. Byrd, Carlo M. Croce, Ernest Hawk, Fadlo R. Khuri, Raphael E. Pollock, Apostolia M. Tsimberidou, Christopher G. Willett, and Cheryl L. Willman.
© 2023 John Wiley & Sons, Inc. Published 2023 by John Wiley & Sons, Inc.

Clinical presentation

The clinical signs and symptoms of ALL are quite variable. The disease can develop insidiously and persist for months prior to diagnosis, but symptoms occur suddenly in most cases and relate to the expansion of the leukemic cells in the marrow, and the involvement of peripheral blood and extramedullary sites such as lymph nodes, liver, spleen, and the central nervous system (CNS). Common symptoms include fatigue, lack of energy, constitutional symptoms (fever, night sweats, and weight loss), easy bruising or bleeding, and dyspnea. Extremity and joint pain may be the only presenting symptoms in children, especially when very young. T-lineage ALL can present with a mediastinal mass, causing stridor, wheezing, pericardial effusions, and superior vena cava syndrome. Testicular involvement occurs with a low frequency, predominantly in infant and adolescent boys. Less than 10% of patients have overt CNS involvement at diagnosis, although CNS disease occurs more often in patients with mature B-cell ALL (Burkitt's leukemia/lymphoma). Cranial nerve palsy (especially cranial nerves III, IV, VI, and VII) can lead to double vision, abnormal ocular movements, facial dysesthesias, and facial droop. Nausea and vomiting, headaches, or papilledema may point toward meningeal infiltration and increased intracranial pressure. Chin numbness due to mental nerve involvement may be subtle and can be easily missed unless sought. Diagnosis of CNS involvement is made from cytospin slides from the cerebrospinal fluid (CSF). Whereas previous guidelines required the presence of >5 WBC/µL of CSF plus identifiable blasts, controversy arose around cases with <5 WBC/µL, with blasts. A more recent approach defined three diagnostic scenarios: (1) no detectable blast cells in CSF regardless of the white blood cell (WBC) count (CNS 1), (2) <5 WBC/µL and presence of blasts (CNS 2), (3) ≥5 WBC/µL and presence of blasts or cranial nerve palsies (CNS 3).[14] On physical examination, pallor, ecchymoses, petechiae, generalized lymphadenopathy, and hepatosplenomegaly can be observed. Tumor lysis syndrome is common in patients with mature B-cell ALL but can also occur in any other subtypes of ALL. Disseminated intravascular coagulation (DIC) is a frequent laboratory finding, but rarely clinically relevant. Hyperleukocytosis syndrome is also less common in ALL than acute myeloid leukemia (AML).

Diagnosis of ALL

The diagnosis of ALL requires the identification of blast cells either in the blood, marrow, or tissue section. A thorough morphologic, cytochemical, and immunologic assessment of ALL blasts remains essential in each patient's workup. The identification of distinct ALL cytogenetic-molecular abnormalities has contributed to a more precise classification of the leukemic blasts and enabled a more accurate assessment of prognosis. Ongoing efforts are focused on genomic profiling leading to a new definition of ALL subtypes and, through it, to the identification of subgroups of patients requiring different treatments and with different prognoses that are only partially distinguished by currently available diagnostic tools (Figure 1).[15,16]

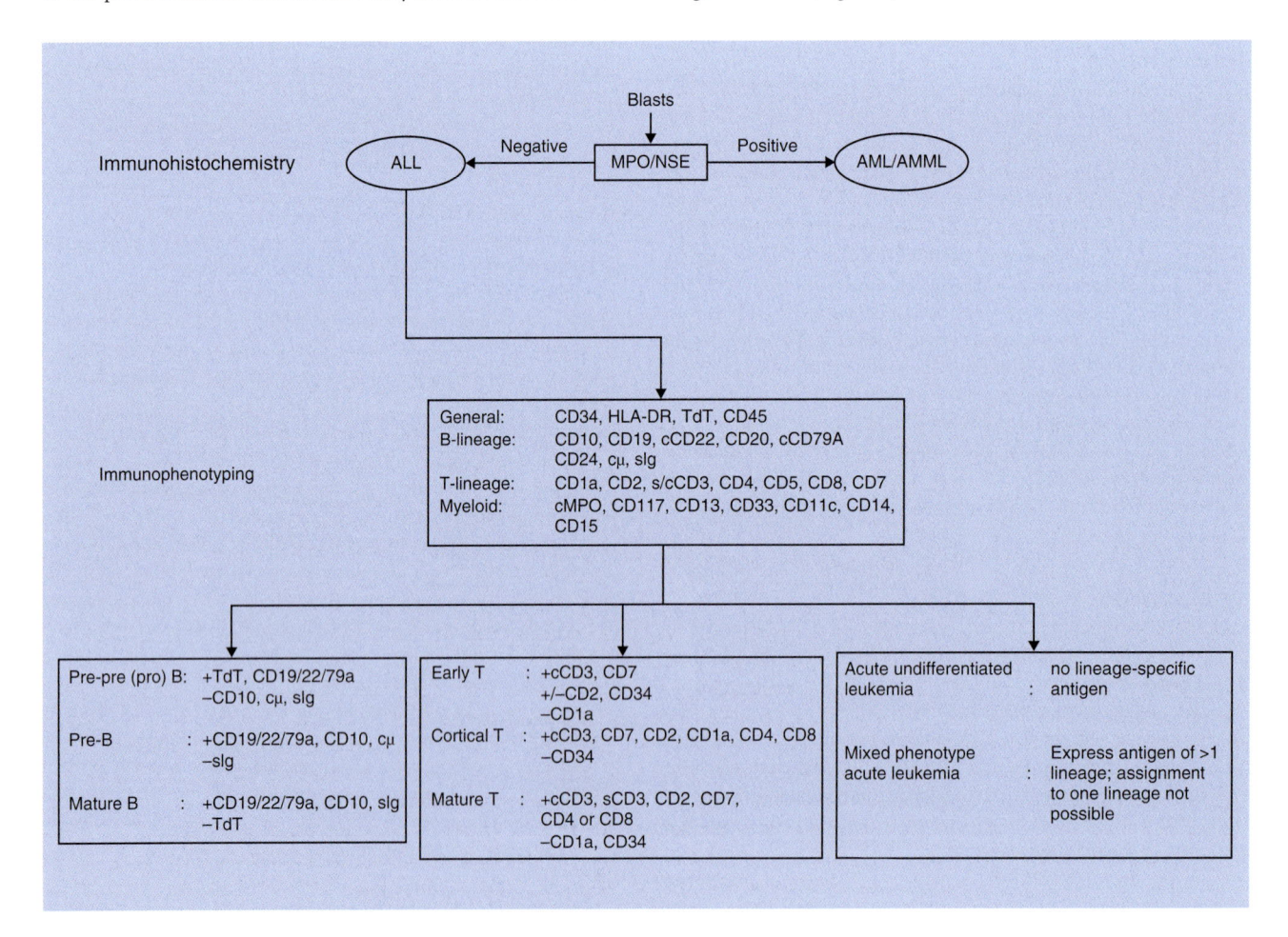

Figure 1 ALL immunophenotyping.

The revised World Health Organization (WHO) classification recognizes three types of ALL: B-ALL, T-ALL, and natural killer (NK)—cell ALL. ALL can involve predominantly bone marrow or predominantly extramedullary sites. In patients with extramedullary lymphoblastic lymphoma, an arbitrary cut-off of 25% blasts in the bone marrow was applied to distinguish lymphoblastic leukemia from lymphoma in the past. The current WHO classification uses a combined term "lymphoblastic leukemia/lymphoma." In contrast to AML, there is no agreed-upon minimal blast percentage required for a diagnosis of ALL. The current WHO classification states that the diagnosis of ALL "should be avoided when there are <20% blasts," but at the same time does recognize that cases of ALL with blasts <20% do exist.[17]

Morphology and cytochemistry

ALL blasts are heterogeneous in size and shape, and one of the first attempts to classify ALL was based on this observation. The French American British (FAB) Cooperative Group thus distinguished three subgroups of lymphoblasts. The L1 blasts are smaller, have a high nuclear-to-cytoplasmic ratio, and inconspicuous nucleoli; the cytoplasm is sparse and variably basophilic. The L2 blasts are larger and more pleomorphic, have moderately abundant cytoplasm, a lower nuclear-to-cytoplasmic ratio, and more prominent nucleoli. The L1 morphology is more common in children than in adults, whereas the L2 morphology is more common in adults. The L3 blasts are more homogenous, medium in size, with dispersed chromatin, prominent nucleoli, typically deep blue cytoplasmic basophilia, and sharply demarcated vacuoles. The L3 morphology is mostly associated with mature B-cell ALL or Burkitt's lymphoma. Mature B-cell ALL is characterized by a high rate of cell turnover, which is reflected morphologically by the so-called "starry sky appearance" in marrow biopsy specimens. The distinction into L1, L2, and L3 morphologies has been largely abandoned, as with the exception of L3 and its association with mature B-cell ALL, it is no longer of prognostic or therapeutic relevance.

Although no cytochemical stain is diagnostic for ALL, the key diagnostic cytochemical feature is the lack of myeloperoxidase (MPO) and nonspecific esterase (NSE) activity. Low-level MPO positivity (3–5%) can occur in patients with lymphoid blast phase of chronic myeloid leukemia and other rare cases.[18] Sudan black B staining closely resembles that of MPO itself, but the lack of specificity and the ease with which MPO stains can be applied has limited its use. Terminal deoxynucleotidyl transferase (TdT) is a useful marker to distinguish between reactive versus malignant lymphocytosis and is usually positive in ≥40% of ALL blasts. L3 ALL is characteristically TdT-negative.[19]

Immunophenotyping

Immunophenotyping by flow cytometry is essential to accurately diagnose ALL, resolve difficult differential diagnoses, and define subtypes further. Although there is no uniformly accepted panel, commonly used markers as listed in Figure 1 are usually sufficient to establish the diagnosis and confirm lineage affiliation in >95% of the cases.

The majority of cases of ALL (75–80%) are of B-lineage. Based on their stage of maturation, they can be divided into (1) pre-pre-B ALL (pro-B-ALL), (2) early pre-B (common acute lymphoblastic leukemia [cALL]), (3) pre-B ALL, and (4) mature B-ALL. In their earliest identifiable stage, pre-pre-B-ALL blasts are positive for CD19, CD79a, or CD22, but no other B-cell differentiation antigens. CD19-positive, CD10-negative, cytoplasmic immunoglobulin (Ig)-negative B-lineage ALL with myeloid marker co-expression is common among infants with ALL, is typically associated with translocation t(4;11) and *KMT2A* gene rearrangements, and has a poor prognosis. cALL (early pre-B-ALL) represents an intermediate stage in blast development and is the most common immunophenotype in adults and children. It is characterized by the expression of CD10 (common acute lymphoblastic leukemia antigen, CALLA) and is a frequent immunophenotype with Philadelphia chromosome (Ph)-positive ALL. In their more mature stages, pre-B-ALL blasts express TdT, HLA-DR, CD19, CD79a, and cytoplasmic Igs. A high fraction of pre-B-ALL cases have the translocation t(1;19). Mature B-cell ALL (Burkitt's leukemia) blasts express surface immunoglobulins (sIg, usually IgM), are clonal for κ or λ light chains, and lack expression of TdT. Expression of CD20 is almost ubiquitous in mature B-cell ALL, whereas it occurs in only about 40–50% of other ALL subtypes.

In contrast to B-ALL, the immunophenotypic classification of T-ALL has acquired a critical clinical importance since the concept of early T-cell precursor lymphoblastic leukemia (ETP-ALL) was introduced.[20] T-cell ALL accounts for 20–25% of cases and can be further stratified into four subtypes based on different stages of intrathymic differentiation. T-cell ALL expresses various levels of CD1a, CD2, CD3, CD4, CD5, CD7, and CD8. CD7 is the most sensitive T-cell marker but lacks specificity because cases of AML or NK-cell leukemia are sometimes CD7-positive. Expression of cytoplasmic CD3 (cCD3) is the most lineage-specific marker for T-cell differentiation. Mature T-ALL expresses both surface CD3 (sCD3) and cCD3, CD2, and either CD4 or CD8 but not both. T-cell ALL of the earlier stages of differentiation expresses cCD3 but not sCD3. Cortical (thymic) T-cell ALL is characterized by expression of CD1a and is positive for both CD4 and CD8; it is thought to have a favorable outcome.[21] The recently identified ETP-ALL is characterized by CD1a negativity, CD8 negativity, weak/absent expression of CD5, and the presence of one of more myeloid markers (CD117, CD34, HLA-DR, CD13, CD33, CD11b, CD65);[20] it is associated with poor outcome.[22]

NK-cell ALL was recently added to the WHO classification as a provisional entity.[17] The entity remains ill-defined and extremely challenging to diagnose,[17] in part due to the limited knowledge about early stages of NK cell development (with most information coming from *ex vivo* analyses of normal CD34-positive progenitor populations[23] and sparse information regarding its malignant counterpart. The true frequency of NK-ALL remains unknown. The neoplastic cells are reported to express cytoplasmic CD56, CD94, and CD161 and could express cCD3, CD2, and CD7; CD16 is usually absent.[17]

Co-expression of myeloid-associated markers is common (15–50% in adult ALL; 5–35% in children) but does not automatically indicate a bilineage potential.[24] Myeloid-associated marker expression is more frequent in ALL with translocation t(9;22), t(4;11), and t(12;21), and is generally absent in mature B-cell ALL. Myeloid-associated marker expression has no prognostic significance in B-ALL[25] but can be used to distinguish leukemic cells from normal progenitor cells, thereby enabling the detection of minimal residual disease.

Cytogenetic and molecular abnormalities

Cytogenetic-molecular abnormalities are common in ALL (Table 1).[3,26] Their identification is important as they provide pathobiological insights, serve as targets for drug development, and furnish prognostic information, which has been translated into risk-adapted therapies.[26] Conventional karyotype analysis remains a cornerstone for the detection of chromosome abnormalities. In

Table 1 Cytogenetic and molecular abnormalities in ALL.

Cytogenetics	Gene involved	Frequency (%)	
		Adult	Child
t(1;14)(p32;q11)	TAL-1	10–15	5–10
del(5)(q35)	HOX11L2	<2	<2
t(5;14)(q35;q32)	HOX11L2	1	2–3
del(6q), t(6;12)	?	5	<5
del(7p)	?	5–10	<5
+8	—	10–12	2
t(8;14), t(8;22), t(2;8)	c-MYC	5	2–5
t(9;22)(q34;q11)	BCR-ABL	15–25	2–6
del(9)(p21-22)	CDKN2A and CDKN2B	6–30	20
del(9)(q32)	TAL-2	<1	<1
Extrachromosome 9q	NUP214/ABL	<5	?
t(10;14)(q24;q11)	HOX11	5–10	<5
del(11)(q22)	ATM	25–30[a]	15[a]
del(11)(q23)	MLL/AF4	5–10	<5
del(12p) or t(12p)	ETV6-AML1	<1[b]	20–25[b]
del(13)(q14)	miR15/miR16	<5	<5
t(14q11-q13)	TCR α and δ	20–25[c]	20–25[c]
t(14q32)	IGH, BCL11B	5	?
t(1;19), t(17;19)	E2A-PBX1, E2A-HLF	<5	4–5
Hyperdiploidy	—	2–15	10–26
Hypodiploidy	—	5–10	5–10

Abbreviations: IgM, immunoglobulin M; Igκ, immunoglobulin kappa; Igλ, immunoglobulin lambda; TdT, terminal deoxynucleotidyl transferase.
[a] As determined by LOH (loss of heterozygosity).
[b] As determined by PCR (polymerase chain reaction).
[c] In T-ALL, overall incidence <10%.

addition, fluorescence in situ hybridization (FISH) and real-time reverse transcriptase-polymerase chain reaction (RT-PCR) assays of mRNA are applied to detect minimal residual disease and to monitor patients after therapy.

Numerical abnormalities
Numerical karyotypic abnormalities have an important prognostic impact in ALL. Hypodiploidy defines a karyotype with less than 44 chromosomes, is seen in <5% of patients, and is associated with a poor outcome.[27,28] A recent study of genomic profiling of 124 hypodiploid ALL identified two subtypes: (1) Near-haploid ALL with 24–31 chromosomes harboring alterations targeting receptor tyrosine kinase signaling and RAS signaling in the majority of the cases; and (2) low-hypodiploid ALL with 32–39 chromosomes characterized by alterations in TP53 in >90% of the cases.[28]

Hyperdiploidy is defined by chromosome numbers of more than 46. It is detected more commonly in children than in adults (~25% vs 5%). The range of added chromosomes is not random. Most commonly increased chromosomes are 4, 8, 10, and 21 followed by chromosomes 5, 6, 14, and 17. Gene expression profiles in pediatric patients demonstrated that 70% of the genes that defined this group belonged to either chromosomes X or 21, irrespective of whether or not these chromosomes were increased in the leukemic blasts.[24] Hyperdiploid blasts from patients with ALL have been shown to accumulate more methotrexate and methotrexate polygluatamate, and to be more sensitive to other drugs such as mercaptopurine, thioguanine, cytarabine, and L-asparaginase.[29–43]

Structural abnormalities translocation t(9;22)
This translocation between the long arms of chromosome 9 and 22, t(9;22)(q34;q11) is the most common abnormality in adult ALL (15–30%) but is rare in children (<5%).[31] While $p210^{BCR-ABL}$ is the most frequent oncoprotein in CML, $p190^{BCR-ABL}$ occurs in the majority of patients with Ph-positive ALL. ALL with t(9;22) typically affects older patients, involves higher WBC and blast counts at diagnosis, is of a pre-B-cell immunophenotype, and often demonstrates coexpression of myeloid markers. Ph-positive ALL used to be one of the subtypes with the worst long-term outcome. The use of novel tyrosine kinase inhibitors (TKIs) (reviewed below) in combination with multiagent chemotherapy and or immunotherapy is now achieving significantly better outcomes.

Translocation t(12;21) and del(12p)
Abnormalities of the short arm of chromosome 12 involve ETV6 (TEL), a transcription regulating the gene of the Ets family of transcription factors. In t(12;21), ETV6 is fused to RUNX1 (AML1, CBFA2) on chromosome 21q22.[32] The fusion protein recruits histone deacetylases, induces closure of the chromatin structure, and inhibits transcription, thereby altering both self-renewal and differentiation capacity. The cryptic translocation can be identified in up to 30% of children with ALL using molecular assays, making it the most frequent recurring cytogenetic-molecular abnormality in pediatric pre-B ALL; it is, however, rare in adults.[33] ETV6-RUNX1-positive ALL has been associated with an excellent outcome in children, although late relapses may occur.[3] ETV6-RUNX1-positive blasts were shown to have suppressed expression of the multidrug resistance-1 (MDR-1) gene, decreased de novo purine synthesis, and suppressed genes involved in purine metabolism.[34]

del(9p21)
Abnormalities of 9p21 occur in up to 15% of patients with ALL.[35] The prognosis in these patients is generally unfavorable, and it is characterized by higher rates of relapse and shorter survival. The prognostic associations are stronger in childhood ALL and are less well-defined in adult ALL.[36] Commonly involved genes with del(9p21) include the cyclin-dependent kinase inhibitor genes CDKN2A (MTS1, p16INK4a) and CDKN2B (MTS2, p15INK4b). Using FISH or PCR, heterozygous and/or homozygous deletions of CDKN2A have been described in up to 80% of children with T-ALL and 20% of those with pre-B ALL.[36]

KMT2A rearrangements (11q23)
The common denominator of 11q23 abnormalities is involvement of the mixed-lineage leukemia gene KMT2A (ALL-1, HRX, HTRX1). KMT2A encodes a nuclear protein that maintains the expression of particular members of the HOX family. It is frequently involved in reciprocal rearrangements with other genes located on chromosomes 4q21, 9p22, 19p13, 1p32, and many others.[37] The fusion of KMT2A with AF4 on chromosome 4q21 is a frequent abnormality in infant ALL, accounting for up to 85% of the cases, but is detected in only 3–8% of adults.[38] Adults with this translocation tend to be older, have higher WBC counts and organomegaly; sanctuary sites such as the CNS are involved more frequently. CD10-negative, cytoplasmic Ig-positive pre-B ALL has a high KMT2A rearrangement rate.[39] Prognosis of KMT2A leukemia is poor in infants and adults but is intermediate in children over 1 year of age.[40]

E2A rearrangements (19p13)
The two known translocations with E2A rearrangements on chromosome 19p13 are t(1;19)(q23;p13) and t(17;19)(q21;p13). The t(1;19) is strongly associated with the pre-B ALL phenotype expressing cytoplasmic Ig. The translocation juxtaposes E2A with the homeobox-containing gene PBX1. The E2A-PBX1 functions as a potent transcriptional activator; in vitro, it transforms a variety of cell types including fibroblasts, myeloid progenitors, and

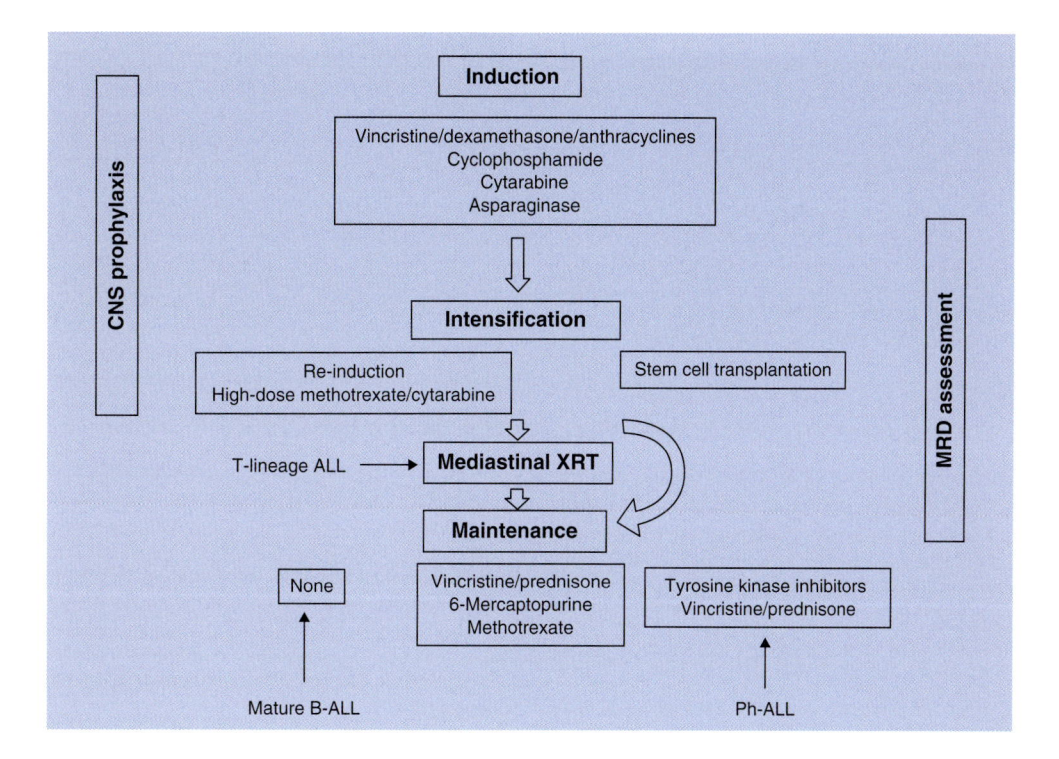

Figure 2 ALL treatment algorithm.

lymphoblasts. E2A-PBX1-positive ALL has a worse prognosis with standard or less aggressive therapy but does better with the more aggressive approaches.[41]

8q24 rearrangements

The c-MYC gene, located on 8q24, is involved in one of the three translocations with the kappa or lambda Ig light chain loci in mature B-ALL: (1) The t(8;14)(q24;q32), with a frequency of 80%, is the most common translocation.[42] In this translocation, c-MYC is juxtaposed to the immunoglobulin heavy chain (IgH) gene locus on 14q32, (2) The t(8;22)(q24;q11) occurs in about 15% of B-ALL patients and involves the Ig lambda gene locus on 22q11, and (iii) The t(2;8)(p12;q24) is the least frequent of the three translocations and involves the Ig kappa gene locus on 2p12.

Other molecular abnormalities and gene expression profiling

Next-generation sequencing (NGS), expression proteomics, and oligonucleotide microarrays have transformed our understanding of the genomic landscape of ALL and are yielding new molecular subgroups with actionable defects.[15,43] Activating mutations in NOTCH1 are detected in around 70%, and FBXW7 in about 25% of cases of T-ALL.[44] The presence of NOTCH1/FBXW7 mutations in the absence of KRAS/NRAS or PTEN abnormalities, seen in approximately 50% of adult T-ALL, is associated with a favorable outcome.[45] On the other hand, the absence of NOTCH1/FBXW7 mutations, the presence of KRAS/NRAS mutations, or the presence of PTEN mutations are associated with a poor prognosis in T-ALL.[46]

Recently, using genome-wide gene expression arrays, a Ph-like signature has been identified in 10% of children with standard-risk ALL and in 25–30% of young and older adults with ALL. This subgroup lacks the expression of the BCR-ABL1 fusion protein but has a gene expression profile similar to that seen in BCR-ABL1 ALL.[47,48] The vast majority of these patients have deletions in genes encoding key transcription factors involved in B-cell signaling, such as IKZF1, TCF3, EBF1, PAX5, and VPREB1, as well as kinase-activating alterations involving ABL1, ABL2, cytokine receptor-like factor 2 (CRLF2), CSF1R, EPOR, JAK2, NTRK3, PDGFRB, PTK2B, TSLP, or TYK2 and sequence mutations involving FLT3, IL7R, or SH2B3. The most common alterations (~60% in adults) are rearrangements of CRLF2, which activates downstream signaling through JAK kinases; and approximately half of these cases have activating mutations in JAK1 or JAK2. CRLF2 expression can be rapidly detected by flow cytometry, and CRLF2 expression by flow cytometry is highly concordant with CRLF2 rearrangement by FISH (Figure 2).[49] Importantly, Ph-like ALL cells with ABL1, ABL2, CSF1R, and PDGFRB expression fusions were sensitive *in vitro* and *in vivo* human xenograft models to ABL class TKIs (e.g., dasatinib or ponatinib).[16] This has been also confirmed clinically: patients with these fusions respond to single-agent TKIs and to combination of TKIs and chemotherapy. Cells with rearrangements in EPOR, IL-7R, and JAK2 mutations and fusions were sensitive to JAK kinase inhibitors (e.g., ruxolitinib); and the ETV6-NTRK3 fusion cells were sensitive to ALK kinase inhibitors (e.g., crizotinib),[16] further expanding therapeutic options in this subgroup with poor outcome. The latter findings are being tested in clinical trials.

The therapy of ALL

Combination chemotherapy with steroids has been the mainstay of management of both pediatric and adult ALL.[31,50–69] The design was based on a combination of all multiple antileukemia drugs delivered in a sequence of extended courses of therapy. The goal was to prevent emergence of resistant leukemic subclones and to restore normal hematopoiesis. Therapeutic strategies in adult ALL have been patterned after the pediatric regimens and although

Table 2 Tips to optimize the hyper-CVAD regimen.

Even courses	MTX 750 mg/m²; ara-C 2 g/m². Dose adjust for older age
Renal monitoring after MTX clearance	If creatinine increase (>1.4), hold ara-C (avoid renal failure and cerebellar toxicity)
Vincristine	VCR 2 mg flat dose (not 2 mg/m²). If constipation or neuropathy, omit VCR
Prophylaxis	Triple: levofloxacin, posaconazole, and valacyclovir
Azoles and VCR interactions	Hold azoles day −1,0,+1 of VCR (avoid excess neurotoxicity)
IT chemotherapy	Switch IT day 2 from MTX to ara-C in even courses (neurotoxicity with IT MTX and HD systemic MTX)

MTX, methotrexate; ara-C, cytarabine; VCR, vincristine; IT, intrathecal; HD, high-dose.

Table 3 Frontline treatment by subsets and outcome.

Entity	Management	% Long term survival
Ph-positive ALL	Chemotherapy + TKI; TKI maintenance; ASCT in CR1 if no CMR; IT × 12	50–70
Adolescents and young adults ALL	Pediatric based regimen; hyper-CVAD-based regimen	60+
Burkitt leukemia	Hyper-CVAD-R × 8 or dose adjusted EPOCH-R; IT × 16; no maintenance	80–90
CD20-positive ALL	ALL chemotherapy + anti-CD20 mAb	50–60
T-ALL	High doses cyclophosphamide; high doses cytarabine; asparaginase; nelarabine?	50–60
Elderly ALL	Low dose chemotherapy plus inotuzumab ozogamicin and/or blinatumomab	45

Ph, Philadelphia-chromosome; TKI, tyrosine kinase inhibitor; ASCT, allogeneic stem cell transplantation; CR1, first complete remission; CMR, complete molecular remission; ALL, acute lymphocytic leukemia.

various combinations with differences in treatment sequence and choice of agents are being used, the same basic principles apply induction therapy followed by early intensification and consolidation, specific CNS treatment, and a prolonged maintenance phase.[31,50–69] Table 2 summarizes tips to optimize the use of the hyper-CVAD regimen.[51]

Primary CNS involvement at diagnosis is uncommon (<10%), but CNS relapse may be as high as 75% without CNS prophylaxis.[31,52,53] Thus, CNS prophylaxis is essential to prevent CNS relapse. High doses of methotrexate and cytarabine provide good CNS penetration, but alone, they are unable to eradicate all leukemic cells in the brain. Therefore, intrathecal (IT) chemotherapy with methotrexate or cytarabine alone (generally in alternating schedule) or triple agents (methotrexate, hydrocortisone, and cytarabine) must be given. Standard risk patients receive a total of eight IT chemotherapy doses while high-risk patients such as those with Philadelphia-positive ALL and Burkitt's leukemia receive 12 and 16 doses, respectively.[51] With effective IT and systemic therapy, prophylactic cranial/craniospinal irradiation, once considered standard treatment for high-risk ALL, has been successfully eliminated in adult and pediatric patients with ALL.[54] This substantially improved the quality of life of the survivors and avoided radiation-associated neurologic and cognitive dysfunctions and secondary cancer.

Patients with CNS involvement (mostly of the leptomeninges) at diagnosis are treated with the standard chemotherapy regimen, and additional triple IT therapy (hydrocortisone 50 mg, cytarabine 40 mg, methotrexate 12 mg [6 mg if intra ommaya]) twice per week until the CSF is negative for malignant cells on two occasions, then weekly IT for 4–8 doses, followed by every other week for four doses, then the normal prophylaxis schedule is resumed with the remaining chemotherapy treatment. Following this, consolidative craniospinal irradiation is considered in selected patients with a curative intent, particularly prior to allogeneic stem cell transplantation (ASCT). Their survival is identical to the CNS-negative cohort of patients, or slightly inferior.[55]

The focus of current ALL treatments is concentrated on improvement of the remission duration and survival of adult patients and to improve the quality of life of pediatric patients. With this goal in mind, validation of subtype-specific prognostic models and the development of risk-adapted and targeted therapy designs have become the major objectives of the clinical trials.

Treatment of newly diagnosed patients

As complex as ALL treatment programs are, and as much variations are found in many of its details, an easily recognizable framework is common to all of them. Because therapy is becoming increasingly subset-specific and depends on proper risk-stratification, the section on prognostic factors is discussed prior to proceeding to sections on therapy programs by disease subset (Table 3).

Prognostic factors and measurable residual disease

Efforts to describe risk models for ALL date back to the 1980s and have since experienced continued improvements as a result of the accumulating experience from a sequence of clinical trials. Although remission rates are high with current induction regimens, prognostic models are still useful for risk-directed postremission therapy to improve outcomes in adults and children with high-risk ALL and to avoid overtreatment of those with favorable disease. It should be noted that improved targeted and immune therapies have abolished the prognostic impact of many clinical, laboratory, or biological variables. For example, once associated with poor prognosis, T-cell ALL has long-term survival rates of over 50% in adults and 80% in children with current therapies including cyclophosphamide, asparaginase, and cytarabine.[3,31] Mature B-cell ALL is now highly curable with short-term dose-intense regimens plus rituximab (complete remission (CR) rates 90%; and survival rates >60% in adults and >80% in children).[56] Information from morphological assessment, immunophenotyping, karyotype analysis, molecular genetics, and, increasingly, the presence of minimal or measurable residual disease (MRD), has contributed to a more comprehensive risk-stratification of patients. Established adverse risk factors include age >60 years; elevated WBC count at diagnosis (>30,000/μL in B-cell ALL, >100,000/μL in T-cell ALL); ETP-ALL immunophenotype; the presence of t(4;11)(q21;q23) and other KMT2A rearrangements; and hypodiploidy or complex karyotype.[31] Furthermore, patients with Ph-like ALL have a poorer outcome when compared to other patients with B-cell ALL; it remains unclear whether they should receive upfront ASCT or only when there is MRD persistence.

Monitoring of MRD after induction and during consolidation has emerged as one of the most powerful predictors of relapse and has been most helpful to further stratify standard-risk patients.[46,57] The significant prognostic value of MRD spans across all subtypes of ALL and supersedes that of historical parameters such as age, WBC count, and cytogenetics. A meta-analysis of 13,637 pediatric and adult patients showed that, across all subgroups and covariates, MRD undetectability has a hazard ratio (HR) of 0.23 in pediatric patients and 0.28 in adults for event-free survival (EFS); and a HR of 0.28 in both pediatric patients and adults for overall survival

(OS).[58] In adult patients, this translated into 10-year OS rates of 60% for patients who were MRD-undetectable and of 15% for those who were MRD-positive.

The time to achieve MRD undetectability is also a strong prognostic factor, particularly in Ph-negative ALL.[57] A study from the MD Anderson Cancer Center analyzed 215 patients with newly diagnosed Ph-negative B-ALL who received intensive chemotherapy and had available MRD assessment at CR and around 12 weeks. Early responders, defined as MRD undetectability at CR had better outcomes with 3-year EFS rates of 65% versus 42% in late responders ($P < 0.001$), and 3-year OS rates of 76% versus 58% ($P = 0.001$). On multivariate analysis, the KMT2A rearrangement and MRD positivity at CR were the only factors correlated with worse OS.[57]

Adolescent and young adults (AYA) with ALL

The age requirements to fit this population have varied considerably in clinical trials and most investigators would consider ages 13–39 years as AYAs. The biology of ALL differs between children, AYAs, and older adults, which is the rationale behind tailoring ALL therapy to the different populations. Such differences include: (1) a higher T-cell phenotype in patients aged 10–40 years old; (2) a near absence of the two favorable subgroups of ALL (hyperdiploidy and t(12;21)/ETV6-RUNX1) during the second decade of life compared to 60% prevalence in children; (3) an increasing prevalence of high-risk Ph-positive ALL with age, from 3% in children to almost 50% in the elderly.[31] In the US intergroup trial C10403, of 295 AYA patients (17–39 years of age) treated with a pediatric regimen, the estimated 5-year OS rate was approximately 60%.[59]

One concern is the tolerability of pediatric regimens in adults ≥40 years. The Group for Research on Adult Acute Lymphoblastic Leukemia (GRAALL) examined this issue in patients aged 15–60.[60] The outcomes, compared to those seen in historical controls treated with an adult regimen, showed the pediatric regimen resulted in a survival improvement for younger patients <45 years old (66% vs 44%; $P < 0.001$). However, among patients 46–60 years, the cumulative incidence of chemotherapy-related death was 15%, negating the benefit of enhanced antileukemic activity. Patel and colleagues[61] reported from the UKALL14 protocol using pegylated-asparaginase at the dose of 1000 IU/m^2 on Days 4 and 18 during induction in 91 adults 25–62 years (median 47 years). The CR rate was 66% and induction mortality 20%; the hepatotoxicity rate was 56%. Patients aged over 40 years had more than a 10-fold increase in risk of death during induction. This prompted the suggestion to exclude pegylated-asparaginase in patients over 40 years.

At the MD Anderson Cancer Center, a nonrandomized study including AYA patients showed no difference in outcomes between the pediatric asparaginase-containing augmented Berlin–Frankfurt–Münster (ABFM) regimen and the non-asparaginase-containing hyper-CVAD regimen.[62] The 5-year CR duration rate was 53% with hyper-CVAD and 55% with ABFM. The 5-year OS rates were 60% in both groups. The ABFM regimen had a higher incidence of asparaginase adverse effects such as hepatotoxicity (41%), pancreatitis (11%), and thrombosis (19%); myelosuppression-related complications were more common with hyper-CVAD.[62] More recently, the hyper-CVAD and ofatumumab combination reported a 4-year OS rate of 74% in the AYA population.[63]

In summary, pediatric regimens and the HCVAD regimen showed similar CR rates, remission duration, and survival outcomes.

CD20-positive precursor B-ALL

The addition of rituximab to the hyper-CVAD regimen was evaluated in newly diagnosed patients with Philadelphia-negative, CD20-positive ALL.[64] Two doses of rituximab were added to each of the first four cycles of intensive chemotherapy (total eight doses of rituximab). It was also incorporated into early and late intensification cycles (months 6 and 18 of maintenance therapy). Among patients <60 years old, the addition of rituximab improved the 3-year CR duration (70% vs 38%; $P < 0.001\%$) and survival rates (75% vs 47%; $P = 0.003$). The German Multicenter Study Group for ALL (GMALL) reported an improvement of the rate of MRD undetectability, and of the 5-year remission duration and survival rates with the addition of rituximab to standard induction and consolidation chemotherapy in patients <55 years old.[65] The addition of rituximab to chemotherapy in the GRAAL-R 2005 randomized study improved the 2-year EFS rates (primary endpoint) from 52 to 65% ($P = 0.038$) and the OS rates from 64 to 71% ($P = 0.095$; censoring for ASCT, $P = 0.018$).[66]

To further improve outcomes of younger patients with newly diagnosed B-cell ALL, a phase 2 trial investigated the sequential use of HCVAD and blinatumomab with promising safety and efficacy.[67] The regimen consists of four cycles of HCVAD followed by four cycles of blinatumomab. Earlier incorporation of blinatumomab after two cycles of chemotherapy is allowed for patients at high risk for early relapse, particularly those with Ph-like ALL, complex karyotype, t(4;11), low-hypodiploidy/near triploidy, or persistent MRD. Four cycles of blinatumomab are also incorporated in the 12 cycles of POMP maintenance (each three cycles of POMP followed by one cycle of blinatumomab) for a total of 18 months of maintenance therapy. Among 34 patients treated (median age 36 years [range 17–59]), the CR rate was 100% and MRD undetectability rate 96% with no induction death. One-third of patients underwent ASCT for high-risk features. With a median follow-up of 22 months, 88% are alive; two patients died of disease progression, one patient died after ASCT of a transplant-related complication, and one died of sepsis during re-induction after relapse. The 2-year relapse-free survival (RFS) and OS rates were 79% and 86%, respectively.[67]

Mature B-cell and Burkitt lymphoma/leukemia

The addition of rituximab to short-term intensive dose-chemotherapy has improved outcomes in adult Burkitt and Burkitt-type lymphoma or ALL.[56] Its addition to hyper-CVAD resulted in a 3-year survival rate of 89% compared to 53% with chemotherapy alone.[56] This was confirmed in a randomized, open-label, phase III trial, in which 260 patients with newly diagnosed Burkitt lymphoma/leukemia received intensive chemotherapy with or without rituximab. The addition of rituximab improved EFS (3-year rate 75% vs 62%; $P = 0.024$) and OS (3-year rate 83% vs 70%; $P = 0.011$).[68]

To further reduce early morbidity and mortality, a pilot study investigated dose-adjusted EPOCH in combination with rituximab in 30 patients (median age 33 years; age >40 years, 40%) diagnosed with Burkitt lymphoma. The treatment was safe and highly effective. The progression-free and OS rates were 95–100% and 90–100%, respectively.[69] Of note, the majority of patients (90%) had low- and intermediate-risk disease; only 13% had marrow involvement and 3% had CNS involvement, both being known adverse factors.[69] The results of a multicenter phase 2 study of DA-EPOCH-R in 113 adults with Burkitt leukemia (BL) were recently reported.[70] The 5-year EFS and OS rates for patients with low-risk disease were 100% and 85%, respectively. These rates for patients with high-risk disease (Stage ≥ 3, or performance status ≥2, or elevated LDH, or tumor ≥ 7 cm) were 82% and 87%, respectively. Patients with baseline bone marrow involvement (25%) and baseline CNS disease (10%) had a significantly inferior outcome with 4-year EFS rates of 67% and 46%, respectively.[70] Therefore, DA-EPOCH-R, which omitted drugs traditionally used for CNS prophylaxis (e.g., high-dose methotrexate and cytarabine) may not be suitable for patients with baseline CNS and medullary disease. In a recent exploratory multivariate model among 557 patients with newly diagnosed BL, baseline CNS involvement and poor performance status predicted subsequent CNS recurrence, an outcome that is associated with a dismal prognosis.[71] Furthermore, treatment with DA-EPOCH was associated with a significantly increased risk of CNS recurrence (cumulative incidence of 13% compared with 2–4% with dose-intense regimens.[71] Regimens such as the hyper-CVAD that employs high doses of methotrexate and cytarabine and highly penetrant of the blood–brain barrier need to be compared with DA-EPOCH-R in patients with higher-risk disease, mainly those with baseline marrow and CNS disease.

Philadelphia chromosome-positive ALL

Combinations of cytotoxic chemotherapy with TKI are the standard of care in Ph-positive ALL. The best results are achieved when TKIs are incorporated early and continuously.[72,73] Imatinib was the first TKI evaluated in Ph-positive ALL.[72] Its addition to intensive chemotherapy led to CR rates >90% and 5-year RFS and OS rates of 43% and 43%, respectively.[72] Dasatinib is a more potent and selective second-generation TKI.[74] In a single-institution study, among 72 patients with newly diagnosed Ph-positive ALL treated with hyper-CVAD and dasatinib, the CR rate was 96%, the complete cytogenetic response (CCyR) rate after one course was 83%, and the complete molecular response (CMR) rate was 65%. The 5-year survival rate was 46%.[74] A confirmatory Southwest Oncology Group (SWOG) study in 94 patients yielded a response rate of 88% and 3-year survival rate of 71%.[75] Patients who underwent ASCT in first CR (CR1) had a better outcome.[75]

In the European Working Group for ALL-Ph (EWALL-Ph)-01 study, patients ≥55 years with newly diagnosed Ph-positive ALL treated with dasatinib and low-intensity chemotherapy had a CR rate of 96%.[76] The estimated 5-year RFS rate was 28%, and the OS rate 36%.[76] Among patients who relapsed, 75% had a T315I mutation. Interestingly, 25% of patients who had baseline sequencing had a T315I mutation. Similar results were reported by the Gruppo Italiano Malattie Ematologiche LAL (GIMEMA LAL) 1509 study combining dasatinib with glucocorticoids in 60 patients (median age 42 years).[77] After 3 months, 97% of patients were in complete hematologic remission, but only 19% achieved CMR. The 3-year disease-free and OS rates were 49% and 58%, respectively. In a multivariate analysis, CMR was an independent predictor of better survival.

Because many patients with Ph-positive ALL relapse with a T315I clone,[74–76] ponatinib (third-generation BCR-ABL1 TKI that suppresses T315I clones) was added to hyper-CVAD in a phase 2 single-arm trial of patients with previously untreated Ph-positive ALL.[78] Ponatinib was given orally at 45 mg daily for the first 14 days of cycle 1 then continuously at 45 mg daily for the subsequent cycles. After treating 37 patients, the protocol was amended after the occurrence of two fatal myocardial events, to reduce the dose of ponatinib to 30 mg daily at cycle 2, with further reduction to 15 mg once a CMR (defined as absence of quantifiable BCR-ABL1 transcripts) was achieved. After the protocol amendment, no further vascular events occurred. A recent update of 86 patients treated with hyper-CVAD and ponatinib was reported with a median follow-up of 43 months.[79] The 3-month CMR rate was 74% and cumulative CMR rate was 84%. Only 19 patients (21%) underwent ASCT in CR1. With a median follow-up of 44 months, 71% of patients remain alive in remission, and only three relapses were observed in patients while still on ponatinib. The 5-year CR duration and OS rates were 68% and 74%, respectively. A landmark analysis performed at 6 months showed a trend toward better OS in patients who did not undergo ASCT in first remission (5-year OS rate of 66% for patients who underwent ASCT compared to 83% for patients who did not [$P = 0.07$]).[79] A propensity score matching analysis comparing the efficacy of hyper-CVAD-ponatinib with hyper-CVAD-dasatinib showed a superior outcome with ponatinib: the 3-month CMR rates were 82% versus 65% ($P = 0.03$); the 3-year event-EFS and OS rates were 69% versus 46% ($P = 0.04$) and 83% versus 56% ($P = 0.03$), respectively.[80]

Blinatumomab was shown to be safe and effective in heavily pretreated relapsed-refractory (R/R) Ph-positive ALL in a single-arm multicenter phase 2 trial.[81] Among 45 patients treated (50% with prior exposure to ponatinib, 44% with prior ASCT, and 27% with T315I mutation), the overall response rate (ORR; defined as CR or CR with incomplete count recover [CRi]) was 36%, with 88% of responders achieving MRD negativity. Responses were observed regardless of T315I mutation status. Half of the patients were able to undergo ASCT, and the median OS was 7.1 months.

The combination of blinatumomab with TKI (mainly ponatinib) has been shown to be safe and effective in a small case series of 15 patients from MDACC with 50% CR rate and 75% molecular response.[82] The GIMEMA group has recently presented early results from D-ALBA, the first trial investigating the sequential use of TKI/steroid (in induction) and blinatumomab (in consolidation).[83] Sixty-three patients have been treated thus far with this regimen of prednisone, dasatinib, and blinatumomab. The CR rate was 98% and the 1-year DFS rate was 88%. Deep molecular response increased throughout therapy (29% after induction, 60% after two cycles of blinatumomab, and 80% after four cycles). T315I mutation was noted in 6/15 patients with rising MRD in induction phase; all cleared after blinatumomab.

The combination of blinatumomab and ponatinib and the sequential combination of ponatinib combined to low-intensity chemotherapy followed by blinatumomab and ponatinib in patients with newly diagnosed Ph-positive ALL are under investigation.

ASCT has improved the outcome in Ph-positive ALL. There is currently a debate over suitable candidates in CR1. We evaluated the predictive value of MRD assessment in patients treated with chemotherapy and TKIs who did not undergo ASCT.[84] At 3 months, the achievement of CMR was associated with longer median OS (127 months vs 38 months, $P = 0.009$) and RFS (126 months vs 18 months, $P = 0.007$). By multivariate analysis, achievement of 3-month CMR was favorable for OS (HR 0.42, $P = 0.01$).[84] Molecular MRD monitoring could identify patients who may not need ASCT, particularly if they are receiving ponatinib therapy.[85]

Older patients with ALL

In older patients with ALL (defined as older than 55–60 years), intensive chemotherapy results in CR rates of 70–80% with high rate of toxicities.[86] One-third of patients achieving CR may die of myelosuppression-associated complications. The long-term cure rate among such patients is only 15–20%.[86] Among 727 older patients (>65 years; 2007–2012) treated under Medicare, median survival was 10 months.[87] In the National Cancer Institute Surveillance, Epidemiology, and End Results database, among 1675 adults (age ≥60 years) with ALL (1980–2011), the median survival was 4 months, and the 3-year survival rate 12.8%.[88] The goal with modern regimens is to maintain or increase efficacy and reduce toxicity.

Thus strategies to de-intensify treatment regimens have been investigated in this population. Inotuzumab ozogamicin (detailed later) with mini-hyper-cyclophosphamide, vincristine, dexamethasone (CVD) (i.e., a lower intensity version of the hyper-CVAD regimen without anthracycline), with or without blinatumomab, is one such promising strategy in the older population.[89,90] Among 64 patients treated with this regimen, the median age was 68 years (range, 60–81 years) and 42% of patients were ≥70 years of age. The CR rate was 98% and the MRD undetectability rate 95%. The 3-year CR duration and OS rates were 76% and 54%, respectively. A propensity-matched analysis showed that this regimen significantly improved survival compared with a historical 3-year OS rate of 32% with hyper-CVAD in this older population ($P = 0.007$).[90] The SWOG 1318 study evaluated chemotherapy-free induction and consolidation with blinatumomab (total of 4–5 cycles) followed by POMP maintenance (prednisone, vincristine, methotrexate, and 6-mercaptopurine). Thirty-one patients (median age of 73 years; range 66–84) were treated. Early results showed no induction death, CR rate of 66% (among them 92% with undetectable MRD), a 1-year OS rate of 65%, and a 1-year DFS rate of 56%.[91] Preliminary results of the combination of venetoclax with low-intensity chemotherapy in newly diagnosed older patients unfit for intensive chemotherapy are promising with objective response and MRD undetectability rates of 91% and 100%, respectively.[92]

T-cell ALL

Treatment of adult T-cell ALL and T-cell lymphoblastic lymphoma (T-LL) results in long-term survival rates of 40–60%. The outcome is strongly associated with the T-cell immunophenotype.[20] Regimens for T-cell ALL are similar to those for B-cell ALL. In the pediatric experience, the addition of nelarabine to frontline regimen in patients with T-cell ALL up to 31 years of age improved the 4-year DFS rate from 83% to 89% ($P = 0.03$).[93] These results have not been replicated in adult patients yet. A single-arm phase II study from the MD Anderson Cancer Center evaluated nelarabine in combination with the frontline hyper-CVAD regimen in 67 patients.[94] Nelarabine was administered after or during consolidation. The estimated 3-year survival rate was 65%. This combination failed to improve CR duration or OS rates compared to that seen with historical controls treated with hyper-CVAD alone. For patients with ETP-ALL and mature T-ALL, the rates were 38% and 70%, respectively.[94] This therapy followed by ASCT should be considered in CR1 in adult patients with ETP-ALL as reported by Bond and colleagues.[95]

Recent insights into the biology of ETP-ALL have revealed BCL-2 dependence which perhaps explains the sensitivity to BCL-2 antagonism.[96] The addition of venetoclax or venetoclax + navitoclax (low dose) to lower-intensity chemotherapy in older patients with newly diagnosed or refractory ALL has yielded encouraging early results.

Salvage therapy

The prognosis of adults with R-R ALL was historically associated with a dismal prognosis and a cure rate of less than 10%.[97,98] The CR rates were 30–40% in Salvage 1 and 20–25% in Salvage 2 with standard chemotherapy regimens, with transition to ASCT in only 10–30% of patients.[97,98] The recent advent of conjugated monoclonal antibodies, bispecific antibodies, and chimeric antigen receptor T (CAR T)-cell therapies has revolutionized the treatment of ALL and resulted in a number of Food and Drug Administration (FDA) approvals for the treatment of ALL in the salvage setting: blinatumomab in 2014, inotuzumab ozogamicin and tisagenlecleucel in 2017 (Table 4).[31] These agents are currently the subject of investigation in different schemas and combinations.

Anti-CD19 Bi-specific T-cell engager: blinatumomab

Blinatumomab is an anti-CD19-directed CD3 bispecific T-cell engager constructed using BiTE® antibody technology.[99] It consists of a recombinant monoclonal antibody composed of an anti-CD19 fragment antigen-binding (Fab) region joined by a short linker to an anti-CD3 Fab region.[99] In the confirmatory

Table 4 Seminal trials for the treatment of relapsed/refractory B-cell acute lymphoblastic leukemia.

Clinical trial	Disease setting	No of patients	Response	Median overall survival (mo)	MRD negativity (%)
Inotuzumab ozogamicin					
INO-VATE [106]	R/R ALL	109	ORR: 81% CR: 35.8%	7.7	78
Mini-hyper-CVD + inotuzumab ozogamicin ± blinatumomab	R/R ALL	84	ORR: 80% CR: 58%	S1: 25 S2: 6 S3: 7	82
Blinatumomab					
TOWER	R/R Ph− ALL	271	ORR: 44% CR: 34%	7.7	76
ALCANTARA	R/R Ph+ ALL	45	ORR: 36% CR: 31%	7.1	88
CAR T-cell therapy					
ELIANA	R/R ALL (age <26 yr)	79	ORR: 82% CR/CRi: 62%	NR	98
Anti-CD19 CAR T-cells	R/R ALL (adults)	53	CR: 83%	12.9	67

No, number; MRD, measurable residual disease; R/R, relapse or refractory; Ph, Philadelphia; ORR, objective response rate; CR, complete remission; CVD, cyclophosphamide, vincristine, dexamethasone; S1, salvage 1; S2, salvage 2; S3, salvage 3; CAR, chimeric antigen receptor; CRi, complete response with incomplete hematologic recovery; NR, not reported.

phase II study of 189 patients with Ph-negative ALL, blinatumomab was associated with an ORR of 43%. The median response duration was 9 months, and median OS was 6 months.[100]

Following these results, a phase III trial (TOWER study) was conducted in more than 400 patients with relapsed/refractory Ph-negative ALL randomized (2 : 1) to blinatumomab ($n = 271$) or standard of care ($n = 134$).[101] The rate of CR with full, partial, or incomplete hematologic recovery was significantly higher in the blinatumomab group than in the chemotherapy group, 44% and 25%, respectively ($P < 0.001$). Molecular remission rates among responders, defined as MRD $< 10^{-4}$ in the first 12 weeks, were 76% and 48%, respectively. Blinatumomab prolonged survival, the primary study endpoint: the median OS was 7.7 months versus 4.0 months ($P = 0.01$). Twenty-four percent of the patients in each group underwent ASCT.[101]

A recent report from a phase III study with 1 : 1 randomization of 208 children and AYAs in first salvage to blinatumomab or standard of care showed that blinatumomab induced a higher rate of MRD undetectability (79% with blinatumomab compared with 21% with standard of care; $P < 0.001$) and a better 2-year OS rate (79% with blinatumomab compared with 59% with standard of care; $P = 0.005$).[102]

In R-R Ph-positive ALL, blinatumomab also demonstrated a positive effect. In the phase II ALCANTARA trial, 45 patients with relapsed/refractory Ph-positive ALL were treated. Thirty-six percent achieved a response. The median RFS and OS were 6.7 and 7.1 months, respectively; 44% of patients received ASCT.[81]

Gökbuget et al.[103] assessed blinatumomab in 113 patients with ALL in MRD positive CR. The MRD clearance rate was 80% after two courses of blinatumomab. The 4-year OS rate was 45%, which compares favorably to expectations of outcomes in MRD-positive patients.[103,104] This has led to the approval of blinatumomab for this indication, the first such approval of an MRD-directed therapy. However, new questions have emerged regarding optimal therapy following MRD clearance with blinatumomab, such as the role of ASCT, or the relative benefit of TKI in patients with positive MRD in Philadelphia-positive ALL.[105]

Anti-CD22 antibody–drug conjugate: inotuzumab ozogamicin

Inotuzumab ozogamicin is an anti-CD22 monoclonal antibody conjugated to the toxin calicheamicin.[106] In a single-institution phase II study in patients with relapsed/refractory ALL, inotuzumab ozogamicin was administered at a starting dose of 1.3–1.8 mg/m^2 IV every 3–4 weeks. Forty-nine patients were treated. The ORR was 57%, and median survival was 5.1 months. Nearly half of the patients treated with inotuzumab ozogamicin proceeded to ASCT.[107] To minimize toxicities and based on pharmacokinetic and pharmacodynamic data, inotuzumab ozogamicin was administered on a weekly basis at 0.8 mg/m^2 IV on day 1 followed by 0.5 mg/m^2 IV on days 8 and 15, every 3–4 weeks in 40 patients. The study yielded a similar response rate as inotuzumab ozogamicin given every 3–4 weeks (59% vs 57%) with a median survival of 9.5 months. Weekly administration of inotuzumab ozogamicin resulted in fewer adverse events, including lower rates of veno-occlusive disease (VOD).[108] In a separate, multicenter phase II trial in heavily pretreated patients with relapsed/refractory ALL, inotuzumab ozogamicin therapy resulted in a remission rate of 66%, with 78% of patients who achieved CR becoming MRD undetectable. The median survival was 7.4 months.[109]

These results led to a randomized trial comparing inotuzumab ozogamicin to physician's choice of chemotherapy in relapsed ALL. The CR rate was 81% with inotuzumab ozogamicin and 29% with standard of care ($P < 0.0001$). Among responders, the MRD undetectability rates were 78% and 28% ($P < 0.0001$), respectively. The median survival was 7.7 versus 6.7 months ($P = 0.02$; HR 0.77).[110] The 2-year survival rates were 23% and 10%, respectively.[111] Serious toxicities included VOD post-ASCT, mainly in patients who received double alkylating agents in pretransplant conditioning. Age was also a risk factor for VOD.[110,111]

Recently, inotuzumab ozogamicin was assessed in 48 children and AYAs (median age 9 years; [1–21]). The ORR and MRD negativity rates were 62% and 65%, respectively. The 12-month OS rate was 40%.[112]

The combination of inotuzumab with bosutinib is being evaluated in a phase 1/2 trial in R/R Ph-positive ALL. Patients with T315I mutation were excluded. Early results on 18 patients reported ORR and CMR rates of 83% and 56%, respectively.[113] The median EFS and OS were 8 and 15.4 months, respectively.

Combination immunotherapies

Inotuzumab ozogamicin was evaluated with mini-hyper-CVD in relapsed/refractory B-cell Ph-negative ALL.[114,115] Among the initial 59 patients with relapsed/refractory ALL treated, the response rate was 78%, with 82% of responders achieving MRD undetectability.[114] The 1-year relapse-free and OS rates were 46% and 41%, respectively. The median OS and RFS were 11 and 8 months, respectively. Almost half of the patients were able to receive subsequent ASCT with an estimated 1-year survival rate of 63% among these patients. The rate of VOD was 15%, mainly in patients with prior or subsequent ASCT (23%).[114] When compared with a historical cohort of patients treated with inotuzumab ozogamicin monotherapy in the salvage setting, the results of the combination were significantly better (median survival: 9.3 vs 5.6 months, $P = 0.02$).[114] To further improve these outcomes, the study was amended to investigate the addition of four cycles of blinatumomab following four cycles of the combination of weekly lower doses of inotuzumab ozogamicin and mini-hyper-CVD. The hypothesis was that the addition of blinatumomab may allow for the use of less chemotherapy and lower doses of weekly inotuzumab ozogamicin, a better eradication of MRD, as well as the distancing of AHSCT from the last dose of inotuzumab ozogamicin, thereby leading to less treatment-related morbidity, less VOD and less mortality. In fact, the incidence of VOD was significantly reduced (from 15% to 5%) by using lower and fractionated dose of inotuzumab ozogamicin (first dose of 0.6 mg/m^2 then 0.3 mg/m^2 for each subsequent dose), and by spacing the last dose of inotuzumab ozogamicin from ASCT by 3–6 months.[31] In the overall cohort of patients treated with mini-hyper-CVD with inotuzumab ozogamicin ($n = 59$), and those treated with sequential combination with blinatumomab ($n = 29$), the 2-year survival rate was 39% and the median survival 13 months. Among the 62 patients treated in first salvage with mini-hyper-CVD and inotuzumab ozogamicin with or without later blinatumomab, the CR/CRi rate was 92%, the MRD undetectability rate was 86%, the median survival was 25 months, and the 3-year OS rate was 42%. The 60-day mortality rate was 3%.[115] These results compare favorably with the results obtained with single-agent inotuzumab ozogamicin and blinatumomab and with historical salvage chemotherapy (median survivals of only 6–12 months).

SWOG 1312 study is a phase I trial of inotuzumab ozogamicin and CVP (cyclophosphamide, vincristine, and prednisone) for relapsed/refractory ALL.[116] Fifty patients (median age of 43 years) were treated. The CR/CRi rate was 61% in the 23 evaluable patients treated at the maximal tolerated dose (MTD), and 60% (3/5) in patients with the Ph-like signature. The median OS was 7.7 months for all patients, and 10.9 months for patients treated at the MTD.[116]

Chimeric antigen receptor T-cell therapies

CAR T-cells are genetically modified autologous T lymphocytes engineered to express variable binding sites of antibodies, such as a receptor against CD19 that are attached to an activating domain intracellularly. These T-cells, harnessed from the patients' own immune system, target the malignant cells.

In a phase 2 multicenter study, 79 children and young adults with relapsed or refractory CD19+ B-ALL received a single infusion of tisagenlecleucel, CD19 CAR T-cells.[117] Among 79 evaluable patients, the ORR was 81% with all responding patients achieving undetectable MRD. The 24-month RFS and OS rates were 62% and 66%, respectively. The CAR T-cells persisted for a median of 168 days (from 20 to 617 days) suggesting that immunosurveillance with these products may be long lasting. Grades 3 and 4 cytokine release syndrome (CRS) and neurotoxicities were encountered in 49% and 40%, respectively, with 48% requiring intensive care unit stay. This led to the approval of tisagenlecleucel for relapsed/refractory ALL in patients up to age 25 postfailure of two prior therapies.[117] In 53 adults with heavily pretreated B-ALL who received the CAR T-cell infusion, the CR rate was 83% including 32 of 48 (67%) evaluable patients achieving undetectable MRD.[118] Better outcomes were observed in patients with low disease burden (≤5% bone marrow blasts) at the time of CAR T-cell infusion with a median EFS of 10.6 months compared to 5.3 months and median OS of 20.1 months compared to 12.4 months in patients with a high disease burden.[118]

There are two main safety concerns with CAR T-cell therapy, CRS and neurotoxicity, occurring in 77–83% and 40–43% of patients, respectively. These were more common in patients with a higher disease burden at baseline.[119] Grade ≥3 CRS (including one death) was observed in 26% of patients and grade ≥3 neurotoxicity in 42% of patients; most required treatment with the anti-interleukin-6 monoclonal antibody, tocilizumab.[118,119] For older adults, CRS and neurotoxicity have limited broad application.

Strategies to improve the safety of CAR-T cells while preserving their efficacy are an active area of basic and translational research. A novel anti-CD19 CAR-T cell product with a lower affinity to CD19 and fast-off rate showed improved in vitro proliferation and cytotoxic activity and enhanced proliferation and *in vivo* antitumor effect.[120] To circumvent CD19 antigen escape as a mechanism of resistance, CD22-targeted CAR-T cells and dual CD19 and CD22 CAR T-cells have also been developed.[121]

There have also been tremendous efforts to develop new platforms of "off-the-shelf" CAR-based therapies to decrease the high cost, manufacturing complexity, and delays associated with currently approved CAR-T cells.[122] Allogeneic CAR-T cells manufactured from healthy donors have been investigated. For example, UCART19 is an allogeneic, genetically modified second-generation CAR-T cell product manufactured from healthy donor T cells, in which TRAC and CD52 genes have been knocked out to allow its administration to patients without increasing the risk of graft-versus-host disease. "Off-the-shelf" NK cells derived from umbilical cord blood and modified to express CAR (CAR-NK cells) are also being developed in B-lymphoid malignancies.[123]

BH3 mimetics

The BH3-mimetics venetoclax and navitoclax demonstrated promising preclinical activity in cell lines of B-cell and T-cell ALL.[124,125] Navitoclax inhibits BCL-2, BCL-xL, and BCL-W with encouraging antileukemic activity in ALL cells.[124] A particularly strong activity was seen in KMT2A-rearranged B-cell ALL; both single-agent activity and synergistic killing in combination with chemotherapy were observed due to the upregulation of BCL-2 in these cell lines.[124,125] In a phase I trial, 47 patients with R-R ALL (median age 27 years; range, 6–72 years) were treated with venetoclax and navitoclax in combination with chemotherapy. The ORR was 60%; the MRD undetectability rate was 58%. The median duration of response was 4.2 months and the median OS was 7.8 months.[126] Preliminary BH3 profiling analysis revealed a trend in BCL-2 dependency at baseline in T-ALL cells versus both BCL-2 and BCL-XL dependency in B-ALL cells.

The evolving role of allogeneic stem cell transplantation

Historically, nearly all patients with ALL were considered to be high risk for relapse, and ASCT was offered as consolidation for all fit candidates with suitable donors. Over the past two decades, the unprecedented progress in our understanding of the disease biology and the improvement of frontline and salvage therapies have resulted in more accurate risk stratification, which is primarily based on unique biological features (cytogenetics, genomic, and MRD status). This has allowed for better refinement of consolidation strategies in CR1. Thus ASCT is now largely reserved for higher-risk patients. High-risk cytogenetic features in adult patients include: low hypodiploidy/near triploidy, t(4;11) (KMT2A rearrangement), and complex karyotype (≥5 abnormalities).[127] Furthermore, adults with Ph-like ALL treated with both hyper-CVAD and ABFM regimens, not only have low rates of MRD undetectability (30% vs 70%), but their outcomes are equally poor regardless of MRD status (assessed at CR by flow cytometry), particularly if JAK2 mutated.[128] Whether the addition of novel agents (inotuzumab or blinatumomab) or ASCT are superior to intensive chemotherapy remains uncertain and this represents an area of active research.

Among T-cell ALL, the ETP subtype and lack of NOTCH1 or FBXW1 mutations are high-risk groups that may derive benefit from ASCT in CR1.[21,95] The presence of NRAS/KRAS mutations or PTEN gene alteration are other high-risk molecular features in T-cell ALL.[63] However, there are no definitive data on the effect of ASCT in this subgroup.[15,22]

The advent of MRD assessment has refined the treatment landscape of ALL. Persistent MRD is generally considered an indication for ASCT in CR1.[114] However, outcomes remain poor for MRD-positive patients even when ASCT is performed. It is currently unclear whether patients who achieve a negative MRD status with blinatumomab or other novel agents would still derive benefit from ASCT. A *post hoc* analysis of the BLAST trial showed no difference in OS rates among patients who underwent ASCT after receiving blinatumomab and those who did not.[103] However, the numbers were small and the equivalent survival outcome may be explained, at least partly, by the fact that ASCT-related mortality may have offset the decreased relapse risk seen with ASCT. The role of consolidative ASCT after CAR T-cell therapy is under evaluation, although it is favored by most experts, especially in ASCT-naive and fit patients.[129]

In Ph-positive ALL, the added benefit of ASCT with the achievement of deep molecular remissions with more potent TKIs is now being questioned. Among patients treated with HCVAD plus a TKI without ASCT, the 4-year OS rate was 66% in patients who achieve CMR at 3 months, suggesting that ASCT may not be needed for these patients.[84] This may be particularly true if patients are treated with a ponatinib-based regimen, which is capable of achieving high rates of CMR.[85] For example, the 5-year OS survival of patients treated with HCVAD plus ponatinib who did not undergo ASCT was 83% in the most recent update.[79] In contrast, patients who do not achieve at least an MMR may benefit from ASCT in CR1.[130] When imatinib was combined with HCVAD or a lower-intensity version of HCVAD in a randomized fashion, the benefit of ASCT was restricted to patients who did not achieve MMR after two cycles.[131] Taken together, these findings suggest that patients with Ph-positive ALL who achieve early deep molecular remissions may have excellent long-term outcomes and may potentially be spared the need of ASCT.

In summary, the role of ASCT in CR1 remains currently valid in certain high-risk circumstances such as (1) KMT2A-rearranged ALL; (2) ETP-ALL; and (3) ALL with complex cytogenetics and low hypodiploidy (including TP53 mutations). Patients with Ph-like ALL with undetectable MRD and those in CR1 who achieve MRD undetectability after blinatumomab may not need ASCT. Patients with Ph-positive ALL with 3-month CMR may not benefit from ASCT; in contrast, patients with positive MRD should be considered for blinatumomab or other MRD-targeted therapy and eventually ASCT, particularly patients who remained positive for MRD. Patients with ALL in CR2 should be referred for ASCT.

> **Summary**
>
> Progress in the understanding of the biology of ALL and refinements of prognostic systems have led to increasing sophistication of therapy. Therapeutic capabilities in adult ALL have rapidly reached new heights over the past decade with the introduction of highly promising monoclonal antibodies, immune conjugates, CAR-T cells, and new-generation TKIs. Genomic profiling has identified new prognostic and predictive markers as well as new therapeutic targets to improve the adverse prognosis of some ALL subsets such as Ph-like ALL. Ph-like ALL and ETP ALL represent two recently defined high-risk subtypes of ALL and may be targetable with TKIs. Patients with mature B-cell ALL do best with short-term dose-intensive therapies. It is now well-established that treatment for Ph-positive ALL should include TKIs, ideally from the start and probably best maintained for many years thereafter. The role of transplantation is modified according to better and more predictable risk-stratification. Transplantation should be considered in first remission in any high-risk patients without prohibitively serious comorbidities, and in any patients beyond a first remission. As many of the newer agents advance through the final stages of development, ongoing clinical trials aim to determine optimal combinations and order of delivery, and the role of cytotoxic chemotherapy to achieve safely high cure rates. The introduction of these effective therapies into frontline regimens may increase the rate of MRD negativity, optimize responses and close the outcome gap separating pediatric and adult ALL. Harnessing the full potential of the immune system with the durable presence of autologous or allogeneic T-cell constructs may ultimately lead to reducing the need of ASCT in adult ALL.

Key references

The complete reference list can be found on Vital Source version of this title, see inside front cover.

1 Siegel RL, Miller KD, Jemal A. Cancer statistics, 2020. *CA Cancer J Clin.* 2020;**70**(1):7–30.

7 Mullighan CG, Goorha S, Radtke I, et al. Genome-wide analysis of genetic alterations in acute lymphoblastic leukaemia. *Nature.* 2007;**446**(7137):758–764.

16 Roberts KG, Li Y, Payne-Turner D, et al. Targetable kinase-activating lesions in Ph-like acute lymphoblastic leukemia. *N Engl J Med.* 2014;**371**(11):1005–1015.

20 Coustan-Smith E, Mullighan CG, Onciu M, et al. Early T-cell precursor leukaemia: a subtype of very high-risk acute lymphoblastic leukaemia. *Lancet Oncol.* 2009;**10**(2):147–156.

22 Jain N, Lamb AV, O'Brien S, et al. Early T-cell precursor acute lymphoblastic leukemia/lymphoma (ETP-ALL/LBL) in adolescents and adults: a high-risk subtype. *Blood.* 2016;**127**(15):1863–1869.

29 Moorman AV, Richards SM, Martineau M, et al. Outcome heterogeneity in childhood high-hyperdiploid acute lymphoblastic leukemia. *Blood.* 2003;**102**(8):2756–2762.

31 Jabbour E, Pui CH, Kantarjian H. Progress and innovations in the management of adult acute lymphoblastic leukemia. *JAMA Oncol.* 2018;**4**(10):1413–1420.

46 Beldjord K, Chevret S, Asnafi V, et al. Oncogenetics and minimal residual disease are independent outcome predictors in adult patients with acute lymphoblastic leukemia. *Blood.* 2014;**123**(24):3739–3749.

47 Den Boer ML, van Slegtenhorst M, De Menezes RX, et al. A subtype of childhood acute lymphoblastic leukaemia with poor treatment outcome: a genome-wide classification study. *Lancet Oncol.* 2009;**10**(2):125–134.

48 Mullighan CG, Su X, Zhang J, et al. Deletion of IKZF1 and prognosis in acute lymphoblastic leukaemia. *N Engl J Med.* 2009;**360**(5):470–480.

51 Rausch CR, Jabbour EJ, Kantarjian HM, Kadia TM. Optimizing the use of the hyperCVAD regimen: clinical vignettes and practical management. *Cancer.* 2020;**126**(6):1152–1160.

54 Pui CH, Campana D, Pei D, et al. Treating childhood acute lymphoblastic leukemia without cranial irradiation. *N Engl J Med.* 2009;**360**(26):2730–2741.

58 Berry DA, Zhou S, Higley H, et al. Association of minimal residual disease with clinical outcome in pediatric and adult acute lymphoblastic leukemia: a meta-analysis. *JAMA Oncol.* 2017;**3**(7):e170580.

63 Jabbour E, Richard-Carpentier G, Sasaki Y, et al. Phase II study of the hyper-CVAD regimen in combination with ofatumumab (HCVAD-O) as frontline therapy for adult patients with CD20-positive acute lymphoblastic leukemia. *Lancet Hematol.* 2020;**7**(7):e523–e533.

67 Richard-Carpentier G, Kantarjian HM, Short NJ, et al. Updated results from the phase II study of hyper-CVAD in sequential combination with blinatumomab in newly diagnosed adults with B-cell acute lymphoblastic leukemia (B-ALL). *Blood.* 2019;**134**:3807.

68 Ribrag V, Koscielny S, Bosq J, et al. Rituximab and dose-dense chemotherapy for adults with Burkitt's lymphoma: a randomised, controlled, open-label, phase 3 trial. *Lancet.* 2016;**387**(10036):2402–2411.

78 Jabbour E, Kantarjian H, Ravandi F, et al. Combination of hyper-CVAD with ponatinib as first-line therapy for patients with Philadelphia chromosome-positive acute lymphoblastic leukaemia: a single-centre, phase 2 study. *Lancet Oncol.* 2015;**16**(15):1547–1555.

83 Chiaretti S, Bassan R, Vitale A, et al. Dasatinib-blinatumomab combination for the front-line treatment of adult Ph+ ALL patients. updated results of the gimema LAL2116 D-Alba trial. *Blood.* 2019;**134**(Supplement_1):740.

89 Kantarjian H, Ravandi F, Short NJ, et al. Inotuzumab ozogamicin in combination with low-intensity chemotherapy for older patients with Philadelphia chromosome-negative acute lymphoblastic leukaemia: a single-arm, phase 2 study. *Lancet Oncol.* 2018;**19**(2):240–248.

101 Kantarjian H, Stein A, Gokbuget N, et al. Blinatumomab versus chemotherapy for advanced acute lymphoblastic leukemia. *N Engl J Med.* 2017;**376**(9):836–847.

103 Gökbuget N, Dombret H, Bonifacio M, et al. Blinatumomab for minimal residual disease in adults with B-precursor acute lymphoblastic leukemia. *Blood.* 2018;**131**(14):1522–1531.

110 Kantarjian HM, DeAngelo DJ, Stelljes M, et al. Inotuzumab ozogamicin versus standard therapy for acute lymphoblastic leukemia. *N Engl J Med.* 2016;**375**(8):740–753.

114 Jabbour E, Ravandi F, Kebriaei P, et al. Salvage chemoimmunotherapy with inotuzumab ozogamicin combined with mini–hyper-CVD for patients with relapsed or refractory Philadelphia chromosome–negative acute lymphoblastic leukemia: a phase 2 clinical trial. *JAMA Oncol.* 2018;**4**(2):230–234.

117 Maude SL, Laetsch TW, Buechner J, et al. Tisagenlecleucel in children and young adults with B-cell lymphoblastic leukemia. *N Engl J Med.* 2018;**378**:439–448.

120 Ghorashian S, Kramer AM, Onuoha S, et al. Enhanced CAR T cell expansion and prolonged persistence in pediatric patients with ALL treated with a low-affinity CD19 CAR. *Nat Med.* 2019;**25**(9):1408–1414.

126 Pullarkat VA, Lacayo NJ, Jabbour E, et al. Venetoclax and navitoclax in relapsed or refractory acute leukemia and lymphoblastic lymphoma. *Cancer Discov.* 2021;**11**(6):1440–1453.

114 Chronic lymphocytic leukemia

Jacqueline C. Barrientos, MD, MS ■ Kanti R. Rai, MD ■ Joanna M. Rhodes, MD, MSCE

> **Overview**
>
> There has been a significant progress, in the past two decades in our understanding of pathobiology of chronic lymphocytic leukemia (CLL) and in the treatment of this disease. CLL is a monoclonal B-cell lymphoproliferative disorder derived from antigen-experienced B lymphocytes that differ in their level of immunoglobulin heavy chain variable region (IGHV) gene mutations. The understanding of CLL biology has advanced with the discovery of chromosomal abnormalities and genetic mutations that contribute to the heterogeneity of the disorder and help predict its clinical course. Equally important has been the discovery of the role of the microenvironment and of the signaling mechanisms that play a key role in CLL pathogenesis.[1-4] This knowledge has led to the development of agents that specifically target dysregulated pathways. A major shift in the treatment paradigm of CLL took place with the approval of several new targeted agents with unprecedented clinical activity, particularly in patients with high-risk disease or with poor prognostic markers. Despite these rapid advances, CLL remains incurable and patients who initially achieve a remission will eventually develop disease recurrence. Current efforts are geared toward the development of novel therapeutics that target the complex biology of CLL with the goal of achieving a cure.

Incidence and epidemiology

CLL is the most common type of leukemia in adults in the United States accounting for more than a third of all leukemias. Approximately 21,040 new cases of CLL and 4060 deaths are expected in the United States in 2020.[5] For the most part, CLL is a disease of the elderly, with a median age of 70 years at diagnosis. The male : female incidence ratio of CLL is approximately 1.5 : 1. CLL is more common in western Europe,[6] Australia,[7] and North America[8] than in Asia[9,10] or Africa.

Diagnosis of CLL

The World Health Organization (WHO) classification of hematopoietic tumors describes CLL as a leukemic, lymphocytic lymphoma, distinguishable from small lymphocytic lymphoma (SLL) only by its leukemic presentation.[11] The International Workshop on CLL (iwCLL) established the diagnosis of CLL as requiring the presence of at least 5×10^9/L clonal B lymphocytes/L (5000/μL) in the peripheral blood confirmed by flow cytometry and sustained for at least 3 months.[12] Peripheral blood smear review reveals small, mature lymphocytes with a narrow border of cytoplasm. Gumprecht nuclear shadows, a.k.a. "smudge cells" can be found as debris (Figure 1). The disease frequently involves the bone marrow (Figure 2).

Pathogenesis and causation

Monoclonal B-cell lymphocytosis and familial CLL

The absence of cytopenias, lymphadenopathy, organomegaly, or disease-related symptoms ("B symptoms") in the presence of fewer than 5×10^9 clonal B lymphocytes/L in the peripheral blood is defined as "monoclonal B-lymphocytosis" (MBL).[13] MBL was further subclassified into "low count" ($<0.5 \times 10^9$/L clonal B cells) and "high count" ($\geq 0.5 \times 10^9$/L clonal B cells) based on the observation of a bimodal distribution with notable differences in progression to CLL requiring treatment and risk of hospitalizations.[14,15] Rawstron and colleagues[16] found MBL among 13.5% of normal first-degree relatives of people known to have CLL. That incidence is much higher than the 3.5% prevalence amongst adults with normal blood counts without a first-degree relative with CLL.[17] There is an increased incidence of CLL and/or related disorders amongst family members of people with a CLL diagnosis,[18,19] though a specific gene or inheritance mechanism has yet to be identified. CLL requiring therapy develops in patients with CLL-phenotype MBL and lymphocytosis at the rate of 1.1–1.4% per year.[14,16]

Immunobiology and immunophenotype of CLL cells

Morphologically, CLL cells resemble mature lymphocytes in the normal peripheral blood but co-express the T-cell antigen CD5 with in addition to the B-cell surface antigens CD19, CD20, and CD23. The levels of surface immunoglobulin, CD20, and CD79b are characteristically low compared with those found on normal B cells,[20] with the clones restricted to expression of either kappa or lambda immunoglobulin light chains. Several other malignancies of mature-appearing lymphocytes present with clinical features overlapping those of CLL, hence flow cytometry and genomic mutations are required to distinguish CLL from other diseases (Table 1).[21,22]

Clinical presentation

By iwCLL criteria,[12] the presence of at least 5×10^9/L B clonal lymphocytes per liter (5,000/L) with the phenotype CD19+, CD20+, CD23+, and CD5+ is required to diagnose CLL, as lymphocytosis may occur with infectious, inflammatory, reactive, or other neoplastic conditions (e.g., leukemic phase of lymphomas, hairy cell leukemia, prolymphocytic leukemia (Figure 3), and large granular lymphocytic leukemia).

Holland-Frei Cancer Medicine, Tenth Edition. Edited by Robert C. Bast, John C. Byrd, Carlo M. Croce, Ernest Hawk, Fadlo R. Khuri, Raphael E. Pollock, Apostolia M. Tsimberidou, Christopher G. Willett, and Cheryl L. Willman.
© 2023 John Wiley & Sons, Inc. Published 2023 by John Wiley & Sons, Inc.

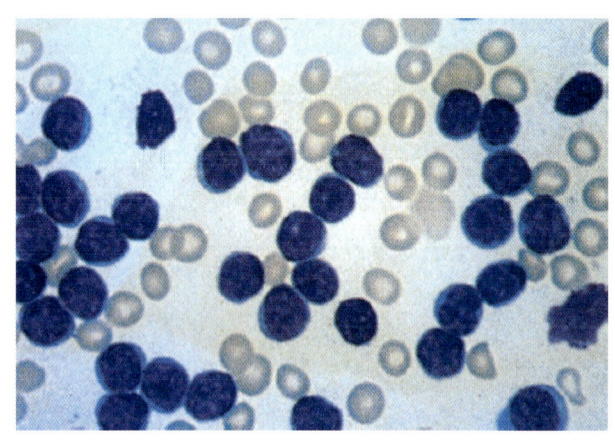

Figure 1 Chronic lymphocytic leukemia morphology in peripheral blood smear. Leukocyte count: 100×10^9/L. Most of the lymphocytes are mature-appearing. One smudge cell is present. Platelets are absent in this thrombocytopenic patient (Wright-Giemsa stain; ×100 original magnification).

Table 1 Phenotypes of lymphoproliferative disorders.

Disease	Typical phenotypes
CLL	**CD20 (d)**, CD19+, CD22 (d), **sIg (d)**, **CD23+**, FMC-7−, **CD5+**, CD10−, CD38, **CD200**
Mantle cell lymphoma	CD20 (i), **sIg (i)**, CD23+/−, FMC-7+/−, **CD5+**, CD10−, **cyclin-D1**
B-prolymphocytic leukemia	CD20 (+i), **sIg (+i)**, FMC-7+/−, CD5+/−, CD10−, CD19+
Marginal zone B-cell lymphoma	**CD23−**, CD11c+/−, CD103+/−, **CD5+/−**, **CD10−**, CD19+, **CD79a+**, CD138 (b)
Lymphoplasmacytic lymphoma	**CD23(−/d)**, sIg+/−, **cIg+**, CD5+/−
Follicular lymphoma	CD20 (+i), CD5−, **CD10+**, CD19+, **bcl-2+**, CD43−
Diffuse large B-cell lymphoma	**CD20 (+i)**, **CD5−** CD10+/−, bcl-2+/−, CD43+/− CD5+/−
Burkitt's lymphoma	Bcl-2−, CD10 (+b), CD43+ CD5−
Hairy cell leukemia	CD20 (b), CD22 (b), **CD11c (b)**, **CD25+**, **CD103+**, sIg (i), **CD123+**, **CD5−**

Abbreviations: +, usually positive; −, usually negative; +/−, may be positive or negative; d, dim; i, intermediate; b, bright; sIg, surface immunoglobulin; cIg, cytoplasmic immunoglobulin.

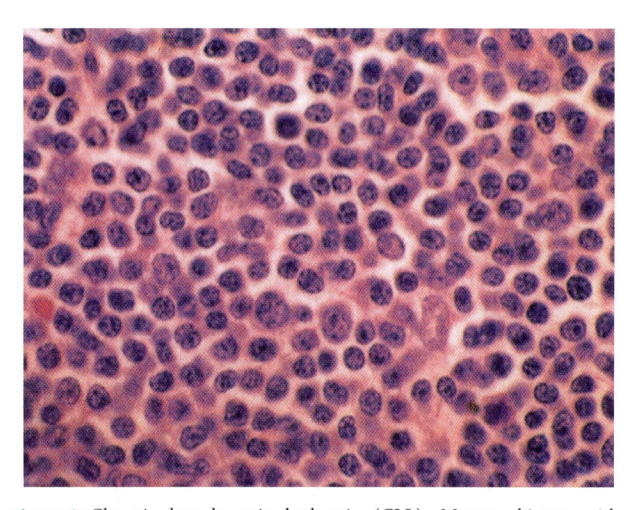

Figure 2 Chronic lymphocytic leukemia (CLL). Marrow biopsy with diffuse infiltration by CLL cells (hematoxylin and eosin stain; ×600 original magnification).

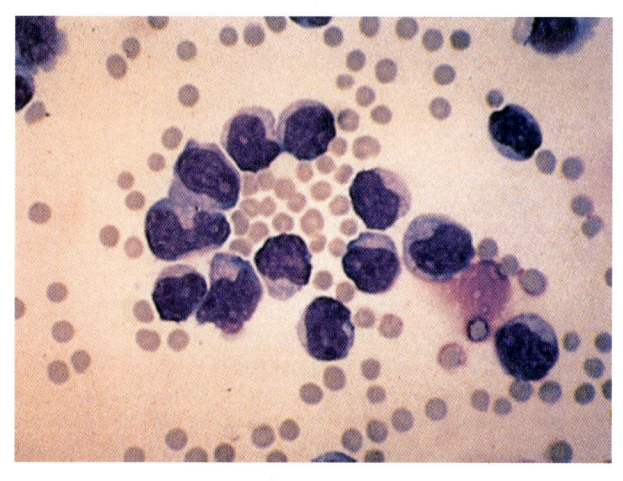

Figure 3 Prolymphocytic leukemia. Peripheral blood smear shows cells with prominent nucleoli and abundant cytoplasm (Wright-Giemsa stain; ×1000 original magnification).

CLL patients infrequently present with constitutional symptoms at the time of diagnosis. The onset of the classic symptoms known as "B symptoms" (unintentional weight loss of 10% or more, fevers higher than 100.5 °F (38 °C), or night sweats for more than one month without evidence of infection) requires work-up to rule out other underlying conditions such as infections or rheumatological conditions. The presence of severe fatigue should always be investigated and not attributed to the CLL diagnosis.

Upon physical examination, a patient may have enlarged nodes in CLL are firm, rounded, discrete, nontender, and freely mobile upon palpation. The most consistent abnormal finding on physical examination is lymphadenopathy, but palpable splenomegaly or hepatomegaly may also be present. Lymph node enlargement may be generalized or localized, and the degree can vary widely leading to obstruction of adjacent organs. Similar to several histopathologic subtypes of non-Hodgkin's lymphomas, the lymph nodes frequently wax and wane. In addition to palpably enlarged peripheral lymph nodes, liver, and spleen, virtually any other lymphoid tissue in the body—for example, Waldeyer's ring or the tonsils—may be enlarged at diagnosis. CLL cells may infiltrate any organ or tissue and cause symptoms. Leptomeningeal involvement is extremely unusual.

Radiologic findings

Radiologic examinations are neither required nor recommended as part of an evaluation at the time of initial diagnosis or during routine follow-up unless there is an area of concern per iwCLL guidelines.[12] Computed tomography (CT) scans or chest films, if performed, often reveal adenopathy not detected on examination, but these findings do not change the clinical Rai or Binet stage. In the setting of a research protocol, imaging may be obtained for specific protocol-related purposes. The justification for radiation exposure should be weighed against the potential benefits that could derive from obtaining the imaging study.

Laboratory abnormalities

Although the absolute blood lymphocyte threshold for diagnosing CLL was arbitrarily placed at 5×10^9/L, clinical MBL and CLL fall upon a continuum with most patients presenting with considerably higher counts of lymphocytes. Upon examination of a peripheral blood smear, mature-appearing small lymphocytes may be the prominent leukocytes, ranging from 50% to 100%.

Asymptomatic anemia and/or thrombocytopenia may be observed at the time of initial diagnosis, but usually these are relatively mild. Although direct antiglobulin (Coombs) test may be positive, overt autoimmune hemolytic anemia at diagnosis is not frequent. Autoimmune cytopenias are diagnosed on the basis of the presence of adequate numbers of precursors in the bone marrow with an abnormally low cell count.

Hypogammaglobulinemia is the most predominant inherent immune defect in CLL patients. All three immunoglobulin classes (IgG, IgA, and IgM) are usually decreased, though in some patients only one or two classes may be reduced. Concurrent hypogammaglobulinemia and neutropenia result in increased vulnerability of CLL patients to severe bacterial, viral, and opportunistic infections. Since a large proportion of cells are B lymphocytes, the normal lymphocyte T : B ratio (2 : 1) is altered. As these patients are not immunocompetent, they should avoid inoculation of live vaccines (varicella, measles, etc.) due to the possibility of viral replication after administration leading to an active infection.[23]

No abnormalities in blood chemistry are characteristic of CLL, but increased levels of serum lactate dehydrogenase, uric acid, hepatic enzymes [alanine aminotransferase (ALT) or aspartate aminotransferase (AST)], and (rarely) calcium may be observed. Pseudohyperkalemia can occur occasionally in patients with leukocytosis or when blood is not processed promptly.

Natural history

It is a generally held belief that CLL is an indolent disease with a prolonged chronic course and that the eventual cause of death may be co-morbidities unrelated to CLL; however, this observation is true for fewer than 30% of all CLL cases. The natural history is heterogeneous in most patients, with many patients living for 5–10 years with an initial benign course until they develop indications to start CLL directed therapy. During the initial asymptomatic phase, the patients are able to maintain their usual lifestyle. In the era of chemotherapy-free regimens, patients can have an improvement in quality of life[24] while on active treatment. The sequencing of novel agents has also allowed for improvement in progression free survival (PFS) while avoiding the use of chemoimmunotherapy.[25] Despite these advances in patients with progressive disease, the cause(s) of death are related to CLL.

Patients with high risk MBL and CLL have been found to have over twice the risk of developing another malignancy compared to the general population[26–29] Skin cancers and other neoplasms occur with considerably greater frequency among CLL patients. We recommend that all CLL patients (including treatment-naive) adhere to age-appropriate cancer screening guidelines.

Clinical staging and other prognostic features

Historically, two staging criteria, the Rai[30] system and the Binet[31] system, are widely used in clinical practice due to their simplicity (only a physical exam and a complete blood count are needed) and accuracy in predicting outcomes. The Rai staging system is based on the presence of lymphocytosis, lymphadenopathy, splenomegaly, anemia (hemoglobin <11 g/dL), and thrombocytopenia (platelets <100 × 10^9/L), with the score increasing (Stage 0–4) with each additional clinical feature. Binet's method classifies all patients with anemia (defined as hemoglobin below 10 g/dL) and/or thrombocytopenia (platelets <100 × 10^9/L), or both, as stage C. All of the remaining (non-C) patients are divided

Table 2 Molecular and cytogenetic markers of prognosis in CLL.

	Markers of	
	Good prognosis	Worse prognosis
IGHV mutation status	Mutated	Unmutated
FISH cytogenetics	13q del	11q del[a], 17p del
Karyotype		Complex (>3–5 abnormalities)
Next generation sequencing		TP53, ATM, SF3B1, NOTCH1

[a]Based on long-term data from chemoimmunotherapy trials.

into two groups, depending on the presence of fewer than three (stage A) or three or more (stage B) sites of palpable enlargement of lymphoid organs. This staging takes into consideration five sites: cervical, axillary, and inguinal lymph nodes (whether unilateral or bilateral, each area is counted as one), and the spleen and liver. This system has been found to be of great value in dividing patients into three types of survival curves, with A, B, and C corresponding, respectively, to Rai's low-, intermediate-, and high-risk groups.

Major prognostic markers

Major prognostic markers of considerable importance to stratify risk in this heterogeneous disease include chromosomal aberrations, IGHV mutation status, complex karyotype (≥3 abnormalities) and genetic mutations (Table 2). Additional prognostic factors that have been tested and found to be useful in predicting the course of disease include age, gender, comorbidities,[29] and β-2-microglobulin.

IGHV gene mutation

Two main subgroups of CLL are recognized based on the presence or absence of mutations in the IGHV gene that is expressed by leukemic B cells.[32] Patients with IGHV mutated genes tend to have a milder form of the disease, better progression-free and overall survival (OS).[33,34] This may be explained in part by the fact that B-cell receptors (BCRs) of unmutated CLL cases transduce stimulatory downstream signals with greater capacity than those of mutated cells.[35] Patients with or without IGVH mutations may be further subclassified based on other significant findings, such as the presence or absence of mutations in TP53,[36] NOTCH1,[37] SF3B1,[29] ZAP-70 protein expression,[38] and CD38,[33] all of which have been shown to have an impact on the clinical course of the disease.

Cytogenetics

Cytogenetic analysis of CLL used to be limited because of an inability to induce metaphases in the leukemic cells with conventional banding techniques. Using interphase fluorescence in situ hybridization (FISH) technique, chromosomal aberrations can be detected in 82% of cases.[36] A seminal study by Döhner and colleagues found the following common lesions and frequencies in CLL patients: deletion in 13q14 (55%), deletion in 11q (18%), trisomy of 12q (16%), deletion in 17p (7%), and deletion in 6q in 7%.[39] In the same study, normal karyotypes were present in 18% of patients. Among the abnormalities, del(13q), del(11q), and del(17q) were considered to have the greatest significance. Deletion in 13q correlates with the best median OS at 133 months. Patients with deletion of either 11q or 17p have the poorest prognosis with a median OS of 79 and 32 months, respectively. Loss of 11q and 17p are believed to involve alteration of the gene encoding for the ataxia-telangiectasia mutation, and inactivation of the tumor suppressor gene p53, respectively. Other genes are deleted from these regions and may contribute to the pathogenesis as well. These high-risk lesions were found to be associated with aggressive disease and resistance to chemotherapy.[40] Patients with normal karyotypes and patients with trisomy 12 have similar survival times of 111 and 114 months, respectively. Recent studies with targeted agents have confirmed deletion 17p continues to confer a poor prognosis,[41] though other cytogenetic markers carry less prognostic value with these treatments.

Molecular genetics

A range of genetic mutations has been found to have prognostic implications in CLL. Somatic mutations in the tumor suppressor gene TP53 are one of the most frequent alterations in several human cancers. This mutation is known to be associated with poor prognosis. The German CLL Study Group (GCLLSG) found that 8.5% of previously untreated CLL patients had the p53 mutation, and some of these even in the absence of a 17p deletion.[36] Patients with a p53 mutation have a poor prognosis regardless of whether 17p is deleted, and its presence is associated with poor response to therapy, short PFS and OS. Moreover, in a multivariate analysis, TP53 mutations analysis provided prognostic value beyond the recognized adverse genetic factors mentioned earlier in the chapter.[42] Additional mutations with prognostic significance in CLL include those in NOTCH1[43] and SF3B1 genes,[29] both of which have been associated with a shortened survival.[44] NOTCH1 is also associated with a higher risk of Richter's transformation.[45]

Treatment

Though early intervention is considered crucial in most malignant diseases, this is not the case in CLL. Early intervention with chemoimmunotherapy has not demonstrated an improvement in survival, and thus the current standard remains "active surveillance"[46] that is follow- approximately every 3–4 months (sooner if there are indications of progressive disease) with a history, physical exam, and complete blood counts. Early intervention trials are underway to determine if chemotherapy-free regimens will lead to improved outcomes in patients with asymptomatic high-risk disease.[47] Currently this approach is not recommended outside of a clinical trial.

Chemoimmunotherapy with the regimens fludarabine/cyclophosphamide/rituximab (FCR) and bendamustine/rituximab (BR) were considered the standard of care up until recently. The approval of small molecules targeting the BCR signaling pathway and the BCL2 inhibitor venetoclax have changed the treatment landscape.

Treatment options available for frontline and salvage therapy in CLL are shown in Tables 3 and 4, respectively.

iwCLL guidelines to initiate therapy

Indications to initiate CLL directed therapies are summarized in Table 5. Enlarging lymph nodes and/or rapid lymphocyte doubling should be assessed cautiously given that such events can be transient. No data exist establishing a particular threshold of lymphocyte count that warrants treatment as leukostasis events are rare in CLL.

Table 3 Front-line regimens for chronic lymphocytic leukemia.

Patient population	Treatment options
Patients ≤70 years of age or older fit patients without significant comorbidities and without del(17p)	• Ibrutinib ± rituximab • Ibrutinib ± obinutuzumab • Acalabrutinib + obinutuzumab • Venetoclax ± obinutuzumab • Fludarabine + cyclophosphamide + rituximab • Clinical trial
Patients aged ≥70 years or younger patients with comorbidities without del(17p)	• Ibrutinib ± rituximab • Ibrutinib ± obinutuzumab • Venetoclax + obinutuzumab • Acalabrutinib ± obinutuzumab • Clinical trial
Patients with del(17p)	• Clinical trial • Ibrutinib ± rituximab • Ibrutinib ± obinutuzumab • Acalabrutinib + obinutuzumab • Venetoclax ± obinutuzumab

Table 4 Salvage therapy for relapsed chronic lymphocytic leukemia.

Patient population	Treatment options
Frontline treatment with chemoimmunotherapy	• Ibrutinib • Acalabrutinib • Venetoclax ± rituximab • Idelalisib ± rituximab • Duvelisib • Clinical trial
Frontline treatment with BTK inhibitor	• Venetoclax ± anti-CD20 antibody • Idelalisib ± rituximab • Alternative BTKi (if discontinuation not due to progression; e.g., BTK and/or PLCγ mutations present) • Duvelisib (after two prior lines of therapy) • Clinical trial
Frontline treatment with venetoclax-based regimen	• Ibrutinib ± anti-CD20 antibody • Acalabrutinib ± anti-CD20 antibody • Idelalisib ± rituximab • Duvelisib • Clinical trial

Goals of therapy

Choosing the optimal treatment for an individual patient depends on the age, functional status, and genetic aberrations. Traditionally, treatment of CLL continued until symptoms resolved or troubling lymphadenopathy was controlled. With the advent of the anti-CD20 monoclonal antibody rituximab (and its addition to a chemotherapy backbone) came the observation that undetectable minimal residual disease–negative (uMRD) complete responses (CRs) improved PFS and OS[48]; therefore criteria to define complete remission and uMRD were developed.[12]

Nevertheless, creating a clear algorithm for CLL treatment is difficult because of the heterogeneity of the disease, the prevalence of comorbidities in the CLL population, and evolving therapeutic endpoints. Although a complete remission and uMRD may be desirable endpoints, in some cases these are not appropriate goals. Clinicians must match the profiles of the patient to one of the available therapies and set a realistic therapeutic goal.

Table 5 iwCLL 2018 indications for treatment.

Progressive marrow failure as evidenced by development or worsening anemia <10 g/dL or thrombocytopenia <100,000/L
Massive or progressive symptomatic splenomegaly
Massive lymph nodes (>10 cm) or progressive, symptomatic lymphadenopathy
Rapidly increasing lymphocytosis defined as an increase in 50% over a 2-month period or a lymphocyte doubling time of <6 months
Autoimmune complications (anemia, thrombocytopenia) poorly responsive to corticosteroids
Symptomatic extranodal involvement
Constitutional symptoms: • Unintentional weight loss >10% within 6 months   • Progressive fatigue   • Fevers >100.5 °F for >2 weeks without another cause   • Night sweats for >1 month without alternative etiology   • ECOG >2 if progressive/worsening

Table 6 iwCLL 2018 response criteria.

Response	Clinical (factors)	Laboratory parameters
Complete response	• No lymph nodes ≥1.5 cm • Spleen <13 cm; normal liver size • Absence of constitutional symptoms	• Normal circulating lymphocyte count • Platelet count ≥100 × 10^{-9}/L • Hemoglobin ≥11.0 g/dL (untransfused without erythropoiten) • BMBX: normocellular marrow without CLL cells or B-lymphoid nodules
Partial response	• Decrease in lymphadenopathy ≥50% from baseline • Decrease in hepatosplenomegaly by ≥50% from baseline • Presence of constitutional symptoms	• Decrease ≥50% in circulating lymphocyte count from baseline • Platelet count ≥100 × 10^{-9}/L or increase ≥50% from baseline • Hemoglobin ≥11.0 g/dL increase ≥50% from baseline • BMBX: presence of CLL cells, B-lymphoid nodules or marrow not performed
Stable disease	• Change in lymphadenopathy of −49 to +49% from baseline • Change of −49 to +49% in hepatosplenomegaly from baseline • Presence of constitutional symptoms	• Change of −49 to +49% of Circulating lymphocyte count from baseline • Circulating lymphocyte count from baseline • Platelet count change of −49 to +49% • Hemoglobin ≥11.0 g/dL increase ≤50% from baseline or decrease <2 g/dL • BMBX: no change in marrow infiltrate
Progressive disease	• Increase in lymph node size ≥50% from baseline or from response • Increase in hepatosplenomegaly ≥50% from baseline or from response • Presence of constitutional symptoms	• Increase in circulating lymphocytosis ≥50% from baseline • Decrease in platelets ≥50% from baseline secondary to CLL • Decrease of ≥2 g/dL from baseline secondary to CLL • BMBMX: increase in CLL ells by ≥50% on successive biopsies

Small molecules that target the BCR pathway required a recent update of the previously established response criteria in order to incorporate the "redistribution phenomenon" seen with these novel agents.[49] BCR inhibitors exert their effects by mobilizing CLL cells from the bone marrow and the lymph nodes into the peripheral blood with increased lymphocytosis. The BCL-2 inhibitor venetoclax has been approved for therapy in CLL, which exerts its mechanism by increasing apoptosis of CLL cells, thus tumor lysis syndrome (TLS) can occur and requires close monitoring.[50]

Response criteria to treatment

Response criteria are summarized in Table 6.

The new concept of "partial response with lymphocytosis" (PRL) requires that all PR criteria are met except for the blood lymphocyte count. In the absence of other objective evidence of progression of disease (PD), lymphocytosis alone should not be considered an indicator of PD. Patients with lymphocytosis and no other evidence of PD should continue therapy until they develop definitive signs of PD.[49]

Minimal residual disease (MRD) eradication refers to the complete eradication of leukemic cells by either flow cytometry (four up to ten color), allele-specific oligonucleotide polymerase chain reaction (PCR), or by next generation to level of 10^{-4}/L.[12] This determination is made at different intervals depending on treatment, but usually is measured at the end of fixed duration treatments. MRD testing is still under study and should be used in the setting of clinical trials. Whereas absence of MRD may indicate a more favorable prognosis in the setting of chemoimmunotherapy and several targeted agents, it's use as both a prognostic tool and therapeutic endpoint is still under study.

Chlorambucil

Chlorambucil is a treatment option for frail and older patients given its ease of use and tolerability.[51] Despite this, it is associated with lower response rates and shorter remission durations compared to other available agents. It can be used as a monotherapy or in combination with an anti-CD20 antibody which has shown improved outcomes and has been used as the control arm for several landmark clinical trials (as detailed in sections below).

Fludarabine–cyclophosphamide–rituximab (FCR)

FCR remains a standard of care for upfront treatment of medically fit CLL patients who have mutated IGHV (M-IGHV).

A single-arm study successfully treated 224 treatment-naïve patients with FCR.[52] The overall response rate (ORR) was 95% with 72% of these patients achieving CR and many achieving MRD negativity. Long term follow-up has demonstrated that patients with mutated IGVH who have uMRD have a prolong PFS, over a decade later.[53,54]

A well-designed, phase III trial of 817 previously untreated patients by the GCLLSG evaluated the benefit of adding rituximab to fludarabine-cyclophosphamide (FC) establishing FCR's superiority.[55] At a median of 47 months follow-up, a superior PFS was maintained in patients receiving FCR compared with FC (57.9 vs 32.9 months, respectively; $p < 0.001$). The FCR arm had a greater incidence of neutropenia, but not of grade 3 or 4 infections. FCR as well as other purine analog-alkylator-rituximab regimens should be given with antibiotic prophylaxis against *Pneumocystis*, varicella, and *Candida*. Recently, FCR was compared to ibrutinib–rituximab (IR) for untreated CLL in patients <70 years in the E1912 study. In shorter follow-up, IR demonstrated an improvement in progression free and OS (see details under section titled "Ibrutinib").

Bendamustine–rituximab

The Food and Drug Administration (FDA) approved bendamustine in 2008 for relapsed/refractory CLL.[56] The Phase III CLL10 trial tested frontline BR compared to FCR in fit patients except 17p deletion patients. Although the ORR was identical in both treatment arms (97.8%), CR was greater in FCR-treated patients and correlated with longer PFS. No difference in OS was observed. Patients receiving FCR experienced significantly greater rates of grade 3/4 adverse events (AEs) including severe neutropenia, myelosuppression, and infections compared with patients receiving BR. Given the milder toxicity profile of BR, this combination may have a role in the upfront treatment of medically unfit CLL patients.[57] In the Phase III A047102 trial, BR was compared to ibrutinib and IR. Both ibrutinib and IR demonstrated an improvement in PFS compared to BR[58] (although there was no difference between the two ibrutinib-containing arms). (Further details under the section titled "Ibrutinib.")

Anti-CD20 monoclonal antibodies

Rituximab is the first anti-CD20 antibody used for management of CLL and its autoimmune complications. It's use for the treatment of CLL has decreased after being shown to be less effective than obinutuzumab in the CLL11 trial. Obinutuzumab is a humanized monoclonal antibody targeting CD20 indicated in combination with chlorambucil for the treatment of previously untreated patients with CLL. Previously untreated patients with CLL were randomized to receive chlorambucil against chlorambucil plus rituximab against chlorambucil plus obinutuzumab.[59] Goede and colleagues found that, in patients with multiple debilitating coexisting conditions, the combination of obinutuzumab with chlorambucil was associated with a significant and clinically meaningful prolongation of PFS, increased CR, and an increased rate of uMRD, as compared with the results with a combination of rituximab and chlorambucil. Moreover, treatment with obinutuzumab plus chlorambucil resulted in a significant OS benefit as compared with chlorambucil alone suggesting that the induction of deeper remissions could translate into a survival advantage even in frail patients. Studies in combination with Bruton's tyrosine kinase (BTK) inhibitors will be discussed in the next section.

BTK inhibitors

Ibrutinib

Ibrutinib is a first in class, orally bioavailable, small-molecule, irreversible inhibitor of BTK that has been shown to induce rapid lymph node responses in patients with CLL. As with other kinase inhibitors developed to treat patients with CLL, ibrutinib inhibits several signaling pathways, including BCR, Toll-like receptors, B cell activating factor (BAFF), and CD40, as well as interfering with the protective effect of stromal cells.[2] In an early phase Ib/II clinical trial, treatment with ibrutinib as monotherapy for patients with relapsed/refractory CLL resulted in a high ORR of 71% and durable remissions (estimated PFS at 26 months: 75%) for all groups of patients tested, including elderly patients and those with high-risk disease.[60] Seven-year follow-up indicated long-lasting response to ibrutinib.[61] In the phase III RESONATE trial, ibrutinib was compared with ofatumumab in patients with relapsed/refractory CLL/SLL.[62] The ORRs were 4.1% and 42.6% in patients receiving ofatumumab and ibrutinib, respectively. Outcomes were independent of 17p status and were seen even in patient's refractory to purine analogs. At a median follow up of 44 months, PFS was significantly longer for ibrutinib compared to ofatumumab (hazard radio [HR] 0.133; 95% confidence interval [CI] 0.099–0.178) and median PFS was not reach for the ibrutinib arm compared to 8.1 months for ofatumumab. The most recent update of this data has confirmed the PFS benefit at >5 years of follow up. Minimal toxicities were reported.

In the largest prospective trial dedicated to the study of del 17p, ibrutinib demonstrated marked efficacy in terms of ORR and PFS, with a favorable risk-benefit profile.[63] At a median follow up of 13 months, 79.3% of patients remained progression-free at 12 months, consistent with efficacy observed in earlier studies.[64] The PFS in this previously treated population compares favorably to that of treatment-naïve del 17p CLL patients receiving FCR with a median PFS of 11 months. Long-term follow-up has confirmed these results, supporting ibrutinib as an effective therapy for patients with deletion 17p CLL/SLL.[65]

Two pivotal trials confirmed the benefit of upfront treatment with ibrutinib in older patients (age ≥65–70 years) compared to chemotherapy. The A047102 trial compared ibrutinib to IR and to BR in patients over the age of 65.[58] PFS was longer for both ibrutinib-containing arms compared to BR, though OS is similar for the three cohorts. The iLLUMINATE trial tested ibrutinib in combination with obinutuzumab versus chlorambucil–obinutuzumab in patients older than 65 or in patients younger than 65 with comorbidities making them unsuitable for fludarabine-based regimens.[66] Similar to A047102 trial, PFS was longer for ibrutinib–obinutuzumab, with higher overall and CR rates in the ibrutinib–obinutuzumab arm. These two trials have led to the recommendation in the United States to use ibrutinib for first line treatment of CLL in older patients or those with medical comorbidities.

The Eastern Cooperative Oncology Group (ECOG) 1912 trial randomized IR to FCR in younger patients (age <70 years) fit to receive intensive chemoimmunotherapy in a 2 : 1 ratio [IR ($n = 354$), FCR ($n = 175$)].[67] Patients with del17p were excluded from the study given the anticipated poor outcomes with FCR. After a median follow-up of 48 months both PFS and OS favored ibrutinib-based therapy, with the majority of deaths in the FCR cohort attributed to CLL progression. The majority of progression events were noted in patients who have unmutated IGHV.[68] E1912 established that young patients, especially those with unfavorable prognostic markers, should be prioritized for treatment with ibrutinib when compared to chemoimmunotherapy.

Common toxicities with ibrutinib treatment include self-limited diarrhea, arthralgias/myalgias, hypertension, cytopenias, and increased bruising. More serious complications with ibrutinib include cardiac arrythmias and increased risk of bleeding, including gastrointestinal bleeding, central nervous systems (CNS) bleeding, and retroperitoneal bleeds. Sudden cardiac deaths have also been reported. Cardiac comorbidities do not preclude treatment with ibrutinib, though there is no consensus about optimizing its use, hence careful consideration and co-management with cardiology is recommended.

Acalabrutinib

Acalabrutinib is a second generation non-covalent oral BTK inhibitor. It is more specific for BTK and has fewer alternative target effects, including less inhibition of interleukin-2-inducible T cell kinase (ITK), TEC protein kinase (TEC), and epidermal growth factor receptor (EGFR).[69,70] In the ELEVATE-TN trial,[71] patients were randomized to receive acalabrutinib monotherapy, acalabrutinib–obinutuzumab, or chlorambucil–obinutuzumab. At a median follow up of 28.3 months, the median PFS was not reached for both acalabrutinib arms. The estimated 24-month PFS was 93% in the acalabrutinib–obinutuzumab arm, 87% for acalabrutinib, and 47% for chlorambucil–obinutuzumab. Best ORR/CR was 94%/13% for acalabrutinib–obinutuzumab, 86%/1% for acalabrutinib, and 79%/5% for chlorambucil–obinutuzumab.

The Phase 3 ASCEND trial, patients with relapsed/refractory CLL who had received a minimum of two prior lines of therapy were randomized to receive acalabrutinib or investigator's choice (idelalisib–rituximab or BR).[72] Patients were randomized to acalabrutinib ($n = 155$), idelalisib–rituximab ($n = 119$), and BR ($n = 36$). At a median follow up of 16.1 months, median PFS was not reach with acalabrutinib compared to investigators choice (16.5 months). OS was not reached in either arm. Headaches, neutropenia, anemia, and pneumonia were the most common AE for patients treated with acalabrutinib. Patients also had fewer serious AEs compared to patients treated with idelalisib–rituximab.

Like ibrutinib, acalabrutinib is overall well-tolerated. In clinical trials, the most common side effects were headache, diarrhea, bruising, arthralgias/myalgias, and neutropenia. There were few severe infections. Rates of atrial fibrillation have been reported ~3%. A Phase 3 non-inferiority trial comparing ibrutinib versus acalabrutinib is ongoing, which will help answer whether there is a difference in the toxicity profile.

PI3K inhibitors

Idelalisib

Idelalisib is a targeted, highly selective oral inhibitor of phosphoinositide 3-kinase delta, an isoform with selective leukocyte expression that promotes the survival and proliferation of malignant B cells.[73,74] A randomized, double-blind, placebo-controlled phase III trial of rituximab with or without idelalisib in patients with relapsed/refractory CLL was stopped early following recommendations by an independent data and safety monitoring committee. Patients receiving idelalisib plus rituximab had an ORR of 81% compared with rituximab monotherapy ORR of 13%.[73,75] Idelalisib plus rituximab was effective for patients regardless of the presence of 17p, TP53, or IGHV mutational status.

Based on this study, idelalisib was approved for relapsed/refractory patients. Clinical trials for its use in frontline treatment were halted early due to toxicity, including colitis, transaminitis, infections (including *Pneumocystis jirovecii* pneumonia), and febrile neutropenia.[76]

Duvelisib

Duvelisib is an oral PI3K inhibitor that targets both the δ and γ isoforms. By blocking both isoforms, duvelisib is able to disrupt the growth and survival of malignant B cells, while also inhibiting the recruitment and differentiation of T cells which support the tumor microenvironment.[77] In the Phase 3 DUO trial, patients with relapsed refractory CLL (treated with a minimum two prior lines of therapy) were randomized to receive duvelisib ($n = 160$) or ofatumumab ($n = 159$).[78] At a median follow up of 22.4 months, median PFS for the duvelisib arm was longer than the comparator, with a higher ORR in the duvelisib arm (73.8% vs 45.3%), though this was associated to more toxicity. The most common AEs for duvelisib were diarrhea (including colitis), neutropenia, anemia, thrombocytopenia.

BCL2 inhibitor

Venetoclax

Venetoclax is a specific, potent, oral inhibitor of BCL-2. In the early phase clinical trials, venetoclax demonstrated impressive responses in high risk CLL, leading to its initial approval for relapsed/refractory CLL with deletion 17p.[79,80] Significant tumor lysis was seen early in development leading to a dose escalation strategy over the course of 5 weeks with a starting dose of 20 mg.[81] This strategy has helped to mitigate the risk of both laboratory and clinical tumor lysis. Tumor lysis risk stratification (Table 7) was developed to determine risk of tumor lysis and guide if therapy can be started as an outpatient or if patients require hospitalization.

The Phase 3 MURANO trial which compared venetoclax-rituximab to BR. Three hundred and eighty-nine patients were randomized to receive 6 months of BR or 2 years of venetoclax plus 6 months of rituximab therapy.[82] At a median of 23.8 months, 2-year PFS was 84.9% in the venetoclax rituximab group versus 36.3% in the BR group. At 4 years, the estimated PFS were 57.3% versus 4.6%, demonstrating that time-limited treatment with venetoclax could induce deep, durable remissions. At 4 years, the median OS favor venetoclax–rituximab (85.3% vs 66.8%). uMRD at end of treatment predicts for longer 18-month PFS (90.3%) compared to low MRD (64.4%) or high MRD (8.33%). Further follow up and data is needed to determine which patients are at high risk for early relapse after fixed duration therapy.

Table 7 Tumor lysis risk stratification for venetoclax therapy.

Risk category	Tumor burden
Low	ALC $<25 \times 10^9$/L AND
	All LN <5 cm diameter
Medium	ALC $\geq 25 \times 10^9$/L OR
	Any LN 5 to <10 cm diameter
High	Any LN ≥ 10 cm diameter OR
	Any LN ≥ 5 cm diameter AND ALC $\geq 25 \times 10^9$/L

Abbreviations: ALC, absolute lymphocyte count; LN, lymph node; cm, centimeter.

CLL14 randomized patients with significant medical comorbidities to receive a fixed duration of 1 year of treatment with venetoclax–obinutuzumab or chlorambucil-obinutuzumab.[83] At a median follow up of 28.1 months, 24-month PFS was 88.2% in the venetoclax–obinutuzumab group and 64.1% in the chlorambucil–obinutuzumab group (HR 0.39, 95% CI 0.22–0.44 $p < 0.0001$). Median OS was unreached in both arms. Three patients treated with venetoclax–obinutuzumab had laboratory evidence of TLS during treatment with obinutuzumab, and there were no clinical TLS events during venetoclax ramp up. The most common hematologic toxicity with venetoclax was neutropenia, with few episodes of febrile neutropenia. Further follow-up to determine the duration of remission and time to next treatment is needed.

Corticosteroids

Currently, the major indication for prednisone is for the management of autoimmune hemolytic anemia and immune thrombocytopenia. Steroids can also be effective for end of life palliation and treating tumor flare that can arise when BTK inhibitors are discontinued.

Cellular therapies

Hematopoietic stem cell transplant

Although allogeneic hematopoietic stem cell transplantation (allo-HSCT) is the treatment of choice for many aggressive hematologic malignancies, the role of HSCT in CLL remains limited.[84,85] Autologous stem cell transplantation (SCT) has no clear benefit in CLL.[86] Allo-HSCTs should be reserved for very specific cases for patients with high risk disease given the high treatment-related morbidity and mortality associated with the procedure, particularly with the availability of novel targeted therapies.[87,88]

Chimeric antigen receptor T cells

Chimeric antigen receptor modified T (CART) cells were initially studied in relapsed/refractory CLL and demonstrated its ability to produce long term responses.[89,90] Several different CAR T-cell products have been studied, both with and without ibrutinib [91–94] demonstrating deep and durable responses. Further long-term follow-up is needed to determine response duration and how this approach will fare amongst an increasing number of approved regimens.

How to select a frontline therapy

Several factors are important when determining frontline treatment for CLL including age, CLL prognostic factors, comorbidities, concomitant medications, and patient preferences on treatment duration (see Table 4). The majority of patients should be offered chemotherapy-free approaches, especially those with high risk disease, as outcomes are improved with these therapies. For patients with M-IGHV, chemoimmunotherapy with FCR should be considered, as these patients could have long durations of response, although chemotherapy-free approaches are also an option. It is important to discuss long-term toxicities, including the potential of secondary leukemias. There are no data available to determine best frontline therapy, although there are ongoing trials that will address this question.

How to sequence therapies for relapsed CLL

Given the number of new therapies, one of the key unanswered questions is how to best sequence their use. Factors including prior lines of therapy, comorbid conditions, and side effect profile. There are limited prospective data to aid in these decisions, and it is unlikely that large scale trials will be performed in the near future to specifically answer these questions. A Phase 2 study demonstrated significant responses to venetoclax after progression on ibrutinib with an ORR 65% and median PFS was 24.7 months.[95] In several multicenter retrospective studies, ibrutinib and venetoclax have demonstrated similar PFS and OS when used as the first targeted agent in the relapsed refractory setting.[96] In contrast, ibrutinib has demonstrated improvement in PFS compared to idelalisib as the initial targeted agent for relapsed refractory CLL.[25]

Richter's syndrome and prolymphocytoid transformation

In 5–16% of CLL patients, a transformation to a diffuse large B-cell lymphoma occurs[97] ["Richter's transformation" or "Richter's syndrome"; (Figure 4)]. It can also rarely transform to Hodgkin lymphoma. The diagnosis of Richter's syndrome requires histopathologic examination of a lymph node which shows large B cells with high proliferative rate (high Ki-67). Positron emission tomography (PET)/CT can be utilized to guide biopsy of suspected area of transformation.[98] Richter's syndrome is associated with a rapidly progressive course with no standard of care treatment. Outcomes are poor with traditional chemoimmunotherapy including rituximab-etoposide-prednisone-vincristine-cyclophosphamide-doxorubicin (DA-R-EPOCH). Many studies are looking at the role of novel agents like venetoclax, ibrutinib, and pembrolizumab in the treatment of this disease.

Additionally, a small proportion of patients with CLL undergo "prolymphocytoid transformation," and peripheral blood morphology reveals the presence of a mixture of small mature CLL cells and prolymphocytes. Similar to a Richter's transformation, prolymphocytoid transformation has an aggressive clinical course.[99] However, PLL transformation can be treated effectively with targeted therapies for CLL (ibrutinib, acalabrutinib, and venetoclax) with good disease control.

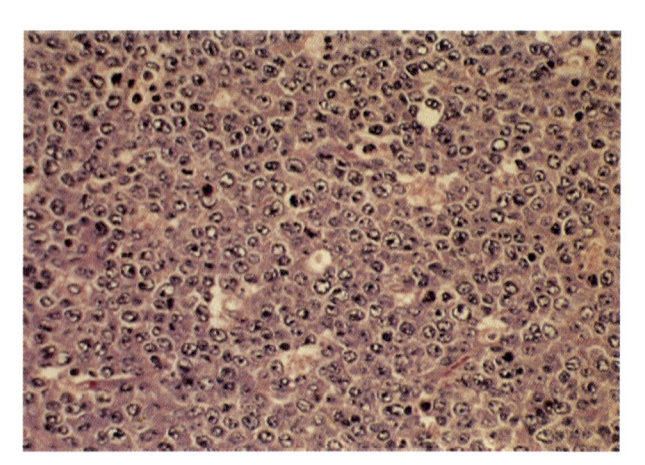

Figure 4 Chronic lymphocytic leukemia, Richter's syndrome. Section of lymph node with immunoblastic proliferation consisting of large cells with prominent nucleoli (hematoxylin and eosin stain; ×600 original magnification).

Psychosocial aspects of CLL

A diagnosis of leukemia is a major emotional challenge to patients. Careful explanation of the natural history of the disorder, emphasizing that some patients never need treatment and that early treatment has not been shown to be beneficial, is required at the time of diagnosis. Patients need to be reassured that effective treatments are available when treatment becomes necessary because of progressive disease or symptoms. Knowledge that survival in some early-stage CLL patients is the same as in the age- and gender-matched general population is comforting to patients. Explanation of newer prognostic factors must also be made with care. Favorable markers can reassure that observation is appropriate, but many patients have difficulty accepting this initial approach when the markers indicate high risk. Development of a close relationship with patients, particularly those in the early phases of disease, and careful responses to questions raised are important in providing psychological and emotional support to the patient and family. The rapidly increasing range of options for therapy, particularly for younger patients, provides a basis for optimism when treatment becomes necessary.

Unmet needs and future directions

Multiple clinical trials have proven targeted therapies improve outcomes for patients with both treatment-naive and relapsed/refractory CLL and have been incorporated into our treatment paradigm. FCR can still be considered for young patients who are M-IGHV. Cellular therapies, particularly CART cells, are under study and have the ability to further alter our treatment paradigm in the relapsed/refractory setting.

Despite the success of targeted treatments, patients with deletion 17p or TP53 mutation remain at high risk for progressive CLL. The incorporation of BTK inhibitors and venetoclax has improved outcomes (PFS and OS) in this group, but response durations and PFS are shorter compared to patients who lack these high-risk markers. Additionally, it is unclear if these patients derive more benefit from BTK inhibitors or venetoclax in the frontline setting, and this decision remains controversial. The utility of fixed-duration therapy in this subgroup is also unknown. Further studies targeting these high-risk patients are ongoing. It is important to mention that stem cell transplant evaluation should be discussed with young fit patients with high risk disease (17p deletion, failure after a novel targeted agent, short PFS after initial therapy).

The goal and duration of therapy for CLL continues to evolve that is the long-term benefit of achieving a CR or uMRD remains unproven in the era of targeted agents. Although combination strategies may offer the opportunity to overcome remaining challenges in certain CLL subgroups, individualized therapy should remain the primary endpoint. The dictum "less is more" may be the best approach for the majority of the patients affected by this disease.

Acknowledgments

Jacqueline Barrientos' work is supported in part by the 2015 American Society of Hematology-Harold Amos Medical Faculty Development Program (ASH-AMFDP) Fellowship.

Joanna Rhodes' work is supported in part by a Conquer Cancer Foundation Young Investigator Award (#15029).

Kanti Rai has been supported by grants from the Nash Family Foundation and the Karches Family Foundation.

Key references

The complete reference list can be found on Vital Source version of this title, see inside front cover.

11. Swerdlow SH, Campo E, Pileri SA, et al. The 2016 revision of the World Health Organization classification of lymphoid neoplasms. *Blood*. 2016;**127**(20):2375–2390.
12. Hallek M, Cheson BD, Catovsky D, et al. iwCLL guidelines for diagnosis, indications for treatment, response assessment, and supportive management of CLL. *Blood*. 2018;**131**(25):2745–2760.
13. Marti GE, Rawstron AC, Ghia P, et al. Diagnostic criteria for monoclonal B-cell lymphocytosis. *Br J Haematol*. 2005;**130**(3):325–332.
14. Shanafelt TD, Kay NE, Rabe KG, et al. Brief report: natural history of individuals with clinically recognized monoclonal B-cell lymphocytosis compared with patients with Rai 0 chronic lymphocytic leukemia. *J Clin Oncol*. 2009;**27**(24):3959–3963.
16. Rawstron AC, Bennett FL, O'Connor SJ, et al. Monoclonal B-cell lymphocytosis and chronic lymphocytic leukemia. *N Engl J Med*. 2008;**359**(6):575–583.
21. Pangalis GA, Angelopoulou MK, Vassilakopoulos TP, et al. B-chronic lymphocytic leukemia, small lymphocytic lymphoma, and lymphoplasmacytic lymphoma, including Waldenstrom's macroglobulinemia: a clinical, morphologic, and biologic spectrum of similar disorders. *Semin Hematol*. 1999;**36**(2):104–114.
23. Morrison VA. Infectious complications of chronic lymphocytic leukaemia: pathogenesis, spectrum of infection, preventive approaches. *Best Pract Res Clin Haematol*. 2010;**23**(1):145–153.
24. Rogers KA, Huang Y, Ruppert AS, et al. Phase II study of combination obinutuzumab, ibrutinib, and venetoclax in treatment-naive and relapsed or refractory chronic lymphocytic leukemia. *J Clin Oncol*. 2020;**38**:JCO2000491.
29. Wang L, Lawrence MS, Wan Y, et al. SF3B1 and other novel cancer genes in chronic lymphocytic leukemia. *N Engl J Med*. 2011;**365**(26):2497–2506.
30. Rai KR, Sawitsky A, Cronkite EP, et al. Clinical staging of chronic lymphocytic leukemia. *Blood*. 1975;**46**(2):219–234.
31. Binet JL, Auquier A, Dighiero G, et al. A new prognostic classification of chronic lymphocytic leukemia derived from a multivariate survival analysis. *Cancer*. 1981;**48**(1):198–206.
33. Damle RN, Wasil T, Fais F, et al. Ig V gene mutation status and CD38 expression as novel prognostic indicators in chronic lymphocytic leukemia. *Blood* 1999;**94**(6):1840–1847.
34. Hamblin TJ, Davis Z, Gardiner A, et al. Unmutated Ig V(H) genes are associated with a more aggressive form of chronic lymphocytic leukemia. *Blood*. 1999;**94**(6):1848–1854.
36. Zenz T, Eichhorst B, Busch R, et al. TP53 mutation and survival in chronic lymphocytic leukemia. *J Clin Oncol*. 2010;**28**(29):4473–4479.
39. Dohner H, Stilgenbauer S, Benner A, et al. Genomic aberrations and survival in chronic lymphocytic leukemia. *N Engl J Med*. 2000;**343**(26):1910–1916.
41. Ahn IE, Tian X, Wiestner A. Ibrutinib for chronic lymphocytic leukemia with TP53 alterations. *N Engl J Med*. 2020;**383**(5):498–500.
45. Rossi D, Rasi S, Fabbri G, et al. Mutations of NOTCH1 are an independent predictor of survival in chronic lymphocytic leukemia. *Blood*. 2012;**119**(2):521–529.
48. Bottcher S, Ritgen M, Fischer K, et al. Minimal residual disease quantification is an independent predictor of progression-free and overall survival in chronic lymphocytic leukemia: a multivariate analysis from the randomized GCLLSG CLL8 trial. *J Clin Oncol*. 2012;**30**(9):980–988.
53. Thompson PA, Tam CS, O'Brien SM, et al. Fludarabine, cyclophosphamide, and rituximab treatment achieves long-term disease-free survival in IGHV-mutated chronic lymphocytic leukemia. *Blood*. 2016;**127**(3):303–309.
54. Fischer K, Bahlo J, Fink AM, et al. Long-term remissions after FCR chemoimmunotherapy in previously untreated patients with CLL: updated results of the CLL8 trial. *Blood*. 2016;**127**(2):208–215.
57. Eichhorst B, Fink AM, Bahlo J, et al. First-line chemoimmunotherapy with bendamustine and rituximab versus fludarabine, cyclophosphamide, and rituximab in patients with advanced chronic lymphocytic leukaemia (CLL10): an international, open-label, randomised, phase 3, non-inferiority trial. *Lancet Oncol*. 2016;**17**(7):928–942.
58. Woyach JA, Ruppert AS, Heerema NA, et al. Ibrutinib regimens versus chemoimmunotherapy in older patients with untreated CLL. *N Engl J Med*. 2018;**379**(26):2517–2528.
59. Goede V, Fischer K, Engelke A, et al. Obinutuzumab as frontline treatment of chronic lymphocytic leukemia: updated results of the CLL11 study. *Leukemia*. 2015;**29**(7):1602–1604.
61. Byrd JC, Furman RR, Coutre S, et al. Up to 7 years of follow-up of single-agent ibrutinib in the phase 1b/2 PCYC-1102 trial of first line and relapsed/refractory patients with chronic lymphocytic leukemia/small lymphocytic lymphoma. *Blood*. 2018;**132**(Supplement 1):3133.
62. Byrd JC, Brown JR, O'Brien S, et al. Ibrutinib versus ofatumumab in previously treated chronic lymphoid leukemia. *N Engl J Med*. 2014;**371**(3):213–223.

63 Burger JA, Tedeschi A, Barr PM, et al. Ibrutinib as initial therapy for patients with chronic lymphocytic leukemia. *N Engl J Med*. 2015;**373**(25):2425–2437.

66 Moreno C, Greil R, Demirkan F, et al. Ibrutinib plus obinutuzumab versus chlorambucil plus obinutuzumab in first-line treatment of chronic lymphocytic leukaemia (iLLUMINATE): a multicentre, randomised, open-label, phase 3 trial. *Lancet Oncol*. 2019;**20**(1):43–56.

67 Shanafelt TD, Wang XV, Kay NE, et al. Ibrutinib–rituximab or chemoim. *N Engl J Med*. 2019;**381**(5):432–443.

70 Byrd JC, Harrington B, O'Brien S, et al. Acalabrutinib (ACP-196) in relapsed chronic lymphocytic leukemia. *N Engl J Med*. 2016;**374**(4):323–332.

71 Sharman JP, Egyed M, Jurczak W, et al. Acalabrutinib with or without obinutuzumab versus chlorambucil and obinutuzumab for treatment-naive chronic lymphocytic leukaemia (ELEVATE-TN): a randomised, controlled, phase 3 trial. *Lancet*. 2020;**395**(10232):1278–1291.

72 Ghia P, Pluta A, Wach M, et al. ASCEND: phase III, randomized trial of acalabrutinib versus idelalisib plus rituximab or bendamustine plus rituximab in relapsed or refractory chronic lymphocytic leukemia. *J Clin Oncol*. 2020;**38**(25):2849–2861.

75 Furman RR, Sharman JP, Coutre SE, et al. Idelalisib and rituximab in relapsed chronic lymphocytic leukemia. *N Engl J Med*. 2014;**370**(11):997–1007.

77 O'Brien S, Patel M, Kahl BS, et al. Duvelisib (IPI-145), a PI3K-δ,γ inhibitor, is clinically active in patients with relapsed/refractory chronic lymphocytic leukemia. *Blood*. 2014;**124**(21):3334.

78 Flinn IW, Hillmen P, Montillo M, et al. The phase 3 DUO trial: duvelisib vs ofatumumab in relapsed and refractory CLL/SLL. *Blood*. 2018;**132**(23):2446–2455.

79 Roberts AW, Davids MS, Pagel JM, et al. Targeting BCL2 with venetoclax in relapsed chronic lymphocytic leukemia. *N Engl J Med*. 2016;**374**(4):311–322.

82 Seymour JF, Kipps TJ, Eichhorst B, et al. Venetoclax–rituximab in relapsed or refractory chronic lymphocytic leukemia. *N Engl J Med*. 2018;**378**(12):1107–1120.

83 Fischer K, Al-Sawaf O, Bahlo J, et al. Venetoclax and obinutuzumab in patients with CLL and coexisting conditions. *N Engl J Med*. 2019;**380**(23):2225–2236.

88 Gribben JG. How and when I do allogeneic transplant in CLL. *Blood*. 2018;**132**(1):31–39.

90 Porter DL, Hwang WT, Frey NV, et al. Chimeric antigen receptor T cells persist and induce sustained remissions in relapsed refractory chronic lymphocytic leukemia. *Sci Transl Med*. 2015;7(303):303ra139.

91 Turtle CJ, Hay KA, Hanafi LA, et al. Durable molecular remissions in chronic lymphocytic leukemia treated with CD19-specific chimeric antigen receptor-modified T cells after failure of ibrutinib. *J Clin Oncol*. 2017;**35**(26):3010–3020.

115 Hodgkin lymphoma

David J. Straus, MD ■ Anita Kumar, MD

> **Overview**
>
> This article provides a historical perspective on the marked advances in radiotherapy and chemotherapy that have contributed to significant improvements in the curability of Hodgkin lymphoma (HL) over the past several decades. The classic features and new insights into the epidemiology, biology, and pathologic characteristics of HL are described. With emphasis on the modern clinical approach to the staging, imaging, and treatment of HL, the article highlights how current management approaches, such as refined risk stratification, use of PET imaging, and the reduction of radiation field and dose, seek to limit long-term toxicities of therapy while maintaining excellent cure rates. Finally, the authors describe how novel, biologically targeted therapies have contributed to significant changes in the therapeutic landscape for patients with relapsed/refractory HL.

Introduction

Classical Hodgkin lymphoma, cHL, is now potentially curable in at least 80% of patients. Well-defined diagnostic criteria, prognostic factors, improved imaging, emphasis on systemic therapy first, and selective limited-field radiotherapy consolidation have all contributed to this outcome. An increased appreciation of curability/quality of survivorship has now added the important goal of reducing the intensity of initial treatment when possible, without compromising cure rates; and, such changes in chemotherapy and radiation dose/field have resulted in reduction of long-term toxicities such as infertility, cardiopulmonary toxicity, and secondary malignancy.

History

In his historic paper of 1832, "On Some Morbid Appearances of the Absorbent Glands and Spleen," Thomas Hodgkin described the clinical history and postmortem findings of massive lymph node and spleen enlargement in patients studied at Guy's Hospital, London. Hodgkin recognized that these patients had suffered from a disease that started in the lymph nodes located along the major vessels in the neck, chest, or abdomen.[1] Sir Samuel Wilks, and later W.S. Greenfield, described the microscopic lymph node appearance. Carl Sternberg, in 1898, and Dorothy Reed, in 1902, are credited with the first definitive microscopic descriptions of Hodgkin lymphoma.[2,3] The early treatment of Hodgkin lymphoma with crude X-rays in 1901 followed the discovery of radiographs by Roentgen, radioactivity by Becquerel, and radium by the Curies at the end of the nineteenth century. Before this time, serum and other biologic preparations, arsenic, iodine, and surgery were ineffective in cHL. These first reports of successful X-ray radiograph treatments produced great excitement and premature predictions for the curability of Hodgkin lymphoma.[4,5]

Modern radiation therapy (RT) techniques began in the 1920s with the work of Gilbert, who was one of the first to point out the predictable clinical patterns of cHL. He advocated treatment of apparently uninvolved adjacent lymph node chains that might contain suspected microscopic disease in addition to the involved nodal sites.[6] In 1950, Vera Peters extended this approach, reporting 5- and 10-year survivals of 88% and 79%, respectively, for patients with stage I.[7] However, the concept that early-stage Hodgkin lymphoma might be curable with RT was slow to be accepted. Henry Kaplan developed the linear accelerator and successfully applied this technology to curing cHL. He defined radiation field sizes and doses, refined and improved diagnostic staging techniques, developed models for translating laboratory findings into clinical practice, and, with Saul Rosenberg, promoted early randomized clinical trials in the United States.[8–10]

Advanced-stage cHL was uniformly fatal until the development of combination chemotherapy. Mechlorethamine was shown to be an active drug in the 1940s, and in the mid-1960s Vincent DeVita and colleagues first treated patients with an effective four-drug regimen termed MOPP (mechlorethamine, vincristine, procarbazine, and prednisone).[11] MOPP provided a high rate of complete remission and prolonged survival, resulting in curative outcomes.[12]

Like radiotherapy, randomized trials were also pivotal to the development of combination chemotherapy. These studies demonstrated no benefit of maintenance chemotherapy, established that treatment durations could be relatively short, and, ultimately, showed that ABVD (doxorubicin, bleomycin, vinblastine, and dacarbazine) was associated with reduced toxicity and similar efficacy compared to MOPP (or MOPP-containing regimens), thus confirming ABVD as the standard regimen.[13,14]

Epidemiology and etiology

In 2019, there were expected to be 8110 new cases of cHL in the United States. The incidence is 2.59 per 100,000 per year and has remained relatively constant for decades (http://seer.cancer.gov/statfacts/html/hodg.html). In the United States, the median age for all new cases is 39 years, with 31% occurring between the ages of 20 and 34. Somewhat more men than women (3.1 to 2.4 per 100,000) develop HL. Although a bimodal distribution was previously apparent in economically developed countries, the second peak is less apparent but persistent, as better pathology classification has found many of these cases to be non-Hodgkin lymphomas.

The etiology of Hodgkin lymphoma remains unknown. Epidemiologic data suggest both infectious and genetic components.[15,16] A viral etiology is suggested by an association between cHL in younger patients and childhood factors that decrease exposure to infectious agents at an early age, including

---

Holland-Frei Cancer Medicine, Tenth Edition. Edited by Robert C. Bast, John C. Byrd, Carlo M. Croce, Ernest Hawk, Fadlo R. Khuri, Raphael E. Pollock, Apostolia M. Tsimberidou, Christopher G. Willett, and Cheryl L. Willman.
© 2023 John Wiley & Sons, Inc. Published 2023 by John Wiley & Sons, Inc.

increased maternal education, decreased numbers of siblings and playmates, early birth order, and single-family dwellings in childhood for economically developed countries.[17,18] This association has led to the proposal that cHL appears to mimic a viral illness that has an age-related host response to infection (such as seen with polio and infectious mononucleosis). Supporting this theory is the infrequent occurrence of cHL in children younger than 10 years in economically developed countries.

Epstein–Barr virus (EBV) is the leading viral candidate.[18-20] EBV is the causative agent in African Burkitt lymphoma, and EBV-associated lymphomas are documented in patients with immune deficiency disorders and following organ transplantation. There is a two- to threefold excess in the incidence of cHL among patients with a prior history of mononucleosis. In addition, there is an altered antibody response pattern to EBV in patients who later develop cHL.

Recent cellular and molecular biology data have provided additional support for the association of EBV and cHL. Through the use of sensitive molecular probes, 30–50% of Hodgkin lymphoma specimens have been found to contain EBV genome fragments in the diagnostic Reed-Sternberg (R–S) cells.[21] EBV genome status appears to be stable over time when studied in initial biopsies and at relapse. EBV genome-positive R–S cells express the so-called type II latency profile, with expression of latent membrane protein (LMP)-1, LMP-2a, EBV nuclear antigen (EBNA)-1, and EBV-encoded ribonucleic acid (EBER). LMP-1 is critical in transformation and acts as an oncogene in transfection studies, whereas EBNA-1 is essential for the replication of the episomal viral genome.

A genetic predisposition is evident with increased incidence among first-degree relatives, in some sibling studies, in monozygotic twins, and among parent–child pairs but not among spouses. In addition, cHL has been linked with certain human leukocyte antigens (HLAs) that are associated with EBV status; and genome-wide association studies have identified, but not proven, non-HLA susceptibility genes.[15]

Immunologic abnormalities in patients

Classical HL is characterized by functional deficits in cellular immunity and in T-cell-mediated immune responses that exist before treatment. These deficits persist in cured patients[22] and include impairment of delayed cutaneous hypersensitivity, depressed proliferative responses to T-cell mitogen stimulation, enhanced immunoglobulin production, and decreased natural killer cell cytotoxicity. These abnormalities suggest an immunosuppression secondary to chronic overstimulation by cytokines. In patients with active cHL, these findings are consistent with increased cytokine secretion by R–S cells. However, it has been difficult to explain the persistence of these abnormalities in patients after successful treatment.

Treatment-induced immunosuppression returns toward normal after treatment but has its greatest effect over the first few years.[23] For example, there is an excess of herpes zoster infections, and more than 75% of such cases occur within the first year. Few occur after the third year (6%). The risk of herpes zoster infection appears highest as the intensity of therapy increases.[22]

Unlike their deficits in delayed hypersensitivity, most patients with cHL at diagnosis appear to have relatively normal B-cell number and function, which may be adversely affected by treatment.[22] Patients should be encouraged to keep vaccinations up to date.

Pathology

Hodgkin lymphoma is unique among lymphomas for its histologic diversity.[24] Involved lymph nodes contain varying degrees of normal reactive and inflammatory cells, fibrosis, and a scattering of the characteristic malignant cHL cells, the R–S cells, and their mononuclear variants. The typical R–S cell has abundant cytoplasm and two to three nuclei, each with a single prominent nucleolus. The large size and unusual appearance of the R–S cell sets it apart from the adjacent smaller background cells. The mononuclear variants have nuclear and cytoplasmic features of R–S cells but have only a single nucleus. The diagnosis of cHL should rarely be made in the absence of R–S cells but also cannot be made on the basis of their presence alone. R–S-like cells have been found in infectious mononucleosis, non-Hodgkin lymphoma, and in some carcinomas and sarcomas. Thus, criteria for a cHL diagnosis include the presence of the R–S cells and the characteristic background of normal lymphocytes, plasma cells, and eosinophils.

The pathology classification includes cHL: nodular sclerosis (NSHL), mixed cellularity (MCHL), lymphocyte-rich (LRHL), and lymphocyte depletion (LDHL) subtypes; as well as nodular lymphocyte-predominant Hodgkin lymphoma (NLPHL). The subtyping of cHL does not affect clinical management, prognosis, or therapy. Nevertheless, the histologic subtypes are associated with different presentations and distinct natural histories. These differences are most evident in NLPHL.

Hodgkin lymphoma subtypes

Two histologic features of NSHL help to differentiate this cHL subtype: (1) a proliferation of collagenous bands dividing the lymph node into circumscribed nodules which contain (2) a variant R–S cell called the lacunar cell. In formalin-fixed tissue, this cell's abundant pale cytoplasm often retracts and gives the appearance of a cell in space (Figures 1–3). Molecular profiling studies have shown a close relationship between primary mediastinal large B-cell lymphoma and NSHL, and a "gray-zone" neoplasm that combines features of both neoplasms rarely may be identified.[25-27]

NSHL is the only subtype of cHL as common in women as in men. It occurs in adolescents and young adults and is unusual in patients older than 50 years. It has a striking propensity to involve lower cervical, supraclavicular, and mediastinal lymph nodes with an orderly pattern of spread.[28] It makes up 60–70% of cHL in economically developed countries but is less commonly seen in underdeveloped countries.

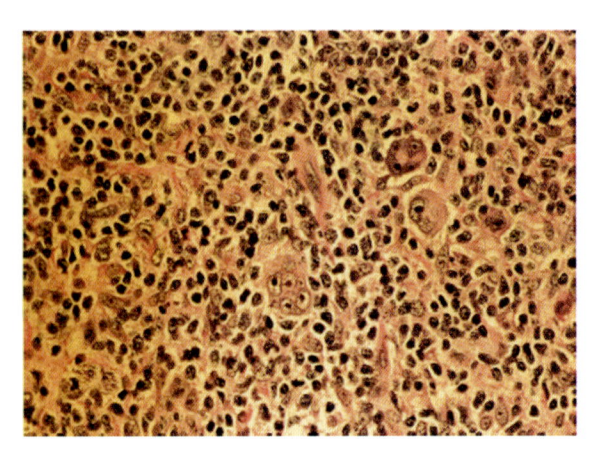

Figure 1 Reed–Sternberg cells and variants in Hodgkin lymphoma of the nodular sclerosis type. Large multinucleated or multilobulated cells and a few mononuclear cells with macronucleoli stand apart from cellular background elements.

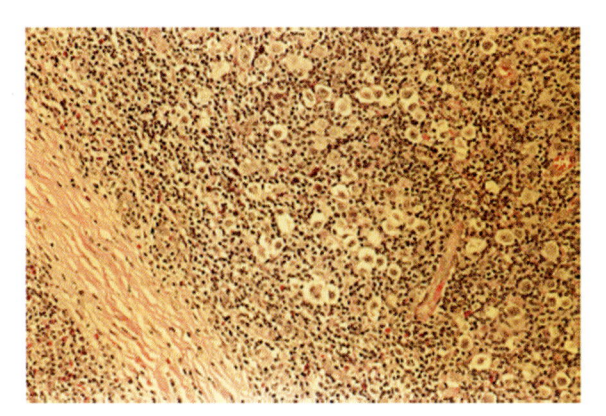

Figure 2 Hodgkin disease, nodular sclerosis. A fibrous band is present in the left lower part of the field. Neoplastic lacunar cells having abundant, clear cytoplasm stand out against the lymphocytic background.

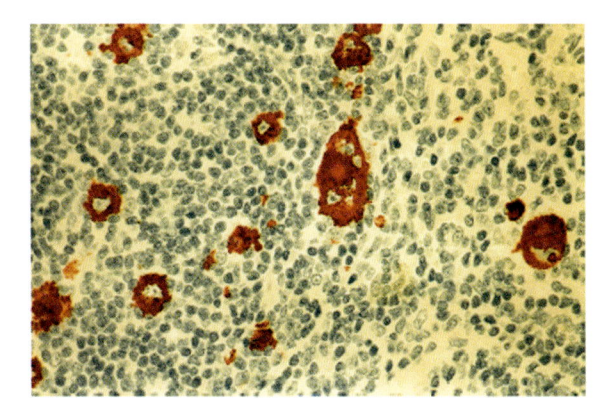

Figure 3 Immunostain for CD15 in Hodgkin disease, nodular sclerosis type. Neoplastic Reed–Sternberg cells and mononuclear Hodgkin cells show positive immunoreactivity.

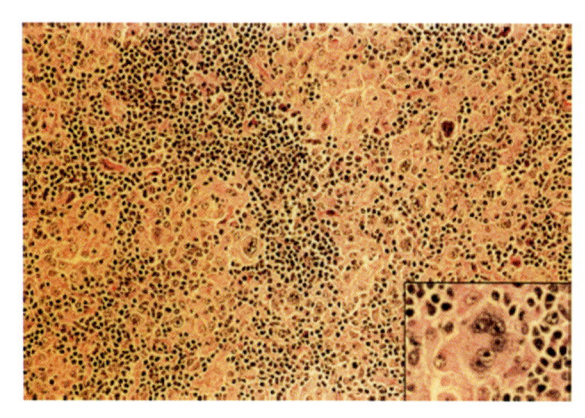

Figure 4 Hodgkin disease, mixed cellularity type. Reed–Sternberg cells in histiocyte-rich cellular background. Inset: Multinucleated Reed–Sternberg cell at higher magnification.

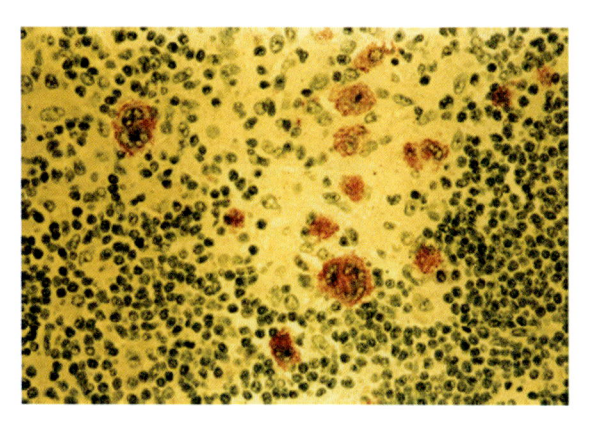

Figure 5 Immunostain for Epstein–Barr virus-latent membrane protein in Hodgkin disease, mixed cellularity type (same biopsy as Figure 4).

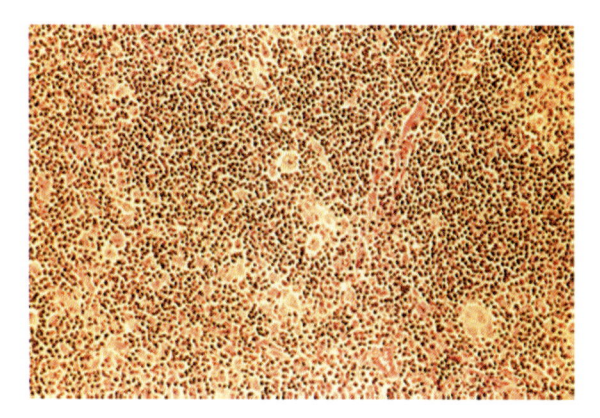

Figure 6 Lymphocyte-rich classic Hodgkin disease. Reed–Sternberg cells and mononuclear Hodgkin cells are relatively rare within the background proliferation of small lymphocytes and histiocytes.

MCHL has an inflammatory background abundant in normal cells as well as 5–15 R–S cells and variants per high-power field (Figures 4 and 5). These patients are older, more likely to have B symptoms, and often have abdominal involvement or advanced disease. Approximately 25% of patients with cHL in the United States have MCHL, and it is more common in underdeveloped countries. MCHL can be confused with peripheral T-cell lymphoma, and the antigen PAX5, a B-cell marker, may be particularly helpful to distinguish it.

LRHL may resemble other histologic subtypes and may be nodular or diffuse. R–S cells are relatively rare, and the background is dominated by small mature lymphocytes (Figures 6 and 7). Eosinophils and neutrophils are usually restricted to blood vessels.

LDHL is rarely diagnosed, accounting for less than 1% of cHL in economically advanced countries. Generally, these patients present with advanced disease and B symptoms. R–S cells and "pleomorphic" variant cells are frequent, and most cases have only sparse normal lymphocytes.

In NLPHL, the lymph node architecture is usually effaced, although a remnant of normal nodal architecture may remain. Diagnostic R–S cells are not seen, but variant lymphocyte predominance (LP) cells are typical (Figures 8 and 9). These cells often have multilobated nuclei and have been called popcorn cells because of their resemblance to a popped kernel of corn. Fibrosis is not usually seen. The LP or "popcorn" R–S variants occur in a background of polyclonal B lymphocytes (Figure 9).[29,30] LP cells are usually positive for the B-cell marker CD20, but negative for the cHL markers of CD15 and CD 30 (Figures 10 and 11).[31,32] EBV is rarely detected in NLPHL.[33] The benign disorder progressive transformation of germinal centers (PTGCs) is often associated with NLPHL. R–S cells and LP variants are absent in PTGC, which can also be seen in association with NLPHL in the same or an adjacent node.[31]

NLPHL makes up 5–10% of Hodgkin lymphomas in the United States. It is often localized to a single peripheral nodal region (high

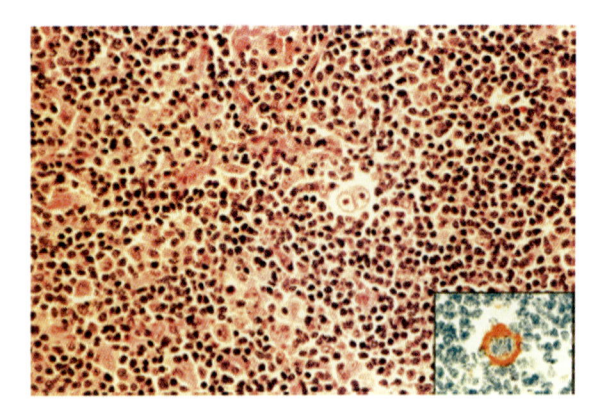

Figure 7 Lymphocyte-rich classic Hodgkin disease. Binucleated Reed–Sternberg cell in center of field. In same biopsy, Reed–Sternberg cells immunostained positively for CD15 (inset).

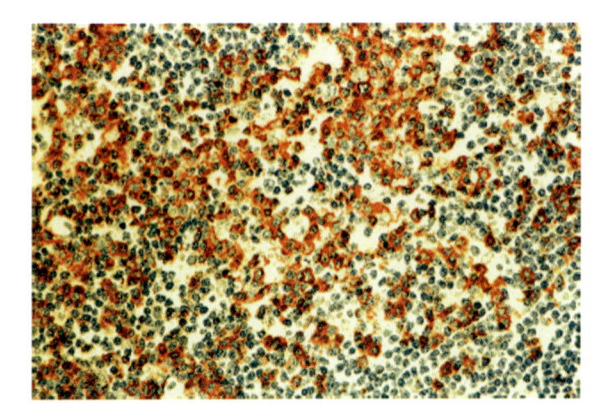

Figure 8 Lymphocyte-predominant Hodgkin lymphoma (same biopsy as Figures 9–11). Immunostain for CD57 reveals a marked increase in immunoreactive cells showing localization around nonimmunoreactive L and H cells within a nodule. The CD3 immunostain showed a similar distribution of immunoreactive cells.

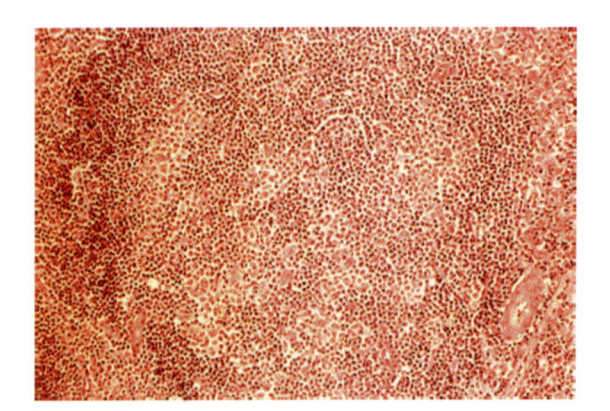

Figure 9 Lymphocyte-predominant Hodgkin disease. The vaguely nodular histologic pattern is apparent.

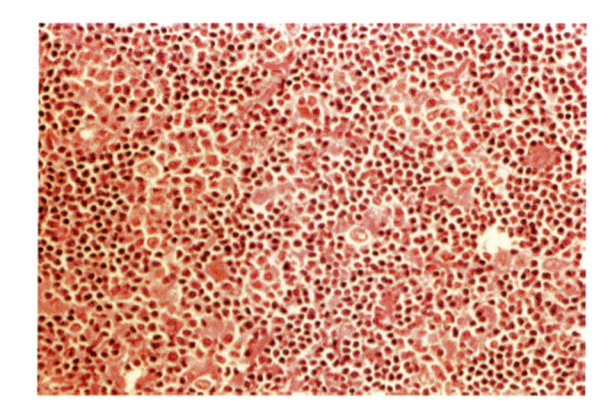

Figure 10 Lymphocyte-predominant Hodgkin lymphoma at higher magnification (same biopsy as Figure 9). Within the background of lymphocytes and histiocytes are scattered large lobated cells having a fine chromatin pattern, relatively small nucleoli, and sparse cytoplasm so-called L and H cells.

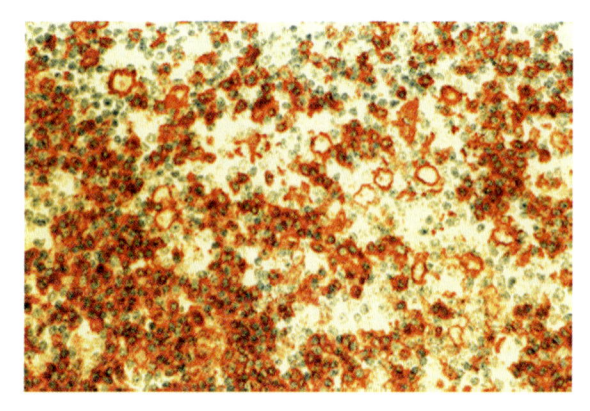

Figure 11 Lymphocyte-predominant Hodgkin lymphoma (same biopsy as Figures 9 and 10). Immunostain for CD20 demonstrates positive staining of L and H cells as well as a high percentage of lymphocytes within a nodule.

cervical, submandibular, epitrochlear, inguinal, or femoral nodes) and infrequently involves mediastinal or abdominal sites.

Immunophenotype and biology

The R–S cell is of B-lymphocyte origin.[24] These cells may express antigens found on resting or activated lymphocytes, most often B cell: usually positive for PAX5, and infrequently, CD20 or CD79a; and rarely positive for T-cell surface antigens (CD3, CD4, and CD8). The LP cells of NLPHL consistently express B-cell antigens. In cHL, the surface antigens CD30 and CD15 are present on most R–S cells, nearly all cases are CD30+, and approximately 80% are CD15+, whereas CD45 (leukocyte common antigen) is usually negative. In contrast, the LP cells of NLPHL are CD15 and CD30 negative and CD45 positive.[32]

Microdissection studies of single R–S cells demonstrate clonal immunoglobulin gene rearrangements in the vast majority of cases, confirming the clonality of the cells and establishing their B-cell lineage, despite their aberrant lack of immunoglobulin gene expression.[34,35] Moreover, R–S cells possess somatically mutated V genes, implying a germinal center or postgerminal center origin. The mutational pattern suggests that this may account for the lack of immunoglobulin expression. Other possible mechanisms include epigenetic silencing of heavy chain gene transcription or constitutive expression of Notch 1 and STAT 5.[24] Normal germinal center B cells that lack functional immunoglobulin receptors are usually eliminated within the germinal center via apoptosis; and therefore, R–S cells appear resistant to this usual apoptotic mechanism. This apoptosis pathway via FAS/CD95 is inhibited by c-FLIP, a gene that is constitutively expressed by R–S cells.[34] Several hypotheses have been generated to explain this phenomenon, including activation of the NF-κB pathway, general lineage promiscuity, and Epstein–Barr infection. Evidence favoring the NF-κB pathway includes the observation of constitutive expression of NF-κB in Hodgkin lymphoma-derived cell lines, the finding that suppression of NF-κB impairs tumor growth in severe combined immunodeficient mice and growth of cell lines,[35] and an epidemiology study showing that regular aspirin use is associated with a reduced risk of developing Hodgkin lymphoma, presumably through inhibition of NF-κB transcription.[33] The cause of the constitutive activation of NF-κB may include amplification of the REL gene, mutations in NF-κB inhibition, and somatic mutations in TNFA1P3.[24] LMP-2a expression may substitute for a functional B-cell receptor in EBV-associated cases.

Microdissection studies of LP cells also demonstrate clonal immunoglobulin gene rearrangements, again establishing clonality and confirming B-cell lineage.[36] In addition to demonstrating somatically mutated V genes, intraclonal sequence diversity can also be detected, providing strong evidence that NLPHL is a germinal center lymphoma. In contrast to cHL, in NLPHL the mutations are compatible with functional antigen receptors.

Cytogenetic abnormalities are common in R–S cells; however, no consistent pattern has been described. Rarely, the $t(14:18)$ translocation, common in follicular B-cell lymphomas, may be detected. Comparative genomic hybridization studies demonstrate recurrent gains on chromosomal arms 2p (the site of NF-κB, REL, and BCL1 1a), 9p (the site of JAK2), and 12q (the site of MDM2), and amplifications on chromosomal bands 4p16, 4q23–q24, and 9p23–p24 (associated with high level of PD-L1 protein expression). Recurrent imbalances have been demonstrated in a majority of cHL using genome-wide GeneScan technology.[37]

The tumor microenvironment has been found to have an important role in the pathogenesis, associated manifestations, and prognosis of Hodgkin lymphoma.[38,39] It has been hypothesized that cytokines are responsible for the marked inflammatory component, fibrosis, and diverse histologic patterns of cHL, as well as the associated clinical symptoms of fever, weight loss, and night sweats.[33,40] Many cases are associated with upregulation of tumor necrosis factor receptor (TNFR) and ligand family members, Th2 and to a lesser extent Th1 cytokines, and other chemokines. Necrosis factor receptor (NFR) members may lead to constitutive activation of NF-κB, an important factor in proliferation and survival of B lymphocytes. Preferential expression of Th2 cytokines and chemokines may explain the frequent presence of eosinophils and fibroblasts, as well as local suppression of the cellular immune response. EBV may contribute to the production of cytokines, for example, via LMP-1-induced activation of NF-κB and stimulation of interleukin (IL)-10, a potent inhibitor of cellular immunity. In some cases, specific cytokines may be associated with specific histologic features. For example, transforming growth factor (TGF), a known stimulus for fibroblast proliferation and collagen formation, is associated with NSHL,[41] and TARC (CCL27), a lymphocyte-directed CC chemokine secreted by Hodgkin cells, may be responsible for the infiltration by CD4+ T cells.[38] Tissue eosinophilia may be due to expression of IL-5, IL-9, CCL11, and CCL28; and IL-13 may play a role in autocrine stimulation of R–S cells.[39]

Staging

Most patients with cHL have a central pattern of lymph node involvement (cervical, mediastinal, and paraaortic) with >80% presenting initially above the diaphragm. In contrast, certain nodal chains (mesenteric, hypogastric, presacral, epitrochlear, and popliteal) are seldom, if ever, involved. Spleen involvement is associated with adenopathy below the diaphragm and systemic symptoms. Isolated liver disease is rare; bone and bone marrow involvement are usually focal. Staging has recently been updated with the Lugano classification, incorporating the original Ann Arbor Stage and the later Cotswolds revision (Table 1).[42] PET imaging is now recognized as the most accurate means of identifying all sites of cHL involvement, and routine bone marrow biopsy is no longer recommended. See Table 2 for pretreatment evaluation.

Table 1 The Lugano classification.[a]

Stage	
Stage I	A single lymph node or a group of adjacent nodes. Stage IE: A single extralymphatic site; Tonsils, Waldeyer's ring, and spleen are considered nodal tissue
Stage II	Two or more lymph node groups on the same side of the diaphragm. Stage IIE: Stage I or II nodal extent and limited contiguous extranodal involvement on the same side of the diaphragm
Stage III	Involvement of nodal tissue on both sides of the diaphragm
Stage IV	Noncontiguous extranodal involvement with or without associated lymph nodes
Designations applicable to any disease stage	
A:	No symptoms
B:	Fever (temperature, >38 °C [100.4 °F]), drenching night sweats, and unexplained loss of >10% of body weight within the preceding 6 months
X:	Bulky disease (a single nodal mass with a maximal dimension of 10 cm or greater, as measured by CT)

[a]Source: Based on Cheson et al.[42]

Table 2 Recommended staging.[a]

Adequate biopsy reviewed by an experienced hematopathologist (surgical excisional biopsy is preferred, and core needle biopsy may be sufficient in some cases; fine needle aspiration is inadequate)
History with attention to the presence or absence of systemic symptoms
Physical examination, emphasizing node chains, size of liver and spleen, and Waldeyer ring inspection
Laboratory tests: complete blood count with differential, erythrocyte sedimentation rate, comprehensive metabolic panel including liver function tests, and HIV, hepatitis B, and C serologies
PET scan
Selected CT imaging of neck, chest, abdomen, and pelvis, if required for radiotherapy
No bone marrow biopsy unless PET scan is equivocal and result of biopsy will change treatment
Evaluation of ejection fraction for doxorubicin-containing regimens
Evaluation of pulmonary function for bleomycin-containing regimens
Counseling: fertility preservation

[a]Source: Based on Cheson et al.[42]

Principles of treatment in classical Hodgkin lymphoma

The initial treatment of cHL is determined by stage at presentation and clinical prognostic category. In general, there are three groups with unique treatment considerations: early stage, favorable risk; early stage, unfavorable risk; and advanced stage.

Radiotherapy

In the earliest years, RT alone was used for treatment, and maximal doses/field sizes were applied. Since then, the RT extent has been dramatically reduced. Several randomized studies confirmed that, in the setting of combined modality therapy (CMT, chemotherapy + radiotherapy), replacing the extended radiation fields (extended-field radiation therapy [EFRT], mantle/inverted Y) with involved-field radiotherapy (IFRT) was equivalent, with disease control and survival remaining similar.[43,44] Consolidative RT could be limited to the initial macroscopically involved volume and radiation doses could be reduced.[45] Such reductions in dose and volume may lessen late RT effects.[46]

IFRT significantly reduced the size of treatment portals to include fewer uninvolved adjacent sites compared with EFRT. Recent iterations of IFRT, involved nodal (INRT)[47,48] and involved site (ISRT),[49] continue to treat all the prechemotherapy sites of involvement while decreasing the size of the postchemotherapy fields. As a result, ISRT and INRT both treat large fields and involve substantial off-target radiation exposure to adjacent organs.[49] Current treatment guidelines limit fields to postchemotherapy disease extent in the lateral dimension to account for tumor regression during chemotherapy and to reduce lung exposure. However, involved prechemotherapy sites are still treated in the longitudinal dimension. Thus, for example, initial pericardiac sites that resolve following chemotherapy are included in ISRT fields, resulting in substantial cardiac exposure. In addition, a young woman who presents with axillary disease that resolves with chemotherapy will still have the axilla included in ISRT fields, leading to a considerable risk of secondary breast cancer. This treatment strategy is suboptimal for patients with bulky mediastinal disease, often female adolescents or young adults who are among the most vulnerable to the late morbidity and mortality associated with RT.

A question for future clinical research is whether a CMT approach could potentially include a safer form of RT, which could reduce the small excess of relapses anticipated with chemotherapy only. There is no evidence that lowering the RT dose further, to below 21 to 25 Gy in CMT, will remain therapeutic. Meeting the current standards of treating all initial nodal sites of involvement makes it difficult to substantially further reduce off-target radiation exposure, even with new techniques such as three-dimensional conformal RT, intensity-modulated RT, deep inspiratory breath-hold, or even proton beam RT. Thus, it may be necessary to treat only a *subset* of all initial nodal sites of involvement when administering adjuvant RT following adequate chemotherapy. It is unclear whether initial nodal sites that have completely resolved with chemotherapy are at increased risk for recurrence, so clinical trials are needed to test the efficacy of only treating the PET-negative *residual* remaining masses on CT imaging following chemotherapy (residual-site RT, RSRT).[50] Most initially bulky sites will have a smaller residual mass after chemotherapy. Importantly, PET-positive residual masses would be biopsied to document persistent refractory disease for appropriate salvage treatment. Combined-modality trials with this design would be particularly useful for patients with initial bulky mediastinal presentations of HL, as these patients routinely continue to receive adjunctive RT. This approach might provide an opportunity to preserve the high rates of progression-free survival (PFS) with CMT without substantially increasing the risk of RT-related toxicity.

A clinical trial employing reduced treatment volume RT with brentuximab vedotin (BV) and AVD (doxorubicin, vinblastine, dacarbazine) is in progress for patients with bulky, unfavorable early-stage cHL at Memorial Sloan Kettering Cancer Center (MSK), Stanford University Medical Center, City of Hope, and the University of Rochester (NCT01868451). Patients receiving this treatment who are PET-negative after four cycles of chemotherapy receive consolidation-volume RT consisting of RT to residual abnormal volumes ≥1.5 cm but not to all initial sites of involvement.[49,51]

Chemotherapy

The introduction of combination chemotherapy facilitated the reduction of RT dose/field, and chemotherapy is now the cornerstone of cHL therapy. Prior toxic regimens, such as MOPP, which were associated with infertility and secondary acute leukemia, have been supplanted by the equally efficacious but less toxic regimen ABVD,[13,52] the treatment standard in the United States. Many regimens have been developed to further improve outcomes. Dose intensification with escalated BEACOPP (bleomycin, etoposide, doxorubicin, cyclophosphamide, vincristine, procarbazine, and prednisone) led to improved rates of freedom from treatment failure (FFTF), but with increased acute and late toxicities and without overall survival benefit.[53–55] Recently, a large randomized clinical trial compared ABVD with a new regimen substituting an antibody–drug conjugate, BV, for bleomycin in the ABVD regimen. This international phase 3 trial of 1334 patients compared six cycles of ABVD with six cycles of BV + AVD in newly diagnosed patients with stages III and IV Hodgkin lymphoma.[56] At 2 years of follow-up, a primary endpoint, the modified progression-free survival (mPFS) was significantly better for BV + AVD compared with ABVD (82.1% vs 77.2%; $P = 0.03$). PFS rates at 3 years of follow-up were 83.1% and 76.0%, respectively ($P = 0.005$). The benefit for BV + AVD in this intent-to-treat population was independent of disease stage and prognostic factors.[57] Primary prophylactic growth factor support is recommended for all patients treated with BV + AVD but not necessarily recommended for those treated with ABVD, and the toxicity profile of BV + AVD is not greatly higher. The United States Food and Drug Administration (FDA) has approved BV + AVD for the treatment of newly diagnosed cHL, a new treatment option for these patients.

Risk-adapted interim PET

To optimize outcome and minimize toxicity, early response assessment with an interim FDG-PET (PET) scan is often performed. This PET is done before completion of treatment, often after the second or fourth cycle of chemotherapy. After two cycles of ABVD, interim PET has been found to predict treatment response and clinical outcomes.[58–60] Thus, in "response-adapted therapy," treatment intensity may be de-escalated with a good early response, or escalated if early response is inadequate.[61]

The cHL criteria for PET response utilize the "five-point scale" (FPS) or Deauville Criteria. Baseline and interim PET scans are scored according to uptake in sites initially involved by lymphoma: (1) no uptake, (2) uptake ≤ mediastinum, (3) uptake > mediastinum but ≤ liver (4) moderately increased uptake > liver, or (5) markedly increased uptake > liver and/or new lesions.[62] A score of 1–3 is usually interpreted as negative for lymphoma, while a score of 4 or 5 is considered positive. In clinical trials, negativity may be more stringently defined as a score of 1–2 in cases where treatment may be substantially reduced for interim PET-negative patients.[63]

Early-stage cHL

In early-stage cHL, favorable and unfavorable risk groups have been defined.[64–66] Common unfavorable features include bulky mediastinal mass, B symptoms, elevated ESR, and involvement of multiple lymph node groups. Bulky disease is variably defined: >1/3 of the mediastinal mass ratio (MMR, maximum width of the mass divided by the maximum intrathoracic diameter), >1/3 of the mediastinal thoracic ratio (MTR, maximum width of the mass divided by the intrathoracic diameter at T5–T6), or any mass >10 cm. Three risk systems have been retrospectively analyzed in early-stage cHL following four cycles of ABVD + IFRT, and the common poor prognostic feature was tumor burden (bulky mass or greater number of nodal sites).[66] In the United States, clinical trials have usually separated patients according to stage I and II nonbulky, stages I and II bulky, and stages III and IV. Some clinical trials have included bulky stage II with stages III and IV.[63,67–69]

Favorable risk

Many studies in early-stage, favorable risk cHL have focused on reducing late effects without compromising cure. The GHSG HD10 study included 1131 patients with stage IA–IIB disease without any risk features.[70] Four treatment arms were randomized: ABVD × 2 cycles + 30 Gy IFRT, ABVD × 2 cycles + 20 Gy IFRT, ABVD × 4 cycles + 30 Gy IFRT, and ABVD × 4 cycles + 20 Gy IFRT. The 5-year FFTF rates were 91.1% versus 93% for two versus four cycles of ABVD, respectively. Similarly, the 5-year FFTF rates in the two radiotherapy arms were not significantly different, at 92.9% (20 Gy) versus 93.4% (30 Gy). Adverse events and acute toxic effects were more frequent in patients who received ABVD × 4 cycles + 30 Gy of IFRT. The authors recommended two cycles of ABVD followed by 20 Gy IFRT in these favorable patients.

The elimination of radiotherapy altogether in selected early-stage cHL emerged as a standard of care. In 2004, MSK reported a study of 152 nonbulky cHL patients with stages I, II A or B, and IIIA randomized to six cycles of ABVD + RT versus six cycles of ABVD alone.[71] At 5 years, failure-free survival (FFS) and OS for ABVD + RT versus ABVD alone were 86% versus 81% ($P = 0.61$) and 97% versus 90% ($P = 0.08$), respectively. The National Cancer Information Center (NCIC) and Eastern Cooperative Oncology Group (ECOG) HD.6 trial randomized stage IA or IIA nonbulky cHL patients to receive ABVD alone or ABVD + subtotal nodal radiation therapy (sTLI).[72] Patients in the RT group who had a favorable risk profile received sTLI alone, whereas patients with an unfavorable risk profile (any of the following: age >39 years, an ESR ≥ 50 mm/h, mixed cellularity or lymphocyte deplete histology, or ≥4 sites of disease) received two cycles of ABVD + sTLI. Patients who received ABVD only received four to six cycles, based on interim CT. At 12 years there was a significant survival benefit favoring ABVD over ABVD + sTLI, with 94% versus 87% OS rates, respectively ($P = 0.04$), and excess secondary malignancies in the CMT arm. This study was criticized because sTLI was outdated; nevertheless, it demonstrated the value of ABVD alone and emphasized concerns regarding CMT.

ABVD alone has been studied with interim PET.[73,74] The UK RAPID study was a randomized noninferiority study including 602 nonbulky stage IA or IIA cHL patients with both favorable and unfavorable risks. All received three cycles of ABVD followed by PET imaging. If interim PET-negative (Deauville 1 or 2), patients were randomized to no further treatment versus one cycle ABVD + 30 Gy IFRT. If interim PET-positive, patients received one cycle ABVD + 30 Gy IFRT. With median follow-up of 60 months, the 3-year PFS was 94.6% for CMT versus 90.8% for three cycles of ABVD alone, with an absolute risk difference of 3.8% points. The EORTC/LYSA/FIL H10 trial, a randomized noninferiority study of both favorable and unfavorable risk early-stage cHL patients utilizing ABVD and interim PET after two cycles, concluded after a preplanned interim futility analysis that, when compared to CMT, the chemotherapy alone arms should be discontinued. However, the 1-year PFS in the ABVD arms were excellent, approximately 95%, raising the question of whether conclusions were made prematurely.[63]

Another phase 2 trial confirmed an excellent PFS for most patients treated with a short course of ABVD alone. CALGB 50604 treated patients with stages I/II nonbulky cHL with two cycles of ABVD. Interim PET/CT was performed and centrally reviewed. Patients whose interim PET/CT was negative, defined as Deauville scores of 1–3 (FDG uptake less than liver), received two more cycle of ABVD (total four cycles) and no irradiation (135/149; 91%). Patients whose interim PET/CT was positive received two cycles of more intensive chemotherapy with escalated BEACOPP, and IFRT to a dose of 3060 cGy (13/149; 9%). Estimated PFS was 91% at 3 years for the interim PET-negative group. The estimated 3-year PFS for the interim PET-positive group was significantly lower, at 66%, than for the interim PET-negative group ($P = 0.011$), suggesting that the intensive treatment regimen did not provide benefit.[63] In the HD16 trial of the German Hodgkin Study Group, patients with early-stage, favorable cHL were randomized to CMT with two cycles of ABVD + 20 Gy IFRT (standard as per HD10 study) versus PET-guided treatment, omitting IFRT after a negative second PET (PET2). With a median follow-up of 45 months, projected 5-year PFS was 93.4% for CMT and 86.1% for ABVD alone. This did not meet the study's noninferiority primary objective of excluding inferiority of 10% or more in 5-year PFS of ABVD alone compared with CMT in a per protocol analysis among PET2-negative patients.[75]

There is no dispute that, compared with ABVD + RT, ABVD alone (two cycles,[75] three cycles,[73] four cycles,[63] or six cycles[72]) for newly diagnosed nonbulky diagnosed cHL will result in an approximately 5–10% lower PFS without lower survival when patients receive appropriate salvage treatment. However, opinions differ as to whether it is necessary to expose approximately 90% of the PET2-negative patients to the late potential risks of IFRT or ISRT to achieve a slightly superior PFS.

Unfavorable risk

The standard of care for patients with early-stage, unfavorable risk cHL is CMT with a 5-year PFS of 80–85%.[64,65] Some patients with nonbulky disease and unfavorable risk may have good outcome with early-interim PET negativity and may be candidates for chemotherapy alone.[76] With bulky disease, however, the addition of RT appears particularly important, and PET-adapted studies omitting radiotherapy have generally excluded such patients.[77]

Several randomized trials have examined dose and schedule of combined modality therapy in early-stage, unfavorable risk cHL.[78–81] The GHSG HD11 trial compared four CMT regimens in 1570 patients: ABVD × 4 cycles + 20 Gy IFRT, ABVD × 4 cycles + 30 Gy IFRT, BEACOPP × 4 cycles + 20 Gy IFRT, BEACOPP × 4 cycles × 30 Gy IFRT. Stage IIB was considered advanced-stage and excluded. Five-year FFTF was 81% (4 ABVD + 20 Gy), 85% (4 ABVD + 30 Gy), 87% (4 BEACOPP + 20 Gy), and 87% (4 BEACOPP + 30 Gy).[78] When combined with 20 Gy IFRT, results favored BEACOPP; however, with 30 Gy IFRT, ABVD + RT was equivalent and had less toxicity. The authors recommended four cycles of ABVD + 30 Gy IFRT in early unfavorable cHL.

The GHSG HD14 trial compared four cycles of ABVD + 30 Gy IFRT versus two cycles of escalated BEACOPP followed by two cycles of ABVD (2 + 2) + 30 Gy IFRT.[79] The "2 + 2" arm had 5-year FFTF of 94.8% versus 87.7% with 4 ABVD + IFRT ($P = <0.001$); however, there were significantly increased acute toxicities in the "2 + 2" arm. At a median follow-up of 43 months, there were no differences in treatment-related mortality or secondary malignancies, however.

The Intergroup Trial E2496 compared six to eight cycles of ABVD + 36 Gy IFRT versus Stanford V.[82] For patients with stage I or II bulky disease (bulk defined as MMR of greater than one third on chest radiography or ≥10 cm on CT), the 5-year FFS was 85% for ABVD + IFRT versus 79% for Stanford V (HR, 0.68; 95% CI, 0.37–1.25), with no significant difference between the two treatment approaches. More patients got IFRT (bulk defined as >5 cm) with Stanford V and more patients on ABVD received long-course chemotherapy.[80,82] Although consolidation RT was the standard of care in these trials, recent randomized data suggest that it may be unnecessary in patients whose PET2 and end-of-treatment PET are negative after six cycles of ABVD.[69]

Advanced-stage cHL

The International Prognostic Score (IPS) identifies seven independent prognostic factors associated with inferior progression-free and overall survival in advanced cHL: serum albumin <4 g/dL; hemoglobin <10.5 g/dL; male gender; stage IV disease; ≥45 years old; white cell count ≥15,000/mm³; lymphocyte count <600/mm³ or 8% of total white cell count.[83] The highest risk group (five or more risk factors) had a 5-year FFP of 42% as compared to 80% for patients without risk factors. The IPS analyzed data before 1990, prompting a new evaluation. This study included 740 patients treated with ABVD or ABVD-like regimens in the British Columbia Cancer Agency (BCCA) database.[82,84] The IPS was still found to be prognostically significant, but with a narrower difference between outcomes: 5-year FFP of 70% for patients with >4 IPS factors compared to 88% with no adverse factors, and 5-year OS of 73% and 98%, respectively. These results demonstrate improved outcomes likely owing to uniform anthracycline-containing chemotherapy (ABVD), growth factor support, improved accuracy of staging, and more accurate pathologic diagnosis.

Treatment

Standard therapy for advanced cHL is six cycles of ABVD. Dose-intensive treatment regimens have been studied. Although phase 2 trials suggested that Stanford V might have superior efficacy as compared to ABVD, the Intergroup Study for advanced-stage cHL patients found no difference in FFS: 74% for ABVD and 71% for Stanford V at 5 years.[82,85–87] Moreover, the Stanford V arm was associated with a higher incidence of lymphopenia and neuropathy.

The GHSG-escalated BEACOPP regimen is widely used in Europe; however, it has failed to gain popularity in the United States owing to excess toxicities and no clear survival benefit. Three GHSG phase 3 trials—HD9, HD12, and HD15—have examined BEACOPP. In the HD9 study, 1196 patients were randomized to COPP-ABVD, standard-dose BEACOPP, or escalated BEACOPP.[53] All were eight cycles + RT to initial sites ≥5 cm. The 5- and 10-year analyses showed that escBEACOPP was significantly better than BEACOPP or COPP-ABVD for FFTF (82%, 70%, and 64%) and OS (86%, 80%, and 75%). The escBEACOPP regimen appeared to have the greatest clinical benefit for IPS scores 4–7 but had greater myelosuppression, infertility, and secondary myelodysplasia/acute leukemia.[53,54]

HD12 compared eight cycles of escBEACOPP to four cycles of escBEACOPP + 4 baseline BEACOPP (4 + 4).[88] Patients were then randomized to no further therapy versus 30 Gy RT consolidation. 5-year FFTF was 86.4% for escBEACOPP versus 84.8% for "4 + 4", and OS was 92% versus 90.3%. The FFTF was better in the RT arm, although OS was not significantly improved.[88]

HD15 trial included 2182 patients who received eight cycles of escBEACOPP, six cycles of escBEACOPP, or eight cycles of a time-intensified standard-dose BEACOPP.[55] RT (30 Gy) was restricted to patients with PET-positive residual sites (≥2.5 cm). 5-year FFTF was 84.4%, 89.3%, and 85.4%; and 5-year OS 91.9%, 95.3%, and 94.5%, respectively. The authors recommended six cycles of escBEACOPP as having significantly better outcomes, less treatment-related mortality, and fewer secondary cancers.

A subset of cHL is CD20+, with expression of this B-cell antigen on the R–S cell. Phase 2 studies adding rituximab (anti-CD20 monoclonal antibody) administered weekly for 6 weeks to ABVD in advanced-stage CD20+ cHL have been reported.[89,90] In one study, 5-year event-free survival (EFS) and OS rates of 83% and 96%, respectively, were reported for this histologic subset.[89]

Risk-adapted interim PET imaging is also being applied in advanced-stage cHL. A phase 2 study from Israel suggests that risk- and response-adapted treatment may be effective. In this study, 45 poor-risk (IPS ≥3) advanced-stage cHL patients received two cycles of escBEACOPP, followed by a PET scan. If PET was negative, patients were subsequently treated with four cycles of ABVD. For the 31 patients who achieved a negative early-interim PET scan, the 4-year PFS was 87%.[61]

Two recent trials have employed interim PET after two cycles of chemotherapy to tailor treatment for patients with advanced-stage cHL. S0816, a phase 2 trial conducted by the US Intergroup, treated stage III and IV patients with two cycles of ABVD followed by interim PET/CT. Interim PET-negative patients received four more cycles of ABVD, while those who were interim PET-positive received six cycles of escBEACOPP. The estimated 2-year PFS was 82% for interim PET-negative patients and 64% for interim PET-positive patients. With additional follow-up (median 5.9 years), estimated 5-year PFS was 76% for interim PET-negative patients and 66% for interim PET-positive patients. Estimated 5-year overall survival was 94%. Of note, there were two treatment-related deaths (4%) among the 49 interim PET-positive patients who receive escBEACOPP and a high rate of second cancers.[67,91]

The Response-Adapted Trial in Advanced Hodgkin Lymphoma (RATHL) treated patients with stages IIB, III, IV, and high-risk IIA with two cycles of ABVD followed by interim PET/CT. Patients who were interim PET-negative were randomized to treatment with four cycles of ABVD or four cycles of AVD without bleomycin. Patients who were interim PET-positive were treated with escBEACOPP or BEACOPP-14 depending on results of further interim PET/CT studies. For postcycle two interim PET-negative patients, the 3-year PFS was 85.7% for the ABVD and 84.4% for the ABVD/AVD groups, respectively. For the interim PET-positive patients treated with BEACOPP, the 3-year PFS was 67.5%. These findings justify reducing exposure to bleomycin with its attendant pulmonary toxicity for patients with advanced-stage cHL who are interim PET-negative after two cycles of ABVD.[68]

As described above, BV + AVD is a new treatment option for patients with stages III and IV cHL,[56] with a 7% higher PFS compared with ABVD at 3 years.[57]

Management of relapsed/refractory Hodgkin lymphoma

The standard treatment approach for relapsed/refractory (r/r) cHL is salvage chemotherapy to achieve remission status, followed by myeloablative chemotherapy and autologous stem-cell transplant (ASCT). Various groups have developed prognostic models to predict the outcome of r/r cHL completing ASCT.[92–96] Unfavorable risk factors include presence of extranodal disease, abbreviated remission duration after frontline therapy (generally <1 year), and presence of B symptoms. In addition, a powerful independent prognostic factor is pretransplant functional imaging status. In one study with median follow-up of 51 months, patients with a negative PET scan before ASCT had superior outcomes with EFS >80% versus 29% for patients with a positive scan.[97]

There are many salvage regimens for r/r cHL including ICE (ifosfamide, carboplatin, and etoposide), DHAP (dexamethasone, high-dose cytarabine, and cisplatin), ESHAP (etoposide, methylprednisolone, high-dose cytarabine, and cisplatin), IGEV (ifosfamide, gemcitabine, and vinorelbine), and GVD (gemcitabine, vinorelbine, and pegylated liposomal doxorubicin).[93,98–101] These regimens have not been prospectively compared, but nevertheless appear to have similar efficacy in phase 2 studies.

The goal of salvage treatment is to achieve a PET-negative remission before consolidative ASCT, as patients with persistent disease at the time of transplant have poor outcomes. This aim may be achieved by one or more salvage regimens, with or without radiotherapy. The potential curative role and significant survival benefit of ASCT in r/r cHL have been established by two large randomized trials comparing chemotherapy alone to chemotherapy followed by ASCT.[102,103]

New agents in Hodgkin lymphoma

Approximately 15% of cHL patients will fail both first- and second-line therapy and require novel therapy. BV was FDA-approved in 2012 for r/r cHL after failure of ASCT or for those not deemed ASCT candidates after failure of at least two multiagent regimens.[104,105] Other agents with demonstrated activity include histone deacetylase inhibitors, PI3-kinase/Akt/mTOR pathway inhibitors, lenalidomide, and bendamustine.[106] Most recently, immune checkpoint inhibitors targeting the programmed death-1/programmed death-1-ligand (PD1/PDL1) pathway have shown promise in cHL. The PD1/PDL1 pathway dampens immune responses, and inhibition of this pathway results in augmentation of host immune response against tumor cells. Preliminary data (2014 American Society of Hematology) has revealed overall response rates ranging from 50% to 89% for two of these agents, pembrolizumab and nivolumab.[107,108]

BV is an antibody–drug conjugate (ADC) consisting of the chimeric anti-CD30 monoclonal antibody (cAC10) chemically conjugated to monomethyl auristatin E (MMAE).[109] MMAE is internalized into the Reed–Sternberg cell, where it is a tubulin inhibitor resulting in cell cycle arrest and apoptosis.[110] The initial phase 1 study enrolled 45 patients with r/r CD30-positive hematologic malignancies. BV was administered intravenously every 3 weeks at doses ranging from 0.1 to 3.6 mg/kg. Dose-limiting toxicities included grade-4 thrombocytopenia, grade-3 hyperglycemia, and febrile neutropenia. The maximum tolerated dose (MTD) was 1.8 mg/kg every 3 weeks. Promising responses were seen, and a phase 2 study in 102 patients with r/r cHL after ASCT confirmed these results.[111] Patients received 1.8 mg/kg BV every 3 weeks for up to 16 cycles. The overall response rate was 75%, with complete remissions in 34 of 102 (33%). The median PFS was 5.6 months and OS 40.5 months. Moreover, 14 patients remained in durable remission after BV and of these, 9 had not started new therapy and 5 had proceeded to consolidative allogeneic SCT. BV is now FDA-approved in combination with AVD for newly diagnosed stage III and IV patients and as maintenance treatment in patients following ASCT.[112] Similar BV combinations regimens are under investigation for early-stage[51] and elderly cHL.[113] Another strategy is BV before ASCT in place of, or in addition to, standard salvage therapy, such as ICE. Following initial treatment,[114,115] approximately one-third of relapsed/refractory cHL patients will achieve a complete remission by PET and can proceed to ASCT without receiving more toxic regimens like ICE.[115] With the addition of nivolumab, this percentage of PET-negative CR patients avoiding more toxic regimens prior to ASCT is increased to approximately two-thirds.[116] Post-ASCT, a phase 3 study of BV maintenance versus placebo demonstrated a significant improvement in median PFS favoring maintenance BV versus placebo (42.9 months vs 24.1 months) in high-risk cHL. This PFS benefit was sustained at 5 years.[112]

Special populations

NLPHL

This rare subset of lymphoma (see pathology discussion) is now recognized to be highly treatable but likely not curable with standard cHL therapy.[117–119] It was recognized 76 years ago by Jackson and Parker that "Hodgkin's paragranuloma" (now nodular lymphocyte-predominant Hodgkin lymphoma [NLPHL] in the modified Lukes and Butler classification) patients "may live unembarrassed by their disease—if the pathologic picture does not change—for many years."[120] Management options include excision only; IFRT or CMT in early stage; and active surveillance;[121] rituximab alone or with chemotherapy, or palliative IFRT for relapsed/advanced-stage disease. Most importantly, survival remains excellent but can be negatively affected by the late effects of active therapy.[121] Thus, in this lymphoma, it is important to be mindful when treating young patients of the intensity of treatment utilized and the likely good outcomes achievable with initial active surveillance or limited therapy. Like indolent lymphoma, NLPHL is associated with the late development of histologic transformation (T-cell-rich B-cell lymphoma, a subtype of DLBCL, or DLBCL). This may be a life-threatening development and requires a multiagent chemotherapy regimen, as in management of DLBCL.

Elderly

In the elderly, the curative aim of cHL treatment remains realistic, although the management approach may be modified for tolerability. ABVD is the standard regimen, although bleomycin may be more lung-toxic, and other regimens are often considered (without doxorubicin or bleomycin). As previously discussed, BV + AVD is a current treatment option that omits bleomycin for newly diagnosed stage III and IV patients. Sequential use of BV before and after AVD has been associated with good outcomes and acceptable toxicity in a phase 2 trial in a newly diagnosed older cHL population.[113] In unfit older patients, combination of BV with dacarbazine was effective and well-tolerated.[122] Relapsed/refractory cHL may still be approached with salvage chemotherapy and ASCT in selected patients, generally those with physiologic age of 70 or lower. Without second-line ASCT, most patients do not have a curative option at this time and are managed with phase 1–2 clinical trials, palliative chemotherapy, and/or RT.

Pregnancy

cHL may occur in young women, and not infrequently, may present during pregnancy. Details of management are discussed elsewhere. Most importantly, cHL is generally a slowly progressive lymphoma and its treatment can often be delayed until delivery, or ABVD can be safely administered during the second and/or third trimesters. Imaging during pregnancy should be minimized with use of MRI, and no PET should be performed.

HIV

Classical HL may be seen in association with HIV, and in this context, the pathology is more likely mixed cellularity or lymphocyte-depleted histologic subtypes, and the stage more advanced with unusual sites such as skin. Treatment regimens remain the same as for non-HIV patients, when the CD4 count exceeds 200 and patients receive concurrent combination antiretroviral therapy (cART) and prophylactic antibiotics as indicated. Results with HIV-associated, newly diagnosed cHL when patients have preserved immune function on ART show good outcomes with standard treatment similar to those without HIV infection.[123–127] A more selective approach is needed in more immunosuppressed patients where infectious complications may be greater.[127]

Posttreatment surveillance

The ability to predict sustained remission and curability has increased with PET imaging, raising the important question of when, how frequently, and for how long surveillance imaging should be continued postremission. All agree that, in the surveillance setting, PET is too sensitive, identifying excess false positives. Selective CT or MRI imaging can be alternatives when needed. As most relapses occur in the first 2–3 years posttreatment, routine imaging after this timeframe may be unnecessary.[128]

References

1. Hodgkin. On some morbid appearances of the absorbent glands and spleen. *Med Chir Trans*. 1832;**17**:68–114.
2. Sternberg C. Uber eine Eigenartige unter dem Bilde der Pseudoleuktiie verlaufende Tuberculose des lymphatischen apparates. *Ztschr Heilk*. 1898;**19**:21–90.
3. Reed DM. On the pathological changes in Hodgkin's disease, with especial reference to its relation to tuberculosis. *J Johns Hopkins Hosp Rep*. 1902;**10**:133–196.
4. Pusey WA. Cases of Sarcoma and of Hodgkin's disease treated by exposures to X-rays—a preliminary report. *JAMA J Am Med Assoc*. 1902;**XXXVIII**(3):166–169.
5. Senn N. Therapeutical value of röntgen ray in treatment of pseudoleukemia. *New York Med J*;**77**:665–668.
6. Gilbert R. Radiotherapy in Hodgkin's disease (malignant granulomatosis): anatomic and clinical foundations; governing principles: results. *Am J Roentgenol*. 1939;**41**:198–241.
7. Peters MV. A study of survivals in Hodgkin's disease treated radiologically. *J Roentgenol Radium Therapy*. 1950;**63**:299–311.
8. Kaplan HS. The radical radiotherapy of regionally localized Hodgkin's disease. *Radiology*. 1962;**78**:553–561.
9. Kaplan HS. Role of intensive radiotherapy in the management of Hodgkin's disease. *Cancer*. 1966;**19**:356–367.
10. Jacobs C. *Henry Kaplan and the story of Hodgkin's Disease*. Stanford, CA: Stanford University Press; 2010.
11. Devita VT Jr, Serpick AA, Carbone PP. Combination chemotherapy in the treatment of advanced Hodgkin's disease. *Ann Intern Med*. 1970;**73**:881–895.
12. DeVita VT Jr, Simon RM, Hubbard SM, et al. Curability of advanced Hodgkin's disease with chemotherapy. Long-term follow-up of MOPP-treated patients at the National Cancer Institute. *Ann Intern Med*. 1980;**92**:587–595.
13. Canellos GP, Anderson JR, Propert KJ, et al. Chemotherapy of advanced Hodgkin's disease with MOPP, ABVD, or MOPP alternating with ABVD. *N Engl J Med*. 1992;**327**:1478–1484.
14. Bonadonna G, Zucali R, Monfardini S, et al. Combination chemotherapy of Hodgkin's disease with adriamycin, bleomycin, vinblastine, and imidazole carboxamide versus MOPP. *Cancer*. 1975;**36**:252–259.
15. Vockerodt M, Yap L-F, Shannon-Lowe C, et al. The Epstein-Barr virus and the pathogenesis of lymphoma. *J Pathol*. 2015;**235**:312–322.
16. Kushekhar K, van den Berg A, Nolte I, et al. Genetic associations in classical hodgkin lymphoma: a systematic review and insights into susceptibility mechanisms. *Cancer Epidemiol Biomarkers Prev*. 2014;**23**:2737–2747.
17. Gutensohn N, Cole P. Childhood social environment and Hodgkin's disease. *N Engl J Med*. 1981;**304**:135–140.
18. Mueller N. Hodgkin's disease. In: Schnottenfeld D, Fraumeni J, eds. *Cancer Epidemiology and Prevention*. New York, NY: Oxford University Press; 1992.
19. Mueller N, Evans A, Harris NL, et al. Hodgkin's disease and Epstein-Barr virus. Altered antibody pattern before diagnosis. *N Engl J Med*. 1989;**320**:689–695.
20. Glaser SL, Lin RJ, Stewart SL, et al. Epstein-Barr virus-associated Hodgkin's disease: epidemiologic characteristics in international data. *Int J Cancer*. 1997;**70**:375–382.
21. Weiss LM, Movahed LA, Warnke RA, et al. Detection of Epstein-Barr viral genomes in Reed-Sternberg cells of Hodgkin's disease. *N Engl J Med*. 1989;**320**:502–506.
22. Cunningham J, Mauch P, Rosenthal DS, et al. Long-term complications of MOPP chemotherapy in patients with Hodgkin's disease. *Cancer Treat Rep*. 1982;**66**:1015–1022.
23. Fisher RI, DeVita VT Jr, Bostick F, et al. Persistent immunologic abnormalities in long-term survivors of advanced Hodgkin's disease. *Ann Intern Med*. 1980;**92**:595–599.
24. King RL, Howard MT, Bagg A. Hodgkin lymphoma. *Adv Anat Pathol*. 2014;**21**:17–30.
25. Calvo KR, Traverse-Glehen A, Pittaluga S, et al. Molecular profiling provides evidence of primary mediastinal large B-cell lymphoma as a distinct entity related to classic Hodgkin lymphoma: implications for mediastinal gray zone lymphomas as an intermediate form of B-cell lymphoma. *Adv Anat Pathol*. 2004;**11**:227–238.
26. Hoeller S, Copie-Bergman C. Grey zone lymphomas: lymphomas with intermediate features. *Adv Hematol*. 2012;**2012**:460801.
27. Wilson WH, Pittaluga S, Nicolae A, et al. A prospective study of mediastinal gray-zone lymphoma. *Blood*. 2014;**124**:1563–1569.
28. Mauch PM, Kalish LA, Kadin M, et al. Patterns of presentation of Hodgkin disease. Implications for etiology and pathogenesis. *Cancer*. 1993;**71**:2062–2071.
29. Poppema S, Brinker MGL, Visser L. *Evidence for a B-Cell Origin of the Proliferating Cells*. Springer US: Cancer Treatment and Research; 1989:5–27.
30. Pinkus GS, Said JW. Hodgkin's disease, lymphocyte predominance type, nodular—further evidence for a B cell derivation. L & H variants of Reed-Sternberg cells express L26, a pan B cell marker. *Am J Pathol*. 1988;**133**:211–217.
31. Burns BF, Colby TV, Dorfman RF. Differential diagnostic features of nodular L & H Hodgkin's disease, including progressive transformation of germinal centers. *Am J Surg Pathol*. 1984;**8**:253–261.
32. Mason DY, Banks PM, Chan J, et al. Nodular lymphocyte predominance Hodgkin's disease. A distinct clinicopathological entity. *Am J Surg Pathol*. 1994;**18**:526–530.
33. Küppers R. Molecular biology of Hodgkin's lymphoma. *Adv Cancer Res*. 2002;**84**:277–312.
34. Mathas S, Lietz A. Anagnostopoulos I, et al.: c-FLIP mediates resistance of Hodgkin/Reed-Sternberg cells to death receptor-induced apoptosis. *J Exp Med*. 2004;**199**:1041–1052.
35. Hinz M, Lemke P, Anagnostopoulos I, et al. Nuclear factor kappaB-dependent gene expression profiling of Hodgkin's disease tumor cells, pathogenetic significance, and link to constitutive signal transducer and activator of transcription 5a activity. *J Exp Med*. 2002;**196**:605–617.
36. Thomas RK, Re D, Wolf J, et al. Part I: Hodgkin's lymphoma—molecular biology of Hodgkin and Reed-Sternberg cells. *Lancet Oncol*. 2004;**5**:11–18.
37. Re D, Starostik P, Massoudi N, et al. Allelic losses on chromosome 6q25 in Hodgkin and Reed Sternberg cells. *Cancer Res*. 2003;**63**:2606–2609.
38. Skinnider BF, Mak TW. The role of cytokines in classical Hodgkin lymphoma. *Blood*. 2002;**99**:4283–4297.
39. Kadin M, Butmarc J, Elovic A, et al. Eosinophils are the major source of transforming growth factor-beta 1 in nodular sclerosing Hodgkin's disease. *Am J Pathol*. 1993;**142**:11–16.
40. Chang ET, Zheng T, Weir EG, et al. Aspirin and the risk of Hodgkin's lymphoma in a population-based case-control study. *J Natl Cancer Inst*. 2004;**96**:305–315.

116 Clonal hematopoiesis in cancer

Philipp J. Rauch, MD ■ David P. Steensma, MD

Overview

Clonal hematopoiesis represents a precursor syndrome to development of hematologic malignancy. The discovery of clonal hematopoiesis resulted from improvement in next-generation sequencing that allows identification of low-variant allele frequency mutations in select genes that provide hematopoietic stem cells a growth advantage over time as compared to un-mutated stem cells. Clonal hematopoiesis results from acquisition of mutations over time in hematopoietic stem cells as individuals age. Clonal hematopoiesis is not only a risk factor for the development of hematologic malignancies but also to many other processes involving inflammation that ultimately have the potential to impact patient survival. Strategies to both utilize the presence of clonal hematopoiesis in risk assessment for cancer, cardiovascular mortality, and to potentially intervene to prevent these outcomes yet to be developed.

Clonal hematopoiesis: discovery and definitions

Normal hematopoiesis represents the orderly contribution to healthy blood cell production of numerous self-renewing hematopoietic stem cells (HSC), which reside in specialized bone marrow niches and give rise to hierarchically organized differentiated progeny.[1] The exact number of functional—in contrast to immunophenotypic—HSCs that contribute to the circulating blood pool at any given time has long been debated. While extrapolation from animal studies performed several decades ago suggested the human long-term pluripotential HSC population might number around 10,000,[2] a more recent study applied population genetic approaches to patterns of somatic mutations in order to reconstruct clonal dynamics of native human hematopoiesis, which resulted in a revised estimate of 50,000–200,000 functional HSCs throughout adult life.[3] These quantitative insights added to an existing body of evidence establishing healthy hematopoiesis as a dynamic and highly polyclonal system, and also inferred that a somatic "passenger" mutation in an HSC conferring no clonal advantage (such mutations arise at a frequency of 1.2 exonic mutations per stem cell per decade[4]) should be present at a variant allele frequency (VAF) on the order of $\sim 10^{-5}$.

In 1960, Peter Nowell and David Hungerford at the University of Pennsylvania cultured cells from patients suffering from what was then called chronic granulocytic leukemia, now known as chronic myeloid leukemia (CML), and observed presence of an abnormal minute chromosome—later identified as chromosome 22, and now known as the "Philadelphia" chromosome—in all leukemic cells.[5] This discovery marked the first demonstration of a clonal marker of abnormal hematopoiesis. With evolving diagnostic capabilities and biological understanding, clonality was subsequently discovered to be a characteristic feature of all hematologic malignancies.[6]

The term "clonal hematopoiesis" is now used as shorthand to describe the presence of one or several blood cell clones, each derived from a single mutated ancestor HSC, that has acquired a somatic variant conferring a competitive advantage (survival, proliferation, or both) compared to cells retaining a germline configuration. This advantage allows the mutant HSC and its progeny to expand and to disproportionately contribute to the circulating blood cell pool.[7] While this definition does not necessarily describe a disease, but rather a biological state of somatic mosaicism,[8] clonal hematopoiesis had long been thought to be predominantly associated with presence of overt hematologic malignancy.

Already in the 1990s, however, there were clues that clonal hematopoiesis might also be common outside the context of malignancy. When studying the blood of healthy women with informative polymorphisms that allowed assessment of myeloid series X-chromosomal inactivation patterns, two independent studies found a surprisingly high proportion of older women to have skewed inactivation of the X chromosome in at least 3 : 1 ratio in terminally differentiated white blood cells.[9,10] The presence of nonrandom X inactivation seemed to correlate with the age of the individual and was much more common in women over 65 years of age. While clonal hematopoiesis in healthy individuals was discussed as a potential hypothesis to explain the experimental findings, other possible causes such as nonrandom stem cell depletion could not be ruled out, and the molecular basis for X-inactivation skewing remained obscure. In the same era, individuals were found to have *BCR-ABL* fusion—the molecular basis of the Philadelphia chromosome—transiently detectable using sensitive molecular techniques, and others were noted to have immunoglobulin translocations characteristic of lymphoma briefly detectable in the absence of malignancy.[11,12]

In 2012, Lambert Busque and colleagues in Quebec performed exome sequencing on three apparently healthy older women with X-inactivation skewing and found all three women to harbor mutations in the gene *TET2*, an epigenetic regulator that had been described a few years earlier as recurrently mutated in hematologic malignancies. The investigators then expanded their studies to a larger group of individuals, detecting *TET2* mutations in 10 out of 182 tested individuals with X-inactivation skewing but in none of the control women without skewing.[13] This work showed that clonal hematopoiesis, defined by the presence of a somatic mutation associated with neoplasia, can be stably present in normal individuals without overt hematologic malignancies. Also in 2012, analysis of single nucleotide polymorphism array genome-wide association studies performed for other reasons indicated that somatic mosaicism at the chromosome level is detectable in 1–2% of healthy people above age 50, and this finding confers an increased risk for subsequently evolving hematologic neoplasia.[14]

In 2014, three independent studies firmly established clonal hematopoiesis as a highly prevalent, age-dependent phenomenon in otherwise healthy individuals.[15–17] All three efforts made use of preexisting whole-exome sequencing data from large, clinically annotated cohorts unselected for hematological phenotypes to characterize the prevalence and mutational spectrum of clonal hematopoiesis. Clonal hematopoiesis was found to be strongly associated with age (Figure 1), and surprisingly common in the general population: as an example, approximately 10% of individuals in the age bracket of 70–79 years turned out to carry a somatic mutation in their blood at a VAF of at least 1–2%. What stood out further was the fact that the mutant clones comprised a fairly large portion of the blood leukocyte pool, with an average of 18% of blood cells being part of the clone (corresponding to an average VAF of 9% with a copy-neutral mutation such as *TET2* present in heterozygous state), and these clones persisted over years, indicating the process likely affected long-lived HSCs or other cells that had acquired self-renewal properties.

Since studied cohorts included tens of thousands of individuals, these repurposed genome-wide association studies were informative with respect to the mutational spectrum of clonal hematopoiesis, showing that mutations occurred primarily in genes that are commonly mutated in cancers of the myeloid lineage, and most commonly in genes that are known to be epigenetic regulators, with mutations in the genes *DNMT3A*, *TET2*, and *ASXL1* being most common. As could be expected, individuals with clonal hematopoiesis had a substantially increased risk of developing a hematologic malignancy. Arguably the most consequential finding, however, was an approximately 40% relative increase in all-cause mortality in individuals over age 70 years carrying a mutation,[15] much more than could be accounted for by relative rare hematological malignancy diagnoses, which is discussed in greater detail below.

These insights led to the definition of clonal hematopoiesis of indeterminate potential (CHIP) as a clinical entity in 2015, which was distinguished from myelodysplastic syndromes (MDS). MDS can be diagnosed in the absence of morphologic evidence if an unexplained cytopenia plus one of a limited repertoire of MDS-associated karyotypes such as deletion of chromosome 5q is detected. In contrast, CHIP is defined as presence of a somatic mutation (recurrently) associated with a hematologic neoplasia at a VAF of at least 2%, in the absence of cytopenias or definitive morphological evidence of a hematological neoplasm. The VAF cutoff of 2% reflected technical limitations of typical next-generation sequencing panels commonly used in clinical practice. Further, individuals with CHIP by definition cannot meet diagnostic criteria for paroxysmal nocturnal hemoglobinuria (PNH), monoclonal gammopathy of undetermined significance (MGUS), or monoclonal B-cell lymphocytosis (MBL), with the latter two representing precursor conditions involving lineage-committed cells, while CHIP affects the HSC compartment.[18] The risk of progression from CHIP to a hematological neoplasm diagnosable using 2016 World Health Organization (WHO) criteria (Figure 2)

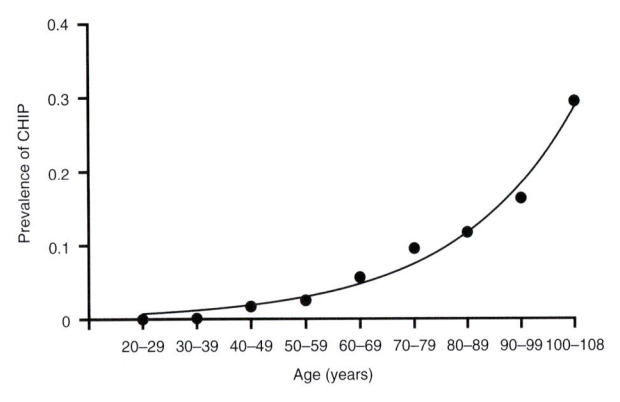

Figure 1 Prevalence of somatic mutations, by age bracket, detected by whole-exome sequencing, with data from Jaiswal et al.[15] (dots). Nonlinear curve fit (exponential regression model), $R^2 = 0.984$. The prevalence is higher if sensitive error-corrected sequencing techniques that can detect clones with a variant allele frequency <1% are used. Source: Data from Jaiswal et al.[15]

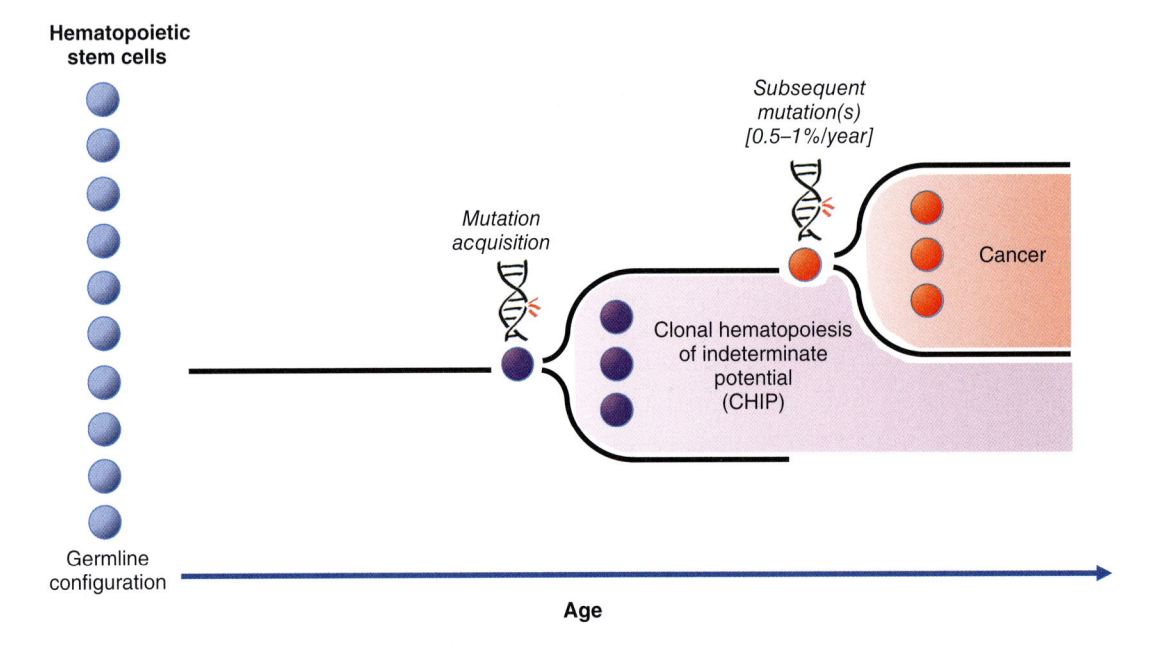

Figure 2 Model depicting the emergence of clonal hematopoiesis of indeterminate potential (CHIP) during aging and subsequent progression to hematologic malignancy at the time of subsequent secondary mutation acquisition.

Table 1 Definitions of clonal hematopoiesis of indeterminate potential (CHIP) and distinction from other disorders of myelopoiesis.[a]

	ICUS	CHIP	CCUS	Lower-risk MDS	Higher-risk MDS/AML
Clonality	–	+ (>2% VAF)	+	+	+
Cytopenia	+	–	+	+	+
Dysplasia	–	–	–	+	+
Blast count	Normal	Normal	Normal	Normal	Elevated
Approximate progression risk at 10 years	10%	5%	90%	n/a	n/a

Abbreviations: ICUS, idiopathic cytopenia(s) of undetermined significance; CCUS, clonal cytopenia(s) of undetermined significance; MDS, myelodysplastic syndromes; AML, acute myeloid leukemia; MDS-EB, MDS with excess blasts; VAF, variant allele frequency.
Estimates of progression risk into WHO-defined malignancy derived from Jaiswal et al.[15] (CHIP) and Malcovati et al.[21] (ICUS, CCUS).
[a]Source: Adapted from Jaiswal et al.[15]; Steensma et al.[18]; Malcovati et al.[21]

has been estimated to be 0.5–1% per year, similar in magnitude to the risk of progression of MGUS and MBL to multiple myeloma or a lymphoid malignancy, respectively. The term aging-associated or aging-related clonal hematopoiesis (ARCH) has also been used to describe any type of acquired clonal event with no defined cut-off for VAF or allele requirement.[19,20]

Detection of recurrent somatic mutations was further used to refine the term idiopathic cytopenia(s) of undetermined significance (ICUS), which had been in use since 2007 to describe the presence of unexplained cytopenia(s) in patients who do not fulfill WHO criteria for MDS or another neoplasm (Table 1).[22] Patients with unexplained cytopenias and a recurrent mutation can now be subclassified as having either ICUS if there is no known somatic mutation or clonal cytopenias of undetermined significance (CCUS) if a mutation is detected.[23] This distinction is clinically relevant, as patients with CCUS have a risk of progression to hematological malignancy meeting WHO diagnostic criteria that reaches approximately 80% at the 5-year mark, compared to less than 10% progression risk at 5 years for patients with nonmutated ICUS. Additionally, overall survival of CCUS patients was shown to be essentially indistinguishable from patients with lower-risk MDS, indicating that many such patients effectively have "MDS without dysplasia."[21]

Risk factors for clonal hematopoiesis

The initial studies showing that clonal hematopoiesis was a highly prevalent phenomenon established aging as the dominant risk factor for developing CHIP. However, the association with age is not exclusive, as CHIP can occur in younger individuals as well,[24] while smaller clones below the CHIP VAF threshold that are detectable only with sensitive error-corrected barcoding sequencing methods are virtually universal by middle age.[25,26] (Even though these mutations may be detectable only on the order of a VAF of 0.1%, the mutant HSCs are still >100-fold expanded compared to HSCs without a clonal advantage.) The initial datasets further suggested a modestly increased risk of developing CHIP in males, individuals of Hispanic ethnicity, and smokers.

Additionally, several germline predispositions to development of clonal hematopoiesis have been identified. A prominent example that is intimately linked to the pathogenesis of CHIP involves germline loss of the *MBD4* gene encoding methyl-CpG binding domain 4 deoxyribonucleic acid (DNA) glycosylase. This enzyme is involved in the repair of DNA mutations resulting from spontaneous deamination of methylated cytosine at CpG dinucleotides, generating thymine, which is the dominant, aging-related mutational event giving rise to ARCH/CHIP. A germline defect in this enzyme leads to an increased likelihood of both clonal hematopoiesis and myeloid malignancy, and a high mutational burden dominated by C to T transitions when neoplasia does arise.[27]

In the Icelandic deCODE genomic study of >10,000 persons, a noncoding telomerase (*TERT*) polymorphism was strongly associated with clonal hematopoiesis, including both clonal hematopoiesis associated with a putative leukemia "driver" gene mutation and that defined by outlier status in terms of overall somatic mutation burden in the absence of a recognized driver mutation.[28] At the chromosome level, several genes including *MPL* copy number variation predispose to somatic mosaicism as well as development of chronic lymphoid leukemia and myeloproliferative neoplasm, while polymorphisms at more than 150 loci were associated with somatic loss of the Y chromosome in a study of >800,000 men in the United Kingdom and Japan.[29,30] A higher than expected prevalence of CHIP in sibling donors in the context of allogeneic hematopoietic cell transplantation specifically for myeloid malignancies further suggests presence of a common germline (or possibly environmental) predisposition to clonal hematopoiesis in donor and recipient, given the myeloid bias in hematologic malignancies secondary to CHIP.[31] Lastly, recent reports suggest that aging-associated inflammation in the bone marrow microenvironment may favor outgrowth of mutated clones, but the exact molecular mechanisms remain to be elucidated.[32]

Emerging evidence suggests that the phenomenon of clonal expansion through somatic mutations in the absence of overt malignancy is not limited to the hematopoietic system. As an example, a study mapping mutant clones in esophagus epithelium from healthy donors found accumulation of somatic mutations with age and selective expansion of clones carrying mutations in cancer-associated genes.[33] Similar processes of age-related somatic mosaicism have been described in many tissues, including colon, brain, and liver, albeit with anatomical constraints that do not apply to the blood.[34–37] Future studies may ultimately lead to the conclusion that this represents a universal aging-associated phenomenon across all tissues.

Clinical consequences of clonal hematopoiesis

While not a disease state *per se*, the most consequential finding in the initial reports characterizing CHIP as a common aging-associated phenomenon was its striking association with adverse mortality outcomes (Figure 3), which was consistent across the different cohorts studied.[15,16]

As one might expect, the presence of CHIP substantially increases the risk of developing a hematological malignancy:

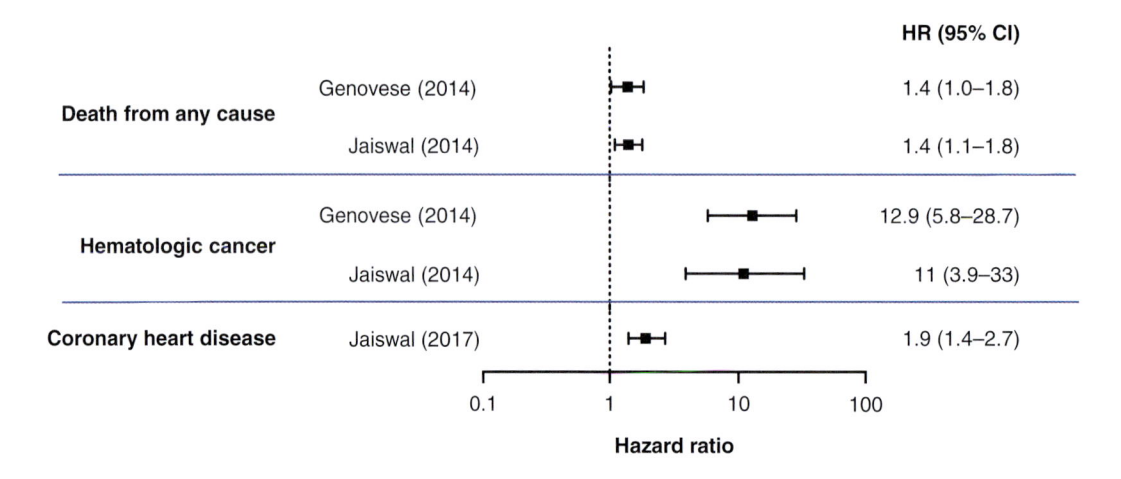

		HR (95% CI)
Death from any cause	Genovese (2014)	1.4 (1.0–1.8)
	Jaiswal (2014)	1.4 (1.1–1.8)
Hematologic cancer	Genovese (2014)	12.9 (5.8–28.7)
	Jaiswal (2014)	11 (3.9–33)
Coronary heart disease	Jaiswal (2017)	1.9 (1.4–2.7)

Figure 3 Hazard ratios for the development of specific clinical outcomes in individuals with clonal hematopoiesis (CH) compared to individuals without CH in three major studies.

a relative risk of more than 100-fold for myeloid neoplasia, and around 10-fold for lymphoid and plasma cell malignancies.[15] There is little doubt that this association reflects causation,[7] establishing CHIP as a precursor state, although it is unclear whether CHIP is a universal precursor state like MGUS is for myeloma or just a common pathway. While meaningful for the affected individuals, the excess mortality attributable to neoplasia can account for only a fraction of the observed increase in all-cause mortality, owing to the relatively low baseline incidence of hematological malignancies.

However, the hematopoietic system is unique in the sense that circulating cells interact with all other tissues in an organism, and as such, has the potential to impact disease states that one would not immediately associate with mutations arising in hematopoietic cells. The prototypic example of such an interaction is the striking finding that presence of CHIP increases the risk of developing events related to atherosclerotic cardiovascular disease, the leading cause of death globally, by approximately twofold, thereby accounting for the lion's share of the increased mortality risk.[38,39] This relationship is consistent across the three most commonly mutated genes, *DNMT3A*, *TET2*, and *ASXL1*, although may vary in magnitude in an allele-specific fashion. In a multivariate analysis, presence of a clonal mutation carried similar weight as traditional cardiovascular risk factors such as hyperlipidemia and hypertension and was synergistic with these risk factors.[40]

A causal relationship between clonal hematopoiesis and atherosclerosis has thus far only been established for loss of function mutations in one gene, *TET2*, which led to increased inflammation in terminally differentiated myeloid cells, namely macrophages, in an NLRP3 inflammasome-dependent manner, and increased atherosclerosis in mouse models.[40,41] The mechanisms by which mutations in other genes, including in the most commonly affected gene *DNMT3A*, may increase the risk for cardiovascular disease are the subject of active investigation. In a placebo-controlled study of an anti-interleukin-1β monoclonal antibody canakinumab in 10,061 patients who had experienced myocardial infarction and still had an elevated C-reactive protein >2 ng/mL, patients with clonal hematopoiesis experienced greater benefit in terms of recurrent myocardial infarction, stroke, or need for angioplasty than the population without *TET2* or *DNMT3A* mutations.[42,43]

More fundamentally, the ubiquitous presence of terminally differentiated mutant hematopoietic cells throughout an organism during aging and their influence on local inflammation leads us to predict that clonal hematopoiesis will be found to influence other age-associated pathophysiological processes, especially those associated with dysregulated inflammation. Studies to establish such associations are ongoing.

Additional clinical consequences of clonal hematopoiesis in the context of aplastic anemia, hematopoietic cell transplant, treatment for acute leukemia, and radiation or chemotherapy for a nonmyeloid tumor are discussed further below.

Determinants of transformation into overt malignancy

The majority of patients with clonal hematopoiesis will never experience progression to a neoplasm. One of the most puzzling aspects of CHIP is why, if somatic mutations confer a clear clonal advantage to HSCs, "clonal sweeping" of the marrow with replacement of all hematopoiesis by mutant cells is not more common than it is.[8] In many cases, clones with *DNMT3A* or *TET2* mutations conferring a growth or survival advantage to HSCs advantage will remain at stable VAFs in the 5–10% range for years. It is possible that certain areas of the hematopoietic niche within the marrow microenvironment are less hospitable to emergent mutant clonal cells than residual wild-type HSCs and cannot be occupied until a secondary mutation occurs, or that clones are constrained by endogenous immunity until downregulation of an immune checkpoint or evolution of a secondary mutation that allows immune evasion, but this remains speculative.[44]

The risk of progression to overt neoplasia likely depends on numerous factors, including the specific mutated allele(s), the number of mutations, the size of the abnormal clone (for which VAF is a surrogate marker), and the clinical context in which mutations are detected. For example, in CCUS, a VAF >20% and the presence of multiple mutations inclusive of a mutation in a gene encoding a component of the ribonucleic acid (RNA) spliceosome is associated with higher progression risk than single epigenetic mutations at VAF <10%.[21] In another series that looked at premorbid blood samples from patients who developed AML (samples were analyzed from a median of 6.3 years prior to diagnosis), certain mutations including splicing mutations were predictive of subsequent clonal progression to AML, as was an increased red cell distribution width (RDW).[45] An altered RDW may be a marker for a greater disruption of erythropoiesis by an emerging clonal process.

After a patient has already developed a malignancy, the persistence of somatic mutations during treatment may help predict relapse, but such assessments must be informed by knowledge of the high frequency of CHIP in aging populations. Persistent clones after completion of AML therapy—so-called "measurable residual disease" or "minimal" residual disease (MRD)—are associated with increased relapse risk, although there is variation in the risk depending on the specific scenario. For example, in one series of patients with AML who underwent intensive induction and consolidation chemotherapy, persistence of *DNMT3A, ASXL1,* or *TET2* mutations (most likely representing an antecedent clone on which the AML either arose or developed in parallel with) was not associated with subsequent leukemia recurrence.[46] However, an abnormal flow cytometry pattern consistent with MRD and presence of other more closely AML-associated mutations such as *FLT3* or *NPM1* was associated with an increased risk of relapse.

In the setting of aplastic anemia, clonal hematopoiesis is quite common, as HSCs with certain mutations may be relatively resistant to a T-cell mediated autoimmune attack.[47] Mutations including *BCOR, BCORL1,* or *PIGA* (the latter associated with PNH clones) predict a greater likelihood of favorable response to immunotherapy and better prognosis. Other mutations including *KRAS, NRAS, TP53,* or *DNMT3A* predict a higher likelihood of immunotherapy resistance and greater risk of clonal progression to MDS or AML. However, this risk is not absolute and even Ras-mutant or other high-risk clones that emerge in the aplastic anemia milieu may disappear over time.[48]

Although there is a myeloid bias in the neoplasms that evolve in the context of CHIP, lymphoid, and plasma cell neoplasms have also frequently been described. This likely reflects the fact that the stem cell that underlies CHIP is a true HSC with lymphoid and myeloid differentiation potential. In one exemplary case of "extensive CHIP," a patient with a high VAF (>40% VAF) clone with *TET2* and *ASXL1* mutations developed a *RHOA* mutation and was diagnosed with angioimmunoblastic T cell lymphoma, was successfully treated, and then subsequently developed an *NPM1* mutation and evolved AML.[49] Effectively in this case the "branches" of the clonal tree had been trimmed during the lymphoma therapy, but the root and trunk remained to branch anew.

Clonal hematopoiesis and chemotherapy

It has long been known that cytotoxic agents with the inherent potential to induce, or select for (Figure 4), mutations in hematopoietic cells can lead to the development of therapy-associated myeloid neoplasms.[50,51] Two major mutational patterns are observed in these neoplasms. In the first, which is most commonly associated with DNA alkylating agents or ionizing radiation, t-MDS/AML arises at a peak of 5–7 years after initial therapy and often involves complex cytogenetic changes, *TP53* mutation or loss, and extensive myelodysplasia.[52] The second pattern is observed after treatment with topoisomerase inhibitors, and is characterized by shorter latency (usually <3 years), specific genetic abnormalities involving *KMT2A(MLL), EVI1* or *RUNX1*, and more frequent presentation as frank AML rather than MDS.[53]

The extent to which mutations causing clonal hematopoiesis and therapy-related MDS/AML are actually induced by DNA-damaging cytotoxic agents versus cytotoxic agents permitting outgrowth of preexisting clones by selectively suppressive healthy wild-type HSCs has been an area of uncertainty.[54] This question was studied prospectively in a large single-center cohort of patients with nonhematologic cancers for whom paired tumor and blood samples were collected prior to therapy.[55] The samples were then assessed for presence of mutations by a targeted next-generation approach, allowing for more sensitive detection of clones compared to whole-exome sequencing approaches, down to a VAF of 1%. The prevalence of clonal hematopoiesis in this cohort

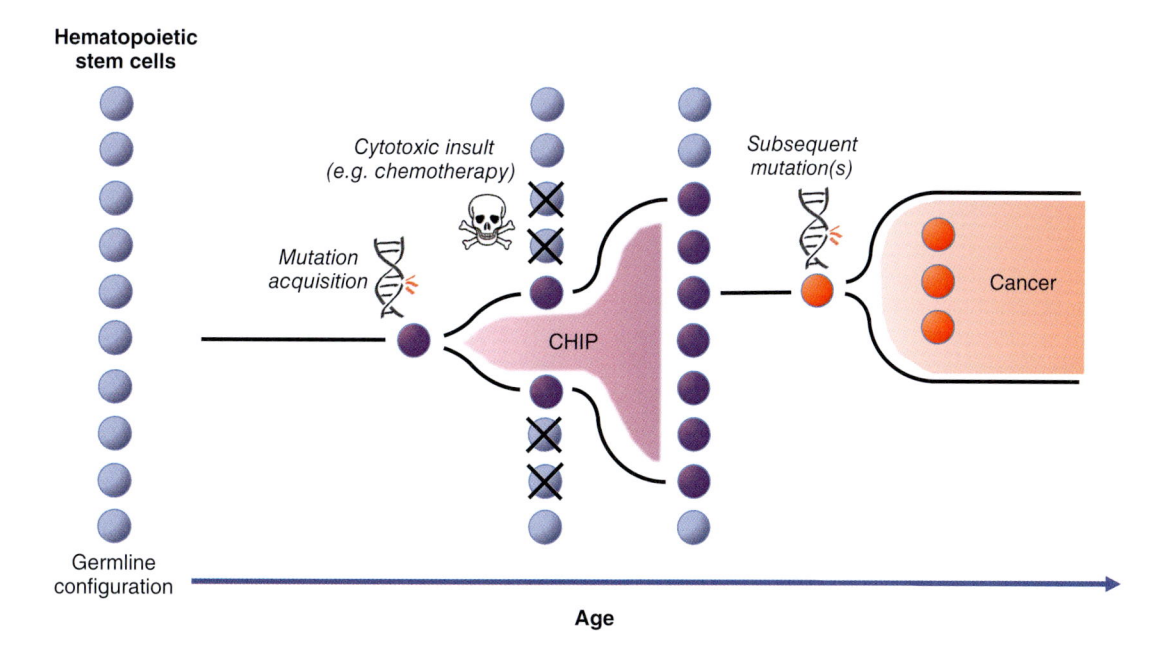

Figure 4 Model depicting the pathogenesis of clonal hematopoiesis of indeterminate potential (CHIP) related to a cytotoxic insult. Preexisting mutant clones can expand at the expense of healthy wild-type clones during hematopoietic stress. When subsequent mutations are acquired (and often in the absence of such mutations), a therapy-related neoplasm may result.

was found to be 25% with about 5% meeting the definition of CHIP (i.e., blood-restricted mutations in putative leukemia driver genes), and age, radiation therapy, and tobacco use were identified as additional risk factors. Presence of clonal hematopoiesis was associated with adverse outcomes, including increased risk of developing a hematological malignancy and, in the subset of patients with putative leukemia driver mutations, decreased overall survival and increased risk of therapy-related MDS/AML. Importantly, the main cause of death in this study was progression of the primary nonhematologic malignancy, suggesting a possible interaction between the presence of CH and cancer progression. The presence of clonal hematopoiesis did not increase transfusion requirements or need for growth factor support.

Two retrospective case-control studies from other large cancer centers showed similar findings, including an increased risk of mortality in patients with clonal hematopoiesis and non-myeloid neoplasms.[56,57] With the increasing use of highly sensitive cell-free/circulating tumor DNA assays,[58] germline cancer predisposition DNA testing (which may detect somatic mutations in TP53 or other genes), and increased survival of patients with nonmyeloid neoplasms, the incidence of t-MDS/AML and of clonal hematopoiesis detection is expected to rise.

Biologically, clonal hematopoiesis arising in the context of cytotoxic therapy is distinct from CH arising in other contexts,[24] including enrichment for alterations in TP53 and PPM1D. Intriguingly, there is data from the t-AML context that these TP53 mutations are likely preexisting and selected for, rather than caused by, cytotoxic therapy,[59] which is thought to apply analogously to the emergence of clonal hematopoiesis.

Clonal hematopoiesis and hematopoietic cell transplantation

HCT involves the reconstitution of the entire hematopoietic system from a hematopoietic stem and progenitor cell (HSPC) graft of autologous (self) or allogeneic (donor) origin. This process involves niche engraftment and dramatic expansion of a limited number of HSPC to supply staggering numbers of terminally differentiated blood cells to the organism: in the case of red blood cells, the required amount is approximately 2 million new red blood cells per second in an adult human at steady state,[60] with even higher numbers needed under conditions of stress. In the transplantation setting, the presence of mutations conferring an inherent competitive advantage to a stem cell, that is, clonal hematopoiesis in the graft, has the potential to exert decisive consequences over a relatively short time scale.

This was demonstrated in a retrospective study of 401 patients who underwent autologous HCT for non-Hodgkin lymphoma. In approximately 30% of patients in this cohort, CHIP was detectable in the autologous stem cell product by targeted sequencing. Presence of CHIP at time of transplant translated into adverse clinical outcomes, including increased risk of death from therapy-associated myeloid neoplasm, cardiovascular disease, and profoundly decreased overall survival.[61] In this cohort, presence of mutations in PPM1D, a gene encoding a protein phosphatase involved in the response to DNA damage and part of the p53 feedback loop, were associated with a particularly grave prognosis.

In the context of allogeneic HCT, the effects of the presence of donor CHIP seem to be more nuanced, providing an intriguing glimpse into the unique biology of allotransplantation. In a comprehensive study of 500 older (>55 years) healthy related stem cell donors in Germany, donors were assessed for the presence of CHIP at time of donation, and the effect of donor CHIP on recipient outcomes was examined. The overall prevalence of CHIP in the donors was 16% and was higher if the related recipient was suffering from a myeloid malignancy compared to a lymphoid neoplasm. The presence of donor CHIP had no effect on overall survival at a median follow-up time of more than 3 years, even though most CHIP clones stably engrafted in the recipient.[31] The presence of CHIP seemed to increase the incidence of chronic graft-versus-host disease (cGVHD) and decrease the incidence of relapse or progression of the original malignancy. Donor cell leukemia was observed in 2 out of 80 recipients of a CHIP-containing graft in this study. Overall, the investigators reasoned that allotransplantation from donors with CHIP appeared safe and resulted in similar survival outcomes, such that many programs have elected not to routinely screen older donors for CHIP.[62]

Clonal mutations are regularly present even in younger donors, although most clones in the young donor population are small (i.e., VAF <1%). In an analysis of 25 donor-recipient pairs with a median age of 28 years (range, 20–58 years), small clones were present in almost one-half of donors (median age of donors with clonal hematopoiesis was 36, median VAF 0.247%) and these clones stably engrafted and expanded over the first year post allografting.[63] Clonal hematopoiesis in the donor was associated with a nonsignificant (given the small size of the study) increase in the incidence of chronic GVHD but no effect on mortality. However, donor-derived leukemia was not observed in this series, and in general donor-derived leukemia is rare after allografting, suggesting that in most cases these clones do not acquire the full repertoire of mutations to cause frank neoplasia.

CHIP-associated inflammation may enhance the graft-versus-leukemia or -lymphoma effect, balancing out any adverse effects at least in the short term, even though this remains to be proven mechanistically. Additionally, although the marrow microenvironment of recipients has already proven itself capable of supporting malignancy, CHIP transplanted from healthy donors is different in terms of biology and mutational spectrum compared to CHIP arising in the context of prior chemotherapy, as is seen in autologous HCT. One study that examined unexplained cytopenias in patients who underwent allogeneic HCT found donor CHIP to be a common occurrence in these patients.[64]

Current management approaches

At present, although patients with CHIP are increasingly identified (Figure 5), there is relatively little that can be done for individuals in whom CHIP is detected. Since anxiety may be great for patients who are told they have a mutation that can progress to leukemia, but is statistically more likely to contribute to a heart attack or stroke, frank individualized counseling of patients about their specific risk and appropriate reassurance is essential.[65,66] Monitoring with serial blood counts seems reasonable, though the optimal interval is unclear and may vary based on presence or absence of cytopenias, number of mutations, specific alleles, and VAF. For patients with small (<10%) DNMT3A or TET2 single-mutant clones, an annual CBC may be reasonable, while those with high-risk clones such as TP53 mutant or clones with multiple high-VAF mutations may need to be monitored every 3–6 months.

Given the cardiovascular risk associated with CHIP, control of modifiable established cardiac risk factors such as hypertension,

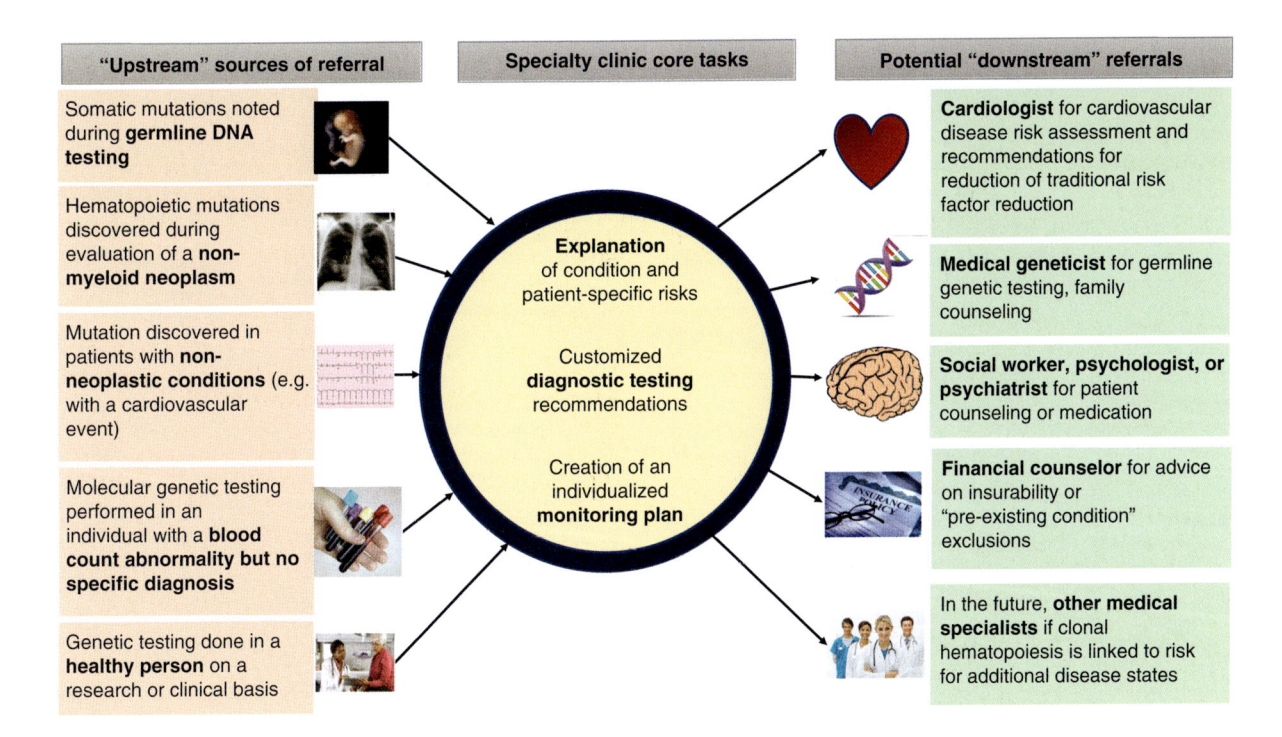

Figure 5 Hematologists may see patients with CHIP who are identified via germline testing, cell-free/circulating tumor DNA assays, genetic testing for nonmyeloid neoplasms. Serial blood count monitoring is appropriate. Downstream referrals may need to include cardiologists for risk factor management and other clinicians if risks for other disease. Source: Reprinted from Steensma and Bolton,[65] with permission.

hyperglycemia, hyperlipidemia, and cigarette smoking is important, but the optimal goals for blood pressure and low-density lipoprotein cholesterol in the setting of CHIP and whether these should differ from the general population are unclear.[38] It is also unknown whether there is any value in additional screening tests such as stress tests or coronary calcification.

Since clonal mutations are increasingly incidentally detected during evaluation of nonhematologic or nonmyeloid cancers or as part of general health evaluation, many institutions have begun to create clinics specializing in counseling patients with clonal hematopoiesis. Population estimates are that more than 20 million persons in the United States meet the definition of CHIP. Reimbursement of molecular testing by third-party payers is inconsistent, so the vast majority are undetected.

At present, there is no approach that is known to cytoreduce abnormal clones. However, given the observation that high dose vitamin C restored the function of certain TET2 mutants in a murine model, an ongoing trial is testing ascorbic acid in TET2-mutant CCUS and MDS.[67] Anti-inflammatory approaches that target interleukin 1β with cardiovascular endpoints are appealing, as are NLRP3 inflammasome inhibitors, given the role such signaling appears to play in clonal hematopoiesis-mediated atherogenesis as well as MDS.[68,69] Clonal mutations that are targetable with currently available precision medications, such as IDH mutations that might be amenable to therapy with IDH inhibitors, are rare, and whether clonal reduction with precision medications actually leads to improved clinical outcomes is unclear.

in the future we may be able to identify populations that may benefit from screening for clonal hematopoiesis. However, this is not yet appropriate in clinical practice since so much uncertainty remains. Additional information is needed about determinants of clonal hematopoiesis progression into overt blood cancer as well as specific determinants of heightened cardiovascular risk before broad-based screening such as is currently done for blood pressure or cholesterol can be considered.

Detection of clonal hematopoiesis at the time of planned cytotoxic therapy for nonmyeloid neoplasia may prove to be important in reducing the risk. For example, if an adjuvant treatment for locally advanced breast cancer is expected to improve the overall survival of a patient by 2–4%, but the patient was found to have a high VAF somatic *TP53* variant or *PPM1D* variant, the risk of developing t-MDS/AML is considerable and that should be part of the discussion of risks and benefits of chemotherapy.

As discussed above, it seems doubtful that the importance of clonal hematopoiesis will be limited to cardiovascular disease and neoplasia, and the relevance of CHIP for other inflammatory conditions is an important area of investigation. Most important is the development of novel therapeutics targeting emergent clones and preserving wild-type hematopoiesis. Only with such approaches can morbidity and mortality from this common aging-related genotype and phenotype be ameliorated.

Future directions

Given the high prevalence of clonal hematopoiesis in the general population and the potential for modifying morbidity and mortality outcomes with an anti-inflammatory or other approach,

Key references

The complete reference list can be found on Vital Source version of this title, see inside front cover.

2 Abkowitz JL, Catlin SN, McCallie MT, Guttorp P. Evidence that the number of hematopoietic stem cells per animal is conserved in mammals. *Blood.* 2002;**100**(7):2665–2667.
4 Welch JS, Ley TJ, Link DC, et al. The origin and evolution of mutations in acute myeloid leukemia. *Cell.* 2012;**150**(2):264–278.

7. Jaiswal S, Ebert BL. Clonal hematopoiesis in human aging and disease. *Science*. 2019;**366**(6465):eaan4673.
8. Steensma DP, Ebert BL. Clonal hematopoiesis as a model for premalignant changes during aging. *Exp Hematol*. 2019;**83**:48–56.
13. Busque L, Patel JP, Figueroa ME, et al. Recurrent somatic TET2 mutations in normal elderly individuals with clonal hematopoiesis. *Nat Genet*. 2012;**44**(11):1179–1181.
14. Jacobs KB, Yeager M, Zhou W, et al. Detectable clonal mosaicism and its relationship to aging and cancer. *Nat Genet*. 2012;**44**(6):651–658.
15. Jaiswal S, Fontanillas P, Flannick J, et al. Age-related clonal hematopoiesis associated with adverse outcomes. *N Engl J Med*. 2014;**371**(26):2488–2498.
16. Genovese G, Kähler AK, Handsaker RE, et al. Clonal hematopoiesis and blood-cancer risk inferred from blood DNA sequence. *N Engl J Med*. 2014;**371**(26):2477–2487.
17. Xie M, Lu C, Wang J, et al. Age-related mutations associated with clonal hematopoietic expansion and malignancies. *Nat Med*. 2014;**20**(12):1472–1478.
18. Steensma DP, Bejar R, Jaiswal S, et al. Clonal hematopoiesis of indeterminate potential and its distinction from myelodysplastic syndromes. *Blood*. 2015;**126**(1):9–16.
20. Shlush LI. Age-related clonal hematopoiesis. *Blood*. 2018;**131**(5):496–504.
21. Malcovati L, Galli A, Travaglino E, et al. Clinical significance of somatic mutation in unexplained blood cytopenia. *Blood*. 2017;**129**(25):3371–3378.
22. Wimazal F, Fonatsch C, Thalhammer R, et al. Idiopathic cytopenia of undetermined significance (ICUS) versus low risk MDS: the diagnostic interface. *Leuk Res*. 2007;**31**(11):1461–1468.
25. Young AL, Wong TN, Hughes AE, et al. Quantifying ultra-rare pre-leukemic clones via targeted error-corrected sequencing. *Leukemia*. 2015;**29**(7):1608–1611.
26. Young AL, Challen GA, Birmann BM, Druley TE. Clonal haematopoiesis harbouring AML-associated mutations is ubiquitous in healthy adults. *Nat Commun*. 2016;**7**:12484.
28. Zink F, Stacey SN, Norddahl GL, et al. Clonal hematopoiesis, with and without candidate driver mutations, is common in the elderly. *Blood*. 2017;**130**(6):742–752.
29. Thompson DJ, Genovese G, Halvardson J, et al. Genetic predisposition to mosaic Y chromosome loss in blood. *Nature*. 2019;**575**:652–657.
30. Loh PR, Genovese G, Handsaker RE, et al. Insights into clonal haematopoiesis from 8,342 mosaic chromosomal alterations. *Nature*. 2018;**559**(7714):350–355.
31. Frick M, Chan W, Arends CM, et al. Role of donor clonal hematopoiesis in allogeneic hematopoietic stem-cell transplantation. *J Clin Oncol*. 2019;**37**(5):375–385.
33. Martincorena I, Fowler JC, Wabik A, et al. Somatic mutant clones colonize the human esophagus with age. *Science*. 2018;**362**(6417):911–917.
38. Jaiswal S, Libby P. Clonal haematopoiesis: connecting ageing and inflammation in cardiovascular disease. *Nat Rev Cardiol*. 2020;**17**(3):137–144.
40. Jaiswal S, Natarajan P, Silver AJ, et al. Clonal hematopoiesis and risk of atherosclerotic cardiovascular disease. *N Engl J Med*. 2017;**377**(2):111–121.
41. Fuster JJ, MacLauchlan S, Zuriaga MA, et al. Clonal hematopoiesis associated with TET2 deficiency accelerates atherosclerosis development in mice. *Science*. 2017;**355**(6327):842–847.
42. Ridker PM, Everett BM, Thuren T, et al. Antiinflammatory therapy with canakinumab for atherosclerotic disease. *N Engl J Med*. 2017;**377**(12):1119–1131.
45. Abelson S, Collord G, Ng SWK, et al. Prediction of acute myeloid leukaemia risk in healthy individuals. *Nature*. 2018;**559**(7714):400–404.
46. Jongen-Lavrencic M, Grob T, Hanekamp D, et al. Molecular minimal residual disease in acute myeloid leukemia. *N Engl J Med*. 2018;**378**(13):1189–1199.
47. Yoshizato T, Dumitriu B, Hosokawa K, et al. Somatic mutations and clonal hematopoiesis in aplastic anemia. *N Engl J Med*. 2015;**373**(1):35–47.
49. Tiacci E, Venanzi A, Ascani S, et al. High-risk clonal hematopoiesis as the origin of AITL and NPM1-mutated AML. *N Engl J Med*. 2018;**379**(10):981–984.
54. Hsu JI, Dayaram T, Tovy A, et al. PPM1D mutations drive clonal hematopoiesis in response to cytotoxic chemotherapy. *Cell Stem Cell*. 2018;**23**(5):700–13 e6.
55. Coombs CC, Zehir A, Devlin SM, et al. Therapy-related clonal hematopoiesis in patients with non-hematologic cancers is common and associated with adverse clinical outcomes. *Cell Stem Cell*. 2017;**21**(3):374–82 e4.
56. Gillis NK, Ball M, Zhang Q, et al. Clonal haemopoiesis and therapy-related myeloid malignancies in elderly patients: a proof-of-concept, case-control study. *Lancet Oncol*. 2017;**18**(1):112–121.
57. Takahashi K, Wang F, Kantarjian H, et al. Preleukaemic clonal haemopoiesis and risk of therapy-related myeloid neoplasms: a case-control study. *Lancet Oncol*. 2017;**18**(1):100–111.
59. Wong TN, Ramsingh G, Young AL, et al. Role of TP53 mutations in the origin and evolution of therapy-related acute myeloid leukaemia. *Nature*. 2015;**518**(7540):552–555.
61. Gibson CJ, Lindsley RC, Tchekmedyian V, et al. Clonal hematopoiesis associated with adverse outcomes after autologous stem-cell transplantation for lymphoma. *J Clin Oncol*. 2017;**35**(14):1598–1605.
65. Steensma DP, Bolton KL. What to tell your patient with clonal hematopoiesis and why. *Blood*. 2020;**136**(14):1623–1631.
66. Bolton KL, Gillis NK, Coombs CC, et al. Managing clonal hematopoiesis in patients with solid tumors. *J Clin Oncol*. 2019;**37**(1):7–11.

117 Non-Hodgkin's lymphoma

Arnold S. Freedman, MD ■ Ann S. LaCasce, MD

Overview

The malignant lymphomas are neoplastic transformations of cells that reside predominantly within lymphoid tissues. Although Hodgkin and non-Hodgkin lymphomas (NHLs) both infiltrate lymphohematopoietic tissues, their biologic and clinical behaviors are distinct. They differ with neoplastic cells of origin, sites of disease, presence of specific symptoms, and response to treatment. Although both are among the most sensitive malignancies to radiation and cytotoxic therapy, their cure rates markedly differ. Hodgkin lymphomas are cured in nearly 80% of all patients employing both conventional and salvage treatment strategies whereas NHLs are cured in fewer than 50% of patients.

Epidemiology and etiology

Incidence and mortality

In 2019, 74,200 new cases of non-Hodgkin lymphoma (NHL) were diagnosed in the United States with 19,970 deaths predicted.[1] Cases rise steadily with age. There is a slight male predominance and the incidence is higher in Caucasians than in African Americans. Although the rate of increase has slowed since the mid-1990s, the incidence continues to rise by 1.5–2% each year. The incidence of NHL subtype varies significantly by age. In children, Burkitt, lymphoblastic, and diffuse large B-cell lymphoma (DLBCL) predominate. With increasing age, rates of follicular lymphomas (FLs) and aggressive lymphomas continue to rise. Small lymphocytic and FLs are most commonly diagnosed in patients over age 60.

Exposures and diseases associated with increased risk of developing NHL

Infectious agents are involved in the pathogenesis of some NHLs (Table 1). Epstein–Barr virus (EBV) has a strong association with development of Burkitt lymphoma (BL), Natural killer cell lymphoma, and human immunodeficiency virus-related (HIV-1) lymphoma.[2,3] About 45–70% of HIV-associated NHLs are EBV-related, as are nearly, 100% of the primary central nervous system (CNS) lymphomas in HIV-1 positive individuals. Human T-cell leukemia virus (HTLV)-1 is responsible for adult T-cell leukemia/lymphoma (ATLL), endemic to the Caribbean and southern Japan.[4] Gastric marginal zone lymphoma (MZL) is associated with *Helicobacter pylori* infection.[5] Splenic MZL is associated with hepatitis C infection.[6] Chronic hepatitis B infection carries an increased risk of NHL.[7] In Europe, ocular adnexal MZL is linked with *Chlamydia psittaci* infection[8] and MZL involving the skin with *Borrelia burgdorfer*. Immunoproliferative small intestinal disease (Mediterranean lymphoma, alpha heavy chain disease) has been associated with *Campylobacter jejuni*.[9] Kaposi sarcoma-associated herpes virus, also known as HHV-8, has been isolated from the neoplastic cells in patients with primary effusion lymphomas.[10,11]

An increased risk of NHL has been associated with a number of exposures and/or disease states. Controversial evidence suggests certain chemical exposures, including the herbicides phenoxyacetic acid and glyphosate, arsenic, pesticides, fungicides, chlorophenols, or organic solvents, halomethane, lead, vinyl chloride, or asbestos increase the risk of NHL.[12-15] Occupational exposures associated with an increased risk include agricultural work, welding, and work in the lumber industry.[16,17]

Diseases of inherited and acquired immunodeficiency as well as autoimmune diseases are associated with an increased incidence of lymphoma.[18,19] The association between immunosuppression and NHLs is compelling given a percentage of lymphomas will regress with the withdrawal of immunosuppression.[20] Patients undergoing organ transplantation necessitating chronic immunosuppression have a nearly 100-fold risk of NHL, greatest in the first year posttransplant. DLBCL is most common NHL in this setting and is frequently associated with EBV.[21] The rare inherited immunodeficiency diseases like X-linked lymphoproliferative syndrome, Wiskott–Aldrich syndrome, Chédiak–Higashi syndrome, ataxia-telangiectasia, and common variable immunodeficiency syndrome are complicated by highly aggressive lymphomas. An increased risk of NHL has been observed in first-degree relatives with NHL and CLL.[22,23]

Pathology, immunobiology, and natural history of NHL

The World Health Organization (WHO) classification of tumors of the hematopoietic and lymphoid tissues (Table 2) integrates morphology, immunotyping, genetic features, and clinical syndromes. To provide a context for this classification, the large numbers of entities will be grouped in "indolent," "aggressive," and "highly aggressive" categories (Table 2).[24,25]

Given the mechanism of Ig and TCR gene rearrangements in normal lymphoid cells, lymphomas are frequently found to have chromosomal translocations that involve the activation of an oncogene or inactivation of a tumor suppressor gene. The former is more common, whereby a proto-oncogene is brought under the control of a constitutively active promoter, resulting in overexpression of the oncogenic gene and its protein product. Examples include the (8;14)(q24;q32) translocation in BL, involving the *MYC* proto-oncogene and the IgH gene; the (14;18)(q32;q32) translocation in FL, involving the *BCL2* proto-oncogene and the IgH gene; and the (11;14) (q13;q32) translocation in mantle cell lymphoma (MCL), involving the gene encoding cyclin D1 (*CCDN1*) and the IgH gene. Less commonly, chromosomal translocations produce fusion genes that encode chimeric oncogenic proteins. Examples

Table 1 Risk factors for the development of lymphoma.

Inherited immunodeficiency states	Acquired immunodeficiency states	Autoimmune and inflammatory disorders	Infectious agents (other than HIV)	Chemicals and drugs
Autoimmune lymphoproliferative disease	HIV-1 infection	Rheumatoid arthritis	Epstein–Barr virus	Herbicides, pesticides, organic solvents
Ataxia telangiectasia	Iatrogenic	Systemic Lupus Erythematosus	HTLV-1	Ionizing radiation
Chediak–Higashi syndrome	Tumor necrosis factor agonists	Sjögren's syndrome	HHV-8	Chemotherapy, radiation therapy
Common variable immunodeficiency		Celiac disease	*Helicobacter pylori*	
Wiskott–Aldrich syndrome		Hashimoto's thyroiditis	*Campylobacter jejuni*	
X-linked lymphoproliferative disease		Inflammatory bowel disease	*Chlamydia psittaci*	
			Borrelia burgdorferi	
			HCV	

Abbreviations: HIV-1, human immunodeficiency virus-1; HTLV-1, human T-cell lymphotropic virus-1; HHV-8, human herpes virus-8; HCV, hepatitis C virus.

Table 2 World Health Organization Classification of Lymphoid Neoplasms 2008: selected B- and T-cell neoplasms.

Precursor B- and T-cell neoplasms
- Precursor B-lymphoblastic leukemia/lymphoma
- Precursor T-lymphoblastic leukemia/lymphoma

Mature B-cell neoplasms
- Chronic lymphocytic leukemia/small lymphocytic lymphoma
- B-cell prolymphocytic leukemia
- Lymphoplasmacytic lymphoma
- Splenic marginal zone lymphoma
- Hairy cell leukemia
- Splenic B-cell lymphoma, unclassifiable
- Plasma cell neoplasms
- Extranodal marginal zone lymphoma
- Nodal marginal zone lymphoma
- Follicular lymphoma
- Primary cutaneous follicle center lymphoma
- Mantle cell lymphoma
- Diffuse large B-cell lymphoma (DLBCL)
  - T-cell/histiocyte-rich large B-cell lymphoma
  - Primary DLBCL of the central nervous system
  - Primary cutaneous DLBCL, leg type
  - EBV-positive DLBCL of the elderly
- DLBCL associated with chronic inflammation
- Lymphomatoid granulomatosis
- Primary mediastinal large B-cell lymphoma
- Intravascular large B-cell lymphoma
- ALK-positive large B-cell lymphoma
- Plasmablastic lymphoma
- Burkitt's lymphoma (BL)
- B-cell lymphoma, unclassifiable, with features intermediate between DLBCL and BL
- B-cell lymphoma, unclassifiable, with features intermediate between DLBCL and Hodgkin lymphoma

Mature T-cell neoplasms
- T-cell prolymphocytic leukemia
- T-cell large granular lymphocytic leukemia
- Adult T-cell leukemia/lymphoma
- Extranodal NK/T-cell lymphoma, nasal type
- Enteropathy-type T-cell lymphoma
- Hepatosplenic T-cell lymphoma
- Subcutaneous panniculitis-like T-cell lymphoma
- Mycosis fungoides
- Sézary syndrome
- Primary cutaneous CD30+ T-cell lymphoproliferative disorders
- Primary cutaneous peripheral T-cell lymphomas, rare subtypes
- Peripheral T-cell lymphoma, not otherwise specified
- Angioimmunoblastic T-cell lymphoma
- Anaplastic large-cell lymphoma, ALK+
- Anaplastic large-cell lymphoma, ALK−

Abbreviations: MALT, mucosal-associated lymphoid tissue; ALK, anaplastic lymphoma kinase; HHV8, human herpes virus-8; NK, natural killer; EBV, Epstein–Barr virus; HIV, human immunodeficiency virus.

of this include the (2;5)(p23;q35) translocation involving the *ALK* and *NPM1* genes in anaplastic large cell lymphoma (ALCL) and the t(11;18)(q21;q21) translocation involving the *API2* and *MLT* genes in mucosal associated lymphoid tissue (MALT) lymphoma. These translocations and rearrangements can be detected by polymerase chain reaction (PCR) using probes that span the chromosomal breakpoints, reverse transcriptase-polymerase chain reaction (RT-PCR) to detect the ribonucleic acid (RNA) product of the fusion gene, or fluorescence *in situ* hybridization (FISH) using probes to specific chromosomal segments. In cases where

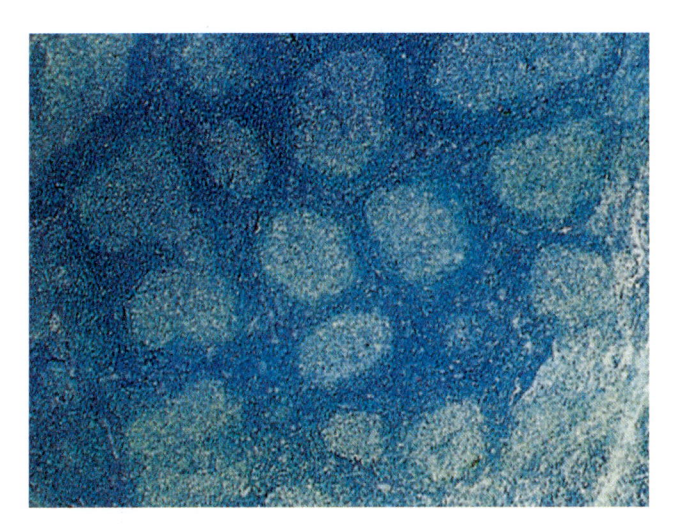

Figure 1 Follicular lymphoma grade I (low power).

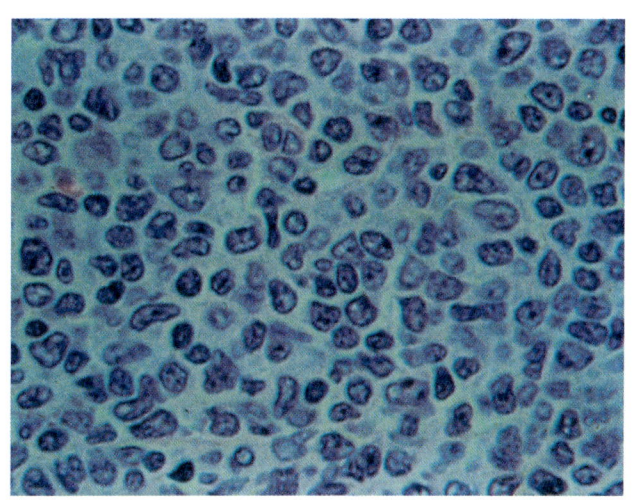

Figure 2 Follicular lymphoma grade I (high power).

the translocation results in expression of a protein or portion of a protein that is never expressed in normal lymphocytes (e.g., ALK kinase), immunohistochemistry can be used to detect the protein.

Indolent lymphomas

The indolent NHLs are generally associated with longer survival, measured in years, even if left untreated but are typically incurable with conventional treatment. Indolent lymphomas represent 35–40% of the NHLs diagnosed in Western countries. The most common subtypes are FL, small lymphocytic lymphoma, and MZL, comprising 22%, 6%, and 5% of all NHLs, respectively. In comparison, lymphoplasmacytic lymphoma (LPL), mycosis fungoides/Sézary syndrome, and splenic MZL are rare diseases, comprising 1% or less of all NHLs.

Follicular lymphoma

FL is the most common indolent NHL, and morphologically recapitulates normal germinal centers of secondary lymphoid follicles (Figure 1). The WHO classification of grade is based on the number of large cells per high power field; grade 1-2 (≤15) (Figure 2) and grade 3 (>15), Grade 3 has been subdivided into grade 3A, in which centrocytes are present, and grade 3B, in which there are sheets of centroblasts. Grade 1-2, and many cases of grade 3A FLs are approached similarly. FL grade 3B frequently harbors BCL6 rearrangements and is an aggressive disease, typically grouped with diffuse large B-cell lymphoma.[24,26]

FL and normal follicular center B cells both express cell surface antigens including monoclonal immunoglobulin and the B-cell antigens CD19, CD20, CD10, CD79a, but lack CD5. Cytoplasmic bcl-2 protein is overexpressed in essentially all cases of grade 1-2, whereas nuclear bcl-6 is expressed by at least some of the neoplastic cells. The most common cytogenetic abnormality in FL is t(14;18) that leads to overexpression of the anti-apoptotic protein bcl-2 in over 85% of cases. Recent sequencing studies have found that the most common mutations in FL (90% of tumors) involve MLL2, a gene encoding a histone H3 methylase. Other less common recurrent mutations involve other genes involving epigenetic modifying genes, such as EZH2, CREBBP, and EP300.[27,28]

FL accounts for about 22% of NHL.[29] Uncommon before the fourth decade, the median age at diagnosis is 60 years. FL is less common in Asians and blacks. Patients usually present with painless peripheral adenopathy, which are often longstanding and may wax and wane. Patients may present with asymptomatic large abdominal masses, though bulky mediastinal disease is rare. Staging studies usually demonstrates widely disseminated disease with involvement of spleen (40%), liver (50%), and bone marrow (70%). Marrow involvement in FL reveals a unique pattern of paratrabecular infiltration. Few patients present with extranodal extramedullary disease, and only 20% present with B symptoms or lactate dehydrogenase (LDH) elevation. Intestinal only presentation may occur and has a favorable prognosis.[30] CNS involvement is uncommon although peripheral nerve compression and epidural tumor masses causing cord compression may develop.

The course of FL is quite variable. Some patients can be observed with waxing and waning disease for 5 years or more without the need for therapy.[31] Others present with more disseminated disease and rapid growth, and require treatment due to organ enlargement, lymphatic obstruction, or organ obstruction. Histologic transformation to aggressive lymphoma, usually DLBCL in approximately 2–3% per year, of patients with FL and is characterized by rapid progression of lymphadenopathy, extranodal disease, B symptoms, elevated LDH, and often a poor prognosis.[32,33]

Small lymphocytic lymphoma and B-cell chronic lymphocytic leukemia

Small lymphocytic lymphoma and B-cell chronic lymphocytic leukemia are viewed as the same entity by the WHO classification. The disease is topic of **Chapter 114** (Figure 3).

Lymphoplasmacytic lymphoma

LPL is an indolent lymphoma composed of diffuse proliferation of small lymphocytes with evidence of maturation to plasma cells.[34] Evidence of immunoglobulin is seen in these cells by special stains or inclusions. These tumors express B-cell antigens CD19, CD20, and surface immunoglobulin M isotype, and in general do not express CD5, CD10, or CD23. Deletions of 6q21 have been identified in 40–60% of patients with Waldenström macroglobulinemia. Activating mutations in MYD88, a protein involved in signaling pathways downstream of the Ig receptor is present in nearly all cases.[35]

LPL represents about 1% of all NHLs. Clinically this disease is similar to small lymphocytic lymphomas. The median age is early 60s, and virtually all patients have stage IV disease by virtue of bone marrow involvement and lymph nodes and spleen are commonly involved. B symptoms and elevated serum LDH are rare. A serum M component is common. As with B-CLL, the paraprotein may

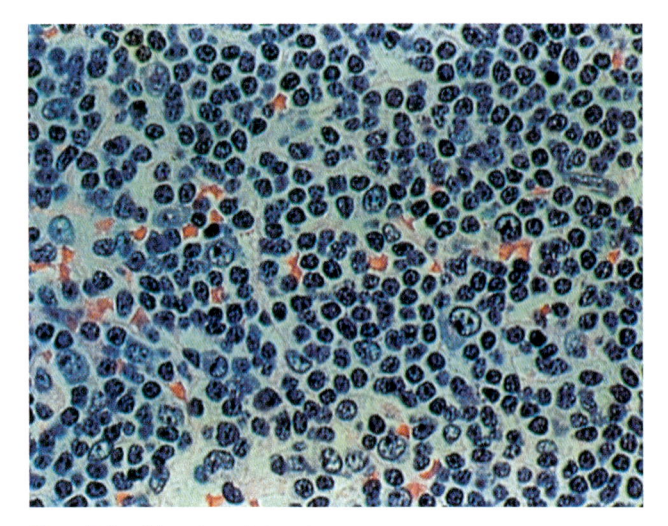

Figure 3 Small lymphocytic lymphoma.

have autoantibody or cryoglobulin activity. However, most cases with mixed cryoglobulinemia have been shown to be related to concurrent hepatitis C virus (HCV) infection.[36] In the WHO clinical study, 5-year overall survival (OS) (58%) and failure-free survival (25%) were identical to that of small lymphocytic lymphomas.

Marginal zone lymphomas

MZLs are a group of distinct entities including nodal MZL; extranodal MZL also known as the lymphomas of mucosal-associated lymphoid tissues; and the splenic MZL.[37,38] In the nodal MZL, the tumor cells cytologically resemble "normal" monocytoid B cells and often involve lymph node sinuses. Phenotypically, tumor cells express surface immunoglobulin M and B-cell antigens (CD19, CD20). Similar to other indolent lymphomas, MZL can transform into a higher-grade lymphoma. The nodal MZLs constitute 1% of all NHLs. Over 70% of patients present with stage III/IV disease and the majority are asymptomatic. Bone marrow involvement is less common than in most indolent lymphomas. The 5-year survival for patients with nodal MZL is 55–79%.

The extranodal MZL tumor cells resemble monocytoid B-cells, express CD19, CD20, and surface immunoglobulin M and are thought to arise from memory B cells. Lymphoepithelial lesion may be seen associated with centrocytes. The disease does not form follicles but the malignant cells surround reactive follicles. When extranodal MZL spreads to lymph nodes, the neoplastic cells involve the marginal zones. The most common cytogenetic abnormality is trisomy 3, occurring in up to 60% of cases (particularly the gastric extranodal MZL) and t(11;18) occurring in 25–40% of cases.[39]

Extranodal MZLs constitute about 5% of all NHLs and almost 50% of all gastric lymphomas. B symptoms are uncommon and most patients present with stage I or II disease. There is no age predilection. The gastrointestinal tract (stomach most commonly), lung, dura, lacrimal and salivary glands, skin, thyroid, and breast may be involved. MZL has been associated with autoimmune diseases and infections with *H. pylori*, *B. burgdorferi*, *Chlamydophila psittaci (C. psittaci)*, *C. jejuni*, and HCV.[40–43] Fewer than 25% of cases have lymph node or bone marrow involvement. Patients can present with peptic ulcer disease, abdominal pain, and sicca syndrome, or a mass at the site of involvement. These lymphomas can disseminate to other mucosal-associated lymphoid tissue sites or bone marrow in about 30% of cases, typically later in the course of the disease. This is more commonly seen in nongastric MZLs.[44]

Complete remission (CR) rates are high, as is OS, as high at 80% at 10 or more years.[45] Like all indolent NHLs these can transform to DLBCL.

Splenic MZL constitutes less than 2% of all NHLs, with a median age of 65, uncommon before age 50.[29] Histologically, there is expansion of marginal zones in the spleen. Bone marrow and peripheral blood involvement (referred to as splenic lymphoma with villous or nonvillous lymphocytes) can also be present. In splenic MZL trisomy, 3 is present in 39% of cases. The survival of patients is in excess of 70% at 10 years. Sequencing studies demonstrate recurrent somatic mutations in genes involved in the NOTCH, NF-kB, and Bcell receptor pathways, as well as mutations in TP53.[46]

Aggressive lymphomas

Mantle cell lymphoma

MCL is generally an aggressive disease.[47,48] The neoplastic cells are counterparts of naive "mantle zone" B cells and are medium sized with irregular nuclei. The disease may have either diffuse architecture or a vaguely nodular appearance. Some cases of MCL have a predominance of "blastoid" cells with a high mitotic rate. The cells express B-cell antigens, surface immunoglobulin M with or without immunoglobulin D, CD5, and CD43, but lack CD10 and CD23, respectively with overexpression of cyclin D1. Approximately 70% of MCLs have t(11;14)(q13;q32) that is rearrangements of *bcl-1* (cyclin D1) gene. Eight percent of MCL cases are cyclin D1-negative and overexpress cyclin D2 and 4 or cyclin D3, without chromosomal rearrangements[49] and are clinically similar to cyclin D1-positive cases.[50] Deep sequencing[27] has identified NOTCH1 mutations in a minority of cases, which may be associated with poor prognosis. SOX11, which is expressed in the majority of cases, is also associated with a worse prognosis.[49,51]

MCL constitutes about 7% of all NHLs. About 75% of patients are males, with median age of 63. Approximately 70% of patients have stage IV disease and B symptoms are observed in approximately one-third of patients. Typical sites of involvement are lymph nodes, spleen, liver, Waldeyer ring, and bone marrow. Peripheral blood involvement is present in 25–50% of patients at presentation. MCL can involve any region of the gastrointestinal tract, occasionally presenting as multiple intestinal polyposis. The median survival of patients with MCL has improved over recent years to 8–10 years with intensive therapy and the introduction of novel therapies. Blastoid transformation can present de novo or as transformation, occurring in 35% of patients, with a risk of 42% at 4 years, and the median survival is 3.8 months.[52] Mutations and deletions of p53 which are commonly seen in the blastoid variant are also associated with a worse prognosis.[53]

Diffuse large B-cell lymphoma

DLBCL consists of a diffuse proliferation of large cells with a high mitotic rate. The cells have a moderate amount of cytoplasm with either cleaved or noncleaved nuclei often with multiple nucleoli, although there can be great variability in the morphology (Figure 4). DLBCL represents many distinct disease entities[24] (Table 2). Gene expression profiling has been applied to DLBCL.[54–57] These studies have subdivided DLBCL into distinct genetic entities. DLBCLs correspond to germinal center B cells or activated B cells. The tumor cells generally express B-cell antigens (CD 19, CD20), monoclonal surface immunoglobulin M, but occasionally other heavy chain isotypes CD5-positive cases are uncommon and may have a worse prognosis.[58] CD10 and bcl-6

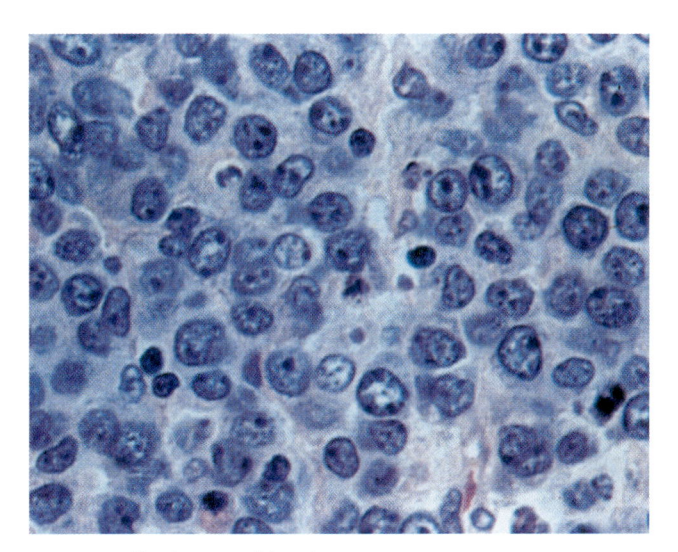

Figure 4 Diffuse large B-cell lymphoma.

support a GC origin, whereas expression of MUM1 a non-GC origin. Approximately 70% express bcl-6 protein, consistent with a germinal center origin.[59]

Several chromosomal abnormalities have been observed in DLBCL. Bcl-6 is associated with chromosomal rearrangements involving 3q27.[60] Rearrangements occur in 20–40% of diffuse aggressive lymphomas. t(14;18) has been observed in approximately 30% of patients with DLBCL. Some of these cases may represent histologic transformations of prior FL. By GEP, the GCB type is often associated with the t(14;18) and amplifications of the REL oncogene on chromosome 2. In contrast, the ABC type is associated with loss of 6q21, trisomy 3, gains of 3q and 18q21-22, and mutations of EZH2.[61,62] ABC cases also have high-level activation of NF-kB.[63] Overexpression of MYC and with BCL2, known as a double protein expressor lymphoma, is associated with inferior outcomes.[64,65]

DLBCL constitutes 31% of all NHL and is the most common histologic subtype. Patients who are generally middle-aged or older (median age 64 years) present with either nodal enlargement or extranodal disease. DLBCL presents in a localized (stage I or IE) manner approximately 20% of the time and 30–40% of patients will have I or II disease. Stage IV disease is seen in approximately 40% of patients. B symptoms occur in 30% of patients, and unlike most NHLs, LDH is elevated in over half the patients. The disease may involve nearly any extranodal site including the liver, kidneys, lung, bone and peripheral nerves, and CNS. Bone marrow involvement is initially found in 10–20% of patients. Extranodal disease, specifically testicular, renal or adrenal involvement, breast, and epidural disease, is associated with increased risk of CNS dissemination, as is elevated LDH in concert with multiple extranodal sites of disease.[32,66] Rare cases of DLBCL present with a disseminated intravascular proliferation of large lymphoid cells, involving small blood vessels, without an obvious tumor mass,[67–69] most commonly involving the CNS, kidneys, lungs, and skin.

High-grade B-cell lymphoma with MYC and BCL2 and/or BCL6 rearrangement

MYC is rearranged in 10% of DLBCLs with the partner gene being one of the Ig genes in 60% of cases and alternative genes in 40% of cases. Approximately 20% of MYC-rearranged cases have concurrent BCL2 and/or BCL6 rearrangements, and now comprise a distinct entity known as high-grade B-cell lymphoma with BCL2 and/or BCL6 rearrangements, commonly referred to as "double hit or triple hit lymphoma"[25] MYC translocation alone in the absence of BCL2 or BCL6 is not associated with inferior outcomes. Additionally, large retrospective analysis revealed that the poor prognosis associated with double hit lymphoma is driven by MYC translocations with immunoglobulin gene partners.[66]

Primary mediastinal large B-cell lymphoma

Primary mediastinal large B-cell lymphoma is a distinct subtype of large B-cell lymphoma (7% of all cases).[70] Histologically, the cellular infiltrate is heterogeneous, and sclerosis is frequently present. The immunophenotype includes B-cell antigens (CD19, CD20), but they are often negative for surface and cytoplasmic immunoglobulin. Gene expression profile studies suggest that this is a distinct entity from germinal center or activated B-cell types of DLBCL and closely resembles classic Hodgkin lymphoma (HL).[47,71] Copy number gains in the region on chromosome 9p containing the genes for JAK2 and programmed cell death ligand 1 and 2 (PDL1 and PDL2), ligands for the programmed cell death receptor-1 (PD-1), which has a role in suppressing Tcell function, are common.[47,61] Primary mediastinal large B-cell lymphoma has a female predominance, with median age of 40. Over 70% of these patients present with stage I/II bulky disease involving the mediastinum, pleural, and pericardial effusions in about one-third of the patients. Superior vena cava syndrome is common. Similar to DLBCL, an elevated LDH is present in the majority, whereas bone marrow involvement is infrequent. The prognosis of patients with primary mediastinal large B-cell lymphoma is favorable.

High-grade B-cell lymphoma, NOS

In high-grade B-cell lymphoma, not otherwise specified (NOS), the neoplastic cells are intermediate to large size, may have a very high Ki67 index, and are CD10+.[25] Cells are more variable size than BL cells, often BCL2-positive may be BCL6-negative, and may have a Ki67 index lower than 100%. GEP has shown these to be heterogeneous.[48] MYC with BCL2 and/or BCL6 are not present. High-grade B cell lymphoma NOS often presents with extranodal disease with high International Prognostic Index (IPI) and generally has a poor prognosis.

Gray zone lymphoma

B-cell lymphoma, unclassifiable, with features intermediate between DLBCL and cHL (B-UNC/cHL/DLBCL), has features intermediate between PMBCL and cHL, or B-UNC/cHL/DLBCL.[25] This rare disease presents commonly in men with a mediastinal mass. Histologically, cells resemble both the HRS cell of cHL and the large cells of DLBCL or PMLBCL. Fibrous stroma and an inflammatory infiltrate are seen. Malignant cells express CD45, CD20, CD79a, and CD30, but often are CD15-; other B-cell markers like PAX5, OCT-2, and BOB1 are often positive. The prognosis of these patients is inferior to both cHL and primary mediastinal large B-cell lymphoma and the optimal therapy has not been demonstrated.[72]

Peripheral T-cell lymphomas

The category of peripheral T-cell lymphomas (PTCLs) includes a large number of entities, which constitute 15% of all NHLs in adults.[73] Among these, in decreasing frequency, are PTCL, not otherwise unspecified (NOS); anaplastic large-cell lymphoma

(ALCL); angioimmunoblastic T-cell lymphoma (AITL), extranodal NK/T-cell lymphoma, nasal type; and much rarer entities such as panniculitis-like T-cell lymphoma; enteropathy type T-cell lymphoma; and hepatosplenic γ/δ T-cell lymphoma.

PTCLs can be nodal or extranodal-based diseases. The diffuse cellular infiltrates range from a mixture of small and large cells; infiltrates of pleomorphic cells, often with a background of epithelioid histiocytes, plasma cells, eosinophils, and Reed–Sternberg-like cells; or predominantly large cells. In contrast to B-cell lymphomas, the pattern of expression of T-cell surface antigens is highly variable. The majority express CD2, CD3, and CD4, with a subset of expressing CD8.[74] In most cases, one or more "mature" T-cell antigens, such as CD5 or CD7, are lost. Some cases of PTCL express are EBV-positive, especially the extranodal NK/T-cell lymphomas, nasal type.[75] EBV positivity is associated with a poor prognosis.

Abnormal metaphases are seen in 90% of T-cell lymphomas. The most commonly seen translocations in PTCLs are t(7;14), t(11;14), inv(14), and t(14;14). AITL is associated with trisomy 3 and or 5.[35] These translocations involve genes for the T-cell receptor (TCR) at 14q11, 7q34-35, and 7p15. AITL is also associated with mutations in TET2, IDH2, DNMT3A, and RHOA.[76,77] Young patients with ALCL have t(2;5), and less commonly t(1;2).[57] ALCL in adults generally lack t(2;5). Hepatosplenic γ/δ T-cell lymphomas are associated with isochromosome 7q and trisomy 8.[78]

Patients with PTCL have a similar median age as patients with DLBCL. However, 80% of patients with PTCL have stage III/IV disease, and more frequently have B symptoms, hepatosplenomegaly, and extranodal disease, such as the skin. PTCLs generally have a worse prognosis than DLBCL.[79,80] A number of uncommon subtypes of PTCL have unique histologic features. AITL is derived from follicular helper T-cells. In addition to a pleomorphic heterogeneous cellular infiltrate, the disease is characterized by increased numbers of high endothelial venules present, giving a hypervascular appearance. In this subtype, Ig heavy chains may be rearranged in 10% cases, and EBV genomes are detected in most cases and may be in either T or B cells.[81] AITL typically affects older adults who present with the acute onset of generalized lymphadenopathy, hepatosplenomegaly, skin rash, and B symptoms.[81] Immunologic abnormalities are common and include plasmacytosis, polyclonal hypergammaglobulinemia, and a positive Coombs test. The median survival is 30 months. Infection is the most common cause of death, followed by the T-cell lymphoma or development of EBV-positive DLBCL.

ALCL is a T-cell NHL that can present as primary systemic ALCL, ALK-positive; primary systemic ALCL, ALK-negative; and primary cutaneous ALCL. When involving nodes, ALCL characteristically involves the sinusoids of lymph nodes with bizarre large cells. Neoplastic cells derived from patients with ALCL also generally express the phenotype of mature activated T cells (HLA-DR, CD30, CD25). The ALK protein (anaplastic lymphoma kinase) is detected in 40–60% of cases using the ALK1 monoclonal antibody, showing both nuclear and cytoplasmic staining in cases with the t(2; 5).[82] The resulting fusion gene encodes a chimeric NPM-ALK fusion protein with constitutive tyrosine kinase activity. ALK-positive cases are more common in children and younger adults and have a better prognosis than ALK-negative cases.[83] In addition, a small subset of patients with ALCL harbor DUSP22 rearrangements which is associated with favorable outcomes.[84] Conversely, rearrangements in TP63 are associated with inferior survival.

ALCL constitutes 2% of all NHLs in adults but is the second most common T-cell lymphoma. The median age of patients with

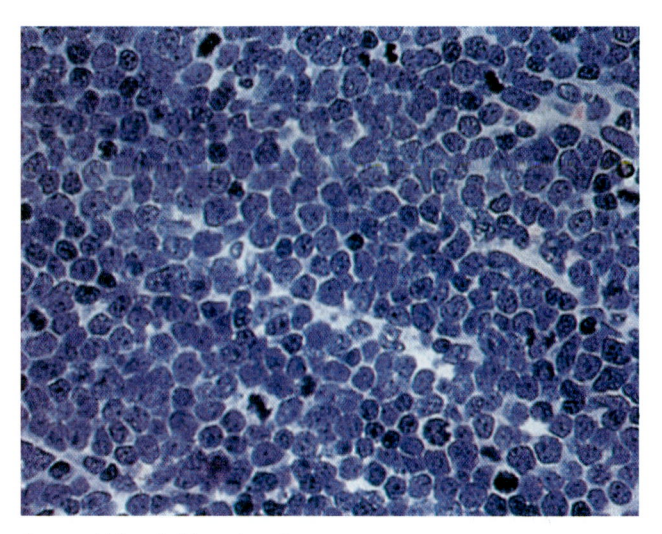

Figure 5 T-lymphoblastic lymphoma.

ALCL is 34 with a male predominance. There is a bimodal distribution of this disease, with peaks in childhood, young adults, and late adulthood. In adults, B symptoms, peripheral and retroperitoneal adenopathy is common. Skin is a frequent site of extranodal disease (about 25% of patients), whereas bone marrow involvement is uncommon. An unusual form of ALCL arises within the breast associated with breast implants.[85] When ALCL, PTCL NOS, and angioimmunoblastic T-cell NHL are compared, ALCL has the highest OS, whereas AITL had the lowest.[86]

Highly aggressive lymphomas

Precursor T- or B-lymphoblastic leukemia/lymphoma
Lymphoblastic lymphoma (LBL) and acute lymphoblastic leukemia ALL (see **Chapter 113**) represent two presentations of the same disease with LBL defined as having less than 25% bone marrow involvement. The neoplastic cells have a high nuclear to cytoplasmic ratio, scant cytoplasm, and nuclei with fine chromatin with multiple small nucleoli, and have a high mitotic rate. The nuclei can have folds or convolutions. Typically, nodes involved with LBL are effaced by malignant cells (Figure 5).

The vast majority of LBLs are of T-cell lineage. Several investigators have noted that most T-cell LBLs correspond to stages of thymocyte differentiation (see **Chapter 113**). Although LBLs represent a major subgroup of childhood NHLs, they are unusual in adults (2% of adult NHLs). Patients are usually males in their 20s or 30s who present with lymphadenopathy in cervical, supraclavicular, and axillary regions (50%) or with a mediastinal mass (50–75%) and may be associated with superior vena cava syndrome, tracheal obstruction, and pericardial effusions. Less commonly, patients present with extranodal disease (e.g., skin, testicular, or bony involvement). More than 80% of patients present with advanced-stage disease, almost 50% have B symptoms, and the majority have elevated LDH. Although the bone marrow is frequently normal at presentation, virtually all patients develop bone marrow infiltration and a subsequent leukemic phase. Patients with bone marrow involvement have a very high incidence of CNS infiltration. B-cell LBL is a very rare variant, affecting patients with a median age of 39.[87] B-cell LBL presents without a mediastinal mass but instead involves lymph nodes and extranodal sites.

Burkitt lymphoma

BL cells resemble the small noncleaved cells within normal germinal centers of secondary lymphoid follicles. Because of the high mitotic rate, frequent mitotic figures are seen and, analogous to normal germinal centers, tingible body macrophages are seen, giving the classical "starry sky" appearance. It is generally agreed that the fraction of Ki-67 (proliferating cells) in Burkitt-like lymphoma should be 99% or greater.[24]

BL is a tumor of B-lineage derivation identified by the expression of a variety of B-cell-restricted antigens including CD19, CD20, surface immunoglobulin M, CD10, and nuclear bcl-6 protein.[88] The endemic BL is EBV-positive, whereas the vast majority of nonendemic BL is EBV-negative. BL cells lack BCL2 protein.

BL involves a translocation of chromosome 8q24 in over 95% of the cases studied with either chromosome 14, 2, or 22.[24] Pathologically identified Burkitt or histologically atypical Burkitt had gene expression profile associated with overexpression of *myc* target genes, differential expression of normal germinal center genes, and decreased expression of MHC class I and NF-kB target genes. These studies will help refine the histologic diagnosis of difficult to classify cases.[14,48,89]

BL is, in general, a pediatric tumor that has three major clinical presentations. The endemic (African) form presents as a jaw or facial bone tumor that spreads to extranodal sites including ovary, testis, kidney, breast, and especially to the bone marrow and meninges. The nonendemic form has an abdominal presentation with massive disease, ascites, renal, testis, ovarian involvement, and, like the endemic form, also spreads to the bone marrow and CNS. Immunodeficiency-related cases more often involve lymph nodes and peripheral blood. BL has a male predominance and is typically seen in patients less than 35 years of age. These tumors have a high propensity to invade the bone marrow and CNS.

Adult T-cell leukemia/lymphoma

ATLL is a rare disease associated with infection by the human T-cell lymphotropic virus, type 1 in 100% of cases.[90–92] ATLL is endemic in southern Japan, the Caribbean basin, Africa, and the southeastern United States. The neoplastic cells' normal counterparts are activated CD4+ T cells, expressing CD2, CD3, CD5, and CD25. The median age of patients is 60.[93] The disease can present as four variants: acute (most common and highly aggressive), lymphomatous, chronic, and smoldering. The median survival of these variants is 6 months, 10 months, 24 months, and not reached, respectively.[94] Patients present with BM and peripheral blood involvement, high white blood cell count, hypercalcemia (due to PTH-related protein, TGF-β, RANK ligand), lytic bone lesions, lymphadenopathy, hepatosplenomegaly, skin lesions, and interstitial pulmonary infiltrates.

Differential diagnosis and sites of disease at presentation

More than two-thirds of patients with NHL present with persistent painless peripheral lymphadenopathy. At the time of presentation, differential diagnosis of generalized lymphadenopathy includes infectious etiologies. A firm lymph node larger than 1.5×1.5 cm not associated with a documented infection and persisting longer than 4–6 weeks and progressing, should be considered for biopsy. However, lymph nodes in indolent NHLs frequently wax and wane. In teenagers and young adults, infectious mononucleosis and HL should be placed high in the differential diagnosis. Involvement of Waldeyer ring, epitrochlear, and mesenteric nodes is more frequently observed in patients with NHL than HL. Forty percent of all patients with NHL present with systemic complaints. B symptoms are more common in patients with aggressive subtypes approaching 50%. Less frequent presenting symptoms, occurring in less than 20% of patients, include complaints such as fatigue, and malaise.

NHLs also present with thoracic, abdominal, and/or extranodal symptoms. Approximately 20% of patients with NHL present with mediastinal adenopathy. These patients most frequently present with persistent cough, chest discomfort, and rarely superior vena cava syndrome. Differential diagnosis of mediastinal presentation includes infections, sarcoidosis, HL, as well as other neoplasms. Involvement of retroperitoneal, mesenteric, and pelvic nodes is common in most subtypes of NHL and the majority of patients are asymptomatic. Aggressive NHLs can present with primary cutaneous lesions, testicular masses, acute spinal cord compression, solitary bone lesions, and rarely lymphomatous meningitis. Symptoms of primary NHL of the CNS include headache, lethargy, focal neurologic symptoms, seizures, and paralysis.

When NHL presents in an extranodal site, the differential diagnosis is more difficult. NHL uncommonly presents in the lung.[95] Between 25% and 50% of patients with NHLs present with hepatic infiltration although relatively few present with large hepatic masses, that are almost always associated with aggressive lymphoma. Of the advanced stage indolent lymphomas, nearly 75% of patients have microscopic hepatic infiltration at presentation. Primary lymphoma of bone occurs in less than 5% of patients, presenting as a painful bony site, most commonly involving the femur, pelvis, and vertebrae. Approximately 5% of NHLs present as primary gastrointestinal lymphoma. These patients present with hemorrhage, pain, or obstruction since the stomach is most frequently infiltrated followed by small intestine and colon, respectively. Most gastrointestinal lymphomas are of the aggressive subtypes, specifically DLBCL, MCL, and the intestinal T-cell lymphoma, and may present rarely with bleeding, obstruction, or perforation. The most common site for extranodal MZL is the stomach. A subset of MCLs presents as multiple intestinal polyposis involving any sites in the gastrointestinal tract. 2–14% of NHL present with renal infiltration, and even less common is localized presentation in the prostate, testis, or ovary. The typical histologic subtypes of these sites are DLBCL, BLs. Rare sites of primary lymphoma include the orbit, heart, breast, salivary glands, thyroid, and adrenal gland.

Staging and disease detection

The Lugano classification[96] is the current staging system used for patients with NHL. It is derived from the Ann Arbor staging system, which was originally developed for HL in 1971, Table 3 summarizes the essential features. Because NHLs most frequently disseminate hematogenously, this staging system has proven to be much less useful than for HL. The Lugano modification requires documentation of size of bulk disease. Systemic "B" symptoms (fever, sweats, weight loss) are no longer included into the staging system for NHL, because these symptoms are not independent prognostic factors for these patients.

The concept of staging has less impact in NHL than in HL. Multiple studies demonstrate that prognosis is more dependent on lymphoma subtype and clinical parameters than stage at presentation. Staging is undertaken in NHLs to identify the small number of patients who can be treated with local therapy or combined modality treatment and to stratify within subtypes to determine prognosis and assess the impact of treatment.

Table 3 Revised staging system for primary nodal lymphoma.

Stage	Involvement	Extranodal (E) status
Limited		
I	One node or a group of adjacent nodes	Single extranodal lesions without nodal involvement
II	Two or more nodal groups on the same side of the diaphragm	Stage I or II by nodal extent with limited contiguous extranodal involvement
II bulky[a]	II as above with "bulky" disease	Not applicable
Advanced		
III	Nodes on both sides of the diaphragm; nodes above the diaphragm with spleen involvement	Not applicable
IV	Additional noncontiguous extralymphatic involvement	Not applicable

[a]Whether stage II bulky disease is treated as limited or advanced disease may be determined by histology and a number of prognostic factors.

Diagnosis and initial evaluation

Staging must be undertaken in the context of the histology. After the initial biopsy, blood tests should be obtained, including complete blood count, routine chemistries, renal function, liver function tests, and serum protein electrophoresis to document the presence of circulating monoclonal paraproteins. HIV, hepatitis B (which may reactivate with lymphoma therapy) and C serologies should be performed. Serum beta-2 microglobulin can be useful as a surrogate marker of disease burden in indolent NHLs. Serum concentrations of LDH are an important independent predictor of survival in NHL. Isolated Waldeyer ring involvement is associated with intestinal involvement in 20% of cases and endoscopy should be considered. Chest, abdominal, pelvic computed tomography scan is essential for accurate staging. Unilateral bone marrow biopsies are performed in some subtypes of lymphoma, particularly in the setting of cytopenias or if involvement will influence therapy. The role of BM biopsy in DLBCL has been questioned.[96] Positron emission tomography (PET) scanning for marrow involvement is more sensitive than bone marrow biopsy, though discordant involvement by an indolent lymphoma may not be evident. In patients with aggressive lymphomas with marrow involvement, paranasal sinus involvement, paraspinal masses, testicular or if clinically indicated, examination of the cerebral spinal fluid (CSF) by lumbar puncture should be performed. PET using 18F-fluorodeoxyglucose is a highly sensitive and specific scanning modality for detecting NHL in both nodal and extranodal sites. PET scanning is very useful for DLBCL, MCL, and FL, and is now recommended in the initial staging of these entities. PET scanning is not as sensitive in SLL and MZL.[97] Magnetic resonance imaging is most valuable for evaluation of the brain and spinal cord.

PET/CT after all therapy is completed can be done at least three but preferably 6–8 weeks after chemotherapy and 8–12 weeks after radiation or chemoradiotherapy. There is no evidence that long-term follow-up should include PET scanning.[98] The role of surveillance scanning in indolent and aggressive NHLs is being reconsidered since the impact and utility of identifying asymptomatic recurrences is of unclear long-term benefit and the associated radiation exposure has been linked to an increased risk of secondary malignancies.[99]

Immunologic and molecular studies

Biologic studies including cell surface markers, cytogenetics, and molecular techniques are used in diagnosis, staging, and minimal disease detection. Monoclonal antibodies directed against cell surface antigens expressed on lymphoid cells, and molecular techniques to define immunoglobulin and TCR gene rearrangements are sensitive tools with which to assess tumor cell infiltration. Immunophenotypic and cytogenetic studies can help to determine histologic subtypes of lymphomas. For those NHLs with known chromosomal translocations, it is possible to identify unique chromosomal breakpoints that can be studied with fluorescent in situ hybridization (FISH), cytogenetics, and PCR. Studies of minimal disease may provide important prognostic information.

Disease parameters that influence prognosis and assessment of disease response

Prognostic factors in NHL

Aggressive NHLs
Clinical prognostic models have been developed for a number of NHL subtypes. The analysis of a large group (2031 patients) with diffuse aggressive NHLs treated with an anthracycline-containing regimen led to the establishment of a prognostic model of predicting outcome known as the IPI (Table 4).[101] Of a large number of factors examined for all patients, age (≤60 vs >60); serum LDH (≤normal vs >normal); performance status (0 or 1 vs 2–4); stage (I or II vs III or IV); and extranodal involvement (≤site vs >1 site) were independently prognostic for OS. The 5-year OS rates for patients with scores of 0 to 1, 2, 3, and 4 to 5 were 73%, 51%, 43%, and 26%, respectively. The IPI has been adapted following treatment with rituximab plus cyclophosphamide, doxorubicin, vincristine, prednisone (CHOP) therapy for DLBCL. Within that model, the 4-year progression-free survival is 94%, 80%, and 53% for 0 and 1, 2, or 3 or more risk factors, respectively.[102]

Follicular NHL
A predictive model based on over 4000 patients with follicular NHL in the prerituximab era, known as the FLIPI score identified the following prognostic factors: age >60; stage III/IV, more than four nodal sites; elevated serum LDH concentration; and hemoglobin less than 12. The 10-year survival rates for patients with zero to one, two, or three or more risk adverse factors averaged 71%, 51%, and 36%, respectively (Table 5).[103] The FLIPI remains clinically relevant with rituximab-based therapy.[104]

Table 4 International Prognostic Index (IPI).[a]

International Prognostic Index (IPI)				
Age >60 years				
LDH > upper limit normal				
ECOG performance status ≥2				
Ann Arbor stage III or IV				
Number of extranodal disease sites >1				
# Factors	Risk group	3-Year EFS (%)	3-Year PFS (%)	3-Year OS (%)
0–1	Low	81	87	91
2	Low-intermediate	69	75	81
3	High-intermediate	53	59	65
4–5	High	50	50	59

Abbreviations: LDH, lactate dehydrogenase; ECOG, Eastern Cooperative Oncology Group; EFS, event-free survival; PFS, progression-free survival; OS, overall survival.
[a]Source: Adapted from Ziepert et al.[100]

Table 5 Follicular Lymphoma International Prognostic Index (FLIPI).[a]

Age >60 years
LDH > upper limit normal
Hgb <12 g/dL
Ann Arbor stage III or IV
Number of involved nodal areas >4

# Factors	Risk group	5-Year OS (%)	10-Year OS (%)
0–1	Low	91	71
2	Intermediate	78	51
3–5	High	52	36

Abbreviations: LDH, lactate dehydrogenase; Hgb, hemoglobin; OS, overall survival.
[a]Source: Adapted from Solal-Celigny et al.[103]

For other NHLs, prognostic models have been developed from uniformly treated patient populations. The mantle cell lymphoma international prognostic index (MIPI) includes age; PS; LDH; WBC as prognostic factors.[52] The proliferation index alone as well as when incorporated into the MIPI provides additional prognostic utility.[105] Several prognostic models for peripheral T cell lymphoma NOS have been reported, but generally, the IPI provides a reasonable stratification of outcome, with low-risk patients having a 55% 2-year OS and high-risk patients a less than 15% 2-year OS.[106]

Gene expression profiling as prognostic factor

Gene expression profiling using deoxyribonucleic acid (DNA) microarrays has been used to examine DLBCL to identify prognostic subgroups.[54–56,107] DLBCLs may be subclassified into "germinal center" or "activated" B-cell types. Patients with germinal center B-like DLBCL had significantly better OS than those with the activated B-like variant. Based on finding from gene expression profiling, immunohistochemistry using tissue microarrays has been used for a limited number of gene products as prognostic markers.[107] Germinal center and nongerminal center B-cell derivation can be determined by expression of CD10 and bcl-6, and MUM1. Using tissue microarrays, 42% of DLBCLs are considered germinal center B-cell derivation and 58% are nongerminal center B-cell derivation.

Gene expression profiling in MCL patients has identified the proliferation signature and high expression of cyclin D1 are associated with unfavorable prognosis.[105]

Therapeutic approaches according to WHO classification

Indolent lymphomas

Therapy of early-stage follicular lymphoma
Fewer than 30% of patients with FL present with stage I/II disease.[108] Radiation therapy (RT) has generally the treatment of choice for limited-stage FL and results in 10-year OS rates of 60–80%; with a median survival is approximately 19 years.[109] A dose of 24 Gy appears to be highly effective, with no benefit of higher doses.[110,111] The freedom from progression is higher when patients are staged with FDG-PET prior to RT.[112] However, most patients with stage I disease treated in the United States do not receive RT, instead, they receive single-agent rituximab or chemoimmunotherapy.[108] Adjuvant chemotherapy has not been demonstrated to add additional survival benefit after local radiotherapy.[113,114] In a large review of over 6000 patients with stage I or stage II FL diagnosed from 1973 to 2004, 34% of whom were initially treated with RT, patients who received initial RT had higher rates of disease-specific survival at 5 (90 vs 81%), 10 (79 vs 66%), 15 (68 vs 57%), and 20 (63 vs 51%) years.[115]

If significant morbidity is possible from radiotherapy based on the location of the disease area or if the patient chooses to not receive radiation, observation may be a reasonable alternative, especially for stage II patients.[116]

In one report, the median OS of selected untreated patients was 19 years. At a median follow-up of 7 years, 63% of patients had not required treatment.[116] The prognosis of patients who relapse after RT is excellent. In an analysis of early-stage patients staged with FDG PET prior to RT reported a 3-year OS of 91.4% after recurrence.[117] The OS was worse for patients who relapsed ≤12 months from diagnosis versus those who relapse >12 months (88.7% vs 97.6%, respectively).

Therapy of early-stage marginal zone lymphoma

The extranodal MZLs often present with localized disease involving the gastrointestinal tract, salivary glands, thyroid, orbit, conjunctiva, breast, and lung. In patients with *H. pylori*-associated gastric MALT, therapy with antibiotics and a proton pump inhibitor induces disease regression in over 80% of patients with long-term disease control and OS in a subset.[118–120] The presence of bcl-10 nuclear expression and/or t(11;18) may be useful to prospectively identify those patients with gastric MZL lymphomas who do not benefit from anti-*H. pylori* treatment.[121] Antibiotic therapy (doxycycline) against *Chlamydophila* has been reported with variable results in ocular MZLs.[8]

For patients with localized disease who progress after antibiotic therapy or are *H. pylori*-negative, involved-field radio-therapy with or without surgical resection has a 10-year disease-free survival of over 90%.[122,123] For other sites of extranodal MZL, since these diseases tend to remain localized for long periods of time prior to systemic spread, surgery remains a highly effective approach, often with adjuvant involved-field radiotherapy. In a retrospective study of patients with stage IE or IIE MZL, most were treated with involved-field RT alone.[124] The 5-year disease-free and OS for the entire group was 76% and 96%, respectively. Patients with gastric and thyroid disease had 5-year disease-free survival of 93%, whereas disease-free survival for other sites of involvement was 69%. The response rate for chemotherapy with alkylating agents, fludarabine or rituximab alone, for MZL is high.[125,126]

Treatment of advanced-stage follicular NHL
The overwhelming majority of patients have advanced-stage disease at diagnosis. Patients with asymptomatic FL do not require immediate treatment unless they have symptomatic nodal disease, compromised end organ function B symptoms; symptomatic extranodal disease, or cytopenias. This approach is supported by randomized prospective trials of observation versus immediate treatment. One of the largest trials compared immediate treatment with chlorambucil to observation.[127] At a median follow-up of 16 years, no difference in OS and cause-specific survival was seen.

A prospective study compared observation to rituximab alone or rituximab followed by maintenance in previously untreated FL. No difference in OS or incidence of histologic transformation was demonstrated.[128] A trial in a similar patient population randomized patients following four doses of weekly rituximab to either observation and retreatment at progression, or rituximab maintenance for 2 years, the RESORT trial. No difference in time to treatment failure, histologic transformation, or OS was seen, but more rituximab was administered to the maintenance arm. There was a difference in time to cytotoxic therapy, in favor of the maintenance rituximab receiving patients.[129] Close observation remains an appropriate recommendation for many newly diagnosed patients.

Rituximab has changed the paradigm of treating FL.[61] The benefit of adding rituximab to combination chemotherapy for the initial treatment has been demonstrated in multiple randomized trials of chemotherapy with or without rituximab.[17,130-132] All of these trials demonstrated improved PFS and OS.

Bendamustine plus rituximab (BR) has been compared to CHOP-R in a randomized phase III trial in 513 patients with advanced follicular, indolent, and MCL.[133] BR had superior median progression-free survival (69.5 vs 31.2 months) at 45 months, with less toxicity, including lower rates of grade 3 and 4 neutropenia and leukopenia was observed. There was no difference in OS at a median follow-up of 45 months. The BRIGHT study found BR to be noninferior to CHOP-R and CVP-R, with BR having a similar complete, overall response rates, PFS, and OS to the other regimens.[129] More second malignancies were observed in the BR patients.[134] These studies provide support for BR as the primary therapy for indolent FL. However, in low tumor burden patients over age 60, and based on a medicare database review, an unacceptable treatment-related mortality has been reported with bendamustine.[62]

The optimal chemotherapy backbone for FL patients has been debated. A randomized phase III trial compared initial treatment in previously untreated stage II–IV FL patients with R-CHOP or R-CVP or R-fludarabine-mitoxantrone. Both R-FM and R-CHOP were superior to R-CVP in 3 year PFS and TTF but there was no difference in OS. The current impact of this study is uncertain given the results of the BR-containing studies.[135] Other anti-CD20 monoclonal antibodies have been evaluated in patients with FL. Obinutuzumab has been evaluated in a phase III study comparing chemoimmunotherapy with either obinutuzumab or rituximab for previously untreated patients with FL.[136] The chemotherapy options were either bendamustine, CHOP, or cyclophosphamide, doxorubicin, vincristine (CVP), followed by 2 years of maintenance with either obinutuzumab or rituximab. The response rates and OS were similar with either obinutuzumab or rituximab, however, the progression-free survival was higher for patients receiving obinutuzumab.[136] Grade 3–5 adverse events, (cytopenias), were most frequent with CHOP, whereas grade 3–5 infections and second malignancies were most frequent with bendamustine, Deaths were more frequent in patients treated with bendamustine.[136]

Rituximab alone has been used as the first therapy in patients with indolent lymphoma, with overall response rates of around 70% and CR rates of over 30% reported.[137-139] In the SAKK trial patients received four weekly doses, then patients with stable disease or better were randomized to observation or four doses of maintenance with one dose every 2 months.[140] Patients with responding or stable disease at week 12 were randomized to no further treatment or rituximab maintenance every 2 months for 4 doses. At a median follow-up of 35 months, patients who received rituximab maintenance had a twofold increase in event-free survival (23 vs 12 months). Now with longer follow-up, 35% of all responders remain in remission at 8 years with 45% of newly diagnosed patients in this study in remission at 8 years with the additional maintenance rituximab. An increase of rituximab maintenance to 5 years was without benefit.

The use of maintenance rituximab after chemoimmunotherapy in patients with FL has been examined in a large randomized trial.[141] While maintenance rituximab appears to improve progression-free survival rates, toxicities, albeit tolerable, are increased and the effect on OS is to date unclear. The Primary Rituximab and Maintenance (PRIMA) phase III intergroup trial in 1018 patients with previously untreated FL responded to chemoimmunotherapy (CVP-R, CHOP-R, or FCM-R) randomly assigned maintenance with rituximab every 8 weeks for 24 months or placebo.[141] At 10 years of follow up the PFS is significantly better with maintenance but no difference in OS has been seen.[142]

A study of rituximab and lenalidomide (R^2) in previously untreated patients reported an overall response rate of 95%. The CR rate was 72%. The 2- and 5-year progression-free survival were 86% and 70%, respectively, and the 5-year OS was 100%.[143] In a phase III trial comparing chemoimmunotherapy to R^2, similar response rates, and similar 3-year PFS were observed in both arms.[144,145] R^2 is a chemotherapy-free alternative for previously untreated patients with FL.

Radioimmunotherapy alone has been used as the initial treatment in a limited number of patients with FL.[146,147] A randomized trial of CHOP plus rituximab to CHOP followed by 131I tositumomab did not yield any differences in PFS between the two arms.[148] Radioimmunotherapy is not widely used in patients with FL.

High-dose therapy and autologous stem cell transplantation (ASCT) has been used to consolidate first remission for selected patients with FL.[149-153] The majority of these studies have demonstrated a significant improvement in PFS, but no impact on OS.[154] One reason for the lack of impact on OS has been the excess number of second malignancies. Although allogeneic stem cell transplantation (HCT) can potentially lead to cure for patients with FL, due to the significantly higher treatment-related mortality than ASCT, this is largely reserved for patients with relapsed and more refractory disease.

Initial treatment of other indolent lymphomas

Patients with MZL not on a clinical trial are often treated in a similar fashion to those with the more common indolent lymphoma FL. Because of the rarity of these diseases, all MZL histologies are often combined in clinical trials. Initial treatment can include rituximab alone. A randomized trial found superior PFS with the use of chlorambucil plus rituximab versus rituximab or chlorambucil alone.[155] In a randomized trial of R-CHOP or R-CVP to BR, no difference in disease free survival (DFS) was seen in patients with MZL.[133] The combination of rituximab plus lenalidomide is very active as initial treatment of MZL of all subtypes. Rituximab alone or with chemotherapy is effective for frontline treatment of splenic MZL, when treatment is indicated and has replaced splenectomy in most settings. Initial treatment for LPL treatment can include rituximab alone or chemoimmunotherapy such as BR. Other regimens include dexamethasone cyclophosphamide, rituximab as well as bortezomib plus rituximab. BTK inhibitors are highly active in Waldenstrom's macroglobulinemia. In 150 treatment naïve and relapsed patients randomized to receive treated ibrutinib plus rituximab versus placebo plus rituximab, PFS at 30 months was 82% versus 28%, respectively.[156] Benefit was independent of the presence MYD88 mutation which correlates with higher response rates in patients treated with BTK inhibitors alone.[157]

Treatment of relapsed FL

When patients with relapsed FL require treatment, there are many options, ranging from rituximab alone to combination chemotherapy plus rituximab, radioimmunotherapy, and for selected patients stem cell transplantation. For rituximab alone, 35% of patients with relapsed or refractory FL treated with rituximab and abbreviated maintenance were progression free at 8 years.[140]

Several humanized anti-CD20 monoclonal antibodies have been studied in patients with relapsed FL. Obinutuzumab is the first type II, glycoengineered, and humanized monoclonal anti-CD20 antibody.[158] In rituximab refractory pts in the high-dose cohort, the response rate was 55% with median PFS of 11.9 months. Studies of obinutuzumab combination with chemotherapy, have shown 93–98% response rates in relapsed and refractory FL patients.[159]

A number of phase II trials of other agents plus rituximab associated with quite high response rates included BR with 90% RR and median PFS of 2 years.[160,161] Bendamustine plus obinutuzumab for six cycles followed by 2 years of maintenance obinutuzumab was superior to 6 cycles of bendamustine alone, with PFS of 26 months versus 14 months, respectively.[162] Moreover, there was a significant OS advantage to the combination.

As already discussed for untreated patients lenalidomide plus rituximab has been studied in relapsed and refractory FL patients. The overall response rate is higher with the combination (70 vs 53%), and the time to progression was 1 year longer for the combination.[163] The results of a phase III randomized trial of lenalidomide plus rituximab versus rituximab alone has been reported in patients with previously treated FL.[12] Improved median PFS was seen in the combination (39%, vs 14%, respectively), with a nonstatistically significant improvement in OS. Anti-CD20 radioimmunotherapy agents have been used for treatment of patients with relapsed and refractory FL.[164] These radioimmunoconjugates have not received widespread use, and the 131I agent has been taken off the market. FL is extremely responsive to RT. Low-dose RT (e.g., total dose of 4 Gy) can be used for the palliation of patients who have symptoms related to a single disease site, with CR rates of 57% and ORR of 82%.[165]

The use of either autologous or allogeneic hematopoietic cell transplantation (HCT) in FL is controversial and the subject of numerous trials.[166] A large number of phase II studies prior to the availability of rituximab, involving high-dose therapy and autologous HCT have shown that for approximately 40% of patients with good performance status and chemosensitive relapsed disease may experience prolong progression-free and OS rates.[167-170] The only phase III randomized trial (the CUP trial) comparing autologous HCT to conventional chemotherapy in relapsed FL patients demonstrated a higher PFS and OS for autologous SCT and no benefit for purging the stem cell graft.[171] An retrospective analysis of patients undergoing autologous SCT following rituximab-based salvage therapy did not suggest a benefit of autologous SCT as compared to conventional therapy. Unfortunately, as has been seen in autologous SCT in first remission, second malignancies both solid tumors and MDS/AML are reported post autologous SCT. An National Comprehensive Cancer Network (NCCN) database retrospective analysis found significantly higher 3 year OS for autologous SCT versus allogeneic SCT (87% vs 61%).[172] Certainly for younger patients with more resistant disease, allogeneic SCT remains a potentially curative option for relapsed FL.[173]

A "revival" of interest in autologous SCT has occurred focused on patients with early relapse. Several retrospective analyses have reported 5-year OS of 70% following autologous SCT in this patient population.[174] Using data from the Center for International Blood and Marrow Transplant Research and the National LymphoCare Study patients with early treatment failure undergoing early autologous SCT had higher 5-year OS than those without auto SCT (73% vs 60%).[175]

There are a multitude of new approaches that have been studied in patients with FL and MZL. This includes monoclonal antibodies, immunomodulatory agents, and novel drugs such as kinase inhibitors. Bcell receptor kinases are logical targets for therapy in FL. To date, kinase inhibitors targeting PI3 kinase and BTK. In relapsed and refractory FL patients, idelalisib an inhibitor of PI3 kinase delta isoform, was the first of these kinase inhibitors to be studied with overall response rate of 57%, and median duration of response was 12.5 months.[129] Another PI3 kinase inhibitor, copanlisib, in patients with relapsed FL has similar responses to idelalisib.[176] This intravenously delivered agent targets PI3 kinase alpha and delta isoforms. A third PI3 kinase inhibitor, duvelisib, targeting the gamma and delta isoforms is also an active oral agent in patients with relapsed FL, with similar activity to idelalisib and copanisib.[177] To date there is no compelling data showing superiority of one over another. Although highly active in CLL and MZL, the Bruton's tyrosine kinase (BTK) ibrutinib has only limited activity in FL (ORR 21%).[178,179]

CD19 CART cells look very promising in patients with relapsed FL. A 71% response rate has been reported in 14 patients treated.[180] With median follow-up of 29 months, 89% of the responders were progression free. Another study of eight patients with relapsed FL receiving CD19 CAR T cell immunotherapy also reported favorable results. Encouraging results have also been reported in tFL.[181] The CR rate was 88%, and all patients who achieved CR remain in remission with a median follow-up of 24 months.

Treatment for relapse of other indolent lymphomas

Patients with other indolent NHLs besides FL, including nodal and extranodal MZL, are generally treated similarly to FL. Patients with SLL are treated with agents used for CLL (see **Chapter 113**). Lenalidomide plus rituximab is approved in relapsed MZL given improvement in PFS compared to rituximab alone.[12] Ibrutinib is also approved for the treatment of patients with recurrent MZL with an ORR of 48% and PFS of 14.2 months.[182]

Aggressive lymphomas

Therapy of early-stage aggressive lymphoma

Fewer than 20% of patients with diffuse large-cell lymphoma have truly localized disease. The recommended treatment for localized disease outside of clinical trials is abbreviated chemotherapy plus involved-field radiotherapy, or combination chemotherapy alone. In the prerituximab era, the Southwest Oncology Group (SWOG) randomized trial of patients with localized diffuse aggressive lymphoma compared eight cycles of CHOP to three cycles of CHOP plus involved-field radiotherapy.[183] Patients treated with three cycles of CHOP plus radiotherapy had a significantly better 5-year progression-free survival and OS than patients treated with eight cycles of CHOP (77% vs 64% for progression-free survival, 82% vs 72% for OS).[183] With longer follow-up, however, the progression free and OS were not different given late recurrences in the radiotherapy containing arm.[184] In addition, the addition of radiotherapy after eight cycles of CHOP in one study and 4 cycles in another in patients over 60 did not improve OS, though disease-free survival was superior in the first.[116,185]

A phase II trial of patients with early-stage DLBCL with at least one risk factor (age >60; increased serum LDH; stage II disease; or performance status ≥1) utilized three cycles of CHOP-R followed by involved field radiation therapy.[186] The PFS and OS at 2 and 4 years was 93% and 88%, and 95% and 92%, respectively. A phase III study in patients age 60 or under with IPI score or 0 or 1 compared 6 cycles of CHOP to CHOP-R, with all patients with bulk disease (masses greater than 7.5 cm) or extranodal sites receiving involved field radiation.[187] The patients with IPI score of 0, with no bulk which includes early-stage patients, the 5-year EFS is approximately 90% with CHOP-R alone, suggesting chemoimmunotherapy alone is an option for early-stage disease. However, bulky disease, defined as masses greater than 7.5 cm, was associated with inferior outcome. In the MiNT trial of CHOP versus CHOP-R, all patients (IPI 0 or IPI 1) with masses greater than 7.5 cm received 30–40 Gy of involved field radiation to those sites. Those patients with IPI of 0 and bulk disease had a 10–15% lower PFS than patients without bulk.[187]

More recently, a noninferiority study compared six cycles of rituximab, cyclophosphamide, doxorubicin, vincristine, prednisone (RCHOP) versus four cycles of CHOP with six doses of rituximab in patients under the age of 60 without bulky disease, increased LDH or ECOG performance status of >1. There was no difference between the two arms in this favorable group of patients.[66] In a PET risk-adapted study, 158 patients with nonbulky, stage I/II DLBCL underwent restaging after three cycles of RCHOP. PET negative patients received one additional cycle of chemotherapy only, while PET-positive patients received IFRT followed by ibritumomab tiuxetan. The 5-year PFS for the entire group was 87% with PET negative and PET-positive patients having similar outcomes.[188]

Primary mediastinal large Bcell lymphoma patients often present with early stage, bulky disease, and historically patients have received combined modality therapy. In the MInT trial, 87 patients with PMLBCL[189] received 6 cycles of CHOP-R, 75% of whom also received radiation therapy; only 7% of patients who received radiation subsequently progressed or relapsed. A study of 51 patients treated with dose-adjusted EPOCH plus rituximab (DA-EPOCH-R), and no radiotherapy, reported an outstanding PFS (93%) and OS (100%).[190] In PET/CT scan at the end of therapy, a subset of had residual uptake from inflammation that resolved over time.

Extranodal NK/T-cell lymphomas present with early-stage disease in 97% of cases. The 5-year OS and PFS for patients with stage IE disease is 78% and 63%, respectively, and for stage IIE the OS and PFS is 46% and 40%, respectively, with no difference between combined modality and RT alone.[16] For patients with stage IE/IIE, early use of radiotherapy (50–55 Gy) is critical, whereas chemotherapy initially followed by radiotherapy yields inferior results. More recent studies suggest that combined modality treatment may yield more favorable results. Phase II trials of concurrent radiation therapy and weekly cisplatin followed by etoposide, ifosfamide, cisplatin, and dexamethasone reported overall response rate of 83% and 3-year PFS and OS of 85 and 86%, respectively.[191,192]

Therapy of advanced-stage aggressive lymphoma

The current recommendation for treatment of advanced-stage DLBCL or PTCL, outside a clinical trial, is combination chemotherapy with CHOP plus rituximab or CHOP with or without etoposide, respectively. In patients with DLBCL ages 60–80, the Groups d'Etude des Lymphomes de L'Adulte (GELA) group reported that eight cycles of CHOP plus rituximab was superior to CHOP alone in terms of PFS, DFS, and OS.[193,194] In a US Intergroup study of CHOP versus R-CHOP in patients over 60[195] responding patients were randomly assigned to receive either rituximab maintenance therapy or no maintenance. A beneficial impact of rituximab added to CHOP chemotherapy on event-free and OS was observed; however, no benefit was seen for maintenance rituximab following R-CHOP induction. Similarly, in patients less than 60, CHOP-R with IPI of 0 and 1, the addition of rituximab to CHOP improved time to treatment failure and OS. This benefit was greater in the patients with an IPI of 1.[187]

In the RICOVER trial, in patients over age 60, R-CHOP was superior to CHOP given for six or eight cycles (70% vs 57%) and there was no benefit of eight cycles of CHOP-R over six cycles.[196] In another study CHOP-R given every 21 days (CHOP-R 21) for eight cycles was compared to six cycles of CHOP-R 14 with no difference in PFS or OS.[197] This supports CHOP-R 21 for six cycles as the standard of care. Alternatives to R-CHOP have been examined in phase III trials. The aggressive regimen R-ACVBP followed by consolidation with methotrexate and leucovorin[144] was compared to CHOP-R plus intrathecal methotrexate in patients under age 60 with IPI score of 1. R-ACVBP plus methotrexate and leucovorin led to higher PFS and OS. The benefit was seen in the non-GCB subgroup of patients.[99]

Given promising results with a single-center phase 2 trial, dose-adjusted REPOCH was compared to RCHOP in patients with DLBCL in a multicenter study and did not demonstrate benefit in progression free or OS.[198] Given the inferior outcomes in patients with nongerminal center-derived DLBCL, multiple studies have added novel agents with activity in this subset of patients to RCHOP with promising results. In each of the randomized studies, however, adding bortezomib, ibrutinib, and lenalidomide to RCHOP compared to RCHOP alone, there was no benefit in PFS or OS.[163,199,200]

Historically, the long-term results of treatment of primary testicular DLBCL are worse for than predicted by the IPI.[126,201] Current therapy has been defined by a report of 53 patients with untreated stage I or II primary testicular lymphoma treated with six to eight cycles of CHOP-R 21, four weekly doses of intrathecal methotrexate (12 mg), and radiation therapy to the contralateral testis (30 Gy) for all patients and (30–36 Gy) to regional nodes for patients with stage II disease.[201] With a median follow-up of 65 months, the OS and PFS at 5 years was 85% and 74%, respectively.

Prophylaxis for CNS disease in DLBCL is highly controversial.[197] In the prerituximab era, the risk of CNS involvement was 2.8%, with intraparenchymal and intraspinal disease occurring in 66%, and isolated leptomeningeal disease in 26%.[202] Risk factors include sites of disease (testis, ovary, bone marrow, breast, epidural space, kidneys, adrenals, and paranasal sinuses); high-intermediate or high IPI score; multiple extranodal sites; and "double hit" cytogenetics and the nongerminal center subtype. The CNS IPI includes the five IPI risk factors (age, stage, >1 extranodal site of disease, ECOG performance status of >1, and elevated LDH) plus renal or adrenal involvement.[66] For patients with 4–6 risk factors, the 2-year rate of CNS was over 10%. With the significant number of parenchymal relapses, intrathecal chemotherapy alone may be inadequate prophylaxis, making high-dose methotrexate a potentially more effective therapy. However, there is no strong evidence that high-dose methotrexate is superior to intrathecal.

The treatment of both high-grade B-cell lymphoma with MYC and BCL2 and/or BCL6 rearrangements and high-grade B-cell lymphoma NOS is uncertain.[201,203] Retrospective evidence suggests that intensive regimens such as modified Magrath regimen with CODOX-M/IVAC (cyclophosphamide, vincristine, doxorubicin, high-dose methotrexate with ifosfamide, cytarabine, etoposide, and intrathecal methotrexate), HyperCVAD, and DA-EPOCH-R are associated with better outcomes than CHOP-R (ORR 86% vs 57%, 4-year PFS approximately 50–65% vs 0–30%).[204] Data of MYC translocation-positive DLBCL treated with DA-EPOCH-R in multi-center phase II studies yielded 71% event-free survival at 48 months.[205] This study, however, included patients with MYC with and without BCL2 and/or BCL6 rearrangements. In a large, international retrospective analysis poor outcome in MYC rearranged aggressive lymphoma was seen only with BCL2 with or without BCL6 translocation with an immunoglobulin partner gene.[66]

For PTCL, similar treatment approaches to DLBCL have been taken for patients with localized and advanced-stage disease. When patients are stratified by the IPI, the disease-free survival and OS are generally inferior for patients with PTCL than for patients with DLBCL. There is presently no overwhelming evidence to support superiority of different treatment regimens for PTCL.[206] A retrospective subset analysis of a phase III study in PTCL patients of CHOP versus CHOEP showed a significant improvement in EFS for PTCL patients younger than age 60 with a normal LDH at diagnosis, but there was no difference in OS.[106] ALCL has the most favorable prognosis of the T-cell lymphomas.[86] The prognosis for patients who express the ALK protein is particularly favorable with 5-year OS of 79%.[83] In CD30 positive PTCL, defined as expression of greater than or equal to 10% by immunohistochemical staining, the anti-CD30 monoclonal antibody–drug conjugate brentuximab vedotin was combined with cyclophosphamide, doxorubicin, and prednisone (BV+CHP) and compared to CHOP.[207] With more than 3 years of median follow-up, BV-CHP was associated with improved median PFS of 48.2 months compared to 20.8 months in the CHOP arm. Improved OS was seen in subset of patients with ALCL.

Autologous stem cell transplantation for NHL in first remission
A number of studies have examined the role of high-dose therapy and ASCT in first CR/PR for patients with aggressive NHL, without clear evidence for a survival benefit.[208,209] A meta-analysis of 3079 patients treated in the prerituximab era on 15 randomized trials with either conventional therapy or ASCT in first CR, showed no difference in EFS, OS, or treatment-related mortality.[210] Given the generally inferior prognosis of patients with PTCL, autologous SCT has been investigated in first remission in several phase II studies with encouraging results.[211,212]

Mantle cell lymphomas (MCL)
With the advent of intensive chemoimmunotherapy, the median survival of patients with MCL is now 8–10 years. CHOP-R was historically the regimen of choice for MCL. A randomized trial comparing CHOP-R to BR reported superior PFS with BR with less toxicity (35 months vs 22 months).[133] Another study of CHOP-R versus FCR (fludarabine, cyclophosphamide, rituximab)[213] in patients over age 60 yielded similar CR rates, but CHOP-R had less toxicity, and the OS at 4 years was 62% versus 47% in favor of CHOP-R.[213] A second randomization of maintenance with interferon-α or rituximab was given until progression. For the patients who received CHOP-R, a survival benefit from maintenance rituximab was observed (OS rate at 4 years of 87% vs 63%).

Autologous transplant for patients less than 65, in first CR or PR, has shown improvement in PFS as compared to interferon-α maintenance, but a nonstatistically significant improvement in OS.[214]

Many phase II studies have intensified the induction therapy prior to ASCT. Incorporation of high-dose cytarabine[215] has given excellent results, with median OS and response duration longer than 10 years, and a median event-free survival (EFS) of 7.4 years. In addition, a randomized trial of 3 years of maintenance rituximab versus observation after ASCT demonstrated improvement in progression free (83% vs 64% at more than 4 years after randomization) and OS (89% vs 80%).[216]

HyperCVAD is an intensive regimen, with escalated doses of cyclophosphamide, high-dose methotrexate and cytarabine is an alternative to ASCT in first remission as a way to prolong remissions in MCL. The M.D. Anderson reported a median OS not reached at 8 years, and a median time to failure 4.6 years.[217] Two multi-institution trials of R-Hyper-CVAD reported excellent disease control but a significant proportion of patients could not complete the proscribed treatment due to toxicity.[33,218]

Highly aggressive lymphomas

Lymphoblastic
The treatment of LBL is detailed in **Chapter 113**.

Burkitt lymphoma
BL is typically treated with aggressive multi-agent chemotherapy with CNS-directed agents. The addition of rituximab to CODOX-M/IVAC, HyperCVAD, and the French LMB regimen is associated with 2 year OS of approximately 75%.[219-221] These regimens, however, are associated with significant toxicity and not appropriate for older patients. A multi-center study of 113 patients treated with DA-EPOCH-R with intratracheal methotrexate reported excellent results with EFS and OS of 84.5% and 87%, respectively at a median follow-up of 59 months.[222] CNS involvement at baseline was associated with inferior outcomes, likely given the lack of systemic CNS prophylaxis. There is presently no evidence that first remission autologous transplant is indicated for adult BL.[223]

Adult T-cell leukemia/lymphoma
ATLLs are approached with intensive multiagent chemotherapy regimens.[224] Antiviral therapy with zidovudine and interferon-α should be considered upfront for the smoldering, chronic subtype.[224,225] For the acute leukemia/lymphoma type, a phase III randomized trial[226] reported that an intensive regimen (VCAP-AMP-VECP) had a 3-year OS of 24% compared to only 13% with CHOP. With the poor results of chemotherapy, both myeloablative and reduced intensity alloSCT has been applied to ATLL, with limited success.[227,228]

Treatment of recurrent aggressive NHL
The majority of recurrences from chemoimmunotherapy are within the first 2 years after treatment.[99] Following relapse, about 60% of patients' disease remains sensitive to conventional treatment, but fewer than 10% of patients with aggressive NHL experience prolonged disease-free survival with second-line treatment regimens. Following relapse, the current curative approach for patients with relapsed NHL involves high-dose therapy and stem cell transplantation.

Several combination chemotherapy regimens have been compared in randomized trials with equivalent results. Specifically, R-ICE yields similar results to R-DHAP which is equivalent to

R-GDP.[106,229–231] The goal is to identify patients with chemosensitive disease who have the greatest likelihood of benefiting from high-dose therapy and ASCT.[232–234]

Disease sensitivity at the time of ASCT has remained the most significant prognostic variable for predicting treatment outcome.[189] Several large series have shown that patients who undergo ASCT with primary refractory have less than 10% probability of disease-free survival. Those relapsed patients whose disease remains sensitive to chemotherapy have a 30–60% probability of long-term disease-free survival. In contrast, only 10–15% of patients with resistant disease are long-term survivors.

ASCT has been compared to conventional salvage therapy for relapsed aggressive NHL in the PARMA trial.[235] Patients with relapsed aggressive NHL (largely DLBCL) received two cycles of cisplatin, cytarabine, solumedrol, and if responsive, were randomized to continued chemotherapy for four additional cycles or high-dose chemotherapy and autologous bone marrow transplantation. With median follow-up in excess of 5 years, patients randomized to the high-dose arm had superior event-free survival (46% vs 12%) and OS (53% vs 32%).

Investigators have to date failed to improve on these results with the addition of maintenance therapy posttransplant with rituximab,[208] an anti-CD19 immunotoxin, the oral kinase inhibitor enzastaurin, or adding radioimmuntherapy[236] to the conditioning regimen. For patients with relapsed or refractory DLBCL, high-dose therapy and ASCT remains the treatment of choice for patients with chemosensitive disease. If the recurrence is localized adjuvant RT either before or after high-dose therapy and ASCT may be beneficial in terms of disease control but may not impact on OS. For patients with chemorefractory disease, clinical trials or palliative therapy, but not stem cell transplantation, should be considered.

CD19 directed chimeric antigen receptor T cell (CAR-T) therapy has emerged as an effective treatment option for patients with relapsed and refractory aggressive B-cell lymphoma. Two products, axicabtagene ciloleucel and tisagenelecluecel, have been approved by the Food and Drug Administration (FDA) after two or more prior lines of therapy. In the pivotal study of axicabtagene, the complete response rate was 54% with 52% OS rate at 18 months.[232] For patients treated on the tisagenelecluecel study, the CR rate was 40% with relapse-free survival of 65% at 12 months after initial response.[233] Both products are associated with largely reversible cytokine release syndrome and neurologic toxicity.

For patients who relapse after ASCT or CAR-T cell therapy or for those who are not candidates, the CD79B-directed antibody–drug conjugate polatuzumab was recently approved in combination with BR for patients with relapsed or refractory based on an OS benefit compared to BR alone, median 12.4 versus 4.7 months.[234] In addition, tafasitamab plus lenalidomide was studied predominantly in patients in first relapse who were not eligible for ASCT. The ORR was 60% with 43% CR and median PFS was approximately 1 year.[237]

Recurrent PTCL has a very poor prognosis, with a median OS of 6.7 months.[238] Gemcitabine and other conventional chemotherapies are with limited benefit.[239] Newer agents for relapsed PTCL, including the antifolate agent pralatrexate, and high dose cytarabine (HDAC) inhibitors romidepsin and belinostat, all of which have a 25–30% response rate with median duration of response of less than 18 months.[204,240] Nonmyeloablative alloSCT for highly selected patients has a 5 year OS and PFS of 50% and 40%, respectively.[241]

Recurrent mantle cell lymphoma

The vast majority of patients with MCL relapse. Agents that are FDA approved for relapsed MCL: bortezomib, lenalidomide, and the BTK inhibitors ibrutinib, acalabrutinib, and zanabrutinib. Bortezomib has a 29% overall response rate (5% CR) with a median duration of 7 months.[242] Lenalidomide, approved for bortezomib failures, has a 26% response rate (7% CR), and median duration of response of 17 months.[154] Ibrutinib was the first BTK inhibitor approved in relapsed MCL and has a 68% response rate, (21% CR), with a median duration of 17.5 months.[178] In phase 2 studies, acalabrutinib and zanabrutinib yielded overall remission rates of 81% and 84% with CR rates of 40% and 59% respectively.[175,243] Autologous stem cell transplantation for relapsed MCL patients is of limited benefit.[32] Nonmyeloablative alloSCT can be considered for select relapsed patients. The 3 year PFS and OS are 30% and 40%, respectively.[32] CD19 CAR-T cell therapy, brexucabtagene autoleucel, was recently approved in relapsed/refractory MCL. About 74 patients were treated in the pivotal study.[244] ORR and CR rates were 85% and 67%, respectively with 12-month PFS of 61%. Grade 3 or higher CRS and neurotoxicity occurred in 15% and 31% of patients.

Allogeneic bone marrow transplantation in NHL

Allogeneic stem cell transplantation has been applied to patients with relapsed and refractory NHL. Nearly all patients had relapsed disease, many of whom were resistant to conventional-dose therapy. In the European Bone Marrow Transplant Registry, the recurrence rate after allogeneic transplantation for aggressive NHL was lower than for autologous transplantation without difference in OS, due to the associated higher transplant-related mortality.[186] The EFS and OS at 5 years was 43%, with treatment-related mortality 25% at 1 year. Patients with recurrent disease following ASCT or CAR-T cell therapy who have good performance status and chemosensitive disease are considered for alloSCT usually with reduced-intensity conditioning. Studies have reported 40–60% year PFS, but with treatment-related mortality of 20% for RIC alloSCT and up to 40% for myeloablative transplants.[245,246]

New therapeutic approaches for NHL

Significant improvements have been made in the treatment of NHL, with a major impact on B-cell malignancies. However, less progress has occurred in therapy of many disease entities, particularly PTCLs. There are a vast number of new, rational targeted agents under evaluation. including antibody–drug conjugates, kinases inhibitors, and immunotherapies that enhance T cell cytotoxicity (chimeric antigen receptor T cells and checkpoint blockade antibodies). The most significant advance is our understanding of the genetic events and aberrant pathways driving lymphomagenesis. This knowledge drives the development of agents directed against novel targets, thereby limiting toxicity to normal cells.

Key references

The complete reference list can be found on Vital Source version of this title, see inside front cover.

1. Siegel RL, Miller KD, Jemal A. Cancer statistics, 2020. *CA Cancer J Clin.* 2020;**70**(1):7–30.
25. Swerdlow SH, Campo E, Pileri SA, et al. The 2016 revision of the World Health Organization classification of lymphoid neoplasms. *Blood.* 2016;**127**(20):2375–2390.

35 Treon SP, Xu L, Yang G, et al. MYD88 L265P somatic mutation in Waldenstrom's macroglobulinemia. *N Engl J Med*. 2012;**367**(9):826–833.

52 Geisler CH, Kolstad A, Laurell A, et al. The mantle cell lymphoma international prognostic index (MIPI) is superior to the international prognostic index (IPI) in predicting survival following intensive first-line immunochemotherapy and autologous stem cell transplantation (ASCT). *Blood*. 2010;**115**(8):1530–1533.

54 Rosenwald A, Wright G, Chan WC, et al. The use of molecular profiling to predict survival after chemotherapy for diffuse large-B-cell lymphoma. *N Engl J Med*. 2002;**346**(25):1937–1947.

57 Shipp MA, Ross KN, Tamayo P, et al. Diffuse large B-cell lymphoma outcome prediction by gene-expression profiling and supervised machine learning. *Nat Med*. 2002;**8**(1):68–74.

96 Cheson BD, Fisher RI, Barrington SF, et al. Recommendations for initial evaluation, staging, and response assessment of Hodgkin and non-Hodgkin lymphoma: the Lugano classification. *J Clin Oncol*. 2014;**32**(27):3059–3068.

99 Maurer MJ, Ghesquieres H, Jais JP, et al. Event-free survival at 24 months is a robust end point for disease-related outcome in diffuse large B-cell lymphoma treated with immunochemotherapy. *J Clin Oncol*. 2014;**32**(10):1066–1073.

101 International Non-Hodgkin's Lymphoma Prognostic Factors Project. A predictive model for aggressive non-Hodgkin's lymphoma. *N Engl J Med*. 1993;**329**(14):987–994.

108 Friedberg JW, Taylor MD, Cerhan JR, et al. Follicular lymphoma in the United States: first report of the national LymphoCare study. *J Clin Oncol*. 2009;**27**(8):1202–1208.

127 Ardeshna KM, Smith P, Norton A, et al. Long-term effect of a watch and wait policy versus immediate systemic treatment for asymptomatic advanced-stage non-Hodgkin lymphoma: a randomised controlled trial. *Lancet*. 2003;**362**(9383):516–522.

132 Salles G, Mounier N, de Guibert S, et al. Rituximab combined with chemotherapy and interferon in follicular lymphoma patients: results of the GELA-GOELAMS FL2000 study. *Blood*. 2008;**112**(13):4824–4831.

140 Martinelli G, Schmitz SF, Utiger U, et al. Long-term follow-up of patients with follicular lymphoma receiving single-agent rituximab at two different schedules in trial SAKK 35/98. *J Clin Oncol*. 2010;**28**(29):4480–4484.

144 Morschhauser F, Fowler NH, Feugier P, et al. Rituximab plus Lenalidomide in advanced untreated follicular lymphoma. *N Engl J Med*. 2018;**379**(10):934–947.

180 Schuster SJ, Svoboda J, Chong EA, et al. Chimeric antigen receptor T cells in refractory B-cell lymphomas. *N Engl J Med*. 2017;**377**(26):2545–2554.

187 Pfreundschuh M, Trumper L, Osterborg A, et al. CHOP-like chemotherapy plus rituximab versus CHOP-like chemotherapy alone in young patients with good-prognosis diffuse large-B-cell lymphoma: a randomised controlled trial by the MabThera International Trial (MInT) Group. *Lancet Oncol*. 2006;**7**(5):379–391.

190 Dunleavy K, Pittaluga S, Maeda LS, et al. Dose-adjusted EPOCH-rituximab therapy in primary mediastinal B-cell lymphoma. *N Engl J Med*. 2013;**368**(15):1408–1416.

191 Yamaguchi M, Tobinai K, Oguchi M, et al. Concurrent chemoradiotherapy for localized nasal natural killer/T-cell lymphoma: an updated analysis of the Japan clinical oncology group study JCOG0211. *J Clin Oncol*. 2012;**30**(32):4044–4046.

194 Feugier P, Van Hoof A, Sebban C, et al. Long-term results of the R-CHOP study in the treatment of elderly patients with diffuse large B-cell lymphoma: a study by the Groupe d'Etude des Lymphomes de l'Adulte. *J Clin Oncol*. 2005;**23**(18):4117–4126.

195 Habermann TM, Weller EA, Morrison VA, et al. Rituximab-CHOP versus CHOP alone or with maintenance rituximab in older patients with diffuse large B-cell lymphoma. *J Clin Oncol*. 2006;**24**(19):3121–3127.

198 Bartlett NL, Wilson WH, Jung SH, et al. Dose-adjusted EPOCH-R compared with R-CHOP as frontline therapy for diffuse large B-cell lymphoma: clinical outcomes of the phase III intergroup trial alliance/CALGB 50303. *J Clin Oncol*. 2019;**37**(21):1790–1799.

199 Younes A, Sehn LH, Johnson P, et al. Randomized phase III trial of ibrutinib and rituximab plus cyclophosphamide, doxorubicin, vincristine, and prednisone in non-germinal center b-cell diffuse large B-cell lymphoma. *J Clin Oncol*. 2019;**37**(15):1285–1295.

200 Vitolo U, Witzig T, Gascoyne RD. ROBUST: first report of phase III randomized study of lenalidomide/R-CHOP (R2-CHOP) vs placebo/R-CHOP in previously untreated ABC-type diffuse large B-cell lymphoma. *Hematol Oncol*. 2019;**37**(S2):36–37.

202 Bernstein SH, Unger JM, Leblanc M, et al. Natural history of CNS relapse in patients with aggressive non-Hodgkin's lymphoma: a 20-year follow-up analysis of SWOG 8516–the Southwest Oncology Group. *J Clin Oncol*. 2009;**27**(1):114–119.

207 Horwitz S, O'Connor OA, Pro B, et al. Brentuximab vedotin with chemotherapy for CD30-positive peripheral T-cell lymphoma (ECHELON-2): a global, double-blind, randomised, phase 3 trial. *Lancet*. 2019;**393**(10168):229–240.

208 Gisselbrecht C, Schmitz N, Mounier N, et al. Rituximab maintenance therapy after autologous stem-cell transplantation in patients with relapsed CD20(+) diffuse large B-cell lymphoma: final analysis of the collaborative trial in relapsed aggressive lymphoma. *J Clin Oncol*. 2012;**30**(36):4462–4469.

214 Dreyling M, Lenz G, Hoster E, et al. Early consolidation by myeloablative radiochemotherapy followed by autologous stem cell transplantation in first remission significantly prolongs progression-free survival in mantle-cell lymphoma: results of a prospective randomized trial of the European MCL Network. *Blood*. 2005;**105**(7):2677–2684.

215 Geisler CH, Kolstad A, Laurell A, et al. Nordic MCL2 trial update: six-year follow-up after intensive immunochemotherapy for untreated mantle cell lymphoma followed by BEAM or BEAC + autologous stem-cell support: still very long survival but late relapses do occur. *Br J Haematol*. 2012;**158**(3):355–362.

216 Le Gouill S, Thieblemont C, Oberic L, et al. Rituximab after autologous stem-cell transplantation in mantle-cell lymphoma. *N Engl J Med*. 2017;**377**(13):1250–1260.

221 Ribrag V, Koscielny S, Bosq J, et al. Rituximab and dose-dense chemotherapy for adults with Burkitt's lymphoma: a randomised, controlled, open-label, phase 3 trial. *Lancet*. 2016;**387**(10036):2402–2411.

224 Bazarbachi A, Suarez F, Fields P, Hermine O. How I treat adult T-cell leukemia/lymphoma. *Blood*. 2011;**118**(7):1736–1745.

229 Gisselbrecht C, Glass B, Mounier N, et al. R-ICE versus R-DHAP in relapsed patients with CD20 diffuse large B-cell lymphoma (DLBCL) followed by autologous stem cell transplantation: CORAL study. *J Clin Oncol*. 2009;**27**:8509.

230 Crump M, Kuruvilla J, Couban S, et al. Randomized comparison of gemcitabine, dexamethasone, and cisplatin versus dexamethasone, cytarabine, and cisplatin chemotherapy before autologous stem-cell transplantation for relapsed and refractory aggressive lymphomas: NCIC-CTG LY.12. *J Clin Oncol*. 2014;**32**(31):3490–3496.

232 Neelapu SS, Locke FL, Bartlett NL, et al. Axicabtagene ciloleucel CAR T-cell therapy in refractory large B-cell lymphoma. *N Engl J Med*. 2017;**377**(26):2531–2544.

233 Schuster SJ, Bishop MR, Tam CS, et al. Tisagenlecleucel in adult relapsed or refractory diffuse large B-Cell lymphoma. *N Engl J Med*. 2019;**380**(1):45–56.

237 Salles G, Duell J, Gonzalez Barca E, et al. Tafasitamab plus lenalidomide in relapsed or refractory diffuse large B-cell lymphoma (L-MIND): a multicentre, prospective, single-arm, phase 2 study. *Lancet Oncol*. 2020;**21**(7):978–988.

244 Wang M, Munoz J, Goy A, et al. KTE-X19 CAR T-cell therapy in relapsed or refractory mantle-cell lymphoma. *N Engl J Med*. 2020;**382**(14):1331–1342.

118 Mycosis fungoides and Sézary syndrome

Walter Hanel, MD, PhD ∎ Catherine Chung, MD ∎ John C. Reneau, MD, PhD

Overview

Mycosis fungoides (MF) and its leukemic variant, Sézary syndrome (SS), are the most common cutaneous T-cell lymphomas. MF/SS originates in the skin and presentation may vary from limited patches to erythroderma and/or widespread cutaneous tumors. Although patients with limited patch-plaque disease generally have an indolent course with favorable prognosis and survival similar to age-matched control populations, patients who present with cutaneous tumors or extracutaneous disease have a relentless progressive course of disease. Treatments for patients with limited disease are primarily skin-directed and include various topical therapies including steroids, chemotherapy (nitrogen mustard), retinoids (bexarotene), immunomodulators (imiquimod), radiation therapy, and phototherapy. When the disease is advanced, skin-directed therapies are still often needed, but systemic treatment becomes essential. Conventional chemotherapy (single agent or combination) is frequently not effective. However, nonchemotherapeutic systemic agents such as retinoids, extracorporeal photopheresis, histone deacetylase inhibitors, the interferons, mogamulizumab, brentuximab vedotin, alemtuzumab, and checkpoint inhibitors may achieve responses. Durable responses are not normally observed and patients will typically require multiple sequential therapies with different mechanisms of action to maintain adequate disease control. Allogeneic hematopoietic cell transplant can be curative in select cases.

Introduction

Mycosis fungoides (MF) was first described by the French dermatologist Alibert in 1806. MF and its leukemic variant, Sézary syndrome (SS), are the most common subtypes of cutaneous T-cell lymphoma (CTCL) accounting for around 50% of all cutaneous lymphomas.

Incidence and epidemiology

Greater than 1000 cases of MF/SS are diagnosed in the United States annually. The median age is 55–60 years; however, younger patients may be affected.[1] There is a 2 : 1 male predominance, without racial predilection. The etiology is unknown. Although various exposures including chemicals and viral infections have been proposed as etiologic agents, the current evidence does not support causality.[2,3]

Pathogenesis and natural history

MF may present first in a premycotic phase with nonspecific, slightly scaling skin lesions that wax and wane over time without a clear diagnosis. Later, patches, plaques, tumors, or generalized erythroderma may develop. The disease is often in a "bathing trunk" distribution, with lesions favoring sun-protected sites. Pruritus is a common symptom. Infiltrated plaques may eventually develop into ulcerating or fungating tumors. Infected tumors may lead to sepsis, a common cause of death for patients with CTCL due to inadequate skin barrier protection from pathogens and impaired immune function.[4]

MF is usually indolent but 15–20% of patients develop advanced disease, most commonly cutaneous tumors or erythroderma.[5] Regional nodes are the most common site of extracutaneous disease, but the spleen, liver, lungs, and other organs may be affected. Patients with erythroderma frequently have intense pruritus. Other presentations include folliculotropic,[6] pagetoid reticulosis,[7] granulomatous,[8] and hypopigmented.[9]

Diagnosis and staging

Diagnosis

Histopathology from classic cutaneous patches and plaques typically consists of a superficial perivascular to lichenoid lymphocytic infiltrate containing atypical lymphocytes with hyperchromatic and angulated nuclei that align the dermal–epidermal junction and infiltrate into the overlying epidermis as single cells (epidermotropism) or clusters (so-called Pautrier microabscesses).[10] The majority have a helper T-cell phenotype (CD4+), although cytotoxic/suppressor T-cell phenotype (CD8+) variants may also occur. Immunohistochemistry demonstrating an aberrant loss of T cell antigens such as CD7 and/or CD5 may be helpful in establishing the diagnosis.[11] Clonal T-cell receptor gene rearrangements can often be detected by Southern blot analysis or by methods utilizing polymerase chain reaction (PCR) amplification.[12] These are positive in the majority of skin specimens, although early-stage lesions may demonstrate a polyclonal pattern.[13] Additionally, clonal populations can be found in nonmalignant conditions and should not be used as the sole test for defining malignancy.[14] Newer methods of determining clonality like high-throughput sequencing of the T cell receptor β gene can also be used; tumor clone frequency using these methods may also have prognostic value.[15] Flow cytometry studies of the blood may show expansion of the CD4+CD7− or CD4+CD26− population reflective of circulating atypical lymphocytes of Sézary type.[11,16] PCR methods can also be helpful in determination of blood or lymph node involvement, especially if matching clones are found in these sites and the skin.[17]

Patients may develop cutaneous tumors with large, atypical lymphocytes comprising >25% of the dermal infiltrate. This is referred to as large-cell transformation. These cells often express CD30, have a high proliferation rate, and share a clonal origin with the preexisting MF. These large cells can exhibit variable loss of one or more T-cell-associated antigens.[18] Large-cell transformation can occur at any stage and these patients may have more rapid disease progression requiring earlier initiation of more intensive systemic therapy.

Table 1 Tumor-node-metastasis-blood classification for MF.[a]

Skin (T)	
T1	Limited patches,[b] papules, and/or plaques[c] covering <10% of the skin surface; may further stratify into T1a (patch only) versus T1b (plaque ± patch)
T2	Patches, papules, or plaques covering ≥10% of the skin surface; may further stratify into T2a (patch only) versus T2b (plaque ± patch)
T3	One or more tumors[d] (≥1 cm diameter)
T4	Confluence of erythema covering ≥80% body surface area
Node (N)	
N0	No clinically abnormal lymph nodes[e]; biopsy not required
N1	Clinically abnormal lymph nodes; histopathology Dutch grade 1 or NCI LN0-2
N1a	Clone negative[f]
N1b	Clone positive[f]
N2	Clinically abnormal lymph nodes; histopathology Dutch grade 2 or NCI LN3
N2a	Clone negative[f]
N2b	Clone positive[f]
N3	Clinically abnormal lymph nodes; histopathology Dutch grades 3-4 or NCI LN4; clone positive or negative
NX	Clinically abnormal lymph nodes; no histologic confirmation
Visceral (M)	
M0	No visceral organ involvement
M1	Visceral involvement (must have pathology confirmation[g] and organ involved should be specified)
Blood (B)	
B0	No significant blood involvement: ≤5% of Sézary cells. For clinical trials, B0 may also be defined as <250/microL Sézary cells; CD4+CD26− or CD4+CD7− cells or CD4+CD26− and CD4+CD7− cells <15% by flow cytometry.
B0a	Clone negative
B0b	Clone positive
B1	Low blood tumor burden: does not meet the criteria of B0 or B2
B1a	Clone negative
B1b	Clone positive
B2	High blood tumor burden: positive clone[h] plus one of the following: ≥1000/microL Sézary cells; CD4/CD8 ≥10; CD4+CD7− cells ≥40%; or CD4+CD26− cells ≥30%. For clinical trials, B2 may also be defined as >1000/μL CD4+CD26− or CD4+CD7− cells

[a] Source: Olsen et al.[19]
[b] Patch = any size lesion without significant elevation or induration. Presence/absence of hypo- or hyperpigmentation, scale, crusting, and/or poikiloderma should be noted.
[c] Plaque = any size skin lesion that is elevated or indurated. Presence or absence of scale, crusting, and/or poikiloderma should be noted. Histologic features such as folliculotropism or large-cell transformation (>25% large cells), CD30+ or CD30−, and clinical features such as ulceration are important to document.
[d] Tumor = at least one 1 cm diameter solid or nodular lesion with evidence of depth and/or vertical growth. Note total number of lesions, total volume of lesions, largest size lesion, and region of body involved. Also note if histologic evidence of large-cell transformation has occurred. Phenotyping for CD30 is encouraged.
[e] Abnormal lymph node(s) indicates any lymph node that on physical examination is firm, irregular, clustered, fixed, or 1.5 cm or larger in diameter or on imaging is >1.5 cm in the long axis or >1 cm in the short axis. Node groups examined on physical examination include cervical, supraclavicular, epitrochlear, axillary, and inguinal.
[f] A T cell clone is defined by polymerase chain reaction or Southern blot analysis of the T-cell receptor gene.
[g] For viscera, spleen and liver may be diagnosed by imaging criteria alone.
[h] The clone in the blood should match that of the skin. The relevance of an isolated clone in the blood or a clone in the blood that does not match the clone in the skin remains to be determined.

Table 2 Clinical staging system for MF/SS.[a]

Clinical stage	TNMB classification			
IA	T1	N0	M0	B0 or B1
IB	T2	N0	M0	B0 or B1
IIA	T1 or T2	N1 or N2	M0	B0 or B1
IIB	T3	N0–N2	M0	B0 or B1
IIIA	T4	N0–N2	M0	B0
IIIB	T4	N0–N2	M0	B1
IVA1	T1–T4	N0–N2	M0	B2
IVA2	T1–T4	N3	M0	B0–B2
IVB	T1–T4	N0–N3	M1	B0–B2

[a] Source: Modified from Olsen et al.[19]

Staging and workup

The T (skin), N (node), M (visceral), B (blood) classification and staging system for MF/SS is summarized in Tables 1 and 2.

Patients with limited disease require a thorough physical examination including palpation of lymph nodes, careful mapping of skin lesions, complete blood count, Sezary cell detection by flow cytometry and peripheral blood T-cell gene rearrangement studies (optional for T1 disease), and serum chemistries including lactate dehydrogenase (LDH). If these are within normal limits, additional studies are unnecessary. Patients with generalized disease should undergo CT (computed tomography) or PET/CT (positron emission tomography and computed tomography) imaging. PET is the preferred modality for systemic staging as it is more sensitive than CT for the detection of lymph node involvement.[20] Enlarged nodes may be biopsied but bone marrow is not routinely sampled.

Prognostic factors and biomarkers

Age, T-classification, and overall stage are the most important prognostic factors for survival. In addition to these factors, the presence of large-cell transformation in the skin and elevated LDH has been associated with worse outcomes. Patients with limited patch/plaque (T1; stage IA) disease have an excellent survival, similar to an age-, sex-, and race-matched control population.[21] Median survival is >33 years and <10% progress to a more advanced stage.

Patients with generalized patch/plaque disease without evidence of extracutaneous involvement (T2; stage IB, IIA) have a median survival >11 years.[22] Twenty-four percent develop progressive disease and ~20% die from their disease. Patients with cutaneous tumors (T3; stage IIB) or generalized erythroderma (T4; stage III) without extracutaneous disease have median survivals of 3–5 years and the majority will die from their disease.[21]

Patients with extracutaneous disease in lymph nodes (stage IVA) or viscera (stage IVB) have a median survival of <1.5 years.[23] The presence of Sézary cells in the peripheral blood usually correlates with more advanced T-classification (usually T4) and the presence of extracutaneous disease.

Treatment

MF and SS are treatable but not curable except in rare cases when allotransplantation is employed. The symptoms of the disease have a considerable impact on the quality of life experienced by patients; therefore, the goals of therapy are to control disease burden, improve quality of life, and extend duration of life. The National Comprehensive Cancer Network (NCCN) has established consensus guidelines for the therapy of MF/SS (see https://www.nccn.org for most up-to-date version). Treatment

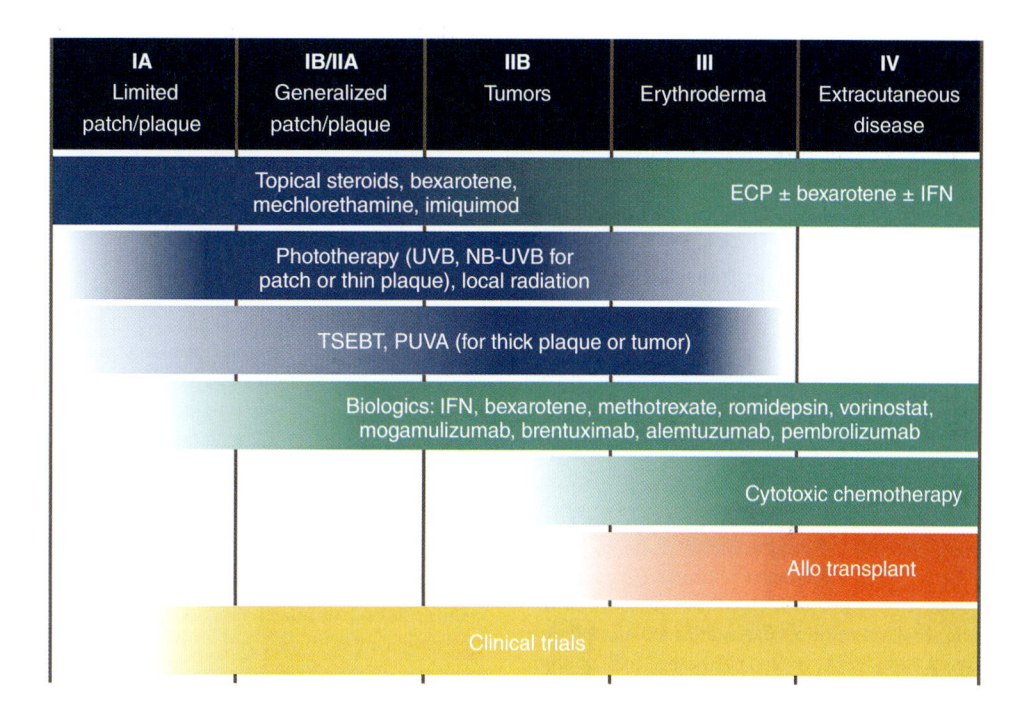

IA Limited patch/plaque	IB/IIA Generalized patch/plaque	IIB Tumors	III Erythroderma	IV Extracutaneous disease
Topical steroids, bexarotene, mechlorethamine, imiquimod			ECP ± bexarotene ± IFN	
Phototherapy (UVB, NB-UVB for patch or thin plaque), local radiation				
TSEBT, PUVA (for thick plaque or tumor)				
	Biologics: IFN, bexarotene, methotrexate, romidepsin, vorinostat, mogamulizumab, brentuximab, alemtuzumab, pembrolizumab			
			Cytotoxic chemotherapy	
				Allo transplant
Clinical trials				

Figure 1 Algorithm for the management of patients with MF/SS.

selection is based on clinical stage (Figure 1). Despite the large number of systemic therapies available for use, few of these have been evaluated in randomized trials and clinical trials are recommended when available and appropriate. Due to the rarity of these diseases and the need for an individualized treatment approach, it is recommended that patients diagnosed with MF/SS be evaluated in a specialized center with expertise in the management of these diseases.

Skin-directed therapies

The majority of patients with early-stage disease are treated with skin-directed therapies with reasonable disease and symptom control. Common skin-directed therapies include topical steroids, chemotherapy (nitrogen mustard), retinoids (bexarotene), immunomodulators (imiquimod), phototherapy, and radiation therapy. Only if skin-directed therapies are exhausted without adequate disease control or if disease progresses to an advanced stage should systemic therapy be considered.

Topical corticosteroids

Topical steroids are the most common treatment for early-stage MF. Detailed instructions on proper application techniques have been previously published. Patients can initially apply a class I steroid, such as clobetasol, twice daily to affected areas. High response rates in both T1 and T2 disease are seen with overall response rates (ORR) at 94% and 82%, respectively.[24] If a response is not seen within 3 months of regular application, an alternate therapy should be considered. Side effects include irritant dermatitis, purpura, skin atrophy, and striae.

Topical chemotherapy

Topical nitrogen mustard (mechlorethamine, HN2) is an effective treatment, especially for T1 or T2 disease. The mechanism of action may be its alkylating agent properties together with immune mechanisms/interaction with the epidermal cell—Langerhans cell—T-cell axis. HN2 may be applied locally or to the entire skin. It may be mixed in water, but most often is in a gel or an ointment base. Topical HN2 is applied at least once daily during the clearing phase. Skin clearance may require 6 months or longer and is followed by maintenance. The gel preparation is available commercially in a concentration of 0.02%.[25]

If response is particularly slow, the concentration of the ointment-based HN2 may be increased or the frequency of application may be increased. The complete response (CR) rate for T1 to T2 disease is ~15% and the partial response (PR) rate is ~50%.[25] The median time to skin clearance is 6–8 months, and response may be maintained for >10 months. Treatment is well tolerated. The primary acute complications include cutaneous hypersensitivity, contact dermatitis, skin irritation, and erythema. There is no systemic absorption and it is safe to use even in children.

Topical retinoids

Bexarotene 1% gel is an retinoid-X receptor (RXR)-selective synthetic retinoid. It is applied thinly to the patches/plaques twice daily. Owing to its irritant effect, it is used to treat only limited areas. Responses are seen in the majority of patients with stage IA to IB disease.[26] The most common toxicity is local irritation, which occurs in most patients. It may be necessary to withhold therapy for a few weeks to assess disease activity. Bexarotene gel is approved for patients with stages IA to IB disease who have refractory or persistent disease after other therapies or who have not tolerated other therapies.

Topical imiquimod

Imiquimod is a nucleoside analog with activity mediated through Toll-like receptor 7 (TLR7) and TLR8.[27] An inflammatory response leads to elevated local levels of IFNα, TNFα, IL-1, and IL-6. CRs have been seen in multi-treatment resistant early-stage disease.[28] Side effects are mild and mainly limited to irritation or pruritis at the application site, thus this agent should be used only on limited, localized areas.

Phototherapy

Phototherapy includes ultraviolet (UV) radiation in the UVA or UVB wavelengths. The long-wave UVA has the advantage over UVB in its greater depth of penetration. For limited disease, UVB alone or home UV phototherapy (UVA + UVB) may be effective.[29] UVB is initiated daily or three times per week with gradual increase in dose. The frequency is gradually reduced during the maintenance period. Narrow-band UVB (nb-UVB) phototherapy is associated with less toxicity than broadband UVB and achieves a CR rate of 54–68% in stage IA–IIA disease with higher response rates in patch stage disease.[30,31] The clinical efficacy of nb-UVB may be superior to broadband UVB.[30]

UVA may be used with a photosensitizing agent, psoralen, as PUVA, referred to as photochemotherapy.[31,32] In the presence of UVA, psoralen intercalates with deoxyribonucleic acid (DNA), forming monofunctional and bifunctional adducts, which inhibit DNA synthesis. This results in cytotoxic and antiproliferative effects and potential immunomodulatory effects. Patients ingest the psoralen (8-methoxypsoralen) followed by controlled exposure to UVA 1–2 h later. Only the eyes are shielded routinely, but other selected areas can be shielded to minimize undesired photodamage. "Shadowed" areas such as the scalp, perineum, axillae, and other skin folds will not receive adequate exposure.

PUVA treatment is initiated three times weekly until skin clearance, then the frequency is decreased. Maintenance therapy is discontinued within a year to minimize risks of cutaneous carcinogenesis. The time to skin clearance is 2–6 months. The CR rate is 62–72% and PR rate 25% in stage IA to IIA disease.[32] The duration of response averages 12 months. PUVA is a primary therapy in stage IA to IIA or a secondary therapy following the failure of other treatments. In patients with SS, PUVA may be supplemented by systemic therapies such as interferon-alpha or systemic retinoids.[33,34]

The primary acute complication of PUVA is a phototoxic reaction, with erythroderma and blistering, occurring in ~20% of patients. Patients should shield their skin and eyes for at least 24 hours following psoralen ingestion. The potential long-term complications of PUVA include cataracts and cutaneous malignancies.

PUVA and nb-UVB have not been directly compared in a prospective manner, but retrospective data suggest that nb-UVB is at least as effective as PUVA but with less toxicity.[31]

Radiation therapy

MF is extremely radiosensitive. Plaques or tumors may be treated with doses of ≥8 Gy with >90% likelihood of local control.[35–38] For unilesional disease, higher doses of 20–24 Gy may be used with curative intent.[35,39,40] Techniques have been developed to treat the entire skin with electrons (total skin electron beam therapy, or TSEBT). Patients are treated while standing in multiple positions at an extended distance. ORR with doses of 30–36 Gy in 4–10 weeks are nearly 100%, with CR rates of 40–98%, depending on the extent of skin involvement.[41] TSEBT is most useful for patients with IB to IIB disease but can be used even in erythrodermic disease, although with a lower response rate. In order to reduce toxicity and duration of therapy and to allow repeat application of TSEBT, low-dose (12 Gy) TSEBT programs have been introduced with an ORR of ~88% and CR rate ~27%.[41] The duration of clinical benefit is shorter with low dose TSEBT when compared to conventional dosing.

The complications of high-dose TSEBT include erythema, desquamation, and temporary epilation. Patients also experience temporary loss of their fingernails and toenails and an impaired ability to sweat for up to 12 months. There is an increased risk of secondary skin malignancy. Patients treated with 12 Gy TSEBT will experience temporary epilation but generally retain their fingernails and toenails, and all other cutaneous effects are much less severe than with high-dose TSEBT programs.

In patients who have lymph node involvement, traditional megavoltage (4–15 MeV) photon irradiation may be used with doses of 30 Gy in 3–4 weeks to achieve local control.[42]

Systemic therapy

In patients with limited-stage disease who continue to have disease progression despite local therapies or in patients who present with advanced-stage disease in which localized therapy is not practical, systemic therapies are generally required for disease control. In the next section, we will discuss systemic therapies used for MF/SS. It is important to note that, given the nonrandomized nature of the vast majority of MF/SS clinical trials in addition to the highly heterogenous patient populations enrolled, it is difficult to compare the efficacy of different systemic treatments. Thus, there is currently no standard approach to the order in which systemic treatments are administered. Only brentuximab vedotin (BV) and mogamulizumab have been evaluated against standard therapies in randomized clinical trials. Bexarotene, vorinostat, romidepsin, mogamulizumab, BV, and extracorporeal photopheresis are the only agents approved by the US Food and Drug Administration (FDA) for MF/SS, all other systemic agents discussed would be considered off label use.

In general, systemic therapies with lower toxicity that can be used for longer periods of time (interferon, bexarotene, extracorporeal photopheresis) are used before systemic therapies with more cumulative toxicity or risk of immunosuppression [histone deacetylase (HDAC) inhibitors, mogamulizumab, BV, pralatrexate, alemtuzumab, pembrolizumab, lenalidomide, cytotoxic chemotherapy, allogeneic stem cell transplant]. It should also be noted that responses to certain agents can be disparate between compartments (blood, skin, lymph nodes, viscera); for example, mogamulizumab has a high response rate in blood (68%), but almost no response in visceral disease.[43] Predictive biomarkers correlating with response to available treatments would be extremely valuable but are lacking at the present time.

Systemic biologic therapies

Interferon

Interferon-α (IFN-α) is a subcutaneously administered cytokine with a number of pleiotropic effects including direct CTCL cytostatic effects, promotion of cell-mediated toxicity by T-cells and NK cells, and suppression of Th2 interleukins IL-4, IL-5, and IL-10. Recommendations on clinical dosing have been previously published.[44] Side effects include flu-type symptoms such as fever, chills, body aches which are typically short term while other side effects such as mood changes, depression, and cognitive disturbances can be persistent and may require cessation of therapy. IFN-α may be used alone, but more often with other topical or systemic therapies. Reported ORRs when used as monotherapy are 53–74%, with CR rates of 21–35%.[33,45] The response rate and duration appear better when combined with phototherapy.[33]

Bexarotene

Systemic retinoid therapy with bexarotene can be effective and may be combined with PUVA (Re-PUVA), IFN-α, or TSEBT.[46] The response rate is 45–55% (10–20% CR).[34,47,48] Bexarotene is typically initially dosed at 150 mg daily and dose adjusted based on clinical response and toxicity to a maximum of 300 mg/m² daily (off label dosing). The most common complications include central hypothyroidism requiring levothyroxine and hypertriglyceridemia requiring lipid-lowering medications and frequent lab monitoring. Other side effects include photosensitivity, xerosis, myalgia, arthralgia, headaches, and possible teratogenic effects. Toxicities are normally reversible after cessation of therapy. Other retinoids with activity in CTCL include acitretin and isotretinoin.

Histone deacetylase inhibitors
Two HDAC inhibitors, vorinostat and romidepsin, have been approved for use by the FDA in MF/SS. Vorinostat, an oral agent that inhibits HDAC class I and II enzymes, has an ORR rate of 24–30% but only rare CRs.[49] The median time to response is 12 weeks, and the median duration of response is 15–26 weeks. Vorinostat is effective in relieving pruritus which can significantly improve the quality of life for patients. The most common side effects include fatigue, diarrhea, nausea, anorexia, dysgeusia, and thrombocytopenia.

Romidepsin, an intravenously administered HDAC class I inhibitor, is associated with an ORR of 34%. A clinically meaningful improvement in pruritus is observed in 43% of patients, including patients who do not achieve an objective response.[50] The primary adverse effects include nausea, vomiting, fatigue, thrombocytopenia, and granulocytopenia with treatment discontinuation the highest after the first cycle of treatment. Patients should be monitored for QTc prolongation while on romidepsin, particularly when used concomitantly with antiemetics that can also prolong QTc.

Moagmulizumab
Mogamulizumab targets the C-C chemokine receptor 4 (CCR4) resulting in direct antibody-dependent CTCL cytotoxicity in addition to promoting a more favorable immune microenvironment by depletion of regulatory T-cells.[51] The MAVORIC study was a randomized phase III study comparing mogamulizumab to vorinostat showing a significant prolonged median PFS of 7.7 months vs 3.1 months in favor of mogamulizumab.[43] Of note, the response rate in various compartments varied significantly with the highest response rate noted in the blood (68%), followed by skin (42%), and lymph nodes (17%), but no responses in visceral disease. The trial led to FDA approval of mogamulizumab for relapsed/refractory MF/SS after failure of one prior systemic therapy. The most common adverse events with mogamulizumab include infusion reactions, cutaneous reactions, diarrhea, and fatigue.

Brentuximab vedotin
BV is an anti-CD30-monomethyl auristatin E antitubulin conjugate with potent and selective antitumor activity against CD30 positive malignancies. Its efficacy in CD30+ MF has been demonstrated in the randomized phase III ALCANZA trial.[52] In this trial, BV was compared to investigator's choice of either oral methotrexate or bexarotene in patients with previously treated MF or primary cutaneous anaplastic large-cell lymphoma. At a median follow-up of 23 months, an objective global response lasting at least 4 months (ORR4) was 56.3% with BV versus 12.5% with physician's choice. Of note, SS was excluded from this trial and CD30 positivity was defined as ≥10% malignant cells positive. Prior studies showed that even negligible CD30 expression can result in responses, although with a lower likelihood.[53] The most common adverse events related to BV are peripheral neuropathy, fatigue, nausea, alopecia, and neutropenia.

Alemtuzumab
Alemtuzumab, a humanized monoclonal antibody directed against CD52, has an overall response rate of 38–85%.[54] Low dose schedules have been developed to reduce the risk of serious infectious complications and other toxicities.[55,56] Alemtuzumab is particularly effective in reducing the peripheral blood Sézary count in patients with SS. In addition to serious infectious complications, alemtuzumab may cause infusion reactions, autoimmune reactions, cytopenias, and increased risk of secondary malignancies. Alemtuzumab is no longer commercially available and can only be obtained for compassionate use under a Risk Evaluation Mitigation Strategy (REMS) Program.

Pembrolizumab
Pembrolizumab has an ORR and CRR of 38% and 8% in a phase II single-arm study of 24 patients with heavily pretreated MF/SS.[57] Of responding patients, 88% were still on treatment at a median follow-up of 58 weeks suggesting pembrolizumab may provide durable responses in certain patients, but further follow-up is needed. A transient increase in erythroderma and pruritus occurred in 53% of patients, exclusively in those with SS, but did not result in treatment discontinuation in any patient. Immune-related side effects resulting in discontinuation were seen in 17% of patients.

Lenalidomide
Lenalidomide is an oral immunomodulatory drug with an ORR of 28% in MF/SS.[58] Primary complications included fatigue, infection, and leukopenia.

Extracorporeal photopheresis
Photopheresis [extracorporeal photopheresis (ECP)] is a method of delivering PUVA systemically using an extracorporeal technique. The patient's white blood cells are collected via leukapheresis, exposed to a photoactivating drug (8-methoxypsoralen, Uvadex), and then irradiated with UVA. The irradiated cells are then returned to the patient intravenously. The mechanism of action of photopheresis remains unclear but may be related to tumor antigens released from apoptotic Sézary cells subsequently being processed by peripheral dendritic cells leading to the augmentation of systemic antitumor responses.[59] The treatment is most effective for patients with blood involvement (SS). Response rates are 69–83%[60] and may be higher when combined with biologic agents such as interferons or retinoids or skin-directed therapies such as topical steroids, topical nitrogen mustard, or TSEBT.[61] ECP has minimal adverse effects. Some patients may experience nausea, mostly due to the ingested psoralen, and some have a transient low-grade fever or slight malaise after treatment. There are no reports of significant organ damage or bone marrow or immune suppression.

Systemic cytotoxic chemotherapy

Systemic chemotherapy is appropriate for patients with extracutaneous, advanced, or refractory disease who have progressed through more effective and better-tolerated biologic therapies. Virtually, all drugs effective in other lymphomas have been tested in MF/SS. Unfortunately, they often result in only temporary palliative responses. In a retrospective study of 198 patients with MF/SS receiving systemic therapy, the time to next therapy was only 3.9 months, and there were few durable remissions.[62] Additionally, the use of chemotherapy as first-line treatment has been associated with an increased risk of death.[63] It is expected that only a minority of patients with MF (10–20%) will require systemic cytotoxic chemotherapy. When used, single-agent cytotoxic chemotherapy should generally be used over combination therapy. Combined chemotherapy and TSEBT were once considered a preferred treatment. However, a prospective randomized trial at the NCI failed to show an improvement compared to sequential conservative therapies.[64]

In 526 patients reported in single-agent chemotherapy trials, the response rates were 20–80% and the median duration of responses was 3–22 months.[65] Single agents include the antifolates methotrexate and pralatrexate, gemcitabine, pegylated liposomal doxorubicin, chlorambucil, the purine analogs pentostatin, cladribine, and fludarabine, temozolomide, and bortezomib. Of these agents, gemcitabine and liposomal doxorubicin are most commonly used in advanced stages, and low dose oral methotrexate (5–50 mg weekly) can be used in early stages of disease.

The largest experience with combination chemotherapy is with cyclophosphamide, vincristine, and prednisone with or without doxorubicin (CHOP).[66] CR rates are generally about 25% and response duration 3–20 months. Given the higher risk of toxicity without significant improvement in efficacy using combination chemotherapy, sequential single-agent therapy is often recommended.

Hematopoietic stem cell transplant (HSCT)

Although autologous transplantation has been used successfully in many lymphomas, this has not been the case for MF/SS. The responses are short lived, with a median time to progression <3 months, thus it is not recommended for patients with MF/SS.[67] Allogeneic transplantation, on the other hand, is more effective presumably because of an allogeneic graft-versus-tumor effect. Eligibility and preparatory regimens have varied. Early reports of patients who received allografts from human leukocyte antigen (HLA)-matched siblings following myeloablative therapy suggested that complete and sustained remissions could be achieved and that the presence of mild graft versus host disease (GVHD) suggested a possible graft versus lymphoma effect.[68]

These results for allogeneic transplant are encouraging, but it has limited applicability owing to transplant-related morbidity and mortality, especially in older patients. Nonmyeloablative approaches with reduced-intensity conditioning regimens are effective and less toxic than myeloablative regimens.[67] International registries report PFS as high as 54% at 3 years.[69] Recent systematic reviews and meta-analyses showed pooled OS and PFS rates of 59% and 36% respectively with a pooled nonrelapse mortality rate of 19%.[70] A novel approach combining TSEBT, total lymphoid irradiation, and antithymocyte globulin as a nonablative preparatory regimen seems to have a lower risk for GVHD. In a series of 35 patients with MF/SS transplanted using this regimen, the incidence of grade II to IV GVHD was 16% and the 2-year OS was 68%.[71]

It appears that allogeneic HSCT (especially with reduced-intensity conditioning regimens) may result in durable long-term remissions. Larger prospective studies will be required to identify the optimal timing of transplant and the best conditioning regimen. With numerous biological agents showing promising activity and tolerability, there may also be a role for maintenance therapy.

Conclusions

MF/SS is a challenging disease. It has a variety of clinical presentations and although often pursues an indolent course, in many patients, it has an aggressive behavior. It responds to topical therapies and systemic biologic treatments, but chemotherapy plays only a minor role in its management. Allogeneic stem cell transplantation may be a curative treatment in selected patients. Patients with multiply relapsing disease should be strongly encouraged to enroll in clinical trials with novel agents.

Key references

The complete reference list can be found on Vital Source version of this title, see inside front cover.

2 Bunn PA, Schechter GP, Jaffe E, et al. Clinical course of retrovirus-associated adult T-cell lymphoma in the United States. *N Engl J Med*. 1983;**309**(5):257–264.

3 Wood GS, Salvekar A, Schaffer J, et al. Evidence against a role for human T-cell lymphotrophic virus type I (HTLV-I) in the pathogenesis of american cutaneous T-cell lymphoma. *J Investig Dermatol*. 1996;**107**(3):301–307.

5 Kim YH, Liu HL, Mraz-Gernhard S, et al. Long-term outcome of 525 patients with mycosis fungoides and sézary syndrome. *Arch Dermatol*. 2003;**139**(7):857.

6 van Doorn R, Scheffer E, Willemze R. Follicular mycosis fungoides, a distinct disease entity with or without associated follicular mucinosis. *Arch Dermatol*. 2002;**138**(2):191.

7 Lee J, Viakhireva N, Cesca C, et al. Clinicopathologic features and treatment outcomes in Woringer–Kolopp disease. *J Am Acad Dermatol*. 2008;**59**(4):706–712.

8 LeBoit PE. Granulomatous slack skin. *Dermatol Clin*. 1994;**12**(2):375–389.

10 Willemze R, Cerroni L, Kempf W, et al. The 2018 update of the WHO-EORTC classification for primary cutaneous lymphomas. *Blood*. 2019;**133**(16):1703–1714.

14 Delfau-Larue MH, Laroche L, Wechsler J, et al. Diagnostic value of dominant T-cell clones in peripheral blood in 363 patients presenting consecutively with a clinical suspicion of cutaneous lymphoma. *Blood*. 2000;**96**(9):2987–2992.

16 Vonderheid EC, Hou JS. CD4(+)CD26(−) lymphocytes are useful to assess blood involvement and define B ratings in cutaneous T cell lymphoma. *Leuk Lymphoma*. 2018;**59**(2):330–339.

17 Thurber SE, Zhang B, Kim YH, et al. T-cell clonality analysis in biopsy specimens from two different skin sites shows high specificity in the diagnosis of patients with suggested mycosis fungoides. *J Am Acad Dermatol*. 2007;**57**(5):782–790.

22 Kim YH, Chow S, Varghese A, Hoppe RT. Clinical characteristics and long-term outcome of patients with generalized patch and/or plaque (T2) mycosis fungoides. *Arch Dermatol*. 1999;**135**(1):26.

23 de Coninck EC, Kim YH, Varghese A, Hoppe RT. Clinical characteristics and outcome of patients with extracutaneous mycosis fungoides. *J Clin Oncol*. 2001;**19**(3):779–784.

24 Zackheim HS, Kashani-Sabet M, Amin S. Topical corticosteroids for mycosis fungoides. Experience in 79 patients. *Arch Dermatol*. 1998;**134**(8):949–954.

28 Lewis DJ, Byekova YA, Emge DA, Duvic M. Complete resolution of mycosis fungoides tumors with imiquimod 5% cream: a case series. *J Dermatol Treat*. 2017;**28**(6):567–569.

30 Boztepe G, Sahin S, Ayhan M, et al. Narrowband ultraviolet B phototherapy to clear and maintain clearance in patients with mycosis fungoides. *J Am Acad Dermatol*. 2005;**53**(2):242–246.

32 Vieyra-Garcia P, Fink-Puches R, Porkert S, et al. Evaluation of low-dose, low-frequency oral psoralen-UV-A treatment with or without maintenance on early-stage mycosis fungoides: a randomized clinical trial. *JAMA Dermatol*. 2019;**155**(5):538–547.

33 Kuzel TM, Roenigk HH, Samuelson E, et al. Effectiveness of interferon alfa-2a combined with phototherapy for mycosis fungoides and the Sézary syndrome. *J Clin Oncol*. 1995;**13**(1):257–263.

34 Thomsen K, Hammar H, Molin L, Volden G. Retinoids plus PUVA (RePUVA) and PUVA in mycosis fungoides, plaque stage. a report from the Scandinavian Mycosis Fungoides Group. *Acta Derm Venereol*. 1989;**69**(6):536–538.

36 Thomas TO, Agrawal P, Guitart J, et al. Outcome of patients treated with a single-fraction dose of palliative radiation for cutaneous T-cell lymphoma. *Int J Radiat Oncol Biol Phys*. 2013;**85**(3):747–753.

37 Piccinno R, Caccialanza M, Cuka E, Recalcati S. Localized conventional radiotherapy in the treatment of Mycosis Fungoides: our experience in 100 patients. *J Eur Acad Dermatol Venereol*. 2014;**28**(8):1040–1044.

38 Neelis KJ, Schimmel EC, Vermeer MH, et al. Low-dose palliative radiotherapy for cutaneous B- and T-cell lymphomas. *Int J Radiat Oncol Biol Phys*. 2009;**74**(1):154–158.

39 Micaily B, Miyamoto C, Kantor G, et al. Radiotherapy for unilesional mycosis fungoides. *Int J Radiat Oncol Biol Phys*. 1998;**42**(2):361–364.

40 Wilson LD, Kacinski BM, Jones GW. Local superficial radiotherapy in the management of minimal stage IA cutaneous T-cell lymphoma (Mycosis Fungoides). *Int J Radiat Oncol Biol Phys*. 1998;**40**(1):109–115.

45. Chiarion-Sileni V, Bononi A, Fornasa CV, et al. Phase II trial of interferon-alpha;-2a plus psolaren with ultraviolet light A in patients with cutaneous T-cell lymphoma. *Cancer*. 2002;**95**(3):569–575.
47. Duvic M, Hymes K, Heald P, et al. Bexarotene is effective and safe for treatment of refractory advanced-stage cutaneous T-cell lymphoma: multinational phase II-III trial results. *J Clin Oncol*. 2001;**19**(9):2456–2471.
48. McGinnis KS, Junkins-Hopkins JM, Crawford G, et al. Low-dose oral bexarotene in combination with low-dose interferon alfa in the treatment of cutaneous T-cell lymphoma: clinical synergism and possible immunologic mechanisms. *J Am Acad Dermatol*. 2004;**50**(3):375–379.
51. Ni X, Langridge T, Duvic M. Depletion of regulatory T cells by targeting CC chemokine receptor type 4 with mogamulizumab. *Oncoimmunology*. 2015;**4**(7):e1011524.
56. Querfeld C, Mehta N, Rosen ST, et al. Alemtuzumab for relapsed and refractory erythrodermic cutaneous T-cell lymphoma: a single institution experience from the Robert H. Lurie Comprehensive Cancer Center. *Leuk Lymphoma*. 2009;**50**(12):1969–1976.
59. Edelson RL. Cutaneous T cell lymphoma: the helping hand of dendritic cells. *Ann N Y Acad Sci*. 2001;**941**:1–11.
61. Horwitz SM, Olsen EA, Duvic M, et al. Review of the treatment of mycosis fungoides and sézary syndrome: a stage-based approach. *J Natl Compr Cancer Netw*. 2008;**6**(4):436–442.
67. Duarte RF, Schmitz N, Servitje O, Sureda A. Haematopoietic stem cell transplantation for patients with primary cutaneous T-cell lymphoma. *Bone Marrow Transplant*. 2008;**41**(7):597–604.
69. Duarte RF, Canals C, Onida F, et al. Allogeneic hematopoietic cell transplantation for patients with mycosis fungoides and Sezary syndrome: a retrospective analysis of the Lymphoma Working Party of the European Group for Blood and Marrow Transplantation. *J Clin Oncol*. 2010;**28**(29):4492–4499.

119 Plasma cell disorders

Andrew J. Yee, MD ■ Teru Hideshima, MD, PhD ■ Noopur Raje, MD ■ Kenneth C. Anderson, MD

Overview

Plasma cell disorders have in common a proliferation of monoclonal plasma cells associated with the production of a monoclonal protein. These disorders range from the common, indolent condition of monoclonal gammopathy of undetermined significance to malignancies such as multiple myeloma characterized by the presence of hypercalcemia, anemia, renal dysfunction, and/or lytic bone lesions. Progress in the understanding of the molecular underpinnings of myeloma has led to remarkable advances in its treatment. High-dose melphalan and autologous stem cell transplant have been a mainstay of treatment. Now, highly effective and well-tolerated drug classes such as the proteasome inhibitors (e.g., bortezomib, carfilzomib), immunomodulatory drugs (e.g., lenalidomide, pomalidomide), and anti-CD38 monoclonal antibodies (e.g., daratumumab, isatuximab) have rapidly transformed treatment and significantly improved overall survival. Newer therapies targeting B-cell maturation antigen (BCMA) have the potential to further improve outcomes.

Multiple myeloma

Multiple myeloma (MM) is a malignant proliferation of plasma cells in the bone marrow (BM) characterized by the presence in the serum and/or urine of a monoclonal immunoglobulin or light chain.[1] This disease has probably been recognized since 1845, when the first patient presented with bone pain and heat soluble "animal matter" in urine.[2,3] The term MM was coined in 1873, reflecting distinct sites of BM involvement. The plasma cell was later discovered in 1890, and MM associated with plasmacytosis shortly thereafter in 1900. The application of electrophoresis in 1939 and immunoelectrophoresis in 1953 allowed for the identification of the monotypic immunoglobulin characteristic of MM.[4,5]

Diagnostic criteria

Active MM is both a clinical and a pathological diagnosis that has traditionally been defined by the presence of a monoclonal protein in the serum and/or urine; ≥10% monoclonal plasma cells in the BM; and hypercalcemia, renal dysfunction, anemia, and/or bone disease (also known as the "CRAB" criteria, see Figure 1 and Table 1).[6] Active MM needs to be distinguished from other disorders characterized by monoclonal gammopathy, both malignant and otherwise, in particular monoclonal gammopathy of undetermined significance (MGUS) and smoldering MM (see below). Other conditions associated with a monoclonal protein include, for example, AL amyloidosis, Waldenström macroglobulinemia, and lymphoma. Smoldering multiple myeloma is defined by the presence of a monoclonal protein ≥3 g/dL and/or ≥10% plasma cells in the bone marrow and the absence of end organ involvement. In 2014, the International Myeloma Working Group (IMWG) introduced myeloma-defining biomarkers to the definition of symptomatic myeloma, where the following conditions upstage the diagnosis to active disease, even in the absence of CRAB features: ≥60% marrow infiltration with plasma cells; an involved/uninvolved serum free light chain ratio of ≥100; or >1 focal lesion on an MRI.[7]

Imaging to assess for bone involvement plays an increasingly important role in differentiating MM from other plasma cell disorders. Imaging with CT and MRI is significantly more sensitive than conventional skeletal survey for detecting lytic bone lesions. In one study, low-dose whole-body CT (LDWBCT) detected lytic lesions that were not visualized on conventional skeletal survey in 22.5% of SMM and MM patients.[8] In recent IMWG guidelines, LDWBCT, where available, is now recommended over the conventional skeletal survey as the screening modality in plasma cell disorders.[9] Whole-body MRI or spine and pelvis MRI are also incorporated in these imaging guidelines, for example, when evaluating patients with smoldering MM.

Epidemiology

MM is the second most common hematologic malignancy, accounting for 32,270 new cases in the United States in 2020 and 2% of cancer-related deaths.[10] In the SEER database, the median age of diagnosis is 69 years, and the incidence in African–Americans is twice that in Caucasians; in African–Americans, it is the most common hematologic malignancy.[11,12] Monoclonal gammopathy of undetermined significance is a precursor condition to MM, and MGUS nearly always precedes the onset of MM.[13,14] Risk factors for development of MGUS and/or MM include obesity,[15] Agent Orange exposure,[16] and exposure to the World Trade Center disaster among firefighters.[17] Chronic antigen exposure, as in the case of lysolipids and Gaucher's disease or chronic infections, has also been postulated.[18,19]

Occupational exposures and risk of MM have shown variable levels of risk, with a stronger association for farming than for radiation or benzene.[20,21] There also can be an inherited predisposition to MM.[22] A study of the Swedish Family-Cancer Database found that the standardized incidence ratio of MM among first-degree relatives for MM was 2.13.[23]

Clinical features

The presenting features of 1027 cases of newly diagnosed MM evaluated from 1985 to 1998 at the Mayo Clinic are summarized

---

Holland-Frei Cancer Medicine, Tenth Edition. Edited by Robert C. Bast, John C. Byrd, Carlo M. Croce, Ernest Hawk, Fadlo R. Khuri, Raphael E. Pollock, Apostolia M. Tsimberidou, Christopher G. Willett, and Cheryl L. Willman.
© 2023 John Wiley & Sons, Inc. Published 2023 by John Wiley & Sons, Inc.

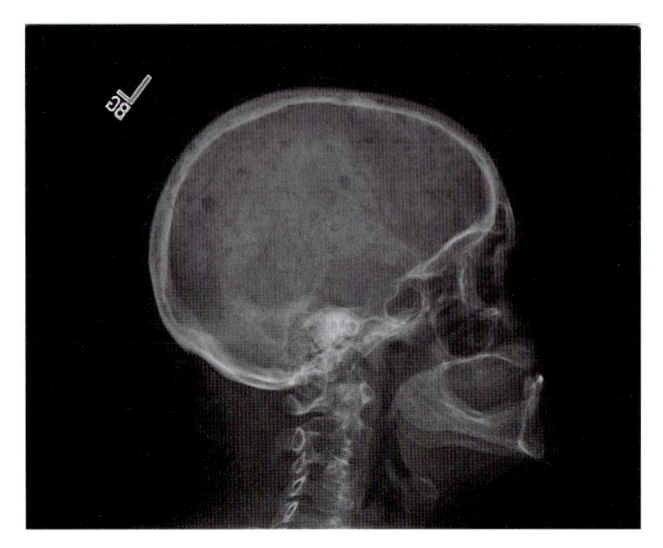

Figure 1 Characteristic lytic bone lesions in multiple myeloma. Note this is the same skull film as the previous edition.

Table 1 Classification of monoclonal gammopathies.[a]

Monoclonal gammopathy of undetermined significance
Non-IgM MGUS
- Serum monoclonal protein <3 g/dL and
- Clonal bone marrow plasma cells <10% and
- Absence of end-organ damage (CRAB criteria) or amyloidosis

Progression to multiple myeloma, solitary plasmacytoma, or AL amyloidosis: 1%/year
IgM MGUS
- Serum IgM monoclonal protein <3 g/dL and
- Bone marrow lymphoplasmacytic infiltration <10% and
- No evidence of anemia, constitutional symptoms, hyperviscosity, lymphadenopathy, hepatosplenomegaly, or other end-organ damage that can be attributed to the underlying lymphoproliferative disorder

Progression to Waldenström macroglobulinemia or AL amyloidosis: 1.5%/year
Light-chain monoclonal gammopathy of undetermined significance
- Abnormal free light chain ratio with elevation in involved free light chain and
- Negative immunofixation for immunoglobulin heavy chain and
- Absence of end-organ damage (CRAB criteria) or amyloidosis

Progression to light chain multiple myeloma or AL amyloidosis: 0.3%/year
Smoldering multiple myeloma
- Serum monoclonal protein (IgG or IgA) ≥3 g/dL or 24 h urine monoclonal protein ≥500 mg and/or clonal bone marrow plasma cells 10–60% and
- No myeloma defining events (see below) or amyloidosis

Multiple myeloma
- Clonal bone marrow plasma cells ≥10% or biopsy-proven plasmacytoma and
- Myeloma defining event:
  o End-organ damage (CRAB criteria) or
  o Biomarker of malignancy (one or more of the following):
    ▪ Clonal bone marrow plasma cell percentage ≥60% or
    ▪ Involved/uninvolved free chain ratio ≥100 (with involved free light chain ≥100 mg/L or
    ▪ >1 focal lesion on MRI (≥5 mm)

End-organ damage (CRAB criteria) includes:
- Hypercalcemia: calcium >1 mg/dL higher than the upper limit of normal or >11 mg/dL or
- Renal insufficiency: creatinine clearance <40 mL/min or creatinine >2 mg/dL or
- Anemia: hemoglobin >2 g/dL below the lower limit of normal or hemoglobin <10 g/dL or
- Bone lesions: one or more osteolytic lesions on skeletal radiography or CT

[a]Source: Adapted from Rajkumar et al.[6]

Table 2 Presenting features of multiple myeloma.[a]

Presenting feature	
Anemia (hemoglobin ≤12 g/dL)	73%
Calcium ≥11 mg/dL	13%
Creatinine ≥2 g/dL	19%
Radiographic abnormality (on plain film)[b]	79%
Bone pain	58%
Fatigue	32%
Weight loss	24%

[a]Source: Adapted from Kyle et al.[24]
[b]Lytic lesions are present in 67% of patients. Other abnormalities include osteoporosis, compression fractures, pathologic fractures.

in Table 2.[24] Anemia (73%) and bone pain (58%) are the most common presenting sign and symptom. Laboratory evaluation typically consists of serum protein electrophoresis and immunofixation, urine protein electrophoresis and immunofixation, and serum free light chains. The SPEP by itself can detect a monoclonal protein in the 0.05 g/dL range.[25] The immunofixation of the serum is used to identify the heavy and light chain of the monoclonal protein and increases the sensitivity for detecting a monoclonal protein. Of note, monoclonal proteins can also be detected in conditions beyond plasma cell disorders, such as B cell lymphoproliferative conditions. The serum free light chain assay was introduced in the early 2000s and is particularly valuable in identifying the 16% of MM that only produces a light chain (Bence Jones protein). This assay decreases the reliance on the conventional 24 h urine collection for protein electrophoresis that was traditionally used to identify light chain only myeloma cases.[24,26] Moreover, the serum free light chain assay can measure disease in patients who were previously classified as "nonsecretory" disease by traditional serum and urine studies. In one study, elevated serum free light chain was found in 19 of 28 patients with nonsecretory multiple myeloma.[27] Overall, the combination of serum protein electrophoresis, immunofixation, and serum free light chain assay has a sensitivity of 100% for detecting multiple myeloma.[28] Instead of electrophoresis, mass spectrometry is now emerging as another way to measure monoclonal proteins that is more sensitive.[29] These parameters such as SPEP and serum free light chains are followed over the course of treatment, to assess for response. The IMWG has defined criteria for response assessment (Table 3).[30,31]

In the Mayo Clinic series, the conventional skeletal survey showed abnormalities in 79% of patients, with lytic lesions in 67% and osteoporosis in 23% of patients.[24] With more sensitive imaging modalities, an even higher percentage of patients show bone involvement. In the IMAJEM substudy of newly diagnosed patients enrolled in the IFM 2009 trial, the MRI (spine and pelvis) or PET CT were abnormal in 95% and 91% of patients, respectively.[32]

Historically, infection and renal failure account for 52% and 21% of deaths, respectively, in patients with MM.[33] This continues to be true when a more recent cohort of patients was evaluated. In this more recent cohort, second primary malignancy related to melphalan exposure accounted for 3.5% of causes of death.[34]

Biology

Cell surface phenotype

B-cell-restricted and associated antigens have been utilized to delineate stages of normal and malignant B-cell differentiation.[35] Antigenic profiles are useful not only to identify stages of malignant B-cell differentiation but also to categorize B-cell tumors. MM cells

Table 3 Uniform response criteria from the International Myeloma Working Group.[a]

Response subcategory	Response criteria
CR	Negative immunofixation of the serum and urine and disappearance of any soft-tissue plasmacytomas and <5% plasma cells in marrow
sCR	CR as defined above plus Normal FLC ratio and Absence of clonal cells in marrow by immunohistochemistry or immunofluorescence[b]
VGPR	Serum and urine M-protein detectable by immunofixation but not on electrophoresis or ≥90% reduction in serum M-protein plus urine M-protein <100 mg per 24 h
PR	≥50% reduction of serum M-protein and reduction in 24-h urinary M-protein by ≥90% or to <200 mg per 24 h If the serum and urine M-protein are unmeasurable, ≥50% decrease in the difference between involved and uninvolved FLC levels is required in place of the M-protein criteria If serum and urine M-protein are unmeasurable, and serum free light assay is also unmeasurable, ≥50% reduction in plasma cells is required in place of M-protein, provided baseline marrow plasma cell percentage was ≥30% In addition to the above-listed criteria, if present at baseline, a ≥50% reduction in the size of soft-tissue plasmacytomas is also required
SD	Not meeting criteria for CR, VGPR, PR, or progressive disease

Abbreviations: CR, complete response; FLC, free light chain; PR, partial response; sCR, stringent complete response; SD, stable disease; VGPR, very good partial response; M-protein, monoclonal protein.
[a]Source: Adapted from Rajkumar et al.[30] and Kumar et al.[31]
[b]Presence/absence of clonal cells is based upon the κ/λ of >4:1 or <1:2. An abnormal κ/λ ratio by immunohistochemistry and/or immunofluorescence requires a minimum of 100 plasma cells for analysis.

share cell surface expression of some antigens, for example, CD38 and PCA-1 (plasma cell-associated antigen-1), which are also present on normal plasma cells, suggesting that the normal cellular counterpart of MM is the normal plasma cell. However, a number of other antigens to date have been described on the surface of MM cells, which in some cases react with B-cells at stages of differentiation earlier than the plasma cell, but also react with non-B cells.[36–41] Harada and colleagues have shown that normal plasma cells are CD19+CD56−, whereas MM cells generally do not have this phenotype.[42] The core protein of MUC-1 antigen is expressed on MM cells[43] and its inhibition triggers MM cell death.[44]

Cellular origin of MM

The cells that accumulate in the bone marrow of patients with MM have plasma cell or plasmablast morphology. However, it has been known since the 1970s, based on studies using anti-idiotypic antibodies, that unique idiotypic determinants can identify clones of peripheral blood lymphocytes in patients with macroglobulinemia, MM, MGUS, and chronic lymphocytic leukemia.[45] The presence of idiotypic determinants on cytoplasmic μ-containing pre-B cells in MM bone marrow provided further evidence that the oncogenic event may occur at the pre-B-cell stage. However, monoclonal B lineage cells in peripheral blood of MM patients, which are late-stage B cells (low CD19 and CD20, moderate CALLA and PCA-1, with strong CD45RO antigen expression) are continuously progressing toward the plasma cell stage.[39] It remains unclear as to which cell within the malignant clone is "clonogenic" and capable of self-renewal. Some evidence suggests that pre-B and naive B cells migrate from the BM to the lymph node (LN) where antigen recognition, selection, and somatic hypermutation occur. The memory B-cell compartment is thought to contain the cytoplasmic μ-positive precursor cell of MM, which then undergoes Ig class switching in the LN.[46] Ig variable (VH) gene sequence analysis has shown MM tumor cells to be postfollicular, with the mutated homogeneous clonal sequences indicating no continuing exposure to somatic hypermutation mechanism.[47] VH gene analysis of IgM MM indicates an origin from a memory cell undergoing isotype switch events.[48] Mutated heterogeneous sequences in MGUS suggest that tumor cells remain under the influence of the mutator.[49] Abnormalities of 14q (the location of IgH) are most common in MM. Since proto-oncogenes are translocated to this region and overexpressed in B cell malignancies including follicular lymphoma, Burkitt's lymphoma, and chronic lymphocytic leukemia, they may also play a role in the oncogenesis of MM. In addition, translocations involving switch regions indicate that the final oncogenic molecular event in MM occurs late in B-cell ontogeny.[49] More recently, CD138− cells with a memory B cell phenotype are thought to be the clonogenic MM "stem" cells, although this concept needs further validation.[50]

Role of adhesion molecules, cytokines, and BM stromal cells in MM

Laboratory and animal models of MM in the BM microenvironment have shown how tumor cell interactions with extracellular matrix proteins, cytokines, and accessory cells promote MM cell growth, survival, and drug resistance as well as confer immunosuppression. For example, adhesion molecules mediate both homotypic and heterotypic adhesion of tumor cells to either extracellular matrix (ECM) proteins or BM stromal cells (BMSCs) that are characterized as progenitors of skeletal tissue components such as bone, cartilage, the hematopoiesis-supporting stroma, and adipocytes (Figure 2).[51,52] Moreover, they play a critical role in pathogenesis of disease progression. After class switching in the LN, adhesion molecules such as CD44, VLA-4 (very late antigen-4), VLA-5, LFA-1 (leukocyte function-associated antigen-1), CD56, syndecan-1 (CD138), and MPC-1 (mitochondrial pyruvate carrier 1) mediate homing of MM cells to the BM.[51,53–56] Subsequently, MM cells bind to BMSCs and localize tumor cells in the BM microenvironment. This interaction stimulates interleukin-6 (IL-6) transcription and secretion from BMSCs with related paracrine growth of MM cells.[57–59] Other factors such as CD40 found on tumor cells also induces IL-6 transcription and secretion, with related autocrine MM cell growth.[60] TNF-α upregulates IL-6 secretion from BMSCs as well as adhesion molecules on MM cells and BMSCs, thereby promoting and increasing binding and cell adhesion-mediated drug resistance (CAM-DR), respectively.[61] Syndecan-1 is a multifunctional regulator of MM cell growth and survival as well as of bone cell differentiation, and elevated serum syndecan-1 correlates with increased tumor cell burden, decreased metalloproteinase-9 activity, and poor prognosis.[62–64]

As the disease progresses, the development of plasma cell leukemia (PCL) is characterized by decreased expression of certain adhesion molecules (e.g., CD56, VLA-5, MPC-1, and syndecan-1), which in turn facilitates tumor cell mobilization. Furthermore, the acquisition of other adhesion molecules on PCL cells, such as CD11b, CD44, and RHAMM (Receptor for HA Mediated Motility), assists transit through endothelium during egress from the BM. Extramedullary spread of MM cells is facilitated by the reappearance of CD56, VLA-5, MPC-1, and syndecan-1. MM cells resistant to melphalan and doxorubicin typically overexpress VLA-4, and adherence to ECM proteins like fibronectin induces CAM-DR, with up-regulation of p27Kip1 in tumor cells.[65] Immunomodulatory drugs (IMiD) such as thalidomide,

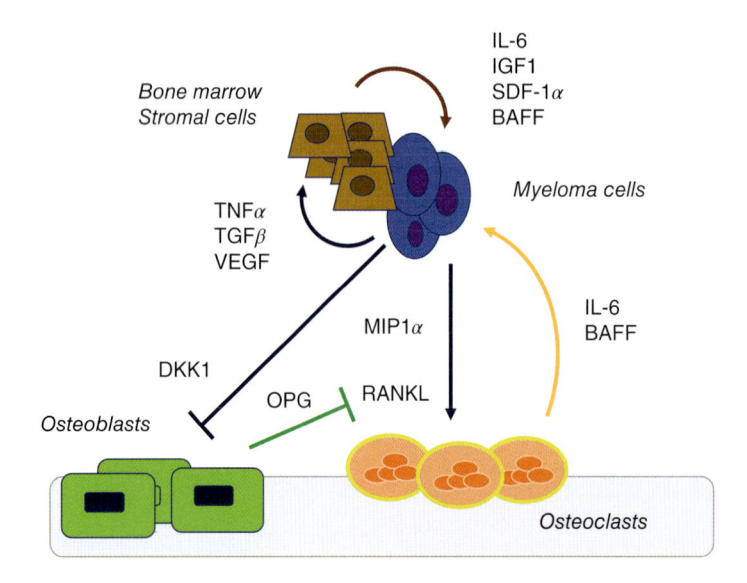

Figure 2 Multiple myeloma cells and the bone marrow microenvironment. There is a complex interplay between myeloma cells and their environment including bone marrow stromal cells, osteoblasts, and osteoclasts, leading to a cycle that promotes myeloma cell growth. Several of the key factors are shown.

lenalidomide, pomalidomide as well as the proteasome inhibitors bortezomib and carfilzomib (see below) can target both the tumor cell and its BM microenvironment and thereby at least partially overcome CAM-DR.[66–70]

Our studies also show that BMSCs secrete other cytokines, such as insulin-like growth factor-1 (IGF-1),[71] vascular endothelial growth factor (VEGF),[72,73] stromal cell-derived growth factor (SDF-1α)[74] and B-cell activating factor (BAFF),[75,76] which augment MM cell growth, survival, drug resistance, and migration in the BM milieu. Besides localizing tumor cells in the BM microenvironment, adhesion of MM cells to BMSCs also triggers the paracrine NFκB dependent transcription and secretion of IL-6 in BMSCs, survival, and resistance to dexamethasone-induced apoptosis via activation of p42/44 mitogen-activated protein kinase MAPK, Janus kinase 2 (JAK2)/signal transducer and activator of transcription 3 (STAT3), and phosphoinositide 3-kinase PI3K/AKT signaling cascades.[57,59,71,77–88] Recombinant IL-1β stimulates MM cells to produce IL-6, which consequently augments proliferation of MM cells.[89] Transforming growth factor-β (TGF-β) is secreted by MM cells and triggers IL-6 secretion in BMSCs, thereby augmenting paracrine IL-6 mediated tumor cell growth.[90] TGF-β secreted by MM cells likely also contributes to the immunodeficiency characteristic of MM by downregulating B cells, T cells, and natural killer cells, without similarly inhibiting the growth of MM cells. IL-10 is a proliferation factor, but not a differentiation factor, for human MM cells.[91] Macrophage inflammatory protein-1α (MIP-1α) is an osteoclast stimulating factor in MM.[92,93] BAFF is produced by BMSCs and osteoclasts. It signals through several receptors including BAFF-R, transmembrane activator, calcium modulator and cyclophilin ligand interactor (TACI), and B-cell maturation antigen (BCMA).[75,76] The level of TACI gene expression in MM cells is associated with microenvironment dependence.[94] This signaling cascade has a prosurvival effect on MM cells. Autocrine growth mediated by IL-15,[95] and more recently IL-21,[96] has been demonstrated in both MM cell lines and patient cells. Of these factors, BCMA has emerged in recent years as a target of great therapeutic interest (see below).

Wnt signaling regulates various developmental processes, can lead to malignant formation, and has been studied in the context of MM. Wnts are a family of secreted glycoproteins that bind to frizzled seven-transmembrane span receptors. Intracellularly, the Wnt signaling cascade blocks degradation of β-catenin in proteasomes, thereby leading to accumulation of β-catenin in the cytoplasm. In MM, a canonical Wnt signaling pathway is activated, associated with accumulation of β-catenin and significant morphological changes in MM cells with rearrangement of the actin cytoskeleton.[97] Derksen et al.[98] demonstrated that MM cells overexpress β-catenin, including its N-terminally unphosphorylated form, consistent with active β-catenin/T-cell factor-mediated transcription. Further accumulation and nuclear localization of β-catenin and/or increased cell proliferation were achieved by stimulation of Wnt signaling with either Wnt-3a, LiCl, or a constitutively active mutant form of β-catenin. Wnt signaling has also been shown as an important regulatory pathway in the osteoblast differentiation of mesenchymal stem cells. Interestingly, MM cells in BM biopsy specimens contained detectable dickkopf 1 (DKK1), a negative regulator of Wnt signaling cascade and a target of the β-catenin/TCF pathway.[99] Moreover, elevated DKK1 levels in BM plasma and peripheral blood from patients with MM correlated with the DKK1 gene-expression patterns and was associated with the presence of focal bone lesions.[100]

Exosomes are a subfraction of extracellular vesicles, ranging in size from 35 to 120 nm. They are actively secreted and transfer their cargo to the target cells, either by endocytosis or by direct fusion with the cell membrane. Importantly, exosomes from BMSCs and MM cells enhance MM progression by the induction of drug resistance, angiogenesis, and/or host immune suppression.[101] Previous data suggests MM BM-mesenchymal stromal cell (MSC)-derived exosomes promoted MM tumor growth via downregulation of a tumor suppressor miR-15a; in contrast, normal BM-MSC exosomes inhibited the growth of MM cells.[102]

Immune microenvironment in MM

An impairment of immune response has been commonly observed in MM patients.[103] The MM-related immunological dysfunction is also able to modulate plasma cell activity.[104] Conversely, the plasma cell-induced modulation of the BM microenvironment also impacts host immune effectors.[105] Levels of B-, T-, and

NK-cells are affected by these interactions. Dendritic cells, specifically, plasmacytoid dendritic cells are a subset of DC possessing toll-like receptor 9 receptors and we have shown that these cells in the BM microenvironment mediate immune deficiency characteristic of MM and promote MM cell growth, survival, and drug resistance.[106]

We have shown that IMiD like lenalidomide inhibit VEGF and IL-6, which are known to downregulate antigen-presenting function of dendritic cells in MM.[107] Moreover, lenalidomide directly activates CD28 on T cells, thereby stimulating transcription and secretion of IL-2, with resultant upregulation of T and NK cell anti-MM activity.[107,108] Lenalidomide can upregulate antibody-dependent cellular cytotoxicity (ADCC).[109] IMiD also affect the cytokine signaling stimulated by the interaction of effector cells with MM cells and BMSCs, and this is via regulation of SOCS1, a member of the suppressor of cytokine signaling genes.[110]

Molecular pathogenesis of MM

The malignant plasma cells in MM are localized to the BM in close association with BMSCs. They are long-lived cells with a very low (1–2%) labeling index that provides a measure of the proliferative rate of the malignant BMPC predicting survival in patients with newly diagnosed MM. The rearranged immunoglobulin genes are extensively somatically hypermutated in a manner compatible with antigen selection, with no evidence that the process of hypermutation is continuing.[47] However, MM cells have a significantly lower rate of immunoglobulin secretion than normal plasma cells. Thus, it appears that the critical oncogenic events in MM cells either occur after or do not interfere with most of the normal differentiation process involved in generating a long-lived plasma cell. Gene expression profiling has recently been utilized to characterize changes associated with the progression from normal plasma cells to MGUS to MM.[111,112]

MM may be broadly classified into hyperdiploid (HD) which generally involve trisomies versus nonhyperdiploid (NHD) disease, which is enriched for recurrent translocations (Table 4).[113,115] Nearly half of MM tumors are HD and the remaining are NHD, which also includes hypodiploid, pseudodiploid, or subtetraploid. Hyperdiploidy is characterized by trisomies of chromosomes 3, 5, 7, 9, 11, 15, 19 and is associated with a favorable prognosis.[116] (The majority of patients (79%) with exceptionally prolonged responses to lenalidomide-dexamethasone have disease with trisomies.[117]) The hallmark genetic lesion in many B-lymphocyte tumors involves dysregulation of an oncogene due to a translocation involving the IgH locus (14q32.3); this is also true in MM. In about 40% of MM cases, there are several recurrent translocations that involve IgH: t(11;14) which results in increased expression of CCND1; t(4;14) leading to overexpression of NSD2 and FGFR3; t(14;16), which involves MAF; t(14;20) which involves MAFB; and t(6;14) involving CCND3.[113,115] NHD myeloma is more strongly associated with these recurrent translocations.[118] The incidence of these translocations is significantly higher in the extramedullary phase of the disease and in myeloma cell lines.

Hyperdiploidy and these recurrent IgH translocations are considered primary cytogenetic abnormalities.[113] They occur early during the transition from a normal plasma cell to a clonal premalignant plasma cell, are present in monoclonal gammopathy of undetermined significance, and do not overlap. Secondary abnormalities occur later and may drive the transition from the premalignant stage to multiple myeloma and tend to be subclonal. These include monosomy 13, del(17p) (associated with lose of TP53), gain of 1q, del(1p32), and rearrangements involving

Table 4 Chromosomal alterations in multiple myeloma.[a]

	Percentage of patients	Gene(s) affected
Primary cytogenetic abnormalities		
Hyperdiploid (trisomies)	45%	
Nonhyperdiploid	40%	
t(11;14)	16%	CCND1
t(6;14)	2%	CCND3
t(4;14)	15%	MMSET; FGFR3 in 75%
t(14;16)	5%	MAF
t(14;20)	2%	MAFB
Secondary cytogenetic abnormalities		
Del(13)	44%	RB1, DIS3
Gain(1q)	35–45%	CKS1B, ANP32E
Del(1p)	30%	CDKN2C, FAF1, FAM46C
8q24 rearrangement	15%	MYC
Del(17p)	7%	TP53

[a]Source: Table adapted from Fonseca et al.[113] and Sonneveld et al.[114]

MYC.[119,120] In one prognostic model, del17p had the largest negative impact on prognosis, followed by del(1p32) and 1q gain.[121] Gain of 1q is one of the most common abnormalities, occurring in 35–45% of patients.[122–124]

FISH is an important tool for identifying these translocations, given the telomeric location of IgH and the low yield of conventional cytogenetics.[125] Many of these translocations are not identified by conventional karyotyping due to the low mitotic index of MM and the karyotypic "silence" of some of these translocations such as t(4;14).[126] On the other hand, the plasma cell labeling index and degree of bone marrow involvement correlate with finding abnormalities on conventional cytogenetics.[127] Another method for classifying multiple myeloma is expression profiling, based on work initially developed at the University of Arkansas.[128] There is significant overlap between classifications based on translocations and hyperdiploidy and the molecular classifications determined by expression profiling.

Cytogenetic and FISH abnormalities such as t(4;14), del(17p), t(14;16), t(14;20), nonhyperdiploidy, and gain of 1q are associated with worse prognosis.[113,114,121] The FISH abnormalities t(4;14), t(14;16), and del(17p) are traditionally considered "high risk" by the IMWG and should be part of the core FISH panel for estimating prognosis.[113] Moreover, these three FISH abnormalities are used in the Revised International Staging System.[129] Alterations in 17p can range from deletion or mutation in one allele of the TP53 gene or involve both alleles. In particular, biallelic inactivation of the TP53 gene ("double hit") is associated with a very poor prognosis.[130] A cancer clonal fraction >0.55 for del17p is also associated with a worse prognosis.[131]

The translocation t(11;14) is the most commonly detected translocation. This translocation is associated with several unique clinical features including increased frequency in rarer variants of multiple myeloma, such as plasma cell leukemia,[132] IgD and IgM MM, nonsecretory disease,[133] lymphoplasmacytic morphology,[134] and expression of CD20.[135] Of particular relevance is that MM with t(11;14) has unique sensitivity to the BCL-2 inhibitor venetoclax (see below). In t(4;14), the apparent oncogene dysregulated is fibroblast growth factor receptor 3 (FGFR3), and it is possible that dysregulated expression of FGFR3, as a result of t(4;14), receives an FGFR3-mediated signal from FGF produced by stromal cells in the BM microenvironment.[136] In addition to FGFR3, the t(4;14) translocation in MM regulates a novel gene, MMSET, resulting in IgH/MMSET hybrid transcripts.[137] Ectopic expression of FGFR3 promotes MM cell proliferation and prevents apoptosis, and its oncogenic potential has been tested in a murine model, confirming its capacity to transform hematopoietic cells.[138,139]

Somatic mutations and interclonal diversity

Multiple myeloma is preceded by MGUS or smoldering myeloma transforming to overt myeloma.[13,14] This is characterized by accumulation of mutations conferring growth advantage (driver mutations) or functionally irrelevant mutations (passenger mutations). Frequently mutated genes identified by whole genome or exome sequencing in myeloma include *KRAS*, *NRAS*, *FAM46C*, *DIS3*, and *TP53*.[140-142] Other significant genes are *BRAF*, *TRAF3*, *CYLD*, *RB1*, *PRDM1*, and *ACTG1*. *TRAF3* and *CYLD* mutations, together with homozygous deletions in *BIRC2/BIRC3*, *NIK* overexpression, and mutations in other genes (*CARD11* and *MYD88*) contribute to constitutively activating the NFκB pathway. Genes involved in protein homeostasis, unfolded protein response, or lymphoid/plasma cell development, such as *PRDM1* involved in plasmacytic differentiation, and *XBP1*, *IRF4*, *LRRK2*, *SP140*, and *LTB* form a cluster of genes mutated in myeloma. Other recurrent mutated genes are *ROBO1*, a transmembrane receptor involved in β-catenin and MET signaling, *EGR1* transcription factor, FAT3, a transmembrane protein belonging to cadherin superfamily, and histone-modifying genes (*MLL*, *MLL2*, *MLL3*, *WHSC1/MMSET*, *WHSC1L1*, and *UTX* among others).[140,141] Recent data support the concept of intratumor heterogeneity in myeloma, where different subclones can emerge and become predominant following different mechanisms of evolution, including linear, branching, parallel, or convergent evolution.[141,143] Clonal diversity similar to Darwinian-like selection, favors cancer progression and adaptation to therapy. Next-generation sequencing analyses show that most patients have a subclonal structure at diagnosis, with one predominant clone and several others which can re-appear at different stages of disease evolution or following treatment.[141,144,145] Recent studies show that many of the genetic abnormalities present in MM are already present at the smoldering myeloma stage and that early progression to myeloma is associated with expansion of a clone already present, whereas later progression is associated with clonal evolution.[146] Moreover, Bustoros et al.[147] have shown that alterations in MAPK pathway, DNA repair pathway, *MYC*, and APOBEC-associated mutations are independent risk factors for progression of smoldering to active myeloma.

Prognostic factors

The Durie-Salmon system, which uses parameters such as anemia, hypercalcemia, amount of monoclonal protein, and degree of bone involvement on skeletal survey, was historically used for prognosis.[148] However, a limitation of the Durie-Salmon system is that assessment of bone involvement may be subjective. Thirty years later, this staging system was replaced by the International Staging System (ISS) based on a multivariate analysis of several variables including serum β2 microglobulin (B2M), platelet count, hemoglobin, creatinine, degree of bone marrow involvement, size of monoclonal component (Table 5).[149] This determined that a three stage system using B2M and albumin provided the most significant prognostic value. B2M represents the light chain of the major histocompatibility complex of the cell membrane, and increased B2M levels are due to release by tumors with high growth fraction and cell turnover rates. In patients with MM and normal renal function, rising serum B2M predicts for progression.[150] The ISS was revised to incorporate serum LDH and high-risk FISH to create the Revised International Staging System. High-risk FISH was defined by the presence of del(17p), t(4;14), or t(14;16).[113]

Treatment

While MM is not considered curable at this time, the treatments for MM are effective and tolerated well, including in the older, frailer patient population. The adoption of high-dose melphalan with autologous stem cell transplant (SCT) and the introduction of three new drug classes in the past decade—IMiD such as thalidomide, lenalidomide, pomalidomide; proteasome inhibitors such as bortezomib, carfilzomib, and ixazomib; and anti-CD38 monoclonal antibodies such as daratumumab and isatuximab—have resulted in dramatic improvements in outcomes. A retrospective study comparing patients diagnosed since 1997 to those diagnosed before 1997 found a significant improvement in overall survival, 44.8 versus 29.9 months, respectively.[151] This was recently updated to an overall survival of 6.1 years for the cohort diagnosed between 2006 and 2010.[152]

A core question is when to initiate treatment for patients with MM. There is uniform consensus recommending treatment for active MM as defined by the presence of one of the CRAB criteria of end organ involvement or one of the myeloma-defining biomarkers.[7] For patients with asymptomatic, smoldering multiple myeloma, the current practice is close observation.[153] This continues to be an area of active investigation (see below).

The treatment of multiple myeloma has advanced considerably since the initial use of oral melphalan and prednisone (MP) over 50 years ago.[154,155] Initial attempts at improving MP by adding additional conventional chemotherapy drugs were not beneficial.[156] Escalating the dose of melphalan[157] followed by improving marrow recovery with autologous stem cell transplant[158] allowed patients to achieve deeper responses. The next and perhaps most significant breakthroughs in MM therapy came with the introduction of IMiD like thalidomide (approved in 2006), lenalidomide (2006), pomalidomide (2013), and proteasome inhibitors such as bortezomib (2003), carfilzomib (2012), and ixazomib (2015). This reflected the rapid translation of findings from the bench to the bedside. In the past, drugs like lenalidomide and bortezomib were considered novel; now they are a routine part of MM care.

Newly diagnosed multiple myeloma

Traditionally, the choice of initial therapy for treatment of newly diagnosed patients was divided between patients eligible for intensive, high-dose melphalan and auto SCT versus patients who were older and not robust enough for intensive therapy. Over time, this distinction in guiding initial therapy has become less prominent due to the improved tolerability and effectiveness of newer therapies. The evolution of therapy for newly diagnosed patients reflects the adoption of drugs that first established efficacy in relapsed disease followed by combinations of these newer therapies (Tables 6 and 7). Typically, initial therapy is based on combination of three drug classes, such as the RVd regimen, which combines an IMiD (lenalidomide), proteasome inhibitor (bortezomib), and dexamethasone.[163,168] Newer regimens incorporate the anti-CD38 monoclonal antibody daratumumab, for example, with lenalidomide and dexamethasone.[170] Four drug combinations, such as daratumumab with RVd, are under active investigation, and may become standard practice soon.[167]

Immunomodulatory drugs

IMiD are a pivotal treatment class in MM. Thalidomide was infamous as a teratogen in the 1950s and 1960s until it emerged that this drug class was beneficial in multiple myeloma.[171] The initial motivation behind using thalidomide in MM was its anti-angiogenic properties.[172] However, the actual mechanism

Table 5 International staging system and revised international staging system.[a]

ISS stage	Criteria	Median overall survival
International Staging System		
I	Serum β2 microglobulin <3.5 mg/L and serum albumin ≥3.5 g/dL	62 months
II	Serum β2 microglobulin <3.5 mg/L and serum albumin <3.5 g/dL OR serum β2-microglobulin 3.5 to <5.5 mg/L	44 months
III	Serum β2 microglobulin ≥5.5 mg/L	29 months
Revised International Staging System		
R-ISS stage	Criteria	Median overall survival
I	ISS stage I and standard-risk FISH and normal LDH	Not reached; 5-year OS 82%
II	Not R-ISS stage I or III	83 months
III	ISS stage III and either high-risk FISH OR high LDH	43 months

High-risk FISH defined as del(17p), t(4;14), or t(14;16).
[a]Source: Palumbo et al.[129] and Greipp et al.[149]

Table 6 Selected trials in newly diagnosed transplant-ineligible patients.

Reference	Name of trial	Arm	N	PFS	HR	ORR	≥VGPR	≥CR
Facon et al.;[159] Bahlis et al.[160]	MAIA	Dara Rd	368	68% at 3 years	0.56	93%	79%	48%
		Rd	369	33.8		81%	53%	25%
Mateos et al.;[161] Mateos et al.[162]	ALCYONE	Dara VMP	318	36.4	0.42	91%	71%	43%
		VMP	263	19.3		74%	50%	24%
O'Donnell et al.[163]	RVD lite	RVd	50	35.1		86%	60%	44%
Benboubker et al.[164]	FIRST	Continuous Rd	535	25.5	0.7[a]	75%	44%	15%
		Rd 18	541	20.7		73%	43%	14%
		MPT	547	21.2		62%	28%	9%
San Miguel et al.[165]	VISTA	VMP	344	24[b]	0.48	74%	41%	33%
		MP	338	16.6[b]		39%	8%	4%

Abbreviations: D, dexamethasone; dara, daratumumab; M, melphalan; P, prednisone; R, lenalidomide; T, thalidomide; V, bortezomib.
PFS is in months.
[a]Hazard ratio of continuous Rd versus Rd for 18 months.
[b]Time to progression.

Table 7 Selected trials for newly diagnosed transplant-eligible patients.

Reference	Name of trial	Arm	N	PFS	HR	ORR	≥VGPR	≥CR
Kumar et al.[166]	ENDURANCE	KRd	545	34.6	1.04	87%	74%	18%
		RVd	542	34.4		84%	65%	15%
Voorhees et al.[167]	GRIFFIN	Dara RVd	99	2 yr, 95.8%		99%[a]	91%	52%
		RVd	97	2 yr, 89.8%		92%[a]	73%	42%
Durie et al.[168]	SWOG S0777	VRd	242	43	0.712	82%	44%	16%
		Rd	229	30		72%	32%	8%
Attal et al.[169]	IFM 2009	RVd + upfront auto SCT	350	50	0.65	98%	88%	59%
		RVD + deferred auto SCT	350	36		97%	77%	48%

Median PFS is in months.
[a]Response rates are at end of consolidation.

of action of IMiDs in MM and their teratogenicity have recently been elucidated. Drugs in this class bind to cereblon (CBN).[173] Binding of IMiDs to CBN prevents autoubiquitylation of CBN, which then enhances CBN-dependent proteasomal degradation of transcription factors IKZF1 (Ikaros) and IKZF3 (Aiolos) that are important to MM proliferation.[174–176] (The teratogenicity of IMiDs has been recently determined to be due to the cereblon-mediated degradation of the zinc finger transcription factor SALL4. Moreover, thalidomide induces degradation of SALL4 in humans and primates but not in rodents or fish, due to differences in cereblon and SALL4 between the species.[177])

The introduction of thalidomide was the first in a series of improvements over the MP regimen. Thalidomide was the first IMiD to establish efficacy in MM, beginning with relapsed disease as a single agent.[172] In newly diagnosed patients eligible for high-dose melphalan and autologous SCT, thalidomide, and dexamethasone showed higher response rates than the standard at the time, VAD (vincristine, doxorubicin, dexamethasone).[178] Moreover, the combination of thalidomide and dexamethasone was superior to dexamethasone alone.[179] In older patients not eligible for intensive therapy, thalidomide was added to the combination of melphalan, pred-nisone, thalidomide (MPT), resulting in a 76% complete or partial response rate compared to 47% in the MP arm. This translated into a doubling of the 2-year event-free survival to 54% versus 27%.[180] The main limitations with thalidomide include peripheral neuropathy and thrombotic events, along with teratogenicity.[181]

Lenalidomide (CC-5013) was the next IMiD to be evaluated and is a core drug in MM. Compared to thalidomide, lenalidomide is associated with significantly less peripheral neuropathy, sedation, and constipation but is associated with more myelosuppression. The efficacy of lenalidomide was initially demonstrated in relapsed disease. Two large phase III trials comparing lenalidomide and dexamethasone versus dexamethasone were unblinded because of statistically significantly higher response rates, as well as increase in time to progression and overall survival, in the lenalidomide and dexamethasone-treated cohort, providing the basis for its FDA approval in 2006 to treat relapsed MM after one prior therapy.[182,183]

The FIRST trial established the role of lenalidomide and dexamethasone in newly diagnosed, transplant-ineligible patients. This phase III trial compared continuous lenalidomide and low-dose dexamethasone (Rd) against 72 weeks of lenalidomide and low-dose dexamethasone and 72 weeks of MPT.[164] The continuous Rd arm compared with the MPT arm had better overall responses (81% vs 67%), superior PFS (26 vs 21.9 months), and OS (59.1 vs 49.1 months).[184] Notably, the incidence of hematological second primary malignancies was lower with continuous Rd than MPT.

Thrombotic complications are a known adverse event of IMiDs. When used as single agents, the risk of venous thromboembolic events (VTEs) with thalidomide or lenalidomide is less than 5%.[185,186] The risk of thrombosis increases in combinations with dexamethasone, anthracyclines, or erythropoietin, and reduction in dexamethasone dose significantly lowers the risk.[187] Two phase III trials of lenalidomide with dexamethasone in relapsed MM showed that the VTE rate was significantly higher with the combination, 11–15%, than with dexamethasone alone 4–5% respectively.[182,183] Aspirin can lower the risk of thrombosis and is commonly used as prophylaxis in treatments which use IMiD.[188] Another significant adverse event is risk of second primary malignancy. Rash is another common side effect of lenalidomide that can be supportively managed with antihistamines.[189] Finally, diarrhea can adversely affect quality of life, which is more of a concern since lenalidomide is increasingly given on a continuous basis as maintenance therapy (see below); this can be managed with bile acid sequestrants.[190]

Proteasome inhibitors

Proteasome inhibitors emerged around the same time as the introduction of the IMiD drug class, and they were similarly transformational in MM treatment. The regulated degradation of proteins by the proteasome, a cylindrical, multienzyme complex found in all eukaryotic cells, is key to normal cell homeostasis.[191,192] This is accomplished by the proteasome, a cylindrical, multienzyme complex found in all eukaryotic cells that manages the disposal of misfolded proteins and obsolete proteins. The ubiquitin-ligase pathway flags proteins for disposal by attachment of ubiquitin polypeptides. The proteasome is composed of a 20S core cylindrical complex with proteolytic activity and capped on each end by two 19S regulatory units, for a total size of 26S. The 19S subunit recognizes ubiquitinated proteins, which are then unfolded and delivered to the 20S subunit. The 20S subunit has several enzymatic sites, categorized as trypsin-like, chymotrypsin-like, and caspase-like. While normal cells are universally dependent on proteasome function, malignant cells are even more dependent on proteasome function and thus more vulnerable to its inhibition.

Bortezomib is a peptide boronic acid that reversibly and potently binds to the chymotrypsin-like subunit of the 20S subunit. The bench to bedside translation of bortezomib and subsequent FDA approval was rapid. The initial rationale to use bortezomib in MM was to block NFκB activity by stabilizing IκB and preventing the translocation of NFκB to the nucleus.[193,194] NFκB was initially identified as a therapeutic target in MM, conferring drug resistance, modulating adhesion molecule expression on MM cells and BMSCs, and modulating constitutive and MM binding-induced transcription and secretion of cytokines.[57] However, additional studies in MM established that bortezomib actually triggers NFκB activation via the canonical pathway but inhibits NFκB in bone marrow stromal cells.[195] This suggests that bortezomib-induced cytotoxicity in MM cells cannot be fully attributed to inhibition of canonical NFκB activity. Rather, in MM, where the malignant plasma cells produce large amounts of monoclonal immunoglobulin, bortezomib leads to the accumulation of unfolded proteins and endoplasmic reticulum stress, followed by activation of the unfolded protein response and arrest of the cell cycle.[196]

Phase I trials of bortezomib showed tolerability and early evidence of enhanced activity in MM compared with other tumors.[197] In relapsed disease, the phase II SUMMIT trial of bortezomib as a single agent demonstrated responses, including complete responses, forming the basis for accelerated FDA approval in 2003.[198] The APEX trial compared bortezomib versus dexamethasone in relapsed MM and was unblinded due to a statistically significant prolongation in time to progression in the bortezomib-treated cohort and overall survival.[199,200] Moreover, bortezomib was added to the standard regimen at the time of MP. In newly diagnosed patients not eligible for intensive therapy, the VISTA trial compared the regimen of bortezomib, melphalan, prednisone (VMP) to MP.[165] Responses (71% vs 35%) and time to progression (24 vs 16.6 months) were improved with the upfront addition of bortezomib, and overall survival was significantly improved in the VMP group versus MP group, with three-year overall survival of 68.5% versus 54% respectively.[201] The VISTA trial led to the FDA approval of bortezomib as initial therapy.

A key limitation of bortezomib is peripheral neuropathy. In the initial studies, peripheral neuropathy was common, occurring in 35% of patients, including 13% where it was grade ≥3.[202] Dose modifications can reduce the frequency of grade ≥3 peripheral neuropathy to 8% in the APEX study[203] along with a weekly schedule.[204,205] Historically, based on its initial approval, bortezomib is given intravenously as a bolus. Subcutaneous administration was studied in a randomized study with significant reduction in grade ≥3 peripheral neuropathy from 12% when given intravenously to 6% when given subcutaneously,[206] with comparable long-term outcomes.[207] Given these findings, bortezomib is given subcutaneously now instead of intravenously. Bortezomib is associated with a significantly higher risk of herpes zoster; in the phase III APEX trial, the incidence of herpes zoster was 13% compared to 5%.[208] Consequently, prophylaxis with acyclovir is standard. Finally, thrombocytopenia is a common hematologic adverse event with bortezomib. In the APEX trial, grade 3–4 thrombocytopenia occurred in 30% of patients. However, unlike the thrombocytopenia seen in traditional cytotoxic chemotherapy, the thrombocytopenia with bortezomib may be due to reversible effects on megakaryocyte function and is not cumulative.[209]

Combination therapy

Importantly, bortezomib has been successfully combined with the IMiD class, based on preclinical data showing synergistic activity.[210] This includes combinations with thalidomide (VTD)[211,212] and lenalidomide (RVd) in newly diagnosed patients, and where with RVd, there was an unprecedented overall response rate of 100% in a pivotal phase II trial.[213] A recent phase III trial, SWOG S0777, confirmed this finding, demonstrating superior outcomes with RVd compared to the standard of lenalidomide and dexamethasone (Rd).[168] RVd improved both progression-free survival (PFS) 43 versus 30 months ($p = 0.0018$) and median overall survival 75 versus 64 months ($p = 0.025$). RVd is now a standard front-line regimen in the United States. Modifications in dosing and schedule of RVd, such as in the RVD lite regimen, allow this triplet regimen to be effectively used in older and frailer patients, with an ORR of 86% and median PFS was 35.1 months.[163] Indeed, an earlier ECOG E4A03 study demonstrated the benefit of reducing the dose of dexamethasone.[187] This study evaluated the dosing of dexamethasone when combined with lenalidomide in newly diagnosed disease. Low-dose dexamethasone (where dexamethasone is given weekly) improved overall survival compared to conventional high-dose, with reduction in grade ≥3 thromboembolism and infections.

Cyclophosphamide, bortezomib, and dexamethasone (CyBorD or VCD) is another combination with comparable activity to RVD based on the phase II EVOLUTION trial.[214] A randomized trial showed that VTD was superior to VCD for induction in depth of response and myelosuppression.[215] There has been no trial directly comparing RVD versus VTD. Nevertheless, an integrated analysis of patients treated on the GEM 2005 and 2012 trials showed that RVD compared with VTD had deeper responses (VGPR rate 66.3% vs 51.2%) and less peripheral neuropathy (grade 2 or higher, 20.7% vs 44.6%).[216] Overall, a meta-analysis from 2013 of several phase III trials showed that bortezomib-based inductions regimens compared to nonbortezomib regimens had superior response rates (posttransplant near complete response rate or better, 38% vs 24%), median progression-free survival (35.9 months vs 28.6 months), and 3 year overall survival (79.7% vs 74.7%), emphasizing the value of incorporating a proteasome inhibitor for induction therapy.[217]

Daratumumab

Daratumumab is a human IgG1κ monoclonal antibody that targets CD38. Initially approved in relapsed disease in 2015, it is now used across all stages of MM from newly diagnosed disease to relapsed disease and in various combinations. CD38 is a type II transmembrane glycoprotein that is expressed highly in MM cells and also expressed to a lower extent on lymphoid and myeloid cells. Indeed, the idea of targeting CD38 was proposed over 25 years ago.[218] Daratumumab was identified in preclinical studies based on its complement-dependent cytotoxicity and antibody-dependent cellular cytotoxicity against MM cells.[219] In addition, daratumumab also has immunomodulatory effects by suppressing CD38+ immune-suppressor cells.[220]

Once the efficacy of daratumumab was established in relapsed disease as a single agent and in combination with bortezomib and dexamethasone or with lenalidomide and dexamethasone (see below), it was evaluated in newly diagnosed patients. For older, transplant-ineligible patients, the ALCYONE study randomized patients to receive daratumumab with VMP versus VMP.[161] In both arms, VMP was given for a fixed duration of nine six-week cycles; the arm with daratumumab received daratumumab until progression. The addition of daratumumab improved progression-free survival (36.4 vs 19.3 months; HR 0.42, $p < 0.0001$) and overall survival (HR 0.6, $p = 0.0003$).[162] The MAIA study evaluated the addition of daratumumab to the lenalidomide and dexamethasone (dara Rd) backbone in transplant-ineligible patients.[159] Similar to ALCYONE, in the MAIA study, the incorporation of daratumumab improved overall response (93% vs 82%) and increased PFS (median not reached vs 33.8 months; HR 0.56, $p < 0.0001$) compared to the control Rd arm.[160] For younger patients eligible for intensive therapy, the addition of daratumumab also has comparable benefit. The CASSIOPEIA study evaluated daratumumab in combination with VTd given as induction for four cycles, followed by high-dose melphalan and autologous stem cell transplant, and with two additional cycles of VTd (at the time, VTd was commonly used for induction in Europe).[221] The primary endpoint was stringent complete response 100 days after transplantation, which was higher in the dara VTd arm (29%) versus the control VTd arm (20%). Daratumumab also improved PFS (HR 0.47, $p < 0.0001$). Similarly, the GRIFFIN study evaluated daratumumab with RVd, which is more commonly used in the United States.[167] The addition of daratumumab yielded deeper, higher quality responses with higher stringent CR rates (62.6% vs 45.4%, $p = 0.0177$) and higher minimal residual disease (MRD) negative rates (10^{-5}) (51% vs 20.4%, $p < 0.0001$). Daratumumab has also been combined with CyBorD as well.[222]

Infusion-related reactions are common with daratumumab, with grade 1–2 reactions ranging from 28% to 56% and grade 3–4 reactions 4–8.6% across various trials.[223] Nearly all reactions occurred during the first infusion, and the incidence decreases sharply with subsequent infusions. Consequently, the first infusion can average 7 h. The risk of IRR can be reduced with the addition of montelukast to standard premedications with corticosteroids, antihistamines, as well as splitting the first dose of daratumumab across 2 days.[224,225] Because of the low incidence of reactions after the first infusion, a 90 min infusion protocol is increasingly used with subsequent infusions.[226]

To help improve the administration of daratumumab, a subcutaneous form of daratumumab was developed. It is co-formulated with hyaluronidase and given over 5 min. The COLUMBA study showed that this subcutaneous form of daratumumab when given as a single agent had equivalent outcomes to conventional intravenous administration in a relapsed patient population.[227] Consequently, the FDA approved this subcutaneous form in 2020, which simplifies the logistics of using daratumumab.

High-dose melphalan and autologous stem cell transplant

The use of high-dose melphalan with autologous stem cell transplant has been a mainstay of MM therapy for nearly four decades, beginning with its initial description in 1983,[157] showing that significantly escalating the dose of melphalan leads to deeper responses than with conventional dosing of melphalan. The IFM 90 study showed that this intensive approach with high-dose melphalan and total body irradiation followed by autologous stem cells was superior to conventional cytotoxic chemotherapy, which consisted of VMCP (vincristine, melphalan, cyclophosphamide, prednisone) alternating with BVAP (vincristine, carmustine, doxorubicin, and prednisone).[228] The complete response rate (22% vs 5%), event-free survival (27 vs 18 months), and 10 year overall survival (30% vs 8%) favored the more intensive approach.[229] This approach has been taken further with tandem autologous stem cell transplant. In a French randomized trial comparing a single versus double high-dose therapy and stem cell transplantation, there was no significant difference in the CR rate between single and double transplantation arms, and EFS and OS curves separated only after 3 years.[230] The Bologna 96 study also showed that double autografting mainly helped patients who did not achieve near-complete response.[231] At present, double autografting is utilized primarily in patients with high-risk disease, based on the results of the EMN02/HO95 and StaMINA trials (see below).[232,233]

Past attempts to improve the outcome of high-dose therapy followed by autografting included the depletion of tumor cells from the graft[234,235] or selection by CD34 expression to select normal hematopoietic progenitor cells.[236] However, these additional steps have not improved outcomes.

In patients where stem cell collection is planned, combinations that include alkylating agents such as melphalan should be avoided, since damage to normal hematopoietic stem cells may occur and affect the ability to collect stem cells. Lenalidomide may also hamper the collection of stem cells, although stem cell mobilization with growth factors and chemotherapy may overcome the myelosuppressive effects of lenalidomide.[237–240] Consequently, the number of cycles of induction treatment, especially with lenalidomide-containing regimens, has traditionally been limited to roughly four cycles. With the increasing use of plerixafor, prior lenalidomide therapy is less of an issue for stem cell collection.[241,242]

Combination therapy with at the time, "novel agents" such as lenalidomide and bortezomib achieves responses comparable to those with high-dose melphalan and autologous stem cell transplant, and higher than that achieved with prior conventional cytotoxic chemotherapy. This reopens the question of the role of high-dose melphalan in newly diagnosed patients, given the higher quality responses with newer agents compared to the traditional cytotoxic chemotherapy studied in IFM 90. The IFM 2009 study randomized patients to upfront autologous stem cell transplant versus delaying transplant to time of relapse.[169] All patients received contemporary induction therapy with RVd for three cycles and all patients received lenalidomide maintenance for one year (see below on maintenance therapy). In patients randomized to upfront transplant, two additional cycles of RVd were given for consolidation; patients in the RVd alone arm went on to receive a total of eight cycles prior to maintenance. Patients who received upfront transplant had significant improvement in PFS (50 vs 36 months) as well as deeper responses (complete response rate 59% vs 48%). However, at this time, no difference in overall survival has been reported. MRD assessment (see below) may be able to provide better risk stratification and help identify patients who benefit the most from high-dose therapy. In the IFM 2009 trial, measurement of MRD at a sensitivity of 1×10^{-6} by next-generation sequencing of samples from patients starting maintenance therapy showed that depth of response by MRD level could stratify outcomes, even among patients in CR.[243] Moreover, outcomes were comparable in patients with MRD negative status, regardless of whether they received high-dose therapy or not. The DETERMINATION study (NCT01208662) shares the same trial design as IFM 2009 and enrolled patients in the United States. However, in DETERMINATION, maintenance lenalidomide is given until disease progression compared to a fixed duration of one year in IFM 2009. The DETERMINATION trial has completed accrual, and results of this trial are pending.

Allogeneic stem cell transplantation

Similar to other hematologic malignancies, allogeneic stem cell transplant has been evaluated in MM. However, a significant limitation is the high treatment-related mortality with conventional myeloablative conditioning, 40–60%.[244] Conditioning regimens have shifted to a nonmyeloablative approach, with more reliance on graft versus myeloma effect.[245] However, trials have shown conflicting results. For example, the BMT CTN 0102 compared autologous stem cell transplant followed by nonmyeloablative allogeneic stem cell transplant versus tandem autologous stem cell transplant.[246] Assignment was based on the availability of an HLA-matched sibling donor. There was no difference in outcomes in terms of PFS or OS. On the other hand, a study with a similar trial design conducted in Italy had different outcomes, with results favoring the allogeneic stem cell arm, with median OS not reached versus 4.25 years.[247] With the increasing availability of newer, better-tolerated therapies, allogeneic stem transplantation is now mainly undertaken as part of a clinical trial in patients with high-risk disease. Syngeneic transplantation is a consideration for patients with an identical twin donor. A case-matched comparison showed that the relapse rate with syngeneic stem cell transplantation was significantly lower than autologous stem cell transplantation.[248]

Maintenance therapy

Maintenance regimens are used to extend the duration of response following initial therapy with high-dose melphalan and autologous stem cell transplant. The increased tolerability and efficacy of newer antimyeloma agents have increased the attractiveness and the applicability of this approach. Previous attempts at maintenance therapy with older conventional chemotherapy agents such as melphalan or interferon were not beneficial.[249] Thalidomide has been evaluated for maintenance, though its use as maintenance is limited by risk of thrombosis and peripheral neuropathy.[250] Moreover, in the Medical Research Council Myeloma IX study, while thalidomide maintenance improved PFS, OS was unexpectedly worse in patients with high-risk FISH.[251]

Several trials have explored the use of lenalidomide as a single agent as maintenance therapy following autologous stem cell transplant. A meta-analysis of three trials, CALGB100104, the Italian study RV-MM-PI-209, and IFM 2005-02, showed a doubling in PFS (52.8 vs 23.5 months) and improvement in median overall survival (not reach vs 86 months).[252] Maintenance therapy was associated with risk of second primary malignancies over 5%, though the risk of progressive disease is higher than the risk of developing a second primary malignancy. Secondary cancers included both hematologic malignancies such as acute myelogenous leukemia as well as solid tumors. A fourth study presented after the meta-analysis, Myeloma XI, also evaluated lenalidomide maintenance after autologous stem cell transplant and corroborated the findings of the meta-analysis.[253] Based on these findings, lenalidomide was approved by the FDA for maintenance.

Proteasome inhibitors have also been evaluated as maintenance therapy. In the HOVON-65/GMMG-HD4 study, bortezomib was given every two weeks and was associated with increasing the near CR and CR rate from 31% to 49%.[254] The benefit of bortezomib maintenance was more pronounced in patients with deletion 17p. Ixazomib is an oral proteasome inhibitor given weekly for three out of our weeks (see below). The TOURMALINE-MM3 study evaluated ixazomib as maintenance therapy compared with placebo in patients following autologous stem cell transplant.[255] The study showed that ixazomib improved PFS (26.5 vs 21.3 months, HR = 0.72) and is another option as maintenance.

The StaMINA trial (BMT CTN 0702) compared maintenance lenalidomide with tandem autologous stem cell transplant or consolidation.[232] In this trial, all patients received high-dose melphalan followed by autologous stem cell transplant along with maintenance lenalidomide. Patients were randomized following autologous stem cell transplant to proceed with maintenance lenalidomide versus a second course of high-dose melphalan and autologous stem cell transplant versus consolidation with four additional cycles of RVd. This trial found that all arms had similar PFS and OS, suggesting that additional treatment did not provide additional benefit. In contrast, the EMN02/HO95 trial also evaluated the role of a second autologous transplant and found benefit with a second transplant.[233] In this study, the European Myeloma Network evaluated several questions, including autologous stem cell transplant versus VMP, consolidation with RVd, and in centers that routinely performed double stem cell transplants, single versus double stem cell transplants. The EMN02/HO95 trial found that a double transplant significantly improved PFS and OS. In patients with high-risk FISH, the benefit was significantly more, with PFS of 46 months with double stem cell transplant versus 26.7 months with single-cell transplant and improvement in overall survival with HR 0.7. Some of the differences between the StaMINA and the EMN092/HO95 findings likely reflect differences in treatment patterns between the United States and Europe. In the United States, initial therapy with lenalidomide and bortezomib was more routine and longer, whereas in the European study, patients received induction with VCD, and exposure to lenalidomide was later on as consolidation and/or as maintenance.

For patients with high-risk disease, maintenance therapy can also be interpreted as continuous therapy with the same agents used as induction, beyond single-agent lenalidomide. The group at Emory evaluated 45 patients with high-risk disease, defined as del(17p), del(1p), t(4;14), t(14;16), or presentation as plasma cell leukemia.[256] After autologous stem cell transplant, these patients continued with RVd as maintenance therapy. Median PFS was 32 months, which compares favorably to what has been previously observed in high-risk disease, including plasma cell leukemia.

Minimal residual disease (MRD)

Sequencing-based platforms and multiparametric flow cytometry are now being used to measure MRD in bone marrow aspirates, especially as patients are achieving deeper responses with newer therapies. Using these modalities, sensitivity for detecting disease can be as low as 1×10^{-6} cells, and MRD negativity rates are beginning to be explored as a surrogate endpoint. Meta-analyses have shown significant improvement in OS in patients with MRD negative status.[257,258] Moreover, importantly, this applies to patients who achieved CR by conventional criteria, where OS was 112 versus 82 months for MRD-positive versus MRD-negative patients.[257] Next-generation sequencing (NGS), which is now available commercially, allows for more sensitive measurements than methodologies based on conventional flow cytometry. Improvements in flow cytometry, next-generation flow, have increased the sensitivity for MRD detection to levels approaching NGS, with the advantage of speed, not requiring a baseline sample, and also having the ability to assess for the quality of the bone marrow aspirate.[259]

NGS was able to show in the IFM 2009 study of upfront v. deferred autologous stem cell transplant that patients who were able to achieve MRD negative status at 10^{-6} had superior outcomes compared to responses at 10^{-5} and 10^{-4}.[243] Indeed, as long as a deep response is achieved, the method of achieving the response may not be as important. For example, in the CASSIOPEIA study, which evaluated daratumumab-VTd versus VTd in newly diagnosed patients as induction and as consolidation following autologous stem cell transplant, patients who achieved CR and MRD negative status were more common in the daratumumab-VTd arm but had similar PFS, irrespective of treatment arm.[260] The GRIFFIN trial compared daratumumab with RVd versus RVd as induction and consolidation in patients undergoing autologous stem cell transplant and similarly showed higher MRD negative rates in the daratumumab arm.[167] This opens the possibility for using MRD assessment to guide decisions regarding use of high-dose melphalan and autologous stem cell transplant and duration and type of maintenance therapy.

A limitation in MRD assessment is the reliance on measuring disease involving the bone marrow. Bone marrow involvement can be heterogeneous, and this does not take into account extramedullary disease outside of the bone marrow. For example, in the IMAJEM study of the IMF 2009 trial, 25% of patients with MRD negative disease had positive PET CT findings.[32]

Relapsed disease

While significant gains have been made with upfront treatment, disease relapse continues to be a central issue in MM. A challenge in relapsed disease is decreasing effectiveness and shorter durability of response with each successive line of treatment.[261,262] A better understanding of the molecular architecture of myeloma may help explain the difficulties with relapsed disease. Comprehensive molecular profiling of MM samples shows multiple heterogeneous clonal populations that evolve with treatment.[141,263] The presence of this clonal heterogeneity and evolution with relapsing disease emphasizes the importance of achieving deep responses both upfront and at time of relapse.

While patients who have symptoms from disease progression, that is, clinical relapse, generally require treatment at that time, for asymptomatic patients, the IMWG provides guidelines for initiating treatment or changing treatment based on significant paraprotein relapse (e.g., doubling of the monoclonal protein in two consecutive measurements in ≤2 months).[30] Some patients with an asymptomatic rise in monoclonal protein may do well with observation. A series examining patterns of relapse in 211 patients after autologous stem cell transplant noted that there was a wide range between onset of asymptomatic relapse (or biochemical relapse) and progression and treatment, varying from 0 to 5.6 years, with a median of 5.6 months.[264] The clinical features of relapse were generally similar to the features at time of presentation, for example, patients who relapsed with renal impairment tended to have renal impairment at time of diagnosis. Notably, 26% of patients with asymptomatic relapse did not require treatment for at least 2 years, suggesting that there is a group of patients with biochemical relapse who may follow a more indolent course. However, the challenge is how to prospectively identify these patients with more indolent relapses.

Moreover, the landscape of patients with relapsing disease is changing, as patients increasingly are treated with lenalidomide upfront and are on maintenance therapy with lenalidomide. Several pivotal trials in relapsed disease excluded patients with lenalidomide-refractory disease—carfilzomib, elotuzumab, and ixazomib—which is a consideration in applying the results of these trials to current practice (Table 8).

Carfilzomib

Carfilzomib is a second-generation proteasome inhibitor. It is an epoxyketone that irreversibly binds to the proteasome through a covalent bond. Compared with bortezomib, carfilzomib has greater selectivity for chymotrypsin-like protease β5 subunit and lower affinity for trypsin- and caspase-like proteases.[192] In contrast, bortezomib binds to the proteasome reversibly and also inhibits other serine proteases (and which may account for its neurotoxicity).[280]

The initial approval of carfilzomib in July 2012 was based on a phase II trial, PX-171-003, that studied carfilzomib as a single agent in heavily pretreated MM patients.[281,282] Carfilzomib was given 20 mg/m² intravenously on days 1, 2, 8, 9, 15, 16 of a 28 day cycle; with cycle 2, the dose was increased to 27 mg/m². Dexamethasone 4 mg was only given as premedication. The patients in this trial received a median of 5 prior lines of treatment, and the regimen showed an ORR of 23.7% and median PFS 3.7 months. The ENDEAVOR trial directly compared carfilzomib with bortezomib in patients with relapsed disease.[274] This phase III study randomized patients with 1–3 prior lines of treatment to the combination of carfilzomib and dexamethasone or bortezomib and dexamethasone. Carfilzomib was given on days 1, 2, 8, 9, 15, and 16 with dexamethasone 20 mg on the days of carfilzomib plus

Table 8 Selected trials in relapsed/refractory multiple myeloma.

Reference	Name of trial	Arm	N	PFS	HR	ORR	≥VGPR	≥CR	Len. ref.	Prior lines
Dimopoulos et al.[265]	APOLLO	Dara Pd	151	12.4	0.63	69%	51%	25%	79%	2 (1–5)
		Pd	153	6.9		46%	20%	4%	80%	
Grosicki et al.[266]	BOSTON	SVd	195	13.93	0.7	74%	45%	24%	NR[a]	2 (1–3)
		Vd	207	9.46		62%	32%	11%	NR[a]	
Dimopoulos et al.[267]	CANDOR	Dara Kd	312	Not reached	0.63	84%	69%	29%	32%	2 (1–3)
		Kd	154	15.8		75%	48%	10%	36%	
Attal et al.[268]	ICARIA	Isa Pd	154	11.5	0.596	60%	32%	5%	94%	3 (2–11)
		Pd	153	6.5		35%	9%	2%	92%	
Richardson et al.[269]	OPTIMISMM	PVd	281	11.2	0.61	82%	53%	16%	71%	2 (1–3)
		Vd	278	7.1		50%	18%	4%	69%	
Dimopoulos et al.[270]	ELOQUENT-3	Elo Pd	60	10.3	0.54	53%	20%	8%	90%	3 (2–8)
		Pd	57	4.7		26%	9%	2%	84%	
Dimopoulos et al.;[170] Bahlis et al.[271]	POLLUX	Dara Rd	286	44.5	0.44	93%	76%	43%	NA	1 (1–11)
		Rd	283	17.5		76%	44%	19%	NA	
Palumbo et al.;[272] Spencer et al.[273]	CASTOR	Dara Vd	251	16.7	0.39	83%	59%	19%	18%	2 (1–10)
		Vd	247	7.1		63%	29%	9%	24%	
Dimopoulos et al.[274]	ENDEAVOR	Kd	464	18.7	0.53	77%	54%	13%	24%	2 (1–3)[b]
		Vd	465	9.4		63%	29%	6%	26%	
Moreau et al.[275]	TOURMALINE-MM1	Ixa Rd	360	20.6	0.74	78%	48%	12%	NA	1 (1–3)
		Rd	362	14.7		72%	39%	7%	NA	
Lonial et al.[276]	ELOQUENT-2	Elo Rd	321	19.4	0.7	79%	33%	4%	NA	2 (1–3)[b]
		Rd	325	14.9		66%	28%	7%	NA	
Stewart et al.[277]	ASPIRE	KRd	396	26.3	0.69	87%	70%	32%	NA	2 (1–3)
		Rd	396	17.6		67%	40%	9%	NA	
San Miguel et al.[278]	PANORAMA 1	Pano Vd	387	12.71	0.63	61%	28%	11%	NR	1 (1–3)
		Vd	381	8.54		55%	16%	6%	NR	
San Miguel et al.[279]	NIMBUS (MM-003)	Pd	302	3.8	0.41	31%	6%	1%	95%	5 (2–17)
		D	153	1.9		10%	1%	0%	92%	

Abbreviations: D, high-dose dexamethasone; d, low-dose dexamethasone; dara, daratumumab; elo, elotuzumab; ixa, ixazomib; isa, isatuximab; K, carfilzomib; P, pomalidomide; pano, panobinostat; R, lenalidomide; S, selinexor; V, bortezomib.
Median PFS is in months. Median number of prior lines of therapy and the range are shown.
NA, not applicable; patients with disease refractory to lenalidomide were excluded from the trial; NR, not reported.
[a]In the BOSTON study, 39% and 37% of the SVd and Vd arms respectively had prior lenalidomide treatment.
[b]Due to a protocol deviation, a patient in the bortezomib arm of ENDEAVOR and one patient in each arm of ELOQUENT-2 received 4 prior lines of treatment.

days 22 and 23 on a 28 day cycle. The dosing of carfilzomib was higher than the initial studies, starting with 20 mg/m² on days 1 and 2 of cycle 1 and then 56 mg/m² thereafter. Bortezomib was given according to the traditional schedule of 1.3 mg/m² on days 1, 4, 8, 11 on a 21-day cycle, with dexamethasone 20 mg the day of bortezomib and the day after. Bortezomib was administered either IV or SC according to the investigator; most patients (79%) received SC bortezomib throughout the study. The ORR was significantly higher in the carfilzomib arm, 77% versus 63% in the bortezomib arm ($p < 0.0001$), and median PFS was also higher, 18.7 versus 9.4 months ($p < 0.0001$). Of note, while 54% of patients had prior bortezomib, in a subgroup analysis, patients who were bortezomib-naïve also showed significantly improved PFS in the carfilzomib arm. An updated analysis showed improvement in overall survival with carfilzomib, 47.8 versus 38.8 months, with a HR 0.761 (0.633–0.915).[283]

Subsequent studies have evaluated combinations with carfilzomib. Notably, the ASPIRE trial was a phase III trial that examined the combination of carfilzomib with lenalidomide and dexamethasone (KRd) compared to lenalidomide and dexamethasone in relapsed MM.[277] Patients were eligible to participate if they received 1–3 prior lines of therapy. Prior lenalidomide and bortezomib treatment were permitted if there was no disease progression with these drugs; the majority of patients (80.2%) had not received prior lenalidomide therapy. Carfilzomib was given on the same schedule as described above in the PX-171-003 trial. From cycles 13–18, the second week of carfilzomib was omitted. After cycle 18, carfilzomib was discontinued. Lenalidomide was given 25 mg on days 1–21 with dexamethasone 40 mg weekly; the same schedule of lenalidomide and dexamethasone was given in the control group. The ORR was significantly higher in the carfilzomib arm compared to the control arm, 87.1% versus 66.7% ($p < 0.001$). The median progression-free survival was 26.3 versus 17.6 months ($p = 0.001$). An updated analysis showed improvement in overall survival with carfilzomib, 48.3 versus 40.4 months (one-sided $p = 0.0045$).[284]

A practical limitation of carfilzomib treatment is the twice/week schedule, especially since patients may be on therapy for a prolonged duration. The ARROW study compared a once-weekly schedule where carfilzomib is given at 70 mg/m² on days 1, 8, 15 with twice-weekly carfilzomib at 20 and 27 mg/m² on the conventional schedule in patients with relapsed disease and 2–3 prior lines of treatment.[285] The once-weekly schedule showed higher responses (overall response rate 62.9 vs 40.8%, $p < 0.0001$) and progression-free survival (11.2 vs 7.6 months, $p = 0.0029$).

While both are proteasome inhibitors, the side effects of carfilzomib are different than bortezomib. Carfilzomib has significantly less peripheral neuropathy than bortezomib. For example, in the ENDEAVOR study, grade ≥2 peripheral neuropathy was significantly higher in the bortezomib compared to the carfilzomib group, 32% versus 6% respectively; grade ≥3 peripheral neuropathy was 8% versus 2%. This was true even though the majority of patients (79%) in the bortezomib arm received it subcutaneously. However, cardiovascular adverse events are more common with carfilzomib. In an analysis of 11 phase 1–3 trials with carfilzomib, cardiovascular events (all grade/grade ≥3) included hypertension (18.5/5.9%), dyspnea (31.9/4.5%), and cardiac failure (6.7/4.4%).[286] However, the frequency of discontinuation or death due to these events was comparable between carfilzomib and the control arms. A prospective study of cardiac events during treatment with carfilzomib or bortezomib found that elevated natriuretic peptides occurring mid-first cycle of treatment was associated with a substantially higher risk of these adverse events.[287]

A substudy of the ENDEAVOR study focusing on echocardiography did not show a reduction in ejection fraction.[286] This suggests that the heart failure related to carfilzomib is not from direct cardiotoxicity, as seen with trastuzumab or anthracyclines. The mechanism of cardiovascular side effects is not understood, though endothelial toxicity has been proposed as a possible mediator.[288] Thrombotic microangiopathy has also been described with carfilzomib and proteasome inhibitors in general.[289]

Carfilzomib in newly diagnosed disease
Carfilzomib has been evaluated in newly diagnosed disease. For example, a phase II study of extended treatment carfilzomib with lenalidomide and dexamethasone (KRd) along with high-dose melphalan and transplant showed rapid achievement of impressive responses and a 5 year PFS of 72%.[290] Moreover, the FORTE trial, which has two of its three arms randomized to KRd with autologous stem cell transplant versus KRd for 12 cycles without upfront transplant, showed comparable outcomes between both arms.[291]

However, despite carfilzomib showing superiority over bortezomib in relapsed disease based on the ENDEAVOR study, a similar level of benefit has not been demonstrated in two randomized studies, CLARION and ENDURANCE. The CLARION study compared in transplant-ineligible patients the combination of carfilzomib, melphalan, prednisone (KMP) with the established standard of VMP from the VISTA trial.[292] There was no difference in PFS with KMP. While the grade ≥2 peripheral neuropathy rate was lower with KMP (2.5% vs 35.1%), there were more episodes of all grade acute renal failure (13.9% vs 6.2%) and cardiac failure (10.8% vs 4.3%) with KMP compared to VMP. In transplant-eligible patients, the ENDURANCE trial (ECOG E1A11) compared carfilzomib, lenalidomide, dexamethasone (KRd) with the standard triplet regimen of bortezomib, lenalidomide, and dexamethasone (RVd) that is widely used in the United States, with the goal of informing clinical practice.[166] Notably, patients with high risk disease (e.g., t(14;16), t(14;20), or del(17p), LDH >2 × upper limit of normal) were excluded from participation. Carfilzomib was given on the conventional twice/week schedule at 36 mg/m^2. The trial found no significant difference in PFS or OS. There was more grade 3–4 neuropathy with bortezomib compared to the carfilzomib (8% vs <1%). On the other hand, there was more dyspnea (7% vs 2%); thromboembolic grade 3–4 events (5% vs 2%); and worsening renal function (1.3% vs 0.38%) in the carfilzomib arm. Interestingly, while there were more cardiac and renal adverse events with carfilzomib, the rate of discontinuation due to adverse events, complication, or death was actually higher in the bortezomib arm (17.9% vs 12.3%). Overall, given the similar PFS, the authors of the study concluded that RVd should be the preferred regimen. However, one limitation in the interpretation of ENDURANCE is that patients with high-risk disease were not evaluated in this trial, and it is possible that high-risk disease is where more of the benefit of carfilzomib may be seen.

Pomalidomide
Pomalidomide (CC-4047) is the third IMiD that was developed, with efficacy in MM refractory to lenalidomide. While its structure is similar to both thalidomide and lenalidomide, compared with thalidomide, pomalidomide is more tumoricidal and has greater immunomodulation and anti-inflammatory effects.[293] *In vitro*, pomalidomide degrades substrates of cereblon more rapidly and completely than lenalidomide or thalidomide.[294] Clinically, its side effect profile is notable for neutropenia and fatigue; rash is not as common as with lenalidomide.[295]

A phase III European study compared pomalidomide and low-dose dexamethasone with monotherapy with high-dose dexamethasone.[279] This study enrolled patients with refractory disease who received at least two previous consecutive cycles of bortezomib and lenalidomide, alone or in combination, and who had adequate alkylator treatment (e.g., as part of an autologous stem cell transplant). Patients in the trial had received a median of five prior lines of treatment. The median PFS with pomalidomide plus low-dose dexamethasone was 3.8 versus 1.9 months ($p < 0.0001$). Adjusting for crossover, the median OS was 12.7 versus 5.7 months.[296]

While high-dose dexamethasone by itself is not typically used in the United States, this study showed that pomalidomide and low-dose dexamethasone was effective in disease refractory to lenalidomide and bortezomib. Based on these findings, pomalidomide with low-dose dexamethasone was approved by the FDA in February 2013 for patients with refractory disease and who have received at least two prior therapies including lenalidomide and a proteasome inhibitor.

The OPTIMISMM study evaluated the addition of pomalidomide to the doublet of bortezomib and dexamethasone.[269] This phase III study randomized patients with relapsed disease, prior lenalidomide treatment, and 1–3 prior lines of therapy to pomalidomide, bortezomib, dexamethasone versus bortezomib, and dexamethasone. The addition of pomalidomide significantly improved PFS (11.2 vs 7.1 months, HR 0.61, $p < 0.0001$), though with higher rates of grade 3–4 neutropenia (42% vs 9%) and infections (31% vs 18%). This randomized trial is notable as one of the initial phase III trials in a lenalidomide-refractory or exposed patient population, which is increasingly relevant given the widespread use of lenalidomide upfront and as maintenance therapy. Overall, these studies with pomalidomide set the stage for several pomalidomide combinations used in relapsed disease (see below).

Ixazomib
Ixazomib (previously known as MLN9708) is an oral proteasome inhibitor where preclinical data demonstrated superior pharmacodynamics, a shorter dissociation half-life, and greater antitumor activity compared to bortezomib.[297] In preclinical models, ixazomib showed activity in bortezomib-resistant MM cells.[298] TOURMALINE-MM1 was a phase III study that compared the combination of ixazomib with lenalidomide and dexamethasone (IRd) versus lenalidomide and dexamethasone (Rd) in patients with relapsed disease and 1–3 prior lines of treatment.[275] The majority of patients (69%) had prior bortezomib treatment, and only 12% had prior lenalidomide treatment. The median PFS was significantly higher in the IRd arm, 20.6 versus 14.7 months in the Rd arm ($p = 0.012$). The toxicity profile between both arms was generally similar, including peripheral neuropathy. However, rash was higher in the ixazomib arm versus the control arm: all grades, 36% versus 17%; grade 3–4 rash 5% versus 2% in the control arm. Based on these encouraging findings in the TOURMALINE-MM1 study, the FDA-approved ixazomib in November 2015 as part of a combination with lenalidomide and dexamethasone in patients with relapsed disease who have received at least one prior therapy. This was an important advance as an all oral triplet combination for relapsed disease.

Ixazomib has been evaluated in newly diagnosed multiple myeloma in the TOURMALINE-MM-2 study.[299] Patients who were not candidates for high-dose therapy were randomized to ixazomib, lenalidomide, and dexamethasone versus lenalidomide and dexamethasone. While there was an improvement in PFS from 21.8 to 35.3 months (HR = 0.83), the finding was not statistically significant ($p = 0.073$).

Histone deacetylase (HDAC) inhibitors

Histone deacetylase (HDAC) inhibitors are another class of drugs with activity in relapsed, refractory myeloma. By increasing histone acetylation, HDAC inhibition activates transcription and other nuclear events. There are several classes of HDACs, and there are also substrates of HDACs in the cytoplasm that are not related to histones. These nonhistone effects may be key to their efficacy, such as effects on protein degradation via the aggresome, protein–protein interactions, and protein localization. In MM, preclinical work with proteasome and HDAC inhibitors showed synergistic activity with accumulation of polyubiquitinated proteins and activation of apoptosis.[300,301] Combinations are necessary, since HDAC inhibitors do not have significant activity in MM as single agents.

Panobinostat (LBH589) is an oral pan-HDAC inhibitor. PANORAMA 1 was a phase III trial comparing panobinostat, bortezomib, and dexamethasone to bortezomib and dexamethasone in patients with 1–3 prior lines of therapy.[278] Patients with disease refractory to bortezomib were excluded. Panobinostat 20 mg was given orally on Monday, Wednesday, Friday for 2 weeks, and bortezomib was given intravenously on a conventional 21 day schedule on days 1, 4, 8, and 11. The median PFS was significantly longer in the panobinostat arm, 11.99 months versus 8.08 months in the control arm ($p < 0.0001$). However, there was more grade 3-4 diarrhea in the panobinostat arm (25%) than in the control arm (8%). Deaths due causes other than disease progression were also higher in the panobinostat arm (7% vs 3%). Given some of these concerns, the FDA in November 2014 deferred accelerated approval of panobinostat as second-line therapy. Panobinostat was later re-evaluated in patients with a median of two prior therapies. The median PFS was 10.6 months in the panobinostat arm versus 5.8 months in the control arm. In this setting, the FDA gave panobinostat accelerated approval in February 2015 in patients who received at least two prior lines of therapy, including bortezomib and an IMiD.[302]

With the increasing number of options for relapsed disease, where panobinostat fits in the sequence of treatment is under evaluation. PANORAMA 3 evaluated lower doses of panobinostat with subcutaneous bortezomib and dexamethasone.[303] This trial found significant improvements in the adverse event profile with less diarrhea and myelosuppression when bortezomib was given subcutaneously compared to PANORAMA-1.

Elotuzumab

Elotuzumab is a humanized recombinant monoclonal IgG1 antibody that targets signaling lymphocyte activation molecule (SLAMF7), also known as CS1 (CD2-subset-1). SLAMF7 is a cell surface glycoprotein that is highly expressed on both normal and MM plasma cells, as well as at a lower level on natural killer (NK) cells.[304,305] Elotuzumab flags myeloma cells for recognition by NK cells for antibody-dependent cellular cytotoxicity and enhances NK cell activity against MM cells by binding to SLAMF7 found on NK cells.[306]

By itself, elotuzumab did not show significant clinical activity in a phase I trial.[307] Elotuzumab enhances the activity of lenalidomide or pomalidomide doublets with dexamethasone. A phase III study, ELOQUENT-2, compared the combination of elotuzumab, lenalidomide, and dexamethasone to lenalidomide and dexamethasone in patients with relapsed disease and 1–3 prior lines of therapy.[276] Of note, the trial limited enrollment of patients with prior lenalidomide treatment to 10%. Elotuzumab 10 mg/kg was given weekly for the first two cycles and then every other week. Lenalidomide and dexamethasone were given according to the conventional 28-day schedule. This trial enrolled 646 patients with a median of two prior lines of therapy. A significant proportion had high-risk FISH (32% with del(17p) and 9% with t(4;14)). The elotuzumab-containing arm had superior progression-free survival (19.4 vs 14.9 months in the control group, hazard ratio 0.7, $p < 0.001$), and the ORR was also higher (79% vs 66%, $p < 0.001$). Moreover, elotuzumab improved median overall survival (48.3 vs 39.6 months, HR 0.82, $p = 0.0408$).[308] The addition of elotuzumab was tolerated well as adverse effects were similar between both arms, except for infusion reactions with elotuzumab (10% grade 1–2). ELOQUENT-2 is the first study to show the benefit in progression-free and overall survival of adding a monoclonal antibody to conventional treatment in MM. In November 2015, the FDA approved elotuzumab in combination with lenalidomide and dexamethasone in patients who have received one to three prior lines of treatment.

Elotuzumab has been evaluated in more advanced disease in combination with pomalidomide and dexamethasone in the randomized phase II study, ELOQUENT-3.[270] Eligible patients had received two or more prior lines of treatment as well as prior treatment with lenalidomide and a proteasome inhibitor. Patients were randomized to elotuzumab with pomalidomide and dexamethasone versus pomalidomide and dexamethasone. Adding elotuzumab significantly improved median PFS, 10.3 versus 4.7 months (HR 0.54, $p = 0.008$) along with doubling the response rate (53% vs 26%). Interestingly, grade 3–4 neutropenia was lower in the elotuzumab arm (13% vs 27%). Finally, three patients in the study (2.6%) had received prior daratumumab, though the numbers are too small to make any conclusions about use of elotuzumab after prior daratumumab treatment. While the benefit with elotuzumab seems greater in this more pretreated population in ELQOUENT-3, in contrast, in newly diagnosed patients, the efficacy of elotuzumab awaits demonstration. In the ELOQUENT-1 trial, newly diagnosed patients not eligible for high-dose therapy were randomized to elotuzumab and lenalidomide and dexamethasone versus lenalidomide and dexamethasone.[309] However, preliminary results showed that the addition of elotuzumab did not improve PFS.

Daratumumab

Daratumumab is a human IgG1κ monoclonal antibody that targets CD38. Two initial phase I/II studies of daratumumab as a single agent in patients with a median of four prior lines of treatment showed an ORR of 31% and 29.2% and median PFS of 5.6 and 3.7 months.[310,311] Based on this single-agent efficacy, the FDA gave accelerated approval to daratumumab in November 2015. Daratumumab was then evaluated in combinations with bortezomib and dexamethasone (CASTOR)[272] or lenalidomide and dexamethasone (POLLUX) in relapsed disease.[170] Both studies showed that the addition of daratumumab significantly improved median PFS with either combination: with bortezomib and dexamethasone, 16.7 versus 7.1 months (HR 0.31, $p < 0.0001$)[273] and with lenalidomide and dexamethasone, 44.5 versus 17.5 months

(HR, 0.44, $p < 0.0001$)[271] in patients with a median of two and one prior line of therapy, respectively. Responses were deep, with patients achieving high rates of negative minimal residual disease at 10^{-5}, 30.4% versus 5.3% in the POLLUX study, which was a significant achievement, given that these patients had relapsed disease. Based on these trials, the FDA approved these combinations in November 2016.

Daratumumab has also been evaluated in combination with pomalidomide and dexamethasone in the EQUULEUS study.[312] This study enrolled patients with a median of three prior lines of treatment, all with prior lenalidomide treatment, with a median PFS of 8.8 months and ORR of 60%. This combination was approved by the FDA in June 2017. The APOLLO study is a randomized study evaluating subcutaneous daratumumab with pomalidomide and dexamethasone versus pomalidomide and dexamethasone.[265] PFS was longer in the daratumumab arm, 12.4 versus 6.9 months in the control arm, (HR = 0.63, $p = 0.0018$) along with higher ORR, 69% versus 46%. Finally, daratumumab has also been studied in combination with carfilzomib and dexamethasone. The CANDOR study was a randomized phase III study that compared the combination of daratumumab with carfilzomib and dexamethasone versus carfilzomib and dexamethasone.[267] Carfilzomib was given on a twice/week schedule at 56 mg/m². The addition of daratumumab improved the median PFS, not reached versus 15.8 months (HR 0.63, $p = 0.0027$). This regimen with carfilzomib was approved by the FDA in August 2020.

Isatuximab

Isatuximab (SAR650984) is a chimeric IgG1 kappa monoclonal antibody that targets CD38, similar to daratumumab. Antibody-dependent cellular cytotoxicity is the primary mechanism by which isatuximab eliminates myeloma cells.[313] Additional mechanisms of action include pro-apoptotic activity that is independent of cross-linking, as well as inhibition of CD38 ectoenzyme function. In contrast to daratumumab, there is less complement-dependent cytotoxicity.[220]

Initial studies evaluated isatuximab as a single agent in relapsed/refractory multiple myeloma. In a phase II study of patients with a median of 5 prior lines of therapy, the overall response rate was 24.3%, with a median progression-free survival of 4.6 months.[314] These findings were similar to the first approved anti-CD38 monoclonal antibody, daratumumab, in a similar patient population. A phase III, randomized study, ICARIA, evaluated isatuximab in combination with pomalidomide and dexamethasone versus pomalidomide and dexamethasone in relapsed and refractory disease.[268] This study enrolled patients with a median of 3 prior lines of therapy, and it showed that the addition of pomalidomide improved ORR to 60% versus 35% in the control arm. Moreover, there was an improvement in PFS to 11.53 months versus 6.47 months (HR 0.596, $p = 0.001$). The findings in this study led to the FDA approval of isatuximab with pomalidomide and dexamethasone in March 2020. Similar to the CANDOR study with daratumumab, isatuximab has been studied in a phase III, randomized study, IKEMA, with carfilzomib and dexamethasone versus carfilzomib and dexamethasone.[315] This study evaluated patients with a median of two prior lines of treatment. The addition of isatuximab improved PFS: the median PFS was not reached in the isatuximab arm versus 19.15 months in the control arm, HR 0.531 ($p = 0.0007$).

Selinexor

Selinexor (KPT-330) is an oral inhibitor of exportin 1 (XPO1), a nuclear exporter of tumor suppressor proteins and messenger RNAs that are involved with proliferation.[316] By inhibiting XPO1, selinexor reactivates tumor suppressor proteins and glucocorticoid receptor signaling, in the presence of dexamethasone.[317] The STORM trial evaluated the combination of selinexor and dexamethasone in a heavily pretreated, relapsed, refractory patient population that had prior treatment with lenalidomide, pomalidomide, bortezomib, carfilzomib, and daratumumab, and was refractory to an IMiD, proteasome inhibitor, and daratumumab.[318] In this patient population, patients with disease refractory to daratumumab have a median overall survival of 8.6 months.[319] Selinexor was given 80 mg twice/week. In the STORM study, the median PFS was 3.7 months with an ORR of 26%. Selinexor is associated with grade 3–4 gastrointestinal adverse events such as nausea (10%), diarrhea (7%), and vomiting (3%). Attention to supportive care and use of, for example, olanzapine can be helpful in managing these adverse events.[320] Based on this trial, the FDA gave accelerated approval to selinexor with dexamethasone in this patient population in July 2019. Selinexor was then evaluated in the BOSTON study, a randomized study of selinexor, bortezomib, dexamethasone versus bortezomib and dexamethasone in patients with 1–3 prior lines of therapy.[266] In this trial, selinexor is given less frequently, weekly, at a dose of 100 mg. In the selinexor arm, bortezomib was only given weekly, whereas in the control arm, bortezomib was given on the conventional twice/week schedule. The addition of selinexor significantly improved median PFS: 13.93 versus 9.46 months (HR 0.7, $p = 0.0075$), even though the dosing of bortezomib and dexamethasone was less in the selinexor arm. Selinexor is currently being evaluated with various partners in the STOMP trial (NCT02343042), such as carfilzomib, pomalidomide, and daratumumab.

B-cell maturation antigen (BCMA)

B-cell maturation antigen (BCMA) is one of the newest and more promising targets in MM, following the flurry of activity targeting CD38 with daratumumab and isatuximab. BCMA is a transmembrane protein, also known as tumor necrosis factor receptor superfamily member 17 (TNFRSF17), which plays a key role in B-cell proliferation and survival, as well as maturation and differentiation into plasma cells.[321] BCMA is expressed in nearly all bone marrow samples, with no difference between newly diagnosed or relapsed disease.[322] Significantly higher levels of BCMA expression are seen in myeloma and plasma cells compared to other tissues. Ligands for BCMA include BAFF (B-cell activating factor) and APRIL (a proliferation-inducing ligand). Membrane-bound BCMA is cleaved by gamma-secretase to release soluble BCMA.

Belantamab mafodotin (GSK2857916) is an antibody–drug conjugate that is the first approved drug to target BCMA. It is a humanized and afucosylated anti-BCMA antibody conjugated to the microtubule inhibitor, monomethyl auristatin F (MMAF).[323] The initial DREAMM-1 study evaluated belantamab mafodotin in a relapsed, refractory patient population with a median of 5 prior lines of treatment, dosed at 3.4 mg/kg intravenously every 3 weeks. The study showed a response rate of 60% and a median PFS of 12 months.[324,325] The subsequent DREAMM-2 study evaluated belantamab mafodotin in a more relapsed and refractory population, as all patients had prior therapy with anti-CD38 monoclonal antibody.[326] Patients were randomized to two different doses, 2.5 and 3.4 mg/kg given every 3 weeks. In this study, patients had received a median of 7 and 6 prior lines of therapy, respectively, and all had prior treatment with lenalidomide and nearly all with bortezomib. The ORR was 30% and 34%, respectively, with a median PFS of 2.9 and 4.9 months, respectively. Ocular toxicity is one of the key limitations of belantamab mafodotin. This study required ophthalmology evaluation prior to each treatment. Grade 3 or higher keratopathy occurred in 27% and 20% of patients in the 2.5 and 3.4 mg/kg cohorts. The 2.5 mg/kg dose was selected for future studies based on its more favorable safety profile. Belantamab mafodotin received accelerated approval by the FDA in August 2020, with a REMS program to help manage the ocular toxicities.

There are ongoing studies evaluating belantamab mafodotin in various combinations. This includes a combination with bortezomib (DREAMM-6);[327] a platform protocol to evaluate belantamab mafodotin in combination with novel agents, for example, an OX40 agonist antibody or a gamma-secretase inhibitor, nirogacestat (DREAMM-5).[328] Pivotal studies that are ongoing or pending include DREAMM-7, which evaluates belantamab mafodotin, bortezomib, dexamethasone versus daratumumab, bortezomib, dexamethasone; DREAMM-8, belantamab, pomalidomide, dexamethasone versus pomalidomide, bortezomib, and dexamethasone; and DREAMM-9, which evaluates in newly diagnosed patients, belantamab mafodotin with bortezomib, lenalidomide, dexamethasone versus bortezomib, lenalidomide, and dexamethasone.[329]

Bispecific antibodies and chimeric antigen receptor T-cell (CAR T-cell) therapies targeting BCMA are under active investigation in MM.[330] Bispecific antibodies bring together T-cells and malignant cells that express the target of interest, leading to T-cell activation and lysis of the targeted cell. Blinatumomab is an example of an approved bispecific T-cell engager, in this case targeting CD19, in relapsed acute lymphoblastic leukemia.[331] In MM, AMG 420 is a bispecific T-cell engager targeting BCMA. In a first in human study of AMG 420, at a maximum tolerated dose of 400 mcg/day, the overall response rate was 70% in a relapsed population with a median of 3.5 prior lines of therapy.[332] However, the main limitation with AMG 420 is its administration as a continuous infusion for 4 weeks without interruption. AMG 701 is an extended half-life bispecific antibody that may be given weekly and is under investigation. Other bispecific antibodies under investigation include CC-93269 and teclistamab (JNJ-7957). In the phase I study, CC-93269 is given weekly intravenously for the first three cycles, then every other week for cycles 3–6, and then once every 4 weeks thereafter; each cycle is 4 weeks long. Preliminary data in patients with a median of 5 prior lines of treatment, including anti-CD38 therapy in 96.7%, showed an ORR of 43.3% across all doses, and 88.9% at the higher 10 mg dose, including MRD negative responses.[333] Cytokine release syndrome (CRS) occurred in 76.7% of patients, including 3.3% grade ≥3; tocilizumab was used in 43.3% of patients. Teclistamab was evaluated in patients with a median of 6 prior lines of therapy and achieved an ORR of 67% at a dose 270 mcg/kg.[334] CRS occurred in 56% of patients, with no grade 3 CRS; tocilizumab was given in 26% of patients. Dose escalation of teclistamab is ongoing.

Cellular therapies using chimeric antigen receptor T-cells (CAR T) have emerged as one of the more promising new developments in MM therapy. T-lymphocytes are genetically modified *ex vivo* to express a CAR that targets a tumor antigen of interest, such as BCMA in MM.[330] CAR constructs generally consist of a single-chain variable fragment (scFv) connected to the CD3ζ intracellular signaling domain along with a costimulatory domain such as CD28 or 4-1BB. Based on unprecedented results across several B-cell lymphoproliferative malignancies, CAR T-cells targeting CD19 are now approved in acute lymphoblastic leukemia in 2017 (tisagenlecleucel);[335] diffuse large B cell lymphoma in 2017 and 2018 (axicabtagene ciloleucel and tisagenlecleucel);[336,337] and mantle cell lymphoma in 2020 (brexucabtagene autoleucel).[338]

Building on the progress with CAR T-cells in B-cell malignancies, application of CAR T-cells in MM is rapidly moving forward. The furthest along in clinical development is idecabtagene vicleucel (ide-cel; bb2121). Ide-cel is a second-generation CAR consisting of a scFv targeting BCMA with a CD3ζ signaling domain and 4-1BB costimulatory domain. (Of note, the majority of anti-BCMA CAR T-cell therapies under evaluation have a 4-1BB costimulatory domain.) In a phase I study of 33 patients with a median of 7 prior lines of treatment (prior carfilzomib, 91%; pomalidomide, 94%; daratumumab, 82%), the ORR was 85%.[339] For the 30 patients who received $\geq 150 \times 10^6$ cells, the median PFS was 11.8 months. The responses were deep in this cohort, and in 16 of these 30 patients, no MRD could be detected (10^{-4}). Cytokine release syndrome occurred in 76%, with grade 3 in 6% of patients. Neurotoxicity occurred 42% of patients, with one grade 4 event (3%). There is an ongoing phase III study, KarMMa-3, comparing ide-cel with standard of care. At the time of this writing, the FDA has set a Prescription Drug User Fee Act (PDUFA) goal date of 27 March 2021. Ciltacabtagene autoleucel (cilta-cel; JNJ-68284528) is following closely in clinical development. Cilta-cel is the same construct as LCAR-B38M, which was evaluated in one of the earlier phase I trials of anti-BCMA CAR in China.[340] Initial results from the CARTITUDE-1 phase 1–2 study of cilta-cel in 29 patients with a median of 5 prior lines of treatment and 100% prior daratumumab showed a 100% ORR, with 100% of 17 evaluable patients MRD negative (10^{-4}).[341] CRS occurred in 93% of patients, with 6% grade 3 or higher, and 10% neurotoxicity with 3% grade 3. Updated results show a 9 month PFS of 86%.[342] A third CAR T-cell study is the EVOLVE study of orvacabtagene autoleucel (orva-cel). A potentially differentiating feature of this product is that the manufacturing is designed to yield a specified ratio of CD4+ and CD8+ CAR T-cells to enrich for central memory phenotype. Updated results of the phase 1–2 EVOLVE of 62 patients treated at dose levels of $\geq 300 \times 10^6$ cells showed 89% all grade CRS and 3% grade ≥3; 13% all grade neurotoxicity and 3% grade ≥3.[343] Overall response rate was 92% and median PFS was 9.3 months for 300×10^6 cells (and median PFS not reached at the higher dose levels). Ongoing anti-BCMA CAR T-cell studies of note include a phase III study, KarMMa-3, comparing ide-cel with standard of care, ide-cel after induction therapy in high risk newly diagnosed patients with R-ISS III (KarMMa-4), and ide-cel in patients with early relapse (KarMMa-2).

Choosing therapy in relapsed disease

The choice of therapy for patients with relapsed disease depends on a number of factors, as is true with the initial treatment. These include host factors, such as the performance status or frailty of the patient, and disease-specific factors. A patient presenting with extramedullary disease or acute onset of hypercalcemia and renal dysfunction may warrant more aggressive treatment than a patient with a slowly rising monoclonal protein (who may be closely observed). The timing of the relapse is also important too, as patients who relapse early, for example, less than a year after an autologous SCT (which occurs in 24% of patients undergoing autologous SCT), have a worse prognosis.[344] Recent analysis of early relapse (e.g., within 18 months from start of therapy), even with the availability of more effective salvage regimens, also continues to show worse outcomes.[345,346]

Options for treatment at time of relapse include the regimens listed above and will depend on what treatment the patient has previously received. Other combinations in use include carfilzomib, pomalidomide, dexamethasone;[347,348] carfilzomib, cyclophosphamide, dexamethasone;[349] and pomalidomide, cyclophosphamide, dexamethasone.[350] Bendamustine has also been evaluated for treatment of relapsed disease, for example, in combination with bortezomib,[351] carfilzomib,[352] or lenalidomide.[353] The choice of regimen depends on what agents are available as well as local practice.

In select patients who are experiencing an aggressive, rapid relapse for example, with a high burden of extramedullary disease and where there is an urgent need for cytoreduction, a salvage infusional regimen combining traditional cytotoxic drugs may be appropriate. These regimens include DCEP (dexamethasone, cyclophosphamide, etoposide, cisplatin), VTD-PACE (bortezomib, thalidomide, dexamethasone, cisplatin, doxorubicin, cyclophosphamide, etoposide), and CVAD (dexamethasone, cyclophosphamide, vincristine, and doxorubicin).[354]

Under investigation

Venetoclax

Dysregulation of the apoptotic pathway mediated by anti-apoptotic proteins such as BCL-2, BCL-XL, and MCL-1 plays an important role across a range of malignancies.[355] Venetoclax (ABT-199) is an oral selective inhibitor of BCL-2 and is the first drug of this class approved in chronic lymphocytic leukemia and acute myelogenous leukemia. In MM, targeting BCL-2 began with preclinical work showing activity of venetoclax in MM cell lines, especially in cell lines with the t(11;14) translocation or a high BCL-2/MCL-1 ratio.[356] The increased activity in t(11;14) MM may reflect a higher BCL-2/MCL-1 ratio compared to other subgroups, based on gene expression profiling and not necessarily from cyclin D1.[357] Motivated by early clinical trial data showing activity of venetoclax as a single agent in patients with t(11;14)[358] and in combination with bortezomib and dexamethasone,[359] venetoclax was evaluated in a randomized trial, BELLINI.

In BELLINI, patients with 1–3 prior lines of treatment were randomized to venetoclax, bortezomib, dexamethasone versus bortezomib and dexamethasone.[360] Unexpectedly, while the venetoclax arm was superior to the control arm for the primary PFS endpoint PFS (22.4 vs 11.5 months, HR 0.6, $p=0.01$), overall survival was unexpectedly worse (HR 2.03, $p=0.034$). However, in the t(11;14) subset (12% of overall population), there was a marked improvement in PFS, median not reached versus 9.3 months (HR 0.09, $p=0.003$), and OS was not worse (not reached vs not reached, $HR = 0.68$, $p = 0.647$).[361] Similar benefit was seen in patients with BCL2^{high} expression without t(11;14) with improvement in PFS (not reached vs 10.2 months, $HR = 0.41$, $p=0.011$) without compromise in OS, HR 0.92 ($p=0.866$). These findings suggest that a biomarker-driven approach by selecting patients with t(11;14) or BCL2^{high} may identify patients who benefit the most from venetoclax. There is an ongoing phase III study, CANOVA (NCT03539744), evaluating venetoclax plus dexamethasone versus pomalidomide and dexamethasone in patients with relapsed multiple myeloma with t(11;14).

Cereblon E3 ligase modulators (CELMoDs)

Cereblon modulators (CELMoDs) represent a new class of drugs that bind to cereblon to promote degradation of specified substrates similar to lenalidomide and pomalidomide, and in the case of new CELMoDs, may include additional substrates beyond Ikaros and Aiolos.[362,363] Iberdomide (CC-220) and CC-92480 are CELMoDs in clinical development that could be viewed as the next generation of IMiDs. Iberdomide binds to cereblon with higher affinity than lenalidomide or pomalidomide and leads to more rapid degradation of Ikaros and Aiolos, with greater efficacy in lenalidomide-sensitive and -resistant cell lines.[364,365] Initial studies of iberdomide and dexamethasone in patients with a median of 5 prior lines of therapy, all with prior treatment with lenalidomide (and prior anti CD38 antibody exposure, 74.2%) showed an ORR of 32.2%.[366] Iberdomide is currently under evaluation in combinations with daratumumab, bortezomib, or carfilzomib. CC-92480 was identified through a strategy that selected cereblon modulators based on speed of Aiolos degradation.[367] Initial studies of CC-92480 with dexamethasone in patients with a median of 6 prior lines of treatment showed an ORR of 21.1%, and at the recommended phase II dose where 7 out of 11 patients were triple class refractory, the response rate was 54.8%.[368]

Melflufen

Melflufen is a melphalan-containing prodrug where aminopeptidase N (which is found at higher levels in malignant cells) converts the prodrug to melphalan, allowing for higher concentrations of intracellular melphalan than achievable by free melphalan.[369] Preclinical work showed that melflufen is effective in melphalan- and bortezomib- resistant cell lines.[369] In a phase I/II trial, melflufen given intravenously with dexamethasone achieved an ORR of 31% and a median PFS of 5.7 months in patients with a median of 4 prior lines of treatment.[370] Thrombocytopenia and neutropenia were the main reported adverse events, and notably gastrointestinal toxicities were not common; alopecia was not reported. In the phase II HORIZON study, melflufen and dexamethasone were evaluated in patients with disease refractory to daratumumab and/or pomalidomide, with a response rate of 28%.[371] The ANCHOR study evaluated melflufen and dexamethasone in combination with daratumumab or bortezomib, where it showed an ORR of 76% and 67%, respectively.[372] There is an ongoing study, OCEAN, that is evaluating melflufen plus dexamethasone versus pomalidomide plus dexamethasone in patients who have received 2–4 prior therapies (NCT03151811).

Checkpoint inhibition

Another area of interest and therapy development is blocking the interactions between the tumor cells and immune cells.[373] PD-1 and PD-L1 are two targets of interest. PD-1 is a receptor present on T-cells that interacts with PD-L1 expressed on tumor cells. MM cells have increased levels of PD-L1,[374] providing the rationale for anti-PD1 therapy in MM. Anti-PD1 antibodies are being used in hematological malignancies,[375] and nivolumab is approved in Hodgkin's disease. However, randomized studies with combinations of pembrolizumab with the IMiDs lenalidomide in newly diagnosed MM[376] or pomalidomide in relapsed MM showed unexpectedly worse outcomes.[377,378] However, it is possible that other modalities or drugs may partner better with checkpoint inhibitors than IMiDs. For example, DREAMM-4 is evaluating pembrolizumab in combination with belantamab mafodotin (NCT03848845). There are ongoing clinical trials exploring PD-1 blockade in combination with dendritic cell/myeloma fusion vaccine.[379,380]

Targeting specific mutations

The RAS/MAPK pathway is the most frequently mutated pathway in MM. For example, in one study mutations occurred as follows: KRAS (23%), NRAS (20%), and BRAF (6%).[142]

In newly diagnosed patients, mutations occurred in this pathway in 43.2% of patients.[123] Initial case reports of BRAF inhibition with vemurafenib suggest that mutations in *BRAF* are driver mutations.[381,382] A basket study of vemurafenib showed responses in 22.2% patients.[383] A retrospective study of the MEK inhibitor trametinib in patients with mutations in *KRAS*, *NRAS*, or *BRAF* showed a response rate of 40%.[384] There is an ongoing study of dabrafenib and trametinib in patients with mutations in *KRAS*, *NRAS*, or *BRAF* (NCT03091257). The Multiple Myeloma Research Foundation is leading the MyDRUG trial (NCT03732703), which evaluates a mutation-driven approach to high-risk relapsed disease.[385] This uses a backbone regimen of pomalidomide, ixazomib, and dexamethasone. Based on the results of sequencing, patients are assigned to an arm of the trial that combines the backbone regimen with a specific drug based on the results of sequencing. Some examples include CDK activating mutation, abemaciclib; IDH activating mutation, enasidenib; RAF or RAS mutation, cobimetinib; FGFR3 activating mutation, erdafitinib; t(11;14), venetoclax. Patients without an actionable mutation receive daratumumab in combination with the backbone regimen.

Complications

Bone disease

The presence of osteolytic bone lesions, bone pain, pathological fractures, or generalized bone loss (or osteoporosis) is a well-defined feature of myeloma.[386] Myeloma bone disease is characterized by an imbalance between osteoblast and osteoclast activities, with suppression of bone formation by osteoblasts and uncoupled activation of osteoclasts (Figure 2).[387,388] The ligand for receptor activator of NFκB (RANKL) binds to RANK receptor to stimulate osteoclast differentiation, formation, and survival;[389] myeloma cells produce RANKL and up-regulate RANKL expression in bone marrow stromal cells and osteoblasts via direct contact, signal induction, or production of IL-7.[390-393] Moreover, myeloma cells promote suppression of osteoprotegerin (OPG),[394-396] a decoy receptor which normally prevents RANK-RANKL interaction,[397] via soluble factors, integrin $α_4β_1$-VCAM1 interaction,[398] production of dickkopf-1 (DKK1),[399] or inactivation by syndecan-mediated internalization into myeloma cells.[400] OPG levels are decreased in the serum of myeloma patients and correlate with the presence of lytic bone lesions;[401] a high RANKL/OPG ratio is associated with a poor prognosis.[402]

Bisphosphonates play a key role in the supportive management of MM by inhibiting osteoclast activity, improving pain related to lytic bone disease, and decreasing skeletal-related events, beginning with pamidronate[403] and then zoledronic acid.[404] Bisphosphonates are drugs that share a P-C-P backbone and accumulate in the mineral phase of bone. They not only reduce osteoclast activity by inhibiting farnesyl pyrophosphate synthase[405] and modulate osteoblast activity but also have an effect on tumor burden;[406] a similar response is reported with OPG peptidomimetics and RANKL constructs using *in vivo* xenograft models.[407]

A randomized trial showed that pamidronate reduced skeletal-related events, including pathologic fractures, radiation therapy to bone, and spinal cord compression in patients with Durie–Salmon stage III MM and ≥1 lytic bone lesion.[403] Moreover, pamidronate significantly improved quality of life, with decreases in pain scores seen within a month. Zoledronic acid is more potent than pamidronate, and it has the advantage of a shorter infusion time with similar efficacy compared to pamidronate for preventing skeletal-related events (SRE).[408] The MRC Myeloma IX trial demonstrated the superiority of zoledronic acid compared with the oral bisphosphonate clodronate in patients with MM, with an OS benefit favoring zoledronic acid.[404] Zoledronic acid reduced mortality by 16% and increased median overall survival from 44.5 to 50 months ($p = 0.04$).[404] At a median follow-up of 3.7 years, there was a lower incidence of SREs with zoledronate, 27%, versus 35% ($p = 0.0004$) with clodronate.[409] Moreover, patients without bone lesions at baseline also derived benefit of zoledronate with skeletal morbidity,[409] although the benefit in survival was seen only in patients with bone disease on study entry.[410]

Denosumab is a fully human monoclonal antibody given subcutaneously that binds to and inhibits RANKL, a cytokine that mediates the formation, function, and survival of osteoclasts.[411] A randomized study compared denosumab to zoledronic acid in newly diagnosed MM patients with at least one bone lesion.[412] Denosumab was noninferior to zoledronic acid in time to SRE, and OS was similar in both arms (HR = 0.98 (0.84–1.14), $p = 0.01$ for noninferiority). Interestingly, PFS, an exploratory endpoint, was longer in the denosumab arm (46.1 months) compared to the zoledronic acid arm (35.4 months), with HR 0.82 ($p = 0.036$). Notably, renal toxicity was significantly lower with denosumab, 10% vs 17.1% ($p < 0.001$). This was especially true in patients with renal insufficiency at baseline (creatinine clearance ≤60 mL/min), where renal toxicity was reduced by half with denosumab compared to zoledronic acid: 12.9% versus 26.4%, respectively. Hypocalcemia was more common in the denosumab arm (all grades, 17% vs 12%). Denosumab is thus another option for managing bone disease in MM, especially in patients with renal dysfunction and where convenience of s.c. administration may be helpful.

Osteonecrosis of the jaw (ONJ) is one of the most serious complications of bisphosphonates.[413,414] ONJ is traditionally defined as exposed, necrotic bone in the jaw that does not heal after 8 weeks and is generally painful. In the Myeloma IX trial, the cumulative incidence of ONJ with zoledronic acid was 3–4% at a median follow-up of 3.7 years.[409] Denosumab has a similar rate of ONJ; in the randomized study comparing denosumab versus zoledronic acid, ONJ occurred in 4% versus 3% of patients, respectively.[412] Dental extractions are a major risk factor for development of ONJ.[415,416] Attention to dental hygiene and minimizing invasive procedures (such as tooth extractions or dental implants) may reduce the risk of ONJ.[417] The IMWG have provided guidelines for managing bisphosphonate and denosumab therapy.[418]

Local therapy with radiation therapy or kyphoplasty

Radiation therapy for MM is used for palliation of localized disease where symptoms may range from pain to neurological compromise from cord compression. About 40% of patients will be expected to receive radiation according to one calculation.[419] MM cells in preclinical studies were found to be among the most sensitive tumors to radiation therapy.[420] The majority of patients who receive radiation therapy (>85%) have palliation of pain in doses ranging from 8 to 40 Gy.[421-424] While painful lytic bone lesions are frequently the primary reason for radiation therapy, other indications include impending fracture, cord compression, or relief of symptoms associated with a mass (i.e., cranial nerve palsies, cosmesis, or organ or joint dysfunction). The International Lymphoma Radiation Oncology Group has provided guidelines.[425]

Pathologic compression fractures are another cause of morbidity in MM. Kyphoplasty is a procedure where methyl methacrylate is percutaneously injected into a collapsed vertebral body, and this is an important tool for managing pain due to this complication. In the CAFE (Cancer Patient Fracture Evaluation) study, 134 patients with malignancy and painful compression fracture were randomly assigned to kyphoplasty versus supportive care alone.[426] In this study, 38% of the patients had MM, and overall, there was significant improvement in pain and function.

Hyperviscosity

Hyperviscosity is characterized clinically by spontaneous bleeding with neurologic and ocular disorders. Hyperviscosity is seen more often in Waldenström macroglobulinemia, due to the larger size of the pentameric IgM paraprotein, in 10–30% of patients.[427] In MM, historically, hyperviscosity occurred in 4.2% of 238 patients with IgG MM and in 22% of 46 patients with serum IgG monoclonal components >5.0 g/dL.[428] The IgG3 subclass produces hyperviscosity at lower levels than other IgG paraproteins.[429] The severity of the syndrome is not directly related to the serum viscosity. Clinical findings improve with plasmapheresis, which reduces both MM protein concentration and serum viscosity.

Infections

Infections are a major cause of morbidity and mortality in patients with MM, stemming from both the adverse effects of MM on humoral and cellular immunity and myelosuppression from treatment.[430] Patients with MM have functional hypogammaglobulinemia coupled with decreased diversity in the antibody repertoire, along with immunosuppression related to treatment. Older data described a biphasic pattern to bacterial infections, with encapsulated bacteria such as *S. pneumoniae* and *H. influenzae* early in the course of illness and *S. aureus* and gram-negative organisms later on.[431] A survey of the Swedish cancer registry from 1998 to 2004 found a sevenfold risk of any infection compared to the general population, with the highest risk during the first year after diagnosis.[432] Indeed, infections may contribute up to 50% of early deaths.[433]

With the use of newer agents such as bortezomib, the type of infections has changed compared to older melphalan-based regimens and historical induction chemotherapy regimens. Bortezomib is associated with a significantly higher risk of herpes zoster; in the phase III APEX trial, the incidence of herpes zoster was 13% compared to 5% ($p = 0.0002$).[208] Using a lower dose of dexamethasone, when combined with lenalidomide, is associated with significantly decreased risk of infections, including pneumonia, 9% vs 16% ($p = 0.04$).[187]

The evidence of increased clinical infections in MM has led to attempts at prevention. Using a high-dose booster vaccination strategy may lead to higher rates of seroprotection for influenza.[434] The TEAMM trial evaluated prophylaxis with levofloxacin or placebo in 977 newly diagnosed patients in the UK.[435] This study found reduction in febrile episodes or deaths from 27% to 19% with the use of levofloxacin prophylaxis, without an increase in health care-associated infections ($p = 0.0018$). The magnitude of this benefit may be less pronounced outside the UK where different regimens may be used for newly diagnosed MM.

Given the functional hypogammaglobulinemia seen in MM, immunoglobulin replacement (IVIG) has been considered. An older randomized study of IVIG in newly diagnosed patients did not find benefit.[436] In patients with stable disease, a randomized, placebo-controlled trial studied the use of IVIG given monthly for a year in 82 MM patients.[437] The IVIG arm did not experience any episodes of septicemia or pneumonia compared to 10 events in the placebo arm ($p = 0.002$). While the findings in this latter study showed benefit, the routine use of IVIG as prophylaxis has not been generally adopted. However, IVIG may be considered in selected patients with severe, recurrent infections and hypogammaglobulinemia.[438]

Renal failure

Renal failure in MM can predict for adverse outcome. One series found that 22% of patients had a serum creatinine ≥ 2 mg/dL at diagnosis; renal function normalized with treatment in 48% of those with creatinine <4 mg/dL.[439] The causes of renal failure in MM are often multifactorial and include hypercalcemia; MM kidney, with distal and proximal tubules obstructed by large, laminated casts containing albumin, IgG, and κ and λ light chains surrounded by giant cells; hyperuricemia; dehydration; plasma cell infiltration; pyelonephritis; and amyloidosis. The most important predisposing factor is dehydration; aggressive hydration is therefore crucial to avoid irreversible renal dysfunction. Otherwise, treatment is for the underlying disease, along with avoidance of intravenous contrast, though the risk of contrast in patients with normal renal function has been undergoing re-evaluation.[440]

Rapid reduction of nephrotoxic free light chain is critical to renal recovery in patients with acute kidney injury from MM. There have been conflicting results on using high-cutoff dialyzers (which are currently only available in Europe) to physically remove free light chains from circulation in patients with cast nephropathy. The MYRE study did not show a difference in hemodialysis independence at three months with use of high-cutoff dialyzer,[441] and in the EuLITE study, there was worse survival.[442] On the other hand, there is general agreement supporting the use of bortezomib-based regimens, given the activity of bortezomib and lack of renal toxicity or effects on clearance due to kidney dysfunction. In one series, 49% of patients achieved dialysis independence using a bortezomib-based regimen.[443] A recent study randomized patients with cast nephropathy and acute kidney injury to cyclophosphamide, bortezomib, dexamethasone versus Bortezomib, and dexamethasone.[444] This study though did not find benefit to adding cyclophosphamide, although there was a trend toward improved renal response rates with the triplet combination in patients with severe kidney injury, 46.7% versus 24.2% ($p = 0.07$).

Other plasma cell dyscrasias

Monoclonal gammopathy of undetermined significance

MGUS is a precursor condition to multiple myeloma and other lymphoproliferative conditions. MGUS is a common condition, present in 3.2% of individuals ≥ 50-years-old, with prevalence increasing with age, 6.6% in ≥ 80-years-old,[445] and rarely seen under the age of 50, where the prevalence is 0.3%.[446] MGUS may be divided into three categories: non-IgM MGUS, IgM MGUS, and the more recently appreciated light chain MGUS.[447] Non-IgM MGUS is more closely associated with risk of progression to MM or AL amyloidosis, whereas IgM MGUS is more associated with risk of progression to lymphoma, especially Waldenström macroglobulinemia. While MGUS is common, the risk of progression to disease that requires treatment is unlikely. The rate that MGUS evolves to one of these conditions is 1.1%/year with IgM MGUS and 0.8%/year in non-IgM MGUS[448] and lower with light-chain MGUS, 0.3%/year.[447] Well-defined risk factors for progression of MGUS include monoclonal protein ≥1.5 g/dL, abnormal free light chain ratio, and non-IgG type monoclonal protein.[449] The rate of progression over 20 years can vary from 7% in patients with no risk factors to 20% with one risk factor and 30% with two risk factors.[448] Currently, patients are not screened for MGUS as part of routine primary care. There is an ongoing Icelandic trial evaluating population screening for MGUS, iStopMM (Iceland Screens, Treats or Prevents Multiple Myeloma (NCT03327597)).

Monoclonal gammopathy of renal significance

Monoclonal gammopathy of renal significance (MGRS) is a recently defined entity where a monoclonal plasma cell clone causes kidney injury. The term MGRS was developed in 2012 to describe disorders where there is renal injury due to the plasma cell clone and monoclonal protein but where the disorders do not meet the traditional "CRAB" criteria for multiple myeloma or other lymphoproliferative condition.[450] MGRS includes a diverse range of conditions including monoclonal immunoglobulin deposition disease and proliferative glomerulonephritis with monoclonal immunoglobulin deposits, among others.[451] Typically, these conditions are treated with plasma cell-directed therapy, with the goal of preserving and/or restoring renal function.

Smoldering multiple myeloma

SMM was initially described in 1980 and is a plasma cell disorder that lies in between MGUS and MM, with higher disease burden but without the clinical sequelae of the CRAB criteria or myeloma defining biomarkers (see below).[452] SMM is less common than MGUS, representing an estimated 13.7% of MM patients with 4100 new cases per year.[453] The rate of progression to active MM is 10% per year for the first 5 years, declines to 3% per year for the next 5 years, and is then 1% per year for the following 10 years. The IMWG have recently described a "2/20/20" risk stratification model to help identify patients with high-risk SMM.[454] Components of the model include serum M-protein >2 g/dL; involved to uninvolved free light chain ratio >20; and marrow plasma cell infiltration >20%. Patients with two or more risk factors are considered high risk, with a 2-year progression risk of 44%. Next-generation sequencing of SMM samples by Bustoros et al.[147] have shown that alterations in the MAPK pathway, DNA repair pathway, *MYC*, and APOBEC-associated mutations were independent risk factors for progression of SMM to active myeloma.

The availability of well-tolerated, effective myeloma therapy has motivated studies examining treatment in SMM, prior to the onset of symptoms and progression to active MM. The Spanish myeloma group conducted a randomized study of active treatment with lenalidomide and dexamethasone versus observation in patients with high risk smoldering MM.[455,456] High risk was defined by the presence of both bone marrow involvement and elevated serum monoclonal protein or flow cytometry criteria and suppressed immunoglobulins (immunoparesis). The study found that 3 year OS was superior in the group undergoing active treatment, 94% versus 80%, and this was the first time improvement in was seen in a SMM trial. However, the generalizability of the trial was limited by several factors. While it showed improvement in OS, it brought into focus several limitations with the diagnosis and follow-up of SMM. Assessment for bone disease was limited to conventional skeletal survey, reflecting the practice at that time; current practice includes more sensitive imaging based on CT or MRI. Progression events occurred early on in the observation arm, raising the possibility that some of these patients may actually have had active MM rather than true SMM. Some of the patients in the trial would likely now be reclassified as active MM, based on the updated 2014 criteria, and therefore excluded from the trial. Moreover, while all patients in the treatment arm received lenalidomide (by definition), only 11% of patients in the observation arm who progressed were treated with lenalidomide (reflecting its limited availability at the time where the trial was conducted), which in turn may negatively affect the overall survival of the control arm.

Treatment of SMM was revisited with the E3A06 trial, evaluating lenalidomide (as a single agent) versus observation.[457] Compared to the Spanish trial, the majority of patients satisfied the updated definition of SMM with exclusion of myeloma defining events. The primary endpoint was PFS, where progression was defined by the presence of both biochemical disease progression as defined by the IMWG and evidence of end organ damage by the traditional CRAB criteria. Patients were randomized to lenalidomide 25 mg on the conventional 21 out of 28 days schedule versus observation. While the number of patients in the individual cohorts is small, the improvement in PFS is best demonstrated in the 20/2/20 high-risk category with HR 0.09 ($N = 56$). However, no difference in OS has been reported to date, reflecting the limited follow-up. The AQUILA study (NCT03301220) is evaluating subcutaneous daratumumab for 3 years versus observation in high-risk SMM. Alternatively, other approaches under evaluation include a more intensive approach with KRd and high-dose melphalan and autologous stem cell transplant (GEM-CESAR)[458] and myeloma peptide vaccination with PVX-410 and lenalidomide[459] and both with the selective HDAC6 inhibitor citarinostat (NCT02886065).

Plasmacytomas

Plasmacytomas are collections of monoclonal plasma cells originating either in bone (solitary osseous plasmacytoma, SOP) or in soft tissue (extramedullary plasmacytoma, EMP). They comprise <10% of plasma cell dyscrasias. MM must be excluded before the diagnosis of either SOP or EMP can be made. MRI can be useful to show additional marrow abnormalities consistent with MM.[460] The median age of diagnosis of either SOP or EMP is approximately 50 years, nearly 10 years younger than that for MM.[461–463] Although patients with SOP and EMP can both progress to MM, patients with SOP progress in the majority of cases, in contrast to EMP, where only up to 50% eventually develop MM. The median survival of 86.4 and 100.8 months for patients with SOP and EMP, respectively, is similar; however, 10 year PFS is markedly different, 16% for SOP patients versus 71% for EMP patients.[462] A more recent analysis showed similar findings, where survival for solitary extramedullary plasmacytoma (132 month) was longer than solitary plasmacytoma of the bone (85 months).[464] The persistence of stable monoclonal immunoglobulin in serum and/or urine after primary treatment of plasmacytoma does not necessitate additional therapy, since it does not influence survival or disease-free survival.[461] In contrast, rising monoclonal immunoglobulin levels in a patient with a history of either SOP or EMP should trigger a work-up for either recurrent plasmacytoma or MM. It has been suggested, as is true for MM, that serum β2M has prognostic value in patients with SOP. Specifically, 17 of 19 patients with elevated serum β2M had transformation to MM and shorter survival (31 months) than those with normal serum β2M levels.[465]

Treatment of SOP and EMP is local therapy, primarily radiotherapy with surgery as needed for structural anatomic support.[461–463] The benefit of chemotherapy, either alone or in combination with radiotherapy and surgery, as primary therapy for SOP or EMP has not been proven. Moreover, the benefit of adjuvant chemotherapy, given to prevent recurrent disease and/or progression to MM, is also undefined. Disappearance of protein after involved-field radiotherapy predicts for long-term disease-free survival and possible cure.[466]

AL amyloidosis

Amyloidosis refers to conditions caused by either localized or systemic deposition of misfolded amyloid proteins, which may lead to symptoms from organ damage and organ failure, with more severe manifestations depending on the organ involved, such as the heart. The major forms of amyloidosis include AL amyloidosis (historically known as primary amyloidosis), which is due to misfolded light chain from a clonal plasma cell disorder; AA amyloidosis, which results from chronic inflammation leading to the production of the acute phase reactant serum amyloid A protein; and ATTR amyloidosis which is related to transthyretin (wild type or mutant).[467]

Establishing the correct diagnosis and type of amyloid is critical, as monoclonal gammopathy of unknown significance is common, and in a series of 350 patients with suspected AL amyloidosis, 9.7% of patients actually had mutations in the fibrinogen A alpha-chain or transthyretin.[468] Direct classification of the amyloid protein through laser microdissection and mass spectrometry has significantly improved the accuracy of diagnosis of AL amyloidosis.[469]

In AL amyloidosis, amyloid involves the heart (75%), leading to heart failure; kidney (65%), leading to proteinuria and nephrotic syndrome; liver (15%) with hepatomegaly; nervous system (10%), and gastrointestinal tract (5%).[470,471] Macroglossia and periorbital purpura are classic features of AL amyloidosis, but these are uncommon manifestations. Cardiac involvement is a major determinant of prognosis, and this is reflected in the revised Mayo Clinic 2012 staging system that uses a combination of NT-pro BNP ≥ 1800 ng/L, troponin $T \geq 0.025$ mcg/L, and difference in free light chain ≥ 18 mg/dL.[472] For patients with three of these risk factors, the overall survival was 6 months.

The treatment of AL amyloidosis overlaps with the treatment of MM. Bortezomib is used as a backbone in treatment, such as the combination of cyclophosphamide, bortezomib, and dexamethasone.[473,474] The combination of bortezomib, melphalan, and dexamethasone was compared to melphalan and dexamethasone in newly diagnosed AL amyloidosis.[475] The study showed higher hematologic response rate, 79% versus 52% as well as higher OS, with median OS not reached versus 34 months (HR 0.46) in the bortezomib cohort. In some institutions, high-dose melphalan and autologous stem cell transplant is also used.[476]

Given the efficacy of daratumumab in multiple myeloma, daratumumab is now being evaluated in AL amyloidosis. An initial retrospective study at Stanford of 25 patients with relapsed AL amyloidosis and a median of 3 prior lines of treatment showed a hematologic response of 76%.[477] These findings were confirmed in several larger studies in relapsed AL amyloidosis with overall responses ranging from 64% to 90%, very good partial response or better 56–86%; including renal (24–67%) and cardiac responses (22–50%).[478–480]

Motivated by the activity of daratumumab in relapsed AL amyloidosis, there is an ongoing randomized study (ANDROMEDA) in newly diagnosed AL amyloidosis evaluating the addition of daratumumab to the standard triplet of cyclophosphamide, bortezomib, and dexamethasone (CyBorD). In the 28 patient safety run-in of the trial, the overall hematologic response was 96%, with an organ response rate of 64%.[481]

Key references

The complete reference list can be found on Vital Source version of this title, see inside front cover.

9. Hillengass J, Usmani S, Rajkumar SV, et al. International myeloma working group consensus recommendations on imaging in monoclonal plasma cell disorders. *Lancet Oncol.* 2019;**20**:e302–e312.
24. Kyle RA, Gertz MA, Witzig TE, et al. Review of 1027 patients with newly diagnosed multiple myeloma. *Mayo Clin Proc.* 2003;**78**:21–33.
30. Rajkumar SV, Harousseau JL, Durie B, et al. Consensus recommendations for the uniform reporting of clinical trials: report of the International Myeloma Workshop Consensus Panel 1. *Blood.* 2011;**117**:4691–4695.
31. Kumar S, Paiva B, Anderson KC, et al. International Myeloma Working Group consensus criteria for response and minimal residual disease assessment in multiple myeloma. *Lancet Oncol.* 2016;**17**:e328–e346.
69. Hideshima T, Richardson P, Chauhan D, et al. The proteasome inhibitor PS-341 inhibits growth, induces apoptosis, and overcomes drug resistance in human multiple myeloma cells. *Cancer Res.* 2001;**61**:3071–3076.
119. Kumar SK, Rajkumar SV. The multiple myelomas - current concepts in cytogenetic classification and therapy. *Nat Rev Clin Oncol.* 2018;**15**:409–421.
128. Zhan F, Huang Y, Colla S, et al. The molecular classification of multiple myeloma. *Blood.* 2006;**108**:2020–2028.
129. Palumbo A, Avet-Loiseau H, Oliva S, et al. Revised international staging system for multiple Myeloma: a report from International Myeloma Working Group. *J Clin Oncol.* 2015;**33**:2863–2869.
149. Greipp PR, San Miguel J, Durie BG, et al. International staging system for multiple myeloma. *J Clin Oncol.* 2005;**23**:3412–3420.
157. McElwain TJ, Powles RL. High-dose intravenous melphalan for plasma-cell leukaemia and myeloma. *Lancet.* 1983;**2**:822–824.
158. Barlogie B, Hall R, Zander A, et al. High-dose melphalan with autologous bone marrow transplantation for multiple myeloma. *Blood.* 1986;**67**:1298–1301.
159. Facon T, Kumar S, Plesner T, et al. Daratumumab plus Lenalidomide and Dexamethasone for Untreated Myeloma. *N Engl J Med.* 2019;**380**:2104–2115.
163. O'Donnell EK, Laubach JP, Yee AJ, et al. A phase 2 study of modified lenalidomide, bortezomib and dexamethasone in transplant-ineligible multiple myeloma. *Br J Haematol.* 2018;**182**:222–230.
165. San Miguel JF, Schlag R, Khuageva NK, et al. Bortezomib plus melphalan and prednisone for initial treatment of multiple myeloma. *N Engl J Med.* 2008;**359**:906–917.
166. Kumar SK, Jacobus SJ, Cohen AD, et al. Carfilzomib or bortezomib in combination with lenalidomide and dexamethasone for patients with newly diagnosed multiple myeloma without intention for immediate autologous stem-cell transplantation (ENDURANCE): a multicentre, open-label, phase 3, randomised, controlled trial. *Lancet Oncol.* 2020;**21**:1317–1330.
167. Voorhees PM, Kaufman JL, Laubach J, et al. Daratumumab, lenalidomide, bortezomib, and dexamethasone for transplant-eligible newly diagnosed multiple myeloma: the GRIFFIN trial. *Blood.* 2020;**136**:936–945.
168. Durie BG, Hoering A, Abidi MH, et al. Bortezomib with lenalidomide and dexamethasone versus lenalidomide and dexamethasone alone in patients with newly diagnosed myeloma without intent for immediate autologous stem-cell transplant (SWOG S0777): a randomised, open-label, phase 3 trial. *Lancet.* 2017;**389**:519–527.
169. Attal M, Lauwers-Cances V, Hulin C, et al. Lenalidomide, bortezomib, and dexamethasone with transplantation for myeloma. *N Engl J Med.* 2017;**376**:1311–1320.
170. Dimopoulos MA, Oriol A, Nahi H, et al. Daratumumab, lenalidomide, and dexamethasone for multiple Myeloma. *N Engl J Med.* 2016;**375**:1319–1331.
178. Cavo M, Zamagni E, Tosi P, et al. Superiority of thalidomide and dexamethasone over vincristine-doxorubicindexamethasone (VAD) as primary therapy in preparation for autologous transplantation for multiple myeloma. *Blood.* 2005;**106**:35–39.
179. Rajkumar SV, Blood E, Vesole D, et al. Phase III clinical trial of thalidomide plus dexamethasone compared with dexamethasone alone in newly diagnosed multiple myeloma: a clinical trial coordinated by the Eastern Cooperative Oncology Group. *J Clin Oncol.* 2006;**24**:431–436.
182. Weber DM, Chen C, Niesvizky R, et al. Lenalidomide plus dexamethasone for relapsed multiple myeloma in North America. *N Engl J Med.* 2007;**357**:2133–2142.
183. Dimopoulos M, Spencer A, Attal M, et al. Lenalidomide plus dexamethasone for relapsed or refractory multiple myeloma. *N Engl J Med.* 2007;**357**:2123–2132.
187. Rajkumar SV, Jacobus S, Callander NS, et al. Lenalidomide plus high-dose dexamethasone versus lenalidomide plus low-dose dexamethasone as initial therapy for newly diagnosed multiple myeloma: an open-label randomised controlled trial. *Lancet Oncol.* 2010;**11**:29–37.
199. Richardson PG, Sonneveld P, Schuster MW, et al. Bortezomib or high-dose dexamethasone for relapsed multiple myeloma. *N Engl J Med.* 2005;**352**:2487–2498.

201 Mateos MV, Richardson PG, Schlag R, et al. Bortezomib plus melphalan and prednisone compared with melphalan and prednisone in previously untreated multiple myeloma: updated follow-up and impact of subsequent therapy in the phase III VISTA trial. *J Clin Oncol.* 2010;**28**:2259–2266.

206 Moreau P, Pylypenko H, Grosicki S, et al. Subcutaneous versus intravenous administration of bortezomib in patients with relapsed multiple myeloma: a randomised, phase 3, non-inferiority study. *Lancet Oncol.* 2010;**12**:431–440.

213 Richardson PG, Weller E, Lonial S, et al. Lenalidomide, bortezomib, and dexamethasone combination therapy in patients with newly diagnosed multiple myeloma. *Blood.* 2010;**116**:679–686.

232 Stadtmauer EA, Pasquini MC, Blackwell B, et al. Autologous transplantation, consolidation, and maintenance therapy in multiple myeloma: results of the BMT CTN 0702 trial. *J Clin Oncol.* 2019;**37**:589–597.

252 McCarthy PL, Holstein SA, Petrucci MT, et al. Lenalidomide maintenance after autologous stem-cell transplantation in newly diagnosed multiple myeloma: a meta-analysis. *J Clin Oncol.* 2017;**35**:3279–3289.

258 Munshi NC, Avet-Loiseau H, Anderson KC, et al. A large meta-analysis establishes the role of MRD negativity in long-term survival outcomes in patients with multiple myeloma. *Blood Adv.* 2020;**4**:5988–5999.

265 Dimopoulos MA, Terpos E, Boccadoro M, et al. Apollo: phase 3 randomized study of subcutaneous daratumumab plus pomalidomide and dexamethasone (D-Pd) versus pomalidomide and dexamethasone (Pd) alone in patients (Pts) with relapsed/refractory multiple myeloma (RRMM). *Blood.* 2020;**136**:5–6.

267 Dimopoulos M, Quach H, Mateos MV, et al. Carfilzomib, dexamethasone, and daratumumab versus carfilzomib and dexamethasone for patients with relapsed or refractory multiple myeloma (CANDOR): results from a randomised, multicentre, open-label, phase 3 study. *Lancet.* 2020;**396**:186–197.

268 Attal M, Richardson PG, Rajkumar SV, et al. Isatuximab plus pomalidomide and low-dose dexamethasone versus pomalidomide and low-dose dexamethasone in patients with relapsed and refractory multiple myeloma (ICARIA-MM): a randomised, multicentre, open-label, phase 3 study. *Lancet.* 2019;**394**:2096–2107.

270 Dimopoulos MA, Dytfeld D, Grosicki S, et al. Elotuzumab plus pomalidomide and dexamethasone for multiple myeloma. *N Engl J Med.* 2018;**379**:1811–1822.

274 Dimopoulos MA, Moreau P, Palumbo A, et al. Carfilzomib and dexamethasone versus bortezomib and dexamethasone for patients with relapsed or refractory multiple myeloma (ENDEAVOR): a randomised, phase 3, open-label, multicentre study. *Lancet Oncol.* 2016;**17**:27–38.

277 Stewart AK, Rajkumar SV, Dimopoulos MA, et al. Carfilzomib, lenalidomide, and dexamethasone for relapsed multiple myeloma. *N Engl J Med.* 2015;**372**:142–152.

279 San Miguel J, Weisel K, Moreau P, et al. Pomalidomide plus low-dose dexamethasone versus high-dose dexamethasone alone for patients with relapsed and refractory multiple myeloma (MM-003): a randomised, open-label, phase 3 trial. *Lancet Oncol.* 2013;**14**:1055–1066.

282 Herndon TM, Deisseroth A, Kaminskas E, et al. U.S. Food and drug administration approval: carfilzomib for the treatment of multiple myeloma. *Clin Cancer Res.* 2013;**19**:4559–4563.

310 Lokhorst HM, Plesner T, Laubach JP, et al. Targeting CD38 with daratumumab monotherapy in multiple myeloma. *N Engl J Med.* 2015;**373**:1207–1219.

312 Chari A, Suvannasankha A, Fay JW, et al. Daratumumab plus pomalidomide and dexamethasone in relapsed and/or refractory multiple myeloma. *Blood.* 2017;**130**:974–981.

315 Moreau P, Dimopoulos M-A, Mikhael J, et al. Isatuximab plus carfilzomib and dexamethasone vs. carfilzomib and dexamethasone in relapsed/refractory multiple myeloma (IKEMA): interim analysis of a phase I randomized, open-label study, European Hematology Association, 2020

318 Chari A, Vogl DT, Gavriatopoulou M, et al. Oral selinexor-dexamethasone for triple-class refractory multiple myeloma. *N Engl J Med.* 2019;**381**:727–738.

326 Lonial S, Lee HC, Badros A, et al. Belantamab mafodotin for relapsed or refractory multiple myeloma (DREAMM-2): a two-arm, randomised, open-label, phase 2 study. *Lancet Oncol.* 2020;**21**:207–221.

333 Costa LJ, Wong SW, Bermúdez A, et al. First clinical study of the B-cell maturation antigen (BCMA) 2+1 T cell engager (TCE) CC-93269 in patients (Pts) with relapsed/refractory multiple myeloma (RRMM): interim results of a phase 1 multicenter trial. *Blood.* 2019;**134**:Abstract 143.

339 Raje N, Berdeja J, Lin Y, et al. Anti-BCMA CAR T-cell therapy bb2121 in relapsed or refractory multiple myeloma. *N Engl J Med.* 2019;**380**:1726–1737.

341 Madduri D, Usmani SZ, Jagannath S, et al. Results from CARTITUDE-1: a phase 1b/2 study of JNJ-4528, a CAR-T cell therapy directed against B-cell maturation antigen (BCMA), in patients with relapsed and/or refractory multiple myeloma (R/R MM). *Blood.* 2019;**134**:Abstract 577.

403 Berenson JR, Lichtenstein A, Porter L, et al. Efficacy of pamidronate in reducing skeletal events in patients with advanced multiple myeloma. Myeloma Aredia Study Group. *N Engl J Med.* 1996;**334**:488–493.

404 Morgan GJ, Davies FE, Gregory WM, et al. First-line treatment with zoledronic acid as compared with clodronic acid in multiple myeloma (MRC Myeloma IX): a randomised controlled trial. *Lancet.* 2010;**376**:1989–1999.

412 Raje N, Terpos E, Willenbacher W, et al. Denosumab versus zoledronic acid in bone disease treatment of newly diagnosed multiple myeloma: an international, double-blind, double-dummy, randomised, controlled, phase 3 study. *Lancet Oncol.* 2018;**19**:370–381.

456 Mateos MV, Hernandez MT, Giraldo P, et al. Lenalidomide plus dexamethasone versus observation in patients with high-risk smouldering multiple myeloma (QuiRedex): long-term follow-up of a randomised, controlled, phase 3 trial. *Lancet Oncol.* 2016;**17**:1127–1136.

457 Lonial S, Jacobus S, Fonseca R, et al. Randomized trial of lenalidomide versus observation in smoldering multiple myeloma. *J Clin Oncol.* 2020;**38**:1126–1137.

473 Mikhael JR, Schuster SR, Jimenez-Zepeda VH, et al. Cyclophosphamide-bortezomib-dexamethasone (CyBorD) produces rapid and complete hematologic response in patients with AL amyloidosis. *Blood.* 2012;**119**:4391–4394.

481 Palladini G, Kastritis E, Maurer MS, et al. Daratumumab plus CyBorD for patients with newly diagnosed AL amyloidosis: safety run-in results of ANDROMEDA. *Blood.* 2020;**136**:71–80.

120 Myeloproliferative disorders

Jeanne Palmer, MD ■ Ruben Mesa, MD

> **Overview**
>
> Myeloproliferative neoplasms (MPNs) are a diverse group of blood disorders that include essential thrombocythemia (ET), polycythemia vera (PV), and myelofibrosis (MF). These disorders share several features, including "driver mutations," thrombotic risk, and symptom burden. The driver mutations, which are usually mutually exclusive, include Janus kinase 2 (JAK2), calreticulin (CAL-R), and myeloproliferative leukemia virus oncogene (MPL). JAK2 mutations include JAK2 V617F, JAK exon 12, and JAK exon 16. CAL-R mutations are divided into type 1, which is a 52-bp deletion (L367fs*46), and type 2, a 5-bp insertion (K385fs*47). The thrombotic risk is present in all three disorders; however, it varies based on age, mutation status, and the history of the thrombotic events. The symptom burden for these disorders includes constitutional symptoms, such as fevers, night sweats, and weight loss; microvascular symptoms such as itching, headache, and peripheral neuropathy; and spleen symptoms such as abdominal discomfort and early satiety. The prognosis and treatment of these is very dependent on the risk factors, symptom burden, and disease presentation and is reviewed in this chapter.

Background

Myeloproliferative neoplasms (MPNs) include a variety of diseases that manifest as excessive growth in the myeloid system. This article will focus on the *BCR-ABL* negative MPNs such as essential thrombocythemia (ET), polycythemia vera (PV), and myelofibrosis (MF), including both primary MF (PMF) and secondary MF, arising following ET or PV. We will cover the basic biology of the diseases, diagnosis, as well as treatment options.

Biology of MPN

There is a shared biology of MPN, in that they share three common driver mutations. These mutations are mutually exclusive, and introduction of the mutations into murine systems results in the manifestation of the disease. The most common driver mutations include *Janus kinase 2 (JAK2), calreticulin (CAL-R),* and *myeloproliferative leukemia virus oncogene (MPL)*. JAK2 mutation include *JAK2 V617F, JAK exon 12,* and *JAK exon 16. CAL-R* mutations are divided into type 1, which is a 52-bp deletion (L367fs*46) and type 2, a 5-bp insertion (K385fs*47).[1] There are also different nondriver mutations which may impact outcomes, including *ASXL1, SRSF2, IDH1/2, EZH2, U2AF1* (see Summary in Table 1).

The biology of MPNs not only results of an increase in blood counts, as seen in PV and ET, but also an increase in inflammatory cytokines which result in a significant symptom burden.[9–13] The symptom burden of MF has been well established.[9,11,14,15] Symptoms such as fatigue, abdominal pain, weight loss, pruritis, anorexia, bone pain, fever, and night sweats are very common in MPNs,[14] and appear to be worse in patients with MF.[9,14] The myeloproliferative neoplasm symptom assessment form (MPN-SAF) was established as a means of capturing MF specific symptoms.[16] In its initial inception, it was administered with the brief fatigue inventory (BFI).[17] The MPN-SAF has been validated internationally.[10] However, subsequently this form has been modified to include the 10 most pertinent symptoms, and is called MPN-total symptom score (MPN-TSS) or MPN-10.[11,18] This score includes nine pertinent symptoms from the MPN-SAF, concentration, early satiety, inactivity, night sweats, itching, bone pain, abdominal discomfort, weight loss, and fever, as well as queries on the worst fatigue from the BFI.[17,18] This score has gained acceptance as a strong measure of quality of life in patients with MF, and is also included as part of the International Working Group (IWG) response criteria.[19]

Presentation of MPN

Patient with MPNs may present with a number of different symptoms. Frequently, they are found with an abnormal complete blood count during routine blood work. They may have an elevated hemoglobin in PV, platelet count in ET, or may present with anemia and elevated leukocytes in the setting of MF. Some patients are discovered when they have an enlarged spleen on routine exam or imaging for another complaint. In rare cases, patients may prevent with a hemorrhagic or thrombotic event. Patients with ET may develop a secondary von Wiillebrand's deficiency which can result in hemorrhage. Patients with PV sometimes present with a portal vein, or splanchic vein thrombosis, and further evaluation shows a *JAK2* mutation, even in the setting of a normal hemoglobin. Finally, patients can present with constitutional symptoms, ranging from fevers, night sweats, and weight loss to more micro-circulatory symptoms such as headaches, visual changes, peripheral neuropathy, erythromelalgia, and difficulty with concentration.

Essential thrombocythemia

Background and presentation

Essential thrombocytosis is the most common MPN, with an incidence of 1.2–3 per 100,000 persons.[20] This disease is characterized by an elevated platelet count and the absence a secondary cause (see Table 2). The diagnosis is generally made when a patient presents with an elevated platelet count. However, patients may present with either a thrombotic or hemorrhagic event.

Work up and diagnosis

Elevated platelets are seen in many clinical situations, many of which do not represent a myeloproliferative disorder. Common causes of secondary platelet elevation include an inflammatory state, postsurgical patients, asplenia, and in the setting of iron deficiency.[23] When a patient is seen in the clinic with elevated

Table 1 Common mutations in MPN and clinical significance.

Mutation	Clinical implication
Driver mutations	
JAK2 V617F	Higher risk of thrombosis in patients with ET[2]
	Intermediate prognosis in patients with PMF[3,4]
MPL W515L/K	Intermediate prognosis in patients with PMF[3,4]
CALR	Improved survival in patients with PMF[3,4]
CALR type1/type1 like	Improved survival compared to CALR type2/type2 like and JAK2V617F[5]
"Triple-negative" absence of a driver mutation	Inferior survival in patients with PMF compared to JAK2 and/or CALR mutated PMF[4]
Somatic mutations	
ASXL1	Independently associated with inferior overall survival and leukemia-free survival[6]
EZH2	Independently associated with worse overall survival in PMF[6]
SRSF2	Associated with worse overall and leukemia-free survival in PMF[6]
TP53	Associated with leukemia transformation[7]
U2Af1 Q157	Inferior overall survival[8]

Table 2 WHO diagnostic criteria 2016.[21a]

| | Polycythemia vera | Essential thrombocythemia | Myelofibrosis | |
			Prefibrotic MF	Overt MF
Major criteria				
Peripheral blood count abnormalities	Hemoglobin >16.5 g/dL (men) >16 g/dL (women) or hematocrit >49% (men) > 48% (women) or increased red cell mass (RCM)	Platelet count >450 × 10^9/L	—	—
Bone marrow findings	BM with hypercellularity (age-adjusted) and trilineage myeloproliferation with pleomorphic, mature megakaryocytes	BM with megakaryocyte proliferation with large and mature morphology. Very rarely minor (grade 1) increase in reticulin fibers	Megakaryocyte proliferation and atypia,[b] without reticulin fibrosis > grade 1,[c] AND increased age-adjusted bone marrow cellularity, granulocytic proliferation, and often decreased erythropoiesis	Megakaryocyte proliferation and atypia[b] accompanied by either reticulin and/or collagen fibrosis (grade 2 or 3)
Molecular	Presence of JAK2 mutation	Megakaryocyte proliferation and atypia[b] accompanied by either reticulin and/or collagen fibrosis (grade 2 or 3) Not meeting WHO criteria for BCR-ABL1+ CML, MDS, or other myeloid neoplasm (including another MPN)	Presence of JAK2, CALR, or MPL mutation or presence of another clonal marker[d] or absence of a reactive bone marrow process	Presence of JAK2, CALR, or MPL mutation or presence of another clonal marker[d] or absence of a reactive bone marrow process
Minor criteria				
	Subnormal erythropoietin	Presence of a clonal marker (e.g., abnormal karyotype) or absence of evidence for reactive thrombocytosis	Presence of one or more of the following:	Presence of one or more of the following:
			Anemia not attributed to a comorbid condition	Anemia not attributed to a comorbid condition
			Palpable splenomegaly	Palpable splenomegaly
			Leukocytosis ≥ 11 × 10^9/L	Leukocytosis ≥ 11 × 10^9/L
			Elevated LDH[j]	Elevated LDH[j]
				Leukoerythro-blastosis
Needed for diagnosis	PV diagnosis requires meeting either all three major criteria or the first two major criteria and one minor criterion	ET diagnosis requires meeting all major criteria or first three major criteria and one minor criterion	prePMF diagnosis requires all three major criteria and at least one minor criterion.	Overt PMF diagnosis requires meeting all three major criteria and at least one minor criterion

[a] Source: Adapted from Barbui et al.[22]
[b] Small-to-large megakaryocytes with aberrant nuclear/cytoplasmic ratio and hyperchromatic and irregularly folded nuclei and dense clustering.
[c] In cases with grade 1 reticulin fibrosis, the megakaryocyte changes must be accompanied by increased marrow cellularity, granulocytic proliferation, and often decreased erythropoiesis (i.e., prePMF).
[d] In the absence of any of the three major clonal mutations, the search for the most frequent accompanying mutations (ASXL1, EZH2, TET2, SRSF2, SF3B1) are of help in determining the clonal nature of the disease.

platelets, secondary causes must be ruled out. However, in the absence of a clear cause of secondary thrombocytosis, a MPN must be ruled out.

Initially testing should be done to evaluate for *JAK2*, *MPL*, and *CAL-R* mutations. Additionally, elevated platelets may be the only finding in patients with *BCR-ABL* positive chronic myelogenous leukemia (CML), therefore, it is recommended to check for evidence of a BCR-ABL mutation as well. A bone marrow biopsy is recommended in all patients, even if a driver mutation is identified, as some patients will have elevated platelets as the only finding in PMF (either prefibrotic or overt). Patients with a very high platelet count are at higher risk of bleeding due to a secondary von Willebrand's deficiency, therefore, evaluating von Willebrand's activity is recommended.

Risk assessment and therapy

In patients with newly diagnosed ET, it is important to evaluate their thrombotic risk. Historically, risk was determined by age and

Table 3 Thrombotic risk in patients with essential thrombocythemia.

Risk	Clinical features	Risk of thrombosis	Treatment
Very low risk	JAK2 neg, <60, no thrombosis	No CV risk: 0.44% patients/year + CV risk: 1.05% patients/year	Observation[a]
Low risk	JAK2 pos, <60, no history of thrombosis	No CV risk: 1.59% patients/year + CV risk: 2.57% patients/year	ASA
Intermediate risk	JAK2 neg, >60, no history of thrombosis	No CV risk: 1.44% patients/year + CV risk: 1.64% patients/year	ASA +/− cytoreduction
High risk	+ history of thrombosis at any age, OR JAK2 pos, >60	No CV risk: 2.36% patients/year + CV risk: 4.17% patients/year	ASA + cytoreduction[b]

[a]One study showed increased bleeding risk with ASA in very low-risk patients.
[b]If venous thrombosis: lifelong anticoagulation.

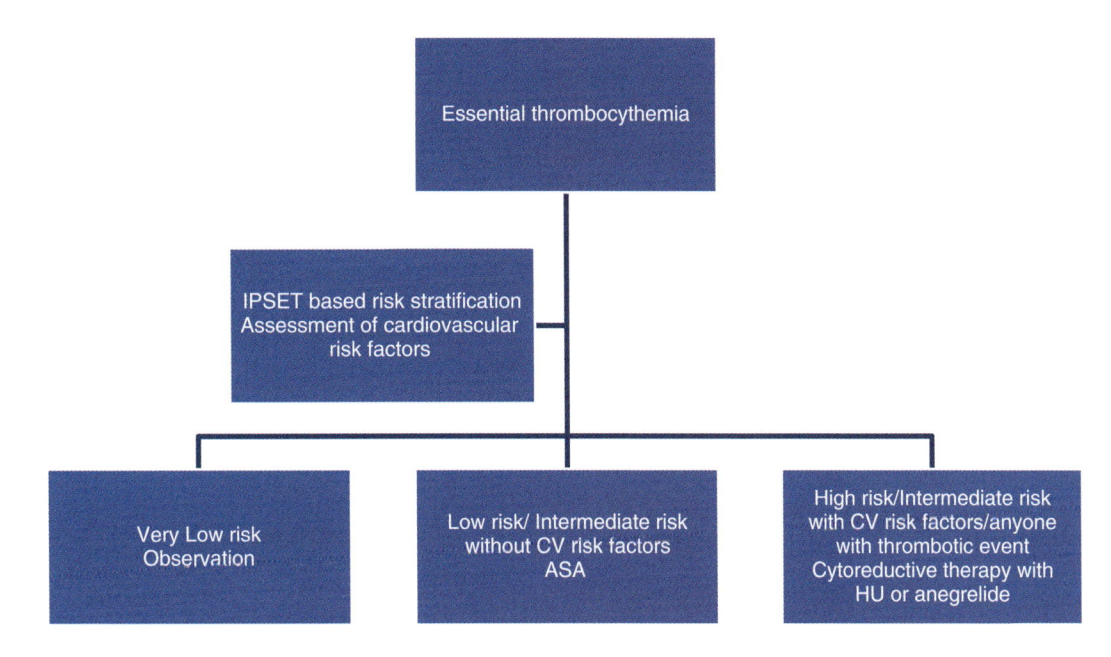

Figure 1 Treatment algorithm for essential thrombocythemia.

history of thrombosis.[24] In this case, low risk (i.e., no history of thrombosis and age <60) the risk of thrombosis was 0.95%/year, however, with either age >60 OR history of thrombosis, the risk increased to 2.86%/year. However, in 2012, Barbui et al. revised IPSET taking into account driver mutation, and created three risk categories, low risk, intermediate risk, and high risk, based on a scoring system that takes into account 3 risks, age >60 (1 point), history of thrombosis (2 points), cardiovascular disease (1 point), and *JAK2V617F* mutation (2 points).[2] This ultimately was developed into a scoring system including very low risk, low risk, intermediate risk, and high risk, based on age, *JAK2V617F* mutation, and history of thrombosis (see Table 3).

Therapy for ET is determined by the risk of the disease (see Figure 1). Historically, anyone with ET was given cytoreduction therapy. However, the current NCCN guidelines recommend basing treatment with aspirin (ASA) and cytoreductive therapy based on the risk of thrombosis based on IPSET criteria.[25] In very low-risk patients, observation alone is recommended. In these patients, the risk of thrombotic events is quite low, and ASA may actually increase the risk of bleeding.[26] In low-risk patients, ASA is recommended. Intermediate patients should take ASA, however, the decision to initiate cytoreductive therapy is based on symptom burden and cardiovascular risk. The only group where cytoreduction is routinely used is in the high-risk group. Other indications for cytoreduction include history of a thrombotic event and secondary von Willebrand's disease. In patients with a symptom burden or microvascular-related issues, cytoreduction can be considered as well.[27]

The choice of cytoreductive therapy is very dependent on the patient. Upfront therapy most commonly is hydroxyurea (HU); however, interferon-alfa2a, and anagrelide can also be considered upfront.[20,28] Cytoreduction is geared to reduce the thrombotic risk for patients. In a retrospective population study done,[29] there was a survival advantage appreciated in patients who took HU. In older patients, busulfan can be considered, however, long-term use may be associated with an increased risk of transformation to acute leukemia.[27] For a summary of the different cytoreductive agents frequently used in MPN, please see Table 4.

Polycythemia vera

Background and presentation

PV is a bone marrow disorder characterized by a high red blood cell mass. The most common presentation of PV is a patient with an elevated hemoglobin, though approximately a third of patients will present with a thrombotic event. The prevalence of this disease is estimated at 1.9 per 100,000.[30,31]

At presentation, many patients will express a number of symptoms. These symptoms are as a result of both vasomotor disturbances, as well as inflammation.[11] Patients may experience

Table 4 Pros and cons of different cytoreductive therapies.

Cytoreductive therapy	Pros	Cons	Who?
Hydroxyurea	• Control in myeloproliferation • Reduction in thrombosis in high-risk ET	• Mucocutaneous toxicity • Increased risk of skin cancer • Decreased blood counts	• Older patients • High-risk ET/PV
Pegylated interferon	• Possible anticlonal activity • Control of counts	• Tolerability long-term • Impact on QoL • Minimal impact on splenomegaly	• Younger patients • Limited co-morbidity • Avoid if patient has history of depression
Ruxolitinib (PV)	• Control of hemoglobin • Reduction in thrombotic risk • Control of symptom burden • Reduction in splenomegaly	• Cost • Infection • Weight gain	• Intolerant to HU • High symptom burden • Splenomegaly
Ruxolitinib (MF)	• Reduction of spleen size • Reduction of symptom burden	• Cost • Infection • Weight gain • Increased risk of infections • Increased cholesterol	• High symptom burden • Splenomegaly

headache, visual changes, erythromelalgia, peripheral neuropathy, night sweats, spleen symptoms, night sweats, aquagenic pruritus, and gastrointestinal disturbances.[11] They will often have elevated platelets, as well as white blood cells noted on the complete blood count.

Work up and diagnosis

When a patient presents with erythrocytosis, it is important to utilize a systematic approach to correctly identify an etiology. A detailed history is critical, specifically inquiring about a history of cardiopulmonary disease, smoking, exogenous testosterone use, sleep apnea, and any evidence of a malignancy.[32] Additionally, patients who have had a renal transplant frequently will have a short-lived polycythemia.[33] At the initial evaluation, it is important to check for JAK2V617F mutations, JAK exon 12 mutations, and erythropoietin level (EPO). If the JAK2 mutation is present, then it is most likely PV. However, in the event these mutations are negative, the likelihood of having PV is quite small. The EPO level can help determine the next steps. If the EPO level is low, a bone marrow biopsy may help identify JAK2 negative PV. A cardiovascular evaluation including overnight pulse oximetry, pulmonary function tests, and echocardiography can be helpful in identifying cardiac or pulmonary disease. If the EPO level is high, one may consider CAT scans of the brain, neck, chest, abdomen, and pelvis to evaluate for evidence of a malignancy. The most common erythropoietin secreting malignancies include cerebellar hemangioblastoma, hepatocellular carcinoma, renal cell carcinoma, and uterine leiomyoma. If the patient is young, or there is a family history of erythrocytosis, one may consider evaluating for a hereditary erythrocytosis.[32]

The risk of thrombosis is dependent on age and history of thrombotic event, and ranges from 1.9% person/year—6.8% person/year.[34] There is also a risk of progression to MF and acute myeloid leukemia (AML). The risk of conversion to AML is 0.4% person/year. The risk of progression to MF is dependent on age as well as duration of time with the disease. A recent meta-analysis, the odds of MF transformation were found to increase on average 6% (95%CI: 1–11%) for each year of age, while those of mortality increase by 21% (95%CI: 9–33%).[34]

Risk assessment and treatment

The cornerstone of treating PV is to reduce the risk of thrombosis, as well as mitigate any symptom burden. When diagnosing a patient with PV, one must assess for any cardiovascular risk factors, or history of thrombosis. Risk stratification is essential in determining upfront therapy. The risk stratification of patients with PV was derived from the data in the ECLAP study, in which patients greater than 65 and with a history of thrombosis were considered high risk for thrombotic events.[35] In patients considered low risk, who are less than 60 years of age, and have no history of thromboembolic disease, they should be started on ASA and initiate therapeutic phlebotomy. In patients who are considered higher risk, based on age greater than 60 and/or a history of a thromboembolic event, it is recommended to use ASA, phlebotomy, and cytoreduction. The hematocrit goal of less than 0.45 was established in the cytoreductive therapy in PV (CYTO-PV), where a more stringent control of hematocrit was associated with a reduced risk of cardiovascular events.[36] Response is measured as hematologic response, which is normalization of the hemoglobin, as well as spleen response, is normalization of spleen size.[37] Newer concepts revolve around molecular response as well as symptom response. Molecular complete response is defined as eradication of the molecular clone, whereas partial response is a 50% reduction.[37] Symptom response is defined as a decrease in at least 10 points in the MPN-TSS.[37]

Phlebotomy is the always initiated at diagnosis, even if systemic therapy is also pursued (see Figure 2). Upfront cytoreductive therapy for PV is recommended in higher-risk patients. Choices for upfront therapy include HU or interferon.[28] HU is a therapy that has been used for many years in the treatment of PV.[34,38,39] The major side effects people experience include mouth sores, nonhealing ulcers on the extremities, and gastrointestinal distress. Another therapy that is used is interferon. Interferon has been used for decades to treat MPNs and was a mainstay of treatment of CML prior to the introduction of imatinib.[40] Its use in non-CML MPNs has been explored.[41,42] It is effective in reducing blood counts but may also have a disease modifying effect. In several studies, including a large randomized study comparing interferon and HU, some patients experienced either reduction in the clonal burden, or a complete molecular remission. The original form of interferon alpha was very difficult to tolerate, however, with the introduction of pegylated formulations of interferon, such as pegylated interferon-2a, the side effect profile is much more manageable.[42] A novel monopegylated interferon ropeginterferon alfa-2b was studied in a large randomized study, divided into the PROUD-PV study (first 12 mo) and CONTINUATION-PV (12–36 mo). In this study, 257 patients were randomized, 127 were treated in each group (three patients withdrew consent in the HU group). Median follow-up was 182.1 weeks (IQR 166.3–201.7

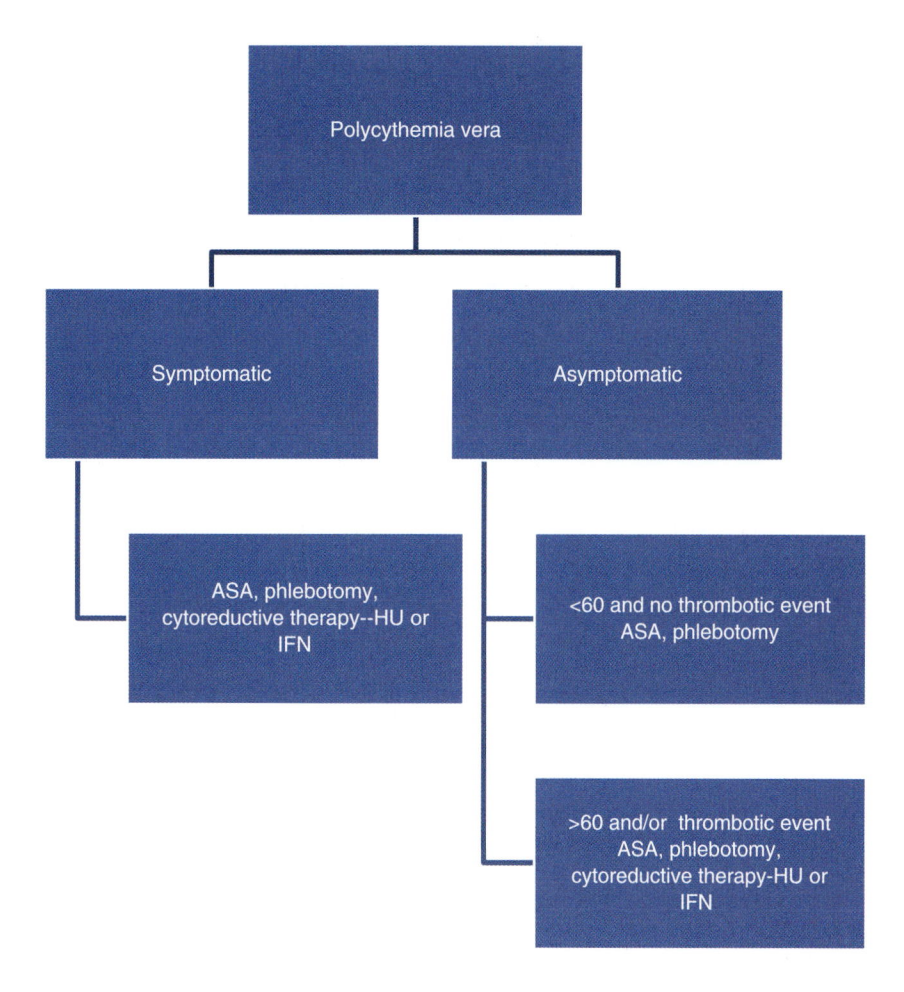

Figure 2 Treatment algorithm for polycythemia vera.

in the ropeginterferon alfa-2b and 164.5 weeks (144.4–169.3) in the standard therapy group. In PROUD-PV, 26 (21%) of 122 patients in the ropeginterferon alfa-2b group and 34 (28%) of 123 patients in the HU group met the composite primary endpoint of complete hematological response with normal spleen size. In CONTINUATION-PV, the primary endpoint was met in 50 (53%) of 95 patients in the ropeginterferon alfa-2b group versus 28 (38%) of 74 patients in the HU group, $p = 0.044$ at 36 months, suggesting ongoing response even after 12 months. Complete hematological response, without meeting spleen criterion, in the ropeginterferon alfa-2b group versus standard therapy group were: 53 (43%) of 123 patients versus 57 (46%) of 125 patients, $p = 0.63$ at 12 months (PROUD-PV), and 67 (71%) of 95 patients versus 38 (51%) of 74 patients, $p = 0.012$ at 36 months (CONTINUATION-PV).

In patients who are not effectively controlled or intolerant of HU, ruxolitinib is an option.[43] The RESPONSE study was a randomized study comparing ruxolitinib with BAT (which was HU in over half the patients) in patients who were intolerant or resistant to HU. The primary endpoint was hematocrit control as well as spleen response (35% reduction in spleen volume reduction). The primary endpoint was met in 28% of patients in the ruxolitinib arm, and 1% in best available therapy (BAT) arm. Hematologic response was observed in 60% of patients in the ruxolitinib arm, and 20% of patients in the BAT arm. Impressively, 49% of patients in the ruxolitinib arm had 50% reduction in their symptom burden, as assessed by MPN-TSS, as compared to 5% of the patients in the BAT arm.[44]

Myelofibrosis

Background and presentation

MF is a disease characterized by bone marrow fibrosis, anemia, elevated WBC, splenomegaly and constitutional symptoms such as fevers, night sweats, unexplained weight loss, and fatigue.[14,45,46] This disease can develop *de novo*, PMF or can be progressive disease after ET (Post-ET MF) or PV (Post-PV MF). The incidence of MF is approximately 1.5 per 100,000 population.[47]

Patients who present with MF may present with a variety of symptoms. In some patients, they will present with debilitating constitutional symptoms, anemia, and elevated WBC. Others may present with pancytopenia and no splenomegaly. At initial diagnosis, patients with PMF can be diagnosed with prefibrotic MF, or overt MF (Table 2). In the case of secondary MF, patients followed for PV or ET start to develop worsening splenomegaly, a leukoerythroblastic picture in their blood, and an elevated lactate dehydrogenase (LDH). To formally receive the diagnosis of secondary MF, patients need a bone marrow biopsy which shows increase increased reticulin fibrosis, and have at least two of the following: splenomegaly, a leukoerythroblastic peripheral blood film, elevated LDH, constitutional symptoms, or not otherwise explained anemia.[48]

At initial diagnosis, it is critical to have a bone marrow aspirate and biopsy, as well as identify whether a driver mutation is present or not. In patients with MF, there are 20% who will not have a driver mutation such as *CAL-R, MPL,* or *JAK2V617F*.

```
                    ┌─────────────────┐
                    │  Myelofibrosis  │
                    └────────┬────────┘
                             │
        ┌────────────────────┤
        │                    │
┌───────────────┐            │
│Risk assessment│            │
│Mutation       │            │
│analysis       │            │
└───────────────┘            │
                             │
              ┌──────────────┴──────────────┐
              │                             │
      ┌───────────────┐            ┌──────────────────┐
      │   Treatment   │            │Transplant        │
      │               │            │evaluation        │
      └───────┬───────┘            └────────┬─────────┘
              │                             │
```

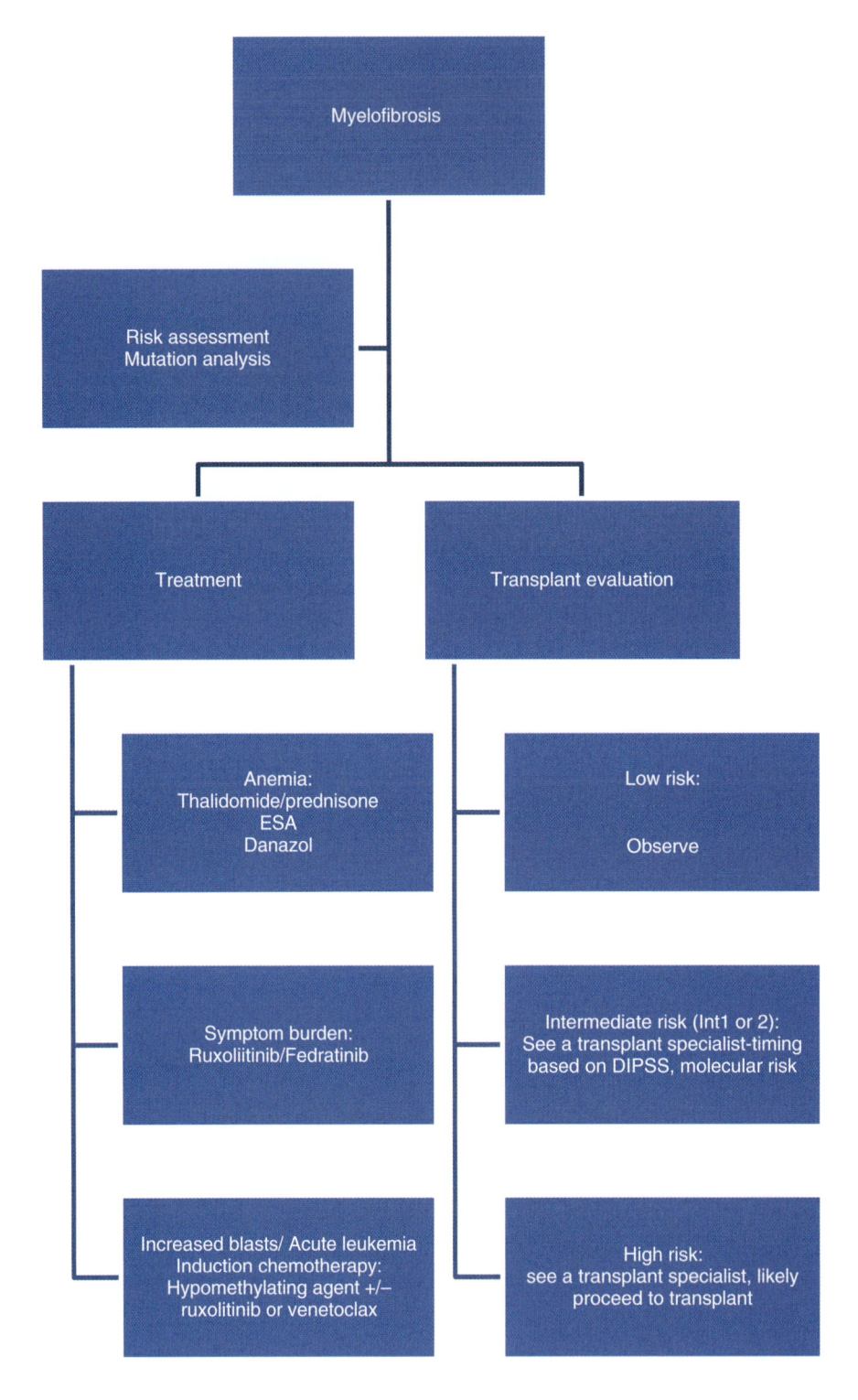

Figure 3 Algorithm for myelofibrosis.

Treatment branches:
- Anemia: Thalidomide/prednisone, ESA, Danazol
- Symptom burden: Ruxoliitinib/Fedratinib
- Increased blasts/ Acute leukemia Induction chemotherapy: Hypomethylating agent +/− ruxolitinib or venetoclax

Transplant evaluation branches:
- Low risk: Observe
- Intermediate risk (Int1 or 2): See a transplant specialist-timing based on DIPSS, molecular risk
- High risk: see a transplant specialist, likely proceed to transplant

Risk assessment and treatment

Prognosis

Risk assessment of patients with MF is critical to determining both therapy, as well as allogeneic stem cell transplantation (alloSCT) (see Figure 3). Prognosis of MF can be evaluated through a number of different prognostic scoring systems (see Table 5). The most commonly used is Dynamic International Prognostic Scoring System (DIPSS), which takes into account laboratory and clinical variables such as anemia, leukocytosis, constitutional symptoms, increased peripheral blasts, and age.[49] This was expanded upon by including transfusion dependence, thrombocytopenia, and poor-risk cytogenetics in the DIPSS plus.[50] The driver mutation can also contribute to risk; patients who are lacking a mutation are considered "triple negative" and carry a worse prognosis. Patients who have a *CAL-R* mutation

Table 5 Prognostic scoring systems for primary myelofibrosis.

Risk scoring system	Factors contributing to risk	Median survival
DIPSS[49]	Anemia (2 pt) Circulating blasts ≥2% Constitutional symptoms Age >65 WBC >25	• *Low risk:* (0 pt) not reached • *Intermediate-1:* (1–2 pt) 14.2 yr • *Intermediate-2:* (3–4 pts) 4 yr • *High risk:* (5–6 pts) 1.5 yr
DIPSS plus[50]	DIPSS score Platelets <100 RBC transfusion dependent Poor risk cytogenetics[a]	• *Low risk:* 185 mo • *Intermediate-1:* 78 mo • *Intermediate-2:* 35 mo • *High risk:* 16 mo
MIPSS70/MIPSS70 plus[51]	Clinical risk factors: • Severe anemia (men: hemoglobin [Hgb] <9 g/dL; women: Hgb <8 g/dL): 2 points • Moderate anemia (men: Hgb 9–10.9 g/dL; women: Hgb 8–9.9 g/dL): 1 point • Circulating blasts ≥2%: 1 point • Constitutional symptoms: 2 points • Cytogenetic risk factors[a]: • Very high risk (VHR): 4 points • Unfavorable: 3 points Mutations: • ≥2 high molecular risk (HMR)[b] mutations: 3 points • One HMR mutation: 2 points • Absence of type 1-like CAL-R: 2 points	• *Very low risk:* (0 pt) median survival not reached • *Low risk:* (1–2 pt) 10.3 yr • *Intermediate risk:* (3–4 pt) 7 yr • *High risk:* (5–8 pts) 3.5 yr • *Very high risk:* (≥9 pts) 1.8 yr
GIPSS[52]	Cytogenetics[a]: • Very high risk (VHR) = 2 points • Unfavorable = 1 point Driver mutations: • Absence of type 1-like CALR = 1 point High molecular risk (HMR) mutations: • ASXL1 mutation = 1 point • SRSF2 mutation = 1 point • U2AF1Q157 mutation = 1 point	• *Low risk:* (0 pt) 26.4 yr • *Int-1:* (1 pt) 10.3 yr • *Int-2:* (2 pt) 4.6 yr • *High risk:* (≥3 pts) 2.6 yr
MYSEC[51]	• Anemia hgb <11 = 2 points • Circulating blasts ≥3% = 2 pt • Non-CALR driver mutation = 2 pts • Plt <150 = 1 pt • Constitutional sx = 1 pt • Age × 0.15	• *Low risk:* (<11 pts) Not reached • *Int-1:* (11–14 pts) 9.3 yr • *Int-2:* (14–16 pts) 4.4 yr • *High risk:* (>16 pts) 2 yr

[a]Single or multiple abnormalities of −7, i(17q), inv(3)/3q21, 12p−/12p11.2, 11q−/11q23, or other autosomal trisomies not including +8/+9 (e.g., +21, +19).
[b]*ASXL1, SRSF2, U2AF1*Q157, *EZH2, IDH1/2*.

have a better prognosis, which appears to hold true in both primary and secondary MF.[3,4,51] There are also many somatic mutations which have been associated with myeloid diseases, some of which are predictive of outcomes with PMF.[4,6,8,53–56] For example, mutations such as *ASXL1, SRSF2, U2AF1*Q157, *EZH2, IDH1/2, p53* have been associated with a worse leukemia free and overall survival.[4,6–8,53–57] With the discovery of the somatic mutations, two more scoring systems were evaluated, Molecular International Prognostic Scoring System (MIPSS70) and Genetically Inspired Prognostic Scoring System (GIPSS). GIPSS is a scoring system which takes into account somatic mutations, driver mutation, and cytogenetics.[52] MIPSS70 is a comprehensive system which includes both clinical and mutational data to help predict outcomes.[51]

Medical treatment

Treatment of MF is dependent on several factors: symptom burden, presence of anemia, and splenomegaly (see Figure 3). If a patient is low risk, and does not have anemia, symptoms, or splenomegaly, it is very appropriate to observe. Treatment for MF historically (prior to the advent of JAK inhibition) included such drugs as HU, thalidomide, interferon alpha, and supportive measures such as erythropoietin simulating agents, and prednisone. To address splenomegaly, patients often underwent splenectomy, a procedure which carries significant morbidity, or splenic radiation.

Treating anemia in patients with MF is a challenge. JAK inhibitors can be challenging as they result in more anemia. The approach to anemia may include agents such as immunomodulators (lenalidomide, pomalidomide, and thalidomide), erythropoiesis-stimulating agents (ESAs), androgens such as danazol.[58] ESAs are most effective when erythropoietin level is <125.[59] Danazol can be considered in patients who have a high erythropoietin. Danazol should be started at 600 mg daily and demonstrated a favorable response rate in 37% of patients, 27% had a CR. It may take up to 3–6 mo to observe a response.[60] Finally, combination therapy of a immunomodulatory such as thalidomide, lenalidomide, or pomalidomide combined with prednisone may achieve 36–70% response.[61–64]

With the discovery of the pathologic mutation of *JAK2* in 2005 (*JAK2 V617F*), a new class of drugs developed, Janus Kinase inhibitors (JAK-is). Janus Kinases are a family of protein-tyrosine kinases that are critical in signaling pathways to promote cell growth. The JAK family includes JAK1, JAK2, JAK3, and TYK2 (tyrosine kinase 2). JAK1/2 and TYK2 are found in many cells throughout the body, and JAK3 appears to be confined to hematopoietic cells. In hematopoietic cells, JAK proteins bind to the juxtamembrane region of specific cytokine receptors and are involved in the generation of thousands of proteins involved in cell growth and differentiation.[65]

Ruxolitinib, a JAK1/2 inhibitor, was the first drug developed in this class. It was approved for MF in 2011. This latter approval arose from the positive results of two phase III studies in MF, COMFORT1,[66] and COMFORT2.[67] Response criteria in MF is defined by the following criteria: the spleen response as defined by spleen volume reduction (SVR) of 35%, and symptom response, which is a reduction of MPN-TSS of 50%. In COMFORT1, ruxolitinib was compared to placebo, and the primary endpoint of 35% SVR, was met in 41.9% of patients, and maintained for 48 weeks in 67% of those patients.[66] Reduction of symptom burden, as measured by a 50% reduction in MF-SAF 2.0, was observed in 45.9% of patients, and a mean improvement of 41.8% was appreciated in all patients who received ruxolitinib.[66] The COMFORTII study, which compared ruxolitinib to BAT, showed equal success, with 28% of the ruxolitinib treated patients experiencing at least 35% SVR, or 50% reduction in palpable splenomegaly at 48 weeks.[67] MPN specific symptoms were was not assessed in this study, but using EORTC-30 and FACT-Lym an improvement in quality of life was appreciated.

Ruxolitinib has been a very successful drug impacting splenomegaly, symptoms, and likely improving survival; however, it is not a cure, and the median time of response is 3.2 years.[68] When patients progress through ruxolitinib, the median survival is 14 months, and may be less in the setting of clonal evolution.[69] Additionally, many patients are intolerant of ruxolitinib due to side effects, such as anemia and thrombocytopenia. Therefore there is a critical need for treatments for patients with MF.

Fedratinib is a JAK-i which was approved in fall of 2019. JAKARTA-1 study randomized to one of three groups: 400 mg daily, 500 mg daily, or placebo.[70] The primary endpoint was reduction in spleen size by at least 35%, which lasted at least 4 weeks.[70] The secondary endpoint was reduction in symptom burden by 50% based on MPN-SAF 2.0. A total of 289 patients were enrolled from December 2011 to September 2012, randomly assigned to fedratinib 400 mg, 500 mg, and placebo. The spleen response observed at week 24, which was durable 4 weeks later, was in 35 (36%), 39 (40%), and 1 (1%) in the fedratinib 400-mg, 500-mg, and placebo groups respectively.[70] The symptom response at week 24 were 33 of 91 (36%), 31 of 91 (34%), and 6 of 85 (7%) in the 400-mg, 500-mg, and placebo groups, respectively. The most common hematologic toxicity was anemia, which had a nadir at 12–16 weeks. The most common nonhematologic adverse event was gastrointestinal symptoms.[70] Unfortunately, four cases of encephalopathy were noted in the patients who were in the Fedratinib 500 mg arm.[70] These were felt to be consistent with Wernike's Encephalopathy (WE), and the study was discontinued. There was also a phase II study, JAKARTA II study which evaluated fedratinib in patients who were ruxolitinib experienced. This study showed 50% reduction of SVR in 40% of the patients. The study was prematurely closed due to the WE observed in other studies.[71] Re-analysis of the JAKARTA- 2 data was done earlier this year, which applied more stringent criteria of ruxolitinib failure. In this new analysis, more specific definitions were applied including treatment >3 mo with regrowth of spleen, or failure of an adequate response specifically defined by less than 10% reduction of SVR or <30% reduction in spleen size. In this re-analysis, 30% of patients experienced a reduction in spleen size, therefore providing an option for those progressing through ruxolitinib.[72]

There are two other new JAK-i which have (1) completed successful phase III trials and (2) are completing additional steps seeking FDA approval: momelotinib[73] and pacritinib.[74] These medications are beneficial to specific groups of patients: momelotinib has mechanisms that make it attractive for patients with anemia, and pacritinib is targeted for patients with low platelets. For a summary of all the JAK inhibitors that are approved, or close to approval, see Table 6.

Future of treatment for MF

It is an exciting time for MF as the landscape of therapeutic options continues to expand. In addition to having two approved medications, as well as another two close to approval, different therapeutic options are becoming available. One area of interest is addressing the fibrosis in patients with MF, for which two antifibrotic agents have been examined. The first is PRM-151, a recombinant human pentraxin-2 molecule,[75] and AVID200, a TGF-beta antibody (NCT03895112),[76] both of which show promising results. Addition of agents to a JAK-i is a promising approach that is being tested with many agents, with the hopes of resurrecting a response. Examples of agents that have been published in the public domain include, umbralisib (PI3Kδ inhibitor, NCT02493530), CPI-0160 (BET-I, NCT02158858),[77] Navitoclax (BCL-2/BCL-xL antagonist,[78] NCT02493530), and Paraclisib (PI3Kδ inhibitor, NCT02718300), all of which show promising results.[79] There are several agents being used as monotherapy, including LC-161 (SMAC mimetics/IAP antagonists),[80] bomedemstat (LSD1 antagonist, NCT03136185),[81] have also shown promise. One other example is a drug that specifically targets anemia, such as luspatercept.[82] All of these represent novel concepts which will improve the treatment options for patients with MF.

Allogeneic stem cell transplantation for myelofibrosis
Hematopoietic stem cell transplant (alloSCT) is a potentially curative option for patients who have PMF, post-PV-MF, and ET-MF.[83-92] Patients who are young, and have a good performance status are considered for transplant, though increasing data suggest that older patients may benefit as well.[93]

Timing of transplant remains a difficult decision, however frequently is based on risk of disease. Transplant is felt to provide the most benefit when patients have DIPSS intermediate-2 or high-risk disease.[90] With the advances made in understanding the biology of the disease based on cytogenetics and somatic mutations, younger patients who have intermediate-1 risk disease and high-risk features may also experience a benefit.[93,94] The process of deciding exactly when to proceed with alloHCT is a shared decision-making process between the physician and the patients.

There are several issues that are unique to MF when considering transplantation. First, donor selection is critical. In transplantation for most diseases, it has become easier to identify a donor due to the use of haploidentical (half-matched) donors. However, in the setting of MF, this has not been well studied, therefore, should only be done after careful consideration.[95] Another issue is management of JAK inhibitors in the transplant setting. There is emerging data that use of peri-transplant JAK inhibition may improve transplant outcomes.[96]

Table 6 Clinical trials of JAK inhibitors in treatment of myelofibrosis.

	Study design	Number of patients	% with SVR >35%	% with ≥50% reduction in MPN-TSS
COMFORT1	**Phase III:** Ruxolitinib (RUX) vs placebo	Total: 309 RUX: 155 Placebo: 154	RUX: 41.9% Placebo: 0.7%	RUX: 45.9% Placebo: 5.3%
COMFORT2	**Phase III:** RUX vs BAT	Total: 219 RUX: 146 BAT: 73	RUX: 32% Placebo: 0%	Not measured
JAKARTA1	**Phase III:** Fedratinib (FEDR) vs Placebo RUX naïve	N= 289 FEDR 400 mg: 96 FEDR 500 mg: 97 Placebo: 96	FEDR 400 mg: 36% FEDR 500 mg: 40% Placebo: 1%	FEDR 400 mg: 36% FEDR 500 mg: 34% Placebo: 7%
JAKARTA2	Phase II FEDR RUX failure	N = 97	83 Evaluable for spleen response: 55%	90 evaluable for symptom response: 26%
SIMPLIFY1	Phase III Momelotinib (MMB) vs RUX	N = 432 MMB: 215 RUX: 217	MMB: 26.5% RUX: 29.0%	MMB: 28% RUX: 42.2%
SIMPLIFY2	**Phase II** MMB	N = 156 MMB: 104 BAT: 52	MMB: 7% BAT: 6%	MMB: 26% BAT: 6%
PERSIST1	**Phase III** Pacritinib (PAC) versus BAT JAK-i naïve	PAC: n = 220 BAT: n = 107	PAC: 19% BAT: 5%	PAC: 36% BAT; 14%
PERSIST2	**Phase III** PAC versus BAT RUX failure	PAC: 400 mg daily : 75 PAC: 200 mg twice daily: 74 BAT: 72	PAC: 18% (both arms) BAT: 3%	PAC: 25% BAT: 10%

Historically, survival at 5 years ranges has been reported between 38% and 75%,[97,98] treatment-related mortality (TRM) ranges from 25% to 40%,[94] and disease relapse occurs in 15–20% of patients.[94] However, this likely represents patients going to transplant at very advanced stages. In more recent years, there is a greater understanding of the importance of proceeding to transplant earlier in the disease course, which has resulted in better outcomes.

MF blast phase

As MF progresses, there is the possibility of conversion to AML. The definition for AML is ≥20% blasts in either the peripheral blood, or bone marrow.[21] However, when blasts are in the range of 10–20%, that is considered blast phase of MF, and caries a worse prognosis.[99] Median survival is only 3–5 months.[99,100]

Risk factors for progression can be divided into clinical characteristics and molecular characteristics. Clinical characteristics that may predict an increased risk of transformation to AML include peripheral blood blast percentage ≥3%, platelet count <100,[101] as well as a high DIPSS score.[49] Molecular characteristics include high-risk cytogenetics, such as monosomal karyotype[50,102]. There are somatic mutations as well that predict progression including *SRSF2, ASXL1,* and *IDH1/2*.[6,8,52,53,57] Interestingly, in a study done on patients who had failed ruxolitinib, clonal evolution was clearly identified, and predicted a shortened survival, however, in this cohort 12.6% had AML.

Treatment for secondary AML can vary widely. In young, fit patients, induction chemotherapy with 7 + 3 is often considered. Another option of induction chemotherapy includes liposomal daunorubicin and cytarabine, which has recently been approved for secondary AML.[103] However, with the advent of less toxic therapies for AML, the options are improving. Use of hypomethylating agents, usually along with another agent, has been effective in treating MF in blast phase.[99,100] One example of a combination therapy is a hypomethylating agent plus ruxolitinib, which had a 53% overall response rate in patients with MF in blast phase.[104] Another combination therapy which has been very effective in treatment of AML is a hypomethylating agent plus venetoclax, a BCL-2 inhibitor.[105] Patients who have proceeded to blast phase may have an IDH2 mutation, in which case they may be eligible for Enasidenib.[106] In patients who are appropriate for alloSCT, it should be considered if they have an appropriate donor and achieve a remission.

Special situations

Patients with MPN must be treated somewhat differently in the setting of pregnancy and surgery.

Pregnancy

The estimated frequency of MPNs during pregnancy is quite low, 3.2/100,000 maternities per year.[107] ET in the setting of pregnancy poses several potential challenges. Key concerns include the impact on the mother, including hemorrhagic and thrombotic events, as well as potential issues with the fetus, including early and late fetal loss, intra-uterine growth retardation, and preterm labor. In retrospective studies, the likelihood of a successful pregnancy outcome is around 60%.[108–111] there has been one prospective study evaluating outcomes of patients with MPNs,[107] which showed improved pregnancy outcomes, in 58 pregnancies (56 singleton and 2 twins) there was 58 live births. This study, however, was done using obstetrics data, so may have missed first trimester pregnancy loss.

Management of pregnancy in patients with ET has no standard guidelines. Griesshammer et al.[109] have suggested risk stratification

Table 7 Pregnancy and essential thrombocythemia.

	Risk factors	Recommended treatment
Low risk	IF NONE are present: 1. No prior ET-related complications, and 2. Absence of hereditary thrombophilic factors, and 3. Age <35 yr 4. Platelet count <1000 × 10⁹/L	ASA
High risk	IF ANY ONE is present 1. Previous microcirculatory disturbances, or 2. Presence of two or more hereditary thrombophilic factors (e.g., Factor V Leiden mutation plus a positive lupus anticoagulants, etc.), or 3. Severe complications in a previous pregnancy (⩾3 first trimester losses or ⩾1 second or third-trimester pregnancy loss, birth weight <5th centile for gestation, intrauterine death or stillbirth, stillbirth and preeclampsia necessitating preterm delivery <37 wk, or development of any such complication in the index pregnancy, or 4. Platelet count >1000 × 10⁹/L, or 5. Age >35 yr	ASA Consider LMWH during pregnancy Consider IFN
Highest risk	1. Actual thrombosis, or thromboembolic event during the last 6 mo, or 2. Previous maternal major thromboembolic or major hemorrhagic complications	ASA IFN Consider LMWH during pregnancy

of patients to low risk, high risk, and highest risk (see Table 7). It is recommended that all patients receive ASA, unless their platelet count is $>1000 \times 10^6$ and they are at risk for bleeding. In some patients, it is recommended that either interferon-α (IFN) is given for cytoreduction or low molecular weight heparin (LMWH) is given prophylactically. Postpartum LMWH and ASA are recommended for 6 weeks.[109]

Pregnancies during PV are rare, as only 15% of patients with PV are less than 40 years of age. There are a couple of reports of patients with pregnancy in the setting of PV that suggests patients have a high risk of poor fetal outcomes, with about 62–66% of pregnancies ending with favorable outcomes.[112,113] One study, which reported 18 pregnancies with PV who had pregnancy, suggested that careful management of hematocrit and anticoagulation may improve outcomes.[113] The NCCN guidelines endorses similar recommendations in both ET and PV with regards to control of blood counts, and use of ASA and LMWH.[28]

Surgery

There are two major risks in MPN patients who are going to undergo surgery: risk of bleeding as well as thrombotic events.[28] In a retrospective multicenter study, patients with PV and ET who underwent surgical evaluations were reviewed. A high proportion of patients experienced a thrombotic event, including 7.7% who had a vascular occlusion, and 7.3% who had a hemorrhagic event. There were 29 hemorrhagic events, 23 major, and 7 minor, and 5 deaths. Patients with ET were more likely to experience arterial thrombosis, and patients with PV were more likely to experience venous events. Bleeding events did not have appear to correlate with type of diagnosis, thrombosis prophylaxis, or type of surgery. A high proportion of PV and ET surgeries was complicated by vascular occlusion (7.7%) or by a major hemorrhage (7.3%).[114] In the event of an urgent need to proceed with surgery, platelet pheresis, and red cell pheresis may be considered. More work needs to be done to understand the optimal strategy for peri-operative management for these patients.

Summary

Management of MPNs is complex and rapidly changing. Understanding the complex clinical and molecular landscape of these diseases is critical to appropriate management. The assessment of thrombotic risk is the cornerstone to choosing therapy in ET and PV. Understanding the various clinical and molecular risk models is important in determining timing for alloSCT; however, therapy is generally driven by clinical presentation. Carefully evaluating both the thrombotic risk and hemorrhagic risk must be done, especially in the setting pregnancy and surgical settings.

Key references

The complete reference list can be found on Vital Source version of this title, see inside front cover.

1 Nangalia J, Massie CE, Baxter EJ, et al. Somatic CALR mutations in myeloproliferative neoplasms with nonmutated JAK2. *N Engl J Med*. 2013;**369**:2391–2405. doi: 10.1056/NEJMoa1312542.
2 Barbui T, Finazzi G, Carobbio A, et al. Development and validation of an International Prognostic Score of thrombosis in World Health Organization–essential thrombocythemia (IPSET-thrombosis). *Blood*. 2012;**120**:5128–5133. doi: 10.1182/blood-2012-07-444067.
3 Rumi E, Pietra D, Pascutto C, et al. Clinical effect of driver mutations of JAK2, CALR, or MPL in primary myelofibrosis. *Blood*. 2014;**124**:1062–1069. doi: 10.1182/blood-2014-05-578435.
4 Tefferi A, Lasho TL, Finke CM, et al. CALR vs JAK2 vs MPL-mutated or triple-negative myelofibrosis: clinical, cytogenetic and molecular comparisons. *Leukemia*. 2014;**28**:1472–1477. doi: 10.1038/leu.2014.3.
6 Vannucchi AM, Lasho TL, Guglielmelli P, et al. Mutations and prognosis in primary myelofibrosis. *Leukemia*. 2013;**27**:1861–1869. doi: 10.1038/leu.2013.119.
9 Mesa RA, Niblack J, Wadleigh M, et al. The burden of fatigue and quality of life in myeloproliferative disorders (MPDs). *Cancer*. 2007;**109**:68–76. doi: 10.1002/cncr.22365.
10 Scherber R, Dueck AC, Johansson P, et al. The myeloproliferative neoplasm symptom assessment form (MPN-SAF): International Prospective Validation and Reliability Trial in 402 patients. *Blood*. 2011;**118**:401–408. doi: 10.1182/blood-2011-01-328955.
16 Mesa RA, Schwager S, Radia D, et al. The myelofibrosis symptom assessment form (MFSAF): an evidence-based brief inventory to measure quality

of life and symptomatic response to treatment in myelofibrosis. *Leuk Res.* 2009;**33**:1199–1203. doi: 10.1016/j.leukres.2009.01.035.
19. Tefferi A, Cervantes F, Mesa R, et al. Revised response criteria for myelofibrosis: International Working Group-Myeloproliferative Neoplasms Research and Treatment (IWG-MRT) and European LeukemiaNet (ELN) consensus report. *Blood.* 2013;**122**:1395–1398. doi: 10.1182/blood-2013-03-488098.
21. Arber DA, Orazi A, Hasserjian R, et al. The 2016 revision to the World Health Organization classification of myeloid neoplasms and acute leukemia. *Blood.* 2016;**127**:2391–2405. doi: 10.1182/blood-2016-03-643544.
22. Barbui T, Tefferi A, Vannucchi AM, et al. Philadelphia chromosome-negative classical myeloproliferative neoplasms: revised management recommendations from European LeukemiaNet. *Leukemia.* 2018;**32**:1057–1069. doi: 10.1038/s41375-018-0077-1.
24. Barbui T, Barosi G, Birgegard G, et al. Philadelphia-negative classical myeloproliferative neoplasms: critical concepts and management recommendations from European LeukemiaNet. *J Clin Oncol.* 2011;**29**:761–770. doi: 10.1200/jco.2010.31.8436.
25. Barbui T, Vannucchi AM, Buxhofer-Ausch V, et al. Practice-relevant revision of IPSET-thrombosis based on 1019 patients with WHO-defined essential thrombocythemia. *Blood Cancer J.* 2015;**5**:e369–e369. doi: 10.1038/bcj.2015.94.
26. Alvarez-Larrán A, Pereira A, Guglielmelli P, et al. Antiplatelet therapy *versus* observation in low-risk essential thrombocythemia with a *CALR* mutation. *Haematologica.* 2016;**101**:926–931. doi: 10.3324/haematol.2016.146654.
28. Network NCC (2020) *Myeloproliferative Neoplasm*, Version 3/2019, https://www.nccn.org/professionals/physician_gls/pdf/mpn.pdf (accessed 23 July 2021).
34. Ferrari A, Carobbio A, Masciulli A, et al. Clinical outcomes under hydroxyurea treatment in polycythemia vera: a systematic review and meta-analysis. *Haematologica.* 2019;**104**:2391–2399. doi: 10.3324/haematol.2019.221234.
35. Marchioli R, Finazzi G, Landolfi R, et al. Vascular and neoplastic risk in a large cohort of patients with polycythemia vera. *J Clin Oncol.* 2005;**23**:2224–2232. doi: 10.1200/jco.2005.07.062.
36. Marchioli R, Finazzi G, Specchia G, et al. Cardiovascular events and intensity of treatment in polycythemia vera. *N Engl J Med.* 2013;**368**:22–33. doi: 10.1056/NEJMoa1208500.

PART 12

Management of Cancer Complications

121 Neoplasms of unknown primary site

John D. Hainsworth, MD ■ Frank A. Greco, MD

> **Overview**
>
> Cancer of unknown primary site (CUP) is a clinical syndrome accounting for 2–3% of all cancer diagnoses. This heterogeneous group is comprised of patients with metastatic cancer who have no anatomic primary site identified after a standard clinical evaluation. Using specialized pathologic techniques, including immunoperoxidase staining and molecular cancer classifier assays, identification of the tissue of origin is possible in most patients, even when an anatomic primary site cannot be located. For treatment planning, patients are divided into two groups. The first group includes a number of favorable subsets, identified by clinical and/or pathologic findings. Recently, new subsets have been identified, so that now approximately 40% of all CUP patients belong to a favorable subset. These various subsets require specific treatments, as detailed in the chapter. The remaining 60% of CUP patients do not fit into any of the favorable subsets; however, a tissue of origin can be predicted in most. These patients have traditionally received empiric chemotherapy, with modest efficacy. Increasing evidence suggests that site-specific treatment, based on the predicted tissue of origin, improves treatment results, particularly in patients predicted to have responsive tumor types. Current studies are also addressing the use of comprehensive tumor molecular profiling to identify actionable molecular alterations in CUP patients.

Cancer of unknown primary site (CUP) is a common clinical syndrome, accounting for 2–3% of all cancer diagnoses.[1,2] Patients with CUP are heterogeneous with respect to clinical features, pathology, response to treatment, and prognosis. The typical patient develops symptoms at a metastatic site, but routine history, physical examination, imaging studies, and laboratory studies fail to identify a primary site. Biopsy shows carcinoma in most patients; however, histologic examination is insufficient to fully characterize most of these tumors.

Optimal management of patients with the CUP syndrome requires the identification of patients within this heterogeneous group who have potentially treatment-responsive cancers and then using the appropriate treatment. Several favorable patient subsets can be identified by clinical and/or pathologic criteria and require specific treatment. With the recent recognition of several new favorable subsets, these groups now include approximately 40% of all CUP patients. Standard treatment for the remaining 60% of patients with CUP has been a trial of empiric chemotherapy, which produces modest benefit. However, as treatments improve and become more tumor-specific for many types of solid tumors, the idea that a single empiric chemotherapy regimen can provide optimum treatment for a heterogeneous group of CUP patients seems increasingly outdated.

Improvements in diagnosis have recently allowed re-evaluation of the role of empiric chemotherapy in CUP. Accurate prediction of the site of tumor origin is now possible for most patients with CUP, using improved immunohistochemical (IHC) stains and/or molecular cancer classifier assays (MCCA) based on tumor gene-expression profiling. Although clinical studies are continuing, most accumulated evidence indicates that site-specific treatment, guided by IHC or MCCA predictions, improves treatment efficacy for patients with potentially treatable cancer types.

In the first section of this chapter, the clinical evaluation of the CUP patient is reviewed. Although the basic evaluation is similar for all patients, specific additional tests based on clinical presentation or initial biopsy results are emphasized. In the second section, the pathologic evaluation for these patients is outlined, with emphasis on improved diagnostic capabilities using IHC and MCCA. In the final section, treatment for CUP is reviewed. Favorable patient subsets are reviewed separately, followed by a discussion of the evolving treatment approach to the patients traditionally treated with empiric chemotherapy.

Clinical evaluation

Most patients with CUP develop signs or symptoms at the site of a metastatic lesion and are diagnosed with advanced cancer. Common metastatic sites include the liver, lungs, lymph nodes, and bones; most patients have metastatic cancer at more than one site. The subsequent clinical course is usually dominated by symptoms related to the sites of metastases. During the clinical course, the primary site becomes obvious in only 5–10% of patients.

At autopsy, primary sites can be found in approximately 70% of patients, and are usually less than 2 cm in size. It is likely that many of the remaining 30% of patients also have small primary sites that are not palpable and remain undetected during the routine autopsy tissue sectioning. Since the largest autopsy series were reported prior to the routine availability of current imaging techniques, the results may not be representative of the current CUP population. The most common primary sites identified in historical autopsy series included the pancreas, hepatobiliary tree, and lung, accounting for approximately half of all cases.[3–5] Adenocarcinomas of the breast and prostate were identified infrequently, despite being common cancer types.

Initial clinical evaluation

When patients first come to the attention of an oncologist, they have had enough evaluation to demonstrate the presence of metastatic cancer, usually in multiple sites. Most have already undergone a biopsy, and have a histologic diagnosis. Almost all patients have carcinoma; categories of histologic diagnosis (in descending order of frequency) include adenocarcinoma, poorly differentiated carcinoma, poorly differentiated neoplasm, squamous carcinoma, and neuroendocrine carcinoma. Initial clinical evaluation is the same for all patients, but then varies based on initial results and histology.

Holland-Frei Cancer Medicine, Tenth Edition. Edited by Robert C. Bast, John C. Byrd, Carlo M. Croce, Ernest Hawk, Fadlo R. Khuri, Raphael E. Pollock, Apostolia M. Tsimberidou, Christopher G. Willett, and Cheryl L. Willman.
© 2023 John Wiley & Sons, Inc. Published 2023 by John Wiley & Sons, Inc.

Table 1 Recommended initial clinical evaluation.

- Complete medical history—includes detailed review of systems
- Complete physical examination—includes pelvic examination, stool for occult blood
- Laboratory evaluation—complete blood count, comprehensive metabolic panel, lactate dehydrogenase, urinalysis
- Computed tomography—chest, abdomen, and pelvis
- Mammography (women)
- Serum prostate-specific antigen (men)
- Positron emission tomography scan in selected patients
- Pathologic evaluation—includes initial IHC evaluation (CK7, CK20, TTF-1, CDX2)

All patients with the presumptive diagnosis of CUP should undergo initial clinical evaluation as outlined in Table 1. This evaluation includes a complete medical history, physical examination, complete blood counts, chemistry profile, and computed tomography of the chest, abdomen, and pelvis. (Many of these procedures may have already been done in the process of arriving at the presumptive CUP diagnosis.) In addition, specific signs and symptoms should be evaluated with directed radiologic or endoscopic studies.

Subsequent directed clinical evaluation

Additional evaluation should be directed by the location of metastases and the initial biopsy results.

Adenocarcinoma or poorly differentiated carcinoma
If the histology from the initial biopsy is adenocarcinoma or poorly differentiated carcinoma, all men should have a serum prostate-specific antigen (PSA) level measured, and all women should have mammography and/or breast magnetic resonance imaging (MRI). At one time, routine positron emission tomography (PET) scanning was recommended for all patients with adenocarcinoma of unknown primary site; however, a prospective comparative study showed that the routine use of PET scanning produced no added benefit when compared to CT scanning alone.[6]

Several subgroups of patients with adenocarcinoma or poorly differentiated carcinoma and specific clinical presentations are shown in Table 2. Additional clinical and pathologic testing is recommended for patients in these subgroups; in some cases, a primary site can be identified, and other patients may fit into a favorable treatment subset (see section titled "Favorable Subsets").

Squamous carcinoma
Squamous carcinoma of unknown primary site usually presents with isolated metastases in the cervical or inguinal lymph nodes. Since curative therapy is available for many of these patients, the initial clinical evaluation is critical for purposes of (1) identifying a regional primary site, and (2) delineating the extent of local tumor involvement.[7]

The cervical lymph nodes are the most common metastatic site for squamous CUP. Patients are often middle-aged or elderly, and many have a history of substantial tobacco and alcohol use. A second group of patients (approximately 25%) have human papillomavirus (HPV)-associated cancers[7-9]; biopsies of involved lymph nodes should be routinely tested for HPV. In addition to standard CUP evaluation, patients should have a thorough examination of the oropharynx, hypopharynx, nasopharynx, larynx, and upper esophagus by direct endoscopy, with biopsy of suspicious areas. Computed tomography of the neck is useful in defining the extent of disease and occasionally in identifying the primary site. PET scanning identifies a primary site in 25% of patients even after other procedures are unrevealing, and should be included as a standard diagnostic procedure.[10] When the lower cervical or supraclavicular lymph nodes are involved, a primary lung cancer should be suspected. Fiber-optic bronchoscopy is indicated if computed tomography and head/neck evaluations are unrevealing.

Ipsilateral or bilateral tonsillectomy has been advocated as a diagnostic modality if the primary site remains unidentified after the evaluation described above.[11,12] In one series, tonsillectomy identified a tonsillar primary site in 23 of 87 patients (26%).[13]

Most patients with squamous carcinoma involving inguinal lymph nodes have a detectable primary site in the genital or anorectal area. In women, careful examination of the vulva, vagina, and cervix is important, with biopsy of suspicious areas. Men should undergo a careful inspection of the penis and perineal areas. Digital rectal examination and anoscopy should be performed in both sexes to exclude lesions in the anorectal area. Identification of a primary site in these patients is important, since potentially curative therapy is available for carcinomas of the vulva, vagina, cervix, and anus, even after metastasis to regional lymph nodes.

Metastatic squamous carcinoma in areas other than the cervical or inguinal nodes usually represents metastasis from a primary lung cancer. Computed tomography of the chest and fiber-optic bronchoscopy should be performed if other clinical features suggest the possibility of lung cancer. A MCCA can also be used to clarify the site of origin. Patients with a lung cancer "profile" should be considered for specific treatment (see section titled "Favorable subsets").

Neuroendocrine carcinoma
The initial clinical evaluation of patients with neuroendocrine carcinoma is the same as described in Table 1; additional evaluation is based on the pathologic characteristics.

Low-grade neuroendocrine tumors (NETs) have the histologic appearance of typical carcinoid or islet cell tumors. When presenting with an unknown primary site, these tumors most frequently involve the liver. The presence of mesenteric masses on CT scan is highly suggestive of a primary tumor location in the small intestine. Some patients have clinical syndromes produced by tumor secretion of bioactive substances.

Approximately 80% of well-differentiated NETs have high concentrations of somatostatin receptors and can be detected using somatostatin receptor imaging. PET scanning with newer somatostatin-receptor analogs (68-Ga-DOTATATE or 68-Ga DOTATOC) is more sensitive than somatostatin receptor scintigraphy with indium-111 pentetreatide (OctreoScan) and is preferred if available.[14,15] Patients who have clinical symptoms or signs of a functioning tumor should have appropriate tests for blood and/or urine tumor markers. Elevated urine 5-hydroxyindoleacetic acid levels (5-HIAA) are highly specific for serotonin-producing NET, most of which originate in the small intestine.[16]

High-grade neuroendocrine carcinomas include typical small-cell or large-cell neuroendocrine carcinomas, as well as poorly differentiated carcinoma that is only recognized as neuroendocrine by IHC staining or MCCA. Patients with high-grade neuroendocrine carcinoma usually have multiple metastatic sites at the time of diagnosis, and rarely have syndromes mediated by secretion of bioactive peptides. Patients with a history of cigarette smoking should be suspected of having an occult lung primary site, and bronchoscopy should be considered. Patients with IHC staining for thyroid transcription factor-1 (TTF-1) should also be considered for bronchoscopy. Extrapulmonary small-cell carcinomas arising from various primary sites (salivary glands, esophagus,

Table 2 Additional evaluation of specific patient subsets identified by initial evaluation.

Patient group	Clinical evaluation	Pathologic evaluation
Women with features of breast cancer (axillary adenopathy, bone, lung, liver metastases; CK7+)	Breast MRI	IHC: ER, GCDFP-15, GATA 3 FISH: HER2 MCCA (if necessary)
Women with features of ovarian cancer (pelvic/peritoneal metastases; papillary/serous adenocarcinoma; CK7+, CK20−)	Pelvic/intravaginal ultrasound	IHC: WT-1, PAX8 MCCA (if necessary)
Features of lung cancer (hilar/mediastinal adenopathy; TTF-1 +)	Bronchoscopy	IHC: Napsin A, thyroglobulin-negative FISH: ALK/ROS-1 Mutation: EGFR MCCA (if necessary)
Features of colon cancer (liver/peritoneal metastases; CK20+/CK7−, CDX2+)	Colonoscopy	Mutation: KRAS MCCA (if necessary)
Features of renal cancer (retroperitoneal/lung/bone metastases; clear cell or papillary histology; CK7 + or CK20+)		IHC: RCC, PAX8, CD10 Mutation: MET (papillary) MCCA (if necessary)
Mediastinal/retroperitoneal mass	Testicular ultrasound Serum HCG, AFP	IHC: OCT4, PLAP FISH: i(12p) MCCA (if necessary)
Poorly differentiated carcinoma, with or without clear cell features	68-Ga Dotatate PET scan (if neuroendocrine stains +)	IHC: chromogranin, synaptophysin, RCC, Hepar-1, HMB-45, Melan-A, serum AFP (if Hepar-1 +) Mutation: BRAF (if melanoma stains +) MCCA (if necessary)

pancreas, bladder, prostate, colon/rectum, uterus, cervix) are occasionally identified during clinical evaluation. Patients with IHC staining for CDX2 should be considered for colonoscopy.

The origin of these high-grade neuroendocrine carcinomas remains unclear. Some patients may have small-cell lung cancer with an occult primary site. However, many of these patients have no smoking history, and the absence of pulmonary involvement makes this diagnosis unlikely in most patients. It has been speculated that high-grade neuroendocrine carcinomas share the same origin as well-differentiated NETs, but represent the opposite ends of a "spectrum" of tumor biology. However, it now seems more likely that high-grade neuroendocrine carcinomas have a different oncogenesis: many share the same chromosomal alterations commonly seen in small-cell lung cancer (deletions of 3p, 5q, 10q, and 17p), while there are no shared molecular alterations with low-grade NETs.[17,18]

Pathologic evaluation

Histologic examination

Examination of tumor histology by light microscopy is the critical first procedure in the pathologic evaluation and provides a practical classification system to direct subsequent evaluation. Almost all patients with CUP have carcinoma, which can be divided into five categories by light microscopic evaluation: (1) poorly differentiated neoplasm, (2) poorly differentiated carcinoma, (3) adenocarcinoma, (4) squamous carcinoma, and (5) neuroendocrine carcinoma. Occasionally, melanoma or sarcoma is identified at the initial examination.

Since histologic examination rarely results in the identification of the site of tumor origin, additional pathologic evaluation is important in almost every patient with CUP. For this reason, the initial biopsy should be planned so as to yield an adequate amount of tissue for all required pathologic studies; material produced from a fine needle aspiration biopsy is insufficient in these patients. Close communication between the oncologist and the pathologist is necessary so that the available biopsy material can be "managed" judiciously, ensuring that the most critical studies are obtained.

Poorly differentiated neoplasm

The diagnosis of poorly differentiated neoplasm is made when histologic features do not allow the pathologist to distinguish between carcinoma and other cancers, such as sarcoma, melanoma, and hematopoietic neoplasms. This diagnosis occurs in approximately 5% of CUP patients after standard histologic examination, but only rarely after specialized tests (IHC staining, MCCA) are performed.[19] Establishing a more precise diagnosis is essential in this group of patients, because highly treatable cancers (e.g., germ cell carcinoma, non-Hodgkin lymphoma, poorly differentiated neuroendocrine carcinoma, melanoma) are common.[20–22]

Poorly differentiated carcinoma

Patients with poorly differentiated carcinoma account for approximately 20% of patients with CUP; an additional 10% of patients have poorly differentiated adenocarcinoma. Examination of poorly differentiated carcinoma using routine light microscopy alone is inadequate to assess these tumors optimally. Panels of IHC stains and MCCA are both useful in establishing more specific diagnoses in this group of patients.

Adenocarcinoma

Adenocarcinoma is the most frequent light microscopic diagnosis in patients with neoplasms of unknown primary site and accounts for approximately 70% of cases. Because various adenocarcinomas share histologic features, the site of the primary tumor cannot usually be ascertained. Certain histologic features are typically associated with a particular cancer type (e.g., "papillary features" with ovarian and thyroid cancer, "signet ring cells" with gastric cancer); however, none of these is specific enough to be used as definitive evidence of the primary site.

Table 3 Poorly differentiated neoplasms: IHC staining patterns useful in determining tumor lineage.

Tumor type	Cytokeratin	Epithelial membrane antigen	Leukocyte common antigen	S-100 Protein, HMB45, melan-A	Vimentin	Desmin	OCT4, HCG, AFP, PLAP	Chromogranin/ synaptophysin
Carcinoma	+	+[a]	−	−	−	−	−	+/−
Lymphoma	−	+/−[b]	+	−	−	−	−	−
Melanoma	−	−	−	+	+	−	−	−
Sarcoma	−	+/−[c]	−	−	+	+[d]	−	−
Neuroendocrine tumor	+	+	−	−	−	−	−	+
Germ cell tumor	−	−	−	−	−	−	+	−

[a] Adenocarcinoma.
[b] Anaplastic large cell lymphoma (Ki-1 or CD30-positive lymphoma).
[c] Epithelioid sarcoma, synovial sarcoma.
[d] Leiomyosarcoma, rhabdomyosarcoma.

In recent years, the ability to accurately predict the site of origin in patients with adenocarcinoma of unknown primary site has improved. The identification of relatively cell-specific proteins by IHC staining allows accurate prediction of the primary site in 35–55% of patients.[23,24] Panels of IHC stains are most useful and are often directed by clinical features (e.g., gender, sites of metastases). In addition, currently available MCCAs accurately predict the site of origin in most patients with adenocarcinoma of unknown primary site, including those in which IHC stains are nondiagnostic (see section titled "Molecular Cancer Classifier Assays"). Complete evaluation of adenocarcinoma of unknown primary site, therefore, requires the use of these specialized pathologic techniques.

Squamous carcinoma
Squamous carcinoma accounts for approximately 5% of patients with CUP. The large majority of these patients have specific clinical syndromes for which effective treatment is available. A definitive diagnosis of squamous carcinoma can usually be made by histologic examination. Squamous carcinomas from various primary sites can often be distinguished using a MCCA.[25,26]

Neuroendocrine carcinoma
A broad spectrum of neuroendocrine neoplasia is now recognized, due in part to improved pathologic diagnosis. Approximately 3% of CUP patients have neuroendocrine carcinoma, and can be divided into three groups including low-grade tumors (carcinoid/islet cell type), high-grade NETs (small-cell carcinoma, atypical carcinoid, large-cell neuroendocrine carcinoma), and poorly differentiated carcinoma (neuroendocrine features apparent only with specialized pathologic tests). The distinction between low-grade and high-grade carcinoma is critical in determining treatment.

Immunohistochemical Staining

IHC staining is the most widely available adjunctive tool for the classification of neoplasms. Specific IHC staining patterns can usually establish the tumor lineage of poorly differentiated neoplasms (Table 3).[23,27–29] Examples include the distinction between carcinoma and lymphoma, the identification of poorly differentiated neuroendocrine carcinoma, and the occasional identification of melanoma and sarcoma.[22,23,30–32]

When used to evaluate CUP, the accuracy of IHC staining in identifying the tissue of origin has improved. Table 4 shows typical staining patterns for a number of carcinomas. These results must be interpreted in the context of clinical and histologic features, since staining patterns overlap and few IHC stains are entirely specific. The PSA stain is an exception and is specific for prostate adenocarcinoma.[29] For other carcinomas, panels of IHC stains have been shown to improve specificity. Four IHC stains (CK7, CK20, CDX2, TTF-1) form the basis of several diagnostic patterns and are appropriate initial stains in the evaluation of most CUP biopsies. Additional stains may be indicated based on clinical features and results of the initial IHC panel.[33–36] A few classic staining patterns have been described that are usually diagnostic (e.g., CK7+/CK20−/TTF-1+ for lung adenocarcinoma, CK7−/CK20+/CDX2+ for colorectal adenocarcinoma). However, specific cancers do not all stain with classic patterns, and false-positive and negative IHC staining are not uncommon. Even with these limitations, IHC stains enable the prediction of a single primary site (as opposed to being inconclusive or being compatible with two or more primary sites) in 35–50% of CUPs.[24,37–40]

Electron microscopy

The identification of specific ultrastructural features by electron microscopy enables a definitive diagnosis in some poorly differentiated neoplasms. Because it is less widely available, requires special tissue fixation at the time of biopsy, and is relatively expensive, electron microscopy should be reserved for the study of neoplasms with uncertain lineage after routine light microscopy, IHC staining, and MCCA.

Table 4 Carcinoma of unknown primary site: IHC staining patterns useful in identifying the tissue of origin.

Specific carcinomas	Immunohistochemical (IHC) staining
Bladder (transitional cell)	CK20 (+), CK5/6 (+), p63 (+), GATA3 (+), urothelin (+)
Breast	CK7 (+), ER (+), PR (+), GCDFP-15 (+), Her2 (+), mammaglobin (+), GATA3 (+)
Colorectal	CK20 (+), CK7 (−), CDX2 (+)
Germ cell	PLAP (+), OCT4 (+), HCG (+), AFP (+)
Liver	Hepar1 (+), CD10 (+), CK7 (−), CK20 (−)
Lung: adenocarcinoma	TTF1 (+), CK7 (+), CK20 (−)
Lung: neuroendocrine (small cell/large cell)	TTF1 (+), chromogranin (+), synaptophysin (+)
Lung: squamous	CK7 (+), CK20 (−), P63 (+), CK5/6 (+), P40 (+)
Ovary	CK7 (+), ER (+), WT1 (+), PAX8 (+), mesothelin (+), CK20 (−)
Pancreas	CK7 (+), CA19-9 (+), mesothelin (+)
Prostate	PSA (+), CK7 (−), CK20 (−)
Renal	RCC (+), PAX8 (+), CD10 (+), pan-cytokeratin AE 1/3 (+)
Thyroid (follicular/papillary)	Thyroglobulin (+), TTF1 (+), PAX8 (+)

Tumor-specific chromosomal abnormalities

Several tumor-specific chromosomal abnormalities are occasionally important in the diagnosis of CUP. Most B-cell and T-cell lymphomas are associated with tumor-specific rearrangements of immunoglobulin genes or T-cell antigen-receptor genes.[41] In the unusual case when the diagnosis of lymphoma cannot be definitively established with either IHC staining or flow cytometric immunophenotyping, the detection of these specific gene rearrangements provides definitive diagnostic information. Specific abnormalities associated with solid tumors include a chromosomal translocation (rcp [11:22][q24; q12]) present in all peripheral neuroepitheliomas and most Ewing tumors,[42,43] t (15 : 19) in children and young adults with carcinoma of midline structures or uncertain histogenesis,[44] and an isochromosome of the short arm or chromosome 12 (i12p) in a large percentage of testicular and extragonadal germ cell tumors.[45] Most of the neoplasms identifiable by specific chromosomal abnormalities can now be identified using methods that are more widely available, including IHC staining and MCCA.

Molecular cancer classifier assays

MCCAs can accurately identify the tissue of origin in most patients with CUP. The diagnostic efficacy of MCCAs is based on the distinct gene expression profiles present in different normal body tissues. When cancers arise from normal tissues, the distinct gene expression profiles are usually retained, at least in part, by the neoplastic cells, allowing identification of the tumor site of origin.[46]

The application of reverse transcriptase-polymerase chain reaction (RT-PCR), gene microarray, or epigenetic techniques, coupled with improved bioinformatics systems, has allowed the development of MCCAs capable of detecting more than 40 tumor types/subtypes.[25,26,47–54] In validation studies, blinded tumor biopsies from patients with advanced cancer (primary site known) were assayed and MCCAs accurately predicted the tissue of origin in 85–90% of cases.[26,53] Accuracy was high regardless of the biopsy site (primary site vs metastasis) or tumor grade (well differentiated vs poorly differentiated).

Accuracy of MCCAs in predicting CUP tissue of origin

The accuracy of MCCAs in CUP has been difficult to assess, since an anatomic primary site is not identified in most patients. However, evidence from several studies strongly suggests that accuracy in CUP is similar to that previously demonstrated in the validation studies using advanced cancers of known primary site. The most direct evidence comes from a study using the 92-gene RT-PCR MCCA (CancerTYPE ID, BioTheranostics, Inc.) in patients with CUP who subsequently had primary sites identified during their disease course (9–314 weeks after initial evaluation).[24,55] In 18 of 24 such patients (75%), MCCA performed on the original biopsy specimen resulted in correct prediction of the anatomic primary site. Despite concerns regarding the unique biology of CUP, most of these cancers apparently retain enough of the gene expression profile of their tissues of origin to allow identification with current assays.

It is of interest to compare the anatomic primary sites identified at autopsy[4] with the primary sites predicted by MCCA in a large group of CUP patients[56] (Table 5). Since these studies were performed more than 30 years apart, it is likely that the composition of the CUP groups differed. However, primary sites in the gastrointestinal tract (hepatobiliary, pancreas, colon/rectum) and lung were common in both series. Within the GI tract, biliary site of origin was more common in the MCCA series; perhaps the clinical and pathologic difficulty in distinguishing intrahepatic cholangiocarcinoma from liver metastases or primary hepatocellular carcinoma provides a partial explanation for these differences. In addition, the urothelium was predicted as a primary site more frequently by MCCA; the identification of breast and ovarian cancers was also more common. It is likely that small primary sites in the breast, ovary, fallopian tubes, and urothelial system may not have been during a routine postmortem examination. These differences may have practical importance, since breast and ovarian cancers are relatively sensitive to treatment.

MCCAs have also been evaluated in patients with poorly differentiated neoplasms of unknown primary site who had undefined tumor lineage after standard pathologic evaluation (which included a median of 18 IHC stains).[19] MCCA gave lineage predictions in 25 of 30 patients (carcinoma 10, melanoma 5, sarcoma 8, hematopoietic malignancy 2), and predicted a tissue of origin for all 10 carcinomas, including germ cell carcinomas. Additional studies and/or response to treatment supported the MCCA results in most patients.

Since MCCAs are not 100% accurate, diagnoses should always be interpreted in conjunction with clinical features and results of other pathologic studies. In particular, two features of MCCAs may cause inaccurate diagnoses. First, several cancer types have overlapping gene expression profiles (e.g., breast, salivary gland, and skin adnexal cancers share similar gene expression profiles); clinical and pathologic features may be critical in determining the correct diagnosis. Second, cancer types that are not included in the particular MCCA being used cannot be diagnosed. When this situation occurs, the cancer is either considered unclassifiable or misdiagnosed as a cancer type with an overlapping gene expression profile.

Table 5 Sites of origin—comparison of historical autopsy results and molecular tumor profiling predictions.

Primary site	Molecular tumor profiling predictions[54] (N = 252)	Autopsy results[a, 4] (N = 133)
Biliary tract	52 (21%)	0
Urothelium	31 (12%)	0
Lung	28 (11%)	29 (22%)
Colon/rectum	28 (11%)	6 (2%)
Pancreas	12 (5%)	28 (22%)
Breast	12 (5%)	1 (1%)
Ovary	11 (4%)	4 (3%)
Gastric/gastroesophageal	10 (4%)	8 (6%)
Kidney	9 (4%)	8 (6%)
Liver	8 (3%)	16 (12%)
Sarcoma	6 (2%)	0
Cervix	6 (2%)	0
Neuroendocrine	5 (2%)	0
Prostate	4 (2%)	4 (3%)
Skin	4 (2%)	0
Germ cell	4 (2%)	0
Carcinoid, gastrointestinal	3 (1%)	0
Mesothelioma	3 (1%)	0
Other (1 each)	3 (1%)	6 (6%)
Thyroid	2 (1%)	1 (1%)
Endometrium	2 (1%)	0
Melanoma	2 (1%)	0
Skin, basal cell	2 (1%)	0
Unlocated/unclassifiable	5 (2%)	23 (17%)

[a] Three patients who had primary sites located antemortem are included.

Table 6 Summary of favorable treatment subsets.

Subset	Typical histology	Therapy
Women, isolated axillary LN	Adenocarcinoma	Treat as stage II breast cancer
Women, axillary LN + other metastases	Adenocarcinoma	Treat as metastatic breast cancer
Women, peritoneal carcinomatosis	Adenocarcinoma (often serous) or poorly differentiated carcinoma	Treat as stage III ovarian cancer
Men, blastic bone metastases or high serum PSA or PSA tumor staining	Adenocarcinoma	Treat as metastatic prostate cancer
Colon cancer profile (intra-abdominal metastases + typical histology/IHC)	Adenocarcinoma	Treat as metastatic colon cancer
NSCLC profile (hilar/mediastinal metastases + typical IHC)	Adenocarcinoma or squamous	Treat as metastatic NSCLC
Renal cancer profile (retroperitoneal/lung/bone metastases + typical IHC)	Clear cell or papillary	Treat as metastatic renal cancer
Thyroid cancer profile (cervical/mediastinal nodes/lung/bone metastases + typical histology + typical IHC)	Follicular or papillary adenocarcinoma	Treat as metastatic thyroid cancer
Isolated inguinal LN	Squamous	Definitive local therapy (inguinal node dissection and/or radiation therapy) +/− chemotherapy
Extragonadal germ cell syndrome	Poorly differentiated carcinoma	Treat for poor prognosis germ cell tumor
Neuroendocrine carcinoma, low grade	Carcinoid/islet cell features	Treat as advanced neuroendocrine tumor (NET)
Neuroendocrine carcinoma, aggressive	Small cell or poorly differentiated carcinoma	Treat as small cell lung cancer

Comparisons of IHC Versus MCCA

Two large studies have compared the accuracy of IHC staining panels versus MCCA in patients with metastatic cancer of known origin.[57,58] In both studies, pathologists were provided with formalin-fixed biopsy specimens; patient gender and biopsy site were the only clinical details provided. Both methods showed considerable accuracy in these patients with advanced cancer. In both studies, MCCA provided the correct diagnosis more often than did IHC staining (79% vs 69%; 89% vs 83%, respectively). The accuracy of IHC staining decreased in patients with poorly differentiated histology.[58]

Performing similar comparative studies in patients with CUP is not possible, since the primary site usually remains unknown. In one study, IHC staining suggested a single site of origin in 52 of 149 patients (35%).[59] In these 52 patients, MCCA predicted the same site of origin in 77%. However, when IHC did not allow prediction of a single site of origin, the correlation between IHC and MCCA predictions was poor.

Four smaller studies also demonstrated good correlations between MCCA and IHC staining when a single diagnosis is suggested by IHC.[37–40] Overall, 78% of 117 patients reported in these five studies had matching diagnoses when IHC staining predicted a single tissue of origin. However, the ability of IHC staining to make a single diagnosis occurred in <55% of patients in all studies.

Summary

Improved diagnostics are able to accurately identify the site of origin in most patients with CUP. IHC panels identify a primary site in 35–50% of patients; these predictions correlate well with MCCA predictions. MCCAs provide accurate predictions in up to 85% of CUP patients, including cancers with nondiagnostic IHC results. Since the identification of treatable tumor types can improve the efficacy of treatment (see next section), panels of IHC stains and/or MCCA should be included in the pathologic evaluation of must CUPs.

Treatment

Following the initial diagnostic evaluation, several groups of patients emerge. In a few patients, evaluation leads to the identification of an anatomic primary site; these patients no longer have CUP and should be treated appropriately for their defined cancer type. A second group of patients (approximately 40%) fit into various favorable subgroups based on clinical and/or pathologic features, even though an anatomic primary site is not identified (Table 6). This group has increased in size with the recent addition of patient subgroups with colon, lung, and renal "profiles". The management of each of these subsets is detailed in this section. Although definitive data are now lacking, it is anticipated that several other cancer types within the CUP syndrome will also be considered as favorable subsets in the near future (e.g., ovarian, urothelial, gastroesophageal junction/gastric). Even with the recognition of additional favorable subsets, about 60% of CUP patients do not fit into any favorable subset. Empiric chemotherapy has been the treatment standard for this unfavorable group for many years and will be briefly reviewed. However, recent and ongoing clinical studies are focused on personalizing treatment based on predicted tumor type (by IHC and/or MCCA) and presence of targetable molecular alterations (identified by comprehensive molecular profiling (CMP)). These new data will also be reviewed.

Favorable subsets

Women with peritoneal carcinomatosis

In women, adenocarcinoma causing diffuse peritoneal involvement usually originates in the ovary, although carcinomas arising in the gastrointestinal tract, breast, or fallopian tubes can occasionally produce this syndrome (Table 6). However, peritoneal carcinomatosis also occurs in women with normal ovaries and no other evident primary site. This syndrome occasionally develops in women from families at high risk for ovarian cancer despite prophylactic oophorectomy[60] and is increased in incidence in women with BRCA1 mutations.[61] Many of these patients have histologic features typical of ovarian carcinoma, such as papillary configuration or psammoma bodies. Clinical features are typical of advanced ovarian cancer, with tumor involvement usually limited to the peritoneal surfaces and elevated serum levels of CA 125 antigen. When histologic features suggest ovarian carcinoma, this syndrome has been termed "multifocal extraovarian serous carcinoma" or "peritoneal papillary serous carcinoma".

Patients with this syndrome should receive the same treatments recommended for advanced ovarian carcinoma. Successful initial surgical cytoreduction is therapeutic and defines a favorable subgroup. Combination chemotherapy as used in advanced ovarian cancer has response rates of 39–66%, with long-term remissions in 15–20%.[62–65] Incorporation of new treatments for advanced ovarian cancer (e.g., poly adenosine diphosphate ribose polymerase [PARP] inhibitors) should also be strongly considered, even though these treatments have not been evaluated specifically in this uncommon subgroup of CUP patients.

Women with axillary lymph node metastases

Metastatic breast cancer should be suspected in women who have axillary lymph node involvement with adenocarcinoma.[66] Breast MRI or PET scanning may identify a primary site even when mammography is normal and should be performed.[67,68] Pathologic evaluation of the axillary lymph node biopsy should include measurement of estrogen and progesterone receptors, HER2 expression, and other IHC breast markers (Table 2). When positive, these findings provide strong evidence for the diagnosis of breast cancer.

Women with isolated axillary lymph node metastases are potentially curable and should be managed according to standard guidelines for stage II breast cancer. Primary therapy should include either modified radical mastectomy or axillary lymph node dissection followed by radiation therapy to the breast.[69–71] When mastectomy is performed, an occult breast cancer is identified in 44–82% of patients, even when physical examination and mammograms are normal.[71] Primary tumors are usually less than 2 cm in diameter; in occasional patients, only carcinoma in situ is identified in the breast.[72] Selection of adjuvant therapy should follow standard guidelines for node-positive breast cancer.

Women with metastatic sites in addition to axillary lymph nodes may also have metastatic breast cancer. These women should receive a trial of systemic therapy using guidelines for the treatment of metastatic breast cancer, particularly if IHC stains or MCCA support a breast cancer diagnosis. Hormone receptor status and HER2 expression should guide therapy, as in patients with metastatic breast cancer.

Men with skeletal metastases

Serum PSA levels should be measured in all men with adenocarcinoma of unknown primary site. Men with elevated serum PSA levels (or positive tumor staining with PSA) should be treated according to guidelines for metastatic prostate cancer, even if clinical features are atypical.[73,74] Osteoblastic bone metastases are also an indication for a trial of prostate cancer treatment, even in the absence of PSA findings.

Colorectal cancer profile

Current treatment has markedly improved the median survival of patients with metastatic colorectal cancer.[75] Identifying patients with occult colorectal primary sites from among the heterogeneous group of CUP patients is therefore potentially important, since many of the standard agents used for colorectal cancer are not contained in the empiric chemotherapy regimens used for CUP.

CUP patients with a colorectal cancer "profile," defined by clinical and pathologic features, are likely to have a colorectal site of tumor origin.[76,77] The colon cancer profile includes (1) typical clinical features (liver, peritoneal metastases), (2) histology compatible with lower gastrointestinal tract adenocarcinoma, and (3) typical IHC staining (CK20+/CK7− or CDX2+). Sixty-eight such patients, all with normal colonoscopies, had median survival of 28 months when treated according to standard guidelines for metastatic colorectal cancer.[77] Although this approach has not been formally compared to standard empiric CUP therapy, the favorable median survival (as compared to the usual median survival of 8–10 months with empiric chemotherapy) strongly suggests the merit of this approach.

Patients with CUP predicted to have colorectal cancer by MCCA should also be considered for colon cancer-specific therapy, regardless of IHC results. In two retrospective series, CUP patients who had a colorectal site of origin predicted by MCCA and received standard regimens for advanced colon cancer had median survival > 20 months.[78,79] In both series, approximately 45% of patients predicted to have colorectal cancer by MCCA had atypical IHC staining, and would not have been identified as having a colon cancer "profile."

CUP patients with a colorectal cancer profile should also have tumor tissue tested for microsatellite instability: high microsatellite instability (MSI-H) predicts efficacy of checkpoint inhibitor therapy (see section titled "Comprehensive Molecular Profiling").

Non-small-cell lung cancer (NSCLC) profile

In autopsy series, primary sites are found in the lung in approximately 20% of patients with CUP.[3–5] More recently, 28 of 252 CUP patients (11%) were predicted to have a lung primary site when tumors were tested with MCCA.[56] Therefore, lung cancer is one of the most common cancers represented in the heterogeneous CUP population.

When empiric chemotherapy regimens were developed for CUP, the use of platinum-based regimens (e.g., paclitaxel/carboplatin, gemcitabine/cisplatin) provided "coverage" for patients with occult NSCLC. However, current optimum treatment of advanced NSCLC may also include immunotherapy, various targeted therapies, and maintenance therapy. Second- and even third-line treatments are routinely administered. None of these therapeutic improvements is included in the empiric treatment for CUP.

CUP patients with a NSCLC "profile" often exhibit the following features: (1) mediastinal and/or hilar adenopathy, often accompanied by metastases at other sites, (2) adenocarcinoma or squamous histology, and (3) typical adenocarcinoma IHC staining pattern (TTF–1 +, CK7 +, CK20 -, thyroglobulin −).[29] MCCA prediction of a lung cancer primary provides additional strong evidence.[26,53,80–82] Standard first-line NSCLC chemotherapy regimens produced a median survival of 16 months in a small group of patients identified by MCCA.[56] However, no prospective studies have applied current NSCLC treatment in its entirety to these CUP patients.

Although further evidence from clinical trials is needed, strong consideration should be given to treating CUP patients with a NSCLC "profile" or a prediction of NSCLC by MCCA according to current guidelines for advanced NSCLC.[81] This includes early testing for critical molecular alterations (EFGR, ALK, ROS-1, BRAF, RET, MET exon 14 skipping mutation, neurotrophic tyrosine receptor kinase [NTRK], TMB, MSI) to guide selection of first-line and subsequent treatment.

Renal cancer profile

Renal cell carcinoma (RCC) accounts for approximately 5% of CUP in autopsy series and in MCCA series.[3–5,56] Improvements in the treatment of advanced RCC include immunotherapy and agents targeting VEGF or mTOR. None of these therapies is included in the empiric chemotherapy regimens for CUP. In addition, the empiric chemotherapy regimens used for CUP have no activity in the treatment of RCC.

Although advanced RCC has diverse clinical presentations, the diagnosis can often be suspected based on pathologic findings: (1) clear cell or papillary histology, (2) IHC staining for RCC marker, CD10, and PAX8, and (3) MCCA diagnosis of RCC.[81] (Since the renal-specific IHC stains are not included in the standard IHC panels, the opportunity to diagnose RCC with specific IHC stains can be missed unless RCC is considered as a possible diagnosis.)

In a retrospective series, 24 CUP patients predicted to have RCC by MCCA were reviewed.[83] Papillary histology was overrepresented in this patient group (11 of 24). Twenty patients received treatment with VEGFR or mTOR-targeting agents; response rate was 19% and median OS was 16 months (range 2–43+ months).

In a second retrospective series, 10 patients predicted to have RCC by histology and IHC (9 of 10) were treated with targeted RCC site-specific therapy. Half these patients were in the poor-risk category, but 40% responded to therapy and a few patients with intermediate risk had a median OS of 18.5 months.[84] In addition to these small series, a number of case reports document efficacy of RCC-specific treatments in CUP patients with a renal cancer "profile"[81,84] Further experience with this treatment approach is necessary in this patient subgroup, particularly with immunotherapy agents.

Thyroid carcinoma profile

Although rare, follicular/papillary thyroid carcinoma can present as a CUP. Metastases are usually in cervical or mediastinal lymph nodes, lungs, or bones. Tumor IHC staining for thyroglobulin is typical and provides strong support for the diagnosis; otherwise, IHC staining is similar to lung adenocarcinoma (TTF-1 +, CK7 +, CK20 −). Serum thyroglobulin levels are usually elevated. Treatment with I-131 is often effective. Treatment should follow guidelines for metastatic follicular/papillary thyroid carcinoma.

Carcinoma presenting as a single metastatic lesion

Occasionally, only a single metastatic lesion is identified after a complete clinical evaluation. Single lesions have been described in a variety of sites, including lymph nodes, brain, lung, adrenal gland, liver, bone, and skin. The possibility of an unusual primary site (e.g., primary cutaneous apocrine, eccrine, or sebaceous carcinoma) mimicking a metastatic lesion should be considered, but this possibility can usually be excluded on the basis of clinical or pathologic features.

In most of these patients, other metastatic sites become evident within a relatively short time. However, local treatment sometimes results in long disease-free intervals, and occasional patients have prolonged survival.[85] Prior to initiating local treatment, a PET scan is useful to rule out the presence of other metastatic sites.[86] If no other metastases are detected, the solitary lesion should be resected, if technically feasible, or irradiated. In some instances (e.g., after resection of a solitary brain metastasis), local radiation therapy may also be appropriate to maximize the chance of local control. The role of systemic chemotherapy in addition to definitive local therapy is undefined; however, adjuvant or neoadjuvant chemotherapy should be considered if a sensitive tumor type is suggested by IHC staining or MCCA.

Extragonadal germ cell tumor syndrome

A few patients with poorly differentiated carcinoma of unknown primary site have extragonadal germ cell tumors that are unrecognizable by standard histologic criteria.[45,87,88] These patients are usually young males with predominant tumor location in the mediastinum or retroperitoneum. Some also have marked elevations of the serum tumor markers HCG or α-fetoprotein. In most of these patients, the diagnosis can be confirmed using IHC, MCCA,[19] or identification of the i(12p) chromosomal abnormality specific for germ cell tumors.[45]

These patients should receive treatment for extragonadal germ cell tumor with four cycles of cisplatin-based chemotherapy followed by resection of residual tumor masses. Treatment results are similar to those achieved in the treatment of typical extragonadal germ cell tumors.[45]

Squamous carcinoma involving cervical or supraclavicular lymph nodes

Squamous carcinoma of unknown primary site most frequently presents with unilateral involvement of the cervical lymph nodes. The recommended clinical evaluation (previously described) results in the identification of a head and neck primary site in 85% of patients.[89]

When no primary site is identified, patients should be treated according to guidelines for locally advanced squamous carcinoma of the head and neck; approximately 50% have long-term disease-free survival.[90–92] As in patients with known primary sites in the head and neck, extensive involvement in neck nodes and poorly differentiated tumor histology are poor prognostic features.[90,93]

Patients with low cervical or supraclavicular lymph nodes are more likely to have a primary lung cancer, and treatment results are inferior. Nevertheless, patients with no detectable disease below the clavicle should be treated with the same approach as are patients with higher cervical nodes, since occasional patients will have long-term survival. Patients predicted by MCCA to have a lung site of origin should be considered for site-specific treatment (see section titled "Non-small-cell Lung Cancer (NSCLC) Profile").

Squamous carcinoma involving inguinal lymph nodes

Most patients with squamous carcinoma involving inguinal lymph nodes have a detectable primary site in the anogenital area. For the occasional patient in whom no primary site is identified, definitive local therapy with inguinal node dissection or radiation therapy sometimes results in long-term survival.[94] Because combined modality therapy has improved survival of patients with squamous cancer arising in this region (e.g., cervix, anus), the addition of chemotherapy should be considered in patients with an unknown primary site.

Low-grade neuroendocrine tumor (NET)

Carcinoid or islet cell tumors of unknown primary site usually exhibit an indolent biology, and management should follow guidelines established for metastatic tumors of these types with known primary sites. Treatment with a long-acting somatostatin agonist (octreotide, lanreotide) lengthens the time to tumor progression with low toxicity.[95] Depending on the clinical situation, appropriate management may also include local therapy (resection of isolated metastasis, radiofrequency ablation, cryotherapy, or hepatic artery chemoembolization). Single-agent treatment with everolimus or sunitinib prolongs PFS in patients with nonfunctioning well-differentiated NETs or pancreatic NETs, respectively.[96,97] For patients with somatostatin-receptor-expressing tumors, radiolabeled somatostatin analogs such as lutetium Lu-177 dotatate should also be considered.[98] The role of chemotherapy (e.g., capecitabine/temozolomide) is debated but may be useful in patients with clinically aggressive tumors.

High-grade neuroendocrine carcinoma
This group of patients includes small-cell and large-cell neuroendocrine carcinomas (histologic diagnoses) and patients with poorly differentiated carcinoma recognized to have neuroendocrine carcinoma by IHC staining. These patients should receive treatment with combination chemotherapy used for small-cell lung cancer; high response rates and a minority of long-term survivors (10–15%) have been reported.[99–101]

Poorly differentiated carcinoma
Patients with poorly differentiated carcinoma of unknown primary site form a large and heterogeneous group. The recognition that some of these patients had highly chemotherapy-sensitive neoplasms first occurred in the 1970s.[87,88,102] However, it is likely that currently available diagnostic methods identify the highly responsive patients in this group. The remaining patients with poorly differentiated CUP have a prognosis similar to patients with adenocarcinoma of unknown primary site. These patients should be evaluated using recommendations for adenocarcinoma.

Patients not included in any favorable subset

Empiric chemotherapy for CUP
Approximately 60% of patients with CUP do not fit into any of the favorable subsets outlined above. For many years, empiric chemotherapy has been the treatment of choice for most of these patients, since their tissue of origin could not be determined. At the time empiric chemotherapy regimens were designed, treatments were poor for many types of solid tumors. In addition, similar cytotoxic agents and regimens were used in the therapy of a variety of cancers. Therefore, it was possible to design "broad spectrum" regimens with reasonable activity against most sensitive tumor types.

Combination regimens containing most of the commonly used cytotoxic agents (taxanes, gemcitabine, topoisomerase I inhibitors, anthracyclines, vinca alkaloids) have been evaluated in the empiric treatment of patients with CUP. Combinations containing a platinum agent and a taxane have been most widely studied, and are commonly used.[103–108] Several other combinations (i.e., gemcitabine/platinum, gemcitabine/taxane) have similar activity.[109–111] Randomized phase II trials have compared various two-drug combinations and have usually yielded similar results.[110,112–116] The addition of a third drug has not improved efficacy.[114,117–120] Although response rates have varied, most trials have reported median survivals within a narrow range of 8–11 months, with two-year survival rates of 14–24%. In larger trials (containing 100 or more patients), the median survival is consistently about nine months.[112,117,119,121,122]

Empiric second-line therapy has been evaluated in a few phase II trials. Single-agent gemcitabine and the combinations of gemcitabine/irinotecan, capecitabine/oxaliplatin, and bevacizumab/erlotinib have had modest activity.[122–126]

Although no definitive studies have compared survival with empiric chemotherapy versus best supportive care alone, evidence from several large tumor registries suggests that current treatment results in an improved survival.[127–131] The Swedish Cancer Registry documented an improved median survival for patients with CUP during the years 2001–2008 (six months) versus 1987–1993 (4 months).[131]

Site-specific treatment directed by the predicted tissue of origin
The tissue of origin can now be accurately predicted in most patients with CUP. Although it is logical to assume that site-specific treatment based on the predicted tissue of origin would be superior to empiric chemotherapy, clinical data to support this assumption have only recently accumulated, and remain incomplete. One cause for skepticism regarding a site-specific approach relates to the unique biology of CUP (evidenced by the fact that the primary site does not become apparent). This fundamental clinical difference has led to the speculation that these cancers may also respond differently to systemic therapy. However, increasing evidence indicates that most cancers of unknown primary site retain the characteristics of cancers with known primary arising from the same site.

Several biological and clinical observations now support these similarities. First, gene expression profiles in CUP remain similar to advanced cancers from the same tissue of origin. Second, no unique molecular "signature" common to CUP has been identified. Third, successful treatments for patients in several of the clinically recognized favorable CUP subsets are based on the presumption that they have specific cancer types (e.g., women with axillary nodes are treated for breast cancer, women with peritoneal carcinomatosis are treated for ovarian cancer, etc.). Fourth, retrospective studies containing CUP patients predicted to have a colorectal site of origin by either IHC staining[76,77] or MCCA[78,79] and treated with standard colorectal cancer therapy documented median survivals >20 months, similar to the survival of patients with metastatic colon cancer.

In spite of these considerations, the superiority of site-specific treatment versus empiric chemotherapy has been difficult to demonstrate definitively. Several factors contribute to the difficulties of designing definitive studies. It is well known from autopsy series and MCCA that a large percentage of CUP patients (>60% in some series) have tumor types that remain poorly treated, and are therefore unlikely to benefit much from any treatment (e.g., pancreas, biliary, hepatic, gastric). Inclusion of such patients in clinical trials makes it difficult to demonstrate an overall benefit for site-specific treatment. In addition, increasing numbers of patients with potentially treatable tumor types are being recognized (e.g., patients with profiles of colorectal, NSCLC, renal cancers) and removed from this population, further skewing the group towards poorly treated tumor types.

The strongest support for site-specific therapy comes from a large, prospective trial in which biopsies from CUP patients were tested with a MCCA (RT-PCR CancerTYPE ID) prior to any treatment.[56] In this trial, a tissue of origin was predicted by MCCA in 242 of 253 patients (98%). Twenty-six different tissues of origin were diagnosed (Table 5). Patients received site-specific therapy based on the MCCA predictions and had a median survival of 12.5 months. Forty-one percent of all patients had treatment-resistant tumor types; these patients had a median survival of only 7.6 months. In contrast, patients predicted to have treatment-sensitive tumor types had a median survival of 13.4 months with site-specific therapy ($p = 0.04$). Although the numbers of patients with individual cancer types were small, median survivals within most of these groups were similar to those expected for the predicted tumor types (median survivals, months: ovary 30, breast 28, NSCLC 16, colorectal 13, pancreas 8, biliary tract 7).

A recent prospective phase II trial used next-generation sequencing (NGS) to identify the site of origin as well as any potential molecular targets; patients then received site-specific treatment.[132] Of the 97 patients treated, 66 (68%) were predicted to have treatment-sensitive cancers; 62% had colon, kidney, breast, ovarian, or lung cancer. The median OS was 13.7 months.

Several retrospective, observational studies also suggest the superiority of site-specific therapy, particularly in specific treatment-sensitive tumor types (colorectal, NSCLC, renal, poorly differentiated neoplasms).[19,54,76-80,83,133,134]

Two recent randomized trials have compared site-specific treatment directed by MCCA results versus empiric chemotherapy.[135,136] Neither trial demonstrated any difference between treatment approaches. In both trials, >60% of patients had treatment-resistant tumor types predicted. In one of the studies, a group of 60 patients with tumor types unlikely to respond to empiric chemotherapy was identified; in this small cohort, 1-and 2-year survival advantages were suggested in patients randomized to site-specific therapy (1-year 39% vs 30%; 2-year 24% vs 10%).[135] The small numbers of patients in these studies who had potentially treatment-sensitive cancer types was, therefore, not sufficient to allow conclusions regarding the best treatment approach.

Although the data remain incomplete, the following recommendations are currently appropriate:

1. For patients with cancer types predicted to be resistant to treatment (e.g., pancreas, biliary, gastric, hepatocellular, squamous carcinomas, others), empiric chemotherapy provides results that are equivalent to site-specific therapy, although both approaches have relatively poor efficacy. (Future improvements in the treatment of specific cancer types may result in a change from "treatment-resistant" to "treatment-sensitive.")
2. Randomized trials have not adequately addressed the subset of patients predicted to have treatment-sensitive tumor types. Based on the considerable evidence from nonrandomized trials, site-specific treatment is currently the best choice for this group. Site-specific treatment includes (1) use of site-specific first-line and subsequent-line chemotherapy, (2) molecular testing for molecular alterations pertinent to the specific tumor type, and (3) use of immunotherapy if indicated for the tumor type identified.

Comprehensive molecular profiling

CMP using a tumor biopsy specimen or a blood/liquid sample (cell-free deoxyribonucleic acid [cfDNA]) involves assaying a broad group of genes for the purpose of identifying potentially actionable oncogenic molecular alterations (e.g., HER2, BRAF, EGFR, others). CMP, therefore, differs from an MCCA, which measures differential expressions of normal genes to enable identification of a tissue of origin.

Testing for specific oncogenes is already a part of the standard management of several cancer types (e.g., HER2 in breast, gastric cancer; EGFR and others in NSCLC). The use of broader molecular testing has become much more common for several reasons: (1) cfDNA liquid biopsy platforms are becoming more common and accepted, (2) additional targetable molecular alterations have been recognized, (3) the activity of targeted agents frequently extends across many tumor types, as long as the specific target is present, and (4) efficacy of immunotherapy drugs can also be predicted based on the presence of specific alterations (MSI-H, high TMB).

In patients with CUP, retrospective CMP studies have identified a substantial number of targetable alterations. In a group of 200 CUP patients, 18% had molecular alterations for which approved targeted agents existed (HER2, BRAF, EGFR, ALK, RET, BRCA, ROS1).[137] The rare TRK mutation (not assessed in this group of CUP patients) is another tumor-agnostic targetable alteration responsive to currently available treatment.[138] Predictors of immunotherapy responsiveness have also been examined in CUP. In one study, high TMB (>20 muts/mb) was found in 8% of adenocarcinomas, 11% of carcinomas, and 23% of squamous carcinomas.[139] PD-L1 overexpression is also common; however, PD-L1 amplification and MSI-H are seen in only 1–2%.[140]

Recently, results of liquid biopsies (cfDNA) from 2022 patients with CUP were reported.[141] In this large group, 527 cancers had potentially actionable genetic alterations (Level 1 or 2) including the following selected examples: BRAF V600E (2.1%), BRCA1/2 (4.2%), MSI-H (2.4%), ERBB2 (2.1%), and MET exon 14 skipping mutation (0.6%). None of these patients had a tissue of origin diagnosed; therefore, the context of these data are uncertain but likely represent many of the specific cancer types within the CUP syndrome and emphasize the importance of cancer type diagnosis.

At present, the efficacy of targeted therapy or immunotherapy in CUP is documented in a few phase II studies[142,143] and several case reports.[80–82,84,144–149] Pembrolizumab produced an overall response rate of 23% in 22 previously treated CUP patients[142]; 3 responses were durable (16.7, 17.6, and 21.3 months). Nivolumab produced an overall response rate of 21% in a group of 56 CUP patients (11 previously untreated).[143] The median OS of all patients was 15.9 months, with several durable responses. Patients in both studies experienced substantial clinical benefits; although the specific cancer types were not diagnosed, they likely represent cancer types within the CUP syndrome that are sensitive to immune checkpoint inhibitors.

More experience is required to fully assess the benefits of these therapies. Even if targetable alterations are identified in a sizable minority of patients (as suggested by retrospective CMP studies), optimal treatment for the majority of these patients will continue to require the identification of a likely tissue of origin/primary site. Combination chemotherapy continues to play an important role in the treatment of many cancer types; targeted agents and immunotherapy are often added to site-specific chemotherapy, and are seldom used as single agents in the first-line setting.

Management of patients with CUP—overview and summary

Figure 1 diagrams the recommended management of patients with CUP. After initial clinical and pathologic evaluations (including IHC staining), patients in whom the anatomic primary site is identified do not have CUP and should be treated accordingly. Patients who fit into a favorable treatment subset should receive appropriate therapy. Patients not included in any favorable subgroup should have a MCCA, unless a single site of origin is predicted by IHC. Patients with treatment-sensitive tumor types (by IHC and/or MCCA) should receive site-specific treatment. In patients with treatment-resistant tumor types, empiric chemotherapy and site-specific treatment produce similar outcomes, so either approach is acceptable. Although further data are required, CMP to identify actionable molecular alterations should be considered in all patients who do not fit into a favorable subset.

The integration of molecular diagnostics into the management of CUP is already supported by clinical data, but continued investigation is necessary to refine management recommendations. The mechanisms of the CUP syndrome remain obscure but are likely related to genetic/epigenetic alterations; an understanding of these mechanisms may help explain the metastatic process and provide further data to develop specific therapies. Further improvements in the treatment for CUP patients will be linked to improvements in therapy of other specific cancer types, particularly those that are currently treatment-resistant. Better definition of the role of

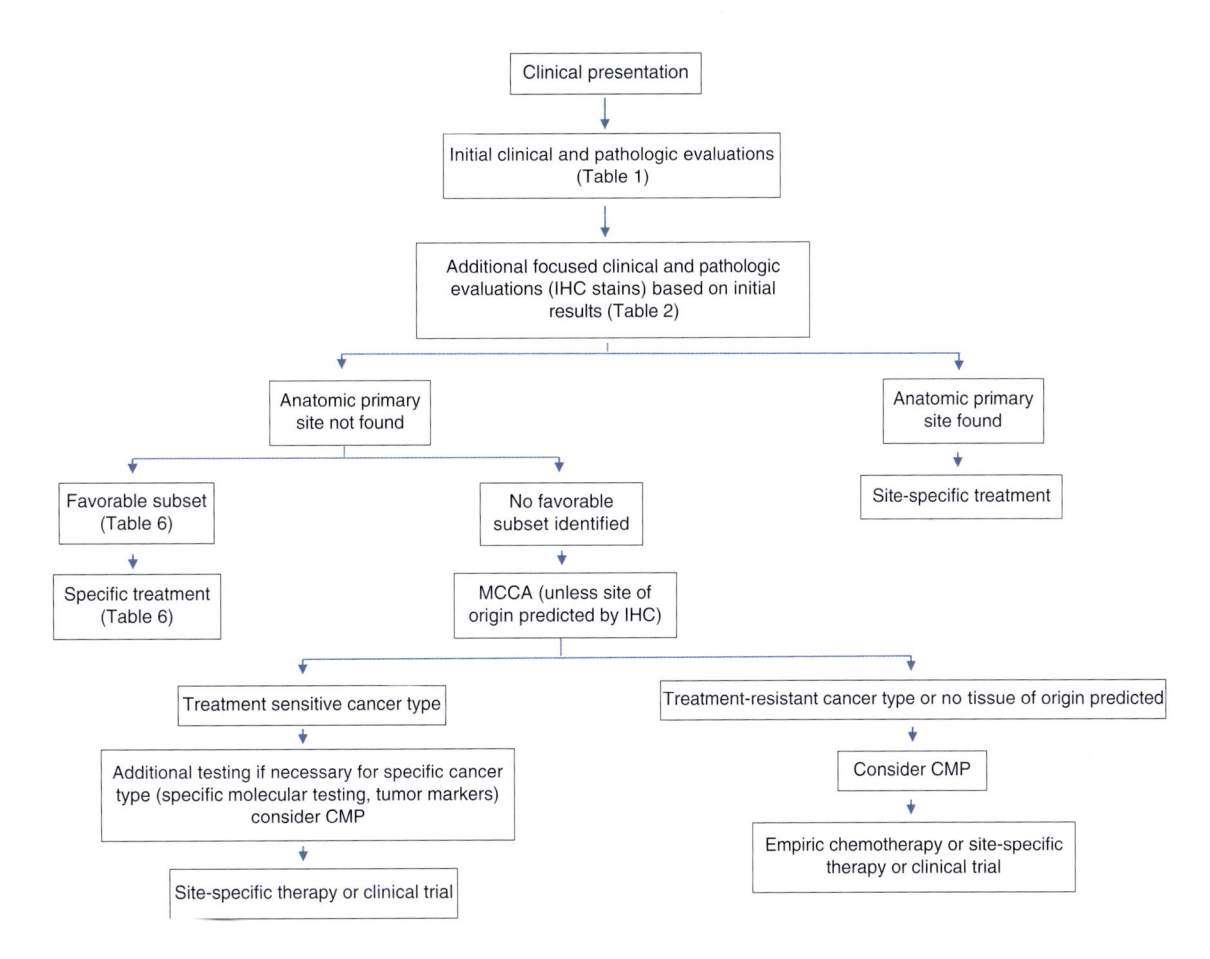

Figure 1 Management of patients with carcinoma of unknown primary site: overview.

molecular testing and molecularly-directed therapy in CUP will be critical in facilitating the rapid incorporation of future treatment advances from specific cancers to the appropriate counterparts in the CUP population.

Key references

The complete reference list can be found on Vital Source version of this title, see inside front cover.

5 Pentheroudakis G, Golfinopoulos V, et al. Switching benchmarks in cancer of unknown primary: from autopsy to microarray. *Eur J Cancer.* 2007;**43**:2026–2036.

6 Moller AK, Loft A, Berthelsen AK, et al. A prospective comparison of 18F-FDG PET/CT and CT as diagnostic tools to identify the primary tumor site in patients with extracervical carcinoma of unknown primary site. *Oncologist.* 2012;**17**:1146–1154.

7 Maghami E, Ismaila N, Alvarez A, et al. Diagnosis and management of squamous cell carcinoma of unknown primary in the head and neck: ASCO guideline. *J Clin Oncol.* 2020;**38**:2570–2596.

8 Compton AM, Moore-Medlin T, Herman-Fernandez L, et al. Human papillomavirus in metastatic lymph nodes from unknown primary head and neck squamous cell carcinoma. *Otolaryngol Head Neck Surg.* 2011;**145**:51–57.

10 Rusthoven KE, Koshy M, Paulino AC. The role of flourodeoxyglucose positron emission tomography in cervical lymph node metastases from an unknown primary tumor. *Cancer.* 2004;**101**:2641–2649.

12 Cianchetti M, Mancuso AA, Amdur RJ, et al. Diagnostic evaluation of squamous cell carcinoma metastatic to cervical lymph nodes from an unknown head and neck primary site. *Laryngoscope.* 2009;**119**:2348–2354.

14 Sadowski SM, Neychev V, Millo C, et al. Prospective study of 68Ga-DOTATATE positron emission tomography/computed tomography for detecting gastroentero-pancreatic neuroendocrine tumors and unknown primary sites. *J Clin Oncol.* 2016;**34**:588–596.

19 Greco FA, Lennington WJ, Spigel DR, et al. Poorly differentiated neoplasms of unknown primary site: diagnostic usefulness of a molecular cancer classifier assay. *Mol Diagn Ther.* 2015;**19**:91–97.

23 Oien KA, Dennis JL. Diagnostic work-up of carcinoma of unknown primary: from immunohistochemistry to molecular profiling. *Ann Oncol.* 2012;**23**(Suppl 10):271–277.

24 Greco FA, Lennington WJ, Spigel DR, Hainsworth JD. Molecular profiling diagnosis in unknown primary cancer: accuracy and ability to complement standard pathology. *J Natl Cancer Inst.* 2013;**105**:782–790.

26 Erlander MG, Ma XJ, Kesty NC, et al. Performance and clinical evaluation of the 92-gene real-time PCR assay for tumor classification. *J Mol Diagn.* 2011;**13**:493–503.

29 Oien K. Pathologic evaluation of unknown primary cancer. *Semin Oncol.* 2009;**36**:8–37.

34 Dennis JL, Hvidsten TR, Wit EC, et al. Markers of adenocarcinoma characteristic of the site of origin: development of a diagnostic algorithm. *Clin Cancer Res.* 2005;**11**:3766–3772.

35 Park SY, Kim BH, Kim JH, et al. Panels of immunohistochemical markers help determine primary sites of metastatic adenocarcinoma. *Arch Pathol Lab Med.* 2007;**131**:1561–1567.

36 Anderson GG, Weiss LM. Determining tissue of origin for metastatic cancers: meta-analysis and literature review of immunohistochemistry performance. *Appl Immunohistochem Mol Morphol.* 2010;**18**:3–8.

46 Su AI, Welsh JB, Sapinoso LM, et al. Molecular classification of human carcinomas by use of gene expression signatures. *Cancer Res.* 2001;**61**:7388–7393.

53 Meiri E, Mueller WC, Rosenwald S, et al. A second-generation microRNA-based assay for diagnosing tumor tissue origin. *Oncologist.* 2012;**17**:801–812.

54 Moran S, Martinez-Cardus A, Savols S, et al. Epigenetic profiling to classify cancer of unknown primary: a multicenter, retrospective analysis. *Lancet Oncol.* 2016;**17**:1386–1395.

55 Greco FA, Spigel DR, Yardley DA, et al. Molecular profiling in unknown primary cancer: accuracy of tissue of origin prediction. *Oncologist.* 2010;**15**:500–506.

56 Hainsworth JD, Rubin MS, Spigel DR, et al. Molecular gene expression profiling to predict the tissue of origin and direct site-specific therapy in patients with carcinoma of unknown primary site: a prospective trial of the Sarah Cannon Research Institute. *J Clin Oncol.* 2013;**31**:217–223.

57. Weiss LM, Chu P, Schroeder BE, et al. Blinded comparator study of immunohistochemical analysis versus a 92-gene cancer classifier in the diagnosis of the primary site in metastatic tumors. *J Mol Diagn.* 2013;**15**:263–269.
58. Handorf CR, Kulkarni A, Grenert JP, et al. A multicenter study directly comparing the diagnostic accuracy of gene expression profiling and immunohistochemistry for primary site identification in metastatic tumors. *Am J Surg Pathol.* 2013;**37**:1067–1075.
59. Hainsworth JD, Greco FA. Gene expression profiling in patients with carcinoma of unknown primary site: from translational research to standard of care. *Virchows Arch.* 2014;**464**:393–402.
66. Pentheroudakis G, Lazaridis G, Pavlidis N. Axillary nodal metastases from carcinoma of unknown primary (CUPAx): a systematic review of published evidence. *Breast Cancer Res Treat.* 2010;**119**:1–11.
77. Varadhachary GR, Karanth S, Qiao W, et al. Carcinoma of unknown primary with gastrointestinal profile: immunohistochemistry and survival data for this favorable subset. *Int J Clin Oncol.* 2014;**19**:479–484.
78. Greco F, Lennington W, Spigel DR, et al. Carcinoma of unknown primary site: outcomes in patients with a colorectal molecular profile treated with site-specific chemotherapy. *J Cancer Ther.* 2012;**3**:37–43.
79. Hainsworth JD, Schnabel CA, Erlander MG, et al. A retrospective study of treatment outcomes in patients with carcinoma of unknown primary site and a colorectal cancer molecular profile. *Clin Colorectal Cancer.* 2012;**11**:112–118.
81. Rassy E, Parent P, et al. New rising entities in cancer of unknown primary: is there a real therapeutic benefit? *Crit Rev Oncol/Hematol.* 2020;**147**:102882. doi: 10.1016/j.critrevonc.2020.102882.
83. Greco FA, Hainsworth JD. Renal cell carcinoma presenting as carcinoma of unknown primary site: recognition of a treatable patient subset. *Clin Genitourin Cancer.* 2018;**16**:e293–e298.
84. Overby A, Duval L, et al. Carcinoma of unknown primary site with metastatic renal cell histologic and immunohistochemical characteristics: results from consecutive patients treated with targeted therapy and review of literature. *Genitourinary Cancer.* 2019;**17**:e32–e37.
86. Rades D, Kuhnel G, Wildfang I, et al. Localised disease in cancer of unknown primary (CUP): the value of positron emission tomography (PET) for individual therapeutic management. *Ann Oncol.* 2001;**12**:1605–1609.
90. Grau C, Johansen LV, Jakobsen J, et al. Cervical lymph node metastases from unknown primary tumours. Results from a national survey by the danish society for head and neck oncology. *Radiother Oncol.* 2000;**55**:121–129.
94. Guarischi A, Keane TJ, Elhakim T. Metastatic inguinal nodes from an unknown primary neoplasm. A review of 56 cases. *Cancer.* 1987;**59**:572–577.
99. Hainsworth JD, Johnson DH, Greco FA. Poorly differentiated neuroendocrine carcinoma of unknown primary site. A newly recognized clinicopathologic entity. *Ann Intern Med.* 1988;**109**:364–371.
100. Hainsworth JD, Spigel DR, Litchy S, et al. Phase II trial of paclitaxel, carboplatin, and etoposide in advanced poorly differentiated neuroendocrine carcinoma: a Minnie Pearl Cancer Research Network Study. *J Clin Oncol.* 2006;**24**: 3548–3554.
102. Hainsworth JD, Johnson DH, Greco FA. Cisplatin-based combination chemotherapy in the treatment of poorly differentiated carcinoma and poorly differentiated adenocarcinoma of unknown primary site: results of a 12-year experience. *J Clin Oncol.* 1992;**10**:912–922.
103. Briasoulis E, Kalofonos H, Bafaloukos D, et al. Carboplatin plus paclitaxel in unknown primary carcinoma: a phase II Hellenic Cooperative Oncology Group Study. *J Clin Oncol.* 2000;**18**:3101–3107.
109. Pouessel D, Culine S, Becht C, et al. Gemcitabine and docetaxel as front-line chemotherapy in patients with carcinoma of an unknown primary site. *Cancer.* 2004;**100**:1257–1261.
110. Culine S, Lortholary A, Voigt JJ, et al. Cisplatin in combination with either gemcitabine or irinotecan in carcinomas of unknown primary site: results of a randomized phase II study—trial for the French Study Group on Carcinomas of Unknown Primary (GEFCAPI 01). *J Clin Oncol.* 2003;**21**:3479–3482.
116. Gross-Goupil M, Fourcade A, Blot E, et al. Cisplatin alone or combined with gemcitabine in carcinomas of unknown primary: results of the randomised GEFCAPI 02 trial. *Eur J Cancer.* 2012;**48**:721–727.
122. Lee J, Hahn S, Kim DW, et al. Evaluation of survival benefits by platinums and taxanes for an unfavourable subset of carcinoma of unknown primary: a systematic review and meta-analysis. *Br J Cancer.* 2013;**108**:39–48.
131. Riihimaki M, Hemminki A, Sundquist K, Hemminki K. Time trends in survival from cancer of unknown primary: small steps forward. *Eur J Cancer.* 2013;**49**:2403–2410.
132. Hayashi H, Takiguchi Y, Minami H, et al. Site-specific and targeted therapy based on moleclar profiling by next-generation sequencing for cancer of unknown primary site. *JAMA Oncol.* 2020;**6**:1931–1938.
134. Gross-Goupil M, Massard C, Lesimple T, et al. Identifying the primary site using gene expression profiling in patients with carcinoma of an unknown primary (CUP): a feasibility study from the GEFCAPI. *Onkologie.* 2012;**35**:54–55.
135. Fizazi K, Maillard A, Penel N, et al. A phase III trial of empiric chemotherapy with cisplatin and gemcitabine or systemic treatment tailored by molecular gene expression analysis in patients with carcinomas of an unknown primary (CUP) site (GEFCAPI 04). *Ann Oncol.* 2019;**30**(Suppl 15):V851.
136. Hayashi H, Kurata T, Takiguchi Y, et al. Randomized phase II trial comparing site-specific treatment based on gene expression profiling with carboplatin and paclitaxel for patients with cancer of unknown primary site. *J Clin Oncol.* 2019;**37**:570–579.
137. Ross JS, Wang K, Gay L, et al. Comprehensive genomic profiling of carcinoma of unknown primary site: new routes to targeted therapies. *JAMA Oncol.* 2015;**1**:40–49.
141. Weipert C, Kato S, Saam J, Kurzrock R. Utility of circulating cell-free DNA (cfDNA) analysis in patients with carcinoma of unknown primary (CUP) in identifying alterations with strong evidence for response or resistance to targeted therapy. *J Clin Oncol.* 2020;**38**(15):105.
143. Tanizaki J, Yonemori K, Akiyoshi K, et al. NivoCUP: an open-label phase II study on the efficacy of nivolumab in cancer of unknown primary. *J Clin Oncol.* 2020;**38**(15):106.

122 Cancer cachexia

Assaad A. Eid, DSc., MBA ■ Rachel Njeim, MSC, PharmD ■ Fadlo R. Khuri, MD ■ David K. Thomas, MD

> **Overview**
>
> Cachexia is a systemic wasting syndrome of progressive muscle and, usually, adipose loss, multi-organ dysfunction, and wide metabolic derangement, often exacerbated by anorexia and diminished nutritional intake. More than half of all cancer patients develop cachexia, which directly causes profound morbidity and substantially reduced survival. New large-scale high-dimensional clinical and experimental studies are revealing unexpected ground truths that cachexia frequently occurs in early stages of many cancers; has several distinct clinical phenotypes; increases complications of and reduces response to cancer-directed therapies. More precise tools for early assessment, diagnosis, and multi-modal interventions, including quantitative image-based body composition analysis, molecular biomarkers, and new targeted therapeutics are in advanced development. These advances, with rapidly expanding basic research into causal molecular mechanisms, are transforming our fundamental understanding of this complex disease as being integral with cancer biology, treatment response, and patient outcomes.

Introduction

Cancer cachexia is a disease of systemic wasting of muscle and adipose tissues, multi-organ dysfunction, and broad metabolic derangement, leading directly to increased complications of cancer-directed treatments, profound morbidity, and significantly higher cancer-related mortality. The disease process is further characterized by broad inflammation, excessive tissue catabolism, impaired anabolism, and elevated resting energy expenditure (REE). Historically, unexplained weight loss of varying degrees has been used to identify patients with cachexia, but monitoring its progression was often limited as it was assumed to be the inevitable consequence of late-stage cancers. While more than 50% of all cancer patients develop cachexia, its prevalence and dynamics vary greatly across cancer types and molecular subtypes. The range spans from 85% of pancreas and stomach cancers with very early onset and rapid progression to 50% of lung and colon cancers with variable onset and progression to 25% of breast and prostate cancers predominantly in ER(−)/PR(−) and AR-independent subtypes, respectively, and with relatively late onset and slow progression. Hematologic malignancies generally exhibit low prevalence of apparent cachexia with the exception of myelofibrosis, where 70% of patients have significant weight loss at diagnosis.[1] Generally, the onset and rate of cachexia progression correlate with the aggressiveness of the underlying cancer, but not necessarily with tumor burden, which is most notable in melanoma and pancreatic cancer. Following response to anti-cancer treatments, cachectic weight loss is frequently an early sign of recurrent or progressing cancers, often preceding evidence of tumor growth in re-staging imaging studies. In addition to cancer, cachexia is also associated with other diseases, such as heart failure, chronic obstructive pulmonary disease, kidney failure, autoimmune diseases, and serious systemic infections, which likely share some of the cascade of danger signals, following systemic stress. Importantly, cachexia is differentiated from malnutrition as it cannot be reversed by nutritional repletion alone, including total parenteral nutrition (TPN). While new anticancer therapies, such as genomically targeted and immune checkpoint inhibitors, provide dramatic responses for some, the majority of cancer patients lack eligibility or durable responses,[2,3] necessitating attending to cachexia. Fortunately, recent large-scale and high-dimensional clinical and experimental research efforts are deepening our understanding of the molecular mechanisms of cachexia, its varied dynamics, broad impact, and the molecular features of cancers that induce it. This remarkable progress is providing the critical resolving power necessary for effective cachexia treatment.

In assessing therapeutic potential for cachexia, an essential question is whether muscle loss can not only be inhibited but reversed. There is broad experimental evidence of impaired components of skeletal muscle's anabolic capacity.[4–6] Yet, there is striking evidence that the regenerative capacity of muscle is preserved in numerous animal models of cachexia, when the inciting mediators are inhibited, improving mass, function, and survival, despite tumor progression.[5,7–9] Additionally, there is evidence for a modest gain of muscle mass in humans from international Phase 2 and 3 clinical trials of anamorelin, a ghrelin mimetic, in lung and GI cancer patients. These trials did not target direct mediators of muscle atrophy, but rather a central orexigenic pathway, yet demonstrated a modest increase of approximately 1.5 kg in lean body mass (LBM) compared to placebo along with improved quality of life (QoL) scores, which served as the basis for recent regulatory approval in Japan.[10-12] Together, these data provide optimism that skeletal muscle retains the ability to recover from cachectic atrophy, if targeted appropriately.

Cachexia etiology: a multi-organ disorder

Cachexia is ultimately a multifactorial syndrome,[13] leading to multi-organ dysfunction (Figure 1).[14] To better understand cachexia, it is important to apply a systemic approach to define the contributions of the tumor, tumor microenvironment, and each affected organ, in the cachectic process, in order to identify critical therapeutic targets. This complexity leads to inherent challenges in translating mechanistic discoveries in animal models of cancer cachexia, either allogenic or genetically engineered, to patients beyond rough, often contradictory, correlations. Fortunately, capabilities in high-dimensional reverse translational discovery in patients are beginning to address these limitations.

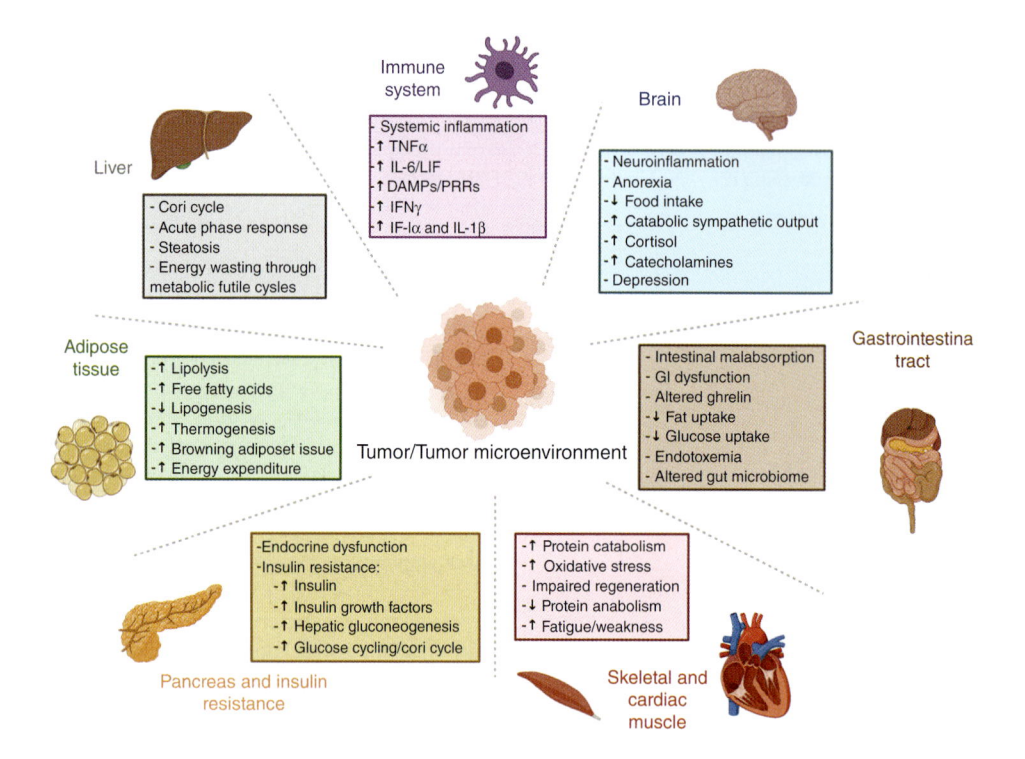

Figure 1 Multi-organ involvement in cancer cachexia. Source: Based on Argilés et al.[14]

Immune system

Systemic inflammation contributes to many aspects of cancer cachexia.[15] Tumors secrete proinflammatory cytokines, eicosanoids, heat shock protein 70 (HSP70), and HSP90 among other danger-associated molecular pattern (DAMP) ligands,[16] members of the transforming growth factor-β (TGFβ) superfamily (activins, myostatin, and GDF15) and adrenomedullin (ADM), which induce catabolism and suppress anabolism in various tissues. Interactions between tumor cells and the host tissue stroma further exacerbate this process, triggering a cascade of signals affecting multiple organs to mediate complex biological responses, such as proteolysis, lipolysis, high sympathetic tone, and anorexia, leading to the systemic tissue wasting[17–19] and distinct disease phenotypes.

Pro-cachectic cytokines and factors

Cytokines produced by the cancer, stroma, and immune cells that are associated with cachexia include tumor necrosis factor-alpha (TNF-α), IL-1, IL-6, interferon-gamma (IFNγ), leukemia inhibitory factor (LIF), growth/differentiation factor 15 (GDF15), and TNF-related weak inducer of apoptosis (TWEAK; also known as TNFSF12). These cytokines, through their surface receptors, have been associated with pathologically activated autophagy and the ubiquitin–proteasome pathway (UPP), while suppressing anabolic processes.

TNF-α

TNF-α was the first cytokine to be to associated with cachexia,[20] though its exact role in adipose and muscle wasting still requires further investigation.[21–24] TNF-α is suggested to exert its effect on white adipose tissue (WAT) wasting through inhibition of fatty acid (FA) uptake by downregulation of FATP, FAT, and FABP4, promotion of lipolysis, and stimulation of thermogenesis via increased expression of uncoupling protein two and three (UCP2 and UCP3).[25,26] TNF-α is also described to stimulate production of oxidative stress and nitric oxide species (NOS). Antioxidants and NOS inhibitors increased body weight and prevented muscle wasting in mice through inhibition of TNF-α.[27] Data from experimental models and human studies have shown that TNF-α activation induces anorexia, increased energy expenditure, and insulin resistance with adipose and muscle wasting.[20,28–31] Of note, most TNF-α systemic effects are mediated through the activation of nuclear factor-κB (NF-κB), which activates the UPP[32] and autophagy. Despite the involvement of TNF-α in systemic inflammation,[33] the hypothesis that increased TNF-α levels is solely responsible for cancer cachexia is not well supported. In fact, some animal studies and clinical trials failed to reduce the cachectic process upon TNF-α inhibition alone.[33–35] Furthermore, recent data described TNF-α to correlate with stage of disease or tumor size rather than the degree of weight loss.[36]

TRAF6

TNF-α receptor adaptor protein 6 (TRAF6),[37–40] which functions as an E3 ubiquitin ligase, was also found to be involved in the murine LLC model of cachexia.[38] TRAF6 mRNA and protein levels, as well as ubiquitin mRNA and protein levels, were upregulated in skeletal muscle tissue of gastric cancer patients, correlating with both disease stage and degree of weight loss.[41] The positive correlation between TRAF6 and ubiquitin expression suggests that TRAF6 may regulate ubiquitin activity in human cachexia.[42]

TWEAK

Another cytokine implicated in muscle wasting is TWEAK, which binds to the surface receptor FN14 (also known as TNFRSF12A), leading to the activation of NF-κB.[43] TWEAK causes myotube atrophy through coordinated activation of the UPP, autophagy, and caspases. Intriguingly, blockade of TNFRSF12A using a neutralizing antibody inhibited weight loss and increased lifespan in experimental models of cachexia.[8] However, significant correlative human data in cancer patients has yet to be reported.

IL-6

IL-6 levels often correlate with weight loss and death in cancer patients.[44,45] IL-6 signals through the ubiquitously expressed heterodimer receptor IL6-R/glycoprotein 130 (gp130).[46] Binding of IL-6 to its receptor phosphorylates Janus kinases (JAK), leading to the activation of signal transducer and activator of transcription (STAT) proteins.[47] The latter translocate to the nucleus, increasing the transcription of genes involved in immune function, cell proliferation, cell differentiation, and apoptosis.[47] IL-6 increases autophagy in myotubes and induces muscle atrophy,[46] while its inhibition can attenuate cachexia progression in different cancer mouse models.[44] Besides, IL-6 trans-signals through the soluble IL-6R and mediates crosstalk between tumor, muscle, and adipose tissue in genetic mouse models of pancreatic cancer cachexia. In these models, tumor-derived IL-6 induced soluble IL-6R production by skeletal muscle, increasing lipolysis via IL-6 trans-signaling and exacerbating muscle wasting.[47] IL-6 has been considered the key cytokine that regulates the hepatic acute phase response (APR) in patients with pancreatic cancer cachexia.[48] Despite these findings, IL-6 inhibitors failed to demonstrate sufficient efficacy in clinical trials of cancer cachexia. The use of anti-IL6 antibody (ALD 518) in patients with non-small-cell lung cancer (NSCLC) resulted in a trend toward reduced loss of LBM compared with controls, yet was not statistically significant.[49] IL-6 remains a potential therapeutic target in cancer cachexia, though a better understanding of its direct and indirect effects, and tissue-specific actions, is required.

IL-1α and IL-1β

The pro-inflammatory cytokine IL-1α is produced mainly by macrophages and endothelial cells and is thought to play a role in cancer pathogenesis.[50] IL-1α levels were increased in animal models of cachexia,[51] yet similar to TNF-α, its role in cachexia remains controversial. For instance, IL-1α-treated tumor-bearing rats demonstrated increased loss of body weight, yet this was not reversed by the administration of IL-1α receptor antagonist (IL-1rα).[52] Furthermore, following direct tumor injection with IL-1rα, colon-26 (C-26) carcinoma-bearing mice had significant reduction in weight loss without an observed effect on tumor burden when compared to mice who had systemic IL-1rα injection.[53] Moreover, IL-1α has been described to inhibit LPL activity and stimulate lipolysis in cultured adipocytes.[54] Besides, IL-1α affects the central nervous system and plays an important role in anorexia, early satiety, and hunger suppression.

IL-1β is a proinflammatory cytokine released by the tumor and macrophages. IL-1β regulates the expression of other cytokines, including IL-6 and IL-12, and participates in mediating systemic inflammation.[55,56] In experimental models of breast cancer, WNT ligands stimulate tumor-associated macrophages (TAMs) to produce IL-1β, driving systemic inflammation. Blockade of WNT secretion by pharmacological and genetic means prevented IL-1β secretion by macrophages and decreased neutrophilic inflammation and metastasis formation.[56] In tumor samples from patients undergoing surgical resection for upper gastrointestinal malignancy, IL-1β and IL-6 mRNA and protein levels were significantly overexpressed, positively correlating with CRP levels.[55] In patients with advanced cancers, IL-1β better correlated with clinical features of cachexia, such as anorexia, weight loss, and sarcopenia, than other cytokines including IL-6.[57] Patients with gastric cancer cachexia were shown to have an increased prevalence of IL-1B+3954 T allele, indicating that patient's genotype may play a role in the immunological regulation of cancer cachexia.[58]

Interferon-gamma (IFNγ)

In cancer, tumor-infiltrating lymphocytes (TILs) are the main source of IFNγ.[59] The involvement of IFNγ in the pathogenesis of cachexia has been established in cancer animal models. IFNγ overexpression induced body weight loss, adipose tissue wasting via the inhibition of LPL and glycerol phosphate dehydrogenase activities and reduced appetite. These homeostatic alterations were reversed upon pretreatment with anti-IFNγ antibodies in experimental models of cachexia.[60–62] Of interest, central administration of rat interferon decreased food intake, whereas peripheral administration failed to do so.[63]

Myostatin and activin A

In addition to inflammatory cytokines, other circulating factors, such as TGFβ family members including myostatin and activin A, possess pro-cachectic activity in skeletal muscles. Enhanced production of myostatin by skeletal muscle leads to muscle atrophy, whereas its genetic inhibition leads to enhanced muscle mass and fiber size.[64] Myostatin is suggested to enhance muscle loss and prevent protein synthesis by the inhibition of rapamycin complex 1 pathway (mTORC1). In pancreatic cancer patients with stage II–IV disease, palliative treatment with antimyostatin antibody in patients with <5% weight loss resulted in better performance-related results, whereas no significant difference was noted in patients with >5% weight loss.[65] These findings suggest that inhibition of myostatin merely reduces muscle loss rather than fully reversing the cachectic process in patients with advanced cachexia.[65]

Activin A, another member of the TGFβ superfamily of growth factors produced by both tumor and immune cells,[66] is increased following activation of the TNFα/TGFβ-activated kinase-1 signaling pathway. When activin A is overexpressed in mice, it promotes weight loss and skeletal muscle wasting with greater potency than IL-6.[67–69]

Myostatin and activin A signal through the ActRIIB receptor. Blockade of the ActRIIB receptor in a rodent model of cancer cachexia effectively reversed muscle wasting and prolonged mice survival.[70] Clinical trials on patients with body myositis, sarcopenia, and disuse atrophy following fracture reported increased muscle volume upon blockade of ActRIIB; however, functionality endpoints were not improved.[71–73]

Brain inflammation, anorexia, and lipolysis

One of the most common and earliest clinical symptoms of cancer is decreased appetite, anorexia, which often leads to decreased food intake, nutritional deficit, negative energy balance, adipocyte lipolysis, and secondary skeletal muscle catabolism. Anorexia is often concomitant with and exacerbates cachexia, making it challenging to disambiguate them and confounding many clinical research studies. This is especially problematic when study designs dichotomize the study population into those with or without cachexia, often comparing the extreme ends of the spectrum of this complex continuous disease. To start addressing these limitations, an international research collaborative conducted a multi-center cross-sectional study of 885 patients with diverse malignancies to determine the explained variance among appetite loss, reduced food intake, and weight loss.[74] Having assessed for impact of cancer type, site of metastasis, concurrent cancer therapy, and other symptoms associated with cancer, age, and sex, multivariate regression modeling determined the explained variance (adjusted R^2) was 44% for appetite loss, 27% for decreased food intake, and only 13% for weight loss. The authors concluded that factors other than reduced nutritional intake were mainly responsible for cachexia, indicating that these were distinct and separable pathophysiologic processes. The study also found that the correlation between anorexia and decreased food intake was 0.50; thus, we cannot assume that anorexia leads to diminished food intake for every patient.

Despite the challenges these overlapping disorders present, remarkable progress has been made recently in identifying mechanisms that cause anorexia and tissue wasting in murine models with likely relevance to patients. A growing number of signaling molecules, including IL-1β/IL-1R, growth differentiation factor-15 (GDF-15)/GFRAL-RET, and LIF/LIFR-gp130, demonstrate pronounced suppression of food intake directly. These factors activate their cognate receptors located in the hypothalamus, which centrally regulates orexigenic–anorexigenic homeostasis. A common theme is emerging of multiple forms of systemic inflammation transducing CNS inflammation with specific effects on pro-opiomelanocortin (POPMC) and Agouti-related protein (AgRP) neurons located in the arcuate nucleus, which ultimately stimulate anorexic and suppress orexigenic behaviors and stimulate sympathetic output. Decreased food intake increases adrenergic tone, activating adipocyte triglyceride lipase (ATGL) and hormone-sensitive lipase (HSL) to drive lipolysis in adipocytes (and potentially myocytes).[75,76] Additionally, normal regulatory processes eventually activate skeletal muscle catabolism to maintain systemic energy homeostasis for vital organ function, though to a significantly lesser degree than in typical cachexia. This overlap is a potential significant confounder in cachexia research, though pair-fed control animals have been useful in quantifying the contribution of diminished food intake to adipose and muscle loss in various experimental contexts. CNS inflammation via IL-1β in mouse models stimulated the hypothalamic-pituitary-adrenal axis to cause a higher release of glucocorticoids. The latter was sufficient to generate modest skeletal muscle atrophy in specific muscle groups, an effect that was completely ablated by adrenalectomy.[75] Representing a parallel pathway of CNS appetite regulation, GDF-15, a distant member of the TGF-β superfamily, is expressed by a wide variety of normal tissues under stress conditions and several human cancer cell types.[77] GDF-15 signals via the heterodimer receptor GFRAL-RET, exclusively expressed in the area postrema and nucleus of the solitary tract of the brain stem. Activation of this pathway causes dramatic anorexia and weight loss, which merges with sympathetic upregulation to drive rapid adipocyte lipolysis through the actions of ATGL and HSL and modest indirect skeletal muscle atrophy as seen in other mechanisms of neuroinflammation.[9,77] Orexigenic and anorexigenic modulators of this pathway are currently in clinical development by large pharmaceutical companies for indications involving appetite at either end of the spectrum.

Intriguingly, obese patients are at higher risk for developing malignancies presumably due to chronic higher exposure to glucose, insulin, and insulin-like growth factor (IGF) signals, but generally have better overall survival—the "obesity paradox." Possible explanations include that cancers arising in the context of obesity are inherently less aggressive or restricted in some way, and/or higher fat reserves provide a buffer from the compensatory loss of muscle mass, which is most deleterious for survival. Ongoing clinical studies are harnessing serial CT-based body composition analyses with deep cancer profiling approaches to help clarify how systemic host factors impact cancer biology and patient outcomes.[78]

Alimentary tract dysfunction: gut and intestinal homeostasis

Ghrelin
Ghrelin, the "hunger hormone," is an orexigenic gut hormone secreted primarily by endocrine cells of the gastric mucosa and acts centrally to regulate hunger, gastric acid secretion, gastrointestinal motility, white and brown adipose tissue function, and glucose metabolism.[79] Serum levels of ghrelin are elevated in several but not all cancers associated with cachexia.[80-83] Increased ghrelin secretion in cancer cachexia was associated with anorexia[84] and is thought to be a compensatory mechanism to buffer cachexia since ghrelin increases adiposity, reduces REE, and impairs muscle atrophy.[85-87] However, in some instances, increased ghrelin levels in cachexia failed to induce appetite and energy storage, a phenomenon explained by ghrelin resistance observed in experimental model of cachectic rats.[82,88] Despite these contradictory data, a ghrelin receptor agonist has been proven to be beneficial for patients with cachexia, on anorexia, weight gain, modest increased lean mass, and reduced loss of adipose tissue.[89] The therapeutic potential of ghrelin can be explained by increasing energy intake,[90] stimulating the release of growth hormone (GH) and IGF-I[91,92] reducing inflammation and p38/CEBP-b/myostatin, and activating Akt, myogenin, and myoD in muscle cells.[92,93]

Malabsorption and leakage
Intestinal malabsorption has been correlated with reduced metabolic efficiency, leading to alteration in whole-body energy metabolism (reduction in lipid and carbohydrate uptake) and wasting especially in cancer patients with gastrointestinal malignancy.[94-97] The exact mechanisms involved in gut malabsorption are speculative but thought to involve altered expression or localization of the intestinal glucose and lipid transporters.[98] Besides malabsorption, gut barrier dysfunction induced by radiotherapy or chemotherapy can play a role in cachexia. Leakage through the gut epithelial tight junctions, damage of which correlates with tumor aggressiveness and survival, results in systemic inflammation and endotoxemia.[99-101]

Gut microbiota
Dysbiosis has been extensively studied in several metabolic diseases[102] and was recently described in cancer-associated cachexia. Gut microbiota composition and diversity were altered in mouse models of cancer cachexia displaying muscle atrophy and loss of fat mass, when compared to control littermates.[103-106] Thus, variations in gut flora due to undernutrition and chemotherapy likely affect specific metabolite availability and absorption.[102-107] Treatment of these mice with probiotics reduced accumulation of tumor cells in the liver, reduced muscle atrophy, decreased adipose wasting, and improved morbidity.[104] Gut microbiota has been described to influence amino acid bioavailability, participate in the release of various metabolites (such as bile acids), and modulate the production of pro-inflammatory cytokines leading to muscle metabolism alteration.[107-109] Pathological intestinal bacteria are associated with the release of several highly inflammatory compounds including lipopolysaccharide, flagellin, and peptidoglycan that stimulate Toll-like receptor 4 (TLR4) in skeletal muscle triggering NF-κB, resulting in muscle wasting.[110] Furthermore, gut microbiota plays a role in WAT browning.[111,112] Macrophages infiltrate the WAT of cachectic mice and colonize the intestine. These observations establish a strong rationale that targeting microbiota homeostasis may be a potential therapeutic approach for the treatment of cachexia.

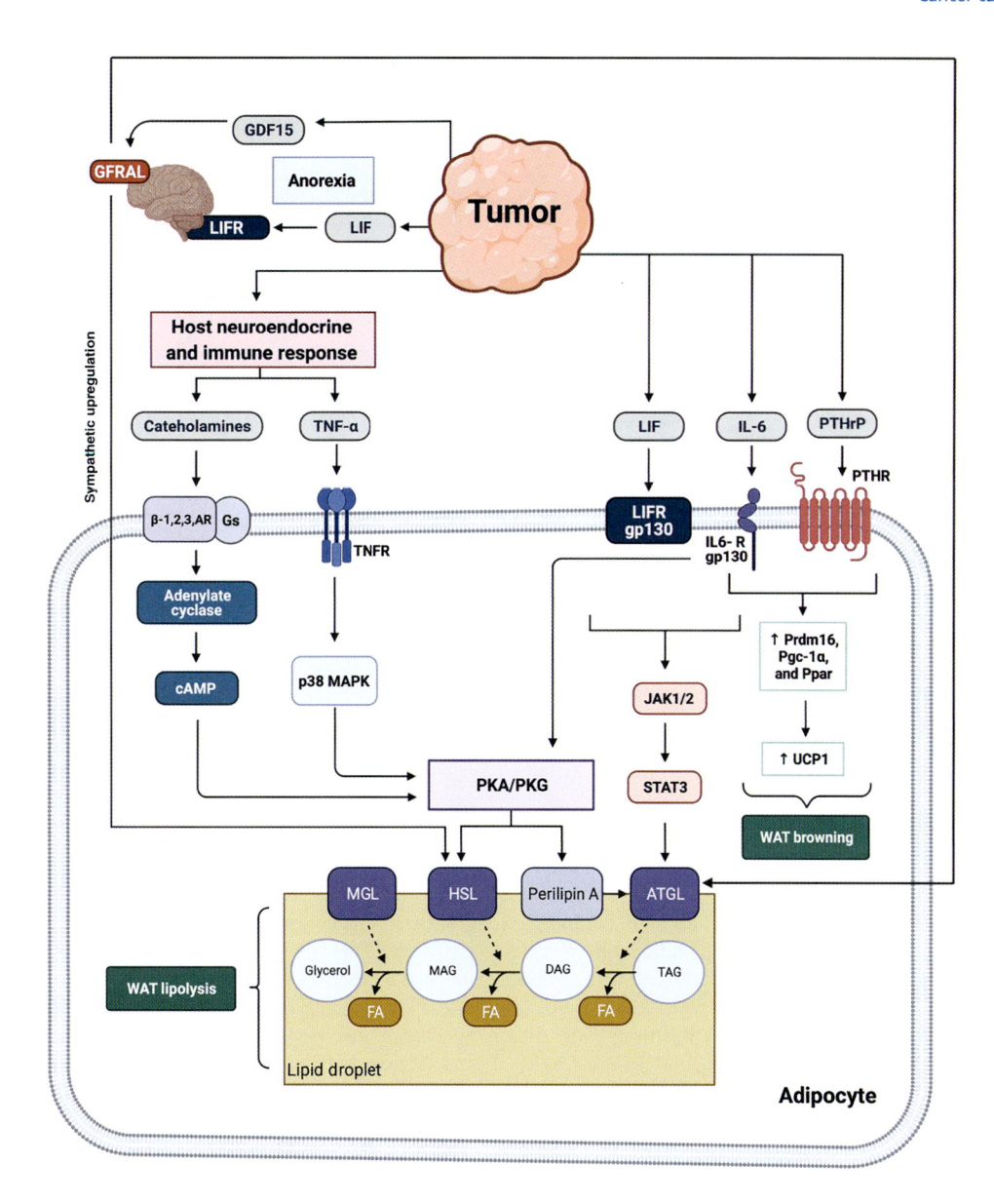

Figure 2 Key cachexia mediator signaling in adipocytes.

Adipose tissue wasting

Fat tissue wasting is an important component in the cachectic process, as it leads to the propagation of cachexia. The main derangements include the activation of lipolysis and browning in WAT, along with the role of brown adipose tissues (BAT) in thermogenesis (Figure 2). These modifications contribute to overwhelming adipose lipolysis and the exacerbation of cachexia.[113,114] Cachexia-induced adipose tissue loss has been attributed to higher lipolytic activity, lipid utilization,[115] and impaired lipogenesis and adipogenesis.[116] Lipolysis is a sequential process orchestrated by three lipases, ATGL, HSL, and MGL. Lipolytic rate is assessed by increased fasting plasma glycerol or FAs levels in relation to body fat.[76,117,118] Excess FAs are oxidized by mitochondria with an upregulation in genes regulating mitochondrial lipid oxidation.[115,119]

WAT wasting is caused by the activation of fat mobilization and conversion into beige adipocytes expressing UCP1.[120,121] Beige adipose tissue eventually acts like BAT, expending energy and thus contributing to energy imbalance. HSL mRNA and protein levels in WAT were elevated in cachectic cancer patients.[117,118,122] As anticipated, knockout of ATGL or HSL in mice partially protects against cancer-induced adipose wasting.[123] While adipose lipolysis is up-regulated, adipogenesis is down-regulated, triggered by peroxisome proliferator-activated receptor-α (PPARα).[124] Several tumor and/or host-derived factors have been implicated in adipose tissue depletion during progressive cachexia.[76,116,125] Inflammatory cytokines such as TNFα, IL-6, and IL-1β contribute to adipose loss by directly activating lipolysis and by impairing insulin sensitivity.[126] Many other factors released by some tumors also promote lipolysis, for example, lipid mobilizing factor zinc-α2-glycoprotein (ZAG),[127] catecholimines, and natriuretic peptides.[117] Expression of the lipolytic receptor β1-AR was high in WAT of cachectic cancer patients and positively correlated with HSL.[118] Several studies using murine cancer models have shown that lipolysis enhances the activation of interscapular BAT during cancer cachexia, leading to energy uncoupling in mitochondria with the subsequent energy imbalance positively correlating with cancer stage.[128] A study has reported that increased BAT

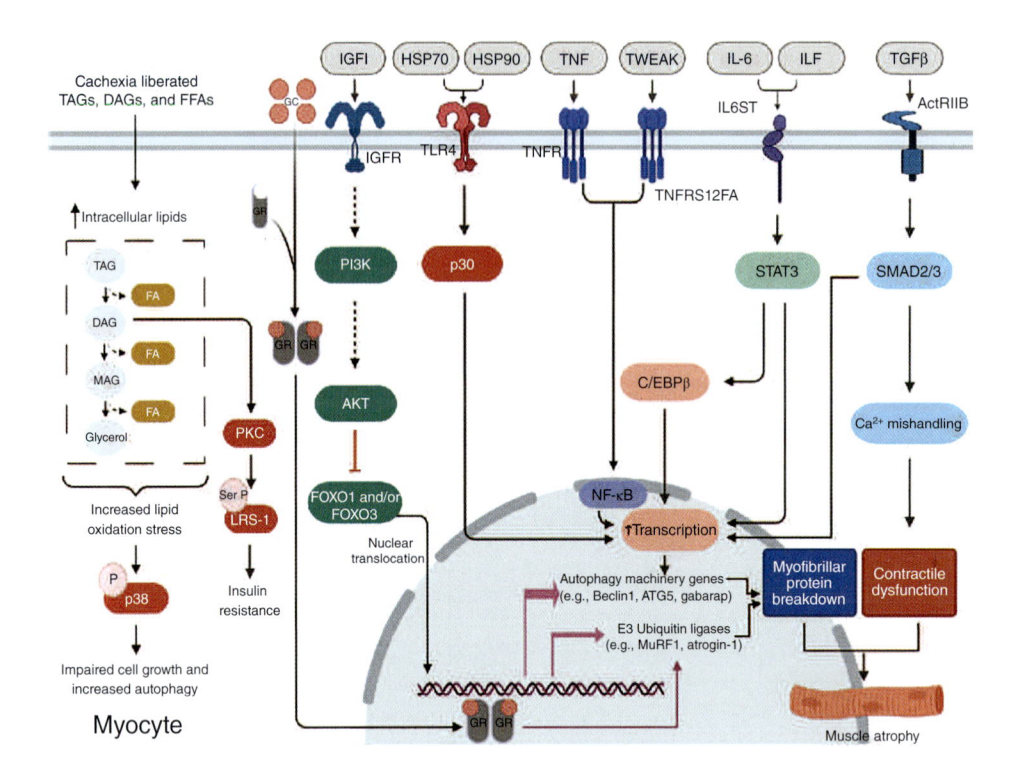

Figure 3 Key cachexia mediator signaling in myocytes.

thermogenesis in cachectic tumor-bearing mice was due to increased UCP1 and STAT3 activation, via an IL-6 dependent mechanism.[129] Pharmacologic blockade of β3-adrenergic receptors also significantly reduced the onset of cachexia in mice, due to lower levels of UCP1 in beige cells.[130]

Several tumor-derived cytokines correlate positively with the induction of adipose browning and thus increased energy expenditure. PTH-rp and ADM are pleiotropic peptide signals that activate their receptors, PTHR and ADMR, expressed on human adipocytes, leading to rapid lipolysis, steady weight loss, but little to no reduction in muscle mass.[131,132] PTH-rp activates a thermogenic gene program in WAT approximating that in BAT, with elevated expression of UCP1 and PPAR gamma co-activator 1a (PGC1a), leading to a futile cycle, thermogenesis, and high lipid turnover. ADM, released by patient-derived pancreatic cancer cells, stimulates lipolysis via ERK1/2 and p38 phosphorylation of HSL. Additionally, LIF has been shown to directly stimulate LIFR-gp130 in peripheral adipocytes, causing dramatic lipolysis, in addition to its central anorexic effects.[133]

Skeletal and cardiac muscle wasting

Skeletal muscle wasting

Muscle homeostasis is sustained through a tightly controlled balance between protein synthesis and protein degradation.[134] This homeostatic balance is controlled by anabolic and catabolic factors, which are extensively dysregulated by tumors.[134,135] A number of studies have shown that levels of proinflammatory mediators including IL-6,[136,137] IL-1β,[75,138] activin A,[67] myostatin,[139,140] IFNγ, and TNFα[141,142] are increased to varying degrees in cancer cachexia. Perplexingly, some cancer patients with cachexia present with a decrease in circulating levels of the anabolic factor IGF-1, which is associated with insulin resistance.[135,143–148]

The UPP, autophagy, and calcium-activated protease calpains are three major degradation pathways described in skeletal muscle.[134,149,150] During cancer cachexia, skeletal muscle atrophy is induced by increased protein degradation mediated by activation of the UPP[151] and/or autophagic–lysosomal system[152] (Figure 3). Specifically, two E3 ligases, muscle ring finger protein 1 (MuRF1) and muscle atrophy Fbox-1 protein (MAFbx or atrogin-1), are considered markers of muscle atrophy. Pro-cachectic cytokines including IL-1, TNFα and TWEAK signal through the NF-κB pathway and p38 MAP kinase to increase the expression of MURF1 and muscle Atrogin-1,[153–157] thus mediating proteolysis.[140,158] MuRF1 and Atrogin-1, which are both significantly upregulated in mouse models of cancer cachexia,[150,159,160] also inhibit protein synthesis and mediate sarcomere breakdown.[150,159–161] TWEAK also signals through NF-κB to increase MuRF1 expression, which in turn mediates ubiquitination and loss of the thick filament of the sarcomere–MyHC.[162] Intriguingly, inhibition of NF-κB significantly decreased muscle loss, partially by inhibiting the increase in MuRF1.[163] Atrogin-1 induces skeletal muscle atrophy through the degradation of eIF3f, which inhibits S6K1 activation by mTOR as well as myoblast determination protein 1 (MyoD) breakdown. This ultimately blocks differentiation and prevents myotube formation.[164] FoxO3a (Forkhead Box (Fox) O), one of several transcription factors that regulate the UPP, upregulates the expression of ubiquitin ligase Atrogin-1.[165] Studies have shown that PI3K/AKT signaling phosphorylates and subsequently inhibits Foxo3a transport to the nucleus, which in turn prevents upregulation of E3 ligases.[165,166] Indeed, the inhibition of Foxo prevented muscle loss in a mouse model of cancer cachexia,[167] whereas overexpression of FoxO3a reduced the size of skeletal muscle fibers, in vivo and in vitro.[165] Moreover, the expression of constitutively active AKT significantly increased myotube formation and the expression levels of MyoD, creatine kinase, MyHC, and desmin.[168]

Autophagy is increasingly gaining attention as a dominant form of skeletal muscle wasting that is upregulated in cancer cachexia.[152,156,169] Enhanced autophagy has been shown to play a role in muscle atrophy in Apc(Min/+), C26,[152] and Lewis lung carcinoma (LLC) tumor-bearing mice.[170] This proteolytic pathway was activated in the muscle of the three different models of cancer cachexia and in glucocorticoid-treated mice.[152] More importantly, a significant increase in autophagic markers, including ATG5, Beclin1, and GABARAP, were found in skeletal muscle of cachectic patients with pancreatic, esophageal, and gastric cancer.[171,172] In a cohort of patients with lung cancer, elevated levels of autophagy mediators BNIP3 and LC3B and of the autophagy-promoting transcription factor FOXO1 were reported.[173] Additionally, studies have reported a predominant loss of type II fibers in cachectic mouse models.[174] Type II skeletal muscle fiber atrophy associated with dysregulated autophagy was reported in atrophic conditions caused by sarcopenia and Pompe disease.[175] Collectively, these findings suggest that dysregulated autophagy contributes significantly to muscle fiber atrophy during cachexia.

It has long been appreciated that substantial weight loss tracks closely with complications of cancer treatments and higher mortality, but the recent use of imaging techniques to quantify LBM has allowed a more specific correlation with sarcopenia. Common cancer drugs, including cisplatin, carboplatin, paclitaxel, and gemcitabine, have demonstrated grade ≥3 or dose-limiting toxicities (DLT) in patients with measurably low skeletal muscle mass (LSMM). A recent meta-analysis of 31 clinical studies in multiple cancer types and anticancer drugs determined that patients with low muscle mass have significantly higher risk for severe toxicity (OR 4.08; $p < 0.001$) and DLT (OR 2.24; $p < 0.001$).[176] A sub-group analysis for sorafenib monotherapy determined significantly higher risk for patients with versus without LSMM (OR 5.60; $p = 0.001$). In early breast cancer, patients with low LBM have higher toxicity risk with anthracycline and taxane-based regimens (RR = 1.48 $p = 0.002$).[177] Another meta-analysis focused on tyrosine kinases, including gefitinib, imatinib, lenvatinib, regorafenib, sorafenib, and sunitinib, that qualified for pooled analysis determined higher risk of DLT in various cancer patients with low muscle mass (OR 2.40 $p = 0.008$).[178] This broad range of drug toxicities is thought to be due to a reduced volume of distribution in patients with low muscle mass, causing higher than expected plasma drug levels and higher risk of toxicities. Perioperative sarcopenia also conveys a higher risk of major grade ≥3 surgical complications by Clavien–Dindo classification (OR 5.46; $p = 0.01$, R 1.40; $p < 0.001$).[179,180] Ultimately, loss of muscle mass conveys an independent higher mortality, even at early cancer stages across multiple cancers: stage I and II NSCLC (HR 3.23),[181] nonmetastatic colon cancer (HR, 1.42),[182] and stage II-III breast cancer (HR, 1.41).[183]

Cardiac muscle wasting
It is understood but underappreciated that the heart atrophies alongside skeletal muscle during cachexia. Heart failure and arrhythmia are prominent causes of death in patients with cachexia.[184] Mechanisms of cachexia-related cardiac wasting parallel those of skeletal muscle wasting. There is evidence of UPP-mediated protein turnover playing a role in cardiac wasting.[185] In a murine model of colon cancer, chronic heart failure was associated with a significant decrease in heart weight and loss of cardiac function.[186] In a C26 model of cachexia, inhibition of NF-κB reduced cardiac tissue atrophy and improved cardiac function.[187] Increased autophagy has also been suggested to play a key role in mediating cardiac muscle atrophy in cancer cachexia. These findings suggest that increased autophagy and AKT-independent suppression of anabolic signaling mediate cardiac mass loss during cachexia progression. Increased energy expenditure in patients with cachexia can be associated with chronic heart failure, which usually correlates with increased REE,[188] and was further validated in a study on tumor-bearing rats whose hearts exhibited an increased oxidative rate *ex vivo*.[189]

Liver in cancer cachexia
Liver hypertrophy is intimately connected to the muscle and adipose responses and may be influenced by the activation of acute-phase responses (APR). Hepatic dysfunction associated with hypermetabolism and elevated REE has been well-documented in cancer cachexia.[13,113,125,190–194] APR, energy-wasting through metabolic futile cycles, and steatosis are the main hepatic energy-consuming processes observed in cachexia.

When the hepatic effect of APR is prolonged, it results in accelerated loss of skeletal muscle and excess morbidity and mortality.[195] This process can be driven by IL-6 and TNFα and involves a series of changes in liver protein synthesis, which shifts from production of albumin to acute-phase proteins (APPs), such as CRP, fibrinogen, serum amyloid A, α2-macroglobulin, and α1-antitrypsin.[125] This eventually results in muscular protein breakdown and adipocyte lipolysis.[173,196–200] Enhanced liver inflammation during cancer cachexia is due to the increased infiltration of macrophages.[191] Activated macrophages secrete IL-6, which stimulates the hepatic synthesis of APP.[201] In addition, hepatic energy wasting can be due to an increase in hepatic mitochondrial cardiolipin phospholipid composition and accumulation,[193] leading to a reduction in the efficiency of oxidative phosphorylation,[200,202–204] and enhanced production of ROS.[194]

Clinical investigations have shown that hepatic gluconeogenesis is increased in cancer patients.[205] Glycolysis in tumors generates lactate, which is reconverted to glucose via hepatic gluconeogenesis. This is referred to as the Cori cycle[125,206,207] and may account for an additional loss of energy in cancer patients of almost 300 kcal/day.[208] Besides, tumor lactate levels are associated with metastasis, tumor recurrence, and death.[209] Hepatic gluconeogenesis can also be fueled by amino acids derived from breakdown of myofibrillar proteins in skeletal muscle and glycerol released by hydrolysis of triglycerides in adipose tissue.[210,211] Furthermore, insulin resistance occurs in patients with cancer and is negatively associated with APR.[212] The resulting glucose is scavenged by glycolytic tumors, supporting their high metabolic rates.[205,213–215]

Hepatic steatosis has also been documented in cancer-associated cachexia patients[216] and is associated with muscle loss.[217] It develops due to a decrease in very-low-density lipoprotein (VLDL) secretion and hepatic triglyceride usage leading to lipid accumulation used as a fuel for liver gluconeogenesis.[218] Increased liver lipogenesis may further contribute to hyperlipidemia.[95] Steatosis is accompanied with cirrhosis which causes a hypermetabolic state, leading to increased energy expenditure, insulin resistance, and increased fat turnover.[219]

Insulin resistance and cachexia
Insulin resistance plays a major role in the development of cancer cachexia as a consequence of tumor byproducts, chronic inflammation, and endocrine dysfunction.[220] In cachexia, glucose intolerance emerges due to increased hepatic glucose production with reduced peripheral utilization upon a decrease in glucose

transporters.[221] Consequently, hyperglycemia promotes insulin secretion in addition to excess IGF-1 release,[222] leading to insulin resistance in cachectic patients.[223] Induction of insulin secretion, increased hepatic gluconeogenesis along with impairment of glucose uptake in skeletal muscle and adipose tissue, make glucose more available for the tumor, thus promoting its growth.[224] Of note, the abnormal increase in hepatic glucose production contributes to the elevated REE associated with cachexia and correlates with weight loss severity.[225]

In cachectic skeletal muscle, insulin resistance promotes muscle wasting by abolishing the anabolic effect of insulin.[226,227] In fact, insulin resistance reduces insulin and IGF-1 binding to IR and IGF1R, respectively, and deactivates PI3K/Akt/mTOR signaling, inhibiting protein synthesis and promoting muscle wasting.[144,220,228,229] In addition, insulin resistance disturbs energy handling by adipose tissue by decreasing glucose uptake, hence promoting its wasting. Similar to skeletal muscle, adipose wasting can also be induced by inactivation of the PI3K/Akt/mTOR pathway.[230] Furthermore, IL-6 and TNF-α in adipose tissue cause insulin resistance by increasing NF-κB-mediated IRS-1 phosphorylation. Tumor cells secrete IL-6 that leads to insulin resistance by reducing GLUT-4 expression in muscles and adipose tissues through activation of the JAK/STAT pathway.[13]

Other signaling pathways have also been implicated as potential mediators of skeletal muscle wasting, lipolysis, and gluconeogenesis which themselves can be regulated in response to FA provision. Cachexia mobilizes FA from the adipose tissue via increased ATGL and HSL activity to various organs, which causes insulin resistance, mitochondrial dysfunction, and apoptosis.[231] Multiple studies have linked lipid metabolites such as TAG, DAG, FFAs, and ceramides to lipotoxicity. Skeletal muscle is one of the main sites of lipid uptake and oxidation. Elevated plasma FAs can be converted into DAGs, which along with ceramides, increase ROS production causing insulin resistance via PKC and/or NF-kB signaling.[232] That results in protein degradation through activation of the proteasome complex. FAs released by adipocytes due to increased lipolysis are transported into myocytes by FA transporters such as FATP1 and CD36.[233] In cancer cachexia, there is marked decrease in fat and carbohydrate uptake in the GI tract due to intestinal dysfunction.[94,234] In addition, elevated hepatic DAG levels upon lipolysis in adipose tissue recruit and promote activation of PKCε which directly inhibits insulin signaling via PKCε/θ[235] dependent phosphorylation of the insulin receptor at Thr1160 and insulin receptor substrates (IRSs) at serine residue 1101.[27,236,237] Activation of JNK by PKC promotes insulin resistance because of decreased PI3K/Akt activity.[6,238,239] At the onset of insulin resistance, GLUT4 does not translocate to the plasma membrane, leading to increased blood glucose levels making glucose more available for tumor cells which exhibit overexpression of glucose transporters in their plasma membranes to meet energy needs.[240] DAG synthesis can also activate PKC, which inhibits downstream effector signaling and GLUT4-dependent glucose uptake.[241]

Diagnosis, assessment, and screening

Diagnostic criteria

Essential to progress in identifying, understanding, and treating cancer cachexia have been efforts to develop robust and validated diagnostic definitions relative to clinical outcomes. A landmark international consensus definition for cancer cachexia based on weight change and body composition was developed in 2011, which provides diagnostic criteria and a conceptual framework for classifying stages of severity.[242] The process integrated systematic literature review with iterative international expert assessment and consensus. Cachexia is described as a multifactorial disease with loss of muscle mass as a key feature due to its particularly strong correlation to adverse outcomes. The consensus statement defines cachexia by weight loss >5% in the past 6 months, or weight loss >2% and evidence of body depletion based on low BMI or sarcopenia (Table 1). There was specific consensus that cachexia is not merely the result of nutritional deficit from any cause, though it frequently exacerbates the condition. The statement classifies cachexia into three stages: precachexia, cachexia, and refractory cachexia, in recognition of distinct risk groups. It was explicitly recognized that special patient populations based on age, sex, ethnicity, genetics, or other factors may require different thresholds. Importantly, the consensus definition and classification concept provide the basis for validation through analyses of clinical outcomes in defined patient populations. Subsequently, a large patient cohort study ($n = 8160$ of diverse cancer types) correlated BMI, weight loss, and overall survival and corroborated the 2011 thresholds for weight loss and BMI.[169] Given the advances in clinical investigation across this field a decade after the original consensus statement, the process of refining definitions has begun; results are anticipated in late 2022.

These proposed diagnostic criteria have brought greater consistency to defining cachexia, which previously had been quite heterogeneous. However, serial measurements of weight are inherently low in accuracy and precision, prone to both noisy measurement (inter- and intra-scale variance) and numerous confounding variables (hydration status, retained fluids, time of day/fed state, even clothing) that can obscure a true change of 2–5% from baseline. Weight is also fairly insensitive to variable changes in composition of different body compartments: LBM, visceral adipose tissue (VAT), and subcutaneous adipose tissue (SAT) both in quantity and quality (e.g., intra- and extramyocellular lipid content). This has significantly limited progress in disambiguating the complex underlying disease processes.

Table 1 2011 consensus diagnostic criteria and features for cachexia.[a]

Weight change (from 6 mo. previous baseline)	Evidence of low body reserves (@ diagnosis of cachexia)	Initial thresholds
>5% loss, or	—	—
>2% loss, and	Low BMI, or	<20 kg/m²
>2% loss, and	Sarcopenida	ASMI: males < 7.26 kg/m², females < 5.45 kg/m²
Key feature: loss of skeletal muscle mass with or without loss of fat mass		
Frequently associated features: negative protein and energy balance, systemic inflammation, and nutritional deficit		
Cachexia cannot be reversed by conventional nutritional supplementation		

Abbreviation: ASMI, Appendicular Skeletal Muscle Index.
[a]Source: Data from Fearon et al.[242]

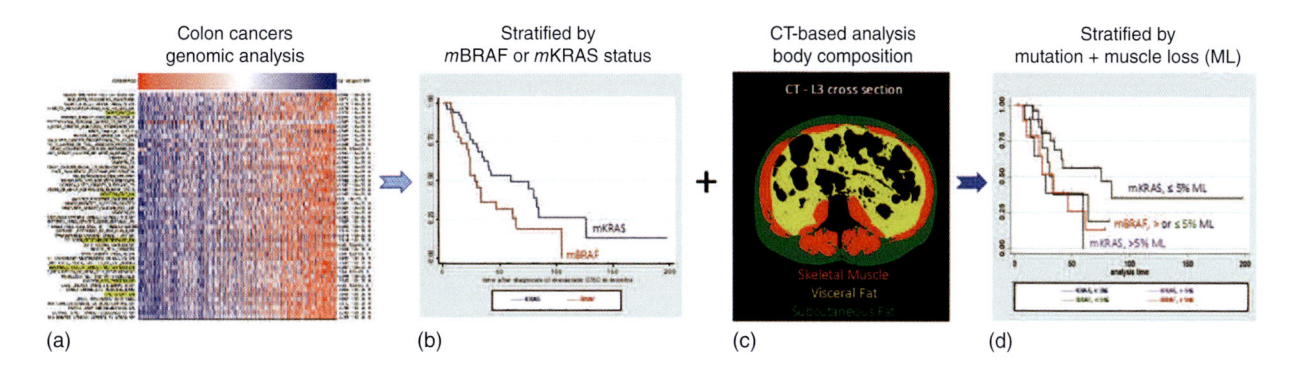

Figure 4 Integration of high-dimensional cancer and host data significantly increases disease resolution. (a) Genomic analyses of clinical colorectal cancer samples. (b) Metastatic colorectal cancer Kaplan–Meier estimates of survival ($n = 78$) stratified based on mutational status (HR 1.94, $p = 0.029$). (c) Longitudinal CT-based body composition changes from the initiation of treatment. (d) Kaplan–Meier estimates of survival stratified based on mutational status and skeletal muscle loss (ML) > or ≤5% (HR 2.25, $p = 0.029$).

Why does this level of detail matter for patients with cancer? We are learning of the surprising connections between detailed cachexia biology and specific drug-resistant cancer biology, which can provide early insight into the cancer's functional evolution under treatment distinct from circulating tumor cells or cell-free tumor DNA (a.k.a. liquid biopsies) and potential new targetable dependencies. Importantly, powerful high-resolution clinical data is becoming routinely available across practice settings at minimal cost. Detailed body composition analyses that quantitate LBM, muscle lipid content, VAT, and SAT from routinely acquired re-staging CT or MRI studies are becoming automated and essentially instantaneous through widely used medical imaging software packages (e.g., TomoVision SliceOMatic V5.0). Tumor sequencing platforms are now widely commercial and gaining penetrance in community-based oncology practices as an ever-increasing variety of mutation-targeting drugs are developed. All of these factors point to the need and feasibility for developing even more precise diagnostic features, criteria, and biomarkers (Figure 4).

Assessment and screening

Clinically relevant cachexia can frequently start at early stages of many cancers but may not be grossly evident; when it is, it is usually fairly late. Therefore, it is essential to leverage readily available information about: **risks** (cancer type, stage, and anticancer treatment toxicities), **confounding conditions** (malabsorption, GI track dysmotility, or obstruction), **interfering symptoms** (nausea, vomiting, diarrhea, dysgeusia, pain, or depression), anticancer treatment **toxicities and complications** (direct chemotherapy muscle toxicity, stomatitis from radiation, or prolonged inactivity following surgery), and **early body composition changes** by imaging studies and weight. Early consultation with nutrition services with attention paid to cachexia-related function and symptoms can help qualify, quantify, and track specific nutritional deficits and needs. The European Organization for Research and Treatment of Cancer (EORTC) QLQ-CAX-24, a patient-reported screening questionnaire, is being developed specifically to facilitate screening and ongoing assessment of cachexia-related symptoms and QoL. Finally, clinically validated digital assessment tools, like actigraphy and EKG monitors, are becoming widely adopted, which provide significantly more detailed functional assessments of patients in real-world settings.

Cachexia phenotypes

While the image of a severely cachectic patient is clear to most clinicians and patients, the ability to identify and characterize clinically significant cachexia in most patients is more subtle. The increasing prevalence of obesity obscures significant early body composition changes. Detailed morphometric studies of varied animal models of cachexia and the expanding use of imaging-based body composition analyses in patient cohorts are revealing frequent occult and distinct cachexia phenotypes, separable from BMI, in diverse disease contexts. The *adipose predominant* phenotype involves early and preferential loss of adipose mass over muscle mass. The prevalence is ~15% but likely varies significantly in different disease contexts. This phenotype involves predominance of anorexia, nutritional deficit, high adrenergic tone, and direct activation of lipolysis (e.g., via LIF, adrenomedullin, PTH-rp, catecholamines). It is likely associated with better survival in some contexts and more likely to respond to nutritional repletion and anti-inflammatory treatment. The *muscle predominant* phenotype is found in ~10% of patients. It involves early preferential loss of muscle mass over adipose mass and is exemplified by sarcopenic obesity. This phenotype likely involves direct mediators of muscle atrophy (e.g., myostatin, activin A, TWEAK, HSP70/90) and is potentially exacerbated by cancer drug-mediated muscle toxicities. There are no specific treatments, and this phenotype is associated with worse survival and drug toxicities than indicated by BMI. The *mixed muscle and adipose* phenotype involves early muscle loss followed by adipose loss and includes the vast majority of patients. It likely involves a combination of nutritional deficit, elevated adrenergic tone, direct lipolytic and direct proteolytic mediators. There is a nearly linear correlation of survival with muscle loss; therapeutic management will likely require all modalities in addition to development of anti-catabolic interventions.

These phenotypes have been underappreciated in previous experimental and clinical assessments as analyses tended to compare the end of the disease spectrum, where there is eventual, if disproportionate, loss of both tissue types. Routine longitudinal image-based body composition analysis can provide real-time dynamic assessment of the degree and composition of body compartment changes that make up each phenotype to guide risk evaluation for adverse events and improved treatment planning.

Among other potential mediators of tissue crosstalk, the profound flux in plasma lipid metabolites from adipose depots undergoing lipolysis due to cachectogenic processes provides a large and powerful biological signal. Mass spectroscopy analysis of plasma from cancer patients with or without cachexia demonstrates that tri-, di-, and monoacylglycerides (TAGs, DAGs, and MAGs), lysophospholipids (LPLs), sphingomyelins (SMs), nonesterified or free fatty acids (NEFA or FFAs), and glycerol are all elevated several-fold in early to mid-stages of cachexia, and fall as lipid stores are eventually depleted in later stages. This significantly elevated lipid metabolite load is systemically available to and taken up by other normal tissues, particularly muscle and liver, and cancer cells. In human skeletal muscle, the high lipid load eventually exceeds intramyocellular storage capacity, leading to elevated concentrations of specific species of DAGs and eventual insulin resistance.[243] Excessive β-oxidation of FFAs in skeletal muscle, as a result of direct activation by various cytokines and increased substrate delivery, causes overwhelming oxidative stress, activation of the p38 stress response, and significant muscle atrophy in human myotubes and xenograft models.[5] Cancer cells have also been shown to avidly take up specific exogenous MAGs, LPLs, and NEFAs promoting cancer growth, progression, stem cell-like features, and broad drug resistance.[244–248] These remarkable discoveries, among others, are beginning to bring detailed mechanistic specificity to the powerful connections between cachexia and fundamental cancer biology.

Cachexia and cancer drug-resistance

It is broadly appreciated that cachexia is associated with advanced and often recurrent cancers. Certainly, decreases in body composition reserves diminish tolerance of patients to a wide variety of challenging treatments, distinct from specific toxicities and complications. Less appreciated is that the cachectic state (cachectic mediators and metabolites, altered cytokines, adipokines and myokines, altered immune cell functioning, and altered pharmacokinetics) can lead to diminished responses or even resistance to potent cancer therapies. The meta-analysis of clinical studies of toxicities to tyrosine kinase inhibitors also assessed clinical responses in cachectic patients.[178] Muscle loss at diagnosis of various cancers correlated significantly with lower OS/PFS in treatments with sorafenib (HR 1.45, $p = 0.02$), sunitinib (HR 4.53, $p < 0.0001$), lenvatinib (adjusted OR 2.25, $p = 0.028$), or regorafenib (HR 2.87, $p = 0.03$) compared to noncachectic patients within each study. Even more unexpected were the results from several recent studies evaluating the efficacy of immune checkpoint inhibitors (ICIs) in RCC and NSCLC patients stratified by BMI or cachectic weight loss. In a retrospective multivariable analysis of 735 patients with RCC stratified by BMI > versus <25 (a previously determined significant cut point for cachexia risk), patients with BMI >25 (63%) had significantly better response to ICI treatment (HR 0.75, $p = 0.03$).[249] In a subset analysis, tumor genomic alteration frequencies and mutational burden were similar between the two groups. Two groups in Japan analyzed the response of NSCLC patients with or without cachectic-defined weight loss to PD-1/PD-L1 inhibitors. The first group found that 48% of these advanced NSCLC patients met diagnostic criteria for cachexia at the initiation of treatment and had dramatically lower PFS compared to noncachectic patients (2.3 mo vs 12.0 mo, $p < 0.001$), regardless of tumor proportion score (TPS) for PD-L1 and PS of 0–1.[250] Surprisingly, cachexia status was as strong a predictor of (poor) treatment efficacy as PD-L1 TPS <50% in both univariate and multivariate analyses. Controlling for drug plasma levels, the second study confirmed the trend of these significant findings.[251] A potential mechanistic explanation comes from the finding that tumor-derived cytokines (G-CSF, GM-CSF, and IL-6) induce myeloid-derived suppressor cells through active uptake of high concentration extracellular lipids (available via cachexia); inhibition of myeloid cell lipid uptake by CD36 gene knockout inhibits MDSC immunosuppression, resulting in $CD8^+$ effector T-cells tumor repression *in vivo*.[252] Collectively, these truly remarkable findings demonstrate cachexia's large impact on and predictive power for the efficacy of potent anticancer therapies.

Another intriguing area of developing research into intrinsic cancer cell therapy resistance involves reprogramming cancer cell lipid metabolism. Antiangiogenesis drugs, for example, bevacizumab, induce hypoxic stress in colorectal cancers, causing increased FFA transport through upregulation of HIF-1α and eventual drug resistance.[253] Inhibition of CPT1, the rate-limiting enzyme of FA oxidation, leads to re-sensitization to AADs. Resistance to lapatinib, a dual Her2/EGFR inhibitor, in HER2+ breast cancers causes upregulation of the multi-lipid transporter, CD36, and increased uptake of exogenous FFA, which when inhibited causes a significantly reduced tumor growth in animal models. In HER2+ breast cancer patients treated with lapatinib, CD36 expression increases, independently predicting significantly reduced survival (HR 3.84, $p = 0.007$).[254] Contemporarily, ferroptosis, an iron-dependent, nonapoptotic form of programmed cell death, was described as a unique vulnerability in diverse therapy-resistant cancer cells. Under stress from chemo, targeted, or radiation therapies, persister cells undergo lipid metabolic rewiring, resulting in high levels of lipid peroxidation and dependence on glutathione peroxidase 4, which leads to a nonmutational EMT-like drug-resistant state.[255,256] The increase in specific polyunsaturated FA oxidative flux from both internal (HIF-2α-dependent) and exogenous sources makes these cancer cells exquisitely GPX4-dependent for detoxification and escape.[247] Our unpublished experiments demonstrated that all tested GPX4-dependent cancer cell clones are highly cachexia-inducing in human skeletal muscle and adipocyte assays and that all tested cachexia-inducing cell lines are among the most sensitive to GPX4 inhibition in cell viability assays. Furthermore, mass-spectroscopy analysis of plasma from cachectic versus noncachectic patients demonstrated a several-fold increase in these specific LPCs which are actively taken up by aggressive and drug-resistant cancer cells. These experimental data are beginning to connect both the induction of cachexia and the resulting systemic lipid metabolites in support of cancer drug-resistant states.

Cachexia management: multimodal intervention

Given the cascade of potential tumor and host-derived mediators of tissue wasting that could be active in any given patient, effective therapeutic intervention should be guided by the risks and clinical features of the individual patient and cachectic phenotype.

Nutritional support

Most cancer patients either present with or develop net energy and protein balance deficits due to diminished intake and elevated total energy expenditure and catabolism, which restrict the impact of all other therapeutic interventions. This may be especially the case in adipose-predominant cachexia. Preventing and repleting these deficits is a major challenge in the face of frequent anorexia, dysgeusia, GI symptoms, mechanical obstruction, and malabsorption, which all must be addressed at the outset. Given the high risk and often occult nature of early cachexia, early dietary counseling with a clinical nutritionist is recommended for all patients.[257] Patients who cannot meet their nourishing requirements through oral diet are advised to take one of the diversely formulated parenteral nutritional supplements best suited to their nutritional requirements and tastes. Orexigenic medications can also be used to mitigate loss of appetite. Supplemental omega-3 FAs, especially eicosapentaenoic acid (EPA) and docosahexaenoic acid, are recognized for their anti-inflammatory effects and have been used in therapeutic interventions to treat or prevent cancer cachexia.[258] Notably, ESPEN guidelines recommend 1.0–1.5 g protein/kg/day for cancer patients.[259] If voluntary eating and oral nutritional supplements are inadequate, artificial TPN is not recommended given the low utility and potential harm, unless the etiology is temporary or expected to be reversible.

Pharmacological treatment

Ghrelin agonists

Ghrelin has been investigated in cancer cachexia and other conditions such as end-stage renal disease, COPD, and anorexia nervosa. Acylated ghrelin increase appetite in both healthy volunteers and cancer patients and is generally well tolerated. Intriguingly, cancer patients with cachexia can present with hyperghrelinemia, which may be explained by the short 30 min half-life of ghrelin.[80,260] The ghrelin receptor agonist anamorelin is primarily orexogenic but also stimulates the secretion of GH, IGF, and IGF-binding protein 3 (IGFBP-3), which also impact LBM. In Phase 1 and 2 trials, anamorelin improved appetite and modestly increased LBM, but did not significantly improve function.[93,146] Two multinational Phase 3 trials in NSCLC patients with cachexia, ROMANA 1 and ROMANA 2, showed that anamorelin (100 mg daily for 12 weeks) increased LBM and body weight and improved cachexia-related QoL.[261] The extension study ROMANA 3, which assessed long-term use of anamorelin over 24 weeks in patients who completed ROMANA 1 and 2, found that anamorelin modestly increased body weight, but failed to improve functional endpoints. Anamorelin was generally well-tolerated and did not show any significant increase in adverse effects compared to the placebo group.[262] Intriguingly, anamorelin did not improve physical functions as measured with hand-grip strength[146,261–266] or a 6-min walk[265] compared to placebo. Similarly, Japanese Phase 2 and 3 studies in advanced NSCLC and GI cancer patients, respectively, taking 100 mg daily of anamorelin over 12 weeks reported improved appetite and QoL metrics and modest gains in body weight and LBM.[265,266] Notably, on 11 December 2020, anamorelin received its first approval for the treatment of weight loss and anorexia in cancer cachexia in Japan. Two ongoing clinical trials [NCT03743064 and NCT03743051] are investigating anamorelin in treating cachexia in patients with NSCLC and will report a "composite clinical response" including a patient-reported anorexia scale and changes in weight.

Nonsteroidal anti-inflammatory drugs (NSAIDs) and Omega-3 FAs

Inflammation is a common component of cachexia, and pharmacologic agents that target inflammatory cytokines have been investigated, but studies remain inconclusive.[267] Celecoxib, a cyclooxygenase-2 (COX-2) inhibitor, was found to play a significant role in improving QoL and BMI in patients with cachexia.[268] In patients with advanced cancer, celecoxib was reported to significantly increase LBM and ameliorate handgrip strength and QoL.[136] The ongoing MENAC trial [NCT 02330926] is investigating a multimodal intervention that includes exercise, nutrition, and ibuprofen in adults with cancer cachexia. Eicosapentaenoic acid (EPA) also appears to stabilize weight in cancer patients by decreasing proinflammatory cytokines[269] and inhibiting proteasome-induced muscle proteolysis.[270] Treating cachexia with EPA increased weight gain, LBM and QoL, but the small absolute difference from the isocaloric control supplement indicates that the majority of benefit was achieved by simple caloric repletion.[271]

Appetite stimulants

Appetite stimulants are the oldest and most extensively studied drugs for cachexia. They include progesterone agents, such as megestrol acetate and medroxyprogesterone acetate, steroids, and cannabinoids. Megestrol acetate improves appetite and increases body weight via fat accrual but is associated with serious adverse events: venous thromboembolism, hypogonadism, adrenal insufficiency, and increased mortality in the elderly.[146] Another progesterone derivative, medroxyprogesterone, improved anorexia, QoL and body weight gain through adipose accrual without lean mass.[272] Corticosteroids can lead to significant improvements in appetite and QoL but are usually avoided due to their significant side effects.[267] Cannabinoids are considered less effective than steroids but remain a viable option.[273] These compounds bind to cannabinoid receptors, such as CB1 and CB2, in the CNS, GI system, skeletal muscle, and adipose tissue among others.[274] Interestingly, the endocannabinoid Δ-9-tetrahydrocannabinol, THC, did not show any significant alterations in appetite or QoL in a Phase III trial.[275] In a Phase II clinical trial, however, nabilone, the synthetic analog of THC, significantly improved appetite, increase caloric intake and QoL in patients with NSCLC and cachexia without eliciting any major adverse effects.[276] Despite the beneficial role of appetite stimulants in helping cachexia patients gain weight, such stimulants have not yet shown any benefit in improving other outcomes including physical performance or survival.[273,277,278]

Beta-blockers

Beta-blockers inhibit catecholamine-dependent lipolysis, induce vasodilation, enhance oxygenation and decrease REE. The use of beta-blockers in cachectic rats inhibited weight loss and improved survival.[279] In ACT ONE, a randomized double-blind parallel-group placebo-controlled Phase II trial, he mixed-effect beta-blocker, espindolol, maintained fat mass and modestly increased LBM in patients with stages III or IV colorectal cancer or NSCLC-related cachexia. These changes were paralleled with significant improvement in handgrip strength.[280] Espindolol is suggested to exhibit its anticachectic effects by reducing catabolism through nonselective β receptor blockade,[280] reducing thermogenesis and fatigue through central 5-HT1a receptor antagonism[280] and increasing anabolism through partial β2 receptor agonism.[281]

TNFα, IL-6, and IL-1 inhibitors

Given their association with and potential role in cancer cachexia, TNFα, IL-6, and IL-1α have received much attention in the development of anticachectic therapies. However, in two randomized controlled trials of advanced cachectic patients, anti-TNFα therapy such as etanercept, a TNFα receptor blocker,[282] and infliximab, a TNF-α blocking monoclonal antibody,[24] were unable to improve appetite or to hinder muscle atrophy. Infliximab actually worsened fatigue and increased treatment-related mortality.[24] Furthermore, thalidomide[283–285] and pentoxifylline,[286,287] which can both decrease TNFα expression, were studied in five randomized control trials and showed no significant benefits or were linked to a worsening in QoL despite a slight recovery in muscle mass.

Anti-IL-6 and anti-IL-1α therapies demonstrated promising trends in the treatment of cachexia in various clinical trials.

However, the results were inconclusive with respect to clinical benefit. A multinational Phase 3 study of the IL-1α-specific monoclonal antibody MABp in patients with advanced colorectal cancer did not find any significant differences in LBM or QoL change.[288] Another Phase 3 study designed to compare overall survival between MABp1 and megestrol acetate in patients with metastatic colorectal cancer and cachexia was terminated early because the study crossed the prospective futility boundary of the primary endpoint [NCT01767857]. The anti-IL-6 monoclonal antibody, clazakizumab, reversed fatigue, increased hemoglobin and albumin, and was well tolerated by patients with advanced cancer who participated in a Phase I clinical trial. Unfortunately, in Phase II, clazakizumab was associated with a slight decrease in loss of lean mass in NSCLC patients.[49]

Androgens/SARMs
Androgenic steroids can increase muscle mass, even in cachectic patients, though with limited clinically functional benefit. Oxandrolone is an oral synthetic testosterone derivative that has been approved for treatment of weight loss. Oxandrolone has generally very few side effects, one of which is hypogonadism in men. It has been used in the treatment of HIV- and COPD-related weight loss and of catabolic conditions such as burns, surgery, and chronic infections.[289] Selective androgen receptor modulators (SARMs) are tissue-specific nonsteroidal androgenic agents that have greater anabolic effects than testosterone, but minimal androgenic effects. Enobosarm is a SARM with anabolic effects in muscle and bone. Enobosarm was associated with a significant increase in total LBM in cancer patients in a recent Phase II randomized controlled trial.[290–292] However, two Phase III studies, POWER I and II, did not meet their primary endpoints of meaningful functional improvement, despite increased muscle mass.

Emerging treatment options

MEK/ERK inhibitors
Overactivation of MEK and ERK1/2 signaling is a convergent signaling hub for many cachexia mediators in both muscle and adipose, leading to pathological activation of ATGL, HSL, autophagy, and proteolysis. As important components of cancer growth programs, they are also the target of multiple safe and potent drugs approved to treat various cancers. Critically, the degree of inhibition to reset signaling homeostasis in normal tissues is significantly lower than that sought in anticancer treatments, where the objective is maximally tolerated inhibition of this pathway. The therapeutic window for MEK/ERK1/2 inhibition is, therefore, significantly lower for the treatment of cachexia-associated muscle and adipose loss and is likely why overt recovery of these tissues has been underappreciated in cancer clinical trials of these inhibitors. That said, a Phase 2 trial of selumetinib in metastatic cholangiocarcinoma, a cancer with frequent and rapid cachexia, found in a secondary analysis a surprising nonfluid weight gain in all 25 evaluable patients, averaging 8.6 pounds.[293] This effect was postulated to be explained through MEK/ERK-inhibition leading to diminished tumor secretion of IL-6, IL-1, and TNF. However, multiple studies suggest direct inhibition of pathological levels of MEK/ERK signaling in cachectic muscle and fat cells is a more compelling mechanism. Specifically designed clinical trials are required of any given MEK/ERK inhibitor to assess optimal dosing through dose-de-escalation, as safety can be reasonably imputed from previous single-agent cancer trials that included a high proportion of cachectic patients.

JAK2 inhibitors
LIF is a signaling protein secreted by tumors and normal tissues that can induce adipose-predominant cachexia.[294] Analysis of The Cancer Genome Atlas (TCGA) database shows that LIF is highly expressed in gastrointestinal, thoracic, and genitourinary cancers that are strongly associated with cachexia.[294] LIF, a member of the IL-6 family of cytokines, binds to the heterodimer, LIF receptor-α and gp130, which then activates the JAK–STAT pathway.[295] Recombinant LIF (r-LIF) administered to mice resulted in dramatic adipose and body weight loss via its action on the JAK/STAT pathway both centrally in the hypothalamus and peripherally in adipose tissue, independent of IL-6.[294] Despite only a transient decrease in food intake with continuous r-LIF infusion, the mice still exhibited a profound loss of adipose from LIF's direct action on adipocyte-expressed LIFR, driving lipolysis.[296] In $IL\text{-}6^{-/-}$ mice, LIF still resulted in adipose loss, which indicates that LIF and IL-6 act by independent mechanisms.[133] Administration of tofacitinib or ruxolitinib, two FDA-approved JAK inhibitors, to r-LIF-driven or tumor-driven models of cachexia resulted in decreased phosphorylation of STAT3 in adipose tissue and in the hypothalamus. This resulted in an improvement in LIF-induced anorexia, adipose, and weight loss and survival.[133] Even more intriguing, LIF (but not IL-6) has been shown to be a powerful dependency in pancreatic cancer: (1) KRAS activates expression of LIF, (2) LIF blockade abrogates tumor progression via suppression of the Hippo signaling pathway, and (3) LIF knockdown or inhibitory antibody dramatically sensitizes multiple patient-derived xenograft tumors to gemcitabine, extending survival.[297] This a compelling example of the direct and specific systemic effects of aggressive cancer biology that can be exploited therapeutically. In sum, the effect of inhibiting JAK 1/2 and subsequently halting cachexia-associated adipose wasting was found to have long-lasting survival benefits in cancer cachexia models and provides clear rationale for testing approved JAK-inhibitors in carefully selected cancer cachexia contexts.

GDF15 Signaling Inhibition: Levels of circulating GDF15 demonstrate a strong positive correlation with cachexia and a negative correlation with survival in patients with cancer.[298–301] GDF15-induced weight loss in mice was found to be regulated by a GFRAL–RET signaling complex in brainstem neurons.[302–304] 3P10, a monoclonal antibody that targets GFRAL, was described to inhibit RET signaling by blocking the cell surface interaction of GFRAL with RET.[9] Intriguingly, administration of 3P10 to tumor-bearing mice protected against cancer adipose-predominant cachexia and reversed excessive lipid oxidation. Mechanistically, activation of the GFRAL–RET pathway increases the expression of lipid metabolism genes in adipose tissue via increased adrenergic tone. GDF15's indirect lipolytic activity in adipose tissue of tumor-bearing mice resulted in impaired muscle function, as measured by forelimb grip strength, but only modest reduction in muscle mass relative to the loss in adipose mass.[9] Thus, inhibition of GFRAL by 3P10 represents a novel mechanism for the treatment of cancer cachexia by preventing GDF15-induced anorexia, lipid oxidation, and muscle atrophy.

Physical activity

Exercise is beneficial in improving muscle strength, fatigue, bone health, psychosocial distress, depression, overall QoL, and in decreasing overall mortality.[305] Exercise is also essential in minimizing the compounding effects of disuse atrophy. A systematic review of 16 trials conducted on patients with cancer under active treatment reported an improvement in upper and lower body muscle strength after undertaking resistance exercise.[306] Progressive resistance training effectively increased LBM and muscle strength in cancer patients with cachexia following radiotherapy.[307] Numerous studies have shown that moderate exercise improves cachexia through optimizing aberrant muscle and adipose metabolism, as well as improving insulin sensitivity. Of note, the anti-inflammatory effects of exercise in adipose and skeletal muscle are due to the upregulation of anti-inflammatory cytokines.[305,308] Exercise is being evaluated as a nonpharmacological therapy to offset muscle wasting and fatigue by reducing oxidative stress, which is thought to play a pivotal role in many pathological processes associated with cancer. Moreover, recent studies have focused on the role of exercise in reducing the toxic effects of chemotherapeutics on skeletal muscle as most cancer treatments, such as doxorubicin, trigger substantial oxidative stress, which leads to muscle wasting and atrophy.[309,310] Combining exercise with other therapies (anti-iatrogenic therapies, nutritional repletion, anti-inflammatories) is essential for maximizing therapeutic benefit of other modalities.

Cachexia biomarkers

While current weight-based diagnostic criteria are important for bringing consistency in defining the complex disease state of cachexia, they are not sufficiently precise to enable new therapeutic development. For this purpose, it would be ideal to have highly specific and sensitive prognostic, diagnostic, and pharmacodynamic biomarkers. Prognostic markers predict which patients are more likely to develop the disease, enriching patient selection for earlier intervention and more focused clinical trials. Two information domains that can provide predictive power are cancer features and host features. Many cancers are now molecularly characterized (e.g., growth factor receptor status, metabolic alterations, or driver mutations) that can provide risk stratification in large patient cohorts. Our own work leveraged multiple large clinical sample profiling datasets to identify the molecular features of cachectogenic cancers, then mapped these features across cancer types to specific molecular subtypes in lung, colon, gastric, pancreatic, renal, ovarian, melanoma, breast, and prostate cancers. These correlations were confirmed in an independent cohort of >2000 diverse cancer patients, collectively presenting a novel approach to biomarker discovery. For a deeper analysis in NSCLC, a collaboration with the precision-medicine-guided therapeutic clinical trial, Lung-MAP, merges the prognostic genomic mutations we identified in lung cancer with an exploration of CT body composition, plasma laboratories, and additional bio-samples for diagnostic biomarker discovery. Host-specific factors that convey higher risk of cachexia could come from GWAS or candidate gene studies, though adequate cohort numbers are usually quite high to achieve adequate power to make significant findings. More precise diagnostic biomarkers would aid in higher-resolution analyses of therapeutic efficacy. Quantification of body composition by CT or MRI-based imaging analysis can be quite sensitive to quantity and quality changes in specific tissue compartments but may not be highly specific to etiology (cachexia, starvation, or toxicity). With the addition of a disease-specific marker or markers, the composite biomarker would improve overall performance. An example of combinatorial power is the addition of neutrophil-to-leukocyte ratio (NLR ≥ 3), a marker of inflammation, to a CT-based sarcopenia threshold that moved the CRC-related death HR from **1.28** (95% CI 1.10–1.53) to **2.43** (95% CI 1.79–3.29) compared to neither.[182] Other possible biomarker types could include other specific markers of inflammation, routine plasma laboratories, lipid metabolites, proteomic features, or specific disease mediator. Pharmacodynamic biomarkers, more proximal to the therapeutic target than a clinical endpoint, would allow early assessment of effective target engagement. These could overlap with certain diagnostic markers, if they are in direct line of a target mechanism.

Conclusions and perspectives

Despite the remarkable progress in targeted and immune-mediated cancer therapies, cachexia remains one of the most significant challenges facing cancer patients in symptom burden, adverse complications, and deleterious impact on treatment response. Historically, it has been viewed as the inevitable manifestation of terminal cancers, for which little could be done. Fortunately, we are at an inflection point where much of that fatalism is fundamentally changing. This shift has resulted from improved scientific and clinical tools to disambiguate complex and dynamic pathophysiology of two intertwined diseases—the cancer and the body's multi-dimensional response. The large-scale use of routine imaging studies for precise and longitudinal body composition analyses is bringing tremendous clarity to a mostly occult disease process in its true prevalence, initiation, evolution, and impact. We now know that: (1) most patients with clinically significant muscle loss do not appear grossly wasted (2) the process of cachexia often starts at even the earliest stages of cancers, (3) cachexia is strongly correlated with toxicities and complications of cancer-directed therapies and worse outcomes at cancer diagnosis, and (4) cachexia directly supports cancer-therapy resistance of many types. So, we should pay attention (e.g., automated calculation of body composition reported with every re-staging imaging study at minimal effort and cost), because cachexia can provide uniquely powerful insight into the plasticity of the underlying cancer with new therapeutic opportunities (e.g., GPX4-dependency). Integration of high-resolution molecular profiling of many patients' cancers and clinical information is providing a deeper understanding of cachexia-inducing cancers. These technological advances will enable the discovery of robust disease mechanisms and more precise prognostic, diagnostic, and pharmacodynamic biomarkers. New therapeutic modalities are being developed and approved, including the real potential to quickly re-purpose currently approved safe and potent medications to treat cachexia, guided by the clinical phenotypes of cachexia.

Key references

The complete reference list can be found on Vital Source version of this title, see inside front cover.

2 Marquart J, Chen EY, Prasad V. Estimation of the percentage of US patients with cancer who benefit from genome-driven oncology. *JAMA Oncol.* 2018;**4**(8):1093–1098.

3 Haslam A, Prasad V. Estimation of the percentage of US patients with cancer who are eligible for and respond to checkpoint inhibitor immunotherapy drugs. *JAMA Netw Open.* 2019;**2**(5):e192535.

5 Fukawa T, Yan-Jiang BC, Min-Wen JC, et al. Excessive fatty acid oxidation induces muscle atrophy in cancer cachexia. *Nat Med.* 2016;**22**(6):666–671.

7 Zhou X, Wang JL, Lu J, et al. Reversal of cancer cachexia and muscle wasting by ActRIIB antagonism leads to prolonged survival. *Cell.* 2010;**142**(4):531–543.

9 Suriben R, Chen M, Higbee J, et al. Antibody-mediated inhibition of GDF15–GFRAL activity reverses cancer cachexia in mice. *Nat Med.* 2020;**26**(8):1264–1270.

10 Wakabayashi H, Arai H, Inui A. The regulatory approval of anamorelin for treatment of cachexia in patients with non-small cell lung cancer, gastric cancer,

25 Cawthorn WP, Sethi JK. TNF-α and adipocyte biology. *FEBS Lett*. 2008;**582**(1):117–131.
27 Lyu K, Zhang Y, Zhang D, et al. A membrane-bound diacylglycerol species induces PKC-mediated hepatic insulin resistance. *Cell Metab*. 2020;**32**(4):654–664 e5.
37 Paul PK, Kumar A. TRAF6 coordinates the activation of autophagy and ubiquitin-proteasome systems in atrophying skeletal muscle. *Autophagy*. 2011;**7**(5):555–556.
49 Rigas J, Schuster M, Orlov S, et al. Efect of ALD518, a humanized anti-IL-6 antibody, on lean body mass loss and symptoms in patients with advanced non-small cell lung cancer (NSCLC): Results of a phase II randomized, double-blind safety and efficacy trial. *J Clin Oncol*. 2010;**28**(15_suppl):7622.
56 Wellenstein MD, Coffelt SB, Duits DEM, et al. Loss of p53 triggers WNT-dependent systemic inflammation to drive breast cancer metastasis. *Nature*. 2019;**572**(7770):538–542.
74 Solheim TS, Blum D, Fayers PM, et al. Weight loss, appetite loss and food intake in cancer patients with cancer cachexia: three peas in a pod? - analysis from a multicenter cross sectional study. *Acta Oncol*. 2014;**53**(4):539–546.
75 Braun TP, Zhu X, Szumowski M, et al. Central nervous system inflammation induces muscle atrophy via activation of the hypothalamic–pituitary–adrenal axis. *J Exp Med*. 2011;**208**(12):2449–2463.
76 Das SK, Eder S, Schauer S, et al. Adipose triglyceride lipase contributes to cancer-associated cachexia. *Science*. 2011;**333**(6039):233–238.
84 Blauwhoff-Buskermolen S, Langius JA, Heijboer AC, et al. Plasma ghrelin levels are associated with anorexia but not cachexia in patients with NSCLC. *Front Physiol*. 2017;**8**:119.
118 Cao DX, Wu GH, Yang ZA, et al. Role of beta1-adrenoceptor in increased lipolysis in cancer cachexia. *Cancer Sci*. 2010;**101**(7):1639–1645.
120 Vaitkus JA, Celi FS. The role of adipose tissue in cancer-associated cachexia. *Exp Biol Med (Maywood)*. 2017;**242**(5):473–481.
133 Arora G, Gupta A, Guo T, et al. JAK inhibitors suppress cancer cachexia-associated anorexia and adipose wasting in mice. *JCSM Rapid Commun*. 2020;**3**(2):115–128.
144 Asp ML, Tian M, Wendel AA, Belury MA. Evidence for the contribution of insulin resistance to the development of cachexia in tumor-bearing mice. *Int J Cancer*. 2010;**126**(3):756–763.
152 Penna F, Costamagna D, Pin F, et al. Autophagic degradation contributes to muscle wasting in cancer cachexia. *Am J Pathol*. 2013;**182**(4):1367–1378.
156 McClung JM, Judge AR, Powers SK, Yan Z. p38 MAPK links oxidative stress to autophagy-related gene expression in cachectic muscle wasting. *Am J Physiol-Cell Physiol*. 2010;**298**(3):C542–C549.
169 Martin L, Senesse P, Gioulbasanis I, et al. Diagnostic criteria for the classification of cancer-associated weight loss. *J Clin Oncol*. 2015;**33**(1):90–99.
178 Rinninella E, Cintoni M, Raoul P, et al. Prognostic value of skeletal muscle mass during tyrosine kinase inhibitor (TKI) therapy in cancer patients: a systematic review and meta-analysis. *Intern Emerg Med*. 2020;**18**:1–6.
179 Jones KI, Doleman B, Scott S, et al. Simple psoas cross-sectional area measurement is a quick and easy method to assess sarcopenia and predicts major surgical complications. *Colorectal Dis*. 2015;**17**(1):O20–O26.
181 Yang M, Shen Y, Tan L, Li W. Prognostic value of sarcopenia in lung cancer: a systematic review and meta-analysis. *Chest*. 2019;**156**(1):101–111.
182 Feliciano EMC, Kroenke CH, Meyerhardt JA, et al. Association of systemic inflammation and sarcopenia with survival in nonmetastatic colorectal cancer: results from the C SCANS study. *JAMA Oncol*. 2017;**3**(12):e172319.

123 Antiemetic therapy

Michael J. Berger, PharmD, BCOP ■ David S. Ettinger, MD, FACP, FCCP

> **Overview**
>
> Dramatic progress has been made in the prevention and treatment of chemotherapy-induced nausea and vomiting (CINV), especially since the introduction of the 5-HT3 receptor antagonists (5HT3 RAs) in the early 1990s and the 2003 introduction of the NK-1 receptor antagonist (NK1 RA), aprepitant. Recent surveys indicate the need for heightened awareness of the frequency and severity of acute and especially delayed CINV. Fortunately, new agents have been added to the antiemetic arsenal to further enhance the efficacy of antiemetic prophylaxis. Complementary therapies such as acupuncture, and mind–body interventions appear promising in controlling nausea, and are being explored further. Appropriate implementation of guidelines for prophylaxis based on patient risk factors and the specific chemotherapy agents used will ensure that fewer patients experience these most distressing of side effects.

Overview

Chemotherapy-induced nausea and vomiting (CINV) remains a significant problem for many cancer patients despite recent advances in pharmacologic therapy.[1] It may have a dramatic impact on a patient's quality of life, in addition to physical consequences including dehydration, nutritional compromise, and metabolic disturbances.[2] Despite the publication of guidelines for preventive antiemetic therapy, some patients continue to receive suboptimal prophylaxis against CINV. Nausea and vomiting occurring after chemotherapy may be more difficult to manage than if the symptoms had been prevented with appropriate prophylactic pharmacologic intervention. In addition, patients may develop a psychological component to their nausea and vomiting as a result of inadequate management in the past. Thus, optimal control of CINV is a crucial aspect of symptom management among cancer patients.

Historically, approximately 70–80% of all cancer patients receiving chemotherapy experienced emesis,[3] and fortunately, there have been dramatic improvements since the introduction of effective antiemetic therapy.[1] Studies over the last 25 years have attempted to quantify the impact of chemotherapy side effects on cancer patients. Repeatedly, nausea and vomiting are mentioned as the "major physical," and the "most troublesome and unpleasant" side effects associated with chemotherapy.[4,5] Although there have been recent advances in pharmacologic prevention of CINV, patients continue to rank nausea and vomiting as one of the most distressing side effects of chemotherapy.[6] Grunberg and colleagues surveyed patients, medical oncologists, and oncology nurses in 2001–2002 to assess the frequency and provider perception of CINV.[1] Although improvements in the prevention of acute nausea and vomiting were seen (acute nausea in approximately 35% and acute emesis in 13%), delayed symptoms were seen more frequently (50–60% with nausea and 30–50% with emesis, depending on the chemotherapy used). Strikingly, more than 75% of physicians and nurses underestimated the occurrence of delayed nausea and vomiting. A more recent patient survey revealed a widespread lack of CINV understanding; many patients believe it is a side effect they must live with, or that the presence of CINV is a sign that chemotherapy was working, or that their CINV was under control as long as they were not vomiting.[7] Progress in relieving the symptoms of CINV will only come with greater awareness of the problem and more aggressive use of current medications.

This chapter highlights the pathophysiology of CINV, the emetogenic potential of common chemotherapeutics, classes of antiemetic therapy, guidelines for prevention of CINV, and the management of breakthrough CINV.

Pathophysiology of nausea and vomiting

Vomiting is controlled by the central nervous system via a complex pathway of varied afferent inputs and neurotransmitters (Figure 1). In the 1950s, studies by Borison and Wang identified two areas of the brainstem involved in nausea and vomiting: the chemoreceptor trigger zone (CTZ) and the emetic center.[8] The CTZ is located in the area postrema in the floor of the fourth ventricle. Because it lies outside the blood–brain barrier, the CTZ is susceptible to emetogenic stimuli from the bloodstream, such as chemotherapeutic drugs or, more likely, their metabolites.[9] Muscarinic, dopamine D2, serotonin (5-HT3), neurokinin 1 (NK-1), and histamine H1 receptors have been identified in the CTZ. Impulses from the CTZ are then transmitted to the emetic center. In addition to those from the CTZ to the emetic center, afferent pathways from the gastrointestinal tract and pharynx via the vagus and splanchnic nerves are coordinated in the emetic center.[10] Inputs from the cerebral cortex may also be involved, especially in anticipatory emesis. The emetic center receives afferent impulses and coordinates the efferent activities of the salivation center, abdominal muscles, respiratory center, and autonomic nerves that result in vomiting. The emetic center, composed of these indistinct receptors and effector nuclei, is located in the nucleus tractus solitarius of the brainstem.[9]

The most critical neurotransmitters involved in these afferent and efferent pathways are serotonin (5-HT3), dopamine, and substance P. Others include acetylcholine, corticosteroid, histamine, cannabinoid, opiate, and gamma-aminobutyric acid (GABA).[11] Blockade of these neurotransmitters and their receptors form the basis of action of various antiemetic drugs. However, it is not fully known how and where along these pathways chemotherapy and its metabolites have their emetic effects. Metabolites may stimulate the CTZ directly. Serotonin and other neurotransmitters may be released from intestinal cells damaged by chemotherapy. Sensory

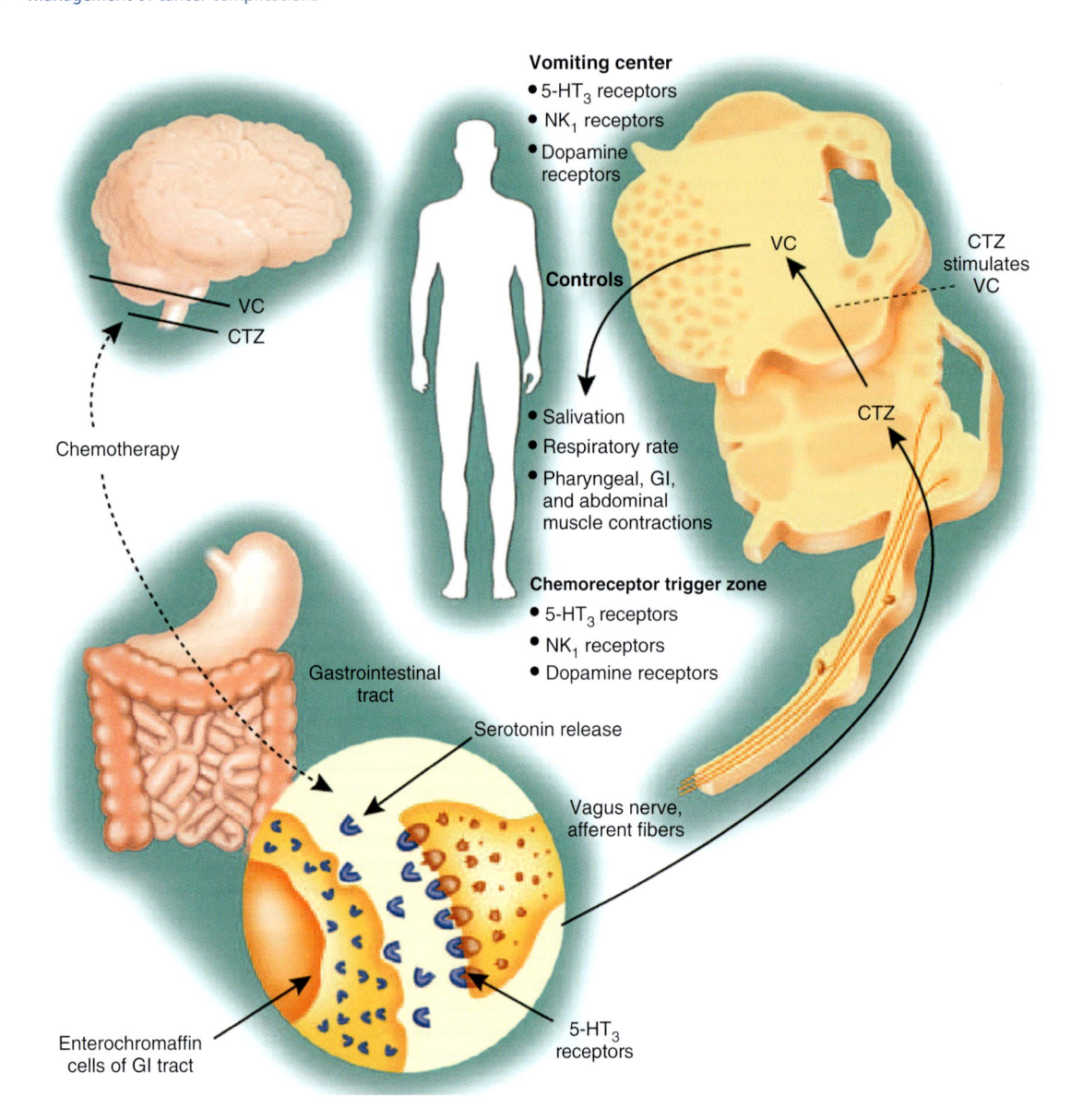

Figure 1 Two sites in the brainstem—the vomiting center and the chemoreceptor trigger zone—are important to emesis control. The vomiting center consists of an intertwined neural network in the nucleus tractus solitarius that controls patterns of motor activity. The chemoreceptor trigger zone, located in the area postrema, is the entry point for emetogenic stimuli. Entero-chromaffin cells in the gastrointestinal tract respond to chemotherapy by releasing serotonin. Serotonin binds to 5-hydroxytryptamine 3 (5-HT3) receptors, which are located not only in the gastrointestinal tract but also on vagal afferent neurons and in the nucleus tractus solitarius and area postrema. The activated 5-HT3 receptors signal the chemoreceptor trigger zone via pathways that may include the afferent fibers of the vagus nerve. Serotonin may also bind with 5-HT3 receptors in the brainstem. Other neurotransmitters, including dopamine and substance P, also influence the chemoreceptor trigger zone. Afferent impulses from the chemoreceptor trigger zone stimulate the vomiting center, which initiates emesis. Source: Modified from Wood et al.[79] Reproduced with permission of MGI Pharma.

neurons release substance P, and numerous NK-1 receptors have been identified in both the CTZ and the nucleus tractus solitarius. Despite increasing knowledge of the central nervous system and pathways involved in control of vomiting, no single common pathway has been discovered, and it is unlikely that any single agent will be able to provide complete antiemetic protection from chemotherapy.

Types of nausea and vomiting

There are several distinct types of chemotherapy-induced emesis that have been identified.

- *Acute emesis* is defined as nausea and vomiting within 24 h of chemotherapy. It has its onset within 1–2 h of chemotherapy and peaks in the first 4–6 h without adequate prophylaxis.
- *Delayed emesis* refers to symptoms that start more than 24 h after chemotherapy. It typically peaks at 48–72 h and may last for 6–7 days. Although delayed emesis may be less frequent and less severe than acute emesis, it is less well controlled than acute emesis. Cisplatin is most frequently associated with delayed emesis, although it is also seen with carboplatin, cyclophosphamide, and anthracyclines.
- *Anticipatory emesis* is seen in patients whose symptoms develop as a conditioned response before the chemotherapy is administered. It may be triggered by sights and activities associated with

Table 1 Emetogenic potential of parenteral anticancer agents.[a–d]

Level	Agent			
High emetic risk (>90% frequency of emesis)[e–g]	• AC combination is defined as any chemotherapy regimen that contains an anthracycline and cyclophosphamide • Carboplatin AUC ≥4 • Carmustine >250 mg/m²	• Cisplatin • Cyclophosphamide >1500 mg/m² • Dacarbazine • Doxorubicin ≥60 mg/m² • Epirubicin >90 mg/m² • Ifosfamide ≥2 g/m² per dose	• Mechlorethamine • Melphalan ≥140 mg/m² • Sacituzumab govitecan-hziy • Streptozocin	
Moderate emetic risk (>30–90% frequency of emesis)[e–g]	• Aldesleukin >12–15 million IU/m² • Amifostine >300 mg/m² • Azacitidine • Bendamustine • Busulfan • Carboplatin AUC[h] <4 • Carmustine[h] ≤250 mg/m² • Clofarabine • Cyclophosphamide[h] ≤1500 mg/m² • Cytarabine >200 mg/m² • Dactinomycin[h]	• Daunorubicin[h] • Dual-drug liposomal encapsulation of cytarabine and daunorubicin • Dinutuximab • Doxorubicin[h] <60 mg/m² • Epirubicin[h] ≤90 mg/m² • Fam-trastuzumab deruxtecan-nxki • Idarubicin • Ifosfamide[h] <2 g/m² per dose • Irinotecan[h] • Irinotecan (liposomal)	• Lurbinectedin • Melphalan <140 mg/m² • Methotrexate[h] ≥250 mg/m² • Oxaliplatin[h] • Temozolomide • Trabectedin[h]	

[a]Source: Reproduced with permission from the NCCN Guidelines® for **Antiemesis V.1.2021**. © 2020 National Comprehensive Cancer Network, Inc. All rights reserved. The NCCN Guidelines and illustrations herein may not be reproduced in any form for any purpose without the express written permission of the NCCN. NCCN makes no warranties of any kind whatsoever regarding their content, use or application and disclaims any responsibility for their application or use in any way.
[b]Hesketh et al.[80]
[c]Grunberg et al.[81]
[d]Potential drug interactions between antineoplastic agents/antiemetic agents and various other drugs should always be considered.
[e]Proportion of patients who experience emesis in the absence of effective antiemetic prophylaxis.
[f]Continuous infusion may make an agent less emetogenic.
[g]The emetic risk is expected to be the same for biosimilars as for the parent compound unless otherwise noted.
[h]These agents may be highly emetogenic in certain patients.

the chemotherapy (e.g. driving to the treatment center or actual CINV experienced in previous cycles). As anticipatory emesis is a conditioned reflex, it is predominantly mediated by the cerebral cortex. As control of CINV has improved, the incidence of anticipatory emesis has declined.[12]
- *Breakthrough emesis* refers to symptoms that occur despite prophylactic treatment and therefore require rescue therapy. This is a difficult clinical problem to manage and there is little clinical trial data to guide antiemetic selection in this setting.[13,14] The breakthrough drug prescribed should be from a different pharmacological class than that used as prophylactic treatment. Several agents are used empirically including haloperidol, olanzapine, and prochlorperazine.[13,14]
- *Refractory emesis* refers to symptoms that occur during a chemotherapy cycle after prophylactic treatment and/or rescue therapy have failed.[14]

In addition to chemotherapy-induced emesis, other potential causes of nausea and vomiting in cancer patients include partial or complete bowel obstruction, brain metastases, uremia, electrolyte disturbances (i.e., hyperglycemia, hypercalcemia, hyponatremia), and gastroparesis. Other medications commonly prescribed in cancer patients, such as opiates, may cause emesis as well.

Emetogenic chemotherapy
The severity and frequency of CINV are affected by both patient-specific and treatment-related risk factors. Patient-related factors predicting a higher incidence of CINV include a history of chemotherapy, a history of CINV, female sex, younger age (<50 y.o.), a history of motion sickness, anxiety, and no/minimal history of alcohol use. Treatment-related factors include the route and rate of administration (IV bolus more emetogenic than IV infusion), chemotherapy drug dosage, and the number of previous chemotherapy cycles received (risk can increase over subsequent cycles). The most predictive factor is the inherent emetogenicity of the specific chemotherapy agent used.[15]

There is no universally accepted classification system of chemotherapy agents by emetogenic potential, although several clinical practice guidelines including the National Comprehensive Cancer Network (NCCN), the American Society of Clinical Oncology (ASCO), and the Multinational Association for Supportive Care in Cancer (MASCC) utilize a classification system using four risk categories of emetogenicity based on the percentage of patients who will experience CINV if no prophylaxis were administered[14,16–18]:

- *High risk*. More than 90%
- *Moderate risk*. 30–90%
- *Low risk*. 10–30%
- *Minimal risk*. Less than 10%

For multi-agent chemotherapy regimens, the emetic risk of the regimen is based upon the individual drug with the highest emetic risk. See Tables 1–3 for the emetogenic potential of parenteral and oral anticancer agents. It should be noted that these classification systems were developed with a focus on acute emesis. It is clear from recent data that the frequency and severity of delayed emesis are often underestimated and remain a significant problem for many patients.[1]

Classes of antiemetics
Our knowledge of the known neurotransmitters involved in the central nervous system pathways that regulate the vomiting response has provided targets for antiemetic therapy (Table 4). In return, successful clinical application of these agents has confirmed the importance of these neurotransmitters and receptors in the vomiting pathway. Neuroreceptors involved in the control

Table 2 Emetogenic potential of parenteral anticancer agents.[a–d]

Level	Agent			
Low emetic risk (10–30% frequency of emesis)[e–g]	• Ado-trastuzumab emtansine • Aldesleukin ≤12 million IU/m^2 • Amifostine ≤300 mg/m^2 • Arsenic trioxide • Axicabtagene ciloleucel[h] • Belinostat • Brexucabtagene autoleucel[h] • Brentuximab vedotin • Cabazitaxel • Carfilzomib • Copanlisib • Cytarabine (low dose) 100–200 mg/m^2	• Docetaxel • Doxorubicin (liposomal) • Enfortumab vedotin-ejfv • Eribulin • Etoposide • 5-Fluorouracil (5-FU) • Floxuridine • Gemcitabine • Gemtuzumab ozogamicin • Inotuzumab ozogamicin • Isatuximab-irfc • Ixabepilone • Methotrexate >50–<250 mg/m^2	• Mitomycin • Mitomycin pyelocalyceal solution • Mitoxantrone • Mogamulizumab • Moxetumomab • Necitumumab • Olaratumab • Omacetaxine • Paclitaxel • Paclitaxel-albumin • Pemetrexed • Pentostatin • Polatuzumab vedotin	• Pralatrexate • Romidepsin • Tafasitamab-cxix • Tagraxofusp • Talimogene laherparepvec • Thiotepa • Tisagenlecleucel[h] • Topotecan • Ziv-aflibercept
Minimal emetic risk (<10% frequency of emesis)[e–g]	• Alemtuzumab • Atezolizumab • Avelumab • Asparaginase • Bevacizumab • Bleomycin • Blinatumomab • Bortezomib • Cetuximab • Cemiplimab • Cladribine • Cytarabine <100 mg/m^2 • Daratumumab	• Daratumumab hyaluronidase-fihj • Decitabine • Denileukin diftitox • Dexrazoxane • Durvalumab • Elotuzumab • Fludarabine • Ipilimumab • Luspatercept-aamt • Methotrexate ≤50 mg/m^2 • Nelarabine • Nivolumab	• Obinutuzumab • Ofatumumab • Panitumumab • Pegaspargase • Pembrolizumab • Pertuzumab • Pertuzumab/trastuzumab/hyaluronidase-zzxf • Ramucirumab • Rituximab • Rituximab/hyaluronidase	• Siltuximab • Temsirolimus • Trastuzumab • Trastuzumab/hyaluronidase • Valrubicin • Vinblastine • Vincristine • Vincristine (liposomal) • Vinorelbine

[a] Source: Reproduced with permission from the NCCN Guidelines® for **Antiemesis V.1.2021**. © 2020 National Comprehensive Cancer Network, Inc. All rights reserved. The NCCN Guidelines and illustrations herein may not be reproduced in any form for any purpose without the express written permission of the NCCN. NCCN makes no warranties of any kind whatsoever regarding their content, use or application and disclaims any responsibility for their application or use in any way.
[b] Hesketh et al.[80]
[c] Grunberg et al.[81]
[d] Potential drug interactions between antineoplastic agents/antiemetic agents and various other drugs should always be considered.
[e] Proportion of patients who experience emesis in the absence of effective antiemetic prophylaxis.
[f] The emetic risk is expected to be the same for biosimilars as for the parent compound unless otherwise noted.
[g] For some low emetic risk agents, factors related to dosing schedule (particularly continuous dosing) and clinical experience suggest routine premedication is not required. An individualized approach is appropriate for whether to premedicate each dose or prescribe antiemetics as needed.
[h] Corticosteroid antiemetic premedication should be avoided for 3–5 days prior to and 90 days after CAR T-cell therapies. Antiemetic regimens used during lymphodepleting chemotherapy regimens should also employ corticosteroid-sparing approach to antiemetic prophylaxis.

of emesis include muscarinic (M1, receptor site for acetylcholine), dopamine (D2, receptor site for dopamine), histamine (H1, receptor site for histamine), 5-HT3 (receptor site for serotonin), NK-1 (receptor site for substance P), and GABA (receptor site for benzodiazepines).[19,20] The most effective antiemetics that form the cornerstone of clinical practice guidelines include olanzapine, 5-HT3 receptor antagonist (5HT3 RAs), NK-1 receptor antagonists (NK1 RAs), and corticosteroids.

Serotonin/5-HT3 receptor antagonists

Beginning in the early 1990s, these agents revolutionized the antiemetic prophylaxis of highly emetogenic chemotherapy (HEC) and moderately emetogenic chemotherapy (MEC). Studies of 5HT3 RAs used alone demonstrated superior efficacy compared with high-dose metoclopramide alone[21] and equivalence to the combination of high-dose metoclopramide and dexamethasone, the previous standard of care for these patients.[22] However, the combination of 5HT3 RAs and dexamethasone was the most effective combination tested.[23] The 5HT3 RAs remain the cornerstone of prophylaxis for both HEC and MEC.

Before 2003, there were three "first generation" 5HT3 RAs approved by the US Food and Drug Administration (FDA): ondansetron, granisetron, and dolasetron. Numerous subsequent clinical trials demonstrated the clinical equivalence of these three agents, despite differences seen in preclinical models.[24–29] A single-dose prechemotherapy was shown to be as effective as repeat dosing.[30–32] In addition, there was no significant difference whether the agent was given orally or intravenously.[33,34]

In July 2003, a new 5HT3 RA, palonosetron, was approved by the FDA for antiemetic prophylaxis. Palonosetron may have advantages over the first-generation 5HT3 RAs because of its higher binding affinity to the 5-HT3 receptor and its longer half-life. Two phase 3 randomized clinical trials demonstrated the superiority of palonosetron compared with ondansetron and dolasetron, particularly in preventing delayed nausea and vomiting.[35,36]

Granisetron is also available as a transdermal system for the prevention of CINV. In a phase 3 study, the transdermal granisetron patch was not inferior to repeat doses of oral granisetron.[37]

More recently, granisetron has been formulated as an extended-release subcutaneous injection. The unique polymer drug delivery system uses different ester linkages to control early versus later drug release, resulting in therapeutic drug levels for more than 5 days. A phase III trial compared a single dose of granisetron extended-release subcutaneous injection with a single dose of IV ondansetron, in combination with a steroid and an NK-1 receptor antagonist for the prevention of CINV associated with HEC. All patients also received dexamethasone for 3 days after chemotherapy. The primary endpoint was complete response (CR)—defined as no emesis and no use of rescue medication in

Table 3 Emetogenic potential of oral anticancer agents.[a–d]

Level	Agent			
Moderate to high emetic risk[e,f] (≥30% frequency of emesis)	• Altretamine • Avapritinib • Azacytidine • Binimetinib • Bosutinib >400 mg/day • Busulfan (≥4 mg/day) • Capmatinib • Ceritinib	• Crizotinib • Cyclophosphamide ≥100 mg/m²/day • Dabrafenib • Enasidenib • Encorafenib • Estramustine	• Etoposide • Fedratinib • Imatinib >400 mg/day • Lenvatinib >12 mg/day • Lomustine (single day) • Midostaurin • Mitotane	• Niraparib • Olaparib • Procarbazine • Rucaparib • Selinexor[g] • Temozolomide (>75 mg/m²/day)
Minimal to low emetic risk[e] (<30% frequency of emesis)	• Abemaciclib • Acalabrutinib • Afatinib • Alectinib • Alpelisib • Axitinib • Bexarotene • Brigatinib • Bosutinib ≤400 mg/day • Busulfan (<4 mg/day) • Cabozantinib • Capecitabine • Chlorambucil • Cobimetinib • Cyclophosphamide <100 mg/m²/day • Dacomitinib • Dasatinib • Decitabine and cedazuridine	• Duvelisib • Entrectinib • Erdafitinib • Erlotinib • Everolimus • Fludarabine • Gefitinib • Gilteritinib • Glasdegib • Hydroxyurea • Ibrutinib • Idelalisib • Imatinib ≤400 mg/day • Ixazomib • Ivosidenib • Lapatinib • Larotrectinib • Lenalidomide • Lenvatinib ≤12 mg/day	• Lorlatinib • Melphalan • Mercaptopurine • Methotrexate • Nilotinib • Neratinib • Osimertinib • Palbociclib • Panobinostat • Pazopanib • Pemigatinib • Pexidartinib • Pomalidomide • Ponatinib • Pralsetinib • Regorafenib • Ribociclib • Ripretinib • Ruxolitinib • Selpercatinib	• Sonidegib • Sorafinib • Sunitinib • Talazoparib tosylate • Tazemetostat • Temozolomide ≤75 mg/m²/day[h] • Thalidomide • Thioguanine • Topotecan • Trametinib • Tretinoin • Trifluridine/tipiracil • Tucatinib • Vandetanib • Vemurafenib • Venetoclax • Vismodegib • Vorinostat • Zanubrutinib

[a]Reproduced with permission from the NCCN Guidelines® for **Antiemesis V.1.2021**. © 2020 National Comprehensive Cancer Network, Inc. All rights reserved. The NCCN Guidelines and illustrations herein may not be reproduced in any form for any purpose without the express written permission of the NCCN. NCCN makes no warranties of any kind whatsoever regarding their content, use or application and disclaims any responsibility for their application or use in any way.
[b]Hesketh et al.[80]
[c]Grunberg et al.[81]
[d]Potential drug interactions between antineoplastic agents/antiemetic agents and various other drugs should always be considered.
[e]Proportion of patients who experience emesis in the absence of effective antiemetic prophylaxis.
[f]For some moderate to high emetic risk agents, factors related to dosing schedule (particularly continuous dosing for prolonged periods), and clinical experience suggests routine premedication is not required. An individualized approach is appropriate for whether to premedicate each dose or prescribe antiemetics as needed.
[g]Emerging data and clinical practice suggest adding low-dose olanzapine and/or NK1 RA or 5-HT3 RA for nausea prevention.
[h]Temozolomide ≤75 mg/m²/day should be considered moderately emetogenic with concurrent radiotherapy.

the delayed phase (24–120 h after chemotherapy). Patients in the granisetron extended-release group experienced higher rates of CR (65%) versus 57% of patients receiving ondansetron, $p = 0.014$. This is the first randomized phase III study comparing a single dose of two different 5HT3 RAs (when used in combination with a steroid and NK1 RA) for the treatment of delayed CINV associated with HEC.[38] All of the 5HT3 RAs are well tolerated; the most common adverse effects include headache, constipation, and dizziness.

Dopamine receptor antagonists

Three classes of dopamine receptor antagonists are available for the treatment of CINV: phenothiazines (including promethazine and prochlorperazine), butyrophenones (haloperidol), and benzamides (metoclopramide). In the 1960s, the phenothiazines were the first drugs proven to have efficacy in the treatment of CINV. Prochlorperazine is the most commonly agent used in this class and is used most frequently for the treatment of breakthrough CINV.[39] Extrapyramidal effects, including dystonia, may be seen. These are treated with diphenhydramine and cessation of the drug. The butyrophenones, including haloperidol, may be effective in the treatment of breakthrough nausea and vomiting and have adverse effects similar to those of the phenothiazines.

Of the benzamides, metoclopramide is the best studied and most widely used in CINV. It blocks central and peripheral dopamine (D2) receptors at low doses and exhibits weak 5-HT3 inhibition at high doses. In addition, it speeds gastric emptying and increases sphincter tone at the gastroesophageal junction. Prior to the introduction of the 5HT3 RA, a combination of high-dose intravenous metoclopramide and dexamethasone was the most effective antiemetic prophylaxis for HEC.[40] Because metoclopramide crosses the blood–brain barrier, side effects, including dystonia and tardive dyskinesia, may be seen, particularly at high doses and in aged patients. Diphenhydramine was commonly given as part of the combination regimen to prevent these adverse effects. This regimen has been replaced by a combination containing a 5HT3 RA because of its improved efficacy and safety profile.[21–23]

Corticosteroids

Corticosteroids, most commonly dexamethasone, are effective in preventing nausea and vomiting when used alone or in combination for all emetogenic classes of chemotherapy. For both MEC and HEC, dexamethasone plus a 5HT3 RA ± an NK1 RA or olanzapine is used. A meta-analysis of 32 randomized clinical trials including 5613 patients from 1984 to 1998 demonstrated the efficacy of dexamethasone in both MEC and HEC either alone or in combination

Table 4 Classes and recommended doses of selected antiemetics.

Agent	Class	Route	Dose
Ondansetron	5-HT3 receptor antagonist	IV	8–16 mg
		PO	8–24 mg
Granisetron	5-HT3 receptor antagonist	IV	1 mg or 0.01 mg/kg
		PO	2 mg
			Transdermal patch 3.1 mg/24 h
			Granisetron extended-release subcutaneous injection 10 mg
Dolasetron	5-HT3 receptor antagonist	PO	100 mg
Palonosetron	5-HT3 receptor antagonist	IV	0.25 mg
Aprepitant	NK-1 receptor antagonist	PO	125 mg day 1
			80 mg day 2, 3
Aprepitant emulsion	NK-1 RA	IV	130 mg
Fosaprepitant	NK-1 RA	IV	150 mg
Fosnetupitant/Palonosetron	NK-1 + 5-HT3 RA	IV	230 mg/0.25 mg
Netupitant/Palonosetron	NK-1 + 5-HT3 RA	PO	300 mg/0.5 mg
Rolapitant	NK-1 RA	PO	180 mg
Olanzapine	Atypical antipsychotic	PO	5–10 mg
Dexamethasone	Steroid	IV	8–20 mg
		PO	8–20 mg
Prochlorperazine	Dopamine receptor antagonist	IV	10 mg
		PO	10 mg
		Rectal suppository	25 mg
Metoclopramide	Dopamine receptor antagonist	IV	10–20 mg
		PO	10–20 mg
Haloperidol	Dopamine receptor antagonist	IV	0.5–2 mg
		PO	0.5–2 mg
Dronabinol	Cannabinoid	PO	5–10 mg
Nabilone	Cannabinoid	PO	1–2 mg

Abbreviations: IV, intravenous; 5-HT3, 5-hydroxytryptamine 3; NK, neurokinin; PO, orally.

with other agents.[41] Later studies revealed the superiority of a combination of a 5HT3 RA and dexamethasone compared with either agent alone in HEC.[42] The site of action of corticosteroids along the vomiting reflex pathway is unknown. Side effects may include insomnia, increased energy, hyperglycemia, and mood disturbances. Given these frequent and oftentimes unpleasant side effects, additional research has focused on the efficacy of using lower dexamethasone doses or using different agents for delayed nausea (olanzapine). The Italian Group for Antiemetic Research performed a dose-finding study which looked at four different doses of dexamethasone used on day 1 of HEC. In terms of complete protection from vomiting, 20 mg was superior to 4 and 8 mg, but not better than 12 mg. In terms of complete protection from nausea, 20 mg was not statistically better than 12, 8, or 4 mg. Given these results, many clinicians preferred an individualized approach when it comes to the dose of dexamethasone for the prevention of CINV.[43]

NK-1 receptor antagonists

NK-1 receptors are found in the nucleus tractus solitarius and the area postrema and are activated by substance P.[44] Inhibitors of the NK-1 receptor have demonstrated antiemetic effects and represent a new target for antiemetic therapy. Two randomized phase III trials demonstrated the efficacy of a three-drug combination regimen consisting of aprepitant, a 5HT3 RA, and dexamethasone versus a two-drug regimen of a 5HT3 RA and dexamethasone for the prevention of CINV associated with HEC.[45,46] These data led to the FDA approval of aprepitant in 2003, the first approved medication in this class.

Aprepitant is a substrate for and moderate inducer and moderate inhibitor of the cytochrome P-450 enzyme 3A4 (CYP3A4).[47] Chemotherapy and other drugs are metabolized by this enzyme, and caution must be used when adding aprepitant in these patients. Docetaxel, paclitaxel, etoposide, irinotecan, ifosfamide, imatinib, vinorelbine, vinblastine, and vincristine are metabolized by CYP3A4. Although, in clinical trials, aprepitant was given to patients receiving these agents without any alteration in dose and no observed adverse effect or decreased efficacy, caution is urged. In addition, aprepitant may interact with other, nonchemotherapy agents. It may induce metabolism of warfarin, leading to reduced levels. Aprepitant appears to increase the active levels of oral dexamethasone and methylprednisolone, and reduced dosing of prophylactic dexamethasone is recommended when used in combination with aprepitant. Other drugs with interactions include oral contraceptives, midazolam, ketoconazole, erythromycin, carbamazepine, rifampin, and phenytoin.

Fosaprepitant is a water soluble phosphoryl prodrug for aprepitant. A single dose of fosaprepitant 150 mg has been approved by the FDA as a parenteral alternative on day 1 in place of a 3 day, oral aprepitant regimen.[48]

Aprepitant emulsion was recently FDA approved for the prevention of MEC and HEC when used in combination with a 5HT3 RA and dexamethasone. Aprepitant emulsion is formulated without polysorbate-80 or other synthetic surfactants, resulting in less infusion hypersensitivity and less infusion site pain than fosaprepitant.[49] Aprepitant emulsion 130 mg was found to be bioequivalent to fosaprepitant 150 mg when studied in healthy subjects.[50]

Netupitant is a novel NK1 RA which has a high binding affinity and long half-life (90 h).[51] In a recently reported phase 3 study, 1455 patients receiving MEC (AC or EC) were randomized in a 1:1 ratio to either a single fixed-dose oral combination of netupitant and palonosetron (NEPA) plus standard oral dexamethasone or oral palonosetron plus standard oral dexamethasone.[52] Efficacy endpoints included acute (0–24 h), delayed (25–120 h), and overall (0–120 h) CR; CR was defined as no emesis and no requirement for rescue medication. The results of this study favored the combination of netupitant and palonosetron for all endpoints with a statistically significant 7–14% absolute increase in CR from 67–75% to 74–84% over the planned four cycles of chemotherapy. Rates of adverse events did not differ significantly between the two arms. Recently, a prospective randomized trial comparing oral NEPA to an intravenous formulation of fosnetupitant and palonosetron was published. The overall incidence and intensity of treatment-related adverse events were similar between the two treatment groups in cycle 1 and throughout the study.[53] The fixed combination product of fosnetupitant and palonosetron has been FDA approved for the prevention of CINV associated with HEC. It contains no polysorbate 80 or other surfactants and is associated with a decreased risk of infusion-related hypersensitivity reactions.

Rolapitant is another novel NK1 RA with a high binding affinity and the longest half-life (180 h) of the NK1 RAs. Rolapitant is available as a 90 mg capsule, the dose is 180 mg given orally 1–2 h prior to chemotherapy. In a prospective, randomized, phase III study in patient receiving HEC, patients were randomized to granisetron and dexamethasone, or rolapitant, granisetron, and dexamethasone. The primary endpoint was CR (no emesis, no use of rescue medication) in the delayed phase. Patients in the rolapitant arm had better control 71% (rolapitant) versus 60% (control), $p = 0.0001$.[54] Rolapitant is the only NK1 RA that does not cause an increased serum level of dexamethasone when given concurrently. Rolapitant does however inhibit CYP2D6, P-glycoprotein, and BCRP (breast cancer resistance protein) and so caution is required when rolapitant is used concomitantly with drugs that are substrates of these enzymes, including thioridazine, pimozide, digoxin, irinotecan, topotecan, methotrexate, and rosuvastatin.

Other classes of antiemetics

Additional classes of antiemetic agents that may provide clinical benefit include the benzodiazepines, cannabinoids, and the atypical antipsychotic olanzapine. The most commonly used benzodiazepines, lorazepam, and alprazolam, block GABA receptors, particularly in the cerebral cortex, and have their greatest utility in the treatment of anticipatory nausea, or as an adjunct with other antiemetics to help reduce CINV when anxiety is associated with chemotherapy.

The cannabinoids are likely to become an increasing focus of attention given the legalization of medical marijuana in several parts of the United States. It should be noted that while synthetic cannabinoids have some evidence to support their use for intractable nausea, in general, they should be reserved for refractory cases and further research is required before their use can be recommended on a general basis.[55,56]

Olanzapine, a thiobenzodiazepine atypical antipsychotic that blocks dopamine, serotonin, histamine, and acetylcholine receptors has been found to be effective in preventing acute and delayed emesis. Olanzapine can cause sedation, fatigue, and orthostatic hypotension, and should be used with caution in the elderly. In a prospective, randomized, phase III trial, olanzapine was used as part of a three-drug prophylactic regimen for the prevention of CINV associated with HEC. Olanzapine 10 mg (once daily on days 1–4), palonosetron, and dexamethasone were found to be noninferior to a three-drug regimen containing an NK1 RA, palonosetron, and dexamethasone. While the primary endpoint of CR (no emesis and no use of rescue medicine in the overall period) was similar between both groups in both the acute and delayed phases, the secondary endpoint of no nausea in the delayed phase found better control with the olanzapine regimen (69% vs 38%).[57] More recently, a prospective, randomized, placebo controlled phase III trial comparing a four-drug prophylactic regimen containing olanzapine to placebo to prevent CINV associated with HEC was published. Patients received olanzapine 10 mg (once daily on days 1–4) or placebo, in combination with an NK1 RA, a 5HT3 RA, and dexamethasone. Olanzapine was superior to placebo in all three co-primary endpoints: no nausea in the acute period (74% vs 45%, $p = 0.002$), no nausea in the delayed period (42% vs 25%, $p = 0.002$), and no nausea in the overall period (37% vs 22%, $p = 0.002$). The authors concluded that a four-drug regimen consisting of olanzapine, NK1 RA, 5HT3 RA, and dexamethasone is superior to a three-drug regimen.[58] For patients experiencing excessive fatigue with 10 mg, there is published data to suggest a 5 mg prophylactic dose is also effective for the prevention of CINV but with less sedation.[59] It is included in the NCCN guidelines to treat both HEC and MEC, as well as for the treatment of breakthrough CINV if it was not part of the prophylactic regimen given prior to chemotherapy.[14,60]

Complementary and alternative medicine (CAM) therapies

The past decade has witnessed a great interest in CAM therapies, particularly among cancer patients. Various CAM therapies such as acupuncture, hypnosis, massage, music, and herbal supplements such as ginger have been tried to control nausea. Of these, acupuncture and certain mind–body therapies appear promising, but further research is needed before they can be recommended in routine clinical practice.

Acupuncture has been traditionally used in China for symptom management of various conditions, including nausea. A recent meta-analysis involving 11 randomized trials ($N = 1247$), evaluated the effect of acupuncture in controlling CINV among patients receiving MEC and HEC.[61] The study found that patients receiving acupuncture had lower acute vomiting than the control group (22% vs 31%, $p = 0.04$). There was no benefit for delayed CINV. It should be noted that all these studies were done before the era of NK1 RAs and olanzapine, and thus utility of acupuncture in the current era is not well established.

Mind–body therapies such as hypnosis, guided imagery, and progressive muscle relaxation therapy (PMRT) have been reported to significantly reduce CINV.[62–65] In a randomized clinical trial in Hong Kong, 71 breast cancer patients receiving antiemetic therapy with metoclopramide and dexamethasone were randomized to progressive muscle relaxation training and imagery (1 h before chemotherapy and then daily for 5 days), versus no intervention. Patients in the intervention arm had decreased duration of CINV ($p = 0.05$) and lower frequency of CINV ($p = 0.07$) as compared to controls. However, the study participants did not receive standard prophylaxis with either 5HT3 RAs or NK1 RAs, limiting the clinical applicability of the study.

Other relaxation therapies such as music and massage have also been reported to be successful as adjunct antiemetic therapies, in small clinical trials involving about 30 patients.[66,67] These relaxation therapies affect the cerebral cortex, and thus are particularly helpful for decreasing the perception of nausea and in anticipatory nausea.

On the other hand, two trials evaluating efficacy of ginger for treatment of CINV were negative.[68,69] A number of clinical trials assessing various CAM therapies are currently underway and would provide further useful information regarding efficacy of these therapies (or lack thereof), facilitating optimal inclusion of these therapies in traditional clinical oncology practice (integrative oncology).

Table 5 Guidelines for prevention of acute and delayed nausea and vomiting in patients depending on emetic risk.

Emetic risk	Acute	Delayed
High (>90%)	Olanzapine + NK-1 receptor antagonist + 5-HT3 receptor antagonist + dexamethasone	Olanzapine + dexamethasone
Moderate (30–90%)	5-HT3 receptor antagonist + dexamethasone, ±NK-1 receptor antagonist	Dexamethasone
Low (10–30%)	Dexamethasone or phenothiazine or metoclopramide or 5-HT3 receptor antagonist	None
Minimal (<10%)	None	None

Abbreviation: 5-HT3, 5-hydroxytryptamine 3.

Recommendations for prevention and treatment of chemotherapy-induced emesis

The goal of antiemetic therapy is complete prevention of CINV. In patients receiving MEC and HEC, the period of risk for nausea and vomiting following chemotherapy lasts at least 3 days for MEC and 4 days for HEC. Protection with scheduled antiemetics is needed throughout this period (Table 5). Although the choice of antiemetic prophylaxis is largely driven by the emetogenic potential of the specific chemotherapy agents as outlined below, additional patient-related risk factors may warrant escalation to a higher level of prophylaxis.[14]

Highly emetogenic chemotherapy

Cisplatin and anthracycline/cyclophosphamide combinations are the agents most frequently associated with HEC. Nausea and vomiting are virtually ensured without adequate prophylaxis. Current supportive care guidelines suggest the combination of olanzapine, an NK1 RA, a 5HT3 RA, and dexamethasone given prior to chemotherapy on day 1, followed by olanzapine and dexamethasone given once daily on days 2, 3, and 4. Variations of this backbone, such as continuing only one drug (olanzapine) on days 2, 3, and 4, or using different dosages of olanzapine and dexamethasone, are reasonable as clinically indicated.[14,17]

Moderately emetogenic chemotherapy

A combination of a 5HT3 RA and dexamethasone is recommended in all patients receiving MEC. For select patients with additional risk factors, or who have failed previous therapy with a 5HT3 RA and dexamethasone alone, an NK1 RA or olanzapine should be added on day 1. Given recent data, their extended half-lives and their efficacy in preventing delayed symptoms, palonosetron (0.25 mg on day 1 only), or granisetron extended-release subcutaneous injection (10 mg on day 1 only) may be the preferred 5HT3 RAs especially when not combined with a NK1 RA. Dexamethasone may be given as 12 mg IV or PO on day 1 and then at a daily dose of 8 mg on days 2–3 (either 8 mg daily or 4 mg in divided doses twice daily).

Low-risk chemotherapy

Options for antiemetic prophylaxis in patients receiving chemotherapy of low emetogenic potential include a single dose of a first-generation 5HT3 RA (ondansetron, granisetron, dolasetron), or dexamethasone (8–12 mg PO or IV), prochlorperazine (10 mg PO or IV), or metoclopramide (10–20 mg PO or IV). All prophylaxis should be given prior to the administration of chemotherapy. No scheduled antiemetics are required in the delayed setting but a rescue agent from a different pharmacologic class should be provided.

Minimally emetogenic chemotherapy

No routine prophylaxis is recommended. If CINV does occur, the use of a 5HT3 RA, dexamethasone, prochlorperazine, or metoclopramide is recommended as prophylaxis prior to the next cycle of therapy.

Special situations

Breakthrough nausea and vomiting

Ideally, the best strategy for breakthrough CINV is to prevent it from occurring in the first place by employing an appropriate, aggressive prophylactic regimen. Despite adequate prophylaxis, breakthrough symptoms still occur. The best therapy for breakthrough symptoms is the addition of agents from another class of antiemetics. If not used as part of the prophylactic regimen, olanzapine is the preferred agent for the use of breakthrough CINV, as it was found to be superior to metoclopramide in this setting.[60] In addition, an alternative route other than oral, such as intravenous, transdermal, or rectal, may need to be used. These medications work best if taken on a schedule rather than on an as-needed basis. When breakthrough CINV occurs, the prophylactic antiemetic regimen should be reevaluated and enhanced prior to the next cycle of therapy.

Anticipatory nausea and vomiting

The key to preventing anticipatory nausea and vomiting is preventing symptoms from occurring with each cycle of chemotherapy. Once the symptoms have developed, agents such as the benzodiazepines may be added to the prophylactic regimen.[14] As outlined above, mind–body therapies such as behavioral therapy, systemic desensitization, and hypnosis have also been proven useful.[62–65]

Multiple day chemotherapy-induced nausea and vomiting

Patients receiving multiple-day chemotherapeutic regimens to treat a variety of malignancies (e.g., germ cell tumors, lymphoma, multiple myeloma with stem cell transplantation, etc.) are at risk for both acute and delayed nausea and vomiting. Although the NCCN has a section in their guidelines entitled "Principles of managing multiday emetogenic chemotherapy regimens," they state that the antiemetic therapy each day should be selected based on the chemotherapy drug with the highest emetic risk.[14] The risk of delayed nausea and vomiting will depend on the specific chemotherapeutic regimen used and the emetogenic potential of the last chemotherapeutic drug used in the regimen.

Studies have evaluated the use of repeat dosing of palonosetron in managing multiple-day emetogenic chemotherapy regimens, however, no definitive conclusions can be made and further studies are needed to answer whether a need exists for repeat dosing of palonosetron.[70,71]

With regard to aprepitant, it has been evaluated in the antiemetic management of multiple drug chemotherapeutic regimens.[72–74] While it may be used in such situations, it is difficult to recommend a specific antiemetic regimen for each day that a multiple drug emetogenic chemotherapeutic regimen is utilized.

The NCCN in their Antiemesis Guidelines outline the general principles for using corticosteroids (dexamethasone), 5HT3 RAs, and NK1 RAs in managing multiday chemotherapy regimens.[14]

Radiation-induced nausea and vomiting

Radiation-induced nausea and vomiting (RINV) is seen in nearly all patients receiving total body irradiation prior to bone marrow transplantation and in more than 80% of those receiving radiation to the upper abdomen.[75] Studies have demonstrated the efficacy of prophylactic 5HT3 RAs compared with placebo[76] or with combinations of metoclopramide and prochlorperazine.[77,78] The recommendation is for all patients undergoing either upper abdominal radiation therapy or total body irradiation to receive prophylaxis with an oral 5HT3 RA dosed either two or three times daily with or without oral dexamethasone.[14]

Conclusions

Prevention and treatment of CINV have advanced significantly in recent years. Recent surveys indicate the need for heightened awareness of the frequency and severity of acute and especially delayed CINV. Fortunately, new agents have been added to the antiemetic arsenal to further enhance the efficacy of antiemetic prophylaxis. Complementary therapies appear promising in controlling nausea, and are being explored further. Appropriate implementation of guidelines for prophylaxis based on patient-related risk factors and the specific chemotherapy agents used will ensure that fewer patients experience these most distressing of side effects.

Key references

The complete reference list can be found on Vital Source version of this title, see inside front cover.

1. Grunberg SM, Deuson RR, Mavros P, et al. Incidence of chemotherapy-induced nausea and emesis after modern antiemetics. *Cancer.* 2004;**100**(10):2261–2268.
7. HOPA CINV Tool Kit - Eisai Inc and Helsinn Therapeutics (U.S.) IHOPA (2017) *Time to Talk CINV [PDF File].* http://www.hoparx.org/images/hopa/resource-library/patient-education/Survey_Infographic.pdf
13. Roila F, Herrstedt J, Aapro M, et al. Guideline update for MASCC and ESMO in the prevention of chemotherapy- and radiotherapy-induced nausea and vomiting: results of the Perugia consensus conference. *Ann Oncol.* 2010;**21**(Suppl 5):v232–v243.
14. National Comprehensive Cancer Network (2020) *Antiemesis Version 1.2020*, www.nccn.org
17. Hesketh PJ, Kris MG, Basch E, et al. Antiemetics: American Society of Clinical Oncology Clinical Practice Guideline update. *J Clin Oncol.* 2017;**35**(28):3240–3261.
18. Roila F, Molassiotis A, Herrstedt J, et al. 2016 MASCC and ESMO guideline update for the prevention of chemotherapy- and radiotherapy-induced nausea and vomiting and of nausea and vomiting in advanced cancer patients. *Ann Oncol.* 2016;**27**(suppl 5):v119–v133.
34. Gralla RJ, Navari RM, Hesketh PJ, et al. Single-dose oral granisetron has equivalent antiemetic efficacy to intravenous ondansetron for highly emetogenic cisplatin-based chemotherapy. *J Clin Oncol.* 1998;**16**(4):1568–1573.
35. Eisenberg P, Figueroa-Vadillo J, Zamora R, et al. Improved prevention of moderately emetogenic chemotherapy-induced nausea and vomiting with palonosetron, a pharmacologically novel 5-HT3 receptor antagonist: results of a phase III, single-dose trial versus dolasetron. *Cancer.* 2003;**98**(11):2473–2482.
36. Gralla R, Lichinitser M, Van Der Vegt S, et al. Palonosetron improves prevention of chemotherapy-induced nausea and vomiting following moderately emetogenic chemotherapy: results of a double-blind randomized phase III trial comparing single doses of palonosetron with ondansetron. *Ann Oncol.* 2003;**14**(10):1570–1577.
37. Grunberg, S.M., Gabrial, N.Y. and Clark, G. (eds) (2007) *Phase III Trial of Transdermal Granisetron Patch (Sancuso) Compared with Oral Granisetron in the Management of Chemotherapy-Induced Nausea and Vomiting (CINV).* Multinational Association of Supportive Care in Cancer (MASCC), June 27–30, 2007, St. Gallen, Switzerland.
38. Schnadig ID, Agajanian R, Dakhil C, et al. APF530 (granisetron injection extended-release) in a three-drug regimen for delayed CINV in highly emetogenic chemotherapy. *Future Oncol.* 2016;**12**(12):1469–1481.
43. Italian Group for Antiemetic Research. Double-blind, dose-finding study of four intravenous doses of dexamethasone in the prevention of cisplatin-induced acute emesis. *J Clin Oncol.* 1998;**16**(9):2937–2942.
45. Poli-Bigelli S, Rodrigues-Pereira J, Carides AD, et al. Addition of the neurokinin 1 receptor antagonist aprepitant to standard antiemetic therapy improves control of chemotherapy-induced nausea and vomiting. Results from a randomized, double-blind, placebo-controlled trial in Latin America. *Cancer.* 2003;**97**(12):3090–3098.
46. Hesketh PJ, Grunberg SM, Gralla RJ, et al. The oral neurokinin-1 antagonist aprepitant for the prevention of chemotherapy-induced nausea and vomiting: a multinational, randomized, double-blind, placebo-controlled trial in patients receiving high-dose cisplatin—the Aprepitant Protocol 052 Study Group. *J Clin Oncol.* 2003;**21**(22):4112–4119.
47. Shadle CR, Lee Y, Majumdar AK, et al. Evaluation of potential inductive effects of aprepitant on cytochrome P450 3A4 and 2C9 activity. *J Clin Pharmacol.* 2004;**44**(3):215–223.
48. Lasseter KC, Gambale J, Jin B, et al. Tolerability of fosaprepitant and bioequivalency to aprepitant in healthy subjects. *J Clin Pharmacol.* 2007;**47**(7):834–840.
49. Ottoboni T, Lauw M, Keller MR, et al. Safety of HTX-019 (intravenous aprepitant) and fosaprepitant in healthy subjects. *Future Oncol.* 2018;**14**(27):2849–2859.
50. Ottoboni T, Keller MR, Cravets M, et al. Bioequivalence of HTX-019 (aprepitant IV) and fosaprepitant in healthy subjects: a Phase I, open-label, randomized, two-way crossover evaluation. *Drug Des Devel Ther.* 2018;**12**:429–435.
51. Spinelli T, Calcagnile S, Giuliano C, et al. Netupitant PET imaging and ADME studies in humans. *J Clin Pharmacol.* 2014;**54**(1):97–108.
52. Aapro M, Rugo H, Rossi G, et al. A randomized phase III study evaluating the efficacy and safety of NEPA, a fixed-dose combination of netupitant and palonosetron, for prevention of chemotherapy-induced nausea and vomiting following moderately emetogenic chemotherapy. *Ann Oncol.* 2014;**25**(7):1328–1333.
53. Schwartzberg L, Roeland E, Andric Z, et al. Phase III safety study of intravenous NEPA: a novel fixed antiemetic combination of fosnetupitant and palonosetron in patients receiving highly emetogenic chemotherapy. *Ann Oncol.* 2018;**29**(7):1535–1540.
54. Rapoport BL, Chasen MR, Gridelli C, et al. Safety and efficacy of rolapitant for prevention of chemotherapy-induced nausea and vomiting after administration of cisplatin-based highly emetogenic chemotherapy in patients with cancer: two randomised, active-controlled, double-blind, phase 3 trials. *Lancet Oncol.* 2015;**16**(9):1079–1089.
55. Hill KP. Medical marijuana: more questions than answers. *J Psychiatr Pract.* 2014;**20**(5):389–391.
56. Sharkey KA, Darmani NA, Parker LA. Regulation of nausea and vomiting by cannabinoids and the endocannabinoid system. *Eur J Pharmacol.* 2014;**722**:134–146.
57. Navari RM, Gray SE, Kerr AC. Olanzapine versus aprepitant for the prevention of chemotherapy-induced nausea and vomiting: a randomized phase III trial. *J Support Oncol.* 2011;**9**(5):188–195.
58. Navari RM, Qin R, Ruddy KJ, et al. Olanzapine for the prevention of chemotherapy-induced nausea and vomiting. *N Engl J Med.* 2016;**375**(2):134–142.
59. Hashimoto H, Abe M, Tokuyama O, et al. Olanzapine 5 mg plus standard antiemetic therapy for the prevention of chemotherapy-induced nausea and vomiting (J-FORCE): a multicentre, randomised, double-blind, placebo-controlled, phase 3 trial. *Lancet Oncol.* 2020;**21**(2):242–249.
60. Navari RM, Nagy CK, Gray SE. The use of olanzapine versus metoclopramide for the treatment of breakthrough chemotherapy-induced nausea and vomiting in patients receiving highly emetogenic chemotherapy. *Support Care Cancer.* 2013;**21**(6):1655–1663.
61. Ezzo J, Vickers A, Richardson MA, et al. Acupuncture-point stimulation for chemotherapy-induced nausea and vomiting. *J Clin Oncol.* 2005;**23**(28):7188–7198.
62. Bardia A, Barton DL, Sood A, Loprinzi CL. Integrative medicine in symptom management and palliative care. In: Abrams D, Weil A, eds. *Integrative Medicine.* New York: Oxford University Press; 2008.
64. Yoo HJ, Ahn SH, Kim SB, et al. Efficacy of progressive muscle relaxation training and guided imagery in reducing chemotherapy side effects in patients

65. Molassiotis A, Yung HP, Yam BM, et al. The effectiveness of progressive muscle relaxation training in managing chemotherapy-induced nausea and vomiting in Chinese breast cancer patients: a randomised controlled trial. *Support Care Cancer*. 2002;**10**(3):237–246.
66. Ezzone S, Baker C, Rosselet R, Terepka E. Music as an adjunct to antiemetic therapy. *Oncol Nurs Forum*. 1998;**25**(9):1551–1556.
67. Grealish L, Lomasney A, Whiteman B. Foot massage - a nursing intervention to modify the distressing symptoms of pain and nausea in patients hospitalized with cancer. *Cancer Nurs*. 2000;**23**(3):237–243.
68. Manusirivithaya S, Sripramote M, Tangjitgamol S, et al. Antiemetic effect of ginger in gynecologic oncology patients receiving cisplatin. *Int J Gynecol Cancer*. 2004;**14**(6):1063–1069.
69. Zick SM, Ruffin MT, Lee J, et al. Phase II trial of encapsulated ginger as a treatment for chemotherapy-induced nausea and vomiting. *Support Care Cancer*. 2009;**17**(5):563–572.
70. Einhorn LH, Brames MJ, Dreicer R, et al. Palonosetron plus dexamethasone for prevention of chemotherapy-induced nausea and vomiting in patients receiving multiple-day cisplatin chemotherapy for germ cell cancer. *Support Care Cancer*. 2007;**15**(11):1293–1300.
71. Giralt SA, Mangan KF, Maziarz RT, et al. Three palonosetron regimens to prevent CINV in myeloma patients receiving multiple-day high-dose melphalan and hematopoietic stem cell transplantation. *Ann Oncol*. 2011;**22**(4):939–946.
72. Jordan K, Kinitz I, Voigt W, et al. Safety and efficacy of a triple antiemetic combination with the NK-1 antagonist aprepitant in highly and moderately emetogenic multiple-day chemotherapy. *Eur J Cancer*. 2009;**45**(7):1184–1187.
73. Olver IN, Grimison P, Chatfield M, et al. Results of a 7-day aprepitant schedule for the prevention of nausea and vomiting in 5-day cisplatin-based germ cell tumor chemotherapy. *Support Care Cancer*. 2013;**21**(6):1561–1568.
74. Albany C, Brames MJ, Fausel C, et al. Randomized, double-blind, placebo-controlled, phase III cross-over study evaluating the oral neurokinin-1 antagonist aprepitant in combination with a 5HT3 receptor antagonist and dexamethasone in patients with germ cell tumors receiving 5-day cisplatin combination chemotherapy regimens: a hoosier oncology group study. *J Clin Oncol*. 2012;**30**(32):3998–4003.

124 Neurologic complications of cancer

Luis Nicolas Gonzalez Castro, MD, PhD ■ Tracy T. Batchelor, MD ■ Lisa M. DeAngelis, MD

> **Overview**
>
> Neurologic complications of cancer and its therapy are common and being seeing with increasing frequency as many patients survive longer with better systemic disease control. Cancer-related complications can be metastatic or nonmetastatic. Metastases in the nervous system can involve multiple anatomical sites (brain, meninges, spinal cord, nerve roots, and nerves), leading to a variety of clinical presentations, including focal weakness, sensory changes, and seizures. Nonmetastatic complications include metabolic derailments, hypercoagulability, and paraneoplastic syndromes, as well as complications due to cancer therapy, such as chemotherapy-induced neuropathy, radiation toxicity, and immunotherapy-related neurologic syndromes.

Introduction

Disorders of the central or peripheral nervous system affect approximately 15% of patients with cancer.[1] The disorders usually appear in patients with advanced metastatic disease, but sometimes the neurologic disorder is the first symptom of cancer. Regardless of whether neurologic complications occur early or late in the course of the patient's cancer, they uniquely threaten the patient's survival and quality of life by causing distressing symptoms such as cognitive decline, weakness, incontinence, and pain.

Neurologic complications of cancer are increasing in frequency. Metastases to the nervous system develop more frequently because systemic tumors are better controlled for longer periods.[1,2] Part of the increase also results from more vigorous treatment of the primary tumor with modalities that cause toxicity to the nervous system. Because these toxic effects are often delayed (e.g., radiation-induced dementia), the longer the patient lives, the more likely toxicity is to appear. Early diagnosis and appropriate treatment of the neurologic symptoms can significantly lessen their impact.

Neurologic complications of cancer can be either metastatic or nonmetastatic (Table 1). Metastatic lesions affect the nervous system by direct invasion (e.g., brachial plexus metastasis), compression (e.g., epidural spinal cord compression [SCC]), or compromise of vascular supply (e.g., sagittal sinus occlusion from skull metastases). Brain metastases are discussed in "Brain Metastases". Although any tumor can metastasize to the nervous system, certain tumors have a predilection for causing particular central or peripheral nervous system disorders. Leukemias frequently metastasize to the leptomeninges, but rarely to the brain. Prostate cancer commonly causes epidural SCC because of its tendency to metastasize to the vertebral bodies, but leptomeningeal or brain involvement is much less common.[1,2]

Nonmetastatic neurologic complications are often tumor specific. Metabolic derangements are more likely to occur with tumors that metastasize widely to vital organs, such as liver (colon cancer), or that cause changes in fluid and electrolyte balance, such as hypercalcemia (breast cancer) or inappropriate antidiuretic hormone secretion (small-cell lung cancer). Central nervous system (CNS) infections are more common in patients whose cancer is associated with immune suppression, as in Hodgkin disease. Vascular complications are more common in hematologic malignancies than in solid tumors. Paraneoplastic syndromes affecting the nervous system are much more frequent with certain tumors, such as small-cell lung and ovarian cancers.[3] Clinically, identifying the site of neurologic dysfunction by the patient's symptoms and signs will help to determine the diagnosis (Table 2).

Metastases

Spinal metastases

Metastatic lesions compressing the spinal cord or cauda equina are, after brain metastases, the most common symptomatic neurologic complication of metastatic cancer.[1,2,4] The spinal cord ends at the L-1 or L-2 vertebral body but compression of the cauda equina below that level is usually also considered SCC because the diagnosis and treatment are identical.[1] SCC causes pain and, if untreated, paralysis and incontinence. Patients who become paraplegic as a result of cancer usually die within a matter of months; however, studies indicate that early diagnosis and treatment maintain a patient's independent ambulation, and usually result in longer survival.

Approximately 5% of patients dying of cancer have evidence of SCC at autopsy, suggesting 18,000–20,000 new cases of SCC annually in the United States.[1,5] Breast, lung, prostate, and lymphoma are the most common primary cancers causing SCC (Table 3). SCC usually occurs in the late stages of metastatic cancer, but in up to 20% of patients, cancer was unsuspected prior to the neurologic symptoms.

Vertebral metastases are common in patients with metastatic cancer, but skeletal complications, including SCC, have been reduced by the use of bisphosphonates.[6] SCC usually results when a vertebral body metastasis extends into the spinal canal or paraspinal tumor invades the epidural space through a neural foramen (Figure 1). Lymphomas may invade the spinal canal through neural foramina without destruction of bone. Epidural lesions may also result when tumors in the colon, kidney, prostate, or head and neck area grow directly into the spinal bony structures.

The thoracic spine is the most common location of SCC, followed by the lumbosacral and cervical spine in a ratio of about 4:2:1. Two or more contiguous vertebral bodies are involved by metastatic disease in approximately 25% of patients with SCC, but,

---

Holland-Frei Cancer Medicine, Tenth Edition. Edited by Robert C. Bast, John C. Byrd, Carlo M. Croce, Ernest Hawk, Fadlo R. Khuri, Raphael E. Pollock, Apostolia M. Tsimberidou, Christopher G. Willett, and Cheryl L. Willman.
© 2023 John Wiley & Sons, Inc. Published 2023 by John Wiley & Sons, Inc.

Table 1 Neurologic complications of cancer

Metastatic
Intracranial (usually to brain; see **Chapter 73**)
Spinal (usually epidural)
Leptomeningeal (usually base of brain and cauda equina)
Cranial nerves (usually from base of skull lesions)
Peripheral nerves and plexus (usually brachial or lumbosacral plexus)
Muscle (rare)
Nonmetastatic
Complications of treatment (radiation, chemotherapy)
Vascular disorders (hemorrhage, infarcts)
Metabolic, nutritional disorders
Paraneoplastic syndromes
Infections

Table 3 Primary cancer-causing symptomatic spinal cord compression in 583 patients at Memorial Sloan-Kettering Cancer Center (MSKCC).

Primary tumor	Number of patients (%)
Breast	127 (22)
Lung	90 (15)
Prostate	58 (10)
Lymphoreticular	56 (10)
Sarcoma	52 (9)
Kidney	39 (7)
Gastrointestinal	29 (5)
Melanoma	23 (4)
Unknown primary	21 (4)
Head and neck	19 (3)
Miscellaneous	69 (12)
Total	583

unlike infection, the intervertebral disc is preserved. As many as 32% of patients have other sites of SCC in addition to the clinically suspected location, emphasizing the importance of imaging the entire length of the spinal canal when evaluating a patient for suspected epidural disease.

Pathophysiology of spinal cord compression

Epidural tumor is found both anterior and posterior to the spinal cord in almost 50% of patients; in approximately 20%, the tumor is circumferential. Histologic studies commonly show demyelination with infiltration by lipid-laden macrophages, interstitial edema, and focal axonal swelling, but infarction is rare, even in patients who develop the sudden onset of paraplegia. Compression of the epidural venous plexus (possibly contributing to spinal cord edema) occurs early in SCC, whereas decreased spinal cord blood flow takes place much later; therefore, venous infarction may contribute to the acute paraplegia which can happen unpredictably, making SCC a neurologic emergency. The release of potentially neurotoxic substances, including prostaglandins and serotonin, by compressed neural tissue, may also play a role in neurologic disability.

Clinical findings and diagnosis

The symptoms and signs depend on the level of compression (e.g., cervical versus thoracic). Back pain is the first symptom of SCC in nearly all patients (Table 4).[5] The pain may be local (at the involved area of the spine), radicular (radiating into arm, trunk, or leg), or both. Local pain is dull, aching, progressive, and usually localizes to the involved area of the spine. Local pain aggravated by movement implies spinal instability. In the cervical and lumbosacral regions, radicular pain is often unilateral, but in the trunk, it is usually bilateral (band-like), a finding highly suggestive of epidural disease. Pain from SCC is typically worse when the patient is supine which helps to distinguish SCC from a herniated disc where the pain improves with recumbency. The pain of SCC is exacerbated by coughing, straining, or Valsalva. Pain may be absent in patients whose SCC is identified incidentally

Table 2 Neurologic complications in cancer patients by site.

Site	Usual causes	Typical symptoms and signs
Brain	Metastasis Leptomeningeal metastasis Metabolic/toxic encephalopathy Infection (meningitis, brain abscess) Radiation encephalopathy Cerebral hemorrhage or infarction Paraneoplastic (limbic encephalopathy)	Headache Confusion Hemiparesis Seizures Ataxia
Spinal cord and cauda equina	Epidural metastasis Leptomeningeal metastasis Intramedullary metastasis Epidural abscess or hematoma Radiation myelopathy Myelopathy following intrathecal chemotherapy Paraneoplastic myelopathy	Back pain Paraparesis Sensory level Incontinence
Cranial and peripheral nerves	Extrinsic compression by tumor or other mass (e.g., hematoma) Direct infiltration by tumor Drug toxicity Varicella-zoster infection Radiation plexopathy Paraneoplastic neuropathy Drugs (aminoglycoside antibiotics)	Focal pain, Sensory loss Motor weakness Decreased reflexes in nerve distribution (focal lesion) or distally in hands and feet (polyneuropathy) Weakness without sensory loss
Neuromuscular junction	Paraneoplastic disorders (Lambert–Eaton myasthenic syndrome, myasthenia gravis)	Respiratory insufficiency
Muscle	Metastasis Steroid myopathy Cachectic myopathy Paraneoplastic polymyositis or dermatomyositis	Proximal weakness Weakness without sensory loss

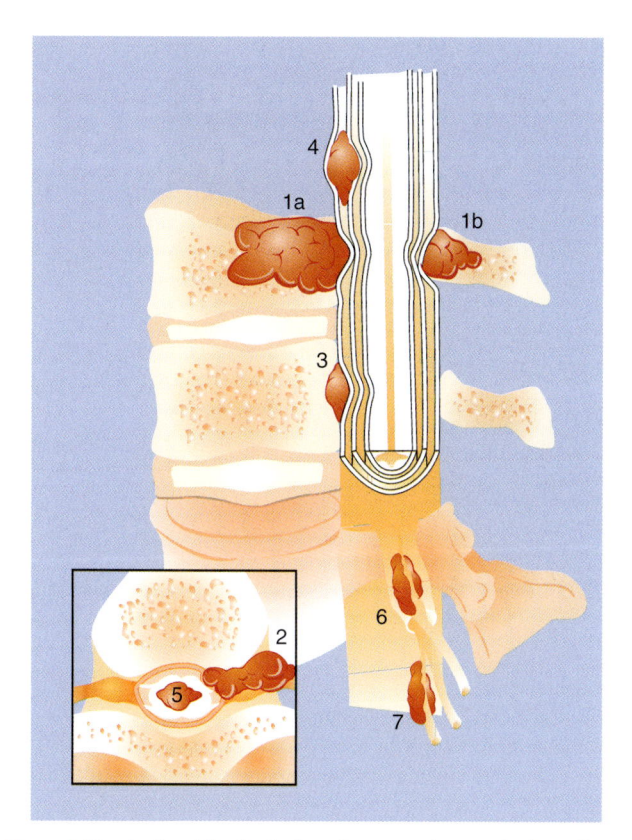

Figure 1 Neoplastic epidural spinal cord compression results from direct extension of a bony metastasis to the vertebral body (1a) or posterior elements (1b), by paraspinal neoplasm infiltrating through neural foramina (2), or a direct metastasis to the epidural space (3). Unusual causes of spinal metastases include subdural metastasis (4), intramedullary metastasis (5), and paraspinal metastasis to the radicular vessels (6) or root (7).

Table 4 Symptoms and signs of spinal cord compression in 213 patients at Memorial Sloan-Kettering Cancer Center (MSKCC).[a]

	First symptom		Present at diagnosis	
	No.	%	No.	%
Pain	201	94	207	97
Weakness	7	3	157	74
Autonomic dysfunction	0	0	111	52
Sensory loss	1	0.5	112	53
Ataxia	2	0.9	8	4

[a]Source: Based on Cole and Patchell.[5]

Table 5 Differential diagnosis of epidural spinal cord compression.[a]

Diagnosis	Example(s)	Diagnostic test
Intramedullary tumor	Glioma Metastasis	MRI with gadolinium
Extramedullary-intradural tumor	Meningioma Neurofibroma	MRI with gadolinium
Leptomeningeal tumor	Metastasis Primary lymphoma	MRI with gadolinium, CSF cytology
Radiation myelopathy	Previous RT to spine	MRI with gadolinium
Arteriovenous malformation	Post-RT cavernous angioma	MRI with gadolinium, myelogram, arteriogram
Transverse myelopathy	Postinfectious myelopathy, multiple sclerosis	MRI with gadolinium
Epidural hematoma	Thrombocytopenia (history of lumbar puncture)	MRI or CT
Epidural abscess	Sepsis, epidural catheter	MRI with gadolinium/culture
Degenerative spinal disorder	Herniated disc, spinal stenosis	MRI
Osteoporosis	Vertebral collapse	MRI/biopsy

Abbreviations: CSF, cerebrospinal fluid; CT, computed tomography; MRI, magnetic resonance imaging; RT, radiation therapy.
[a]Source: Adapted from DeAngelis and Posner.[1]

on chest or abdominal CT or MRI done to evaluate the patient's primary cancer.

Weakness is the second most common feature of epidural SCC; it usually follows the onset of pain by weeks to months and is most obvious in proximal muscles of the legs. By the time weakness occurs, tone in the lower extremities is usually increased, reflexes are hyperactive, and the plantar responses are extensor. If the SCC occurs below the cord involving the cauda equina, hyporeflexia or areflexia is found. If pain limits strength testing, analgesics should be administered to permit adequate evaluation.

Bowel and bladder dysfunction usually occurs late in SCC. However, when the conus medullaris is the site of compression (vertebral lesions from T-10 to L-1), bladder dysfunction may be the first and only sign. The patient may be unaware of urinary retention because bladder sensation is lost; examination reveals a distended bladder, and a postvoid ultrasound reveals urinary retention. The anal sphincter is usually flaccid. Sensory symptoms include numbness and paresthesias that begin in the toes and spread proximally. Except in conus medullaris compression, the sacral segments may be spared, even when a sensory level is found on the trunk. In a few patients, gait or truncal ataxia may be the only neurologic finding although back pain usually precedes the ataxia. Varicella-zoster eruption may occur at the dermatomal level of epidural metastasis and can delay the recognition of SCC.

None of the clinical symptoms or signs of epidural SCC are specific (Table 5). Some disorders that mimic SCC such as herniated disc or spinal stenosis, are common and may confuse the initial evaluation of an individual cancer patient. Others, such as epidural hematomas and abscesses, may be directly related to the cancer or its treatment.

Patients with cancer who develop back pain are presumed to have SCC until proved otherwise. Evaluation should proceed urgently because high-grade compression may cause abrupt compromise of the spinal cord and severe neurologic dysfunction. The only necessary diagnostic test for spinal lesions caused by cancer is an MRI (Figure 2). The entire spinal axis should be imaged. Although contrast is not necessary to detect spine metastasis or epidural tumor, contrast is essential to identify intramedullary or leptomeningeal metastasis (LM). Patients unable to have an MRI (e.g., pacemaker) should be imaged by CT-myelography.

Treatment

SCC requires urgent therapy directed at reduction of tumor mass and prevention of regrowth.[1,4] Radiation therapy (RT) is the primary treatment for most patients, but surgery and chemotherapy are important modalities in individual patients. The initial treatment for all patients is corticosteroids which can have an oncolytic effect, relieving SCC by shrinking tumors, especially lymphoma, but in most instances, their salutary effects result from the reduction of spinal cord edema.

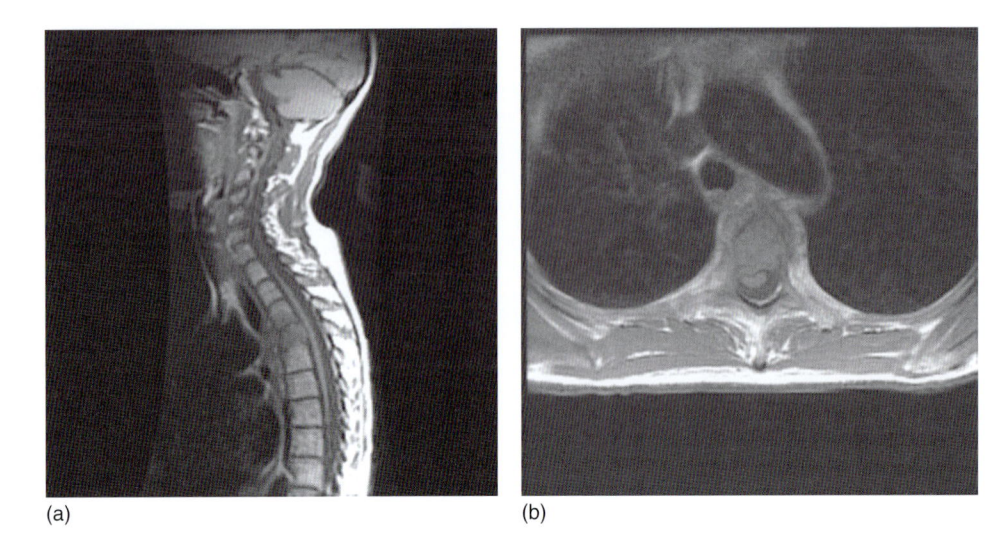

Figure 2 MRI demonstrating spinal cord compression from metastatic breast cancer. (a) Tumor in the vertebral body compressing the spinal cord arteriorly. (b) Axial image at the same level demonstrating anterior and lateral compression and distortion of the cord.

For patients with pain only, dexamethasone at 4 mg every 6 h can be started increasing the dose if pain persists or new symptoms develop.[7,8] For patients with severe pain, or evidence of myelopathy, an intravenous bolus of 100 mg of dexamethasone should be administered, followed by 100 mg every 24 h in divided doses. The drug should be tapered as the patient is treated with more definitive modalities. Corticosteroids may cause adverse effects, and some may be more prominent in patients with epidural SCC. Perforation of the gastrointestinal (GI) tract may occur in as many as 1% of patients; constipation, a frequent complication of SCC, appears to increase the risk of GI rupture. Thus, a rapid taper, particularly of high initial doses, is essential.

RT is the most common treatment for patients with SCC, many of whom are poor surgical candidates because of advanced cancer or multiple vertebral body metastases.[1,5] RT to a total dose of 3000 cGy (300 cGy × 10 fractions) is administered to the site of compression and one or two vertebral bodies above and below that level. Multiple courses of RT for patients who respond initially but then relapse may be helpful and carries only modest risk.[9] Intensity-modulated stereotactic radiotherapy (IMRT) is effective and safe and can be administered with good results to a previously irradiated site or in place of standard external beam RT.[10-12]

Surgery plays an increasingly important role in SCC treatment. Traditionally, surgery was restricted to: (1) patients who developed SCC at sites already irradiated, (2) patients in whom a diagnosis of cancer had not been established, (3) when epidural defects result from displaced bone or disc fragments, (4) when spinal instability results from bone destruction, and (5) patients with radio-resistant tumors (e.g., renal cancer). However, a randomized phase III trial demonstrated the superiority of surgery plus RT versus RT alone for SCC.[13,14] Tumor resection which usually required resection of the vertebral body had a superior outcome with significantly better neurologic function for longer, including a greater proportion of patients who regained ambulation and continence. Length of survival was not significantly different between the two groups, but there was a trend towards longer survival with surgery (129 days vs 100 days, $p = 0.08$). These data suggest that surgery should be a consideration in all patients with SCC. However, the patients enrolled in the study were highly selected and it is not clear that the excellent outcome reported can be expected for all patients with SCC.

Patients with cauda equina compression were excluded from this study. Alternatives to surgery including vertebroplasty and kyphoplasty have proven effective for selected patients with SCC, especially those with vertebral compression fractures and severe pain.[15]

Chemotherapy, with or without RT, is useful in some patients with tumors that are sensitive, especially lymphoma and occasionally other solid tumors.[16] Excellent responses of SCC from chemosensitive tumors to appropriate chemotherapy are observed, but this approach is limited to those who have minimal to no neurologic compromise. If myelopathy is present, urgent RT or surgery must be the primary therapy. Regardless of treatment type, the majority of patients who are ambulatory at the beginning of therapy remain ambulatory. Some paraparetic patients will recover sufficient function to walk again, but only a few who are paraplegic recover useful function.

Leptomeningeal metastasis

LM is less frequent than brain metastasis or SCC but is becoming more common, particularly in patients with small-cell lung, breast, and ovarian cancers. Quality of life and duration of survival are both severely compromised by LM, and fewer than one-half of those treated by currently available therapy receive benefit.

Reliable estimates of the incidence of LM are difficult to obtain, but LM is found in approximately 5% of patients with metastatic cancer. Few studies of LM give incidence figures and the diagnosis is heavily dependent on the diligence with which it is pursued. Recognizing these limitations, the frequency of LM in different cancers varies widely (Table 6).

Pathophysiology

Malignant cells may enter the subarachnoid space by several routes (Figure 3). Subarachnoid invasion can occur via infiltration of the wall of veins and of the marrow trabeculae; malignant cells can attach to leptomeningeal capillaries and move directly into the subarachnoid space. Brain parenchymal lesions can erode into the ventricle or subarachnoid space or be spilled at surgery, causing LM. LM developed in 40% of patients following resection of a cerebellar metastasis but in only 2–3% of those who had resection of a supratentorial lesion. The choroid plexus is a rare route of entry.

Table 6 Frequency of leptomeningeal metastases (LM) in various cancers.

Cancer	Percent developing LM	Features
Carcinoma		
Breast	5	Incidence may be increasing, more common with infiltrating lobular carcinoma
SCLC	9–25	Incidence is increasing, risk increases with duration of survival
NSCLC	?	Less common than breast
Melanoma	23	50% at autopsy
Leukemia		
AML	<5	10% without prophylaxis; associated with high WBC count, elevated LDH, extramedullary disease at diagnosis, and monocytic morphology
ALL	11	30% without prophylaxis; associated with T-cell phenotype, Burkitt morphology, and high WBC count
CLL	Rare	May occur during blast crisis
Lymphoma		
NHL	4–10	Associated with diffuse large B-cell and lymphocytic histology, bone marrow involvement
HD	Rare	
Overall	8.6	LM present at autopsy in 56 of 649 brains examined at Memorial Sloan-Kettering Cancer Center

Abbreviations: ALL, acute lymphocytic leukemia; AML, acute myelogenous leukemia; CLL, chronic lymphocytic leukemia; HD, Hodgkin disease; LDH, lactic acid dehydrogenase; NHL, non-Hodgkin lymphoma; NSCLC, non-small-cell lung cancer; SCLC, small-cell lung cancer; WBC, white blood cell.

Malignant cells may invade the subarachnoid space by direct infiltration along nerve roots, and possibly via epineural lymphatics.

LM causes nervous system dysfunction by several mechanisms: (1) direct infiltration of malignant cells into the brain, spinal cord, cranial nerves, or spinal roots which interferes with neural function; (2) interruption of CSF flow leading to increased intracranial pressure (ICP) with or without hydrocephalus; and, (3) infiltration of tumor along the Virchow–Robin spaces reducing blood supply to the brain causing cerebral ischemia and infarction.

Symptoms and signs
LM is strongly suggested by the patient having symptoms or signs at multiple sites of the neuraxis.[1,2] These include (1) headache, particularly early in the morning or posturally induced headache in the absence of brain metastases; (2) cranial nerve palsies, particularly, diplopia or facial weakness; (3) neck pain in the absence of cervical spine metastases; (4) radicular pain in the arms or legs, particularly when accompanied by weakness but without local spine pain; (5) unexplained constipation, impotence, or urinary incontinence or retention; (6) asymmetric leg weakness and diminished reflexes in the absence of pain or sensory changes; and (7) confusion, memory loss, or other cognitive abnormalities.

Diagnosis
The diagnostic gold standard of LM is the demonstration of malignant cells in the CSF. However, imaging is a much more common means of diagnosis in the modern era.[17] A cranial MRI may reveal enhancing cranial nerves or enhancing tumor in cortical sulci; communicating hydrocephalus may suggest LM. A gadolinium-enhanced spine MRI may demonstrate tumor nodules on spinal roots, particularly in the cauda equina, even when symptoms of nerve root dysfunction are absent (Figure 4).

The whole neuraxis should be imaged to identify sites of bulky disease. When characteristic findings are identified, this suffices to establish the diagnosis. MRI is 76% sensitive and 77% specific for the diagnosis of LM. Occasionally, FDG-PET imaging may identify LM.[18] However, negative imaging does not exclude the diagnosis in a patient with typical features. A lumbar puncture should be performed and the opening pressure, cell count, protein, glucose, and bacterial and fungal studies should be obtained; the cytology specimen should contain at least 10 mL of CSF optimally, and should be processed quickly according to the laboratory's protocol.

Malignant cells are found in the initial CSF sample in 50–60% of patients with LM. Cytologic examination is 75% sensitive, but almost 100% specific; additional samples increase the yield, and occasionally cisternal CSF may be positive when lumbar CSF is negative. Likewise, cytology may be positive in ventricular fluid but negative in lumbar fluid or vice versa. Rare cell capture technology may enhance the identification of malignant cells in CSF over routine cytology.[19]

Tumor markers, deoxyribonucleic acid (DNA) studies, and immunocytochemistry may help confirm LM when cytologic studies are negative. In the presence of a normal blood–brain barrier (suggested by a normal CSF protein concentration), the level of tumor antigens, such as carcinoembryonic antigen (CEA), beta-human chorionic gonadotropin (βHCG), cancer antigen (CA) 125, CA 27.29, CA 19-9, and prostate-specific antigen (PSA), should be no greater than 1% of the serum level. When that amount is exceeded, and particularly if the CSF level is higher than the serum level, the diagnosis is established, even without a positive cytology. When LM is suspected in patients with lymphoma or leukemia, flow cytometry, or molecular markers may demonstrate a clonal excess of cells similar to the systemic neoplasm, suggesting LM.

Treatment
If untreated, LM usually causes relentless progression of neurologic dysfunction and death within weeks. Treatment is not very effective, and it usually does not reverse fixed neurologic deficits. Nevertheless, therapy alters the clinical course in about one-half of patients and often improves symptoms.[1,20] Occasionally, the course may be indolent especially in patients with LM from lymphoma or breast cancer.

The type of primary cancer is the best predictor of response to treatment; the majority of lymphoma and breast cancer patients respond because these tumors are relatively sensitive to RT and systemic and intrathecal chemotherapy. Patients with lung cancer or melanoma respond in about one-third and one-fifth of cases, respectively. Patients with severe neurologic disability from LM are less likely to derive benefit because neural damage is often irreversible. Unlike brain metastases, dexamethasone provides little symptomatic relief unless there is elevated ICP.

Among patients receiving therapy for LM, survival is prolonged only in those whose disease responds to treatment; however, the inability to predict which patients will respond to treatment makes prognostication difficult. In addition to surviving longer (4–6 months median versus 1–2 months median in nonresponders), patients who respond to therapy are less likely to die from their LM than are patients whose disease progresses despite therapy.

Radiation therapy
RT should be administered to symptomatic sites even if subarachnoid tumor is not evident radiographically at the symptomatic location. Entire neuraxis RT is rarely used because of its acute

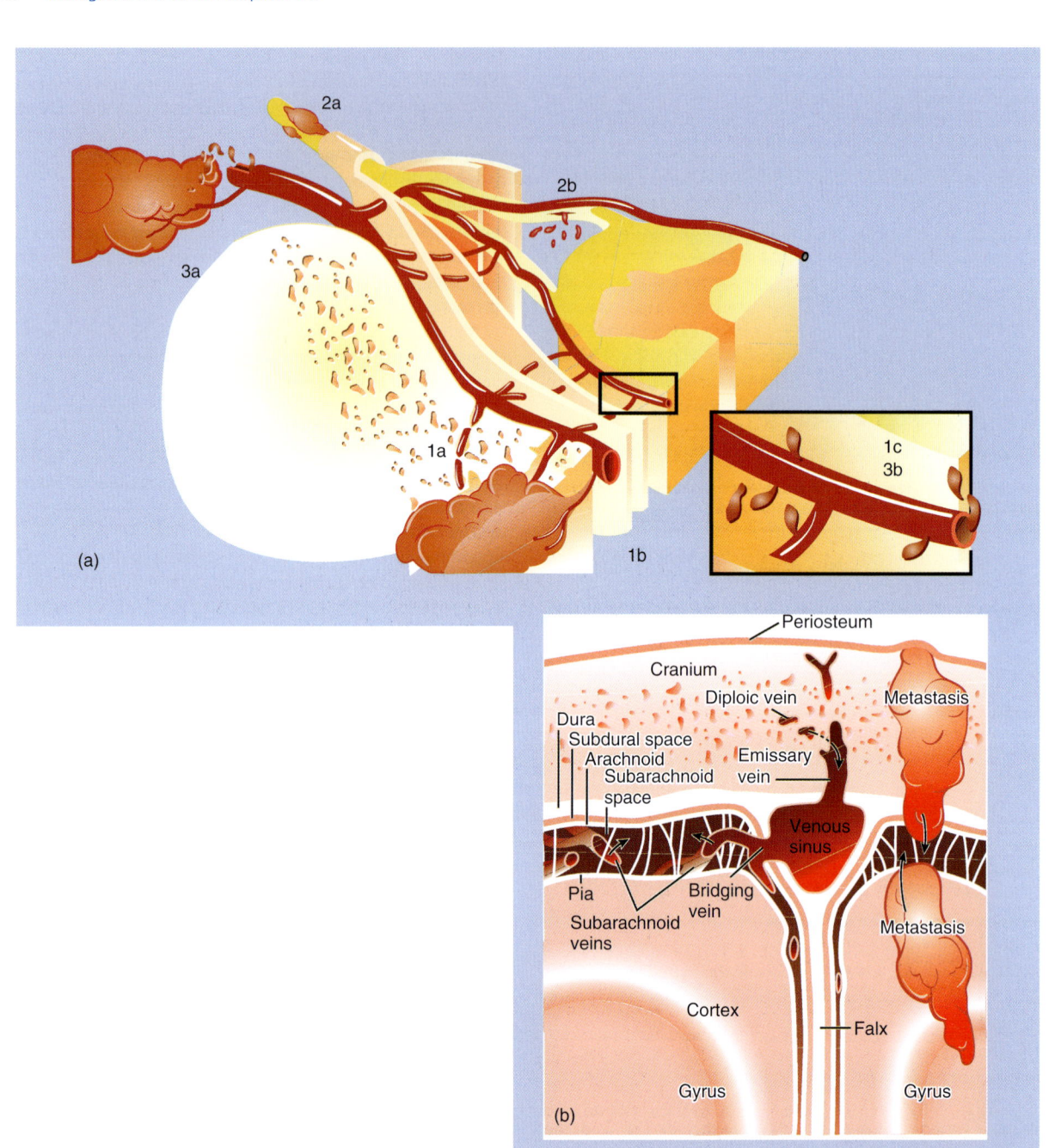

Figure 3 Pathophysiology of leptomeningeal metastases. (a) Mechanisms of tumor cell entry into the spinal subarachnoid space. Tumor may invade the vertebral body (1a) and grow along vertebral veins (1b) into the subarachnoid space (1c). Tumor may invade peripheral nerves or nerve roots outside the vertebral canal (2a) and grow along the nerve sheath into the spinal canal to seed the leptomeninges (2b). The tumor can invade blood vessels outside the central nervous system (3a) and transverse subarachnoid veins into the subarachnoid space (3b). Source: DeAngelis and Posner.[1] (b) Possible mechanisms of tumor entry into the cerebral subarachnoid space. Tumor may enter the cranial subarachnoid space via metastases either to the skull or brain, to the diploic veins of the skull, or directly from subarachnoid veins. The choroid plexus (not shown) is also an occasional site for the formation of leptomeningeal tumor.

morbidity and myelosuppression that interferes with subsequent chemotherapy. Neuraxis RT is not used even when bulky LM is seen on MRI along the entire spinal axis. The brain is the most common site to which RT is administered, usually in a dose of 3000 cGy, but the cauda equina also requires RT frequently.

Chemotherapy

Historically, intrathecal chemotherapy is commonly used to treat LM and when it is administered intraventricularly through a surgically implanted reservoir, there is better distribution and greater ease and reliability of delivery than when a drug is administered by lumbar puncture. The most commonly used agent is methotrexate (MTX), which is active against breast cancer, lymphoma, and leukemia but has poor activity against some of the other common cancers that cause LM. An Ommaya reservoir is usually placed to access the right lateral ventricle. MTX is administered intrathecally to adults in doses of 12–15 mg, diluted in preservative-free saline. With this dose, MTX levels in the CSF

CSF, but its active conversion product, 5-methyltetra-hydrofolate (5-methylTHFA), does; however, the CSF levels of 5-methylTHFA are very low after oral leucovorin and are incapable of rescuing tumor cells in the CSF. Intrathecal MTX as a single agent is equal in efficacy to multiagent intrathecal chemotherapy and has less toxicity.[22] Patients treated with MTX plus RT respond more often than those treated with either alone. As discussed below, intravenous high-dose MTX (HD MTX) is an alternative to intrathecal MTX, particularly for breast and lung LM.[7,23]

Cytarabine (cytosine arabinoside [ara-C]) and thiotepa may also be useful, particularly in LM from lymphoma, leukemia, or breast cancer. Intrathecal liposomal cytarabine has a long CSF half-life and can be given every 14 days; it has been reported effective against LM from solid tumors not usually considered sensitive to cytarabine,[24] and has been shown to improve progression-free survival when added to systemic therapy in patients with breast cancer LM.[25] However, intrathecal liposomal cytarabine can cause a severe chemical meningitis and patients must receive prophylactic steroids (dexamethasone 6 mg daily) beginning one day before a dose is administered and continued for 4 days following the dose.[1] Intrathecal antibodies such as rituximab and trastuzumab have been effective in LM from lymphoma and HER2+ breast cancer, respectively.[26] There are few data to guide decisions regarding the duration of therapy in patients who are clinically stable and whose CSF remains free of malignant cells after 6 months of therapy. Neurotoxicity from intrathecal drug can occur and is discussed later in this article.

Because LM disrupts the blood–brain barrier, systemic chemotherapy, particularly when administered in high doses, may also be effective. HD-MTX (e.g., $3-8\,g/m^2$) with leucovorin rescue after 24 h may result in CSF MTX levels that exceed 10^{-6} M and may represent an alternative to intrathecal delivery, particularly in patients with impaired CSF flow.[7,23] Systemic drugs may also treat bulky LM, whereas intrathecal chemotherapy has insufficient penetration into tumor nodules. Other agents that can reach the CSF or have been reported effective for LM include high-dose cytarabine for hematologic malignancies and capecitabine for breast cancer.[27] Newer agents, including the tyrosine kinase inhibitors and bevacizumab, have been reported effective in individual patients and should be chosen on the basis of the likely sensitivity of the primary to a given drug.[28–30] In a phase I study, patients with EGFR-mutated NSCLC who had LM were treated with osimertinib and demonstrated radiologic, cytologic, clinical, and overall survival improvements with a median duration of response of 8.3 months.[30] Programmed cell death protein 1 (PD-1) immune checkpoint inhibition also shows promise for the treatment of LM of multiple different primary cancers, albeit with a high rate of toxicity (see section on Immunotherapy under Nonmetastatic Complications of Cancer Therapy).[31]

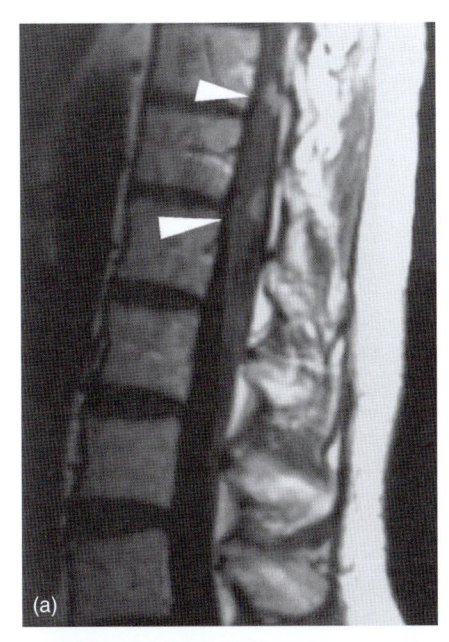

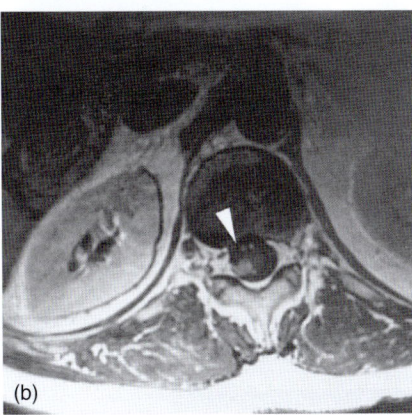

Figure 4 Gadolinium-enhanced MRI demonstrating leptomeningeal metastases from lung cancer. (a) Sagittal and (b) axial images demonstrating enhancing nodules within the thecal sac. This patient had a positive cerebrospinal fluid cytology for malignant cells.

exceed the therapeutic concentration of 10^{-6} M and remain above this level for 36–48 h.

Studies of CSF flow dynamics using indium[111]-DPTA (diethylenetriamine penta-acetic acid) cisternography have found impaired CSF flow in a high percentage of patients with LM. Indium[111] studies predict CSF MTX distribution and indicate that drug reaches all areas of the subarachnoid space unless a complete block is present.[21] Patients with impaired CSF flow have a worse prognosis, and increased incidence of leukoencephalopathy. If a patient has symptoms of elevated ICP with or without hydrocephalus, this takes priority and requires placement of a ventriculoperitoneal shunt; no patient with hydrocephalus or a shunt should receive intrathecal chemotherapy, even if a valve can turn off drainage temporarily. Obstruction of CSF flow should be suspected in patients with LM who develop focal leukoencephalopathy around the ventricular catheter track of an Ommaya reservoir (see MTX).

MTX appears in the serum for prolonged periods following intrathecal administration, and myelosuppression and stomatitis may result. Oral leucovorin can avert these complications starting 12 h after MTX injection. Leucovorin does not appear in the

Cranial and peripheral nerve metastases

Lesions of cranial or peripheral nerves often cause severe pain and, depending on the nerve involved, substantial neurologic disability. The frequency of metastatic disease-causing cranial and peripheral nerve dysfunction is unknown because only a few studies address this issue in particular tumors. For example, facial nerve paralysis occurs in 5–25% of malignant parotid neoplasms, the lower figure associated with acinous cell carcinomas, and the higher with undifferentiated neoplasms. Primary lung cancer arises in the superior sulcus in approximately 3% of patients, the vast majority

---

[1] Liposomal cytarabine is not currently available in the United States.

presenting with pain caused by infiltration of the brachial plexus (pancoast syndrome). Individual nerves either alone or in combination (mononeuritis multiplex) may be compressed or invaded by tumor.

Pathogenesis
Tumors affect cranial and peripheral nerves either by compression or invasion along perineurial and endoneurial planes. Pancoast tumors and breast carcinoma metastatic to supraclavicular lymph nodes compress the brachial plexus but usually do not invade it, whereas squamous cell carcinoma of the face, certain melanomas, and prostate cancer can be neurotropic, tracking microscopically along the course of a nerve, often reaching the spinal canal or even the brainstem.[32] A blood–nerve barrier similar to the blood–brain barrier may exclude water-soluble chemotherapeutic agents from nerve and provide a "sanctuary" for tumor cells.

Symptoms
The specific symptoms and signs of cranial and peripheral nerve dysfunction depend on the nerves involved and the mechanism of involvement. With compressive lesions, pain at the site of compression or more distantly in the sensory distribution of the nerve or plexus involved is usually the first symptom. In invasive lesions of nerves, pain and neurologic dysfunction develop simultaneously. In general, when mixed nerves are involved, motor function is affected out of proportion to sensory loss, no matter what the mechanism of nerve involvement. Compressive lesions of nerves can generally be identified by MRI directed at the area of dysfunction (Figure 5).[1,32] When the lesion is infiltrative, imaging studies may be normal and the diagnosis must be established clinically or by biopsy. Occasionally infiltration of large nerves such as a plexus or root can be imaged by an enhanced MRI or PET.

Cranial and peripheral neuropathies also occur as side effects of radiation, chemotherapy, or as paraneoplastic syndromes. It is frequently difficult to distinguish these nonmetastatic peripheral nerve lesions from those caused by metastases, but in general, the former are usually painless, whereas the latter tend to be painful. Furthermore, most paraneoplastic and drug-induced neuropathies are bilateral and symmetric, whereas metastatic neuropathies are unilateral or at least asymmetric.

Cranial neuropathies
Cranial nerves may be affected by metastases at any point from within the brainstem to their end organ (Table 7). Brainstem metastases occasionally cause isolated cranial nerve dysfunction, but usually, other signs reveal the central location of the lesion. LM is a common cause of cranial neuropathies that are often multiple. Base of skull metastases often causes recognizable patterns of cranial nerve dysfunction that localize the lesion.[1,2] Finally, the cranial nerves may be damaged after exiting their foramina.

Evaluation should include an enhanced MRI to visualize the involved cranial nerve along its entire course. Lumbar puncture should be performed even when an appropriately placed skull base metastasis is discovered, because LM may coexist. Nonmetastatic causes of cranial neuropathies are also common in cancer patients (Table 8). RT is usually employed for skull base

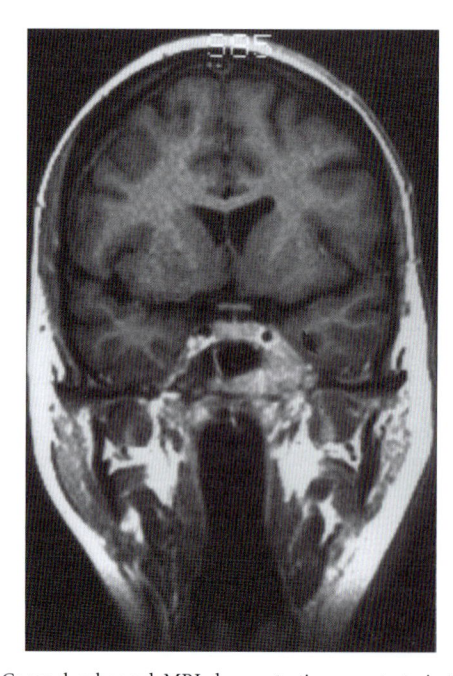

Figure 5 Coronal-enhanced MRI demonstrating a metastasis to the left cavernous sinus (*arrowhead*) from breast carcinoma. Patient presented with retro-orbital pain and had evidence of a partial third, sixth, and V1 palsy.

Table 7 Metastatic lesions causing cranial neuropathies.

Lesion site	Findings	Comments
Eye	Decreased visual acuity; retinal detachment	Choroidal lesions are more common than retinal: pain, proptosis, and diplopia are rare; breast and lung cancer are common causes
Orbit	Pain, proptosis, diplopia; sensory loss V1; decreased visual acuity in one-third of cases, usually late	As common as choroidal metastases; breast and prostate cancer and lymphoma are common causes
Parasellar	Unilateral frontal headache, oculomotor palsies (CN III, IV, VI), sensory loss V1	Vision rarely affected, no proptosis; lymphoma common
Sella	Diabetes insipidus	Anterior pituitary insufficiency and visual loss are rare; when present, they suggest a primary pituitary tumor. Breast cancer is a common cause
Middle cranial fossa	Facial numbness (V2, 3), VI palsy in some	Lightning-like facial pains (trigeminal neuralgia) rare in patients with neoplastic compression
Jugular foramen	Hoarseness, dysphagia, pain in pharynx (IX, X), sternocleidomastoid weakness (XI), occasionally tongue weakness (XII)	Papilledema may occur if dominant jugular vein is compressed. Glossopharyngeal neuralgia is uncommon
Occipital condyle	Unilateral occipital pain and neck stiffness, unilateral tongue weakness (XII)	Pain may radiate to forehead
Mandible	Unilateral numb chin and gum ("mental neuropathy")	Also results from meningeal or skull base metastases; breast cancer and lymphoma are common causes
Carotid sinus or glosso-pharyngeal nerve	Syncope, pharynx, or neck pain on swallowing	Cardioinhibitory, vasodepressor syncope, or both; head and neck cancer, indicates recurrent tumor; may be life-threatening
Left upper mediastinum	Recurrent laryngeal paralysis	Hoarseness; lung, breast, and head and neck cancers

Table 8 Nonmetastatic causes of cranial neuropathy in cancer patients.

Cranial nerve (symptom)	Causes
II (unilateral vision loss)	Gallium, interferon-alpha, RT, temporal arteritis, retinal diseases including hemorrhage
III (diplopia, ptosis)	Diabetes (usually spares pupil), aneurysm, increased intracranial pressure (uncal herniation); myasthenia gravis and Grave disease[a]
V (jaw pain; facial pain)	Vincristine, trigeminal neuralgia (sudden, lancinating pains without sensory loss)
VI (diplopia)	Vincristine, increased intracranial pressure, head trauma, diabetes, drug toxicity (e.g., narcotics, anticonvulsants), strabismus
VII (facial weakness)	Bell's palsy (idiopathic), varicella-zoster infection (Ramsay Hunt syndrome), diabetes
VIII (hearing loss, dysequilibrium)	Cisplatin, aminoglycosides, degenerative disease, acoustic neuroma, RT-induced serous otitis
X (weak phonation, laryngeal paralysis)	Vincristine

Abbreviation: RT, radiation therapy.
[a]Common causes of diplopia, but are not cranial nerve diseases.

and orbital metastases. Chemotherapy can be used in appropriate circumstances.

Brachial plexopathy

Brachial plexopathy in cancer patients usually results from metastatic cancer in axillary or cervical lymph nodes, local bony structures (e.g., clavicle), or from superior sulcus lung tumors.[1,2] Because most metastatic tumors compress the plexus from below, the initial symptom is usually pain in the posterior shoulder or pain radiating down the medial aspect of the arm, elbow, and forearm to the fourth and fifth fingers (C-8 or T-1 distribution). Weakness usually begins in the hand and sensory loss begins in the fourth and fifth fingers; both may progress to affect the entire arm. This initial presentation is helpful in distinguishing tumor from the more common cervical disc herniation where pain commonly affects the outer arm and dorsal surface of the forearm, with weakness in the triceps and wrist extensors (C-7 radiculopathy). Tumor masses are occasionally palpable in the axilla or supraclavicular area. When present, an ipsilateral Horner syndrome (ptosis, miosis, and anhydrosis) indicates the tumor has involved the stellate ganglion in the paraspinal region and, therefore, epidural extension must be sought on cervical MRI.

The differential diagnosis includes radiation-induced plexopathy, trauma (e.g., intraoperative positioning, or following central line placement), idiopathic plexopathy, and radiation-induced malignant peripheral nerve sheath tumor. A common diagnostic dilemma is the differentiation of metastatic from radiation-induced plexopathy. Clinical features that distinguish these two conditions include (1) initial symptom of pain in metastatic plexopathy, and paresthesias in RT-induced plexopathy; (2) Horner syndrome, which is more consistent with metastatic plexopathy; (3) more rapid progression of symptoms and signs in metastatic plexopathy; (4) supraclavicular fullness in metastatic plexopathy; and (5) lymphedema, which suggests RT-induced plexopathy. CT or MRI may demonstrate a mass in the plexus (metastatic plexopathy) or loss of soft-tissue planes from fibrosis (RT-induced plexopathy). When findings are equivocal, a PET scan may help.

RT is the best available treatment for metastatic plexopathy; chemotherapy may be useful for some previously irradiated patients (e.g., those with breast cancer or lymphoma). There is no satisfactory treatment for radiation-induced plexopathy. Surgical lysis of fibrotic tissue surrounding the nerves has not been helpful, nor has systemic corticosteroid, local steroid injection, hyperbaric oxygen, or bevacizumab. Treatments for pain include carbamazepine, opioids, gabapentin, pregabalin, and neurosurgical ablative procedures.

Lumbosacral plexopathy

The lumbosacral plexus is formed from spinal nerve roots L-2 to S-5. The upper lumbar portion (L-2 to L-4) exits the pelvis mainly as the obturator (adductor muscles) and femoral (quadriceps muscles) nerves, whereas the remainder of the leg is innervated by the sciatic nerve (L-5 to S-1). The bladder, rectum, and anus are innervated by roots S-3, S-4, and S-5. Symptoms are usually unilateral leg weakness and numbness although 25% of metastatic plexopathies may be bilateral. Incontinence requires bilateral loss of innervation and, therefore, its presence suggests central (i.e., cauda equina) or sacral involvement. Clear differentiation requires enhanced spinal MRI and CSF analysis. Local extension of pelvic and abdominal tumors is the predominant cause of metastatic lumbosacral plexopathy. The differential includes herniated lumbar disc, epidural and meningeal metastases to the cauda equina, radiation-induced plexopathy (usually from brachytherapy for pelvic neoplasms), intraoperative trauma, hematoma, abscess, and diabetic or idiopathic lumbosacral plexopathy. The differential features of metastatic and radiation-induced plexopathy are similar to those for brachial plexopathy. CT or MRI often demonstrates a mass in the region of the lumbosacral plexus. Biopsy is indicated if an abscess or a secondary tumor is suspected. RT is the most commonly employed treatment for metastatic lumbosacral plexopathy. If metastatic disease approaches the spine, epidural disease may be present and should be included in the radiation field.

Peripheral neuropathy

Single peripheral nerves are sometimes damaged by metastatic cancer, and more widespread invasion of peripheral nerves, causing either a mononeuritis multiplex or diffuse polyneuropathy, may complicate the course of leukemia or lymphoma; PET imaging of the limbs may be diagnostic.[33] However, when polyneuropathy occurs in cancer patients, it usually results from toxin exposure or paraneoplastic disorders, both of which are discussed below.

Nonmetastatic complications of cancer therapy

Many cancer treatments are neurotoxic (Table 9). Some drugs (e.g., vincristine) cause neurotoxicity even at low doses, whereas others (e.g., cytarabine) cause neurotoxicity only during intensive therapy. Neurologic toxicity is a dose-limiting factor in several cancer treatments, such as RT, and patients may suffer more from these toxicities than from the cancer itself.[1,2,34] The more commonly encountered neurologic toxicities from cancer treatment are discussed below.

Chemotherapy

Vinca alkaloids
Vinca alkaloids cause nerve damage by binding tubulin in peripheral nerves and disrupting the formation of microtubules that mediate fast axonal transport. Neurotoxicity is a dose-limiting side effect of all the vinca alkaloids, but especially of vincristine; vinorelbine can also cause peripheral neuropathy particularly

Table 9 Neurotoxicity of agents commonly used in cancer patients.

Acute encephalopathy/encephalopathy	Headache without meningitis
Asparaginase	Corticosteroids
Blinatumomab	Ondansetron
Cisplatin	Retinoic acid
Corticosteroids	Tamoxifen
Cytarabine (high-dose IV, IT)	Temozolomide
Ifosfamide/mesna	Erlotinib
Interferons	Osimertinib
Ipilimumab	Trametinib
Nivolumab	Cobimetinib
Pembrolizumab	
Atezolizumab	Seizures
Avelumab	Asparaginase
Durvalumab	Busulfan (high-dose)
CAR T cells	Blinatumumab
Methotrexate (high-dose IV, IT)	Carmustine
Nelarbine	CAR T cells
Nitrosoureas (high-dose)	Cisplatin
Procarbazine	Dacarbazine
Vincristine	Etoposide
Bevacizumab (PRES)	5-Fluoracil
Everolimus (PRES)	Ifosfamide
Tacrolimus (PRES)	Methotrexate
Cyclosporin (PRES)	Vincristine
Sunitinib (PRES)	
Sorafenib (PRES)	Myalgias
5-Flourouracil (± levamisole)	Alectinib
	Brigatinib
Chronic encephalopathy (dementia)	Ceritinib
Carmustine	Crizotinib
Cytarabine	Dabrafenib
Fludarabine	Vemurafenib
Methotrexate	Trametinib
Fluorouracil	Cobimetinib
Ophthalmologic toxicity/visual loss	Myelopathy (any intrathecal drug)
Cisplatin	Cytarabine
Erlotinib	Methotrexate
Bevacizumab	Thiotepa
Gallium nitrate	
Interferon alpha	Peripheral neuropathy
Osimertinib	Vinca alkaloids, cisplatin
Tamoxifen	Alectinib
	Brigatinib
Venous sinus thrombosis, ischemic/hemorrhagic stroke	Ceritinib
	Crizotinib
Bevacizumab	Dabrafenib
Sunitinib	Vemurafenib
Sorafenib	Oxaliplatin
	Etoposide
Cerebellar dysfunction/ataxia	Teniposide
5-Fluorouracil (±levamisole)	Paclitaxel
Cytarabine	Docetaxel
Phenytoin	Suramin
Procarbazine	Bortezomib
	Brentuximab vedotin
Aseptic meningitis	Lenalidomide
Bortezomib	Thalidomide
IVIG	Nelarbine
Cetuximab	Ipilimumab
Corticosteroids (IT)	Nivolumab
Cytarabine (IT; especially liposomal preparations)	Pembrolizumab
	Atezolizumab
Methotrexate (IT)	Avelumab
NSAIDs	Durvalumab
Trimethoprim-sulfamethoxazole (Cotrimoxazole)	

Abbreviations: CAR, chimeric antigen receptor; IV, intravenous; IVIg, intravenous gammaglobulin; IT, intrathecal; NSAID, nonsteroidal anti-inflammatory drugs; PRES, posterior reversible encephalopathy syndrome.

when combined with or following other neurotoxic agents. Central neurotoxicity is rare because vincristine does not penetrate the normal blood–brain barrier. Vinca alkaloids should never be given intrathecally.

Vinca alkaloid neurotoxicity is age- (more severe in adults) and dose-dependent, and appears to be more prominent in patients with hepatic dysfunction, and in those who have received other potentially neurotoxic therapies. Tingling paresthesias develop in the fingertips, and usually in the toes, of virtually all patients treated with vincristine, although clinically detectable sensory loss is often absent. Loss of ankle reflexes is an early and almost universal sign, and with continued therapy, all reflexes may diminish or disappear. Weakness occurs as therapy continues and is of two types: (1) A generalized distal neuropathy that preferentially affects the foot and hand extensors, causing impairment of fine motor function and foot drop. Weakness can become severe enough to render the patient immobile or bed-bound, but the drug should be discontinued prior to severe weakness. Preexisting peripheral nerve diseases, especially Charcot–Marie–Tooth neuropathy and probably other neuropathies (e.g., diabetic polyneuropathy), increase the severity of vincristine neuropathy. (2) Some patients develop focal weakness, (e.g., unilateral foot drop or cranial nerve palsies, such as ptosis or extraocular muscle, facial, or laryngeal paralysis. Although symptomatic toxicity is usually reversible after discontinuation of the drug, significant weakness may persist in severely affected patients. Autonomic dysfunction, particularly abdominal cramping and constipation, often occurs within hours to days of each dose. Adynamic ileus may result and can be life-threatening; a prophylactic bowel regimen is essential for all patients. Impotence has been reported.

Less common complications of vincristine administration include aching bone pain, sharp stabbing pain in the jaw or throat, or an increase in any preexisting pain; this typically occurs within hours of injection and subsides over several days. The symptoms appear with the first or second dose and rarely recur with subsequent doses. Hyponatremia from inappropriate secretion of antidiuretic hormone occurs within days of drug administration and may recur with subsequent doses.

Methotrexate

There are several clinically distinct forms of MTX toxicity.[1,2] An acute reaction with meningismus, confusion, fever, and CSF pleocytosis often occurs 4–6 h after intrathecal injection and resolves over several days. This syndrome is frequently confused with infectious meningitis, but the onset is too rapid after the injection for bacterial contamination; antibiotics are unnecessary unless Gram stain or cultures demonstrate organisms. Dexamethasone relieves or prevents some of these symptoms. Mild acute toxicity occurs in as many as 10% of patients, but further doses of intrathecal MTX are usually uneventful.

Paraplegia may follow instillation of MTX or cytarabine by lumbar puncture. The disorder is characterized by weakness and sensory loss in the legs, which evolves over several days to complete transverse myelopathy. Some patients recover, but most remain paraplegic. Extensive necrosis of the spinal cord is found at autopsy. The pathogenesis is unknown, but it appears to be idiosyncratic rather than dose related.

An early delayed reaction follows high-dose systemic MTX in about 4% of patients. The disorder usually occurs 7–10 days after the third or fourth treatment and is characterized by stupor or coma, often associated with lateralizing neurologic signs that change from hour to hour. MRI may show diffusion positive lesions suggestive of ischemia. Most patients recover completely and the disorder usually does not recur with subsequent doses of MTX. MTX leukoencephalopathy can occur in patients who have received a high cumulative dose of intrathecal or systemic MTX or MTX in combination with cranial RT. In adults, progressive cognitive impairment in the absence of lateralizing signs may be seen in patients who survive >6 months following treatment. Leukoencephalopathy, when clinically present, is always found on neuroimaging, but occasionally it may be found on MRI in asymptomatic patients. The neuropathologic findings consist of multifocal areas of coagulative necrosis and calcification in the white matter, often with a periventricular predominance. Unlike cerebral radionecrosis, fibrinoid necrosis of blood vessels is absent.

Alternatively, focal leukoencephalopathy may develop around an Ommaya reservoir catheter track. When MTX is injected into ventricles with elevated pressure, the drug tracks along the outside of the catheter, producing focal leukoencephalopathy seen on MRI as an enhancing mass (Figure 6); this may resolve on its own or require removal of the catheter.

Platins

Peripheral neuropathy is a dose-limiting toxicity of some platins, particularly cisplatin and oxaliplatin.[1,35] Neuropathic symptoms begin as tingling paresthesias in the toes and fingers; loss of reflexes and reduced vibratory and position sensation are characteristic but pain, temperature sensation, and strength are preserved. Severe, disabling sensory ataxia may result. Symptoms are often mild during treatment but they progress for months before stabilizing, making dose adjustment during treatment difficult. Gradual resolution follows, although some patients are permanently disabled. Lhermitte sign, an electric sensation in the arms, back, or legs upon neck flexion, is an occasional manifestation of platin neurotoxicity. Oxaliplatin may cause cold-induced paresthesias either during or shortly after an infusion and may also cause a sensory neuropathy. Magnesium infusions do not prevent oxaliplatin neurotoxicity.[36]

Ototoxicity caused by cisplatin is a result of damage to the organ of Corti. Toxicity severe enough to interfere with speech perception is uncommon, but hearing loss may or may not resolve. Seizures and encephalopathy have been reported in patients receiving cisplatin, independent of the magnesium and calcium wasting commonly caused by the drug. Vascular disease-producing neurologic symptoms have been reported as a late delayed effect of cisplatin-based chemotherapy. Many such patients develop Raynaud phenomenon, and a few have developed transient ischemic attacks or cerebral infarctions. Other platin drugs are less neurotoxic.

Taxanes

Paclitaxel and docetaxel both bind tubulin, stabilizing and promoting microtubular assembly. Both cause a predominantly sensory peripheral neuropathy, beginning with paresthesias of the toes and then fingers.[1,37] More severe sensory impairment and loss of reflexes develop with increasing duration of drug administration. Symptoms usually recover with drug discontinuation. Weakness is seen occasionally; it can be predominantly proximal, mimicking a myopathy, but this is likely secondary to neuropathy. Because taxanes are often used concurrently with or following other neurotoxic agents such as cisplatin, patients may develop significant symptoms with the first few doses because of additive neurotoxic

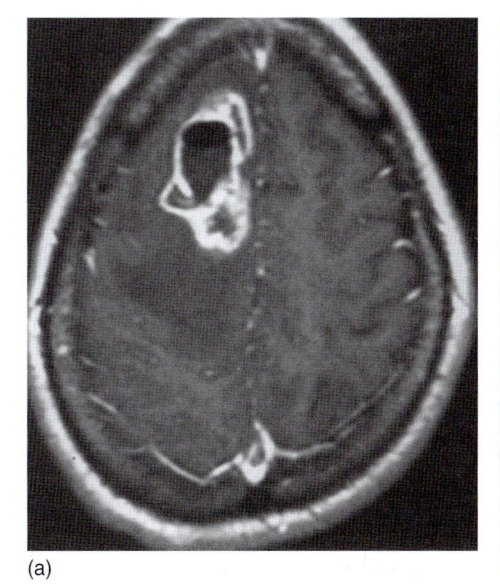

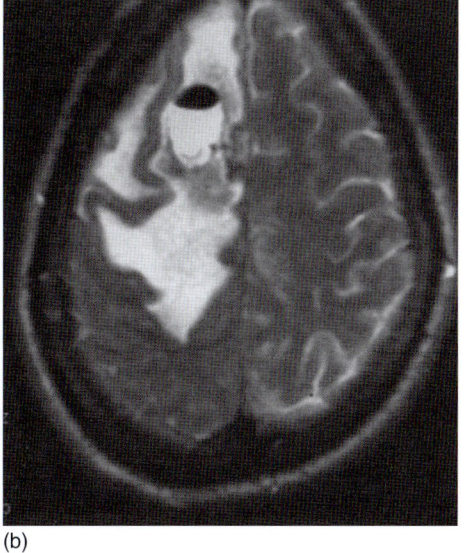

Figure 6 Gadolinium-enhanced T1-weighted (a) and T2-weighted (b) MRIs of focal leukoencephalopathy in a patient with a malfunctioning Ommaya reservoir. This reservoir was obstructed but unrecognized. Multiple courses of methotrexate were instilled into the catheter. The drug dissected around the catheter and into the frontal lobe, causing a region of necrosis with prominent surrounding edema. Air can be seen in the central cavity of the lesion after a recent instillation. The patient presented with seizures and a left hemiparesis, both of which resolved with corticosteroids.

effects. Nab-paclitaxel, the taxane bound to nano particles of albumin, is less neurotoxic than the standard drug.

5-Fluorouracil
Encephalopathy has been seen in association with severe systemic toxicity during therapy and may indicate an inherited deficiency of dihydropyrimidine dehydrogenase, the enzyme responsible for pyrimidine catabolism.[38] Capecitabine, doubly esterified fluorouracil for oral use, appears to be less neurotoxic than intravenously administered fluorouracil.

Cytosine arabinoside
Intrathecal cytarabine can cause an acute chemical meningitis with confusion, fever, and CSF pleocytosis. This occurs in almost all patients who receive the liposomal preparation and requires dexamethasone prior to and after every administration.[24]

Intravenous high-dose cytarabine (e.g., $3\,g/m^2$ every 12 h for six doses) causes neurotoxicity in 10–25% of patients; the risk is increased with older age and poor renal function. Neurotoxicity has been documented with minimum cumulative doses of $18\,g/m^2$, but higher cumulative doses (e.g., $30–40\,g/m^2$) are associated with a higher incidence and more severe toxicity. Commonly, a pancerebellar dysfunction starts several days after the initiation of therapy and worsens for several more days. Gradual recovery begins about 2 weeks after onset, but recovery may be incomplete especially in those with severe dysfunction. Pathologic changes include loss of cerebellar Purkinje cells and neurons in the deep cerebellar nuclei. Encephalopathy and seizures also occur, usually in the setting of cerebellar toxicity. A recrudescence of neurologic symptoms may occur with retreatment.

Other drugs
High-dose busulfan therapy, used to prepare patients for stem cell transplantation, can cause seizures; at standard doses, the drug is not neurotoxic. Gemcitabine, with or without radiation, has been reported to cause myositis with acute muscle pain and tenderness; it is responsive to steroids.[1,39]

Small molecule and antibody targeted therapies

The epidermal growth factor receptor (EGFR) inhibitors erlotinib and osimertinib can cause headache and keratitis. Anaplastic lymphoma kinase (ALK) inhibitors, such as alectinib, brigatinib, ceritinib, and crizotinib, can cause myalgias and neuropathy.[40] The B-Raf proto-oncogene serine/threonine kinase (BRAF) inhibitors dabrafenib and vemurafenib can cause myalgias, and peripheral neuropathy; they can also act as radiation sensitizers, increasing the risk of radiation necrosis in patients receiving drug and concurrent RT. The mitogen-activated protein kinase (MEK) inhibitors such as trametinib and cobimetinib can cause headache and myalgias. Selumetinib, another MEK inhibitor, can cause focal neck extensor weakness causing the dropped head syndrome.[41]

Bortezomib, a first-generation proteasome inhibitor, can cause a painful peripheral neuropathy, and it can also predispose to compression neuropathies superimposed on the diffuse neuropathy.[42] A second generation proteosome inhibitor, carfilzomib, causes less severe peripheral neuropathy. Thalidomide causes peripheral neuropathy, but lenalidomide and pomalidomide are less neurotoxic. Chronic use of rituximab, an anti-CD20 antibody used in NHL and CLL, can induce persistent immunosuppression which may lead to progressive multifocal leukoencephalopathy (PML) due to reactivation of JC virus in the brain.[43] MRI shows multiple, usually nonenhancing, white matter lesions. Restoration of immune function is the only effective therapy of this otherwise lethal disease which presents with confusion and lateralizing signs such as hemiparesis. A case series suggests a role of PD-1 immune checkpoint inhibition in the restoration of immune function in PML, with a reduction of JC virus viral load and clinical improvement in 5 of 8 patients.[44] A recent case report describes clinical and radiographic improvement in a patient with PML after hematopoietic stem cell transplant, when treated with the interleukin-15 (IL-15) superagonist N-803.[45]

Bevacizumab, an antivascular endothelial growth factor (VEGF) agent, can cause optic neuropathy, as well as hypertension which may lead to confusion and seizures from posterior reversible encephalopathy syndrome (PRES).[46] PRES can be identified on MRI by the presence of white matter lesions best seen on MRI T2-FLAIR sequence (see Figure 7). PRES warrants immediate attention to blood pressure management. PRES has also been associated with other agents, such as everolimus, tacrolimus, cyclosporin, and mycophenylate used after allogeneic stem cell transplantation along with many conventional chemotherapeutics such as the platins and gemcitabine. In addition to PRES, bevacizumab and the small molecule VEGF inhibitors sunitinib and sorafenib are associated with venous sinus thrombosis, as well as ischemic and hemorrhagic strokes. Blinatumomab, a bispecific T cell receptor-engaging (BITE) antibody used to treat B-cell acute lymphocytic leukemia (ALL), is associated with encephalopathy, seizures, and ataxia in approximately 20% of patients.[43]

Brentuximab vedotin, a CD30 antibody–drug conjugate, can cause a predominantly sensory neuropathy which improves when the drug is held; it can be restarted when the neuropathy has improved.[43] Myalgias are also common with brentuximab vedotin.

Immunotherapy

Immune checkpoint inhibitors
Immune checkpoint inhibitors (ICIs) are approved for multiple cancers. A number of neurologic and nonneurologic immune-related toxicities have been recognized in patients treated with ICIs. Ipilimumab, an anti-CTLA4 antibody can cause aseptic meningitis as well as encephalitis when given concurrently with an anti-PD1 antibody.[47] Ipilimumab can also cause hypophysitis with enhancing lesions seen in the hypothalamus on MRI. In the peripheral nervous system, ipilimumab can cause cranial neuropathies, acute or chronic immune demyelinating polyneuropathy (AIDP, CIDP), myasthenic syndromes, and myositis.[47,48] Anti-PD1 (nivolumab, pembrolizumab) or anti-PD1-Ligand 1 (anti-PD1-L1; atezolizumab, avelumab, durvalumab) antibodies can also cause neurologic immune-related toxicities, including encephalitis, peripheral demyelinating neuropathies, myasthenic syndromes, and myositis.[47,48] The concurrent use of an anti-CTLA4 antibody with an anti-PD1/PD1-L1 antibody increases the risk of neurotoxicity. The initial management of ICI-associated neurotoxicities is through discontinuation of ICI treatment and administration of high-dose corticosteroids.[47–49] Treatment with intravenous immunoglobulin (IVIG) or plasmapheresis is warranted if no response is seen to high-dose steroid therapy after 3–5 days. Patients who are rechallenged with ICI therapy after resolution of neurotoxicity are at high risk of toxicity relapse.[48]

Adoptive cell therapies
Adoptive cell therapies (ACTs) are a group of immunotherapies that require the infusion of genetically engineered immune effector cells for the treatment of different malignancies. The most

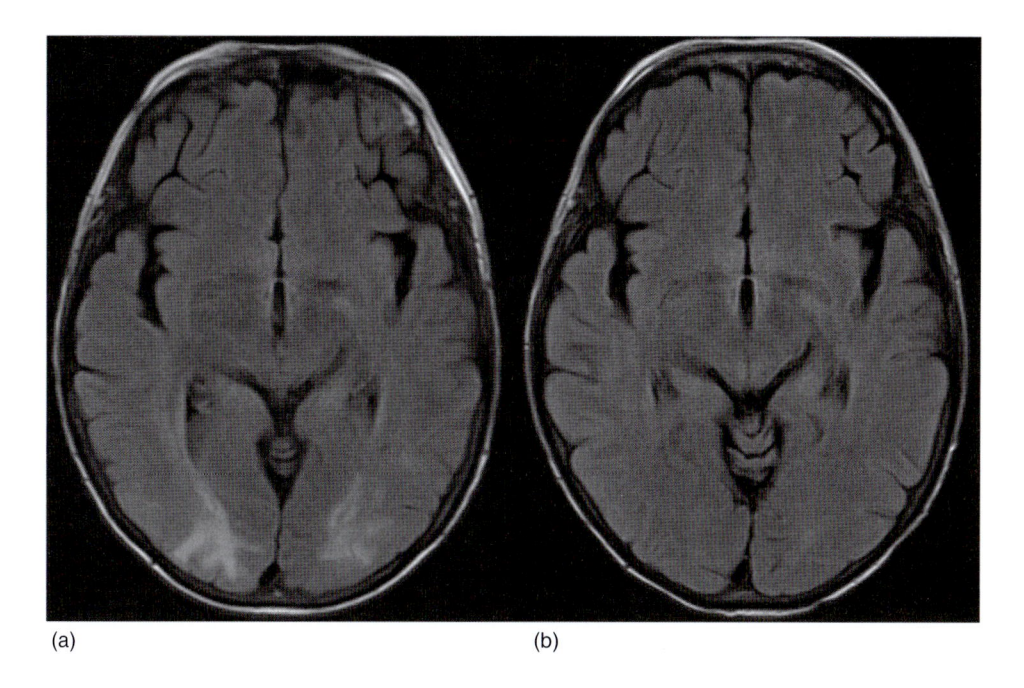

Figure 7 T2-FLAIR axial MRI sequences of a 60-year-old woman on day 20 status post bone marrow transplant presenting with hypertension and headache. (a) Note the occipitoparietal hyperintensities consistent with posterior reversible encephalopathy syndrome. (b) On an interval MRI 5 weeks later, the patient has resolution of the radiographic changes. Source: Images courtesy of Dr. Bruno Di Muzio, Radiopaedia.org.

widely adopted form of ACT involves the infusion of chimeric antigen receptor (CAR) T cells targeting specific tumor antigens, with a number of CAR T cell constructs being approved for the treatment of leukemia and lymphoma and many others being studied in clinical trials.[50,51] CAR T cell therapy is frequently associated with systemic and neurologic toxicity. After infusion, CAR T cells rapidly expand producing an inflammatory state with associated macrophage activation and subsequent release of multiple cytokines—IL-1, IL-2, IL-6, IL-8, IL-10, IL-15, IFN-gamma—leading to endothelial cell activation, increased brain-barrier permeability, and meningeal inflammation.[52,53] Within minutes to hours of CAR T cell administration, 77–96% of patients experience the onset of fever, myalgias, arthralgias, confusion, and in severe cases hypoxia and hypotension. This constellation of symptoms, the cytokine release syndrome (CRS), is accompanied by elevation of acute inflammatory markers (C-reactive protein, ferritin). CRS generally responds to supportive treatment.[49,51] The initial symptoms of CAR T cell neurotoxicity are generally noted on day 3 or 4 postinfusion and sometimes can overlap with the encephalopathy that may be associated with CRS. The clinical presentation most commonly begins with deficits in language and attention, and can rapidly progress to severe encephalopathy with seizures, and in rare cases coma in the setting of cerebral edema.[51,54–56] Characterization of neurologic baseline preinfusion and close follow-up of neurologic function is essential in patients treated with CAR T cells. In symptomatic patients, the neurologic examination is the most useful element in guiding management. Diagnostic studies—MRI brain, EEG, CSF studies—are routinely obtained to evaluate for alternative causes (stroke, seizures, CNS infection) but are generally unrevealing in most cases of *bona fide* CAR T cell neurotoxicity.[54,55] Patients with mild symptoms (inattention, word-finding difficulty) can be monitored with frequent neurologic examinations but patients with severe encephalopathy or ongoing seizures should be managed in an ICU setting. Patients with severe CAR T cell neurotoxicity are treated with high-dose corticosteroids (initial dose of 10–60 mg of dexamethasone, followed by 4–20 mg every 6–12 h). Patients with ongoing seizures should be treated with antiepileptics per status epilepticus protocols. The administration of prophylactic antiepileptics on the day of infusion and continuing for 30 days is commonly advised but the utility of this measure has not been validated. After administration of corticosteroids, neurologic symptoms begin to improve within hours to days. Corticosteroids can be rapidly tapered once patients have returned to their neurologic baseline. In one case series, corticosteroid use for more than 10 days was associated with worse overall survival, but survival or disease response was not affected by shorter courses.[54]

Radiation therapy

Despite the fact that cells in the CNS turn over slowly, the brain, spinal cord, and, to a lesser degree, peripheral nerves are susceptible to damage by ionizing radiation that usually causes symptoms months or years after the radiation has been completed (Table 10).[2] With patients living longer after initial treatment, the problem of delayed radiation injury to the CNS is increasingly important.

Brain toxicity

Acute reactions, occurring within hours of a dose of RT, are rare with current fractionation schedules when patients are pretreated with dexamethasone. Patients with large or multifocal tumors and cerebral edema, especially those with symptoms of increased ICP, are more likely to experience this side effect. Symptoms and signs of acute RT toxicity include worsening of existing neurological deficits, headache, nausea and vomiting, and lethargy. These are usually transient and respond to corticosteroids. The etiology has been ascribed to radiation-induced disruption of the blood–brain barrier with worsening cerebral edema.

Early delayed encephalopathy occurs a few weeks to a few months after RT. Patients being treated for cerebral tumors may develop worsening of lateralizing signs. Symptoms may persist for days to weeks and are often relieved by corticosteroids; complete

Table 10 Neurologic complications of CNS irradiation.[a]

Complication	Latency	Symptoms and signs	Comments
Brain			
Acute	Hours	Increase in existing deficits, headache, nausea, vomiting, confusion, somnolence	Transient, corticosteroids beneficial
Early	Weeks to months	Increase in existing signs, increased seizures, lethargy	Resolves over days to weeks, corticosteroids beneficial
Delayed			
a. Radionecrosis	6 months to years	Focal mass lesion	Treatment includes corticosteroids and surgery, tumor often coexists
b. Dementia	1 year	Loss of cognitive function	May be subtle
c. Endocrine	Years	Hypothyroidism, amenorrhea/galactorrhea, changes in libido, growth failure	Hypothalamic or pituitary in origin
d. Secondary tumors	10–40 years, earlier if radiated as a child	Symptoms of brain tumor	Meningioma, sarcoma, malignant glioma
e. Stroke	Years	Abrupt onset of neurologic dysfunction	Large or branch vessels
Spinal cord			
Early	Weeks to months	Electric shocks with neck movement (Lhermitte symptom)	Usually transient
Delayed			
a. Myelopathy	Weeks to years	Progressive cord dysfunction, starts with sensory symptoms	Often fatal
b. Lower motor neuron syndrome	Months to years	Focal weakness and atrophy	May improve spontaneously

[a]Source: Schiff et al.[2]

resolution is usual. Early delayed encephalopathy is often confused clinically and radiographically with tumor progression and is sometimes called pseudo-progression. MRI reveals an enhancing lesion indistinguishable from progressive tumor. Advanced imaging with PET or perfusion MRI sometimes clarifies the situation; however, gradual resolution of symptoms may be the only confirmation of the cause of the deterioration.

Delayed radiation toxicity is the most serious complication of brain RT, and radionecrosis is its most common manifestation, arising months to years after treatment.[1,2,57] In one study, cerebral radionecrosis occurred in 6% of patients treated with 4500 cGy or more.[57] The total dose is the most important risk factor, and there is a threshold near 6000 cGy above which radionecrosis becomes common. However, high daily fractionation schedules also carry increased risk, and radionecrosis is seen most commonly after stereotactic radiosurgery (SRS) for brain metastases. Headache, focal deficits, and seizures are the usual symptoms. MRI reveals a contrast-enhancing lesion with surrounding edema; PET or perfusion MRI may differentiate tumor that is hypermetabolic and hypervascular from necrosis that is hypometabolic and avascular. However, the differentiation between radionecrosis and tumor is difficult, and biopsy may be required. Marked symptomatic improvement follows treatment with dexamethasone, and some patients remain well after steroids are discontinued. Surgical resection of the necrotic material is often necessary. Reports that anticoagulation or hyperbaric oxygen relieve symptoms require confirmation. Bevacizumab may prove effective.[58]

Brain RT may also cause dementia unassociated with necrosis. The MRI shows ventricular dilatation, sulcal atrophy, and white matter hyperintensity. Some of these patients respond to ventriculoperitoneal shunting albeit incompletely and temporarily.[1] Pre-RT and serial neuropsychological testing can be very useful and enable appropriate patients to receive cognitive rehabilitation or other resources. Cerebral infarction may result from occlusion of cervical or intracranial arteries that have received large doses of RT.[59] Vascular malformations may appear and bleed many years after brain RT. Complicated migraine-like episodes may occur in patients after cranial irradiation, this is termed SMART syndrome (stroke-like migraine attacks after RT).[60]

Endocrinologic dysfunction may arise years after RT, resulting from either hypothalamic or pituitary failure. Serial monitoring of hypothalamic-pituitary axis function via endocrinology can be useful in long-term survivors after brain RT. Brain tumors may occur decades after cranial RT or radiosurgery administered in adulthood, but latency is often much shorter (median 6 years) in those irradiated in childhood. Radiation-induced brain tumors include meningioma, sarcoma, and malignant glioma.

Spinal cord toxicity

Spinal cord damage caused by RT is uncommon. Lhermitte symptoms may occur weeks to months after RT to the cervical cord, including mantle RT for Hodgkin disease. Spontaneous resolution is the rule. Progressive radiation myelopathy, on the other hand, is a devastating, progressive, often irreversible complication with onset months to years (median 20 months) following spinal cord RT. The incidence of radiation myelopathy is affected by the total RT dose and dose per fraction; an estimate of the ED5 (5% incidence of complication) is between 5700 and 6100 cGy for RT delivered in 200 cGy fractions. Symptoms of radiation myelopathy usually begin with sensory changes in the legs and gradually progress to sensory loss, weakness, and sphincter dysfunction. Pain may be present at the level of the cord damage. Unlike SCC, sensory and motor findings are often asymmetric at onset and a Brown-Séquard syndrome is often present, paralysis and loss of proprioception on one side of the body ipsilateral to the lesion and loss of pain and temperature sensation on the opposite side of the body, contralateral to the lesion. The MRI reveals either a normal, enlarged, or atrophic cord that may contrast enhance, but extrinsic compression is absent (Figure 8). Steroids do not reverse the deficits. Anticoagulants and hyperbaric oxygen have been reported to be effective, but this has not been verified, and myelopathy is usually permanent.

Seizures and tumor-related epilepsy

Seizures are common in patients with primary and metastatic brain tumors but can also occur in cancer patients without brain lesions as a result of adverse effects of systemic therapies, infections,

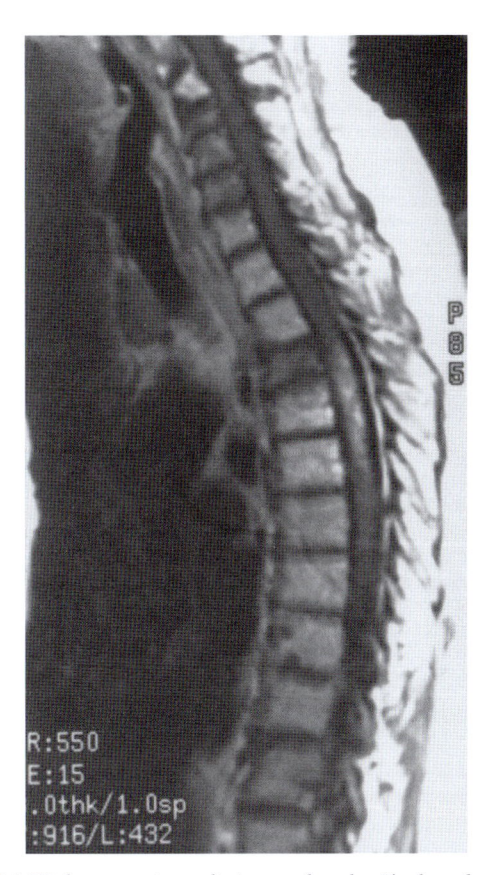

Figure 8 MRI demonstrating radiation myelopathy. The hypodense thoracic vertebral body is the site of a bone metastasis from breast cancer for which the patient was radiated. Some months later, the patient developed a myelopathy, and the contrast-enhancing lesion seen in the spinal cord represents radiation damage.

or metabolic derangements.[61] Uncontrolled seizures can lead to physical and psychological harm, reducing quality of life in cancer patients.

Pathophysiology

Seizures are most common in patients with brain lesions, ranging from 10% to 100% in patients with primary brain tumors (for gliomas, incidence is inversely proportional to grade) and 10–30% in patients with brain metastases.[61,62] Lesions involving the cerebral hemispheres, particularly those affecting the cortical surface or those associated with hemorrhage or edema are most likely to cause seizures. In addition, seizures in patients with brain lesions can be a byproduct of surgical, radiation, or systemic treatment. In cancer patients without brain lesions, systemic therapies (see Table 9 for systemic cancer therapies commonly associated with seizures), metabolic derangements (e.g., hyponatremia, hypocalcemia, hyperglycemia), or CNS infections (particularly in immunosuppressed patients) can lead to seizures.

Evaluation

The evaluation of a cancer patient presenting after a first seizure should include a detailed history of the event noting any abnormal sensations or symptoms reported by the patient before the event; their state of consciousness and motor activity if the event was witnessed; loss of urinary or stool continence; the duration of the event; and the presence of confusion or agitation after the event. Current medications and recent treatments should be carefully reviewed. Neurologic examination should try to detect possible postictal deficits or evidence of ongoing seizure activity (persistent deficits in language, focal motor seizures). Brain MRI is the preferred imaging modality but head CT without contrast should be obtained to rule out hemorrhage if there is delay in obtaining MRI. Investigations should include a complete blood count with differential, a complete metabolic panel, toxicology studies, and urinalysis. Blood cultures and chest X-ray should be obtained when infection is suspected. In patients with meningeal signs or concern for infection in the setting of persistent altered mental status, lumbar puncture with opening pressure, glucose, total protein, cell count, cell culture, Gram stain, and cytology, is indicated but only after obtaining brain imaging (head CT suffices) to exclude a significant brain mass which is usually a contraindication to performing a lumbar puncture. Imaging or CSF studies should not delay the start of empiric antimicrobial therapy if infection highly suspected. Electroencephalogram (EEG) is indicated in the setting of unexplained neurologic symptoms to evaluate for nonconvulsive status epilepticus or subclinical seizures.

Management

The treatment of brain metastases with surgery, RT, and systemic therapies, which might contribute to seizure control, is discussed in *Chapter 73*. In terms of antiepileptic drug (AED) therapy, a single, unprovoked seizure in a patient with a brain tumor establishes the diagnosis of tumor-related epilepsy (TRE) warranting the indefinite use of an AED. However, in patients without a history of seizures, prophylactic AED use is not recommended, as prophylaxis does not decrease the risk of seizure and can lead to side effects.[63–66] In a high-risk patient, such as a patient with multiple hemorrhagic cortical metastases, there may be a benefit from prophylaxis with newer AEDs that lead to fewer side effects.[67] There are no randomized trials that have established the superiority of one AED over others for the treatment of TREs. Older, first-generation AEDs have more drug interactions and side effects and should be avoided if possible. Phenytoin, carbamazepine, and phenobarbital induce cytochrome p450 enzymes and can decrease the effectiveness of chemotherapy. Valproate is a cytochrome p450 enzyme inhibitor and can increase the levels of certain chemotherapeutic agents as well as contribute to hepatotoxicity and thrombocytopenia. Levetiracetam is often favored as the first line AED for TRE, given its absence of chemotherapy interactions and its overall good tolerability, although it can cause fatigue, irritability, and worsening of depression. Lacosamide is another AED with no induction or inhibition of hepatic enzymes, few drug interactions, and a low incidence of side effects (it can, however, cause PR interval prolongation and should not be initiated in patients with PR > 200 ms). AEDs should be titrated to their lowest effective dose in consultation with a neurologist to minimize their side effects.

Cerebrovascular complications of cancer

Cerebrovascular lesions are the second most common neuropathologic finding, after metastases, in postmortem studies of cancer patients. Hemorrhage into a metastasis is the most common cause of intracranial hemorrhage in cancer patients;[68] it is most common in lung cancer, but occurs proportionately more frequently in melanoma, thyroid, renal, and germ cell metastases. Nonmetastatic intracerebral hemorrhages are seen in patients with leukemia, thrombocytopenia, or coagulopathy.[1] Subdural hemorrhage may occur in association with dural metastases or coagulopathy.[69] A hemorrhage may cause abrupt neurologic symptoms with headache, vomiting, lethargy, and focal deficits, or may be unsuspected prior to obtaining a brain scan. For patients with intracerebral hemorrhage resulting from coagulopathy or thrombocytopenia, the underlying problem should be treated and the patient observed. Subdural hematomas and some hemorrhages into metastases may benefit from surgical evacuation.

Cerebral infarction is as common as hemorrhage.[70,71] Infarctions secondary to accelerated atherosclerosis take place decades following RT that has included cervical or cerebral vessels in the irradiated field. RT for head and neck cancer predisposes to carotid stenosis and intracranial arterial stenosis with subsequent cerebral infarction. Septic cerebral infarction is usually secondary to Aspergillus, Candida, or Mucor. These opportunistic organisms produce a vasculitis, and the infarctions are often multiple and hemorrhagic. Aspergillus is the most common causative agent and is always associated with pulmonary infection. Antifungal therapy is usually unsuccessful, and the outcome is often fatal.

Cerebral venous thrombosis (e.g., superior sagittal sinus thrombosis) may result from compression or invasion of vascular structures by a metastasis, or from a coagulopathy. Clinical features include headache, focal deficits, and seizures. The diagnosis can be made by MRI combined with magnetic resonance venography. Lumbar puncture reveals an elevated opening pressure, and frequently red cells in the CSF. Anticoagulation is generally safe and should be considered for progressive neurologic symptoms, even when due to hemorrhage from venous infarction. Consultation with a neurologist is advised in these complicated cases.

Cerebral embolism accounts for more than one-half of strokes in patients with cancer.[70,71] Nonbacterial thrombotic endocarditis (NBTE) is an established cause of cardioembolism which is most common with lung and GI carcinomas. Infarctions in patients with NBTE are often multiple and hemorrhagic. Diffuse encephalopathy and focal deficits usually coexist. Approximately one-third of patients with NBTE also have laboratory evidence of disseminated intravascular coagulation (DIC). DIC alone may result in cerebrovascular thrombosis. Neurologic symptoms usually begin abruptly with diffuse encephalopathy and fluctuating multifocal deficits. Two-dimensional echocardiography is rarely helpful, but transesophageal echocardiography may demonstrate valvular vegetations. Contrast-enhanced brain MRI is typically negative, although small foci of ischemia are seen occasionally on diffusion-weighted sequences. After obtaining a head CT without contrast to rule out hemorrhagic lesions, anticoagulation with heparin may prevent progressive neurologic dysfunction. Hypercoagulability of malignancy is also a recognized cause of cardioembolic stroke.[72] In these patients, anticoagulation with enoxaparin or direct oral anticoagulants (DOACs; apixaban, rivaroxaban, edoxaban, dabigatran) is indicated.

Paraneoplastic neurologic syndromes

Paraneoplastic syndromes refer to disorders of unknown etiology that occur with increased frequency in patients with cancer (Table 11).[3] Compared with known complications of cancer, paraneoplastic syndromes are rare, seen in less than 1% of patients with cancer. As paraneoplastic syndromes precede the diagnosis of cancer in about two-thirds of cases, prompt recognition may lead to early diagnosis and cure of the underlying neoplasm. These disorders often debilitate the patient to a greater degree than the malignancy, but some of the syndromes improve with successful treatment of the cancer.

The etiologies of these syndromes are not well understood, but most are suspected to have an autoimmune basis. The strongest evidence for an autoimmune disorder is for the Lambert–Eaton myasthenic syndrome (LEMS) in which autoantibodies inhibit the function of presynaptic calcium channels at the neuromuscular junction, resulting in weakness. Examination demonstrates an increase in muscle power after repetitive muscle contraction (the opposite of myasthenia gravis), and absent deep tendon reflexes. These findings, along with autonomic and sensory complaints of dry mouth, impotence, and thigh paresthesias, point to a nerve

Table 11 Paraneoplastic neurologic syndromes.[a]

Syndrome	Associated cancer[b]	Clinical features
Brain		
Limbic encephalopathy[c]	SCLC	Depression, memory loss, confusion, abnormal CSF
Brainstem encephalopathy[c]	SCLC	Ataxia, cranial nerve dysfunction, corticospinal dysfunction, abnormal CSF
Subacute cerebellar degeneration	Breast, ovary, SCLC, Hodgkin	Ataxia, dysarthria, nystagmus, normal CSF
Opsoclonus, myoclonus	Lung	Jerky, irregular movements of eyes and skeletal muscles
Optic neuritis, retinal degeneration	SCLC	Painless loss of vision, transient visual obscuration
NMDA receptor encephalitis	Teratoma	Seizures, psychosis, rhythmic movements, impaired cognition
Spinal cord		
Necrotizing myelopathy	SCLC, lymphoma, leukemia	Ascending myelopathy
Subacute motor neuronopathy	Hodgkin and NHL	Patchy weakness, atrophy, and fasciculations
Dorsal root ganglia		
Subacute sensory neuronopathy[c]	SCLC	Dysesthesias, sensory ataxia, areflexia
Peripheral nerve		
Gammopathy associated neuropathy	Myeloma	Sensory loss, weakness, reflex loss
Acute polyradiculitis (Guillain–Barré)	Lymphoma	No cells in CSF; high CSF protein
Neuromuscular junction		
LEMS	SCLC	Proximal weakness, decreased reflexes, ocular muscles spared
Myasthenia gravis	Thymoma	Weakness, ocular muscles often involved
Muscle		
Dermatomyositis, polymyositis	Lung, breast, ovary, GI	Weakness, elevated CPK

Abbreviations: CPK, creatine phosphokinase; CSF, cerebrospinal fluid; GI, gastrointestinal; LEMS, Lambert–Eaton myasthenic syndrome, NHL, non-Hodgkin lymphoma; NMDA, N-methyl D-aspartate; SCLC, small-cell lung cancer.
[a]Source: Based on Darnell and Posner.[3]
[b]The most commonly associated tumors are listed.
[c]Often occur in association with each other.

disorder. Several other paraneoplastic syndromes are associated with the presence of specific antibodies, including subacute sensory neuronopathy, limbic encephalitis, subacute cerebellar degeneration, and gammopathy-associated neuropathies. These specific antibodies serve as markers that not only identify the syndrome as paraneoplastic but suggest the site of the underlying tumor.[3]

A variety of therapies directed at immunomodulation, including plasmapheresis, corticosteroids, and intravenous immunoglobin, have failed to reverse the neurologic impairment associated with most paraneoplastic disorders. However, some syndromes, such as the LEMS and anti-NMDA receptor Ab encephalitis, respond to immunosuppressive treatments. Some patients with paraneoplastic neurologic disorders have reversal or stabilization of their neurologic dysfunction when the underlying malignancy is treated effectively and this should be a therapeutic priority for all of these patients.

Key references

The complete reference list can be found on Vital Source version of this title, see inside front cover.

1. DeAngelis LM, Posner JB. *Neurologic Complications of Cancer*, 2nd ed. New York: Oxford University Press; 2008.
2. Schiff D, Kesari S, Wen PY. *Cancer Neurology in Clinical Practice. Neurologic Complications of Cancer and Its Treatment*. Totowa, New Jersey: Humana Press; 2007.
3. Darnell RB, Posner JB. Paraneoplastic syndromes affecting the nervous system. *Semin Oncol*. 2006;33(3):270–298.
5. Cole JS, Patchell RA. Metastatic epidural spinal cord compression. *Lancet Neurol*. 2008;7:459–466.
7. National Comprehensive Cancer Network. *NCCN Clinical Practice Guidelines in Oncologoy: Central Nervous System Cancers*. 2019.
8. Sørensen PS, Helweg-Larsen S, Mouridsen H, et al. Effect of high-dose dexamethasone in carcinomatous metastatic spinal cord compression treated with radiotherapy: a randomised trial. *Eur J Cancer*. 1994;30(1):22–27.
12. Bydon M, De La Garza-Ramos R, Bettagowda C, et al. The use of stereotactic radiosurgery for the treatment of spinal axis tumors: a review. *Clin Neurol Neurosurg*. 2014;125:166–172.
13. Patchell RA, Tibbs PA, Regine WF, et al. Direct decompressive surgical resection in the treatment of spinal cord compression caused by metastatic cancer: a randomised trial. *Lancet*. 2005;366(9486):643–648.
14. Bilsky M, Smith M. Surgical approach to epidural spinal cord compression. *Hematol Oncol Clin North Am*. 2006;20:1307–1317.
16. Grommes C, Bosl GJ, Deangelis LM. Treatment of epidural spinal cord involvement from germ cell tumors with chemotherapy. *Cancer*. 2011;117(9):1911–1916.
17. Clarke JL, Perez HR, Jacks LM, et al. Leptomeningeal metastases in the MRI era. *Neurology*. 2010;74(18):1449–1454.
22. Kim DY, Lee KW, Yun T, et al. Comparison of intrathecal chemotherapy for leptomeningeal carcinomatosis of a solid tumor: methotrexate alone versus methotrexate in combination with cytosine arabinoside and hydrocortisone. *Jpn J Clin Oncol*. 2003;33(12):608–612.
23. Lassman AB, Abrey LE, Shah GG, et al. Systemic high-dose intravenous methotrexate for central nervous system metastases. *J Neurooncol*. 2006;78:255–260.
24. Glantz MJ, LaFollette S, Jaeckle KA, et al. Randomized trial of a slow-release versus a standard formulation of cytarabine for the intrathecal treatment of lymphomatous meningitis. *J Clin Oncol*. 1999;17(10):3110–3116.
25. Le Rhun E, Wallet J, Mailliez A, et al. Intrathecal liposomal cytarabine plus systemic therapy versus systemic chemotherapy alone for newly diagnosed leptomeningeal metastasis from breast cancer. *Neuro Oncol*. 2020;22(4):524–538.
30. Yang JCH, Kim S-W, Kim D-W, et al. Osimertinib in patients with epidermal growth factor receptor mutation-positive non-small-cell lung cancer and leptomeningeal metastases: the BLOOM study. *J Clin Oncol*. 2020;37:538–547.
31. Brastianos PK, Lee EQ, Cohen JV, et al. Single-arm, open-label phase 2 trial of pembrolizumab in patients with leptomeningeal carcinomatosis. *Nat Med*. 2020;1–5. doi: 10.1038/s41591-020-0918-0.
37. Argyriou AA, Koltzenburg M, Polychronopoulos P, et al. Peripheral nerve damage associated with administration of taxanes in patients with cancer. *Crit Rev Oncol Hematol*. 2008;66:218–228.
40. Zukas AM, Schiff D. Neurological complications of new chemotherapy agents. *Neuro-Oncol*. 2018;20:24–36.
42. O'Connor OA, Wright J, Moskowitz C, et al. Phase II clinical experience with the novel proteasome inhibitor bortezomib in patients with indolent non-Hodgkin's lymphoma and mantle cell lymphoma. *J Clin Oncol*. 2005;23(4):676–684.
43. Magge RS, DeAngelis LM. The double-edged sword: neurotoxicity of chemotherapy. *Blood Rev*. 2015;29(2):93–100.
44. Cortese I, Muranski P, Enose-Akahata Y, et al. Pembrolizumab treatment for progressive multifocal leukoencephalopathy. *N Engl J Med*. 2019;380(17):1597–1605. doi: 10.1056/NEJMoa1815039.
46. Tlemsani C, Mir O, Boudou-Rouquette P, et al. Posterior reversible encephalopathy syndrome induced by anti-VEGF agents. *Target Oncol*. 2011;6(4):253–258.
48. Dubey D, David WS, Reynolds KL, et al. Severe neurological toxicity of immune checkpoint inhibitors: growing spectrum. *Ann Neurol*. 2020;87(5):659–669.
49. Thompson JA, Schneider BJ, Brahmer J, Andrews S. Management of immunotherapy – related toxicities. *NCCN Clin Pract Guidel Oncol*. 2020;18(3):230–241.
51. Neelapu SS, Tummala S, Kebriaei P, et al. Chimeric antigen receptor T-cell therapy-assessment and management of toxicities. *Nat Rev Clin Oncol*. 2018;15: 47–62.
52. Neelapu SS. Managing the toxicities of CAR T-cell therapy. *Hematol Oncol*. 2019; 37(S1):48–52.
54. Karschnia P, Jordan JT, Forst DA, et al. Clinical presentation, management, and biomarkers of neurotoxicity after adoptive immunotherapy with CAR T-cells. *Blood [Internet]*. 2019;133(20):2212–2221.
55. Rubin DB, Danish HH, Ali AB, et al. Neurological toxicities associated with chimeric antigen receptor T-cell therapy. *Brain*. 2019;142(5):1334–1348.
57. Ruben JD, Dally M, Bailey M, et al. Cerebral radiation necrosis: incidence, outcomes, and risk factors with emphasis on radiation parameters and chemotherapy. *Int J Radiat Oncol Biol Phys*. 2006;65(2):499–508.
58. Boothe D, Young R, Yamada Y, et al. Bevacizumab as a treatment for radiation necrosis of brain metastases post stereotactic radiosurgery. *Neuro Oncol*. 2013;15(9):1257–1263.
60. Black DF, Morris JM, Lindell EP, et al. Stroke-like migraine attacks after radiation therapy (SMART) syndrome is not always completely reversible: a case series. *Am J Neuroradiol*. 2013;34(12):2298–2303.
61. Gonzalez Castro LN, Milligan TA. Seizures in patients with cancer. *Cancer*. 2020;126(7):1379–1389.
62. Louis DN, Ohgaki H, Wiestler OD, et al. In: Louis DN, Ohgaki H, Wiestler OD, Cavenee WK, eds. *World Health Organization Classification of Tumours of the Central Nervous System*, 4th ed. Lyon: International Agency for Research on Cancer; 2016:1–403.
63. Glantz MJ, Cole BF, Forsyth PA, et al. Practice parameter: Anticonvulsant prophylaxis in patients with newly diagnosed brain tumors: Report of the Quality Standards Subcommittee of the American Academy of Neurology. *Neurology*. 2000;54(10):1886–1893.
64. Sirven JI, Wingerchuk DM, Drazkowski JF, et al. Seizure prophylaxis in patients with brain tumors: a meta-analysis. *Mayo Clin Proc*. 2004;79(12):1489–1494.
68. Navi BB, Reichman JS, Berlin D, et al. Intracerebral and subarachnoid hemorrhage in patients with cancer. *Neurology*. 2010;74(6):494–501.
71. Navi BB, Singer S, Merkler AE, et al. Recurrent thromboembolic events after ischemic stroke in patients with cancer. *Neurology*. 2014;83(1):26–33.
72. Selvik HA, Thomassen L, Bjerkreim AT, et al. Cancer-associated stroke: the Bergen NORSTROKE study. *Cerebrovasc Dis Extra*. 2015;5:107–113.

125 Dermatologic complications of cancer chemotherapy

Anisha B. Patel, MD ■ Padmavathi V. Karri, MD ■ Madeleine Duvic, MD

> **Overview**
>
> Dermatologic complications of cancer chemotherapy have become increasingly significant, especially with the continued development of new targeted antineoplastic agents. The frequency of mucocutaneous complications in cancer chemotherapy is often a reflection of the increased proliferative nature of affected tissues, such as the mucous membranes, skin, hair, and nails, which renders them particularly susceptible to the actions of chemotherapeutic drugs. This article reviews the specific side effects associated with newer targeted and immune therapies as well as the more classic side effects of cytotoxic chemotherapies and their associated drugs.

Diagnosis of cutaneous reactions in the cancer patient is complicated by the degree of their malignancy, concomitant diseases, polypharmacy, and immunosuppression. With the advances in bone marrow transplantation, graft-versus-host disease (GVHD), opportunistic infections, and malignancies are also being seen more frequently and may mimic and complicate the diagnosis of chemotherapy-induced reactions. The major cutaneous reactions and a variety of miscellaneous reactions are discussed in this article and are listed in Table 1. As seen in Table 2, these reactions occur in varying degrees of frequency and severity among the classes of chemotherapeutic drugs. Although dermatologic complications are rarely fatal, it is important to recognize potential reactions as they may result in significant morbidity, chemotherapy cessation or dose reduction, cosmetic disfigurement, and psychological distress. Proper treatment of potentially dose-limiting cutaneous toxicity may also allow ideal schedules of chemotherapy administration and optimization of response.

Drug hypersensitivity reactions

"Traditional" drug reactions have been categorized into immunologic and nonimmunologic or toxic. Of the immunologic drug reactions, there are four subtypes, formerly Types I–IV, that are outlined in Table 3. The most common reactions are delayed-type, T-cell-mediated drug reactions and include the morbilliform or exanthematous drug eruptions. They clinically present as erythematous macules and thin papules on the face and upper trunk spreading to the extremities. They are usually asymptomatic but may itch. When the rash is painful, the differential diagnosis includes erythema multiforme (EM), Stevens–Johnson Syndrome (SJS), and toxic epidermal necrolysis (TEN). EM is characterized by erythematous targetoid urticarial lesions with a darker center, involving the palms and soles. Advanced disease forms central bullae and spreads to the oral and genital mucosa. SJS and TEN, however, start with centrally distributed dusky papules and plaques that coalesce and vesiculate and have severe mucosal involvement. SJS involves less than 10% of body surface area and TEN involves greater than 30% of body surface area. The mortality rate of SJS is 1–5% and that of TEN is 25–35%.[1]

Drug reaction with eosinophilia and systemic syndrome (DRESS) and acute generalized exanthematous pustulosis (AGEP) have unclear pathogeneses. The cutaneous findings in DRESS resemble hypersensitivity drug rash, however, the peripheral edema, lymphadenopathy, and liver transaminitis are characteristic. AGEP presents with abruptly-appearing sheets of cutaneous pustules. It usually begins on the face or intertriginous areas, with burning and itching. It can be accompanied by fever, neutrophilia, and eosinophilia.[2] Ninety percent of cases are drug-induced, mostly with antibiotics but are also reported with imatinib, lapatinib, and erlotinib.[3,4] Other reported triggers include the histone deacetylase inhibitor bryostatin,[5] mercury, thallium, iohexol, patch testing, pseudoephedrine, diltiazem, furosemide, and viral infections.[6] These two reactions are less common than the exanthematous eruption and can be more severe.

Targeted cancer therapeutics

Targeted antibodies, fusion proteins, and small molecules first appeared in the mid-1990s, and we are still delineating all of their side effects. Although the systemic toxicities are decreased, many of the signaling mediators targeted also affect the epithelium, and these effects are much more specific than previous chemotherapy cutaneous reactions, which are usually described as the general term "toxic erythema of chemotherapy." This change is reflected in the literature of clinical trials, where adverse events were previously described as a "rash" or "lesion." Descriptions have become more specific making it easier to anticipate and track different reactions.

Numerous targeted therapies are available; however, only those with specific cutaneous reactions occurring at high incidences are discussed below.

Epidermal growth factor receptor (EGFR) inhibitors

Epidermal growth factor receptor (EGFR) is a significant regulator of cancer cell proliferation, apoptosis, angiogenesis, and metastasis. Ligand binding to the receptor causes receptor dimerization, which

Table 1 Major cutaneous reactions associated with chemotherapy.

Acral reactions (acral erythema/toxic erythema of chemotherapy, hand-foot skin reaction)
Antibody-mediated (bullous pemphigoid, dermatomyositis, lupus erythematosus)
Cutaneous eruption of lymphocyte recovery
Drug hypersensitivity reactions (morbilliform, erythema multiforme/Stevens–Johnson/toxic epidermal necrolysis)
Extravasation reactions (irritant, vesicant)
Hair (anagen effluvium, scarring alopecia, change in quality, telogen effluvium)
Inflammatory dermatoses (eczematous, psoriatic, lichenoid, granulomatous)
Mucosal reactions (stomatitis, aphthae)
Nail reactions (pigment changes, dystrophy, nail fold changes)
Neoplasms (actinic keratosis recall, benign keratoses, squamous cell carcinoma, lentigines, melanoma, mycosis fungoides)
Neutrophilic dermatoses (Sweet's syndrome, erythema nodosum, pyoderma gangrenosum, neutrophilic eccrine hidradenitis)
Pigmentary changes (hyperpigmentation, vitiligo)
Radiation-associated reactions (radiation enhancement, radiation recall, photosensitivity)
Superinfection/colonization

Table 2 Most common mucocutaneous reactions of the major classes of cytotoxic chemotherapeutic drugs.

Alkylating agents	Antibiotics
Hyperpigmentation	Hyperpigmentation
Morbilliform eruption	Morbilliform eruption
	Radiation recall
Vinca alkaloids	**Antimetabolites**
Alopecia	Acral erythema
Chemical cellulitis	Alopecia
Inflammation of keratosis	Hyperpigmentation
Neutrophilic eccrine hidradenitis	Photosensitivity
Photosensitivity	Photo recall

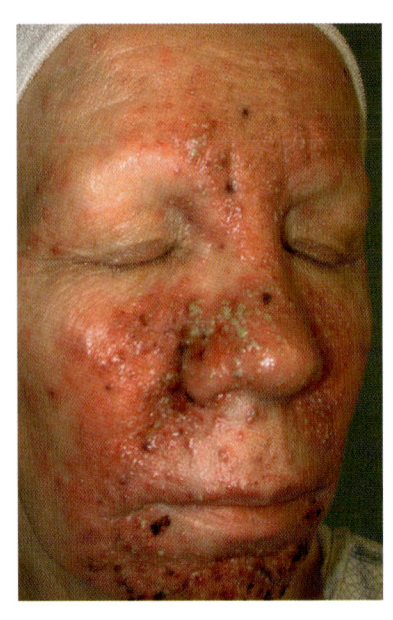

Figure 1 Severe acneiform eruption of the face associated with cetuximab therapy.

activates the intracellular tyrosine kinase domain.[7] EGFR also plays a significant role in normal skin homeostasis.[8] Activation of EGFR in epidermal keratinocytes promotes cell cycle progression, differentiation, and migration, which are all critical for normal skin function and wound healing.[9] The most common cutaneous side effects for EGFR inhibitors are an acneiform eruption, paronychia, xerosis, eczema, mucositis, and geographic tongue. Acne folliculitis appears on the face and upper trunk 8–10 days after treatment initiation. In phase I trials, erlotinib at the maximally tolerated dose induced a pustular acneiform eruption in 50% of cases during the second week of therapy.[10] The eruption can be extremely pruritic and EGFR inhibitors have cutaneous side effects that lead to dose alteration in greater than 75% of patients.[11] The presence and severity of acne folliculitis have been correlated with tumor response and survival.[12] This reaction has been reported with cetuximab, panitumumab, nimotuzumab, erlotinib, and gefitinib.[13–15] Oral tetracyclines combined with topical steroids are the gold standard treatment. For recalcitrant cases, oral retinoids have proven useful in these patients.[16] Epithelial dysregulation with *Staphylococcus* colonization can worsen the eruption and cultures and antibiotics are recommended if lesions are pustular or crusted (Figure 1).

The human epidermal growth factor receptor (HER)1/2 blockers have the same side effects as EGFR inhibitors but are milder. Trastuzumab, lapatinib, dacomitinib, and afatinib all have had reported acneiform eruptions.[17–20] Similarly, the vascular endothelial growth factor receptor (VEGFR) inhibitors have overlap between the EGFR inhibitors, with mucositis and geographic tongue, and the multikinase inhibitors, with hand-foot skin reaction (HFSR), which is discussed below.[21]

BCR-ABL tyrosine kinase inhibitors

Imatinib mesylate targets the *BCR-ABL* gene and has been used in the treatment of chronic myeloid leukemia and acute lymphoblastic leukemia. It frequently causes dose-dependent cutaneous reactions, including facial edema, morbilliform eruption, urticaria, eczematous dermatitis, and AGEP.[22,23] One patient developed an eczematous rash with histologic features of mycosis fungoides.[24]

Second and third-generation Bcr-Abl specific TKIs, dasatinib, nilotinib, and ponatinib have been associated with follicular lichenoid eruptions of the scalp, face, and body that can be pruritic and lead to scarring alopecia.[25] This alopecia is irreversible, even upon dose cessation.

Multikinase inhibitors

Sunitinib and sorafenib are the multikinase inhibitors targeting VEGF receptor, platelet-derived growth factor receptor (PDGFR), c-Kit, and FLT-3. Sorafenib also inhibits RAF kinase. They were developed for advanced renal cell carcinoma but have also been used for hepatocellular carcinoma, gastrointestinal stromal tumors, and thyroid cancer. They are most associated with the HFSR as well as mucositis, alopecia, xerosis, and xerostomia. However, because they overlap with multiple groups of targeted therapies, the cutaneous squamous cell carcinoma (SCC) of BRAF inhibitors and the acneiform eruption of VEGFR inhibitors can be seen as well.[26]

HFSR appears within 2–4 weeks of starting the therapy and is present in one-fifth to one-third of patients, with sorafenib having a slightly higher incidence. Patients develop a focal keratoderma at points of friction and pressure, which can vesiculate, leading to painful blisters. The risk of developing HSFR depends on which drug the patient is on and which cancer type is being treated. The originally proposed mechanism was that the VEGFR blocking

Table 3 Immunologically—mediated drug hypersensitivity reactions.

Hypersensitivity type	Drug	Reaction
IgE-dependent drug reactions (formerly type I)	Cisplatin (intravesical) Docetaxel L-Asparaginase Paclitaxel Teniposide	Anaphylaxis Angioedema Urticaria
Cytotoxic drug-induced reactions (antibody against a fixed antigen; formerly type II)		Petechiae secondary to drug-induced thrombocytopenia
Immune complex-dependent drug reactions (formerly type III)		Serum sickness Urticaria (certain types) Vasculitis
Delayed-type, cell-mediated drug reactions (formerly type IV) versus undefined	Cytarabine Immune checkpoint inhibitors (CTLA-4, PD-1, and PD-L1) Nucleoside analogs (both can also have IgE-dependent and immune-complex mediated drug reactions) Procarbazine	AGEP DRESS Exanthematous/morbilliform eruption Fixed drug eruption Lichenoid drug reaction SJS/TEN
No reported immunologically mediated reactions	Altretamine Dactinomycin Nitrosoureas Vinca alkaloids	

Table 4 Chemotherapeutic agents associated with acral reactions.[a]

Acral erythema most common		Acral erythema least common		Hand-foot skin reaction	Keratoderma
Capecitabine	Doxorubicin	Floxuridine	Mitotane	Axitinib	Dabrafenib
Cisplatin	Etoposide	Idarubicin	Paclitaxel	Pazopanib	Vemurafenib
Cyclophosphamide	Fluorouracil	Lomustine	Pegylated liposomal doxorubicin	Regorafenib	
Cytarabine	Hydroxyurea	Melphalan	Suramin	Sorafenib	
Daunorubicin	Sorafenib	Mercaptopurine	Tegafur	Sunitinib	
Docetaxel	Sunitinib	Methotrexate	Troxacitabine	Vemurafenib	
Doxifluridine		Mitomycin	Vincristine		

[a]Source: Adapted from Seynaeve et al.[30]

capabilities of these drugs caused the patients to have a poor response to damage caused by pressure and trauma.[27,28] More recently, the Fas/Fas ligand response was implicated, proven by blocking the reaction by administering anti-Fas ligand antibody. These are the same mediators of Stevens–Johnson and TEN.[29] There are no FDA-approved treatments for HFSR, and potent topical steroids combined with drug holidays or dose reduction are commonly used for management.

Although more common in multikinase inhibitors such as sorafenib and sunitinib, HFSR has been reported with BRAF inhibitors among other drugs outlined in Table 4.[31] These are distinct from the more common hand-foot syndrome/acral erythema/toxic erythema of chemotherapy seen with cytotoxic chemotherapies. HFSR does not have the diffuse erythema and edema of hand-foot syndrome and also has a longer latency period before appearing (2–4 weeks). HFSR usually self-resolves with continued treatment with the multikinase inhibitors.[32]

mTOR inhibitors

Overlapping with the EGFR signaling pathway is the PI3K/AKT pathway, which activates mammalian target of rapamycin (mTOR). This molecule is associated with cell growth and angiogenesis. Sirolimus or rapamycin was the original drug in this category, followed by everolimus and temsirolimus. All are associated with the papulopustular rash of EGFR inhibitors, which has an incidence of 45.8% in the most recently developed drug, temsirolimus. They all also can induce the more classic morbilliform drug eruption and oral mucositis. As opposed to cytotoxic chemotherapies, individual deeper oral ulcerations more similar to aphthous stomatitis are present as well. Finally, everolimus and temsirolimus also had a population with eczematous dermatitides.[33] PI3K inhibitors, including idelalisib and alpelisib, have overlapping side effects, most commonly an erythematous morbilliform rash.[34]

BRAF inhibitors

BRAF inhibitors, first introduced in metastatic melanoma patients, have significant cutaneous side effects that include inflammatory, follicular, and neoplastic eruptions. These side effects lead to dose cessation or reduction in less than 10% of patients as management of these toxicities is well-established.[35] Of the inflammatory cutaneous toxicities, neutrophilic dermatoses, including acute febrile neutrophilic dermatosis (Sweet's syndrome) and neutrophilic panniculitis, have been attributed to the use of BRAF inhibitors.[36–43]

Three patients with the erythematous pseudovesicular papules and plaques of Sweet's syndrome of the trunk and extremities presenting with systemic symptoms of fever and arthralgias have been reported.[41–43] The patients with neutrophilic panniculitis presented with tender nodules of the legs and occasionally arms mimicking erythema nodosum, and had histology consistent with a neutrophilic lobular panniculitis.[37–40] Vitiligo,[44] cutaneous sarcoidosis,[45] Grover's disease,[46] and hidradenitis suppurativa[47] have been reported less commonly.

Patients on BRAF inhibitors also have increased radiation sensitivity to UV light and radiation therapy with quicker and more severe sunburns and acute radiation dermatitis, respectively.[48,49] Further, cases of radiation-recall dermatitis have been reported as well.[50,51]

Epidermal and follicular dysregulation contribute significantly to BRAF inhibitor cutaneous side effects. Palmoplantar hyperkeratosis or keratoderma (Table 4) is a thickening of the epidermis without inflammation presenting as thick yellow plaques of the palms and soles similar to a large callus. Most commonly, the keratoderma is seen on the feet in pressure points, without vesiculation.[52] A superficial keratotic plugging of the follicle results in a keratosis pilaris eruption. This is seen frequently on the trunk and extremities and is more often asymptomatic than pruritic. It was noted in 5–9% of patients in Phase 2 and 3 trials,[53,54] although probably underreported.[55–57]

Neoplastic lesions cause the highest morbidity in these patients. Actinic keratoses represent precancerous epithelial lesions typically associated with chronic sun damage. The incidence of actinic keratoses is 6–16% in vemurafenib patients[53–55] and 5–10% in dabrafenib patients.[52,58–60] Wart-like keratoses are hyperkeratotic papules that are often inflamed and appear in an eruptive nature during BRAF inhibitor therapy about 3–4 months after starting therapy.[60] These lesions are not true verruca as human papillomavirus testing has been negative in multiple reports.[61,62] Prompt treatment of both types of lesions with cryotherapy, photodynamic therapy, curettage, and topical 5-fluorouracil (5-FU) helps prevent cutaneous SCC formation.

Patients with SCC usually present with dome-shaped, well-demarcated, hyperkeratotic, erythematous papules, and nodules. They are quickly growing and more prevalent in older patients with chronic sun damage.[52]

The incidence of SCC is 4–31% in vemurafenib patients[53,54,63] and 6–11% in dabrafenib patients.[58,59,64,65] Sosman et al. showed that they are predominantly well-differentiated or keratoacanthoma-type SCC, which are less aggressive than the normal array of sun-induced SCC (Figure 2). The median time to occurrence is 8 weeks. HRAS upregulation has been implicated in a portion of BRAF-induced SCC causing a paradoxical upregulation of the MAP kinase pathway.[53]

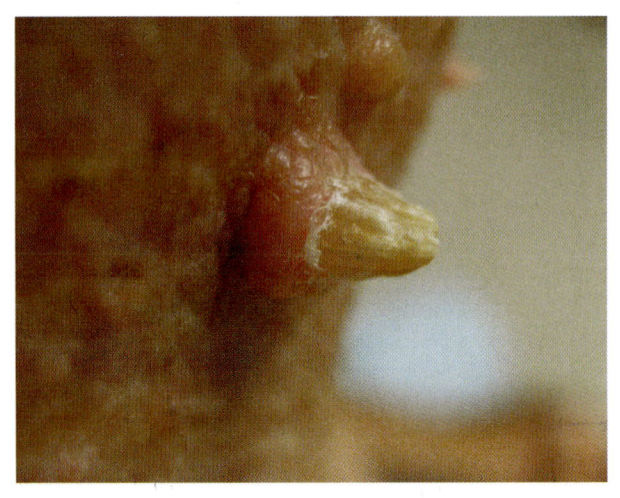

Figure 2 Squamous cell carcinoma with vemurafenib therapy.

Patients have been reported to have involution of nevi as well as new and darkening nevi.[66] The new nevi have shown wild-type BRAF and lack the V600E mutation and appear in 8 to 14 weeks.[67] These lesions have been biopsied as common nevi, dysplastic nevi, and new primary cutaneous melanomas. Five of 464 patients in the Phase 2 and 3 clinical trials with vemurafenib had a new melanoma occurring after start of therapy.[68]

MEK inhibitors

Selumetinib, trametinib, cobimetinib, and binimetinib are FDA-approved MEK inhibitors, and function downstream of BRAF inhibitors and have similar side effects to the EGFR inhibitors.[69] Interestingly, the addition of a MEK inhibitor to a BRAF inhibitor decreases the squamous proliferations seen with the BRAF inhibitor alone, possibly addressing the HRAS mutation as well.

Immunomodulators

With advances in biotechnology, there have been increased developments of cytokines and immunotherapeutic agents, which target cancer at the cellular level. This class of drugs is less specific than the targeted therapies described above and works by enhancing the inflammatory response to metastatic and hematologic tumors. The cutaneous side effects are less specific than those described above and generally encompass reactive inflammatory processes.

Immune checkpoint inhibitors

Immunomodulatory drugs used for melanoma include cytotoxic T-lymphocyte-associated protein 4 (CTLA4) inhibitors, programmed cell death protein 1 (PD-1) inhibitors, and programmed death-ligand 1 (PD-L1) inhibitors. Ipilimumab and tremelimumab are monoclonal antibodies targeting CTLA4, which inhibits binding of the costimulatory molecule, CD28. Blocking CTLA4 allows unopposed activation of cytotoxic T cells and stimulates the immune response to metastatic melanoma. The main side effects are morbilliform or eczematous drug eruptions, and vitiligo.[70] Similarly, nivolumab, cemiplimab, and pembrolizumab block PD-1, which, when bound to its ligand, decreases the cytotoxic effects of T cells. This molecule is upregulated in tumor cells and is thought to be more specific than ipilimumab. Finally, atezolizumab, avelumab, and durmalumab inhibit the PD-L1 molecule. The cutaneous side effects are similar to ipilimumab but also include bullous pemphigoid, psoriasis, lichenoid dermatitis, and SCC-like eruptions.[30,71–73] These drugs are being used as mono or combination therapy across many solid organ malignancies and have 30–60% incidence of cutaneous toxicities.

Cytokines

Roles have already been established for interleukin 2 (IL-2) as alternative treatment for advanced metastatic melanoma and renal cell cancer and for interferon-alpha (IFN-α) as standard treatment for chronic myelogenous leukemia, hairy-cell leukemia, cutaneous T-cell lymphoma, melanoma, and Kaposi sarcoma (KS). In addition to significant toxicities (Table 5) such as capillary leak syndrome, there is a 72% incidence of cutaneous reactions reported with IL-2.[74] Commonly, a pruritic diffuse erythroderma occurs 1–3 days after administration and resolves with desquamation two days after cessation of therapy.[74] This reaction is clinically

Table 5 Cytokine reactions.

Other IFN-α reactions	Other IL-2 reactions
Eosinophilic fasciitis	Erosions in surgical scars
Exacerbation of herpes labialis	Hypersensitivity to iodine contrast dye
Increased growth of eyelashes	Linear IgA bullous dermatosis
Necrotizing vasculitis	Pemphigus vulgaris (de novo, recurrent)
Paraneoplastic pemphigus	Poly/dermatomyositis exacerbation
Psoriasis exacerbation and de novo	Psoriasis exacerbation
SLE or cutaneous LE	Staphylococcal infections
	TEN-like bullous desquamation
	Vitiligo

Table 7 Chemotherapeutic agents associated with hair changes.

Hair color change	Hirsutism	Hair texture change
Bleomycin	Diethylstilbestrol	BRAF inhibitors
Cisplatin	EGFRIs	Cyclophosphamide
Cyclophosphamide	Fluoxymesterone	EGFR inhibitors
Methotrexate	Tamoxifen	Taxanes
Tamoxifen		
Anti-PD-1/PD-L1 inhibitors		
Sunitinib		

similar to toxic shock syndrome and has been associated with staphylococcal sepsis in some patients. Intra-arterial IL-2 also causes hypersensitivity to iodine-containing contrast dyes in up to 30% of patients.[75] Of potential importance, one study of IL-2 for metastatic melanoma reported a possible correlation between the development of vitiligo and good prognosis.[76] Although IFN-α is relatively less toxic than IL-2, several cutaneous reactions have been reported. One-third of patients develop a local injection-site reaction. In a study of 1000 patients receiving IFN-α, alopecia and herpes labialis exacerbation were common with 10% and 5% incidence, respectively.[75,77] Similar to nonmodified recombinant IFN-α, pegylated IFN-α has been shown to cause local cutaneous ulcerations at sites of subcutaneous injection.[78] Both IFN-α and IL-2 also induce and/or exacerbate seborrheic dermatitis and psoriasis.[75]

Alopecia

Alopecia is the most common dermatologic complication associated with chemotherapy. Whereas most drug-induced alopecias involve a telogen effluvium pattern by inducing normal hair to synchronize their cycles, the anagen effluvium pattern of hair loss is the most common type of alopecia produced by chemotherapeutic agents (Table 6), with the exception of interleukin-2 (IL-2) and IFN-α therapy. Following chemotherapy, anagen effluvium is caused by the abrupt cessation of the high mitotic activity of hair matrix cells in the anagen phase of hair follicles.[79] Anagen effluvium manifests within 1–2 weeks after the beginning of chemotherapy but is most noticeable 1–2 months later.[80] Hair regrowth can usually be expected 5 months after the end of chemotherapy, although hair color and texture may change (Table 7).[81] Persistent alopecia has been reported with busulfan/cyclophosphamide therapy.[82] More recently described is persistent chemotherapy-induced alopecia (PCIA) and scarring alopecia which can be persistent or permanent and should be noted by the oncology team.[83]

Hair loss often has emotional impact on patients receiving chemotherapy. Unfortunately, there are currently no widely accepted methods of prevention and treatment for alopecia. PCIA has shown some response to spironolactone and minoxidil, but scarring alopecia remains irreversible.[84,85] Scalp hypothermia has shown some benefit as a preventative measure in hair preservation during cancer therapy.[86]

Stomatitis

Stomatitis and other oral complications of cancer chemotherapy are discussed in this article.

Nail reactions

Hyperpigmentation is the most common nail abnormality encountered in patients receiving chemotherapy, particularly in dark-skinned patients.[87] Hyperpigmentation due to chemotherapy-induced melanocyte stimulation should be distinguished from yellow nail syndrome (YNS). YNS nails have increased transverse curvature, absent lunulae, and no cuticle. Suggested etiologies include paraneoplastic process, AIDS association, and drug induction.[88]

Other common nail manifestations include horizontal depressions of the nail plate called Beau's lines (Figure 3), horizontal white discoloration of the entire width of the nail plate called Mees lines, horizontal white discoloration involving partial nail width called leukonychia, onycholysis, and onychodystrophy. Associations between bleomycin and nail loss; hydroxyurea and brittle nails; etoposide and nail bed pigmentation have also been reported.[87,89] With the increased use of EGFR inhibitors,

Table 6 Chemotherapeutic agents associated with alopecia.

Most common		Least common		Persistent alopecia
Bleomycin	Ifosfamide	Amsacrine	Methotrexate	Busulfan
Cisplatin	Interferon-a	Busulfan	Mitomycin	Cyclophosphamide
Cyclophosphamide	Irinotecan	Carboplatin	Procarbazine	Tamoxifen
Cytarabine	Mechlorethamine	Carmustine	Sorafenib	Taxanes
Dacarbazine	Nitrosoureas	Chlorambucil epirubicin	Sunitinib	Vismodegib
Dactinomycin	Paclitaxel	Dabrafenib	Teniposide	
Daunorubicin	Thiotepa	Gemcitabine	Trametinib	
Docetaxel	Topotecan	Hydroxyurea	Vemurafenib	
Doxorubicin	Vinblastine	Melphalan	Vinorelbine	
Etoposide	Vincristine	Mercaptopurine		
Fluorouracil	Vindesine			
Idarubicin	Vismodegib			

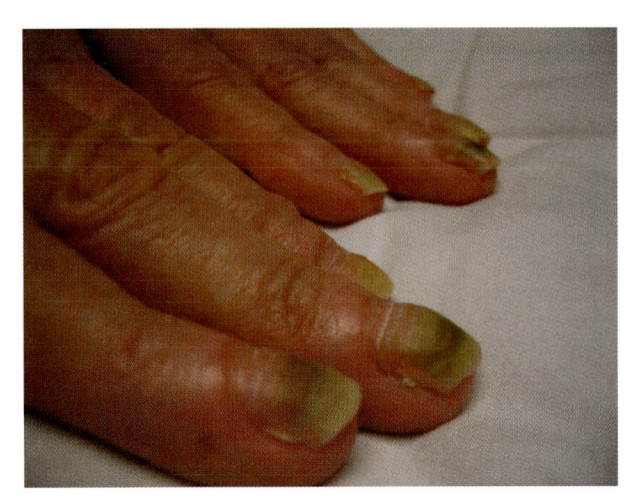

Figure 3 Hyperpigmentation and Beau's lines.

Table 8 Summary of nail abnormalities and associated chemoagents.

Onychopathy	Associated chemoagents
Acute paronychia	EGFR inhibitors, MEK inhibitors, methotrexate, mTOR inhibitors, taxanes
Beau's lines	Bleomycin, cisplatin, doxorubicin, melphalan, taxanes, vincristine
Ischemic changes	Bleomycin, busulfan, cyclophosphamide, doxorubicin, etoposide, melphalan, methotrexate, nitrogen mustard, taxanes
Melanonychia	Aminoglutethimide, bleomycin, busulfan, capecitabine, cisplatin, cyclophosphamide, dacarbazine, daunorubicin, docetaxel, doxorubicin, fluorouracil, hydroxyurea, idarubicin, ifosfamide, imatinib, melphalan, methotrexate, mitomycin, mitoxantrone
Nonmelanotic pigmentation	5-FU, vorinostat
Muehrcke lines	Cyclophosphamide, doxorubicin, leucovorin, levamisole, methotrexate, vincristine
Onycholysis	Bleomycin, capecitabine, doxorubicin, EGFR inhibitors, etoposide, fluorouracil, MEK inhibitors, mitoxantrone, mTOR inhibitors, taxanes
Onychomadesis, defluvium unguium	Bleomycin, fluorouracil, mercaptopurine, mitoxantrone, taxanes
Pyogenic granuloma	Cetuximab, EGFR inhibitors, gefitinib, MEK inhibitors, mTOR inhibitors
Transverse leukonychia	Adriamycin, cyclophosphamide, doxorubicin, vincristine

paronychia, or inflammation of the nail fold, is seen commonly and can be extremely painful—this reaction is also seen with MEK inhibitors, mTOR inhibitors, and PI3K inhibitors. Superinfections with *Staphylococcus aureus* and *Candida albicans* are common. Other onychopathies and their associated chemoagents are summarized in Table 8.[90–94] Patients can be reassured that these nail changes are generally benign and resolve after discontinuation of the causative agent and the affected nails grow out. However, nails damaged by chemotherapy are more susceptible to infection by yeast, dermatophytes, and pseudomonas. Infections may cause lasting damage to the matrix that will not resolve.

Extravasation reactions

Extravasation injury is a well-known adverse event that occurs when offending drugs escape from the veins or intravenous

Table 9 Chemotherapeutic agents associated with chemical cellulitis.

Most common		Least common	
Dactinomycin	Amsacrine	Esorubicin	Plicamycin
Daunorubicin	Bisantrene	Etoposide	Pyrazofurin
Doxorubicin	Bleomycin	Fluorouracil	Streptozocin
Mitomycin	Carmustine	Idarubicin	Vinblastine
	Chlorozotocin	Mechlorethamine	Vincristine
	Cisplatin	Melphalan	Vindesine
	Dacarbazine	Mitoxantrone	Vinorelbine
	Epirubicin	Paclitaxel	

catheters into subcutaneous tissues. Accidental extravasation occurs in approximately 0.1–6% of patients receiving intravenous chemotherapy[95] (Table 9). The cutaneous manifestations of extravasation may range from discomfort and mild erythema to severely painful skin necrosis, ulcerations, and damage to deep tissue structures.

Extravasated cytotoxic agents cause two types of local cutaneous reactions: irritant and vesicant reactions. Irritants cause a short-lived and self-limited phlebitis and tender, warm, erythematous reaction along the vein or at the site of intravenous administration. A variant of this local irritation is an erythematous and urticarial hypersensitivity flare reaction that has been associated with the anthracyclines. Vesicants initially cause a similar reaction; however, the irritation may worsen, depending on the amount of drug that has extravasated, leading to nerve and tendon damage and subsequent neurologic deficits, contractures, and joint stiffness. The extent of tissue damage in extravasation largely depends on the concentration, volume, and vesicant nature of the extravasated agent.[95,96]

Paclitaxel can induce an extravasation recall reaction, in which extravasation of the agent at one site has induced a cutaneous reaction, ranging from erythema to ulcerations, at a previous extravasation site.[97] Central lines may dislodge, or venous vessels may be perforated with potentially disastrous consequences, including mediastinitis presenting with fever, severe pleuritic pain, upper extremity and neck swelling, and a widened mediastinum.

Vesicant injury displays poor healing and often continues to worsen, necessitating surgical intervention. Vesicants delay fibroblastic wound contraction and have the ability to bind to DNA, possibly allowing them to be recycled and retained in the tissue to induce damage for a longer duration.[96] One-third of all vesicant extravasations will develop into ulcerations; vigilant recognition and management of extravasation play a major role in limiting tissue injury.[98] When extravasation is suspected, prompt discontinuation of the infusion is recommended, followed by aspiration of residual drug and removal of the catheter. Local cold application and elevation of the affected extremity are commonly used and helpful.[97] Intermittent local cooling alone has an 89.1% success rate in preventing ulceration.[99] For the vinca alkaloids, heat application is recommended instead, as cold application may actually induce ulceration.[98]

The use of antidotes is controversial, and some antidotes such as sodium bicarbonate may be harmful or ulcerative. Sodium thiosulfate (mechlorethamine), hyaluronidase (vinca alkaloids), granulocyte-macrophage colony-stimulating factor (doxorubicin), and pyridoxine (mitomycin) have been recommended as local injections.[100–102] The success of locally injected corticosteroids has been variable as few inflammatory cells are involved in extravasation reactions.[102] Whether a local antidote has a specific effect or acts as a diluent is hard to determine. Locally injected saline

Table 10 Chemotherapeutic agents associated with hyperpigmentation or pigmentation changes.

Targeted therapy	Alkylating agents	Antibiotics nucleoside analogues	Antimetabolites	Miscellaneous combined regimens
Imatinib	Busulfan	Bleomycin	Brequinar sodium	Bleomycin/doxorubicin/vincristine
Sunitinib (yellow)	Cisplatin	Dactinomycin	Docetaxel	Busulfan/cyclophosphamide
	Cyclophosphamide	Daunorubicin	Fluorouracil	Cyclophosphamide/doxorubicin/vincris-tine/prednisone
	Fotemustine	Doxorubicin	Hydroxyurea	Cyclophosphamide/etoposide/carboplatin
	Ifosfamide	Gemcitabine	Methotrexate	Doxorubicin/bleomycin/vinblastine/dacarbazine
	Thiotepa	Mitoxantrone	Procarbazine	
			Tegafur	
	Topical carmustine	Plicamycin	Vinorelbine	Ifosfamide/carboplatin/etoposide
	Topical mechlorethamine	Troxacitabine		Methotrexate/cytarabine/lasparaginase/daunorubicin/mercaptopurine/cyclophosphamide

alone has proven successful in resolving extravasation reactions and preventing ulceration.[103] Although conservative treatment is preferable for most vesicant extravasations, early excision is sometimes favored, especially when the most potent vesicants are involved.[103,104] For topical therapy, the free-radical scavenger dimethyl sulfoxide (DMSO) has shown consistent therapeutic success. In 1995, an analysis of 96 cumulative patients from multiple studies showed that DMSO protected 98.3% of extravasation cases from ulceration.[105]

Pigmentary changes

Hyperpigmentation is a common cutaneous manifestation that may be of cosmetic and emotional concern to patients. The skin, mucous membranes, hair, teeth, and nails may be affected, and the reaction may be diffuse or localized. Hyperpigmentation most commonly accompanies use of alkylating agents, antitumor antibiotics, and gemcitabine (Table 10).[89,106,107] Among the antimetabolites, methotrexate may produce a characteristic hair "flag sign" with horizontal hyperpigmented bands alternating with normal hair color in light-haired individuals.[89] Tegafur can induce hyperpigmentation of the palms, soles, nails, and glans penis in a third of patients receiving the drug. A flagellate, band-like hyperpigmentation in areas of trauma also occurs with high incidence in 8–20% of patients receiving bleomycin (Figure 4). Busulfan's hyperpigmentation can mimic Addison's disease, with symptoms of weakness, weight loss, and diarrhea, but with normal melanocyte-stimulating hormone and adrenocorticotropic hormone serum levels.[81] The mechanism of chemotherapy-induced hyperpigmentation reactions is unknown but may involve direct toxicity, melanocyte stimulation, and postinflammatory changes. Although these reactions may occasionally be permanent, in most cases, discoloration will gradually resolve after the discontinuation of the chemotherapy.

Vitiligo, a complete absence of melanocytes resulting in depigmentation, is seen with targeted drug therapies, particularly those used in the treatment of metastatic melanoma[44,70,71,108,109] (Table 11). It presents with asymptomatic, depigmented patches,

Table 11 Chemotherapeutic agents associated with depigmentation/vitiligo.

Vemurafenib	Gefitinib
Dabrafenib	Interferon
Labrolizumab	IL-2
Imatinib	Immune checkpoint inhibitors (CTLA-4, PD-1, and PD-L1)

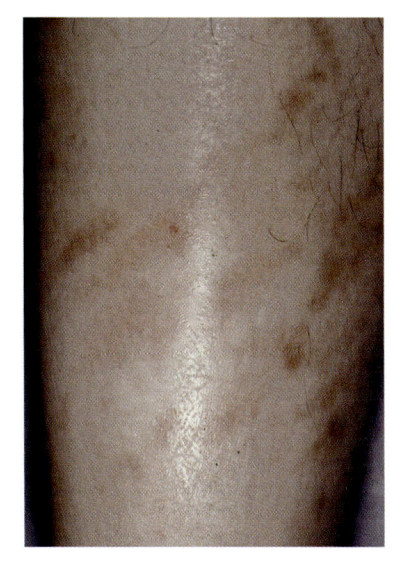

Figure 4 Cutaneous flagellate hyperpigmentation of bleomycin.

often symmetrical in distribution, not necessarily related to sites of disease. Although speculated to be related to disease response, this has not been proven.

Radiation-associated reactions

Radiation can include environmental exposure to ultraviolet rays as well as therapeutic radiation exposure. Three different types of reactions have been noted: enhancement or recall at radiation sites or generalized photosensitivity (Tables 12 and 13).

Radiation enhancement

Enhancement of radiation therapy may occur when both chemotherapy and radiation therapy are given within 1 week of each other. Although other organs are also affected by this potentiation, the skin is the most common site of this toxicity. The reaction may appear as dry or moist desquamation, or as erythema and edema. When bullae, erosions, crusts, and ulcerations accompany erythema, *Staphylococcus* is usually the causative factor, and systemic antibiotics should be given according to culture results.[110] The degree of enhancement of radiation damage depends on and is inversely related to, the time interval between administration of the drug and radiation. The less time there is between chemotherapy and irradiation, the greater the enhancement

Table 12 Chemotherapeutic agents implicated in radiation-associated reactions.

Radiation enhancement	Radiation recall	
Bleomycin	Bleomycin	Hydroxyurea
Camptothecins	Cyclophosphamide	Idarubicin
Chlorambucil	Cytarabine	Lomustine
Cisplatin[a]	Dabrafenib	Melphalan
Cyclophosphamide[a]	Dactinomycin	Methotrexate
Dactinomycin	Daunorubicin	Oxaliplatin
Dabrafenib	Doxorubicin	Paclitaxel
Doxorubicin	Docetaxel	Tamoxifen
Fluorouracil	Edatrexate	Triazinate
Hydroxyurea	Etoposide	Trimetrexate
Interferons	Fluorouracil	Vemurafenib
Mercaptopurine	Gemcitabine	Vinblastine
Methotrexate		
Triazinate		
Vemurafenib		
Vincristine[a]		

[a]Reported only in combination drug regimens.

Table 13 Chemotherapeutic agents associated with phototoxicity.

Brequinar sodium	Methotrexate
Dabrafenib	Mitomycin C
Dacarbazine	Porphyrins
Dactinomycin	Procarbazine
Doxorubicin	Tegafur
EGFR inhibitors	
Fluorouracil	Thioguanine
Flutamide	Vandetanib
Hydroxyurea	Vemurafenib
Imatinib	Vinblastine

effect.[111] Enhancement is also dependent on drug dosage and the pharmacologic mechanism of the drug.[87]

Radiation recall

Radiation recall is an erythematous inflammatory reaction in areas of previously irradiated skin or sunburned skin. This includes the inflammation of actinic keratoses, which are caused by chronic sun exposure. Severe radiation dermatitis can even spread to areas outside the portal as an id reaction. Radiation recall occurs from 8 days up to 15 years after radiation therapy and may also occur in other organs.[89] The radiation dosage and the time interval between radiation and chemotherapy determine the occurrence and severity of recall, respectively.[112] The UV recall reaction is observed with suramin (35% incidence), methotrexate, vemurafenib, and etoposide/cyclophosphamide therapy, which causes a sunburn reactivation if the drugs are administered within 1 week of obtaining a sunburn.[113]

Inflammation of actinic keratoses (AKs), known as an AK recall reaction, is common in elderly patients with fair complexion and history of sun damage and may be confused with a drug rash (Table 14). Suramin and cytarabine-induced inflammation of seborrheic keratosis and fludarabine-induced SCC have also been reported. The association between systemic fluorouracil and the irritation of clinical and subclinical AKs is well-known

Table 14 Miscellaneous reactions of interest.

AGEP	**Erythema nodosum**	**Flushing (cont)**	**Nonmelanoma skin cancer**
Erlotinib	Busulfan	Plicamycin	BRAF inhibitors
Imatinib	BRAF inhibitors	Procarbazine	JAK inhibitors
Lapatinib	Diethylstilbestrol	Suramin	Nitrogen mustard (topical)
Bullous pemphigoid	IL-2	Tamoxifen	Sorafenib
Dactinomycin/MTX	Imatinib	Teniposide	**Porphyria**
PD-1/PD-L1 inhibitors	**Fixed-drug eruption**	Trimetrexate	Busulfan (PCT)
Capillaritis	Dacarbazine	**Folliculitis**	Cisplatin
Aminoglutethimide	Hydroxyurea	Dactinomycin	Chlorambucil (AIP)
Cutaneous adherence, acquired	Paclitaxel (bullous)	Daunorubicin	Cyclophosphamide (PCT)
Doxorubicin/ketoconazole	Procarbazine	Fluorouracil	Diethylstilbestrol (PCT)
Cutaneous ulcers	**Flushing**	MEK inhibitors	Methotrexate (PCT)
Hydroxyurea	L-Asparaginase	Methotrexate	Cyclophosphamide
IFN-α, pegylated IFN-α		EGFR inhibitors	**Pustular psoriasis**
IL-2	Bleomycin	**Inflammation of actinic keratoses**	Aminoglutethimide
Methotrexate	Carboplatin	Dactinomycin/vincristine/dacarbazine	Pegylated liposomal doxorubicin
Dermatitis herpetiformis, flare	Carmustine (BCNU)	Docetaxel	PD-1 inhibitors
Cyclophosphamide/doxorubicin/vincristine	Cisplatin	Doxorubicin/cytarabine/thioguanine	Steroids
Bleomycin	Cyclophosphamide	Doxorubicin/vincristine	**Seborrheic dermatitis, flare**
Cisplatin	Dacarbazine	Fluorouracil	Fluorouracil
Vincristine	Didemnin B (not used anymore?)	Fluorouracil/cisplatin	IL-2
Dermatomyositis-like reaction	Diethylstilbestrol	Pentostatin	IFN-α
Hydroxyurea	Docetaxel		Sorafenib
ICIs	Doxorubicin		**Telangiectasia**
Tamoxifen	Etoposide		Carmustine (BCNU)
Tegafur	Fluorouracil		Fluorouracil (topical)
Bleomycin	Flutamide		Hydroxyurea
Docetaxel	High dose IL-2		IFN-α
Drug-induced SLE	Leuprolide		
Aminoglutethimide	Lomustine		
Diethylstilbestrol	Paclitaxel		
Hydroxyurea			
ICIs			
IFN-α			
Leuprolide			
Tegafur			

and resembles the same effect produced by topical application of 5-FU. AK recall reactions usually appear 1 week following the initiation of drug administration and usually resolve 1–4 weeks following the end of therapy or they may regress during therapy as well.[114] This recall reaction may be due to a process similar to radiation recall or increased DNA synthesis in AK lesions and consequently higher chemo agent uptake.[114,115] Although these lesions are self-limiting, superficial ulceration and staphylococcal colonization can occur and necessitate antibiotics or corticosteroids. The reaction may or may not recur with drug readministration. Similar to the effect of topical 5-FU on AKs, systemic fluorouracil often clears the affected AKs after the inflammatory reaction resolves.[116]

The mechanism of the recall reaction is thought to be similar to 5-FU killing of AKs when applied to skin. It has been theorized that impaired tissue repair may be a result of inadequate stem cell reserve or mutations in cells that survived radiation.[117]

Generally, the treatment for radiation-associated reactions is symptomatic with an effort to avoid or treat secondary infections with appropriate antibiotics. Severe ulcerative and necrotic reactions may necessitate debridement if infection is ruled out. Topical mupirocin and systemic corticosteroids are mainstays in the treatment of radiation recall and may even allow continuation of the offending drug without further recall effects.[117]

Photosensitivity

Finally, cutaneous reactions related to chemotherapy and ultraviolet (UV) light exposure have been well documented, though they are relatively infrequent (Table 13). Generally, most of these reactions involve exogenous phototoxicity with the agents acting as chromophores. Both clinically and histologically, these phototoxic reactions appear as exaggerated sunburns. Phototoxicity has also been reported to affect the nails in the form of mercaptopurine-induced photo-onycholysis, which is tender and usually involves the distal third of the nail.

Another form of photosensitivity is the photoallergy that has been described with flutamide and tegafur, in which the photodistributed cutaneous reaction recurs with readministration of the implicated agent. This has also been observed with vandetanib.[118]

Therapy for photosensitivity reactions is symptomatic with topical corticosteroids and antipruritics. Severe cases may require systemic steroids. Chloroquine and β-carotene have been used for prophylaxis but were not effective in controlled studies.[119] As the agent may remain in the patient's skin for several weeks, patients should be advised to take sun-avoidance measures.

Acral reactions

Three types of acral reactions have been described; the more classical acral erythema (AE), HFSR seen with targeted therapies, and keratoderma seen with BRAF inhibitors (Table 4). Acral erythema has many names, including hand-foot syndrome and toxic erythema of chemotherapy.

AE was first reported in association with chemotherapy by Zuehlke in 1974.[120] Other names include palmoplantar erythrodysesthesia, palmoplantar erythema, hand-foot syndrome, peculiar AE, and Burgdorf reaction. There is a prodrome of dysesthesia of the palms and soles, evolving into painful, tingling, symmetric, well-demarcated swelling, and erythema (Figure 5),

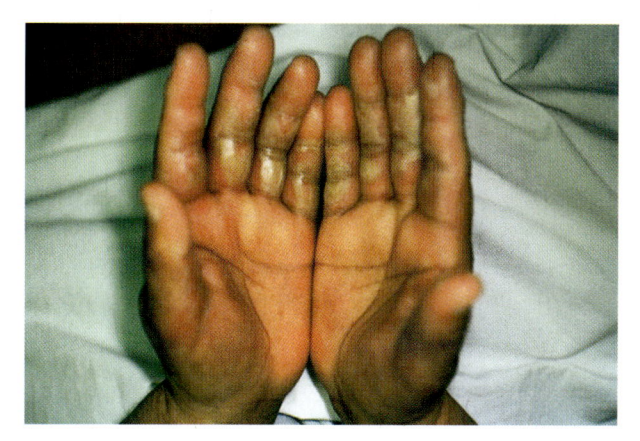

Figure 5 Desquamation phase of hand-and-foot syndrome, secondary to capecitabine.

followed by a desquamative phase on resolution. Erythema and swelling usually appear on the thenar and hypothenar eminences, lateral aspect of the fingers, and the pads of the distal phalanges. The hands are more often affected than the feet. In its various manifestations, AE may appear as alternating bands of erythema and sparing and may also be accompanied by a mild erythema or a morbilliform eruption on the trunk, neck, chest, scalp, and extremities.[121] Methotrexate and cytarabine can reportedly induce a bullous variant of AE, which may progress to full-thickness epidermal necrosis before resolving.[122]

AE occurs with an incidence of 6–42% in different series and occurs mostly in adults.[123] AE appears to be dose-dependent on peak levels and total cumulative dose, as it occurs earlier and more severely after bolus infusions (24 h to 3 weeks), as compared with continuous low-dose administration (2–10 months).[121,124] AE tends to persist and worsen with further continuation of chemotherapy and may be dose limiting, as the associated pain may progress to become physically and functionally limiting. Cessation of the causative agent will allow resolution of AE in 1–2 weeks, with desquamation and re-epithelialization (Figure 6). AE may or may not recur with readministration. The treatment of AE is symptomatic, aimed at increasing tolerability to allow continued chemotherapy. Corticosteroids have shown variable success. Supportive treatment includes topical wound care, elevation, and pain medication. Similar to the concept of scalp hypothermia for alopecia, the cooling of hands and feet may help prevent AE.[124] Celecoxib, a cyclooxygenase 2 (COX-2) inhibitor, was shown to decrease the incidence of AE in a retrospective study of 67 patients with metastatic colorectal cancer who took capecitabine.[125] Celecoxib also attenuated capecitabine-induced diarrhea, increased tumor response, and increased median time to tumor progression compared with capecitabine alone. Pyridoxine may also reduce dysesthesia and pain to allow continuation of therapy.[126]

The pathogenesis of AE is currently unknown, but it is likely multifactorial. Biopsies of AE appear histologically nonspecific but are consistent with a toxic reaction.[124] In the setting of chemotherapy, diagnosis of AE is a relatively simple matter. However, in bone marrow transplant (BMT) patients, it may be difficult to differentiate from acute GVHD. There is a 35% incidence of AE in BMT patients, which may be due to the use of higher doses of chemotherapy and total body irradiation.[127] Histologically and clinically, AE may resemble acute GVHD in the first 3 weeks: As in AE, the palms are commonly affected in acute GVHD

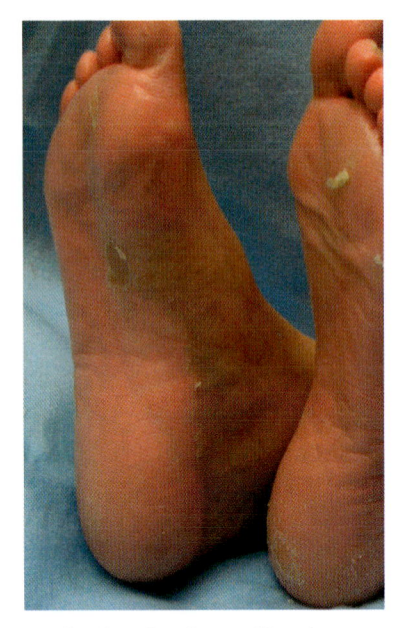

Figure 6 Chemo-induced acral erythema of the soles.

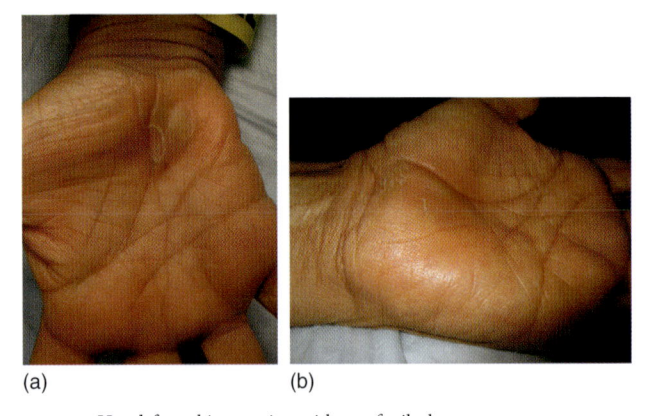

Figure 7 Hand-foot skin reaction with sorafenib therapy.

although it usually progresses with involvement of other areas of the body. Since early biopsies of acute GVHD mimic AE, serial biopsies at 3 to 5-day intervals are helpful in establishing patterns of progression supportive of acute GVHD.[127] Distinguishing AE from acute GVHD is important because the latter requires greater intervention with further immunosuppression; without treatment, it usually progresses and may be fatal.

HFSR is most commonly seen with multikinase inhibitors sorafenib, sunitinib, and regorafenib. It is also seen with VEGFR inhibitors and has been reported with MEK inhibitors. It is distinguished from AE by the focal nature, overlying calluses, and tendency to vesiculate (Figure 7). The keratoderma seen with BRAF inhibitors is a diffuse thickening of the stratus corneum that presents as a large hyperkeratotic plaque of the soles without erythema; it is usually asymptomatic.

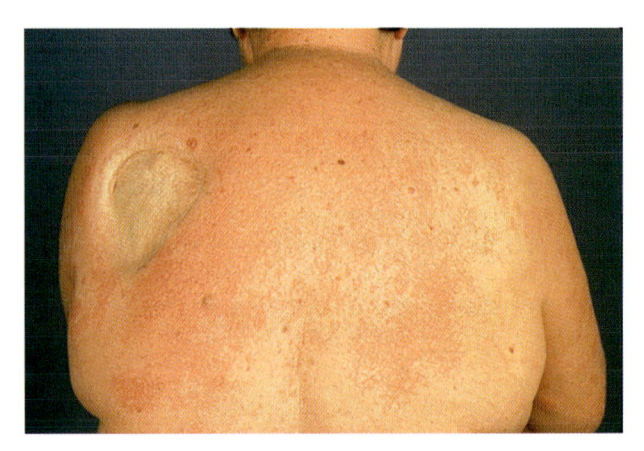

Figure 8 Erythematous rash associated with IL-2 therapy in a melanoma patient.

Cutaneous eruption of lymphocyte recovery

The cutaneous eruption of lymphocyte recovery (ELR) may be seen in patients receiving intensive marrow aplasia-inducing chemotherapy.[128] As with ESS, the ELR phenomenon has been observed with various cytotoxic agents but is not associated with a particular agent. Clinically, ELR has the appearance of variably distributed erythematous and pruritic macules, papules, and plaques, which may become confluent and erythrodermic, and is often associated with a couple of days of fever. In the setting of chemotherapy, this reaction has been found to occur 6–21 days after the chemotherapy-induced nadir of the leukocyte count, which correlates with the time of the initial recovery of peripheral lymphocytes (Figure 8). ELR may reflect the return of highly alloreactive immunocompetent lymphocytes to the peripheral circulation and skin.[128] ELR is self-limited and resolves over several days with desquamation and mild residual hyperpigmentation. The differential diagnosis includes acute GVHD, sepsis, viral exanthem, leukemia or lymphoma cutis, eccrine syringosqumaous metaplasia, and drug hypersensitivity. Of these types of eruptions, acute GVHD is similar in time of onset to ELR in the setting of bone marrow transplantation. The similarity with ELR is especially true in the case of autologous GVHD, as both involve a lymphocytic recovery in which histocompatibility is present. However, acute autologous GVHD cannot be reliably distinguished from ELR by skin biopsy.[129] As theorized by Horn, GVHD may represent a prolonged form of ELR.[130]

Summary

Cutaneous AEs are increasing in incidence and relavence to cancer patients, particularly as combination therapies become more prevalent. A summary of the above major classes of toxicities, diagnostic pearls, and treatment guidance is included in Table 15.

Table 15 Diagnosis and management of cutaneous reactions associated with chemotherapeutic agents.

			Diagnosis	Management
Hair	Changes in color	Hypopigmentation or hyperpigmentation	History and physical	Cessation of treatment if necessary Reversible
	Changes in texture	Kinking or curling of hair	History and physical Brittle, kinky texture Tight curling	Cessation of treatment if necessary Reversible
	Cicatricial alopecia	Not common with systemic cancer therapy.	Pruritus	Topical or intralesional steroids Dose reduction or cessation of treatment
			Erythema and perifollicular scale Scalp biopsy	Irreversible
	Nonscarring alopecia (hair will grow back after cancer treatment)	Immune-mediated alopecia areata	History	Topical or intralesional steroids
			Smooth, round, and irregular areas of hair loss without inflammation	Reversible
			Positive hair pull test at periphery of alopecic patches	
		Telogen effluvium	History	Identify and correct the underlying stressor
			Positive hair pull test	Reversible
		Anagen effluvium (most common)	History and physical	Topical minoxidil solution
				Scalp cooling during chemotherapy Camouflage makeup Reversible
		Persistent chemotherapy-induced alopecia	History	Topical minoxidil
			Incomplete hair growth after postcancer therapy	Spironolactone
		Endocrine therapy associated with alopecia	History	Topical minoxidil
			Positive hair pull test	Spironolactone
Nail	Dystrophy	Onycholysis	Separation of nail plate from nail bed can be caused by fungal infection	Monitor for superinfections, Cessation of treatment if necessary
		Onychomadesis	Nail plate divided in to two parts by a traverse thick groove called sulcus, nail ultimately sheds	Self-limiting, cessation of treatment if necessary
	Periungual changes	Paronychia	Inflammation of nail folds	Initial treatment with warm water and antiseptic soaks Keep hands dry and high-dose topical steroids Topical tacrolimus is an alternative Surgery for recalcitrant disease Manage superinfections
		Pyogenic granuloma	Erythematous dome-shaped friable papule of nail fold	Topical application of liquid nitrogen, topical steroids, weekly 10% aqueous silver nitrate can reduce granulation tissues
			Biopsy	Granulation tissues can also be removed by electrodesiccation 88% phenol or 35% trichloroacetic acid topical are viable treatments
	Pigment changes	Leukonychia	White coloration of the nail plate	Cessation of treatment if necessary
		Melanonychia	Nails can be diffusely black/brown or alternating dark brown and white lines	Cessation of treatment if necessary
		Nonmelanocytic pigmentation	Xanthochromia or orange (subungual hemorrhages)	Cessation of treatment if necessary
Skin	Acral	Acral erythema/hand-foot syndrome	Dysaesthesia, pain, redness, and/or swelling	Cessation of treatment if necessary
				Avoid friction, heat, and pressure
		Hand-foot skin reaction	Hyperkeratotic lesions on erythematous base	Grade 1: Moisturize with urea-based cream and use keratolytic emollients with urea; topical analgesics lidocaine 5%
			Tender to palpation	Grade 2: Continue above in addition to superpotent topical steroids and oral analgesics like NSAIDS and GABA agonists Grade 3: Hold drug, continue recommendations
		Keratoderma	Diffuse or focal thickening of the skin	Emollients Keratolytic agents Topical/oral retinoids Calcipotriol

(continued overleaf)

Table 15 (Continued)

		Diagnosis	Management
Inflammatory dermatoses	Acneiform	Erythematous follicular papules and pustules	Grade 1: topical steroid cream Grade 2: topical steroids and oral tetracyclines Grade 3: topical steroids, oral low dose steroids, and oral tetracyclines Recalcitrant severe rash: isotretinoin or acitretin
	Eczematous	Red rough papules coalescing into plaques	Topical steroids Systemic immunomodulators
	Lichenoid	Violaceous papules with fine silvery scale	Topical steroids Acitretin Systemic immunomodulators
	Psoriatic	Well-demarcated erythematous plaque with adherent scale	Topical steroids Topical vitamin D analogs Topical retinoids Systemic immunomodulators
Neoplastic	Keratoses	Hyperkeratotic papule	Conservative symptomatic removal Reversible
	Lentigines	Well demarcated homogenous hyperpigmented macules and papules Biopsy if suspicious	No treatment Irreversible
	Melanoma	Irregular pigmented macule or papule Biopsy	Wide-local excision Stage-indicated further treatment
	Squamous cell carcinoma	Erythematous hyperkeratotic papule Biopsy	Electrodessication and curettage Surgical removal Intralesional chemotherapy Unknown if reversible as we treat them
Neutrophilic dermatoses	Erythema nodosum	Tender erythematous subcutaneous nodules Biopsy	Pain management Systemic corticosteroids
	Pyoderma gangrenosum	Painful full thickness rapidly enlarging ulcer Positive pathergy test, nonspecific Biopsy to rule out other causes of ulceration	Small ulcers: Potent topical, intralesional, or systemic corticosteroids Cyclosporine Tacrolimus
	Sweet's syndrome	Painful erythematous pseudovesicular papules and plaques Biopsy	Topical steroids Dapsone Colchicine Systemic immunomodulators
Pigmentary changes	Hyperpigmentation	Darkening of skin	Reversible
	Vitiligo	Pigment loss in patches	Topical steroids Topical JAKi UVB light therapy
Toxic	Acute generalized exanthematous pustulosis	Febrile pustular eruption and edematous erythema Culture negative for bacteria Biopsy	Drug discontinuation For symptomatic relief and pruritis, use topical steroids Systemic immunomodulators
	Stevens Johnson Syndrome/toxic epidermal necrolysis	Rapidly progressing painful erythematous papules and plaques, diffuse erythema with vesicles and bullae, mucosal involvement, positive Nikolsky sign Biopsy	Drug discontinuation Supportive care +/− IVIG +/− high dose steroids

Key references

The complete reference list can be found on Vital Source version of this title, see inside front cover.

1 Revuz J, Laurence V-A. Drug reactions. In: Bolognia J et al., eds. *Dermatology*, 3rd ed. Elsevier Saunders; 2012.

6 Tan AR, Steinberg SM, Parr AL, et al. Markers in the epidermal growth factor receptor pathway and skin toxicity during erlotinib treatment. *Ann Oncol*. 2008;**19**(1):185–190.

8 Busam KJ, Capodieci P, Motzer R, et al. Cutaneous side-effects in cancer patients treated with the antiepidermal growth factor receptor antibody C225. *Br J Dermatol*. 2001;**144**(6):1169–1176.

10 Hidalgo M, Siu LL, Nemunaitis J, et al. Phase I and pharmacologic study of OSI-774, an epidermal growth factor receptor tyrosine kinase inhibitor, in patients with advanced solid malignancies. *J Clin Oncol*. 2001;**19**:3267–3279.

11 Boone SL, Rademaker A, Liu D, et al. Impact and management of skin toxicity associated with anti-epidermal growth factor receptor therapy: survey results. *Oncology*. 2007;**72**(3–4):152–159.

12 Saltz LB, Meropol NJ, Loehrer PJ, et al. Phase II trial of cetuximab in patients with refractory colorectal cancer that expresses the epidermal growth factor receptor. *J Clin Oncol*. 2004;**22**:1201–1208.

13 Lacouture ME. Mechanisms of cutaneous toxicities to EGFR inhibitors. *Nat Rev Cancer*. 2006;**6**(10):803–812.

25 Amitay-laish I, Stemmer SM, Lacouture ME. Adverse cutaneous reactions secondary to tyrosine kinase inhibitors including imatinib mesylate, nilotinib, and dasatinib. *Dermatol Ther*. 2011;**24**(4):386–395.

26 Balagula Y, Lacouture ME, Cotliar JA. Dermatologic toxicities of targeted anticancer therapies. *J Support Oncol*. 2010;**8**(4):149–161.

27 Chu D, Lacouture ME, Fillos T, Wu S. Risk of hand-foot skin reaction with sorafenib: a systematic review and meta-analysis. *Acta Oncol*. 2008;**47**(2):176–186.

28. Chu D, Lacouture ME, Weiner E, Wu S. Risk of hand-foot skin reaction with the multitargeted kinase inhibitor sunitinib in patients with renal cell and non-renal cell carcinoma: a meta-analysis. *Clin Genitourin Cancer*. 2009;7(1):11–19.
31. Boyd KP, Vincent B, Andea A, et al. Nonmalignant cutaneous findings associated with vemurafenib use in patients with metastatic melanoma. *J Am Acad Dermatol*. 2012;67(6):1375–1379.
33. Balagula Y, Rosen A, Tan BH, et al. Clinical and histopathologic characteristics of rash in cancer patients treated with mammalian target of rapamycin inhibitors. *Cancer*. 2012;118(20):5078–5083.
35. Lacouture ME, Duvic M, Hauschild A, et al. Analysis of dermatologic events in vemurafenib-treated patients with melanoma. *Oncologist*. 2013;18(3):314–322.
39. Monfort JB, Pagès C, Schneider P, et al. Vemurafenib-induced neutrophilic panniculitis. *Melanoma Res*. 2012;22(5):399–401.
40. Sinha R, Edmonds K, Newton-bishop J, et al. Erythema nodosum-like panniculitis in patients with melanoma treated with vemurafenib. *J Clin Oncol*. 2013;31(19):e320–e321.
41. Yorio JT, Mays SR, Ciurea AM, et al. Case of vemurafenib-induced Sweet's syndrome. *J Dermatol*. 2014. doi: 10.1111/1346-8138.12430.
42. Pattanaprichakul P, Tetzlaff MT, Lapolla WJ, et al. Sweet syndrome following vemurafenib therapy for recurrent cholangiocarcinoma. *J Cutan Pathol*. 2014;41(3):326–328.
49. Satzger I, Degen A, Asper H, et al. Serious skin toxicity with the combination of BRAF inhibitors and radiotherapy. *J Clin Oncol*. 2013;31(13):e220–e222.
55. Huang V, Hepper D, Anadkat M, Cornelius L. Cutaneous toxic effects associated with vemurafenib and inhibition of the BRAF pathway. *Arch Dermatol*. 2012;148(5):628–633.
60. Anforth RM, Blumetti TC, Kefford RF, et al. Cutaneous manifestations of dabrafenib (GSK2118436): a selective inhibitor of mutant BRAF in patients with metastatic melanoma. *Br J Dermatol*. 2012;167(5):1153–1160.
67. Cohen PR, Bedikian AY, Kim KB. Appearance of new vemurafenib-associated melanocytic nevi on normal-appearing skin: case series and a review of changing or new pigmented lesions in patients with metastatic malignant melanoma after initiating treatment with vemurafenib. *J Clin Aesthet Dermatol*. 2013;6(5):27–37.
69. Curry JL, Torres-cabala CA, Kim KB, et al. Dermatologic toxicities to targeted cancer therapy: shared clinical and histologic adverse skin reactions. *Int J Dermatol*. 2014;53(3):376–384.
70. Lacouture ME, Wolchok JD, Yosipovitch G, et al. Ipilimumab in patients with cancer and the management of dermatologic adverse events. *J Am Acad Dermatol*. 2014.
71. Hamid O, Robert C, Daud A, et al. Safety and tumor responses with lambrolizumab (anti-PD-1) in melanoma. *N Engl J Med*. 2013;369(2):134–144.
75. Asnis LA, Gaspari AA. Cutaneous reactions to recombinant cytokine therapy. *J Am Acad Dermatol*. 1995;33:393–410.
80. Hood AF. Dermatologic toxicity. In: Perry MC, ed. *The Chemotherapy Source Book*, 2nd ed. Baltimore: Williams & Wilkins; 1996:595–606.
87. Fischer D, Knobf M, Durivage H. *The Cancer Chemotherapy Handbook*. St. Louis: Mosby; 1997.
88. Skarin A. Diagnosis in oncology: skin lesions in malignancy. *J Clin Oncol*. 2001;19:2098–2102.
89. Susser WS, Whitaker-Worth DL, Grant-Kels JM. Mucocutaneous reactions to chemotherapy. *J Am Acad Dermatol*. 1999;40:367–398.
95. Clamon GH. Extravasation. In: Perry MC, ed. *The Chemotherapy Source Book*, 2nd ed. Baltimore: Williams & Wilkins; 1996:607–611.
96. Rudolph R, Larson DL. Etiology and treatment of chemotherapeutic agent extravasation injuries: a review. *J Clin Oncol*. 1987;5:1116–1126.
111. Houtee PV, Danhier S, Mornex F. Toxicity of combined radiation and chemotherapy in non-small cell lung cancer. *Lung Cancer*. 1994;10:S271–S280.
112. Yeo W, Leung S, Johnson P. Radiation-recall dermatitis with docetaxel: establishment of a requisite radiation threshold. *Eur J Cancer*. 1997;33:698–699.
114. Johnson T, Rapini R, Duvic M. Inflammation of actinic keratoses from systemic chemotherapy. *J Am Acad Dermatol*. 1987;17:192–197.
121. Demircay Z, Gurbuz O, Alpdogan T, et al. Chemotherapy induced acral erythema in leukemic patients: a report of 15 cases. *Int J Dermatol*. 1997;36:593–598.
124. Baack BR, Burgdorf WHC. Chemotherapy-induced acral erythema. *J Am Acad Dermatol*. 1991;24:457–461.
128. Horn TD, Redd JV, Karp JE, et al. Cutaneous eruptions of lymphocyte recovery. *Arch Dermatol*. 1989;215:1512–1517.
129. Bauer DJ, Hood AF, Horn TD. Histologic comparison of autologous graft-vs-host reaction and cutaneous eruption of lymphocyte recovery. *Arch Dermatol*. 1993;129:855–858.

126 Skeletal complications

Michael A. Via, MD ■ Ilya Iofin, MD ■ Jerry Liu, MD ■ Jeffrey I. Mechanick, MD

> **Overview**
>
> The skeletal complications of cancer are highly prevalent. Bone metastases are present in approximately 70% of patients with cancer-related deaths. Skeletal complications can present clinically as pain associated with bone metastases, pathologic fractures, or hypercalcemia. Additionally, several therapies for cancers may have deleterious effect on bone health such as aromatase inhibition in patients with breast cancer. The presence of skeletal metastases often indicates that cure from cancer unlikely. Goals of therapy may shift to palliation and to systemic control with possible prolonged survival. Surgical treatments, medical therapies, including antiresorptive agents, and/or radiation therapy should each be considered to achieve optimal care in patients with skeletal complications of cancer.

Introduction

Cancer represents a major public health concern as 44% of American men and 38% of women develop cancer at some point in their lifetime. As of 1 January 2019, there were 16.9 million Americans with history of cancer living in the United States. It is estimated that there will be 1.8 million new cancer cases in the United States in 2020 of whom 606,520 are expected to succumb to the disease.[1] As cancer treatments evolve and survival of patients with cancer continue to improve, skeletal complications of cancer are becoming more prevalent. These complications include pain associated with metastases to bone, fractures, hypercalcemia of malignancy (HCM), and potential deleterious effects of cancer treatments.

Approximately 70% of patients who die from cancer are found to have skeletal metastases detected on autopsy, making the skeleton to be the most common site of metastatic disease. A significant portion of these metastases will be clinically relevant and require treatment.[2] Once a patient develops skeletal metastases, cure is very unlikely and it must be understood by both the patient and the treating physicians that the goal of treatment is palliation and not cure.[2] The five most common cancer types that metastasize to bone are of breast, prostate, lung, renal, and thyroid (Table 1). Almost any cancer subtype can metastasize to bone, however, multiple myeloma is the most common malignancy originating in bone and is responsible for significant skeletal-associated morbidity. As in cases of metastatic carcinoma, cure is unlikely, though systemic control is possible and survival times are continuing to improve with evolving therapies. In the case of prostate or breast cancer, therapies that target testosterone or estrogen activity are deleterious to bone health, owing to the effect these hormones exert on osteoclast and osteoblast activity.[10] The treatment of problems arising from malignant disease affecting bone requires a multidisciplinary approach involving medical, orthopedic, and radiation oncologists.

Evaluation of a patient with bone lesions

Evaluation of a patient starts with a careful history and physical examination. Location of pain, inciting and alleviating factors, prior history cancer, and of prior treatments are all required to formulate an appropriate treatment plan. In addition to metastases being the potential source of disability, coexisting arthritis, and other orthopedic conditions may be the cause of the patient's pain while the presence of the metastasis may be purely incidental. Imaging of the bone affected by metastatic disease is first done with orthogonal plain radiographs visualizing the entire length bone as the process may be multifocal (Figure 1). Bone lesions may be purely lytic (where only bone destruction is seen, as is typical of lymphoma, multiple myeloma, lung, renal, and thyroid cancer metastases), blastic (where abnormal bone deposition is seen, as is common in metastatic prostate cancer), or mixed (usual for breast cancer metastases). While radioactive technetium bone scans and MRI are very sensitive modalities for detecting metastases, a noncontrast CT is superior for evaluation of bone integrity and is often needed to make decisions regarding potential need for surgical intervention. Again, the entire length of the involved bone should be imaged in order to accurately assess fracture risk and help guide potential surgical intervention.

Solitary lesions of bone

Special attention needs to be drawn to the patient with a solitary bone lesion but no biopsy-proven metastatic disease. While prior cancer history makes it likely that the newly seen lesion is a metastasis of that cancer, there is no guarantee of that, so a thorough evaluation is required prior to any intervention. An important error to avoid is to presume that a patient has metastatic disease, and failing to recognize a primary bone sarcoma, which might be curable. While sarcomas usually affect teenagers and young adults, they can occur in all age groups. The treatment of sarcoma is radically different from treatment of metastatic carcinoma, multiple myeloma, and lymphoma. Bone sarcoma surgery usually entails wide resection of the tumor with curative intent, while most metastatic lesions are treated with intralesional procedures where palliation is the goal. One of the most common orthopedic procedures indicated for metastatic disease is intramedullary nailing. However, an intramedullary nail inadvertently placed through a bone sarcoma leads to contamination of the entire length of the bone as well as the surrounding soft tissues. A patient in whom limb salvage maybe have been possible prior to intramedullary

---

Holland-Frei Cancer Medicine, Tenth Edition. Edited by Robert C. Bast, John C. Byrd, Carlo M. Croce, Ernest Hawk, Fadlo R. Khuri, Raphael E. Pollock, Apostolia M. Tsimberidou, Christopher G. Willett, and Cheryl L. Willman.
© 2023 John Wiley & Sons, Inc. Published 2023 by John Wiley & Sons, Inc.

Table 1 Prevalence of SREs and survival by cancer type.[a]

Primary malignancy	Prevalence of SREs	Common skeletal locations	Median survival when SREs present
Small cell lung	9–16%	Spine, long bones	2–4 months
Non-small-cell lung	15%	Spine, long bones	2 months
Breast	17–37% of patients with distant metastases	Spine, femur, pelvis, limbs, skull	2.1–4 years
Renal cell	22%	Spine, long bones	10 months
Gastric	3%	Long bones, hip, spine	3 months
Prostate	2%	Spine, long bones	9 months
Thyroid, follicular	5–7%	Spine, long bones, skull	4 years
Thyroid, papillary	0.4%	Spine	

[a]Source: Conen et al.[3]; Cetin et al.[4]; Zhang et al.[5]; Santini et al.[6]; Silvestris et al.[7]; Choksi et al.[8]; Broder et al.[9]

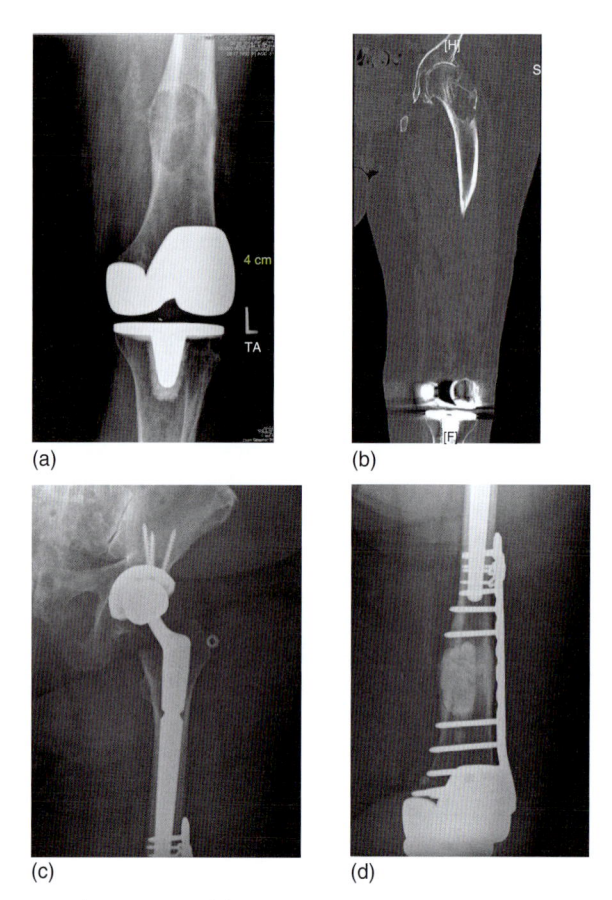

Figure 1 (a) A 81-year-old woman with metastatic breast cancer with a chief complaint of knee pain. Note the destructive lesion in the distal femoral metaphysis above a well-fixed total knee arthroplasty. (b) A non-contrast CT of the entire femur was obtained, demonstrating an additional destructive lesion in the femoral neck. While the lesion was asymptomatic, it was at high risk of sustaining a displaced pathologic fracture. Significant degenerative changes are also seen in the hip joint. (c, d) The distal femoral lesion was treated with intralesional curettage, internal fixation with a locking plate, and packing with PMMA bone cement. A press-fit long stem total hip arthroplasty was performed to treat the femoral neck lesion and the arthritis. Note the overlap of the two implants which minimize the risk of periprosthetic fracture and protects the entire length of the bone.

nailing will require a much more disabling resection at best, and a high-level amputation such as a hemipelvectomy at worst. Additionally, reaming of the medullary canal pushes sarcoma cells into the systemic circulation and the lungs, increasing the risk for metastatic disease and death.[11] Even in the presence of a pathological fracture through a sarcoma, limb salvage with modern chemotherapy and surgical modalities is possible in most cases if fracture healing can be achieved with cast immobilization or minimally invasive fixation methods that do not lead to tissue contamination.[12] Knowledge of the exact tumor diagnosis is required to guide appropriate treatment.

When presented with a patient with an uncertain cancer diagnosis, further staging studies should be undertaken, in addition to evaluating the affected bone. A CT of the chest, abdomen, and pelvis with oral and IV contrast should be performed to look for visceral metastases and a potential primary tumor. Other skeletal metastases can be detected with a technetium-99 whole-body bone scintigraphy while detection of a monoclonal spike on serum and/or urine immunofixation or protein electrophoresis can help establish the diagnosis of multiple myeloma.[13] Bone scintigraphy detects new bone deposition in response to tumor activity, trauma, or degenerative joint disease. Even though bone scintigraphy is a sensitive test for detecting skeletal metastases, these lesions can be missed in patients with multiple myeloma, renal cell carcinoma, and thyroid carcinoma skeletal metastases. This is because these lesions are typically purely lytic in nature with minimal bone deposition. When one of these primaries is suspected, a skeletal survey, consisting of anteroposterior (AP) radiographs of the long bones, chest, and pelvis, as well as lateral radiographs of the spine and skull, should be obtained since it has better sensitivity than bone scintigraphy. Other sites of skeletal involvement identified on bone scintigraphy or skeletal survey should be further evaluated at least with plain radiographs for risk of fracture that may require treatment. PET CT is another sensitive modality for staging, though its exact indications are continuing to evolve. It is routinely used in staging of cancers such as multiple myeloma, breast and lung carcinoma, and lymphoma, but it can also be used as an initial staging modality. Besides looking for additional lesions, the fluorodeoxyglucose (FDG)-avidity can suggest whether the lesion is likely benign or malignant. Caution should be exercised as low-grade chondrosarcomas and some cancers, such as well-differentiated thyroid carcinoma, can have low metabolic activity on PET CT. If not biopsied, solitary lesions should at the very least be followed with serial imaging.[14] All discovered sites of skeletal involvement should be further evaluated for risk of fracture that may require treatment. Prostate-specific antigen levels (total and free), usually elevated in patients with metastatic prostate cancer, should be checked in men where this diagnosis is suspected.

This systematic approach of comprehensive imaging will distinguish patients with multiple bone and visceral lesions in whom metastatic disease or multiple myeloma or lymphoma is suspected from the rare patients with solitary bone lesions, in whom suspicion of primary bone sarcoma is higher. There are additional benefits to this tactic. The most accessible site for biopsy can be found, which may be different from the site of the patient's original complaint. Metastatic renal cell and thyroid carcinomas are well known to be hypervascular and can hemorrhage significantly during biopsy. Prior knowledge of these diagnoses is useful, since preoperative tumor embolization can be performed and preparations made accordingly.

The final diagnosis, though often suspected based on the radiographic evaluation, is confirmed with a tissue biopsy. If the treating physician is confident in the diagnosis even prior to surgical intervention, either based on the radiographic findings or in a patient with known history of metastatic carcinoma or multiple myeloma, then an intraoperative frozen section can be used to confirm that diagnosis. Care must be exercised though as frozen section is not 100% accurate and only provides the correct diagnosis in 86–94% of biopsies of skeletal lesions.[15] If a sarcoma is suspected, then definitive treatment should be delayed until final histological diagnosis is made. Additionally, the reliability of frozen section is dependent on the experience of the pathologist, as most pathologists have limited experience with primary bone tumors. It is important to note that the biopsy tract, especially in cases of an open biopsy, is deemed contaminated by tumor cells and needs to be resected.[16] While that is of little consequence in metastatic disease or multiple myeloma, in cases of sarcoma inappropriate placement of the biopsy has been shown to adversely affect outcomes to the point of even leading to unnecessary amputations in 4.5% of cases.[16] Therefore, biopsy should be performed at a tertiary referral center by, or at least in coordination with, a surgeon with training and expertise in treatment of bone sarcomas.

Options for treatment of skeletal lesions

A range of treatment options exists for skeletal lesions and it spans the spectrum from observation for asymptomatic lesions that do not present a fracture risk, to pharmaceuticals and radiation that target, to operative intervention for displaced and impending pathologic fractures. Of particular interest is the use of bisphosphonates and denosumab. These agents are typically used for osteoporosis but have also been shown to reduce the number of skeletal events, such as spine compression fractures and need for surgery or radiation in patients with metastatic bone disease and multiple myeloma.[17]

Radiation therapy (RT) is a commonly used modality that provides pain relief in about 70% of patients. Sensitivity to systemic and radiation therapies is one of many factors when choosing the most appropriate treatment for a patient with a skeletal lesion. Radiation is most appropriate for lesions that do not present a significant fracture risk. The pelvis, spine, ribs, and scapulae are appropriate sites for radiation treatment in the majority of cases, while lesions of the long bones, especially in the lower extremity, present a higher fracture risk and should be evaluated for potential surgical intervention.

In patients with small lesions that are not structurally significant, where radiation does not usually provide pain relief, radiofrequency ablation (RFA) and cryoablation are useful minimally invasive treatment options. Following both procedures, polymethyl methacrylate (PMMA bone cement) may be injected into the void left by the tumor to provide structural support and additional pain relief.[18,19] Such image-guided thermal ablation techniques are most appropriate for lesions that present a minimal risk of fracture, such as vertebral body, sacral and iliac wing lesions, and many acetabular lesions. Once fracture is present or the bone is at significant risk of fracture due to loss of structural integrity, surgery is usually required.

Principles of pathologic fracture treatment

The goals of pathologic fracture treatment are to improve function and provide pain relief. The patient and his or her family must be informed and will need to understand that the goal of this treatment is palliative in nature and will not result in cure. Risks of complications must be carefully balanced against the potential benefit. Though survival time of cancer patients is difficult to predict, it should exceed the expected surgical recovery time. Pathologic fractures often fail to heal or may be slow to heal. In a series of 123 patients with 129 pathologic fractures, the overall fracture healing rate was only 35%. In patients who survived for more than 6 months, this rate went up to 74%.[20] Moreover, the fact that patients with pathologic fractures have multiple systemic comorbidities should be kept in mind when selecting the optimal treatment modality. Unlike conventional fractures, where union is likely after a relatively short period of restricted weight bearing, in pathologic fractures such an expectation cannot be made. Fixation must be sufficiently durable to allow immediate unrestricted weight bearing and last for the entire lifetime of the patient. Multiple surgeries are not a desirable option. Chemotherapeutic regimens are cytotoxic and are often interrupted to allow wound healing from surgery. As systemic disease can progress during such interruptions of systemic treatment, all efforts should be made to minimize the duration and number of interruptions by minimizing the need for multiple surgeries.

The bone affected by tumor invasion has poor structural integrity, which can lead to fracture. Intralesional resection of the tumor and augmentation of the fixation with PMMA bone cement is often required to both provide sufficient stability to the fixation construct and to obtain better local control of the tumor. Addition of bone cement to internal fixation has been shown to provide pain relief that is superior to internal fixation alone[21] and provides a more biomechanically stable construct.[22] Bone grafting is not used in the treatment of metastatic disease and multiple myeloma since the graft cannot be expected to incorporate with ongoing chemotherapy and radiation. PMMA bone cement provides immediate stability, is inexpensive and easy to use, and preferable to bone grafting. Also, fracture healing can occur in the presence of bone cement (Figure 2). In addition to tumor debulking with curettage and high speed burring to lower risk of recurrence, cryosurgery can be used as a treatment modality in cases of relatively radioresistant tumors where prolonged patient survival is likely, such as in cases of oligometastatic renal cell carcinoma.[23]

Treatment options for pathologic fractures consist of intramedullary nailing, fixation with plates and screws, endoprosthetic replacement, and resection of bone without reconstruction. Choice of treatment depends on tumor biology, location, and surrounding bone integrity. For example, a pathologic fracture of the clavicle due to multiple myeloma, which is chemo- and radio-sensitive, will usually respond well to nonoperative treatment, while the same clavicle fracture due to metastatic renal cell carcinoma is best treated with resection of the clavicle. Radiation treatment is an important adjunct to surgical treatment of bone lesions as it reduces the likelihood of tumor progression that might require reoperation and improves function. In one series, it has been shown to reduce the need for reoperation from 15% seen in

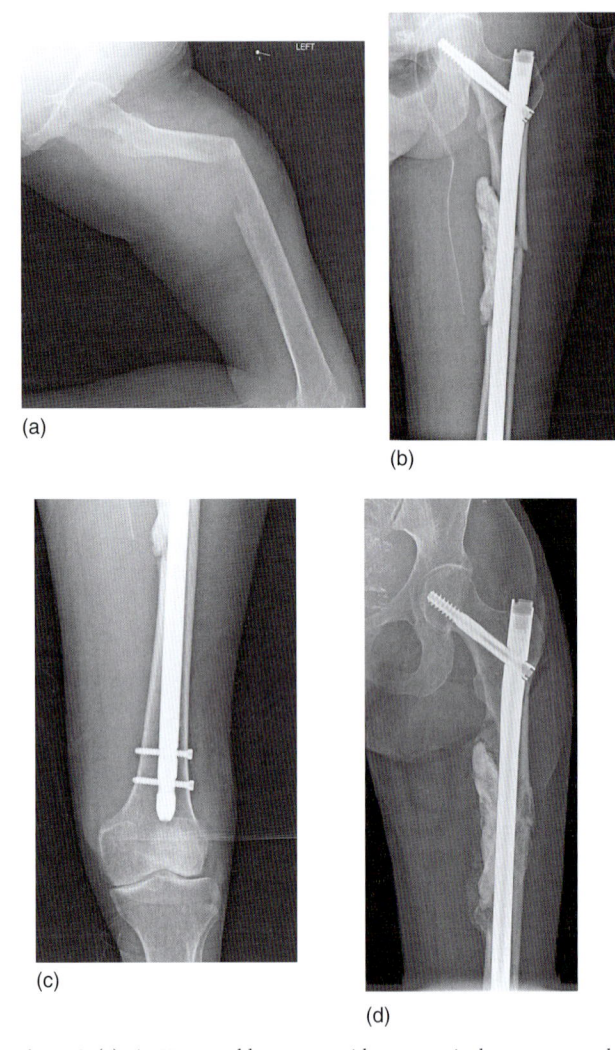

Figure 2 (a) A 57-year-old woman with metastatic lung cancer who sustained a left femoral midshaft diaphyseal fracture. (b, c) The patient underwent resection curettage of the tumor, intramedullary nailing, and packing of PMMA bone cement around the nail into the defect left by the tumor. (d) 4 months later, the fracture line over the lateral cortex is no longer visible and bone callus is seen, indicating healing of the fracture. Note the fracture callus forming on the medial side around the cement.

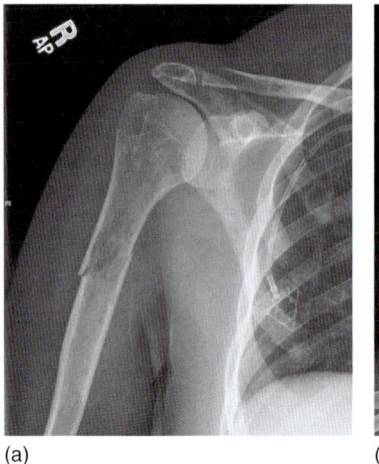

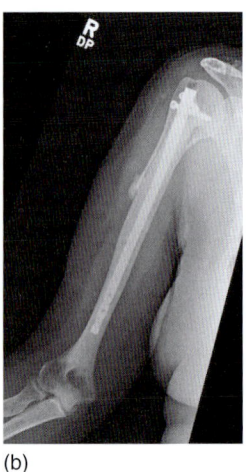

Figure 3 (a) A 49-year-old woman with multiple myeloma who sustained a pathologic right proximal humerus fracture. (b) The fracture was sufficiently distal to allow the use of a cemented intramedullary nail. Note the cement mantle going up to the proximal diaphysis. Distal interlocking screws were not used as the entire nail is supported by bone cement.

the group that received surgery alone, to only 3% in the group that had radiation treatment after surgery.[24]

Intramedullary nailing

Intramedullary nailing is the most commonly used surgical method of treatment of metastatic disease affecting bone due to its many advantages. The entire length of the bone is protected by the length of the nail, so if other lesions develop within the same bone, further surgery may not be necessary. The surgery can be done in a minimally invasive fashion, allowing for a quicker recovery and a lower surgical risk. However, an open approach and placement of PMMA bone cement are required in some cases, depending on fracture characteristics and the sensitivity of the tumor to chemotherapy and radiation. Relatively radiation-resistant tumors, such as metastatic renal cell carcinoma, are more likely to require an open approach to lower risks of complications associated with local tumor progression. The nail can be embedded into the bone cement that has been injected along the entire length of the intramedullary canal to enhance construct stability (Figure 3) or, alternatively, cement can be packed around the nail into the defect left by the tumor (Figure 2).

The femur is the most common bone to be treated with intramedullary nailing. A cephalomedullary nail is preferable as the lag screw provides fixation of the femoral neck (FN), a site that is commonly affected by metastatic disease or multiple myeloma. Metaphyseal and diaphyseal humeral lesions are also amenable to intramedullary nailing. The tibia is rarely affected by metastatic disease or multiple myeloma, but intramedullary nailing can be performed in those rare cases. Even more rare are lesions of the long bones of the forearm, but in selected cases, intramedullary nailing of pathologic forearm fractures can be used safely and effectively instead of the more traditional fixation with plates and screws used in that location.

There must be sufficient bone in both the proximal and distal aspects of the long bone to allow the nail to have sufficient fixation and biomechanical stability. While it is best suited for diaphyseal lesions, intramedullary nailing can be safely used in metaphyseal locations where there is sufficient distance from the joint to allow good fixation. Lesions of the FN are best suited for treatment with arthroplasty and lesions of the humeral head are best suited for treatment with arthroplasty or plate and screw fixation with cement augmentation.

Plate and screw fixation

The locking plate technology has revolutionized fracture fixation in general, and has also become an invaluable tool in the treatment of pathologic fractures. In contrast to traditional plating techniques, which rely on friction of the plate against bone, locking plate technology creates a fixed angle device where the head of each screw is secured into the plate. Thus, for the construct to fail, all the screws need to fail together, requiring far greater force. In conventional plating screws can fail sequentially, requiring less force for failure of the entire construct. Locking plates have been shown to be an excellent choice for treatment of fractures close to joints where traditional fixation methods have not provided optimal results.[25] Locking plates in conjunction with liberal use of PMMA

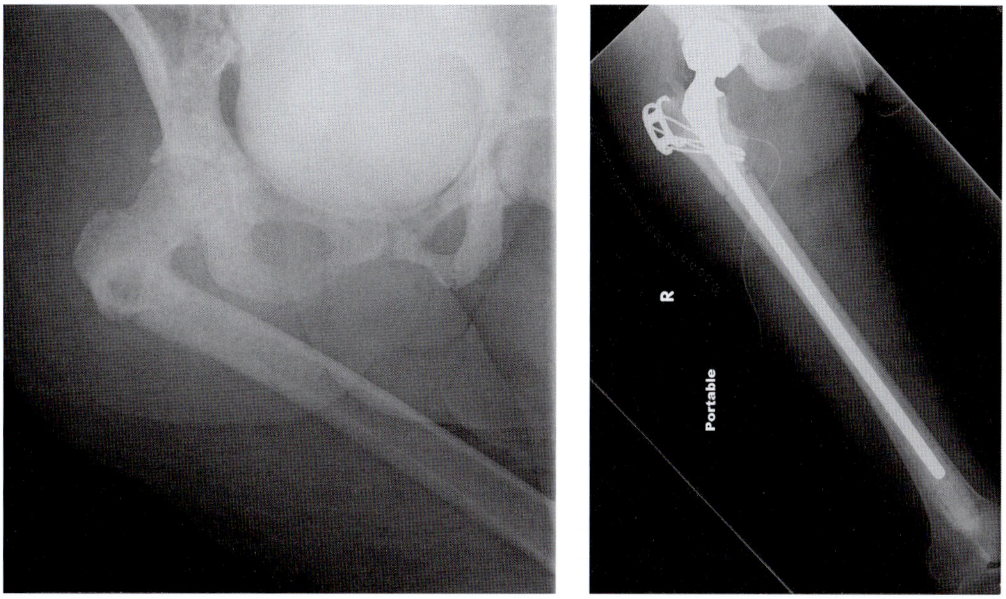

Figure 4 (a) A 40-year-old woman with metastatic breast cancer who sustained a subtrochanteric right femur fracture. Note the mixed lytic and blastic changes seen in the femoral head as well as in much of the pelvis. (b) A long-stem cemented hip hemiarthroplasty was performed. A femoral nail would not have been an appropriate choice for this patient as the bone in the femoral head is compromised by metastatic tumor. With an intramedullary nail, risk of lag screw cut-out would have been unacceptably high. The arthroplasty stem serves the same function as a nail in fixing the fracture while the compromised bone in the head of the femur is replaced with the prosthetic head.

bone cement should be used in preference to conventional plates whenever possible. They are best suited for locations near a joint, such as the distal femur, proximal tibia, and proximal and distal humeri, where there is insufficient fixation for an intramedullary nail. They are preferable to a joint arthroplasty as they potentially provide better functional results.[26] Additionally, this fixation method can be used when another implant, such as a total joint arthroplasty or previous fracture fixation, would interfere with placement of an intramedullary device (Figure 1).

Arthroplasty

Joint arthroplasty is reserved for lesions that are so close to the joint that neither intramedullary nailing nor plate and screw fixation will provide reliable stable fixation. Joint arthroplasty is most commonly used for lesions of the femoral head and neck, especially since even conventional displaced fractures without an underlying oncological process (often found in the geriatric patient) have a low union rate. Arthroplasty has even been shown to have superior results to internal fixation for intertrochanteric and subtrochanteric lesions, though the subgroup of patients in whom tumor was removed and internal fixation was augmented with PMMA bone cement fared much better than those in whom internal fixation alone was performed.[27] In cases of diaphyseal fractures where the tumor involves the point of interlocking screw fixation, use of arthroplasty is preferred over the use of an intramedullary nail, since the interlocking screws will not have sufficient support within bone weakened by tumor and are likely to cut out of the bone (Figure 4). Pain from acetabular wear is not a significant concern in patients with a limited life expectancy from a malignancy, so the higher dislocation risk and the longer surgical time associated with a total hip arthroplasty is not justified. Therefore, a hemiarthroplasty is preferable except in cases of severe preexisting arthritis or an acetabular lesion requiring surgical intervention (Figure 1). Hemiarthroplasty can also be used for lesions of the proximal humerus where there is insufficient bone stock to allow fixation with joint sparing implants.

For isolated lesions of the head and neck of the femur, a conventional arthroplasty is used by some surgeons while others use a cemented long-stem hemiarthroplasty to protect much of the length of the femur from progression of metastatic disease. In lesions affecting much of the proximal femur, a long stem hemiarthroplasty is needed (Figure 4). This procedure uses PMMA bone cement and is associated with a ~2% risk of intraoperative cardiac arrest and ~1% risk of early preoperative or intraoperative mortality.[28] As the risk of such an adverse event can be lowered, communication with the anesthesia team is mandatory prior to and during cementation of the prosthesis. Placement of venting holes in the distal femur prior to cementation has been shown to lower the intramedullary pressure, but unfortunately, no data exists that would demonstrate that this translates into a lower clinical risk of intraoperative cardiac arrest.[29] In addition, the venting hole can theoretically act as a stress riser, leading to a fracture distal to the prosthesis.

Megaprostheses

Large oncological endoprosthetic devices are generally used to reconstruct the large defects that remain after resection of bone sarcomas, as well as occasionally but also in the treatment of metastatic disease and multiple myeloma. Overall there are three main indications for the use of large oncological endoprosthetic devices in cases of metastatic disease and multiple myeloma. The first indication is when the tumor is so extensive and bone stock is so poor, that neither osteosynthetic devices nor conventional arthroplasty is feasible. The second indication is for prior failed fixation due to tumor progression or hardware failure due to a nonunion. The third indication is for the rare patient with a solitary metastatic lesion where resection of the lesion may improve long-term survival. While megaprostheses are an appropriate choice in selected cases, they are associated with a longer operative time, higher complication rate, such as infection and dislocation, and prolonged recovery. Location of the lesion also plays a role as excellent function can be expected in the distal and proximal femoral replacements, while the function of proximal tibial and proximal and distal humeral replacements is inferior. In cases where there is a large diaphyseal defect, an intercalary prosthesis can be used instead of an intramedullary nail. An intercalary prosthesis has been shown to be more biomechanically stable than an intramedullary nail even with cement augmentation.[30] At least 5 cm of diaphysis are required on each side of the intercalary prosthesis to allow the cementation of the stems.

Treatment of periacetabular lesions

Surgical treatment of periacetabular lesions can be associated with significant morbidity, complications, and intraoperative blood loss. Fortunately, many of these lesions respond well to nonoperative measures, such as weight-bearing restrictions and radiation. Small lesions resistant to radiation may be treated with cementoplasty that can be combined with ablative techniques, such as cryosurgery or RFA. However, surgery is required in selected patients with sufficient life expectancy who fail nonoperative treatment. In cases where there is sufficient bone stock and the subchondral plate is preserved, intralesional curettage and PMMA cement packing can be effective. In cases of displaced pathological acetabular fractures, or large lesions affecting the medial wall and/or the subchondral plate, a complex total hip arthroplasty is required. The goal of the reconstruction is to distribute the forces from the acetabulum to the portions of the pelvis, such as ilium and ischium, which are not affected by the disease process. Antiprotrusio acetabular cages, Steinman pins embedded in the ilium, and bone cement to fill the defect left by the tumor are commonly used. Constrained cemented acetabular liners may be required to reduce instances of dislocation when there is not sufficient soft tissue left to reconstruct the capsular structures. In rare cases, where bone destruction is so significant that even a reconstruction with a cage will not provide sufficient mechanical support, use of a partial pelvic prosthetic replacement can be considered, though it is associated with a high complication rate. The last surgical option for treatment of acetabular lesions is resection arthroplasty without reconstruction. It is associated with limb length inequality of about 5 cm and a decline in ambulatory capacity, though ambulation is not precluded, but holds the advantages of having a low complication rate and being a technically quick and relatively simple surgery. This option is most appropriate for patients in whom a more extensive reconstruction would be medically contraindicated or who are nonambulatory at baseline.[31] Periacetabular tumors, especially due to multiple myeloma, renal cell carcinoma, and thyroid carcinoma metastases may be quite vascular, so appropriate preoperative preparation for potential administration of blood products is required and tumor embolization should be considered.

Resection without reconstruction

While metastatic disease most frequently affects the axial skeleton and proximal femora and humeri, there are instances of metastatic disease to smaller bones such as the clavicle, proximal radius, distal ulna, and proximal fibula. These bones are very slender and hardware, even if fixation is augmented with bone cement, has a high risk of failure. Fortunately, excellent function can be obtained with resection of bone from these location without reconstruction. Once the fractured bone segment or the entire bone is resected, there is no fracture to heal and excellent pain relief is obtained. This approach can reduce surgical time and lower the risk of complications while providing results that are equivalent, if not superior, to fracture fixation. As discussed above, resection of the femoral head and hip joint without reconstruction is also a good surgical option for patients with large painful periacetabular lesions whose baseline performance status is very poor, or if there are medical contraindications to performing large periacetabular resections with extensive reconstruction joint reconstruction.

Spine lesions

While the spine is the most common site of metastatic disease, fortunately, most spine metastases do not require surgery. Spinal metastases are usually incidentally detected on staging studies such as bone scintigraphy or CT of the chest, abdomen, and pelvis. Mechanical integrity of the spine is usually not compromised, so RT for axial back pain is usually effective. In cases of compression fractures without neurological compromise, kyphoplasty combined with radiation has been shown to provide pain relief in over 90% of cases.[32] Kyphoplasty is a technique in which a balloon is percutaneously inserted into the vertebral body through the pedicle under image guidance and inflated to restore vertebral body height, which is then maintained by injection of PMMA bone cement into the resultant void. Surgical decompression and fusion are indicated in cases of severe and progressive deformity or neurological compromise from compression of neural structures (Figure 5). In cases of spinal cord or caudal equina compression, surgical intervention provides superior pain relief and is more likely to allow the patient to maintain or even restore ambulatory capacity compared to RT alone.[33] Timely surgical decompression before irreversible neural damage is critical. In cases of neurologic compromise from radiosensitive lesions such as multiple myeloma and lymphoma, emergency radiotherapy is the preferred treatment modality. Corticosteroids should be administered to relieve edema around the spinal cord and attempt to preserve neurologic function while treatment is being instituted.

Treatment of painful metastases and impending fractures

Besides a displaced pathologic fracture, the indications for surgery are impending pathological fractures and painful lesions that are not responsive to radiation or other nonoperative treatments. Prophylactic surgical intervention has been shown to be associated with a quicker recovery and superior functional results, compared to treatment of a fracture that has already occurred.[34,35] Several systems have been devised to identify the patients at risk of fracture. The one used most commonly was described by Mirels in 1989.[36] The lesion is assigned a score of 1 to 3 based on four categories:

1. Location of the lesion. The peritrochanteric femur experiences the highest forces and is assigned a score of 3 while the upper extremity is nonweight bearing and is thus assigned a score of 1;

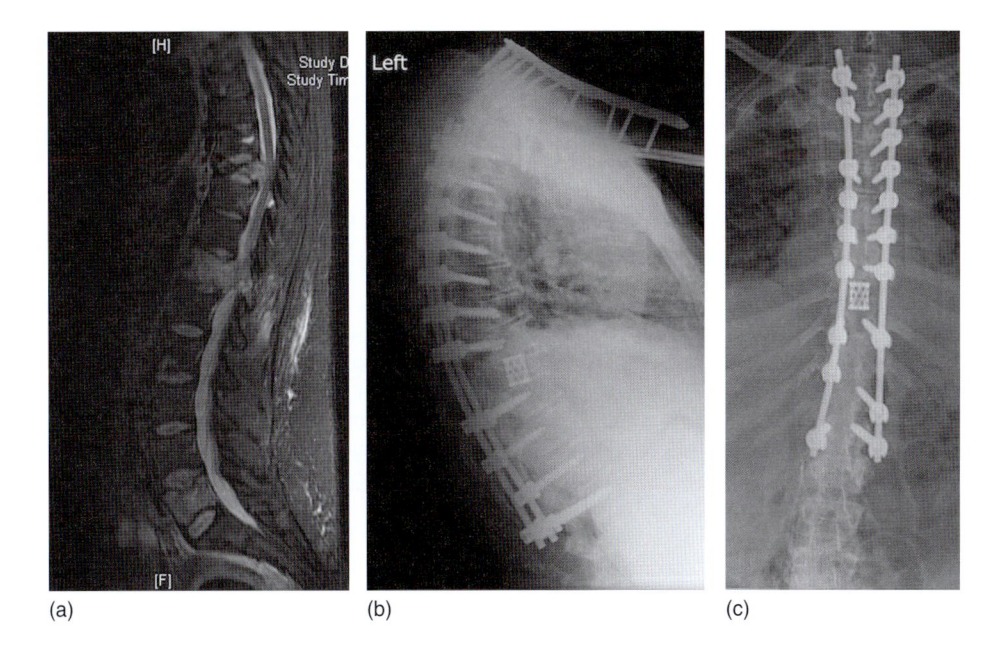

Figure 5 (a) A 56-year-old woman with metastatic endometrial carcinoma who developed significant lower extremity weakness due to spinal cord compression from a pathologic fracture of the T9 vertebral body. Metastatic deposits in other vertebral bodies are seen. (b, c) The patient underwent resection of the T9 vertebral body and fusion with a cage, posterior T8–T10 hemilaminectomy, and instrumentation and fusion from T1 to L1.

2. Pain quality. Pain exacerbated by activity is the most ominous sign as it implies a mechanical instability at the site of the lesion; all of patients with activity-related pain went on to fracture in Mirels' study while only 10% of patients without functional pain sustained fractures;
3. Lesion type. Lytic lesion is the most susceptible to fracture as native bone is destroyed by tumor and not replaced, so a score of 3 is assigned; blastic lesions are composed of abnormal tumor bone that does not undergo normal remodeling, and are therefore weaker than native bone, but stronger than bone affected by purely lytic lesions, so a score of 1 is given; and
4. Size of the lesion as seen on plain radiographs. Larger lesions present a higher fracture risk and therefore get a higher score.[36]

The scores from the four categories are added up to obtain a total score from 4 to 12. A score of 9 is associated with a 33% fracture risk, which is the threshold for recommending surgery for scores of 9 and above, while radiation is recommended for scores of 7 or less.[36] A score of 8 is associated with a 15% fracture risk, so patient factors, such as activity level, body weight, life expectancy, and sensitivity of the tumor to chemotherapy and radiation will need to be considered. While Mirels' system is 91% sensitive, its specificity is only 35%.[37] In a multicenter trial, CT-based structural rigidity analysis (CTRA) was shown to have higher sensitivity (100% vs 66.7% and specificity (60.6% vs 47.9%) when used to predict femoral fracture risk.[38] CTRA is based on computer software which is not yet widely available but shows significant promise in the treatment of patients at risk of pathologic fracture.

Medical management of bone metastases

The optimal management of bone metastases requires the coordinated efforts of various disciplines. In addition to systemic chemotherapy or radiotherapy for bone metastases, endocrine interventions directed at bone metabolism have demonstrated effectiveness in controlling oncogenic bone pain, fracture risk, metastatic growth, and even prolonging survival.

Bone metabolism is governed by a delicate, though highly regulated, balance between bone formation (by osteoblasts) and bone resorption (by osteoclasts). This results in bone remodeling, which confers strength and decreases fracture risk. Antiresorptive agents, including bisphosphonates or denosumab, are the most efficacious therapeutic options for the medical management of metabolic bone disease and tumor-induced skeletal-related events (SREs).

Bisphosphonates

Bisphosphonates are pyrophosphate analogs with a high affinity for bone that inhibit osteoclast function and diminish the recruitment and differentiation of osteoclast precursors.[39] In breast cancer patients, the administration of intravenous bisphosphonates reduced SREs by approximately 30%.[40] Zoledronate or pamidronate demonstrate greater efficacy in reduction for treatment of bone metastases than ibandronate.[40,41] The non-nitrogen-containing bisphosphonates (nBP) (etidronate and clodronate [not available in the United States]) are metabolized into cytotoxic analogs of ATP and are not considered to have antitumoral activity.[42]

Studies in animal models have identified several mechanisms for antitumoral activity of the n-BP (pamidronate, ibandronate, zoledronate, risedronate, and alendronate). These include inhibition of tumor cell adhesion, inhibition of tumor cell invasion through the extracellular matrix, improvement of immune surveillance and macrophage differentiation targeting cancer cells, inhibition of angiogenic effects (via reduction in vascular endothelial growth factor [VEGF], basic fibroblast growth factor [b-FGF], and effects on endothelial cell adhesion) and induction of tumor cell apoptosis.[43–46] n-BPs induce apoptosis of osteoclasts and antagonize osteoclastogenesis via (1) osteoblast secretion of an inhibitor of osteoclast recruitment; (2) altering osteoblast secretion of transforming growth factor-ß (TGF-β), an osteoclast apoptosis signal; (3) inhibition of farnesyl diphosphate synthase, a key enzyme in the mevalonate pathway; (4) impaired isoprenylation (farnesylation) causing interference with small guanosine triphosphatases (GTPases) that regulate cytoskeletal arrangement, vesicular trafficking and activation of intracellular signals such as Ras, Rab, Rho, and Rac (important for cancer cell migration and invasion); and (5) released mitochondrial cytochrome C and caspase activation.[47,48] n-BPs also affect expression of the antiapoptotic protein bcl-2, activate the p38 mitogen-activated protein kinase (MAPK) pathway, down-regulate integrins, and increase expression of osteoprotegerin.[43,49] Furthermore, n-BPs are broad-spectrum matrix metalloproteinase (MMP) inhibitors, which may prevent metastases into soft and hard tissue as well as reduce active circulating levels of TGF-β.[50]

In clinical studies, bisphosphonates are well tolerated with minimal acute side effects.[51] Patients may develop nausea, vomiting, and, with pamidronate, a posterior uveitis. Fever may occur after initial treatment with intravenous bisphosphonates owing to tumor necrosis factor (TNF)-α and interleukin (IL)-6 elaboration by γ/δ T cells, which may also be associated with antitumor activity.[52,53] This acute phase response is either greatly diminished or completely absent in further bisphosphonate challenges.

The majority of an intravenously administered bisphosphonate dose is deposited in the bone, where it remains for extended periods of time. Oral absorption is only 0.6–1% of the administered dose. Bisphosphonates are not metabolized and are eliminated by renal excretion. Recycling of skeletal stores allows for extended periods of pharmacologic activity even after cessation of administration.

Nephrotoxicity may be observed but is uncommon, though bisphosphonate therapy may exacerbate preexisting renal impairment and caution should be taken with bisphosphonate use in patients with impaired renal function (glomerular filtration rate (GFR) < 35 mL/min).[54] In patients with renal failure, pamidronate may be dosed during, or within 24 h before, hemodialysis. In one series, the use of pamidronate was associated with improvement in renal function among critically ill patients at all levels of acute renal impairment.[55] Ibandronate 6 mg IV over 30 min has been given to cancer patients with renal insufficiency resulting in no apparent adverse effects and with an improvement in renal function in some cases.[56] Hypocalcemia and hypophosphatemia may also occur, particularly in patients with a vitamin D deficiency. The safety of long-term bisphosphonate administration (over 2 years) has been well documented.[39,57]

The antiresorptive response to bisphosphonates is best assessed with urine N-telopeptide (NTx) levels or fasting serum C-telopeptide (CTx) levels.[58] NTx and CTx are bone-specific collagen breakdown products that is also highly predictive of skeletal complications from metastatic bone disease, as well as of mortality.[59]

Denosumab

Denosumab, a fully human monoclonal antibody, serves as an alternative antiresorptive agent by directly inhibiting receptor activator of nuclear factor κB ligand (RANKL), thereby inhibiting osteoclast maturation, activation, and recruitment. Cytokines and other paracrine factors secreted locally by skeletal metastases stimulate RANKL release, activating osteoclasts.[60] Consequently, osteoclast activity induces the release of growth factors from bone that may stimulate growth within the metastatic lesion. Through inhibition of RANKL, denosumab is a potent antiresorptive agent and may possess antitumor activity in addition to great therapeutic benefits in metabolic bone disease, including reduction of SREs.[61]

Studies in animal models of malignancy demonstrate reduced overall tumor occurrence rates in RANK knock-out mice, hinting at the potential for antitumor activity of denosumab, in addition to inhibition of bone resorption.[62] Moreover, animal models demonstrate enhanced effector T-cell antitumor activity with denosumab treatment that appears to be synergistic with immune checkpoint inhibitor therapy.[63] These preclinical findings are supported by analysis of several Phase III clinical trials of denosumab in cancer patients that demonstrate either superior or noninferior efficacy compared to bisphosphonates.[64] The antiresorptive activity of denosumab with low rates of serious adverse effects makes this an attractive therapeutic option.

In malignant osteolytic bone disease, administration of antiresorptive agents has been associated with reduced SREs, including pain. Common treatment protocols include (1) Denosumab 120 mg subcutaneous injection every 4 weeks; (2) zoledronate 4 mg IV every 3–4 weeks; or (3) pamidronate 60–90 mg IV every 3–4 weeks.[54,56,65–68] The shorter and more convenient infusion protocols, with comparable safety and potential advantages favor denosumab, or alternatively zoledronate as the bisphosphonate of choice. In a large metareview of 30 randomized controlled trials involving 3682 patients, bisphosphonate use was significantly more effective than placebo in providing pain relief from bone metastases.[56] Direct comparison trials published in the past decade suggest denosumab may be superior to zoledronate for the prevention and treatment of SREs, however, an analysis of published data from a pricing standpoint suggests zoledronate given every 3 months is more cost-effective.[69] Since pain relief can be delayed, the use of antiresorptive agents should be combined with analgesics, radiotherapy, and/or radiopharmaceuticals when appropriate.[70]

The standard of care for the management of osteolytic lesions from breast cancer includes the use of intravenous pamidronate, zoledronate, or denosumab. Pamidronate 45 mg IV every 3 weeks increased the median time to bone progression, improved pain control, reduced the need for radiotherapy, and increased the median time to radiotherapy with no serious adverse effects or worsening of chemotherapy-related toxicities.[71] These results were confirmed in a larger study of stage IV breast cancer patients with at least one lytic bone lesion given pamidronate, 90 mg IV over 2 h every month for 12 cycles.[72] However, clinical trials demonstrate superiority of zoledronate in comparison to pamidronate, and several studies suggest denosumab to be more efficacious in patients with breast cancer than zoledronate. In a study of 1648 patients with either stage III multiple myeloma or advanced breast cancer, zoledronate, 4 mg IV over 15 min, was associated with greater sustained beneficial effects on osteolytic bone lesions than 90 mg of IV pamidronate.[73] In a randomized controlled study of 1130 patients with breast cancer with at least one osteolytic lesion, 4 mg IV zoledronate was more effective than 90 mg IV pamidronate in reducing skeletal complications.[74] A more recent multicenter direct comparison trial demonstrated that patients with evidence of bone metastases from solid tumors, including breast cancer, treated denosumab had a 15% reduction in SREs compared to those treated with zoledronate.[75] Another multicenter trial demonstrated reduced time to SRE with denosumab compared to zoledronate treatment in patients with solid tumors.[17] By these results, denosumab has emerged as a preferable antiresorptive agent, with zoledronate or pamidronate as reasonable alternatives.

Antiresorptive therapies are also used to manage cancer-treatment-induced bone loss (CTIBL). This has particular application to patients undergoing hormonal therapies for breast and prostate cancers, and for adult survivors of childhood cancers, many of which are treated with glucocorticoids, agents that cause hypogonadism, or with cranial radiation that can cause growth hormone deficiency and hypogonadism.[76] Average rates of CTIBL owing to ovarian ablation are 1.4–5.9% (lumbar spine [LS]) and 0.34–2.7% (FN); owing to lutenizing hormone releasing hormone (LHRH) agonist therapy, 5.3% (LS) and 3.2% (FN); owing to aromatase inhibitors, 2.6% (LS) and 1.7% (FN); and owing to androgen deprivation therapy for prostate cancer, 0.98–8% (LS) and 0.92–9.6% (FN).[77] For the treatment of CTIBL oral risedronate, 30 mg/day × 2 weeks followed by 10 weeks of no drug, repeated for 8 12-week cycles, has been associated with prevention of trabecular and cortical bone loss in women with breast cancer.[78] Standard protocols for the use of bisphosphonates in the treatment of postmenopausal osteoporosis include alendronate, 70 mg/week oral or risedronate, 35 mg/week oral, clinical trials have also demonstrated efficacy of pamidronate, 60–90 mg IV every 1–3 months[79,80]; zoledronate, 4 mg IV every 3–6 months[81–83]; or denosumab, 60 mg subcutaneous every 6 months,[84,85] to manage CTIBL. Hormone replacement (testosterone, estrogen, or growth hormone) may be indicated if levels are low in childhood cancer survivors.[86] Supplementation with calcium, 1200–1500 mg/day and vitamin D, 800–1600 units/day, targeting serum level for 25-hydroxy-vitamin D of 30 ng/mL is recommended.[87]

In prostate cancer, metabolic bone disease can result from direct effects of bone metastases, which have osteoblastic and osteoclastic components, or CTIBL. Fractures are an independent and adverse predictor of survival in prostate cancer patients.[79] Prostate cancer bone metastases produce MMPs, which promote osteolysis, and also RANKL, parathyroid hormone related peptide (PTHrp), and IL-6, all of which induce osteoclastogenesis.[88] The process of tumor-mediated local bone resorption can facilitate micrometastasis, tumor cell hiding, and eventual macrometastases.[89] Antiresorptive therapy can target this osteoclastic component of prostate cancer bone metastases as well as promote caspase-dependent apoptosis via G-protein geranylgeranylation.[90] However, pamidronate, 90 mg IV q 3 weeks × 27 weeks, was found to lack significant effects on SREs in men with metastatic prostate cancer.[91] Moreover, while one study demonstrated reduction in SREs in men with metastatic prostate cancer who were given zoledronate, 4 mg over 15 min every 3 weeks for 15 months, another study of patients with progressive prostate cancer demonstrated no benefit with monthly zoledronate infusions.[92] In contrast, a Phase III trial in patients with prostate cancer demonstrated a superior 18% reduction in SREs with denosumab therapy in comparison to zoledronate over a mean follow-up of 11 months.[93] There were also similar complication rates, though hypocalcemia was twice as prevalent in the denosumab group (13%). By these results, denosumab is preferred for the treatment of bone metastases in patients with prostate cancer.

Intravenous pamidronate and zoledronate or subcutaneous denosumab have been used to reduce SREs in patients with multiple myeloma.[94] Bisphosphonates may induce apoptosis in plasma cells; this antitumor effect is enhanced by dexamethasone and thalidomide[95] but may diminish over time because of increased farnesyl pyrophosphate synthase activity.[96,97] Pamidronate, 90 mg over 4 h IV every 4 weeks for nine cycles, was associated with decreased bone pain without deterioration in performance status or quality of life in patients with multiple myeloma.[98] However, pamidronate therapy had no effect on progression-free survival in multiple myeloma.[99] Zoledronate, 2–4 mg over 5 min, demonstrated comparable efficacy in the management of multiple myeloma bone lesions.[100] Zoledronate has also been found to augment the antileukemic activity *in vitro* of several chemotherapeutic agents.[101] The effectiveness of denosumab appears similar to zoledronate. A multicenter international head-to-head comparison trial of denosumab versus zoledronate in patients with multiple myeloma demonstrated similar outcomes with both agents.[102] Similar rates of osteonecrosis of the jaw (ONJ) were also seen in both groups. The use of one of these antiresorptive therapies can augment the chemotherapeutic regimen in multiple myeloma patients.

ONJ represents a potential rare but serious complication of chronic therapy with antiresorptive agents including both bisphosphonates and denosumab. In this condition, areas of the mandible or maxilla are exposed and fail to heal. Patients will present with oral swelling, pain, bleeding of the gums, or loose teeth. If suspected, the diagnosis should be confirmed by biopsy and the patient should be referred for immediate surgical debridement.[103] Antibiotics and hyperbaric oxygen therapy are generally ineffective. Several prospective studies and a review of the SEER database reveal a 5–7% prevalence of ONJ 3 years after bisphosphonate therapy is started in cancer patients, with a higher prevalence in those treated more frequently and in those that received intravenous bisphosphonates, especially zoledronate, or denosumab.[104–106] Other risk factors for ONJ include increasing age, concurrent use of antiangiogenic or chemotherapeutic agents, trauma, oral infections, and dental extractions.[107] Radiation or chemotherapies may also raise the risk of ONJ. This is especially noteworthy among patients treated with antiangiogenic tyrosine kinase inhibitors, such as sunitinib, who demonstrate a 16% incidence of ONJ with bisphosphonate therapy.[108] In a small study of 41 patients with renal cell carcinoma given denosumab and either sunitinib, pazopanib, or axitinib, seven patients (17%) developed ONJ over a median of 12 months exposure.[109] Most authors suggest a complete dental evaluation prior to and during antiresorptive therapy.[107,110]

Atypical fractures of the hip represent another potential adverse outcome that results from the use of antiresorptive agents. Diminished bone remodeling is believed to play a causative role in atypical hip fractures, which may comprise 3–5% of all femoral shaft fractures.[111] Atypical fractures have been described in cancer patients receiving intravenous bisphosphonates (1.2% incidence) and denosumab (1.8% incidence).[112,113] To be classified as atypical, a hip fracture must meet four of five major criteria[114] that include:

1. Minimal or no trauma;
2. The fracture line originates in the lateral cortex and progresses transversely, though it may become oblique as it crosses medially across the femur;
3. Complete fractures extend through both cortices while incomplete fractures extend through only the lateral cortex;
4. Fractures are not comminuted or minimally comminuted;
5. Presence of localized periostial or endostial thickening of the lateral cortex.

Current recommendations for patients that sustain atypical fractures include the cessation of antiresorptive therapy and referral for surgical intervention. In several small studies, risk of atypical fracture of the contralateral hip declined by 60–70% in patients that discontinued bisphosphonates compared to those who were maintained on this therapy after an initial atypical fracture.[115,116]

Several novel therapeutic agents that affect bone physiology may become available in the forthcoming years.[117] Sclerostin and dickkopf-1 are peptide signals secreted by osteocytes that inhibit osteoblast activity. Inhibitors of sclerostin, such as romosozumab or blosozumab, are under active investigation. By enhancing osteoblast activity, these compounds increase bone mineral density and may be beneficial for the treatment of cancer-related skeletal disease.[117] Additionally, as anabolic agents, there may be benefit for combination therapy with antiresorptive agents.[118]

In the case of multiple myeloma, cancer cells induce excessive sclerostin release by osteocytes, which contributes to uncoupling and to the formation of lytic lesions.[119] Animal models of multiple myeloma show promising effects of sclerostin inhibitor therapy. This is further supported by the reports of patients with naturally occurring mutations in sclerostin who are apparently protected from the development of lytic bone lesions of multiple myeloma.[118]

Odanacatib is an orally administered inhibitor of cathepsin K, a lysosomal enzyme produced by osteoclasts that breaks down type 1 collagen. Animal models of malignancy demonstrate potential benefits of this agent in treating SREs.

Hypercalcemia of malignancy

Hypercalcemia associated with skeletal metastases is a common metabolic complication and a life-threatening disorder. Symptoms include weakness, polyuria, nausea, vomiting, anorexia, dehydration, lethargy, confusion, stupor, and coma. HCM is due to direct effects of local osteolytic factors derived from skeletal metastases (IL-1, TNF, TGF, and prostaglandins) or is due to production of systemic factors (PTHrp) secreted by the tumor that influence bone physiology. HCM is most common with multiple myeloma or breast cancer, but it can also occur with renal, ovarian, lung, and other cancers. The hypercalcemia associated with lymphomas is generally due to cytokines that stimulate osteoclastic bone resorption or is due to activation of ectopic 1α-hydroxylase activity, which converts 25-hydroxyvitamin D into the activated 1,25-dihydroxyvitamin D. The resultant hypervitaminosis D state causes increased gastrointestinal (GI) absorption of calcium. Medical management of HCM consists of the following strategies: (1) promoting calciuresis with IV saline and using loop diuretics only if excessive fluid retention occurs; (2) using pamidronate, 90 mg over 4–24 h IV, or denosumab, 120 mg subcutaneous weekly for four doses to inhibit bone resorption[120,121]; (3) discontinuing calcium and vitamin D supplementation (if any); and (4) consideration of glucocorticoids, which increase the effective circulatory volume, GFR, and calciuresis and suppress ectopic vitamin D activation. Calcitonin may also be used and can inhibit bone resorption to a lesser degree.

Corticosteroid-induced osteopenia

When glucocorticoids decrease the intestinal absorption of calcium, the 24-h urinary calcium excretion rate will be low and calcium (1200–1500 mg/day) and vitamin D (800–1600 units/day) may be provided orally. If glucocorticoids are increasing the urinary excretion of calcium, hydrochlorothiazide, 25–50 mg once or twice daily, may be used to reduce calciuresis. Negative calcium balance may be reflected by an elevated parathyroid hormone level (secondary hyperparathyroidism). The suppressive effect of glucocorticoids on osteoblastic bone formation may be reflected by low serum osteocalcin levels. Bisphosphonates can also prevent osteocyte and osteoblast apoptosis induced by glucocorticoids in experimental models.[122] Oral alendronate, 70 mg/week, or risedronate 35 mg/week, retards glucocorticoid-induced bone loss.[123,124]

Tumor-induced osteomalacia

Rarely occurring mesenchymal tumors can secrete fibroblast growth factor-23 (FGF-23), which induces renal phosphorus losses and inhibits vitamin D activation.[125] Hypophosphatemia and secondary hyperparathyroidism develop. These deleterious effects on calcium, phosphorus, and vitamin D metabolism lead to tumor-induced osteomalacia (TIO). Patients experience symptoms of bone pain, weakness, risk of fracture, height loss, impaired growth in children, and gait disturbance.[125] Decreased bone mineralization that is observed does not respond to vitamin D supplementation.

Tumors associated with TIO include osteosarcoma, giant cell tumors, hemangiopericytoma, among other rare mesenchymal tumors.[126] Initial misdiagnosis is reported among 95% of patients with TIO.[125] Biochemical testing should include serum calcium, phosphorus, 25-hydroxy-vitamin D, 1,25-dihydroxy-vitamin D, parathyroid hormone, FGF-23, and 24 h urinary phosphorus. A careful family history can help to differentiate TIO from inherited forms of excessive FGF-23 activity, such as X-linked hypophosphatemic rickets (XLH) or autosomal dominant hypophosphatemic rickets.

Disease localization is recommended using whole body 99-Technicium octreotide scanning[127] or 68-Gadolinium dotatate positron emission tomography.[128] Confirmation and further imaging may be obtained by computed tomography or magnetic resonance imaging, though these modalities are not as useful for initial detection due to poor specificity.[128]

Surgical resection is the preferred treatment, demonstrating a 30–50% increase in bone mineral density.[129] Repeat or debulking procedures can be considered if initial surgery is only partially successful. The use of localized techniques such as radiofrequency, cold, or ethanol ablation for TIO has been reported in small case series, though long-term follow-up is lacking.[130]

Medical treatment includes supportive measures using calcitriol at typical doses of 0.25–1 mcg daily, and phosphate supplementation. Somatostatin analog therapy has shown benefit in early reported cases,[131] but no benefit has been reported in a larger and more recently published series.[132] Future medical therapies for TIO may include therapy with FGF-23 antibodies, which has demonstrated benefit in adults with XLH.[133]

Radiation therapy for bone metastases

RT is one of the effective modalities for addressing bone metastases. Approximately 40% of all palliative RT is delivered for addressing bone metastases. Most commonly, RT is utilized in this setting for the purpose of pain relief with up to 80% of treated patients attaining significant durable analgesia, often for the remaining duration of their lives.[134] Especially when utilized early, RT can help preserve function by preventing spinal cord compression and pathologic fracture, thereby maintaining mobility. Ultimately, when used in careful coordination with other modalities (systemic therapy, surgery, analgesics, osteoclast inhibitors), RT can help optimize the quality of life of patients with bone metastases.

In its most common form, RT for bone metastases is delivered using external beam radiation therapy (EBRT) with high-energy photons generated by a linear accelerator. Other forms include particle-beam EBRT or injectable radioisotopes. Generally, the target volume for EBRT is defined by the anatomic borders of involved bone with margins applied to account for patient motion and setup uncertainty.

The effect of RT on bone metastases is based on several factors. Tumor cell kill results in decreased bulk of treated lesions allowing for osteoblastic repair to restore integrity of bone. Additionally, there seems to be inhibition of osteoclast activity and precursor migration further allowing for regenerative osteoblastic activity. Also, the early symptom relief often seen during palliative RT suggests an initial reduction of inflammatory cells thereby decreasing release of chemical pain mediators partially responsible for metastasis-related pain.[135]

Of note, in up to a third or more of patients, there is a recognized incidence of pain flare: a temporary worsening of pain at site of the irradiated bone within one to 2 weeks following RT. This is likely from an increased inflammatory microenvironment related to RT effect on tumor and normal tissues, resulting in elevated biochemical mediators of pain as well as direct nerve compression from edema. This flare is usually transient, lasting 1–2 days, and should be considered during management of patients getting RT for bone metastases.[136] In addition to analgesics such as nonsteroidal anti-inflammatory drugs (NSAIDs) and opiates, prophylactic dexamethasone may be considered for select patients, as this was found in a Phase 3 randomized controlled trial to significantly decrease the incidence of pain flare when compared with placebo (26% vs 35%, $p = 0.05$) following single-fraction radiation therapy (SFRT) for bone metastases.[137]

In the setting of palliative RT, the toxicity of treatment is an important consideration given the limited life expectancy of most patients with metastatic disease. Patients should be counseled on risks for acute and even late toxicities from RT which depend on location of target volume and dose delivered to adjacent normal tissues. Decisions regarding RT modality, dose fractionation, and technique are made to maximize the therapeutic ratio of treatment and this is particularly important in the setting of re-irradiation.

Dose fractionation

For management of uncomplicated painful bone metastases (no fracture or impending fracture, no significant soft tissue component), the American Society for Radiation Oncology (ASTRO) recently released updated evidence-based guidelines which advocate for SFRT as the most convenient and cost-effective regimen.[138]

Several large randomized trials have demonstrated that SFRT with dose of 8 Gy resulted in similar rates of pain relief (70% response), time to response (<1 month), and treatment-related toxicities when compared with multiple fraction radiation therapy (MFRT) schedules (24–30 Gy in 6–10 fractions).[138–142] In the Radiation Therapy Oncology Group (RTOG) trial 9714, 949 patients were randomized to receiving a single 8 Gy fraction versus 30 Gy in 10 fractions. No significant differences in narcotic analgesic use were seen between treatment arms.[141] A 2014 updated meta-analysis of randomized trials revealed patients undergoing SFRT or MFRT had similar incidences of pathologic fracture and spinal cord compression after treatment. SFRT patients were, however, more than twice as likely to need re-treatment of the same site (20% vs 8%, $p < 0.00001$).[143] In terms of economic impact, a Dutch multicenter trial of 1171 patients demonstrated that SFRT, even after accounting for retreatments, yielded cost savings of 8% and significantly freed radiotherapy capacity at treatment centers allowing more patients to be treated.[139]

Despite evidence-based guidelines advocating SFRT as the most cost-effective regimen for uncomplicated painful bone metastases, there remains underutilization of SFRT in the United States and beyond. In a 2009 survey analysis of three international radiation oncology profession organizations (ASTRO, Canadian Association of Radiation Oncology [CARO], Royal Australian and New Zealand College of Radiologists), 962 respondents detailed a median dose of 30 Gy in 10 fractions utilized in palliative EBRT for bone metastases. Principal factors considered when prescribing were prognosis, risk of spinal cord compression, and performance status.[144] A 2015 National Cancer Database (NCDB) analysis of patients treated for osseous metastases from breast, prostate, and lung cancer showed that from 2005 to 2011 only 5% of all palliative RT was given with single fraction. SFRT utilization was associated with older age, farther travel distance to treatment, nonprivate health insurance, and academic treatment facility ($p < 0.05$).[145] More awareness and supportive data seem to be needed to adjust practice patterns toward utilization of SFRT for uncomplicated painful bone metastases.

Epidural spinal cord compression

One of the most common complications of vertebral metastases is direct extension into the spinal canal causing epidural spinal cord compression (ESCC) which can lead to significant pain and loss of neurologic function (motor, sensory, bowel/bladder control). If there is significant spinal instability (fracture, vertebral body collapse, misalignment) associated with the ESCC, surgical stabilization (decompression, vertebroplasty, kyphoplasty) is generally indicated prior to other treatment interventions in order to reverse deficits and/or preserve remaining neurologic function.

Treatment is dictated by patient characteristics, tumor histology, and extent of ESCC. For tumors sensitive to both systemic and RT (e.g., myeloma, lymphoma, small cell lung cancer), these may respond quickly to systemic therapy (chemotherapy, glucocorticoids) which can be used either before or in lieu of palliative EBRT for rapid alleviation of tumor-related symptoms and risk to function. Less radiosensitive tumors (e.g., prostate, breast, ovarian) may require time for response to EBRT, and depending on extent of ESCC (low vs high-grade) decompressive surgery should be considered to allow for rapid decompression of the spinal cord prior to EBRT. The addition of decompressive surgery improves ambulatory outcomes and decreases need for corticosteroids and opioids when compared with radiation alone.[33] For patients with short expected survival (<3 months), SFRT (8 Gy) is a convenient option for palliation with median duration of response of 4.5 months with minimal toxicity.[146] Longer course MFRT is a better option for patients with more prolonged life expectancy (>6 months) due to more durable tumor control in the setting of ESCC.[147]

For radioresistant tumors (melanoma, renal cell carcinoma, non-small-cell lung cancer, GI cancers, sarcoma) extent of ESCC dictates treatment decisions. For low-grade ESCC, stereotactic body radiation therapy (SBRT) is an ideal noninvasive treatment to deliver high dose RT (18–24 Gy in single fraction, 24–30 Gy in three fractions) with highly conformal technique, yielding high, durable rates of tumor control (85 to >90%) with minimal rates of acute toxicity, no significant incidence of RT-related myelopathy.[148–151] In one large single-institution series with 811 spinal metastases treated with single-fraction SBRT, local control was significantly better with higher dose (>22.4 Gy) regardless of tumor histology.[148] Higher single-dose SBRT, however, as well preexisting fracture or spinal deformity and lytic bone lesions, were associated with higher rates of vertebral compression fracture (up to 10–15%).[152] If SBRT technique is not available, surgical excision followed by MFRT provides the best chance for local control. Patients with radioresistant tumors and high-grade ESCC should undergo decompression surgery followed by SBRT.[153,154]

Reirradiation

Retreatment of osseous metastases with RT can be considered for patients with persistent or recurrent pain more than 1 month after prior palliative RT (SFRT or MFRT) but risks for toxicity must be carefully evaluated. A 2012 systematic review and meta-analysis of clinical trials addressing effectiveness of reirradiation for painful bone metastases revealed that the overall pain response rate was approximately 60%.[155] A multicenter international trial randomized 425 patients between receiving reirradiation with either SFRT (8 Gy) or MFRT (20 Gy in five fractions) regimens showed no clinically significant differences in response rate (45% vs 51%, $p = 0.17$), although there was more GI toxicity (anorexia and diarrhea) with MFRT when retreating below the diaphragm. When looking specifically at spine lesions (limited up to only 20 Gy in five fractions given previously), no incidences of myelopathy were seen after either regimen. No significant differences were seen in rates of pathologic fractures (7% vs 5%, $p = 0.15$) but there seemed to be a trend toward increased spinal cord/cauda equina compression events with use of SFRT (2% vs <1%, $p = 0.094$).[156] For reirradiation of spine in setting of prior EBRT > 20 Gy, SBRT technique should be considered. Based on a systematic review of literature investigating SBRT for spinal reirradiation, overall improvement in patient-reported pain ranged 65–81% with low rates of vertebral body fracture (12%) and RT-induced myelopathy (1.2%).[157]

Radiation technique

Upfront palliative RT for bone metastases is often delivered with 2D technique or 3D conformal radiation therapy (3DCRT) techniques. 2D planning utilizes simple target delineation based on bone anatomy with simple field arrangements (opposed anterior–posterior or opposed lateral fields) without concern for dose conformality around a target volume. In a body location wherein normal tissue toxicity is not a significant concern (e.g., extremities), 2D planning may be the most appropriate for palliative RT. More frequently, especially for axial skeletal sites, 3DCRT planning technique is utilized. 3DCRT allows for more complex beam arrangements and field design to increase conformality of prescription dose around a specified 3D target volume and away from dose-limiting normal tissues, all contoured on CT-based planning software (Figure 6).

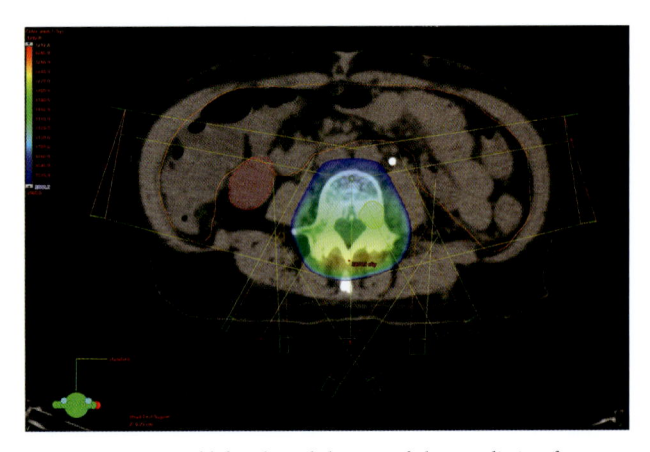

Figure 6 A 62-year-old female with history of chemoradiation for unresectable pancreatic adenocarcinoma developed painful metastasis at L4 vertebra (yellow). A 3D conformal radiation therapy (3DCRT) plan is displayed utilizing several beam angles in order to conform prescription dose (30 Gy in 10 fractions) away from previously irradiated normal structures such as bowel (orange) and right kidney (red).

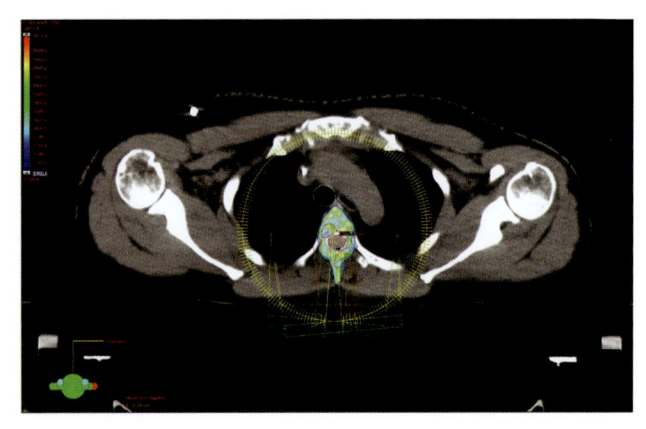

Figure 7 A 43-year-old female with metastatic breast cancer on systemic therapy with progressive T3 vertebral metastasis (red). A stereotactic body radiation therapy (SBRT) plan is displayed utilizing three coplanar arcs via volumetric modulated arc therapy (VMAT) delivery. Notice the adjacent trachea (lavender) and esophagus (dark blue) are well-excluded from prescription dose (27 Gy in three fractions) and the high conformality with VMAT technique allows sparing of spinal cord (orange) within the target volume.

In certain settings, especially with reirradiation, even more highly conformal techniques such as intensity-modulated radiation therapy (IMRT), volumetric modulated arc therapy (VMAT) should be considered. These techniques involve highly complex beam arrangements or rotational arc therapy which produce even greater dose conformality around the target volume while minimizing dose overlap of normal tissues. This is especially helpful in situations where sensitive dose-limiting normal tissues previously received RT. With SBRT, very high dose RT can be given with exact precision in a single or multiple fraction regimen utilizing IMRT or VMAT planning (Figure 7). SBRT is particularly helpful in setting of recurrent tumor when significant dose (>20 Gy in five fractions) has been given previously to adjacent central nervous structures (e.g., brain stem, spinal cord) and other dose-limiting structures (e.g., esophagus, bowel).[138,157] As discussed previously, SBRT may also be appropriate for management of symptomatic bone metastases from radioresistant primary cancers, especially in setting of ESCC from vertebral bone metastases.

SBRT is also being investigated as a more optimal treatment of limited metastatic disease in patients with expected survival >3–6 months. In a Phase II nonblinded noninferiority trial, 160 patients were randomized between single-fraction SBRT (12–16 Gy depending on tumor size) versus MFRT (30 Gy in 10 fractions) for painful bone metastases. Significantly higher rates of pain response (partial and complete) were seen with SBRT at 2 weeks, 3 months, and 9 months demonstrating durable, superior analgesia.[158] In SABR-COMET, an international Phase II randomized, open-label trial, 99 patients with controlled primary cancer and one to five oligometastases were randomized in 1 : 2 fashion to receiving standard of care ($n = 33$) therapies (including systemic therapies and/or conventional EBRT) or standard of care with SBRT to all metastatic lesions ($n = 66$). SBRT regimens included 30–60 Gy in three to eight fractions and high dose single fraction treatments (16–24 Gy) were allowed for brain and vertebral sites. One-third of the metastases were of bone sites and evenly distributed between groups. Use of SBRT demonstrated a trend toward improved overall survival (median 41 months vs 28 months, $p = 0.09$) at the cost of 20% increase in toxicity and three treatment-related deaths (4.5% of SBRT arm).[159] Phase III studies investigating use of SBRT for oligometastatic disease are now accruing (SABR-COMET-3, SABR-COMET-10, NRG-LU002, and NRG-BR002).

Hemibody irradiation

A less-widely utilized RT technique to address diffuse bone pain from osseous metastases is half-body or hemibody irradiation (HBI) which was introduced in the late 1970s in order to allow for comprehensive treatment of multiple symptomatic areas in a short period of time for a patient population with generally limited survival and poor performance. Single-dose HBI (6–8 Gy) was shown to be effective in achieving rapid symptomatic and disease response but came at cost of significant toxicity including acute radiation syndrome, pneumonitis, and prolonged anemia. This usually required a comprehensive pre- and post medication program (antiemetics, fluids, etc.) with intense monitoring.[160] Subsequently, several studies demonstrated fractionated HBI schedules (12–15 Gy in four to five fractions) remained as effective in pain relief while significantly reducing toxicity and need for premedication and hospitalizations.[161,162] The use of HBI for treatment of diffuse, symptomatic osseous metastases has largely been supplanted by the advent of bone-targeting radioisotopes but HBI remains a reasonable and effective option when access to such agents is limited.[163]

Radioisotopes

There has been growing use of bone-targeting radioisotopes (e.g., radium-223, samarium-153 lexidronam, strontium-89) which can localize to sites of predominantly osteoblastic metastases to deliver focal ionizing radiation at a very short range. These are typically utilized in patients with multiple and/or diffuse sites of involvement. Clinical investigations have shown the most promise for patients with bone metastases related to prostate and breast cancer, particularly with radium-223.[164]

Radium-223 mimics calcium, complexing with hydroxyapatite at sites of bone turnover, and emits high-energy, short-range alpha particles. Currently, radium-223 is approved for use treating patients with metastatic castration-resistant prostate cancer and symptomatic bone metastases without visceral metastatic disease. This was based an interim analysis of a landmark international Phase III double-blind randomized placebo-controlled trial investigating radium-223 use for patients with this disease setting.[165] Patients received one injection (intravenous, 50 kBq/kg body weight) every 4 weeks for six cycles. When compared with placebo, radium-223 demonstrated significantly improved overall survival (median 14.1 vs 11 months; $p = 0.001$) with low myelosuppression rates with pain relief in majority of patients by the third dose. Use of radium-223 both reduced total number of symptomatic skeletal event and lengthened time to first symptomatic skeletal events. Additionally, patients getting radium-223 were at lower risk for getting palliative EBRT or developing spinal cord compression.[166] Interestingly, there is emerging data showing that addition of EBRT to symptomatic sites with radioisotope therapy can further increase analgesic benefit without significant added toxicity.[167]

Key references

The complete reference list can be found on Vital Source version of this title, see inside front cover.

2 Coleman RE. Clinical features of metastatic bone disease and risk of skeletal morbidity. *Clin Cancer Res*. 2006;**12**(20 Pt 2):6243s–6249s.

3 Conen K, Hagmann R, Hess V, et al. Incidence and predictors of bone metastases (BM) and skeletal-related events (SREs) in small cell lung cancer (SCLC): a Swiss patient cohort. *J Cancer*. 2016;**7**(14):2110–2116.

4 Cetin K, Christiansen CF, Jacobsen JB, et al. Bone metastasis, skeletal-related events, and mortality in lung cancer patients: a Danish population-based cohort study. *Lung Cancer*. 2014;**86**(2):247–254.

5 Zhang H, Zhu W, Biskup E, et al. Incidence, risk factors and prognostic characteristics of bone metastases and skeletal-related events (SREs) in breast cancer patients: a systematic review of the real world data. *J Bone Oncol*. 2018;**11**:38–50.

6 Santini D, Procopio G, Porta C, et al. Natural history of malignant bone disease in renal cancer: final results of an Italian bone metastasis survey. *PLoS One*. 2013;**8**(12):e83026.

13 Rougraff BT, Kneisl JS, Simon MA. Skeletal metastases of unknown origin. A prospective study of a diagnostic strategy. *J Bone Joint Surg Am*. 1993;**75**(9):1276–1281.

17 Henry DH, Costa L, Goldwasser F, et al. Randomized, double-blind study of denosumab versus zoledronic acid in the treatment of bone metastases in patients with advanced cancer (excluding breast and prostate cancer) or multiple myeloma. *J Clin Oncol*. 2011;**29**(9):1125–1132.

18 Toyota N, Naito A, Kakizawa H, et al. Radiofrequency ablation therapy combined with cementoplasty for painful bone metastases: initial experience. *Cardiovasc Intervent Radiol*. 2005;**28**(5):578–583.

21 Laitinen M, Nieminen J, Pakarinen TK. Treatment of pathological humerus shaft fractures with intramedullary nails with or without cement fixation. *Arch Orthop Trauma Surg*. 2011;**131**(4):503–508.

39 Mundy GR, Martin TJ. The hypercalcemia of malignancy: pathogenesis and management. *Metabolism*. 1982;**31**(12):1247–1277.

40 Wong MH, Stockler MR, Pavlakis N. Bisphosphonates and other bone agents for breast cancer. *Cochrane Database Syst Rev*. 2012;**2**:CD003474.

43 Green JR, Clezardin P. Mechanisms of bisphosphonate effects on osteoclasts, tumor cell growth, and metastasis. *Am J Clin Oncol*. 2002;**25**(6 Suppl 1):S3–S9.

46 Comito G, Pons Segura C, Taddei ML, et al. Zoledronic acid impairs stromal reactivity by inhibiting M2-macrophages polarization and prostate cancer-associated fibroblasts. *Oncotarget*. 2017;**8**(1):118–132.

54 Rosen LS, Gordon D, Tchekmedyian NS, et al. Long-term efficacy and safety of zoledronic acid in the treatment of skeletal metastases in patients with non-small cell lung carcinoma and other solid tumors: a randomized, phase III, double-blind, placebo-controlled trial. *Cancer*. 2004;**100**(12):2613–2621.

57 Ralston SH, Gallacher SJ, Patel U, et al. Cancer-associated hypercalcemia: morbidity and mortality. Clinical experience in 126 treated patients. *Ann Intern Med*. 1990;**112**(7):499–504.

60 Chappard D, Bouvard B, Basle MF, et al. Bone metastasis: histological changes and pathophysiological mechanisms in osteolytic or osteosclerotic localizations. A review. *Morphologie*. 2011;**95**(309):65–75.

63 Ahern E, Harjunpaa H, O'Donnell JS, et al. RANKL blockade improves efficacy of PD1-PD-L1 blockade or dual PD1-PD-L1 and CTLA4 blockade in mouse models of cancer. *Oncoimmunology*. 2018;**7**(6):e1431088.

64 Ahern E, Smyth MJ, Dougall WC, Teng MWL. Roles of the RANKL-RANK axis in antitumour immunity - implications for therapy. *Nat Rev Clin Oncol*. 2018;**15**(11):676–693.

69 Zheng GZ, Chang B, Lin FX, et al. Meta-analysis comparing denosumab and zoledronic acid for treatment of bone metastases in patients with advanced solid tumours. *Eur J Cancer Care (Engl)*. 2017;**26**(6). doi: 10.1111/ecc.12541.

70 Wong R, Wiffen PJ. Bisphosphonates for the relief of pain secondary to bone metastases. *Cochrane Database Syst Rev*. 2002;**2**:CD002068.

73 Rosen LS, Gordon D, Kaminski M, et al. Zoledronic acid versus pamidronate in the treatment of skeletal metastases in patients with breast cancer or osteolytic lesions of multiple myeloma: a phase III, double-blind, comparative trial. *Cancer J*. 2001;**7**(5):377–387.

75 Henry D, Vadhan-Raj S, Hirsh V, et al. Delaying skeletal-related events in a randomized phase 3 study of denosumab versus zoledronic acid in patients with advanced cancer: an analysis of data from patients with solid tumors. *Support Care Cancer*. 2014;**22**(3):679–687.

76 Shao YH, Moore DF, Shih W, et al. Fracture after androgen deprivation therapy among men with a high baseline risk of skeletal complications. *BJU Int*. 2013;**111**(5):745–752.

83 Smith MR, Eastham J, Gleason DM, et al. Randomized controlled trial of zoledronic acid to prevent bone loss in men receiving androgen deprivation therapy for nonmetastatic prostate cancer. *J Urol*. 2003;**169**(6):2008–2012.

84 Ellis GK, Bone HG, Chlebowski R, et al. Randomized trial of denosumab in patients receiving adjuvant aromatase inhibitors for nonmetastatic breast cancer. *J Clin Oncol*. 2008;**26**(30):4875–4882.

93 Fizazi K, Carducci M, Smith M, et al. Denosumab versus zoledronic acid for treatment of bone metastases in men with castration-resistant prostate cancer: a randomised, double-blind study. *Lancet*. 2011;**377**(9768):813–822.

107 Lee SH, Chan RC, Chang SS, et al. Use of bisphosphonates and the risk of osteonecrosis among cancer patients: a systemic review and meta-analysis of the observational studies. *Support Care Cancer*. 2014;**22**(2):553–560.

112 Chang ST, Tenforde AS, Grimsrud CD, et al. Atypical femur fractures among breast cancer and multiple myeloma patients receiving intravenous bisphosphonate therapy. *Bone*. 2012;**51**(3):524–527.

113 Takahashi M, Ozaki Y, Kizawa R, et al. Atypical femoral fracture in patients with bone metastasis receiving denosumab therapy: a retrospective study and systematic review. *BMC Cancer*. 2019;**19**(1):980.

134 Spencer K, Morris E, Dugdale E, et al. 30 day mortality in adult palliative radiotherapy—a retrospective population based study of 14,972 treatment episodes. *Radiother Oncol*. 2015;**115**(2):264–271.

135 Vakaet LA, Boterberg T. Pain control by ionizing radiation of bone metastasis. *Int J Dev Biol*. 2004;**48**(5–6):599–606.

138 Lutz S, Balboni T, Jones J, et al. Palliative radiation therapy for bone metastases: update of an ASTRO evidence-based guideline. *Pract Radiat Oncol*. 2017;**7**(1):4–12.

140 van der Linden YM, Lok JJ, Steenland E, et al. Single fraction radiotherapy is efficacious: a further analysis of the Dutch Bone Metastasis Study controlling for the influence of retreatment. *Int J Radiat Oncol Biol Phys*. 2004;**59**(2):528–537.

146 Maranzano E, Trippa F, Casale M, et al. 8Gy single-dose radiotherapy is effective in metastatic spinal cord compression: results of a phase III randomized multicentre Italian trial. *Radiother Oncol*. 2009;**93**(2):174–179.

154 Redmond KJ, Lo SS, Fisher C, Sahgal A. Postoperative stereotactic body radiation therapy (SBRT) for spine metastases: a critical review to guide practice. *Int J Radiat Oncol Biol Phys*. 2016;**95**(5):1414–1428.

159 Palma DA, Olson R, Harrow S, et al. Stereotactic ablative radiotherapy versus standard of care palliative treatment in patients with oligometastatic cancers (SABR-COMET): a randomised, phase 2, open-label trial. *Lancet*. 2019;**393**(10185):2051–2058.

161 Salazar OM, DaMotta NW, Bridgman SM, et al. Fractionated half-body irradiation for pain palliation in widely metastatic cancers: comparison with single dose. *Int J Radiat Oncol Biol Phys*. 1996;**36**(1):49–60.

162 Scarantino CW, Caplan R, Rotman M, et al. A phase I/II study to evaluate the effect of fractionated hemibody irradiation in the treatment of osseous metastases--RTOG 88-22. *Int J Radiat Oncol Biol Phys*. 1996;**36**(1):37–48.

165 Parker C, Nilsson S, Heinrich D, et al. Alpha emitter radium-223 and survival in metastatic prostate cancer. *N Engl J Med*. 2013;**369**(3):213–223.

167 Baczyk M, Milecki P, Pisarek M, et al. A prospective randomized trial: a comparison of the analgesic effect and toxicity of 153Sm radioisotope treatment in monotherapy and combined therapy including local external beam radiotherapy (EBRT) among metastatic castrate resistance prostate cancer (mCRPC) patients with painful bone metastases. *Neoplasma*. 2013;**60**(3):328–333.

127 Hematologic complications and blood bank support

Roger Belizaire, MD, PhD ■ Kenneth C. Anderson, MD

Overview

Many of the fundamental therapies used to treat cancer (e.g., chemotherapy, stem cell transplantation) disrupt normal hematopoiesis in the bone marrow. As a result, blood transfusion for patients with cancer is an essential supportive modality. The primary focus of this article is on "classical" blood component support: how red cells, plasma, platelets, and granulocytes are collected, tested, stored, and administered to address specific deficiencies in patients with cancer. Particular attention is paid to studies of prophylactic platelet transfusion, which over the past several decades has been critical in allowing myelosuppressive treatments to be applied to a variety of malignant disease states. Current infectious risks of blood products are reviewed.

Table 1 Causes of anemia, thrombocytopenia, and leukopenia in cancer.

Bone marrow replacement by primary tumor (e.g., leukemia)
Bone marrow involvement by metastatic tumor (e.g., breast, prostate)
Derangement of normal physiology

- Nutritional (e.g., folate, iron, negative nitrogen balance)
- Abnormal feedback (e.g., stimulation/inhibition of hematopoiesis)
- Bone marrow reaction (e.g., fibrosis)
- Peripheral destruction (e.g., immune hemolysis, diffuse intravascular coagulation, splenomegaly)
- Blood loss

Myelosuppression by chemotherapy or radiotherapy

Table 2 Characteristic effects of drugs and treatments on bone marrow.

Treatment	Hematologic complication
Most chemotherapeutic agents	Leukopenia and thrombocytopenia at 9–10 days; nadir counts at 14–18 days; recovery of counts at 21–28 days
Nitrosourea	Myelosuppression at 4–6 weeks
Vincristine, 1-asparaginase, bleomycin, myelosuppression methotrexate with leucovorin	No myelosuppression
Gamma irradiation	Chronic lymphopenia
Whole-body irradiation	Profound suppression of humoral and cellular immune response

Hematologic complications occur commonly in patients with cancer, related either to the underlying disease or to its treatment.[1,2] Abnormalities in the red blood cell (RBC), white blood cell (WBC), and platelet number and function require transfusion medicine expertise for the provision of appropriate blood component support.[3,4] Indeed, the therapeutic advances made using high-dose combination chemotherapeutic approaches would not have been possible without the parallel development of technology to support patients through the hematologic complications of therapy.

Causes of pancytopenia

Cancer and its treatment may alter normal hematopoiesis either by direct effects on hematopoietic stem cells or by inhibiting production of and responsiveness to hematopoietic growth factors (Table 1).

Disease related

Bone marrow hematopoietic cells can be replaced either by primary tumor derived from marrow cells or by metastatic spread of tumor to the marrow from neoplasms of other organs. Hodgkin and non-Hodgkin lymphoma (NHL), malignant melanoma, neuroblastoma, as well as carcinoma of the breast, prostate, lung, adrenal, thyroid, and kidney commonly manifest marrow involvement. Ultimately, diffuse involvement of marrow with tumor can lead to either marrow fibrosis or necrosis, which may be associated with splenomegaly, thrombocytopenia, and immature cells of all lineages in the peripheral blood.[5]

Chemotherapy related

The role of treatment in marrow injury and recovery varies both with the drugs employed and with the normal turnover rate of cells of different hematologic lineages. The characteristic effects of several drugs on marrow are shown in Table 2. The bone marrow has a storage compartment that can supply mature cells to the peripheral blood for 8–10 days after the stem cell pool has ceased to function. Events in the peripheral blood are therefore a week behind the events in the bone marrow. In previously untreated patients, leukopenia and thrombocytopenia are described on the ninth or tenth day after treatment, with the nadir of counts on days 14–18. Recovery of counts is evident by day 21 and complete by day 28. The cytotoxic dose–response effect is usually related to the nadir WBC and platelet count, not the duration of cytopenia. This is due to the resting state of the stem cells of normal bone marrow, which protects them from damage.

Gamma radiation related

Cells damaged by irradiation may divide one time or more before all progeny are rendered reproductively sterile; thus, an irradiated cell will not appear damaged until it divides.[6] At the time of the first postirradiation subdivision, the cell may die, divide aberrantly, and produce unusual forms, be unable to divide and remain physiologically functional, or give rise to one or more generation of progeny until cells become sterile. Since bone marrow stem cells have a very low capacity for repair of sublethal irradiation damage, multiple smaller radiation fractions may preserve other normal tissues (e.g., lung, intestine) but will not spare bone marrow.

Associated processes

It is essential to remain cognizant of derangements in normal physiology that may occur in the setting of cancer and/or treatment and that contribute to pancytopenia. These include nutritional factors, such as folate, iron, or vitamin deficiencies. There may be abnormal feedback loops in hematopoiesis, such as cell-mediated suppression of hematopoiesis in aplastic anemia or stimulation of thrombopoiesis in the setting of antibody-mediated platelet destruction.[7] Fibrosis can occur either as part of a disease process or as a reaction to therapy, thereby compromising bone marrow reserve. Immune-mediated destruction of cells and other factors, such as splenomegaly, can result in cytopenias. Moreover, occult bleeding must always be considered as a cause of persistent anemia and refractory thrombocytopenia. These clinical examples emphasize the importance of carefully assessing patients with cancer for treatable medical etiologies of their hematologic complications prior to attributing these effects to their underlying neoplasms.

Abnormalities of red cells and red cell support

Anemia

Anemia in patients with cancer can be mild to severe and may be attributable to many causes. Hematopoiesis in patients with early stages of cancer may be normal. On the other hand, replacement of marrow cells by tumor is not essential for the development of anemia, even in patients with metastatic cancer. Most commonly, the incidence and magnitude of anemia in patients with cancer increase as the disease progresses. This anemia is designated as anemia of chronic disease only if the cellular pattern in the marrow is nearly normal, the serum iron and iron-binding capacity are low, the iron content of the marrow is normal or increased, and the serum ferritin is elevated.[8] The coexistence of low plasma iron levels with adequate amounts of storage iron helps distinguish anemia of chronic disease from iron-deficiency anemia. Moreover, other causes of anemia, for example, overt hemolysis, bleeding, nutritional deficiency, or marrow replacement, must be ruled out. In some patients, such as those with Hodgkin disease (HD), erythrophagocytosis or hypersplenism may account for this decrease in red cell survival, but in others its etiology is unclear.

Red cell transfusion

Red cell transfusions are indicated to increase oxygen-carrying capacity in patients with anemia that is not adequately compensated by normal physiologic mechanisms. Sufficient oxygen-carrying capacity to maintain cardiopulmonary function can be met by a hemoglobin of 7 g/dL (a hematocrit of approximately 21%) when the intravascular volume is adequate for perfusion.[9] In a multicenter randomized trial of critical care patients, a restrictive transfusion strategy (maintaining hemoglobin levels between 7 and 9 g/dL) was demonstrated to be at least as safe as a more liberal transfusion strategy, with the possible exception of patients with acute myocardial infarction or unstable angina.[10] Subsequent randomized trials have compared restrictive versus liberal RBC transfusion strategies in patients with cardiovascular disease having hip surgery[11] or cardiac surgery,[12–14] in patients with sepsis,[15] in patients with upper gastrointestinal bleeding,[16] and in patients with acute myocardial infarction.[17] A restrictive transfusion strategy (hemoglobin transfusion threshold of 7–8 g/dL) appears to be safe and appropriate for the vast majority of hospitalized inpatients. A recent randomized trial in patients undergoing autologous or allogeneic hematopoietic stem cell transplant did not demonstrate a difference in several important transplant-related outcomes, including 100-day survival, when comparing liberal (hemoglobin 9 g/dL) and restrictive (hemoglobin 7 g/dL) transfusion thresholds.[18] Additional high-quality clinical trial data to guide RBC transfusion in patients with malignancy are still awaited. Overall, there is no single hemoglobin level that can be universally applied as a "transfusion trigger." In deciding whether to transfuse a specific patient, the physician should consider the patient's age, degree of anemia, the intravascular volume, and the presence of coexisting cardiac, pulmonary, or vascular conditions.[19] To meet oxygen needs, some patients may require RBC transfusions at higher hemoglobin levels. In particular, hemoglobin levels are commonly maintained at levels of 8 g/dL in the setting of cancer and its therapy. Transfusing one unit of RBC will usually increase the hemoglobin by 1 g/dL and the hematocrit by 2–3% in the average adult weighing 70 kg.

Packed red blood cells (PRBCs) are prepared either from whole blood (WB) by the removal of plasma or by erythrocytapheresis. Red cells can be depleted of leukocytes by filtration to produce leukoreduced red cells (LRBCs). Leukoreduction can prevent a significant percentage of febrile nonhemolytic transfusion reactions and cytomegalovirus (CMV) infection in transfusion recipients.[20] In the United States and internationally, there is a trend to universally transfuse leukoreduced cellular components to avoid the multiple adverse sequelae of leukocytes. Washed RBCs are prepared by further removal of plasma from PRBCs. These products are sometimes indicated to prevent allergic reactions to plasma proteins.[21] PRBCs are currently stored for up to 42 days at 4°C. Retrospective studies have suggested that transfusing older stored PRBC units may be associated with adverse consequences for the recipient.[22,23] However, older RBC units have not been demonstrated to be increase morbidity or mortality when compared with fresher RBC units in multiple randomized controlled trials.[24–29]

Therapeutic antibody treatments interfering with pretransfusion red cell testing

Standard pretransfusion screening for the presence or absence of antibodies reactive with RBC antigens can be complicated by the patient's underlying diagnosis, clinical status, and ongoing therapies. Indeed, intravenous immunoglobulin (IVIg), which is derived from human donor plasma, can contain antibodies recognizing RBC antigens, and patients receiving IVIg may misleadingly appear to have generated RBC-specific antibodies.[30] More recently, the prevalent use of an anti-CD38 monoclonal antibody, daratumumab, and an anti-CD47 antibody, magrolimab, in oncology patients has presented another issue for pretransfusion red cell testing. Both CD38 and CD47 are highly expressed on RBCs, including the reagent RBCs used for laboratory testing. Thus patients treated with either daratumumab or magrolimab typically have pan-reactive antibody screens that cannot be resolved using standard approaches; magrolimab treatment also causes difficulty with ABO typing. Effective laboratory protocols to address the technical challenges of daratumumab and magrolimab have been developed[31,32], though it is probable that additional interferences from new monoclonal antibody therapies will arise in the future.

In this context, it is essential for oncologists to alert blood bank physicians and staff prior to initiating therapies that are likely to affect pretransfusion laboratory testing.

Leukopenia and white cell support

Leukopenia

Leukopenia may occur related to cancer and its treatment. In 1965, Hersh et al.[33] summarized the causes of death in patients with acute leukemia treated at the National Cancer Institute and noted a marked decline in fatal hemorrhage, due to the availability of platelet transfusions, with a concomitant increase in the occurrence of infection alone as a cause of death. A quantitative relationship between circulating leukocytes and infection was established in patients with leukemia; in particular, the probability of being infected is proportional to both the severity and duration of leukopenia.[34]

Granulocyte transfusion

Therapeutic granulocytes were first utilized nearly 30 years ago in leukemic patients with leukopenia and serious infection. The earliest trials, which demonstrated the potential value of granulocyte transfusions, utilized granulocytes harvested from patients with chronic myelogenous leukemia and achieved cell dosages never approached when normal donors were utilized.[35] The importance of dose was defined: less than 10^{10} granulocytes were ineffective whereas greater than 10^{11} cells were effective. Indeed, in an afebrile, uninfected man, the half-life of granulocytes in the circulation is 6.7 (4–10) hours and the daily turnover rate is 230%. Parallel work in canine models had also demonstrated that dogs deliberately made leukopenic by irradiation and given Gram-negative bacteremia and pneumonia could be successfully treated with granulocyte transfusions.[36,37]

There have been several randomized prospective trials of prophylactic leukocyte transfusions, given to prevent infections in leukopenic recipients.[38] However, none of the studies demonstrated improved survival because alloimmunization, transfusion reactions, CMV infection, and pulmonary infiltrates occurred more frequently in the transfused group. These studies have been criticized due to inadequate donor-recipient matching and inadequate doses of granulocytes transfused. A recently completed randomized trial of high-dose granulocytes collected from donors mobilized with a combination of G-CSF and dexamethasone did not observe a difference in survival or microbial response in patients transfused with granulocytes, though the study was underpowered due to low patient enrollment.[39] Currently, the role for granulocyte transfusions remains controversial. When granulocytes transfusions are used, the products must be irradiated to prevent graft-versus-host disease (GVHD) when transfused to an immunocompromised host.

Thrombocytopenia and platelet support

Thrombocytopenia

Thrombocytopenia in cancer patients is usually attributable to treatment with chemotherapy and radiotherapy. Impaired production of platelets due to a decrease or absence of megakaryocytes is therefore the most common cause of thrombocytopenia in patients

Table 3 Causes of thrombocytopenia.

Acute thrombocytopenia due to increased

- Platelet depletion (utilization, sequestration, or destruction)
- Massive blood replacement
- Cardiac surgery
- Splenomegaly

Immune destruction of platelets

- Self-limited acute idiopathic thrombocytopenia purpura (ITP)
- Posttransfusion purpura
- Drug purpura
- Chronic idiopathic thrombocytopenia purpura
- Consumptive thrombocytopenia

Hereditary defects
Thrombocytopenia with decreased platelet production

- Aplastic anemia
- Acute leukemia

Idiopathic megakaryocytic aplasia
Marrow infiltration

- Malignant
- Nonmalignant—Gaucher disease, granulomatous diseases

Following radiation or myelosuppressive drugs
Drugs producing specific suppression of platelet production (e.g., thiazides, ethanol, estrogens)
Nutritional deficiency—megaloblastic anemia, severe iron deficiency (rare)
Viral infections
Paroxysmal nocturnal hemoglobinuria

with cancer (Table 3). However, thrombocytopenia may also be due to splenic sequestration in patients who have splenomegaly as part of their primary neoplastic process. In this setting, increased numbers of megakaryocytes are evident unless extensive marrow infiltration is present. Immune-mediated thrombocytopenia may also occur related to antihuman leukocyte antigen (anti-HLA) or antiplatelet-specific alloantibodies. Finally, thrombocytopenia may be related to diffuse intravascular coagulation (DIC), especially in patients with acute myelocytic leukemias, lymphomas, and carcinoma of lung, breast, gastrointestinal, or urologic origin. DIC commonly complicates acute promyelocytic leukemia due to the presence of both thromboplastic material and fibrinolytic proteases in the promyelocytic subcellular components.[40]

Abnormalities in platelet function

Platelet function can be abnormal in several chronic myeloproliferative disorders. Although most bleeding in patients with AML is related to thrombocytopenia, intrinsic abnormalities in platelet function have been described including decreased platelet pro-coagulant activity and decreased aggregation and serotonin release responses to ADP, epinephrine, or collagen.[41] Platelet dysfunction is evident in a fraction of patients with IgA myeloma or Waldenstrom macroglobulinemia, multiple myeloma, and monoclonal gammopathy of undetermined significance.[42]

Platelet transfusion support

In 1910, fresh whole blood was first transfused to thrombocytopenic patients, resulting in a significant rise in the platelet count, hemostasis, and improvement of the bleeding time.[43] In the 1950s, platelets were first used for the treatment of thrombocytopenia related to combination chemotherapeutic treatments of leukemias.[44] Data from the National Cancer Institute in the early 1960s clearly demonstrated that leukemia patients died of hemorrhage during induction of remission with chemotherapy and established the quantitative relationship between platelet count and hemorrhage.[45] It was shown that platelet therapy could modify the course of hemorrhage in both pediatric and adult settings, the only difference being the doses required. Two randomized trials compared a prophylactic platelet transfusion strategy with a therapeutic platelet transfusion strategy in patients with hypoproliferative thrombocytopenia. Both studies demonstrated a benefit, albeit limited, of platelet prophylaxis, and both showed that prophylaxis has a greater effect on bleeding risk in patients treated with chemotherapy for leukemia compared with autologous stem cell transplant recipients.[46,47]

Single- and multiple-donor platelets

In the United States, one unit of platelet concentrate is obtained from one unit of whole blood by centrifugation and contains approximately 5.5×10^{10} platelets/unit. (This method of preparing platelets is known as the "platelet-rich plasma" (PRP) method. In other countries, platelet concentrates are prepared from whole blood using the alternate "buffy coat" method.) Concentrates from multiple (4–6) donors are pooled to produce a single component for transfusion. Apheresis technology has permitted harvesting the equivalent of several platelet concentrates from a single donor during a single donation. A single-donor platelet unit typically contains at least 3×10^{11} platelets/unit. Single-donor platelets are generally considered to be the platelet product of choice for patients being treated for malignancy. In patients who do not respond to platelet transfusion due to HLA alloantibodies, single-donor HLA-matched platelets may also be utilized. In the United States, platelet units may be stored at room temperature for up to 5 days.

Indications for therapeutic and prophylactic platelet transfusion

Platelets are commonly transfused to patients with cancer. The majority of platelet transfusions are given prophylactically to prevent bleeding, as opposed to therapeutically, to treat active bleeding.[48] The appropriate indications for transfusion of platelets have been the subject of a recent clinical practice guideline from the AABB.[49] At present, one dose of one apheresis platelets (or equivalent pool of random donor platelet concentrates) is routinely transfused to cancer patients with platelet counts less than $10,000/mm^3$ to reduce the risk of hemorrhage. Prospective clinical trials have shown that the risk of major bleeding was similar whether $10 \times 10^9/L$ or $20 \times 10^9/L$ was used as the platelet-transfusion threshold in patients with acute leukemia, and that the lower threshold reduced platelet use.[50–53] In patients with hematologic malignancies, a randomized trial comparing a prophylactic platelet transfusion threshold of $10,000/mm^3$ with a "no-prophylaxis" strategy demonstrated increased bleeding among patients in the "no-prophylaxis" group; interestingly, in the subgroup of patients undergoing autologous hematopoietic stem cell transplant, there was no difference in bleeding between the two groups, suggesting that the underlying diagnosis and/or treatment modify bleeding risk in the setting of severe thrombocytopenia.[54]

There are additional clinical observations indicating that the risk of bleeding at a given platelet count may vary in distinct clinical settings. For example, patients with thrombocytopenia due to AML were reported to have increased bleeding at less than $10,000/mm^3$ platelets, in contrast to patients with ALL, who had similar risk of hemorrhage at less than $20,000/mm^3$ platelets.[55] Patients with chronic thrombocytopenia due to decreased platelet production (i.e., myelodysplastic syndromes) may require transfusions, in contrast to patients with accelerated destruction but active production of platelets (i.e., idiopathic thrombocytopenic purpura), who may not require routine platelet transfusions. Moreover, patients with chronic thrombocytopenia may tolerate lower absolute platelet counts without transfusion. In patients with abnormalities of platelet function, it is not the absolute platelet count but rather the number of functional platelets that is important for the prevention of bleeding. Thus, it is difficult to define an absolute platelet threshold for transfusion for all patients, and both the timing and the dose of prophylactic platelet transfusion must therefore be determined on a clinical basis.[56–58]

The multicenter randomized PLADO (PLAtelet DOsing) study demonstrated that prophylactic transfusion with low-dose platelets does not increase the risk of Grade 2 or higher bleeding as compared with standard-dose prophylaxis among inpatients with hypoproliferative thrombocytopenia. Patients receiving low-dose prophylaxis do require more frequent platelet transfusions, although fewer total platelets are required overall.[59]

Clinical and laboratory assessment of the effectiveness of platelet transfusion

The effectiveness of platelet transfusion can be assessed by laboratory parameters (the platelet count increment 1 hour or 10 to 15 minutes after transfusion) as well as by the observed clinical outcome after transfusion.[60–62] The corrected count increment (CCI) is defined as the increment in platelet counts from pre- to posttransfusion corrected for the number of units transfused and for the body surface area of the recipient. A CCI of $15,000–20,000/\mu L/m^2$ is usual at 18–24 hours, provided fresh, properly stored platelets have been transfused.[63]

Posttransfusion increments in platelet count may be less than expected due to splenic sequestration, especially in the setting of splenomegaly.[64] Drug-induced platelet antibodies, which mediate immune destruction of platelets, have been demonstrated.[65] The survival of transfused platelets can also be compromised if the recipient possesses antibodies against donor antigens of HLA-A and HLA-B loci, the ABO system, or platelet alloantigens. Response to platelet transfusion in recipients of hematopoietic stem cell transplantation has been specifically studied.

Alloimmunization

Platelets bear HLA-A and -B but lack HLA-C and -DR Antigens, and there is a high correlation between the development of lymphocytotoxic anti-HLA antibodies in the recipient and refractoriness to random-donor platelets.[66] Currently, anti-HLA antibodies are most easily detectable using the patient's serum in a flow cytometry assay using HLA antigen-coated beads.

Yankee et al.[67] first demonstrated that platelets obtained from HLA-identical siblings or from unrelated donors matched at the HLA-A and -B loci (grade A or B matches) could result in satisfactory posttransfusion increments in alloimmunized recipients who were refractory to random-donor platelet transfusions. Subsequently, Duquesnoy and colleagues found that donors whose HLA antigens were the same (B match) or cross-reactive with the patient's antigens (BX match) were equivalent.[68]

The recognition of the refractoriness associated with the development of anti-HLA antibodies led to attempts to either avoid or delay alloimmunization by modifying the platelets to be transfused. Since HLA antigens are expressed on leukocytes, and platelets themselves are poor immunogens, investigators have attempted to (1) remove WBCs from platelets or treat platelets with ultraviolet irradiation (UV) to abrogate the leukocyte antigen-presenting function; (2) use single rather than multiple donor platelets to minimize exposure to HLA; and (3) transfuse only HLA-matched or leukocyte-depleted HLA-matched platelets. The multicenter prospective Trial to Reduce Alloimmunization to Platelets (TRAPs) study confirmed that the incidence of anti-HLA and platelet-specific antibodies alone, as well as the incidence of antibodies associated with platelet refractoriness, were reduced in leukemic recipients who received either filtered or UV-treated pooled random-donor concentrates or filtered single-donor platelets compared to similar patients who received nonfiltered pooled random-donor concentrates.[69] Only 13% of patients developed platelet refractoriness associated with lymphocytotoxic antibodies, suggesting that the majority of unresponsiveness to platelet transfusion is related to other factors. When sensitized recipients remain refractory to HLA-matched platelets, cross-matched platelets are sometimes provided. A third method of dealing with HLA immune refractoriness is to provide antigen-negative platelets, analogous to providing antigen-negative RBCs for patients with RBC alloantibodies.

ABO blood group determinants are intrinsic to platelet membranes.[70] Unlike the case with RBC transfusion, ABO mismatch between donor and recipient is not an absolute contraindication to platelet transfusion. That said, ABO-identical platelet transfusions are preferred. Transfused ABO major-incompatible platelets (e.g., A donor, O recipient) demonstrate recoveries that are about 1/3rd lower than those seen with ABO-identical transfusions.[71,72]

Additionally, passively transfused high-titer isohemagglutinins present within the plasma in the transfused platelet concentrates (e.g., donor O, recipient A) have occasionally caused severe hemolysis. The United Kingdom, notably, has instituted routine screening of platelet units for anti-A/B to prevent this problem. Other countries, including the United States, have not adopted a uniform strategy of prevention.[73]

Other therapeutic modalities

Transfusion of fresh frozen plasma
Fresh frozen plasma is the fluid portion of one unit (450 mL) of whole blood that is centrifuged, separated, and frozen at −18°C or lower. It contains physiologic levels of coagulation factors. Fresh frozen plasma is utilized to correct coagulation factor deficiencies; to reverse the effect of warfarin; and to treat thrombotic thrombocytopenic purpura, disseminated intravascular coagulation, coagulopathy of liver disease, thrombolytic agent overdose, and protein C or S deficiency.[74] In addition to the plasma obtained from donated whole blood, it can be collected using plasmapheresis procedures for the production of derivatives: coagulation factors (factors VIII and IX), immunoglobulin, and albumin preparations.

Effects of transfusion on the immune system

Alloimmunization
The most firmly established effect of transfusion is the stimulation of antibodies in the recipient against antigens in the transfused products. Both cellular and plasma antigens in transfused blood expose the recipients to hundreds of known alloantigens.

Over 400 RBC antigens have been identified, yet we routinely ensure compatibility for only three of them: A, B, and D. More than 100 HLA antigens, as well as granulocyte- and platelet-specific antigens, have also been identified. Genetic variants can result in structural and antigenic differences in plasma and cell-associated proteins, leading to recipient immunization against donor alloantigens. The vast majority of RBC transfusions do not result in alloimmunization.[75] A recent analysis of more than 30,000 transfused patients in the United States observed that patients with hematologic or solid malignancies were less likely to develop RBC alloantibodies, which could be explained by the receipt of immunosuppressive or myeloablative therapies;[76] not surprisingly, sickle cell disease patients analyzed as part of the same study showed RBC alloimmunization rates that were significantly higher. In this context, the risk of RBC alloimmunization is almost certainly related to several factors, including patient demographics (e.g., age, sex, ethnicity), diagnosis (e.g., oncologic, medical, surgical, hemoglobinopathy), treatment (e.g., immunosuppressive vs nonimmunosuppressive), clinical presentation (e.g., febrile vs afebrile), and transfusion characteristics (e.g., antigen matching, number of units, number of episodes); however, it remains unclear how the combination of these factors influence the development and persistence of clinically significant RBC alloantibodies. Alloantibodies to RBCs can lead to recipient morbidity and shortened RBC survival; antibodies to leukocytes are associated with febrile transfusion reactions and can impair effectiveness and survival of transfused granulocytes.[77] Anti-HLA-A and -B antibodies, as well as platelet-specific alloantibodies, impair survival of transfused platelets. Finally, anti-IgA can cause anaphylactic reactions in IgA deficient recipients, but anti-IgG or -IgM or antibodies recognizing lipoproteins are not clinically significant in the setting of transfusion.[78]

Transfusion-associated GVHD

Historic perspective
GVHD is commonly observed after allogeneic BMT but is rarely recognized after transfusion or transplantation of other organs. Transfusion-associated (TA)-GVHD usually occurs in the immunosuppressed recipient (e.g., BMT recipients), but it can also occur in immunocompetent recipients in the setting of a one-way HLA mismatch.[79] The clinical manifestations include fever and skin rash, anorexia, nausea, vomiting, and watery or bloody diarrhea with or without elevated liver enzymes and hyperbilirubinemia. Since there are no pathognomonic features of GVHD, this syndrome is sometimes difficult to distinguish from viral infections or drug eruptions. TA-GVHD is usually severe, and, unlike the situation after allogeneic BMT, it frequently results in pancytopenia secondary to marrow aplasia. The majority of reported cases of TA-GVHD have not responded to immunosuppressive therapies and have been fatal.

Definition of those at risk
In 1986, the National Institutes of Health Consensus Development Conference defined patients who have undergone BMT or those with other forms of immunodeficiency as candidates for irradiated platelet concentrates to avoid GVHD. Patients with leukemias and other cancers who may be immunosuppressed secondary to chemotherapy and/or radiation therapy or due to intrinsic immune dysfunction (e.g., HD), may be at risk for TA-GVHD.

Among patients with HD, it had previously been assumed that combined radiation and chemotherapy were necessary as predisposing factors for the development of TA-GVHD, but several cases of TA-GVHD have been documented in patients with HD who were treated with chemotherapy alone. Patients receiving high-dose chemotherapy followed by autologous bone marrow support are also at risk for TA-GVHD.[80] Finally, immunocompetent patients who share an HLA haplotype with HLA-homozygous blood donors are also at risk for TA-GVHD.[81,82] Homozygosity for HLA types is more likely to occur among first-degree family members (e.g., parents, children, and siblings). It has, therefore, recently been recommended that cellular blood components from such donors be irradiated with at least 25 Gy prior to transfusion. Indeed, products from all family member-directed donors should be irradiated, given that TA-GVHD has now been reported after transfusion of blood from a second-degree relative.[83] Reports of TA-GVHD after transfusion of cellular blood components from homozygous blood donors to heterozygous nonblood relatives suggest that indications for gamma irradiation may need to be broadened; the risk of transfusion of blood from HLA homozygous donors to unrelated HLA heterozygous patients is 1 in 874 in Japan and may be as high as 1 in 7174 in the United States.[83–85] Finally, reports confirm that all HLA-matched cellular components should be irradiated.[86–89]

Strategies for prevention

The only currently effective method to prevent TA-GVHD is gamma irradiation of blood products prior to transfusion. Studies suggest that irradiation at 15–20 Gy can reduce mitogen-responsive lymphocytes by 5–6 logs compared to unirradiated controls.[86] The standards of the AABBs (formerly, the American Association of Blood Banks), as well as those of the FDA, now require that blood and cellular components are irradiated with a midplane dose of a minimum of 25 Gy.[87] Studies to date suggest no adverse effects of irradiation on storage of platelets, but the clinical significance of potassium release on storage of irradiated red cells is not yet defined, and posttransfusion red cell recovery of irradiated units may be decreased.[88,89]

Transfusion-related infectious diseases

Hepatitis B

Although hepatitis B (HB) was formerly a common transfusion-related infection, the use of several generations of HB surface antigen assays to screen potential donors and the use of volunteer versus commercial donors has markedly reduced the incidence of HB transmitted by transfusion.[90] Nucleic acid testing (NAT) is now often performed to test for HB as well. The current estimated per-unit risk of HB is approximately 1 in 200,000[91] (Table 4).

Hepatitis C

Following the identification of hepatitis A virus and HB virus, it was quickly appreciated that neither agent was responsible for most cases of posttransfusion hepatitis. Thus, the term non-A non-B Hepatitis (NANBH) was introduced. In the mid-1980s, donors were screened for alanine aminotransferase (ALT) as well as anti-HBc; these served as "surrogate" markers for individuals having a 20% chance of transmitting NANBH.[92,93]

The causative agent of NANBH was finally discovered by cloning a fragment of viral cDNA from a chimpanzee infected with NANBH.[94] Subsequently, the entire genome of what is now called hepatitis C virus (HCV) was cloned. A specific assay was developed for blood-borne NANBH, in which a recombinant HCV polypeptide is used to capture viral antibodies.[95] Subsequent testing using multiple-antigen HCV enzyme assays confirmed that nearly all cases of posttransfusion NANBH are caused by HCV. Uniform screening of blood donors for anti-HCV antibodies was implemented in 1990. NAT is now being employed to enhance sensitivity in detecting infection.[96] Along with HIV (discussed below) all blood donations in the United States are now screened for HCV. By narrowing the preseroconversion window period from about 75 days to less than 30, the use of NAT has reduced the per-unit risk of HCV to approximately 1 in 2,000,000.[91]

Cytomegalovirus

Cellular blood components transfused from CMV-seropositive donors to CMV-seronegative transplant recipients and neonates can cause CMV seroconversion and infection. Although equivalent numbers of autologous and allogeneic BMT recipients either seroconvert to or excrete CMV, recipients of autologous BMT rarely develop clinical sequelae. The traditional CMV-seronegative blood products are red cells and platelets harvested from CMV-seronegative donors. Leukoreduced red cells and platelets have been shown to decrease transfusion-acquired CMV infection in infants, in patients undergoing treatment for acute leukemia, and in autologous and allogeneic BMT recipients.[97–100] A multicenter randomized trial compared seronegative with leukoreduced cellular blood components in CMV-seronegative patients undergoing autologous BMT and seronegative patients receiving allografts from CMV-seronegative donors.[97] Rates of CMV seroconversion and infection were equivalent in recipients of seronegative and leukoreduced components, but significant CMV disease was noted only in those patients receiving leukoreduced, unscreened components. These results suggest that leukoreduction can markedly reduce CMV transmission, and leukoreduced components are now considered "CMV safe"; however, it may be premature to conclude that leukoreduced and seronegative components are exactly equivalent.

Table 4 Risks of transfusion.

Complication	Frequency (Episodes:Unit)
Reactions	
Febrile nonhemolytic	1–4 : 100
Allergic	1–4 : 100
Transfusion-associated circulatory overload	1 : 100
Transfusion-related acute lung injury	1 : 10,000
Acute hemolytic	1 : 250,000
Delayed hemolytic	1 : 1000
Anaphylactic	1 : 150,000
Infections	
Hepatitis C	1 : 2,000,000
Hepatitis B	1 : 200,000
HIV-1	1 : 2,000,000
HIV-2	None reported
HTLV-I and II	1 : 250,000 to 1 : 2,000,000
Malaria	1 : 4,000,000
Bacterial sepsis red cells	1 : 500,000
Bacterial sepsis platelets	1 : 75,000
Other complications	
RBC allosensitization	1 : 100
HLA allosensitization	1 : 10
Graft-versus-host disease	Rare

Abbreviations: HIV, human immunodeficiency virus; HLA, human leukocyte antigen; HTLV, human T-cell leukemia/lymphoma virus; RBC, red blood cell.

West Nile virus

West Nile virus (WNV) is a mosquito-borne flavivirus that can be transfusion transmitted. The vast majority of WNV infections result from mosquito bites. About 80% of individuals infected with WNV are asymptomatic. Of the 20% who manifest symptoms, most will have a mild illness (WNV fever). Less than 1% of infected individuals develop a severe meningoencephalitis, with advanced age being the strongest risk factor.[101] WNV first appeared in the United States in 1999. In 2002, over 4000 clinically significant cases of WNV were reported, including 23 cases determined to have been transfusion-associated. In 2003, nucleic acid testing of blood products was begun nationwide under an FDA investigational new drug (IND) protocol. This testing has eliminated most of the risk of transfusion-transmitted WNV.

Zika virus

Zika virus (ZIKV) is a member of the *Flaviviridae* family that typically results in asymptomatic infection but can cause a self-limited illness in adults, comprising fever, rash, and arthralgias. The majority of ZIKV infections occur via mosquito bites, though it is now well-documented from the ZIKV epidemic of 2015–2016 that maternal-fetal, sexual, and transfusion-related transmission also contribute to infections.[102–104] During ZIKV epidemics in French Polynesia and Puerto Rico, 1–3% of asymptomatic donors were viremic.[105,106] Given the risk of transfusion-transmitted infection, blood donations are now routinely screened for ZIKV by NAT, per FDA recommendations.

Human immunodeficiency virus

Since 1985, all American blood donors have been screened for anti-HIV antibody using ELISA. Transfusion-transmitted HIV is now exceedingly rare; the few cases that do occur result almost exclusively from seronegative window period donations. Following the initial implementation of HIV antibody screening, improvements in the sensitivity of the HIV-1 and HIV-2 ELISA limited the seronegative window period to approximately 22 days.[107] All units donated in the United States are now tested by minipool NAT. NAT (transfusion mediated amplification, TMA, or polymerase chain reaction, PCR) is performed on pools of 16–24 samples; this technology shortens the window period to approximately 10 or 11 days from the time of exposure. It is estimated that the current residual per-unit risk of HIV transmission is less than 1 in 2,000,000.[107]

Human T-cell lymphotropic virus type 1

Human T-cell lymphotropic virus type 1 (HTLV-1) is associated with adult T-cell leukemia/lymphoma (ATL) and tropical spastic paresis (TSP)/HTLV-1–associated myelopathy (HAM), and clusters geographically in endemic areas such as parts of Japan and the Caribbean. In the United States, ATL incidence is similar to that in the Caribbean, since the cases in the United States are all among African Americans or in patients born outside the United States.[108]

In 1988, blood collection agencies initiated testing of all blood donors for anti-HTLV-1 antibodies at the time of all donations, with permanent deferral of individuals with confirmed seropositivity. Studies in the United States document that HTLV-1 has been transmitted via transfusion and demonstrate the efficacy of screening. The risk per unit transfused is between 1 in 250,000 and 1 in 2,000,000.[107]

Bacterial sepsis

Bacteria very rarely survive in whole blood stored at 4°C. In contrast, platelets are stored at room temperature on an agitator and are a potential source of bacterial contamination, which can result in transfusion-related sepsis. Blood collection facilities in the United States are now required by AABB to both detect and limit bacterial contamination of platelets.[107] A variety of screening techniques to address bacterial contamination within platelets, such as automated culture systems, are now in use.[109]

Parasitic diseases

Since there is no practical laboratory screening test for malaria, exclusion of donors who have either traveled to or emigrated from endemic areas is the only effective measure to prevent transfusion-related infection. Other parasitic diseases, such as babesiosis or Lyme disease, can be transmitted by an asymptomatic donor who has been bitten by a tick and may be of particular importance in immunocompromised or asplenic patients. Transfusion-transmitted babesiosis is a regional disease. At this time, there are seven endemic US states: Massachusetts, Connecticut, Rhode Island, New York, New Jersey, Wisconsin, Minnesota.[110] Although transmission of syphilis by transfusion is possible, it requires that blood be drawn during the rather short period of spirochetemia and that the organisms remain viable at the time of transfusion. Although performing a serologic test for syphilis does not prevent transmission of syphilis because this test does not become positive until well after the brief period of infectivity, US federal regulations do require its use as a screening test of potential donors.

Another recognized transfusion-related infection is Chagas disease.[111,112] In the majority of cases, spontaneous resolution occurs, and patients enter the indeterminate phase with lifelong, low-grade parasitemia, antibodies to parasite antigens, and absence of symptoms. Between 10% and 30% of persons in the indeterminate phase eventually develop symptoms. However, in immunocompromised patients, this illness may take a more fulminant course. The diagnosis of acute infection is made by detection of parasites on blood smear and the diagnosis of chronic infection by the detection of serum antibodies.

Pathogen inactivation in blood products

There are several new technologies that inactivate potentially infectious organisms in blood products, including enveloped viruses and organisms that require nucleic acids for reproduction. Notably, specific identification of the target organism(s) is not required, indicating that these approaches may be used to prevent transfusion-transmitted infections by unknown, emerging pathogens.[113] Solvent-detergent treatment and nucleic acid-damaging methods have been shown to effectively reduce or eliminate pathogens in plasma, RBCs, and platelets; nucleic acid-damaging methods have the added benefit of targeting donor leukocytes, thus mitigating the risk of TA-GVHD. To date, several clinical studies evaluating bleeding risk in cancer patients have not observed a significant difference between pathogen-reduced and standard platelets. However, pathogen-reduced platelets have been associated with an increased platelet transfusion requirement and increased risk of platelet transfusion refractoriness.[114,115] Recent clinical trials in cardiac surgery and thalassemia indicated that pathogen-reduced RBCs were noninferior to standard RBCs.[116,117] A comparison of pathogen-reduced and standard RBCs in cancer patients has yet to be performed.

Creutzfeldt–Jakob disease

Prospective donors of blood products who have a familial history of dementia and have undergone corneal or brain surgery are deferred.[118,119] Due to the identification in 1996 of a variant CJD (vCJD), which may be associated with bovine spongiform encephalopathy (BSE), or "mad cow disease," potential donors who resided in the United Kingdom for 3 months from 1980 to 1996 are deferred from donating.[120] Donors residing in Europe for 5 years cumulatively from 1980 onward are also deferred. These travel restrictions are expected to eliminate 90% of person-days of exposure to the causative agent of vCJD at a cost of eliminating 5% of US blood donors. In the United Kingdom, a small number of human cases of transfusion-transmitted vCJD have been reported.[121] Universal use of leukoreduced components for transfusion is recommended in many countries, based on the fact that the vector for transmission of vCJD appears to be the B lymphocyte.

Blood component support posttransplantation

After BMT, there is a period of pancytopenia, when patients require multiple RBC and platelet transfusions. In cases of donor-recipient ABO incompatibility (about one-third of allogeneic transplants), particular care must be paid to blood provision. In these situations, blood products are selected to be ABO-compatible with both the donor and recipient.

ABO incompatibility between marrow donor and recipient may be either major, with isohemagglutinin in the recipient directed against donor RBC antigens, or minor, with isohemagglutinin in the donor directed against recipient RBC antigens. Major ABO incompatibility has the potential risk of severe hemolytic reactions, graft rejection, or delayed engraftment.[122,123] Attempts to overcome major ABO incompatibility have included depletion of RBCs from the bone marrow graft prior to BMT and/or removal of isohemagglutinin from the recipient by large-volume plasma exchanges or immunoadsorption, but these maneuvers are not done routinely.[124,125] Although studies suggest that major ABO incompatible HLA-matched transplants have resulted in no increase in patient mortality, incidence of rejection, delayed reconstitution, or GVHD compared to ABO compatible controls, some reports suggest that RBC reconstitution can be delayed in this setting.[126] Red cell engraftment may be especially delayed in the setting of major ABO-incompatible nonmyeloablative stem cell transplantation, where host antidonor isohemagglutinin levels tend to decrease more slowly than in myeloablative BMT.[127]

Potential adverse outcomes of minor ABO incompatibility between marrow donor and recipient include rapid immune hemolysis at the time of infusion of donor marrow resulting from passive transfer of isohemagglutinin in the marrow plasma, or delayed immune hemolysis caused by anti-RBC antibodies produced by donor lymphocytes.[128,129] There is no effect of minor ABO incompatibility on graft rejection, the incidence, and severity of GVHD, or patient survival. Although exchange transfusion of the recipient before BMT using red cells of the donor's blood group has been utilized to prevent hemolysis caused by passive transfer of isohemagglutinin in the marrow product, this is rarely a clinically significant problem and can more easily be avoided by removing plasma from the marrow prior to infusion. Minor ABO incompatibility can result in adverse reactions due to the production of anti-A and/or anti-B antibodies by donor marrow lymphocytes early (1–3 weeks) following transplantation, particularly in patients on cyclosporine therapy or those receiving T cell-depleted allografts.[130,131] In this setting, transfusions of either group O or donor group RBCs are utilized to dilute the recipient red cells; in some cases, exchange transfusion has been required due to very rapid engraftment of donor lymphocytes and production of anti-RBC antibodies.

Conclusion

The development and implementation of new and aggressive therapies for patients with cancer to date would not have been possible without parallel developments for the provision of blood component support. In the future, the blood component laboratory will provide specialized cellular components to facilitate the use of new and promising transplantation and cellular therapies for patients with hitherto incurable diseases.

Key references

The complete reference list can be found on Vital Source version of this title, see inside front cover.

3. Webb IJ, Anderson KC. Transfusion support in acute leukemias. *Semin Oncol.* 1997;**24**:141–146.
10. Hebert PC, Wells G, Blajchman MA, et al. A multicenter randomized, controlled clinical trial of transfusion requirements in critical care. Transfusion requirements in critical care investigators, Canadian Critical Care Trials Group. *N Engl J Med.* 1999;**340**:409–417.
18. Tay J, Allan DS, Chatelain E, et al. Liberal versus restrictive red blood cell transfusion thresholds in hematopoietic cell transplantation: a randomized, open label, phase III, non-inferiority trial. *J Clin Oncol.* 2020;**38**:1463–1473.
26. Lacroix J, Hebert PC, Fergusson DA, et al. Age of transfused blood in critically ill adults. *N Engl J Med.* 2015;**372**:1410–1418.
28. Heddle NM, Cook RJ, Arnold DM, et al. Effect of short-term vs. long-term blood storage on mortality after transfusion. *N Engl J Med.* 2016;**375**:1937–1945.
29. Spinella PC, Tucci M, Fergusson DA, et al. Effect of fresh vs standard-issue red blood cell transfusions on multiple organ dysfunction syndrome in critically ill pediatric patients. *JAMA.* 2019;**322**:2179–2190.
30. Knezevic-Maramica I, Kruskall MS. Intravenous immune globulins: an update for clinicians. *Transfusion.* 2003;**43**:1460–1480.
31. Chapuy CI, Nicholson RT, Aguad MD, et al. Resolving the daratumumab interference with blood compatibility testing. *Transfusion.* 2015;**55**:1545–1554.
32. Velliquette RW, Aeschlimann J, Kirkegaard J, et al. Monoclonal anti-CD47 interference in red cell and platelet testing. *Transfusion.* 2019;**59**:730–737.
34. Bodey GP, Buckley M, Sathe YS, Freireich EJ. Quantitative relationships between circulating leukocytes and infection in patients with acute leukemia. *Ann Intern Med.* 1966;**64**:328–340.
38. Estcourt LJ, Stanworth S, Doree C, et al. Granulocyte transfusions for preventing infections in people with neutropenia or neutrophil dysfunction. *Cochrane Database Syst Rev.* 2015;**2015**(6):CD005341.
39. Price TH, Boeckh M, Harrison RW, et al. Efficacy of transfusion with granulocytes from G-CSF/dexamethasone-treated donors in neutropenic patients with infection. *Blood.* 2015;**126**:2153–2161.
45. Gaydos LA, Freireich EJ, Mantel N, et al. The quantitative relation between platelet count and hemorrhage in patients with acute leukemia. *N Engl J Med.* 1962;**266**:905–909.
47. Wandt H, Schaefer-Eckart K, Wendelin K, et al. Therapeutic platelet transfusion versus routine prophylactic transfusion in patients with haematological malignancies: an open-label, multicentre, randomised study. *Lancet.* 2012;**380**(9850):1309–1316. doi: 10.1016/S0140-6736(12)60689-8.
49. Kaufman RM, Djulbegovic B, Gernsheimer T, et al. Platelet transfusion: a clinical practice guideline from the AABB. *Ann Intern Med.* 2015;**162**:205–213.
51. Rebulla P, Finazzi G, Marangoni F, et al. The threshold for prophylactic platelet transfusions in adults with acute myeloid leukemia. *N Engl J Med.* 1997;**337**:1870–1875.
54. Stanworth SJ, Estcourt LJ, Powter G, et al. A no-prophylaxis platelet-transfusion strategy for hematologic cancers. *N Engl J Med.* 2013;**368**:1771–1780.
59. Slichter SJ, Kaufman RM, Assmann SF, et al. Dose of prophylactic platelet transfusions and prevention of hemorrhage. *N Engl J Med.* 2010;**362**(7):600–613.

63. Davis KB, Slichter SJ, Corash L. Corrected count increment and percent platelet recovery as measures of post-transplantation platelet response: problems and a solution. *Transfusion*. 1999;**39**:586–592.
64. Aster RH. Pooling of platelets in the spleen: role in the pathogenesis of "hypersplenic" thrombocytopenia. *J Clin Invest*. 1966;**45**:645–657.
65. Aster RH, Curtis BR, McFarland JG, Bougie DW. Drug-induced immune thrombocytopenia: pathogenesis, diagnosis and management. *J Thomb Haemost*. 2009;**7**:911–918.
66. Herzig RH, Terasaki PI, Trapani RJ, et al. The relationship between donor-recipient lymphocytotoxicity and the transfusion of response using HLA-matched platelet concentrates. *Transfusion*. 1977;**17**:657–661.
69. Slichter SJ. Leukocyte reduction and ultraviolet B irradiation of platelets to prevent alloimmunization and refractoriness to platelet transfusions. *N Engl J Med*. 1997;**337**:1861–1869.
72. Kaufman RM. Platelet ABO matters. *Transfusion*. 2009;**49**:5–7.
74. Green L, Bolton-Maggs P, Beattie C, et al. British society of hematology guidelines on the spectrum of fresh frozen plasma and cryoprecipitate products: their handling and use in various patient groups in the absence of major bleeding. *Br J Haematol*. 2018;**181**:54–67.
75. Higgins JM, Sloan SR. Stochastic modeling of human RBC alloimmunization: evidence for a distinct population of immunologic responders. *Blood*. 2008;**112**:2546–2553.
76. Karafin MS, Westlake M, Hauser RG, et al. Risk factors for red blood cell alloimmunization in the Recipient Epidemiology and Donor Evaluation Study (REDS-III) database. *Br J Haematol*. 2018;**181**:672–681.
79. Anderson KC, Goodnough LT, Sayers M, et al. Variation in blood component irradiation practice: implications for prevention of transfusion associated graft versus host disease. *Blood*. 1991;**77**:2096–2102.
85. Charpentier F, Bracq C, Bonin P, et al. HLA-matched blood products and post-transfusion graft-versus-host disease. *Transfusion*. 1990;**30**:850.
88. Read EJ, Kodis C, Carter CS, Leitman SF. Viability of platelets following storage in the irradiated state. A pair-controlled study. *Transfusion*. 1988;**28**:446–450.
89. Davey RJ, McCoy NC, Yu M, et al. The effect of prestorage irradiation on post-transfusion red cell survival. *Transfusion*. 1992;**32**:525–528.
91. Stramer SL. Current risks of transfusion-transmitted agents: a review. *Arch Pathol Lab Med*. 2007;**131**:702–707.
97. Bowden RA, Slichter SJ, Sayers M, et al. A comparison of filtered leukocyte-reduced and cytomegalovirus (CMV) seronegative blood products for the prevention of transfusion-associated CMV infection after marrow transplant. *Blood*. 1995;**86**:3598–3603.
107. Busch MP, Bloch EM, Kleinman S. Prevention of transfusion-transmitted infections. *Blood*. 2019;**133**:1854–1864.
109. Bloch EM. Residual risk of bacterial contamination: what are the options? *Transfusion*. 2017;**57**:2289–2292.
113. Salunkhe V, van der Meer PF, de Korte D, et al. Development of blood transfusion product pathogen reduction treatments: a review of methods, current applications and demands. *Transfus Apher Sci*. 2015;**52**:19–34.
114. Estcourt LJ, Malouf R, Murphy MF. Pathogen-reduced platelets for the prevention of bleeding in people of any age. *JAMA Oncol*. 2018;**4**:571–572.
123. Marmont AM, Damasio EE, Bacigalupo A, et al. A to O bone marrow transplantation in severe aplastic anemia. Dynamics of blood group conversion of early dyserythropoiesis in the engrafted marrow. *Br J Haematol*. 1978;**36**:511–518.
127. Bolan CD, Leitman SF, Griffith LM. Delayed donor red cell chimerism and pure red cell aplasia following major ABO-incompatible nonmyeloablative hematopoietic stem cell transplantation. *Blood*. 2001;**98**:1687–1694.
129. Anderson KC. The role of the blood bank in hematopoietic stem cell transplantation. *Transfusion*. 1992;**32**:272–285.

128 Coagulation complications of cancer patients

Tzu-Fei Wang, MD, MPH ■ Kristin Sanfilippo, MD, MPHS

> **Overview**
>
> Patients with cancer have increased risks of coagulation complications including bleeding and/or thrombotic problems, which can be a result of malignancy itself and/or related to cancer therapies. These complications can lead to increased morbidity and mortality, as well as delays or alterations in cancer treatment. Therefore, identification of risk factors, prevention, and treatment strategies are important priorities in the care of cancer patients. In this chapter, we discussed and summarized relevant literature in common bleeding and thrombotic complications, their presentations, risk factors, prevention and management strategies.

Bleeding complications

Background

Cancer patients have high risk of bleeding complications from many etiologies. Here, we aim to summarize pertinent bleeding complications and management in patients with cancer.

Thrombocytopenia

The most common cause of thrombocytopenia in patients with cancer is secondary to systemic chemotherapy. However, patients with cancer may also develop thrombocytopenia secondary to the underlying cancer directly infiltrating the bone marrow or spleen, cancer-induced immune thrombocytopenia, or as a result of cancer-associated microangiopathies (i.e., disseminated intravascular coagulation, thrombotic thrombocytopenic purpura, or atypical hemolytic uremia syndromes). Patients with thrombocytopenia are at increased risk of bleeding necessitating provider awareness and appropriate management.

Chemotherapy-induced thrombocytopenia, nonmyeloablative
Patients with solid tumors and/or lymphoma commonly receive nonmyeloablative chemotherapy regimens. Studies document a prevalence of chemotherapy-induced thrombocytopenia (CIT) in this population to be at 20–80%, with rates dependent on the types of chemotherapy agents, and the highest rates noted with carboplatin and gemcitabine-based regimens.[1,2] CIT can result in delays and dose reduction of chemotherapy.[3] In patients receiving curative intent therapy, dose delay or reduction could reduce efficacy and affect outcomes in cancer survival. In addition, CIT increases hospitalization and healthcare costs.[4] Fortunately, CIT is associated with low rates of major bleeding.[5,6]

To combat the adverse effects of CIT, several trials have assessed intervention of thrombopoietic agents to reduce the rate of CIT including interleukin-11, recombinant human thrombopoietin (TPO), and TPO receptor agonists. Interleukin-11 was the first agent approved by the United States (US) Food and Drug Administration (FDA) after it was shown to be effective in reducing the need for platelet transfusion in two clinical trials.[7,8] However, its toxicity limited clinical applicability in the United States and it eventually fell out of favor. While initial trials were promising, the development of neutralizing antibodies eventually led to the discontinuation of PEGylated recombinant human megakaryocyte growth factor and development factor (PEG-rHuMGDF) as a candidate treatment for CIT.[9,10] Similarly, the development of antibodies in patients treated with PEG-rHuMGDF led to the discontinuation of production of all first-generation recombinant human TPO agents as well, although initial trials demonstrated success. Subsequently, agonists of TPO receptors, romiplostim, and eltrombopag, have been developed and successfully used for the treatment of immune thrombocytopenia leading to FDA approval in 2008. While these agents are associated with concerns including the generation of marrow reticulin fibrosis and increased risk of portal vein thrombosis, particularly in the setting of high dose and/or overshoot of platelet count, they have a high success rate and good safety profile in a well-controlled patient. Therefore, this has generated interest in using TPO agonists for the treatment of CIT. Small studies have demonstrated success; however, additional studies are needed.[11–14]

Chemotherapy-induced thrombocytopenia, myeloablative
Patients with hematological malignancies have a particularly high risk of severe and prolonged thrombocytopenia. Up to 100% of patients with acute leukemia will develop thrombocytopenia during the course of their disease. Randomized controlled trials (RCTs) showed that in patients with hematologic malignancies, prophylactic platelet transfusion for platelet count $<10 \times 10^9$/L prolonged time to the first World Health Organization (WHO) grade 2 or greater bleed and reduced the duration of bleeding in comparison with therapeutic platelet transfusion (transfusion only for bleeding symptoms).[15,16] Furthermore, in patients with hematologic malignancy or chemotherapy-related thrombocytopenia, transfusion prophylactically for a morning platelet count $<10 \times 10^9$/L showed no more bleeding complications compared with a higher platelet threshold of <20–30×10^9/L.[17–20] Reduction in bleeding risk did not translate into a survival benefit. Therefore, transfusion prophylactically for platelet count $<10 \times 10^9$/L has been the standard of care for cancer patients.

Disseminated intravascular coagulation

Disseminated intravascular coagulation (DIC) is a consumptive coagulopathy associated with an underlying disorder (e.g., cancer, sepsis, trauma, etc.). The phenotype of DIC can vary based on presentation, with acute DIC (i.e., decompensated) more likely to present with a bleeding phenotype and chronic DIC (i.e.,

---

Holland-Frei Cancer Medicine, Tenth Edition. Edited by Robert C. Bast, John C. Byrd, Carlo M. Croce, Ernest Hawk, Fadlo R. Khuri, Raphael E. Pollock, Apostolia M. Tsimberidou, Christopher G. Willett, and Cheryl L. Willman.
© 2023 John Wiley & Sons, Inc. Published 2023 by John Wiley & Sons, Inc.

compensated) more likely to present with a thrombotic phenotype. However, patients with DIC may experience both bleeding and/or thrombosis with thrombosis more common than bleeding.[21] The bleeding phenotype of DIC typically presents with petechiae, ecchymoses, bleeding from mucosal surfaces (i.e., gingival or gastrointestinal), and/or from sites of catheters, and less commonly, intracranial bleeding. The bleeding can be fatal especially in patients with acute promyelocytic leukemia. While the mainstay of therapy is to treat the underlying disease, the International Society on Thrombosis and Haemostasis (ISTH) puts worth guidelines to address the coagulopathy in the setting of cancer-associated DIC.[22] Given that the risk of thrombosis remains elevated in patients with DIC, administration of blood products should be considered judiciously. The following have been recommended in patients with **active** bleeding, in need of surgical interventions, or those with very high risk of bleeding: transfusion of platelets for thrombocytopenia <50,000, fresh frozen plasma (or prothrombin complex concentrate if volume is a concern) for an elevated prothrombin time (i.e., international normalized ratio (INR) of >1.5), and cryoprecipitate for fibrinogen levels <1.5 g/L.[21,22] The routine use of tranexamic acid or recombinant FVIIa in the absence of refractory bleeding is not recommended.[22] The thrombotic presentation in DIC is especially more common in patients with solid tumors and DIC.[23] Given this, the ISTH guidelines recommend prophylactic anticoagulation in patients with cancer-associated DIC.[22] Dosing should be escalated to therapeutic regimens in the setting of acute venous or arterial thrombosis.

Acquired hemophilia

Hematological malignancies such as plasma cell dyscrasias or lymphoproliferative disorders, as well as some solid tumors, can rarely cause acquired hemophilia. The majority of cases of acquired hemophilia are secondary to an acquired deficiency in Factor VIII (FVIII).[24] Patients would present with spontaneous bleeding symptoms or ecchymoses, as well as isolated prolonged activated partial thrombin time (aPTT), reduced FVIII levels, and positive FVIII inhibitors. FVIII inhibitors are quantified using the Bethesda assay, and the titer is reported as Bethesda unit (BU).

Management strategies include: (1) treating the acute bleeding episode, (2) eradication of the inhibitor with immunosuppression. For acute bleeding episodes, treatment depends on the inhibitor titer. In patients with low inhibitor titer (i.e., <5 BU), FVIII concentrates can be used, but often a much larger quantity of factor is needed to overcome the inhibitor, and there is a risk of generating further immune response and raising inhibitor titers. In patients with high inhibitor titers (≥5 BU), bypassing agents are indicated, including recombinant activated Factor VIIa (rFVIIa) or FEIBA® (anti-inhibitor coagulant complex). Recently, porcine FVIII is approved to treat acquired FVIII deficiency and has the advantage of allowing the monitor of FVIII levels and titration of FVIII doses accordingly (which cannot be done with rFVIIa or FEIBA). Emicizumab, a chimeric bispecific antibody against both factor IX and factor X and mimic the co-factor function of FVIII, have been successfully used in case report/series in noncancer patients with acquired FVIII deficiency, although not currently approved for this indication.[25]

For irradiation of inhibitors, various immunosuppressants have been investigated. Corticosteroids are typically the first-line therapy, other immunosuppressant agents including rituximab, cyclophosphamide, vincristine, cyclosporine, and mycophenolate, have been reported in small case series as potentially effective treatment. While the aforementioned therapies may have success, treating the underlying cancer is the cornerstone of management and has resulted in eradication of the inhibitor in up to 22% in some trials.[26] However, patients with more advanced disease (i.e., metastatic disease) are less likely to respond to cancer-directed therapies alone.

Acquired Von Willebrand disease (aVWD)

Hematological malignancies, especially plasma cell dyscrasia or lymphoproliferative diseases, are the most common etiologies for acquired Von Willebrand disease (aVWD). These include monoclonal gammopathy of undetermined significance (MGUS), multiple myeloma, Waldenström macroglobulinemia, chronic lymphocytic leukemia, non-Hodgkin lymphoma, or myeloproliferative diseases such as essential thrombocytosis or polycythemia vera. The clinical presentations are similar to those seen in patients with congenital Von Willebrand disease (VWD), including mucocutaneous or gastrointestinal (GI) bleeding, spontaneous ecchymosis, or postoperative bleeding. Laboratory findings include an elevated aPTT (but not always), reduced Von Willebrand factor (VWF) antigen, and activity (typically with activity reduced out of proportion of antigen).

Treatment of aVWD includes (1) treatment of the underlying malignancy and (2) treatment of the acute bleeding episodes. Unlike acquired hemophilia, inhibitors associated with aVWD cause increased clearance of VWF rather than directly counteract factors. Therefore, for acute bleeding episodes, VWF concentrates can be effective but with shorter half-life due to increased clearance, and intravenous immunoglobulin (IVIG) is commonly used to combat rapid clearance of VWF.[27]

Targeted cancer therapy-associated bleeding

In recent years, there has been a significant shift in cancer therapy, with increasing use of different targeted cancer therapy agents over traditional cytotoxic chemotherapy. Each targeted agent has unique side effect profiles, with bleeding occurring with some. The prototype of targeted cancer therapy-associated bleeding is ibrutinib, an irreversible Burton tyrosine kinase inhibitor approved in the treatment of multiple B-cell malignancies including chronic lymphocytic leukemia, mantel cell lymphoma, marginal zone lymphoma, and Waldenström macroglobulinemia. Ibrutinib can inhibit several other off-target tyrosine kinases including kinase Tec in platelets, which causes platelet dysfunction and easy bleeding/bruising in patients taking ibrutinib. Levade et al.[28] demonstrated that ibrutinib inhibits platelet adhesion to VWF and collagen-induced platelet aggregation. Patients on ibrutinib are commonly elderlies with multiple co-morbidities and potential need for concurrent antiplatelet agents and/or anticoagulants, which can further increase the risks of bleeding or bruising symptoms. Clinicians should be vigilant about the potential complications and be cautious about concurrent use.

Thrombotic complications

Venous thromboembolism (VTE)

Epidemiology

Malignancy accounts for at least 20% of all venous thromboembolism (VTE) in population studies.[29] Approximately 1–15% cancer patients will develop VTE during the course of their cancer treatment, and VTE is the second leading cause of death in cancer patients.[30] Cancer patients have a four- to sevenfold increased

Table 1 Khorana risk score.

Patient characteristics	Risk score
Site of primary cancer	
Very high risk (stomach, pancreas)	2
High risk (lung, lymphoma, gynecologic, bladder, testicular)	1
Prechemotherapy platelet count $\geq 350 \times 10^9$/L	1
Prechemotherapy hemoglobin <10 g/dL or use of erythropoiesis stimulating agent	1
Prechemotherapy leukocyte count $\geq 11 \times 10^9$/L	1
Body mass index ≥ 35 kg/m²	1

risk of VTE and a twofold increased risk of major hemorrhage on anticoagulation when compared with patients without cancer.[31] VTE and its treatments commonly result in morbidity and mortality, delay cancer treatments, and impact quality of life. Therefore, appropriate strategies for prevention and treatment of VTE in cancer patients are crucial.

Risk factors
Risk assessment for first VTE

Cancer patients have many risk factors for VTE, including malignancy itself, cancer treatment, cancer surgery, and central venous catheters (CVCs). In addition, patients' underlying characteristics and comorbidities can increase the risk of VTE. Due to the multitude of risk factors and the complexity in clinical scenarios, several risk assessment tools have been developed to guide risk stratification in cancer patients. The Khorana risk score was developed as a pan-malignancy risk assessment tool and is the most validated.[32] Using the Khorana risk score, patients are categorized into three risk groups: low (0 points), intermediate (1–2 points), and high-risk (≥ 3 points) (Table 1). The risks of symptomatic VTE in three months are 0.3%, 2%, and 6.7% in the validation cohort in the low, intermediate, and high-risk groups, respectively. While the Khorana risk score validates in many studies, other studies found limited predictability in specific tumor types such as lung and hematological malignancies.[33,34] Modifications to include biomarkers such as D-dimer and soluble p-selectin have been proposed to improve the discriminative performance of the score but remain to be with limited applicability in routine clinical practice.[35] In addition, other risk assessment tools have been proposed, such as risk factors including tumor site and d-dimer from the Vienna Cancer and Thrombosis Study (CATS), but require further validation and utility determination.[36] Recent additional studies also focus on developing risk prediction models for specific types of malignancy, such as the IMPEDE VTE and SAVED scores for multiple myeloma,[37,38] or COMPASS-CAT (Prospective Comparison of Methods for thromboembolic risk assessment with clinical Perceptions and Awareness in real-life patients-Cancer Associated Thrombosis) for patients with breast, colorectal, lung or ovarian cancers.[39] These scores require further validation and investigation before their use in clinical practice.

Risk assessment for recurrent VTE

Cancer patients have increased risk for recurrent VTE, and identifying those with high risk of VTE recurrence can help tailor management. However, risk prediction models for recurrent VTE in cancer patients are limited. The Ottawa score, which includes four factors—gender, type of cancer, stage of cancer, and history of VTE dichotomizes patients into two risk groups, low- and high-risk, based on risk scores (≤ 0 and ≥ 1, respectively). The risk of recurrent VTE at six months is $\leq 4.5\%$ in the low-risk group compared to $\geq 19\%$ in the high-risk group.[40] External validations of the model have had conflicting results and the model has not been widely used.[41,42] Additional risk factors for recurrent VTE in cancer patients have been identified in other studies, such as elevated tissue factor, venous compression, and hepatobiliary cancer in the CATCH trial.[43] Further research is needed to identify cancer patients with high risk of recurrent VTE.

Prevention of VTE in cancer patients
Prevention of thrombosis in cancer patients undergoing surgery

A meta-analysis including 39 cohort studies and RCTs compared peri-operative pharmacological thromboprophylaxis in cancer patients undergoing surgery versus no pharmacological prophylaxis (mechanical prophylaxis was permitted).[44] Pharmacological prophylaxis reduced the rate of deep vein thrombosis (DVT) by 50%, but the incidence of all bleeding events increased by 2.5-fold. There was no difference in mortality or the incidence of pulmonary embolism (PE) between the two arms. Another systematic review and meta-analysis of seven RCTs ($N = 4807$) showed that extended thromboprophylaxis (2–6 weeks) after abdominopelvic cancer surgery significantly reduced the risk of proximal DVT by approximately 50%, when compared with a shorter thromboprophylaxis of <2 weeks,[45] with no difference in the incidence of symptomatic PE, major bleeding, or all-cause mortality at 3-months.[45] Based on these data, current guidelines recommend pharmacological thromboprophylaxis for most cancer patients undergoing surgery, with extended prophylaxis (4 weeks) for patients undergoing abdominopelvic cancer surgery.[46,47]

Prevention of thrombosis in the ambulatory outpatient setting

Prophylactic low-molecular-weight heparin (LMWH) has been shown to reduce the risk of VTE in ambulatory cancer patients receiving chemotherapy.[48,49] However, given the high number needed to treat (NNT),[40–50] the burden associated with daily injections, and concerns of bleeding complications, it has not been accepted as standard of care. Subsequent studies have worked to improve the tolerability and effectiveness of primary thromboprophylaxis by targeting high-risk patients identified by the Khorana Risk Score as well as substituting direct oral anticoagulants (DOACs) in place of LMWH.

In 2019, the results of two large, double blind, placebo-controlled RCTs, AVERT, and CASSINI, investigating DOACs as primary VTE prophylaxis in ambulatory cancer patients were published.[50,51] Both studies included cancer patients with moderate to high risk of VTE as defined by a Khorana score ≥ 2. Patients in the AVERT trial received apixaban 2.5 mg twice daily while those in the CASSINI trial received rivaroxaban 10 mg daily.[50,51] Over the study period of 180 days, apixaban significantly reduced the rate of VTE over placebo [4.2% vs 10.2%, hazard ratio (HR) 0.41, 95% confidence interval (CI): 0.26–0.65], with increased risk of major bleeding (3.5% vs 1.8%, HR 2.00, 95% CI: 1.01–3.95) by intention-to-treat analysis. The on-treatment major bleeding rates (events occurred while on study drugs or up to 2 days after last dose) were not statistically different (2.1% vs 1.1%, HR 1.89; 95% CI, 0.39–9.24). The NNT for VTE prevention was 17 and the on-treatment number needed to harm (NNH) was 100. The CASSINI trial has a few notable differences from the AVERT trial. Screening bilateral lower extremity ultrasounds were performed at 8, 16, and 24 weeks with results included in the primary efficacy outcome. Forty-nine patients (4.5%) were found to have incidental DVT on baseline screening ultrasound and thus excluded. Over the study period of 180 days, rivaroxaban was associated with a lower, but nonstatistically significant, VTE

Table 2 Comparison of patient characteristics in randomized trials of cancer-associated thrombosis.

Study	CLOT	Hokusai VTE cancer	Select-D	ADAM VTE	Caravaggio
Number	676	1050	406	300	1155
Age (mean)	62.5	64.0	67 (median)	64.2	67.2
Male	51.5%	51.6%	51%	48.3%	49.2%
Solid tumor	89.6%	89.1%	97%	89%	92.6%
Metastatic disease	67.3%	59%	59%	64.3%	68.0%[a]
ECOG ≥2	36.7%	23.8%	23.5%	10.7%	20.9%
Cancer treatment at enrollment	77.7%	72.4%	69%	72.7%	62.1%
Incidental VTE	0%	32.5%	53%	N/A	20%
History of VTE	11%	10.7%	N/A	6.7%	9.2%

[a]Includes recurrent locally advanced or metastatic disease.
ECOG, Eastern Cooperative Oncology Group; N/A, not available; VTE, venous thromboembolism.

Table 3 Comparison of six-month outcomes in randomized trials of cancer-associated thrombosis.

Study Arms	CLOT		Hokusai VTE cancer		Select-D		ADAM VTE		Caravaggio	
	Warfarin	Dalteparin	Edoxaban	Dalteparin	Rivaroxaban	Dalteparin	Apixaban	Dalteparin	Apixaban	Dalteparin
Recurrent VTE	53/336 (15.8%)	27/336 (8.0%)	34/522 (6.5%)	46/524 (8.8%)	8/203 (3.9%)	18/203 (8.9%)	1/145 (0.7%)	9/142 (6.3%)	32/576 (5.6%)	46/579 (7.9%)
Major bleeding	12/335 (3.6%)	19/338 (5.6%)	29/522 (5.6%)	17/524 (3.2%)	11/203 (5.4%)	6/203 (3.0%)	0/145 (0%)	2/142 (1.4%)	22/576 (3.8%)	23/579 (4.0%)
Mortality	136/336 (40.5%)	130/336 (38.7%)	140/522 (26.8%)	127/524 (24.2%)	48/203 (24%)	56/203 (28%)	23/145 (16%)	15/142 (11%)	135/576 (23.4%)	153/579 (26.4%)

VTE, venous thromboembolism.

rate versus placebo [6.0% vs 8.8%, HR 0.66; 95% CI, 0.40–1.09]. A nonsignificant increased risk of major bleeding was found in the on-treatment analysis with rivaroxaban (2.0% vs 1.0%, HR 1.96; 95% CI, 0.59–6.49). The NNT with rivaroxaban was 35 (26 when considering on-treatment) and NNH was 101. Based on these data, major practice guidelines have been recently updated to include recommendations to consider primary thromboprophylaxis with rivaroxaban, apixaban, or LMWH in ambulatory cancer patients with Khorana score ≥2 starting systemic cancer therapies.[52,53]

Treatment of cancer-associated thrombosis (CAT)
Acute treatment (within 3–6 months)

LMWH LMWH has been the standard of care to treat acute cancer-associated thrombosis (CAT) since the CLOT trial in 2003. The CLOT trial randomized patients with acute CAT to LMWH (dalteparin) versus vitamin K antagonists (VKAs). Dalteparin was associated with a significant reduction in VTE recurrence compared to VKA, with no increased risk of major bleeding events.[54] Several subsequent studies found consistent results. A meta-analysis demonstrated that compared to VKA, LMWH reduced the risks of recurrent VTE by 40% (relative risk [RR] 0.60, 95% CI 0.45–0.80) with no difference in major bleeding events (RR 1.07, 95% CI 0.65–1.75).[55] Therefore, major clinical guidelines have recommended LMWH as one of the first-line therapies for treatment of acute CAT.[56–58]

DOACs Several recently completed RCTs have established the role of DOACs in the treatment of acute CAT: Hokusai VTE Cancer (edoxaban), Select-D (rivaroxaban), ADAM VTE (apixaban), and Caravaggio (apixaban).[59–62] All studies compared DOAC to dalteparin. The ADAM VTE trial was the smallest (N = 300), with notable differences from other studies, such as the inclusion of patients with upper extremity DVT, splanchnic or cerebral vein thrombosis, lower mortality rate, and so on, all of which could affect outcomes.[62] Tables 2 and 3 summarize the patient characteristics and main outcomes in these studies, adding the CLOT trial as a comparison.

The Hokusai VTE Cancer trial was an open-label, randomized, noninferiority study, that included 1050 patients with a cancer diagnosis within the past two years with an acute proximal DVT and/or PE.[59] The primary outcome—the composite of the first recurrent VTE or major bleeding event within 12 months—occurred in 12.8 % versus 13.5% (edoxaban vs dalteparin, HR 0.97, 95% CI 0.70–1.36), indicating that edoxaban was noninferior to dalteparin ($p = 0.006$ for noninferiority). When compared to dalteparin, edoxaban was associated with fewer recurrent VTE events (7.9% vs 11.3%, $p = 0.09$) but significantly more major bleeding events (6.9% vs 4.0%, $p = 0.04$). The majority of major bleeding events on edoxaban were upper GI bleeding in patients with GI cancer and not fatal.[63]

The Select-D pilot trial randomized 406 cancer patients with acute lower extremity DVT or PE to rivaroxaban or dalteparin. The primary endpoint—the six-month VTE recurrence rate—was 4% versus 11% (rivaroxaban vs dalteparin, HR 0.43, 95% CI 0.19–0.99), with major bleeding events of 6% versus 4% (rivaroxaban vs dalteparin, HR 1.83, 95% CI 0.68–4.96). There were more clinically relevant nonmajor bleeding (CRNMB) events associated with rivaroxaban (rivaroxaban vs dalteparin, 13% vs 4%, HR 3.76, 95% CI 1.63–8.69). Similar to the Hokusai VTE Cancer trial, the majority of the bleeding events occurred as GI bleeding in patients with upper GI cancer and recruitment of this population was terminated early due to the concern of bleeding.

The Caravaggio trial randomized patients with cancer diagnosed within the past 2 years with acute lower extremity DVT or PE to apixaban or dalteparin. The primary endpoint—the 6-month VTE recurrence rate—was 5.6% versus 7.9% (apixaban vs dalteparin, HR 0.63, 95% CI 0.37–1.07, $p < 0.001$ for noninferiority), with major bleeding event rate of 3.8% versus 4.0% (HR 0.82; 95% CI, 0.40–1.69). There were numerically more CRNMB events associated with apixaban (9.0% vs 6.0%, HR1.42, 95% CI 0.88–2.30). Despite that one-third of enrolled patients had GI malignancy, there were no increased risks of major bleeding or major GI bleeding events in apixaban arm. This is in contrast with the prior two trials (Hokusai VTE Cancer and Select-D pilot trial). Therefore, apixaban is a promising anticoagulant for patients with CAT, including those with GI malignancy.

Based on data from these RCTs, major practice guidelines have been quickly revised to include edoxaban, rivaroxaban, and apixaban as appropriate treatment for CAT.[53,64,65] However, caution is needed in situations such as potential drug-drug interaction, high risk of GI bleeding, and more.

Vitamin K antagonists (VKA) VKA were less effective than LMWH in the prevention of recurrent VTE in cancer patients and could be associated with increased risk of bleeding events in the CLOT and CATCH trials.[54,66] It also requires frequent laboratory monitoring and dose adjustments, has multiple drug and diet interactions, and slow onset and offset. Therefore, in patients with CAT, VKA is not preferred and would be recommended only when neither a DOAC nor LMWH is feasible.

Extended treatment (beyond 6 months)
The study period of most RCTs in patients with CAT was limited to 3 to 6 months. Therefore, outcomes beyond six months are not well studied, and the optimal duration of anticoagulation in CAT patient is unclear. In the LMWH era, two single-arm prospective cohort studies treating CAT with dalteparin (DALTECAN study) or tinzaparin (TiCAT study) for 12 months,[67,68] showed that the risk of recurrent VTE or major bleeding is the highest during the first 3–6 months, but with an ongoing risk of recurrent VTE between 6 and 12 months (4.1% in the DALTECAN study and 1.1% in the TiCAT study). Therefore, major guidelines recommend to continue long-term anticoagulation as long as the risk factors (active malignancy and/or ongoing cancer treatment) are persistent. The Hokusai VTE Cancer trial was the first to follow patients with CAT on DOAC beyond 6 months. It showed that the risks of recurrent VTE and major bleeding (on anticoagulation) were low during 6–12 months after the initial VTE (0.7% and 1.7%, respectively, in the edoxaban arm).[69] Edoxaban was noninferior to dalteparin in either outcome. This provides evidence that edoxaban is a reasonable option for anticoagulation beyond 6 months for CAT. Other studies are ongoing to evaluate the use of reduced dose DOAC after the initial 6 months of therapeutic anticoagulation.

Treatment in special populations

Incidental VTE Incidental VTE are common in cancer patients, as they frequently have computed tomography (CT) scans for cancer staging. The incidence of incidental PE varies widely in different studies, with an average of 3% found on routine imaging.[70] Previous studies showed that the outcomes (recurrent VTE or survival) after an incidental PE are comparable to those after a symptomatic VTE,[71,72] and therefore the same management including anticoagulation is recommended for incidental VTE in patients with cancer.[73] About 32.5% and 52% of patients enrolled in the Hokusai VTE Cancer and Select-D trials presented with an incidental VTE, respectively.[59,60] The analysis in the Hokusai VTE Cancer study showed that patients with incidental VTE were more likely to have PE and solid tumor and less likely to have extensive PE, as compared to those with symptomatic VTE.[74] There were no statistical differences in recurrent VTE, major bleeding events, or all-cause mortality in patients with incidental compared to symptomatic VTE. Edoxaban was noninferior to dalteparin in the primary composite outcomes in both groups of incidental and symptomatic VTE. On the country, in the Select-D trial, symptomatic VTE was a risk factor for increased risk of recurrent VTE compared to incidental VTE (HR 2.78, 95% CI 1.20–6.41).[60] Overall, both studies support the current recommendations of standard anticoagulation for patients with incidental VTE.

Catheter-related thrombosis Cancer patients commonly have CVCs for frequent blood draws and administration of chemotherapy. One of the most common complications associated with CVCs is catheter-related thrombosis (CRT). The reported incidence of CRT in cancer patients varies widely in studies, but a rate of as high as 20% has been reported.[40] Primary thromboprophylaxis has not been shown to be beneficial and is therefore not routinely recommended.[75] Standard anticoagulation is effective for line preservation and is recommended to continue as long as the catheter is in place.[76] However, the optimal duration of anticoagulation after catheter removal remains unclear. Although CRT is common in cancer patients, there remains limited evidence on the optimal type or duration of anticoagulation. Two prospective single-arm cohort studies, the CATHETER and CATHETER 2 studies, enrolled 74 patients on dalteparin bridged to warfarin and 70 patients on rivaroxaban, respectively, in cancer patients with CRT.[76,77] At three months, the line preservation rates were 100% in both studies, with low rates of recurrent VTE (CATETER: 0%; CATETER 2: 1.43%). The rates of major bleeding were higher, 4% in CATETER study and 10% in CATEHTER 2 study. More studies are needed to guide management in this population.

Patients with recurrent VTE while on anticoagulation Cancer patients have an increased risk of recurrent VTE despite anticoagulation, especially in the setting of progressive cancer. However, there are little data to management thus guidelines are based on expert opinions and small observational studies.[78-80] In the LMWH era, common recommendations included: (1) in patients on VKA, switch to LMWH, (2) in patients on LMWH, increase LMWH intensity to therapeutic dosing (if not on therapeutic dosing), or by 20–25% (if already on therapeutic dosing). Pivotal RCTs including Hokusai VTE Cancer, Select-D, and Caravaggio, all suggest that DOACs are associated with numerically reduced risks of recurrent VTE, and should be considered in cancer patients whom high risk of recurrent VTE is a concern. In addition, the management of patients who develop a recurrent or progressive VTE while on DOACs is unknown, although many clinicians would switch to LMWH or an alternate DOAC empirically. Further studies are needed to address this issue.

Patients with thrombocytopenia The presence of thrombocytopenia commonly complicates the management of cancer patients who require anticoagulation and increases the risk of bleeding.[81] The optimal management in this challenging situation is unclear, as large RCTs investigating the treatment of CAT, mentioned above, all excluded patients with platelet counts $<50 \times 10^9/L$. Available data are from retrospective studies only (mostly with LMWH), and recommendations are based on expert opinions.

ISTH guidance document published in 2018 recommends that in patients with acute VTE (within 30 days) with high risk of thrombus progression (such as proximal DVT or PE) and a platelet count $<50 \times 10^9$/L, to use therapeutic anticoagulation plus platelet transfusion to keep platelet count ≥ 40–50×10^9/L.[82] However, the platelet threshold of 50×10^9/L is not based on high-quality evidence and many debate the need to maintain this threshold. In patients with acute VTE but lower risk of thrombus progression, subacute or chronic VTE (>30 days), a reduced dose LMWH is recommended in those with platelet count of 25–50×10^9/L, and to stop anticoagulation for platelet count $<25 \times 10^9$/L.[82]

Patients with brain tumors Brain tumors, either primary or metastatic, increase the risks of both thrombotic and bleeding complications. A matched cohort study in patients with metastatic brain tumor showed that LMWH did not increase the risk of intracranial hemorrhage (ICH).[83] This result was confirmed by a subsequent meta-analysis of nine retrospective cohort studies.[84] However, the same meta-analysis showed that patients with primary brain glioma had 3.75-fold increased odds of ICH associated with anticoagulation (OR 3.75, 95% CI 1.42–9.95). This was confirmed by another matched cohort study of 133 patients with high-grade glioma, in which LMWH was associated with a 3.37-fold increased hazard of major ICH when compared to no LMWH.[85] However, the lack of anticoagulation was associated with an 11-fold increased hazard of VTE in patients with primary brain tumors (HR 11.2, 95% CI 1.5–86.3) in the same study.[86] A retrospective cohort study compared DOAC versus LMWH in patients with primary brain tumor ($N = 67$) and metastatic brain tumor ($N = 105$), and found that DOACs were not associated with increased incidence of ICH compared to LMWH in either group. While more research is needed, available data showed that in patients with metastatic or primary brain tumor and acute VTE, standard anticoagulation (with either DOAC or LMWH) is recommended, but clinicians should be aware that the risk of ICH is particularly increased in patients with primary brain tumor.

Arterial thrombosis and atrial fibrillation

Epidemiology
Arterial thrombosis is common in developed countries and risk increases with age and in patients with malignancy. An analysis of SEER data revealed that the 6-month cumulative incidence of arterial thromboembolism in cancer patients was 4.7% compared with 2.2% in controls without cancer.[87]

Risk factors
Common risk factors of arterial thrombosis in the general population apply to cancer patients as well, including hypertension, dyslipidemia, smoking, obesity, diabetes, and history of cardiovascular events, as shown in the Vienna CATS.[88] The investigators also found that the risk of arterial thrombosis increased as the number of risk factors increased. In addition, targeted cancer therapies such as ibrutinib can increase the risk of atrial fibrillation by three- to fourfold[89] which is a known risk factor for ischemic strokes. However, ibrutinib also has antiplatelet properties, and a study showed that the risks of arterial and venous thrombosis in patients on ibrutinib are likely to be lower compared to historical controls.[90] More studies are needed. Other cancer therapies such as tamoxifen, bevacizumab, or multitargeted tyrosine kinase inhibitors such as sunitinib and sorafenib are also associated with increased risk of arterial thrombosis, in addition to venous thrombosis.

Management/prevention
The CATS cohort revealed that arterial thrombosis was associated with a threefold increased risk of mortality,[88] thus optimal management is crucial. The management of arterial thrombosis and atrial fibrillation in cancer patients is similar to that in noncancer patients. Treatment and optimization of underlying medical comorbidities and risk factors are important. If anticoagulation for atrial fibrillation is needed, DOAC is preferred over other agents given the available evidence, connivance, and safety.[91]

> **Summary**
>
> Coagulopathy is a common complication in patients with cancer and can result in bleeding and/or thrombotic sequelae. These complications can lead to increased morbidity and mortality, as well as delays or alterations in cancer treatment. Therefore, identification of risk factors, preventative measures, and treatment strategies are important priorities in the care of cancer patients.

Key references

The complete reference list can be found on Vital Source version of this title, see inside front cover.

2 Ten Berg MJ, van den Bemt PM, Shantakumar S, et al. Thrombocytopenia in adult cancer patients receiving cytotoxic chemotherapy: results from a retrospective hospital-based cohort study. *Drug Saf*. 2011;**34**(12):1151–1160.

4 Weycker D, Hatfield M, Grossman A, et al. Risk and consequences of chemotherapy-induced thrombocytopenia in US clinical practice. *BMC Cancer*. 2019;**19**(1):151.

5 Dutcher JP, Schiffer CA, Aisner J, et al. Incidence of thrombocytopenia and serious hemorrhage among patients with solid tumors. *Cancer*. 1984;**53**(3):557–562.

6 Hitron A, Steinke D, Sutphin S, et al. Incidence and risk factors of clinically significant chemotherapy-induced thrombocytopenia in patients with solid tumors. *J Oncol Pharm Pract*. 2011;**17**(4):312–319.

8 Cairo MS, Davenport V, Bessmertny O, et al. Phase I/II dose escalation study of recombinant human interleukin-11 following ifosfamide, carboplatin and etoposide in children, adolescents and young adults with solid tumours or lymphoma: a clinical, haematological and biological study. *Br J Haematol*. 2005;**128**(1):49–58.

9 Li J, Yang C, Xia Y, et al. Thrombocytopenia caused by the development of antibodies to thrombopoietin. *Blood*. 2001;**98**(12):3241–3248.

11 Winer ES, Safran H, Karaszewska B, et al. Eltrombopag with gemcitabine-based chemotherapy in patients with advanced solid tumors: a randomized phase I study. *Cancer Med*. 2015;**4**(1):16–26.

13 Soff GA, Miao Y, Bendheim G, et al. Romiplostim treatment of chemotherapy-induced thrombocytopenia. *J Clin Oncol*. 2019;**37**(31):2892–2898.

14 Zhang X, Chuai Y, Nie W, et al. Thrombopoietin receptor agonists for prevention and treatment of chemotherapy-induced thrombocytopenia in patients with solid tumours. *Cochrane Database Syst Rev*. 2017;**11**:CD012035.

18 Heckman KD, Weiner GJ, Davis CS, et al. Randomized study of prophylactic platelet transfusion threshold during induction therapy for adult acute leukemia: 10,000/microL versus 20,000/microL. *J Clin Oncol*. 1997;**15**(3):1143–1149.

19 Zumberg MS, del Rosario ML, Nejame CF, et al. A prospective randomized trial of prophylactic platelet transfusion and bleeding incidence in hematopoietic stem cell transplant recipients: 10,000/L versus 20,000/microL trigger. *Biol Blood Marrow Transplant*. 2002;**8**(10):569–576.

20 Diedrich B, Remberger M, Shanwell A, et al. A prospective randomized trial of a prophylactic platelet transfusion trigger of 10 x 10(9) per L versus 30 x 10(9) per L in allogeneic hematopoietic progenitor cell transplant recipients. *Transfusion*. 2005;**45**(7):1064–1072.

21 Levi M, Scully M. How I treat disseminated intravascular coagulation. *Blood*. 2018;**131**(8):845–854.

23 Feinstein DI. Disseminated intravascular coagulation in patients with solid tumors. *Oncology (Williston Park)*. 2015;**29**(2):96–102.

26 Sallah S, Wan JY. Inhibitors against factor VIII in patients with cancer. Analysis of 41 patients. *Cancer*. 2001;**91**(6):1067–1074.

27 Bertolino J, Ibrahim M, Seguier J, et al. Intravenous immunoglobulin in patients with acquired Von Willebrand syndrome: a single referral centre experience. *Haemophilia*. 2019;**25**(1):e42–e45.

28. Levade M, David E, Garcia C, et al. Ibrutinib treatment affects collagen and von Willebrand factor-dependent platelet functions. *Blood*. 2014;**124**(26):3991–3995.
29. Timp JF, Braekkan SK, Versteeg HH, Cannegieter SC. Epidemiology of cancer-associated venous thrombosis. *Blood*. 2013;**122**(10):1712–1723.
31. Blom JW, Doggen CJ, Osanto S, Rosendaal FR. Malignancies, prothrombotic mutations, and the risk of venous thrombosis. *JAMA*. 2005;**293**(6):715–722.
33. Mansfield AS, Tafur AJ, Wang CE, et al. Predictors of active cancer thromboembolic outcomes: validation of the Khorana score among patients with lung cancer. *J Thromb Haemost*. 2016;**14**(9):1773–1778.
34. Mulder FI, Candeloro M, Kamphuisen PW, et al. The Khorana score for prediction of venous thromboembolism in cancer patients: a systematic review and meta-analysis. *Haematologica*. 2019;**104**(6):1277–1287.
35. Ay C, Dunkler D, Marosi C, et al. Prediction of venous thromboembolism in cancer patients. *Blood*. 2010;**116**(24):5377–5382.
38. Li A, Wu Q, Luo S, et al. Derivation and validation of a risk assessment model for immunomodulatory drug-associated thrombosis among patients with multiple myeloma. *J Natl Compr Cancer Netw*. 2019;**17**(7):840–847.
39. Gerotziafas GT, Taher A, Abdel-Razeq H, et al. A predictive score for thrombosis associated with breast, colorectal, lung, or ovarian cancer: the prospective COMPASS-cancer-associated thrombosis study. *Oncologist*. 2017;**22**(10):1222–1231.
41. Menapace LA, McCrae KR, Khorana AA. Predictors of recurrent venous thromboembolism and bleeding on anticoagulation. *Thromb Res*. 2016;**140**(Suppl 1):S93–S98.
42. van Es N, Louzada M, Carrier M, et al. Predicting the risk of recurrent venous thromboembolism in patients with cancer: a prospective cohort study. *Thromb Res*. 2018;**163**:41–46.
43. Khorana AA, Kamphuisen PW, Meyer G, et al. Tissue factor as a predictor of recurrent venous thromboembolism in malignancy: biomarker analyses of the CATCH trial. *J Clin Oncol*. 2017;**35**(10):1078–1085.
48. Di Nisio M, Porreca E, Otten HM, Rutjes AW. Primary prophylaxis for venous thromboembolism in ambulatory cancer patients receiving chemotherapy. *Cochrane Database Syst Rev*. 2014;**8**:CD008500.
49. Schünemann H, Ventresca M, Crowther M, et al. An individual participant data meta-analysis of 13 randomized trials to evaluate the impact of prophylactic use of heparin in oncological patients. *Blood*. 2017;**130**(supplement 1):626.
63. Bleker SM, Brekelmans MPA, Eerenberg ES, et al. Clinical impact of major bleeding in patients with venous thrombo-embolism treated with factor Xa inhibitors or vitamin K antagonists. *Thromb Haemost*. 2017;**117**(10):1944–1951.
86. Edwin NC, Khoury MN, Sohal D, et al. Recurrent venous thromboembolism in glioblastoma. *Thromb Res*. 2016;**137**:184–188.

129 Urologic complications related to cancer and its treatment

Omar Alhalabi, MD ■ Ala Abudayyeh, MD ■ Nizar M. Tannir, MD, FACP

Overview

Urologic complications of cancer itself or its treatment often require timely identification and intervention. In patients with early-stage disease, skilled multidisciplinary management of urologic complications is critical to ensure optimal renal function and delivery of adequate doses of chemotherapy that do not compromise the likelihood of cure. Similarly, the management of urologic complications such as urinary obstruction in patients with metastatic disease can have a significant impact on the quality of life. Multiple sites of ureteric obstruction, long occlusions, or a tortuous ureter may be indications to proceed directly with percutaneous nephrostomy instead of ureteral stenting. In contrast to urinary obstruction in newly diagnosed prostate cancer that is likely sensitive to androgen deprivation, castrate-resistant prostate cancer will likely require more permanent relief of obstruction, either by nephrostomy or suprapubic catheter.

Introduction

Anticipation and timely intervention for urologic complications of cancer and its therapy may facilitate treatment of patients with localized disease and expand opportunities for the treatment of patients with metastatic disease. Management of obstructive uropathy and drug-induced renal toxicity allows for the delivery of optimal unreduced doses of chemotherapy without reduction. Renally based dose adjustment and the monitoring of multiple agents with nephrotoxic potential are nuanced yet essential components of oncologic practice, and management of urologic complications often requires coordinated multidisciplinary care. This article reviews the most frequent urologic complications of cancer and its therapy.

Urinary tract obstruction

Obstruction of the urinary tract may occur at multiple levels (ureter, bladder, or urethra) due to direct extension, encasement, or invasion of these structures. Time course (acute versus chronic) and level of obstruction determine its clinical presentation and management. Minimally invasive interventions such as stenting and external drainage of the urinary tract, which are performed by a urologist or an interventional radiologist, may allow early intervention and reduce the need for extensive surgical procedures.

The first clue to an obstructive uropathy may be a rising serum creatinine level, particularly in ureteral obstructions which are often painless. Bladder outlet or urethral obstruction results in a painfully distended bladder that may be palpable on physical exam. Acute unilateral hydronephrosis may cause a renin–angiotensin-mediated hypertension which is often reversible with relief of the obstruction.[1] The cornerstones of diagnostic imaging are ultrasound and computerized tomography (CT) with contrast, with the former often pursued first to avoid the potential nephrotoxicity of intravenous contrast media and exposure to radiation.

If not relieved, urinary obstruction leads to renal tubule atrophy and irreversible injury and may also provide a nidus for infection.[2] The radiographic appearance of the kidney under conditions of acute and chronic obstruction are distinct, with the former appearing as an enlarged kidney with a normal-to-thickened renal cortex, and the latter appearing as a smaller than average kidney with a thinned cortex. Relief of the obstruction is unlikely to result in significant improvement in renal function with chronic obstruction, and the visualization of a small kidney with thinned cortex on ultrasound should usually precludes an optimal outcome of a planned intervention. Return of renal function has been reported following the relief of a chronic obstruction; however, recovery was incomplete.[3] In the period immediately following relief of the obstruction, the renal tubule's concentrating capacity is often abnormal, which may cause a period of postobstructive diuresis. This is most commonly observed with acute high-grade obstructions.

Ureteral obstruction

Located in the retroperitoneum, the ureters are particularly vulnerable to mechanical obstruction by pathologic retroperitoneal lymphadenopathy or retroperitoneal fibrosis. Such obstructive uropathy most frequently is the result of either primary nodal diseases (lymphomas) or periaortic lymph node metastases of urologic neoplasms, particularly prostate cancer and germ cell tumors. In the case of retroperitoneal adenopathy due to highly chemotherapy-responsive malignancies, particularly some germ cell tumors or aggressive lymphomas, the expected prompt response to therapy may allow the clinician to avoid intervention for the obstruction, particularly in the case of unilateral or partial obstruction. The need to administer nephrotoxic curative-intent chemotherapy (e.g., cisplatin) may require intervention to temporarily bypass the obstruction even in chemo-responsive disease. The rate and degree of anticipated response to therapy and the degree of compromise in renal function together govern whether placement of a percutaneous nephrostomy is necessary or whether a reasonable expectation exists that relief of obstruction can be achieved with cytotoxic chemotherapy alone.

When mechanical bypass of a ureteral obstruction is required, a ureteral stent or percutaneous nephrostomy may be employed. Multiple sites of ureteral obstruction, long occlusions, or a tortuous ureter may be indications to proceed directly with percutaneous nephrostomy.[4] While a unilateral percutaneous nephrostomy may preserve adequate renal function for palliative therapy, patients whose long-term disease-free survival is dependent on nephrotoxic therapy require maximal preservation of renal function, and bilateral percutaneous nephrostomy is often required in this setting. Although they may be key to the delivery of therapy, percutaneous nephrostomies are not without risk and are a potential source of infection that may complicate, delay, or even require modification of treatment plans.[5] Placement of appropriately sized catheters to reduce pain, frequent catheter exchanges, and care of the insertion site is essential to reduce complications.

During nephrostomy tube placement, complications are rare and may include hematoma formation, hemorrhage, vascular injury, sepsis, bowel or lung injury, or death.[4] An internal double-J stent may be placed following the relief of the intra-renal pressure by nephrostomy tube placement, which is performed in an antegrade fashion using the nephrostomy as an entry point. While intervention with percutaneous nephrostomy or stenting may allow for delivery of curative-intent treatment in a patient who might not otherwise be able to receive therapy, the risk-benefit analysis may be markedly different in a patient with advanced incurable disease. Recent studies show that percutaneous nephrostomy can be associated with significant morbidity in patients with advanced pelvic malignancy and does not always prolong survival.[6] A patient with severe pain (unrelated to obstruction) and very short life expectancy may be best served by no intervention, but rather implementation of comfort measures. This difficult decision requires careful communication between physician, patient, and the patient's family members.

Bladder outlet and urethral obstruction

Malignant bladder outlet and urethral obstructions are most commonly caused by prostate or bladder cancers and may be seen with ovarian, cervical, and uterine cancers as well. Patients with bladder outlet and urethral obstruction often present with troublesome symptoms resulting from bladder irritation and distension. These may have a significant impact on a patient's perceived quality of life.[7,8] Prostate cancers that arise from the portion of the prostate immediately adjacent to the intra-prostatic urethra need not be large to cause marked symptoms. Urine output may fluctuate, with periods of both relative oliguria and increased urinary output due to overflow incontinence.

The management of obstructions due to prostate cancer is guided by the stage of the prostate cancer. Newly diagnosed prostate cancer is likely to be exquisitely sensitive to androgen deprivation therapy (ADT). Temporary Foley catheter placement may result in relief of the obstruction with prompt removal of the indwelling—Foley after tumor response to ADT. In contrast, castrate-resistant prostate cancer, which nearly invariably develops after a period of response to ADT, will not exhibit this prompt response to therapy and will likely require more permanent relief of obstruction, either by nephrostomy or suprapubic catheter. In addition, very large prostate or bladder tumors, regardless of their anticipated response to therapy, may be indications to proceed directly with placement of percutaneous nephrostomy tubes. Bladder outlet or urethral obstruction may be managed by the placement of a suprapubic urinary catheter. Generally, this technique provides palliation of symptoms and should not be pursued in patients being treated with curative intent as it violates normal anatomic barriers of the genitourinary (GU) tract.

For patients with urethral obstruction, symptoms are often difficult to relieve. Although percutaneous nephrostomies and suprapubic catheters can divert urinary flow, they do not fully relieve symptoms related to urgency, hematuria, dysuria, and frequency. Transurethral resection of the prostate may be considered for palliation of symptoms in advanced disease, and definite prostate surgery may provide significant relief in prostate cancers treated with curative intent. The management of these symptoms remains a therapeutic challenge for clinicians.

Cystitis and nephritis

Cystitis and nephritis usually manifest with hematuria and frequent urination. The management of treatment-induced inflammation, often related to the use of cyclophosphamide, ifosfamide, or radiation, may induce cystitis and bleeding that can be a challenging clinical problem. Embolization of bladder vessels or instillation of steroids has been used with limited success. Other treatments include hyperhydration, bladder irrigation, oral or intra-vesical aminocaproic acid (for lower urinary tract bleeding only), and intravesical prostaglandins.[9–11] Experimental approaches include argon laser coagulation, and conjugated estrogens.[12,13]

Chemotherapy-induced cystitis

Both cyclophosphamide and ifosfamide are metabolized to acrolein, a urothelium-toxic metabolite.[14] Chemotherapy-induced thrombocytopenia may exacerbate bleeding. With conventional doses of cyclophosphamide, cystitis can be prevented by encouraging abundant oral hydration at the time of chemotherapy. With ifosfamide, this complication can be reduced with intravenous hyperhydration and the use of uroprotective mesna, an agent that decreases the risk of bleeding from the bladder following the use of ifosfamide or cyclophosphamide. Mesna is given as an intravenous bolus equal to 20% of the ifosfamide dose 15 min before ifosfamide administration, as well as 4 and 8 h later (the total dose of mesna should be equivalent to 60% of the ifosfamide dose). Mesna may also be given as a continuous infusion at a dose equivalent to the ifosfamide dose. Continuous infusion of mesna should be maintained for 4–8 h after completion of ifosfamide infusion. When given with cyclophosphamide, mesna is predominantly used with high-dose chemotherapy in bone marrow transplantation. The dose of mesna used is approximately 60–160% of the cyclophosphamide dose and is given intravenously in 3–5 divided doses or by continuous infusion.[15] Of note, hemorrhagic cystitis in bone marrow transplantation due to chemotherapeutic regimens must be differentiated from infectious hematuria.[16]

Radiation-induced cystitis

Although relatively uncommon, hemorrhagic cystitis may develop following the treatment of pelvic neoplasms with either external beam radiation or brachytherapy. Cystitis may appear from 6 months to several decades following completion of radiation, and in one study, affected 6.5% of patients receiving pelvic radiation.[17] Total-body irradiation for bone marrow transplantation is associated with hemorrhagic cystitis in 10–17% of patients.[18] Patients who are at highest risk are those receiving concurrent cyclophosphamide or who have undergone urologic interventions.

Delayed radiation cystitis is a diagnosis of exclusion after ruling out urinary tract malignancy.

Radiation nephritis

Modern shielding techniques have dramatically decreased the incidence of this radiation nephritis when delivering therapy to radiation-sensitive tumors (e.g., lymphomas and seminomas). Renal dose tolerance (TD5/5) is estimated to be 20 Gy in adults, with glomerular function declining at 15 Gy and function nearly completely lost at 25–30 Gy. Signs and symptoms often develop 6–12 months after radiation and include hyper-reninemic hypertension, edema, albuminuria, active urinary sediment, and rise in BUN and serum creatinine. Total-body irradiation in bone marrow transplantation has been associated with dose-dependent long-term renal toxicities as well. Pathologic findings include necrosis of vascular structures and disruption of both endothelial and epithelial cells of the basement membrane.[19] In a review of bone marrow transplant patients receiving total-body irradiation with 14 Gy, the incidence of nephropathy decreased with increased renal shielding: 30% of patients treated without shielding developed nephropathy, 15% of patients treated with partial shielding developed nephropathy, and no patients developed nephropathy with 30% shielding.[20]

Table 1 Therapeutic agents associated with nephrotoxicity.

Alkylating agent
AZQ (diaziquone)
Platinums
Oxazaphosphorines (e.g., cyclophosphamide, ifosfamide)
Nitrosoureas (e.g., streptozocin, carmustine, lomustine)
Antitumor antibiotic
Mitomycin C
Plicamycin
Antimetabolite
5-Azacytidine
Clofarabine
Gemcitabine
Antifolates (e.g., methotrexate, pemetrexed)
Targeted therapies
Antiangiogenics (e.g., bevacizumab, sunitinib, cabozantinib, lenvatinib)
mTOR inhibitors (e.g., everolimus)
Immunotherapy agent
Cytokines (e.g., aldesleukin, interferon)
AntiCTLA4 (e.g., ipilimumab)
AntiPD-1/PDL-1 (e.g., pembrolizumab)
Other
Asparaginase
Cyclosporine
Gallium nitrate
Gefitinib
Imatinib
Pentostatin
Tacrolimus

Diagnosis, treatment, and prevention of nephrotoxicity related to cancer therapy

Many widely used chemotherapy agents have the potential for renal toxicity (Table 1 and Figure 1). In addition, nephrotoxicity can occur in the context of tumor lysis syndrome, paraneoplastic glomerulonephritis, and obstructive nephropathy. Nephrotoxicity is more common in the geriatric age group, as well as in the bone marrow transplant population secondary to polypharmacy and comorbid conditions. In the following sections, we describe commonly used agents that cause serious renal toxicity.

Cisplatin

Effective prevention and management of cisplatin's renal toxicity are critical to appropriate delivery of this drug, and development of platinum analogs has, in part, been motivated by cisplatin's renal toxicity. The study of cisplatin, the modification of its delivery, and the anticipation of and screening for nephrotoxicity provide a paradigm for the study of nephrotoxic agents in general. Cisplatin is principally excreted by the kidneys; however, only a small portion of the total cisplatin dose can be identified in the urine in the first few days of therapy.[21] Clearance of the plasma component of cisplatin is triphasic, with nearly all of the administered drug eliminated in 4 h, but with a terminal half-life exceeding 24 h. Cisplatin nephrotoxicity is a result of necrosis of the proximal convoluted tubules (Figure 1), and its severity can be abrogated with aggressive hydration.[22] As cisplatin is a highly emetogenic medication, brisk intravenous fluid administration and aggressive use of antiemetics are central to avoiding dehydration, which may potentiate nephrotoxicity.[23] Clinically, cisplatin-induced nephrotoxicity may be identified by a rise in serum creatinine and a decline in glomerular filtration rate (GFR). Other signs may include hypomagnesemia and moderate proteinuria, which is attributed to a tubular defect.[24] Hemolytic-uremic syndrome (HUS) has also been described, particularly when cisplatin is combined with bleomycin.[25] Routine monitoring of GFR, as well as electrolytes including calcium, magnesium, and phosphorus, is recommended, as is a minimum interval of 7 days between cisplatin doses, as maximal nephrotoxicity frequently does not manifest in less than 7 days. A significant decline in the creatinine clearance should result in a delay of therapy.

Prevention of toxicity with hydration is crucial. Administration of normal saline supplies abundant chloride ions, which diminish the formation of aquated species by mass action, thereby lessening nephrotoxicity. Conflicting reports exist about the role of mannitol and furosemide in cisplatin hydration.[26,27] Coadministration with other nephrotoxic medications including ifosfamide and methotrexate can potentiate renal damage, and adequate hydration is crucial in this setting. Furthermore, concurrent cisplatin and aminoglycoside antibiotic use have been reported to significantly enhance the extent of renal dysfunction.[28] A score-based predication model for acute kidney injury (AKI) in cisplatin exposed patients has been developed and validated where factors associated with AKI were age, cisplatin dose, hypertension, and serum albumin.[29]

Methotrexate

Methotrexate (MTX) is principally excreted by renal glomerular filtration. Renal toxicity due to MTX may be particularly devastating, as prolonged exposure to the drug substantially increases bone marrow toxicity and mucositis. The renal toxicity of MTX is a dose-dependent phenomenon, and as it is highly protein bound, it is not readily cleared by dialysis in case of overdose.[25] The nephrotoxicity of MTX manifests primarily in the renal tubule, where extensive necrosis of the convoluted tubules occurs. The lesion has been termed crystalline hydronephrosis and has been attributed to deposition of the agent. The likelihood of nephrotoxicity may be reduced by pursuing optimal hydration and alkalinizing the urine to pH 7 or higher. Careful balance of the risks and benefits of using this agent, especially in patients who present with impaired

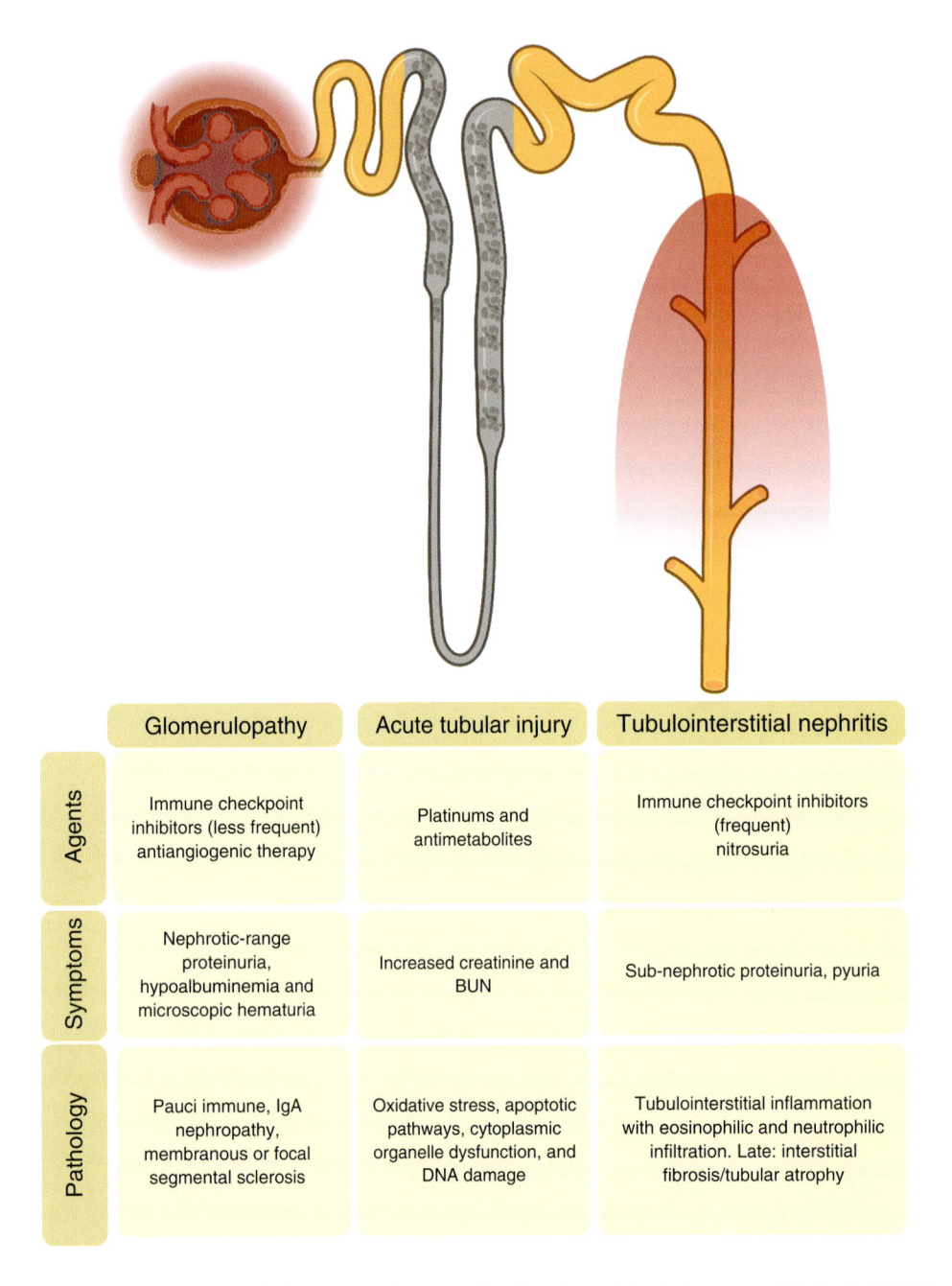

	Glomerulopathy	Acute tubular injury	Tubulointerstitial nephritis
Agents	Immune checkpoint inhibitors (less frequent) antiangiogenic therapy	Platinums and antimetabolites	Immune checkpoint inhibitors (frequent) nitrosuria
Symptoms	Nephrotic-range proteinuria, hypoalbuminemia and microscopic hematuria	Increased creatinine and BUN	Sub-nephrotic proteinuria, pyuria
Pathology	Pauci immune, IgA nephropathy, membranous or focal segmental sclerosis	Oxidative stress, apoptotic pathways, cytoplasmic organelle dysfunction, and DNA damage	Tubulointerstitial inflammation with eosinophilic and neutrophilic infiltration. Late: interstitial fibrosis/tubular atrophy

Figure 1 **Agents, symptoms, and pathology underlying cancer therapy-induced nephrotoxicity.** IgA, immunoglobulin A; BUN, blood urea nitrogen. Source: Figure was created with BioRender.com.

renal function, are a vitally important consideration. Furthermore, prior to administration of MTX, adequate renal function should be ensured (normal serum creatinine and minimum urinary flow of 100 mL/h). Additional protective measures include ensuring alkalinization of urine pH to 7 or higher, and administration of leucovorin starting 24–36 hours after the start of therapy and continuing until plasma methotrexate levels fall to <0.1 micromolar. Monitoring for potential drug–drug interactions is crucial; weak organic acids such as salicylates increase MTX levels by displacing the drug from binding sites on plasma proteins. Additionally, renal tubular transport is diminished by probenecid and salicylates. These agents should be avoided during methotrexate infusion where it can lead to toxic levels of MTX because of delayed renal elimination. In cases where patients develop renal failure and decreased urine output, dialysis would be indicated to mitigate the toxic effects of MTX but need to observe for rebound effects.[30]

Another potential treatment is glucarpidase (carboxypeptidase G2) that can be used in the setting of severe renal failure and elevated levels of methotrexate, as it can lower serum MTX using a single dose of 50 units per kg by bolus IV injection over five minutes.[31] Glucarpidase is a recombinant bacterial enzyme that metabolizes chemically similar antifolates such as MTX to inactive metabolites. Based on the 2018 consensus guideline for its use in patients with MTX-induced AKI, glucarpidase should only be used when other therapies have failed, and certain criteria have been met. In addition, glucarpidase should not to be given after more than 60 h of exposure to high-dose methotrexate.[31]

Nitrosoureas

Significant nephrotoxicity had been predicted and anticipated for the nitrosoureas (lomustine [CCNU], methyl-CCNU, BCNU), a characteristic that has been confirmed in large phase 3 trials.[32–34] Unlike methotrexate and cisplatin, nitrosoureas cause interstitial nephritis (Figure 1). Hydration does not appear to prevent nitrosourea-induced nephrotoxicity, and limiting the cumulative dose administered is the primary method of preventing renal damage.

Mitomycin C

Mitomycin C is an antibiotic isolated from *Streptomyces caespitosus*. Although it has demonstrated significant activity in a variety of tumors, its current use is limited due to adverse effects including prolonged thrombocytopenia and pneumonitis. Mitomycin C has also been associated with hemolytic-uremic syndrome (HUS) with a widely varying interval between drug exposure and onset of HUS.[35] Patients receiving mitomycin C should be carefully monitored for any early signs or symptoms suggestive of HUS (rising creatinine or LDH, anemia). Total cumulative doses of less than 30 mg/m^2 of body surface area are rarely associated with HUS and most cases occur with doses >60 mg/m^2.[36] While steroids can reduce the pulmonary toxicity of this agent, they have demonstrated no clear nephroprotective effect.

Targeted therapies

Mammalian target of rapamycin (mTOR) inhibitors, everolimus, temsirolimus, may produce proteinuria and AKI[37] via a mechanism of biopsy-proven focal segmental glomerulosclerosis as well as acute tubular necrosis (Figure 1).[38,39] Cases of irreversible renal injury requiring dialysis have been reported. AKI due to mTOR inhibitors should prompt drug withdrawal, and guidelines for medication re-challenge are lacking. As the likelihood of irreversible kidney injury is higher in patients over 65 with hypoalbuminemia, hypertension, or preexisting chronic kidney disease (CKD), these patients should not be re-challenged with mTOR inhibitors.[38]

Targeted therapies that inhibit angiogenesis via inhibition of the vascular endothelial growth factor (VEGF) pathway (bevacizumab, sunitinib, sorafenib, pazopanib, axitinib, lenvatinib, and cabozantinib) may produce proteinuria and hypertension due to renal effects. VEGF is expressed by podocyte cells of the glomerulus as well as capillary cells, and VEGF inhibitors are thought to decrease podocyte tight junction expression, leading to proteinuria. The effects are dose dependent and reversible with drug withdrawal. Patients on VEGF inhibitors should have frequent monitoring of blood pressure, and antihypertensive medications should be initiated promptly if hypertension is noted. It is not uncommon to prescribe 2–3 medications for control of blood pressure, however, with aggressive medical management of blood pressure, VEGF therapy usually can be continued. The presence of both hypertension and proteinuria should prompt the use of an ACE-inhibitor as first-line antihypertensive therapy. The management of proteinuria by grade is outlined in the package insert of each individual VEGF inhibitor. In general, therapy is temporarily suspended for moderate proteinuria.[40] Once proteinuria is less than 2 g/day, then VEGF inhibitor may be resumed at a reduced dose.

Immunologic agents

In the last few years, immune checkpoint blockade (ICB) has become a standard of care strategy for an expanding group of malignancies. Ipilimumab, a fully human, IgG1 monoclonal antibody blocking cytotoxic T-lymphocyte-associated antigen 4 (CTLA-4), nivolumab, a fully human IgG4 antibody blocking the programmed death-1 (PD-1) receptor, and pembrolizumab, a humanized monoclonal IgG4–kappa isotype antibody against PD-1, have all achieved approval as options against a variety of cancers. Ipilimumab has been associated with several immune phenomena including colitis, pneumonitis, and rarely nephritis. The injury is associated with infiltration of highly activated CD4 and CD8 T-cells and elevated levels of inflammatory cytokines.[41] The mechanism of renal injury is usually interstitial nephritis, with rare reports of glomerulopathy.[42] Renal function may returns to normal with drug withdrawal, and in some cases, steroids have been used as well. In a multicenter retrospective study, 86% of patients with ICB-induced renal injury received steroids; however, 60% of them did not have complete renal recovery and of the 22% patients re-challenged with ICB, 23% had relapse of AKI.[43,44] Nivolumab and pembrolizumab nephrotoxicity are immune mediated; however, the clinical manifestations of this agent are usually less severe when compared with ipilimumab. A possible explanation is that PD1/PD-L1 checkpoint interaction takes place at the tumor site, whereas the CTLA4/B7 interaction occurs mostly in the lymphoid organs with more systemic effects, which may then spare the kidneys. Combination ICB therapy has been associated with an incidence of grade 3/4 toxicity of 53%, which was higher than reported with monotherapies.[45] Serious AEs related to the treatment were hepatic events (in 15% of patients), gastrointestinal events (in 9% of patients), and renal events (in 6% of patients).[46]

Other agents

Other agents with potential for nephrotoxicity are listed in Table 2.

Monitoring for drug-induced nephrotoxicity

The anticipated mechanism of renal injury should guide what monitoring tests are employed. For example, tubular defects resulting from cisplatin nephrotoxicity may not be immediately reflected in GFR, whereas hypermagnesuria and hypomagnesemia are characteristic of cisplatin nephrotoxicity. Monitoring patients for nephrotoxicity with agents that can cause interstitial nephritis (nitrosoureas) requires routine and frequent urinalyses, whereas agents that may cause HUS (Mitomycin C, gemcitabine) should prompt attention to the relevant laboratory parameters. The appearance of microhematuria should lead physicians to further investigate drug-induced renal injury. The most common renal functional abnormality resulting from cytotoxic therapy is a decline in GFR, and this may prompt a dose adjustment or a change of therapy. Attention should be paid to the correct calculation of renal function by adjusting for weight. The creatinine clearance calculated by the Cockcroft–Gault formula (GC) (Table 3) is accurate in patients of average body habitus but may result in erroneous predictions in patients who are significantly under- or over-weight. The wide fluctuations in weight that may occur in patients undergoing cancer therapy require frequent monitoring of weight and re-calculation of GFR with each chemotherapy dose. There is more evidence in the literature to support the use of the chronic kidney disease epidemiology (CKD-EPI) equation in cancer patients since the CKD-EPI is superior over the CG equation to estimate GFR, CKD-EPI formula estimates GFR, whereas the CG formula estimates CrCl, which is a poor estimation of true GFR. It has been demonstrated in several studies that GC formula underestimates kidney function to a higher degree than either CKD-EPI or MDRD and inadvertently leads to exclusion of patients with

Table 2 Clinical and pathologic features of chemotherapy-associated nephrotoxicity.

Drug	Type of injury	Clinical features	Urine analysis	Time of toxicity	Treatment/outcome	Prevention
5-Azacytidine	Acute tubular	Renal tubular acidosis	Bland, hypoosmolar on therapy	Polyuria and rising creatinine 7–10 d postdose	Replace HCO_3, PO_4, Mg; recovery is complete	Daily creatinine, BUN, and electrolytes
Bevacizumab	Glomerulopathy	Proteinuria	Proteinuria	Increasing with cumulative dose	Discontinue if nephrotic syndrome; hold therapy if urinary protein	Monitor regularly
Carboplatin	Tubular	Mg wasting	Bland	Rising creatinine 5–10 d after therapy	Cessation of drug; dialysis as necessary; recovery usually incomplete	Avoid other nephrotoxic drugs; Mg may increase in patients previously treated with cisplatin
Cisplatin	Acute tubular	Mg wasting	Bland	Rising creatinine with cumulative dose	Cessation of drug; dialysis as necessary; recovery usually incomplete	Vigorous hydration; Cl diuresis, mannitol diuresis, Nathiosulfate; avoid aminoglycosides
Cyclosporine	Tubular and afferent arteriole vasoconstriction	Increased K and decreased Mg; renal tubular acidosis; edema; hypertension	Proteinuria	Rising creatinine from days to months after initiation of therapy	Cessation of drug; dialysis as necessary; recovery usually complete	Periodic drug level; monitor creatinine, BUN, and electrolytes
AZQ (diaziquone)	Tubular and glomerular	Anuria, proteinuria, and renal tubular acidosis	Proteinuria	Rising creatinine 5–10 d after therapy	Cessation of drug; dialysis as necessary; recovery usually complete	Avoid doses >245 mg/m^2
Gallium nitrate	Glomerulopathy	Proteinuria and occasional azotemia	Proteinuria	Proteinuria followed by rising creatinine during and shortly after therapy days	Cessation of drug; recovery usually complete	Daily urine flow >2 L; avoid doses >300 mg/m^2/d for 7 consecutive d
Ifosfamide	Acute tubular	Oliguria	Bland	Rising creatinine within 1–2 d after therapy	Supportive dialysis; recovery usually complete	Oliguria may be increased in patients with prior cisplatin therapy; mesna
Interleukin-2	Prerenal azotemia	Oliguria and hypotension	Proteinuria and hematuria	Rising creatinine during therapy	Stop drug when creatinine ≥4.5 mg/dL or >4 mg/dL with acidosis, fluid overload, or increased K; creatinine >1.5 mg/dL with oliguria; recovery usually within 1–2 weeks	Dopamine at renal doses and fluids
Ipilimumab	Interstitial nephritis	Rising creatinine	Proteinuria, few WBC, few RBC	Weeks	Drug withdrawal, steroids may be necessary	Careful monitoring or serum creatinine
Methotrexate	Acute tubular	Oliguria	Bland	Rising creatinine within 1–2 d of dose	High-dose leucovorin based on methotrexate level; high-volume urine output and alkalinization; recovery is complete	Vigorous hydration and urine alkalinization; dose reduction on renal dysfunction; avoid aminoglycosides and nonsteroidal antiinflammatory; leucovorin
Plicamycin	Acute tubular	Abrupt renal failure	Mild proteinuria	Rising creatinine during dosing	Cessation of drug; re-treat, if recovery complete	Alternate-day dosing; check creatinine and BUN daily
Mitomycin C	Renal vascular lesions	Hypertension, anemia	Hematuria, proteinuria	Rising creatinine after 2 or more doses (12–40 weeks from start)	Permanent cessation of drug; SPA immunoperfusion and dialysis; poor recovery	Stop drug at cumulative dose of 60 mg
mTOR inhibitors	Acute tubular, FSGS	Rising creatinine	Proteinuria	Weeks to months	Cessation of drug; recovery may not be complete in patients with comorbidities	Regular monitoring

(continued overleaf)

Table 2 (Continued)

Drug	Type of injury	Clinical features	Urine analysis	Time of toxicity	Treatment/outcome	Prevention
Nitrosoureas	Interstitial fibrosis, glomerular sclerosis	Late complications	Bland	Rising creatinine months to years after therapy	Supportive dialysis; recovery is complete	Stop BCNU at cumulative dose of 1200 mg/m^2
Streptozocin	Tubular	Proteinuria, occasionally severe	Proteinuria, aminoaciduria	Proteinuria followed by rising creatinine during dosing	Cessation of drug; recovery usually complete	Stop drug at first evidence of proteinuria; hydration will not prevent injury
VEGF inhibitors	Tubular, capillaries	Proteinuria, hypertension	Proteinuria, may be nephrotic range	Weeks to months	Hypertension: aggressive medical management. Proteinuria: hold for moderate proteinuria until resolution. Nephrotic range proteinuria should prompt permanent discontinuation	Regular monitoring

Abbreviations: BCNU, carmustine; BUN, blood urea nitrogen; SPA, staphylococcal protein A; FSGS, focal segmental glomerulosclerosis.

Table 3 Cockcroft formula.

$$\frac{(140-\text{Age}) \text{ weight (kg)}}{72 \times \text{Serum creatinine}}$$

mild kidney impairment from clinical trials.[47] In a recent study evaluating the most accurate GFR estimation in cancer patients, it was concluded that a BSA-adjusted CKD-EPI model improves this estimation of GFR.[48] Drug–drug interaction is another crucial consideration in the administration of potentially nephrotoxic agents; Table 4 highlights some of these drug interactions. These tables are not comprehensive, and careful review of all prescription and over-the-counter medications is essential to the prevention of renal toxicity in the cancer patient. Dose adjustment for several essential chemotherapy agents is summarized in Table 5.

Table 4 Drug interactions that can increase serum levels of antineoplastic agents or add renal toxicity.

Axitinib	CYP3A4/5 inhibitors
Cabozantinib	CYP3A4 inhibitors
Capecitabine	Leucovorin
Carboplatin	Cyclophosphamide, aminoglycosides, topotecan
Cisplatin	Any nephrotoxic agent[a], melphalan, paclitaxel[b], rituximab, topotecan[b]
Cladribine	Cyclophosphamide (high dose)
Cyclophosphamide	Allopurinol
Cyclosporine	Any nephrotoxic agent[a], vancomycin, melphalan, cimetidine, potassium-sparing diuretics, naproxen, sulindac, diclofenac, allopurinol, cytochrome P-450 inhibitors[c], methotrexate
Etoposide	Aprepitant, cyclosporine, valspodar
Everolimus	Selected strong CYP3A4 inhibitors, many antivirals, ketoconazole
Gefitinib	Cytochrome P-450 3A4 inhibitors
Gemcitabine	5-Fluorouracil
Ifosfamide	Cytochrome P-450 inhibitors[c], aprepitant
Interleukin-2	Any nephrotoxic agent[a]
Melphalan	Buthionine
Methotrexate	Organic acids, penicillins, cisplatin, NSAIDs, amiodarone, aspirin, ciprofloxacin, cotrimoxazole, cyclosporine, doxycycline, mercaptopurine, probenecid, procarbazine
Mercaptopurine	Allopurinol, methotrexate, TPMT inhibitors
Mitomycin	5-Fluorouracil-related hemolytic-uremic syndrome
Pazopanib	CYP3A4 inhibitors and inducers
Streptozocin	Any nephrotoxic agent[a]
Sunitinib	CYP3A4 inhibitors and inducers
Temsirolimus	CYP3A4 inhibitors and inducers, many antivirals, dexamethasone
Tacrolimus	Any nephrotoxic agent[a], cyclosporine, cisplatin, drugs metabolized through cytochrome P-450 3A
Thioguanine	TPMT inhibitors
Topotecan	Cisplatin[b], carboplatin[b]
Trimetrexate	Cimetidine, cytochrome P-450 inhibitors[c]

Abbreviations: NSAIDs, nonsteroidal antiinflammatory drugs; TPMT, thiopurine methyltransferase.
[a]For example, aminoglycosides, amphotericin B, intravenous contrast, NSAIDs.
[b]Related to sequence of administration.
[c]Azoles antifungals, macrolides, calcium channel blockers, corticosteroids, grapefruit juice.

Table 5 Adjustment of antineoplastic agents based on renal insufficiency.

Azacytidine	Unexplained increase in creatinine or blood urea nitrogen; delay treatment until back to baseline, then reduce dose by 50%
Bleomycin	Creatinine clearance 10–50 mL/min: reduce dose by 25%
	Creatinine clearance <10 mL/min: reduce dose by 50%
Capecitabine	Creatinine clearance 30–50 mL/min: reduce dose by 25%
	Creatinine clearance <30 mL/min: not recommended
Carboplatin	Adjust according to Calvert formula:
	Total dose (mg) = (target AUC) × (GFR + 25)
Carmustine	Cretinine clearance <60 mL/min: omit dose
Cisplatin	Creatinine clearance 10–50 mL/min: decrease dose by 25%
	Creatinine clearance <10 mL/min: decrease dose by 50%
Clofarabine	Use with extreme caution
Cyclophosphamide	Creatinine clearance 10–50 mL/min: reduce dose by 25%
	Creatinine clearance <10 mL/min: reduce dose by 50%
Cytarabine	Creatinine clearance <60 mL/min, use caution; may decrease dose or change schedule
Daunorubicin	Creatinine >3 mg/dL: decrease dose by 50%
Etoposide	Creatinine clearance 15–50 mL/min: decrease dose by 25%
	Creatinine clearance <15 mL/min: consider 50% dose reduction
Fludarabine	Creatinine clearance 30–70 mL/min: decrease dose by 20-50%
	Creatinine clearance <30 mL/min: not recommended
Gefitinib	Use caution with severe renal impairment
Gemcitabine	Use caution with severe renal impairment
Hydroxyurea	Creatinine clearance <10 mL/min: reduce dose by 80%
Ifosfamide	Creatinine clearance 46–60 mL/min: reduce dose by 20%
	Creatinine clearance 31–45 mL/min: reduce dose by 25%
	Creatinine clearance ≤30 mL/min: reduce dose by 30%
Lomustine	Creatinine clearance <60 mL/min: omit dose
Melphalan	Dose reduction may be necessary; IV: BUN >30 mg/dL or creatinine >1.5 mg/dL: consider 50% dose reduction
Mercaptopurine	Decrease dose or increase interval
Methotrexate	Creatinine clearance 10–50 mL/min: reduce dose by 50%
	Creatinine clearance <10–30 mL/min: avoid use
Mitomycin C	Creatinine clearance <10–60 mL/min: reduce dose by 25%
	Creatinine clearance <10 mL/min: reduce dose by 50%
Oxaliplatin	Use with caution in mild to severe renal impairment
Pemetrexed	Hold therapy if creatinine clearance <45 mL/min: patient with grade 3/4; nonhematologic toxicity should decrease dose by 25%
Pentostatin	Creatinine clearance <30–6 0 mL/min: dose reduction may be necessary
Plicamycin	Creatinine clearance 10–50 mL/min: reduce by 25%
	Creatinine clearance <10 mL/min: reduce dose by 50–70%
Procarbazine	Creatinine clearance <30 mL/min: omit dose
Ralitrexed	Creatinine clearance <25–30 mL/min: reduce dose by 50%
	Creatinine clearance <25 mL/min: omit dose
Streptozocin	Use with caution
Teniposide	Dose reduction may be necessary
Thiotepa	Dose reduction may be necessary
Topotecan	Creatinine clearance 20–39 mL/min: decrease dose to 0.75 mg/m^2
	Creatinine clearance <20 mL/min: insufficient evidence
Tretinoin	Maximum dose of 25 mg/m^2
Trimetrexate	Hold therapy if creatinine >2.5 mg dL; dose adjustment may be necessary

Abbreviations: AUC, area under the curve; BUN, blood urea nitrogen; GFR, glomerular filtration rate; IV, intravenous.

Key references

The complete reference list can be found on Vital Source version of this title, see inside front cover.

1 Weidmann P, Beretta-Piccoli C, Hirsch D, et al. Curable hypertension with unilateral hydronephrosis. Studies on the role of circulating renin. *Ann Intern Med*. 1977;**87**(4):437–440.
2 Wilson DR. Renal function during and following obstruction. *Annu Rev Med*. 1977;**28**:329–339.
3 Better OS, Arieff AI, Massry SG, et al. Studies on renal function after relief of complete unilateral ureteral obstruction of three months' duration in man. *Am J Med*. 1973;**54**(2):234–240.
4 Stables DP. Percutaneous nephrostomy: techniques, indications, and results. *Urol Clin North Am*. 1982;**9**(1):15–29.
5 Bahu R, Chaftari A-M, Hachem RY, et al. Nephrostomy tube related pyelonephritis in patients with cancer: epidemiology, infection rate and risk factors. *J Urol*. 2013;**189**(1):130–135.
6 Misra S, Coker C, Richenberg J. Percutaneous nephrostomy for ureteric obstruction due to advanced pelvic malignancy: have we got the balance right? *Int Urol Nephrol*. 2013;**45**(3):627–632.
8 Donovan JL, Kay HE, Peters TJ, et al. Using the ICSOoL to measure the impact of lower urinary tract symptoms on quality of life: evidence from the ICS-'BPH' study. International continence society–benign prostatic hyperplasia. *Br J Urol*. 1997;**80**(5):712–721.
9 Trotman J, Nivison-Smith I, Dodds A. Haemorrhagic cystitis: incidence and risk factors in a transplant population using hyperhydration. *Bone Marrow Transplant*. 1999;**23**(8):797–801.
10 Lakhani A, Raptis A, Frame D, et al. Intravesicular instillation of E-aminocaproic acid for patients with adenovirus-induced hemorrhagic cystitis. *Bone Marrow Transplant*. 1999;**24**(11):1259–1260.
11 Miller LJ, Chandler SW, Ippoliti CM. Treatment of cyclophosphamide-induced hemorrhagic cystitis with prostaglandins. *Ann Pharmacother*. 1994;**28**(5):590–594.
13 Liu YK, Harty JI, Steinbock GS, et al. Treatment of radiation or cyclophosphamide induced hemorrhagic cystitis using conjugated estrogen. *J Urol*. 1990;**144**(1):41–43.
15 Abudayyeh A, Abdelrahim M. Current strategies for prevention and management of stem cell transplant-related urinary tract and voiding dysfunction. *Curr Bladder Dysfunct Rep*. 2015;**10**(2):109–117.
16 Bedi A, Miller CB, Hanson JL, et al. Association of BK virus with failure of prophylaxis against hemorrhagic cystitis following bone marrow transplantation. *J Clin Oncol*. 1995;**13**(5):1103–1109.
17 Levenback C, Eifel PJ, Burke TW, et al. Hemorrhagic cystitis following radiotherapy for stage Ib cancer of the cervix. *Gynecol Oncol*. 1994;**55**(2):206–210.

18. Lunde LE, Dasaraju S, Cao Q, et al. Hemorrhagic cystitis after allogeneic hematopoietic cell transplantation: risk factors, graft source and survival. *Bone Marrow Transplant*. 2015;**50**(11):1432–1437.
19. Kapur S, Chandra R, Antonovych T. Acute radiation nephritis. Light and electron microscopic observations. *Arch Pathol Lab Med*. 1977;**101**(9):469–473.
20. Lawton CA, Cohen EP, Murray KJ, et al. Long-term results of selective renal shielding in patients undergoing total body irradiation in preparation for bone marrow transplantation. *Bone Marrow Transplant*. 1997;**20**(12):1069–1074.
22. Daugaard G, Rossing N, Rørth M. Effects of cisplatin on different measures of glomerular function in the human kidney with special emphasis on high-dose. *Cancer Chemother Pharmacol*. 1988;**21**(2):163–167.
23. Gonzalez-Vitale JC, Hayes DM, Cvitkovic E, Sternberg SS. The renal pathology in clinical trials of cis-platinum (II) diamminedichloride. *Cancer*. 1977;**39**(4):1362–1371.
25. Berns JS, Ford PA. Renal toxicities of antineoplastic drugs and bone marrow transplantation. *Semin Nephrol*. 1997;**17**(1):54–66.
26. Morgan KP, Buie LW, Savage SW. The role of mannitol as a nephroprotectant in patients receiving cisplatin therapy. *Ann Pharmacother*. 2012;**46**(2):276–281.
27. Santoso JT, Lucci JA, Coleman RL, et al. Saline, mannitol, and furosemide hydration in acute cisplatin nephrotoxicity: a randomized trial. *Cancer Chemother Pharmacol*. 2003;**52**(1):13–18.
28. Gonzalez-Vitale JC, Hayes DM, Cvitkovic E, Sternberg SS. Acute renal failure after cis-dichlorodiammineplatinum(II) and gentamicin-cephalothin therapies. *Cancer Treat Rep*. 1978;**62**(5):693–698.
29. Motwani SS, McMahon GM, Humphreys BD, et al. Development and validation of a risk prediction model for acute kidney injury after the first course of cisplatin. *J Clin Oncol*. 2018;**36**(7):682–688.
30. Howard SC, McCormick J, Pui C-H, et al. Preventing and managing toxicities of high-dose methotrexate. *Oncologist*. 2016;**21**(12):1471–1482.
31. Ramsey LB, Balis FM, O'Brien MM, et al. Consensus guideline for use of glucarpidase in patients with high-dose methotrexate induced acute kidney injury and delayed methotrexate clearance. *Oncologist*. 2018;**23**(1):52–61.
33. Schein P, Kahn R, Gorden P, et al. Streptozotocin for malignant insulinomas and carcinoid tumor: report of eight cases and review of the literature. *Arch Intern Med*. 1973;**132**(4):555–561.
34. Harmon WE, Cohen HJ, Schneeberger EE, Grupe WE. Chronic renal failure in children treated with methyl CCNU. *New Engl J Med*. 1979;**300**(21):1200–1203.
36. El-Ghazal R, Podoltsev N, Marks P, et al. Mitomycin–C-induced thrombotic thrombocytopenic purpura/hemolytic uremic syndrome: cumulative toxicity of an old drug in a new era. *Clin Colorectal Cancer*. 2011;**10**(2):142–145.
37. Hudes G, Carducci M, Tomczak P, et al. Temsirolimus, interferon alfa, or both for advanced renal-cell carcinoma. *New Engl J Med*. 2007;**356**(22):2271–2281.
38. Izzedine H, Boostandoot E, Spano JP, et al. Temsirolimus-induced glomerulopathy. *Oncology*. 2009;**76**(3):170–172.
39. Izzedine H, Escudier B, Rouvier P, et al. Acute tubular necrosis associated with mTOR inhibitor therapy: a real entity biopsy-proven. *Ann Oncol*. 2013;**24**(9):2421–2425.
40. Izzedine H, Rixe O, Billemont B, et al. Angiogenesis inhibitor therapies: focus on kidney toxicity and hypertension. *Am J Kidney Dis*. 2007;**50**(2):203–218.
41. Kaehler KC, Piel S, Livingstone E, et al. Update on immunologic therapy with anti-CTLA-4 antibodies in melanoma: identification of clinical and biological response patterns, immune-related adverse events, and their management. *Semin Oncol*. 2010;**37**(5):485–498.
42. Mamlouk O, Selamet U, Machado S, et al. Nephrotoxicity of immune checkpoint inhibitors beyond tubulointerstitial nephritis: single-center experience. *J Immunother Cancer*. 2019;**7**(1):2.
43. Brahmer JR, Lacchetti C, Schneider BJ, et al. Management of immune-related adverse events in patients treated with immune checkpoint inhibitor therapy: American society of clinical oncology clinical practice guideline. *J Clin Oncol*. 2018;**36**(17):1714–1768.
44. Cortazar FB, Kibbelaar ZA, Glezerman IG, et al. Clinical features and outcomes of immune checkpoint inhibitor-associated AKI: a multicenter study. *J Am Soc Nephrol*. 2020;**31**(2):435.
45. Robert C, Soria JC, Eggermont AM. Drug of the year: programmed death-1 receptor/programmed death-1 ligand-1 receptor monoclonal antibodies. *Eur J Cancer*. 2013;**49**(14):2968–2971.
47. Sprangers B, Abudayyeh A, Latcha S, et al. How to determine kidney function in cancer patients? *Eur J Cancer*. 2020;**132**:141–149.
48. Janowitz T, Williams EH, Marshall A, et al. New model for estimating glomerular filtration rate in patients with cancer. *J Clin Oncol*. 2017;**35**(24):2798–2805.

130 Cardiac complications

Michael S. Ewer, MD, JD, PhD ■ Steven M. Ewer, MD ■ Thomas M. Suter, MD

> **Overview**
>
> Patients with malignant diseases often have coexisting cardiovascular disorders or may face serious cardiovascular complications in the course of their disease.[1] The disorders may result from underlying conditions such as atherosclerosis, hypertension, or valvular abnormalities, or they may result directly from cancer or its treatment (Table 1). In addition, cardiovascular disorders that are unusual in patients not afflicted with cancer may be more common in the cancer patient, and sometimes are unsuspected. Furthermore, cardiovascular diseases common in the general population must not be overlooked in patients with cancer; the presentation of such entities may be unusual, and the diagnosis often is more complex. Increased clinical scrutiny is therefore necessary in this vulnerable population. Multiple clinical problems may also coexist and defy a simple illumination because of the complex interactions between the malignancy, consequences of its treatment, and the status of the cardiovascular system; what affects one of these variables often alters the presentation and course of the others. This article will look at some of the more common cardiovascular complications of cancer and its treatment and will also address some of the dilemmas encountered in cancer patients with concomitant cardiac conditions.

Evaluation of the cardiovascular system in the cancer patient

The importance of a detailed history and a complete physical examination in the evaluation of the cardiovascular system in patients with cancer cannot be overstated. Signs or symptoms suggestive of heart failure, dysrhythmia, ischemia, or pericardial disease—all of which are common in the cancer patient—should trigger a more rigorous cardiovascular assessment. The individual approach should be targeted to include the specific clinical entities that are enumerated in Table 1. If clinical assessment of the patient indicates possible cardiac disease, further evaluation may include chest X-ray and electrocardiogram, which can detect arrhythmias, allow measurement of the QT interval, and aid in evaluation of ischemia or pericardial disease. Additional imaging techniques or invasive modalities such as coronary angiography or electrophysiologic evaluation may be required for specific instances.

The echocardiogram has enjoyed the widest usage in evaluating cancer patients. It plays an important role in evaluating cardiac structure and function, as well as assessing hemodynamics.[2] Transthoracic two-dimensional echocardiography provides a comprehensive structural assessment, including chamber sizes and global and regional function of both ventricles. Localized or loculated pericardial effusions, as well as primary and metastatic tumors, can be appreciated using two-dimensional echocardiography.[3] Where ultrasound images are suboptimal, contrast can be enhanced using perflutren lipid microsphere, an injectable suspension. Contrast agents should be employed generously. However, while generally regarded as safe, rare serious adverse reactions have been reported following perflutren lipid microsphere injection.[4,5]

Spectral and color flow Doppler studies, which are performed routinely as part of a cardiac ultrasound evaluation, show the direction and velocity of blood flow in the cardiac chambers and across the valves. Valvular hemodynamics, intracardiac shunts, turbulent blood flow, and abnormal direction of blood flow are best evaluated using Doppler studies. Doppler studies provide important information regarding diastolic function, an aspect of cardiac physiology that is important in the assessment of patients with suspected heart failure.

Strain (deformation) echocardiography provides quantitative information regarding active and passive repositioning of myocardial segments. Algorithms have been developed to detect acoustic footprints, or speckles, within the myocardial tissue. The distance between speckles is tracked over time within a region of interest in the myocardium and then displayed graphically. Many studies have demonstrated the ability of global longitudinal systolic strain to predict future declines in ejection fraction as well as the development of heart failure during potentially cardiotoxic cancer treatment.[6,7] Many centers now incorporate strain techniques in the assessment of cancer patients; however, the variability of the interpretative algorithms has delayed its broader incorporation into standard practice. Further standardization of the technique should improve evaluation of global and regional left ventricular contractility. These newer techniques improve the predictive value of the ultrasound examination. Their role in the routine management of cancer patients is expanding.

Transesophageal echocardiography provides a higher resolution view of certain cardiac structures than does the transthoracic study. Although the technique is semi-invasive, the increased diagnostic sensitivity of the transesophageal studies often offsets this disadvantage. Transesophageal studies are especially useful in identifying vegetations and other valvular lesions or myocardial involvement of cancer, which may be difficult or impossible to assess on transthoracic studies (Figure 1). The transesophageal study, in part because of the position of the probe, is an important adjunct for the evaluation of posterior accumulations of pericardial fluid, as may be seen postoperatively; they are also of considerable value in defining and monitoring intracardiac masses and thrombi[6] (Figure 2). Intraoperative transesophageal echocardiography is helpful in documenting the extent of a tumor invading the inferior vena cava as well as the result of resection of such tumors[5] (Figure 2). Three-dimensional cardiac ultrasound now is available in many centers and provides enhanced information regarding spatial relationships of intra-cardiac structures including the cardiac valves. The technique allows the two-dimensional image to be rotated around a selected axis, providing perspective and improved spatial orientation.[8]

Holland-Frei Cancer Medicine, Tenth Edition. Edited by Robert C. Bast, John C. Byrd, Carlo M. Croce, Ernest Hawk, Fadlo R. Khuri, Raphael E. Pollock, Apostolia M. Tsimberidou, Christopher G. Willett, and Cheryl L. Willman.
© 2023 John Wiley & Sons, Inc. Published 2023 by John Wiley & Sons, Inc.

Table 1 Important cardiovascular complications of cancer.

- Primary cardiac neoplasia
  - Malignancy
    - Cardiac tumors
    - Pericardial tumors
- Metastatic cancer
  - Pericardial metastasis
    - Pericardial effusion
    - Pericardial tamponade
  - Myocardial metastasis
    - Cardiomyopathy
    - Arrhythmias
      - Tachyarrhythmias
      - Conduction system disease
- Complication of cancer treatment
  - Coronary vasospasm
    - Myocardial infarction
  - Arrhythmias
    - Supraventricular
    - Ventricular
      - QT prolongation
  - Cardiomyopathy
    - Type I dysfunction (irreversible)
      - Chronic heart failure
      - Sudden cardiac death
    - Type II dysfunction (reversible)
    - Disorders of diastolic filling
  - Hypertension
  - Effects of radiation
- Miscellaneous entities
  - Cardiac amyloidosis
  - Carcinoid heart disease
  - Thromboembolic phenomena
  - Pulmonary hypertension
  - Cardiac inflammation

Magnetic resonance imaging (MRI) can delineate intracardiac, pericardial, and great vessel anatomy, and can define intracardiac and pericardial masses.[9] Rapid-acquisition MRI, MR angiography, and contrast-enhanced MRI techniques, while not having usurped cardiac ultrasound, are assuming a broader role in the routine evaluation of cancer patients.[10,11] To some extent, it now can be considered the new gold standard for quantification of ventricular volumes, function, and mass.[12] The cost of MRI remains substantial, and acquisition times are problematic for some patients. Cardiac MRI is increasingly utilized to estimate ejection fractions for patients who cannot be otherwise evaluated. Cardiac computerized tomography is increasingly being used as an imaging modality, and like MRI, allows for excellent visualization of the pericardium and nearby extracardiac structures.

Nuclear imaging techniques provide important information concerning both cardiac function and evaluation of ischemic heart disease. The multi-gated (MUGA) cardiac blood pool scan remains a common assessment tool for following left ventricular ejection fraction in patients being treated with agents known or suspected of being cardiotoxic and continues to be an alternative to echocardiography or MRI in some clinical trials. Nuclear imaging techniques may have a lower intra- and inter-observer variability than do echocardiographic assessments. The technique requires electrocardiographic gating that can be problematic in patients with dysrhythmia; additionally, MUGA scans acquire data over a period of several minutes, and therefore depend on patients being able to remain immobile during acquisition. Once the imaging data is acquired, MUGA provides an estimation of ejection fraction, as well as information regarding wall-motion abnormalities, and parameters of cardiac relaxation (diastolic function). Radiation exposure is a concern and often precludes frequent or sequential measurements. While MUGA scans were previously more widely used, the improvement in cardiac ultrasound imaging and the concerns regarding radiation exposure are providing an impetus toward the wider use of ultrasound in following patients both in and out of clinical trials.[13] Positron emission tomography (PET) has theoretical advantages over more traditional imaging techniques and is increasingly used to evaluate myocardial viability in cancer patients.[14] PET imaging can also assess the metabolic activity of suspicious masses, including cardiac tumors, and help determine the likelihood of malignancy in these cases.

Regardless of the method used, it must be emphasized that the results of any estimation of cardiac function are affected by many noncardiac factors and that alterations in cardiac function for a specific patient must be interpreted with caution. Furthermore, it should be noted that small changes in left ventricular function (LVEF changes of 10 percentage points or less) frequently reflect conditions not associated with the cancer or its treatment but rather by physiological variations in cardiac function or inter-observer variations. False-positive results, that is, a change not related to the consideration under investigation, are an increasingly recognized concern.[15]

Metastatic involvement of cardiac structures

Metastatic involvement of cardiac structures is common and is seen in approximately 8% to 10% of patients with cancer; the incidence is somewhat less in elderly patients.[16] Involvement may constitute an incidental finding at autopsy or may be the initial catastrophic presentation of cancer. There are wide variations among primary disease sites and tumor types. Newer imaging techniques have made it possible to recognize cardiac involvement much earlier than was previously possible, often at a time when intervention can be efficacious. Tumor spread to cardiac structures may be by direct invasion (i.e., lung or esophagus), by retrograde lymphatic spread (i.e., lung, breast), or by hematogenous seeding (i.e., melanoma, leukemia, or lymphoma). In view of the relatively high incidence of lung and breast cancers, these neoplasms are the most common primary sites of metastatic lesions to cardiac structures. Malignant melanoma, once metastatic, is especially likely to involve cardiac structures.[17] While spread to the pericardium is much more common than is spread to other cardiac tissue, metastatic involvement has the potential to involve myocardial and endocardial structures. The heart, therefore, should be included in routine examinations that seek metastatic involvement in patients with Hodgkin and non-Hodgkin lymphomas, leukemias, gastrointestinal and gynecologic cancers (especially ovarian cancer), multiple myeloma, and sarcoma (Figure 2).[18] In addition, renal cell cancer may spread

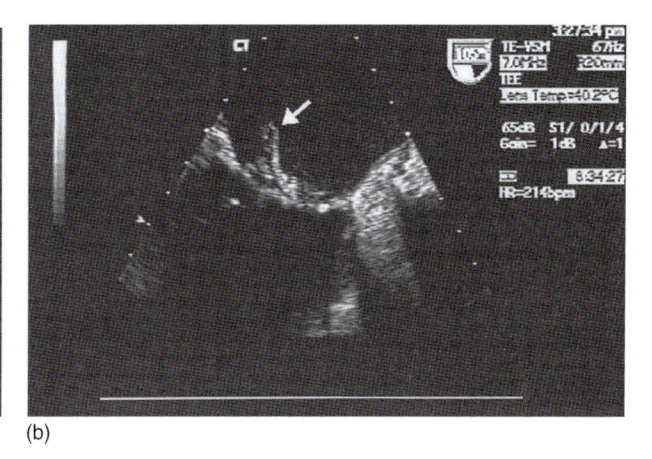

Figure 1 Echocardiogram frames of a patient with infective endocarditis involving the mitral valve. (a) Nonspecific findings often seen on transthoracic studies, although suggestive of thickening of the leaflets, are not diagnostic for the valve infection. (b) Transesophageal image from the same patient recorded the same day, clearly showing the infected mitral valve leaflet.

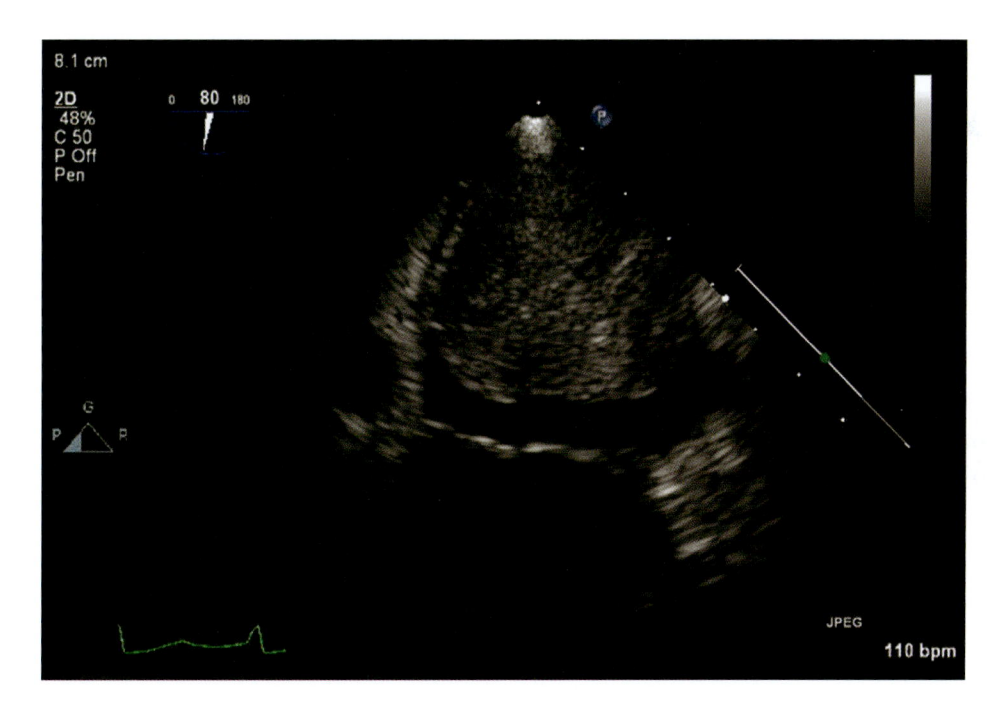

Figure 2 Transesophageal echocardiogram demonstrating a large left atrial mass in a patient who presented with angina. Echocardiographic features were consistent with tumor, and pathology was consistent with a pleomorphic myxoid sarcoma.

to the inferior vena cava and extend into the right atrium and ventricle; these lesions often are amenable to surgical resection.

Pericardial involvement

Pericardial effusion

Pericardial effusion in cancer patients may be malignant or nonmalignant in nature and may be related to the tumor, its treatment, or to underlying cardiac or systemic disease. Malignant pericardial effusion is defined as an effusion associated with pathologic evidence for tumor invasion of the pericardium. A malignant pericardial effusion, however, may still be present even when malignant cells are not demonstrable by routine cytologic examination of the fluid. Pericardial effusion is seen also following radiation, other forms of anticancer treatment, lymphatic obstruction, altered oncotic balance, or infection. Effusions may vary considerably with regard to the quantity of fluid that accumulates, as well as the pressure exerted on the cardiac chambers. The rate of accumulation and the distensibility of the pericardial sac determine the hemodynamic effect and the symptoms of these effusions.[19] As little as 100 mL of fluid may cause symptoms in a patient with a scarred or infiltrated nondistensible parietal pericardium, whereas large effusions containing as much as 1 L may remain relatively indolent when the pericardial sac is elastic and the effusion accumulates gradually. The finding of malignant pericardial effusion generally implies a poorer prognosis.[20]

Generally, pericardial fluid is not static but is in equilibrium with other body fluids. Abnormal fluid build-up occurs when fluid enters the pericardial sac more faster than it can be reabsorbed. This disequilibrium may occur when the efferent lymphatic vessels are obstructed, or when subcarinal lymph node metastases mechanically prevent effective drainage. Malignant effusions are often serosanguinous or frankly bloody and often (but not always) contain cytologically identifiable cancer cells. When chylous effusions are malignant, the most likely cause is lymphoma; chylous effusions also have been reported following radiation for gynecologic malignancy.[21]

The onset of symptoms in patients with malignant pericardial effusion may be insidious. Indeed, many patients with large effusions are totally asymptomatic. Decreased mean electrocardiographic QRS voltage also suggests a pericardial effusion, but other causes of decreased voltage are common in cancer patients, making this finding less useful; a recent drop in voltage should raise suspicion of the presence of pericardial effusion. Pericardial effusions are often first discovered as incidental findings on ultrasound, radionuclide, or other cardiac imaging studies, with the fluid appearing as a relatively inactive area separating the cardiac from the hepatic and pulmonary blood pools. Occasionally, a rocking motion of the heart suggesting hemodynamic compromise (cardiac tamponade) is noted. Computed tomographic (CT) images of the chest also may demonstrate pericardial effusions but are not especially helpful for estimating the fluid volume. Once detected, the diagnosis is usually confirmed by echocardiography and further assessed for hemodynamic significance. Its progression or resolution may be followed with serial studies.[22,23]

Cardiac tamponade

The accumulation of pericardial fluid may lead to an increase in global or localized intrapericardial pressure and compromise cardiac output (cardiac tamponade).[24] Symptoms include dyspnea and exertional intolerance; signs include hypotension, tachycardia, jugular venous distention, hepatomegaly, lower extremity edema, and, as a late manifestation, cardiogenic shock. Heart sounds are often, but not always, distant and difficult to auscultate, and pericardial friction rubs may or may not be present; rubs are often absent in the presence of very large effusions. Vague chest discomfort or fullness is frequently noted. Most patients with significantly increased intrapericardial pressure also demonstrate an exaggeration of the decrease in pulse pressure during inspiration; when the systolic blood pressure decreases more than 10 mmHg with normal inspiration, *pulsus paradoxus* is deemed to be present. A highly characteristic finding of cardiac tamponade is electrical alternans, whereby the electrocardiographic QRS voltage becomes larger and smaller on alternate complexes. This phenomenon is caused by physical movement of the heart toward and away from the electrode as the heart rocks back and forth within the fluid-containing pericardial sac. While electrical alternans is not always seen in cases of cardiac tamponade, when present it is a very helpful finding. Cardiac tamponade can almost always be diagnosed on the basis of physical findings and noninvasive studies. Echocardiography confirms the diagnosis and characterizes the extent, location and may yield important information regarding hemodynamic compromise by the accumulated fluid. Systolic collapse of the right atrium is a sensitive but not specific finding; collapse becomes more specific when it extends for more than one-third of the cardiac cycle. Diastolic collapse of the right ventricular wall becomes more pronounced as hemodynamic compromise progresses and is a much more specific finding. A dilated, incompressible inferior vena cava is uniformly present in the setting of tamponade. Doppler flow studies show exaggerated respiratory variation in aortic outflow and mitral inflow velocities. Cardiac catheterization is usually not required to confirm the diagnosis but may show a graphic representation of pulsus paradoxus, and elevation and equalization of the diastolic pressures in the cardiac chambers ensues as tamponade progresses. With tamponade, the pulse becomes weak or totally absent during inspiration, and patients develop symptoms of low-output cardiogenic shock. Death, sometimes preceded by profound bradycardia, may ensue if tamponade is not resolved promptly.

Management of malignant pericardial effusion and pericardial tamponade

The management of malignant pericardial effusion depends on a number of factors, including the likelihood of the tumor responding to local (surgical, radiotherapeutic, or intracavitary) or systemic anticancer therapy; the extent of and the symptoms attributable to the effusion; and the overall anticipated survival of the patient.[25,26] Patients with tumors highly likely to respond to the systemic therapy may proceed with their treatment; sometimes the malignant effusion resolves in responses to the systemic anticancer therapy alone. Pericardial effusion diagnosed in patients with tumors unresponsive to treatment may require local intervention.

Pericardiocentesis is now almost always undertaken with either echocardiographic or fluoroscopic guidance. Newer instrumentation using smaller penetrating devices and improved imaging techniques have lowered the pericardiocentesis risk.[27] A drain is typically left in place for several days until there is minimal output. Mild inflammation due to the presence of the drainage catheter may encourage adherence of the pericardium to the epicardium and help prevent re-accumulation of fluid. Some patients experience transient left ventricular dysfunction after resolution of cardiac tamponade, and thus a period of careful monitoring is important.[28]

In patients who have a more favorable oncologic prognosis, who have experienced fluid re-accumulation following needle drainage, and who do not have contraindications to general anesthesia and surgery, creation of a pleuropericardial window is effective and may be considered the procedure of choice in some centers. Surgical intervention also allows the removal of pericardial tissue that may provide important prognostic information. Although the transthoracic and the subxiphoid surgical approaches are equally efficacious, in-hospital mortality was significantly greater for patients treated with the subxiphoid approach.[29,30] Using either approach, the communication formed usually remains patent, and the larger surface area available in the pleural space permits more effective reabsorption of the excess fluid. Pericardial needle drainage may be required prior to surgery as a stabilizing measure in patients who have very large effusions or evolving tamponade. Symptoms often resolve dramatically after removal of fluid, allowing patients to once again engage in activities that had become impossible.

The advantages of the pericardial window over percutaneous pericardiocentesis have not been fully evaluated, but some studies suggest little advantage to the more invasive pericardial window procedure. The advisability of routine drainage of large pericardial effusions in patients without tamponade has also been questioned; Merce et al.[31] point out the low diagnostic yield and the lack of therapeutic benefit. The clinical management of such patients should be determined by their overall performance status, oncologic prognosis, and by the expertise available at the treatment center.

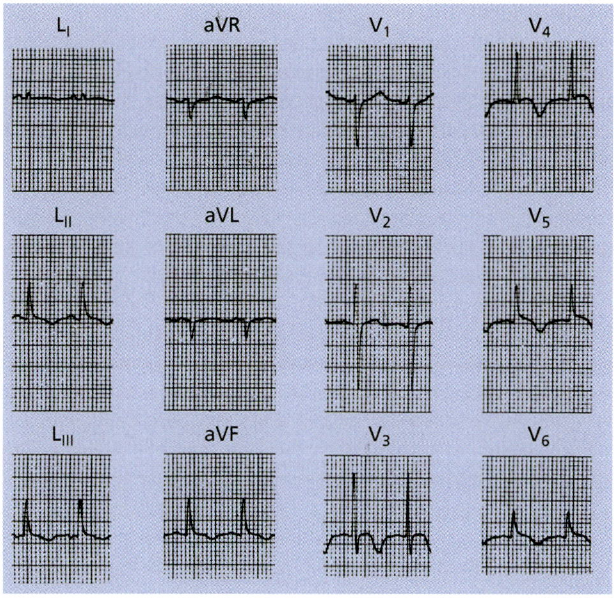

Figure 3 Electrocardiogram suggesting ischemia in a 26-year-old man with documented (by magnetic resonance imaging) myocardial metastatic disease and no history to suggest other causes of the electrocardiographic abnormality. Note T-wave inversions in the inferior leads (LII, LIII, and aVF) as well as in the precordial leads (V4–V6).

Sclerosis was previously undertaken following pericardiocentesis, and a variety of agents, including hyperosmolar glucose, radioactive gold, bleomycin, sterile talc, doxycycline, and triethylenethiophosphoramide (thio-TEPA®) have been studied.[32,33] Doxycycline in particular has received considerable attention as an effective sclerosing agent.[34] Sclerosis is now utilized less frequently and been supplanted by the techniques described above.[35] Balloon pericardiotomy has been largely replaced by surgical pericardiotomy, an intervention that can often be accomplished with minimal invasion and acceptable risk.[36]

Metastatic involvement of the myocardium

The spread of malignant tumors to the myocardium is being increasingly recognized in vivo through the broader use of imaging studies. Many patients with metastatic disease to the myocardium also have evidence of concomitant pericardial involvement. The most dramatic manifestation of myocardial metastatic disease is dysrhythmia that may occur with little or no warning.[37,38] Sudden cardiac death can occur in this setting but is unusual. Cardiac perforation and erosion of the coronary vessels with hemorrhage or infarction may also occur but are exceedingly rare. More commonly, patients with myocardial involvement demonstrate signs of loss of functioning muscle mass and present with progressive shortness of breath or exercise intolerance; a decreased ejection fraction may be seen. The electrocardiographic representation of loss of electrical potential can be seen and may be indistinguishable from changes typically encountered with myocardial infarction due to coronary occlusion (Figure 3). ST segment elevations, T-wave inversions, or Q waves may be seen in such cases, even when the coronary arteries are normal angiographically.[39]

Even with modern imaging techniques, the diagnosis of metastatic involvement of the myocardium may be challenging. A high suspicion may prompt special imaging, and MRI studies may be helpful in determining the presence and extent of metastatic myocardial disease. Although treatment of metastatic disease to the myocardium often is supportive, large lesions or those with impending valvular obstruction should be considered for surgical removal.[40,41]

Cardiac effects of mediator release, high output states, and infiltrative disorders in cancer patients

Metabolically active mediators commonly are associated with some forms of neoplastic diseases and frequently are the immediate cause of a patient's presenting signs and symptoms.[42,43] Such mediator-associated diseases, or paraneoplastic syndromes, may have a direct or indirect effect on the cardiovascular system.

Carcinoid heart disease

Carcinoid tumors arise from enterochromaffin cell-derived neuroendocrine tissue, most commonly in the gut or lungs; oncologic considerations regarding these tumors are considered elsewhere in this text. Carcinoid heart disease results from prolonged release of biologically active mediators from tumor cells that stimulate the formation of a distinctive fibromuscular plaque that destroys the integrity of the cardiac valves.[43–48] The exact mechanism of plaque formation and cardiac injury remains elusive, but a number of possible mediators, most importantly serotonin, but kinins, 5-hydroxytryptophan, histamine, and prostaglandins, have been suggested; other as yet unidentified compounds or combination of compounds may also be involved.[49] These mediators can be cleared by the liver or the lungs. Carcinoid heart disease is seen most commonly in patients who have ileocecal carcinoid tumors that have metastasized to the liver. Rarely, it occurs in patients with bronchial or ovarian carcinoid tumors, and, if blood from the carcinoid drains outside the confines of the portal venous system, carcinoid heart disease may develop in the absence of hepatic metastases.

Mediator release into the hepatic vein from metastatic liver disease predisposes patients to right-sided cardiac lesions. Because these mediators are eliminated by the lungs, the left heart is spared unless a right-to-left shunt or lung metastases are present. The lesions generally appear along the intima of the great veins, the right atrium, and the coronary sinus. The margins and distal (ventricular or downstream) aspect of the tricuspid leaflets are often thickened, and the chordae tendineae may also be involved. The pulmonic valve may be thickened and retracted. The damage appears to be aggravated by turbulent blood flow, which explains the characteristic location of the lesions. When the primary tumor or metastasis is in the lung, the mediators are released directly into the pulmonary venous bed and bypass the inactivating properties of lung tissue; left-sided valvular lesions are seen in such cases.[50] Left-sided lesions are less frequent than right-sided ones but are more likely to result in hemodynamic compromise. A review of surgically excised valves noted considerable variation in the histological appearance of the material.[51–53]

The most important consequence of carcinoid plaques is thickening and fibrosis of the valves with resultant distortion of the valvular apparatus and ring. Tricuspid regurgitation is the primary valve lesion, but pulmonic regurgitation is frequently present as well. Some degree of stenosis may be present earlier in the disease process but is not usually hemodynamically compromising. Right heart failure with elevated central venous pressure and superimposed large V wave from tricuspid regurgitation contribute to the jugular venous distention commonly seen in patients with the carcinoid heart disease. A high-output state, probably due to mediator release, has also been described.[54]

The clinical manifestations of carcinoid heart disease vary considerably. Some patients are able to tolerate the hemodynamic consequences of their valvular lesions well, whereas others develop symptoms early; this is especially so in the elderly or those with predisposing cardiac abnormalities.[55] Early symptoms include fatigue, dyspnea on exertion, and palpitations due to either a high-output state, dysrhythmias, or to both. Later, symptoms of right-sided congestive heart failure, including edema, hepatomegaly, and ascites, predominate. Cardiac murmurs often predate symptoms, and the murmur of tricuspid regurgitation may be an early finding. Most frequently the murmur is appreciated as a loud, holosystolic, blowing sound heard along the left lower sternal border. The murmur may be augmented during inspiration. The murmur of pulmonic stenosis cannot always be distinguished from that of the often-coexisting tricuspid regurgitation; when heard, the pulmonic murmur is usually harsher and is appreciated most prominently in the second left intercostal space.

The chest radiograph may reveal prominence of the right ventricle. Unlike congenital pulmonic stenosis, which often includes poststenotic dilatation of the pulmonary trunk, this finding is usually not seen in carcinoid heart disease. Electrocardiographic findings include changes suggestive of right ventricular volume or pressure overload with or without right atrial abnormalities, right ventricular hypertrophy, right bundle-branch block, and/or right axis deviation; low voltage in the standard (limb) leads may also be seen.

Echocardiography is the most useful noninvasive tool for diagnosing carcinoid heart disease (Figure 4). It not only identifies the valvular abnormality but when coupled with Doppler ultrasonography studies, also provides hemodynamic data for estimating the degree of valvular involvement.[56] Along with the thickening and loss of mobility of the tricuspid leaflets, increased flow velocity across the tricuspid valve during diastole is often evident. A regurgitant jet can be seen in the right atrium during systole. Furthermore, echocardiography can quantify the right atrial and ventricular enlargement that is characteristic of this condition. When of sufficient size, echocardiography is helpful in recognizing metastatic carcinoid tumors that involve the heart.[57]

The management of patients with carcinoid heart disease must be individualized and is often challenging. Although the carcinoid plaque is largely irreversible, controlling or eliminating the offending mediators can delay plaque progression. In this respect, treatment of the primary tumor or metastatic disease is crucial. Once the diagnosis is established, carcinoid heart disease is initially managed pharmacologically with diuretics, afterload reduction, and salt restriction. Surgical intervention in the form of valve replacement is being considered more frequently than heretofore and with improved outcome; some suggest early intervention, as long as the malignancy is under optimal or at least sufficient control.[58]

High-output states and high-output cardiac failure

Increased cardiac output occurs in many cancer patients and is most commonly due to anemia, hyperthyroidism, the syndrome of inappropriate antidiuretic hormone secretion, or the shunting of blood through tumors. High-output states are relatively common in patients with multiple myeloma.[59] Additionally, liver disease (nutritional cirrhosis or infectious hepatitis), fever, emotional excitement, and hypoxemia are also common causes of increased cardiac output and hyperdynamic states. High-output states are seen as well following treatment with a number of biologic response modifiers, including the interferons (possibly related to fever and the influenza-like reaction) and interleukins, in which case the phenomenon usually is of short duration.

High-output states are associated with a moderately increased heart rate (usually 85–110 beats per minute, but sometimes higher) and with increased stroke volume. Physical examination typically reveals neck veins of normal appearance as right-sided pressures are generally not increased. Peripheral pulses, however, are often bounding and have a rapid upstroke and fall; systolic blood pressure is elevated, and diastolic blood pressure often is reduced. Auscultation may reveal a systolic murmur and demonstrate a presystolic (S4) gallop. Pulmonary congestion is not uncommon in severe hyperdynamic states.

Treatment-related high-output states may also result in myocardial ischemia in patients with fixed atherosclerotic lesions that preclude increasing the blood supply because the vessels cannot dilate, a phenomenon known as "coronary steal." The interferons are especially likely to initiate ischemia in this manner. Ischemia may also result from fever, often produced by biologic modifying agents, and from hyperthyroidism. Tumor necrosis factor has been associated with a hypercoagulable state, which suggests vascular occlusion as a possible alternative explanation for the ischemia that occurs in patients being treated with cytokines and other biologic response modifiers. Anemia is an important coexisting factor, as any cause of ischemia can be exacerbated by a diminished oxygen-carrying capacity.

Echocardiography or radionuclide imaging is helpful in establishing the diagnosis. Two-dimensional studies show increased wall motion in all views. In extreme cases, the images appear to suggest an almost total obliteration of the left ventricular cavity during systole; the ejection fraction is increased. Doppler examination reveals uniformly increased flow across all four valves. MUGA scans may also offer important data concerning the left ventricular ejection fraction and cardiac output. Right heart catheterization with the measurement of cardiac output confirms the diagnosis. It is important not to confuse this clinical picture with that of the more commonly encountered low-output congestive heart failure, with which it shares a number of characteristics. The treatment of high-output states should be directed toward the underlying cause; in the cancer patient metastatic disease with or without shunting, hyperthyroidism, hypoxia, anemia, and infection are the most common considerations. High-output states often respond to blood transfusion, diuretics, oxygen administration, or antipyretics. In selected cases, β-adrenergic blockers may be useful. Unless patients are symptomatic, the high-output state does not require specific therapy.

Cardiac amyloidosis

Amyloidosis, or the deposition of amyloid proteins, may occur in a variety of organs including the heart and may be caused by a number of pathologic processes.[60] Amyloid proteins are made up of fibrils consisting of antiparallel beta-pleated sheets that deposit in the interstitial spaces and are resistant to proteolysis. They are formed from a wide variety of precursor proteins.[61] Clinically significant cancer-related amyloidosis is encountered in patients with multiple myeloma and, rarely, in patients with Hodgkin lymphoma. The amyloid protein associated with these diseases is known as AL amyloid and is derived from light chain immunoglobulin (both Igλ and Igκ). AL amyloid accumulates in the atrial and ventricular myocardium and leads to either a restrictive or less commonly a dilated cardiomyopathy. Endocardial deposition resulting in valvular abnormalities has also been described.

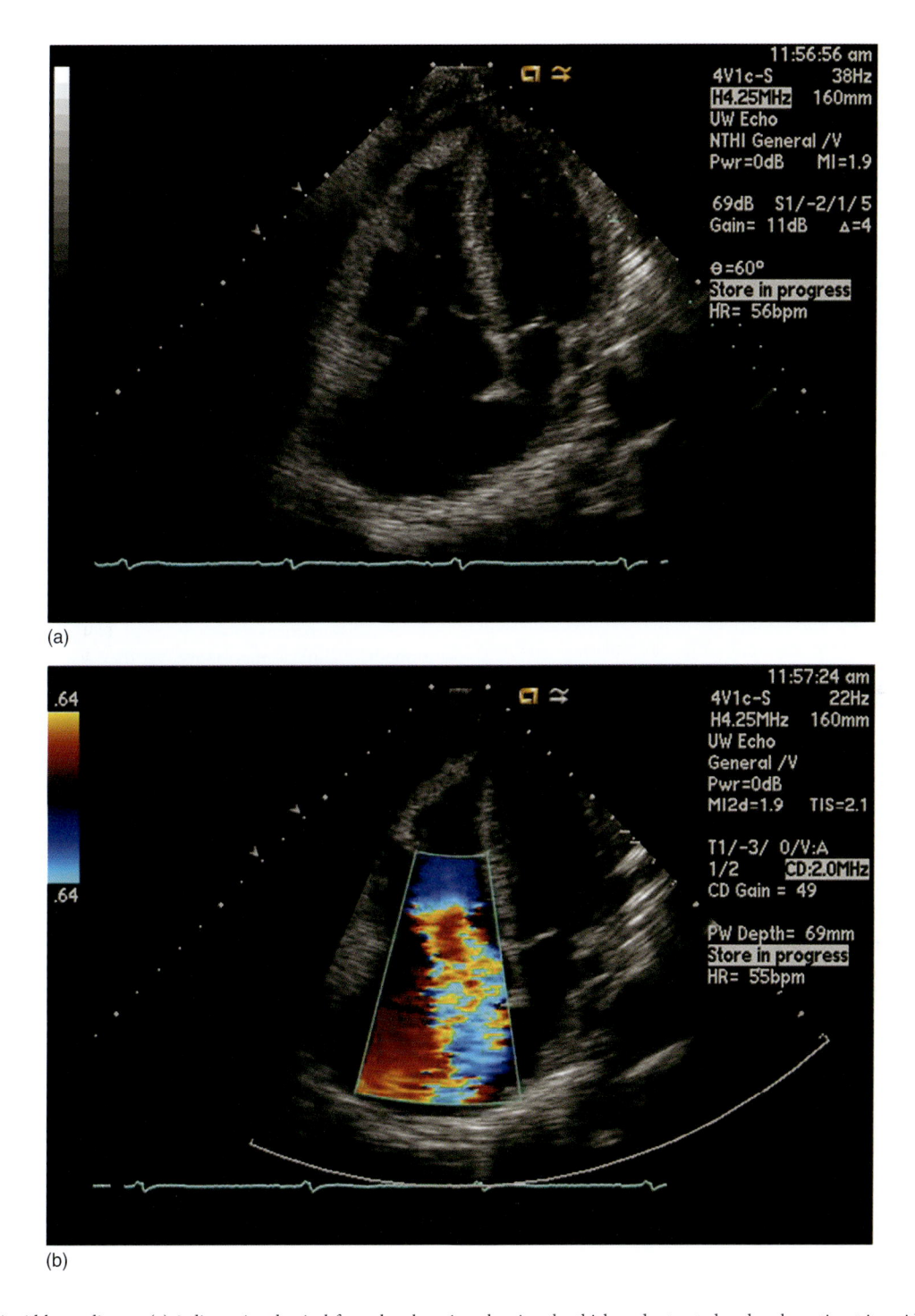

Figure 4 Carcinoid heart disease: (a) 2-dimensional apical four-chamber view showing the thickened retracted and malcoapting tricuspid valve leaflets. (b) image from the same study with color-flow Doppler views showing severe tricuspid regurgitation. Also evident is right atrial and right ventricular chamber enlargement and a small pericardial effusion.

Clinically, patients with cardiac amyloidosis experience fatigue and show signs of decreased cardiac output. Dyspnea and edema are common symptoms, and anorexia, weight loss, and presyncope are also encountered. In addition to heart failure, atrial or ventricular dysrhythmias or cardioembolic events are reported. Physical exam findings include elevated jugular venous pressure, edema, hepatic congestion, ascites, hypotension, macroglossia, and periorbital purpura. Conduction abnormalities are seen and, when associated with low effective heart rates or low-output states, may be symptomatic; stress-precipitated syncope may be a precursor of sudden cardiac death.[62,63] Both systolic and diastolic function may be impaired. Restrictive cardiomyopathy can be difficult to distinguish from constrictive pericarditis clinically; even findings at cardiac catheterization are not always conclusive in establishing the correct diagnosis. The chest radiograph shows a normal-sized or slightly enlarged cardiac silhouette. When cardiac failure appears, pulmonary congestion or pleural effusion may be seen. Electrocardiographic findings can include decreased voltage, a pseudo-infarction pattern, conduction system abnormalities, and atrial arrhythmias.[64] The echocardiogram is often helpful in

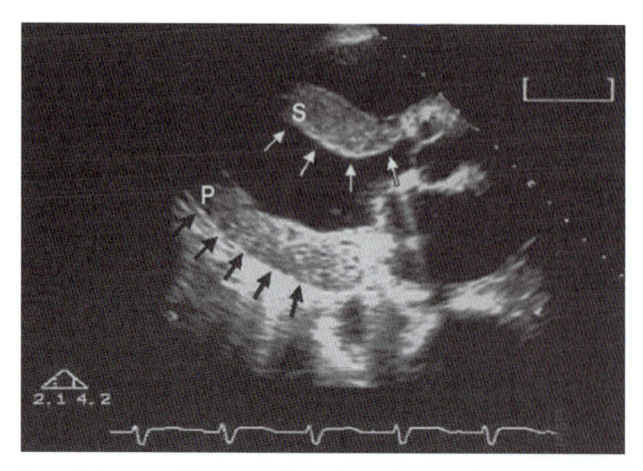

Figure 5 Parasternal long-axis echocardiographic view from a patient with cardiac amyloid infiltration. Note thickened septum (S) and posterior wall (P) with stippled appearance (arrows).

suggesting the diagnosis of amyloidosis (Figure 5). Ultrasonic images may demonstrate a thickened septum and posterior wall with normal internal dimensions of the left ventricle; diastolic function is significantly impaired. Atria are enlarged and may show markedly reduced mechanical function, even in the absence of atrial dysrhythmias. The paradox of increased left ventricular wall thickness on cardiac ultrasound with decreased electrocardiographic voltage should suggest cardiac amyloidosis.[65] Antimyosin scintigraphy, showing left ventricular thickening and diffuse myocardial antimyosin uptake, has been reported to be highly suggestive of amyloid heart disease. Cardiac MRI may be a useful adjunct in diagnosing amyloid infiltration, as a characteristic pattern of late gadolinium enhancement helps distinguish amyloid heart disease from other cardiomyopathies.[66]

Cardiac catheterization demonstrates elevated intracardiac pressures in all chambers, with the minimum left ventricular pressure often increased to at least 10 mm Hg. The "dip and plateau" pattern seen on intraventricular pressure tracings in patients with constrictive pericarditis may be absent. Prominent papillary muscles are demonstrated with angiography. Endomyocardial biopsy with specimens stained with Congo red may be helpful in establishing the diagnosis.[67]

The therapeutic interventions for cardiac amyloidosis are limited. Loop diuretics serve as the mainstay of medical treatment. Cardiac glycosides are dangerous in that they contribute to dysrhythmias; sudden death has been reported following their use.[68] Beta-blockers and nondihydropyridine calcium channel blockers can exacerbate a low cardiac output state and angiotensin-converting enzyme (ACE) inhibitors can precipitate profound hypotension. In instances where malignant dysrhythmia is triggered, implantable defibrillators have been offered, but patient selection and criteria for implantation for such devices have not yet been clearly established.[69] Clinical improvement may parallel control of the underlying process in patients with reactive forms of amyloidosis, and systemic treatment of myeloma may delay or alleviate the symptoms of myeloma-related cardiac amyloidosis.[70] Intracardiac thrombosis is a significant risk in patients with amyloid infiltration. In one autopsy series, thrombosis was encountered in 33% of patients coming to autopsy. Anticoagulation in the presence of significant cardiac amyloidosis has been suggested. Therapy with a number of antineoplastic agents, including melphalan, cyclophosphamide, carmustine, and vincristine, have been attempted, as has hematopoietic stem cell transplantation.[71] Restrictive cardiomyopathy due to light-chain deposition disease may, in rare cases, be reversible. Cardiac transplantation followed by autologous hematopoietic stem cell transplant has been successfully performed in selected patients.[72]

Cardiac dysrhythmia in the cancer patient

Cardiac rhythm disturbances are common in cancer patients. Dysrhythmias may be caused by tumor invasion, but more often they are a consequence of anticancer treatment, the result of metabolic abnormalities, or from stress in a patient with reduced dysrhythmic threshold associated with underlying heart disease. The rhythm disturbances seen in cancer patients are morphologically and functionally identical to those seen in patients without malignancy. In some settings, it is essential to suppress a cardiac dysrhythmia vigorously, whereas in others, rhythm disturbances may be a transient manifestation of a temporary disturbance in homeostasis requiring little or no intervention. Many antineoplastic agents are associated with transient dysrhythmia, and because such rhythm disturbances are often asymptomatic the phenomenon is not fully appreciated. Such chemotherapy-related rhythm disturbances generally are of short duration and of little immediate clinical importance, yet they may be an indication of actual myocardial involvement that may become overtly manifest only at a later time. When associated with cancer treatment, most instances of dysrhythmia do not constitute an absolute indication to alter the chemotherapeutic regimen.

When faced with clinical decisions regarding which patients to treat, at what point in their management to initiate therapy, how long to continue treatment, and what form of therapy (pharmacologic or electrical) to use have been the focus of considerable debate. The wide assortment of antiarrhythmic drugs has not simplified these decisions. One useful approach is to distinguish dysrhythmias resulting from toxic substances or other metabolic abnormalities from those associated with structural abnormalities directly related to cardiac structures.[37]

Categories of dysrhythmia: primary (structural) versus secondary (metabolic)

The structural abnormalities within the heart that can result in cardiac abnormalities encompass a broad group of cardiac disorders. Ischemic heart disease, muscle hypertrophy, valvular disease, and infiltrative processes all fall within this group of disturbances. In cancer patients, tumor infiltration, cell loss following chemotherapy, pharmacologically induced ischemia, and fibrosis following radiation should also be included. Severe dysrhythmias, both supraventricular and ventricular, may appear with little warning and progress to hemodynamic instability and sudden cardiac death. Sudden death is more common in the presence of infiltrative processes such as amyloidosis.

Dysrhythmias in cancer patients also may be the result of nonstructural abnormalities. Most commonly these include alterations in volume status, electrolyte disturbances, drug effects, and hormonal alterations, but other metabolic abnormalities that affect cardiac pacemaker and conduction tissue should also be considered.

Treatment of cardiac rhythm disturbances

Acute rhythm disturbances that result from metabolic abnormalities and that are not life-threatening may be managed conservatively; in such cases, careful observation during treatment

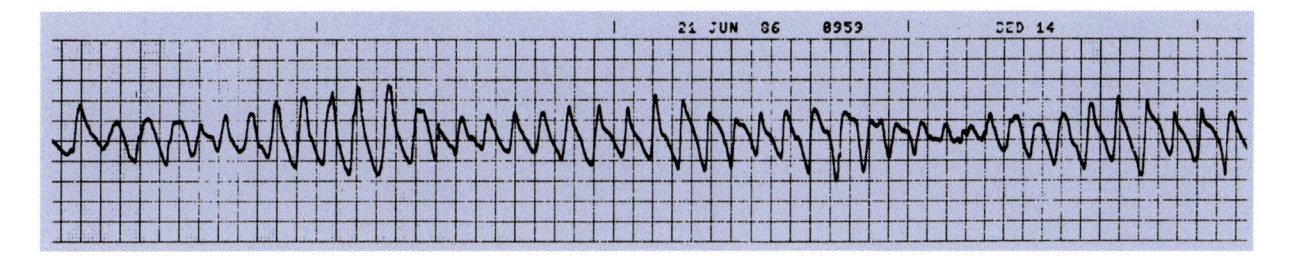

Figure 6 Rhythm strip of a patient with episodes of *torsades de pointes*. A previous rhythm strip (not shown) demonstrated prolongation of the QT interval.

of the underlying abnormality may suffice. Active intervention is required when the dysrhythmia results in significant hemodynamic embarrassment, when the rhythm disturbance is likely to progress and become life threatening, or when a protracted rhythm disturbance is of the type that results in an increased likelihood of a thromboembolic event. Ventricular ectopy is seen commonly and ranges from isolated ventricular extrasystoles and benign accelerated idioventricular rhythm to malignant forms such as ventricular tachycardia or fibrillation. Coexisting conditions, such as fever or debilitation, which may augment tissue hypoxia, especially in anemic patients, predispose patients to ventricular ectopy. Unexpected death in cancer patients is usually attributed to dysrhythmia. Hemodynamic instability, regardless of the underlying cause, constitutes a medical emergency requiring the use of advanced cardiac life-support protocols.

Once the decision has been made to treat a patient experiencing dysrhythmia, the choice between pharmacologic intervention or the use of internal nonpharmacologic therapy such as implantable pacemakers or defibrillators, or the use of ablation therapy, generally follows the usual guidelines for these therapies. In difficult cases, electrophysiologic studies or pharmacologic threshold analysis may be useful. Implantable devices increasingly are being used in cancer patients; malignant disease *per se* should not be considered a barrier to their use but should be balanced with the patient's prognosis.

While much attention has been given to ventricular dysrhythmia, the supraventricular dysrhythmia associated with the Bruton tyrosine kinase inhibitor ibrutinib is of special interest. Atrial fibrillation following ibrutinib administration has been reported in 6–16% of treated patients and is more prevalent in older patients and those with a prior history of atrial fibrillation. Although ibrutinib is associated with an increased risk of bleeding, most patients who develop atrial fibrillation on ibrutinib can tolerate direct oral anticoagulants; some have suggested avoiding antiplatelet agents.[73]

Considerable interest has surrounded the possible cardiac effects of paclitaxel. In one study, asymptomatic bradycardia occurred in 29% of patients treated with maximally tolerated doses of paclitaxel. More severe rhythm abnormalities have also been reported, but they usually are seen in patients with underlying cardiac abnormalities or in the presence of electrolyte imbalance.[74] Serious cardiac problems are rare with paclitaxel, and most patients can be treated without special monitoring. Hypersensitivity reactions are also known to occur.

An ever-increasing number of drugs are being implicated in causing prolongation of the QT interval on the standard electrocardiogram. QT prolongation is associated with ventricular dysrhythmia, which can evolve into a well-recognized variant form of ventricular tachycardia known as *torsades de pointes* (Figure 6). This form of ventricular dysrhythmia is also associated with some antibiotics (erythromycin, clarithromycin, and pentamidine), psychotropic drugs (haloperidol), antiemetics, some forms of high-dose chemotherapy, and bone marrow transplantation.[75,76] Arsenic trioxide, which is most commonly used in the treatment of acute promyelocytic leukemia, also prolongs the QT interval, and patients should be observed carefully for QT prolongation during treatment with this agent.[77,78] Prompt recognition of this potentially malignant dysrhythmia and withdrawal of the offending agent may be the most appropriate therapy. QT prolongation has been reported to be more frequent in male patients as well as in those with hypokalemia. Serial monitoring of the QT interval is advised in high-risk individuals.[79] Table 2 lists the most important agents associated with QT prolongation.

Emergent intervention for unstable patients with *torsades de pointes* may be life-saving and consists of nonsynchronized electrical defibrillation. First-line medical management in a less urgent setting includes intravenous magnesium sulfate, regardless of the serum magnesium level. Isoproterenol infusion or overdrive pacing can suppress *torsades de pointes* by increasing the heart rate and thus shortening the QT interval. Lidocaine and phenytoin are additional treatment options.[80,81] Maintenance of potassium and magnesium homeostasis is crucial in preventing recurrences of this dysrhythmia. The offending QT-prolonging agent should be identified and discontinued, and other potential QT-prolonging drugs carefully avoided.

Table 2 Marketed drugs associated with QT prolongation and known risk of *torsades de pointes*.[a]

Aclarubicin	Hydroquinidine
Amiodarone	Hydroxychloroquine
Anagrelide	Ibogaine
Arsenic trioxide	Ibutilide
Azithromycin	Levofloxacin
Bepridil	Levomepromazine
Cesium Chloride	Levosulpiride
Chloroquine	Methadone
Chlorpromazine	Moxifloxacin
Chlorprothixene	Nifekalant
Cilostazol	Ondansetron
Ciprofloxacin	Oxaliplatin
Citalopram	Papaverine
Clarithromycin	Pentamidine
Cocaine	Pimozide
Disopyramide	Procainamide
Dofetilide	Propofol
Domperidone	Quinidine
Donepezil	Roxithromycin
Dronedarone	Sevoflurane
Droperidol	Sotalol
Erythromycin	Sulpiride
Escitalopram	Sultopride
Flecainide	Terlipressin
Fluconazole	Terodiline
Halofantrine	Thioridazine
Haloperidol	Vandetanib

[a] Adapted from the Arizona Center for Education and Research on Therapeutics. Reference: https://crediblemeds.org/ (accessed 1 July 2020).

Cardiac complications of cancer treatment

Nonsurgical therapies used to treat patients with cancer can impact the heart in a variety of ways. These therapies consist of chemical and biological agents as well as physical agents such as ionizing radiation (Table 3). Individual modalities and combinations may act independently, additively, or synergistically; for example, the combination of cardiac irradiation and anthracyclines produces additive or synergistic toxicity. Damage resulting from cancer treatment may affect the pericardium, the myocardium, the vasculature, the conduction system, and the heart valves. With some modalities, the heart may incur subclinical damage at the time of exposure; later insults or sequential stress may then trigger clinically relevant cardiac dysfunction in the patient with compromised reserve.[82]

Cardiotoxic anticancer agents

Cardiotoxic anticancer agents may cause permanent or temporary contractile dysfunction, ischemia, rhythm disturbances, and fluctuation in blood pressure. The discussion will review the subject of specific cardiotoxic anticancer agents according to this classification.

Agents associated with left ventricular dysfunction

Anthracyclines and their related anthraquinones are the most widely studied agents associated with contractile dysfunction, but other agents may affect cardiac function through different mechanisms. From a functional standpoint, anticancer agents can be divided into two types, Type I and Type II, according to a number of characteristics.[83] Type I agents are associated with primary or direct myocyte cellular injury that progresses to cell death with ongoing exposure or stress. Cardiac damage at the cellular level, once it has progressed beyond the threshold of cell death, is permanent. Type I drugs cause damage that is cumulative and dose-related and is associated with typical endomyocardial biopsy changes. Agents associated with Type II treatment-related cardiac dysfunction may cause myocyte dysfunction that resembles hibernation or stunning, and is therefore more likely to be reversible. Additionally they may contribute to injurious increases in wall stress through other mechanisms such as increased afterload or fluid retention that may compromise vulnerable myocytes, resulting in cell death that can be established or quantified by elevations in cardiac biomarkers. Type II agents do not demonstrate toxicity that is cumulative or dose-related and they are not associated with the typical endomyocardial biopsy changes that are seen with anthracyclines.[81] These differences are summarized in Table 4.

Type I anticancer treatment-related agents: anthracyclines and related agents

The effects of anthracyclines on the heart have been the most extensively studied of all of the cardiotoxic agents; doxorubicin cardiotoxicity serves as a model for understanding anthracycline-associated and related Type I cardiomyopathies.

Doxorubicin cardiotoxicity may be recognized early or late during a course of treatment, or it may present months or even years after the completion of treatment. Early manifestations of toxicity include electrocardiographic abnormalities and elevated cardiac biomarkers; myopericarditis is sometimes seen. Significant early cardiac dysfunction is rare with current dosing regimens, but cases of heart failure occurring within weeks of the first administration of the drug have been reported.[84,85] Early toxicity is more likely to occur in elderly patients or in patients who have received large single doses and has been reported more commonly in patients

Table 3 Anticancer agents associated with cardiotoxicity.[a]

I) Drugs associated with myocardial depression
  a. Anthracyclines and Type I agents
    i. Doxorubicin
    ii. THP Adriamycin
    iii. Idarubicin
    iv. Epirubicin
    v. Daunorubicin
  b. Other anthraquinones
    i. Mitoxantrone
  c. Potential toxicity intensifiers
    i. Cyclophosphamide
    ii. Ifosfamide
    iii. Mitomycin c
    iv. Etoposide
    v. Melphalan
    vi. Vincristine
    vii. Bleomycin
    viii. Paclitaxel
  d. Toxicity inhibitors
    i. Dexrazoxane (Zinocard, ICRF-187)
  e. Type II agents and other drugs associated with myocardial depression
    i. Trastuzumab
    ii. Lapatinib
    iii. Sunitinib
    iv. Imatinib
    v. Antibodies/tyrosine kinase inhibitors
  f. Other cardiodepressant agents
    i. Cyclophosphamide (high dose)
    ii. α-Interferon
II) Antineoplastic agents associated with ischemia
    i. 5-Fluorouracil (5-FU)
    ii. Capecitabine
    iii. Vinblastine
    iv. Vincristine
    v. Bleomycin
    vi. Cisplatin
    vii. Biological response modifiers
III) Antineoplastic agents associated with inflammation
  a. Checkpoint inhibitors
    i. Nivolumab
    ii. Ipilimumab
    iii. Pembrolizumab
    iv. Avelumab
    v. Durvalumab
    vi. Cemiplimab
IV) Antineoplastic agents associated with hypertension
    i. Bevacizumab
    ii. Sunitinib
V) Antineoplastic agents associated with pulmonary hypertension
    i. Dasatinib
VI) Miscellaneous agents with known or suspected cardiac toxicity
    i. Radiation
    ii. Paclitaxel (associated with bradycardia)
    iii. Ibrutinib (atrial fibrillation)
    iv. Arsenic trioxide (prolonged QT interval/torsades de pointes)
    v. Bleomycin actinomycin D
    vi. Mitomycin C
VII) Alkylating agents (cyclophosphamide, Ifosfamide)

[a]This timeliness of the information contained in this table is limited in that the pharmacologic spectrum of agents with suspected or demonstrated cardiotoxicity is expanding rapidly.

Table 4 Type I and Type II treatment-related cardiac dysfunction.

Type I (Primary) (e.g., Doxorubicin)	Type II (Secondary) (e.g., Trastuzumab)
Cellular death	Cellular dysfunction
Damage starts with the first administration	
Biopsy changes (typical of anthracyclines)	No typical anthracycline-like biopsy changes
Cumulative dose-related	Not cumulative dose related
Permanent damage (myocyte death; bad prognosis)	Predominantly reversible (myocyte dysfunction; good prognosis)
Risk factors:	Risk factors:
Combination CT	Prior/concomitant anthracyclines of paclitaxel
Prior/concomitant RT	
Age	Age
Previous cardiac disease	Previous cardiac disease
Hypertension	Obesity (BMI >25 kg/m^2)

Abbreviations: CT, chemotherapy; RT, radiation therapy; BMI, body mass index.

treated with doxorubicin than with daunorubicin.[86] Sudden death following doxorubicin administration also has been reported but is rare. Both ventricular and supraventricular cardiac dysrhythmias may be seen during the administration of doxorubicin but are seldom life-threatening. It is now believed that these phenomena are manifestations of cell injury and death associated with anthracyclines. This is supported by the finding that markers of acute cardiac damage such as troponin T are increased following exposure.[87] Early manifestations, therefore, may be more important than had heretofore been appreciated and troponin release following administration is an important marker and quantifier of early cell death. Early elevation of troponin has also been shown to predict subsequent development of left ventricular dysfunction; higher levels of troponin imply greater injury at the time of exposure, and therefore correlate with diminished reserve that increases risk for subsequent cardiac dysfunction.[88] The initial damage marks the beginning of an ongoing process that may go largely unrecognized in view of the vast ability of the heart to compensate for myocyte loss, and our inability to measure small changes in myocardial reserves with the usually utilized parameter of ejection fraction.[89]

The cumulative dose of anthracycline has been correlated with risk of clinically significant heart failure. Overt clinical manifestations are unusual when the cumulative dose is below 400 mg/m^2, but the risk becomes greater as the cumulative dose exceeds 450 mg/m^2 administered by the usual rapid-infusion schedule.[90] Cardiomyopathy may occur at lower doses when other cardiotoxic drugs are administered concomitantly (see later discussion). Considerable inter-patient variability exists that often cannot be explained by the known risk modifiers of prior cardiac injury or conditions known to increase susceptibility to injury, and genetic differences may play a role—a subject of ongoing interest and research. It follows that if cardiac decompensation occurs early, that is, less than 4 weeks from the last doxorubicin administration, it is much more likely to be serious or have a fatal outcome. Patients who experience early toxicity probably have had more severe initial damage, less baseline cardiac reserves, or a combination of these factors. Doxorubicin cardiomyopathy may become manifest months, and even years, after an uncomplicated course of chemotherapy at or near the usual maximum recommended dose. Sequential stress or injury may explain some of the cases heretofore thought of as late cardiotoxicity. As the anthracyclines have been in use for more than 50 years, some of the patients cured of leukemias, lymphomas, sarcomas, and breast cancer may harbor subclinical cardiac damage that now makes them particularly prone to symptomatic heart failure in the event of additional cardiac insult. The effect of doxorubicin exposure on the genesis of coronary artery disease, myocardial infarction, and other cardiac injuries that occur with aging is unknown. In one older review, 12 of 43 patients with doxorubicin-induced cardiomyopathy died due to progressive cardiac dysfunction.[91] The diminished cardiac reserve in patients who have experienced myocyte apoptosis would suggest that sequential stresses will result in a life-long disproportionately higher clinical expression of cardiac insults.

Mechanism of anthracycline-associated cardiotoxicity

The mechanism of the cardiac damage caused by anthracycline exposure has not been fully elucidated, however free radical formation is believed to be an important factor. Free radicals can injure lipid structures in the myocardial cell, and the resultant peroxidation of these lipid structures impairs the function of the sarcoplasmic reticulum and mitochondria. Cardiac myocytes are more prone to these degenerative changes since they lack catalase and superoxide dismutase and thus are less able to metabolize free radicals than are other cells.[92] Cell necrosis is the end result of this damage. It is evident that the mechanisms for cardiotoxicity are sufficiently different from those of oncologic efficacy that cardioprotection is possible. While the generation of the oxygen free radicals is associated with cardiotoxicity, there is increasing evidence that topoisomerase IIß plays a major role, and that inhibition of topoisomerase, as may be associated with dexrazoxane, is cardioprotective.[93,94]

Clinical manifestations of anthracycline-associated cardiotoxicity

The clinical manifestations of doxorubicin-related cardiomyopathy are indistinguishable from other forms of congestive heart failure. Patients may be asymptomatic in the early stages or may exhibit only minimal signs of cardiac dysfunction. In many patients, the first sign of a cardiac abnormality may be a failure to return to baseline cardiac rate promptly following exertion. Resting tachycardia and loss of respiratory variation in heart rate may also be seen. As cardiac damage progresses, patients experience increasing dyspnea, with dyspnea at rest a poor prognostic sign.

The cardiac examination of a patient with fully developed cardiomyopathy often reveals an S3 gallop, an enlarged area of cardiac dullness, an exaggerated increase in cardiac rate with minimal activity and, when pulmonary congestion ensues, diffuse rales. The chest radiograph shows nonspecific findings of an enlarged cardiac silhouette and engorged vasculature. Pleural effusion may be noted. The electrocardiogram may show nonspecific repolarization changes. B-type natriuretic peptide (BNP), a marker of volume expansion and high ventricular filling pressures is usually elevated, the elevation proportional to the degree of cardiac failure. It has been suggested that the level of natriuretic peptides is increased in at least some patients with doxorubicin-associated cardiotoxicity, and this appears to correlate more with changes in diastolic than with changes in systolic function.[95–97] The left ventricular ejection fraction remains the most widely used parameter with which to monitor the cardiac status in patients receiving doxorubicin or related agents.

The structural changes in myocardial tissue seen on examination of cardiac biopsy specimens have provided vital information concerning the toxicity of doxorubicin and related compounds.[98–100] In highly selected patients, biopsy may provide the essential information and is generally regarded as safe.[101] The cardiac biopsy specimens can be graded according to ultrastructural changes seen by electron microscopy with both the degree and the extent of the abnormalities considered in determining the final grade. With the presently used anthracycline regimens, cardiac biopsy is rarely necessary for anthracycline dosing decisions, but the procedures have regained relevance in the evaluation of patients with suspected myocarditis or infiltrative processes.

Several groups of patients are known to be at greater risk of developing cardiac dysfunction at relatively lower cumulative doses of anthracyclines. Among these are elderly patients, pediatric patients, those with preexisting cardiovascular disease. It is now postulated that any patient with diminished cardiac reserve or where increased oxidative stress is present is at increased risk for anthracycline-associated cardiotoxicity. Despite some reports to the contrary, anthracyclines are generally not considered to be associated with coronary spasm or primary myocardial ischemia. For all patients in whom an increased risk is present, heightened surveillance and consideration of cardiac-sparing regimens should be considered, as should, when feasible, nonanthracycline regimens. Irradiation through portals that include the heart is a well-documented risk factor for cardiomyopathy, and patients who are expected to undergo concomitant or sequential cardiac irradiation should be considered for cardioprotection or additional monitoring.[102,103]

A number of antineoplastic drugs have also been associated with increased anthracycline toxicity. Cyclophosphamide (discussed below) may augment the cardiotoxic effect of doxorubicin toxicity, a matter of particular clinical importance because the drugs are often used together.[104] Dactinomycin, plicamycin, dacarbazine, and mitomycin C, all reportedly augment doxorubicin toxicity, but the evidence for the first three has not been persuasive. Mitomycin C, however, appears to add substantially to the toxicity of doxorubicin, even when given after the completion of doxorubicin therapy.[105] Paclitaxel has also been reported to increase the cardiotoxic effect of doxorubicin. In one study, however, patients receiving the combination at cumulative doses of doxorubicin of below 340 to 380 mg/m^2 did not demonstrate the additive effect.[106] The higher incidence of cardiac toxicity observed when the two drugs are administered within a short time may be due to the fact that paclitaxel interferes with the pharmacokinetics of doxorubicin, leading to higher systemic levels of both doxorubicin and doxorubicinol, a metabolite.[107] Alternatively, the apparent increase in toxicity may simply be the result of increased surveillance using imperfect tests in patients undergoing frequent monitoring of cardiac function. Other anthracyclines and related agents, such as mitoxantrone (an anthraquinone), demonstrate intrinsic cardiac toxicity that is additive; as is noted below, changing from one anthracycline to another does not provide cardioprotection.[108] The interaction between anthracyclines and trastuzumab is discussed below.

Various strategies can lower the extent of doxorubicin cardiotoxicity. Limiting the cumulative dose is a strategy that grew out of the observation that clinically apparent cardiotoxicity is unusual at cumulative doses of less than 300 mg/m^2 and that the incidence is about 5% at a cumulative dose of 400 mg/m^2.[88] Limiting the cumulative dosage to these levels in patients without risk factors helps to keep the cardiotoxicity within an acceptable range. Dose limitation also decreases the need for cardiac monitoring, as the likelihood of cardiotoxicity is lower; the risk of stopping effective therapy early because of false-positive testing results may exceed the benefits of such testing. Dose-limitation, however, does not take into consideration patients who are still responding after receiving the limiting dose. Most patients, including many who are identified as having "risk factors" tolerate 300 mg/m^2 of doxorubicin or the cardiotoxic equivalent of other anthracyclines. Notwithstanding these established considerations, it is now clearly evident that once myocyte loss has occurred, the injury is substantially permanent, and the longer exposed patients are watched, the greater is the likelihood that intercurrent factors and sequential stresses will result in greater appreciation of diminished cardiac reserve evidenced by biomarker elevations or parameters of cardiac systolic or diastolic function. Higher incidences of late toxicity continue to be reported as an acknowledgment of greater oncologic success with longer survival of treated cancer patients.

Encapsulating the parent anthracycline compound in liposomes reduces the incidence and severity of cardiotoxicity.[109,110] Both pegylated and nonpegylated preparations have been studied, and the pegylated preparation is approved for the treatment of Kaposi's sarcoma, ovarian carcinoma, and multiple myeloma in the United States. Pegylated liposomal doxorubicin is also effective in the treatment of breast and ovarian cancer; comparisons of liposome-encapsulated and conventional doxorubicin in the treatment of these diseases confirmed cardioprotection with comparable antitumor activity. Pegylated liposomal doxorubicin appears to have a clinical efficacy similar to its parent compound in a subset of anthracycline-sensitive tumors.[111] Both pegylated and nonpegylated liposomal doxorubicin are clearly cardioprotective.[112] With the pegylated form, cardioprotection has been demonstrated both by cardiac biopsy as well as by noninvasive studies.[113] The degree of cardioprotection is difficult to quantify, but studies suggest that up to twice the number of cycles of pegylated liposomal doxorubicin can be given with the same degree of cardiotoxicity as is seen with the unprotected parent compound (see Table 5). The spectrum of oncologic efficacy may be slightly different for the liposomal-encapsulated preparation; the degree of stomatitis and hand-foot syndrome is higher.[114]

Modification of the dose schedule has been shown to decrease anthracycline cardiotoxicity. A series of trials of continuous-infusion doxorubicin using infusion times of 24 to 96 hours, gauging the cardiotoxicity on the basis of endomyocardial biopsy findings have been undertaken.[115] Patients treated with continuous infusions showed a significantly lower incidence of high-grade endomyocardial pathology in their biopsy specimens despite receiving a significantly higher cumulative dose. Efficacy is not compromised, but infusions longer than 96 hours are limited by increasingly troublesome mucositis and hand-foot syndrome.[116] Continuous infusion has also been evaluated in the pediatric population with conflicting reports as to cardioprotection.[117,118] The relative cardioprotection of various doxorubicin administration schedules is depicted in Table 5. Despite clear evidence of cardioprotection, the inconvenience of using portable infusion pumps and indwelling catheters that are required for continuous infusion, as well as the trend to use lower cumulative dosages of doxorubicin has made many clinicians reluctant to use such schedules.

A number of compounds with possible cardioprotective properties have been investigated. The single approved cardiac protector to date is the iron chelator dexrazoxane. In a study of 92 patients randomly assigned to receive a doxorubicin-containing regimen (50 mg/m^2 doxorubicin with 500 mg/m^2 cyclophosphamide and 500 mg/m^2 fluorouracil given every 21 days) or the same regimen together with dexrazoxane, the investigators found a significant decrease in cardiotoxic effects demonstrated by ejection fraction measurements, biopsy grades, and clinical signs or symptoms of cardiac dysfunction.[119] Other toxicities and antitumor effects were unaffected. However, one subsequent study that confirmed

Table 5 Relative toxicities of anthracycline: a comparison of relative toxicities of different cardiotoxic drugs and dosage schedules.

Drug	Schedule	Relative myelosuppressive potency compared with doxorubicin administered by standard schedule	Approximate relative cardiotoxicity[a]	Cardiotoxicity index compared with doxorubicin administered by standard schedule[b]	Recommended maximum dose (mg/m^2)[c]
Doxorubicin	Rapid infusion (20 min)	1	1	1	400
Doxorubicin	Weekly	1	0.73	0.73	550
Doxorubicin	24-h infusion	1	0.73	0.73	550
Doxorubicin	48-h infusion	1	0.62	0.62	650[d]
Doxorubicin	96-h infusion	1	0.5	0.5	800–1000[d]
Pegylated liposomal doxorubicin	Rapid infusion	1	Uncertain probably <0.7	Uncertain probably <0.7	450–550
Epirubicin	Rapid infusion	0.67	0.66	0.44	900
Mitoxantrone	Rapid infusion	5	0.5	2.5	160
Daunorubicin	Rapid infusion	0.67	0.75[e]	0.5[e]	800[e]
Idarubicin	Rapid infusion	5	0.53	2.67	150
Pirarubicin	Rapid infusion	1	0.62	0.62	650[e]
Doxorubicin + dexrazoxane	Rapid infusion	1[e]	0.5	0.5[e]	800–1000[e]
Doxorubicin, 300 mg/m^2 + dexrazoxane	Rapid infusion	1[e]	0.73[e]	0.73[e]	550[e]

[a]Factor by which the cardiotoxic effects of the cumulative dose of rapid infusion doxorubicin can be compared with the cumulative dose of the agent, combination, and schedule listed, when given at an equivalent myelosuppressive doses.
[b]Derived by dividing 400 mg/m^2, the recommended maximum dose of rapid-infusion doxorubicin, by the recommended maximum dose for the agent in question. The cardiotoxicity index represents a factor by which to multiply the cumulative dose of a drug administered to obtain an approximation of toxicity that might be expected had the resultant amount of doxorubicin been given by rapid infusion. For example, if a cumulative dose of 120 mg/m^2 mitoxantrone had been administered, the patient would be expected to demonstrate cardiac damage approximately equal to 300 mg/m^2 of doxorubicin given by rapid infusion (120 × 2.5 = 300). This value is useful when changing from one cardiotoxic regimen to another. When the sum of the products of the indexes and the cumulative dosages administered exceeds 400, the risk of clinically significant cardiotoxicity exceeds 5%.
[c]Dose producing clinically significant congestive heart failure in 5% of patients.
[d]Less toxic by endomyocardial biopsy.
[e]Inadequate data.

the cardioprotective activity of dexrazoxane showed a decrease in antitumor effect as well.[120] There was no suggestion of diminished antineoplastic activity, however, in patients given dexrazoxane after they had received 300 mg/m^2 of doxorubicin.[121] Other studies have not found the efficacy of anthracyclines to be decreased by dexrazoxane. Dexrazoxane also has been studied in conjunction with epirubicin and mitoxantrone.[122] These studies suggest that dexrazoxane also reduces the cardiotoxicity of agents other than doxorubicin. Dexrazoxane also is used in children where there are special concerns regarding late toxicity.[123] Recent investigations suggest that dexrazoxane interferes with or inhibits topoisomerase II complexes, providing a possible explanation as to why dexrazoxane is cardioprotective while other antioxidants have not been shown to do so.[124]

A number of studies have looked at cardioprotection of agents that affect cardiac contractility or afterload, namely beta-blockers and ACE inhibitors. These studies have looked at the protection of both Type I and Type II agents and have reported substantial variation in the extent of protection. Protection during and after exposure of Type I agents would be expected, especially in instances of higher cumulative dosages. Reduced oxidative stress at the time of exposure should mitigate the extent of cell injury. Following exposure, reduced work-load would be expected to delay remodeling and forestall development of clinically relevant heart failure and has been shown, in some studies where Type I agents were used, to do so.[125] Cardioprotection using statins has also been explored, albeit not in large populations. Statins reduce oxydative stress, and so their role in cardioprotection of Type I agents should be anticipated.[126]

Cardiac monitoring of patients receiving doxorubicin

Most patients undergoing treatment for cancer, even elderly patients and those with known cardiac disease, can tolerate at least some doxorubicin. Patients with significant dilated cardiomyopathy and patients who have experienced cardiotoxicity from the prior use of an anthracycline or related drugs are the major exceptions. Most patients with reduced ejection fractions as the result of prior myocardial infarctions tolerate doxorubicin when it is given with some form of cardioprotection, and when the cumulative dose remains below 300 to 400 mg/m^2; increased monitoring in those settings is prudent. Patients being considered for doxorubicin therapy generally undergo a cardiac evaluation including a determination of ejection fraction and a standard (12-lead) electrocardiogram to provide a basis for later comparison.[127,128]

Patients without risk factors and who are without signs or symptoms suggesting cardiac compromise generally tolerate cumulative dosages of doxorubicin in the range of 300 to 350 mg/m^2 by standard infusion or its equivalent (see Table 5). When higher cumulative dosages are administered increased surveillance is prudent. At any dose level, patients with increased risk factors for early toxicity should be monitored more closely. At dosages suggested in Table 5, the risk of heart failure approaches 5% in the absence of other cardiac risk factors.

Patients whose ejection fractions fall below 50% are at increased cardiac risk. If the ejection fraction has not changed they usually tolerate cumulative dosages up to 350 mg/m^2 with careful monitoring. For those whose ejection fraction has either fallen by more than 15 percentage points, or has fallen by 10 percentage points to a value below 50%, consideration should be made to stop doxorubicin and substitute alternative therapy using

Table 6 Summary of cardiotoxicity in adjuvant trials involving trastuzumab.[a]

Trial	Number of patients	Entry criteria	Arms	Reported cardiac events (%)	Reported reversibility	Follow-up (year)
NSABP B-31	2043	Node+	(A) AC-T (B) AC-TH	(A) 0.8 (B) 4.1	Yes	7
BCIRG 006	3222	Node+ or high-risk node Age < 70	(A) AC-T (B) AC-TH (C) TPH	(A) 0.4 (B) 1.9 (C) 0.4	N/A	3
NCCTG N9831	1944	Node+ or high-risk node	(A) AC-T (B) AC-T-H (C) AC-TH	(A) 0.3 (B) 2.8 (C) 3.3	Yes	3
HERA	3386	Node+ or high-risk node	(A) Std (B) Std-H	(A) 3.6 (B) 0.6	Yes	8
FinHer	232	Node+ or high-risk node Age < 66	(A) V/T-FAC (B) V/T(H)-FAC	(A) 3.4 (B) 0	N/A	5

Abbreviations: A, anthracycline; C, cyclophosphamide; T, taxane; H, trastuzumab; P, carboplatin; Std, standard (neo)adjuvant regimen (94% contained anthracycline); V/T, vinorelbine or taxane; F, 5-fluorouracil; N/A, not applicable; Follow-up time reflects most recently reported data.
[a]Source: Based on Tan-Chiu[135]; Suter et al.[136]; Joensuu et al.[137]

noncardiotoxic agents. The rare patients requiring extreme dosages of anthracyclines may be considered for enhanced surveillance; in very rare instances cardiac biopsy may be considered to quantitate structural changes, whereby a biopsy grade of 1.5 or higher constitutes a contraindication to continued treatment with any form of anthracycline.

Other anthracyclines and related (type I) agents

Clinically, the cardiotoxic effects of daunorubicin, idarubicin, epirubicin, pirarubicin, and mitoxantrone are identical to those of doxorubicin. As is the case with oncologic efficacy of these agents, the cumulative dosages, expressed in mg/m^2 that causes cardiotoxicity, differ between the different agents. The cardiotoxicity of these agents has not been studied as extensively as has that of doxorubicin. Nevertheless, on the basis of ejection fractions and findings from cardiac biopsy specimen evaluation at equivalent oncologic doses, some data has emerged. Epirubicin is associated with a decrease in the incidence of cardiac toxicity compared with that seen for doxorubicin given by rapid infusion (see Table 5).[129] The cardioprotection afforded by epirubicin, which is being used increasingly for the treatment of breast cancer, allows an additional margin of safety that may be especially important in populations at increased cardiac risk. A Cochrane review noted the relative cardioprotection of epirubicin but suggested that the degree of protection may not be as high as was previously thought.[130] Some investigations have suggested that the combination of paclitaxel and epirubicin causes less cardiotoxicity than the combination of doxorubicin and paclitaxel, and they attribute this to the fact that paclitaxel interferes less with the metabolism of epirubicin than with the parent compound.[131] Available data regarding idarubicin suggest that $150 mg/m^2$ is a safe cumulative dose for patients who have not yet been exposed to anthracyclines.[132] Data for pirarubicin (THP doxorubicin), a doxorubicin analogue used extensively in Japan and France, but not approved for use in the United States, suggest that the agent is significantly less cardiotoxic than doxorubicin given by standard-infusion schedules.[133] Mitoxantrone, an anthraquinone, is considered less cardiotoxic than doxorubicin in equivalent myelosuppressive dosages.[134]

Switching from one agent to another does not offer cardioprotection, and considerable care must be exercised when considering a new cardiotoxic treatment in a patient who has previously been treated with other Type I cardiotoxic agents, even remotely. Converting the various cardiotoxic drug doses to the corresponding doses of rapidly administered doxorubicin allows approximate, albeit useful comparisons (see Table 5).

Type II anticancer treatment-related agents: trastuzumab

Type II agents by definition do not demonstrate cumulative dose-related toxicity, and therefore the cardiotoxic expression is much less predictable. The best studied of these agents is trastuzumab, but other agents should also be considered in this grouping as well. Trastuzumab, a humanized monoclonal antibody directed against HER2, is effective for the treatment of breast cancers and other cancer types that overexpress this antigen (approximately 20–25% of breast cancers). Concerns regarding cardiotoxicity led to a number of large multi-center trials that included more than 10,000 patients who received trastuzumab. A summary of the trials and their respective treatment arms is shown in Table 6.[135–137] Several important conclusions have emerged. The most important from the perspective of cardiotoxicity are (1) cardiac dysfunction in treatment arms that include an anthracycline followed by trastuzumab are higher than similar arms without trastuzumab; the difference, however, is less than 4% but has, nevertheless, been of concern; (2) cardiac toxicity is largely but not invariably reversible; (3) cardiac deaths following trastuzumab, when given as a single agent, are rare; (4) regimens that include trastuzumab without pretreatment with an anthracycline have a smaller incidence of cardiac dysfunction; and (5) the cardiotoxicity associated with trastuzumab, while different from that of doxorubicin, is clinically indistinguishable using MUGA or echocardiographic parameters of decreased systolic function.

Although the precise mechanism of trastuzumab-induced cardiomyopathy is not well understood, its specific binding to HER2 and its disruption of the HER2 signaling pathway in the heart are thought to be the primary mechanisms. ErbB-2 (HER2/neu) belongs to the epidermal growth factor receptor (EGFR) family of receptor tyrosine kinases, of which there are four members: EGFR, HER2, HER3, and HER4. These receptors are activated by the EGF family of ligands, including EGF itself, heregulin, and neuregulins, all of which are expressed in the heart. Binding of these EGF ligands to EGFR, HER3, or HER4 induces heterodimer formation with HER2, triggers receptor autophosphorylation, and initiates downstream signaling. Among those pathways activated are Ras/Raf, PI3K/Akt, JNK, and MAPK, all important regulators of transcription in cardiac myocytes. An extensive body of work has implicated these pathways in cardiac development, maintenance of normal cardiac function, response to stress, hypertrophy, and regulation of apoptosis. Indeed, targeted deletion of HER2 in murine models has demonstrated a specific role for this receptor in mediating the growth, repair, and survival of cardiomyocytes after

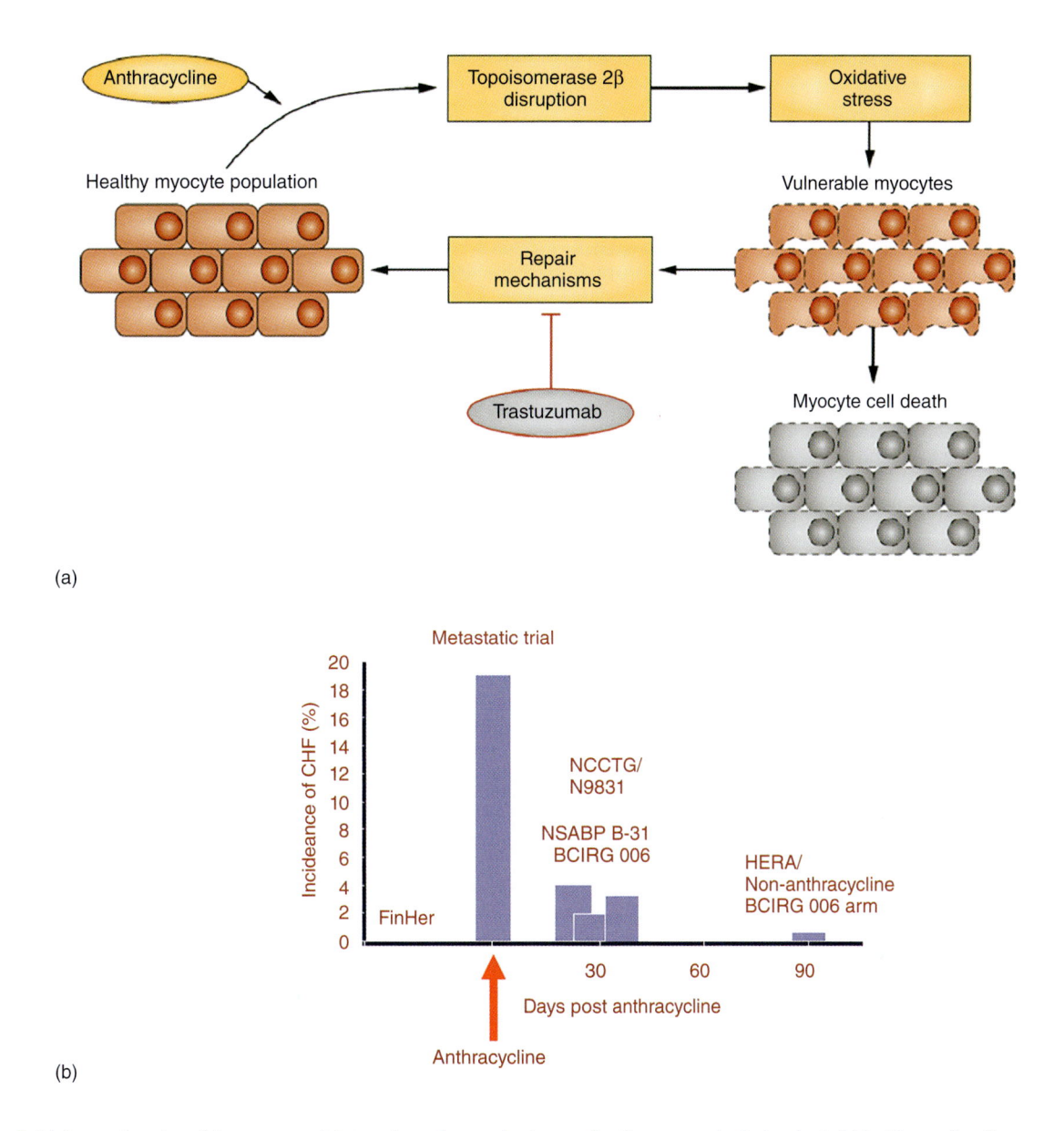

Figure 7 (a) One explanation of the trastuzumab interaction; other mechanisms and pathways may also be involved. (b) Incidence of cardiac events plotted against the interval between the conclusion of anthracycline therapy and the start of trastuzumab in adjuvant trials. *Abbreviations*: NSABP, National Surgical Adjuvant Breast and Bowel Project; NCCTG/N9831, North Central Cancer Treatment Group/Intergroup; BCIRG, Breast Cancer International Research Group; HERA, Herceptin Adjuvant. Source: Based on Ewer and Ewer.[141]

stress.[138] Temporary disruption of the HER2 signaling pathway by trastuzumab thus results in an inadequate or even maladaptive response to cardiac stress that can lead to systolic dysfunction and congestive heart failure.[139]

Cardiac dysfunction related to trastuzumab appears to be largely reversible.[140] However, some instances of assumed reversibility may be an artifact related to the sub-optimal predictive value of cardiac ultrasound.[12] As trastuzumab-related dysfunction presents as an insult to an organ often previously damaged by exposure to an anthracycline, the question as to how great a portion of the observed dysfunction is attributable to trastuzumab arises. It has been observed that Erb-B2 is upregulated in the heart after anthracycline exposure, and it is known that ErbB-2 signaling pathways play an important role in the cardiac myocyte's response to injury. Furthermore, interruption of HER2 signaling in mice augmented anthracycline cardiotoxicity. Similarly, in humans, it appears that prior anthracycline exposure represents a significant risk factor for the development of trastuzumab-associated cardiomyopathy in a synergistic manner. Thus, it is plausible that trastuzumab interferes with cellular recovery following anthracycline damage.[130] The administration of trastuzumab during a vulnerable window when anthracycline injury is potentially reversible may trigger additional apoptosis (Figure 7a). The longer the interval between anthracycline and trastuzumab during the vulnerable period, the less likely is a finding of cardiac dysfunction (Figure 7b).[141] The dilemmas of whether and when to temporarily hold or permanently stop trastuzumab, how to assess the risk of restarting after functional recovery, and how to monitor such patients remains controversial. Several groups have suggested guidelines, which are generally based on expert opinion as well as published supporting data; data derived from prospective clinical trials is often lacking.[100]

Other type II agents
In addition to trastuzumab, lapatinib, sunitinib, imatinib, osimertinib, pertuzumab, and other agents have raised concerns of possible cardiotoxicity. Myocardial dysfunction has been reported with these agents, but the incidence is generally low; reversibility is often acknowledged.[142,143] To date, none have shown biopsy changes that are characteristic for anthracyclines, although some alterations in mitochondrial structure have been reported. Interestingly, these agents do not exhibit cumulative dose-related toxicity and can be given for extended periods of time in many patients. With regard to myocardial depression, a secondary effect may be implicated; in the case of sunitinib, significant hypertension is noted, and in the case of imatinib fluid retention may be the crucial factor.[144–146]

Other drugs that demonstrate a decrease in cardiac function
Significant decreases in myocardial function are occasionally noted for other agents that do not clearly fit within either the Type I or Type II classification. Rarely α-interferon has been associated with a dramatic decrease in ejection fraction. The mechanism is unknown; however, inflammation and increased metabolic requirements have both been implicated; patients who survive the initial episode usually go on to recover cardiac function.[147] An unusual form of cardiac damage is associated with high-dose cyclophosphamide administration. When severe, the damage takes the form of a hemorrhagic myocarditis.[148] The process is often acute, is related to high individual doses (usually 4.5 g/m² or more) rather than to the cumulative dose, and is associated with decreased ejection fractions and mean QRS voltage. Although severe hemorrhagic myocarditis may be fatal, milder presentations may be asymptomatic and reversible.

Treatment considerations of patients with treatment-related cardiac failure or dysfunction

The most important treatment consideration in patients who develop anthracycline-associated cardiac dysfunction is the avoidance of additional anthracyclines. Once established, anthracycline-associated cardiac dysfunction differs little from other forms of cardiomyopathy and it is treated in a similar way. The American College of Cardiology and The American Heart Association have issued guidelines for the diagnosis and management of chronic heart failure in adults.[149] Patients who have been treated with anthracyclines but show no symptoms of cardiac dysfunction should have other conditions that exacerbate cardiac dysfunction aggressively treated. Hypertension should be controlled and lifestyle changes encouraged. Pharmacological intervention should also be considered for those who have ejection fractions below 45–50%. Evidence suggests that medical therapy is most effective when given early, and therefore should be initiated as soon as LV dysfunction is appreciated.[150] ACE inhibitors, beta adrenergic blockers, and aldosterone antagonists are indicated for patients with LV dysfunction. For patients with symptomatic heart failure, salt restriction and diuretics may be added. There is no specific therapy for anthracycline-related cardiomyopathy. An underlying malignancy should not, however, be considered a contraindication to aggressive heart failure therapy and, in selected patients, mechanical assist devices and cardiac transplantation may be considered for those who have achieved oncologic stability or cure.[151]

Agents associated with myocardial ischemia, thromboembolic disease, and myocarditis

A number of agents have the potential to cause myocardial ischemia, with or without frank myocardial infarction. The most extensively studied such agent is 5-fluorouracil (5-FU), especially when the agent is administered in combination with cisplatin.[152] Capecitabine is an orally administered prodrug which is enzymatically converted to 5-FU. Myocardial infarction and dysrhythmia have been reported with both drugs.[153] Ischemia is triggered through coronary artery vasospasm. Isolated cases of myocardial ischemia have also occurred after the administration of vinblastine, vincristine, bleomycin, cisplatin, and biologic response modifiers. The wide spectrum of ischemic responses suggests that ischemia accompanying anticancer treatment is more common than is generally appreciated. Nonspecific electrocardiographic changes may be seen in nearly half the patients treated with 5-FU and as many as 16% show electrocardiographic evidence of ischemia including ST-segment depression or elevation and changes suggesting myocardial infarction (Figure 8). Many of the affected patients have underlying coronary artery disease, which suggests that preexisting coronary artery abnormalities augment the ischemic potential of 5-FU and related agents. The use of a calcium channel blocker has been reported to prevent the ischemia.[154] Selected patients may also be treated with intravenous nitroglycerin while receiving 5-FU to prevent myocardial ischemia or infarction. When ischemia can be controlled treatment may be continued, albeit with increased monitoring and caution.

Patients with evidence of myocardial ischemia, regardless of the mechanism, should be observed closely for rhythm disturbances, although the level of observation and intervention depends on the overall prognosis. Individuals with known preexisting coronary artery disease can be treated with beta-adrenergic blockers and/or a long-acting nitrate to help reduce the likelihood of an ischemic event. Controlled underlying ischemia or evidence of ischemia associated with a particular therapy should not be considered an absolute contraindication to further treatment with the implicated agent or agents. Cancer patients with underlying coronary artery disease are often candidates for revascularization, which can significantly improve the patient's ability to tolerate therapy and their overall quality of life.

The immunomodulatory agents thalidomide, lenalidomide, and pomalidomide, used to treat multiple myeloma, have been associated with significantly increased risk of venous thromboembolic disease. The risk is highest when these agents are used in conjunction with high-dose corticosteroids, doxorubicin, or multi-agent chemotherapy. Prophylaxis should be considered in this setting, with aspirin for lower-risk patients and anticoagulation (warfarin or direct oral anticoagulant) for higher-risk cohorts.[155] Antiangiogenic agents, including bevacizumab, sunitinib, and sorafenib, have been associated with arterial thromboembolic events. The mechanism likely involves perturbations in endothelial function. Events can include stroke and myocardial infarction.[156]

The cardiac events associated with hormonal therapy have been studied in large groups of postmenopausal breast cancer patients. Tamoxifen is associated with a significantly decreased cholesterol and low-density lipoprotein cholesterol (LDL-C); when used in the setting of breast cancer prevention, tamoxifen was not shown to have cardiovascular effects. However, an increased risk of cardiovascular adverse events with aromatase inhibitors when compared with tamoxifen has been demonstrated; a review and metanalysis has drawn attention to the likelihood that the lower incidence of these events is related to the probable cardioprotective effect of tamoxifen.[157,158]

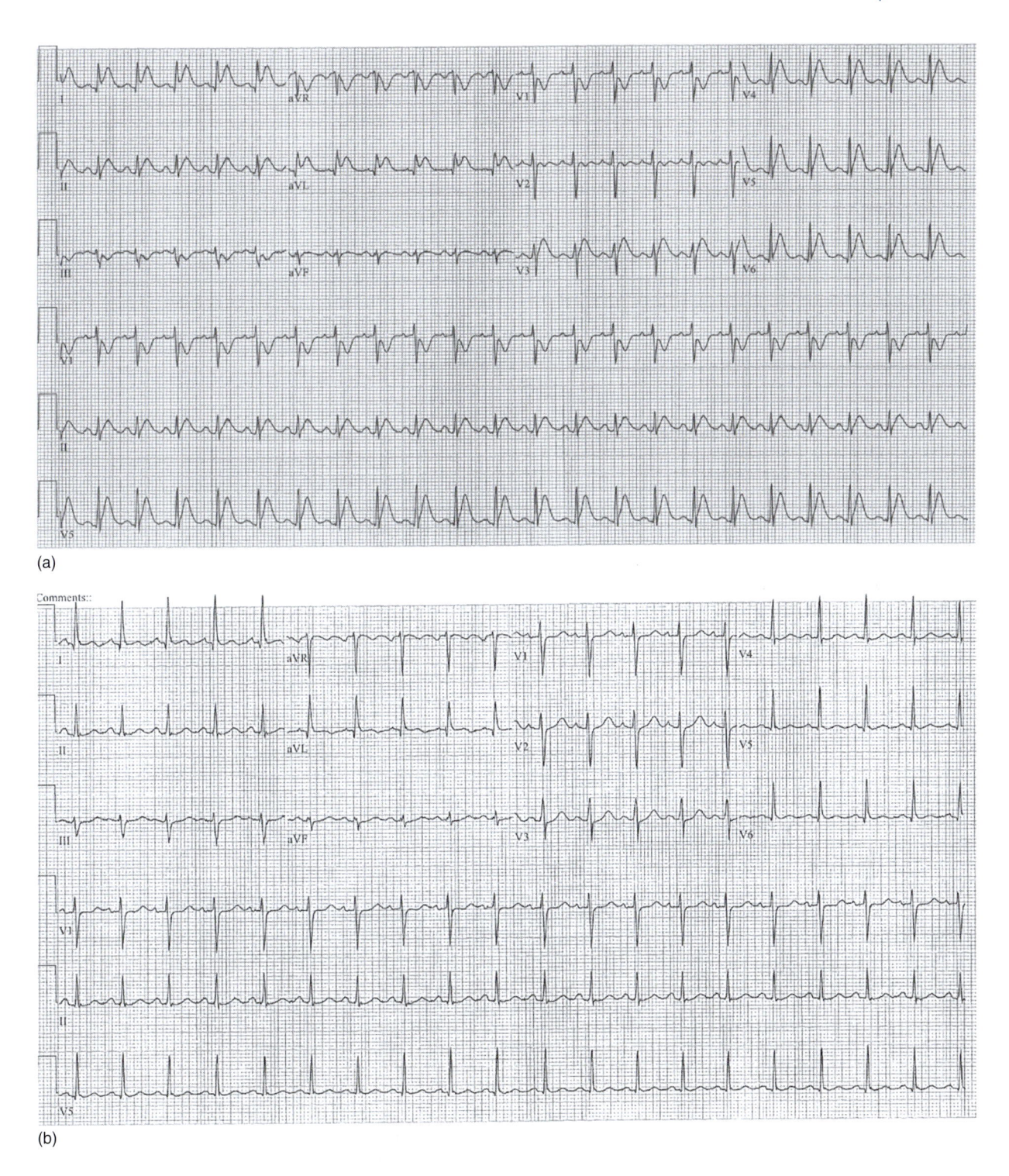

Figure 8 (a) Electrocardiogram in a 44-year-old woman experiencing chest pain while receiving 5-fluorouracil. Acute anterolateral ST elevation was due to coronary vasospasm. (b) Chest pain and ECG changes resolved with nitroglycerin.

Immune checkpoint inhibitors cause an unusual form of autoimmune myocarditis. These agents target cytotoxic T-lymphocyte-associated protein 4 (CTLA-4), programmed death-1 (PD-1), and programmed death-ligand 1 (PD-L1), and have emerged as front-line therapies for a number of tumors.[159] The mechanisms involved in immune checkpoint-inhibitor myocarditis are not yet well elucidated but are suspected to involve shared antigens between myocytes and the tumor. In its most severe form, patients experience rapid onset of fulminant inflammation with profound hemodynamic compromise and shock.[160] Other manifestations include ventricular tachycardia, heart block, and pericardial involvement.[161] The true incidence of immune checkpoint inhibitor-associated myocarditis is uncertain, as the entity is likely to represent a spectrum whereby those most seriously affected come to the attention of the treating physicians. Clinically, serious or life-threatening disease has been reported in about 1% of those treated. The diagnosis is supported by clinical symptoms, troponin elevation, reduced left ventricular ejection fraction,

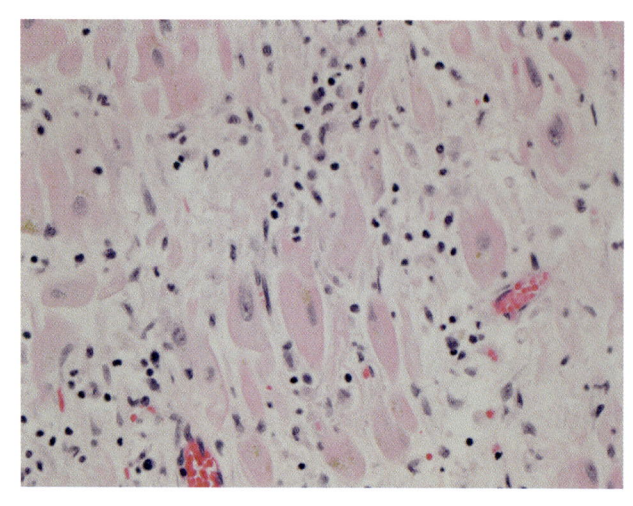

Figure 9 Hematoxylin and eosin-stained section demonstrating lymphocyte infiltration of the myocardium in a patient who succumbed to nivolumab-associated autoimmune myocarditis (400×).

and electrocardiographic alterations that include ST-segment elevation, conduction abnormalities, rhythm abnormalities. Cardiac magnetic resonance imaging and endomyocardial biopsy are helpful in establishing or confirming the diagnosis. Specific treatment is not available, but eliminating further exposure to the offending agent along with high-dose steroids, antithymocyte globulin have been proposed.[162] Autopsy examination of the heart shows lymphocytic infiltration and necrosis (Figure 9).

Agents associated with hypotension or hypertension

Some degree of hypotension develops in many patients as a consequence of their chemotherapy. The most frequent cause is volume depletion, often as a result of nausea and/or vomiting. Other causes of hypotension related to chemotherapy are decreased cardiac output, loss of vascular tone, and increased permeability of the small vessels and capillaries (capillary leak). Most instances of hypotension in patients receiving chemotherapy are transient and can be managed with careful monitoring and the administration of fluids or vasopressor agents. Rare instances of life-threatening and profound hypotension have been reported.

Interleukin-2 use is associated with significant, but usually transient, hypotension, frequently requiring pressor agents. Capillary leakage has been implicated. Interleukin-2-related myocardial ischemia is possibly related to the hypotension, although a direct toxic effect has not been excluded. Interleukin-2 is also associated with an increased incidence of supraventricular dysrhythmias and myocarditis. The vasodilation that occurs in response to interleukin-2 appears to be mediated by the release of nitric oxide.[163] Evidence has suggested that NG-monomethyl-L-arginine, an inhibitor of nitric oxide synthase, reverses the hypotension caused by interleukin-2, lending support to the role of nitric oxide in the production of hypotension and indicating the therapeutic potential of NG-monomethyl-L-arginine as well.[164]

Omacetaxine mepesuccinate, previously called homoharringtonine, is approved for the treatment of refractory chronic myeloid leukemia. The drug is associated with dose-related, sometimes severe, hypotension arising immediately after its intravenous administration.[165] Intravenous epinephrine has been helpful in stabilizing patients in this setting.

Cisplatin, an agent widely used to treat genitourinary malignancy, head and neck tumors, and non-small-cell lung cancer is known to induce hypertension. Thalidomide and paclitaxel may induce hypotension. Bevacizumab, a monoclonal antibody against vascular endothelial growth factor, has been associated with significant increases in blood pressure in more than 25% of treated patients. Serious and sometimes permanent hypertension has been reported in up to 14% of treated patients; rarely patients develop hypertensive crises. Patients with baseline hypertension are at increased risk and should be monitored during therapy.[166] Control of underlying hypertension prior to initiating treatment with bevacizumab is important; mild ongoing hypertension is generally not considered a contraindication to the use of bevacizumab.[167] Treatment is often initiated with amlodipine, with the addition of an ACE inhibitor, an angiotensin II receptor blocker (ARB) or beta-blocker added as needed.[168] Severe or malignant hypertension with hypertensive encephalopathy is an absolute contraindication to the use of bevacizumab, and dose reductions are not recommended in those circumstances. Other antiangiogenic agents, including sunitinib, alemtuzumab, gemtuzumab, infliximab, muromanoab-CD3, rituximab, and sorafenib are likewise associated with increased incidence of hypertension, usually reversible upon holding or stopping the medication. Once hypertension is controlled re-challenge may be initiated, and many patients are able to continue treatment with acceptable cardiac risk.

Cardiac complications of radiation therapy

Links between radiation to the chest in the treatment for malignancy and subsequent heart disease have been clearly established. Inclusion of cardiac tissue in the radiation portals can lead to a broad spectrum of disease, which often presents decades after exposure. Recognition of these risks has led to dramatic improvements in radiation techniques over the years, but the degree to which the heart can be spared has not been fully determined, as long-term follow-up studies in patients treated with modern techniques are still underway.

The pathophysiology of ionizing radiation's cardiotoxic effects involves both DNA damage and generation of reactive oxygen species. Cells with higher turnover are more susceptible, particularly the vascular endothelium. Small vessel damage then leads to inflammation and ultimately fibrosis of cardiac tissue. All layers of the heart are involved, leading to acute and chronic pericardial disease, accelerated coronary artery disease, cardiomyopathy, valvular disease, and conduction system abnormalities. Secondary cardiac malignancies attributed to radiation therapy are well recognized.[169] The heart responds to the radiation insult over time with late-presentation and chronic progressive functional decline showing a direct correlation with the radiation fraction to the heart. Animal models have demonstrated a radiation dose-dependent chronic congestive myocardial failure with damage to the myocardial microvasculature; histological examination shows a marked reduction in capillary density, myocardial degeneration, and necrosis with interstitial fibrosis.[170] Cell kinetic studies show increased endothelial cell proliferation about 30 to 100 days postradiation. The morphologic changes in animal models parallel the drops in cardiac output and left ventricular ejection fraction.

Human data on cardiac effects of radiation therapy have come mostly from patients with Hodgkin's lymphoma and breast cancer, who historically received significant doses of cardiac radiation and who also are available for long-term follow-up studies. In contrast, survival in lung cancer is generally too poor to allow significant development of cardiac complications. Risk factors include total

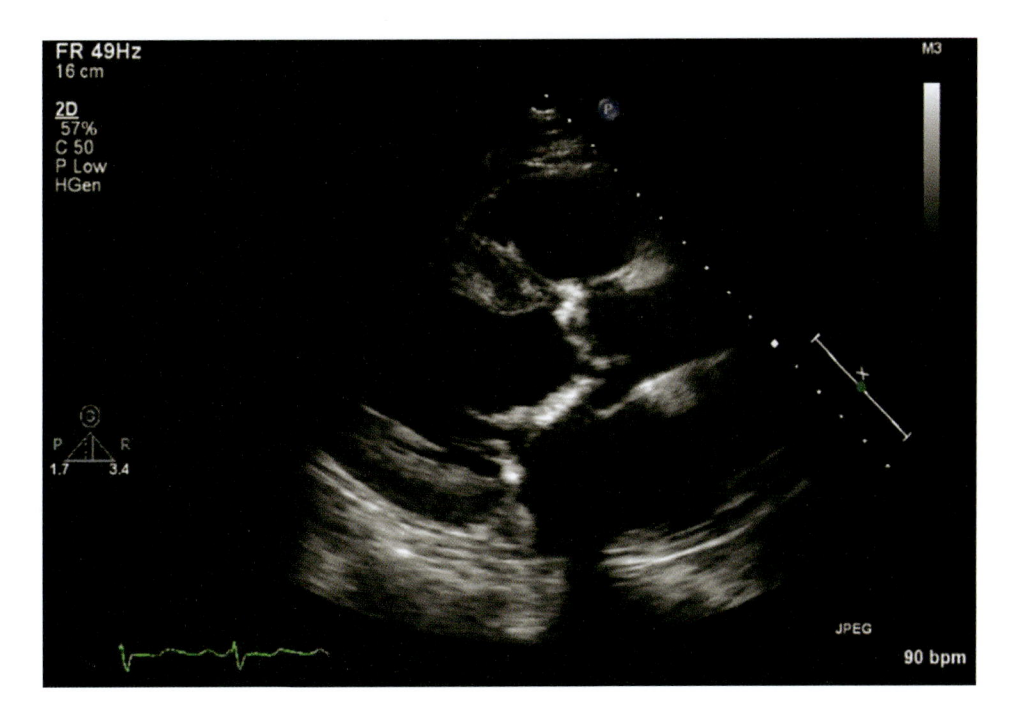

Figure 10 Parasternal long-axis echocardiographic view from a 40-year-old patient who received mantle radiation for lymphoma two decades prior. Note the severe thickening and calcification of the aortic and mitral valves. This patient also had severe coronary artery disease, cardiomyopathy, and abnormal pericardial thickening, all likely sequelae of his prior cancer treatment.

radiation dose, volume of the heart exposed, and specific techniques used, but other factors play a role, including age at the time of exposure (younger patients are at higher risk), concurrent treatment with anthracycline-containing chemotherapy regimen, and traditional cardiac risk factors. Although exposure of the heart to >35 Gy is commonly considered to increase risk, recent studies have shown risk with lower doses as well. The Childhood Cancer Survivor Study found a greater than two-fold increase in risk of heart failure, myocardial infarction, pericardial disease, and valve disease at radiation doses of 15–35 Gy.[171] Another smaller study found a relative risk of 12.5 for cardiac death in those exposed to cardiac doses of 5–15 Gy, and relative risk of 25 at >15 Gy.[172]

Radiation treatment for Hodgkin's lymphoma carries the highest risk of cardiac complications due to proximity of mediastinal nodes to the heart, younger age at diagnosis, and good potential for long-term survival. The relative risk of fatal cardiac events has been reported to be 2.2–7.2 after radiation for Hodgkin's disease.[173] Because it may take decades for radiation-related heart disease to become clinically manifest, the discovery of major complications may not appear until late follow-up assessments are undertaken. The most common complications are valvular lesions and myocardial infarction but also seen are restrictive cardiomyopathy, dysrhythmia, and autonomic dysfunction. Pericardial disease has become less prevalent with better cardiac shielding and other technical improvements (Figure 10).[174]

Breast cancer cohorts provide us with the richest body of evidence regarding radiation effects on the heart, due both to overall disease prevalence and to the opportunity to compare right-sided versus left-sided disease. Several studies have utilized this natural control group to distinguish between systemic effects of chemotherapeutics and those of localized cardiac radiation. A strong correlation between radiation therapy and increased cardiovascular mortality was established by many early randomized trials. Improved techniques, including better cardiac shielding, tangential fields, and respiratory gating have certainly reduced or delayed cardiac morbidity and mortality, yet significant risk probably remains, especially for left-sided cancers. Inclusion of the right or left internal mammary lymph node chain in the radiation field increases cardiac exposure and has been shown to increase subsequent cardiovascular complications. Similar to the data for Hodgkin's lymphoma, risk of cardiac events after radiation therapy increases with duration of follow-up, treatment with anthracyclines, and the presence of traditional cardiovascular risk factors.

Clinical manifestations of radiation cardiotoxicity are broad. Acute pericarditis can occur at the time of radiation treatment, and pericardial effusion is commonly seen in the acute and subacute setting but can also be chronic. Distinction from malignant pericardial effusion can be difficult and occasionally necessitates fluid analysis by cytology. Cardiac tamponade is rare. Chronic inflammation can manifest as constrictive pericarditis, which can be challenging to diagnose and carries a grave prognosis unless the patient is well enough to undergo surgical pericardiectomy.

Coronary artery disease after radiation can present as angina, myocardial infarction, or sudden death; the risk increases with time. At least two mechanisms appear to be involved in macrovascular disease. First, radiation induces thickening of the arterial wall secondary to intimal and adventitial proliferation; the luminal area is thereby reduced. Second, radiation greatly accelerates atherosclerosis and acts synergistically with that process to enhance cholesterol deposition and luminal ulceration.[175] Thus, as noted above, traditional cardiac risk factors such as smoking and dyslipidemia play a key cooperative role in the pathogenesis. Because of its location, the left anterior descending artery is the most frequently affected.

The treatment of radiation-associated vascular injury is similar to the conventional treatment of ischemic cardiac disease; nitrates, beta-adrenergic blockers, platelet inhibitors, and calcium channel blockers are the mainstays of pharmacological therapy. Invasive approaches for the management of ischemic heart disease are also often helpful; balloon angioplasty, however, often requires inflation pressures that are higher than those ordinarily used, and longer periods of balloon inflation may be required. Bypass surgery may prove more difficult than usual from a technical standpoint because of the smaller vascular lumens and because the surgeon must work in a previously irradiated field. Nevertheless, bypass surgery remains an important option for these patients.

The spectrum of radiation-induced cardiomyopathy includes diastolic dysfunction, restrictive cardiomyopathy, and systolic dysfunction. Small vessel ischemic disease and fibrosis are the predominant underlying pathology, with subsequent ventricular remodeling possible. Restrictive cardiomyopathy can be very difficult to distinguish from pericardial constriction—especially since both may be present in the same patient. Endomyocardial biopsy is sometimes employed prior to pericardiectomy to rule out coexisting myocardial disease, which carries a prohibitive operative mortality.

Valvular involvement, while common, is usually not severe. Nevertheless, valve injury is progressive and can contribute to significant morbidity that accompanies the irradiated heart. The most common lesions found are tricuspid regurgitation, mitral regurgitation, and aortic regurgitation, but aortic stenosis is occasionally encountered. Histologically, the valves show endocardial thickening resembling fibroelastosis.

Radiation injury to the cardiac conduction system has also been noted and is usually suggested by abnormalities on the electrocardiogram. Prolongation of the PR interval is often seen, as are intranodal and infranodal atrioventricular blocks. Complete heart block is occasionally encountered, and pacemaker implantation may prove lifesaving for such patients. Autonomic dysfunction typically causes elevation of the resting heart rate and exaggerated heart rate response to physical exertion.

Key references

The complete reference list can be found on Vital Source version of this title, see inside front cover.

1 Ewer MS, Ewer SM, Suter T. Cardiac complications. In: Holland J, Frei E, eds. *Cancer Medicine*, 9th ed. Wiley-Blackwell.
2 Armstrong WF, Ryan T. *Feigenbaum's Echocardiography*, 8th ed. LWW; 2019: 816. ISBN-13:978-1451194272.
7 Plana JC, Galderisi M, Barac A, et al. Expert consensus for multimodality imaging evaluation of adult patients during and after cancer therapy: a report from the American Society of Echocardiography and the European Association of Cardiovascular Imaging. *J Am Soc Echocardiogr*. 2014;**27**:911–939.
9 Francone M, Dymarkowski S, Kalantzi M, Bogaert J. Magnetic resonance imaging n the evaluation of the pericardium. A pictoral essay. *Radiol Med*. 2005;**109**:64–74.
12 Kramer C. Current and future applications of cardiovascular magnetic resonance imaging. *Cardiol Rev*. 2000;**8**(Jul–Aug):216–222.
13 Ritchie J, Bateman T, Bonow R. Guidelines for clinical use of cardiac radionuclide imaging. Report of the American College of Cardiology/American Heart Association Task Force on Assessment of Diagnostic and Therapeutic Cardiovascular Procedures (Committee on Radionuclide Imaging), developed in association with the American Society of Nuclear Cardiology. *J Am Coll Cardiol*. 1995;**25**:521–547.
15 Ewer MS, Herson J. False positive cardiotoxicity events in cancer-related clinical trials: risks related to imperfect noninvasive parameters. *Chemotherapy*. 2018;**63**:324–329.
20 Garcia-Riego A, Cuinas C, Vilanova J. Malignant pericardial effusion. *Acta Cytol*. 2001;**45**:561–566.
29 Liberman M, Labos C, Sampalis J, et al. Ten-year surgical experience with nontraumatic pericardial effusions: a comparison between the subxyphoid and transthoracic approaches to pericardial window. *Arch Surg*. 2005;**140**:191–195.
30 Tsang T, Seward J, Barnes M, et al. Outcomes of primary and secondary treatment of pericardial effusion in patients with malignancy. *Mayo Clin Proc*. 2000;**75**:248–253.
38 Jafferani A, Yusuf SW, Ewer SM. Cardiac Arrhythmia in the cancer patient. In: Ewer MS, ed. *Cancer and the Heart*, 3rd ed. Shelton, CT: Medical Publishing House-USA; 2019:197–218.
46 Patel C, Mathur M, Escarcega RO, Bove AA. Carcinoid heart disease: current understnading and future directions. *Am Heart J*. 2014;**167**:789–795.
48 Bhattacharyya S, Toumpanakis C, Caplin ME, Davar J. Analysis of 150 patients with carcinoid syndrome seen in a single year at one institutino in the first decade of teh twenty-first century. *Am J Cardiol*. 2008;**101**:378–381.
53 Hassan SA, Banchs J, Iliescu C, et al. Carcinoid heart disease. *Heart*. 2017;**103**: 1488–1495.
61 Di Giovanni B, Gustafson D, Delgado DH. Amyloid transthyretin cardiac amyloidosis: diagnosis and management. *Expert Rev Cardiovasc Ther*. 2019;**17**(9): 673–681.
66 Fontana M, Pica S, Reant P, et al. Prognostic value of late gadolinium enhancement cardiovascular magnetic resonance in cardiac amyloidosis. *Circulation*. 2015;**132**(16):1570–1579.
71 Tuzovic M, Yang EH, Baas AS, et al. Cardiac amyloidosis: diagnosis and treatment strategies. *Curr Oncol Rep*. 2017;**19**:46.
72 Falk RH, Alexander KM, Liao R, Dorbala S. AL (Light-Chain) cardiac amyloidosis: a review of diagnosis and therapy. *J Am Coll Cardiol*. 2016;**68**:1323–1341.
73 Brown JR, Moslehi J, Ewer MS, et al. Incidence of and risk factors for major haemorrhage in patients treated with ibrutinib: an integrated analysis. *Br J Haematol*. 2019;**184**(4):558–569.
75 Kim PY, Ewer MS. Chemotherapy and QT prolongation: overview with clinical perspective. *Curr Treat Options Cardiovasc Med*. 2014;**16**:303–308.
81 European Heart Rhythm Association, Heart Rhythm Society, Zipes DP, et al. ACC/AHA/ESC 2006 guidelines for management of patients with ventricular arrhythmias and the prevention of sudden cardiac death: a report of the American College of Cardiology/American Heart Association Task Force and the European Society of Cardiology Committee for Practice Guidelines (Writing Committee to Develop Guidelines for Management of Patients With Ventricular Arrhythmias and the Prevention of Sudden Cardiac Death). *J Am Coll Cardiol*. 2006;**48**:247–346.
83 Ewer MS, Lippman S. Type II chemotherapy-related cardiac dysfunction: time to recognize a new entity. *J Clin Oncol*. 2005;**23**(13):2900–2902.
87 Herman E, Lipshultz S, Rifai N, et al. Use of cardiac troponin T levels as an indicator of doxorubicin-induced cardiotoxicity. *Can Res*. 1998;**38**:195–197.
90 Swain S, Whaley F, Ewer M. Congestive heart failure in patients treated with doxorubicin: a retrospective analysis of three trials. *Cancer*. 2003;**97**:2869–2879.
98 Ewer MS, Ali MK, Mackay B, et al. A comparison of resting and exercise ejection fractions with cardiac biopsy grades in patients receiving adriamycin. *J Clin Oncol*. 1984;**2**:112–117.
102 Armenian SH, Lacchetti C, Barac A, et al. Prevention and monitoring of cardiac dysfunction in survivors of adult cancers: American Society of Clinical Oncology Clinical Practice Guideline. *J Clin Oncol*. 2017;**35**(8):893–911.
104 Yeh ET, Bickford CL. Cardiovascular complications of cancer therapy: incidence, pathogenesis, diagnosis, and management. *J Am Coll Cardiol*. 2009;**53**: 2231–2247.
110 Ewer M, Martin F, Henderson I, et al. Cardiac safety of liposomal anthracyclines. *Semin Oncol*. 2004;**31**(Suppl 13):161–181.
118 Berrak S, Ewer M, Jaffe N, et al. Doxorubicin cardiotoxicity in children: reduced incidence of cardiac dysfunction associated with continuous-infusion schedules. *Oncol Rep*. 2001;**8**:611–614.
120 Swain S, Whaley F, Gerber M, et al. Cardioprotection with dexrazoxane for doxorubicin-containing chemotherapy in advanced breast cancer. *J Clin Oncol*. 1997;**15**(4):1318–1332.
121 Swain S, Whaley F, Gerber M, et al. Delayed administration of dexrazoxane provides cardioprotection for patients with advanced breast cancer treated with doxorubicin-containing chemotherapy. *J Clin Oncol*. 1997;**15**(4):1333–1340.
123 Lipshultz SE, Scully RE, Lipsitz SR, et al. Assessment of dexrazoxane as a cardioprotectant in doxorubicin-treated children with high-risk acute lymphoblastic leukaemia: long-term follow-up of a prospective, randomised, multicentre trial. *Lancet Oncol*. 2010;**2010**:950–961.
124 Ky B, Veipongsa P, Yeh ETH, et al. Emerging paradigms in cardiomyopathies associated with cancer therapies. *Circ Res*. 2013;**113**:754–764.
128 Ewer MS. Anthracycline cardiotoxicity: clinical aspects, recognition, monitoring, treatment, and prevention. In: Ewer MS, ed. *Cancer and the Heart*, 3rd ed. Cary, North Carolina: People's Medical Publishing House-USA; 2019:47–78.
130 de Korte MA, de Vries EG, Lub-de Hooge MN, et al. 111Indium-trastuzumab visualises myocardial human epidermal growth factor receptor 2 expression shortly after anthracycline treatment but not during heart failure: a clue to uncover the mechanisms of trastuzumab-related cardiotoxicity. *Eur J Cancer*. 2007;**43**(14):2046–2051.
135 Tan-Chiu E, Yothers G, Romond E, et al. Assessment of cardiac dysfunction in a randomized trial comparing doxorubicin and cyclophosphamide followed by paclitaxel, with or without trastuzumab as adjuvant therapy in

136 Suter T, Procter M, Van Veldhuisen D, et al. Trastuzumab-associated cardiac adverse effects in the Herceptin Adjuvant Trial. *J Clin Oncol.* 2007;**25**:3859–3865.

137 Joensuu H, Bono P, Kataja V, et al. Fluorouracil, epirubicin and cyclophosphamide with either docetaxel or vioorelbine, with or without trastuzumab as adjuvant treatment of breast cancer. Final results of the FinHer Trial. *J Clin Oncol.* 2009;**27**:5685–5692.

140 Ewer MS, Vooletich M, Durand J, et al. Reversibility of trastuzumab-telated cardiotoxicity: new insights based on clinical course and response to medical treatment. *J Clin Oncol.* 2005;**23**:7820–7827.

141 Ewer MS, Ewer SM. Cardiotoxicity of anticancer treatments. *Nat Rev Cardiol.* 2015;**12**(9):547–558.

142 Ewer MS, Tekumalla SH, Walding A, Atuah KN. Cardiac safety of osimertinib: a review of data. *J Clin Oncol.* 2021;**39**(4):328–337.

143 Piccart M, Procter M, Fumagalli D, et al. APHINITY steering committee and investigators. Adjuvant pertuzumab and trastuzumab in early HER2-positive breast cancer in the APHINITY trial: 6 Years' follow-up. *J Clin Oncol.* 2021;**39**(13):1448–1457.

145 Ewer MS, Suter TM, Lenihan DJ, et al. Cardiovaxcular events among 1090 cancer patients treated with sunitinib, interferon or placebo: a comprehensive adjudicated database analysis demonstrating clinically meaningful reversibility of cardiac events. *Eur J Cancer.* 2014;**50**:2162–2170.

150 Cardinale D, Colombo A, Lamantia G, et al. Anthracycline-induced cardiomyopathy: clinical relevance and response to pharmacologic therapy. *J Am Coll Cardiol.* 2010;**55**:213–220.

160 Tajiri K, Aonuma K, Sekine I. Immune checkpoint inhibitor-related myocarditis. *Jpn J Clin Oncol.* 2018;**48**(1):7–12.

161 Tajiri K, Ieda M. Cardiac complications in immune checkpoint inhibition therapy. *Front Cardiovasc Med.* 2019;**6**:3.

166 Zhong J, Ali AN, Voloschin AD, et al. Bevacizumab-induced hypertension is a predictive marker for improved outcomes in patients with recurrent glioblastoma treated with bevacizumab. *Cancer.* 2015;**121**(9):1456–1462.

131 Respiratory complications

Vickie R. Shannon, MD ■ George A. Eapen, MD ■ Carlos A. Jimenez, MD ■ Horiana B. Grosu, MD ■ Rodolfo C. Morice, MD ■ Lara Bashoura, MD ■ Ajay Sheshadre, MD ■ Scott E. Evans, MD ■ Roberto Adachi, MD ■ Michael Kroll, MD ■ Saadia A. Faiz, MD ■ Diwakar D. Balachandran, MD ■ Selvaraj E. Pravinkumar, MD, FRCP ■ Burton F. Dickey, MD

Overview

The respiratory system is particularly susceptible to complications of cancer and cancer therapy. This vulnerability arises from the stringent architectural requirements for gas exchange, the continuous exposure of the respiratory tract to the external environment, and the severe symptoms that can accompany respiratory compromise. Gas exchange requires patent airways, an effective musculoskeletal ventilatory pump, a thin alveolocapillary membrane, and adequate blood flow through the pulmonary circulation. In cancer patients, primary and metastatic tumors of the chest compromise major airways; pleural effusions externally compress the lungs and impair diaphragmatic function; direct, hematogenous or lymphangitic spread of tumor replaces functioning lung parenchyma; resectional surgery reduces parenchymal volume; nonresectional surgery can transiently impair lung function; radiotherapy, chemotherapy, stem cell therapy, and infection injure the vulnerable alveolocapillary membrane; tumors directly or indirectly compromise the musculoskeletal pump; venous thromboembolism and pulmonary vasculopathy obstruct pulmonary blood flow.

The normal respiratory system contains considerable physiologic reserve, such that surgical loss of one lung is generally well tolerated. However, in cancer patients, insults to multiple components of the respiratory system may result in progressive loss of physiologic reserve and increasing dyspnea. Dyspnea, cough, wheezing, stridor, chest pain, and hemoptysis are common symptoms in the cancer setting that lead to pulmonary consultation.

In this article, we will discuss the pathophysiology, diagnosis, and management of the major respiratory complications of cancer and its therapy. We begin with the direct effects of cancer and cancer therapies on the lungs, review major indirect effects of cancer on the lungs, and end with respiratory failure in the cancer patient.

Malignant airway obstruction

Malignant airspace disease may be central or peripheral, focal or diffuse, endoluminal, extraluminal, or both.

Common cancer types and clinical presentation

The most common cause of malignant airway obstruction is direct extension from an adjacent tumor, particularly bronchogenic carcinoma. Esophageal and thyroid malignancies also frequently extend directly into the airways. Primary tumors of the major airways are relatively rare, with squamous cell carcinoma, adenoid cystic carcinoma, and carcinoid tumors most often implicated.[1] Airway compromise can also occur from metastatic renal and breast carcinomas or intrathoracic lymphomas. Both endoluminal disease and extrinsic compression by tumor may severely compromise airway luminal diameter. Reduction in airway caliber and architectural distortion synergistically impair airflow obstruction and mucus clearance, leading to increased work of breathing and dyspnea.[2] Luminal narrowing of the trachea and mainstem bronchi typically manifests as dyspnea, cough, wheeze, stridor, and atelectasis. Airway obstruction beyond the mainstem bronchi usually results in atelectasis, postobstructive pneumonitis, cough, and dyspnea. Individual patient presentations range from asymptomatic discovery on staging work-up to frank respiratory failure due to critical airway obstruction.[3] Exertional dyspnea typically occurs when tracheal diameter is reduced below 8 mm. Further reduction in tracheal diameter to <5 mm is usually associated with dyspnea at rest.[4] Chronic obstructive pulmonary disease (COPD) exacerbations or mucosal edema and increased secretions that accompany superimposed pneumonias may precipitate respiratory failure, even in patients with only moderate tumor-related airflow limitation. Symptoms may thus improve with measures directed at treating the infection or COPD exacerbation.

Differential diagnosis

While critical airway obstruction is not usually a diagnostic challenge, the clinical presentation of subcritical obstruction can be. Stridor indicates significant tracheal obstruction. Other findings, including dyspnea and wheezing, are prominent but nonspecific clinical symptoms that denote airflow limitation. Concurrent conditions, such as congestive heart failure, pleural effusions, and pulmonary emboli may produce similar symptoms, obscuring the diagnosis.

Diagnostic evaluation

The diagnostic workup is aimed at establishing a definitive diagnosis, quantifying airflow limitation, and delineating anatomic extent in an effort to optimize therapeutic strategies. The characteristic blunting noted in the flow-volume loop upon pulmonary function testing often provides an indication of tracheal obstruction. However, this is a relatively insensitive test, with positive findings noted only with tracheal diameters below 10 mm.[5] Spirometry may also precipitate frank respiratory failure in patients with severe airway obstruction and should be used with caution in this subgroup of patients. Rarely, deviation or compression of the trachea may be seen on plain chest radiographs. Plain chest X-rays otherwise are not helpful in defining the anatomic extent of tumor or therapeutic options. Standard chest computed tomography as well as the latest iterations of low dose, multidetector scanners and advanced airway imaging techniques that allow multiplanar and three-dimensional

---

Holland-Frei Cancer Medicine, Tenth Edition. Edited by Robert C. Bast, John C. Byrd, Carlo M. Croce, Ernest Hawk, Fadlo R. Khuri, Raphael E. Pollock, Apostolia M. Tsimberidou, Christopher G. Willett, and Cheryl L. Willman.
© 2023 John Wiley & Sons, Inc. Published 2023 by John Wiley & Sons, Inc.

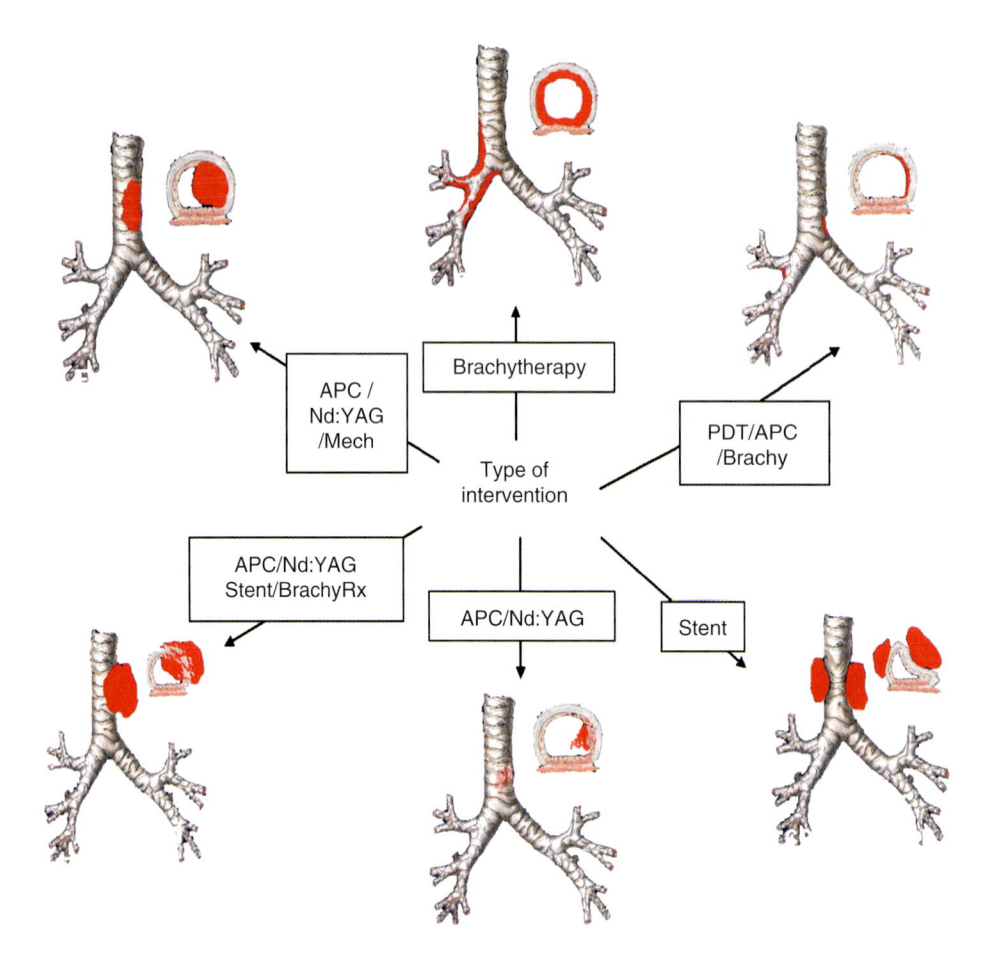

Figure 1 Approach to airway obstruction using interventional bronchoscopic therapy. Source: Courtesy Dr R. Morice.

reconstruction provide valuable additional information regarding the extent of the lesion and guidance in optimizing therapeutic strategies.[6] Bronchoscopy, either flexible or rigid, remains the gold standard in the work-up of airway obstruction. Histologic confirmation of malignancy can be obtained at the time of the examination. Furthermore, bronchoscopy offers direct visualization of the lesion, which permits precise characterization of tumor vascularity and the extent of obstruction, as well as the degree of obstruction attributable to endoluminal versus extraluminal disease. Recent reports have also supported the use of endobronchial ultrasonography as an adjunctive tool in treatment planning.[7]

Management of malignant airway obstruction

Tumor characteristics, including histologic type, stage and location, and patient attributes, such as urgency of presentation and performance status, dictate management. Therapeutic strategies vary based on the location and type of obstruction, as well as the local expertise and available institution-specific resources. Surgical resection provides the best prospect for long-term disease control and should be considered in all patients during the initial evaluation. Localized involvement of the small airways and lung parenchyma is best treated by surgical resection, if feasible. In many cases, however, external beam radiotherapy or systemic chemotherapy may be the only treatment options. Patients with central airway obstruction often present with either medically or surgically unresectable disease. While a comprehensive review of the various modalities is beyond the scope of this article, some basic principles are outlined (Figure 1). In emergent cases, the barrel of the rigid bronchoscope may be used to mechanically core out the tumor and dilate the airways, providing palliation. Flexible bronchoscopy and balloon bronchoplasty may be used to dilate the airways in less urgent cases.[8] Electrocautery, argon plasma coagulation, laser therapy, cryotherapy, brachytherapy, and photodynamic therapy are reasonable approaches for predominantly endoluminal disease (Figure 2). Extraluminal-predominant disease may be best treated with external beam radiotherapy and endobronchial stent placement (Figure 3). Since most lesions are mixed with endo- and extraluminal components, multimodality therapy, using endobronchial laser therapy with mechanical debulking followed by stent placement and subsequent consolidation with external beam radiotherapy, for example, is quite common. Symptom palliation, resulting in reduction in levels of care, may be accomplished in most instances with the judicious application of endoscopic techniques.[9] Patients should be carefully evaluated with an early referral to an experienced bronchoscopist who can match the various therapeutic modalities available to the individual patient.

Malignant pleural effusions

Malignant pleural effusions (MPEs) are a common clinical problem in the cancer setting that signifies advanced disease. In the United States, the incidence approaches 150,000 cases annually. Malignant pleural involvement without effusion occurs in up to 45% of patients with metastatic disease to the pleura.[10] In primary pleural malignancies, such as malignant mesothelioma, pleural

Respiratory complications 1781

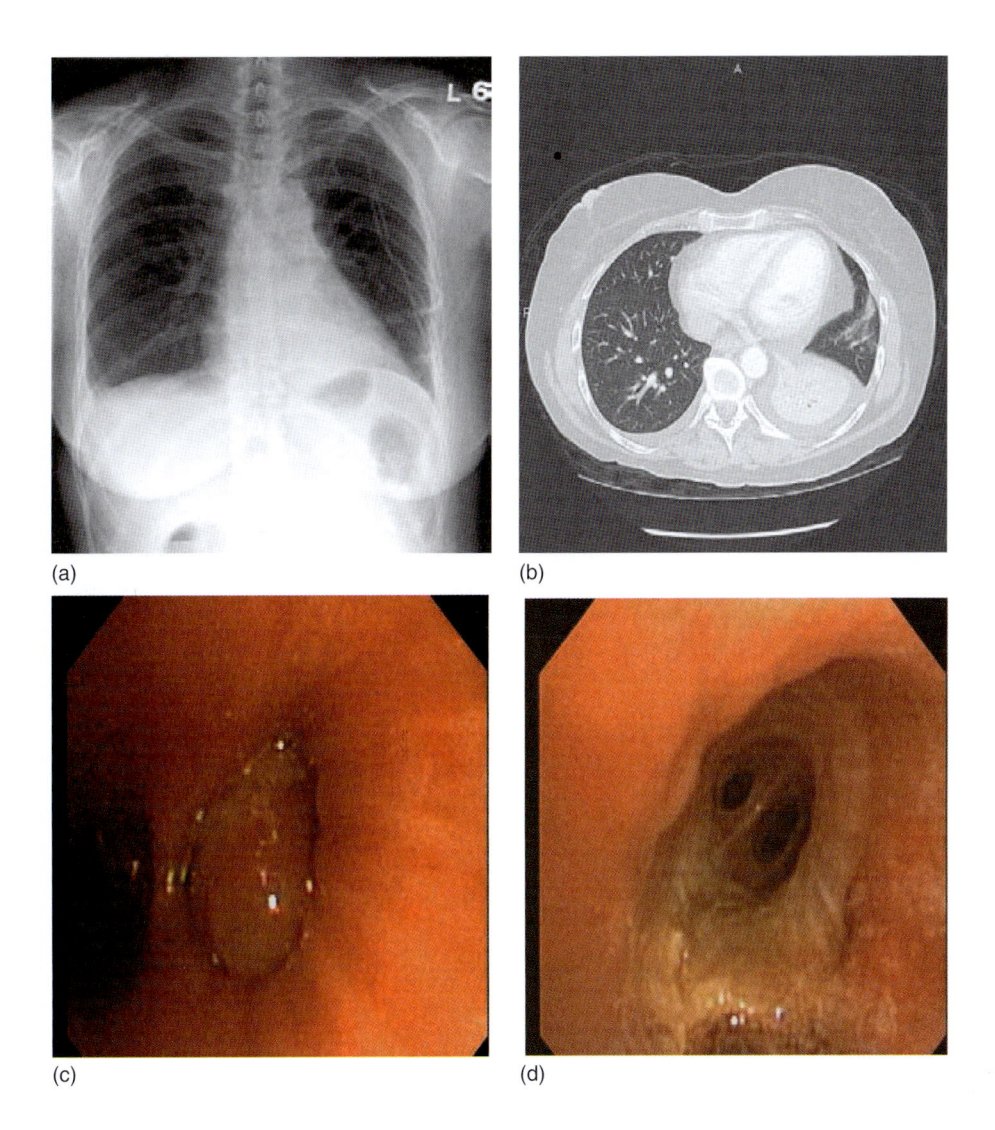

Figure 2 Left lower lobe collapse secondary to metastatic sarcoma (a and b). Complete obstruction of the LLL basilar segments due to a large obstructing tumor was noted at bronchoscopy (c) which was removed using snare forceps and argon plasma coagulation, revealing a patent distal airway (d).

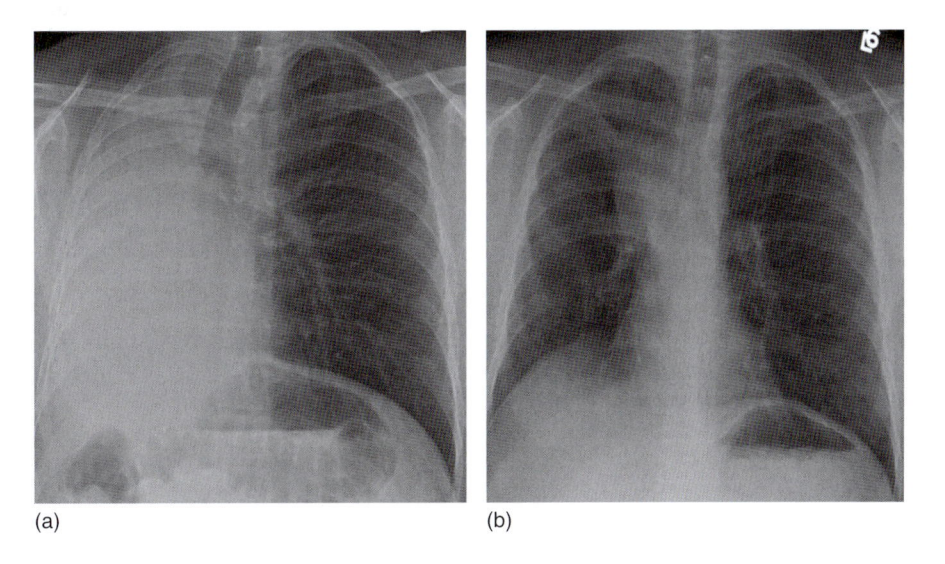

Figure 3 Complete opacification of the right thorax secondary to obstruction of the right mainstem bronchus by a large, predominantly extraluminal mass (a). A wire stent was placed into the bronchus intermedius (b), resulting in partial reexpansion of the right lung.

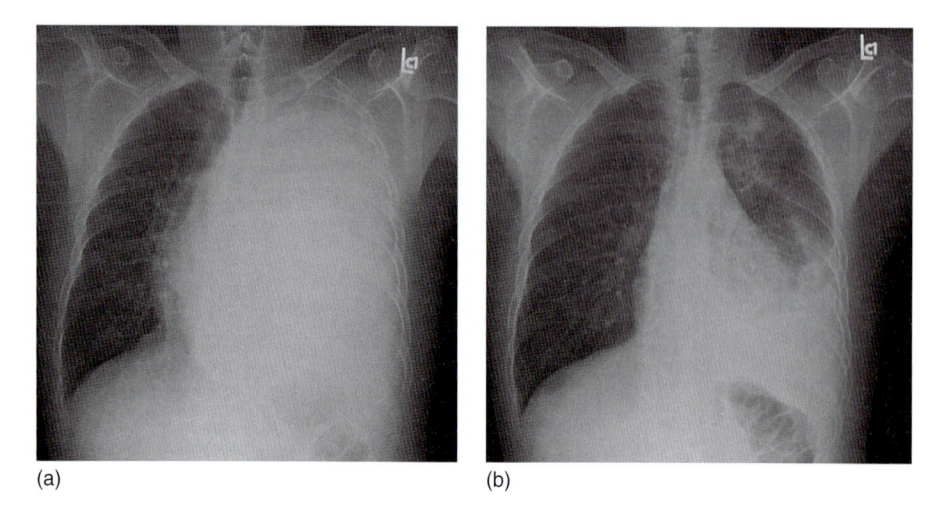

Figure 4 Large left-sided pleural effusion causing opacification of the left hemithorax and contralateral shift of the mediastinum (a). Following thoracentesis (b) the mediastinum shifted back the midline.

effusions may be absent. Almost any type of neoplasm can affect the pleura. Lung cancer accounts for up to half of all MPEs, followed in frequency by breast carcinoma and lymphoma. Pleural effusions may occur with leukemias and myelodysplastic syndrome. In patients with leukemia, pleural effusions are most often due to infection and, to a lesser extent, leukemic infiltration of the pleura.[11] Unfortunately, in 5–10% of patients, a primary tumor cannot be identified.[12,13] Most MPEs arise from tumor emboli to the visceral pleura, with secondary parietal pleural involvement, presumably as a result of seeding from the visceral pleura. Direct extension of tumor from the lung, chest wall, mediastinal structures, or diaphragm and hematogenous metastasis to the parietal pleura are other mechanisms that contribute to the genesis of MPE formation.[14] In addition to direct tumor involvement of the pleura, MPEs can result from lymphatic blockage anywhere between the parietal pleura and the mediastinal lymph nodes.[15] Elevations in the local production of vascular endothelial growth factor (VEGF), a potent mediator of increased vascular permeability, also play a significant role in the formation of MPEs.[16] Among VEGF homologs, VEGF-D showed a 92.6% rate of positive expression in a study of MPE and may be a useful marker in the diagnosis.[17] Seventeen percent of all pleural effusions in patients with cancer are "paramalignant," a term used for effusions that occur in the setting of cancer that is not caused by direct malignant involvement of the pleural space.[14] These effusions develop as a result of local or systemic effects of the tumor, complications of cancer therapy, or concurrent nonmalignant disease.[18] Lymphatic obstruction is associated with both malignant and paramalignant effusions and is the most common cause of paramalignant effusions. Other common causes include bronchial obstruction, trapped lung, and pulmonary embolism (PE).

Clinical manifestations, imaging studies, and diagnosis

Constitutional symptoms are common signals of advanced disease, and thus malaise, weight loss, and poor appetite may become more frequent as the performance status worsens. Hemoptysis and chest wall pain are less common symptoms and may indicate malignant endobronchial disease and tumoral invasion of the chest wall. Standard chest X-rays and ultrasonography of the chest provide critical information in the initial evaluation of pleural effusions, including effusion size, position of the mediastinum and diaphragms, presence of loculations, and air–fluid levels within the pleural space, and characteristics of the underlying lung parenchyma. Knowledge regarding the position of the mediastinum is imperative in therapeutic decision-making. Large pleural effusions with contralateral mediastinal shift typically require prompt therapeutic thoracentesis, while those with a centered mediastinum or ipsilateral shift of the mediastinum should be approached cautiously (Figures 4 and 5). In addition to pleural effusions, other disease processes that may cause an ipsilateral shift of the mediastinum or a centered mediastinum with hemithorax opacification include a frozen mediastinum associated with malignant mesothelioma or lymphoma, atelectasis related to occlusion of the ipsilateral central airway, or extensive tumoral infiltration of the ipsilateral lung simulating a large effusion.[19]

Computer tomography (CT) is helpful in identifying loculated effusions; it offers more detailed anatomical information of the chest wall, parietal and visceral pleurae, mediastinal structures, and lung parenchyma, and is especially valuable in delineating alternate diagnoses.[19] Ultrasonography provides guidance in locating the optimal site for thoracentesis and is particularly helpful in the setting of loculated pleural effusions. The identification of entrapped lung by ultrasonography using tissue movement may permit deformation (strain) analysis prior to thoracentesis.[20,21] Positron emission tomography (PET) with ^{18}F-fluorodeoxyglucose (FDG) and magnetic resonance imaging (MRI) are both helpful in highlighting extrapleural extension of disease.[22] PET imaging provides valuable information associated with malignant mesothelioma; however, its utility in the evaluation of other malignant pleural diseases has not been established.

Chemical analysis reveals an exudative effusion in most cases, with only 5% of MPEs being transudates.[18] Positive pleural fluid cytology, noted in 62% of cases, represents the diagnostic cornerstone of MPEs.[22] Tumor marker measurements improve the diagnostic yield of cytologically negative effusions by 33% and are particularly valuable when lymphoma, leukemia, or multiple myeloma is suspected.[23,24] The role of flow cytometry in the study of mesotheliomas remains controversial.[25] Pleuroscopic pleural biopsies have a 95% sensitivity in the diagnosis of pleural malignancies, and diagnostic yield increases only incrementally (1%) when combined with pleural fluid cytology. Image-guided pleural biopsies have similar high sensitivity.[21,26] By contrast, closed

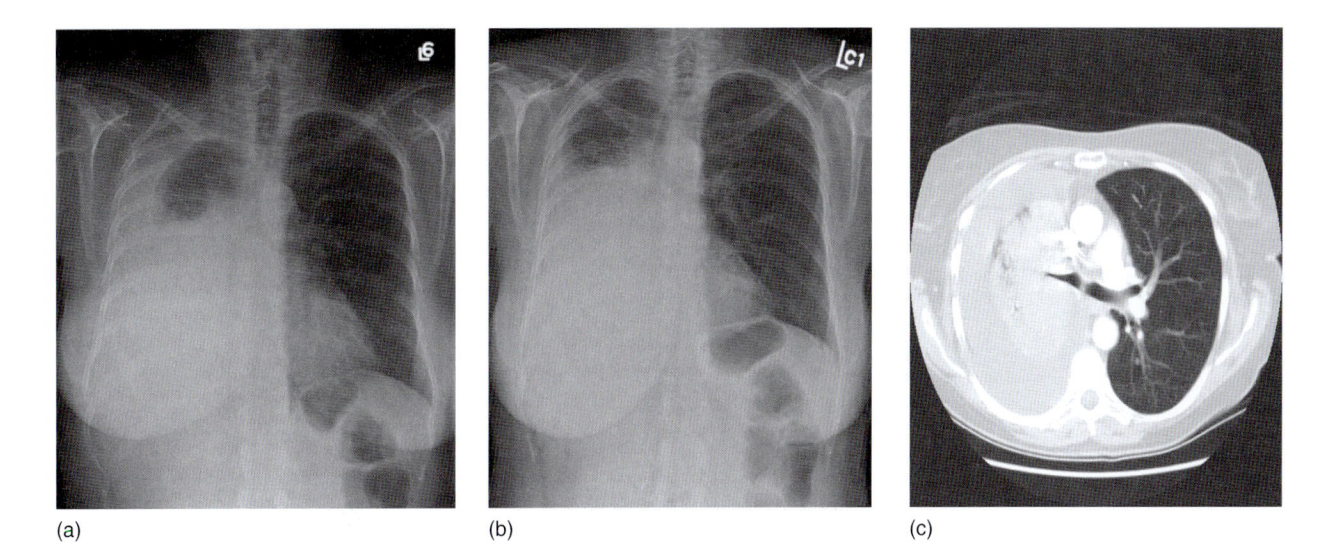

Figure 5 Large right-sided pleural effusion (a) with ipsilateral shift of the mediastinum following thoracentesis (b), indicating volume loss secondary to atelectasis or mass. A CT scan of the chest (c) demonstrates a large mass compressing the right mainstem bronchus.

pleural biopsy has a diagnostic yield of only 44% but improves to 77% when combined with an analysis of pleural fluid cytology.[22]

Management of malignant pleural effusions

Because MPEs often signal advanced disease and incurability, treatment efforts are frequently directed toward palliation. Hence, awareness of available therapeutic options tailored to individual patient needs is important. The patient's performance status and information regarding prior thoracenteses, including the volume of fluid evacuated, whether lung reexpansion and symptom palliation were obtained, and the time interval between repeated taps, are important components of the evaluation that help to guide further therapy. Performance status is the best predictor of survival in patients with recurrent MPEs.[27] The presence of local chest wall abnormalities, future cancer treatment plans, the patient's preferences, and the availability of family support influence the approach to these patients. Palliation with simple therapeutic thoracentesis represents a reasonable approach to patients with newly diagnosed chemo- or radiosensitive tumors, such as lymphoma, breast, small-cell lung, germ cell, ovarian, prostate, and thyroid neoplasms, while awaiting response to definitive therapy. After the initial clinical and chest X-ray evaluation, a symptom-limited therapeutic thoracentesis is recommended. A recent consensus statement by the American Thoracic Society and the European Respiratory Society recommends that not more than 1.0–1.5 L of fluid be slowly evacuated from the pleural space in one sitting and that drainage should be discontinued if the patient develops symptoms of dyspnea, cough, or chest discomfort.[28] However, in our experience, patients can safely tolerate the removal of 1.5 L or more of fluid in one sitting as long as there are no procedure-related symptoms of chest pain, cough, or dyspnea. We have also observed that symptom-limited, large-volume thoracentesis appears to be safe in patients with ipsilateral mediastinal shift on preprocedure chest imaging studies.[29]

Measurement of pleural pressure by manometry during large-volume thoracentesis does not alter procedure-related chest discomfort.[30] In addition, thoracentesis via vacuum bottle system and gravity drainage are both safe and result in comparable levels of procedural comfort and dyspnea improvement. Active vacuum bottle suction requires less total procedural time.[31]

Lung re-expansion following thoracentesis may be assessed with posterior–anterior (PA) and lateral chest X-rays. In 97% of patients, MPEs will recur within 1 month, with most of these effusions reappearing within 1–3 days following fluid evacuation.[32] Patients with limited life expectancies (<30 days) and poor performance status or those in which pleural fluid reaccumulation is slow are best treated with repeated therapeutic thoracentesis. Repeated thoracentesis is a reasonable approach for patients with malignancies that are expected to respond to chemotherapy and/or radiation therapy (RT). However, frequent thoracentesis may trigger the production of local cytokines and fibrin, resulting in pleural fluid loculation, which not only complicates further thoracenteses but also limits future modes of palliation.[33]

The use of indwelling pleural catheters (IPCs) has been accepted over the past few years as an alternative palliative option for patients with recurrent MPEs. Ideal candidates for this palliative modality include patients with life expectancies in excess of 30 days and in whom prior thoracenteses affected symptomatic relief. Considerations for IPC implantation are valid in this group of patients regardless of lung re-expansion following thoracentesis. IPCs may be placed in an outpatient setting. Following documentation of proper catheter position, the patient, trained family members, or caregivers may drain the fluid intermittently at home. When evaluated in prospective fashion daily drainage of pleural fluid via an IPC led to a higher rate of autopleurodesis and faster time to liberation from catheter.[34] Drainage should be continued until the patient develops cough or chest discomfort, or the fluid stops flowing spontaneously, presumably because the pleural space has been emptied. In an unpublished study at our institution, 92% of patients treated with IPCs reported significant relief of dyspnea, and 52% achieved effective pleurodesis. The mean time from catheter insertion to catheter removal was 32 days. Catheter-related complications were observed in only 4% of the patients, including one patient with empyema and two patients with persistent pain at the insertion site. In another study, only 6% of patients required additional drainage of fluid following removal of the catheter.[35] Patients who have chemotherapy or radiation after catheter placement and those who are more short of breath at baseline have greatest improvements in utility.[36] In a subgroup analysis, patients meeting criteria for a pleurodesis procedure achieved 70% effective pleurodesis after insertion of IPC.[37]

Traditionally, chemical pleurodesis has been the most widely used method to control recurrent MPE. Unfortunately, the lack of prospective studies precludes comparative analyses of efficacy, safety, and cost of the existing chemical agents and pleurodesis techniques. The results from available literature suggest that nonchemotherapeutic agents are more efficacious and the most cost-effective sclerosants.[28] Sterilized, asbestos-free talc is the preferred pleurodesing agent. Complications vary with the surface characteristics of the talc particles. The use of talc particles that are less than 5 μm in size has been associated with pulmonary injury, including acute pneumonitis and respiratory failure associated with adult respiratory distress syndrome, and should be avoided.[38] The safety of large-particle talc for pleurodesis was recently confirmed in a European multicenter trial in which no association with adult respiratory distress syndrome was identified.[39]

The superiority of thoracoscopic talc insufflation over talc slurry as a method of administration of the sclerosant is a matter of debate. Success rates of >90% have been reported for both techniques, without significant differences in the rate of overall complications or disease recurrence.[28] The largest published prospective randomized trial comparing thoracoscopic talc insufflation and talc slurry included 501 patients with a performance status of 1 or 2. Results showed no difference in 30-day survival rates and pleurodesis success rates between chest tube talc slurry and thoracoscopic talc poudrage. Unexpected high morbidity and mortality rates were reported in both groups. A subset analysis suggested that thoracoscopic talc insufflation may be advantageous for patients with lung or breast cancer.[40] Comparing IPCs vs talc pleurodesis in prospective fashion among patients with MPE and no previous pleurodesis, the authors found no significant difference between IPCs and talc pleurodesis in relieving patient-reported dyspnea.[41] In addition, there was no significant difference in the mean cost of managing patients with IPCs compared with talc pleurodesis, however, for patients with limited survival, IPC appears less costly.[42] In 2018, Bhatnagar et al. published the first randomized controlled trial demonstrating significantly higher success rates of pleurodesis in the outpatient setting using medical-grade talc administered through the IPC.[43] Based on the available information, our group considers all patients with a good performance status (ECOG 0, 1, or 2), and in whom symptomatic relief and lung re-expansion is achieved after initial drainage of the pleural fluid, for either IPC placement or pleurodesis with pleuroscopic talc poudrage as the preferred palliative modalities. Rarely, alternative modalities such as pleuroperitoneal shunts and parietal pleurectomy are used in the management of recurrent symptomatic effusions following pleurodesis failures or effusions associated with trapped lung.

Chylous effusions associated with malignancy are controlled by treating the primary tumor. Prolonged loss of chyle, a protein-rich, fat-laden, and lymphocyte-predominant fluid, may result in lymphopenia, severe nutritional depletion, and water and electrolyte loss. Mortality due to chylothorax can be as high as 50%. Among those patients with recurrent symptomatic chylothorax and cancer relapse or progressive disease despite adequate treatment, parenteral alimentation and talc pleurodesis and IPC placement represent reasonable treatment alternatives.[44,45] Pleuroperitoneal shunt placement appears to be an attractive option, however, pleuroperitoneal shunt pump mechanism displaces only 1.5–2.5 mL at a time, making its use cumbersome and the incidence of obstruction of the pump is high. Embolization of the thoracic duct represents an alternative strategy in the management of recurrent chylous effusions. This procedure appears to be well tolerated, but definitive evidence of its efficacy in the cancer population is not available.

Parietal pleurectomy, decortication, and pleuro-pneumonectomy are associated with high mortality rates and do not provide better symptom control than other palliative options.[28] The utilization of compounds to block VEGF either alone or in combination with other palliative modalities appears promising. However, the final results of a single-arm phase II clinical trial of the VEGF receptor inhibitor, vandetanib, combined with intrapleural catheter placement in patients with non-small-cell lung cancer (NSCLC) and recurrent MPE did not significantly reduce time to pleurodesis.[46]

In summary, in patients with limited life expectancies, modalities that offer the best chance for palliation of symptoms, the lowest procedure-related morbidity and mortality, and the shortest hospital stay represent a reasonable approach to the management of recurrent malignant effusions. A multidisciplinary approach (Figure 6), involving oncology, pulmonary medicine, interventional radiology, and thoracic surgery, offers optimal opportunities to achieve these goals.

Postsurgical respiratory insufficiency

Diagnostic evaluation

The initial approach to the patient with an anatomically resectable tumor includes strategies to determine the patient's functional operability and the predicted long-term pulmonary disability following the loss of the resected lung. This may be accomplished through pulmonary-specific testing as well as a general assessment aimed at identifying and optimizing control of any coexisting systemic diseases. The pulmonary evaluation consists of three sequential steps: (1) measurement of baseline pulmonary function; (2) quantitative radionuclide regional ventilation-perfusion pulmonary studies to estimate expected postoperative lung function; and (3) exercise testing for patients that do not meet acceptable results on the two previous steps.[47] Among the pulmonary function tests that have been used as predictors of postoperative outcome, reduced values of forced expiratory volume in 1 second (FEV_1) and diffusing capacity for carbon monoxide (DLCO) are the most reproducible and most frequently used parameters for predicting complications of lung resection.[48] For decision-making, values of FEV_1 reported as percent of predicted that take into account variations in patients' height, gender, and race are preferred over values reported in absolute units (L). In our laboratory, more than half of patients with an FEV_1 between 60% and 80% of predicted have an estimated postpneumonectomy FEV_1 by radionuclide studies that are below acceptable values for safe resection (<40% of predicted). Therefore, we recommend that only those patients with baseline FEV_1 and DLCO ≥ 80% of predicted and no clinical evidence of contralateral pulmonary disease be considered for resection without further testing. All other patients should undergo a "split function" evaluation, which is a quantitative radionuclide assessment of regional lung ventilation and/or perfusion. In split function studies, the uptake of radioactive ions by various regions in each lung is measured by inhalation of ^{133}Xe or by intravenous administration of ^{133}Xe dissolved in saline or ^{99}Tc macroaggregates. In practice, estimates of lung perfusion alone are easiest and most commonly measured. The percentage of radioactivity contributed by each lung correlates with the contribution to the overall function of that lung. The predicted postoperative FEV_1 (FEV_1ppo) and predicted postoperative DLCO (DLCOppo) are calculated by subtracting the percent functional uptake of

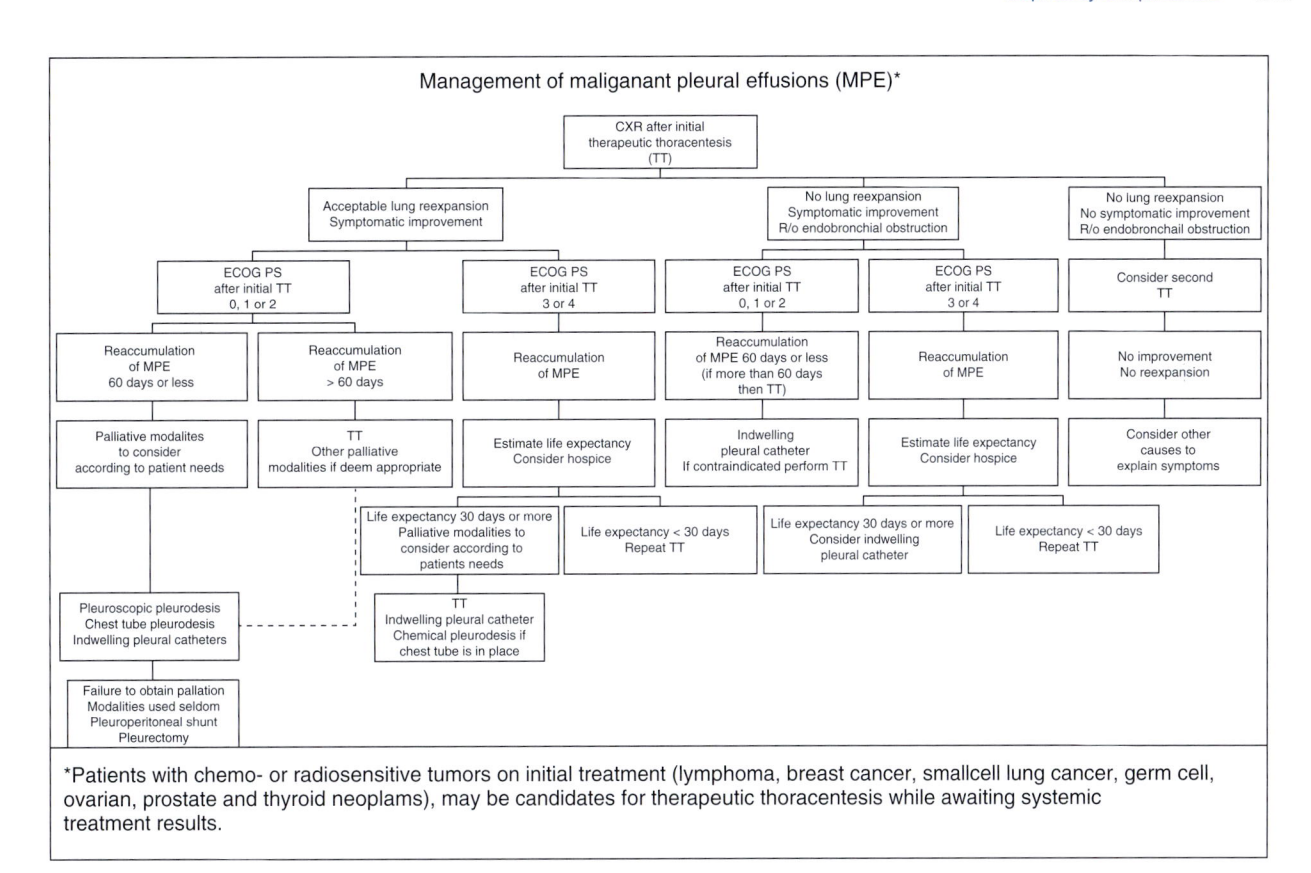

Figure 6 Management of malignant pleural effusions (MPE).

the region to be resected from the total uptake. Several investigators have documented the usefulness of split function studies for predicting both the risk of complications and the loss of pulmonary function after pulmonary resection.[49,50] In these studies, preoperative predicted values are close to measured postoperative values for pneumonectomy and for resections involving more than three segments.[51] Pulmonary function remains relatively stable after pneumonectomy. Predictions for a smaller resection, such as a lobectomy, however, are less reliable, owing to a disproportionate early loss, followed by significant functional improvement with time.[52] Kearney et al. also described a low FEV_1ppo as the only significant independent predictor of complications.[53] Other variables, including age ≥60, male sex, history of smoking, pneumonectomy, hypercarbia ($pCO_2 \geq 45$ mm Hg), desaturations on exercise oximetry ($SaO_2 \leq 90\%$), and a preoperative $FEV1 \leq 1L$ were not predictive of complications. Markos et al.[54] reported that a DLCOppo <40% of predicted was associated with higher morbidity and mortality and was the best predictor of postoperative respiratory failure. In summary, an FEV_1 ppo and DLCO ppo of ≥40% of predicted on split function studies represent safe preoperative criteria for lung resection, including pneumonectomy. Patients that do not meet these criteria but are candidates for lesser surgeries, such as a lobectomy or segmentectomy should undergo further evaluation with exercise testing.

The rationale for using exercise testing in these high-risk patients is based on two concepts: (1) lung function is not the only determinant of performance and, (2) losses for lobectomies or lesser resections improve over time and tend to be overestimated by radiospirometric studies.[47] Exercise testing also offers the advantage of examining cardiopulmonary and musculoskeletal interactions during stress in a single study. The most validated form of exercise testing is cycle ergometry with incremental workloads to the symptom-limited maximum ($\dot{V}O_{2peak}$). Using this method, Smith et al found that only 1 of 10 patients with a $\dot{V}O_{2peak} > 20$ mL/kg/min developed complications postoperatively, whereas all patients with a $\dot{V}O_{2peak} < 15$ mL/kg/min had complications.[55] We conducted two studies on patients that had been considered inoperable because of $FEV_1 \leq 40\%$ of predicted, FEV_1 ppo $\leq 33\%$ of predicted, and/or arterial $PCO_2 \geq 45$ mm Hg. Patients that reached a $\dot{V}O_{2peak} \geq 15$ mL/kg/min underwent surgical treatment; others were referred to radiation and/or chemotherapy. All surgically treated patients were extubated within 24 h and the median time to discharge following surgery was 8 days. There were no in-hospital deaths, although reversible postoperative complications occurred in 40% of the patients. Moreover, a survival benefit among these high-risk patients treated surgically was noted.[56,57] More recently, we determined that values of $\dot{V}O_{2peak}$ expressed as percent of predicted more accurately estimated surgical risk and helped to maximize the number of patients that can safely undergo lung resection. We concluded that high-risk patients that achieve a $VO_{2peak} \geq 60\%$ of predicted during exercise have an acceptable outcome after lung resection, even if $VO_{2peak} < 15$ mL/kg/min.[35] An approach to preoperative assessment for lung resection is summarized in Figure 7. In addition to an estimation of surgical risk and postoperative function, the goals of preoperative assessment include the development of strategies to reduce the risk and maximize the number of patients that can benefit from surgical therapy. Finally, one must keep in mind that there is no test that will predict all complications and that the patient and the surgeon should make the final decision regarding the risk–benefit balance of surgical versus nonsurgical treatment.

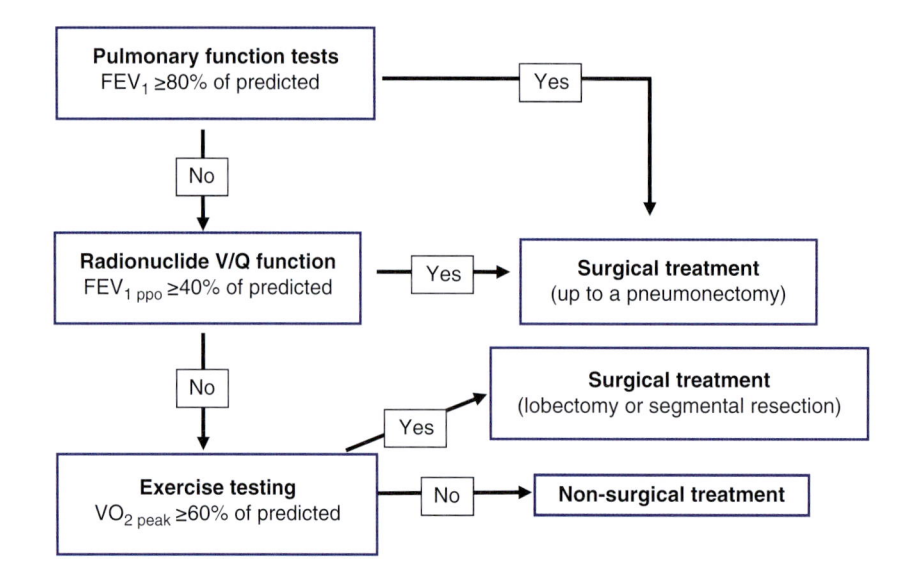

Figure 7 Approach to preoperative evaluation for lung resection.

Chemotherapy-induced lung injury

Systemic pharmacotherapeutic interventions in cancer management may be broadly divided into three major categories: conventional chemotherapy, molecular targeted agents, and immunotherapy. Recognition of immune checkpoints as modifiable targets in cancer therapy represents the newest pharmacotherapeutic tier in the management of a growing list of diverse cancers. Although the mechanism of cancer killing among each major category of systemic cancer therapy is vastly different, each form of intervention can produce adverse effects on normal host tissues. Compared to other organ systems, the lungs are a less frequent target of drug-induced injury but nonetheless highlighted because of the potential for severe and life-threatening events. The pathogenesis of drug-induced lung injury (DiLI) is poorly understood. Proposed mechanisms include direct cytotoxicity to type II pneumocytes and/or the alveolar-capillary endothelium; cytokine release resulting in endothelial dysfunction and capillary leak syndrome; oxidative injury associated with the release of free oxygen radicals; and/or cell-mediated lung mechanisms.[58–60]

Treating clinicians are often confronted with the dilemma of withholding potentially effective and life-saving therapy, based on a clinical suspicion of drug-related lung injury, as no pathognomonic clinical or histopathologic features of drug-induced lung disease (DILD) exists. Moreover, the clinical and histopathologic patterns of lung injury may vary broadly within a specific drug category as well as across drug classes. Thus, knowledge of key features of DILD is critical and may facilitate early recognition and aversion of potentially catastrophic outcomes while avoiding premature withdrawal of potentially effective therapy.

Lung injury may be confined to a single specific intrathoracic site, such as pulmonary interstitium, alveoli, pleura, pulmonary circulation, or airways or, alternatively, involve multiple intrathoracic structures. Across drug categories, the pulmonary interstitium and alveolar-capillary membrane are the major targets of toxicity, resulting in stereotyped patterns of interstitial lung diseases (ILD), including organizing pneumonia (OP) and nonspecific interstitial pneumonitis (NSIP).[61–64] Other lung injury patterns associated with this diverse group of diffuse lung diseases include hypersensitivity pneumonitis (HP), diffuse alveolar hemorrhage (DAH), acute interstitial pneumonia (AIP), eosinophilic pneumonias (EP), alveolar proteinosis (AP), vasculitis, noncardiogenic pulmonary edema, acute respiratory distress syndrome/diffuse alveolar damage (ARDS) and sarcoid-like reactions. If left unchecked, many of these histologic correlates of lung injury may lead to irreversible pulmonary fibrosis (PF). Differentiation syndrome, another cause of diffuse lung disease, gives rise to capillary leak and noncardiogenic pulmonary edema. Infusion reactions and airway-centric forms of drug-induced ILD (DiILD), such as bronchiolitis obliterans, have also been described. DiLD involving the pleura, mediastinum, and pulmonary vasculature are less common but troubling sequelae of all three categories of cancer pharmacotherapies. Finally, drug-related immune suppression may trigger pneumonias caused by a variety of opportunistic pathogens. These recalcitrant lung infections may be life-threatening and are discussed elsewhere. DiLD is often designated as pneumonitis or interstitial lung disease without further histopathologic description.

This section highlights drugs from the three major classes of cancer pharmacotherapy that cause predictable and unusual forms of lung disease. General features of DiLI caused by conventional cytotoxic drugs and molecular targeted therapies are discussed first followed by a discussion of specific pulmonary syndromes and histopathological lung injury patterns associated with these two drug categories. Lung injury associated with immunotherapies is discussed separately.

Lung injury associated with conventional cytotoxic chemotherapy

Bleomycin, busulfan, BCNU, methotrexate, and cyclophosphamide are the most well-studied cytotoxic agents causing lung injury. The clinical characteristics of lung injury within the cytotoxic class of drugs are very heterogeneous with histopathologic findings varying from one cytotoxic drug class to another. Bleomycin-related lung injury occurs in up to 20% of patients, with the higher rates associated with total cumulative doses above 400 units, age greater than 70 years, uremia, bolus administration, multiagent therapy, and multimodality therapy with concomitant or sequential radiation. Anecdotal reports suggest that high-inspired fractions of oxygen in bleomycin-exposed patients may provoke severe acute lung injury, although the threshold fraction of inspired oxygen, duration of oxygen therapy, or the interval between bleomycin and hyperoxia that confers an increased risk has not been defined (Figure 8).[58,65,66] Acute and late forms of cytotoxic

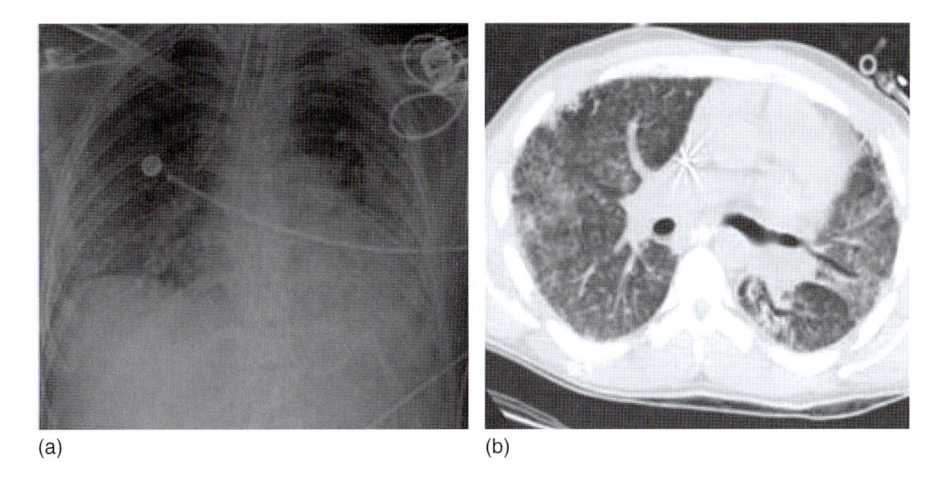

Figure 8 A 24-year-old woman developed respiratory distress following abdominal surgery for an unrelated illness 3 months after completing bleomycin-based treatment for Hodgkin's lymphoma. CXR (a) and CT scan (b) showed bilateral patchy reticulonodular and airspace disease. Work-up was consistent with ARDS associated with bleomycin toxicity, presumably triggered by hyperoxia during surgery.

lung injury occurring years after exposure have been described, particularly following busulfan exposure. A reported 8–10% of busulfan-treated patients develop lung injury which tends to be dose dependent (threshold dose above 500 mg). Symptoms of cough and progressive dyspnea typically develop insidiously, 4 years or more (range 2–10 years) after drug exposure. Acute symptoms, occurring 6 weeks after busulfan therapy, have also been reported.[67,68] Early and late-onset pneumonitis associated with cyclophosphamide therapy has also been described. Histopathologic patterns of lung injury associated with this agent include diffuse alveolar damage/ARDS, usual interstitial pneumonia with PF, and DAH. Fortunately, lung disease is rare and has typically been described with long-term and high-dose use of the drug.[69] In addition to NSIP and HP, the nitrosoureas, BCNU and CCNU, may provoke an acute and sometimes fulminant illness similar to ARDS, occurring days to weeks after treatment initiation. The nitrosoureas have also been implicated as causal in the development of pleuroparenchymal fibroelastosis (PPFE), a subtype of PF with predilection for the lung apices.[70] Patients with this form of PF may present with progressive cough, dyspnea, and pleuritic chest pain 17–20 years after a treatment-free interval, which underscores the need to remain clinically vigilant years after therapy. A list of cytotoxic chemotherapies and their associated patterns of lung injury is provided in Table 1.

Lung injury associated with molecular targeted therapies

The identification of aberrant proteins that are either overexpressed or dysregulated in cancer cells has resulted in a rapidly growing class of molecularly targeted antineoplastic agents. This class of agents comprises an extensive list of small-molecule tyrosine kinase inhibitors (TKIs) and monoclonal antibodies (mAbs). Despite their narrow spectrum of inhibition, many of these agents are associated with a variety of end-organ toxicities, including lung toxicity. Interstitial lung disease, infusion reactions (IRs), vasculopathies, and pleural effusions are common lung sequelae of targeted therapies which may arise from on-target (inhibition of the intended targets) or off-target (inhibition of unintended targets) mechanisms (Table 2). Symptoms of dry cough, dyspnea, and fever are most common and typically occur early during the course of treatment. However, the onset of toxicity may be delayed months or even years after the start of therapy.[71,72]

Cytotoxic and molecular targeted therapies: general considerations

Epidemiology and risk factors for drug-induced lung disease

Estimates of the incidence of DILD or DiLI caused by individual agents are hampered by the frequent use of complex multidrug and multimodality regimens given either concomitantly or sequentially. In general, approximately 10–20% of all patients treated with an antineoplastic agent experience lung toxicity. Estimates may be much higher with multidrug and multimodality regimens.[61,62,73,74] The greater susceptibility of the lungs compared to other organs to injury caused by systemic drug therapies is in part attributed to the fact that the entire blood supply flows through the lungs, resulting in greater exposure to potential toxins.[75]

Predisposing factors, such as older age, cumulative dose, concomitant or sequential radiotherapy, oxygen administration, prior lung injury, and the use of multidrug regimens significantly influence both the occurrence and latency periods between drug exposure and the development of clinical symptoms. For example, threshold doses for BCNU (1500 mg/m^2), bleomycin (400U), and busulfan (500 mg), beyond which pulmonary toxicity is increased, are well established.[76] The administration of cytotoxic chemotherapies such as busulfan, gemcitabine, the taxanes, or the nitrosoureas given concurrently or during subsequent administration with other potentially pneumotoxic chemotherapies, particularly other alkylating agents or with lung irradiation, may enhance pulmonary toxicity.[77–79] Preexisting fibrotic lung disease may potentiate severe and accelerated lung toxicity following exposure to a variety of conventional agents, including gemcitabine, the taxanes, and a variety of the TKIs, including agents targeting EGFR and the mTOR inhibitors.[79–90] Hyperoxia following bleomycin- and mitomycin-based therapies may trigger severe ARDS.[91,92]

Clinical presentation

Clinical symptoms of dry cough, dyspnea, and hypoxemia are nonspecific and typically develop insidiously, within weeks to a few months after drug exposure. Rarely, acute fulminant disease associated with ARDS develops within hours to days of exposure and may rapidly progress to respiratory failure. Delayed pneumonitis associated with cyclophosphamide, and gemcitabine, and

Table 1 Histopathologic findings associated with lung injury caused by cytotoxic chemotherapies.

Agent class	Specific agent	NSIP	OP	HP	NCPE DAD ARDS	DAH hemoptysis	EP	Pleural disease	PE VTE	PH	Sarcoid-like reactions	IR	MetHg	Radiation-recall pneumonitis
Alkylating agents	Busulfan	X	X	X	X		X							
	Cyclophosphamide	X	X		X			X					X	X
	Ifosfamide	X	X		X								X	
	Temozolomide	X			X									
	BCNU	X		X	X						X			
	CCNU	X		X	X							X		
	Oxaliplatin	X	X	X	X		X					X		X
	Cisplatin		X		X							X		X
	Carboplatin		X		X									X
	Melphalan	X												
	Chlorambucil	X												
Antimetabolites	Methotrexate	X	X		X		X	X			X			
	Azathioprine	X		X		X								
	Cytarabine	X	X									X		
	Fludarabine	X					X							
	Azacitidine	X			X		X							
	Gemcitabine	X	X	X	X	X								X
	Pemetrexed													
	Pentostatin				X									
	Zinostatin										X			
	Cladribine						X							
	6-Mercaptopurine			X										
Cytotoxic antibiotics	Bleomycin	X	X	X							X	X		
	Mitomyin C[a]	X	X	X								X		
Podophyllotoxins	Etoposide											X		X
	Teniposide											X		
Topoisomerase inhibitors	Irinotecan		X									X		
	Topotecan	X										X		
	Amrubicin													
	Liposomal Doxorubicin													X
	Idarubicin													X
	Mitoxantrone													X
Taxanes, microtubule stabilizers	Paclitaxel	X					X					X		
	Docetaxel	X					X	X				X		
	Nab-paclitaxel	X					X					X		
	Cabazitaxel	X										X		X
	Vincristine[a]													X
	Vinblastine[a]													X
	Vinorelbine[a]													X
	Vindesine[a]													X
	Ixabepilone											X		
Immunomodulatory anti-angiogenic agents	Thalidomide		X	X					X					
	Lenalidomide			X					X					
	Pomalidomide			X					X					
Proteosome inhibitors	Bortezomib	X			X					X				
	Carfilzomib	X	X		X					X		X		
Other	All-trans retinoic acid		X		X	X		X						
	Arsenictrioxide		X		X	X		X						
	Procarbazine		X				X					X		
	L-Asparaginase		X									X		
	Tamoxifen							X		X				

NSIP, nonspecific interstitial pneumonitis; OP, organizing pneumonia; HP, hypersensitivity pneumonitis; NCPE, noncardiogenic pulmonary edema; DAD, diffuse alveolar damage; ARDS, acute respiratory distress syndrome; DS, differentiation syndrome/cytokine release syndrome; DAH, diffuse alveolar hemorrhage; TE fistula, tracheoesophageal fistula; EP, eosinophilic pneumonia; VTE/PE, venous pulmonary embolism/pulmonary embolism; IR, infusion reaction; PH, pulmonary hypertension; IR, infusion reaction; MetHgb, Methemoblobinemia.
[a]In combination with mitomycin C.

late fibrotic disease, occurring 6 months to years after exposure to agents such as bleomycin, busulfan, and the nitrosoureas has also been described.[59,60,67,93–96]

Diagnostic considerations

The diagnosis of DiLD relies on compatible clinical, radiological, and histopathologic features of lung injury occurring in temporal association with the use of the culprit drug. The histopathologic and radiologic features of DiLD can be seen in a variety of non-drug-related causes of lung injury. Competing diagnoses, such as cardiogenic and noncardiogenic pulmonary edema, infections, cancer relapse, aspiration, or RT should be excluded.[97] Imaging studies, including high-resolution computer tomography (HRCT) scans, are important tools in the evaluation of patients with suspected DiLI, although the findings are nonspecific. Interstitial and mixed alveolar-interstitial abnormalities, manifested as ground-glass opacities that localize to the peripheral and lower lung zones, are the most frequent radiographic findings on CT. Upper lung zone predominant infiltrates are also seen, particularly following drug-induced hypersensitivity reactions. Nodular lesions

Table 2 Histopathologic findings associated with lung injury caused by molecular targeted therapies.

Molecular target	Specific agent	Pneumonitis	NCPE DAD ARDS	DS CRS	DAH hemoptysis	Pleural disease	Pneumothorax alveolar-pleural fistula; TE fistula	PE/VTE	PH	Sarcoid-like reactions	IR	Radiation-recall pneumonitis
EGFR	Gefitinib	X	X									X
	Erlotinib	X	X									X
	Afatinib	X										
	Osimertinib	X	X									
	Lapatinib											
	Dacomitinib		X									
	Cetuximab	X						X			X	
	Panitumumab	X						X			X	
EGFR-Her2	Trastuzumab	X	X								X	X
	Pertuzumab	X	X								X	
	Ado-trastuzumab	X	X								X	
	Fam-trastuzumab	X	X								X	
ALK	Crizotinib	X	X								X	
	Ceritinib	X	X									
	Alectinib	X	X									
	Brigatinib	X	X									
	Lorlatinib	X	X									
c-MET	Capmatinib	X	X									
VEGF	Sunitinib	X			X*			X				
	Sorafenib	X	X		X*			X				
	Pazopanib						X	X				
	Vandetanib	X						X				
	Axitinib							X				
	Lenvatinib							X				
	Cabozantinib							X				
	Apatinib							X				
	Regorafenib							X				
	Aflibercept							X				
	Bevacizumab				X		X	X			X	
	Ramucirumab				X		X	X			X	
PI3K	Idelalisib	X										
	Copanlisib	X										
	Duvelisib	X										
	Apelisib	X										
Rapamycin and analogs	Sirolimus	X								X		
	Temsirolimus	X										
	Everolimus	X										
Bcr-Abl	Imatinib	X				X						
	Dasatinib	X				X			X			
	Nilotinib	X							X?			
	Bosutinib	X				X			X?			
	Ponatinib	X										
JAK1/2	Ruxolitinib		X***									
Fms-related TKI (FLT3)	Midosataurin	X	X	X								
	Gilteritinib	X	X	X								
	Quazartinib	X	X	X								
MEK	Trametinib	X	X									
	Cobimetinib	X	X									
	Binimetinib	X	X									
Cyclin-dependent kinase 4/6	Palbociclib	X										
	Ribosiclib	X										
	Abemaciclib	X										
BRAF	Dabrafenib							X**				
	Vemurafenib							X**				
	Encorafenib							X**				
Isocitrate dehydrogenase	Ivosidenib			X								
	Enasidenib			X								
CD20	Rituximab	X	X		X						X	
	Obinutuzumab	X									X	
	Ofatumumab	X									X	
	Tositumomab	X	X								X	
	Ocrelizumab	X									X	
	Ibritumomab	X									X	

(continued overleaf)

Table 2 (Continued)

Molecular target	Specific agent	Pneumonitis	NCPE DAD ARDS	DS CRS	DAH hemoptysis	Pleural disease	Pneumothorax alveolar-pleural fistula; TE fistula	PE/VTE	PH	Sarcoid-like reactions	IR	Radiation-recall pneumonitis
CD22	Moxetumomab	X	X								X	
CD33	Gemtuzumab ozogamicin	X	X		X						X	
CD52	Alemtuzumab	X	X								X	
CD19	Blinatumomab										X	
CD30	Brentuximab	X	X								X	
CD38	Daratumuma Isatuximab										X X	
SLAMF7	Elotuzumab										X	
CCR4	Mogamulizumab										X	

X*: Sunitinib and sorafenib have more often been associated with hemoptysis from primary lung cancers versus metastatic lesions to the lungs.
X**: Increased risk of PE/DVT with BRAF-MEK inhibitor combinations versus BRAF monotherapy.
X***: NCPE/ARDS has been reported with abrupt Ruxolitnib withdrawal.
X?: Bosutinib- and ponatinib-associated PH has only been reported following dasatinib therapy, raising questions regarding the contribution of these drugs to PH development.
EGFR, epidermal growth factor receptor; EGFR-Her2, epidermal growth factor receptor/human epidermal growth factor receptor 2; ALK, anaplastic lymphoma kinase; c-MET, mesenchymal-epithelial transition factor; PI3K, phosphoinositol 3 kinase; Bcr-Abl, breakpoint cluster region-Abelson; JAK 1/2, Janus kinase 1/2; fms-related tyrosine kinase 3/FLT-3, fms-like tyrosine kinase 3; MEK, mitogen-activated protein kinase; NSIP, nonspecific interstitial pneumonitis; OP, organizing pneumonia; HP, hypersensitivity pneumonitis; NCPE, noncardiogenic pulmonary edema; DAD, diffuse alveolar damage; ARDS, acute respiratory distress syndrome; DS, differentiation syndrome/cytokine release syndrome; DAH, diffuse alveolar hemorrhage; TE fistula, tracheoesophageal fistula; EP, eosinophilic pneumonia; VTE/PE, venous pulmonary embolism/pulmonary embolism; IR, infusion reaction; PH, pulmonary hypertension; IR, infusion reaction.

may mimic underlying malignancy. Reticular lines, septal thickening, and mosaic attenuation are also observed. PF associated with traction bronchiectasis and honeycomb patterns may be seen as the disease progresses. Infiltrates are typically mild to moderately FDG-avid on FDG-PET imaging.[98] Derangements on pulmonary function testing are nonspecific, but nonetheless, important in assessing the degree of DLI-related pulmonary impairment. Reductions in the diffusing capacity for carbon monoxide (DLCO) are generally accepted as the most sensitive parameter in the assessment of DiLI, although the predictive potential for the detection of early change has been variable.[97,99–103] With disease progression, a restrictive ventilatory defect may be seen.[104,105] Near-complete normalization of pulmonary function within 2 years of exposure is common following some forms of chemotherapy-induced lung injury. Systemic markers of inflammation, such as leukocytosis, elevated erythrocyte sedimentation rate, and C-reactive protein are common but nonspecific findings.

Bronchoscopy with performance of bronchoalveolar lavage (BAL) may be helpful in excluding competing diagnoses of infection or background disease. Studies have shown diagnostic yields as high as 70–90% for pulmonary infections and 35–70% for lymphoma and lymphangitic spread of lung cancers.[106,107] BAL fluid in DiLI is typically hypercellular with increased numbers of neutrophils or lymphocytes. Decreased CD4/CD8 ratios on BAL fluid are supportive findings, however, ratios vary widely and cannot distinguish sufficiently between drug-induced versus other causes of ILD.[108] Drug-induced HP is suggested by BAL lymphocytosis of greater than 50%, with a low CD4 to CD8 ratio. BAL eosinophilia of greater than 25% is supportive of drug-induced EP. The presence of DAH is supported by progressively bloody BAL samples on sequential saline aliquots and/or cytologic evidence of increased numbers of hemosiderin-laden macrophages on BAL fluid. Transbronchial and surgical lung biopsies may be helpful in documenting IP, DAD, EP, OP, and excluding competing diagnoses such as vasculitis, infection, and underlying malignancy. Histopathologic criteria for DiLD have not been established and no findings are considered pathognomonic. Lung biopsies are, nonetheless, valuable in excluding competing diagnoses and characterizing the histopathologic pattern of lung injury. This information is not only useful in diagnosing DiLI but also in guiding therapeutic options.

General approach to therapy

Treatment of chemotherapy-related DiLI has not been validated in any prospective trials. Strategies are guided by common terminology criteria for adverse events (CTCAE) and based on pneumonitis grades 1 (mild) through 5 (death). Supportive care (including inhaled bronchodilators, supplemental oxygen, and mechanical ventilation) should be initiated, as clinically indicated. Spontaneous improvement may be seen following drug interruption. Current expert opinion advocates close surveillance with high-resolution CT scans and continued therapy with or without dose interruption for asymptomatic (grade 1) ILD. For symptomatic patients (grade 2 or higher), the grade of pneumonitis should be used to guide management decisions, which may include dose modification or interruption, and the institution of corticosteroid therapy.[109] Prior to initiation of corticosteroid therapy, infectious etiologies should be excluded with appropriate stains and cultures obtained from sputum or BAL. The addition of empiric antimicrobial therapy directed at likely pathogens while awaiting the results of diagnostic procedures is reasonable. Evidence supporting the utility of corticosteroids and optimal dosing schedules in the management of DiLD is largely observational. Most experts recommend 0.75–1 mg/kg/day of prednisone or its equivalent with at the higher dose until symptom improvement is established, then tapered over a 1 to 3-month time period, pending the response to therapy. Corticosteroids have been shown to abrogate symptoms of DiLI in certain steroid-responsive lung injury patterns, such as HP, eosinophilic pneumonia, and bronchiolitis obliterans with organizing pneumonia (BOOP). In other entities, including PF and pulmonary vascular disease, corticosteroids have no beneficial role. Histopathologic confirmation of steroid-responsive DILD correlates may therefore be helpful, but lung biopsies are often not feasible due to prohibitive thrombocytopenia. Once sufficient clinical evidence linking an association between symptomatic pneumotoxicity to the suspected drug has

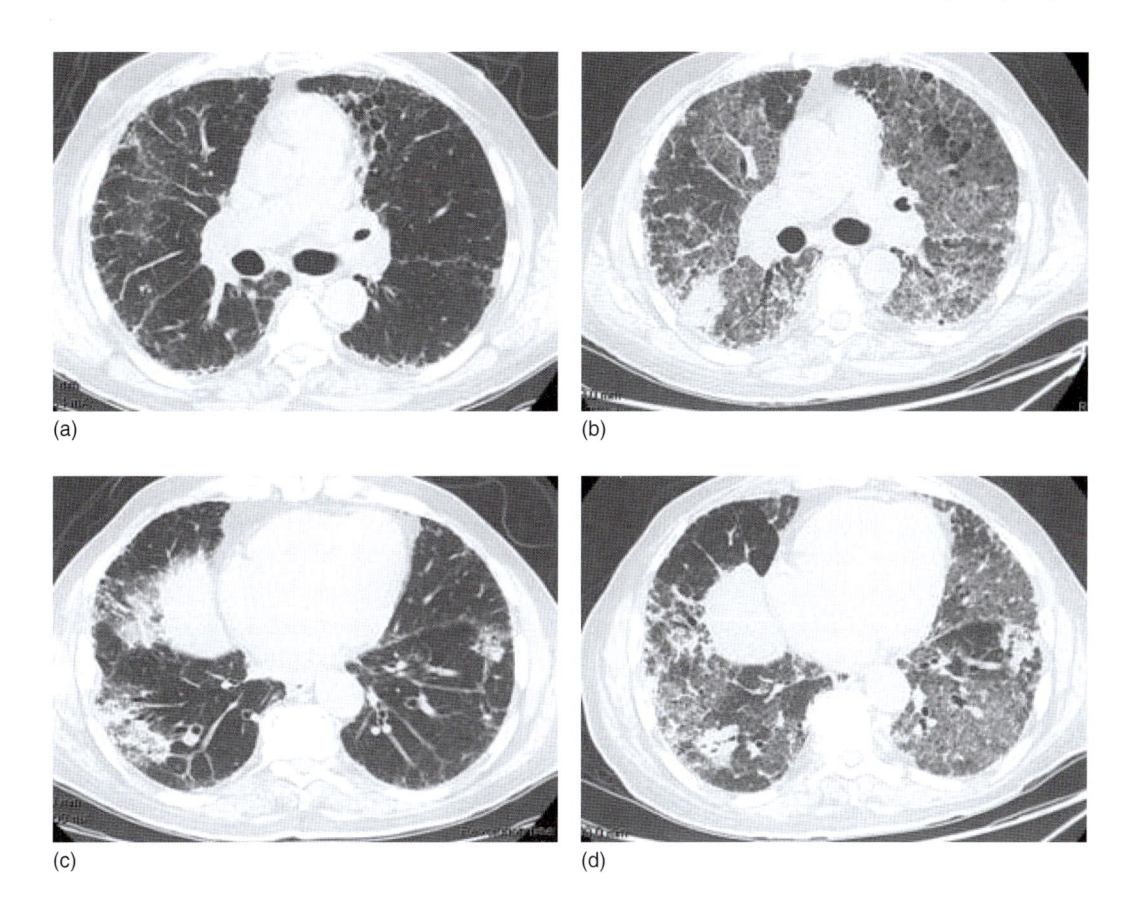

Figure 9 An 80-year-old man developed progressive dyspnea and dry cough 4 weeks after initiation of panitumumab for colon cancer. Chest CT imaging at baseline showed mild interstitial fibrosis (a, c). Four weeks later, diffuse bilateral interstitial thickening and ground glass infiltrates. BAL cultures were negative. Analysis of lung biopsies suggested nonspecific interstitial pneumonitis.

been established, rechallenge with the culprit agent is generally not recommended. The decision to reintroduce the offending agent following resolution of respiratory symptoms must be made on a case-by-case basis and should consider the pneumonitis grade, response to treatment, toxicity profile of the individual agent, and the availability of alternative therapies. One clear exception to this recommendation has been in the setting of the differentiation syndrome (DS) following all-trans-retinoic acid (ATRA)- and arsenic trioxide therapies for treatment of acute promyelocytic leukemia (APL).[110,111] Systemic steroid therapy along with de-escalation of drug dose rather than drug withdrawal has been associated with successful resolution of toxicity in patients with mild to moderate forms of this syndrome.

Specific drug-induced lung syndromes

Nonspecific interstitial lung disease
Nonspecific interstitial pneumonia (NSIP) represents one of the most frequent morphologic patterns of DiLD. Injury is signaled by the insidious development of a nonproductive cough and dyspnea, which typically occurs within weeks to months following drug exposure. Symptom development may precede radiographic findings by days to weeks and tends to be milder than other histologic forms of pneumonitis, although progression to PF can occur. Bilateral interstitial and mixed alveolar-interstitial abnormalities that localize to the peripheral and lower lung zones and often spare the subpleural space are key features on CT imaging. Nodular lesions, reticular lines, septal thickening, mosaic patterns, and ground glass attenuations are also observed (Figure 9).[112] Antineoplastic agents from all three drug categories have been associated with development of NSIP. Specific conventional therapies with the highest incidence include paclitaxel and gemcitabine. NSIP has been reported following treatment with many classes of targeted agents, including mTOR inhibitors (everolimus, temsirolimus); EGFR inhibitors (gefitinib, erlotinib, cetuximab, panitumumab, obinutuzumab); multikinase angiogenesis inhibitors (sorafenib, sunitinib); the HER2 inhibitor, trastuzumab; multikinase Bcr-Abl inhibitors (imatinib, dasatinib, nilotinib, bosutinib); proteasome inhibitors (bortezomib, carfilzomib), the ALK inhibitors (crizotinib, ceritinib, alectinib, and brigatinib); the c-met inhibitor (capmatinib), and immunomodulatory agents (thalidomide, lenalidomide, pomalidomide). Inhibitors of the immune checkpoints are also implicated in the development of NSIP and are discussed in a separate section. Drug interruption and corticosteroid therapy are the mainstay of treatment. Steroid therapy is typically initiated for pneumonitis grades 2 or higher, based on CTCAE criteria, and tapered over 1–3 months, depending on the response to therapy.[63,75,113,114] Clinical features of specific agents causing NSIP deserve a more detailed attention and are discussed below.

Organizing pneumonia
OP is one of the most common patterns of DiLD. Bilateral multifocal areas of mass-like consolidation and bilateral diffuse ground-glass opacities that typically localize to the lung periphery are nonspecific, but common findings on chest CT (Figure 10). This

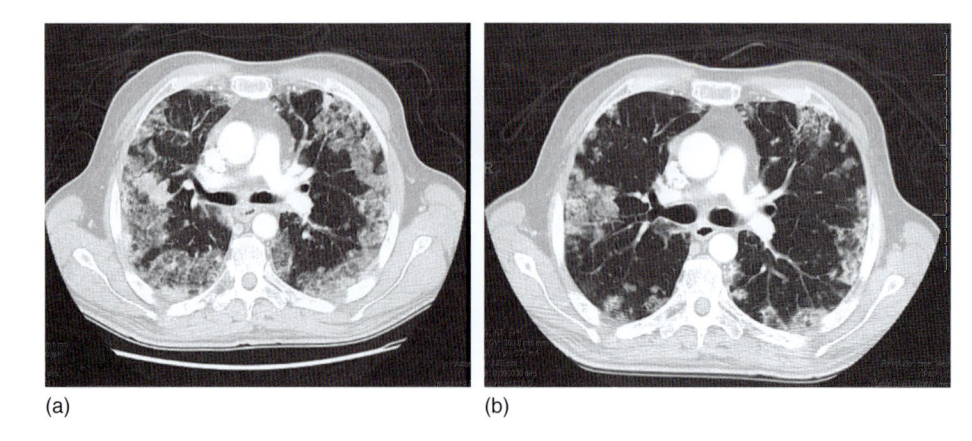

Figure 10 A 60-year-old man presents with a maculopapular rash and progressive dry cough with shortness of breath that developed 12 weeks after starting erlotinib for advanced pancreatic cancer. The extensive, ground glass and nodular pleural-based infiltrate (a) significantly improved within two weeks of discontinuation of erlotinib and initiation of systemic steroid therapy (b). Biopsy of the lung suggested organizing pneumonia.

pattern of ILD has as its histologic hallmark intralumenal fibrin plugs within the distal airways with associated chronic inflammation. BAL lymphocytosis and bilateral areas of consolidation that are often migratory are important clues to diagnosis. PFTs reveal mixed obstructive-restrictive defects in most cases.[115] Agents from every drug category have been implicated in the development of OP. In the lung cancer setting, paclitaxel, gemcitabine, the EGFR inhibitors, ALK antagonists, and m-tor inhibitors are implicated as culprits for OP. Inhibitors of the immune checkpoints, programmed cell death-1 (PD-1), and programmed cell death ligand 1 (PD-L1) are also well described. Early recognition and discontinuation of therapy generally result in a favorable prognosis. OP appears to be steroid-responsive. Initiation of systemic steroids represents standard therapy, although the precise dose and duration of treatment have not been established. A slow steroid taper over 4–6 weeks is generally recommended to avoid disease relapse.

Hypersensitivity pneumonitis

HP reactions are typically characterized by fever, dyspnea, dry cough, headache, fatigue, rash, and BAL lymphocytosis following repeated exposure to the offending agent. Interstitial pneumonitis may evolve over the first 3–4 weeks after drug exposure and wax and wane without adjustments in therapy. Poorly formed granulomas with mononuclear cell infiltration are common histologic findings in subacute and chronic HP. Hilar adenopathy and pleural effusions occur in up to 10% of patients. Histologic evidence of ill-defined granulomas, together with skin rash and radiographic findings of hilar adenopathy or pleural effusions may help to distinguish methotrexate-induced lung injury. Radiographic changes include homogeneous opacities with upper lobe predominance, particularly in chronic forms of the disease. Among the drugs that have been implicated in the development of HP, methotrexate has been the most extensively studied. Lung injury has been reported following oral, intravenous, intrathecal, and intramuscular routes of methotrexate administration. HP has been reported following a variety of other chemotherapeutic agents (bleomycin, busulfan, the taxanes, L-asparaginase, gemcitabine, oxaliplatin, procarbazine, azathioprine, lenalidomide); targeted therapies (imatinib); and inhibitors of the PD-1/PD-L1 and CTLA-4 immune checkpoint axis. Anti-TNF agents and BCG therapy have also been implicated.[116–127] Overall, the prognosis for patients with chemotherapy-induced HP is very favorable. Complete resolution of clinical symptoms and radiographic findings is typical following steroid therapy in early-stage disease.

Noncardiogenic pulmonary edema (NCPE), diffuse alveolar damage (DAD)/acute respiratory distress syndrome (ARDS)

NCPE occurs as a result of injury to the alveolar-capillary membrane, resulting in capillary leak and a noncardiogenic (permeability) pulmonary edema. With disease progression, severe physiological impairment consistent with ARDS and its histologic hallmark, DAD, may ensue. Drug-induced NCPE often occurs as an idiosyncratic reaction, unrelated to drug dosage or duration of therapy. Patients frequently present with acute dyspnea, hypoxia, and alveolar infiltrate in the absence of heart failure. Reactions are typically mild and self-limited, although progression to ARDS with fatal outcomes occasionally occurs. Drug withdrawal, supplemental oxygen, and the judicious use of diuretics usually affect a rapid recovery. Apart from ATRA- and arsenic-induced NCPE (see below), drug rechallenge with the offending drug often results in recrudescence of symptoms and is not recommended. Aggravating factors that potentiate disease progression to ARDS include multiagent protocols and the concomitant or sequential use of radiation or oxygen therapy, particularly following therapy with bleomycin or busulfan.[74,128] Once established, the response of ARDS to drug withdrawal and corticosteroid therapy is variable. Progressive respiratory impairment, leading to respiratory failure and death has been reported with some agents (busulfan, cyclophosphamide, bleomycin) despite drug withdrawal. Among molecular targeted therapies, ARDS has been best described following agents that inhibit EGFR (gefitinib, erlotinib, cetuximab); the antilymphocyte mAbs (rituximab, alemtuzumab, ofatumumab, gemtuzumab ozogamicin); and the rapamycin inhibitors (everolimus, temsirolimus).[82,88,129] Acute withdrawal of the JAK1/2 inhibitor, ruxolitinib, has been associated with the development of ARDS as a result of cytokine rebound. ARDS has also been rarely reported following the immune checkpoint inhibitors (ICIs).[63,130–132] Preemptive use of corticosteroids, along with supportive therapy and a slow taper off this agent is recommended to mitigate this potential problem.[133,134]

Differentiation syndrome and cytokine release syndrome

The earliest reports of DS (formerly known as retinoic acid syndrome) were derived from patients treated with the differentiating agents, all-trans retinoic acid or arsenic trioxide for APL. ATRA and arsenic are thought to trigger the release of inflammatory and vasoactive cytokines by differentiating myeloblasts, causing a cascade of events that lead to endothelial damage and a systemic inflammatory state. These events underlie the development of the DS. Roughly 25% of patients treated with ATRA and/or arsenic trioxide experience DS, which is variably characterized by fever, tachycardia, tachypnea, hypotension, hypoxia, weight gain, pleural and pericardial effusions, and noncardiogenic pulmonary edema associated with capillary leak. Signs and symptoms of DS typically develop 7 to 21 days after drug exposure and may be life-threatening.[135] The FLT3 inhibitors (midostaurin, gilteritinib, and quazartinib) and the IDH inhibitors (ivosidenib and enasidenib) cause induction of terminal myeloid differentiation and an associated DS that is largely analogous to the that seen with ATRA- and arsenic-associated DS. DS has been reported in 20% of patients treated with IDH inhibitors (20%) and up to 12% of patients treated with FLT3 antagonists.[136,137] Concomitant appearance of neutropenic dermatosis (Sweet's syndrome) in FLT3-treated patients may offer a helpful diagnostic clue.[138] The diagnosis of drug-induced DS is supported by clinical presentation and timing, response to treatment, and exclusion of alternate diagnoses such as infection, heart failure, and renal insufficiency. Data from retrospective and prospective studies suggest a reduction in mortality from 9% to <1% with prompt initiation of corticosteroid therapy. Thus, systemic steroids should be initiated as soon as DS is suspected and concurrent with the diagnostic evaluation. In the absence of severe DS, differentiating agents may be continued without interruption. For severe DS, drug withdrawal is recommended with resumption of therapy once clinical findings of DS have resolved. Because of the prolonged half-lives of the FLT3 (113 h) and IDH (97–137 h) inhibitors, drug interruption is not expected to have an immediate impact on the clinical course and prognosis of DS. DS treatment should also include supportive care, empiric antibiotics, and renal replacement therapy, as indicated. The use of corticosteroids as prophylaxis during induction therapy with the differentiating agents remains controversial.[135,139] Severe and potentially fatal capillary leak associated with cytokine release has also been described following gemcitabine, some of the mAbs (rituximab, alemtuzumab), the interleukin therapies, and diphtheria conjugates, including denileukin difitox and tagraxofusp.[140–142]

Diffuse alveolar hemorrhage (DAH) and hemoptysis

Drug-induced diffuse alveolar hemorrhage (DAH) most often occurs as a result of injury to the alveolar-capillary membrane but may occasionally be seen as a consequence of bland alveolar hemorrhage without distortion of the lung architecture. DAH in the absence of DAD is a rare complication of alemtuzumab, gemtuzumab ozogamicin, and nivolumab.[143–145] Acute dyspnea, bilateral alveolar infiltrates, and hemoptysis represent the cardinal features of DAH. Hemoptysis is a supportive clue but is lacking in one-third of cases. Progressively bloody aliquots of BAL fluid are the best diagnostic clue. Tumor cavitation with sometimes fatal hemoptysis has been described during treatment of central airway tumors with bevacizumab therapy.[146]

Eosinophilic pneumonia

Eosinophilic pneumonia (EP) is characterized by fever, dyspnea, hypoxia, and homogeneous ground-glass opacities that have a predilection for the periphery and upper lobes. Alveolar and peripheral blood eosinophils are common features. A leukocyte composition of >20% eosinophils of the total leukocytes recovered by bronchoalveolar lavage is consistent with eosinophilic pneumonia. The "reverse pulmonary edema pattern" is a classic radiographic feature but is seen in only 33% of patients. A growing list of agents that have been implicated in the development of EP, including bleomycin, busulfan, methotrexate, azacytidine, procarbazine, fludarabine, the interleukins and, more recently, oxaliplatin- and taxane-based therapies.[147–150] The ICIs have also been added to the list of drugs that may provoke EP. Drug withdrawal and initiation of high-dose steroids are typically associated with favorable outcomes.[151–154]

Pleural effusions and fibrosis

Drug-induced pleural disease is typically a manifestation of a generalized pleuroparenchymal abnormality but may occur as an isolated event.[155] Isolated pleural effusions are occasionally seen following methotrexate, imatinib, dasatinib, bosutinib, docetaxel, ATRA, arsenic trioxide, and granulocyte-colony stimulating factor (GCSF) administration.[156,157] An exudative, lymphocyte-predominant effusion is typical, which may be unilateral or bilateral and small to moderate in size. Optimal therapy for drug-induced pleural effusions is not well defined, but thoracentesis, diuresis, and steroid therapies have been employed with varying rates of success. Spontaneous resolution of the pleural effusion may occur following drug withdrawal in some cases. Pleural thickening may accompany PF as a late manifestation of cyclophosphamide, BCNU, or bleomycin toxicity.

Thromboembolic disease, pulmonary hypertension, pulmonary veno-occlusive disease

The adverse effects of chemotherapeutic agents on the pulmonary vasculature may result in thrombosis, pulmonary hypertension, or pulmonary veno-occlusive disease (PVOD). The diagnosis of pulmonary vascular disease is suggested by an isolated reduction in DLCO or a DLCO that is disproportionately decreased relative to other lung function parameters on pulmonary function testing. The prothrombotic effects of tamoxifen appear to be related to drug-related decrements in protein C and antithrombin III levels.[158] Combined therapy with tamoxifen and other chemotherapeutic agents, such as cyclophosphamide, methotrexate, and 5-fluorouracil confers a threefold increased risk of thromboembolic phenomenon.[159,160] Thromboembolic events, with rates ranging from 14% to 43% have been reported among recipients of thalidomide-based chemotherapy, given in combination with steroids, doxorubicin, or BCNU.[161–164] The VEGF inhibitors, bevacizumab, sunitinib, and sorafenib are also associated with thromboembolic events (Figure 11).[146,165–168] Pulmonary arterial hypertension (PAH) is a rare complication of antineoplastic agents, suggesting possible individual susceptibility. Severe pulmonary arterial hypertension (PAH) has been reported following treatment with the Bcr-Abl TKI, dasatinib, which in most cases, is only partially reversible after drug withdrawal.[169–172] An off-target mechanism of drug-induced PAH following use of this multikinase inhibitor has been postulated. The Bcr-Abl inhibitors, ponatinib, and bosutinib have rarely been implicated in the development of PAH, however, these associations are confounded by prior use of dasatinib therapy in each of these cases, rendering the specific attributable cause challenging.[173,174] There have been no reports of PAH following exposure to the more selective Bcr-Abl TKIs. In fact, the safe use of selective Bcr-Abl TKIs, such as nilotinib and imatinib following dasatinib-associated PAH is well described.[170,175] Once dasatinib-associated PAH is suspected, the drug should be withdrawn and rechallenge is not recommended.[176] Pulmonary hypertension (PH) following interferon therapy has been attributed to potential interferon-induced endothelial dysfunction.[177,178] Zinostatin, an antitumor antibiotic, causes hypertrophy of the pulmonary vascular wall leading to

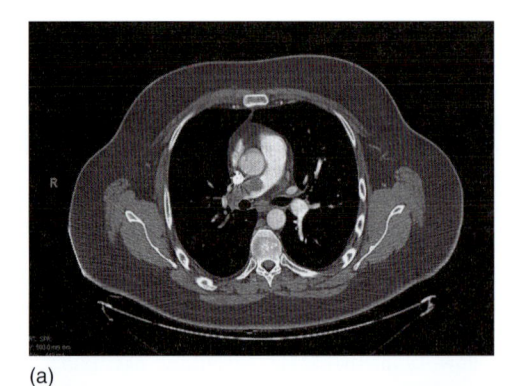

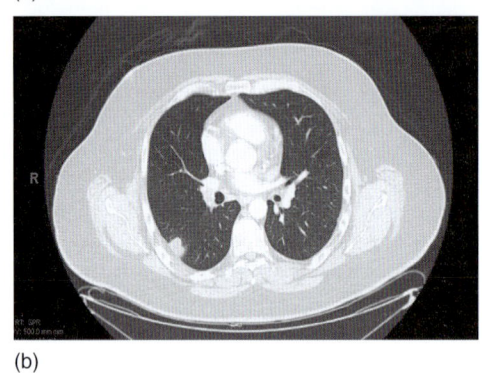

Figure 11 CT angiogram showing large central embolus in a patient treated with bevacizumab-based chemotherapy for cholangiocarcinoma (a). Associated pulmonary infarct is suggested by the wedge-shaped subpleural density overlying the lateral segment of the right middle lobe (b).

pulmonary hypertension, possibly as a result of direct toxicity to the pulmonary endothelium.[179] Chemotherapy-related pulmonary hypertension may also present as PVOD, a process characterized by fibrous obliteration of pulmonary venules and small pulmonary veins (see section titled "Pulmonary hypertension in the cancer patient"). Although several drugs have been implicated in the development of PVOD, bleomycin and BCNU have been associated with the most incriminating data.[180,181]

Infusion reactions
Bronchospasm with associated dyspnea, wheezing, and hypoxia is a common and sometimes life-threatening manifestation of chemotherapy-related acute IRs. Virtually all chemotherapeutic agents may trigger IRs, defined as an adverse reaction that is temporally related to drug infusion with signs and symptoms inconsistent with the known toxicity profile of the drug. Conventional cytotoxic agents with the highest rates of IRs include the taxanes, platinum drugs, pegylated liposomal doxorubicin, procarbazine, etoposide, cytarabine, ixabepilone, cyclophosphamide, cytarabine, and bleomycin.[182–186] Until recently, all adverse events associated with drug infusions were referred to as "hypersensitivity reactions." However, an allergic component may be absent and, thus, "IR" is the preferred term. IRs associated with most conventional cytotoxic chemotherapies typically occur as an IgE-mediated hypersensitivity response to foreign proteins (type 1 hypersensitivity reaction) or as a non-IgE mediated pseudo-allergic response. The latter is caused by cationic drugs that trigger the activation of mast cells and subsequent cytokine release (anaphylactoid reaction).[182,187] Following drug exposure, IgE antibodies are produced and bind mast cells and basophils. Subsequent re-exposure to the drug may trigger an explosive release of vasoactive mediators (histamines, leukotrienes, and prostaglandins) from basophil and mast cells, triggering a type 1-hypersensitivity reaction and anaphylaxis. Acute IRs typically occur within the first few minutes to hours of drug exposure, although late reactions, occurring 10–24 h following drug administration have also been reported. Type 1 reactions typically occur within minutes of infusion. Associated respiratory symptoms include cough, dyspnea, wheezing, and chest tightness. Stridor due to oropharyngeal and laryngeal edema may also occur. As the disease progresses, bilateral pulmonary infiltrates associated with permeability pulmonary edema may develop, which may progress to ARDS. These reactions may occasionally be sufficiently severe, leading to respiratory failure, shock, and death.

Although taxane-related IRs are clinically similar to IgE-mediated type 1 reactions, the proposed mechanism is different. Both paclitaxel and docetaxel are poorly soluble in water and require formulation in Cremophor EL (paclitaxel) and polysorbate 80 (docetaxel) for activity. Cremophor EL, a highly allergenic polyoxyethylated castor oil solvent, triggers mast cell/basophil activation and subsequent hypersensitivity reactions. Polysorbate 80 may induce IRs via similar mechanisms.[188] IRs due to taxane administration are primarily attributed to its solubilizing vehicle, although the drug itself may occasionally trigger IRs. Other antineoplastic agents that are formulated in Cremophor EL (cyclosporine, teniposide, ixabepilone) or polysorbate 80 (etoposide) should be avoided in patients with a history of IRs following taxane administration.[189] Taxane-associated IRs typically occur early during the first or second infusion. Standard prophylaxis with histamine receptor antagonists and steroids has reduced the incidence of paclitaxel-induced bronchospasm from 30% to 2%.[190] Recent studies have shown the presence of BRCA1/2 mutations to be an independent risk factor for the development of IRs among women treated with carboplatin-based chemotherapies for breast or ovarian cancer. Infusion reactions in this setting tend to occur at lower cumulative dose exposure.[191]

mAbs are a frequent cause of IRs. The binding of most mAbs to their target cell provokes the release of cytokines and subsequent cytokine release reactions. These immune-mediated reactions appear clinically similar to cytotoxin-mediated IRs. Dyspnea, wheezing, and "flu-like symptoms" typically occur within the first hours few hours of drug infusion.[192] Symptoms are typically mild, with fatal reactions occurring in a minority of patients. The percentage of mouse protein is felt to roughly correlate with the immunogenic response. Thus, the murine-derived (blinatumomab, ibritumomab, moxetumomab) mAbs are highly immunogenic in humans. One strategy to decrease the immunogenicity of mAbs has been the development of chimeric (30% mouse protein) mouse–human (cetuximab, rituximab, brentuximab), partially (10% mouse protein) humanized (bevacizumab, trastuzumab, alemtuzumab, gemtuzumab, obinutuzumab), and fully humanized (ipilimumab, ofatumumab, panitumumab, ramucirumab) mAbs. Reduced immunogenicity and associated IRs based on murine content of the mAb was suggested in a recent study in which the severity of IRs following panitumumab therapy (0.5%) was fourfold less than that following cetuximab therapy (2%).[193] There are exceptions to this observation, however, as several fully human mAbs (avelumab, durvalumab, ofatumumab) and humanized mAbs (mogamulizumab, trastuzumab, elotuzumab) are associated with rates of IRs that are sufficiently high to warrant premedication therapy.[182,184,185,194] Decisions regarding the need for prophylaxis and safety of drug rechallenge are typically based on the severity of IR and are made on a case by case basis.[195] Risk factors for mAb-induced IRs include a prior

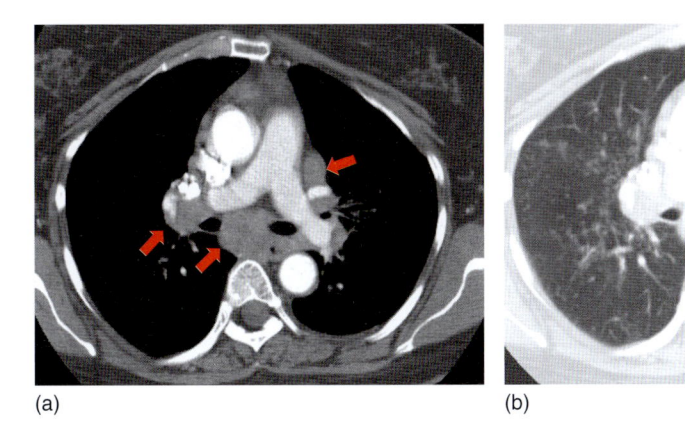

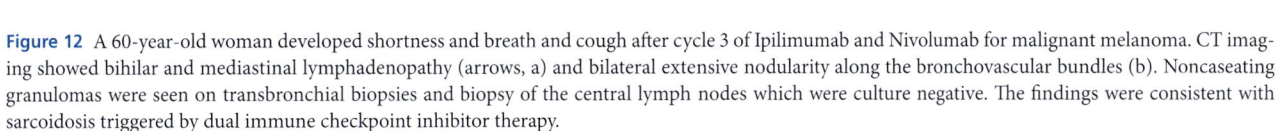

Figure 12 A 60-year-old woman developed shortness and breath and cough after cycle 3 of Ipilimumab and Nivolumab for malignant melanoma. CT imaging showed bihilar and mediastinal lymphadenopathy (arrows, a) and bilateral extensive nodularity along the bronchovascular bundles (b). Noncaseating granulomas were seen on transbronchial biopsies and biopsy of the central lymph nodes which were culture negative. The findings were consistent with sarcoidosis triggered by dual immune checkpoint inhibitor therapy.

history of allergic reaction to the drug, rate of drug administration, drug form, and multiagent therapy. Test-dosing prior to infusion does not reliably predict subsequent IRs. Mild IR events following mAb therapy may be managed with supportive care including supplemental oxygen, antihistamines, steroids, and nebulized β2 agonists. Premedication with antihistamines, corticosteroids, and antipyretics is generally recommended for the chimeric mouse–human mAbs, such as rituximab and cetuximab. Breakthrough IRs may occur despite prophylaxis. Thus, close monitoring during and immediately following drug infusion is recommended.

One other class of agents that has been associated with bronchospasm includes the vinca alkyloids. Although vinorelbine and other vinca alkyloids are rarely associated with lung toxicity, acute reactions characterized by cough, bronchospasm, flushing, dyspnea, abdominal pain, and hypotension have been described when these agents are given either concurrently or sequentially with mitomycin chemotherapy.[196,197]

Granulomatous disease

The development of noncaseating granulomas is a rare manifestation of DiLI that has been described most often following methotrexate and interferon therapy.[198,199] Methotrexate- and interferon-induced granulomatous lymphadenopathy is indistinguishable from sarcoidosis. In addition to methotrexate and interferon, procarbazine, sirolimus, and the ICIs may also incite a granulomatous pneumonitis (Figure 12).[198,200–204] Drug withdrawal may result in disease regression.

Methemoglobinemia

Cyclophosphamide and its structural analog, ifosfamide, may induce methemoglobinemia.[205,206] Clinical cyanosis and hypoxia unresponsive to supplemental oxygen and in the setting of normal arterial PO_2 are important diagnostic clues. The mechanism of methemoglobinemia in this setting has not been elucidated, although glutathione depletion by these agents has been proposed.[205–207] Co-oximetry and spectrophotometric analysis of blood for methemoglobin are important components of the diagnostic workup. Once the diagnosis of methemoglobinemia is established permanent discontinuation of the culprit drug is recommended.

Lung injury associated with immunotherapy

Immune checkpoint inhibitors

The ICIs act by releasing negative regulatory controls involved in T-cell activation at specific regulatory immune checkpoints, thereby effectively tilting immune equilibrium in favor of immune attack and tumor killing. Agents in this drug class target the PD-1 (nivolumab, pembrolizumab, cemiplimab), PD-L1 (atezolizumab, avelumab, durvalumab), and cytotoxic T-lymphocyte antigen-4 [(CTLA-4), ipilimumab, tremelimumab] signaling pathways resulting in an augmented T cell-mediated immune response. The antitumor mechanism of action of ICI therapy differs from cytotoxic therapy and is responsible for both the therapeutic efficacy of this class of agents and the driver behind a diverse spectrum of immune-related adverse events (IrAEs). IrAEs are off-target, T-cell-driven inflammatory responses that affect virtually every organ system, with a variable incidence of 20–90% across ICI regimens and cancer types.[208,209] CTLA-4 and PD-1 mAbs have distinct IrAE profiles and histology-specific IrAE patterns which are possibly driven by different immune microenvironments. For instance, CTLA-4 inhibition is more often associated with colitis, hypophysitis, and dermatitis, whereas with PD-1 and PD-L1 mAbs, IrAEs associated with pneumonitis, hypothyroidism arthralgias, and vitiligo are more frequently reported.[210] Although pneumonitis, the most common form of lung-IrAE, does not occur with the frequency of IrAEs targeting other organ systems, it is a potentially lethal form of ICI-related toxicity and is therefore clinically relevant.[211–216] ICI-related sarcoid-like reactions, pleural effusions, and airway disease have also been observed.[204,217–223]

The incidence of ICI pneumonitis across tumor types for all grades is 3–19% and 0.8–1.4% for ICI pneumonitis grades >3.[131,212,214,224] In addition to ICI class, tumor histology, preexisting fibrotic lung disease, prior radiotherapy, and anti-PD-1/CTLA-4 dual therapies are risk factors that influence both the incidence and severity of disease. For example, anti-PD-1/CTLA-4 dual therapies are associated with a 2- to 3-fold increase in pneumonitis compared to ICI monotherapy.[225–229] Rates of all-grade pneumonitis ranging from 5.8% to 19% have been associated with ICI monotherapies that target the PD-1 or PD-L1 axis, whereas pneumonitis associated with CTLA-4 inhibitor monotherapy is rare (0–0.8%).[230] Pneumonitis rates are highest among patients treated with PD-1 or PD-L1 inhibitors for primary lung or renal

Table 3 Major histopathologic patterns of lung injury associated with immune checkpoint inhibitors.

Agent target/Class	Specific agent	NSIP	OP	HP	NCPE DAD ARDS	DS CRS	DAH	EP	Pleural disease	Sarcoid-like reactions	IR	Radiation recall pneumonitis
PD-1	Nivolumab	X	X	X	X		X	X	X	X	X	X
	Pembrolizumab	X	X	X	X	X		X	X	X	X	X
	Cemiplimab	X	X	X	X			X	X	X	X	X
PD-L1	Atezolizumab	X	X	X	X			X	X	X	X	X
	Avelumab	X	X	X	X			X	X	X	X	X
	Durvalumab	X	X	X	X			X	X	X	X	X
CTLA-4	Impilimumab	X	X	X	X			X	X	X	X	X
	Trimelimumab	X*	X*	X*	X*			X*	X	X	X	X

NSIP, nonspecific interstitial pneumonitis; OP, organizing pneumonia; HP, hypersensitivity pneumonitis; NCPE, noncardiogenic pulmonary edema; DAD, diffuse alveolar damage; ARDS, acute respiratory distress syndrome; DS, differentiation syndrome/cytokine release syndrome; DAH, diffuse alveolar hemorrhage; TE fistula, tracheoesophageal fistula; EP, eosinophilic pneumonia; VTE/PE, venous pulmonary embolism/pulmonary embolism; IR, infusion reaction; PH, pulmonary hypertension; IR, infusion reaction.

carcinomas compared to patients with other tumor types, including melanoma, head and neck squamous cell carcinoma, and urothelial carcinoma.[130,131,226,230–232] Increased cumulative incidence of pneumonitis has not been observed with long-term use of ICI agents. The role of preexisting lung disease and current or prior tobacco use has also been implicated in the development of ICI-related pneumotoxicity, although details of these associations have not been fully established.[224,227,233,234] Other potential risk factors, such as preexisting autoimmune disorders, chronic viral syndromes, and solid organ or hematopoietic stem cell transplantation, are of uncertain significance, as patients with these disorders were excluded from early clinical trials. Since then, information gleaned from several small retrospective studies has suggested that patients with preexisting autoimmune disorders may be safely treated with ICI therapies.[235] Response to ICI blockade in these studies has ranged from the development of new IrAEs, transient flare-ups of preexisting autoimmune disease, or both. New IrAEs and disease exacerbations were mild in most cases, although rare cases of severe and fatal pneumonitis were reported, thus underscoring the need for careful selection of these patients and close monitoring.[236–238]

The spectrum of ICI-related pneumonitis patterns is similar to histopathologic correlates caused by other drugs. OP and NSIP are the most frequently observed patterns. HP, DAD with ARDS, PF, DAH, bronchiolitis, and sarcoid-like reactions have also been reported.[130,214,223,224,227] Lung injury may manifest as a single histopathologic pattern, as more than one pattern simultaneously, or as different patterns with relapsed disease (Table 3).

Low-grade pneumonitis associated with asymptomatic pulmonary infiltrates (CTCAE grade 1) or nonspecific symptoms of dyspnea and dry cough, (CTCAE grade ≤2) are the presenting signs and symptoms in nearly 2/3 of patients. Acute respiratory distress associated with tachypnea, tachycardia, and hypoxia signal more advanced disease, which may be life-threatening.[234] The appearance of IrAEs involving other organ systems may occur concomitantly or sequentially in 60% of patients and should heighten the suspicion for lung-related IrAEs. Although lung-related IrAEs frequently occur within the first 12 weeks after initiation of therapy, events may occur at any time, including after the cessation of immune checkpoint blockade. Symptom onset has been consistently shorter among patients with primary lung cancer (2.9–7.7 weeks) and patients treated with combination therapy regimens (median onset 2.7 months, range 9 days to 6.9 months).[214,227]

The lung examination is typically bland. Bibasilar rales are nonspecific and signify advanced disease. Although no histocytologic findings on bronchoscopically obtained lavage fluid are pathognomonic, the bronchoscopic examination is an important component of the diagnostic workup which may help to exclude alternative diagnoses. BAL fluid cultures are helpful when positive. The yield of bronchoscopy declines with time elapsed after clinical presentation.[107] Thus, bronchoscopic examination to interrogate infection should be performed early in the course of evaluation of all patients with unexplained symptomatic pulmonary infiltrates (CTCAE grade 2 or higher). Predominant CD8-positive lymphocytosis with increased BAL eosinophils is frequent findings on cellular analysis. Transbronchial and surgically obtained lung biopsies may offer additional information, particularly in the setting of unexplained lymphadenopathy or suspicious lesions suggestive of underlying tumor progression. Lung function impairments, including reductions in forced expiratory volume in 1 second (FEV-1) and diffusing capacity of the lung for carbon monoxide (DLCO) are early signs of lung injury that may precede clinical and radiographic findings. However, pulmonary testing has not been proven to be reliably predictive of pneumonitis and threshold changes that presage clinically significant disease have not been determined.[227]

Treatment strategies for ICI-pneumonitis are guided by CTCAE pneumonitis grades and have not been validated in any prospective trials (Table 4). Outpatient monitoring is appropriate for asymptomatic patients with pulmonary infiltrates (grade 1). ICI therapy may continue uninterrupted if the patient remains asymptomatic and there is no evidence of disease progression on subsequent chest CT imaging and/or deterioration in lung function. If symptoms develop, ICI therapy should be interrupted and treatment strategies escalated to grade 2 or higher, depending on the severity of symptoms. For patients with pneumonitis grade 2 or higher, drug interruption is recommended along with initiation of systemic corticosteroids after infection and other competing diagnoses have been excluded. Steroids are usually dosed at 1–2 mg/kg/day and continued over 4–6 weeks. However, the optimal dose and tapering schedule for systemic corticosteroids have not been validated in any controlled trials, and treatment duration is largely dictated by response to steroid therapy. For patients with pneumonitis grade 2, outpatient management and consideration for drug rechallenge with close follow-up after resolution of signs and symptoms is recommended. Permanent withdrawal of ICI therapy and inpatient initiation of corticosteroids at 1–2 mg/kg/day is recommended for patients with pneumonitis grades 3 and 4. Steroid tapers typically occur over 6–12 weeks and should be tailored to the severity of the pneumonitis event. Rapid steroid tapers may precipitate pneumonitis flares in up to 25% of patients.[227]

Consideration for escalation of care is generally recommended after 48 h if there is no clinical improvement. Intensification of immunosuppressive therapy with infliximab, azathioprine,

Table 4 Treatment guidelines for pneumotoxicity associated with immune checkpoint inhibitor therapies.

CTCAE grade	Clinical presentation	Chest imaging findings	Diagnostic work-up	Management	Rechallenge?
1	Asymptomatic	Infiltrates involving <25% of entire lung parenchyma	Chest CT, consider PFTs, BAL (if infection is strongly considered)	Monitor weekly with history and physical examination and pulse oximetry;	Continue ICI therapy without interruption if no clinical or radiographic evidence of disease progression
				Reassess after 3–4 weeks with PFTs (if done at baseline) and repeat CT: if infiltrates have completely resolved or non-drug-related, continue ICI treatment; if no improvement or worsening infiltrates, treat as higher-grade pneumonitis (depending on symptoms and CT findings)	
2	Mild symptoms that do not interfere with ADLs	Multi-lobar infiltrates involving 25–50% of entire lung parenchyma	Chest CT, pulse oximetry; PFTs	Hold ICI therapy until resolution to Grade 1 or less	May rechallenge ICI if no clinical or radiographic evidence of disease progression
			Consider pulmonary consultation for bronchoscopy with BAL ± lung biopsies, if indicated	Empiric antibiotics;	
			Consider infectious disease consultation	Monitor every 2–3 days with history and physical examination and pulse oximetry	
			Check T-spot prior to prolonged immunosuppressive therapy	Prednisone 1–2 mg/kg/day with slow taper over four to six weeks	
				If no clinical improvement after 48–72 h of prednisone, hospitalize and treat as higher-grade pneumonitis	
				Consider GI and PJP prophylaxis with PPI and trimethoprim–sulfamethoxazole (unless contraindicated) with prolonged corticosteroid use	
				Consider calcium and vitamin D supplementation for prolonged steroid use	
3	Severe symptoms that limit self-care and ADLs; oxygen indicated	Multi-lobar infiltrates involving all lung lobes or >50% of lung parenchyma	Chest CT, pulse oximetry; PFTs	Discontinue ICI therapy	No. Permanently discontinue ICI therapy
			Consider pulmonary consultation for bronchoscopy with BAL ± lung biopsies, if indicated	Hospitalize patient for further care	
			Consider infectious disease consultation	Empiric antibiotics	
			Check T-spot prior to prolonged immunosuppressive therapy	Start methylprednisolone IV 1–2 mg/kg/day; no improvement after 48 h, consider addition of other immunosuppressive agents (infliximab 5 mg/kg; mycophenolate mofetil IV 1 g twice a day; IVIG for five days; tocilizumab or cyclophosphamide)	
				Slow steroid taper corticosteroids over four to six weeks	
				Start methylprednisolone IV 1–2 mg/kg/day; no improvement after 48 h, consider addition of other immunosuppressive agents (infliximab 5 mg/kg; mycophenolate mofetil IV 1 g twice a day; IVIG for five days; tocilizumab or cyclophosphamide)	
				Taper corticosteroids over four to six weeks	
				Consider GI and PJP prophylaxis with PPI and trimethoprim–sulfamethoxazole (unless contraindicated) with prolonged corticosteroid use	
				Consider calcium and vitamin D for prolonged steroid use	

(continued overleaf)

Table 4 (Continued)

CTCAE grade	Clinical presentation	Chest imaging findings	Diagnostic work-up	Management	Rechallenge?
4	Life-threatening respiratory compromise; urgent intervention indicated (eg, intubation, tracheostomy)	Multi-lobar infiltrates involving all lung lobes or >50% of lung parenchyma	Chest CT, pulse oximetry; PFTs Consider pulmonary consultation for bronchoscopy with BAL ± lung biopsies, if indicated Consider infectious disease consultation Check T-spot prior to prolonged immunosuppressive therapy	Same as Grade 3	No
5	Death				

mycophenolate mofetil, cyclophosphamide, and/or tocilizumab have not been rigorously studied in this setting, with support primarily derived from anecdotal reports and small case series.[239–241] Pharmacologic prophylaxis against *Pneumocystis jeroveci* pneumonia (PJP) is advocated for patients undergoing prolonged high dose steroids, although the dose and duration of steroids that connote "high dose" and "prolonged" have not been established. In general, PJP prophylaxis is recommended for steroid doses of 20 mg or higher for a duration of 30 days or longer.[242,243] Baseline screening for tuberculosis is suggested for all patients before initiating anti-TNF-α agents, given the known propensity for these agents to increase the susceptibility to serious infections, including reactivation of latent tuberculosis.[244–247] Pharmacologic prophylaxis against steroid-induced gastrointestinal stress ulcers should also be considered. Rapid steroid tapers may precipitate pneumonitis flares in up to 25% of patients which may be earlier in onset than the first event and more severe.[227] Rechallenge is considered absolutely contraindicated among patients with life-threatening toxicities, particularly those involving the lungs, heart, or central nervous system. Approximately 25–33% of patients experience recurrent IrAEs following drug reintroduction after initial resolution of signs and symptoms. If pneumonitis recurs, permanent discontinuation of ICI therapy is recommended. Unprovoked pneumonitis flares occurring months after drug discontinuation have also been reported.[229]

Chimeric antigen receptor T cell therapy (CAR-T)
CAR-T cell therapy is a form of T-cell-engaging immunotherapy in which genetically modified T cells are used to express a chimeric antigen receptor. Tisagenlecleucel and axicabtagene ciloleucel are first-in-class CAR-T agents that target the B lineage molecule, CD19. While these agents have broadened the therapeutic landscape in the management of certain hematologic malignancies, their widespread use is limited by unique toxicities that may be life-threatening. Cytokine release syndrome (CRS), a T-cell-mediated inflammatory response, and CAR-T-associated encephalopathy syndrome are the most common adverse effects associated with CAR-T therapy.[248,249] CRS-related symptoms range in severity from low-grade constitutional symptoms to life-threatening multiorgan dysfunction. Rarely, severe CRS can evolve into fulminant haemophagocytic lymphohistiocytosis (HLH).[250] Direct CAR-T-related lung toxicity has not been reported. Dyspnea, dry cough, and bilateral alveolar infiltrates may occur as sequelae of CRS-induced capillary leak with noncardiogenic pulmonary edema. Infection, pulmonary nodules, mediastinal lymphadenopathy, and noncardiogenic pulmonary edema have also been observed in association with HLH.[251] Symptoms may quickly progress to life-threatening hypotension and hypoxic respiratory failure. The median time to onset of CRS after CAR-T infusion is 3 days (range 1–14 days).[248,252] The duration of CRS is variable, with resolution typically by 2–3 weeks (depending on intervention) after drug infusion. Supportive care and initiation of an IL-6 inhibitor (tocilizumab or siltuximab) is the mainstay of therapy, based on the high correlation of CRS and IL-6 expression.

Pulmonary complications of thoracic radiation

Radiation pneumonitis and fibrosis
One of the many challenges of RT is the precise delivery of the radiation dose to target organs while sparing critical surrounding normal tissues. In thoracic neoplasms, where anatomical changes during treatment and tumor motion associated with respiratory variation are common, clinically significant lung injury following conventional thoracic radiation occurs in 5–20% of patients. Radiation-induced lung injury (RILI) is, in fact, the most common dose-limiting complication following thoracic radiation and chemoradiation regimens. Recent advances in radiation techniques, imaging, and delivery systems, such as proton therapy, three-dimensional conformal radiation therapy (CRT), intensity-modulated radiation therapy (IMRT), and stereotactic body radiation therapy (SBRT) have the potential to achieve higher target doses of radiation while mitigating radiation exposure to adjacent normal tissues. Radiation damage does occur with the newer radiation strategies, however, and the associated radiographic patterns and severity of RILD may differ from lung injury caused by conventional radiotherapy. Factors such as total radiation dose, dose per fraction, the volume of irradiated lung, and beam

characteristics and arrangements all influence the development of RP. Preexisting lung disease, underlying poor pulmonary reserve, prior radiotherapy, and rapid steroid withdrawal also influence the clinical appearance and severity of lung injury.[84,253] Multimodality regimens that combine radiation with chemotherapeutic agents such as mitomycin, cyclophosphamide, vincristine, doxorubicin, bleomycin, gemcitabine, the taxanes, and actinomycin D may not only potentiate radiation pneumotoxicity but shorten the latency period following radiation exposure.[254] Although data regarding optimal dose–fractionation and dose–volume relationships that mitigate lung injury are still evolving, it is generally agreed that a hyperfractionated course of radiation delivered to the smallest lung volume offers the lowest possibility of lung toxicity. Radiographically apparent lung damage is common with total doses of radiation that exceed 40 Gy. At doses >70 Gy, unusual pulmonary complications, including bronchial stenosis, bronchomalacia, mediastinal fibrosis, and injury to the recurrent laryngeal nerve have been reported. Lung injury at radiation doses below 20 Gy, is rare.[255]

Radiation pneumonitis (RP) and radiation fibrosis (RF) represent acute and late phases of RILI, respectively, and are the most frequent forms of radiation toxicity. Acute pneumonitis is heralded by fever, dyspnea, and nonproductive cough which may develop insidiously, 1–3 months after completion of RT and may precede the radiographic changes of RP. Radiographic changes may be seen as early as 3–4 weeks following RT, and discrete ground-glass opacities, ill-defined patchy nodules, or consolidation with air bronchograms and volume loss within the irradiated field. In mild cases of acute RP, these changes may resolve within 6 months, leaving a linear scar. Regional scarring is seen in nearly all patients, including those without clinical symptoms. Measurable changes in pulmonary function tests, including a reduction in lung volumes and diffusing capacity, may be seen as early as 2–3 months after irradiation. Histopathologic features of early RP include interstitial edema, hemorrhage, and fibrinous exudates with reactive type II pneumocytes. With more severe injury, RF develops. RF is signaled by the appearance of a well-demarcated area of volume loss, linear densities, bronchiectasis, retraction of the lung parenchyma, tenting and elevation of the hemidiaphragm, and ipsilateral pleural thickening (Figure 13). Like RP following conventional RT, these changes usually occur within the irradiated field. RF usually evolves over 6–12 months posttreatment and stabilizes within 1–2 years following completion of RT. RP detection methods using 18[F]-2-fluoro-2-deoxyglucose positron emission tomography (FDG-PET) imaging permits quantitative assessment of radiation pneumonitis, which manifests as enhanced FDG uptake. Higher standard uptake values (SUV) derived from PET-CT imaging have been associated with increased risks of symptomatic RP.[256] The utility of this imaging modality in identifying individuals at high risk for developing symptomatic RP is currently being investigated.

Factors such as the location, type, and extension of the primary tumor as well as the corresponding beam configuration and portals directly influence the shape and distribution of radiation-induced lung damage. RILD associated with the newer modes of RT delivery and imaging, such as 3D-CRT and IMRT, may not result in the stereotyped straight-edged infiltrate, but rather, assume a mass-like or whorled appearance or, alternatively, appear as poorly marginated and irregular nodules. Thus, lung injury following newer radiation techniques may be remarkably difficult to distinguish from competing disease entities such as infection or recurrence of the underlying malignancy.[257] Postradiation volume loss, bronchiectasis, and consolidation may occur with these modes of RT delivery, but typically are less extensive than injury patterns

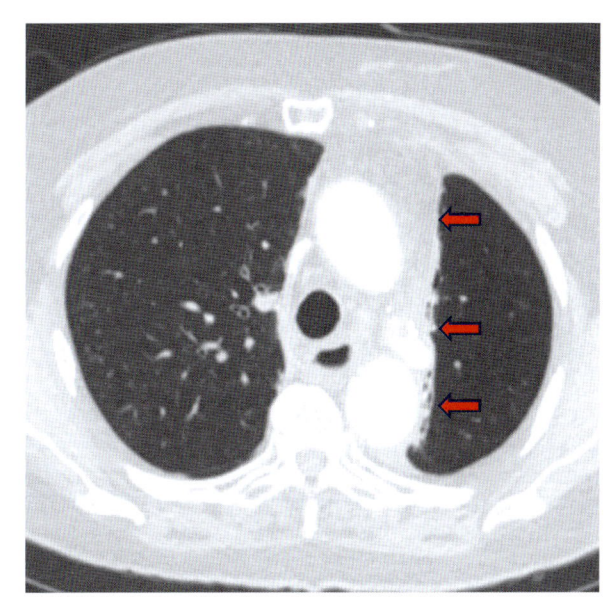

Figure 13 A 76-year-old man who presented with loud snoring, witnessed apneas, and daytime hypersomnolence, 9 years following completion of chemoradiation therapy for tonsillar squamous cell carcinoma. BMI at presentation was 22 kg/m^2. Severe obstructive sleep apnea/hypopnea syndrome with an Apnea-Hypopnea Index of 32 events/hour of sleep and an oxygen saturation nadir of 72% was observed on polysomnography (5-minute view).

following conventional radiation.[258] Proton radiotherapy improves delivery of radiation dose to the tumor with less dispersion before reaching the tumor target. This observation may permit safe escalation of radiation dose to tumoricidal levels while sparing critical normal lung tissues.[259,260] In one small study, patients that received proton therapy for medically inoperable NSCLC, tolerated higher doses of radiation with reduced rates of pneumonitis versus those who underwent conventional radiotherapy.[259] Further studies are needed to investigate these radiation modalities and their true impact reducing the risk of radiation pneumonitis.

Infection, drug toxicity, and recurrent tumor are major mimickers of RILI. Correlation with radiation treatment plans, knowledge of expected patterns of RILI, and temporal correlation with RT are important in the diagnosis of radiation damage. Lung opacities that develop prior to the completion of radiation should suggest an alternative diagnosis. Cavitation within the fibrotic area of irradiated lung may be due to a superimposed infectious, process such as tuberculosis or *Aspergillus* species, recurrent tumor, or postradiation necrosis. The loss of bronchiectasis due to filling of the airways with tumor or infection is also an important radiographic indication of superimposed disease.

It is generally accepted that RILI represents a continuum of changes initiated by an inflammatory pneumonitis, which progresses to fibrosis, although whether pneumonitis and fibrosis represent a continuum or separate entities has not been definitively resolved. Unfortunately, definitive pharmaceutical strategies in the successful prevention and treatment of RILI remain elusive. RP may respond to steroid therapy. Although evidence-based recommendations regarding dosing schedules and strategies are not available, in general, 40–60 mg of daily prednisone over several weeks, followed by a several-week taper provides relief of symptoms in most patients. There is no conclusive evidence that successful treatment of acute pneumonitis mitigates the later development of RF. Once established, steroids have not shown to be of benefit in the treatment of this late sequela of RT.

A less predictable or sporadic form of RP has also been recognized.[171] Sporadic pneumonitis occurs in a minority (5%) of patients and is thought to represent a type of HP characterized by a bilateral CD_4+ T-lymphocytic alveolitis that diffusely involves both lungs. Hence, radiation changes on imaging studies may extend well beyond the irradiated field. Patients present at 1–3 months following thoracic irradiation with symptoms of dyspnea and dry cough that are disproportionate to the volume of lung irradiated. This form of pneumonitis and its associated symptoms typically abate in 6–8 weeks without significant long-term sequelae.[171,261,262]

It is generally accepted that RILI represents a continuum of changes initiated by an inflammatory pneumonitis, which progresses to fibrosis, although whether pneumonitis and fibrosis represent a continuum or separate entities has not been definitively resolved. Unfortunately, definitive pharmaceutical strategies in the successful prevention and treatment of RILI remain elusive. RP may respond to steroid therapy. Although evidence-based recommendations regarding dosing schedules and strategies are not available, in general, 40–60 mg of daily prednisone over several weeks, followed by a several-week taper provides relief of symptoms in most patients. There is no conclusive evidence that successful treatment of acute pneumonitis mitigates the later development of RF. Once established, steroids have not shown to be of benefit in the treatment of this late sequela of RT.

Radiation recall pneumonitis

Radiation recall pneumonitis describes a rare but well recognized inflammatory reaction that occurs within a previously irradiated area of pulmonary tissue after application of certain chemotherapeutic agents. Recall pneumonitis has been observed most often following taxane- and anthracycline-based therapies. Gemcitabine, etoposide, vinorelbine, trastuzumab, and erlotinib have also been implicated as triggers for this disease (Tables 1 and 2).[263,264] Patients typically present with dry cough, low-grade fever, and dyspnea during the initiation of the precipitating agent or following several courses of therapy. Lung injury in recall pneumonitis typically occurs shortly after administration of the inciting antineoplastic agent, which may be weeks to years following completion of radiotherapy. Radiographically, ground-glass opacities and areas of consolidation that conform to the radiation treatment portal are seen. Drug withdrawal and initiation of corticosteroids and supportive care usually result in a favorable outcome. Rechallenge with the offending agent has been successful in some cases.[265]

Radiation-related pleural effusions

Radiation-related pleural effusions may occur as an early complication (within 6 months) of radiation pleuritis or as late sequelae (1–5 years) of mediastinal irradiation with associated mediastinal fibrosis, systemic venous hypertension, or lymphatic obstruction. These effusions are typically small, ipsilateral, and asymptomatic. Occasionally patients may complain of shortness of breath or pleuritic chest pain. Pleural fluid cytology is negative. Reactive mesothelial cells within the pleural fluid are common. Pulmonary veno-occlusive disease has also been reported as a rare complication of radiation-induced lung toxicity. Radiation-induced OP and eosinophilic pneumonia (EP) involving nonirradiated areas of in patients with breast cancer have also been documented.[266,267] Radiation-induced OP is thought to represent an immunologically mediated, lymphocyte-predominant hypersensitivity-like reaction. Both EP and OP may produce migratory pulmonary opacities on chest radiographs, which typically develop 1–3 months following radiotherapy. The presence of blood or tissue eosinophils, coupled with a prior history of asthma or atopy, favors the diagnosis of eosinophilic pneumonia. Corticosteroid therapy is associated with prompt recovery of radiation-induced OP and EP, although relapsed disease may rarely occur after steroid withdrawal. Other intrathoracic complications of RT include pulmonary congestion, which may occur as a sequela of radiation-induced myocardial and/or valvular dysfunction.

Pulmonary complications of hematopoietic stem cell transplantation

Hematopoietic stem cell transplantation (HSCT) is the only curative option for many patients with relapsed and high-risk hematologic malignancies. Despite advances in treatment regimens and supportive care, pulmonary complications occur in up to 60% of HSCT recipients, accounting for significant morbidity and mortality.[268–270] Pulmonary complications of HSCT are divided into "early" (those that occur during the first 100 days posttransplant) and "late" (those that occur > than 100 days posttransplant) (Table 3). These complications are primarily due to direct toxicities from conditioning regimens, delayed bone marrow recovery, prolonged immunosuppressive therapy, and graft-versus-host disease (GVHD). Infectious complications commonly occur after allogeneic HSCT, in part due to the use of immunosuppressive therapy for GVHD. As successful prophylactic treatment strategies have effectively reduced the rates of infectious pulmonary complications, noninfectious pulmonary complications have emerged as a major cause of post-HSCT morbidity and mortality Table 5.

Early onset noninfectious complications of HSCT

Pulmonary edema and pleural effusions
Diffuse pulmonary edema is one of the most common early complications after transplantation. Etiologies include increased hydrostatic capillary pressure from large-volume intravenous fluids, sometimes in combination with cardiac dysfunction and cardiac dysfunction. Increased pulmonary capillary permeability can occur due to conditioning regimens.[268,271] The abrupt onset of dyspnea, hypoxemia, and bilateral pulmonary infiltrates, without clinical evidence of infection, support a diagnosis of pulmonary edema. Pleural effusions, often bilateral, may accompany pulmonary edema and may be managed conservatively, without the need for diagnostic thoracentesis.

Peri-engraftment respiratory distress syndrome (PERDS)
Peri-engraftment respiratory distress syndrome (PERDS) is characterized by fever, noncardiogenic pulmonary edema, an

Table 5 Noninfectious pulmonary complications following hematopoietic stem cell transplantation.

Early (<100 days)	Late (>100 days)
Pulmonary edema	Bronchiolitis obliterans
Idiopathic pneumonia syndrome	Cryptogenic organizing pneumonia
Diffuse alveolar hemorrhage	Post-transplant lymphoproliferative disorders
Engraftment syndrome	
Secondary pulmonary alveolar proteinosis (rare)	Lymphocytic interstitial pneumonitis (rare)
Pulmonary veno-occlusive disease (rare)	

erythematous skin rash, and hypoxemia. PERDS occurs during the neutrophil recovery phase of HSCT. Estimates of incidence vary from less than 3% to nearly 50%, in part due to definitional variations.[269,270] While the pathophysiology is not well understood, proposed mechanisms include the release of pro-inflammatory cytokines during the engraftment period and endothelial damage from conditioning regimens. Risk factors include the use of growth factors, the number of infused mononuclear, high CD34+ cell counts, rapid neutrophil recovery, type of conditioning regimen, underlying disease, and cord blood as the source of stem cells. Most cases show improvement with corticosteroid therapy, though well-controlled studies are lacking.[272,273]

Idiopathic pneumonia syndrome (IPS)
In 1993, a panel convened by the NIH proposed a broad working definition of IPS as widespread radiographic infiltrates in the absence of congestive heart failure or evidence of lower respiratory tract infection.[160] IPS occurs in 3–4% of HSCT recipients, usually 14–90 days following transplantation.[274,275] A substantial proportion of historical IPS cases were found to have other infections, including human-herpesvirus 6. Mortality rates range from 50% to 70%.[276–278] Risk factors include transplantation for malignancy other than leukemia, older age, total body irradiation, type of pretransplant chemotherapy, high-grade GVHD, CMV (cytomegalovirus)-seropositive donor, HLA (human leukocyte antigen) disparity, and lower performance status.[276] Possible etiologies of IPS include direct toxic effects of the chemoradiation conditioning regimen and release of inflammatory cytokines. However, the association of IPS with the presence of acute GVHD after allogeneic transplantation leaves open the possibility that alloreactive T-cell injury could contribute.[276,277] The clinical presentation typically features symptoms of acute dyspnea, cough, and fever associated with diffuse infiltrates on chest radiograph. The diagnosis of IPS relies largely on the exclusion of infection and absence of cardiac, renal, or iatrogenic fluid overload. Treatment includes high-dose intravenous corticosteroids and supportive care with supplemental oxygen and broad-spectrum antibiotics. Earlier preclinical and clinical data suggested a potential role for tumor necrosis factor-α (TNF-α) in the pathogenesis of IPS. However, one randomized trial found high early response rates to systemic corticosteroid therapy but no further increase in response to treatment with the addition of etanercept, a TNF receptor fusion protein.[279]

Diffuse alveolar hemorrhage (DAH)
Posttransplant DAH is characterized by widespread lung injury and diffuse radiographic infiltrates in the absence of identifiable infection following allogeneic and autologous stem cell transplants.[280–282] The Blood and Marrow Transplant Clinical Trials Network includes DAH within the definition of IPS. DAH has also been described in up to one-third of patients during the peri-engraftment period.[283,284] DAH may represent a severe IPS, a distinct entity defined by alveolar capillaritis, or a failure of normal clotting mechanisms, and current definitions do not distinguish between these possible etiologies. Bronchoscopically, DAH appears as progressively bloody returns on lavage fluid taken from three or more subsegmental bronchi. The bronchoscopic criteria for DAH diagnosis have expanded to include cytologic evidence of >20% hemosiderin-laden macrophages in the BAL fluid. Increased hemosiderin-laden macrophages and bloody lavage fluid may be seen in association with diffuse lung injury from a wide variety of causes in the posttransplant setting. Bloody BAL fluid is, thus, neither sensitive nor specific for DAH and may simply represent an index of severity of alveolar injury and concomitant hemostatic defects rather than a separate syndrome. More important, prognosis and therapy are determined by the underlying pathophysiologic process (engraftment syndrome, IPS, sepsis, etc.).[284] There are no associations between the development of DAH and coagulopathy or thrombocytopenia. Furthermore, platelet transfusion does not improve respiratory status. Treatment of DAH includes high-dose intravenous corticosteroids and supportive care, such as supplemental oxygen, mechanical ventilation, and platelet transfusion.[285] Recombinant human factor VIIa (rFVIIa) has been used to enhance hemostasis, but a recent retrospective analysis showed no survival advantage with the addition of rFVIIa to high-dose corticosteroid therapy.[286]

Pulmonary veno-occlusive disease (PVOD)
PVOD is a rare complication of HSCT in which progressive occlusion of pulmonary veins and venules caused by intimal proliferation and fibrosis leads to PH.[287] High-dose chemotherapy, particularly alkylating agents, and infections are implicated as causes of PVOD. The onset is typically insidious, with progressive dyspnea and fatigue occurring several weeks to months after transplant.[288,289] Current treatment options are limited, and mortality rates can reach up to 100% within 2 years.

Late-onset noninfectious complications of HSCT

Bronchiolitis obliterans syndrome (BOS)
Bronchiolitis obliterans syndrome (BOS) is an underrecognized pulmonary complication among long-term survivors of allogeneic HSCT. BOS is a late manifestation of GVHD that leads to progressive respiratory insufficiency and sometimes death. Five-year mortality may be as high as 50%. BOS almost always occurs in the presence of GVHD of nonlung organs in allogeneic HSCT.[269,290,291] The incidence of BOS varies between 5% and 26% depending upon diagnostic criteria.[292] The NIH consensus guidelines for diagnosing PTCB include (1) $FEV_1/FVC < 0.7$ and $FEV_1 < 75\%$ of predicted, residual volume on PFTs > 120% predicted; (2) evidence of air trapping, small airway thickening, bronchiectasis on HRCT, or pathological confirmation of constrictive bronchiolitis; and the (3) absence of any infectious process on radiographic, laboratory, or clinical testing.[293] BOS affects small airways, causing chronic inflammation, epithelial mucous metaplasia, submucosal scarring, smooth muscle hypertrophy, and concentric bronchiolar fibrosis. The most commonly identified risk factors are chronic GVHD, older age, viral infections during the first 100 days after transplant, the presence of airflow limitation before transplant, as well as the use of methotrexate or busulfan in the conditioning regimen.[269,293] Patients may be asymptomatic in early stages of BOS, which delays the diagnosis.[294] Late presentations, including dyspnea, cough, and wheezing, are more common, as airflow obstruction progresses.[290,291] Chest radiographs are usually normal, but high-resolution CT scans may show evidence of air trapping, thickened or dilated small airways, and mosaic attenuation.[274,295] Newer quantitative CT techniques may give more accurate estimates of the degree of small airway obstruction. Bronchoscopy with BAL and transbronchial lung biopsy is generally not helpful in establishing the diagnosis. PFTs are the most important test in the evaluation of BOS. Importantly, NIH diagnostic criteria are useful to confirm clinically evident BOS, but some have proposed revising these criteria to facilitate the diagnosis of BOS at earlier stages (BOS Stage 0p), though this criteria trade increased sensitivity for reduced specificity and a higher false-positive rate in a low-prevalence disease.[293]

BOS treatment typically consists of augmentation of systemic immunosuppression with corticosteroids and calcineurin inhibitors along with the initiation of inhaled corticosteroids. High-dose inhaled corticosteroid therapy is effective in stabilizing FEV_1 in many patients.[296,297] The combination of inhaled corticosteroids, azithromycin, and montelukast was historically the combination of choice to treat BOS based on prospective data, but recent data suggest that azithromycin may be associated with increased rates of hematologic relapse or second neoplasms.[298] Lung transplantation is an option in selected patients with post-HSCT BOS but is associated with higher mortality than most lung transplant recipients. Pulmonary rehabilitation should be considered in all symptomatic patients. Second-line therapies have not been well studied in BOS, although extracorporeal photopheresis, a therapy that improves peripheral tolerance, may improve outcomes.[299] Early detection and properly conducted prospective trials for the management of BOS are crucial to improve survival.

Cryptogenic organizing pneumonitis (COP)

Also known as *bronchiolitis obliterans organizing pneumonia* (*BOOP*), cryptogenic organizing pneumonitis (COP) occurs mostly in allogeneic HSCT recipients with GVHD. COP is a distinct entity that should not be confused with BOS and is not generally considered a form of GVHD. COP is less common than BOS, with an incidence of 1–2% in long-term survivors. Dry cough, dyspnea, and fever accompanied by patchy infiltrate on chest radiograph and CT scan are the predominant presenting signs and symptoms.[300] The diagnosis is made with surgical lung biopsy. COP is usually responsive to corticosteroids with more favorable prognosis; however, no standard treatment guidelines are currently available.

Posttransplant lymphoproliferative disorder (PTLD)

Posttransplant lymphoproliferative disorder (PTLD) is an uncontrolled expansion of donor-derived Epstein–Barr virus (EBV)-infected B lymphocytes that develop in response to inadequate cytotoxic T cell function.[301,302] It occurs in approximately 1% of HSCT patients, usually within the first 4–12 months after transplant. The lung is involved only 20% of the time, most commonly with ill-defined nodular infiltrates. Treatment includes reduction of immunosuppressive therapy anti-CD20 mAbs (rituximab), antiviral drugs, and infusion of EBV-specific cytotoxic T lymphocytes.

Pneumonia

Pulmonary infections frequently complicate cancer and its therapy.[303,304] Classic clinical indicators to suggest the presence of lower respiratory infections include the development of pulmonary parenchymal infiltrates, leukocytosis, fever, and expectoration of purulent secretions. However, as a consequence of impaired immune responses, these typical clinical observations may be absent in cancer patients with pneumonia. Therefore, a high index of suspicion is required to avoid overlooking the diagnosis. Furthermore, early radiographic imaging, often including CT scanning, is indicated in cancer patients with unexplained clinical deterioration or new infiltrates on conventional imaging.[305]

The diagnosis of pneumonia is confirmed by recovery of the likely pathogen from an otherwise sterile source (e.g., blood, urine, pleural fluid) or isolation of a noncommensal organism in respiratory secretions. Although the utility of expectorated sputum in the diagnosis of pneumonia is debated, cytologically confirmed lower respiratory samples appear to be diagnostically useful. Fiberoptic bronchoscopy with BAL is considered the diagnostic tool of choice for obtaining lower respiratory samples. While this procedure is safe for most cancer patients traditional culture methods yield the responsible pathogen in only 25–51% of cases.[306-311] The benefit of BAL may be enhanced by early bronchoscopic evaluation, particularly if obtained before the initiation of antimicrobial therapy. Microscopic examination of transbronchial biopsy specimens can identify angioinvasion of commensal microbes (e.g., *Aspergillus* spp.). Culture of biopsy material, however, has not been proved diagnostically superior to BAL, and is often precluded in cancer patients due to coagulopathy and/or thrombocytopenia.[312] Culture results from BAL or biopsy can be difficult to interpret due to frequent microbial colonization of the upper airway. Conversely, sterile respiratory tract cultures do not exclude an infectious etiology, particularly in the setting of recent administration of broad-spectrum antibiotics. Molecular techniques, including polymerase chain reaction (PCR) testing for pathogen genomic material or antigen detection methods (e.g., serum galactomannan, urinary *Histoplasma* antigen), can also supplement the diagnostic evaluation and are now formally recommended for the evaluation of suspected fungal respiratory infections in immunocompromised cancer patients by the American Thoracic Society.[313]

Early and accurate diagnoses are critical to a successful outcome, although treatment should not be withheld while diagnostic interventions are undertaken. Antimicrobial selections are based on knowledge of the infecting pathogen, if available, pneumonia severity, underlying immune status, and the presence of co-morbid conditions[314,315] (see section titled "Pneumonia"). Delays in appropriate antimicrobial therapy increase the risk of secondary complications and infection-associated deaths, especially in severely immunosuppressed individuals. Therefore, it is common practice to initiate empiric and/or preemptive antimicrobial therapy in patients in which the suspicion of infection is high. However, the clinician is cautioned to recall that cancer patients are prone to numerous causes of fever and pulmonary infiltrates other than infectious pneumonias, including toxicities of therapy, systemic inflammation associated with extrapulmonary infections, heart failure, parenchymal cancer involvement, or intrapulmonary hemorrhage.[316]

Venous thromboembolism

PE and deep venous thrombosis (DVT) are manifestations of venous thromboembolism (VTE). Approximately 20% of all VTEs are associated with cancer, and cancer increases the risk for VTE 4–6-fold. Surgery, chemotherapy, hormonal therapy, growth factors, angiogenesis inhibitors, erythropoietic agents, and central venous catheters (CVC) contribute to cancer-associated VTE.[205] The diagnosis and therapy of VTE may delay, discontinue or preclude many forms of cancer therapy.[317,318] Cancer-related VTE is associated with significant overall mortality but is an infrequent cause of death.[206] One study found that 3.5% of cancer patients die from VTE.[207]

The clinical presentation of VTE is nonspecific. Scoring systems developed to estimate the pretest probability of DVT and PE (such as Well's scores) in combination with D-dimer testing can be used to rule out VTE in cancer patients, however, the likelihood of finding normal D-dimer levels among cancer patients is less than

30%. Furthermore, an elevated D-dimer has no significant positive predictive value in the cancer setting.[208] Doppler/compression ultrasound is the preferred method to diagnose DVT, although MRI and CT may be required in special circumstances, such as internal iliac vein or vena cava thrombosis. High-resolution CT or CT angiography is the best method for diagnosing PE and offers the advantage of providing additional information regarding thoracic pathology that may confound the diagnosis.[209] Urgent bed-side echocardiography should be considered for diagnosis and risk stratification of unstable patients with suspected massive PE.[319]

Pharmacological VTE prophylaxis should be considered in every hospitalized patient with cancer.[210] Cancer patients undergoing abdominal or pelvic surgery should receive low molecular weight heparin (LMWH) prophylaxis extended for 4 weeks.[211] Routine prophylaxis in ambulatory cancer patients undergoing active chemotherapy is recommended only for patients with myeloma receiving thalidomide or lenalidomide as part of combination chemotherapy.[211] There is no evidence that anticoagulation prevents catheter-associated thrombosis, and guidelines recommend against it.[210]

Routine VTE induction therapy is used in cancer patients. LMWH is the preferred drug for initial treatment of VTE in this setting. Unfractionated heparin should be used in patients with impaired renal function. Thrombolytics have not been systematically studied in patients with cancer, but their use may be considered in cases of massive PE. An IVC filter should be placed when anticoagulation is contraindicated.[210,212] Based on limited evidence, VTEs found incidentally should be managed as symptomatic VTE.[320] For maintenance therapy, LMWH rather than vitamin K antagonists (VKA) is preferred because LMWH is better at preventing recurrences.[321] However, warfarin remains the preferred agent in patients with renal insufficiency. The use of edoxaban, apixaban, and rivaroxaban have been studied only in open-label and pilot studies in patients with cancer and VTE.[322–324] These agents seem to be well tolerated, but their use should be individualized. When tolerated, maintenance therapy can be continued indefinitely for patients with active cancer.[325–327]

Pulmonary hypertension in the cancer patient

PH is an under-recognized problem in the cancer setting. Transthoracic Doppler echocardiography (TTE) provides an estimation of pulmonary artery systolic pressure (PASP) and serves as a noninvasive screening tool for PH. In the revised 2019 World Health Organization clinical classification scheme, PH is categorized into five groups which share similar etiologies, hemodynamic characteristics, and therapeutic approaches. These include Pulmonary Arterial Hypertension (PAH, Group 1), PH due to left heart disease (Group 2), PH due to lung diseases and/or hypoxia (Group 3), chronic thromboembolic pulmonary hypertension (CTEPH, Group 4), and PH with unclear multifactorial mechanisms (Group 5).[328] Right heart catheterization (RHC) is required for the diagnosis of PAH and to further classify PH.[208] RHC allows assessment of hemodynamic impairments and evaluation of vasoreactivity of the pulmonary circulation, which may guide subsequent classification and management. PAH denotes a subpopulation of PH characterized by the presence of precapillary PH based on an end-expiratory pulmonary artery wedge pressure (PAWP) ≤ 15 mm Hg and a pulmonary vascular resistance > 3 Woods unit.[207]

PH may precede the cancer diagnosis or occur at any point along the continuum of cancer care. PH occurring after completion of cancer therapy has also been described. Estimates of cancer-related PH vary broadly with specific cancers, associated cancer therapies, and detection methods. Nonspecific signs and symptoms of exertional dyspnea and fatigue early in the disease process render diagnostic evaluations notoriously difficult and result in substantial delays in treatment. Therefore, a high degree of suspicion is needed to detect PH early, when treatments are more efficacious. Syncope, angina, peripheral edema, abdominal distention, and hemodynamic instability are signs of advanced disease which is often refractory to therapy. In acute presentations of PH, secondary causes, such as acute thromboembolic disease, hypoxemic respiratory insufficiency, airway bronchoconstriction, or cardiac dysfunction, must be excluded.

Cancer-related PH is represented in several of these categories. Dasatinib, a TKI, rarely results in moderate to severe precapillary PAH. Cessation of dasatinib may result in improvement or resolution of PAH, however, occasionally vasodilator therapy is required.[170,175] Other therapies including alkylating agents, interferon-α and -β, and bosutinib have also been implicated as potential etiologies of PAH, but further data is needed.[328] PVOD, a rare cause of PH that is characterized by occlusion or narrowing of the pulmonary veins, represents a subgroup of Group I. Infection, chemotoxins, thoracic radiation, and stem cell transplantation are postulated risk factors for PVOD, although no clear causal relationship has been established.[329,330] The prognosis for PVOD is poor. Although some patients may tolerate arterial vasodilators, fatal pulmonary edema precipitated by pulmonary vasodilator therapy has been observed.

Chronic myeloproliferative disorders (MPDs) constitute a rare cause of PH. Several potential mechanisms of MPD-associated PH include high cardiac output, splenectomy, direct obstruction of pulmonary arteries, chronic thromboembolism, portal hypertension, and congestive heart failure.[331] Other cancer- and cancer treatment-related entities that involve the pulmonary vasculature may also cause PH. These include external compression and/or entrapment of large pulmonary veins by adenopathy, neoplasms, or mediastinal fibrosis. Hodgkin's lymphoma and germ cell tumors underlie most causes of PH due to mediastinal compression. Fibrosing mediastinitis related to radiation and infection (*Aspergillus*, *Mycobacterium tuberculosis*, blastomycosis, mucormycosis, and cryptococcosis) has also been reported to cause PH.[332–334]

The principal primary malignancies involving the pulmonary vasculature are sarcomas. Typically, these rare and frequently fatal tumors arise from the main pulmonary arteries, although pulmonary venous sarcomas have also been described.[335] Patients with pulmonary arterial sarcomas often present with signs and symptoms that mimic CTEPH (dyspnea, chest pain, cough, hemoptysis). However, associated findings of unexplained fever, weight loss, clubbing, anemia, and elevated ESR should raise suspicion of malignancy. Secondary tumoral involvement of the pulmonary vascular bed may present as macrovascular central tumor emboli or tumor cell aggregates that occlude small vessels. The latter may occur with or without lymphangitic spread of disease. Choriocarcinomas and mucinous tumors originating in the breast, lung, gastrointestinal tract, and kidneys are associated with the highest rates of tumor embolization.[336] Clinical symptoms of tumor emboli range from the abrupt onset of dyspnea, chest pain, and cardiovascular collapse to subacute symptoms of cough, exertional dyspnea, and exercise intolerance associated with unexplained PH. Pulmonary tumor thrombotic microangiopathy

(PTTM) is an unusual cause of malignancy-related PH that is most often seen in patients with adenocarcinomas, particularly of the stomach.[335] Patients present with severe, refractory PH that rapidly progresses to sudden cardiovascular collapse and death. Findings on pulmonary microvascular cytology are diagnostically useful; however, the diagnosis of PTTM is most often made at necropsy. No definitive treatment has been identified thus far. Although in most major medical centers, CT angiography has replaced V/Q scans in the evaluation of thromboembolic events; in the setting of suspected tumor emboli, V/Q scans may be of greater diagnostic utility than the chest CT. Multiple subsegmental mismatched defects on V/Q scintigraphy are supportive findings. Pulmonary microvascular cytology of samples obtained from a wedged pulmonary artery catheter during RHC may offer additional support for tumor embolization.[337]

The evolution of therapy guidelines for PAH over the past two decades has resulted in evidence-based treatment strategies that favorably impact survival and significantly improve the quality of life of these patients.[338] Treatment of PH should address the underlying cause. The need for supportive therapies, including supplemental oxygen, diuretics, anticoagulant therapy, and exercise should be assessed in all patients. More advanced therapies are directed at PAH itself and should be initiated based on the results of further testing and national guidelines. Current and emerging therapies for PAH target the endothelin, nitric oxide, and prostaglandin pathways. Specific treatment strategies may include monotherapy or, more frequently, combination therapy.[338,339] Unfortunately, no cure exists for this devastating condition. Caution in extrapolating PAH treatment guidelines to other forms of PH is warranted. No studies have addressed the utility of pulmonary vasodilator therapy in the management of cancer-related PH. Dobutamine, milrinone, intravenous prostacyclin, inhaled vasodilators, and extracorporeal life support are accepted therapies for PH with hemodynamic decompensation in the general population.[340] Specific guidelines regarding the optimal use of vasopressor therapy in the critically ill cancer patient with PH and associated hemodynamic deterioration have yet to be delineated.

Sleep disorders in cancer patients

Sleep disturbance and chronobiology have important implications throughout the continuum of care of the cancer patient.

Cancer prevention

Prolonged sleep duration and disturbed circadian rhythms of sleep are associated with an increased risk of cancer. In a large Japanese Cohort Study, sleep durations of less than 5 h or greater than 9 h per night conferred higher cancer prevalence.[341] Chronic sleep disturbance caused by rotating and nocturnal shift work may also increase the risk of cancer. Nurses who worked rotating shifts for more than 30 years had an increased relative risk of breast cancer in one study. Suppression of melatonin, a naturally occurring hormone with oncostatic potential, occurs with nocturnal light exposure and may contribute to the increased cancer risk among patients with chronic sleep disturbance.[342–344] Sleep disruption and abnormal circadian rhythms have been associated with impaired immune system-mediated tumor surveillance which may also increase cancer risk.[345,346] Obstructive sleep apnea (OSA) appears to confer an increased cancer risk, with higher rates associated with more severe nocturnal hypoxia.[347–349] These findings implicate a link between sleep disruption and cancer, and they highlight improvement of sleep hygiene and treatment of sleep disorders as potential targets for cancer prevention.

Cancer treatment

Excessive daytime sleepiness and fatigue are associated with increased plasma cytokines, such as IL-6. A good night's sleep can decrease the levels of this cytokine. Inflammatory mediators produced by specific cancer interventions or the cancer itself may exacerbate sleep disruption. For example, chemotherapy regimens used to treat breast cancer may induce elevations in VEGF which is associated with disturbed sleep.[350] Sleep loss and, in particular, loss of rapid eye movement (REM) sleep, are known to be hyperalgesic. Thus, reduced sleep conditions, including REM sleep deprivation, which is common in many cancer patients, confer increased sensitivity to pain.[351]

Primary sleep disorders, including restless leg syndrome and periodic leg movement disorders, are often associated with insomnia and daytime hypersomnolence. These disorders are more common among certain cancer subgroups, perhaps due to chemotherapy-related anemia and peripheral neuropathy.[352] The OSA syndromes may also be more prevalent in certain cancers. In a study of 56 patients with tumor of the head and neck region, 84% met clinical criteria for OSA (Figure 14).[353] Opioids are known to worsen symptoms of central sleep apnea. This form of sleep-disordered breathing may be problematic in cancer patients, as many are on opioid medications for cancer-related pain.[354]

Chronobiology and chronotherapy attempt to optimize the effects of cancer chemotherapy while minimizing toxicity by taking advantage of the differences in the circadian rhythm of the cell cycle of tumor cells versus host tissues. Clinical and animal studies have shown that dose intensity can be increased while simultaneously reducing toxicities and improving treatment outcomes.[355,356]

Cancer survivorship

Disturbed sleep, fatigue, and insomnia may occur in up to 51% of some cancer survivors.[357] Cognitive and behavioral therapy (CBT) has been shown to improve symptoms of insomnia, decrease sedative-hypnotic medication use, and improve quality of life and is the treatment of choice for insomnia. CBT can also impact immune function in cancer patients by increasing levels of IL-1β and γ-interferon, which are thought to promote sleep.[358]

Pulmonary rehabilitation

Pulmonary rehabilitation (PR) represents a multidisciplinary strategy that incorporates exercise training, patient and family education, psychosocial and behavioral interventions, and outcome assessment in the management of patients with chronic respiratory diseases. Evidence-based support for pulmonary rehabilitation (PR) in the care of patients with COPD has led to the implementation of this treatment strategy as standard of care in the management of this group of patients. The systemic effects and comorbidities associated with cancer, specifically, fatigue, dyspnea, anemia, skeletal muscle impairment, muscle wasting, poor exercise intolerance, depression, deconditioning, and anxiety add substantially to the burden of the disease. PR targets many of these symptoms, resulting in reductions in symptoms of dyspnea and fatigue, and improvements in exercise tolerance and quality of life. Poor exercise tolerance confers worse surgical outcomes following lung resection and limits the ability to withstand the potential toxicities of chemotherapy.[359,360] Thus, the rationale for providing PR to patients with cancer is quite strong, particularly in the setting of lung cancer, where COPD and lung cancer often coexist.

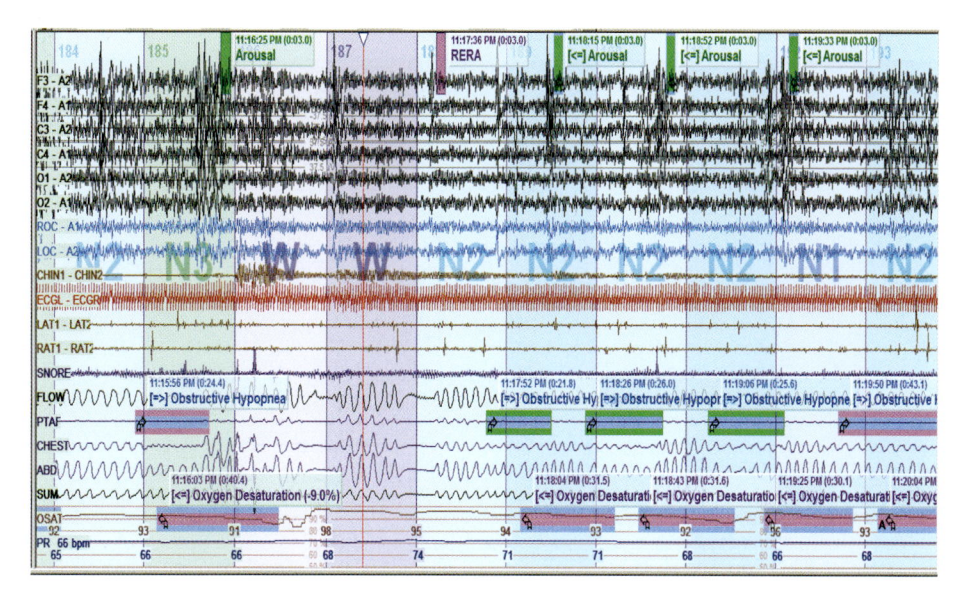

W = awake; N1, N2, N3 = sleep stages

Figure 14 Radiation fibrosis. Well-demarcated linear fibrotic changes along the paramediastinum (arrows) with bronchiectasis and volume loss is noted approximately 9 months after completion of radiation therapy for adenocarcinoma involving the left upper lobe. Source: Based on Faiz et al.[353]

Recent small studies suggest that pulmonary rehabilitation may favorably impact lung cancer management by improving a variety of clinically meaningful outcomes, such as performance status, chemotherapy-related fatigue, oxygen consumption, exercise tolerance, and health-related quality of life.[361] In a study by Bobbio and colleagues, an increase in work rate and oxygen consumption (VO_2max) following a 4-week course of preoperative PR permitted patients who were considered nonoperative based on presurgical VO_2max to undergo successful lung resection.[362] In other investigations, improvements in exercise endurance, muscle strength, and dyspnea scores following 6 to 8 weeks of postsurgical PR have led to reduced hospital stay and increased quality of life among patients that underwent thoracotomy and resection for lung cancer.[362–366] In the nonsurgical setting, several small reports have suggested a beneficial role for PR in countering chemotherapy- and radiotherapy-related fatigue, ameliorating performance status, and reducing the length/frequency of hospitalizations among patients with cancer.[367–370]

Acute respiratory failure

Acute respiratory failure (ARF) is the most common reason for ICU admission among adult patients with cancer. Predisposing conditions for both acute and chronic respiratory insufficiency in cancer patients can be divided into those that cause "lung" failure or "pump" failure. Lung failure is typically associated with ventilation/perfusion abnormalities, shunts, or alterations of alveolar-capillary diffusion and leads primarily to hypoxia, at least in its early stages. A classic example of lung failure is ARDS. Lung failure may also develop in the absence of ARDS as a consequence of ventilation/perfusion mismatch associated with pneumonia, atelectasis, or PE, or as a result of shunt associated with pulmonary edema. Other common causes of lung failure are listed in Table 6. Pump failure, by contrast, results from primary failure of alveolar ventilation and leads to severe hypercapnia and acidosis with only mild hypoxemia. Multifactorial causes of ARF, such as severe COPD exacerbation with superimposed pneumonia may lead to both lung and pump failure. This mixed picture is a common source of respiratory failure in the cancer patient, which requires a systematic approach to each component of respiratory failure in an effort to logically devise treatment strategies.

Causes of pump failure central nervous system disorders: impaired drive

Isolated central depression of ventilatory drive is a rare cause of pump failure that may result from insults to the central nervous system, such as medullary tumors or infarction, and sedating or narcotic medications. Acquired central hypoventilation may occur following neurosurgical procedures for brainstem tumors, particularly those that are close to the fourth ventricle. Radiation to the base of the skull may have similar adverse effects. Occult hypothyroidism may also contribute to central hypoventilation and ventilatory failure, particularly in elderly women and following treatment for head and neck carcinoma. More often, respiratory failure owing to depressed central drive occurs as an additional insult, superimposed on chronic respiratory insufficiency. In this setting small doses of narcotic or sedating medications may have a profound effect on alveolar ventilation. Respiratory muscle fatigue may also contribute to central hypoventilation by sending inhibitory signals to the respiratory center in the CNS to reduce drive, thereby protecting the muscles from injury and mitigating further muscle fatigue.

Peripheral nervous system disorders: inadequate neuromuscular competence

Transmission of signals from the CNS to the respiratory muscles occurs via the spinal cord and peripheral nerves. Hence, conditions causing neuromuscular dysfunction, such as primary neurologic diseases, spinal cord lesions, neuromuscular blocking drugs, and muscle weakness may precipitate ventilatory failure. Systemic anesthetics cause potent neuromuscular blockade and ventilatory depression. Other agents, including sedatives, anxiolytics, hypnotics, and aminoglycosides typically produce severe

Table 6 Lung versus pump failure in acute respiratory failure: characteristics and underlying causes.

	Lung failure	Pump failure
Characteristic features	Hypoxemia	Severe hypercapnia with acidosis mild hypoxemia
Pathogenesis	Ventilation/perfusion mismatch shunts	Exhaustion of ventilatory pump (CNS*, PNS** or respiratory muscles)
	Alterations in alveolar-capillary membrane	
	Acute lung injury/ARDS	Coexisting COPD
Underlying conditions	Pneumonia	Intrinsic or extrinsic airway compression
	Atelectasis	Obstructive sleep apnea associated with head and neck malignancies
	Pulmonary embolism/tumor emboli	
	Lymphangitic spread of tumor	
	Chemotherapy	
	Radiation therapy	
	Pulmonary leukostasis	
	Transfusion-related lung injury	
	Postoperative respiratory insufficiency	

respiratory depression only in the setting of preexisting neuromuscular diseases such as myasthenia gravis and myasthenic paraneoplastic syndrome or after massive overdose. One exception to this principle is methadone, which may cause ventilatory insufficiency with chronic administration. Muscle fatigue, a pervasive problem in the cancer setting, is central to the development of respiratory failure. An extensive list of factors may potentiate cancer-related muscle fatigue, including hypoperfusion states (cardiogenic, septic, or hemorrhagic shock), excess lactate or hydrogen ion production, severe anemia and, thereby, respiratory failure. Malnutrition and cachexia are well-known complications of advanced cancer. One of the most relevant manifestations of cancer cachexia is muscle wasting, which contributes to markedly depressed strength and endurance of the skeletal muscles, including the diaphragm.[371] Overinflation of the thorax and flattened diaphragms associated with COPD, a common co-morbidity of lung cancer, further contributes to compromised respiratory muscle performance and ventilatory failure. Electrolyte disturbances such as hypophosphatemia, hypokalemia, and hypomagnesemia frequently complicate chemotherapy and may cause profound muscle weakness in the cancer patient. In addition, many of the drugs used in the treatment of ventilatory failure, including beta-agonists, diuretics, and corticosteroids may exacerbate hypophosphatemia and aggravate muscle weakness. Chemotherapeutic agents and other drugs used in cancer treatment may also have deleterious effects on the neuromuscular system. Although corticosteroid-induced myopathy has been well described, the role of these drugs in potentiating respiratory muscle dysfunction has only recently been recognized.[372,373] Among the chemotherapeutic agents, vinca-alkyloids, cisplatin, and the taxanes are most frequently associated with peripheral neurotoxicity. The clinical manifestations of these drugs on lung function may be subtle in the absence of predisposing factors, such as preexisting neuromuscular abnormalities. In addition to their CNS effects, the use of anesthetic agents, in particular, halothane, propofol, and nitrous oxide may induce respiratory depression by decreasing diaphragmatic contractility.[374,375] Injury to the phrenic nerve following surgery for head and neck cancer, or surgery to the anterior mediastinum, esophagus, or lungs may cause persistent diaphragmatic dysfunction and ventilatory failure. Loss of diaphragmatic function from direct phrenic nerve invasion by tumor may also be seen, particularly among patients with lymphoma or cancers of the lung, or head and neck. Diffuse neural dysfunction resulting from paraneoplastic syndromes is another cause of respiratory failure in the cancer setting. Lambert–Eaton myasthenic syndrome, which affects about 3% of patients with small-cell lung cancer, myasthenia gravis, which occurs in 10–15% of patients with thymoma, and demyelinating peripheral neuropathy, seen in 50% of patients with the osteosclerotic form of plasmacytoma are the most common types of paraneoplastic disorders of the peripheral nervous system. These disorders typically have a subacute and debilitating course that may lead to ventilatory failure.

Increased work of breathing: increased respiratory system load and chest wall abnormalities

A variety of cancer-related factors may result in acute or chronic escalations in the respiratory system load. Elevations in airway resistive workloads, characterized physiologically by abnormal airway resistance and increased elastance, are cardinal features of COPD, airway inflammation, airway edema, or physical obstruction by mucous, blood, or tumor. Upper airway obstruction caused by tracheal stenosis associated with prior intubation or radiation to the head and neck, and intubation with a small (<7.5 mm internal diameter) endotracheal tube significantly contributes to increased airflow resistance, and respiratory failure. Abnormalities involving the chest wall and thoracic spine caused by tumor, radiation, or surgery may cause increased chest wall elastic loads, increased work of breathing, and respiratory failure.

Lung failure (pulmonary edema, acute respiratory distress syndrome/acute lung injury)

Pulmonary edema/acute respiratory distress syndrome (ARDS)/acute lung injury (ALI)

The predilection for pulmonary edema in the setting of cancer arises from a broad array of insults to the lungs that may be sorted according to the underlying permeability characteristics of the microcirculation, and the presence or absence of diffuse alveolar damage seen histopathologically. In normal permeability pulmonary edema, increased hydrostatic pressure caused by an imbalance in Starling forces leads to fluid filtration into the lungs. Pulmonary edema of cardiogenic and neurogenic etiologies, as well as lung edema caused by lung reexpansion, lymphatic obstruction, and relief of upper airway obstruction, is typically associated with normal microvascular permeability.

The histopathologic hallmark of increased microvascular permeability is the accumulation of proteinaceous fluid within the interstitium and alveoli resulting from a breach in the integrity of the alveolar and microvascular surfaces. Increased permeability pulmonary edema occurring in the absence of diffuse alveolar damage is referred to as capillary leak syndrome. In the cancer setting, this type of pulmonary edema may occur following the administration of cytokines such as interferon, IL_2, and TNF, which disrupt capillary endothelial integrity. These drugs may also cause direct toxicity to the myocardium, resulting in mixed or overlap edema associated with normal and increased permeability etiologies. Neurogenic and re-expansion pulmonary edema represent two other causes of mixed edema, which are frequently observed in the cancer setting. The frequent need for transfused blood products (packed red blood cells, platelets, and granulocytes) in the cancer setting predisposes the cancer patient to the syndrome of transfusion-related lung injury (TRALI), another form of noncardiogenic pulmonary edema. Pulmonary hypertension with normal left ventricular end-diastolic pressures is also a cardinal feature of this syndrome. The treatment is supportive. Resolution of clinical symptoms and radiographic changes typically occurs within 2–3 days of symptom onset without permanent pulmonary sequelae, although in 20% of patients, symptoms and radiographic changes may persist for a week and may be associated with lung injury (ALI/ARDS—see below).[376,377]

Acute lung injury (ALI) and ARDS are terms used for varying severity of pulmonary edema accompanying the histopathologic finding of diffuse alveolar damage. ARDS is reserved for severe lung injury in which bilateral pulmonary infiltrates and severe hypoxemia (as defined by a ratio of the partial pressure of arterial oxygen to the fraction of inspired oxygen < 200) occur in the absence of clinical evidence of left atrial hypertension.[378] ALI is reflective of a lesser injury, as indicated by a PaO_2/FiO_2 ratio between 200 and 300. The list of cancer-related precipitating conditions associated with ARDS is extensive. An etiological dichotomy that sorts the causes of ARDS into conditions that provoke direct lung injury (pneumonia, gastric aspiration) and those that are associated with systemic diseases that promote indirect lung injury (sepsis, transfusion-related lung injury) provides a simplistic approach to ARDS but is confounded by the fact that the inciting events are often multifactorial or unknown. Clinically, patients may present with acute respiratory failure and associated hypoxemia within 24–48 h of the predisposing event. Fever and leukocytosis, owing to the inflammatory response associated with lung injury, may be prominent findings, even in the absence of infection. Although the radiographic changes in ARDS are not distinctive, the CXR is nonetheless important in ruling out competing diagnoses such as pneumothorax, infections, and congestive heart failure. Patchy areas of lung involvement may be seen as ground glass opacifications early on which may progress to diffuse areas of consolidation. Radiographic findings suggestive of cardiogenic pulmonary edema such as Kerley B lines, cardiomegaly, and apical vascular redistribution are typically absent. Progression to the fibroproliferative phase is common, resulting in persistent hypoxemia associated with poor lung compliance, increased dead space, ventilation-perfusion imbalance, and pulmonary hypertension.

Management of respiratory failure: medical therapy

The management of the critically ill cancer patient with respiratory failure involves aggressive supportive care as well as strategies that target the precipitating cause. Standard supportive measures include the provision of supplemental oxygen, inhaled bronchodilators, nutritional support, chest physiotherapy and pulmonary toilet, and the prudent use of diuretics, vasopressors, and antibiotics, where indicated. Although fluid loading augments oxygen consumption and tissue oxygen delivery, careful attention to fluid homeostasis is imperative, as a persistent positive fluid balance has been associated with a poor outcome.[379,380] More specific interventions, such as administration of helium-oxygen (heliox) mixtures may provide temporary relief of acute respiratory distress associated with proximal airway obstruction and serve as a bridge to more definitive therapy. Patients with DAH may benefit from the early use of high-dose steroids, desmopressin acetate (DDAVP®), and aggressive blood and blood product support.[381] Recombinant Factor VII (rFactory VII), and antifibrinolytics, such as aminocaproic acid, have been used to treat transplant-related DAH, although convincing evidence supporting this practice is not available.[382–384] The effect of activated protein C administration in reducing sepsis-related ARDS mortality has been exciting, however, conflicting results in subgroup analysis and concerns regarding serious bleeding have led to removal of this from the market.[385–387]

Advances in supportive care coupled with early identification and management of precipitating condition(s) and strategies that attenuate ventilator-associated lung injury have contributed to significant increases in ARDS-related survival rates over the past decade.[388] Several trials of high-dose corticosteroids for early-phase ARDS failed to demonstrate a survival benefit. A salutary effect of high-dose glucocorticoids given during the fibroproliferative phase of ARDS was suggested in several small studies, though not borne out in a large, multicenter, NIH-sponsored (ARDS-Net), trial.[389–392]

Mechanical ventilation: *noninvasive ventilation (NIV)*

Assisted ventilation is often required to manage ARF that is nonresponsive to conservative medical therapy. Newer modes of mechanical ventilation as well as the use of noninvasive ventilation (NIV) have shown promising results and gained broad acceptance in the management of cancer patients with respiratory failure. The efficacy of NIV has been clearly demonstrated in several randomized, controlled studies in the management of pump failure as well as selected cases of lung failure.[393,394] In a recent retrospective study of the outcome of cancer patients following ICU transfer for ARF, the use of NIV was associated with marked improvements in patient survival.[395] In addition, significant reductions in the need for conventional mechanical ventilation and declines in both ICU and post-ICU hospital mortality have been linked to the use of intermittent NIV during the early stages of hypoxemic ARF (PaO_2/FiO_2 ratio <250).[396–398] Evidence favoring the early use of NPPV for ARF among immunocompromised patients is derived from several small studies which purport reduced rates of endotracheal intubation, length of ICU stay, and ICU mortality.[396,399,400]

Immunocompromised patients with respiratory failure who require mechanical ventilation have notoriously poor prognoses, with an estimated 1% increase of risk for pneumonia per day of mechanical ventilation.[401] Thus, NIV in this setting has quickly gained broad acceptance in the management of cancer patients with respiratory failure.

Invasive mechanical ventilation (IMV)

Intermittent mandatory ventilation (IMV) remains the standard of care for severe ARF and for NIV treatment failures. Overdistension of the lungs at end-inspiration and repetitive collapse of the lungs at end exhalation that occurs with conventional mechanical ventilation at high tidal volumes may trigger further lung injury. This observation prompted the development of lung-protective ventilator strategies that mitigate alveolar overdistension and enhance recruitment of atelectatic alveoli, thereby reducing the incidence of ventilator-induced lung injury. Lung-protective ventilator strategies may be accomplished with conventional modes of ventilation such as assist-control and pressure-controlled ventilation with or without inverse ratio ventilation or alternative methods, such as biphasic positive airway pressure ventilation (BIPAP), airway pressure release ventilation (APRV), jet and high frequency oscillatory ventilation, and differential lung ventilation. None of these modes of ventilation have proven to be superior to conventional ventilatory strategies. Convincing evidence favoring the use of protective ventilator strategies is derived from the National Institute of Health ARDS Network trial where lower tidal volumes (6 mL/kg of predicted body weight) and limited static inspiratory pressures (<30 cm H_2O) resulted in a 22% improved survival compared to patients mechanically ventilated using higher tidal volumes and inflation pressures.[402,403] Other adjuncts to ventilator management of patients with ARF, including extracorporeal membrane oxygenation (ECMO) and partial liquid ventilation (PLV), prone positioning, and surfactant instillation have been proposed; however, the merits of these therapies over conventional treatment strategies have not been definitively proven. Early tracheostomy may be associated with improved outcomes in critically ill patients. Practice guidelines regarding the appropriate timing of tracheostomy in patients that require prolonged mechanical ventilation are based on a consensus statement, nearly 2 decades old, that suggested that tracheostomy be considered after 21 days of mechanical ventilation. Although these recommendations were only based on expert opinion, modern practice broadly continues to follow them. In a recent meta-analysis, an 8.5-day decrease in total mechanical ventilation days and significant reduction in ICU length of stay was seen among patients that underwent early tracheostomy (within 7 days of initiation of invasive mechanical ventilation) compared to those in which tracheostomy was performed late, although mortality was not significantly altered.[404]

Respiratory failure outcomes

The mortality rate of critically ill cancer patients with respiratory failure is at least threefold higher than that of concurrently admitted cancer patients without respiratory failure.[405–407] Conditions common to the critically ill cancer patient such as cardiac, renal, or hepatic dysfunction, disseminated intravascular coagulation, hemodynamic instability, and the need for mechanical ventilation are independent predictive variables that portend a poor outcome.[405,406,408] Early reports documented mortality rates among mechanically ventilated cancer patients with ARF in excess of 90%, especially among patients with hematologic malignancies and recipients of hematopoietic transplants.[409–412] More recent investigations have offered a more favorable perspective, with mortality rates of 69–84/%.[413,414] Survival gains may be attributable to better infection prophylaxis measures, improved transplantation techniques, standard use of preventive measures that mitigate aspiration, more aggressive use of hematopoietic growth factor support following transplantation, and trends toward the use of peripheral stem cells rather than bone marrow as a source of donor stem cells. In addition, the newer ventilation strategies including NIV and lung-protective ventilator strategies may play a role in improved survival.[407] Finally, the implementation of programs for early identification and management of deteriorating patients on general hospital wards and improvements in ICU admission and triage criteria may not only contribute to overall improved ICU survival but also to the appropriate use of hospital resources.[415]

> **Summary**
>
> The unique vulnerability of the respiratory system to cancer and its treatment gives rise to a broad spectrum of respiratory complications that may significantly impact cancer-related morbidity and mortality. The spectrum of respiratory complications continues to evolve as new therapies for cancer emerge. Early recognition, prompt diagnosis, and treatment play a pivotal role in the management of these patients and are essential to optimizing outcomes.

Key references

The complete reference list can be found on Vital Source version of this title, see inside front cover.

21. Salamonsen MR, Lo AK, Ng AC, et al. Novel use of pleural ultrasound can identify malignant entrapped lung prior to effusion drainage. *Chest.* 2014;**146**(5):1286–1293.
34. Wahidi MM, Reddy C, Yarmus L, et al. Randomized trial of pleural fluid drainage frequency in patients with malignant pleural effusions. The ASAP trial. *Am J Respir Crit Care Med.* 2017;**195**(8):1050–1057.
37. Tremblay A, Mason C, Michaud G. Use of tunnelled catheters for malignant pleural effusions in patients fit for pleurodesis. *Eur Respir J.* 2007;**30**(4):759–762.
41. Davies HE, Mishra EK, Kahan BC, et al. Effect of an indwelling pleural catheter vs chest tube and talc pleurodesis for relieving dyspnea in patients with malignant pleural effusion: the TIME2 randomized controlled trial. *JAMA.* 2012;**307**(22):2383–2389.
56. Morice RC, Peters EJ, Ryan MB, et al. Exercise testing in the evaluation of patients at high risk for complications from lung resection. *Chest.* 1992;**101**(2):356–361.
63. Shannon VR. Pneumotoxicity associated with immune checkpoint inhibitor therapies. *Curr Opin Pulm Med.* 2017;**23**(4):305–316.
64. Galie N, Humbert M, Vachiery JL, et al. 2015 ESC/ERS guidelines for the diagnosis and treatment of pulmonary hypertension: The Joint Task Force for the Diagnosis and Treatment of Pulmonary Hypertension of the European Society of Cardiology (ESC) and the European Respiratory Society (ERS): Endorsed by: Association for European Paediatric and Congenital Cardiology (AEPC), International Society for Heart and Lung Transplantation (ISHLT). *Eur Heart J.* 2016;**37**(1):67–119.
72. Anders CK, LeBoeuf NR, Bashoura L, et al. What's the price? Toxicities of targeted therapies in breast cancer care. *Am Soc Clin Oncol Educ Book Am Soc Clin Oncol Annu Meet.* 2020;**40**:55–70.
96. Possick JD. Pulmonary toxicities from checkpoint immunotherapy for malignancy. *Clin Chest Med.* 2017;**38**(2):223–232.
97. Gore EM, Lawton CA, Ash RC, Lipchik RJ. Pulmonary function changes in long-term survivors of bone marrow transplantation. *Int J Radiat Oncol Biol Phys.* 1996;**36**(1):67–75.
107. Shannon VR, Andersson BS, Lei X, et al. Utility of early versus late fiberoptic bronchoscopy in the evaluation of new pulmonary infiltrates following hematopoietic stem cell transplantation. *Bone Marrow Transplant.* 2010;**45**(4):647–655.
130. Naidoo J, Page DB, Li BT, et al. Toxicities of the anti-PD-1 and anti-PD-L1 immune checkpoint antibodies. *Ann Oncol Off J Eur Soc Med Oncol.* 2015;**26**(12):2375–2391.
132. Petri CR, Patell R, Batalini F, et al. Severe pulmonary toxicity from immune checkpoint inhibitor treated successfully with intravenous immunoglobulin: case report and review of the literature. *Respir Med Case Rep.* 2019;**27**:100834.
140. Siddall E, Khatri M, Radhakrishnan J. Capillary leak syndrome: etiologies, pathophysiology, and management. *Kidney Int.* 2017;**92**(1):37–46.
144. Shannon VR, Subudhi SK, Huo L, Faiz SA. Diffuse alveolar hemorrhage with nivolumab monotherapy. *Respir Med Case Rep.* 2020;**30**:101131.
152. Trojan A, Meier R, Licht A, Taverna C. Eosinophilic pneumonia after administration of fludarabine for the treatment of non-Hodgkin's lymphoma. *Ann Hematol.* 2002;**81**(9):535–537.
170. Montani D, Bergot E, Gunther S, et al. Pulmonary arterial hypertension in patients treated by dasatinib. *Circulation.* 2012;**125**:2128–2137.
174. Riou M, Seferian A, Savale L, et al. Deterioration of pulmonary hypertension and pleural effusion with bosutinib following dasatinib lung toxicity. *Eur Respir J.* 2016;**48**(5):1517–1519.
177. Savale L, Sattler C, Gunther S, et al. Pulmonary arterial hypertension in patients treated with interferon. *Eur Respir J.* 2014;**44**(6):1627–1634.

190 Markman M. Management of toxicities associated with the administration of taxanes. *Exp Opin Drug Saf*. 2003;**2**(2):141–146.
192 Maggi E, Vultaggio A, Matucci A. Acute infusion reactions induced by monoclonal antibody therapy. *Exp Rev Clin Immunol*. 2011;**7**(1):55–63.
201 Murphy KP, Kennedy MP, Barry JE, et al. New-onset mediastinal and central nervous system sarcoidosis in a patient with metastatic melanoma undergoing CTLA4 monoclonal antibody treatment. *Oncol Res Treat*. 2014;**37**(6):351–353.
205 Shehadeh N, Dansey R, Seen S, Abella E. Cyclophosphamide-induced methemoglobinemia. *Bone Marrow Transplant*. 2003;**32**(11):1109–1110.
206 Hadjiliadis D, Govert JA. Methemoglobinemia after infusion of ifosfamide chemotherapy: first report of a potentially serious adverse reaction related to ifosfamide. *Chest*. 2000;**118**(4):1208–1210.
210 Khoja L, Day D, Wei-Wu Chen T, et al. Tumour- and class-specific patterns of immune-related adverse events of immune checkpoint inhibitors: a systematic review. *Ann Oncol*. 2017;**28**(10):2377–2385.
219 Nishino M, Sholl LM, Awad MM, et al. Sarcoid-like granulomatosis of the lung related to immune-checkpoint inhibitors: distinct clinical and imaging features of a unique immune-related adverse event. *Cancer Immunol Res*. 2018;**6**(6):630–635.
224 Delaunay M, Cadranel J, Lusque A, et al. Immune-checkpoint inhibitors associated with interstitial lung disease in cancer patients. *Eur Respir J*. 2017;**50**(2): 1700050.
227 Naidoo J, Wang X, Woo KM, et al. Pneumonitis in patients treated with anti-programmed death-1/programmed death ligand 1 therapy. *J Clin Oncol*. 2017;**35**(7):709–717.
229 Nishino M, Chambers ES, Chong CR, et al. Anti-PD-1 inhibitor-related pneumonitis in non-small cell lung cancer. *Cancer Immunol Res*. 2016;**4**(4):289–293.
231 Cadranel J, Canellas A, Matton L, et al. Pulmonary complications of immune checkpoint inhibitors in patients with nonsmall cell lung cancer. *Eur Respir Rev*. 2019;**28**(153). doi: 10.1183/16000617.0058-2019.
260 Mehta V. Radiation pneumonitis and pulmonary fibrosis in non-small-cell lung cancer: pulmonary function, prediction, and prevention. *Int J Radiat Oncol Biol Phys*. 2005;**63**(1):5–24.
271 Afessa B, Peters SG. Major complications following hematopoietic stem cell transplantation. *Semin Respir Crit Care Med*. 2006;**27**(3):297–309.
291 Afessa B, Litzow MR, Tefferi A. Bronchiolitis obliterans and other late onset non-infectious pulmonary complications in hematopoietic stem cell transplantation. *Bone Marrow Transplant*. 2001;**28**(5):425–434.
307 Grosu HB, Morice RC, Sarkiss M, et al. Safety of flexible bronchoscopy, rigid bronchoscopy, and endobronchial ultrasound-guided transbronchial needle aspiration in patients with malignant space-occupying brain lesions. *Chest*. 2015;**147**(6):1621–1628.
317 Timp JF, Braekkan SK, Versteeg HH, Cannegieter SC. Epidemiology of cancer-associated venous thrombosis. *Blood*. 2013;**122**:1712–1723.
319 Torbicki A, Perrier A, Konstantinides S, et al. Guidelines on the diagnosis and management of acute pulmonary embolism: the Task Force for the Diagnosis and Management of Acute Pulmonary Embolism of the European Society of Cardiology (ESC). *Eur Heart J*. 2008;**29**(18):2276–2315.
327 Carrier M, Khorana AA, Zwicker JI, et al. Management of challenging cases of patients with cancer-associated thrombosis including recurrent thrombosis and bleeding: guidance from the SSC of the ISTH: a reply to a rebuttal. *J Thromb Haemost*. 2014;**12**(1):116–117.
385 Bernard GR, Vincent JL, Laterre PF, et al. Efficacy and safety of recombinant human activated protein C for severe sepsis. *N Engl J Med*. 2001;**344**(10): 699–709.
392 Steinberg KP, Hudson LD, Goodman RB, et al. Efficacy and safety of corticosteroids for persistent acute respiratory distress syndrome. *N Engl J Med*. 2006;**354**(16):1671–1684.
402 Acute Respiratory Distress Syndrome Network, Brower RG, Matthay MA, et al. Ventilation with lower tidal volumes as compared with traditional tidal volumes for acute lung injury and the acute respiratory distress syndrome. *N Engl J Med*. 2000;**342**:1301–1308.

132 Gastrointestinal and hepatic complications in cancer patients

Robert S. Bresalier, MD ■ Emmanuel S. Coronel, MD ■ Hao Chi Zhang, MD

> **Overview**
>
> Gastrointestinal and hepatic complications represent some of the most common and potentially life-threatening disorders associated with treatment of cancer patients. The expansion of therapeutic options for these patients has been accompanied by a growing number of direct and indirect consequences which affect the rapidly dividing cells of the GI tract. Cytotoxic, immunologic, and infectious insults often act synergistically to augment toxicity. Recognition of these complications, together with proper evaluation and management are key to the well-being of these patients.

Introduction

A growing spectrum of treatments is available to combat cancer. Chemotherapy, radiotherapy, and molecular targeted therapies including immunotherapies lead to adverse effects in several organ systems, including those of the gastrointestinal (GI) tract. GI complications are very common in patients undergoing cancer treatment. Some of these complications can be life threatening and require prompt and appropriate diagnosis and treatment. This article addresses common GI complications that result from cancer treatment and focuses on the evaluation and management of these problems.

Esophageal disorders

Esophagitis

Esophagitis in patients with cancer may be due to the direct cytotoxic effects of chemotherapy or radiation, or by infections due to immunosuppressive effects of cancer therapy (Table 1). Cell death leads to mucosal atrophy, ulceration, and initiation of the inflammatory response. Reactive oxygen species, pro-inflammatory cytokines, and metabolic byproducts of colonizing organisms may also play a role in amplifying tissue injury.[1,2] Synergy between chemotherapy and radiotherapy may increase the severity and extent of esophagitis observed with combined modality therapy. Esophagitis may also be due to pill-induced injury, acid reflux disease, and graft-versus-host disease (GVHD) in hematopoietic stem-cell transplant recipients. When esophagitis is suspected, particularly in an immunocompromised patient, prompt evaluation with endoscopy with biopsies and/or brushings is indicated to allow for early diagnosis and therapy.

Radiation-induced esophagitis

Radiation-induced esophagitis can occur during external beam radiation treatment of lung, head and neck, and esophageal cancers. Acute radiation esophagitis is primarily due to injury to the rapidly dividing cells of basal epithelial layer, which subsequent thinning and denudation of the esophageal mucosa. The severity of esophagitis depends on radiation dose and is exacerbated by the concurrent use of chemotherapeutic agents such as cisplatin.[3–5] Patients generally complain of odynophagia, dysphagia, and chest pain. Endoscopy findings include erythema, edema friable mucosa, ulcerations, or scarring with stricture formation. Treatment of acute esophagitis includes the use of local anesthetics such as oral viscous lidocaine hydrochloride, systemic narcotic analgesics, and acid suppression with proton pump inhibitors. Symptoms in some patients are so severe as to require temporary percutaneous endoscopic gastrostomy (PEG) placement. Some patients undergoing extensive head and neck surgery and chemoradiation may benefit from PEG placement prior to treatment in anticipation of severe symptoms. A recent consensus statement of the Multinational Association of Supportive Care in Cancer (MASCC) and the International Society of Oral Oncology (ISOO) suggested the use of intravenous amifostine to prevent esophagitis induced by concomitant chemotherapy and radiation in patients with non-small-cell lung cancer.[1] Esophageal strictures are treated by endoscopic dilation. In patients with malignant tracheoesophageal fistulas due to esophageal cancer or bronchogenic carcinoma, endoscopic placement of self-expanding covered metal stents is the palliative treatment of choice.[6]

Fungal infections

Esophageal candidiasis is very common in immunocompromised patients, with *Candida albicans* being the most common causative organism for esophageal and oropharyngeal candidiasis (OPC). Patients complain of odynophagia and/or dysphagia. On endoscopy, esophageal candidiasis is identified by white plaque-like lesions with surrounding erythema on the esophageal wall. Esophageal biopsies or brushings may confirm the presence of invasive yeast or hyphal forms of *C. albicans*. An empiric course of antifungal therapy is recommended in immunocompromised patients with odynophagia or dysphagia. Endoscopy should be performed if symptoms do not improve within 72 h. The general duration of antifungal treatment is 14–21 days. ***Candida*** esophagitis in immunocompromised patients requires systemic antifungal therapy; it cannot be treated with topical agents.[7–10] Patients unable to tolerate oral agents require intravenous therapy. The treatment of esophageal candidiasis includes azoles, echinocandins, or amphotericin B.[7–14] Azoles inhibit cell

Table 1 Common causes of esophagitis in patients receiving cancer therapy.

Infectious agent/injury	Endoscopic appearance	Treatment
Candida albicans	White plaque-like lesions with surrounding erythema on the esophageal mucosa	Systemic antifungal treatment with fluconazole, itraconazole, voriconazole, or echinocandins
Herpes Simplex Virus	Small vesicles, coalescing to form ulcers	Acyclovir, foscarnet sodium
Cytomegalovirus	Linear or serpiginous ulcers	Ganciclovir, foscarnet sodium, valgancyclovir
Varicella-zoster virus	Small vesicles, similar to HSV ulcers	Intravenous acyclovir
Polymicrobial oral flora	Bacteria mixed with necrotic epithelial cells in biopsy samples	Broad-spectrum antibiotics
Injury due to chemotherapy and radiation	Friable mucosa with erythema and edema	Lidocaine hydrochloride, narcotic analgesics, proton pump inhibitors, endoscopic dilation/stents (for strictures), PEG[a]

[a] Percutaneous gastrostomy.

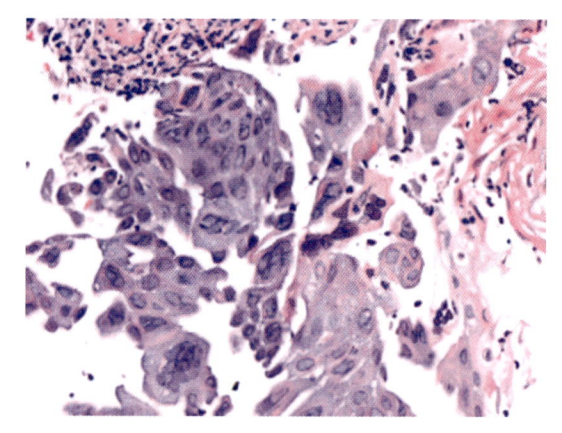

Figure 1 **Herpes simplex virus (HSV) esophagitis.** High power view of esophageal mucosa shows squamous cells with ground glass nuclear viral inclusions and multinucleated giant cells in a background of neutrophilic exudates.

membrane formation by inhibiting the synthesis of ergosterol, a principal component of fungal cell membrane. Fluconazole, an azole, is the recommended first-line agent due to its efficacy, ease of administration, and low cost. For patients with fluconazole-refractory esophageal candidiasis who can tolerate oral therapy, newer azoles (voriconazole and posaconazole) are available. Itraconazole has been found to be as effective as fluconazole for the treatment of esophageal candidiasis however its use is limited by significant nausea and by its potential for drug interactions due to inhibition of the cytochrome p 450 enzymes.

Patients requiring intravenous therapy should be treated with fluconazole or one of the echinocandins (caspofungin, micafungin, or anidulafungin), rather than amphotericin B, because of their better toxicity profiles. Echinocandins inhibit synthesis of $\beta(1,3)$-D-glucan, an essential component of the fungal cell wall. Mammalian cells do not require $\beta(1,3)$-D-glucan, thereby limiting potential toxicity. Relapse rates are higher with echinocandins compared to azoles, and these are used as second-line therapy if treatment with azoles has failed. Amphotericin B is reserved for esophageal candidiasis during pregnancy and in individuals with drug-resistant candidiasis. OPC is a local infection. Risk factors include radiation, chemotherapy, antibiotics, and steroids. Treatment is with local agents such as nystatin or clotrimazole troches. Patients at risk of developing OPC may be given antifungal prophylaxis. Topical antifungals, such as clotrimazole or miconazole, are effective for prophylaxis.[15]

Viral infections

Viral infections of the esophagus are caused by herpes simplex virus (HSV), cytomegalovirus (CMV) and, rarely, varicella-zoster virus (VZV).[9,16] Patients usually present with odynophagia and dysphagia. Less frequent symptoms include nausea, vomiting, heartburn, epigastric pain, and fever. In the case of HSV esophagitis, some patients may have coexistent herpes labialis or oropharyngeal ulcers. Diagnosis is made by endoscopy and biopsy (Figure 1). In the early stage, HSV lesions may appear as small vesicles, although they are rarely seen. The vesicles eventually coalesce to form large ulcers which are usually less than 2 cm in size. The ulcers are well circumscribed with normal-appearing intervening mucosa. CMV will cause ulcers which are linear or serpiginous and deeper than HSV-related ulcers. Exudates may also be present. Biopsies taken from the edge of an HSV-related ulcer will show intranuclear inclusions and multinucleated giant cells. Inclusions can also be detected by immunohistochemistry using monoclonal antibodies to HSV. Viral cultures are helpful in identifying resistant strains in patients who do not respond to acyclovir. VZV can produce esophagitis in adults with herpes zoster, usually in the setting of disseminated infection. Endoscopically, VZV ulcers are similar to those seen with HSV. On biopsy specimens, distinction from HSV will require immunohistochemistry or culture.

CMV infects endothelial cells and fibroblasts, but not epithelial cells as with HSV and VZV. Routine biopsies in a CMV-infected patient show intranuclear inclusions in fibroblasts and endothelial cells. Immunohistochemistry with anti-CMV antibodies is also helpful for diagnosis.

For patients with HSV esophagitis, acyclovir (400 mg orally five times daily for 14–21 days or 5 mg/kg intravenously every 8 h for 7–14 days) is the therapy of choice.[8,9,17,18]

Acyclovir-resistant HSV results from mutations in the thymidine kinase (TK) gene of HSV. Viruses with TK mutations are generally cross-resistant to valacyclovir but remain susceptible to agents that act directly on DNA polymerase such as foscarnet (80–120 mg/kg/day IV in two to three divided doses until clinical response). Cases of severe persistent infection with acyclovir-resistant HSV occur almost exclusively in immunocompromised hosts. Famciclovir or valacyclovir can be considered in patients able to tolerate oral therapy, although there is limited clinical experience with these drugs for the treatment of HSV-associated esophagitis. VZV esophagitis is initially treated with intravenous acyclovir as these patients usually have disseminated infection. After clinical improvement, treatment may be changed to an oral agent used for HSV esophagitis. CMV esophagitis is treated with intravenous ganciclovir (5 mg/kg twice daily) or foscarnet sodium (68 mg/kg IV every 8 h or 90 mg/kg every 12 h) for 3–6 weeks.[9,19–21] Patients may be switched to valganciclovir 900 mg every 12 h once they can absorb and tolerate oral therapy. Valganciclovir is an oral precursor of ganciclovir. Valganciclovir is an oral precursor of ganciclovir. At a dose of 900 mg daily, valganciclovir produces systemic drug exposure equivalent to 5 mg/kg of intravenous ganciclovir. The role maintenance treatment after the clearance of infection is not well defined.

Bacterial infections

Bacterial esophagitis can occur in the immunocompromised patient and is usually polymicrobial and derived from oral flora. The diagnosis is made by endoscopic biopsies and treatment is broad-spectrum antibiotics.

Pill-induced esophagitis

Pill-induced esophagitis can occur in patients taking medication at bedtime with insufficient liquid or in the recumbent position. The most common medications associated with this disorder include potassium chloride, tetracyclines, aspirin, nonsteroidal anti-inflammatory drugs, quinidine, iron, and alendronate. Injury is caused by prolonged contact of the caustic contents of the medication with the esophageal mucosa. Patients will often present with sudden onset of odynophagia which may be severe enough to make even the swallowing of saliva difficult and painful. Endoscopy is helpful in making a diagnosis; but more importantly, it serves to rule out other diagnoses such as infectious esophagitis and malignancy. On endoscopy, there is usually a discrete, single ulcer located in the proximal esophagus. On occasion, the injury appears as a nodular, polypoid lesion suggestive of a neoplasm, or as a stricture (Figure 2). Esophageal biopsies are nonspecific and may show only acute inflammatory changes. There is no specific therapy for this disorder, since pill-induced ulcerations can heal spontaneously within a few days without any intervention. Severe strictures that result in dysphagia may require endoscopic treatment.

Malignant dysphagia Patients with esophageal cancer often present at an advanced, incurable stage. For those who are not candidates for chemoradiation or surgery, and for those who develop recurrent dysphagia after treatment, a variety of endoscopic techniques have been developed to improve esophageal luminal patency. Esophageal dilation can be performed with through-the-scope balloons, mercury-filled rubber bougies, or wire-guided polyvinyl bougies (Savary–Gilliard dilators), but dilation, to be successful, must be repeated every few weeks; the procedure carries a risk of perforation. Self-expanding metal stents (SEMS) are an effective nonsurgical option for the palliation of obstructive, advanced esophageal tumors and are considered the treatment of choice.[22–24] SEMS are made of a variety of metal alloys in different shapes and sizes to adjust to the length and position of the malignant stricture. Furthermore, approved devices are available in the uncovered, partially covered and fully covered design, with no major difference in outcomes[24] (Figure 3).

Ablative techniques such as lasers, photodynamic therapy, and high-dose brachytherapy have been successfully applied for palliation of malignant esophageal obstruction, but for the most part have been supplanted by SEMS.

SEMS are safe, effective, and quicker in palliating dysphagia compared to other modalities; high-dose intraluminal brachytherapy is a suitable alternative and may provide additional survival benefit with a better quality of life. Combinations of brachytherapy and SEMS may reduce the need for re-interventions.[25] Rigid plastic stent insertion, ablative techniques, dilation alone or in combination with other modalities, and chemotherapy alone are not recommended for palliation of malignant dysphagia due to a high incidence of complications and recurrent dysphagia.

Diarrhea

Chemotherapy and radiation

Diarrhea is a common complication of cytotoxic therapy and has been described with fluoropyrimidines (5-fluorouracil and capecitabine), irinotecan, methotrexate (MTX), and cisplatin (Table 2).[26–28] Diarrhea also commonly occurs in patients receiving small molecule epidermal growth factor receptor-tyrosine kinase inhibitors (erlotinib, sorafenib). Diarrhea can be very debilitating and in severe cases, it can lead to treatment delays, reduced quality of life, and diminished compliance. It is the dose-limiting factor and the major toxicity of regimens containing a fluoropyrimidine and/or irinotecan. The severity of chemotherapy-induced diarrhea is often described, particularly for study purposes, using the National Cancer Institute Common Toxicity Criteria (NCI CTC). Grading is based on number of stools per day, presence of nocturnal stools, and the need for parenteral support or intensive care.

The severity of diarrhea with 5-FU is increased by the addition of leucovorin. Moreover, diarrhea can be worse when 5-FU is administered by bolus injection as opposed to intravenous infusion. Irinotecan can cause an early-onset diarrhea accompanied by abdominal cramping, lacrimation, salivation, and other symptoms that appear cholinergic-mediated. The late diarrhea associated with irinotecan is unpredictable and can occur at all dose levels. It is seen less often when given in a three-week schedule compared to every week. Significant diarrhea has been reported with a combination of irinotecan, 5-FU and leucovorin compared to 5-FU and leucovorin alone. Grade 1 to 2 diarrhea has been reported in up to 56% of patients receiving erlotinib, and 34% of patients taking sorafenib.[29,30]

Radiation therapy can produce injury to the GI mucosa. Symptoms typically occur during the third week of fractionated radiotherapy. Pelvic or abdominal radiation can lead to acute enteritis, characterized by abdominal cramping and diarrhea in approximately 50% of patients. These symptoms are made worse by concomitant chemotherapy.[1]

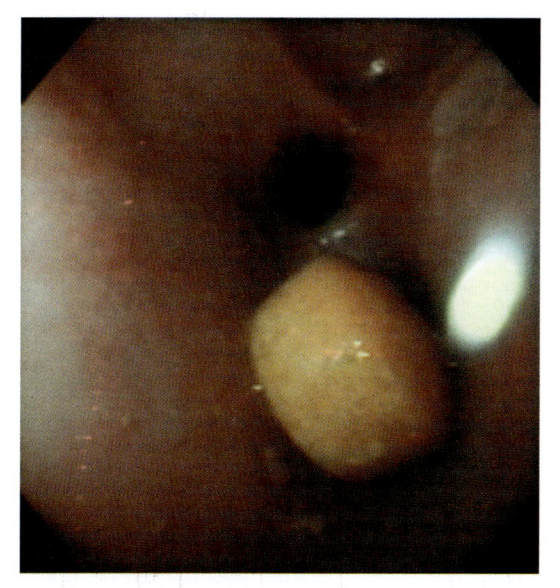

Figure 2 Pill-induced esophageal damage. A pill is seen at endoscopy lodged above an esophageal stricture.

(a)   (b)

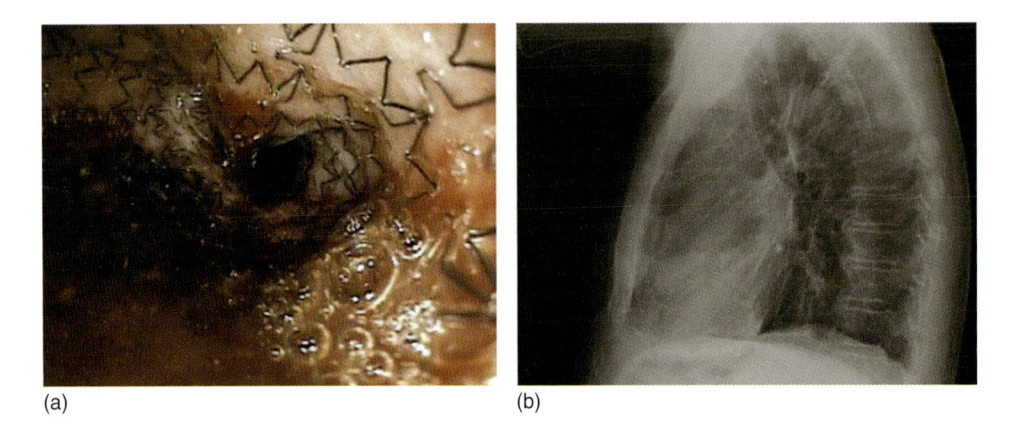

Figure 3 **Self-expanding esophageal stent.** (a) Endoscopic view of a self-expanding stent deployed in the esophagus for treatment of an esophageal stricture. (b) Chest radiograph showing stent deployed in the esophagus.

Table 2 Differential diagnosis of diarrhea in the cancer and hematopoietic cell transplant patient.

Chemotherapy-related (fluoropyrimidines, irinotecan, methotrexate, cisplatin, small molecule epidermal growth factor receptor tyrosine kinase inhibitors: erlotinib, sorafenib), and others
Colitis secondary to immune-modulatory agents (ipilimumab, nivolumab, lambrolizumab, and others)
Radiation therapy
Conditioning regimen
Graft-versus-host disease
Infection
   Bacterial (including *C. difficile*)
   Viral (including CMV)

Opioid agonists are the cornerstone of therapy for chemotherapy-induced diarrhea.[31] Loperamide and diphenoxylate are both widely used and are approved by the US Food and Drug Administration (FDA) for this indication. Loperamide is more effective. For mild-to-moderate diarrhea, an initial dose of 4 mg loperamide hydrochloride may be given, followed by a further 2 mg every 4 h or after every lose stool. Severe diarrhea often requires a more aggressive regimen, with an initial dose of 4 mg loperamide hydrochloride followed by a further 2 mg every 2 h or 4 mg every 4 h until the patient is diarrhea-free for 12 h. This high dose of loperamide has been used effectively for the control of irinotecan-induced diarrhea. Octreotide, a synthetic long-acting somatostatin analog, has been used as second-line therapy in opioid-resistant patients.[1] It decreases the secretion of vasoactive intestinal peptide, prolongs intestinal transit time, and reduces secretion of intestinal fluid and electrolytes. The recommended initial dose of octreotide is 100–150 g given subcutaneously three times per day, or 25–50 g every hour if given as an intravenous infusion. Octreotide can be titrated to higher doses (500–2500 g three times daily) for the treatment of those individuals who do not respond to lower doses.

Other drugs used as adjunctive therapy in chemotherapy or radiation-induced diarrhea include absorbents such as kaolin and charcoal, deodorized tincture of opium, paregoric, and codeine phosphate.

Because of the well-recognized risk of diarrhea associated with irinotecan, several recent studies have investigated prophylactic regimens to prevent chemotherapy-induced diarrhea. Long-acting, slow-release formulation of octreotide (octreotide LAR) can be administered by intramuscular injection once a month. Once steady-state levels have been achieved, a 20-mg intramuscular dose of octreotide LAR every 4 weeks produces the same pharmacologic effects as 150 µg octreotide three times daily by subcutaneous injection and dramatically reduces fluctuations in peak and trough octreotide concentrations. Additionally, octreotide LAR (at a starting dose of 20 mg) effectively controls diarrhea associated with carcinoid syndrome, and monthly doses of 20–30 mg are currently being investigated for the treatment and prevention of chemotherapy-induced diarrhea.[32]

For patients undergoing hematopoietic stem cell transplantation (HCT), diarrhea may be due to the conditioning regimen (total body irradiation and/or high dose chemotherapy). Pretransplant conditioning regimens can injure the GI mucosa, causing secretory diarrhea that resolves after mucosal restitution. After day 20, acute GVHD is the most common cause of diarrhea in these patients. (See below for GVHD discussion.)

Clostridium difficile-associated diarrhea

If diarrhea is not directly the result of chemotherapy or radiation and particularly if it occurs in a hospital setting, *Clostridium difficile* infection should be considered since this is the most common cause of infectious diarrhea in hospitalized patients. Although commonly associated with use of antibiotic therapy, risk factors for *C difficile* diarrhea or colitis also include bowel surgery, immunocompromised state, and any process that suppresses the normal flora including antifungal and chemotherapeutic agents. Cancer patients receiving chemotherapy appear predisposed to *C. difficile*-induced diarrhea even in the absence of antibiotics. MTX, doxorubicin, and cyclophosphamide are the drugs most frequently associated with *C. difficile* infection. Clinical presentation may vary from mild diarrhea without colitis, colitis with systemic manifestations, pseudomembranous colitis with or without protein-losing enteropathy, and fulminant colitis with development of toxic megacolon. Diagnostic testing for *C. difficile* has rapidly evolved.[33,34] Previously rapid EIA tests for toxin A or B were the most widely used diagnostic tests. These tests have a sensitivity of 75–95% and specificity of 83–98%. Two major advances in the laboratory diagnosis of *C. difficile* are the use of glutamate dehydrogenase (GDH; an enzyme produced by *C. difficile*), detection in stool (75% to >90% sensitivity with a negative predictive value of close to 100%), and nucleic acid amplification tests (PCR) for toxin genes. Endoscopically, pseudomembranes

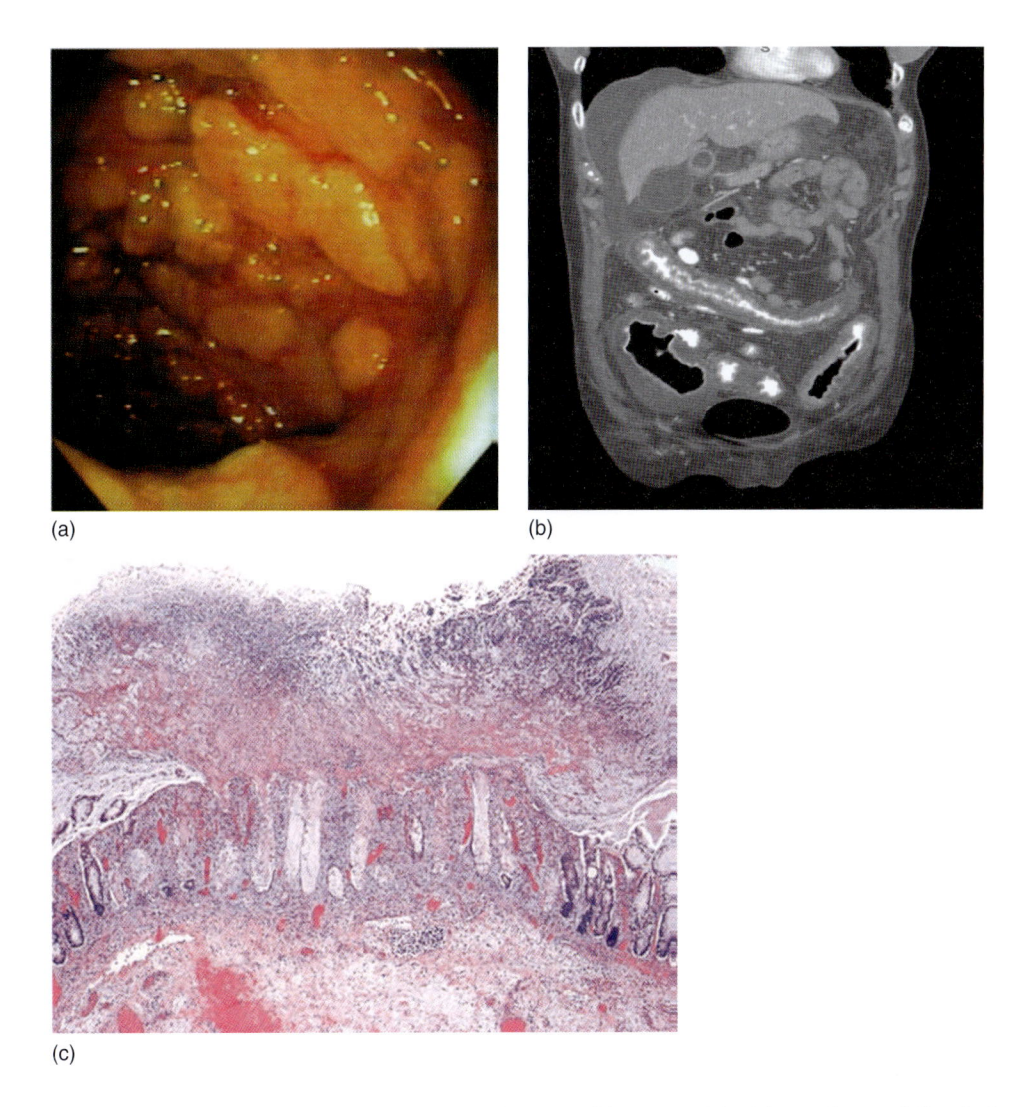

Figure 4 (a) Pseudomembranes adherent to the colonic mucosa seen at colonoscopy. (b) CT scan of the abdomen showing diffuse thickening of the bowel wall due to pseudomembranous colitis. (c) Low power view of colonic mucosa shows a typical volcano (mushroom)-like appearance with luminal inflammatory exudates.

can be seen as adherent yellow plaques that vary in diameter from 2 to 10 mm (Figure 4). The rectum and sigmoid colon are typically involved, but in approximately 10% of cases, colitis is only present in the more proximal colon and can be missed during sigmoidoscopy.

Therapy for C. *difficile* diarrhea depends on disease severity.[33,34] The standard therapy for C. *difficile*-associated diarrhea has changed and the most current IDSA recommends the use of oral vancomycin or fidaxomicin on the initial episode and the use of metronidazole in cases where access to other medications is limited.[33] The lower dose of vancomycin 125 mg four times a day for 10 days is as effective as the higher dose of 250 mg four times a day in nonsevere or severe cases and is less expensive. Fidaxomicin should be administered at a dose of 200 mg given twice daily for 10 days. In patients with fulminant C. *difficile* infection and signs of systemic toxicity, the recommended treatment regimen is initial therapy with vancomycin 500 mg orally four times daily. In patients with severe ileus, vancomycin retention enemas (0.5–1 g of vancomycin dissolved in 1–2 L of normal saline every 4–12 h) should be considered and if this approach is used, intravenous metronidazole can be added to this treatment. The use of antiperistaltic agents is not recommended as they may obscure symptoms and there is evidence that decreased transit time can lead to complications and lengthen the duration of illness. Relapse of CDI is common, occurring in up to 10–25% of all patients with CDI. Relapses usually occur within 1–3 weeks after termination of initial therapy and are probably caused by failure to eradicate the organism rather than development of antibiotic resistance. These patients are likely to relapse repeatedly. First relapses should be treated with a second 10-day course of oral vancomycin or fidaxomicin. This decision may depend on the drug given on the index episode. If a patient relapses after taking a second course of antibiotics, different approaches have been suggested, including tapered or pulsed antibiotic therapy, longer duration of treatment (several weeks), addition of rifaximin, and the use of fecal microbiota transplantation. Two randomized control trials (MODIFY I and MODIFY II) studied two human monoclonal antibodies against C. *difficile* toxin A (actoxumab) and toxin B (bezlotoxumab) and found that among patients receiving antibiotics for primary or recurrent C. *difficile* infection, bezlotoxumab was associated with a substantially lower rate of recurrent infection with a good safety profile. The addition of actoxumab did not improve treatment efficacy.[35]

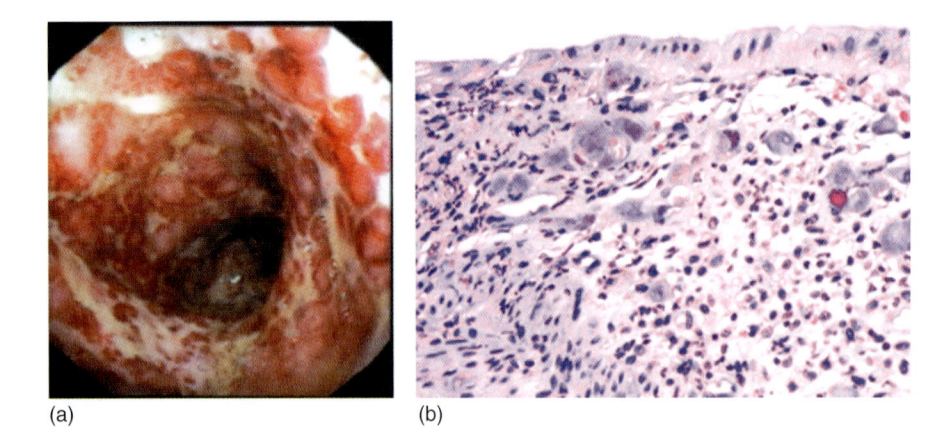

Figure 5 **Cytomegalovirus (CMV) colitis.** (a) CMV colitis as seen at endoscopy. (b) High power view of inflamed colonic mucosa demonstrates multiple viral inclusions in stroma cells.

Other considerations related to infectious diarrhea

In the posthematopoietic cell transplant patient, infectious diarrhea is relatively uncommon. Viruses are the most common organisms found (astrovirus, adenovirus, CMV, and rotavirus), followed by nosocomial-acquired bacteria (*Clostridium difficile* and Aeromonas). CMV deserves a special mention since it can cause diarrhea and bleeding because of mucosal ulceration. The diagnosis of CMV is made by endoscopic biopsy (Figure 5); specimens should be sent for immunohistochemistry and viral culture. Infectious diarrhea related to *Salmonella*, *Shigella*, and *Campylobacter* species is very rare in hospitalized transplant patients. Diarrhea related to parasites (*Cryptosporidium*, *Giardia lamblia*, *Entamoeba histolytica*) is also a rare cause of diarrhea; most of these patients are infected pretransplantation.

Colitis

Neutropenic enterocolitis

Neutropenic enterocolitis is clinically characterized by fever and right lower quadrant pain in neutropenic patients. It is seen in children and adults with hematologic malignancies, aplastic anemia, and after myelosuppressive therapy for solid malignancies.[36–40] Histologic examination of biopsy samples from patients with neutropenic enterocolitis is characterized by bowel wall edema, mucosal ulcerations, focal hemorrhage, and mucosal or transmural necrosis. Numerous bacterial and/or fungal organisms have been identified in surgical specimens and peritoneal fluid from patients with neutropenic enterocolitis; the diagnosis is usually established by computerized tomography (CT). Abnormal findings on CT and ultrasound include a fluid-filled, dilated cecum, a right lower quadrant inflammatory mass, and pericecal fluid or inflammatory changes in the pericecal soft tissues. Treatment consists of bowel rest, intravenous fluids, and broad-spectrum antibiotics. Cytopenias and coagulopathy associated with oncologic treatment should be corrected since neutropenia contributes to the pathogenesis of the disease and coagulopathy can be associated with blood loss from mucosal hemorrhage. Recombinant granulocyte colony-stimulating factor (G-CSF) may be used to hasten leukocyte recovery, which contributes to the resolution of neutropenic enterocolitis. Surgery has been recommended for patients with persistent GI bleeding despite correction of cytopenias, and coagulopathy as well as for patients with perforation or clinical deterioration despite conservative therapy.

Colitis secondary to immune-modulatory, antineoplastic agents

Immune modulatory agents enhance tumor-directed immune responses through modification of immune checkpoint pathways (CPI), T-cell stimulatory pathways, or with adoptive cell therapy.[41] However, this approach has also been associated with intestinal adverse effects, in particular with therapeutic agents targeting immune checkpoint pathways which include inhibitors of cytotoxic T lymphocyte-associated protein (CTLA-4; ipilimumab, tremelimumab), programmed death-1 (PD-1; nivolumab, pembrolizumab, cemiplimab), and its ligand (PD-L1; atezolizumab, avelumab, and durvalumab).[42–46] Checkpoint inhibitors (CPI) target molecules involved in T cell regulation, boosting effector functions in the tumor microenvironment, and thus may lead to off-tumor inflammatory responses or immune-related adverse events (irAEs), including enterocolitis.[41,44] Adverse events are most frequent with anti-CTLA-4 agents or when these drugs are used in combination (nivolumab plus ipilimumab). The majority of immune-related adverse events have been observed during the induction and reinduction periods, but adverse events may have a delayed onset and prolonged duration. The colon is the most frequent site of clinically evident GI toxicity, but inflammation can occur throughout the GI tract. Enterocolitis most commonly presents with diarrhea but abdominal pain, nausea/vomiting, fever, anal pain has been reported as well. Enterocolitis is graded using Common Terminology Criteria for Adverse Events (CTCAE) from grade 1 (mild) to grade 5 (death).[47] The majority of patients who develop enterocolitis do so within 21 days following their last dose. Patients with mild colitis on CPIs are often diagnosed clinically based on new-onset diarrhea in the absence of other factors such as infection, but endoscopic biopsy is the gold standard for diagnosis of CPI enterocolitis. Radiologically, CPI-associated colitis is characterized by mesenteric vessel engorgement, colonic wall thickening, mucosal enhancement, and fluid-filled colonic distension. Colitis can either develop diffusely or as segmental colitis. While pan-enteritis has been described, the colon is the most commonly involved area clinically. Endoscopic presentation of ICI colitis is nonspecific and severity-dependent showing macroscopic findings such as mucosal erythema, friability, edema, and ulcerations (Figure 6).[48] Retrospective analyses suggest that the presence of ulceration at colonoscopy may be

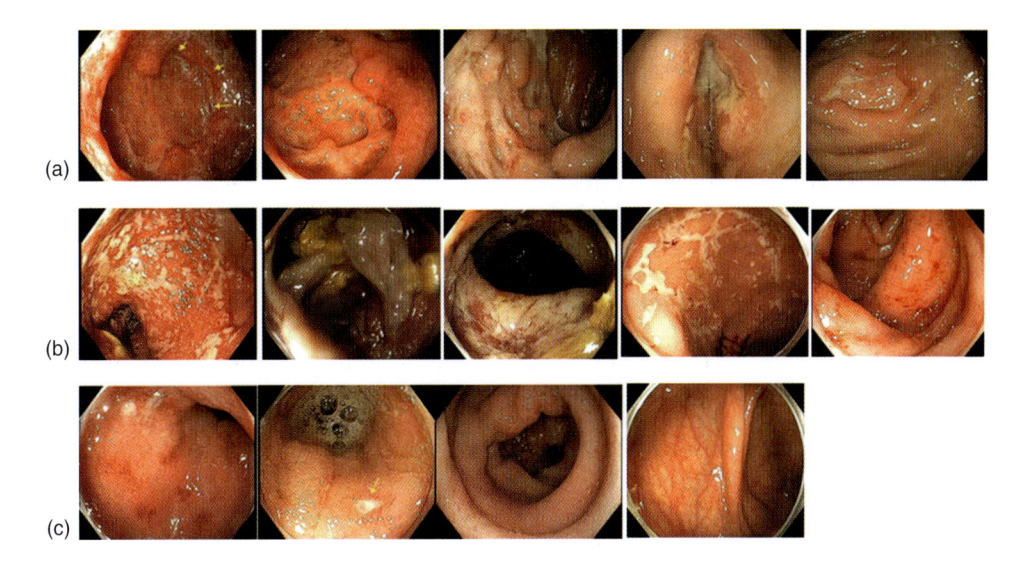

Figure 6 Endoscopic appearance of immune-mediated colitis. The appearance of immune-mediated colitis at colonoscopy may range from mild to severe. (a) Severe inflammation with deeply ulcerated mucosa. (b) Moderate-to-severe inflammation with diffuse erythema, superficial ulceration, and exudate. (c) Mild inflammation with patchy erythema and edema.

predictive of resistance to corticosteroid therapy. In the majority of patients, histologic findings include neutrophilic inflammation with cryptitis and occasional crypt abscesses or depict a mixed neutrophilic-lymphocytic inflammatory picture. In few patients, lymphocytic predominant inflammation is seen with increased numbers of CD8+ T-cells in crypts and CD4+ cells in the lamina propria. Treatment of CPI-associated adverse events is guided by severity (Table 3) but other etiologies need to be ruled out.[45,46] Mild GI symptoms (grade 1) can be treated symptomatically without discontinuation of the CPI; however, frequent reassessment is imperative to identify the development of more severe symptoms or life-threatening complications. In cases of moderate enterocolitis, the offending drug should be withheld but can be restarted after significant symptom-improvement or -resolution. If moderate (grade 2) symptoms persist, initiation of treatment with systemic corticosteroids is recommended (prednisone/methylprednisolone 1–2 mg/kg per day) until improvement to mild symptoms or symptom-resolution is observed. If there is no response to steroids within two to three days, the addition of infliximab or vedolizumab should be considered. After grade 2–3 colitis, once symptoms are ≤grade 1, PD-1/PD-L1 agents can be resumed. Severe enterocolitis and life-threatening complications require permanent discontinuation of anti-CTL4 agents. In these cases, systemic corticosteroids should be administered (1–2 mg/kg/d IV methylprednisolone) once intestinal perforation is ruled out.[49] In corticosteroid-refractory cases, the addition of infliximab or vedolizumab should be strongly considered. Certain microflora in the colon have been associated with the risk of CPI colitis, and in a small number of reported cases, fecal microbiota transplant has been reported to have therapeutic benefit.[50]

Radiation-induced proctitis and colitis

Patients receiving radiation therapy to the abdomen and pelvis for the treatment of gynecologic, genitourinary, GI, and other malignancies are at risk of developing acute or chronic intestinal injury.

Table 3 Management of immune checkpoint inhibitor-related diarrhea and enterocolitis.[a]

Severity	Definition	Management
Mild (Grade 1)	Fewer than four stools/day over baseline and no colitis symptoms	• Consider holding immunotherapy • Symptomatic management. • If no response and infection ruled out, add mesalamine
Moderate (Grade 2)	Increase of 4–6 stools/day over baseline – Abdominal pain – Blood or mucus in stool	• Hold immunotherapy • Prednisone/methylprednisolone (1–2 mg/kg/day) • No response in two to three days, continue steroids, consider adding infliximab or vedolizumab
Severe (Grades 3)	– Increase of >7 stools/day over baseline – Severe abdominal pain – Peritoneal signs	• Discontinue anti-CTL4 • Consider resuming anti-PD-1/PD-L1 after resolution of toxicity • Intravenous methylprednisolone (1–2 mg/kg/d) • No response in 2 days, continue steroids, strongly consider adding infliximab or vedolizumab
Life-threatening (Grade 4)	Life-threatening consequences; urgent intervention indicated	• Permanently discontinue immunotherapy • Intravenous methylprednisolone (1–2 mg/kg/d) • No response in 2 days, continue steroids, strongly consider adding infliximab or vedolizumab

[a]Source: Based on NCCN Clinical Practice Guidelines in Oncology. Management of immunotherapy-related toxicities. Version 1.2020, December 16, 2019. Available at NCCN.org.

Acute radiation injury in the rectum and distal colon usually occurs within 6 weeks of therapy and is characterized by diarrhea, rectal urgency, tenesmus and, occasionally, rectal bleeding. These symptoms usually resolve within 6 months without the need for therapy. Chronic radiation proctitis or coloproctitis has a delayed onset, occurring approximately one year or later after exposure to radiation. It is caused by obliterative endarteritis and chronic mucosal ischemia resulting in epithelial atrophy and fibrosis. It may end in stricture formation and bleeding within the colon and rectum. Patients with radiation proctitis often present with diarrhea, bleeding, tenesmus, urgency, difficulties with defecation, and less commonly fecal incontinence.

The diagnosis of radiation proctitis is made by colonoscopy or sigmoidoscopy. Endoscopic findings include mucosal edema, erythema, friability, and the presence of telangiectasias. In severe cases, mucosal ulcerations and strictures can be observed.

Treatment for radiation proctitis depends on symptoms.[1] In some studies, sucralfate enemas have been used to treat chronic radiation-induced proctitis but may increase the risk of rectal bleeding, other treatments that have shown some benefit in small clinical trials include hyperbaric oxygen and short-chain fatty acid enemas. Various endoscopic therapies can be used to treat bleeding associated with radiation proctitis, including argon plasma coagulation (APC), radiofrequency ablation, heater probe, or bipolar electrocoagulation, there is insufficient evidence to recommend one specific modality.[51] Surgery should be considered for patients with intractable symptoms such as strictures, pain, or bleeding. A detailed discussion of the endoscopic and surgical treatment of radiation proctitis is beyond the scope of this review. The selection of treatment for radiation proctitis should be based on the type and severity of symptoms as well as local expertise. Intravenous amifostine has been recommended at a dose of >340 mg/m^2 to prevent acute radiation proctitis in patients receiving radiation therapy.[52]

Intestinal manifestations of graft-versus-host disease (GVHD)

The use and indications for allogenic hematopoietic cell transplantation (HCT) have significantly increased throughout the last decades with approximately 25,000 procedures per year.[53] The main complication of HCT is GVHD with GI involvement occurring in 54% of those undergoing transplantation.[54,55] GVHD occurs as a response of donor T-cells to genetically defined recipient cell surface proteins. Human leukocyte antigens (HLAs) are class I HLA (A, B, and C) and class II (DR, DQ, and DP) proteins. The former are expressed by all nucleated cells, while the latter are predominantly expressed by hematopoietic cells; however, HLA class II protein can also be expressed by other cell types in the setting of inflammation and injury. HLA class I and II mismatch is positively correlated with the frequency of acute GVHD.[56,57] However, HLA-matched patients can still develop GVHD due to individual differences in ubiquitously expressed minor histocompatibility antigens (i.e., HY and HA-1).[58–60] Interestingly, incidence rates of acute GVHD following mismatched umbilical cord-derived HCT are similar to rates of matched bone marrow-derived HCT, but incidence rates of chronic GVHD are higher after peripheral stem cell versus bone marrow stem cell transplant with a reported incidence of 53% versus 41%.[61,62] Autologous GVHD is a distinct entity describing an autoimmune GVHD-like syndrome that develops after autologous stem cell transplant and has been associated with drugs such as cyclosporine and alemtuzumab.[63,64]

Based upon its chronologic correlation to the time of cell transplantation, GVHD has been classified as acute ($\leq$100 days posttransplant) or chronic (>100 days posttransplant). The latter form can be an extension of acute GVHD, reoccurrence of a successfully treated acute form or can occur *de novo*. However, this classification has been found inaccurate due to changes in condition regimens resulting in later onset of acute GVHD and overlap syndromes.[53,65] Therefore, an expert panel has suggested a new classification for GVHD (Table 4).[66,67]

Acute GVHD

The most common presentation of acute GVHD is high-volume, secretory diarrhea. GI hemorrhage has been associated with a poor prognosis; it can be indicative of mucosal ulceration in the setting of GVHD but other causes have to be considered.[68,69] GVHD-associated diarrhea has been described as an exudative, protein-losing enteropathy; however, sensitivity and specificity of fecal α1-anti-trypsin in the diagnosis of stage 2–3 GI-GVHD is only 79% and 62%, respectively.[70] Occasionally GI-GVHD can also result in pancreatic insufficiency, thereby, potentially contributing to diarrhea. Other common GVHD-associated symptoms include anorexia, nausea, vomiting, abdominal pain, and ileus. The absence of such symptoms does not exclude the presence of GVHD, and the differential diagnoses for these symptoms are broad in HCT patients given the aggressive conditioning regimens, their multidrug use, and their susceptibility to infections due to severe neutropenia following HCT. Hence, a high level of suspicion is required. On physical examination, sequelae of GVHD manifestations and complications should be assessed such as cutaneous GVHD, dehydration and weight loss, and failure to thrive. Occasionally, patients can develop ascites. Oropharyngeal manifestations of GVHD can include gingivitis, mucositis, and erythema.[67] Radiologic features of intestinal GVHD include bowel wall thickening, intestinal dilatation, mucosal enhancement, and gastric wall thickening. Diffuse small bowel wall thickening has been associated with worse prognosis, and any colon involvement on CT correlates with GVHD severity.[71,72] Radiologic findings do not significantly differ between acute and late-onset

Table 4 Modified classification of acute and chronic graft-versus-host disease (GVHD).[a]

Categories	Time of symptom onset post-HCT	Presence of acute GVHD features	Presence of chronic GVHD features
Acute GVHD			
Classic acute GVHD	$\leq$100 days	Yes	No
Persistent, recurrent or late-onset acute GVHD	>100 days	Yes	No
Chronic GVHD			
Classic chronic GVHD	No time limit	No	Yes
Overlap syndrome	No time limit	Yes	Yes

[a]Source: Based on Jagasia et al.[67]

GVHD.[73] Endoscopic findings in GVHD include a spectrum from mild erythema to mucosal edema and diffuse mucosal loss. In particular, mucosal sloughing has been reported to be highly specific.[74] While endoscopy has been shown to be highly predictive for the diagnosis of GVHD, approximately one-fifth of patients with histologically confirmed GVHD have no significant macroscopic findings on endoscopic evaluation.[75] Therefore, a tissue diagnosis is usually required in the diagnosis of acute GVHD. Typical histologic findings include crypt epithelial cell apoptosis, crypt destruction ("exploding crypt cells"), and variable lymphocytic infiltration of the epithelium and lamina propria (Figure 7). Importantly, similar findings can also be observed in the absence of GVHD within the immediate posttransplant period secondary to pretransplant regimens. Non-GVHD-related histologic changes, however, have usually resolved 20 days after transplant.[76] Other differential diagnoses that need to be excluded in the evaluation of GVHD-like symptoms and histologic findings include infectious etiologies (i.e., CMV and cryptosporidium) and iatrogenic adverse effects (i.e., mycophenolate mofetil and proton pump inhibitors). Histologically, GI-GVHD has historically been classified as grades 1–4 based on severity.[65] Controversies around endoscopic evaluation include the extent of endoscopic evaluation. Discordance between upper intestinal biopsies and rectal biopsies has been reported in up to 45% of patients with GI-GVHD. Symptoms are not predictive of site of involvement. While some studies suggested rectal biopsies are sufficient, other studies reported gastric biopsies as providing higher yields in diagnosing GI-GVHD. Distal colonic evaluation (flexible sigmoidoscopy) is frequently sufficient and associated with lower complication rates than total colonoscopy.[77] Reduced-intensity conditioning regimens were effective in reducing tissue injury and were shown to delay onset of acute GVHD to >100 days but have been associated with higher rates of relapse in some patients.[78,79] The main stay of GVHD prevention is pharmacologic calcineurin inhibition (i.e., cyclosporine, tacrolimus, or sirolimus) in combination with other immunosuppressants (i.e., MTX or mycophenolate mofetil) in the early posttransplant phase.[80,81] A recent Cochrane database analysis, however, concluded that high-quality RCTs are needed to define the optimal GVHD prevention strategy.[82] Frequently, patients who develop acute GVHD on calcineurin-inhibitor prophylaxis, do so in the second month after transplant. Any form of visceral GVHD requires high-dose corticosteroid treatment which results in resolution of acute GVHD in up to 60%.[53,54,83] For cases with corticosteroid-refractory cases of GVHD, therapeutic strategies such as extracorporeal photopheresis and anti-TNFα agents (e.g., etanercept) have been evaluated; further studies are required.[53] In addition to immunosuppressive therapy, supportive management is essential, including infection prophylaxis, rehydration, and nutritional supplementation.

Chronic GVHD

The prevalence of chronic GVHD in long-term survivors of HCT is >50%.[66] It is the major cause of late nonrelapse mortality in HCT patients.[53] Risk factors associated with its development include age, prior acute GVHD, time from transplantation to chronic GVHD, donor type, disease status at transplantation, GVHD prophylaxis, and gender mismatch.[84] Unfortunately, the pathophysiology, diagnostic criteria, and optimal management are poorly understood. The National Institute of Health (NIH) developed several consensus documents on criteria for clinical trials in chronic GVHD.[67] In these documents, the diagnosis is based upon signs of chronic GVHD, or distinctive signs (defined as manifestations not typical for acute GVHD but not sufficient to establish the diagnosis of chronic GVHD without further testing), with confirmation by biopsy, laboratory test, or radiologic imaging. Similar to acute GVHD, chronic GVHD can manifest as anorexia, nausea, vomiting, diarrhea, weight loss, and failure to thrive.[67] Oropharyngeal manifestations of chronic GVHD include lichen planus-like changes, hyperkeratotic plaques, xerostomia, mucosal atrophy, mucoceles, pseudo-membranes, and ulcers. Esophageal findings can include esophageal webs, strictures, and concentric rings. Other findings include mucosal erythema, edema, and erosions. Histologic evaluation can also show epithelial apoptosis and crypt cell loss, but these changes are not specific, and therefore not considered diagnostic for chronic GVHD. Supportive care is one of the key elements in the management of chronic GVHD. Patients need to be monitored for infectious complications. Oropharyngeal lesions in HCT patients developing 3 years after transplant should be evaluated for squamous cell carcinoma and other secondary malignancies. Similarly, patients with dysphagia and odynophagia need to be evaluated for other etiologies such as pill or radiation esophagitis, and viral esophagitis. Dysphagia due to strictures can be managed by careful endoscopic dilatation; unfortunately, studies regarding perforation rates are lacking. Patients with diarrhea need to be evaluated for infectious etiologies, malabsorption, pancreatic insufficiency, and nutritional deficiencies. Forty-three percent of patients with chronic GVHD are malnourished and 14% severely malnourished; nutritional assessment and support should be provided.[85,86] A key element in the treatment of chronic GVHD is immunosuppression. Topical corticosteroids can be attempted (i.e., budesonide and beclomethasone) in mild cases of chronic GVHD.[87,88] However, moderate or severe chronic GVHD and GVHD of nonaccessible areas require systemic corticosteroids usually at a dose of 1 mg/kg/day for two weeks followed by a 6–8 weeks taper; patients should be thoroughly reassessed at 3 months to decide on further tapering versus maintenance, or if second-line therapy is indicated.[89]

Hepatic complications of cancer treatment

Chemotherapy-associated liver injury is an unfortunate consequence of the treatment of many cancers. Consequently, it is important to assess liver function carefully before and during therapy (Tables 5 and 6).

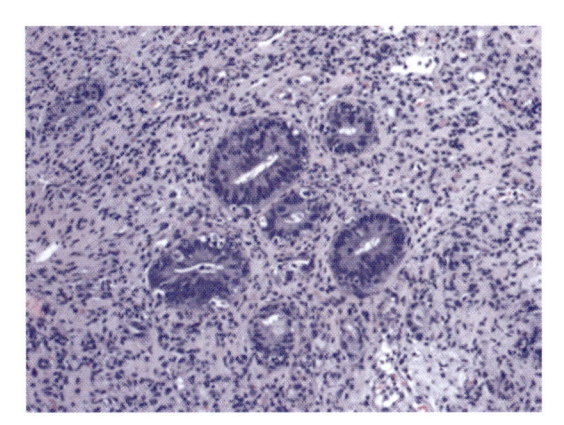

Figure 7 Graft-versus-host disease involving the colon. The colonic mucosa shows prominent crypt apoptosis and focal crypt dropouts in a background of granulation tissue.

Table 5 Causes of hepatic abnormalities in cancer patients.

Preexisting liver disease
Viral hepatitis
Nonalcoholic fatty liver disease
Alcoholic liver disease
Hemochromatosis
Autoimmune hepatitis
Wilson disease
Celiac disease
Alpha-1-antitrypsin deficiency

Direct effects of the tumor
Hepatic metastases
Portal vein thrombosis
Biliary obstruction

Indirect effects of the tumor
Paraneoplastic syndromes

Causes of liver disease during cancer treatment
Drug-induced liver disease
Graft-versus-host disease (acute and chronic)
Sinusoidal obstruction syndrome
Viral hepatitis
Sepsis-induced cholestasis
Ischemic liver injury
TPN

Liver disease affected by cancer treatment
Hepatitis B
Nonalcoholic fatty liver disease
Autoimmune hepatitis

Table 6 Differential diagnosis of hepatic biochemical tests abnormalities associated with cancer therapy.

	AST/ALT	Alkaline phosphatase	Bilirubin
Drug-induced liver disease	2–10 × ULN	2–10 × ULN	2–20 × ULN
Viral hepatitis	2–10 ULN	2–3 × ULN	2–10 × ULN
Sinusoidal obstruction syndrome	2–5 × ULN	2–3 × 2 ULN	2–10 × ULN
Graft-versus-host disease	2–5 × ULN	2–10 × ULN	2–20 × ULN

Effect of preexisting liver disease on cancer therapy

Preexisting liver disease can affect not only the choice of therapeutic options but for drugs that are metabolized by the liver, necessitate dosage modification. Measurement of hepatic enzymes, commonly referred to as "liver function tests," does not assess functional capacity of the liver. They are sensitive indicators of acute liver injury but do not measure the liver's ability to metabolize drugs or synthesize important proteins. The albumin and bilirubin concentrations are surrogate markers of the liver's synthetic and biotransformation potential but are influenced by external factors limiting their sensitivity and specificity. Consequently, a reliable assessment of liver function should not be based on a simple profile of a few laboratory tests, but a composite picture based on clinical, laboratory, and radiographic data. In addition, none of the frequently used hepatic laboratory tests can accurately assess hepatic fibrosis. Common hepatic disorders like nonalcoholic fatty liver disease can progress silently to cirrhosis with normal or minimally elevated transaminases and bilirubin. The only evidence for chronic liver disease might be evidence of portal hypertension on the physical exam or nodularity of the liver on imaging studies.

For some drugs, published guidelines describe usage restrictions and dosing on the basis of readily available hepatic serologic tests. But for many therapeutic agents, the clinician must use subjective data on which to design a treatment regimen. Many treatment protocols require dosage modification based on the bilirubin concentration, but relying on the bilirubin concentration alone can be misleading. Gilbert's syndrome, a benign disorder of bilirubin metabolism, can spuriously raise the total bilirubin concentration leading to an inappropriate modification of a treatment regimen.

Up to 30% of patients undergoing cancer therapy have evidence of preexisting liver disease with nonalcoholic fatty liver the most common. Many drugs can exacerbate fat deposition in the liver; the most common of these are hormonal therapies used to treat breast cancer and prostate cancer. Hepatic steatosis develops in up to one-third of women treated with tamoxifen. It is usually asymptomatic and not associated with progressive liver disease, although elevated transaminases and steatohepatitis can occur, which may affect therapy selection.[90] Antiantigen therapy for prostate cancer can exacerbate components of the metabolic syndrome resulting in accelerated hepatic steatosis.[91]

Chemotherapy or chemoradiation can lead to reactivation of underlying hepatitis B caused by intensification of the immune response to the hepatitis B virus (HBV) when immunosuppressive therapy is withdrawn. While HBV reactivation can occur with any chemotherapy regimen, the risk is highest with anti-CD20 monoclonal antibodies such as rituximab and ofatumumab.[92] Reactivation can occur in patients with inapparent hepatitis B infection manifested only by a positive core antibody (anti-HBc) in the absence of detectable surface antigen (HBsAg). In one report, 5 of 21 HBsAg negative/anti-HBc positive patients receiving rituximab developed reactivation of underlying hepatitis.[93] Several major societies have published guidelines for the evaluation and treatment of HBV infection in patients undergoing cancer treatment.[94-96] Most recommend prophylactic antiviral therapy before the onset of cancer treatment and, depending on the regimen used, for at least 6-12 months after completion of therapy; at least 12 additional months of prophylactic antiviral therapy is recommended in cases where B-cell-depleting treatment regimens were used. Lamivudine can be used in patients with no detectable HBV DNA and with a short duration of immunosuppression (<12 months).[97] However, because of known potential viral resistance with lamivudine, either tenofovir or entecavir is the preferred agent in general for patients who are positive for anti-HBc, when there is detectable HBV DNA, or when anticipated duration of therapy is greater than one year.[98]

Patients with underlying hepatitis C appear to respond differently to chemotherapy compared to those with hepatitis B.[99] Modest increases in transaminase and HCV RNA levels develop in approximately half of HCV-infected patients but a severe hepatitis flare-up is rare. Consequently, dose modification is usually not indicated. Effective oral antiviral regimens for the treatment of HCV that do not require interferon suggest that many more patients with HCV infection who are undergoing cancer therapy will become candidates for antiviral treatment.

The impact of the growing utilization of immune CPI for cancer treatment in patients with chronic viral infections such as hepatitis B (HBV) and hepatitis C (HCV) is largely unknown. In general, treatment has been well tolerated, but case reports have indicated the potential for hepatitis reactivation or flare-ups. It is recommended that patients scheduled to receive ICPIs be screened for HBV by checking HBsAg and anti-HBc, and that primary prophylaxis (lamivudine or entecavir) be considered in those with HBV infection if not already on treatment.[100] In those with resolved HBV infection, careful monitoring with serum ALT and HBV DNA is suggested. A few case reports of HCV activation during ICPI therapy have been reported, and these patients were treated successfully with antiviral therapy. HCV-positive patients should complete curative antiviral treatment with verification of HCV viral load below limits of quantification prior to receiving ICPI therapy.[100]

Hepatotoxicity caused by cancer therapy

Adverse drug reactions occur commonly in patients undergoing cancer treatment. Recognizing hepatotoxicity can be challenging since this population of patients frequently receive multiple medications; there can be many potential causes of abnormal liver function including tumor progression, systemic infection, or the administration of parenteral nutrition.

Most hepatotoxic reactions are idiosyncratic and caused by either metabolic disruption or an immunologic reaction to the drug or one of its metabolites.[101] Typically, these reactions occur in patients without underlying liver disease and resolve when the drug is discontinued without significant fibrosis or impaired synthetic function. With more severe drug toxicity, often manifested by elevations in the serum bilirubin, the offending agent has to be discontinued even when therapeutic alternatives are limited.

The antimetabolites commonly used in cancer therapy include cytosine arabinoside (Ara-C), 5-FU, 6-mercapto purine (6-MP), azathioprine, 6-thioguanine, and MX. Hepatic metabolism plays an important role in the processing of these drugs, and dose reductions are usually necessary for patients with liver dysfunction. Ara-C, used in the treatment of acute myelogenous leukemia (AML), has on rare occasions been associated with cholestasis, which appears reversible.[102] Intra-arterial administration of the 5-FU metabolite floxuridine (fluorodeoxyuridine [FudR]) has been associated with two types of toxicity: one suggestive of hepatocellular injury, and the second one consistent with sclerosing cholangitis, with structuring of the intra- and extra-hepatic bile ducts, and elevations of alkaline phosphatase and bilirubin.[103–105]

Combinations of 5-FU and oxaliplatin or irinotecan are used for neoadjuvant therapy in patients with colorectal cancer prior to the resection of liver metastases. These neoadjuvant regimens, particularly those with oxaliplatin, have been associated with steatosis and injury to the hepatic vasculature causing a disorder with features of chronic sinusoidal obstruction syndrome (SOS).[106–109] This, in turn, may lead to noncirrhotic portal hypertension and its associated complications.

Trastuzumab emtansine (T-DM1), a monoclonal antibody–drug conjugate utilized in the treatment of HER2-positive breast cancer, has the potential for hepatotoxic effects in the form of elevated liver enzymes and development of nodular regenerative hyperplasia (NRH). NRH may be initially identified on abdominal imaging and can be confirmed on liver biopsy. In some cases, patients may even manifest in findings of noncirrhotic portal hypertension.

Maintenance therapy with 6-mercaptopurine (6-MP) is often used in cases of acute lymphoblastic leukemia (ALL). Two patterns of toxicity have been reported: hepatocellular injury and cholestasis.[110] Toxicity occurs more commonly when the daily dose of 2 mg/kg is exceeded. Azathioprine is a nitroimidazole derivative of 6-MP. Its toxicity is less frequent and less dose dependent when compared with 6-MP. Three different patterns of toxicity are described: a hypersensitivity reaction, a cholestatic reaction, and endothelial cell injury with development of elevated portal pressures, SOS, and peliosis hepatis.[111]

High-dose MTX therapy has been associated with reversible elevations in aminotransferases. Patients taking chronic low-dose MTX therapy for psoriasis or rheumatoid arthritis are at risk for developing hepatic fibrosis and cirrhosis. The risk is low in patients who receive less than 1.5 g of MTX as cumulative dose.[112]

Alkylating agents uncommonly cause hepatotoxicity. With the exception of cyclophosphamide and ifosfamide, patients receiving alkylating agents do not require dose reduction. Temozolomide, an alkylating agent used to treat brain tumors, has caused severe hepatotoxicity prompting an FDA recommendation for monitoring hepatic enzymes throughout the course of therapy.[113] Other alkylating agents (including melphalan, chlorambucil, nitrogen mustard, and busulfan) are not dependent upon the liver for their metabolism and are not frequently associated with hepatotoxicity.

The antitumor antibiotics include doxorubicin and daunorubicin. Doxorubicin can cause hepatocellular injury and steatosis. Dose reduction has been recommended in patients with cholestasis to avoid greater toxicity.[114] Similar guidelines are followed for daunorubicin.

Asparaginase, used to treat ALL, causes a form of mitochondrial injury in the liver, particularly in those with underlying fatty liver diseasePegasparaginase is a pegylated form of asparaginase with a longer half-life than its parent compound. Liver biochemistries may manifest themselves in a pattern of hepatocellular injury with or without a mixed cholestatic pattern of injury. Hepatic imaging or histologic analysis may reveal evidence of hepatic steatosis and potentially histologic cholestasis. Patients with asparaginase-induced hepatotoxicity may respond to a combination of L-carnitine with or without vitamin B complex.[115] The breakdown of asparagine can also cause hyperammonemia, which could contribute to clinical signs of hepatic encephalopathy.[116]

Many of the molecularly targeted kinase inhibitors are metabolized in the liver and require dose adjustment in patients with underlying liver disease. Lapatinib, a dual inhibitor of both human epidermal growth factor receptor 2 and EGFR, causes hepatotoxicity in approximately half of the patients receiving the drug with several reports of potentially fatal reactions.[117] The presence of certain HLA alleles is associated with an increased risk for hepatotoxicity.[118] Pazopanib, which may be used for treatment of advanced renal cell carcinoma and soft tissue sarcomas, targets multiple tyrosine kinases and causes severe hepatitis in approximately 20% of patients.[119] Pazopanib administration is also associated with or could unmask a more benign form of hyperbilirubinemia in individuals with underlying Gilbert's syndrome, possibly via inhibition of UGT1A1, and dose modification may or may not be necessary.[120]

Hepatotoxicity associated with immune CPI is a well-recognized irAE.[46,49,121,122] Patients are generally clinically asymptomatic, and the degree of liver injury is typically mild, but can be severe; it is rarely life threatening. Transaminase elevations occur overall in 2–5% of patients treated with CPI monotherapy, with high-grade transaminase elevations (i.e., CTCAE grade 3–4) somewhat more common with anti-CTLA-4 agents (i.e., ipilimumab) compared to anti-PD-1/PD-L1 agents (i.e., nivolumab, pembrolizumab, cemiplimab, atezolizumab, avelumab, and durvalumab). Consequently, the reported incidence of hepatotoxicity may vary depending on the type of CPI used. Moreover, the risk of CPI-mediated hepatotoxicity increases substantially when with immunotherapy is combined with chemotherapy or targeted agents, or when combination CPI is utilized (i.e., ipilimumab with nivolumab), which may increase the incidence to as high as 23%. The onset of new elevations in transaminases is generally detected at a median of 6–14 weeks from initial CPI administration, or after one to three doses of CPI, although this irAE could manifest itself within a few weeks after the first CPI administration; the timing is depending on the agent used.

The role of liver biopsy in distinguishing CPI-mediated hepatitis from other causes is controversial. CPI-mediated hepatitis has been associated with a variety of findings histologically, and no pathognomonic histologic findings have been identified.[122] It has been characterized by lymphocytic infiltration (CD8+ cytotoxic T lymphocytes), but centrilobular necrosis, sinusoidal inflammatory infiltrates, and fibrin ring granulomas have also been described. The histologic inflammatory pattern (including CD3+ and CD8+ findings on immunostaining) stands in contrast to traditional autoimmune hepatitis, where plasma cells and CD20+ and CD4+ predominate. Furthermore, in addition to typically seen hepatocellular-predominant injury, cholestatic, or abnormal cholangiopathic features may present concurrently in some cases of this suspected irAE. It is important for the clinician to distinguish this hepatic irAE from traditional autoimmune hepatitis; autoimmune hepatitis is strongly associated with positive ANA in high titers and/or antismooth muscle antibody tests, in addition to a predilection for affecting females, whereas these associations are not observed in CPI-mediated hepatitis.

Management of CPI-related hepatotoxicity is based on the CTCAE classification for adverse events according to elevations in transaminases and bilirubin.[47] As with other irAEs associated with CPIs, systemic corticosteroids are the mainstay of treatment for moderate-to-severe and life-threatening manifestations.[46] Patients experiencing grade 1 liver injury may continue CPI therapy with close monitoring. However, grade 2–4 liver injury requires cessation of CPI therapy and institution of corticosteroids. Some cases of grade 3–4 liver injury have been observed to improve even without immunosuppression. In steroid-refractory disease, consideration is given to adding mycophenolate mofetil or azathioprine. Infliximab should not be used in this setting due to concerns for its own hepatotoxic potential. Current guidelines recommend permanent discontinuation of CPI in cases where grade 3–4 severity of liver injury occurs.[46] However, in practice, even patients who undergo re-challenge with CPI after recovering from grade 3–4 hepatotoxicity do not necessarily suffer from a recurrent episode of liver injury; a recent analysis suggested that only 26% of such patients exhibited recurrent hepatotoxicity.[123]

Sinusoidal obstruction syndrome

SOS, formerly called veno-occlusive disease (VOD), occurs most commonly after HCT but can also result from exposure to toxins such as alkaloids, nontransplant chemotherapeutic agents, high dose radiation therapy to the liver, or after liver transplantation.[124] It is characterized clinically by tender hepatomegaly, jaundice, and weight gain with ascites. The prevalence of SOS varies widely in published studies but has been estimated at around 20%. The clinical presentation of SOS mimics the Budd–Chiari syndrome, where occlusion of the hepatic veins results in postsinusoidal portal hypertension. However, in SOS, it is the sinusoidal and terminal hepatic venule endothelial cells, not the hepatic veins, that are targeted.[125,126] Following injury to the endothelial cells, there is activation of the coagulation cascade with clot formation. Fibrin plugs, intracellular fluid entrapment, and cellular debris progressively occlude the sinusoids, causing intrahepatic sinusoidal hypertension (Figure 8).

Pretransplant risk factors for the development of SOS include older transplant recipient age, female gender, poor performance status, donor-recipient HLA disparity, advanced malignancy, prior abdominal radiation, second myeloablative transplant,

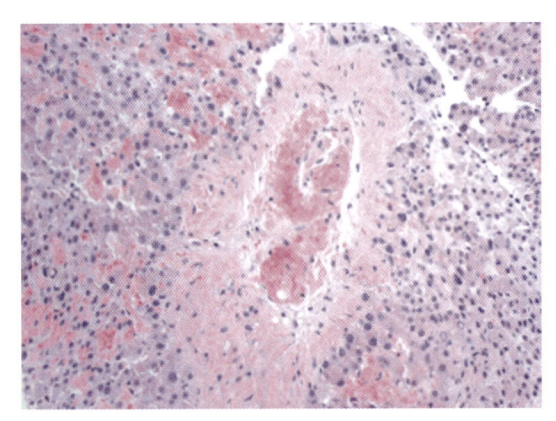

Figure 8 Sinusoidal obstruction syndrome (venoocclusive disease) of the liver. The small hepatic vein demonstrates fibrous obliteration with fibrin deposits. The perivenular hepatocytes show prominent sinusoidal congestion.

reduced pulmonary diffusion capacity (DLCO), and prior liver disease.[127-130]

The type and intensity of the transplant conditioning regimen are the greatest risk factors for developing severe SOS. Risk increases with total body irradiation dose and the use of certain drugs such as 6-MP, 6-thioguanine, actinomycin D, azathioprine, busulfan, cytosine arabinoside, cyclophosphamide, dacarbazine, gemtuzumab-ozogamicin, melphalan, oxaliplatin, and urethane.[125,127]

Typically, the initial presentation of SOS is unexplained weight gain and tender hepatomegaly within the first week posttransplant. Ascites develops in about 25% of patients. Moderate elevations in the transaminases with direct hyperbilirubinemia follow, with peak bilirubin levels less than 20 mg/dl.[131] The diagnosis can be made frequently on the basis of typical signs and symptoms after ruling out other conditions such as viral infection, GVHD, systemic infection, and tumor infiltration. Two systems for the diagnosis of SOS, the Baltimore and Seattle criteria, have been published, but each system has recognized limitations.[129,131,132] Liver biopsy is rarely required for the diagnosis of SOS, but when undertaken, typically shows sinusoidal dilatation with zone 3 hemorrhagic necrosis. Fibrin deposition with congestion is seen in the sinusoids and centrilobular venules. With time, collagen is deposited in the sinusoidal and venular lumens with occlusion of the terminal hepatic veins. If a biopsy is necessary for diagnosis, trans-jugular access is the safest route and can be accompanied by measurement of the hepatic venous gradient (HVPG).[133] Assessing the HVPG can discriminate between GVHD and SOS since the HVPG is greater in the latter.

Prevention of SOS should be a goal in all HCT's. Minimizing the use of potentially hepatotoxic agents and reduced-intensity conditioning regimens can potentially limit the severity of SOS. Pharmacologic prophylaxis is used routinely in many transplant centers. With allogeneic HCT, ursodeoxycholic acid, started before the preparative regimen and continued for three months, resulted in a reduced incidence of SOS when compared with placebo. Some centers use continuous infusion of low-dose heparin in autologous HCT.

Mild to moderate SOS can be treated with supportive therapy including analgesics for right upper quadrant pain relief and diuretics to control extravascular fluid accumulation. Patients with severe SOS rarely respond to supportive therapy alone. Based on the histological presence of microthrombosis and fibrin deposition in the hepatic venules of patients with severe SOS, therapies that promote fibrinolysis with or without anticoagulation have been used. These treatment strategies include the use of alteplase (recombinant tissue-type plasminogen activator or tPA) alone or in combination with heparin, and defibrotide. Treatment with alteplase and heparin resulted in a response rate of about 30% but was associated with a significant risk of life-threatening hemorrhage, particularly in patients with multiorgan failure.[134–136] Defibrotide is a polydeoxyribonucleotide with antithrombotic, anti-ischemic, and thrombolytic properties without causing significant anticoagulation. Defibrotide given intravenously in doses ranging from 5 to 60 mg/kg per day for a minimum of 14 days, results in a response in 42–55% of patients, without significant treatment-related toxicity.[137] Predictors of survival with defibrotide therapy included younger age, autologous stem cell transplantation, and abnormal portal vein flow, while regimens based on busulfan as well as the presence of encephalopathy predicted worse outcomes.[138] Insertion of a trans-jugular intrahepatic portosystemic stent-shunt (TIPS) has been reported in small number of patients with severe SOS. TIPS was effective in improving portal pressure gradient; and in some patients, it was associated with clinical improvement of hepatic and renal symptoms. Nonetheless, these effects may be transient and may not improve overall survival.[139–141] Orthotopic liver transplantation (OLT) has been reported anecdotally as a rescue therapy in patients with SOS after stem cell transplant, when there has been no response to medical therapy. The majority of patients with severe SOS, however, are not candidates for OLT, because of the presence of malignancies and/or multiorgan failure.[142,143]

Graft-versus-host disease of the liver

The liver is the second most commonly involved organ in acute GVHD affecting approximately 50% of patients. Severe hepatic GVHD without other organ involvement is rare. The earliest biochemical findings are elevations in the conjugated bilirubin and alkaline phosphatase concentrations reflecting the underlying pathologic injury.[67] Typically, there is extensive bile duct damage with degeneration and atypia of the bile duct epithelium, cell dropout, and a mixed cellular infiltration of small bile ducts leading to cholestasis.[144] While clinical and laboratory data can be highly suggestive of hepatic GVHD, a liver biopsy may be required for a definitive diagnosis and to rule out confounding diagnoses such VOD, infection, or drug toxicity. In some cases, a percutaneous liver biopsy may not be feasible because of the risk of bleeding due to thrombocytopenia soon after hematopoietic cell transplant. In these instances, if a liver biopsy is deemed to be necessary for diagnosis, a trans-jugular approach may be the preferred option. For acute GVHD, the first and most effective treatment option is the use of corticosteroids alone or in combination with tacrolimus. If this combination is unsuccessful in controlling hepatic GVHD, second-line treatments include antithymocyte globulin and mycophenolate mofetil.[145,146] Chronic hepatic GVHD can develop after previous acute GVHD or de novo, i.e., without a history of previous acute GVHD. Approximately 50% of patients with chronic GVHD have hepatic involvement most often with asymptomatic elevations of the bilirubin and alkaline phosphatase concentrations.[147] The histologic appearance of chronic hepatic GVHD mimics that of another immune-mediated liver disease, primary biliary cirrhosis, with injury to septal and interlobular bile ducts by chronic inflammatory cells.[144,148] The initial treatment of chronic hepatic GVHD is the same as acute GVHD with corticosteroids and tacrolimus. Patients with refractory chronic hepatic GVHD may respond to thalidomide.[149]

Other GI complications of cancer therapy

Constipation

Constipation is a common problem in patients undergoing cancer treatment. In this setting, constipation is usually caused by a combination of poor oral intake, decreased physical activity, antiemetic agents such as ondansetron and opioid analgesics. Opioid-induced constipation (OIC) is one of the most frequent adverse effects of opioid therapy.[150] These agents slow intestinal transit time. Constipation has also been reported in patients taking vinca alkaloids, in particular, vincristine and thalidomide.

Impaction, bowel obstruction, and colonic pseudo-obstruction must be ruled out before initiating pharmacologic therapy for constipation. Constipation should be anticipated in the cancer patient, and steps taken to avoid this complication. Electrolyte abnormalities and other reversible causes of constipation should be corrected. Drugs that can cause constipation should be discontinued if possible. Laxatives, with or without stool softeners, can be used in the initial treatment of constipation. Stimulant laxatives such as bisacodyl and senna alter electrolyte transport by the intestinal mucosa and increase intestinal motor activity. If these agents are not effective, osmotic agents such as lactulose or sorbitol can be effective at improving stool frequency and consistency. Polyethylene glycol solutions are available in powder form and have been found to be effective at improving chronic constipation. The use of drugs to improve colonic transit has been disappointing. Metoclopramide seems to be ineffective. Tegaserod (a 5-hydroxytryptamine receptor agonist) was perceived to have significant cardiovascular adverse effects and was initially withdrawn from the US market. However, a large cohort study based on a US health insurance database showed no increase in the risk of cardiovascular events were found under tegaserod treatment, and in 2019, tegaserod was reintroduced as for use in irritable bowel syndrome with constipation (IBS-C) in women under 65. Lubiprostone a chloride channel activator is FDA approved for the treatment of chronic idiopathic constipation. It is a bicyclic acid that works locally on the apical part of the intestine and helps to increase intracellular fluid and intestinal motility. It may be useful in the patient with constipation whose symptoms are increased with opioid use, and with constipation induced by chemotherapy. It is FDA approved for treatment of OIC related to noncancer pain. Methylnaltrexone and naloxegol, both a micro-opioid-receptor antagonist, are approved in the United States for the treatment of OIC in advanced-illness patients. These agents, selectively antagonize the peripheral micro-receptors in the GI tract without effects on the CNS. In clinical trials, subcutaneous methylnaltrexone reversed OIC after the first dose in approximately 50–60% of the patients.[151] In most of the cases, effective laxation occurred within 1 h. It does not affect opioid analgesic effects or induces opioid withdrawal symptoms. Recent advances in neuro-gastroenterology are leading to the development of new classes of medications which may aid in the treatment of severe constipation.[152] Peripherally active μ-opioid receptor antagonists (PAMORA) allow preservation of the central analgesic effects of these drugs, while antagonizing peripheral effects on the GI tract.[153] Methyltrexone, naldemedine, and naloxegol are prototypes in this class. Naloxegol is an oral PEGylated conjugate of naloxone. Naloxegol is approved to treat OIC in adults with noncancer pain,[152] while in the European Union it is approved for adults who had an inadequate response to laxative therapy. Prucalopride, a selective high affinity 5-HT4 receptor agonist has recently been approved for in the United States for treatment of chronic constipation.

Nausea and vomiting

Nausea and vomiting frequently occur after administration of chemotherapeutic agents (chemotherapy-induced nausea and vomiting or CINV) and may affect not only quality of life, but result in chemotherapy delays, dose reductions, and increased use of health care resources. Several organizations have published antiemesis guidelines including ESMO,[154] ASCO,[155] and NCCN.[156] The likelihood of developing nausea and vomiting following chemotherapy depends on several factors including the chemotherapy dose and the intrinsic emetogenicity of a given agent.[157] The emetogenic potential of intravenously administered antineoplastic agents can be assigned to levels of risk, ranging from minimal or less than 10% risk (e.g., bevacizumab) to a high or greater than 90% risk (e.g., cisplatin). Drugs with the highest emetogenic risk are classified as highly emetogenic chemotherapy or HEC. Emesis can be acute (i.e., occurring within the first 24 h of receiving chemotherapy) or delayed.

Various antiemetic agents are now available for the prevention and treatment of CINV. The choice of an antiemetic should be based on the emetic risk of therapy, prior experience, and patient factors. These include agents with a high therapeutic index such as 5-hydroxytryptamine-3 (5-HT_3) receptor antagonists (5HT3 RA, e.g., ondansetron, granisetron, dolasetron, tropisetron, palonosetron), neurokinin-1-receptor antagonists (NK1 RA, e.g., aprepitant, fosaprepitant, rolapitant), and corticosteroids (usually used in combination with other agents). All guidelines recommend a triple combination regimen of a NK1 RA, 5HT3 RA, and dexamethasone ±olanzapine as an evidence-based approach to HEC. Many antiemetic agents have multiple drug–drug or drug–disease interactions which need to be considered. Agents with a low therapeutic index are also used, such as metoclopramide hydrochloride, butyrophenones, phenothiazines, substituted benzamides, antihistamines cannabinoids, and olanzapine (an atypical antipsychotic agent). The preferred agent and regimen depend on the emetogenic level of a given chemotherapeutic drug. For drugs with a low emetogenic risk, antiemetics are given before chemotherapy, while antiemetics are provided before and after chemotherapy for those chemotherapy drugs with a high emetogenic risk. Prophylactic antiemetic regimens should be chosen based on the drug with the highest emetic risk in the anticancer regimen. Antiemetic agents should be started before administration of anticancer agents and should cover at least the first 24 h. Patients should be protected throughout the entire period of risk.

Gastrointestinal perforation, fistula formation, arterial thrombosis, and bleeding

GI perforation, fistula formation, arterial thrombosis, and bleeding have been reported with bevacizumab, a monoclonal antibody against VEGF. Intestinal perforation has been reported in 1–2% of patients treated with bevacizumab for metastatic colorectal cancer.[158,159] Risk factors associated with perforation include an intact primary tumor, prior irradiation, acute diverticulitis, intra-abdominal abscess, and GI obstruction.

Acute pancreatitis

Acute pancreatitis in patients with cancer or in those who have undergone hematopoietic stem-cell transplantation can be caused by conditions present in the general population, including gallstones and alcohol. However, other etiologies should be taken into consideration when managing cancer patients who have acute pancreatitis, including medications and chemotherapeutic agents.

Drug-induced pancreatitis has no distinguishing clinical features, and therefore taking a careful drug history and excluding other etiologies are essential to make a diagnosis. Some of the most common drugs known to cause acute pancreatitis include metronidazole, sulfonamides, tetracycline, furosemide, thiazides, estrogen, and tamoxifen. During the course of chemotherapy, pancreatitis has been reported with the use of azathioprine, prednisone, cytosine arabinoside, immune CPI, and various regimens of combination chemotherapy including vinca alkaloids, MTX, mitomycin, 5-FU, cyclophosphamide, cisplatin, and bleomycin. The significance of symptomatic amylase or lipase elevations associated with CPIs is unclear. ICI-related pancreatitis if moderate or severe is usually treated with holding (moderate disease) or discontinuing (severe disease) immunotherapy and intravenous hydration; steroids do not appear to prevent adverse outcomes.[160] Associated illnesses and multi-drug regimens often make it difficult to determine a cause and effect relationship.[161]

Oral and gastrointestinal mucositis

Oral mucositis or painful ulceration of the mucosal lining of the oropharynx occurs frequently in individuals undergoing radiation and chemotherapy for solid malignancies. It occurs in 20–40% of patients receiving conventional chemotherapy, 80% of patients receiving high-dose chemotherapy, and has been reported in up to 98% of individuals undergoing hematopoietic stem-cell transplantation. Evidence-based recommendations for prevention and treatment of oral mucositis have been published and recently updated.[1,162,163] Palifermin, a recombinant human keratinocyte growth factor-1 decreases the incidence and duration of mucositis in patients with hematologic malignancies who are receiving chemotherapy and requiring stem-cell transplantation support and has been approved by the FDA for this indication. It is recommended that this agent be used to prevent oral mucositis in patients receiving high-dose chemotherapy and total body irradiation followed by autologous stem cell transplantation for hematologic malignancies.[1] Oral cryotherapy is also recommended to be used to prevent oral mucositis in patients receiving bolus 5-fluorouracil chemotherapy. Low-level laser therapy has been recommended to prevent oral mucositis in patients receiving human stem cell transplantation conditioned with high-dose chemotherapy. Benzydamine mouthwash (but not antimicrobial mouthwash such as chlorhexidine) should be used to prevent oral mucositis in patients with head and neck cancer receiving moderate-dose radiotherapy without concomitant chemotherapy. Zinc supplements may beneficial to prevent oral mucositis in oral cancer patients receiving radiation or chemotherapy. Evidence is lacking to support the use of sucralfate to prevent or treat mucositis in those receiving chemotherapy or radiation for head and neck cancer. Numerous natural products and herbal remedies have been studied for the management of oral mucositis. Evidence supports the use of honey (combined topical and systemic delivery) for this purpose. The use of topical morphine 0.2% is supported to treat mucositis-associated pain in head and neck cancer patients treated with chemo-radiation regimens.

Gastrointestinal mucositis (GIM) refers to mucosal injury and related symptoms distal to the oropharyngeal cavity. The use of probiotics containing *Lactobacillus* species for prevention of chemoradiotherapy and radiotherapy-induced diarrhea in patients with pelvic malignancy, and hyperbaric oxygen therapy to treat radiation-induced proctitis has been recommended, but inadequate or conflicting evidence exists for preventing or treating GIM. Agents under investigation include palifermin, glutamine, sodium butyrate, and dietary interventions.[162]

Abbreviations

ALT   alanine aminotransferase
AST   aspartate aminotransferase
ULN   upper limit of normal

Key references

The complete reference list can be found on Vital Source version of this title, see inside front cover.

7. Pappas PG, Kauffman CA, Andes DR, et al. Clinical Practice Guideline for the Management of Candidiasis: 2016 Update by the Infectious Diseases Society of America. *Clin Infect Dis.* 2016;**62**(4):e1–e50.
9. Masur H, Brooks JT, Benson CA, et al. Prevention and treatment of opportunistic infections in HIV-infected adults and adolescents: updated Guidelines from the Centers for Disease Control and Prevention, National Institutes of Health, and HIV Medicine Association of the Infectious Diseases Society of America. *Clin Infect Dis.* 2014;**58**(9):1308–1311.
23. van Rossum PSN, Mohammad NH, Vleggaar FP, van Hillegersberg R. Treatment for unresectable or metastatic oesophageal cancer: current evidence and trends. *Nat Rev Gastroenterol Hepatol.* 2018;**15**(4):235–249.
24. Didden P, Reijm AN, Erler NS, et al. Fully vs. partially covered selfexpandable metal stent for palliation of malignant esophageal strictures: a randomized trial (the COPAC study). *Endoscopy.* 2018;**50**(10):961–971.
25. Dai Y, Li C, Xie Y, et al. Interventions for dysphagia in oesophageal cancer. *Cochrane Database Syst Rev.* 2014;**10**:Cd005048.
33. McDonald LC, Gerding DN, Johnson S, et al. Clinical Practice Guidelines for *Clostridium difficile* infection in adults and children: 2017 update by the Infectious Diseases Society of America (IDSA) and Society for Healthcare Epidemiology of America (SHEA). *Clin Infect Dis.* 2018;**66**(7):e1–e48.
35. Wilcox MH, Gerding DN, Poxton IR, et al. Bezlotoxumab for prevention of recurrent *Clostridium difficile* infection. *N Engl J Med.* 2017;**376**(4):305–317.
41. Sharma P, Allison JP. Dissecting the mechanisms of immune checkpoint therapy. *Nat Rev Immunol.* 2020;**20**(2):75–76.
42. Dougan M. Gastrointestinal and hepatic complications of immunotherapy: current management and future perspectives. *Curr Gastroenterol Rep.* 2020;**22**(4):15.
43. Pauken KE, Dougan M, Rose NR, et al. Adverse events following cancer immunotherapy: obstacles and opportunities. *Trends Immunol.* 2019;**40**(6):511–523.
44. Postow MA, Sidlow R, Hellmann MD. Immune-related adverse events associated with immune checkpoint blockade. *N Engl J Med.* 2018;**378**(2):158–168.
45. Puzanov I, Diab A, Abdallah K, et al. Managing toxicities associated with immune checkpoint inhibitors: consensus recommendations from the Society for Immunotherapy of Cancer (SITC) Toxicity Management Working Group. *J Immunother Cancer.* 2017;**5**(1):95.
46. Thompson JA, Schneider BJ, Brahmer J, et al. Management of immunotherapy-related toxicities, version 1. 2019. *J Natl Compr Canc Netw.* 2019;**17**(3):255–289.
47. U.S. Department for Health and Human Services NIoH, National Cancer Center (2017) *Common Terminology Criteria for Adverse Events (CTCAE). 5.0 ed2015.*
48. Wang Y, Abu-Sbeih H, Mao E, et al. Endoscopic and histologic features of immune checkpoint inhibitor-related colitis. *Inflamm Bowel Dis.* 2018;**24**(8):1695–1705.
49. Brahmer JR, Lacchetti C, Schneider BJ, et al. Management of immune-related adverse events in patients treated with immune checkpoint inhibitor therapy: American Society of Clinical Oncology Clinical Practice Guideline. *J Clin Oncol.* 2018;**36**(17):1714–1768.
50. Wang Y, Wiesnoski DH, Helmink BA, et al. Fecal microbiota transplantation for refractory immune checkpoint inhibitor-associated colitis. *Nat Med.* 2018;**24**(12):1804–1808.
51. Lee JK, Agrawal D, Thosani N, et al. ASGE guideline on the role of endoscopy for bleeding from chronic radiation proctopathy. *Gastrointest Endosc.* 2019;**90**(2):171–82.e1.
52. Grabenbauer GG, Holger G. Management of radiation and chemotherapy related acute toxicity in gastrointestinal cancer. *Best Pract Res Clin Gastroenterol.* 2016;**30**(4):655–664.
67. Jagasia MH, Greinix HT, Arora M, et al. National Institutes of Health Consensus Development Project on Criteria for Clinical Trials in Chronic Graft-versus-Host Disease: I. The 2014 Diagnosis and Staging Working Group report. *Biol Blood Marrow Transplant.* 2015;**21**(3):389–401.e1.
80. Cutler C, Logan B, Nakamura R, et al. Tacrolimus/sirolimus vs tacrolimus/methotrexate as GVHD prophylaxis after matched, related donor allogeneic HCT. *Blood.* 2014;**124**(8):1372–1377.
85. Carpenter PA, Kitko CL, Elad S, et al. National Institutes of Health Consensus Development Project on Criteria for Clinical Trials in Chronic Graft-versus-Host Disease: V. The 2014 Ancillary Therapy and Supportive Care Working Group Report. *Biol Blood Marrow Transplant.* 2015;**21**(7):1167–1187.
93. Reddy KR, Beavers KL, Hammond SP, Lim JK. Falck-Ytter YT; American Gastroenterological Association Institute. American Gastroenterological Association Institute guideline on the prevention and treatment of hepatitis B virus reactivation during immunosuppressive drug therapy [published correction appears in Gastroenterology. 2015 Feb;148(2):455. Multiple investigator names added]. *Gastroenterology.* 2015;**148**(1):215–e17. doi: 10.1053/j.gastro.2014.10.039.
96. Lampertico P, Agarwal K, Berg T, et al. EASL 2017 Clinical Practice Guidelines on the management of hepatitis B virus infection. *J Hepatol.* 2017;**67**:370–398.
100. Rico GT, Chan MM, Loo KF. The safety and efficacy of immune checkpoint inhibitors in patients with advanced cancers and pre-existing chronic viral infections (hepatitis B/C, HIV): a review of the avaiable evidence. *Cancer Treatment Rev.* 2020;**86**:1–15.
107. Puente A, Fortea JI, Del Pozo C, et al. Porto-sinusoidal vascular disease associated to oxaliplatin: an entity to think about it. *Cells.* 2019;**8**(12):1506.
115. Arora S, Klair J, Bellizzi AM, Tanaka T. L-carnitine and Vitamin B Complex for PEG-L-asparaginase-Induced Hepatotoxicity. *ACG Case Rep J.* 2019;**6**(8):e00194.
121. Suzman DL, Pelosof L, Rosenberg A, Avigan MI. Hepatotoxicity of immune checkpoint inhibitors: an evolving picture of risk associated with a vital class of immunotherapy agents. *Liver Int.* 2018;**38**(6):976–987.
122. De Martin E, Michot JM, Papouin B, et al. Characterization of liver injury induced by cancer immunotherapy using immune checkpoint inhibitors. *J Hepatol.* 2018;**68**(6):1181–1190.
123. Miller ED, Abu-Sbeih H, Styskel B, et al. Clinical characteristics and adverse impact of hepatotoxicity due to immune checkpoint inhibitors. *Am J Gastroenterol.* 2020;**115**(2):251–261.
132. Mohty M, Malard F, Abecassis M, et al. Revised diagnosis and severity criteria for sinusoidal obstruction syndrome/veno-occlusive disease in adult patients: a new classification from the European Society for Blood and Marrow Transplantation. *Bone Marrow Transplant.* 2016;**51**(7):906–912.
150. Siemens W, Gaertner J, Becker G. Advances in pharmacotherapy for opioid-induced constipation — a systematic review. *Expert Opin Pharmacother.* 2015;**16**(4):515–532.
153. Pergolizzi JV Jr, Christo PJ, LeQuang JA, Magnusson P. The use of peripheral μ-opioid receptor antagonists (PAMORA) in the management of opioid-induced constipation: an update on their efficacy and safety. *Drug Des Devel Ther.* 2020;**14**:1009–1025.
154. Herrstedt J, Roila F, Warr D, et al. 2016 Updated MASCC/ESMO consensus recommendations: prevention of nausea and vomiting following high emetic risk chemotherapy. *Support Care Cancer.* 2017;**25**(1):277–288.
155. Hesketh PJ, Kris MG, Basch E, et al. Antiemetics: American Society of Clinical Oncology Clinical Practice Guideline Update. *J Clin Oncol.* 2017;**35**(28):3240–3261.
156. NCCN (2020) *Antiemesis (Version 2.2020).* https://www.nccn.org/professionals/physician_gls/pdf/antiemesis.pdf
157. Hesketh PJ. Chemotherapy-induced nausea and vomiting. *N Engl J Med.* 2008;**358**(23):2482–2494.
160. Abu-Sbeih H, Tang T, Lu Y, et al. Clinical characteristics and outcomes of immune checkpoint inhibitor-induced pancreatic injury. *J Immunother Cancer.* 2019;**7**(1):31.
161. Morgan C, Tillett T, Braybrooke J, Ajithkumar T. Management of uncommon chemotherapy-induced emergencies. *Lancet Oncol.* 2011;**12**(8):806–814.
162. Bowen JM, Gibson RJ, Coller JK, et al. Systematic review of agents for the management of cancer treatment-related gastrointestinal mucositis and clinical practice guidelines. *Support Care Cancer.* 2019;**27**(10):4011–4022.
163. Special Section on the MASCC/ISOO Clinical Practice Guidelines for the Management of Mucositis—2019 Update Part 2: Guest Editor: Sharon Elad, DMD MSc. *Support Care Cancer.* 2020;**28**(5):2443.

133 Oral complications of cancer and their treatment

Stephen T. Sonis, DMD, DMSc ■ *Anna Yuan, DMD, PhD* ■ *Alessandro Villa, DDS, PhD, MPH*

Overview

The oral cavity is uniquely heterogeneous relative to tissue types, microbiome, immunology, and fluidic environment which make it a sentinnental site for manifestations of both acute and late cancer regimen-related toxicities. The rapid turnover of its non-keratinized mucosa is subject to a radiation and chemotherapy initiated biological cascade that results in dramatic epithelial injury. Osteonecrosis of the jaws is associated with bisphosphonate and radiation. A diverse and shifting microflora parallels myelosuppressive treatment or drug- and radiation-induced xerostomia resulting in secondary infections and a bacterial repository for bacteremia and sepsis. Exacerabation of dental caries and periodontal disease is a common consequence of treatment. Virtually every form of current cancer treatment from conventional cytotoxic regimens to the most innovative forms of targeted and immunotherapy are associated with the risk of toxic manifestations in the mouth. Preventive and management strategies can be helpful in attenuating risk and modulating the severity of these complications. Given the potential disproportionate impact of oral complications on patient outcomes, it is incumbent on providers to assure that the mouth is not overlooked in the overall management of the patient being treated for cancer.

Introduction

Oral complications from cancer treatment range broadly in their nature, incidence, severity, and course, but all adversely affect patients' quality of life, ability to tolerate therapy, overall cost of treatment, risk of local and systemic infection, and rehabilitation. Oral toxicities are perceived as common in some cohorts such as patients with head and neck cancer (HNC), but relatively rare in others. This perception has been largely fueled by under-reporting, often by patients concerned that mentioning toxicity symptoms might result in dose de-escalation and subsequent compromise of their optimum anti-cancer therapy. While this phenomenon is not unique to oral complications, data surrounding the under-estimates of oral toxicities are substantial. Additionally, oral side effects have been reported with many forms of developing therapies including cetuximab, antiresorptive medications, mammalian target of rapamycin (mTOR)-inhibitors, and immune check point inhibitors. It has also becoming clear that oral complications rarely occur in isolation. Rather, probably because of common biologic mechanisms, they predictably occur with other regimen-related toxicities.[1]

Overall, about 40% of patients being treated for cancers not of the head and neck develop some form of mouth-related problem, which range from xerostomia to mucositis.[2] This frequency escalates to more than 75% for patients being treated for HNC, those who develop graft-versus-host disease (GVHD), and patients receiving aggressive myeloablative chemotherapy regimens. The symptomatic and functional consequences of oral complications include increases in analgesic and antibiotic use, length of hospital stays, hospitalizations for pain and fluid management, nursing resource use, diagnostic tests, and the need for parenteral feeding. The impact on charges and costs is dramatic. In a study population of patients receiving treatment for HNC and non-small cell lung cancer, the incremental cost of oral mucositis alone, per patient, was found to be $17,244.[3] In the past, oral complications were largely considered to be inevitable, often were not recognized early, and were treated retrospectively rather than in a prospective or preventive manner. Significant progress has been made in the past decade to better define the biology and epidemiology of oral complications of treatment. As a result, interventions that target mechanisms have evolved, as has a better understanding of at-risk populations.

Pretreatment assessment

The risk of many of the side effects that impact the mouth can be successfully reduced by the elimination of existing sites of dental disease before anticancer treatment is initiated.[4-6] A pretreatment dental visit is strongly recommended as it serves a range of purposes. First, it provides an opportunity for the identification and elimination of sources of active and chronic dental or periodontal infections or chronic irritation when the patient is best able to tolerate treatment with the least risk of undesirable post-treatment sequelae, such as infection or osteonecrosis. Second, oral manifestations of the primary cancer may be detected. Third, it provides an opportunity for patient education and discussion regarding the impact of the cancer and its treatment on short- and long-term oral health. Fourth, for the patient about to undergo surgical intervention for tumors in or adjacent to the mouth, pretreatment evaluation is critical to optimize the fabrication of prostheses. The construction of protective appliances prior to the start of radiation therapy may reduce the impact of treatment on scatter-induced injury.

The frequency of dental disease, faulty prostheses or dental restorations reported upon screening of patients with cancer reflects the incidence of these conditions in the general population. While findings of less than optimal oral health were reported in two-thirds of patients evaluated prior to hematopoietic stem cell transplantation (HSCT), pathology severe enough to require intervention was only found in about a third of screened patients.[7] Similarly, of patients with cancers of the head and neck who were screened prior to radiation therapy, between one half to two-thirds required dental extractions, primarily because of diagnoses

Holland-Frei Cancer Medicine, Tenth Edition. Edited by Robert C. Bast, John C. Byrd, Carlo M. Croce, Ernest Hawk, Fadlo R. Khuri, Raphael E. Pollock, Apostolia M. Tsimberidou, Christopher G. Willett, and Cheryl L. Willman.
© 2023 John Wiley & Sons, Inc. Published 2023 by John Wiley & Sons, Inc.

associated with periodontal disease.[8,9] Although elimination of possible oral and dental sites of infection prior to chemotherapy had a significant, favorable impact on morbidity relative to local infection and sepsis, definitive data demonstrating that pre-irradiation elimination of oral foci of infection favorably impacts outcomes is needed.[4,10] Effective dental screening with appropriate treatment, prior to the onset of cancer therapy results in significant cost savings by reducing the incidence of infection during periods of granulocytopenia.[11]

Timing of assessment and dental treatment

If oral screening is performed so close to the initiation of cancer therapy as to preclude dental intervention, the value of the process is nullified. The ideal interval between the completion of dental treatment, particularly extraction, and the initiation of radiation therapy has been the subject of much debate. Nonetheless, given the rate at which wounds of the mouth heal, particularly at extraction sites, it appears that a minimum of 2 weeks is acceptable and 3 weeks desirable.[12] For patients about to undergo chemotherapy, sufficient time between the completion of dental treatment and the patient's anticipated granulocyte nadir (<500 cells/mL) is required. In general, non-emergent dental treatment should not be performed in a typical ambulatory setting if the patient is significantly thrombocytopenic (<50,000 platelets/mL).[13]

Because of the acute onset of some hematologic malignancies and the need for immediate chemotherapy, pretreatment dental and oral screening in this high-risk population may not be possible. In these cases, oral assessment should be performed as close to the initiation of therapy as possible for two reasons: first, such an examination provides an important baseline for oral health; and second, the finding and elimination of active oral infection in this markedly myeloablated group is often critical to their overall clinical course. Eradication of identified sources of odontogenic infection should not be delayed, as there is significant data to support the conclusion that dental extractions may be performed safely in this group if they are managed well, preferably in a hospital setting.[10] The complication rate for extractions in patients with hematologic malignancies is reported to be 13%, with no effect on length of hospital stay or mortality. The most common complications include pain and bleeding. It is important to note that there is no evidence to suggest that an aggressive strategy of extraction of *asymptomatic* teeth has any benefit in the prevention of systemic infection.

Components of the pretreatment assessment include baseline data such as medical and dental histories; laboratory data—such as antibody status relative to herpes simplex type 1 virus—and a clinical assessment that should include an extra-oral examination of the head and neck, intra-oral soft tissue examination, periodontal disease screening, and dental evaluation. Radiographic evaluation should include those images that are necessary to definitively diagnose periodontal disease and caries, periapical pathology, and impacted teeth. It is also important to assess the patient's knowledge of, and motivation for dental maintenance. Teeth that demonstrate evidence of untreated periapical pathology, or advanced caries or periodontal disease should be extracted.

Patients with removable prostheses should be encouraged to minimize their use or leave them out during their cancer therapy since even subtle mucosal trauma accelerates the risk and onset of mucositis. Similarly, the removal of orthodontic bands prior to the start of chemotherapy is an essential component in preventing trauma to atrophied mucosa.[14]

Oral complications of radiotherapy

Oral complications of radiation therapy are primarily the result of acute and chronic local tissue injury. In addition, radiation-induced xerostomia may result in secondary effects on the teeth and periodontium.[15] The dose rate, total dose of radiation, use of concomitant chemotherapy, the size of, and structures within, the radiation field are the major determinants of oral toxicity. As a result, patients being treated for tumors of the mouth, oropharynx, tongue, nasopharynx, and salivary glands are at highest risk. Patients with hypopharyngeal or laryngeal tumors are also often affected, although at a slightly lower rate. Brachytherapy tends to be more stomatotoxic than external beam irradiation. Although intensity-modulated radiation therapy (IMRT) (see **Chapter 79**) may spare some structures; its impact on oral mucosa is significant. Oral tissues that are directly affected by radiation include mucosa (epithelium and tissues in the lamina propria), salivary glands, bone, and muscle. In children, radiation that includes the jaws negatively affects craniofacial and dental development.[16]

Mucositis

Both radiation and chemotherapy can produce significant damage to the oral mucosa as a side effect of treatment. The term mucositis (ICD-10-CM Diagnosis Code K12.30) is preferred over stomatitis when describing mucosal injury caused by antineoplastic therapy as the latter is a generic term and can be associated with a range of infectious or traumatic etiologies unrelated to chemo- or radiotherapy. The severity and kinetics of radiation-induced oral mucositis are related to dose rate and total dose that target the oral mucosa. Local mucosal irritation, secondary infection, and xerostomia are factors that amplify the damaging effects of radiation to the tissue.

Three themes have characterized the mucositis discussion in recent years: first, the pathobiology has been more fully defined; second, the commonality in mechanisms by which mucosal injury occurs has been applied to all parts of the alimentary canal; and third, mucositis rarely occurs as an isolated toxicity.[17] In addition, the impact of genomics on toxicity risk, including mucositis, has become clear and is being more fully defined.

Historically, mucositis was viewed as the result of direct radiation or chemotherapy mediated injury to stem cells in the basal layer of the oral mucosa. It was proposed that these rapidly dividing cells were indiscriminately damaged resulting in atrophy and subsequent ulceration. Simultaneously, connective tissue injury was thought to lead to an increase in vascular permeability and tissue edema. However, studies defining the mechanisms by which mucositis occurs reveal a process that is biologically more complex. Although epithelial stem cells are the ultimate mediators of mucosal injury, it is now clear that their demise occurs by indirect, as well as direct, mechanisms.[18,19] In fact, direct clonogenic cell death of these cells is insufficient to produce the extent of clinical injury that is typically observed. Rather, a sequence of events triggered by the generation of reactive species in cells of the lamina propria produce a cascade of events in the endothelium, connective tissue, and extra-cellular matrix, including inflammatory infiltration.[19] This sequence begins almost immediately, following the initial exposure of the mucosa to radiation, and results in a range of molecular mediators and signals that permeate to the epithelium and cause injury, apoptosis, and necrosis.

Radiation-induced oral mucositis typically begins within the first 2 weeks of therapy, at cumulative doses of 10–20 Gy. Although clinical changes are observed at these doses, the cellular and tissue events producing these changes begin almost immediately following initial dosing (see below). Mucosal erythema, mild epithelial sloughing, and the formation of islands of hyperkeratosis characterize early changes of mucositis. These changes are accompanied by relatively mild symptoms characterized by a painful burning sensation that is analogous to a food burn such as that caused by hot cheese. Patients often have difficulty tolerating spicy foods. With the exception of the dorsal surface of the tongue, hard palate, and the gingiva, any mucosal surface of the mouth is susceptible. Most commonly affected areas are the buccal mucosa (cheeks), ventral and lateral surfaces of the tongue, and the floor of the mouth (Figure 1). The soft palate and oropharynx are also frequently involved and are consistent drivers of symptoms associated with pain on swallowing. Consequently, patients may complain of a sore throat early in their treatment.

At cumulative doses of about 30 Gy, the integrity of the mucosa breaks down and ulceration occurs. Ulcers typically begin as isolated lesions, but then coalesce forming large, contiguous breaks in the mucosa, often covered by a collection of dead cells and bacteria in a pseudomembrane. In severe cases, the lesions may bleed (Figure 2). Ulcerative mucositis is extremely painful. Not only do ulcers cover large mucosal surface areas, but they are also deep. Patients who have undergone radiation therapy and have developed mucositis describe this complication as the most burdensome of their treatment.[20] In many cases, mucositis results in breaks in radiation treatment, hospitalization for fluid support or pain management, and the need for parenteral feeding.[21] The incremental economic cost of oral mucositis in this population is significant.[3] It is important that patients about to begin treatment have some concept of the severity of mucosal injury that they are likely to develop. The typical pretreatment characterization of mucositis as "mouth sores" seems to trivialize their significance to patients. It seems likely that a more realistic description and management plan would be advantageous. In most patients, ulcerative mucositis is self-limiting and resolves spontaneously 4–6 weeks following the completion of radiation. In rare cases ulcerations may persist for months after radiation therapy (chronic oral mucositis).

Evaluation of mucositis
Comparisons of the stomatotoxicity of treatment regimens and efficacy assessments of mucositis interventions have been hindered by the lack of a universally acceptable scoring system for the

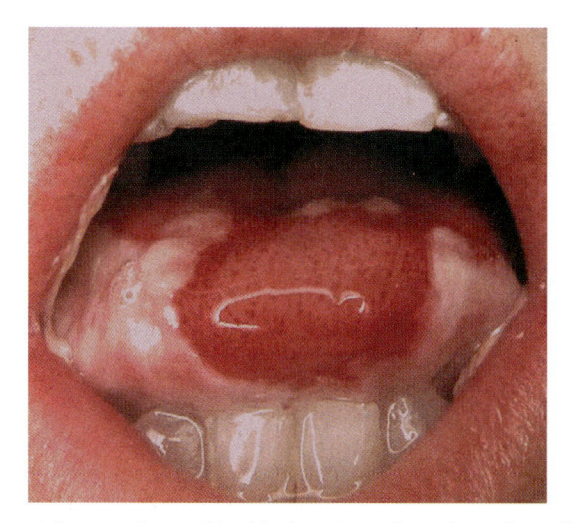

Figure 1 Severe oral mucositis with ulceration and pseudomembrane formation of the lateral and ventral surfaces of the tongue and buccal mucosa induced by myeloablative chemotherapy for conditioning prior to HSCT.

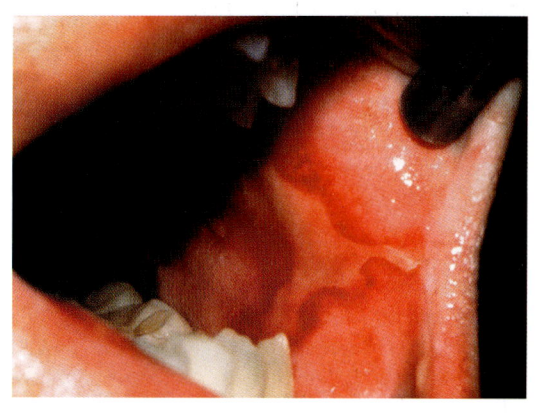

Figure 2 Severe oral mucositis with ulceration, erythema, and pseudomembrane formation of the left buccal mucosa induced by radiation therapy for treatment of an oral carcinoma.

condition. Currently, the grading systems most commonly used to describe oral mucosal toxicity are the World Health Organization (WHO) and National Cancer Institute's common terminology criteria for adverse events (NCI-CTCAE version 5) scales. The WHO scale combines objective findings of erythema and ulceration with the patients' ability to eat solids, liquids, or nothing by mouth (Table 1). The CTCAE scale for oral mucositis relies completely on symptomatic and functional (oral intake) endpoints. While this approach minimizes the clinician's effort to assess mucositis, the dependence on patient-reported symptoms and function is complicated by analgesic use, individual pain perception, and non-mucositis related function modifiers such as edentulism, nausea, and so on.

Prevention and treatment
There is currently no approved, active preventive or treatment intervention for radiation-induced mucositis in the United States. There is consensus that improved oral status may reduce the risk or severity of mucositis. Maintaining a high level of oral hygiene during treatment is thought to be beneficial.

Since mucosal injury is related to the extent of mucosa exposed to radiation, the use of midline radiation blocks and three-dimensional radiation treatment may reduce the extent of stomatotoxicity.[22,23]

Benzydamine hydrochloride is a nonsteroidal rinse with anti-inflammatory, analgesic, and anesthetic properties that is approved for use in the prevention and treatment of radiation-induced mucositis in Canada, Australia, and Europe. Results of a number of studies suggest its efficacy in this application.[24,25] The Multinational Association of Supportive Care in Cancer (MASCC) panel recommended the use of benzydamine among patients receiving moderate dose radiotherapy.[26] There is no data to support its use in patients receiving concomitant chemotherapy.

A number of palliative barrier agents have been suggested to alleviate symptoms associated with oral mucositis. Gelclair, which has Food and Drug Administration (FDA) approval as a device, purportedly forms a barrier on injured mucosa.[27] Sucralfate, an agent that has wide use in the treatment of gastric ulcers, forms a protein-drug complex on the site of ulcerated mucosa. Its use as a rinse in the treatment of mucositis has been reported in a number of studies, although its efficacy seems inconsistent.[28,29] It is specifically not recommended in the MASCC guidelines. MuGard, a hydrogel, demonstrated significant palliation in a multi-institutional, randomized, placebo-controlled trial.[30]

Table 1 Oral mucositis scales.

	Grade 0	Grade I	Grade II	Grade III	Grade IV	Grade V
WHO	None	Erythema and soreness; no ulcers	Oral erythema, ulcers, solid diet tolerated	Oral ulcers, liquid diet only	Not able to tolerate a solid or liquid diet	NA
NCI-CTCAE (chemotherapy induced)	None	Painless ulcers, erythema, or mild soreness in the absence of lesions	Painful erythema, edema, or ulcers but eating or swallowing possible	Painful erythema, edema, or ulcers requiring intravenous hydration	Severe ulceration or requiring parenteral enteral nutritional support or prophylactic intubation	Death related to toxicity

A variety of topical agents exist for mucositis pain management. These include viscous lidocaine, benzocaine in Orabase, and suspensions of Benadryl in Kaopectate or milk of magnesia. Caphosol, a rinse originally developed as a tooth remineralizing solution for patients with xerostomia, is an electrolyte solution of sodium phosphate, calcium chloride, sodium chloride, and purified water, which purportedly lubricates the mucosa and thereby attenuates mucositis. The solution is approved as a device, but the results of clinical trials are inconsistent.[31-33] Oral *Aloe vera* has been available for some time as a palliative agent. However, it failed to demonstrate efficacy in a phase 2, double-blind, randomized, placebo-controlled study.[34] Topical palliative rinses are typically effective only for mild forms of the condition. Systemic pain management following the WHO pain ladder is often necessary. Additionally, cold foods, such as ice cream or Popsicles, may be soothing. Patients should be instructed to remove dental prostheses.

The role of microbes on the severity and course of radiation-induced mucositis is unclear.[35] The strategy of mucosal decontamination as a mucositis intervention has produced conflicting results. Chlorhexidine gluconate rinses do not appear to have a role in mucositis prevention or treatment in radiation mucositis and, in fact, might exacerbate the condition.[36] Lozenges containing polymyxin E, tobramycin, and amphotericin have been studied and seem to of marginal value and are not recommended.[37] Good oral hygiene and multi-agent combination oral care protocols may reduce the risk, severity, and duration of oral mucositis.[38]

Given its importance as an unmet need, the development pipeline for mucositis is rich with agents which target key elements in its pathogenesis. Clinical trials are currently in progress in which drugs targeting oxidative stress, the innate immune response and pro-inflammatory elements are being studied.[39,40] Low level laser therapy (LLLT) is also being investigated for its potential utility as an intervention of oral mucositis. While results of clinical trials are encouraging, the lack of substantive studies defining its biological effects as related to tumor response is troubling. More investigation is clearly needed to assure that its impact on pre-malignant and malignant tissue is benign.[41]

Xerostomia

Xerostomia is one of the most consistent and bothersome side effects of radiation therapy in which the salivary glands are included in the field of treatment, and may be exacerbated by concomitant chemotherapy.[42] The effects of radiation on salivary flow are variable and symptoms of dry mouth may not correspond to observed salivary flow. Xerostomia is caused by the effects of radiation on acinar cells, especially of the serous glands (parotid). Consequently, inflammation, degeneration, and fibrosis of the glandular parenchyma occur. The extent, duration, and degree of recovery are functions of the dose rate, total dose, and radiation port. Onset of xerostomia may be noted as early as 1 week following the start of radiation (cumulative dose of 10 Gy).[43] The saliva turns thick and ropey as serous function is diminished, but mucous production remains. Patients whose radiation to the ear and neck in cumulative doses of 60 Gy more often develop irreversible xerostomia, with an 80% loss in salivary gland function.[44] Spontaneous recovery is unlikely for patients with xerostomia persisting for 12 months or longer.[45] With lesser doses of radiation, however, inflammation and edema of glandular tissue often spontaneously disappear within a year of the completion of treatment.[44]

In addition to functional changes caused by xerostomia, such as dysphasia and alteration in taste, loss of saliva is also associated with a reduction in oral clearance, diminished salivary immunoglobulin A (IgA) levels, and salivary antibacterial enzymes. Consequently, patients with xerostomia are susceptible to increases in local oral infections including caries, periodontal disease, and candidiasis. Aggressive oral hygiene to reduce the tooth-borne bacterial load is critical to reducing the risk of dental disease.

Radiation-induced caries can be a common problem in patients with xerostomia.[46] Changes in salivary composition, decreases in buffering capacity, and loss of the cleansing action of saliva results in the accumulation of bacteria, increases in local cariogenic flora, and tooth decalcification with consequent caries development.[47,48] Typically, radiation caries presents with lesions at the cervical margins of teeth, which then progresses rapidly. Decalcification (white, chalky enamel) of the incisal edges of the teeth may also be noted. In addition to tooth loss, a major consequence of uncontrolled caries may be abscess formation in patients who are at risk for osteoradionecrosis (ORN).

Four goals should be considered for the prevention and treatment of xerostomia. Preservation of salivary function is critical. Whenever possible, tissue-sparing techniques aimed at minimizing the amount of salivary tissues exposed to direct radiation should be utilized. Whereas bilateral field radiation may result in an 80% reduction of salivary flow, mantle irradiation typically causes only a 30–40% decrease. Parotid sparing using three-dimensional treatment or intensity-modulated radiotherapy techniques offers the greatest chance of glandular repair.[49] Stimulation of salivary flow should start simultaneously with radiotherapy (XRT), as should an anticaries regimen to protect the dentition. Replacement of reduced secretions may be introduced as soon as needed. Stimulation of salivary flow may be accomplished through local or systemic means. Sucrose-free lemon drops or sugarless chewing gum may be used. Cinnamon- or mint-flavored mints or gum should be avoided as they may irritate the mucosa.

Drug therapy may also help to stimulate parotid flow.[50] Of the cholinergic agents, pilocarpine has been best studied and found to stimulate parotid function, but not submandibular or sublingual gland function in patients with Sjögren disease and radiation-induced xerostomia.[51,52] Other agents such as bromhexine, anetholtrithion, bethanechol HCl, potassium iodide, neostigmine, and reserpine have been used for salivary stimulation, but data substantiating their efficacy are scant. In contrast, substantial data exist to support the use of pilocarpine HCl tablets to stimulate salivary flow in patients with radiation-induced xerostomia.[53] In cases in which pilocarpine is used after patients have completed radiation treatment and are symptomatic, at least some residual salivary function must be present, and patients should be cautioned that clinically significant improvements in salivary flow may not be realized for up to 3 months following the initiation of treatment. Alternatively, pilocarpine may be prescribed to start simultaneously with radiation therapy. In either case, the typical dose of 5 mg given three times daily may be titrated depending on the patient's response and manifestation of side effects.

Amifostine, a non-protein, free-radical scavenger has been approved as a cytoprotective agent for salivary glands to prevent radiation-induced xerostomia.[54] The recommended dose for amifostine is 200 mg/m^2 administered once daily as a 3-min infusion, starting 15–30 min prior to standard fraction radiation therapy. The need for intravenous infusion, frequency of dosing, cost, and potential side effects have limited amifostine's adoption. Furthermore, the results of a recent meta-analysis suggest that amifostine's efficacy is tempered among patients receiving radiation regimens in which concomitant chemotherapy is also administered.[55]

Salivary replacement can be accomplished with the use of saliva substitutes or artificial saliva.[56] Most of these materials contain carboxymethylcellulose and may provide transient symptomatic relief of mucosal dryness. Saliva substitutes are available as over-the-counter rinses or sprays and are most effective if used before meals and at bedtime. A number of toothpastes and chewing gums have been developed specifically for use in patients with xerostomia. Promising new regenerative approaches to restore salivary gland function have recently been reported, but are still limited to pre-clinical studies.[57]

The most effective protective strategy for radiation-induced caries is the aggressive use of topical fluorides.[58] Topical fluoride supplements should be initiated at the start of radiation treatment. Continuation of fluoride following the completion of radiotherapy is critical, especially in patients who develop xerostomia. Fluorides for dental use come in three forms: rinses, gels applied by tooth brushing or in customized trays, and drops also used in trays molded to fit over patients' teeth. Patients in whom xerostomia is anticipated should have fluoride trays fabricated prior to the initiation of radiotherapy. Fluoride gel or drops are placed in the trays and applied by the patient each day. Use of tray-borne application can be supplemented with acidulated fluoride rinses; generally, the use of rinses in the morning and trays before sleep is most effective and easiest for patients. Acidulated fluorides tend to work best, although neutral fluoride rinses are available for patients with mucositis in whom acidulated material might be irritating, or for patients with porcelain prostheses in whom pitting of the restorations might occur. The supplemental use of a remineralizing toothpaste should also be considered.[59] Aggressive oral hygiene is to be encouraged, and patients should be seen by a dentist frequently. Regular dental visits are critical to insure early detection and intervention of caries and periodontal disease.

For patients who cannot tolerate trays because of gagging or mucositis, fluoride gels may be applied with a toothbrush, either as 1.1% sodium fluoride or as 0.4% stannous fluoride. The latter appears to be more efficacious. Patients should be instructed to avoid sucrose.

Loss of taste is a transient, but bothersome sequelae of head and neck radiation.[60] The severity of taste loss increases rapidly up to doses of 30 Gy, but then usually plateaus. Patients who receive doses of 30 Gy or more may lose their ability to distinguish salt or sweet tastes. Fortunately, hypogeusia is typically transient and taste begins to return within 1–2 months after the completion of treatment. Total recovery may take up to a year. If there does not seem to be progression to improvement following radiotherapy, candidiasis should be ruled out.

Osteoradionecrosis

Of all of the oral complications of head and neck radiation, one of the most significant is ORN.[61] First described in 1927, ORN results in the denudation of soft tissue and exposure and necrosis of bone.[62,63] Although not limited to the jaws, it frequently occurs at this site. ORN causes a painful, chronic, open, and foul-smelling wound that is typically of great distress to the patient. Most cases ultimately heal with conservative treatment, but the course is usually prolonged. ORN was attributed to a triad of trauma (often tooth extractions), radiation, and infection.[64] Subsequent studies suggest, however, that ORN represents a defect in wound healing rather than a true osteomyelitis.[65] The etiology appears to relate to diminished vascularization as a consequence of XRT.[66] Histologic changes of thickened arterial and arteriolar walls substantiate this hypothesis. The finding of cultivable and non-cultivable bacteria may suggest an infectious component.[67]

No consensus exists concerning the overall frequency of ORN. Reported ranges vary between 4% and 44%. While approximately 15% appears to be the preponderant value, a recent meta-analysis reported that only 2% of HNC patients are at risk.[61,65] The mandible is involved more often than the maxilla, which probably reflects the difference in blood supply and vascularity of the two bones. Time until onset of ORN following XRT is variable. Some authors have described ORN as early as 2 weeks after XRT, others report it as a late condition. Most cases occur within the first 3 years after XRT (74%). Equally controversial is the rate at which ORN risk diminishes with time after the completion of XRT, although it seems clear that the risk never reaches zero.[68]

A number of risk factors for ORN have been positively identified.[69,70] Men have been reported to have a risk for ORN that is threefold higher than women.[63] Patients who are edentulous are twice as likely as patients with teeth to develop ORN. Furthermore, the frequency of ORN increases dramatically in individuals with active dental disease (e.g., periodontal disease, caries, periapical disease, poorly fitting prostheses).[61] Fifty percent of cases appear to be associated with tooth extraction following radiation. These findings strongly support pre-XRT dental evaluation and aggressive repair and removal of diseased teeth. The field size, dose rate, and total dose of XRT have a marked effect on the frequency of ORN. Patients who receive cumulative doses of 65 Gy or more to the mandible or maxilla are more likely to develop ORN than are patients receiving lesser doses. Use of three-dimensional radiation techniques has resulted in a slight reduction in ORN risk.[71] Patients with tumors that are adjacent or contiguous with bone are also at higher ORN risk. It is likely that this finding is due to the inclusion of bone in the radiated field since the volume of bone exposed to XRT has a direct impact on ORN risk. Poor nutrition and immune status also appear to predispose to the condition. Diagnosis of ORN is usually based on clinical findings. In cases in which the diagnosis is questionable, magnetic resonance imaging may be of value.[72]

Treatment of ORN is based on the severity and chronicity of the condition.[73] Fortunately, most lesions (up to 60%) eventually heal in approximately 6 months with conservative therapy consisting of local debridement, saliva irrigation, and oral antibiotics.[74] Results of studies in which pentoxifylline, used for its anti-TNF activity, was assessed are inconsistent.[75,76]

Lesions showing no improvement or demonstrate progression require more aggressive therapy. For these cases, surgical debridement and hyperbaric oxygen (HBO) may be indicated.[77,78] In extensive cases, radical resection of involved bone with immediate microvascular reconstruction has been used successfully in patients who have failed more conservative treatment, including HBO.[79] The use of autologous bone marrow aspirate concentrate coupled with allogeneic dental pulp stem cells with platelet rich plasma was recently reported to be successful in patients refractory to conventional approaches.[80]

Because most cases of intra-oral ORN are associated with dental disease and post-XRT extractions, eliminating potential sites of odontogenic pathology before the start of radiation is the basis for prevention. Teeth with periodontal disease, advanced caries with a risk of impingement on the dental pulp, fracture, or periapical disease should be removed before the initiation of XRT. Teeth adjacent to or involved in potential surgical sites (for tumor resection) also should be extracted. Because of the consequences of ORN, even suspiciously diseased teeth, especially in the XRT area, should be eliminated. The timing of dental extractions in patients being treated with XRT has been the subject of much analysis, discussion, and controversy; however, the consensus is that teeth should be extracted before XRT.[16] Ideally, a minimum 21-day healing period is desirable, although a shorter time may be dictated by circumstances. In either instance, extraction before XRT is much more desirable than extraction after the start of therapy, because a number of studies suggest that post-XRT extractions carry significant risk of ORN, no matter how long after XRT they are performed. In all cases, extraction should be performed as atraumatically as possible, with special care given to the soft tissue, primary closure if possible, and good local postoperative wound management. Perioperative use of antibiotics is also recommended.

Aggressive oral hygiene, use of fluorides, and dental care are important components in preventing the development of dental disease once XRT has started. If dental disease develops after XRT and a tooth is restorable, endodontic therapy is more desirable than extraction. Inevitably, extractions are sometimes required of teeth in radiated fields.[81] The risk of ORN in these cases has been reported to be reasonable (5.6%), even without the use of HBO. The efficacy of HBO in these cases is unresolved. One study found that, among patients having teeth removed within the first year following radiation, 98.5% of extraction sites treated pre- and postoperatively with HBO healed without complications. However, the efficacy of HBO reportedly decreased the farther out from where radiation extractions were performed.[82] The utility of HBO, with its incurred cost and multiple visits, warrants additional study.[83,84]

Oral complications of chemotherapy
Oral complications of cancer chemotherapy result from the effects of the drug acting on the oral mucosa (direct or primary stomatotoxicity), the patients' inability to contain local, minor oral disease during myelosuppression (indirect or secondary stomatotoxicity), or some combination of the two.

Risk factors
Not all patients who undergo cancer chemotherapy are at equal risk to develop oral complications. This is especially true of oral mucositis. Although a number of variables have been identified that bear on the frequency and severity of oral problems, their predictive value, in general, has yet to be definitely defined. Risk factors can be divided into those that are associated with the patient and those that are related to the treatment regimen.[85]

Patient-related risk factors include tumor diagnosis, patient age, gender, body mass, genetics, the patient's oral condition before cancer therapy, the level of oral care during therapy, baseline xerostomia, and baseline neutrophil numbers. Patients with hematologic malignancies (i.e., leukemia and lymphoma) are at greater risk of oral complications than are patients with non-head and neck solid tumors. For example, more than 66% of patients with leukemia and 33% of patients with non-Hodgkin lymphoma develop oral problems. It seems likely that tumor-related myelosuppression is at least partly the basis for this observation.[86] Almost all patients with tumors of the head and neck who receive local therapy develop problems after treatment.

The role of age as a risk factor for mucositis is unclear as there are few studies that compare the rate of mucositis among patients of varying ages with similar diagnoses. Among children, nadir of the neutrophil count, lower body weight, and higher peak creatinine levels have been observed to be associated with higher rates of mucositis.[87] Among adult patients with solid tumors being treated with 5-fluorouracil (5-FU), mucositis appears to be more severe and persistent among older persons.

An individual's sex may affect risk, given reports suggesting that women are more likely to have toxicities associated with 5-FU than men.[88] This trend was also reported in patients receiving high-dose chemotherapy (BCNU, etoposide, ara-C, and melphalan [BEAM]) or high-dose melphalan followed by autologous HSCT.[89] A mechanism to explain this phenomenon has yet to be determined. Genetics may affect mucositis risk in at least two ways.[90] Patients with genetic defects, which affect drug metabolism, are at increased risk for mucositis.[91,92] For example, among a population of patients being treated with methotrexate for chronic myelogenous leukemia, increased toxicity (including mucositis) was observed in those individuals with lower methylenetetrahydrofolate reductase activity (TT genotype). Similarly, deficiencies in dihydropyrimidine dehydrogenase (DPD) predispose to toxicities mediated by 5-FU. Alternatively, genetics may affect and regulate the mechanisms, which provide the biological basis for chemotherapy-induced mucosal injury. For example, proinflammatory cytokine production varies among the population and is genetically controlled. These cytokines play a role and track closely with non-hematologic toxicities. Consequently, patients who are predisposed to be high producers of these proteins may also be at increased risk for mucositis and other toxicities. For example, among a cohort of allogeneic HSCT recipients, specific tumor necrosis factor polymorphisms conferred a relative risk (RR) of severe toxicities in excess of 17-fold.[93] The results of a recently reported study in a pediatric cohort being treated for a variety of malignancies suggest an association between ABO blood type. The RR of oropharyngeal mucositis was 2.86 among patients with type O compared to 0.47 for type A and 0.59 for type B.[94] Further study is needed to fully elucidate the impact of functional genes on mucosal injury, but it promises to be important in determining both risk and predicting responsiveness to mechanism-based interventions.[95] It is generally agreed that patients whose pretreatment oral condition is poor are at greater risk for some, but not all, oral complications.[96] Chronic irritation for poorly fitting prostheses or faulty restorations predisposes patients to the development of ulcerative mucositis. Patients with advanced periodontal disease, pulpal disease, or low-grade soft-tissue infections such as those associated with partially erupted third molars (wisdom teeth) are at increased risk for developing sepsis of oral origin once they become myelosuppressed. However, elevated risks of infection are not associated with asymptomatic radiographically demonstrable periapical lesions in endodontically treated teeth.[97]

The level of oral care during therapy has a marked influence on outcome relative to oral complications and infection.[98] The ability of the patients and their healthcare providers to reduce the load of oral bacterial flora favorably affects the risk of both local and systemic infection.[99] Aggressive techniques of oral hygiene, including mechanical debridement of the teeth and soft tissue, and antimicrobial rinses are effective.

Xerostomia prior to and during chemotherapy maybe associated with an increased risk of mucositis.[100] It has been suggested that alterations in the health of desiccated oral mucosa and an overall increase in the resident oral micro-flora may contribute to increasing the probability of mucositis. Studies evaluating treatment strategies aimed at replenishing saliva or mouth moisture have had very mixed results. The favorable effect of pilocarpine on chemotherapy-induced mucositis reported in 1 study was not replicated in a similar trial[100] or among recipients of autologous HSCT.[101]

The extent of mucositis correlates negatively with neutropenia. Baseline neutrophil counts of less than 4000 are associated with higher rates of mucositis.[102] This finding may explain, in part, the observation of increased rates of mucositis among patients with hematologic malignancies.

Risk of complications also relates to the form, schedule, and dose of chemotherapy used.[21] Concomitant radiation, including total body irradiation (TBI), also enhance the risk of oral problems. For example, the incidence of mucositis has been reported to be markedly lower in reduced intensity stem cell transplant recipients (30.9%) compared to patients who received conventional conditioning regimens (90.2%).[102] Significant differences exist in the degree of stomatotoxicity of drugs used for chemotherapy.[21] Drugs or regimens containing anthracyclines, taxanes, platinum, and 5-FU are consistently stomatotoxic. Conditioning regimens in which TBI is used also cause mucositis at high rates. There are 17 specific drugs or combinations in which oral mucositis rates (grade 3–4) affect a significant percentage of patients (>25%). (Table 2):

In considering these drugs or combinations, it is important to remember that the incidence of oral complications, particularly mucositis, tends to be vastly underreported in terms of occurrence and severity. Virtually every chemotherapeutic agent in the current armamentarium has the potential to produce a stomatotoxic response in at least some portion of the treated population.

Repetitive, low-dose regimens tend to be less toxic than do bolus doses of the same agent. Toxicity that is secondary to radiation is dependent on cumulative dose; pulsed application of therapy does not significantly reduce stomatic changes.

Ulcerative mucositis usually occurs 5–8 days following the administration of chemotherapy and lasts approximately 7–14 days. Lesions heal spontaneously and without scar formation. Chemotherapy-induced mucositis is confined to the movable oral mucosa: the mucosa of the cheeks, lateral and ventral tongue, inner aspects of the lips, floor of the mouth, and soft palate. Unlike radiation-induced mucositis, that produced by chemotherapy does not affect the hard palate or gingiva. The dorsal surface of the tongue is also not affected. This observation is likely to be attributable to the differences in the character of the epithelium on each mucosal surface. Of the sites in the mouth, the buccal mucosa (cheeks), lateral and ventral surfaces of the tongue, and the floor of the mouth are the most commonly involved. In patients who receive multiple cycles of chemotherapy, lesions tend to reappear in the same sites. Numerous studies have confirmed that mucositis is not of infectious (particularly viral) origin.

The biologic mechanisms, which underlie chemotherapy-induced mucositis, are currently the topic of intense investigation.[22,103] As noted above, mucositis was viewed as the result of nonspecific toxicity of chemotherapy directed against the rapidly dividing cells of the oral basal epithelium. Although data exist to support the hypothesis, the observation that agents could alter the course of mucositis with little or no epithelial activity suggests a more broadly-based pathogenesis. It appears that mucositis represents a clinical outcome due to a complex interaction of local tissue toxicity (endothelium, connective tissue, and epithelium), the level of myelosuppression, and the local environment. Disruption of connective tissue and endothelial cells initiated by free radical formation likely leads to the activation of a range of transcription factors and increased expression of a number of genes that results in stimulation of proinflammatory cytokine production and tissue damage. Simultaneous activation of other signaling pathways and enzyme activation results in increases in ceramide, proteolytic enzymes, and other mediators of direct and indirect epithelial injury. Thus, in addition to clonogenic death of basal cells caused by direct deoxyribonucleic acid (DNA) injury, secondary pathways produce a barrage of mechanisms that lead to apoptosis or necrosis. Therefore, the epithelium first becomes atrophic, as its renewal ceases, and then eventually completely breaks down to form an ulcer. It is noteworthy that in some patients, the extent of cumulative injury to the basal epithelium does not reach the threshold needed for ulceration to occur. In these patients, the thinned mucosa is mildly to moderately symptomatic (grade 1 mucositis). In cases when ulceration does occur, secondary colonization by oral bacteria (both gram positives and gram negatives) occurs. Cell wall products from these bacteria make their way into the underlying connective tissue where they effectively stimulate additional proinflammatory cytokine production by infiltrating macrophages.

The better understanding of the pathobiology of mucositis has served as the basis for the development of mechanistically based interventions.[41] The first of these agents to gain approval was palifermin (keratinocyte growth factor-1, Kepivance©, Amgen) for the prevention and treatment of oral mucositis in patients receiving conditioning regimens in preparation for HSCT to treat

Table 2 Drugs or combinations associated with significant percentages of patients demonstrating grade 3–4 mucositis.

- Docetaxel/5-FU
- Docetaxel + XRT
- Paclitaxel + XRT
- Docetaxel + 5-FU
- Paclitaxel/5-FU + XRT
- Docetaxel/platinum + XRT
- Paclitaxel/platinum + XRT
- Docetaxel/platinum/5-FU
- Paclitaxel/platinum/5-FU
- Oxaliplatin + XRT
- Platinum/taxane + XRT
- Platinum/methotrexate/leucovorin
- 5-FU/platinum
- 5-FU/leucovorin/taxane
- Irinotecan/5-FU CI + XRT
- Ara-C/idarubicin/fludarabine
- Methotrexate
- Isofamide/etoposide
- Melphalan

hematologic malignancies. In a phase 3 trial in 212 HSCT recipients receiving a stomatotoxic conditioning regimen, palifermin, administered in multiple doses prior to and after transplantation was successful in significantly reducing the duration, incidence, and severity of oral mucositis, favorably affecting patient-reported quality of life outcomes, and in reducing days of opioid use and fever.[104] It seems likely that palifermin's effect was the consequence, not only of its ability to stimulate epithelial proliferation, but also because of its cytoprotective activities mediated through increased expression of mediating transcription factors. Of the 450,000 patients who develop mucositis each year in the United States, the HSCT population comprises only 5%. Consequently, extension of these and other agents to other tumor populations is a major objective.

LLLT (helium–neon) has demonstrated efficacy in reducing the severity and symptoms associated with oral mucositis.[105,106] While additional studies are needed to confirm its value, the cost and logistics of LLLT may limit its overall utility. As more is learned about the ability of photobiomodulation to impact a wide range of cellular and molecular pathways known to be associated with tumor progression and growth mandates studies demonstrating its lack of activity relative to impacting tumor response.[107]

A number of cytoprotective strategies and agents have been suggested as mucositis interventions. Oral cryotherapy is inexpensive and without risk, its use for 30 min starting 5 min before the infusion of bolus 5-FU, edatrexate, or melphalan may be helpful in reducing the severity of mucositis.[26] Pentoxifylline has been evaluated in a number of studies with mixed results. The topical application of trefoil factor was reportedly beneficial in mitigating mucositis in patients with colorectal and HNCs.[39,108] The development of biologics, gene transfers, and other therapies targeting specific biological pathways is also under investigation.[39]

Because the presence of oral micro-organisms is thought to adversely affect the course of mucositis, antimicrobial therapy has been studied extensively as an approach to intervention.[36] In general, the weight of data suggests that reduction of the oral bacterial load through medication does not bear significantly on the incidence or severity of mucositis. The use of topical antimicrobials such as chlorhexidine gluconate has consistently failed to improve the frequency or course of mucositis in randomized, blinded trials.[109,110]

Palliation has been the most widely used approach for the management of mucositis. Saline 0.9% has been used for years and is more effective than hydrogen peroxide, and at least as good as "magic mouthwashes."[111] Barrier type palliatives such as sucralfate suspension and Gelclair are available, although their benefit has not been convincingly shown. Topical lidocaine or Benadryl in Kaopectate or milk of magnesia may offer some topical relief, but often do not eliminate the need for parenteral analgesia.

Effects of targeted therapies

Ulceration associated with mTOR-inhibitor use

Inhibitors of the mTOR have demonstrated encouraging results in clinical trials as an intervention for advanced malignancies. Oral ulceration is among the most significant dose-limiting toxicities associated with these agents and has been reported as mucositis.[112] However, the clinical course, behavior, appearance, and likely pathogenesis mTOR-inhibitor induced oral ulcers strongly suggests that they are profoundly different from mucositis induced by radiation or cytotoxic agents.[113]

Unlike typical chemotherapy-induced mucositis, aphthous lesions present as discrete, ovoid, relatively shallow ulcers, and

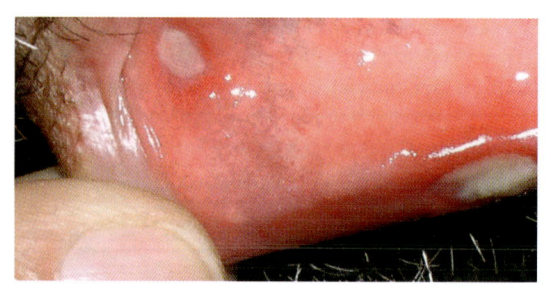

Figure 3 Oral mucosal ulcers associated with the administration of an mTOR inhibitor. Note that the lesions are well-defined and oval with a central area of necrosis and an erythematous periphery reminiscent of aphthous stomatitis.

surrounded by a characteristic erythematous margin (Figure 3).[114] Lesions develop more quickly after drug administration and typically resolve spontaneously after an extremely painful course. Although randomized trials have not yet been performed, treatment approaches similar to those used for major aphthous stomatitis may be effective.

Dysesthesia associated with mTKIs

Multi-targeted tyrosine kinase inhibitors (mTKIs) offer a specifically directed approach to cancer therapy for an increasing number of malignancies. These small molecular inhibitors have been associated with oral discomfort without evidence of physical findings. The term dysesthesia is more precise and descriptive; it is preferred to stomatitis, which is non-specific but was used in previous studies. These dysesthesias can present as mucosal sensitivity, burning, dysgeusia or hypogeusia, xerostomia (with adequate salivary flow), and other altered sensations such as paresthesia and anesthesia. These symptoms can occur in up to 60% of patients on mTKI therapy and can be associated with other side effects of therapy including the development of palmar-plantar erythrodysesthesia.[115]

Calcineurin-induced inflammatory fibrovascular hyperplasia

Calcineurin inhibitors used for immunosuppression can induce inflammatory fibrovascular hyperplasias in the oral cavity. While cyclosporine is associated with a more diffuse, generalized overgrowth of densely fibrous gingival tissue, tacrolimus-induced pyogenic granulomas present as localized fibrous polyps more often seen on the tongue and buccal mucosa.[116]

Oral adverse events associated with immune checkpoint inhibitors

Immune check point inhibitors have been widely used in oncology settings. Oral toxicities associated with immune checkpoint inhibition may present as lichenoid changes, ulcerations, or oral erythema-like lesions. Severe dry mouth has also been reported.[117,118] The median time to oral immuno-related adverse events onset from immunotherapy initiation is approximately 100 days. Concomitant cutaneous, intestinal, and rheumatological immune-related adverse events are common in patients with oral lesions.

Osteonecrosis

Bisphosphonates and the RANK-L inhibitor denosumab have been administered concomitant with chemotherapy as a strategy to reduce metastases to bone. Among patients being treated in this way, osteonecrosis of the jaws, particularly of the mandible (twice as common compared to maxilla) has been reported with increasing frequency.[70] The frequency of the condition has been reported to be between 3% and 8.5%.[119] Newer cases have been reported with angiogenesis inhibitors such as sunitinib and bevacizumab, prompting the nomenclature designation as medication related osteonecrosis of the jaw (MRONJ).[120] The presentation of osteonecrosis in this population varies in symptomatology. Although some patients experience pain, others do not. The majority of cases appear to be associated with dental manipulation, such as extraction, or soft tissue trauma. The mechanism underlying this pathology is yet to be defined, as is a full appreciation of the natural history of the condition. Conservative treatment seems to be most appropriate (Table 3). Presently, the most judicious strategy is to assure aggressive dental screening and treatment prior to the initiation of treatment so that the possible need for dental intervention is minimized.

Infections

Simultaneous with the breakdown of the oral epithelium, the patients' ability to deal with the abundant oral microbial flora is compromised by their myelosuppression. Thus, the mouth becomes an important source of bacteremia and sepsis in the granulocytopenic cancer patient, as well as locoregional secondary infection. These manifestations of indirect stomatotoxicity parallel the bone marrow status; hence, they are maximal at, or just proceeding toward the patient's granulocyte nadir. Systemic invasion of oral viridans streptococci are particularly common. Of these, *Streptococcus mitus* is associated with the most serious sequelae.

Fungal infections

Local oral infections in myelosuppressed patients are attributable to fungal, viral, and bacterial organisms, in order of descending frequency. Candidiasis is the most frequent oral infection and may appear in its characteristic white, curdy form or as erythematous, macular lesions.[121] It most frequently occurs on the palate, tongue, and corners of the mouth. Poorly controlled oral candidiasis increases the risk of aspiration and the development of candidal esophagitis or fungemia. In addition, aspergillosis and mucormycosis are not uncommon in myelosuppressed patients; these lesions can appear as invasive oral ulcerations that are painful and may involve bone.

Since systemic candidiasis is associated with high rates of morbidity and mortality, antifungal prophylaxis may be a reasonable consideration among patients in whom prolonged neutropenia is anticipated, that is, HSCT or stomatotoxic, myeloablative chemotherapy recipients.[122] In general, topical agents are ineffective in this group. Treatment options include fluconazole, caspofungin, and micafungin.[123]

Topical antifungal prophylaxis directed against *Candida* may be beneficial for patients receiving head and neck radiation and promotes xerostomia and in patients who are immunosuppressed with steroids. The polyene antifungal agents (e.g., nystatin) or the imidazole agents, clotrimazole (Mycelex) are equally efficacious. Nystatin is formulated as a thick, cherry-flavored suspension that is not a favorite of chemotherapy-nauseated individuals. Mycelex is dispensed as a troche. For pediatric patients, nystatin popsicles made by putting the drug plus water into an ice cube tray seems to work well. Two other imidazoles also are available: ketoconazole (Nizoral©) and fluconazole (Diflucan©); both have demonstrated efficacy for the prophylaxis and treatment of existing disease. The requirement of an acidic environment for ketoconazole, however, may limit its usefulness in patients who have difficulty eating. Azole resistance may be of relevance in the treatment of fungal infections. Some of the candida species such as *Candida glabriela* and *Candida krusei* are inherently less sensitive to azole antifungal medications.[124]

The efficacy of chlorhexidine gluconate rinses as a topical antifungal agent is unclear.[125] *In vivo* data suggest that chlorhexidine reduces the activity of nystatin.[126] Hence, its simultaneous use with nystatin is not recommended.

While the use of surveillance cultures for predicting the presence or course of fungal infection has long been shown to be of little value, PCR may have a role in the rapid diagnosis and speciation of oral candidal infections.[127]

Viral infections

Herpes simplex virus type (HSV-1) is the most common oral viral infection in patients receiving chemotherapy or head and neck radiation and determination of antibody status is an important part of risk assessment. Oral HSV-1 infection can result from a primary infection with the virus or the reactivation of latent virus in a previously exposed host.[128] It is the latter that is most frequent in patients receiving cancer therapy. Individuals with prior HSV-1 exposure who are seropositive for the virus are at much greater risk than are patients who are negative. The most common manifestation of infection with HSV-1 is oral ulceration. While this may appear to be clinically similar to other forms of mucositis, it usually differs in its course and distribution.

The timing of HSV-1 infection in patients receiving chemotherapy or HSCT typically is quite consistent.[129] Lesions generally are seen approximately 18 days following the start of therapy. This temporal relationship is important in differentiating lesions that likely result from HSV-1 from those that result from direct

Table 3 Staging and management of medication-related osteonecrosis of the jaw.[a]

Stage	Clinical presentation	Management
At risk	No exposed bone	Patient education
0	No clinical evidence of necrotic bone, but non-specific clinical findings, radiographic changes, and symptoms	Systemic management, including the use of pain medication and antibiotics
1	Asymptomatic exposed and necrotic bone, or fistulae that probes to bone with no evidence of infection	Patient education; antibacterial rinses; careful follow-up
2	Exposed and necrotic bone, or fistulae that probes to bone, associated with infection as evidenced by pain and erythema in the region of the exposed bone with or without purulent drainage	Patient education; antibacterial rinses; antibiotics; pain control; superficial debridement of bone to dislodge loose fragments and smooth rough contours; careful follow-up
3	Exposed bone with pain and usually with associated soft tissue inflammation or infection; may see osteolysis extending to the inferior border of mandible or pathologic fracture; may see extraoral fistula	Patient education; antibacterial rinses; antibiotics; pain control; palliative surgery; careful follow-up

[a]Source: Ruggiero et al.[120]

stomatotoxicity, which are noted 5–7 days after the start of treatment, and from secondary surface infection (usually bacterial) that are seen at the patient's maximum myelosuppression (i.e., granulocyte nadir), which occurs around 12–14 days. Lesions can appear on any mucosal surface including the most heavily keratinized tissues of the hard palate and gingiva. Viral culture is the most definitive way to diagnose HSV-1 infection, and aggressive culturing is recommended, especially in patients who are seropositive. Systemic acyclovir remains the treatment of choice for prophylaxis and treatment of HSV infection.[130]

Herpes zoster also may present with oral lesions in patients who receive therapy for cancer.[123] These lesions tend to be crop-like. Although they begin as vesicular lesions, they quickly rupture and form painful, small, ulcerative lesions. Unlike those from HSV-1, these lesions usually are unilateral and linear, often following one of the branches of the fifth cranial nerve.

Bacterial infections
The oral cavity may be a frequent source of local and systemic bacterial infection in the myelosuppressed patient with cancer, as evidenced by the increasing frequency of a-streptococcal infections among patients with granulocytopenic cancer.[123] Bacterial infections may be of soft tissue or gingival or odontogenic origin. Patients receiving cancer therapy often have increased numbers of oral organisms as a consequence of reduced hygiene and xerostomia. Additionally, the composition of the oral flora shifts from one in which gram-positive organisms predominate to one with an abundance of gram-negative pathogens.

Most often, odontogenic infections result from degeneration and infection of the dental pulp subsequent to bacterial invasion secondary to caries. Because of a patient's inability to mount an inflammatory response, conventional signs of dental infection (e.g., abscess formation, swelling) are absent, and patients complain of localized tooth pain. Percussion or thermal sensitivity with clinical and/or radiographic evidence of caries progressing into the pulp is diagnostic. Neurotoxicity may cause dental pain that mimics odontogenic infection in patients receiving plant alkaloids. Odontogenic infections predominantly result from anaerobic species that are similar to those found in dental plaque. Treatment should consist of eliminating the source of infection, and in most cases, this involves tooth extraction. The safety of tooth extraction in the face of myelosuppression has been reported by a number of investigators.[131] These studies indicate that extraction may be performed with antibiotic coverage, platelet transfusion if needed, attention to tissue management, and good closure. Use of hemostatic agents such as Gelfoam in extraction sockets is discouraged, because they may act as foci of infection. Generally, platelet transfusion is not necessary for counts greater than 50,000 cells/mL. Systemic antibiotic coverage is indicated until the wound is epithelialized.

Gingival infections are relatively common in patients receiving myelosuppressive therapy. Some are localized, such as those that are associated with partially erupted third molars (wisdom teeth), whereas others tend to be more diffuse. Acute gingival and periodontal infections are worse in patients with preexisting chronic gingival inflammation or periodontal disease.

The clinical appearance of acute gingival infections, which occur during periods of granulocytopenia, resembles that seen in acute necrotizing ulcerative gingivitis. Pain and loss of the gingival architecture, particularly necrosis of the interdental papillae, are characteristic. These lesions tend to be of a mixed bacterial nature, and include a variety of pathogens, such as *Staphylococcus epidermidis*, *Pseudomonas aeruginosa*, and bacteria typically associated with periodontal disease such as bacteroides and veillonella.

Treatment should include local debridement in addition to systemic antibiotics. Local culture of lesions may more useful than blood culture, because invasion of intact organisms may not occur. Empirical treatment is recommended regardless of culture results.

Mucosal infections in the myelosuppressed patient often are superimposed on ulcerated areas that have broken down as the result of direct stomatotoxicity. Ulcers may appear to be penetrating, with rounded borders and yellowish-white necrotic centers. Because of the lack of an inflammatory response, erythematous borders are usually absent. If the ulcerations are precipitated by trauma, secondary hematoma formation may occur in the patient with thrombocytopenia. Soft-tissue infections tend to be of gram-negative etiology, although HSV-1 must be ruled out. Treatment should include debridement, palliation, and antimicrobial therapy. Bacterial and viral cultures should be performed as well.

Strategies for the prevention of oral infection include eliminating sources of mucosal irritation and reducing the quantity of the local oral flora.[6] In addition, treatment of low-grade, asymptomatic infection before the start of therapy minimizes the risk of acute episodes once myelosuppression occurs. Reduction in the oral flora may be accomplished by mechanical and/or chemical means. Local debridement of the teeth can be accomplished with conventional tooth-brushing; soft brushes should be used. Thrombocytopenia is not a contraindication to mechanical debridement if common sense is used. Brushing should be discontinued in the face of significant bleeding. Alternatively, cotton swabs or a towel-wrapped finger may be used to clean the teeth. Dental floss is an excellent adjuvant for cleaning but may be difficult for patients to use if they are unfamiliar with it. It also may be used until patients become profoundly thrombocytopenic. Essentially, anything that the patient or provider can use to physically wipe debris and microorganisms from the teeth will be beneficial. Cotton swabs, sponges, and rubber tips all may be of use.

Rinses are of varying degrees of help in maintaining oral hygiene. Any fluid that flushes the mouth, including water, will be of some help. Saline and diluted peroxide are frequently used. Generally, mouth rinses containing alcohol as their active agent cause burning of the atrophic mucosa and are not recommended. Mixed results have been reported with chlorhexidine gluconate rinses. If chlorhexidine is used, its administration should be timed to avoid contact with nystatin, because the effects of the latter may be inactivated by chlorhexidine. Similarly, povidone iodine rinses have demonstrated efficacy in reducing the resident oral flora. Other drugs have been tried as preventatives, and fluoride rinses reduce the ability of oral bacteria to adhere to teeth. Consequently, they also may be helpful.

Patients with removable prostheses should be instructed to remove them during periods of myelosuppression. Oral bleeding during such periods most often is of gingival origin. Spontaneous gingival bleeding is a rare occurrence when platelet counts exceed 20,000 cells/mL. Slow oozing may be noted at lower platelet levels, especially in areas with preexisting periodontal disease. Local treatment of gingival bleeding includes initial debridement, nondisturbance of formed clots, and topical application of thrombin under pressure. Gingival bleeding usually is interpreted as evidence that the platelet count is low enough to allow other, more threatening hemorrhage.

Hematoma formation often occurs in areas of trauma, especially the buccal mucosa, alveolar mucosa, or edentulous areas. Areas of submucosal hemorrhage form bluish, blister-like areas, which then form a yellowish-white, tumor-like mass of fibrin.

Epithelialization occurs beneath the mass. If bleeding occurs before healing is complete, topical therapy may include thrombin, microfibrillar collagen, or other hemostatic gel. Before healing is complete, the clot may serve as a focus for microbial growth. It should be checked daily and removed as soon as epithelialization is complete. Unchecked sublingual bleeding may cause respiratory embarrassment by elevating the tongue.

Oral complications associated with HSCT

Mucositis

The risk of mucositis in the HSCT population is largely dependent on the intensity of HSCT conditioning regimen and varies widely to a high incidence of 76%.[131] The inclusion of total-body irradiation also impacts the risk of developing mucositis.[16] As with other forms of chemotherapy-induced mucositis, lesions are localized to the movable oral mucosa and are most frequent in the floor of the mouth, lingual frenum, and labial and buccal mucosae (see Figure 1). There appears to be no significant difference in either the onset of mucositis following transplantation or the duration of mucositis among recipients of autologous or allogeneic HSCT. Woo and colleagues reported a mean time of mucositis onset as 5 days following HSCT for autologous recipients, as compared to 6 days for allogeneic recipients.[132] The mean duration of mucositis for both groups was approximately 6 days, with resolution in 10–12 days. In another study in which autologous HSCT were performed in patients who received cyclophosphamide and TBI, the duration of WHO grade 3/4 mucositis was longer. Mucositis almost always resolves by 3 weeks after transplant, an important diagnostic observation when patients go on to develop GVHD. There is an association between absolute neutrophil count (ANC) and mucositis resolution. Unless patients have extremely severe lesions, mucositis usually spontaneously resolves with an ANC of greater than 500 cells/mL. However, it does not appear that the administration of either granulocyte colony-stimulating factor (GCSF) or GM-CSF prevent or minimize the mucositis development.

The mechanism of mucositis induction is discussed elsewhere in this chapter. It is important to note that the condition occurs independently of oral mucosal infections with either viral or fungal etiology. As noted above, palifermin has recently been approved for the prevention and treatment of oral mucositis in autologous HSCT recipients (see above).

Infection

Oral infection is a major cause of morbidity among HSCT recipients. Of special importance in this patient population is the oral cavity as a source of systemic or distant infection.[133] The incidence of streptococcal infections in HSCT recipients has increased dramatically. Consequently, pretreatment screening to identify and eliminate asymptomatic, dormant, or potential sources of dental infection or irritation should be mandated for HSCT recipients.

In addition to bacterial infections, HSCT recipients are at risk for oral viral and fungal infections during the period of their granulocytopenia. As with other myelosuppressed patients, the clinical presentation of these infections in the BMT population often varies from the classic descriptions typically associated with these lesions. Consequently, early and aggressive culturing is mandated. Members of the herpes group account for most viral infections; herpes simplex, varicella, and herpes zoster are associated with oral infections in HSCT patients. The routine practice of acyclovir prophylaxis, however, generally has been discontinued. In addition, acyclovir resistant mucocutaneous herpes simplex infections have been reported in HSCT populations. Candidiasis is the most common fungal infection, although both mucormycosis and aspergillosis have been reported. Lesions of the deep fungal infections generally present as non-healing gingival ulcerations. Biopsy is the diagnostic method of choice.

Graft-versus-host disease

The mouth is a common site for manifestations of both acute and chronic GVHD.[134,135] Oral features of acute GVHD, include painful extensive erythema and large ulcers of both the non-keratinized and keratinized mucosa; oral lesions have been described and are noted as early as 3 weeks following transplantation and almost 1 week after the onset of skin lesions (Figure 4).[136] Initially, multiple, small, white, papillated lesions present on the movable mucosa. These progress to the development of keratotic, white, lacey lesions that clinically resemble lichen planus and, in fact, have been described as lichenoid in appearance. Desquamative lesions may then develop. These also are similar to the lesions of erosive or bullous lichen planus, and unlike the other two forms, these tend to be symptomatic and require intervention.

The mouth is only second to the skin as a site for manifestations of chronic GVHD. The oral lesions of chronic GVHD appear approximately 3 months or later following transplantation. Approximately 70% of patients with GVHD develop oral lesions, which most typically are lichenoid in appearance. Symptomatic lesions usually present as erosive, vesiculobullous lesions of the oral mucosa, with peripheral areas of keratotic striations. Additionally, xerostomia is a frequent finding among patients with chronic GVHD. Both mucosal and salivary gland changes result from lymphocytic infiltration; the resulting tissue changes are analogous to those seen in other autoimmune changes in the mouth.

Biopsy of the minor salivary glands of the lip appears to be an accurate and sensitive way to confirm the diagnosis of chronic GVHD, and it is more predictive than either biopsy of the buccal mucosa or the parotid gland. Technically, minor salivary gland biopsy is easily performed in an office setting with local anesthesia and a minimum of tissue manipulation. Histologically, one notes acinar atrophy and/or destruction accompanied by a lymphocytic infiltrate that is rich in CD3+ T cells.

Lichenoid lesions generally respond to topical or systemic steroid therapy. Ultraviolet A light therapy reportedly has benefit

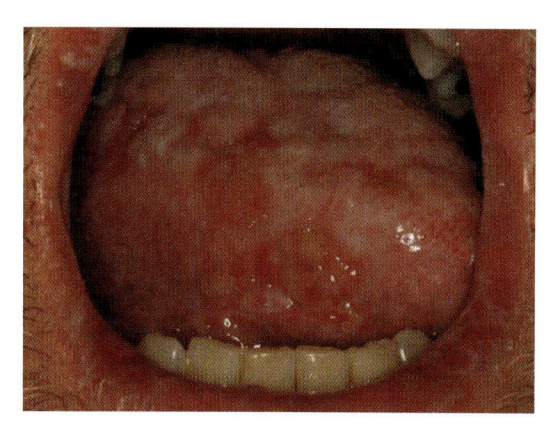

Figure 4 Oral manifestations of graft-versus-host disease characterized by mucosal ulcerations and lichenoid changes. Source: Courtesy of Dr. Nathaniel Treister.

in the treatment of severe, nonresponsive lesions. Therapy for xerostomia was discussed earlier in this chapter. As with other patients having xerostomia, patients with GVHD are at increased risk for caries and should be managed accordingly.

Patients affected by GVHD following HSCT may develop secondary malignancies, with the oral cavity being the second most common affected site. Consequently, patients should receive routine and thorough oral examinations to screen for the development of squamous cell carcinoma and/or dysplasia. Pediatric HSCT has also been reported to be associated with significant long-term oral and craniofacial complications. Early referral and aggressive follow-up care by pediatric dental specialists are recommended.

Key references

The complete reference list can be found on Vital Source version of this title, see inside front cover.

1. Aprile G, Ramoni M, Keefe D, et al. Application of distance matrices to define associations between acute toxicities in colorectal cancer patients receiving chemotherapy. *Cancer*. 2008;**112**:284–292.
2. Epstein JB, Guneri P, Barasch A. Appropriate and necessary oral care for people with cancer: guidance to obtain the right oral and dental care at the right time. *Support Care Cancer*. 2014;**22**:1981–1988.
4. Schuurhuis JM, Stokman MA, Roodenburg JL, et al. Efficacy of routine pre-radiation dental screening and dental follow-up in head and neck oncology patients on intermediate and late radiation effects. A retrospective evaluation. *Radiother Oncol*. 2011;**101**:403–409.
5. Hinchy NV, Jayaprakash V, Rossito RA, et al. Osteonecrosis of the jaw – prevention and treatment strategies for oral health professionals. *Oral Oncol*. 2013;**49**:878–886.
6. Elad S, Raber-Durlacher JE, Brennan MT, et al. Basic oral care for hematology-oncology patients and hematopoietic stem cell transplantation recipients: a position paper from the joint task force for the Multinational Association of Supportive Care in Cancer/International Society of Oral Oncology (MASCC/ISOO) and the European Society for Blood and Marrow Transplantation (EBMT). *Support Care Cancer*. 2015;**23**:223–236.
10. Schuurhuis JM, Stockman MA, Witjes MJ, et al. Evidence supporting pre-radiation elimination of oral foci of infection in head and neck cancer patients to prevent oral sequelae. A sytstematic review. *Oral Oncol*. 2015;**51**:212–220.
11. Mawardi H, Manlove AE, Elting LS, et al. Cost analysis of dental services needed before hematopoietic cell transplantation. *Oral Surg Oral Med Oral Pathol Oral Radiol*. 2014;**117**:59–66.
13. Brennan MT, Woo SB, Lockhart PB. Dental treatment planning and management in the patient who has cancer. *Dent Clin N Am*. 2008;**52**:19–37.
15. Villa A, Akintoye S. Dental management of patients who have undergone oral cancer therapy. *Dent Clin N Am*. 2018;**62**(1):131–142.
22. Jensen SB, Jarvis V, Zadik Y, et al. Systematic review of miscellaneous agents for the management of oral mucositis in cancer patients. *Support Care Cancer*. 2013;**21**:3223–3232.
30. Allison RR, Ambrad AA, Arshoun Y, et al. Multi-institutional, randomized, double-blind, placebo-controlled trial to assess the efficacy of a mucoadhesive hydrogel (MuGard) in mitigating oral mucositis symptoms in patients being treated with chemoradiation therapy for cancers of the head and neck. *Cancer*. 2014;**20**:1433–1440.
35. Donnelly JP, Bellm LA, Epstein JB, et al. Antimicrobial therapy to prevent or treat oral mucositis. *Lancet Infect Dis*. 2003;**3**:405.
37. Stokman MA, Spijkervet FK, Burlage FR, et al. Oral mucositis and selective elimination of oral flora in head and neck cancer patients during radiotherapy: a double-blind clinical trial. *Br J Cancer*. 2003;**88**:1012–1018.
39. Yuan A, Sonis S. Emerging therapies for the prevention and treatment of oral mucositis. *Expert Opin Emerg Drugs*. 2014;**19**:343–351.
40. Villa A, Sonis S. An update on pharmacotherapies in active development for the management of cancer regimen-associated oral mucositis. *Expert Opin Pharmacother*. 2020;**21**(5):541–548.
50. Vissink A, Burlage FR, Spijkervet FKL, et al. Prevention and treatment of the consequences of head and neck radiotherapy. *Crit Rev Oral Biol Med*. 2003;**14**:213.
51. Taylor SE. Efficacy and economic evaluation of pilocarpine in treating radiation-induced xerostomia. *Expert Opin Pharmacother*. 2003;**4**:1489.
56. Villa A, Connell CL, Abati S. Diagnosis and management of xerostomia and hyposalivation. *Ther Clin Risk Manag*. 2015;**11**:45–51.
61. Reuther T, Schuster T, Mende U, Kubler A. Osteoradionecrosis of the jaws as a side effect of radiotherapy of head and neck tumour patients—a report of a thirty year retrospective review. *Int J Oral Maxillofac Surg*. 2003;**32**:289–295.
67. Aas JA, Reime L, Pedersen K, et al. Osteoradionecrosis contains a wide variety of cultivable and non-cultivable bacteria. *J Oral Microbiol*. 2010;**10**:3402.
68. Epstein J, van der Meij E, McKenzie W, et al. Postradiation osteonecrosis of the mandible: a long-term follow-up study. *Oral Surg Oral Med Oral Pathol Oral Radiol Endod*. 1997;**83**:657.
120. Ruggiero SL, Dodson TB, Fantasia J, et al. American Association of Oral and Maxillofacial Surgeons position paper on medication-related osteonecrosis of the jaw – 2014 update. *J Oral Maxillofac Surg*. 2014;**72**:1938–1956.
121. Worthington HV, Clarkson JE, Eden OB. Interventions for treatment of oral candidiasis for patients with cancer receiving treatment. *Cochrane Database Syst Rev*. 2007;**18**:CDO01972.
123. Lerman MA, Laudenbach J, Marty FM, et al. Management of oral infections in cancer patients. *Dent Clin N Am*. 2008;**52**:129–153.
133. Herbers AHE, de Haan AFJ, van der Velden WJFM, et al. Mucositis not neutropenia determines bacteremia among hematopoietic stem cell transplant recipients. *Tanspl Infect Dis*. 2014;**16**:279–285.
135. Kuten-Shorrer M, Woo SB, Treister NS. Oral graft-versus-host disease. *Dent Clin N Am*. 2014;**58**:351–368.
136. Ion D, Stevenson K, Woo SB, et al. Characterization of oral involvement in acute graft-versus-host disease. *Biol Blood Marrow Transplant*. 2014;**20**(11):1717–1721.

134 Gonadal complications

Robert W. Lentz, MD ■ Catherine E. Klein, MD

> **Overview**
>
> Anticancer therapies often cause alterations in gonadal function for both men and women, which can cause infertility. This chapter reviews the assessment of gonadal function in men and women, effects of specific anticancer therapies on gonadal function (including cytotoxic chemotherapy, targeted agents, and radiation), and pregnancy implications of select anticancer therapies. Protective measures for fertility preservation are discussed in detail, including standard of care modalities (sperm cryopreservation in men and embryo or oocyte cryopreservation in women) and experimental techniques.

Gonadal complications of anticancer therapies are common. Women face symptoms of premature ovarian failure (POF), including menopause, sterility, accelerated osteoporosis, and possibly early heart disease. As a group, women who undergo treatment for cancer of any type, compared to the general population, have a 38% lower chance of pregnancy.[1] Men experience oligo-azoospermia and subclinical Leydig cell dysfunction, leading to infertility and long-term effects of "andropause," including decreased bone density, decreased lean muscle mass, decreased libido, and increased risk of coronary artery disease. With recognition has come better documentation of the frequency and severity of these complications, more effective patient counseling, and innovative approaches to attenuate gonadal toxicity. However, several studies have shown that only about half of female cancer survivors recall discussing fertility implications of treatment; this percentage is higher in men (80%).[2,3]

Options for fertility preservation include hormonal manipulation, tissue or cell cryopreservation, surgical interventions, and various experimental methods, but these choices must be offered pretherapy, take time to arrange, and often patients remain uninformed of potential loss of fertility or preventive options. As cancer therapies improve and the number of cancer survivors increases, the practicing oncologist must address these issues in a timely and sensitive manner.

Historical background

The impact of radiation on gonadal function was recognized nearly a century ago. Research published in 1939 demonstrated that 500 cGy to human ovaries was associated with amenorrhea that persisted up to 18 months and all exposed women over the age of 40 became permanently infertile.[4] Atomic Energy Commission studies of healthy men in the 1960s confirmed exquisite sensitivity of spermatogonia to as little as 10 centiGray (cGy) of irradiation.[5] A study in the 1940s showed that 27 out of 30 men who received nitrogen mustard had testicular atrophy and absent spermatogenesis on pathologic evaluation.[6] The first convincing report of menstrual irregularities in women undergoing chemotherapy appeared in 1956, when women treated with busulfan for chronic leukemia developed POF.[7] Gonadal toxicity from other drugs was soon recognized, and the list continues to grow. See Table 1.

Assessment of gonadal function

Assessment in males

Semen analysis has been the cornerstone of assessment of gonadal function in men. Semen volume, sperm concentration, mobility, and morphology are markers of testicular function in adult men. Measurement of gonadotropins (follicle-stimulating hormone, FSH, and luteinizing hormone, LH), anti-Müllerian hormone (AMH), and inhibin-B levels are used in children and prepubertal boys, but fluctuate widely and are not predictive of reproductive outcomes. AMH is produced by Sertoli cells and impacts male sexual differentiation by causing regression of Müllerian ducts. After age 9, AMH levels decline indicating androgen effect on Sertoli cells and early spermatogenesis.[8] In prepubertal boys older than 9 years, inhibin-B and basal testosterone levels assume more relevance. Low or normal testosterone levels and elevated LH levels are seen commonly in adult survivors of cancer but are also subject to inter-individual variability and lack sensitivity to detect small but meaningful changes in testicular function.[9] Novel biomarkers including sperm messenger RNA, micro-RNAs, histone modifications, and DNA methylation patterns are under development. Genetic testing of sperm using fluorescent *in situ* hybridization (FISH) and DNA fragmentation identify chromosomal aneuploidy in the sex chromosomes and assess the extent of DNA damage after gonadotoxic therapy. The future impact of these measurements is potentially intriguing. Leydig cells are more resistant to the effects of chemotherapy than germ cells, thus childhood survivors of cancer may have normal testosterone despite being azoospermic.[10]

Assessment in females

Oocyte numbers are fixed at birth and are not replenished.[11] Advancing age and antineoplastic therapy quantitatively and qualitatively decrease this pool and adversely affect fertility. Assessing ovarian reserve prior to fertility preservation is important, especially in women over 35.

Measurement of FSH, inhibin B, clomiphene citrate challenge test, antral follicular count (AFC), and AMH assess ovarian reserve

Table 1 Probability of decreased gonadal function associated with commonly used antineoplastic agents.

Frequency	Men	Women
Common	Cyclophosphamide	Busulfan
	Nitrogen mustard	Cyclophosphamide
	Nitrosoureas	Melphalan
	Procarbazine	Nitrogen mustard
		Nitrosoureas
		Procarbazine
		Thalidomide
Possible	Carboplatin	Actinomycin D
	Cisplatin	Bevacizumab
	Corticosteroids	Chlorambucil
	Crizotinib	Cisplatin
	Cytosine arabinoside	Cytosine arabinoside
	Etoposide	Docetaxel
	Everolimus	Etoposide
	Hydroxyurea	Everolimus
	Ifosfamide	Hydroxyurea
	Imatinib	Imatinib
	Interferon	Interferon
	Sirolimus	Paclitaxel
	Thioguanine	Sirolimus
	Vinblastine	Tamoxifen
		Thioguanine
		Vinblastine
Rare	5-Fluorouracil	5-Fluorouracil
	Azathioprine	Bleomycin
	Bleomycin	Dacarbazine
	Doxorubicin	Doxorubicin
	Ipilimumab[a]	Ipilimumab[a]
	Methotrexate	Methotrexate
	Nivolumab[a]	Nivolumab[a]
	Pembrolizumab[a]	Pembrolizumab[a]
	Trastuzumab	Trastuzumab
	Vincristine	Vincristine
Inadequate information	Afatinib	Afatinib
	Alemtuzumab	Alemtuzumab
	Bevacizumab	Bevacizumab
	Binimetinib	Binimetinib
	Bosutinib	Bosutinib
	Cetuximab	Cetuximab
	Cobimetinib	Cobimetinib
	Dabrafenib	Crizotinib
	Dasatinib	Dabrafenib
	Docetaxel	Dasatinib
	Encorafenib	Encorafenib
	Entrectinib	Entrectinib
	Erlotinib	Erlotinib
	Gefitinib	Gefitinib
	Gemcitabine	Gemcitabine
	Interleukin	Ifosfamide
	Navelbine	Imatinib
	Nilotinib	Navelbine
	Osimertinib	Nilotinib
	Paclitaxel	Osimertinib
	Panitumumab	Panitumumab
	Pemetrexed	Pemetrexed
	Ponatinib	Ponatinib
	Rituximab	Rituximab
	Sorafenib	Sorafenib
	Sunitinib	Sunitinib
	Trametinib	Trametinib
	Vemurafenib	Vemurafenib

[a] Via hypophysitis.

and predict the oocyte yield with assisted reproduction. Elevated FSH (>20 mIU/mL) in the early follicular phase of the menstrual cycle indicates impaired ovarian reserve and predicts failure of assisted conception.[12] However, the FSH level varies during the menstrual cycle, and neither FSH nor inhibin-B levels are reliable in prepubertal girls. The AFC can be quantified by transvaginal ultrasound to assess ovarian reserve but is not useful in determining oocyte quality or predicting pregnancy outcomes with IVF.[13]

The granulosa cells of ovarian antral follicles produce AMH, and serum levels are a surrogate for the number of developing ovarian follicles. AMH levels decline towards menopause. Unlike FSH and inhibin-B, serum AMH levels do not fluctuate through the menstrual cycle and are valid in children.[11]

Low serum AMH levels were first described in women with prior childhood cancer who still had regular menses, indicating low ovarian reserve.[14] Well-conducted studies have found low AMH levels in breast cancer and childhood HD survivors with a clear dose–response relationship between the number of chemotherapy cycles and serum AMH levels.[15,16] Therapy with alkylating agents and pelvic/total-body irradiation often results in low or undetectable AMH levels.[17] Women with low pretreatment AMH levels are more likely to develop amenorrhea after chemotherapy for breast cancer.[18] Nomograms incorporating age and AMH levels have been developed to predict postchemotherapy ovarian recovery in newly diagnosed breast cancer patients and accurately gauge the need for fertility preservation techniques. AMH levels do not predict spontaneous conception of pregnancy or pregnancy outcomes.

Effects of cytotoxic chemotherapy on gonadal function

Effects in boys

The frequency of testicular dysfunction following chemotherapy varies widely, however some reports suggest that prepubertal and pubertal boys (i.e., those with less mature testicles) are more resistant to chemotherapy toxicity. Three major factors determine the extent of testicular damage among prepubertal boys receiving cytotoxic chemotherapy: the drug, the cumulative drug dose, and the pubertal stage. The majority of boys progress normally through puberty without supplemental androgen.[19,20] Testicular volume may be reduced, however, and elevated LH levels indicate some degree of Leydig cell dysfunction.[10]

Years after treatment with single-agent cyclophosphamide, the prevalence of normal adult sperm counts has been reported in small, heterogeneous case series to range between 0% and 100%.[21,22] Oral cyclophosphamide cumulative doses of 0.7–52 g caused gonadal damage in 16% of prepubertal boys; 67% of pubertal boys had evidence of gonadal dysfunction.[23] A meta-analysis of 30 studies comprising 456 patients who received cyclophosphamide for renal disease, HD, or leukemia found that fewer than 10% of prepubertal boys receiving less than 400 mg/kg (total dose) of cyclophosphamide had gonadal dysfunction, whereas 30% of those over 400 mg/kg did.[24] Gonadal dysfunction ranged from 0% to 24% in prepubertal boys but was 68–95% in sexually mature men. A recent analysis of 214 adult male survivors of childhood cancer treated with alkylating agents found the incidence of oligospermia and azoospermia to be 28% and 25%, respectively. Impaired spermatogenesis was unlikely when the cumulative cyclophosphamide equivalent dose (CED) was less than 4000 mg/m^2 CED was associated with a statistically significant increase in the risk per 1000 mg/m^2 for azoospermia and oligospermia.[25] Unfortunately, poorly understood exceptions to these general trends and lack of reliable predictions for any given patient are problematic. Even small doses of alkylating drugs in prepubertal children can cause permanent sterility.

Whether Leydig cell function is affected in pubertal males is less clear. Gynecomastia with elevated FSH and LH has been reported in pubertal boys receiving MOPP treatment.[20] A study of 17 adult survivors of childhood sarcoma demonstrated azoospermia in 58%, oligospermia in another 30%, but normal testosterone in 94%. LH was elevated in 92% (40% of those with normal testosterone levels) suggesting Leydig cell insufficiency.[10] Although levels of LH, FSH, and serum testosterone following chemotherapy in prepubertal boys may be normal, testicular biopsies after combination chemotherapy for acute lymphoblastic leukemia (ALL) or HD commonly show seminiferous tubular damage and interstitial fibrosis.

Effects in men

Single-agent alkylating drugs induce permanent damage to adult seminiferous epithelium. Cyclophosphamide cumulative doses over 9 g result in universal azoospermia; with doses over 18 g that change is irreversible.[26] Multiple studies of HD patients receiving combination chemotherapy with or without procarbazine indicate this drug is uniquely gonadotoxic. In one study of 19 patients treated with COPP chemotherapy (cyclophosphamide, vincristine, procarbazine, and prednisone), all remained oligospermic 11 years after therapy; 7 of 10 treated with COPP without procarbazine had return of spermatogenesis within 3 years.[27,28] Limited data suggest that ifosfamide may cause less irreversible infertility than its similarity to cyclophosphamide might predict.[29,30]

Methotrexate causes minimal long-term reproductive toxicity. That vincristine may be less toxic than vinblastine is inferred from the slightly lower incidence of infertility following MOPP than MVPP (mechlorethamine, vinblastine, procarbazine, and prednisone). Although studies of single-agent daunorubicin are not available, it appears to have minimal long-term effect when used in combination therapy not containing cyclophosphamide. When used with cyclophosphamide, however, daunorubicin appears to potentiate gonadal toxicity. Long-term administration of azathioprine does not seem to affect semen quality.

Most data have been derived from studies of combination chemotherapy and indicate permanent infertility among HD and nonseminomatous testicular cancer survivors. Complicating the interpretation of these studies is the observation that prior to therapy as many as 30% of men with HD and 50% with germ cell tumors are oligospermic; disorders of sperm motility and morphology are more common.[31–33] Multivariate analysis found that elevated erythrocyte sedimentation rate and advanced stage are predictors of pretherapy infertility in patients with HD.[34] Pretreatment FSH levels may provide a prognostic marker for subsequent spermatogenesis in young men with germ cell cancer.[35] MOPP or MOPP-like regimens to treat HD render all men infertile during therapy, and recovery is unlikely (Table 2). In a prospective study of 37 men receiving MVPP, 12 had low sperm counts before treatment, but all were azoospermic after two cycles and remained so for the first 12 posttreatment months.[41] Longer-term follow-up finds only 5–15% ever regain spermatogenesis. Studies comparing MOPP to ABVD (doxorubicin, bleomycin, vinblastine, and dacarbazine) conclude that the latter combination produces less gonadal toxicity.[23,36] For patients with advanced HD, BEACOPP (bleomycin, etoposide, doxorubicin, cyclophosphamide, vincristine, procarbazine, and prednisone) is increasingly employed. The German Hodgkin study group found the incidence of azoospermia was significantly higher among those treated with eight cycles of BEACOPP or four cycles of COPP/ABVD compared to two cycles of COPP/ABVD (93%, 91%, and 56%, respectively).[45] An update of the Stanford V regimen (vinblastine, doxorubicin, vincristine, bleomycin, mustard, etoposide, and prednisone) reported 19 conceptions in 13 male survivors.[44]

Data on outcomes after treatment for non-Hodgkin lymphoma (NHL) are less robust, but evidence suggests that the cyclophosphamide, vinblastine, and prednisone regimen is less toxic than MOPP.[28] A report of 14 men treated with vincristine, doxorubicin, prednisone, etoposide, cyclophosphamide, and bleomycin suggests this may be an effective, relatively nontoxic regimen for NHL.[47] Leukemia therapy appears less toxic,[53] although both allogeneic and autologous stem cell transplant (SCT) increase the likelihood of long-term infertility.

The majority of men presenting with testicular tumors are oligospermic. In 41 patients studied prospectively, Drasga reported that 77% were oligospermic and 17% were azoospermic; only 6% had adequate sperm counts for cryopreservation.[52] Abnormalities of sperm motility are at least as prevalent. Following two months of therapy with PVB (cisplatin, vinblastine, and bleomycin), with or without doxorubicin, 94% of men in Drasga's study were azoospermic. Recovery of spermatogenesis following chemotherapy for testis cancer is common. Most studies show a time-dependent recovery of spermatogenesis, with nearly 50% of patients recovering some sperm production after 2 years (Table 2).[49,50] Recovery seems to be partly related to the cumulative dose of cisplatin. In those who receive over 400 mg/m^2, permanent infertility should be anticipated.

As in boys, Leydig cell function is more resistant and is usually well compensated; despite frequently elevated gonadotropin levels, few men require androgen replacement.[28,37] However, subclinical Leydig dysfunction may have under-recognized sequelae, including excess cardiovascular morbidity, hypercholesterolemia, and obesity.[72]

Effects in prepubertal girls

Chemotherapy can damage multiple parts of the ovary and may exert different effects based on the stage of development. This includes prenatal loss of oogonia, direct loss of, or accelerated maturation of primordial follicles, damage to stroma or blood vessels, and inflammatory effects.[1] The ovarian effects of chemotherapy in prepubertal girls are variable. Most girls treated with procarbazine or nitrosoureas for brain tumors show biochemical evidence of primary ovarian dysfunction, but progress normally through puberty. Ovarian function returns to normal over a period of years, and elevated gonadotropin levels decrease to baseline in most women. Eighty percent of girls treated for ALL also proceed normally through puberty.[65] In a large study of survivors of childhood cancer, the likelihood of premature menopause was 13-fold higher when compared with siblings, with 8% occurring by age 40.[73] This increase was associated with higher doses of alkylating agents, ovarian radiation, and a diagnosis of HD. In Ewing sarcoma survivors, 67% developed POF at a median follow-up of 5.7 years.[74]

Histologically, however, prepubertal ovaries are significantly damaged by cancer chemotherapy. Follicular maturation arrest, stromal fibrosis, and a partially depleted ova population have all been reported following single-agent cyclophosphamide as well as cytosine arabinoside (ara-C)-based antileukemic therapy.

Effects in women

The frequency of amenorrhea and infertility depends on the drug, its total dose, concomitant radiation, and the patient's age when

Table 2 Gonadal effects of combination chemotherapy.[a]

Disease	Regimen	n	Azoospermia/amenorrhea (%)	References
Males				
Hodgkin disease	MOPP (adults)	150	73–95	24, 36–38
	MOPP (pubertal)	18	78	36, 39
	MOPP (boys)	27	14–80	37, 40
	ABVD	13	0	36, 37
	ChlVPP	13	87	39
	MVPP	210	84–100	41, 42
	PACE BOM	12	0	43
	Stanford V	79	<85	40, 44
Non-Hodgkin lymphoma	BEACOPP	15	93%	40, 45, 46
	COPP	7	66–100	
	VAPEC-B	14	14	47
	MACOP-B	15	0	48
Testis cancer	PVB	112	15–28	29, 49–51
	PVB + Dox	36	17–39	50, 52
	PEB	42	12	52
Acute leukemia	Standard dose	48	3–75	53
	High-dose	104	14–32	54, 55
Sarcomas	Dox/MTX (rt)	222	6–90	56
Females				
Ovarian cancer	P + others	66	0–8	57
Breast cancer	L-pam + FU	98	21–72	38, 58, 59
	CMF	549	54–96	60, 61
Hodgkin disease	MOPP (adults)	95	55–71	62, 63
	MOPP (pubertal)	15	7	42, 62
	MVPP	72	36	42
	ABVD	24	0	64
	PACE BOM	15	0	43
	Stanford V	63	<60	40, 44
Acute leukemia	Various	47	15	54, 55, 65
Non-Hodgkin lymphoma	Various	36	44	46, 48, 62
	High-dose	Case reports of pregnancy		66

Abbreviations: ABVD, Adriamycin (doxorubicin), bleomycin, vinblastine, dacarbazine; ChlVPP, chlorambucil, vinblastine, prednisone, procarbazine; CMF, cyclophosphamide, methotrexate, 5-fluorouracil; COPP, cyclophosphamide, vincristine, prednisone, procarbazine; 5-FU, 5-fluorouracil; MACOP-B, methotrexate, doxorubicin (Adriamycin), cyclophosphamide, vincristine (Oncovin), prednisone, bleomycin; MOPP, mechlorethamine, Oncovin (vincristine), prednisone, procarbazine; MVPP, mechlorethamine, vinblastine, prednisone, procarbazine; NOVP, mitoxantrone, vinblastine, vincristine, prednisone; PACE BOM, doxorubicin, cyclophosphamide, etoposide, bleomycin, vincristine, methotrexate, prednisolone; PEB, cisplatin (Platinol), etoposide, bleomycin; L-PAM, L-Phenylalanine mustard; PVB, Platinol (cisplatin), vinblastine, bleomycin; PVB + dox, cisplatin, vinblastine, bleomycin, doxorubicin; VAPEC-B, vincristine, doxorubicin, prednisone, etoposide, cyclophosphamide, bleomycin.
[a]Source: Based on Williams et al.[67]; Bergeron et al.[68]; Suresh et al.[69]; Brochard et al.[70]; Aneman et al.[71]

treated. Clinically, POF presents with vaginal dryness with dyspareunia, endometrial hypoplasia, decreased libido, hot flashes, oligomenorrhea evolving into amenorrhea, and low serum estrogen levels with compensatory elevations of serum FSH and LH levels.[75,76] Single-agent alkylating drugs are those most consistently associated with POF. Cyclophosphamide was one of the first chemotherapeutic agents associated with ovarian dysfunction, but there is limited data in humans.[1] Small series report that 50–75% of women treated with cyclophosphamide develop amenorrhea within a month of starting therapy, although there is a strong age-related susceptibility. In one study, the total dose of cyclophosphamide received before the onset of amenorrhea was 5.2 g for patients over 40 years old, 9.3 g for those 30–39, and 20.4 g for those 20–29. Menses returned in 50% of women under 40.[58] Return of menstrual function was correlated with the dose administered after the cessation of menses. Single-agent treatment with busulfan or chlorambucil is associated with well-documented age- and dose-related ovarian toxicity.[77,78] One autopsy series of acute leukemia patients showed no difference in the number of primary follicles, but secondary follicles were markedly depleted.[79]

Sarcoma patients treated with high-dose methotrexate rarely report amenorrhea and serum gonadotropin levels remain normal during and after therapy.[80] Lower dose methotrexate for gestational trophoblastic tumors appears to exert no significant toxicity, although one survey from England found that menopause occurred on average three years earlier in chemotherapy-treated women.[81] Fluorouracil, daunorubicin, and bleomycin as single agents are also well-tolerated. Few data are available for etoposide, but ovarian dysfunction has been reported among women receiving the drug for gestational tumors.[82]

Tamoxifen appears to exert a mild estrogenic effect associated with decreased gonadotropin levels in both premenopausal and postmenopausal women treated for breast cancer. Menstrual irregularities are common, but the incidence of persistent amenorrhea is unclear.

Most reported outcomes come from studies of multi-agent therapy. The incidence of amenorrhea in women treated with MOPP, MVPP, or COPP ranges from 15% to 80% (Table 2).[28,46,83–85] Two-thirds of women develop amenorrhea during these treatments. A dose–response relationship is unclear. In one study, there appeared to be no difference between three and six cycles of MOPP.[62] Age at the time of treatment, however, is an important variable affecting the incidence and onset of permanent amenorrhea. Sixty to 100% of patients over age 25 develop permanent amenorrhea during therapy. POF occurs with initiation of therapy in 5–30% of women under 25 and in an additional percentage over the following months.[42] Horning has reported 24 conceptions among 19 women treated with the Stanford V regimen.[85] Women receiving methotrexate, doxorubicin, cyclophosphamide, vincristine, prednisone, and bleomycin for aggressive lymphomas appear, in small series, to maintain fertility.[48] Women treated with four cycles of mega-CHOP (high-dose cyclophosphamide with doxorubicin, vincristine, and prednisone) for NHL had recovery of ovarian function.[63] Eight of these patients conceived spontaneously. In a study of women younger than age 40 receiving standard-dose CHOP therapy for NHL, only 2 of 36 women developed POF.[86] Fifty percent of these women conceived in first remission of their disease.

Women receiving cisplatin-containing therapy for germ cell tumors typically become amenorrhoeic during treatment, but over 90% resume menstruation within a few months after completing treatment.[87-90] Among women with breast cancer, who may already have age-related decreased reproductive potential, 80% receiving adjuvant therapy with cyclophosphamide, methotrexate, and 5-fluorouracil (CMF) become menopausal within 10 months of beginning therapy.[60,61] Adjuvant docetaxel with doxorubicin and cyclophosphamide resulted in a 61% rate of amenorrhea in a patient population whose average age was 49.[91]

Effects of radiation therapy on gonadal function

Effects in men

In adults, single 400–600 cGy doses of testicular radiation may produce azoospermia for five years or longer.[5] Previously, 2400 cGy was delivered to the bilateral testes in boys with testicular cancer to prevent relapse. This dose-induced permanent Leydig cell damage, puberty was delayed, testosterone levels were diminished, and gonadotropin levels were increased in most patients.[92]

Berthelsen evaluated men undergoing prophylactic radiotherapy for seminoma and found that two-thirds became azoospermic from scatter doses of 20–130 cGy.[93] Shapiro has documented oligospermia/azoospermia lasting up to 24 months after as little as 27 cGy.[94] Total body irradiation for SCT conditioning is routinely associated with permanent azoospermia. Secondary infertility has been reported in association with radiation administered to the hypothalamus or pituitary in conjunction with chemotherapy for intracranial neoplasms.[95] Adult Leydig cell dysfunction, with elevated LH values, occurs at radiation doses greater than 2000–3000 cGy, and can require hormone replacement. Fractionated radiation appears to produce tubular damage equivalent to that seen with single doses. Most studies have been unable to document an increase in malignancies in the offspring of men who received testicular radiation.[96]

Effects in women

The radiation sensitivity of the human ovary has not been well defined. Small primordial oocytes are considerably more sensitive than large follicles, and ovarian sensitivity to radiation is dose- and age-dependent. In adult women of all ages, single doses of 500 cGy produce menstrual irregularities. For women over 40,600 cGy reliably induces menopause. Women aged 20–30 can tolerate up to 3000 cGy if fractionated over 6 weeks.[97] Uterine radiation in childhood increases risk for nulliparity, spontaneous abortions, and intrauterine growth retardation, so fertility is not assured even if ovarian function is preserved.

Effects of targeted therapies on gonadal function

In the era of molecularly targeted therapy, multiple new drug classes have entered clinical use, but there is a paucity of data regarding their effects on fertility. Most data on fertility complications come from small animal experiments included in drug labels. Furthermore, cytotoxic agents are often used concurrently, and the effect of combination therapy on gonadal function has not been studied.

Effects of kinase inhibitors

BCR-ABL tyrosine kinase inhibitors

Little is known about fertility complications of tyrosine kinase inhibitors (TKIs), with the exception of TKIs used in chronic myeloid leukemia (CML). Imatinib inhibits c-KIT, crucial for Leydig cell function, and platelet-derived growth factor receptor (PDGFR), essential for gonocyte migration. c-KIT and PDGFR are also expressed in oocytes and have important roles in folliculogenesis and female fertility. Oligozoospermia, gynecomastia, and testicular failure have been described in prepubertal boys.[98] Case reports document oligospermia in men, but most men father normal offspring.[99] Men can consider sperm cryopreservation prior to imatinib treatment, but this may not be necessary.

Women treated with imatinib appear to conceive normally but may have an increased risk of congenital malformations. In animal studies, nilotinib did not impair male or female fertility, and dasatinib did not impair male fertility.[100] The effect of dasatinib on female fertility, as well as fertility implications with bosutinib and ponatinib, are unknown. Thus, it is recommended that women discontinue TKI use prior to pregnancy, if possible, after consulting with their hematologist/oncologist and high-risk obstetrician to discuss this possibility and optimal timing.

Vascular endothelial growth factor (VEGF) TKIs

Ovarian follicular growth is dependent on angiogenesis. A study of sunitinib in mice found that ovulation, but not ovarian reserve, was temporarily reduced during treatment.[101] Sorafenib may reversibly reduce sperm count and motility, as noted in a mouse model.[102] There is a paucity of data for the newer VEGF TKIs. Impairment is likely transient, but long-term effects are not known.

Epidermal growth factor receptor (EGFR) TKIs

Erlotinib did not impair fertility in rats.[103] An animal study suggested that gefitinib may impair female fertility.[104] Afatinib may impair both male and female fertility. An animal model showed decreased sperm count but overall fertility was unaffected. Female rats showed a decrease in number of corpora lutea and increase in postimplantation pregnancy loss. It is not known whether these effects are reversible.[105] Osimertinib caused decreased male rat fertility and corpora lutea degeneration in female rats.[106]

BRAF kinase inhibitors and MEK inhibitors

Little is likewise known about the BRAF and MEK inhibitors. In rats, the BRAF kinase inhibitor dabrafenib reduces corpora lutea and causes testicular degeneration.[107] The MEK inhibitors cobimetinib and trametinib cause similar effects as dabrafenib in women.[107] The effect of combination BRAF/MEK inhibition therapy is not known.

Mammalian target of rapamycin (mTOR) kinase inhibitors
Sirolimus and everolimus alter the hypothalamic–pituitary–adrenal axis. The reproductive side effects of mTOR inhibitors are inferred from organ transplant patients. Men treated with sirolimus and everolimus have low testosterone, with elevated FSH and LH, in addition to quantitative and qualitative defects in spermatogenesis; these effects are likely reversible after discontinuation of therapy, but this is debated.[108,109] Women treated with mTOR inhibitors have increased risk of oligo- and amenorrhea.[109]

Effects of monoclonal antibodies and immunotherapy

Alemtuzumab, a monoclonal antibody against CD52, causes immobilization and agglutination of sperm because CD52 is also expressed on the surface of the sperm, theoretically increasing the risk of male infertility.[110] The VEGF inhibitor bevacizumab appears to impair female fertility, while effects on male fertility are unknown. In a study of 179 premenopausal women randomized to adjuvant chemotherapy with or without bevacizumab for the treatment of solid tumors, amenorrhea developed in 34% of women treated with bevacizumab, compared to 2% who did not receive bevacizumab. Recovery of ovarian function occurred in a subset of women.[111] The EGFR inhibitor cetuximab caused oligo- and amenorrhea in monkeys, with no effect on male fertility.[112] The EGFR inhibitor panitumumab caused menstrual cycle irregularities in monkeys, which were reversible on drug discontinuation.[113] The effect of panitumumab on male fertility is unknown. There is no evidence of fertility impairment with trastuzumab.

Immune checkpoint inhibitors (ICI), which target cytotoxic T-lymphocyte-associated antigen 4 (CTLA-4), antiprogrammed cell death-1 receptor (PD-1), and its ligand (PD-L1), can cause hypophysitis. In a pooled analysis, single-agent immunotherapy (independent of the specific agent used) caused hypophysitis in <2% of patients, whereas with combination ipilimumab and nivolumab this occurred in 7.3% of patients.[114] The incidence of direct gonadal toxicity with ICI is not known but thought to be uncommon. Yet, immunotherapeutic agents can disrupt maternal immune tolerance to the fetus, increasing the risk of abortion. This has been demonstrated in animal models, with some showing a three-fold increase in abortion rate; human data is not available.[115,116] Effective contraception is recommended during treatment with immunotherapy and for four months after therapy completion.

Protective measures

Providers should discuss the possibility of infertility with cancer patients (and their parents, if applicable) as early as possible, to allow the widest array of fertility preservation options to be considered. Interested patients should expeditiously be referred to a reproductive expert. Current standard of care includes cryopreservation of sperm, oocytes, and embryos. Additional methods can be considered and are detailed below. Unresolved medical and ethical issues have fueled debate regarding these techniques.[117] See Table 3.

Protection for men

Men anticipating cancer therapy should consider sperm cryopreservation, which is the standard of care for male fertility preservation.[118] Because of the high prevalence of abnormal pretherapy semen analyses, many patients have been considered poor candidates, but successful impregnation has been achieved following artificial insemination using semen with quite low sperm counts and poor sperm motility.[119] If this is unsuccessful, other methods can be used, including in vitro fertilization (followed by implantation) and intracytoplasmic sperm injection (ICSI, in which a single live spermatozoon is injected into an oocyte and produces a 62% live birth rate in patients with cancer).[120,121] Sperm should be collected prior to initiation of treatment, as genetic damage can otherwise occur.

It has long been speculated that halting spermatogenesis through hormonal manipulation during chemotherapy might ameliorate testicular damage, as most chemotherapy agents are selectively toxic to dividing cells. In clinical trials of men receiving chemotherapy for HD, two attempts using gonadotropin-releasing hormone (GnRH) agonists have been unsuccessful.[122,123] The use of GnRH agonists is not recommended by ASCO Guidelines.[118]

Several additional methods remain experimental, including testicular tissue cryopreservation followed by reimplantation and testicular sperm extraction.[118] Testicular sperm extraction is reported to recover spermatozoa in 55–85% of men with nonobstructive azoospermia of various etiologies. In a series of men azoospermic after chemotherapy, spermatozoa were found in 65%. Gonadal shielding remains the mainstay of protection from therapeutic radiation. Penile vibratory stimulation and electro-ejaculation may provide an option for sperm collection in pubertal boys.[124]

Protection for women

Cryopreservation of embryos and unfertilized oocytes remains the standard of care.[118] The former is preferred for women in stable relationships as it minimizes the risk of multiple pregnancy and maximizes the overall rate of pregnancy.[125] Cryopreservation of unfertilized oocytes can be done if the woman does not have a male partner, declines use of a sperm donor, or has objections to the storage of embryos. Ovarian stimulation can now be done independent of the menstrual cycle, decreasing lengthy delays previously required. It currently takes around 10–12 days to complete cryopreservation.[126] Additionally, aromatase-inhibitor-based stimulation protocols can be effectively used in patients for whom estrogen-based protocols could be problematic (i.e. breast or gynecologic malignancies), without an increased risk of malignancy.[118] With cryopreservation of embryos and unfertilized oocytes, the implantation rate is 8–30% and the cumulative pregnancy rate can be more than 60%.[127]

Cryopreservation of ovarian tissue, followed by tissue reimplantation, remains experimental but may soon become a standard of care option.[118] This can be considered in women who require urgent cancer treatment without waiting for ovarian stimulation and in prepubertal girls. Ovarian cortical tissue also has the advantage of containing large numbers of follicles, thereby increasing the potential for successful future pregnancies. Ovarian tissue can ultimately be transplanted back into the patient, thus restoring ongoing fertility.[128] In 114 Belgian women treated for various malignancies who underwent ovarian tissue cryopreservation, a total of 49 spontaneous pregnancies in 33 patients and 2 induced pregnancies were reported after a mean follow-up of 50 months.[129] Pregnancy rates and live-birth rates may be on the order of 30–40% and 20–30%, respectively.[126] This technique may offer an option for young girls as well as sexually mature young women.

Reversible suppression of ovarian function by oral contraceptives or GnRH agonists might offer gonadal protection to cycling women about to undergo potentially sterilizing radiation or chemotherapy. Overall, the available data are conflicting on

Table 3 Options for preservation of fertility in patients with cancer.

	Males	Status	Females	Status
Children	Testicular tissue cryopreservation	Unproven	Ovarian tissue cryopreservation	Unproven
Adults	Sperm cryopreservation	Accepted	Embryo cryopreservation	Accepted
	Testicular tissue cryopreservation	Experimental	Oocyte cryopreservation	Accepted
	Testicular sperm extraction	Experimental	Ovarian tissue cryopreservation	Experimental
	GnRH agonist	Not recommended	Ovarian transposition (oophoropexy)	Experimental
			GnRH analog	Experimental
			OCP suppression	Unproven

Abbreviations: GnRH agonist, gonadotropin-releasing hormone agonist; OCP, oral contraceptives.

this topic. In a meta-analysis of six randomized controlled trials (RCTs) that examined reproductive outcomes among women with HD, ovarian cancer, and breast cancer, administration of GnRH agonists during chemotherapy was associated with a statistically significant increase in resumption of spontaneous menstruation and ovulation (odds ratio 3.46 and 5.70, respectively).[130] However, conflicting results have been obtained in other trials and the numbers of patients and histologies (primarily breast, ovarian, and lymphoma) that have been studied are small. In one study, women receiving MVPP for HD were given oral contraceptives; 5 out of 6 had resumption of normal menses at a mean follow-up of 26 months.[131] In another study, patients ages 15–20 with lymphoma were given leuprolide, starting prior to treatment and ending one month after cessation of chemotherapy.[132] All 12 patients treated with leuprolide resumed normal menstrual cycling within six months, compared to none of the four women who did not receive leuprolide. Three pregnancies were reported. Contrarily, a randomized trial published in 2016 by Demeestere showed that GnRH agonist use during chemotherapy for lymphoma did not prevent POF in 129 women with 5-year follow-up.[133]

The use of hormonal ovarian suppression in breast cancer patients for fertility preservation is controversial and remains experimental but can be considered if proven methods are not recommended. Guidelines from various professional societies draw different conclusions on the topic.[118] Meta-analyses of RCTs exclusively among patients with breast cancer have yielded conflicting results regarding prevention of POF and spontaneous resumption of menses with use of GnRH agonists.[134–136] In support of GnRH agonist use for this indication, a recent meta-analysis published in 2018 by Lambertini and colleagues compared the rates of POF and posttreatment pregnancy in women with early breast cancer who received neoadjuvant or adjuvant chemotherapy with or without a concurrent GnRH agonist. The rate of POF was 14.1% in the GnRH agonist group and 30.9% in the control group; 10.3% of patients in the GnRH agonist group had a pregnancy compared to 5.5% in the control group.[137]

For patients undergoing pelvic radiotherapy, ovarian transposition (oophoropexy) can be considered. At the time of exploratory or staging laparotomy, the ovaries are moved medially and posteriorly to the uterine fundus or laterally out of the radiation port. Radiation exposure is decreased 90%, and hormonal function is preserved in 55–95% of patients. Another option is transposition of only one ovary and removal of the second for cryopreservation.[138] However, fertility can still be compromised, as transposed ovaries may not be protected from radiation scatter or may migrate back into the radiation field. The abnormal tubo-ovarian anatomy may also reduce fertility. Performing ovarian transposition as close to radiation treatment as possible may reduce risk of migration. Ovarian shielding may be useful in some cases.

Various preventive drug-based strategies have been attempted, however, this has almost exclusively been studied in nonhuman models.[1] Tamoxifen is one of the few agents tested in humans as an ovarian-protectant, hypothesized to reduce inflammation and vasoconstriction. However, in a study where patients were treated with CMF, the use of tamoxifen did not affect ovarian function.[139] The Edinburgh selection criteria for identifying patients at risk for POF after gonadotoxic therapy may be useful in selecting patients for intervention.[140]

Protection for children

No proven methods for protection of future fertility in children are available at this time. Some centers offer ovarian tissue or testicular tissue cryopreservation as an experimental approach, but research in this area is fraught with ethical problems. Many excellent reviews of the technical and ethical issues of fertility preservation are available.[141,142]

Outcomes of pregnancy

Systemic therapy

As a whole, chemotherapy use during the first trimester results in congenital malformation in about 20% of cases, with lower risk during the second and third trimesters.[143–146] Guidelines recommend that all premenopausal women and men who are receiving any form of systemic anticancer therapy should use effective contraception during treatment and for 3–6 months after therapy completion.[147] If pregnancy occurs while a woman is receiving systemic anticancer therapy, she should be informed of possible fetal harm, and pregnancy termination can be considered. However, case reports document successful conception and delivery of normal infants to patients who have received even the most aggressive of chemotherapy regimens during pregnancy; neither male nor female permanent infertility, nor fetal anomalies, can be assumed following chemotherapy. Among women who previously received chemotherapy and later conceived after completing chemotherapy, many studies have documented normal fetal development.[148,149] Offspring of fathers previously treated with chemotherapy likewise appear to be normal Further follow-up suggests that offspring growth, development, and school performance are probably normal, however, there may be an excess of cancers diagnosed in male offspring under age 5.[148]

Risk to the fetus exposed in utero to chemotherapy agents depends on gestational age and the drug and dose administered. Folate antagonists should not be administered during the first trimester. Other antimetabolites have rarely been associated with congenital abnormalities. First-trimester exposure to 5-fluorouracil, cyclophosphamide, busulfan, and chlorambucil has been associated with low birth weight in infants and other abnormalities on rare occasion. Fetal myocardial necrosis has been reported following maternal administration of anthracyclines.[150,151]

Whether the risk to the fetus is further increased with drug combinations is uncertain. Case reports and small series indicate that multi-agent treatment in the second and third trimesters is associated with minimal risk to the fetus and that long-term development of these offspring is normal.[152,153] Nonteratogenic effects including low birth weight and intrauterine growth retardation remain to be defined. In utero exposure to diethylstilbestrol has been linked to the development of genital clear cell carcinomas in the female offspring of these women,[154] but other associations of carcinogenesis from in utero exposure to chemotherapy are lacking. No information is available on the reproductive potential of these children.

The degree to which TKIs cross the placenta during the first trimester remains unclear but may carry some risk of fetal harm. Imatinib has demonstrated teratogenicity in animal models, but case reports have documented successful pregnancies in women who conceive during treatment.[155] Dasatinib and nilotinib cause fetal damage in animal models.[100] There is insufficient data regarding gonadal complications of rituximab. The use of rituximab during pregnancy increases the risk of B-cell depletion in the newborn, temporarily reducing newborn immunity. B-cell count in the infants recovered in all reported cases.[156] ESMO guidelines do not discourage the use of rituximab during pregnancy if doing so would significantly impact maternal outcome.[147] Interferon has been given safely during pregnancy for a variety of malignant and nonmalignant diseases in a small number of women.[157,158] Monoclonal antibodies do not cross the placenta early in pregnancy, therefore the risk of fetal malformation is lower.[147] Small human studies suggest that brief first-trimester exposure to trastuzumab does not cause fetal malformation.[147] However, trastuzumab does carry a boxed warning for oligohydramnios and use during pregnancy is not recommended.

Radiation therapy

Most of what is known about adverse effects of in-utero radiation exposure comes from survivors of atomic bomb exposure. In-utero exposure to radiation can result in prenatal death, growth restriction, microcephaly, organ malformation, and intellectual disability.[159] The highest risk of teratogenesis is during the period of organogenesis (from the second to eighth week). Development of childhood cancer following low-level in-utero radiation exposure is very uncommon.[160] The increase in untoward outcomes of pregnancies (major congenital defects, stillbirth, and death during the first week of life) is small, estimated at 0.00182/gonadal rem (roentgen equivalent man)—the quantity of any ionizing radiation equivalent to the biologic effect of 1 rad (1 cGy). Among women treated with radiation therapy below the diaphragm, preterm delivery in up to 20% of pregnancies and an excess of low birth-weight infants have been reported. That these adverse outcomes are often clustered in the first posttreatment year suggests they may result from local uterine or hormonal factors and may not be due to genetic defects.[153] A safe dose has not yet been defined, but generally, a therapeutic abortion is recommended for any uterine dose of 10 cGy during the first trimester. Supradiaphragmatic radiation is associated with considerable scatter to the fetus, much of which can probably be prevented with abdominal shielding. Local radiation of the neck and axilla may be safe during the first trimester.

Psychosocial issues

Infertility and sexual dysfunction can have significant psychosocial impacts on patients treated for cancer. Detailed discussion of these important issues is beyond the scope of this article, but excellent reviews are available for the interested reader seeking further information.[67,161-165]

Key references

The complete reference list can be found on Vital Source version of this title, see inside front cover.

1. Spears N, Lopes F, Stefansdottir A, et al. Ovarian damage from chemotherapy and current approaches to its protection. *Hum Reprod Update*. 2019;**25**(6):673–693.
3. Armuand GM, Rodriguez-Wallberg KA, Wettergren L, et al. Sex differences in fertility-related information received by young adult cancer survivors. *J Clin Oncol*. 2012;**30**(17):2147–2153.
4. Jacox HW. Recovery following human ovum irradiation. *Radiology*. 1939;**32**:538–545.
8. Josso N, Cate RL, Picard JY, et al. Anti-Müllerian hormone: the Jost factor. *Recent Prog Horm Res*. 1993;**48**:1–59.
9. Dere E, Anderson LM, Hwang K, et al. Biomarkers of chemotherapy-induced testicular damage. *Fertil Steril*. 2013;**100**:1192–1202.
11. Dewailly D, Andersen CY, Balen A, et al. The physiology and clinical utility of anti-Müllerian hormone in women. *Hum Reprod Update*. 2014;**20**(3):370–385.
12. Jain T, Soules MR, Collins JA. Comparison of the basal follicle-stimulating hormone versus the clomiphene citrate challenge test for ovarian reserve screening. *Fertil Steril*. 2004;**82**(1):180.
17. Gracia CR, Sammel MD, Freeman E, et al. Impact of cancer therapies on ovarian reserve. *Fertil Steril*. 2012;**97**:134–140 e131.
19. Shalet SM, Hann IM, Lendon M, et al. Testicular function after combination chemotherapy in childhood for acute lymphoblastic leukaemia. *Arch Dis Child*. 1981;**56**:275–278.
20. Whitehead E, Shalet SM, Jones PH, et al. Gonadal function after combination chemotherapy for Hodgkin's disease in childhood. *Arch Dis Child*. 1982;**47**:287–291.
30. Pont J, Albrecht W. Fertility after chemotherapy for testicular germ cell cancer. *Fertil Steril*. 1997;**68**:1–5.
37. Aubier F, Flamant F, Caillaud JM, et al. Male gonadal function after chemotherapy for solid tumors in childhood. *J Clin Oncol*. 1989;**7**:304–309.
42. Waxman JHX, Terry YA, Wrigley PFM, et al. Gonadal function in Hodgkin's disease: long-term follow-up of chemotherapy. *Br Med J*. 1982;**285**:1612–1613.
50. Hansen PV, Trykker H, Helkjaer PE, Andersen J. Testicular function in patients with testicular cancer treated with orchiectomy alone or orchiectomy plus cisplatin-based chemotherapy. *J Natl Cancer Inst*. 1989;**81**:1246–1250.
52. Drasga RE, Einhorn LH, Williams SD, et al. Fertility after chemotherapy for testicular cancer. *J Clin Oncol*. 1983;**1**:179–183.
65. Quigley C, Cowell C, Jimenez M, et al. Normal or early development of puberty despite gonadal damage in children treated for acute lymphocytic leukemia. *N Engl J Med*. 1989;**321**:143–151.
85. Horning SJ, Hoppe RT, Kaplan HS, Rosenberg SA. Female reproductive potential after treatment for Hodgkin's disease. *N Engl J Med*. 1981;**304**:1377–1382.
86. Elis A, Tevet A, Yerushalmi R, et al. Fertility status among women treated for aggressive non-Hodgkin's lymphoma. *Leuk Lymphoma*. 2006;**47**:623–627.
88. Marchetti M, Romagnolo C. Fertility after ovarian cancer treatment. *Eur J Gynaecol Oncol*. 1992;**13**:498–501.
93. Berthelsen JG. Sperm counts and serum follicle-stimulating hormone levels before and after radiotherapy and chemotherapy in men with testicular germ cell cancer. *Fertil Steril*. 1984;**41**:281–286.
96. Hawkins MM. Is there evidence of a therapy-related increase in germ-cell mutation among childhood cancer survivors? *J Natl Cancer Inst*. 1991;**83**:1643–1650.
114. King GT, Sharma P, Davis SL, Jimeno A. Immune and autoimmune-related adverse events associated with immune checkpoint inhibitors in cancer therapy. *Drugs Today (Barc)*. 2018;**54**(2):103–122.
115. Poulet FM, Wolf JJ, Herzyk DJ, DeGeorge JJ. An evaluation of the impact of PD-1 pathway blockade on reproductive safety of therapeutic PD-1 inhibitors. *Birth Defects Res B Dev Reprod Toxicol*. 2016;**107**(2):108–119.
117. Dudzinski JM. Ethical issues in fertility preservation for adolescent cancer survivors: oocyte and ovarian tissue cryopreservation. *J Pediatr Adolesc Gynecol*. 2004;**17**:97–102.

118 Oktay K, Harvey BE, Partridge AH, et al. Fertility preservation in patients with cancer: ASCO Clinical Practice Guideline Update. *J Clin Oncol.* 2018;**36**(19):1994–2001.

121 Garcia A, Herrero M, Holzer H, et al. Assisted reproductive outcomes of male cancer survivors. *J Cancer Surviv.* 2014;**9**(2):208–214.

125 Argyle CE, Harper JC, Davies MC. Oocyte cryopreservation: where are we now? *Hum Reprod Update.* 2016;**22**(4):440–449.

126 Donnez J, Dolmans MM. Fertility preservation in women. *N Engl J Med.* 2017;**377**(17):1657–1665.

127 Donnez J, Dolmans MM, Demylle D, et al. Livebirth after orthotopic transplantation of cryopreserved ovarian tissue. *Lancet.* 2004;**364**:1405–1410.

128 Tulandi T, Al-Shahrani AA. Laparoscopic fertility preservation. *Obstet Gynecol Clin N Am.* 2004;**31**:611–618.

130 Bedaiwy MA, Abou-Setta AM, Desai N, et al. Gonadotropin-releasing hormone analog co-treatment for preservation of ovarian function during gonadotoxic chemotherapy: a systematic review and meta-analysis. *Fertil Steril.* 2011;**95**(3):906–914.

133 Demeestere I, Brice P, Peccatori FA, et al. No evidence for the benefit of gonadotropin-releasing hormone agonist in preserving ovarian function and fertility in lymphoma survivors treated with chemotherapy: final long-term report of a prospective randomized trial. *J Clin Oncol.* 2016;**34**(22):2568–2574.

137 Lambertini M, Moore HCF, Leonard RCF, et al. Gonadotropin-releasing hormone agonists during chemotherapy for preservation of ovarian function and fertility in premenopausal patients with early breast cancer: a systematic review and meta-analysis of individual patient-level data. *J Clin Oncol.* 2018;**36**(19):1981–1990.

138 Martin JR, Kodaman P, Oktay K, Taylor HS. Ovarian cryopreservation with transposition of a contralateral ovary: a combined approach for fertility preservation in women receiving pelvic radiation. *Fertil Steril.* 2007;**87**:189.e5–189.e7.

140 Wallace HB, Smith AB, Kelsey TW, et al. Fertility preservation for girls and young women with cancer: population-based validation of criteria for ovarian tissue cryopreservation. *Lancet Oncol.* 2014;**15**(10):1129–1136.

141 Burns KC, Hoefgen H, Strine A, et al. Fertility preservation options in pediatric and adolescent patients with cancer. *Cancer.* 2018;**124**:1867–1876.

147 Peccatori FA, Azim HA Jr, Orecchia R, et al. Cancer, pregnancy and fertility: ESMO Clinical Practice Guidelines for diagnosis, treatment and follow-up. *Ann Oncol.* 2013;**24**(Suppl 6):vi160–vi170.

148 Mulvihill JJ, Connelly RR, Austin DF, et al. Cancer in offspring of long-term survivors of childhood and adolescent cancer. *Lancet.* 1987;**2**:813–817.

153 Doll DC, Ringenberg S, Yarbro JW. Management of cancer during pregnancy. *Arch Intern Med.* 1988;**148**:2058–2064.

160 McCollough CH, Schueler BA, Atwell TD, et al. Radiation exposure and pregnancy: when should we be concerned? *Radiographics.* 2007;**27**:909–917.

135 Sexual dysfunction

Leslie R. Schover, PhD

Overview

Sexual problems related to cancer are usually caused by physiological damage from treatment but are exacerbated by psychosocial issues such as poor individual coping, relationship conflict, or preexisting sexual dysfunction. Sexual dysfunction affects almost two-thirds of the estimated 17 million cancer survivors in the United States, including well over 50% of those treated for pelvic or breast cancers and at least 25% for other sites. Optimal treatment is multidisciplinary, addressing both physical damage and behavioral skills. If a committed relationship exists, it is best to include the partner in education and intervention.

Box 1

Although recognition of cancer-related sexual problems began in the 1950s, most men and women still do not seek professional help for their dysfunctions and attempts to modify cancer treatment to spare sexual function have been disappointing.

Historical perspective

Sexual dysfunction has been recognized as a morbidity of cancer treatment since the 1950s. Early publications focused on mutilating surgery for breast cancer, impaired body image, and loss of feminine identity.[1] By the 1990s, it became clear that even with breast conservation, many breast cancer survivors experienced sexual problems related to systemic therapy and psychosocial issues.[2] Attention also was given to sexual function in women with gynecological cancers,[3] particularly the effects of premature ovarian failure and pelvic radiotherapy.[4] Sexual dysfunction in women with cancer remains an area in need of more research and clinical focus.[5]

Surgeons introduced nerve-sparing radical pelvic surgery in the 1980s to prevent erectile dysfunction.[6] However, nerve-sparing radical prostatectomy resulted in a return to baseline erectile function in fewer than 25% of men.[7] More recently, robotic-assisted laparoscopic prostatectomy (RALP) claimed to increase the accuracy of nerve-sparing and enhance recovery of normal erections. However, two large studies using Medicare and Surveillance, Epidemiology, and End-Results (SEER) databases found no superiority of minimally invasive or robotic surgery in preserving sexual function.[8,9] Attempts to minimize sexual consequences of pelvic radiotherapy were also disappointing, with high rates of erectile dysfunction in the long-term after brachytherapy,[10] computerized three-dimensional conformal or intensity-modulated radiation fields,[11] or use of proton beams.[12]

In 2017, both the American Society of Clinical Oncology[13] and the National Comprehensive Cancer Network[14] published practice guidelines on identifying, assessing, and treating cancer-related sexual dysfunction. Guidelines agree that a multidisciplinary team effort is needed, since the problems typically have both physiological and psychosocial aspects. Nevertheless, fewer than half of cancer patients recall even a brief mention of sexual issues from their oncology team.[15] Only 25% of adults in the United States seek professional help for their sexual problems.[16]

Incidence and epidemiology—local and worldwide

An overall estimate is that about 60% of men and women surviving cancer treatment end up with long-term sexual dysfunction, with higher incidence for those with breast or pelvic malignancies[17,18] and rates of at least 25–33% even for survivors of childhood cancer or hematologic cancer. Currently, an estimated 10 million out of 17 million survivors in the United States[19] are affected. Since the prevalence and types of cancer are similar in other industrialized nations, the risk for sexual dysfunction is also likely to be the same.[20] Less information is available on sexual consequences of cancer in countries with low medical resources, but cancers potentiated by the human immunodeficiency virus (HIV) and the human papillomavirus (HPV) such as cervical, vulvar, anal, and penile cancer are more common, with a high likelihood of sexual morbidities.[21,22] Stigmatization of cancer may also lead to social isolation and relationship loss in low- and middle-income countries.[23]

Sexual problems related to cancer are severe and generalized, including loss of desire for sex, inability to get aroused and reach orgasm, and interference from fatigue, pain, or incontinence.[17,18] Without professional treatment, most problems do not resolve with time. Most dysfunctions are caused by cancer treatment,[17,18] including damage to autonomic nerves in the pelvis, reducing genital blood flow during sexual arousal especially for men,[6] and direct damage to genital blood vessels and tissue from pelvic radiation therapy.[4] Male erectile dysfunction also results from decreased genital blood flow after surgical interruption of blood supply. Without regular inflow of oxygenated blood, erectile tissue in the penis atrophies.[24] Orgasm dysfunction, including lack of ejaculation of semen, leakage of urine, weak sensation, and pain with orgasm can occur after radical pelvic surgery.[25]

Although the vagina expands and the clitoris swells with sexual arousal in women,[26] damage to hemodynamics is poorly understood. It is clear that estrogen deprivation plays a major role in female sexual problems,[17,18,27,28] decreasing lubrication produced by the vaginal mucosa during sexual arousal and reducing vaginal size and elasticity. Sexual caressing and penetration become painful, often leading to loss of desire to engage in sex and difficulty reaching orgasm.[29]

In both men and women, loss of desire for sex and sexual avoidance often have multifactorial causes after cancer.[17,18] Painful sex in women and erectile dysfunction in men are common antecedents. Low androgen levels can contribute to loss of desire for men, for example during anti-androgen therapy for prostate cancer[30] or after intensive chemotherapy[31] or radiation that damages the testes.[32]

> **Box 2**
>
> Toxicity from cancer treatment leads to severe and long-term sexual dysfunction affecting desire, arousal, orgasm, and pain.

Risk factors—premorbid sexual function, cancer treatments, and behavioral characteristics

Sexual dysfunction is common regardless of health status,[33] particularly with aging.[34] Erectile dysfunction is strongly associated with cardiovascular disease, hypertension, diabetes, smoking, sedentary lifestyle, and obesity and is a biomarker for increased mortality.[35] At least half of women over age 50 are no longer sexually active because of lack of a functional sexual partner.[36] Although many cancer patients are sexually inactive or dysfunctional at diagnosis, being sexually active and in a relationship are risk factors for increased distress when sexual problems develop posttreatment.[37,38]

Cancer treatments with a high risk of sexual dysfunction include intensive chemotherapy,[31] total body irradiation,[39] graft versus host disease after allogeneic transplant,[40] treatments leading to abrupt ovarian failure in premenopausal women,[28] pelvic radiation therapy,[4] radical pelvic cancer surgery in men[6–9,41,42] and women,[41,42] chemoradiation for pelvic tumors,[43] anti-androgenic therapy for prostate cancer,[30] and aromatase inhibitors for breast cancer.[38] Although penile and vulvar cancers are rare in Western nations, radical surgery removing major areas of genital tissue obviously also causes problems.[44,45] Vaginal reconstruction for advanced cervical or rectal cancer often fails to restore women's sexual pleasure.[46]

Psychosocial or behavioral factors also contribute to cancer-related sexual problems. Patients with a history of sexual abuse or trauma may have difficulty coping with cancer treatment, especially if the malignancy is in the reproductive system.[47] Relationship conflict and poor communication are also associated with poor sexual outcomes.[48] Traditional beliefs on masculinity and suppression of emotion may contribute to deterioration of sexual function after treatment for prostate cancer.[49] Both men and women scoring high on neuroticism, a personality trait involving depression and anxiety, have higher rates of sexual problems after cancer.[50,51]

Prevention—surgical, medical, behavioral

As previously discussed, modifying radical pelvic surgery to spare autonomic nerves near the prostate has been disappointing in preventing erectile dysfunction.[7–9,41,42] Animal research and theoretical models support penile rehabilitation after surgery, using treatments for erectile dysfunction to promote penile blood flow, but benefits on recovery of erections in humans are unclear.[24]

Nerve-sparing in radical hysterectomy has little impact on female sexual function.[52] Tissue-sparing surgery has been used instead of partial penectomy to treat localized penile cancer[44] or substituted for radical surgery in women for vulvar cancer,[45,53] but a majority of patients still have major sexual problems. Breast conservation or reconstruction also have few advantages over mastectomy in preserving women's sexual pleasure and desire.[54]

Cancer treatments that preserve ovarian function in younger women, such as conservative surgery for low-grade ovarian cancer,[55] preserving ovaries in women who have radical hysterectomy,[56] or omitting systemic therapy for ductal carcinoma *in situ* of the breast,[57] leave most women with normal sex lives. Treating early-stage Hodgkin lymphoma with nonalkylating chemotherapy also spares more gonadal function.[58] The trend toward personalized medicine and use of biological response modifiers may eventually lessen sexual morbidity, but early reports suggest that molecular therapies such as anti-angiogenesis inhibitors and immune checkpoint inhibitors also damage sexual function.[59,60]

Behavioral strategies may prevent some cancer-related sexual problems. Promoting genital blood flow and stretching genital tissues through resuming sexual activity, penile rehabilitation, or use of vaginal dilators may prevent atrophy.[24,61,62] Counseling that promotes more open sexual communication and continued, noncoital sexual intimacy may preserve intimacy and sexual self-esteem.[63,64]

> **Box 3**
>
> Risk factors for sexual dysfunction after cancer include:
> - Intensive chemotherapy
> - Radiation damage to the gonads or genitals
> - Hypogonadism due to cancer treatment
> - Removal of genital tissue
> - History of sexual trauma
> - Relationship conflict
> - Personality factors such as neuroticism or traditional gender beliefs
>
> Prevention may include:
> - More conservative cancer surgery
> - Less toxic chemotherapy
> - Behavioral strategies to preserve genital tissue or promote intimacy

Screening

Only half of patients recall their oncology team discussing sexual problems, and even then, it is usually a brief mention during informed consent to treatment.[15] Patients should be screened for sexual concerns and problems across the continuum of cancer care.[5,13] During treatment planning, potential damage to sexuality from cancer treatment should be explained, including a mention of any options to spare function. During treatment and at follow-up visits, sexual function should be monitored, at least with a periodic question, for example: "Sexuality is one important part of quality of life. Do you have any questions or concerns today about changes in your sex life since your cancer treatment?" Even among palliative care patients, about half want to continue sexual activity, despite a very high prevalence of sexual problems.[65] Although some symptom checklists include an item about sexuality, many patients do not check it despite having concerns, and even worse, clinic staff fail to acknowledge it.[66]

To screen for sexual dysfunction repeatedly across time, a good choice is the Patient-Reported Outcomes Measurement Information System (PROMIS) Brief Sexual Function profiles for men and women, multiple choice questionnaires with 8 and 10 items, respectively.[67]

Diagnosis

Because sexual dysfunction is typically measured by self-report, diagnostic nomenclature has been varied and controversial.[68] Many labels do not help clinicians in choosing evidence-based treatments for problems. It is helpful to categorize sexual problems as follows:

- difficulty desiring sex and experiencing subjective arousal
- impaired genital engorgement with blood during sexual arousal (i.e., erection in men and vaginal lubrication and expansion in women)
- difficulty experiencing a satisfying orgasm
- pain interfering with sexual pleasure
- urinary or fecal incontinence during sex

Most people treated for cancer have more than one, specific sexual problem. A woman who had chemoradiation for anal cancer may have vulvovaginal atrophy and vaginal stenosis, causing dryness and acute pain with sexual caressing or penetration. As a result, her desire for sex and ability to reach orgasm are also impaired. A man may be unable to get or keep firm erections after radical prostatectomy. Urine may also drip from his penis during sexual arousal and orgasm. If he uses a medical treatment for erections, he may realize that his penis has shrunk in size or developed a curvature.[69]

Eliciting a full description of the patient's sexual problems remains the most important aspect of diagnosis. For women, a pelvic examination with attention to pain and atrophy on the vulva and inside the vagina is crucial.[70] For men with erectile dysfunction, many urologists prescribe treatments unrelated to etiology, starting with oral medication and proceeding if necessary to penile injection therapy, a vacuum device, or a urethral suppository, with a penile prosthesis as the final step.[71,72] Nevertheless, evaluation should include screening for hypogonadism, cardiovascular risk factors, and genital anatomic changes.

> **Box 4**
>
> Screening and diagnosis should be multidisciplinary, using a verbal screening question, a careful interview, and relevant focused examinations to get a full picture of the type of problem and its medical and psychosocial causes.

Prognostic factors

Only a few prognostic factors for sexual rehabilitation have been identified. Men or women who were not sexually active before cancer diagnosis are unlikely to seek help after cancer, unless they had previously sought treatment for their problems.[38,73] Younger men who start out with normal erections are more distressed and likely to seek help after surgery for prostate cancer.[74] Having a partner who still enjoys sex is also crucial.[75] For women, being in a sexual relationship is key to help-seeking.[73]

Poor general and sexual communication are barriers to success with cognitive-behavioral treatment of sexual problems.[48] Couples with troubled relationships are less likely to enter clinical trials of sexual counseling.[76,77] Research on treatment outcomes is not available for people who are in a same-sex relationship.[78,79]

> **Box 5**
>
> Since research focuses on medical or counseling treatments that are short-term, it is not surprising that barriers to success include a history of sexual problems, lack of a motivated partner, and poor sexual communication.

Multidisciplinary care

Research suggests that a multidisciplinary approach, combining medical and psychosocial care, is the most effective for cancer-related sexual problems.[75,77] Table 1 lists common sexual problems and suggested treatment components. Resuming a satisfying sex life requires good communication,[79,117] acceptance that intimacy may include noncoital sexual stimulation,[75,77,79] and ability to cope with some "performance" limitations. Intervention programs using brief counseling without any medical therapies may reduce distress about sexual problems or improve sexual satisfaction somewhat, but do not resolve sexual dysfunction.[103,117]

Barriers to sexual rehabilitation include a dearth of expert medical or behavioral professionals and very few specialty clinics providing multidisciplinary treatment to cancer survivors.[118]

Psychosocial factors and management

In addition to the psychosocial factors already mentioned, a clinician should also assess the influence of culture and religion,[119] sexual orientation,[78,79] and ethnicity[120–122] on sexual issues. Interventions need to be compatible with patients' sexual attitudes.

Survivorship and follow-up

Continued assessment of sexual problems and referral for treatment is crucial during survivorship, particularly given the long-term nature of cancer-related sexual dysfunction.

Unmet needs, future directions, and conclusions

Although sexual problems have often been dismissed as an unfortunate, but minor side effect of cancer treatment, they affect over 50% of cancer survivors and have negative impacts on quality of life. Improvements are needed in the availability of cost-effective solutions for assessment, patient education, and multidisciplinary care. For patients with reasonable levels of literacy, education and self-help tools can be provided in high quality, online interventions.[75,77] Patients from underserved communities may need additional guidance from peer counselors[121] or patient navigators. When first-line interventions do not resolve sexual problems, a stepped care approach can be used to refer patients for more intensive treatment.

Table 1 Components of multidisciplinary care for common, cancer-related sexual problems in men and women.

Sexual problem	Factors to consider	Brief sexual counseling	Physiological treatments
Male low desire	Problem often multifactorial, not simply hormonal (shame about erections, fatigue, medications, emotional withdrawal)	Help with loss of masculine self-esteem, emotional coping, communication skills, relationship conflict	Androgen replacement only if hypogonadal,[31,32] even after prostatectomy[80]; change medications that may contribute[81]
Erectile dysfunction	Aging, premorbid risk factors, and cancer treatment all can damage erections	Help with decision-making on medical treatments; include partner and enhance sexual communication to increase adherence[82,83]	PDE5-inhibitors, vacuum erection devices, penile injection therapy, urethral suppositories[82]; penile prosthesis surgery[84]
Changes in orgasmic pleasure	Cancer treatment may lead to orgasms without erection or ejaculation, weakened orgasmic sensation, climacturia, inability to reach orgasm (central nervous system damage)[25]	Re-learn how to reach orgasm or intensify sensations, use vibrators or erotica[85]	Treat hypogonadism or hyperprolactinemia, change medications that can interfere with orgasm,[86,87] treat climacturia[88]
Premature ejaculation	Erectile dysfunction sometimes misperceived as premature ejaculation since prolonged stimulation to get erection results in rapid ejaculation	Sex therapy techniques such as stop–start or squeeze[85]	Oral medication, though modestly effective[87]; treatment for erectile dysfunction may correct problem[87]
Penile curvature	Cancer treatment can create penile curvature, understand timeline of pain with erection and changes in curvature[89]	Counseling about depression and body image issues[90]	Use medical treatments and traction to reduce curvature; surgical correction of curvature with or without penile prosthesis[91]
Pain during sex	Causes of genital pain during sex and interference with sex from chronic nongenital pain	Sensate focus exercises or mindfulness to focus on sexual pleasure and away from pain[92]	Treat chronic genital pain with pelvic floor physical therapy[93] or other medical treatments[94]; medication or other modalities; treat nongenital pain syndromes
Incontinence during sex	If has stoma, consult with specialty nurse on minimizing interference with sex; urinary incontinence common after radical prostatectomy	Counsel on coping with incontinence during sex, use of mattress pads and other aids	Oral medications or penile tension loop to prevent urinary leakage during sex[88,95]; surgery to insert artificial sphincter[96]; control of fecal incontinence using diet and medication[97]
Female low desire	Understanding that problem typically multifactorial, not simply hormonal[98,99]	Help with poor body image, relationship conflict, coping with history of traumatic sexual experience,[47] chronic fatigue, and life stress	Treat pain that may lead to avoidance of sex[100]; change medications that may contribute[81]; androgen replacement rarely helpful and may increase breast cancer risk[101]; new medications for premenopausal women need further research[102]
Vulvovaginal dryness and pain with sex	Vulvovaginal atrophy is common after normal menopause and more severe after some cancer treatments[70,100]	Counseling on medical treatment options, optimizing sexual stimulation and communication to maximize sexual arousal, positions for penetration that may help avoid pain[77,103–105]	Regular use of vaginal moisturizers and water- or silicone-based lubricants during sexual activity[104–106]; use of graduated vaginal dilators[62,104]; consider low-dose vaginal estrogen[107]; ospemifene[108]; pelvic floor physical therapy[109]; prescribe options early in women starting aromatase inhibitors[105]
Difficulty reaching orgasm	Women normally reach orgasm more easily with clitoral stimulation, genetic contribution to ease of reaching orgasm[110]; after cancer, problems often secondary to low desire and/or pain with sex	Training on reaching orgasm with self-stimulation or vibrator; transition to partner sex[111]	Change in medications that can interfere with orgasm[81]
Incontinence during sex	If has stoma, consult with specialty nurse on minimizing interference with sex; urinary incontinence commonly interferes with sex[112]; fecal incontinence frequent after pelvic radiation[113]	Behavioral bladder training and pelvic floor therapy[109,114]	Use of oral medications[115]; sacral neuromodulation for neurogenic or overactive bladders[116]; control of fecal incontinence using diet and medication[97,113]

Key references

The complete reference list can be found on Vital Source version of this title, see inside front cover.

4 Incrocci L, Jensen PT. Pelvic radiotherapy and sexual function in men and women. *J Sex Med*. 2013;**10**(Suppl 1):53–64.

7 Nelson CJ, Scardino PT, Eastham JA, Mulhall JP. Back to baseline: erectile function recovery after radical prostatectomy from the patients' perspective. *J Sex Med*. 2013;**10**:1636–1643.

10 Gaither TW, Awad MA, Osterberg EC, et al. The natural history of erectile dysfunction after prostatic radiotherapy: a systematic review and meta-analysis. *J Sex Med*. 2017;**14**:1071–1078.

11 Sheets NC, Goldin GH, Meyer AM, et al. Intensity-modulated radiation therapy, proton therapy, or conformal radiation therapy and morbidity and disease control in localized prostate cancer. *JAMA*. 2012;**307**:1611–1620.

13 Carter J, Lacchetti C, Andersen BL, et al. Interventions to address sexual problems in people with cancer: American Society of Clinical Oncology Clinical Practice Guideline Adaptation of Cancer Care Ontario Guideline. *J Clin Oncol*. 2018;**36**:492–511.

15 Reese JB, Sorice K, Beach MC, et al. Patient-provider communication about sexual concerns in cancer: a systematic review. *J Cancer Surviv*. 2017;**11**:175–188.

17 Schover LR, van der Kaaij M, van Dorst E, et al. Sexual dysfunction and infertility as late effects of cancer treatment. *EJC Suppl*. 2014;**12**:41–53.

18 Schover LR. Sexual quality of life in men and women after cancer. *Climacteric*. 2019;**22**:553–557.

24 Fode M, Ohl DA, Ralph D, Sønksen J. Penile rehabilitation after radical prostatectomy: what the evidence really says. *BJU Int*. 2013;**112**:998–1008.

25 Clavell-Hernández J, Martin C, Wang R. Orgasmic dysfunction following radical prostatectomy: review of current literature. *Sex Med Rev*. 2018;**6**:124–134.

26 Puppo V. Anatomy and physiology of the clitoris, vestibular bulbs, and labia minora with a review of the female orgasm and the prevention of female sexual dysfunction. *Clin Anat*. 2013;**26**:134–152.

28 Schover LR. Premature ovarian failure and its consequences: vasomotor symptoms, sexuality, and fertility. *J Clin Oncol*. 2008;**26**:753–758.

31 Kiserud CE, Schover LR, Dahl AA, et al. Do male lymphoma survivors have impaired sexual function? *J Clin Oncol*. 2009;**27**:6019–6026.

34 Lindau ST, Schumm LP, Laumann EO, et al. A study of sexuality and health among older adults in the United States. *N Engl J Med*. 2007;**357**:762–774.

37 Steinsvik EA, Axcrona K, Dahl AA, et al. Can sexual bother after radical prostatectomy be predicted preoperatively? Findings from a prospective national study of the relation between sexual function, activity and bother. *BJU Int*. 2012;**109**:1366–1374.

40. Hamilton BK, Goje O, Savani BN, et al. Clinical management of genital chronic GvHD. *Bone Marrow Transplant*. 2017;**52**:803–810.
44. Kieffer JM, Djajadiningrat RS, van Muilekom EA, et al. Quality of life in patients treated for penile cancer. *J Urol*. 2014;**192**:1105–1110.
46. Scott JR, Liu D, Mathes DW. Patient-reported outcomes and sexual function in vaginal reconstruction: a 17-year review, survey, and review of the literature. *Ann Plast Surg*. 2010;**64**:311–314.
54. Schover LR, Yetman RJ, Tuason LJ, et al. Partial mastectomy and breast reconstruction. A comparison of their effects on psychosocial adjustment, body image, and sexuality. *Cancer*. 1995;**75**:54–64.
57. Bober SL, Giobbie-Hurder A, Emmons KM, et al. Psychosexual functioning and body image following a diagnosis of ductal carcinoma *in situ*. *J Sex Med*. 2013;**10**:370–377.
59. Rouanne M, Massard C, Hollebecque A, et al. Evaluation of sexuality, health-related quality-of-life and depression in advanced cancer patients: a prospective study in a Phase I clinical trial unit of predominantly targeted anticancer drugs. *Eur J Cancer*. 2013;**49**:431–438.
64. Nelson CJ, Kenowitz J. Communication and intimacy-enhancing interventions for men diagnosed with prostate cancer and their partners. *J Sex Med*. 2013;**10**(Suppl 1):127–132.
66. Bradford A, Fellman B, Urbauer D, Bevers T. Effect of routine screening for sexual problems in a breast cancer survivorship clinic. *Psychooncology*. 2016;**25**:1375–1378.
67. Weinfurt KP, Lin L, Bruner DW, et al. Development and initial validation of the PROMIS(®) Sexual Function and Satisfaction Measures Version 2.0. *J Sex Med*. 2015;**12**:1961–1974.
70. Lindau ST, Abramsohn EM, Baron SR, et al. Physical examination of the female cancer patient with sexual concerns: what oncologists and patients should expect from consultation with a specialist. *CA Cancer J Clin*. 2016;**66**:241–263.
72. Mulhall JP, Giraldi A, Hackett G, et al. The 2018 revision to the process of care model for management of erectile dysfunction. *J Sex Med*. 2018;**15**:1434–1445.
75. Schover LR, Canada AL, Yuan Y, et al. A randomized trial of internet-based versus traditional sexual counseling for couples after localized prostate cancer treatment. *Cancer*. 2012;**118**:500–509.
77. Schover LR, Yuan Y, Fellman BM, et al. Efficacy trial of an internet-based intervention for cancer-related female sexual dysfunction. *J Natl Compr Cancer Netw*. 2013;**11**:1389–1397.
78. Quinn GP, Sanchez JA, Sutton SK, et al. Cancer and lesbian, gay, bisexual, transgender/transsexual, and queer/questioning (LGBTQ) populations. *CA Cancer J Clin*. 2015;**65**:384–400.
81. Gitlin M. Sexual dysfunction with psychotropic drugs. *Expert Opin Pharmacother*. 2003;**4**:2259–2269.
83. Matthew A, Lutzky-Cohen N, Jamnicky L, et al. The Prostate Cancer Rehabilitation Clinic: a biopsychosocial clinic for sexual dysfunction after radical prostatectomy. *Curr Oncol*. 2018;**25**:393–402.
85. McMahon CG, Jannini E, Waldinger M, Rowland D. Standard operating procedures in the disorders of orgasm and ejaculation. *J Sex Med*. 2013;**10**:204–229.
88. Mendez MH, Sexton SJ, Lentz AC. Contemporary review of male and female climacturia and urinary leakage during sexual activities. *Sex Med Rev*. 2018;**6**:16–28.
93. Cohen D, Gonzalez J, Goldstein I. The role of pelvic floor muscles in male sexual dysfunction and pelvic pain. *Sex Med Rev*. 2016;**4**:53–62.
99. Clayton AH, Goldstein I, Kim NN, et al. The international society for the study of women's sexual health process of care for management of hypoactive sexual desire disorder in women. *Mayo Clin Proc*. 2018;**93**:467–487.
104. Carter J, Goldfrank D, Schover LR. Simple strategies for vaginal health promotion in cancer survivors. *J Sex Med*. 2011;**8**:549–559.
105. Advani P, Brewster AM, Baum GP, Schover LR. A pilot randomized trial to prevent sexual dysfunction in postmenopausal breast cancer survivors starting adjuvant aromatase inhibitor therapy. *J Cancer Surviv*. 2017;**11**:477–485.
109. Wallace SL, Miller LD, Mishra K. Pelvic floor physical therapy in the treatment of pelvic floor dysfunction in women. *Curr Opin Obstet Gynecol*. 2019;**31**:485–493.
118. Bober SL, Varela VS. Sexuality in adult cancer survivors: challenges and intervention. *J Clin Oncol*. 2012;**30**:3712–3719.
119. Oberguggenberger AS, Nagele E, Inwald EC, et al. Phase 1-3 of the cross-cultural development of an EORTC questionnaire for the assessment of sexual health in cancer patients: the EORTC SHQ-22. *Cancer Med*. 2018;**7**:635–645.

136 Endocrine complications and paraneoplastic syndromes

Sai-Ching J. Yeung, MD, PhD, FACP ■ Robert F. Gagel, MD

Overview

Transformation of normal cells results in activation and/or suppression of a number of hormonally active genes, resulting in ectopic humoral paraneoplastic syndromes. Treatment of cancer also results in a number of endocrine or metabolic abnormalities, most of which are related to hormone deficiency or drug-related toxicity. Targeted therapy may disrupt signaling pathways involved in endocrine function, and immunotherapy has led to autoimmune endocrine dysfunctions. This article will outline ectopic endocrine paraneoplastic syndromes and the major endocrine toxicities of antineoplastic therapy.

Introduction

This article is divided into two major sections. The first focuses on ectopic endocrine paraneoplastic syndromes, and the second on endocrine complications of cancer treatments. Paraneoplastic syndromes may have immune or humoral etiologies; we shall limit the discussion to ectopic humoral paraneoplastic syndromes. Cancer treatments can lead to endocrine or metabolic dysfunction or clinical and laboratory abnormalities that obscure or mimic endocrine or metabolic diseases. The discussion of these cancer treatment complications will be organized by glandular functions.

Ectopic endocrine paraneoplastic syndromes

Some cancers produce hormones. Production of a hormonal substance by a cell type that normally produces the hormone is orthotopic, for example, parathyroid hormone (PTH) production by a parathyroid cancer, production of calcitonin by medullary thyroid carcinoma, and serotonin by carcinoid tumors. In this situation, the malignant cell type continues to produce its normal product but does so in an unregulated manner. These clinical syndromes are discussed in the relevant chapters for these malignancies. The "ectopic" production of hormones, to be discussed here, is by malignant cells that normally produce the hormones at very low levels or not at all. In some instances (e.g., parathyroid hormone-related protein (PTHrP) production by squamous cell carcinoma),[1] the cells may have produced the hormones early in embryonic development, or ectopic hormone production occurs in neuroendocrine cells whose hormone production machinery has been hijacked to produce another hormone (e.g., adrenocorticotrophic hormone (ACTH) by neuroendocrine tumors). Ectopic production of peptides by neuroendocrine-like tumors comprise most of these syndromes.

Ectopic ACTH production

Ectopic ACTH or ectopic corticotrophin-releasing hormone (CRH) secretion causes an ectopic form of Cushing syndrome. The most common etiology of ectopic ACTH production is expression of proopiomelanocortin (POMC), the precursor of ACTH, by a tumor. POMC is processed posttranslationally via two mutually exclusive proteolytic pathways,[2] one of which produces big melanocyte-stimulating hormone and ACTH. The most common tumor type that ectopically produces ACTH is small-cell lung cancer (SCLC), although a broad spectrum of tumors including pulmonary carcinoid, medullary thyroid carcinoma, islet cell malignancy, pheochromocytoma, and occasional ganglioneuromas may also produce ACTH. The second cause of excessive ACTH is tumor production of CRH.[3] Neoplasms that can produce CRH include medullary thyroid carcinoma, paragangliomas, prostate cancer, and islet cell neoplasms. There are also rare tumors that produce both ACTH and CRH. Cushing syndrome produced by ectopic production of ACTH is characterized by adrenal cortical hyperplasia and hypercortisolemia[4] while ectopic CRH would cause pituitary corticotrope hyperplasia with excessive ACTH production, adrenal cortical hyperplasia, and Cushing syndrome.

Patients with ectopic ACTH syndrome may present with clinical features of Cushing syndrome—easy bruising, centripetal obesity, muscle wasting, hypertension, diabetes mellitus, and metabolic alkalosis. Alternatively, patients with rapidly growing SCLC may present with a clinical syndrome characterized by cachexia, muscle atrophy, profound hypokalemic metabolic alkalosis, and hypertension without the other typical findings of Cushing syndrome.

The hallmark of ectopic ACTH syndrome is an elevated plasma ACTH. However, in the differential diagnosis of hypercortisolemia in a cancer patient with an elevated plasma ACTH concentration, one should also consider an ACTH-producing pituitary tumor.[5] Differentiation between pituitary ACTH production (a primary pituitary tumor) and ectopic tumor production of ACTH or ectopic CRH production is one of the greatest diagnostic challenges in endocrinology.[6] In some cases, such as ectopic ACTH production by a SCLC, the clinical syndrome (hypokalemia, metabolic alkalosis, hypertension, exceedingly high plasma cortisol levels, and a rapidly growing lung cancer) will lead to a straightforward diagnosis.[7] In other cases, full access to interventional radiologic techniques used to differentiate pituitary from nonpituitary sources of ACTH will be needed to make the diagnosis.

The diagnostic evaluation begins by measuring plasma ACTH in a patient with hypercortisolemia. A plasma ACTH concentration >100 pg/mL should prompt investigation for an ectopic source of ACTH.[8] If ACTH <10 pg/mL, a primary adrenocortical source of cortisol (adrenal adenoma or carcinoma) should be considered. In most ectopic ACTH cases, plasma ACTH concentrations fall between 10 and 100 pg/mL. The major differential diagnoses

Table 1 Dynamic testing of the hypothalamic/pituitary axes.

Test	Dose/sampling	Contraindications
Growth hormone axis		
Insulin hypoglycemia	0.075–0.1 U regular insulin/kg IV to achieve glucose <40 mg/dL. Sample for glucose and growth hormone (GH) at 0, 30, 45, 60, and 90 min	Coronary heart disease or seizures—patients should be closely monitored during and given glucose at the conclusion of the study
Arginine	0.5 gm/kg (up to 30 gm) IV over 30 min. Sample for GH at 0, 30, 60, 90, and 120 min	Liver disease or renal disease
L-Dopa	500 mg by mouth. Sample for GH at 0, 30, 60, 90, and 120 min	Systolic blood pressure <100 mmHg or age >60 years
Arginine and growth hormone-releasing hormone (GHRH)	Arginine dose as above. GHRH 1 µg/kg IV push. Sample for GH at 0, 30, 60, 90, and 120 min	Liver disease or renal disease
Clonidine stimulation protocol	Clonidine 0.15 mg/m² by mouth. Collect GH samples at baseline, 30, 60, 90, and 120 min	
Growth hormone-releasing hormone (GHRH) stimulation protocol	GHRH at 1.0 µg/kg body weight IV push. Collect GH samples at baseline, 15, 30, 45, 60, 90, and 120 min	
Growth hormone suppression test	The test should be performed after an overnight fast with the patient maintained at bed rest. The patient should drink a solution of 100 g glucose. Collect GH samples at baseline, 60, and 120 min	
Adrenal axis		
Adrenocorticotropin hormone (ACTH) stimulation test, 1-hour	Synthetic ACTH 1–24 1 µg or 250 µg IM or IV. Draw blood for cortisol at 30 and 60 min after injection	
ACTH stimulation test, 48-hour	Beginning at 9 AM, obtain baseline 24-h urine for 17-hydroxycorticosteroids (17-OHCS) and creatinine. Collect 24-h urine as on day 1. Beginning at 9 AM, start IV and give 250 µg synthetic ACTH 1–24 in 250 mL normal saline over 8 h every 8 h for 48 h. Alternatively, 40 IU of depot formulation of purified bovine ACTH in gelatin IM every 12 h for 48 hours. Repeat 24-h urine as on days 1 and 2. Days 4 and 5: Collect 24-h urine as on previous days	
Corticotropin-releasing hormone (CRH) stimulation test	Fast for at least 4 h prior to the test. Human CRH at 1.0 µg/kg IV bolus over 30 s. Blood samples should be collected at 15 min and 1 min before CRH administration and at 15, 30, 45, 60, 90, and 120 min after for measurements of cortisol and ACTH	
Low-dose dexamethasone test, overnight	Dexamethasone 1.0 mg (adult) or 20 µg/kg (children) PO between 11 PM and midnight. Serum cortisol is collected at 8–9 AM the next morning. A cortisol level <1.8 µg/dL essentially excludes Cushing syndrome	
Low-dose dexamethasone test, 48-hour	Serum cortisol is collected at 8–9 AM. Dexamethasone 0.5 mg (adult) or 10 µg/kg (children) PO immediately after the cortisol is drawn and again every 6 h for 48 h. A second plasma cortisol is drawn at 9 AM, 6 h after the last dexamethasone dose. Serum cortisol concentrations <1.8 µg/dL exclude Cushing syndrome	
High-dose dexamethasone test, overnight	Dexamethasone 8 mg (adult) PO between 11 PM and midnight. Serum cortisol is collected at 8–9 AM the next morning. In patients with ACTH >10 pg/mL, <50% suppression indicates an ectopic source of excess ACTH	
High-dose dexamethasone test, 48-hour	Serum cortisol is collected at 9 AM. Dexamethasone is administered (2.0 mg; 50 µg/kg in children) every 6 hours for 48 h. A second plasma cortisol is drawn at 9 AM, 6 h after the last dexamethasone dose. Patients with functional adrenal adenomas show no suppression of cortisol levels in the 48-h sample relative to the initial (baseline) sample. Seventy-eight percent of patients with pituitary source of excess ACTH showed >50% suppression of plasma cortisol while only 11% of patients with an ectopic source of excess ACTH had a >50% suppression	
Comprehensive, 6-day, low-/high-dose dexamethasone test	This protocol incorporates the low- and high-dose dexamethasone tests in succession. 24-h urinary-free cortisol and/or 17-hydroxycorticosteroid (17-OHCS) measurement can help verify the results of serum cortisol and ACTH	
Gonadotropin-releasing hormone (GnRH) stimulation test	GnRH 100 µg IV. A sample for serum LH should be collected at baseline and 40 min after GnRH administration	
Metyrapone stimulation (overnight) test	At 11 PM, metyrapone 30 mg/kg (maximum 3 g) PO with a snack. On the following morning, at 8 AM, measure serum cortisol and 11-deoxycortisol	

Abbreviations: GH, growth hormone; GNRH, growth hormone-releasing hormone; IV, intravenous; IM, intramuscular; PO, by mouth.

include a central (pituitary), peripheral (ectopic) source of ACTH, or production of ectopic CRH by a tumor (a rare possibility). Differentiation between central and peripheral sources of ACTH is accomplished by MRI of hypothalamic/sella region, dynamic testing, and petrosal venous sinus sampling to differentiate between a central (pituitary) and peripheral (ectopic) source of ACTH.[9] Ectopic CRH production is diagnosed first by suspecting it and then with measurement of plasma CRH. Other approaches to diagnose ectopic ACTH syndrome include the inability to suppress ACTH production in an overnight high-dose dexamethasone test (Table 1).[4]

Surgical removal or cancer chemotherapy are primary treatments for an ACTH- or CRH-producing malignancy. Electrolyte abnormalities, diabetes mellitus, or hypertension should be corrected prior to surgery. Patients with long-standing Cushing syndrome and hypercortisolemia have high perioperative morbidity and mortality. Preoperative treatment options include metyrapone (1–4 g/d orally), aminoglutethimide (250 mg orally four times per day with upward titration), or ketoconazole (200–400 mg twice a day orally).[10,11] Parenteral etomidate, used for sedation and induction of anesthesia, rapidly inhibits cortisol synthesis at sub-hypnotic concentrations,[12] and can be titrated (0.3–4 mg/kg/h) to rapidly reverse hypercortisolemia. After surgical treatment or pharmacologic inhibition of cortisol production, replacement glucocorticoid therapy is needed to prevent adrenal insufficiency. If surgical removal of an ACTH- or

CRH-producing tumor is not possible or inadvisable, chronic therapy with inhibitors of cortisol synthesis may be required.

Patients with rapidly progressive SCLC and ectopic ACTH syndrome form a unique subgroup because of the need to initiate chemotherapy expeditiously. They are highly susceptible to opportunistic infections, and chemotherapy often leads to serious life-threatening infection.[13] One to two weeks may be required to normalize the serum cortisol pharmacologically but normalization of immunity will take longer. If a delay in starting chemotherapy is deemed unacceptable from an oncologic perspective, retroperitoneal laparoscopic adrenalectomy provides a rapid and generally safe approach to rapidly stop corticosteroid secretion. Prophylactic therapy for opportunistic infections caused by pneumocystis carinii or fungi should be considered if chemotherapy is initiated shortly after normalization of the serum cortisol.

Hypercalcemia caused by malignancy

Hypercalcemia is a common cause of morbidity and mortality in cancer patients, having an incidence of about 1%.[14] Hypercalcemia in cancer patients is an indicator of poor prognosis and may be associated with a shortened survival if it cannot be corrected. The most common causes are PTHrP-mediated hypercalcemia, increased production of the active metabolite of vitamin D, calcitriol or 1,25 dihydroxy vitamin D3, and localized osteolytic hypercalcemia.[15,16] Ectopic production of PTH is rare. Other common causes of hypercalcemia, most notably primary hyperparathyroidism, should also be considered in cancer patients with hypercalcemia. Serum intact parathyroid hormone (iPTH) permits differentiation between hyperparathyroidism and a number of other causes of hypercalcemia. Hypercalcemia, increased iPTH and increased urinary calcium excretion constitute prima facie evidence for primary hyperparathyroidism. Suppression of the iPTH is found in PTHrP or calcitriol-mediated hypercalcemia.

Parathyroid hormone-related protein

PTHrP is a small peptide in which 8 of the first 16 amino acids are identical to PTH. This small peptide causes hypercalcemia by binding to the PTH receptor and activating the expression of an osteoblast-specific cell surface protein, RANK ligand (RANKL). Interaction between RANKL and the RANK receptor on the osteoclast precursor causes increased osteoclast differentiation, bone resorption, and hypercalcemia. Other PTH-like actions of PTHrP include hypophosphatemia and increased urinary calcium excretion. PTHrP-mediated hypercalcemia is characterized by a suppressed iPTH level and a low or normal calcitriol level, which contrasts with an elevated iPTH and calcitriol levels in primary hyperparathyroidism. PTHrP production is found commonly in squamous cell carcinomas; other tumors that produce PTHrP include breast, neuroendocrine, renal, melanoma, and prostate cancers.

Calcitriol production by malignant tumors

Lymphoma commonly produces calcitriol, leading to increased gastrointestinal absorption of calcium. Lymphomatous tissue, like granulomatous tissue (e.g., sarcoid, tuberculosis, and fungal infection), expresses 1α-hydroxylase which converts 25-hydroxy vitamin D3 to calcitriol. Clinical studies show that a high percentage of lymphoma patients have hypercalciuria at the time of diagnosis; a smaller percentage have frank hypercalcemia.[17] The characteristic clinical features of hypercalcemia in the context of lymphoma include a suppressed serum iPTH, a normal or slightly increased phosphorus level (caused by the suppression of PTH), hypercalciuria, absence of bone metastasis, and an elevated serum calcitriol level, found in approximately one-half of hypercalcemic patients.[17]

Localized osteolytic bone resorption causing hypercalcemia

Certain malignancies metastasize to bone frequently and some cause hypercalcemia. Hypercalcemia associated with breast cancer and myeloma is common. In contrast, prostate cancer, despite its more frequent presence in bone, rarely produces hypercalcemia. Malignancies that cause hypercalcemia produce cytokines, PTHrP, or other factors that stimulate increased bone resorption.[15,16] In multiple myeloma several factors contribute to localized osteolysis. Increased expression of RANKL causing localized osteoclast proliferation appears to be the most important cause. Other factors that may contribute to osteoclast proliferation in myeloma are interleukin-6 and macrophage inflammatory protein 1α.[16]

Impact of malignancy-related hypercalcemia

Severe hypercalcemia in the context of malignancy is associated with poor survival, measured in weeks to months if severe or if unresponsive to therapy. The causes of death include complications of hypercalcemia (coma, renal failure) and progression of tumor. The development of hypercalcemia is often, although not always, an indicator of tumor progression in the face of adequate therapy. Since it is not always possible to predict which patients will respond to oncologic therapy, it is important to treat hypercalcemia in all newly diagnosed patients with cancer. Whether to continue to treat recurrent and/or refractory hypercalcemia is a decision that should be based on response of the causative tumor to oncologic therapy and the overall prognosis of the patient. Severe hypercalcemia frequently causes depression of cerebral function or coma, a clinical situation that may reduce suffering in a dying patient.

Therapy of hypercalcemia

Dehydration is a common finding in hypercalcemic patients. Increased urine excretion of calcium causes a concentrating defect leading to increased fluid loss. Initial management should focus on the reversal of dehydration by infusion of a solution of normal saline at rates between 100 and 300 mL/h, although caution should be exercised in patients with diminished cardiac function. Hydration will commonly lower the elevation of serum calcium by 10–40% over a period of 6–12 h. Patients with serum calcium >13 mg/dL (3.25 mmol/L), an alteration of mental status, or evidence of renal dysfunction attributable to hypercalcemia should be treated with either intravenous bisphosphonate [zoledronate (4 mg over 30 min), preferred because of increased potency and effectiveness, or pamidronate (60–90 mg over 4 h)] or glucocorticoids (40–60 mg/d prednisone equivalent).[18–21] Calcitonin (3 units/kg subcutaneously twice daily) may lower the serum calcium concentration by 1–2 mg/dL early in the treatment course but is rarely effective long-term. These drugs are sometimes used in combination or sequentially in patients who are poorly responsive. Glucocorticoids, which inhibit calcium absorption, are most commonly used as primary therapy for lymphoma, whereas bisphosphonate therapy is more likely to be effective in hypercalcemia associated with solid tumors. Although bisphosphonates for long-term treatment of bone metastasis have been associated with osteonecrosis of the jaw in 1–2.5% of treated patients, this has not been an issue in patients treated short-term for hypercalcemia of malignancy. A monoclonal antibody against RANKL (denosumab) prevents its interaction with the RANK receptor on osteoclast precursors, thereby reducing osteoclast-mediated bone resorption.[22] Denosumab is an effective inhibitor of bone resorption and is efficacious in patients with hypercalcemia and bone metastasis, particularly those who are unresponsive to bisphosphonate therapy.[22]

Human chorionic gonadotropin

Human chorionic gonadotropin (hCG) is formed from two different protein subunits encoded by separate genes. The first is the α subunit that is shared by all members of the pituitary class of glycoprotein hormones including hCG, luteinizing hormone (LH), follicle-stimulating hormone (FSH), and thyroid-stimulating hormone (TSH). The second, the β-subunit, is unique for each of these hormones. Production of hCG is found in trophoblastic tumors (choriocarcinomas, testicular embryonal carcinomas, and seminomas) and, uncommonly, in tumors of the lung and pancreas. In younger children, precocious puberty, caused by hCG stimulation of ovarian function, is seen. In adult males, gynecomastia is common. Hyperthyroidism may develop from interaction of hCG with the thyroid-stimulating hormone receptor (TSHR) particularly when β-hCG level is very high.

Tumor removal or effective antineoplastic therapy is effective in controlling excessive β-hCG production. Hyperthyroidism can be treated short-term with thionamide therapy if treatments for the underlying malignancy are likely to be effective; in patients with less responsive tumors, thyroidectomy or radioactive iodine may be required.

Hypoglycemia

Tumor-induced hypoglycemia is uncommon; three clinical syndromes have been identified. First, insulin can be produced by islet cell malignancy. Islet cell tumors commonly produce low levels of insulin that are clinically insignificant until the tumor burden is large, more commonly encountered in patients with hepatic metastasis. A second cause is insufficient gluconeogenesis, which is seen in patients with near-complete replacement of hepatic parenchyma by cancer or in lactic acidosis in patients with end-stage leukemic or lymphomatous involvement of the liver.[23] The third is caused by increased insulin-like growth factor II (IGF-II), a peptide that activates the insulin receptor. This syndrome is commonly seen in patients with fibrosarcomas, hemangiopericytomas, or hepatomas. In these patients, IGF-binding protein 3 (IGFBP3) and acid-labile subunit fail to efficiently bind IGF-II and elevated circulating IGF-II causes hypoglycemia by activation of the insulin receptor.[24–26]

The primary manifestation is fasting hypoglycemia, which most likely develops during periods of low caloric intake, particularly during nocturnal hours. Measurement of a plasma insulin, proinsulin, and C-peptide during a period of hypoglycemia is important to distinguish insulin production from replacement of liver by tumor and IGF-II production. Unregulated insulin production as the cause of hypoglycemia is diagnosed by elevated insulin, proinsulin, and C-peptide in the face of hypoglycemia and the absence of any drugs (by a drug screen for sulfonylureas) that might stimulate insulin release from the normal pancreas. In contrast, insulin, proinsulin, and C-peptide levels will be low in tumor replacement of the liver or IGF-II-mediated hypoglycemia. IGF-II-mediated hypoglycemia is diagnosed by an elevated serum IGF-II, low or normal insulin, proinsulin, and C-peptide measurements, low IGF-I levels, and generally normal IGFBP3 or acid-labile subunit measurements in the context of a large sarcoma or retroperitoneal tumor.

Surgical excision or antineoplastic therapy to reduce tumor mass is effective in insulin or IGF-II-mediated hypoglycemia; there is little effective therapy for insufficient hepatic gluconeogenesis other than providing glucose. Hypoglycemia is treated with frequent meals. Patients may be kept symptom-free by being awakened for caloric intake during nocturnal hours or continuous infusion of 20% dextrose through a central venous catheter to maintain normal blood glucose. Glucagon infusion (0.5–2 mg/h) to stimulate gluconeogenesis is also effective, and the response to glucagon can be initially tested by injecting 1 mg subcutaneously with measurement of plasma glucose after 30 and 60 min. It is important to assess hepatic gluconeogenesis in response to glucagon by showing an increase of the blood glucose after injection of the peptide. Glucagon can be administered in small volumes (1–5 mL over 24 h) using micro-infusion pumps.[27] Patients treated with glucagon may develop the characteristic rash associated with glucagonoma, necessitating discontinuance of this treatment modality. Other therapies that have been applied with periodic success include glucocorticoids (20–40 mg prednisone equivalents per day) and diazoxide (3–8 mg/kg/d in 2–3 divided doses; edema may limit the dosage).

Syndrome of inappropriate antidiuretic hormone

Syndrome of inappropriate antidiuretic hormone (SIADH) is a paraneoplastic syndrome seen in approximately 15% of SCLC, 1% of other lung cancers, and 3% of squamous cell head and neck cancers with unregulated vasopressin secretion, and is associated with decreased overall survival.[28] Other neoplasms such as primary brain tumors, hematologic neoplasms, skin tumors, and gastrointestinal, gynecologic, breast, and prostate cancers, and sarcomas can also cause SIADH. In a prospective study of hospitalized cancer patients, the incidence of hyponatremia is 3.7%, with sodium depletion and SIADH each accounting for about one-third of causes.[29]

Figure 1 outlines the algorithm for evaluation and treatment of hyponatremia. SIADH is characterized by low serum osmolality and inappropriately high urine osmolality relative to the serum osmolality in the absence of diuretics, heart failure, cirrhosis, adrenal insufficiency, and hypothyroidism.[30] In cancer patients, SIADH may be caused by vasopressin secreted by tumors (e.g., up to 15% of SCLCs), abnormal secretory stimuli (e.g., intrathoracic infection, positive pressure ventilation), or cytotoxicity affecting paraventricular and supraoptic neurons; these need to be considered before making a diagnosis of paraneoplastic SIADH. It is also possible that chemotherapy-induced lysis of vasopressin-containing cancer cells contributes to or worsens SIADH.

Most patients with SIADH are asymptomatic. When serum sodium falls <120 mEq/L, altered mental status and seizures may develop. In particular, women of reproductive age who develop hyponatremia may develop profound cerebral edema. Acute hyponatremia with neurological changes will require management in intensive care with hypertonic (sodium chloride 3% in water) saline infusion to raise serum sodium by 4–6 mEq/L in 1–2 h followed by slower correction over the next 2 days. In patients with a serum sodium <120 mEq/L, the intravenous vasopressin (V2) receptor antagonist, conivaptan (20 mg intravenously over 30 min followed by 20 mg over 24 h) results in improvement or normalization of the serum sodium over a 24–48 h period. Intravenous urea (0.25–0.50 g/kg/day) is effective for hospitalized patients with SIADH.[31] Fluid restriction (<1.5 L/day) can be first-line management effective for patients with high solute intake and high

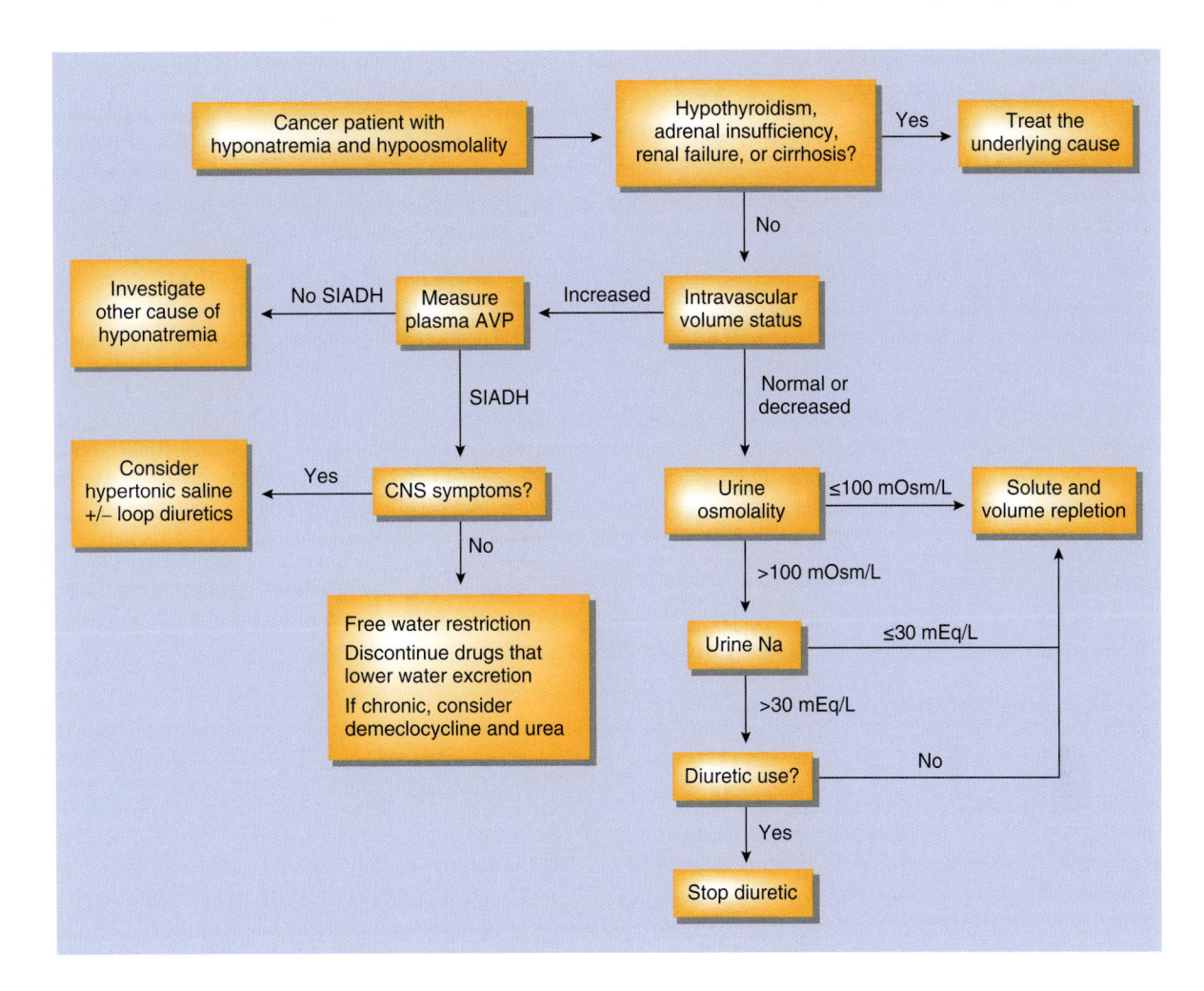

Figure 1 Approach to evaluation of hyponatremia in a cancer patient.

diuresis, Patients with low sodium intake and low diuresis may be treated with oral urea.[32] Adding salt tablets and loop diuretic (furosemide) to fluid restriction may not improve efficacy.[33] The oral V2 receptor antagonist tolvaptan (15–60 mg/day) has shown efficacy.[28] Treatment with demeclocycline (150–300 mg/d), a tetracycline antibiotic that inhibits the effects of vasopressin on the kidney, may be less expensive than V2 receptor antagonists but have more side effects.

Tumor-induced osteomalacia

Severe hypophosphatemia caused by renal phosphate wasting is the hallmark of tumor-induced osteomalacia. This clinical syndrome is characterized by osteomalacia, caused by inadequate mineralization of osteoid, and moderate to severe proximal myopathy.[34] Tumors that produce this clinical syndrome include mesenchymal tumors (osteoblastomas, giant cell osteosarcomas, hemangiopericytomas, hemangiomas, and nonossifying fibromas)[35] and, rarely, malignant tumors such as prostate or lung cancer. There is compelling evidence that fibroblast growth factor-23 (FGF-23), a member of the fibroblast growth factor family that is mutated in autosomal dominant osteomalacia, is overexpressed by some neoplasms causing tumor-induced osteomalacia.[36,37] Oral or intravenous supplementation of phosphate combined with vitamin D therapy is generally effective for eradicating or improving clinical symptoms. Complete surgical resection is generally curative. In patients with incomplete resection or regrowth of a tumor with recurrent FGF-23 production and hypophosphatemia, a monoclonal antibody (burosumab) that targets FGF-23 has recently been approved for treatment of this condition.

Erythropoietin, thrombopoietin, leukopoietin, or colony-stimulating factor production

Polycythemia caused by ectopic erythropoietin production is a rare clinical syndrome. It is found in cerebellar hemangioblastoma, uterine fibroids, pheochromocytomas, and renal cell, ovarian and hepatic cancers.[38,39] Treatment can include surgical reduction of tumor mass, chemotherapy, or phlebotomy. Other less well-defined syndromes include production of thrombopoietin, leukopoietin, or colony-stimulating factor by some tumors. These conditions are treated by appropriate chemotherapy to reduce their size or by surgical removal.

Renin production

Production of renin by renal (Wilms tumor, renal cell carcinoma, or hemangiopericytoma), lung (SCLC, adenocarcinoma), hepatic, pancreatic, or ovarian carcinomas can produce a clinical syndrome characterized by hypertension, hypokalemia, and evidence of increased aldosterone production.[40] Therapy with spironolactone, angiotensin-converting enzyme inhibitors, or angiotensin receptor antagonists may lower the blood pressure and normalize electrolyte abnormalities in patients in whom the tumor cannot be resected.

Growth hormone and prolactin

Acromegaly is a condition characterized by elevated growth hormone (GH) and IGF-1 levels, most commonly caused by a pituitary tumor. There are rare examples of GH production by lung and gastric adenocarcinomas. Ectopic production of growth hormone-releasing hormone (GHRH), the hypothalamic peptide that normally regulates GH production by the pituitary, has been demonstrated for islet cell tumors, bronchogenic carcinoids, and SCLC.[41] It is unlikely that treatment with somatostatin analogs, one of the mainstay therapies for pituitary tumors producing GH, will be effective. However, the GH antagonist, pegvisomant, is likely to be effective for treating GH excess. Ectopic prolactin production is found rarely in gonadoblastoma, lymphoma, leukemia, and colorectal cancer.[40,42–44] The clinical syndrome includes galactorrhea and amenorrhea in women and hypogonadism and gynecomastia in men. Dopamine agonists (bromocriptine, quinagolide, or cabergoline), effective for treatment of pituitary prolactinomas, are generally ineffective for treatment of ectopic prolactin production and it may be necessary to supplement estrogen/progesterone in women and testosterone in men.

Oncologic complications of endocrine functions

Hypothalamic–pituitary dysfunction

Radiotherapy is a cause of hypothalamic–pituitary dysfunction in cancer patients. There is no strong direct evidence to implicate cytotoxic chemotherapy as a cause of hypothalamic–pituitary dysfunction, although some targeted therapies may affect pituitary function. Metastasis to the hypothalamic region or the pituitary gland is uncommon, and endocrine dysfunction due to metastatic disease is rare although pituitary tumors and craniopharyngiomas frequently affect this anatomic region and cause endocrine problems.[45] Cancer immunotherapy by immune checkpoint blockade [anti-CTLA4 antibodies (ipilimumab and tremelimumab), anti-PD-1 antibodies (nivolumab, cemiplimab, and pembrolizumab), and anti-PD-L1 antibodies (avelumab and atezolizumab)] has been associated with development of autoimmune hypophysitis that requires hormonal replacement (corticosteroids or thyroid hormone).

Hormonal deficiency can insidiously manifest years after radiation, and the rapidity of onset and severity of dysfunction depend on the total dose and delivery rate of radiation. The sequence and frequency of dysfunction vary among the hypothalamic–pituitary axes: the somatotropic axis being the most susceptible, and the thyrotropic axis the least susceptible (Figure 1).[46–49]

The diagnosis of hypothalamic–pituitary dysfunction requires vigilance of the physician because most presenting symptoms (e.g., fatigue and weakness) are nonspecific and attributable to other causes common among cancer patients. Signs of overt hypopituitarism include hypoglycemia, hypotension, and hypothermia. In children and adolescents, growth and sexual development should be monitored using serial measurement of height and weight and staging sexual development according to Tanner's criteria. In children treated with spinal and craniospinal irradiation, local rather than general growth abnormalities may be present; foot size and radiographic bone age are reliable indicators of general growth. In adults who have received cranial or head and neck irradiation, detection of hypothalamic–pituitary abnormalities is more challenging. Immune checkpoint inhibitor-induced hypophysitis and hypopituitarism typically occur after the third or fourth dose of immune checkpoint inhibitor. In addition to symptoms of hypopituitarism such as general weakness, fatigue, anorexia, nausea, weight loss, altered mental status, cold intolerance, and arthralgia, hypophysitis cases may also have symptoms of headache and rarely visual defects (typically bitemporal hemianopsia). Morbidity of hypophysitis is predominantly related to central adrenal insufficiency and can be fatal if undiagnosed and untreated.[50]

If initial evaluation of thyroid (free T_4 and TSH), adrenal (ACTH and 8 AM serum cortisol), growth (GH and IGF-1), and gonadal (LH, FSH, and estradiol in females or testosterone in males) axes shows abnormalities, then detailed dynamic testing (e.g., low dose cosyntropin stimulation test) to evaluate the hypothalamic/pituitary axes should be performed (Table 1). Diagnostic MR imaging of the sella-pituitary area is indicated. Patients undergoing immune checkpoint inhibitor immunotherapy should be routinely screened for central hypothyroidism and adrenal insufficiency to facilitate early diagnosis and treatment.

Initial treatment of immunotherapy-induced hypophysitis may include high-dose glucocorticoids (1 mg/kg methylprednisone or equivalent) along with management of hyponatremia and hypotension. Without significant hyponatremia, intense headaches, or optic chiasm compression, physiologic replacement of glucocorticoids may be considered.[51] Hormonal deficiencies are managed by hormone replacement therapy, although the replacement of GH in patients with active cancer is controversial.

Central/secondary hypothyroidism has been caused by bexarotene (a RXR-selective ligand used in the treatment of cutaneous T-cell lymphoma) in a dose-dependent manner.[52] A single dose can rapidly suppress TSH in healthy subjects.[53] In addition to suppressing transcription of TSH by an RXR-mediated thyroid hormone-independent mechanism, bexarotene also increases metabolic clearance of thyroid hormones by a nondeiodinase-mediated pathway.[54] Long-term central hypothyroidism is managed with thyroid hormone replacement. L-Asparaginase, in addition to inhibition of TBG synthesis, may also inhibit TSH synthesis reversibly and lead to temporary hypothyroidism with decreased free T_4 levels.[55] Temporary reversible short-term central hypothyroidism may not need any intervention.

Secondary adrenal insufficiency because of metastasis to the pituitary or hypothalamus may rarely occur. The most common cause of secondary adrenal hypofunction, however, is exogenous glucocorticoid therapy that suppresses hypothalamic–pituitary–adrenal function. A prolonged course of therapy may lead to hypothalamic–pituitary suppression lasting for many months or a lifetime. Short periods of steroid therapy (i.e., 1, 2, or 4 weeks) in patients with leukemia and lymphoma suppress adrenal function for 2–4 days in most patients, and for longer in some patients. In patients who have received glucocorticoids for more than 2 weeks, a tapering period of 10–14 days should be considered. This is especially true for chemotherapy regimens that included high-dose glucocorticoids such as those used in the treatment of acute leukemia, lymphoma, and myeloma. In addition, patients who have been treated within the past year with prolonged glucocorticoid courses should receive stress dosages of glucocorticoid if acute medical or surgical complications occur (e.g., neutropenic fever with hypotension, and acute typhlitis). Irradiation of the hypothalamic–pituitary region causes ACTH deficiency and secondary adrenal insufficiency in 19–42% of treated patients (Figure 2). Several diagnostic approaches have been used to evaluate secondary adrenal insufficiency, including basal 8 am serum cortisol measurements and dynamic tests with 1 µg of synthetic $ACTH_{(1-24)}$, insulin-induced hypoglycemia (not

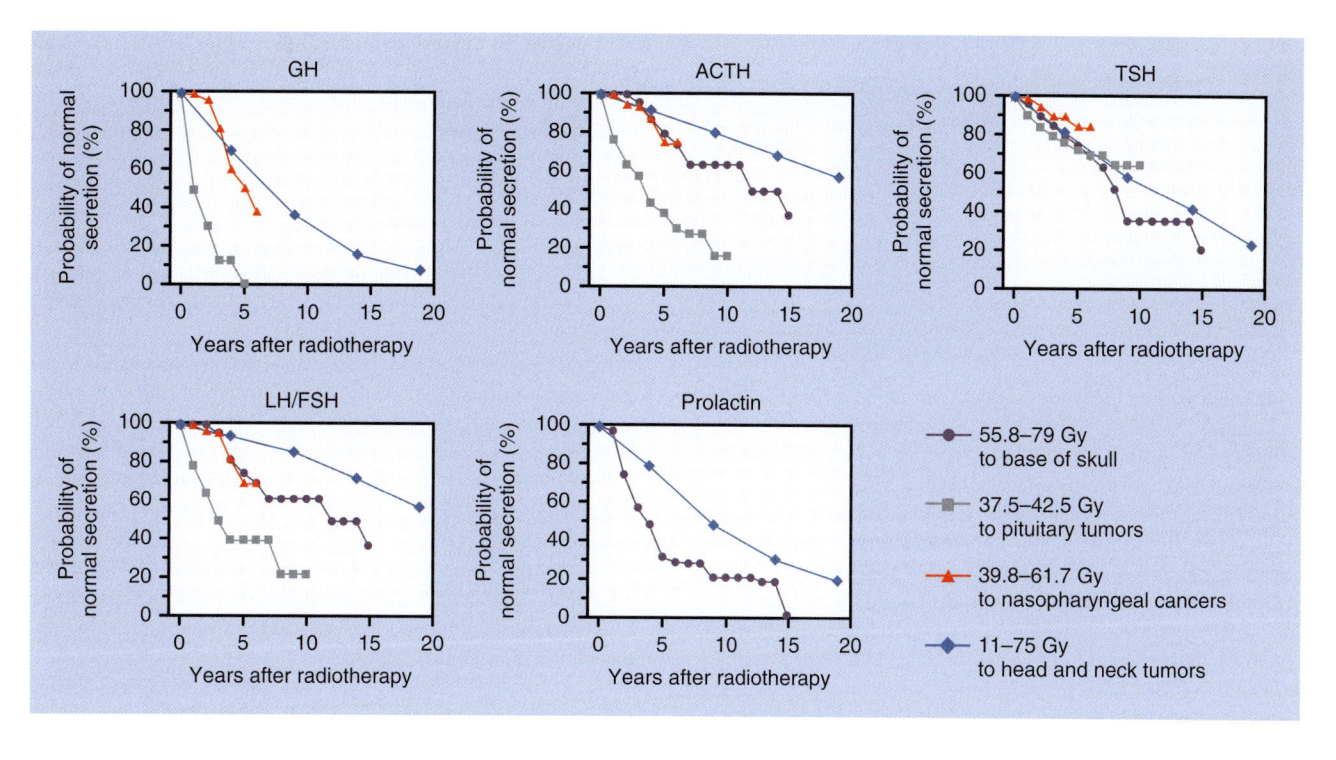

Figure 2 Probability of normal pituitary hormone secretion over time after radiation exposure to the hypothalamic–pituitary areas. Data from four studies were replotted on this single figure. The first set of values (*closed circle*) are from Pai et al.[47] where the patient received 55.8–79 Gy to the base of the skull. The second set of values (*solid square*) are from Shalet et al.,[56] where patients with pituitary tumors were treated with 37.5–42.5 Gy. The third series (*open triangle*), from Lam et al., shows the effect of radiation treatment for nasopharyngeal carcinoma with 39.8–61.7 Gy.[46] The final series (*open diamond*) represents data from Samaan et al.,[48] in which 11–75 Gy was administered to treat of head and neck tumors.

done often because of potential neurologic effects of a low glucose), or metyrapone. Impaired pituitary ACTH secretion also occurs in the setting of immune checkpoint inhibitor-induced hypophysitis as discussed above.

Primary thyroid dysfunction

Therapy-induced hypothalamic–pituitary dysfunction of the thyroid axis has been discussed above. Primary thyroid disorders and abnormalities in thyroid function are commonly associated with antineoplastic therapy. Therapy-induced atrophy/destruction of the thyroid glands through inhibition of angiogenesis and thyroiditis or disruption of thyroid hormone synthesis will cause primary hypothyroidism. Mechanisms that change serum binding and conversion of thyroxine to triiodothyronine may change thyroid hormone test results without true thyroid dysfunction.

Serum thyroid hormone-binding protein abnormalities

The levels of thyroid hormone-binding proteins (thyroxine-binding globulin [TBG], prealbumin, and albumin) can be modified by sex hormone levels and nutritional factors; abnormalities of both are encountered frequently in cancer patients. Several chemotherapy drugs affect thyroid function test results. L-Asparaginase appears to reversibly inhibit synthesis of albumin and TBG, resulting in low total thyroxine (T_4) but normal free T_4 levels.[57] Both 5-fluorouracil and mitotane increase the total T_4 and triiodothyronine (T_3) levels without suppressing TSH, suggesting that these drugs increase thyroid hormone-binding capacity in the serum.[58,59]

Euthyroid sick syndrome

Alterations in thyroid hormone metabolism occur in patients with cancer and other serious systemic illnesses.[60] Low serum T_3 levels, which may be found in up to 70% of moderately to seriously ill cancer patients, are caused by a decrease in the extrathyroidal conversion of T_4 to T_3. Serum concentrations of free T_4 are usually normal or high, while concentrations of free T_3 are below normal or low. The patients are clinically euthyroid, and serum TSH level and TRH stimulation test results are normal. Clinical manifestations of hypothyroidism are usually absent, but assessment may be confounded by obtundation, edema, and hypothermia that may accompany advanced cancer. Low free T_4 levels in the context of euthyroid sick syndrome usually indicate a grave prognosis, with a mortality rate of more than 50%. Although it is generally accepted that thyroid hormone therapy has no benefit, in practice it is sometimes difficult to differentiate between the euthyroid sick syndrome and central hypothyroidism.

Hypothyroidism

Hypothyroid symptoms are often nonspecific.[61] Typical complaints include fatigue, lethargy, constipation, and cold intolerance. However, unrecognized severe hypothyroidism may progress to myxedema coma. Severe hypothyroidism signs and symptoms include slow mentation, lethargy, bradycardia, hyponatremia, or hypothermia. The management involves replacement of thyroid hormone (levothyroxine) and supportive measures.[62]

Radiation

Radiation is an important cause of primary hypothyroidism. Radiation damage induces thyroid follicular cell destruction, inhibition of cell division, vascular damage, and possibly an immune response causing further immune-mediated glandular destruction. Factors that increase the risk of primary hypothyroidism include a high radiation dose to the vicinity of the thyroid, duration since therapy, lack of shielding of the thyroid during radiotherapy, and

Table 2 Incidence of hypothyroidism (including compensated hypothyroidism) after radiotherapy.

Type of malignancy or conditions	Radiation dose	% with hypothyroidism
Hodgkin disease	30–60 Gy	30–50
Head and neck cancer	40–72 Gy	25–50
Lymphoma	20–40 Gy (median 36 Gy)	30–42
Breast carcinoma	?	15–21
Total-body irradiation in BMT	13.75–15 Gy	15–43

Abbreviation: BMT, bone marrow transplantation.

combined irradiation and surgical treatments.[63] The incidences of primary hypothyroidism after radiotherapy vary for various cancers and conditions (Table 2).[48,63–73] A relationship between radiation dose and the prevalence of hypothyroidism is clear and is based on studies of patients with Hodgkin disease.[66,69] Long-term follow-up suggests that the threshold for causing clinically evident hypothyroidism is approximately 10 Gy. For Hodgkin disease patients who received >30 Gy, the actuarial risk was up to 45% 20 years after irradiation.[66] Patients with frank or subclinical hypothyroidism should receive thyroid hormone replacement.

Children who have received either head-and-neck or cranial irradiation should have routine screening for thyroid dysfunction. Early detection of thyroid dysfunction will permit medical intervention before hypothyroidism adversely affects physical and intellectual development and growth. In adults, neck irradiation for treatment of lymphoma and various head and neck tumors is associated with a high incidence of primary hypothyroidism. Patients who have received irradiation should also have regular screening for thyroid dysfunction.

Chemotherapy

The diagnosis of hypothyroidism in 14% of BMT patients who received chemotherapy but did not receive total-body irradiation suggests a causal relation between hypothyroidism and high-dose combination cytotoxic chemotherapy.[74] This observation is also supported by studies that showed an increased incidence of primary hypothyroidism in patients treated with multiple combination drug regimens with or without radiation.[75,76]

Targeted therapy

Tyrosine kinase inhibitors (TKIs) may cause primary hypothyroidism. A number of TKIs target tyrosine kinase receptors with well-defined functions in the thyroid gland, that is, VEGFR, EGFR, RET, KIT, MET, and downstream signaling pathways, for example, BRAF, PI3K, and mTOR pathways. Particularly, RET and BRAF play important roles in thyroid physiology. Nevertheless, primary hypothyroidism occurs at significant incidence rates: sunitinib, 7–85%; pazopanib, 12%; nilotinib, 22%; axitinib, 20–100%; cabozantinib, 15%; sorafenib, 8–39%; dasatinib, 50%; and imatinib, 0–25%. Several of these TKIs interfere with normal thyroid hormone absorption; patients on thyroid replacement therapy for preexisting hypothyroidism should be closely monitored. Monoclonal antibody against VEGFR2 (ramucirumab) also causes hypothyroidism, but antibody against VEGF-A (bevacizumab) does not seem to be associated with thyroid dysfunction. Routine screening for thyroid dysfunction during therapy with TKIs known to cause hypothyroidism is indicated.[77]

The etiologic mechanisms may include the following: (1) Destruction/atrophy of thyroid gland: antiangiogenic effects lead to regression of the gland vascular bed with capillary dysfunction and destruction of thyroid tissue, and if thyroid autoimmunity is triggered, immune thyroiditis may cause further damage. Sunitinib, sorafenib, and nilotinib, but not imatinib, may induce autoimmune thyroiditis; (2) Inhibition of thyroid hormone synthesis (It has been suggested that sunitinib directly inhibits the sodium and iodide symporter or thyroperoxidase); and (3) Inhibition of monocarboxylate transporter 8 (MCT8), the principal thyroid hormone transport protein (MCT8 is inhibited by imatinib and sunitinib). These inhibitors inhibit different targets with varying potencies/selectivity, and the relative contribution of inhibition of specific pathways or specific etiologic mechanisms of specific TKIs will vary.

Agents approved (vandetanib, cabozantinib, sorafenib, lenvatinib, pazopanib, and sunitinib) for treatment of differentiated or medullary thyroid carcinoma increase TSH and decrease thyroid hormone levels in patients previously stable on thyroid hormone replacement at high incidence rates: vandetanib, 49%; cabozantinib, 57%; sorafenib, 41%; lenvatinib, 57%. Increasing the thyroid hormone dosages by as much as one-third generally resolves the problem. This increased dose requirement may be related to increased thyroid hormone clearance. As many of these agents cause diarrhea and malabsorption, another mechanism is reduced absorption of thyroid hormone.

Immunotherapy

Immune thyroiditis is a recognized side effect of immunotherapy using cytokine treatments and immune checkpoint inhibitors. Increased titers of thyroid peroxidase antibodies and antithyroglobulin antibodies may be present and help to diagnose thyroiditis. Thyroiditis typically has a clinical course of transient hyperthyroidism (due to thyroid hormones released by destruction of the thyroid gland) followed by prolonged or permanent hypothyroidism.[78,79] Treatment with interleukin-2 produces thyroid dysfunction in approximately 20–35% of patients.[80] Approximately 10% of interferon-treated patients develop primary hypothyroidism.[81] Patients with antithyroid antibodies before therapy are at higher risk of cytokine-induced thyroid dysfunction.

Immune checkpoint inhibitor-induced immune thyroiditis may destroy enough thyroid tissue to cause hyperthyroidism (caused by inflammatory release of preformed thyroid hormone) followed by primary hypothyroidism.[82] Almost two-third of the patients are asymptomatic during the hyperthyroid phase. Hypothyroidism occurs in over 80% of patients after a median of about 10 weeks after starting immunotherapy. Less than 1% of the hypothyroid patients recover. Increased titers of thyroid peroxidase antibodies and antithyroglobulin antibodies are present in 45% and 33%, respectively when thyroiditis is diagnosed. Immune checkpoint inhibitor combinations induce thyroid dysfunction earlier than monotherapy.

Thyroidectomy

Thyroidectomy may be performed for a variety of oncologic reasons in the management of thyroid cancer, head and neck cancer, or thyroid metastasis. Thyroid hormone replacement is needed in these patients. In thyroid cancer patients, suprahysiologic doses of thyroid hormone are adjusted to suppress TSH with a goal of avoiding hyperthyroid symptoms. In others, the dose should be adjusted to keep TSH normal.

^{131}I-Containing compounds

The use of ^{131}I for the treatment of thyroid cancer requires a high serum TSH level. High TSH level is achieved by either withholding thyroid hormone replacement in a thyroidectomized patient or increasingly by administration of recombinant human TSH. The use of ^{131}I-containing compounds in the treatment of other tumors may result in hypothyroidism. For instance, using high-dose (100–1000 mCi) [^{131}I]-metaiodobenzylguanidine to treat unresectable or malignant pheochromocytoma may result in primary hypothyroidism.[83]

Hyperthyroidism
Thyrotoxicosis may precipitate arrhythmia, such as atrial fibrillation, flutter, and supraventricular tachycardia. Graves disease is autoimmune hyperthyroidism due to stimulation by antibodies for TSHR (thyrotropin receptor antibodies [TrAbs]). Measurements of thyroid peroxidase antibodies, TrAbs, and radioactive iodine uptake can distinguish Graves disease from thyroiditis. Low uptake of radioiodine by the thyroid in most of these cases suggests a diagnosis of silent thyroiditis; high uptake diffusely spread throughout the thyroid gland is most consistent with Graves disease. The clinical presentation of thyrotoxicosis in thyroiditis is usually mild and manageable with β-blockers. However, in patients with Graves disease, serious thyrotoxicosis may qualify as thyroid storms that may require additional treatments (antithyroid agents, glucocorticoids, potassium iodide, iopanoic acid, etc.).[84,85]

Radiation-induced painless thyroiditis with hyperthyroxinemia is an uncommon side effect of external beam radiotherapy to the head and neck area. Transient hyperthyroidism may occur as a result of inflammation and destruction of thyroid tissue with release of thyroglobulin (containing T_4 and T_3). Transient hyperthyroidism has been reported after mantle radiotherapy in Hodgkin disease patients and occurs usually within 18 months of treatment.[86] There have also been examples of TKI-associated hyperthyroidism, including two deaths (sorafenib- and sunitinib-associated).[87] The presumed mechanism of hyperthyroidism is thyroiditis. Almost one-third of the immune checkpoint inhibitor-induced immune thyroiditis patients have symptoms during the hyperthyroid phase.[82]

Graves' disease as an irAE accounts for only a small percentage of thyrotoxic patients after immune checkpoint inhibitor therapy. In one series of Hodgkin disease patients treated with radiation, the risk of Graves' disease after irradiation was estimated to be at least 7.2 times that in a healthy population.[66] Radiation-induced thyroid injury may trigger an autoimmune process leading to Graves' disease. Graves' ophthalmopathy has been reported to occur 18–84 months after high-dose radiotherapy to the neck for lymphoma and various solid tumors. Ophthalmopathy may occur without hyperthyroidism and in the absence of the human leukocyte antigen-B8.[88] However, euthyroid ophthalmopathy is rare after cancer immunotherapy (e.g., interferon and immune checkpoint inhibitors).

Adrenal diseases

Adrenal metastasis
Hematogenous metastasis to the adrenal glands is common, exceeded in frequency by metastasis to the lung, liver, and bone.[89] About one-half to two-thirds of cases with adrenal metastasis are bilateral. Characteristics on CT scan that suggest cancer metastasis rather than primary adrenal disease include heterogeneity, intravenous contrast enhancement, bilaterality, and size >3 cm.[90] Without evidence of metastatic disease elsewhere, whether the adrenal mass is actually a metastasis is critical information in determining cancer therapy. Evaluation of a cancer patient with an adrenal mass should include a history and physical examination to ascertain evidence of adrenal insufficiency, Cushing syndrome, mineralocorticoid excess, or pheochromocytoma. Biochemical assessment should include a standard cosyntropin (250 mcg, intravenously) stimulation test to rule out adrenal insufficiency. A 24-h urine collection should measure urinary free cortisol, aldosterone, catecholamines, and metanephrines. Pheochromocytoma must be excluded, especially if there is hypertension or any planned operative procedure.[91] MRI may help to diagnose pheochromocytoma. Functional scintigraphy using ^{131}I-6-iodomethyl-19-*nor*-cholesterol (NP-59) may be used in conjunction with CT and MRI to aid the diagnosis of a unilateral adrenal mass >2 cm.[92] If there is no evidence of pheochromocytoma, CT-guided fine-needle aspiration of the adrenal mass, which is 85% sensitive in detecting cancer, may be considered.[93]

Adrenal insufficiency
Clinically evident adrenal hypofunction occurs infrequently, except when both adrenal glands are extensively affected by metastases.[94] It is estimated that >80% of adrenal tissue must be destroyed before corticosteroid production is impaired.[95] Because the clinical manifestations of adrenal insufficiency are nonspecific and overlap findings in cancer patients, a high index of suspicion is required to detect this treatable condition. The cachexia and weakness seen in patients with adrenal insufficiency can mimic the general wasting (cancer cachexia) seen in patients with extensive metastatic disease. Electrolyte abnormalities are often attributed to poor intake, malnutrition, side effects of chemotherapeutic agents, or paraneoplastic syndromes without recognition of the contribution by adrenal insufficiency.

Adrenal insufficiency is diagnosed by the cosyntropin (250 mcg of cosyntropin IV with basal, 30 and 60 min cortisol measurements) stimulation test. Glucocorticoid (20 mg of hydrocortisone in the morning and 10 mg in the early afternoon) and mineralocorticoid replacement therapy may be started when adrenal insufficiency is suspected and stopped after normal adrenal function is documented. In the event of circulatory instability, sepsis, emergency surgery, or other major complications, stress dosages of parenteral glucocorticoid should be given (e.g., hydrocortisone succinate 100 mg intravenously every 8 h).

Approximately 20–30% of the patients with bilateral adrenal metastasis will develop adrenal insufficiency.[94] Other causes of primary adrenal insufficiency in cancer patients include autoimmune adrenalitis induced by immune checkpoint inhibitors, adrenal hemorrhage, and granulomatous diseases. Many cancer patients may be immunocompromised (e.g., leukemia patients with prolonged neutropenia), and are susceptible to infection of the adrenal glands by cytomegalovirus, mycobacteria, or fungi, etc., leading to adrenal insufficiency.

Drugs that cause adrenal insufficiency include etomidate, a common intravenous anesthetic, and ketoconazole, an antifungal drug; they inhibit the production of cytochrome P450-dependent enzymes in glucocorticoid synthesis.[94] Aminoglutethimide and metyrapone inhibit enzymes in steroidogenesis and may cause adrenal insufficiency when used for treatment of prostate, breast, and adrenocortical cancers. Mitotane, structurally related to the insecticide dichlorodiphenyltrichloroethane (DDT), has selective toxicity for adrenocortical cells. Adrenal insufficiency is common at mitotane doses used to treat adrenocortical cancer and there may be increased daily requirement of glucocorticoids due to increased binding of glucocorticoids to proteins.[59]

Sexual dysfunction

Sexual function is affected directly by hyperprolactinemia or gonadotropin deficiency, commonly observed in patients treated with >40 Gy of cranial irradiation.

Hyperprolactinemia occurs commonly (up to 50% incidence within 2 years) following head and neck irradiation with a median hypothalamic–pituitary radiation exposure of 50–57 Gy.[48] Hyperprolactinemia inhibits the secretion of gonadotropins by the pituitary and decreases the responsiveness of the pituitary to gonadotropin-releasing hormone, thereby causing secondary hypogonadism. Treatment with dopamine agonists (bromocriptine or cabergoline) inhibits prolactin secretion, and it may be reasonable to proceed with a therapeutic trial, assessing serum prolactin at periodic intervals, if other anterior pituitary functions are normal.

Gonadotropin deficiency occurs commonly (up to 61%) in patients treated with irradiation for brain tumors.[96] In children, delayed puberty, absent menarche, and inadequate sexual development are significant problems related to gonadotropin deficiency. Early or precocious puberty has been reported in patients treated with combined chemotherapy and cranial irradiation for acute lymphoblastic leukemia or brain tumor.[97,98] In adults, gonadotropin deficiency may cause sex hormone deficiency, low libido, and sexual dysfunction (impotence).

Engergy balance and glucose metabolism

Obesity and metabolic syndrome

Cancer treatments may lead to obesity and the metabolic syndrome (a cluster consisting of central obesity, low high-density lipoprotein (HDL) cholesterol, hyperglycemia, hypertriglyceridemia, and hypertension).[99-101] The mechanisms by which obesity promotes cancer include: hyperinsulinemia due to insulin resistance, high IGF-1, adipokines, low adiponectin, increased production of estrogens by adipose tissue and increased inflammation. Obesity in cancer survivors may place them at increased risk for poor disease outcomes and secondary colorectal and genitourinary cancers.[99,102-104] Although low physical activity can contribute to obesity, the pathophysiologic basis of the weight gain in cancer survivors is unclear. Since obesity is an adverse prognostic factor for many cancers and is a modifiable risk factor, secondary obesity after cancer treatment needs to be addressed.

Diabetes mellitus

Diabetes mellitus type 2 (DM2) is associated with an elevated risk of pancreatic, liver, colon, gastric, breast, and endometrial cancer.[105-110] Extensive epidemiologic data suggest important roles of DM2 in carcinogenesis and cancer survival.[105-111] Apart from the frequently coexisting obesity, the mechanisms by which diabetes promotes cancer include hyperinsulinemia, high IGF-1, and hyperglycemia. Evidence-based guidelines for the management of DM2 in cancer patients to optimize patient survival are lacking.

The administration of glucocorticoids (e.g., in combination therapy regimens, for edema of brain metastasis, for prevention of transplant rejection, for graft-versus-host disease in stem cell transplantation, and for nausea/vomiting) is a frequent cause of diabetes mellitus in cancer patients. Therefore, patients who receive glucocorticoids must be periodically screened for diabetes with evaluation of fasting glucose levels during therapy. Treatment with streptozocin or L-asparaginase may result in insulin-deficient diabetes mellitus. Diabetes mellitus may also develop as a consequence of serious pancreatitis secondary to treatment with L-asparaginase.[112,113] Immunotherapy for cancer using cytokines such as interleukin-2 and interferons may cause toxicity to pancreatic β cells and lead to insulin-dependent diabetes.[114] Immunotherapy with immune checkpoint inhibitors can induce type I diabetes mellitus, and diabetic ketoacidosis can occur even after one dose.[115-118] Tacrolimus, an immunosuppressive agent used to prevent graft-versus-host disease, also increases the incidence of diabetes, perhaps by damaging pancreatic β cells.[119] Patients who received allogenic stem cell transplants are likely to be receiving both glucocorticoids, cyclosporine A and tacrolimus, and are particularly at risk for developing diabetes mellitus.[120] Management of the blood glucose levels would depend on the severity of the blood glucose abnormality and on the underlying pathophysiologic mechanism of hyperglycemia. Measurement of C-peptide can determine whether there is endogenous insulinopenia. In general, insulin will be needed in patients who are insulin deficient.

Disorders of lipid metabolism

Short-term lipid abnormalities caused by cancer therapy are generally of little clinical significance. However, major abnormalities can lead to acute complications such as stroke and pancreatitis. Interferons and vitamin A derivatives can cause significant increases in triglycerides that can lead to pancreatitis. Interferons cause hypertriglyceridemia by increasing hepatic and peripheral fatty acid production and by suppressing hepatic triglyceride lipase.[121,122] Long-term treatment with interferon-α_2 causes hypertriglyceridemia in approximately one-third of patients, most of whom had previous serum lipid abnormalities. Serum triglyceride levels of more than 1000 mg/dL are not unusual. All-*trans*-retinoic acid (tretinoin) and derivatives, such as 13-*cis*-retinoic acid (isotretinoin), have been used to treat several malignancies, most notably head and neck cancers and acute promyelocytic leukemia. They are well known to induce hypertriglyceridemia by elevating very-low-density lipoprotein level and hypercholesterolemia by increasing low-density lipoprotein level. Hyperlipidemia may be treated with gemfibrozil or fish oil in combination with diet.

Disorders of electrolyte/mineral metabolism

Hyponatremia

Platinum drugs and alkylating agents such as ifosfamide and cyclophosphamide are toxic to the proximal renal tubules. Although cisplatin has been reported to induce SIADH, the mechanism of cisplatin-induced hyponatremia is unclear. Cisplatin may induce hyponatremia by renal salt wasting due to nephrotoxicity, that is, decreased papillary solute content, and maximal urinary osmolality.[123] In a majority of the patients who have elevated vasopressin levels, the vasopressin levels became suppressed after correction of hypovolemia.[123] Therefore, the stimulus for vasopressin was probably hypovolemia caused by renal salt wasting. High-dose cyclophosphamide may directly affect the hypothalamus, releasing vasopressin.[124] Low-dose cyclophosphamide also causes hyponatremia, urinary hypertonicity, and increased plasma vasopressin levels. Damage to the renal tubules and resulting defects in salt and water transport may be the major cause of hyponatremia associated with low-dose cyclophosphamide.[125] Ifosfamide is structurally related to cyclophosphamide; ifosfamide is rapidly taken up into renal tubular cells through organic cation transporters and metabolized into chloracetaldehyde which is toxic.

Risk factors for hyponatremia include treatment-induced nausea and vomiting, certain chemotherapy agents, hydration with hypotonic fluid, pain, opiates, and stress (both physical and psychological). Drug-induced renal salt wasting or tumor-induced salt wasting (mediated by atrial natriuretic peptide) can also cause hyponatremia, hypoosmolality, elevated urinary sodium, and urinary osmolality.[126] These SIADH-like syndromes are difficult to distinguish from SIADH when signs and symptoms of fluid volume depletion are subtle or absent (Figure 1). For hypovolemia and sodium loss, fluid and sodium replacement is the primary treatment.

Hypernatremia

Hypernatremia secondary to central diabetes insipidus occurs frequently as a complication of neurosurgery or tumor invasion into the supraoptic or paraventricular hypothalamic nuclei or posterior pituitary. Nephrogenic diabetes insipidus (damage to tubular cells) can result from the effects of ifosfamide or streptozocin on tubular reabsorption of water. Ifosfamide has broad nephrotoxic effects, although tubular damage predominates. Distal tubular defects develop in about half of patients treated with ifosfamide. However, frank nephrogenic diabetes insipidus leading to hypernatremia is not common.[127] Streptozocin is another nephrotoxic drug; in addition to causing glomerular defects (proteinuria) and tubular defects (Fanconi syndrome), streptozocin therapy has been reported to cause nephrogenic diabetes insipidus.[128]

Hypocalcemia

Hypocalcemia may be one of the features of tumor lysis syndrome. Hypocalcemia can also be caused by primary hypoparathyroidism after surgical procedures in the neck that sacrifice or damage the parathyroid glands (e.g., total laryngectomy, total thyroidectomy). Primary hypoparathyroidism has also been reported as an immune-mediated adverse effect of immune checkpoint immunotherapy.[129-132]

Chemotherapy-induced hypocalcemia is common.[133] Carboplatin has a 16–31% incidence of hypocalcemia and cisplatin a 6–20% incidence. Platinum drugs have toxic effects on renal tubular function, magnesium metabolism, bone resorption, and vitamin D production, all contributing to development of hypocalcemia. Profound hypomagnesemia causes a decrease in the secretion of PTH and a reduction in the calcium-mobilizing effects of PTH. Hypomagnesemia also inhibits formation of 1,25-dihydroxy vitamin D_3 (1,25-dihydroxycholecalciferol). Cisplatin may inhibit the mitochondrial function in the kidneys and thereby inhibit conversion of 25-hydroxycholecalciferol to 1,25-dihydroxy cholecalciferol by the enzyme 1-alpha-hydroxylase. In addition, platinum drugs may have a direct inhibitory effect on bone resorption. Asymptomatic hypomagnesemia, hypocalcemia, and hypoparathyroidism have also been reported in patients treated with a combination of doxorubicin and cytarabine.

In thyroid cancer or head and neck cancer patients, many TKIs cause diarrheal side effects. It is important to note this may induce malabsorption of calcium, magnesium, and vitamin D, causing worsening hypocalcemia or hypomagnesemia in patients with mild hypoparathyroidism.[134]

Hypercalcemia

The paraneoplastic syndrome of hypercalcemia of malignancy is discussed in the first section of this article. No chemotherapy has been identified as a cause of hypercalcemia. However, there is a clear association between low-dose (usually 2–7.5 Gy) external-beam irradiation of the head and neck area and subsequent development of primary hyperparathyroidism.[135] Among patients who developed primary hyperparathyroidism, 14–30% had prior exposure to radiation. The interval from irradiation to development of hyperparathyroidism ranges from 29 to 47 years. Primary hyperparathyroidism also develops sporadically and in the context of multiple endocrine neoplasia, types 1 and 2. Surgery is the principal treatment for primary hyperparathyroidism. Removal of adenoma is usually curative, but in the context of multiple endocrine neoplasia type 1 (MEN1), the surgical procedure of choice is 3.5-gland parathyroidectomy.[136]

Hypomagnesemia

Long-term hypomagnesemia is linked to increased risks of diabetes, hypertension, coronary artery disease, ischemic stroke, and cardiac arrhythmias. Hypomagnesemia is associated with unfavorable overall survival in ovarian cancer patients.[137] Mild hypomagnesemia is generally associated with no symptoms; in those with very low magnesium levels symptoms may include general weakness and easy fatigue, muscle twitches, tremor, constipation, hyperreflexia, nausea, and vomiting.

Hypomagnesemia may be caused by renal wasting following cyclical glucocorticoid, antiinfective agents (e.g., amphotericin B), nephrotoxic chemotherapy, or targeted therapies. Chemotherapy with cisplatin, carboplatin, and oxaliplatin causes morphologic changes and necrosis in the proximal tubule, an important site of magnesium reabsorption. Hypomagnesemia after platinum chemotherapy is highly prevalent. Alkylating agents such as ifosfamide and cyclophosphamide also have similar nephrotoxicity causing hypomagnesemia. Treatment with monoclonal antibodies that block epidermal growth factor interaction with its receptor on distal convoluted tubule cells reduces renal magnesium reabsorption reversably.[138] The incidence of hypomagnesemia is 17% in patients treated with anti-EGFR antibodies (cetuximab and panitumumab), and the risk of hypomagnesemia increases by about six-fold.[139]

Metabolic bone diseases

Osteoporosis

Four groups of adult cancer patients are at particular risk for accelerated bone loss and osteoporosis: (1) patients with lymphoma, myeloma, or leukemia; (2) breast cancer patients with chemotherapy-induced early menopause; (3) postmenopausal women with estrogen-receptor-positive breast cancer; and (4) men with prostate cancer who are on antiandrogenic therapy.[140] Normal bone remodeling involves a delicate balance between osteoblasts and osteoclasts. Cytotoxic chemotherapy is toxic to osteoblast function and decreases bone formation. Tumor-derived humoral factors (e.g., PTHrP, lymphotoxin, interleukin-1, and interleukin-6) may contribute to bone loss. In most cases, it is not clear whether bone loss is caused by antineoplastic therapy, the underlying malignancy, or nutritional issues (malabsorption, poor calcium and vitamin D intake, etc.). In patients with breast or prostate cancer, sex steroid hormone deficiency induced by cancer therapy is the most important causative factor for bone loss. Bone loss is prominent in malignancies affecting hematopoietic cells (myeloma, leukemia, lymphoma), perhaps because of cytokine production, an intimate relationship of hematopoietic cells with bone-forming cells, and the prolonged/repeated use of high-dose glucocorticords.

A number of drugs can induce osteoporosis in cancer patients.[141] Glucocorticoids, methotrexate and cytotoxic drugs that cause renal loss of calcium, magnesium, or phosphorus (e.g., platinum compounds, cyclophosphamide, and ifosfamide) have significant impact on bone density. Prompt diagnosis of gonadal dysfunction in cancer survivors and prompt replacement of gonadal steroids (in the absence of contraindications) in young hypogonadal men or women are recommended to decrease the risk of bone fractures. The bone mass of long-term cancer survivors should be assessed when the patient is about 30 years old, the age at which most people have attained peak bone mass.[142] If bone mass is abnormal (>2 standard deviations below normal), the patient should be referred for evaluation of the multiple reversible causes of osteoporosis. This is particularly true for therapeutic agents that lower plasma estrogen or testosterone levels, as the use of these agents is clearly associated with increased fracture risk. A key point in the management of osteoporosis in cancer patients is to measure bone mineral density (e.g., by dual-energy X-ray absorptiometry) and assess fracture risk early in the course of cancer management and to monitor the effects of cancer therapy on bone mass. Treatments for osteoporosis include bisphosphonates (e.g., alendronate, risedronate, ibandronate, or zoledronate), teriparatide, calcitonin, selective estrogen receptor modulators (SERMs), romosozumab and denosumab, in addition to a daily intake of 1200–1500 mg elemental calcium and vitamin D supplementation. While osteoporosis in children will frequently reverse as they are in the formative years of bone development, management in adults should be proactive and use a bisphosphonate or denosumab to prevent bone loss rather than waiting for fractures to occur. Nutritional deficiency in teenagers and young adults results in low bone mass. Treatment of hypocalcemia, hypomagnesemia, and vitamin D deficiency is integral to the successful therapy of osteoporosis in cancer patients.

Osteomalacia

Osteomalacia, a condition characterized by unmineralized bone matrix, is a rare complication of chemotherapy but should be considered in osteopenic patients and those with osteomalacic clinical syndrome (bone pain and proximal myopathy). The most common cause is a decrease in the serum calcium and/or phosphorus concentrations caused by nutritional deficiency and renal wasting of phosphorus and calcium. Tumor-induced osteomalacia has been discussed above in the paraneoplastic syndromes section. Patients who have received chemotherapeutic agents that cause hypophosphatemia, hypomagnesemia, or hypocalcemia are particularly at risk. Appropriate replacement therapy of these vitamins and minerals should be instituted once deficiencies have been identified. Other contributing factors include systemic acidosis and drugs such as anticonvulsants and aluminum.[141]

Ifosfamide causes tubular damage leading to renal phosphate wasting, hypophosphatemia, and rickets/osteomalacia.[143] The toxic effects of ifosfamide on renal tubular function include Fanconi syndrome. Tubular damage is common for ifosfamide doses ≥ 50 g/m^2, or when it is used in combination with cisplatin.[144] Rickets is reported most commonly in children. Estramustine, another alkylating agent used for prostate cancer, can cause hypocalcemia, hypophosphatemia, and secondary hyperparathyroidism with increased bone resorption.[145]

Key references

The complete reference list can be found on Vital Source version of this title, see inside front cover.

1. Maioli E, Fortino V. The complexity of parathyroid hormone-related protein signalling. *Cell Mol Life Sci.* 2004;**61**:257–262.
2. Eipper BA, Mains RE. Structure and biosynthesis of pro-adrenocorticotropin/endorphin and related peptides. *Endocr Rev.* 1980;**1**:1–27.
4. Findling JW, Raff H. Diagnosis and differential diagnosis of Cushing's syndrome. *Endocrinol Metab Clin North Am.* 2001;**30**:729–747.
9. Doppman JL, Oldfield EH, Nieman LK. Bilateral sampling of the internal jugular vein to distinguish between mechanisms of adrenocorticotropic hormone-dependent Cushing syndrome. *Ann Intern Med.* 1998;**128**:33–36.
11. Nieman LK, Ilias I. Evaluation and treatment of Cushing's syndrome. *Am J Med.* 2005;**118**:1340–1346.
14. Vassilopoulou-Sellin R, Newman BM, Taylor SH, Guinee VF. Incidence of hypercalcemia in patients with malignancy referred to a comprehensive cancer center. *Cancer.* 1993;**71**:1309–1312.
15. Stewart AF. Clinical practice. Hypercalcemia associated with cancer. *N Engl J Med.* 2005;**352**:373–379.
18. Berenson JR, Rosen LS, Howell A, et al. Zoledronic acid reduces skeletal-related events in patients with osteolytic metastases. *Cancer.* 2001;**91**:1191–1200.
19. Body JJ, Bartl R, Burckhardt P, et al. Current use of bisphosphonates in oncology. International Bone and Cancer Study Group. *J Clin Oncol.* 1998;**16**:3890–3899.
22. Hu MI, Glezerman IG, Lebouleux S, et al. Denosumab for treatment of hypercalcemia of malignancy. *J Clin Endocrinol Metab.* 2014;**99**:3144–3152.
27. Hoff AO, Vassilopoulou-Sellin R. The role of glucagon administration in the diagnosis and treatment of patients with tumor hypoglycemia. *Cancer.* 1998;**82**:1585–1592.
30. Flombaum CD. Metabolic emergencies in the cancer patient. *Semin Oncol.* 2000;**27**:322–334.
33. Krisanapan P, Vongsanim S, Pin-On P, et al. Efficacy of furosemide, oral sodium chloride, and fluid restriction for treatment of syndrome of inappropriate antidiuresis (SIAD): an open-label randomized controlled study (The EFFUSE-FLUID Trial). *Am J Kidney Dis.* 2020.
36. Shimada T, Mizutani S, Muto T, et al. Cloning and characterization of FGF23 as a causative factor of tumor-induced osteomalacia. *Proc Natl Acad Sci U S A.* 2001;**98**:6500–6505.
37. Jonsson KB, Zahradnik R, Larsson T, et al. Fibroblast growth factor 23 in oncogenic osteomalacia and X-linked hypophosphatemia. *N Engl J Med.* 2003;**348**:1656–1663.
41. Doga M, Bonadonna S, Burattin A, Giustina A. Ectopic secretion of growth hormone-releasing hormone (GHRH) in neuroendocrine tumors: relevant clinical aspects. *Ann Oncol.* 2001;**12**(Suppl 2):S89–S94.
45. Fassett DR, Couldwell WT. Metastases to the pituitary gland. *Neurosurg Focus.* 2004;**16**:E8.
46. Lam KS, Tse VK, Wang C, et al. Effects of cranial irradiation on hypothalamic-pituitary function–a 5-year longitudinal study in patients with nasopharyngeal carcinoma. *Q J Med.* 1991;**78**:165–176.
47. Pai HH, Thornton A, Katznelson L, et al. Hypothalamic/pituitary function following high-dose conformal radiotherapy to the base of skull: demonstration of a dose-effect relationship using dose-volume histogram analysis. *Int J Radiat Oncol Biol Phys.* 2001;**49**:1079–1092.
48. Samaan NA, Schultz PN, Yang KP, et al. Endocrine complications after radiotherapy for tumors of the head and neck. *J Lab Clin Med.* 1987;**109**:364–372.
49. Shalet SM. Disorders of the endocrine system due to radiation and cytotoxic chemotherapy. *Clin Endocrinol (Oxf).* 1983;**19**:637–659.
50. Postow MA. Managing immune checkpoint-blocking antibody side effects. *Am Soc Clin Oncol Educ Book.* 2015;**35**:76–83.
51. Faje A. Immunotherapy and hypophysitis: clinical presentation, treatment, and biologic insights. *Pituitary.* 2016;**19**:82–92.
52. Sherman SI. Etiology, diagnosis, and treatment recommendations for central hypothyroidism associated with bexarotene therapy for cutaneous T-cell lymphoma. *Clin Lymphoma.* 2003;**3**:249–252.
54. Smit JW, Stokkel MP, Pereira AM, et al. Bexarotene-induced hypothyroidism: bexarotene stimulates the peripheral metabolism of thyroid hormones. *J Clin Endocrinol Metab.* 2007;**92**:2496–2499.
56. Shalet SM, Clayton PE, Price DA. Growth and pituitary function in children treated for brain tumours or acute lymphoblastic leukaemia. *Hormone Res.* 1988;**30**:53–61.
60. Chopra IJ. Clinical review 86: euthyroid sick syndrome: is it a misnomer? *J Clin Endocrinol Metabol.* 1997;**82**:329–334.
62. IDSCITF, Farooki A, Girotra M, et al. The current understanding of the endocrine effects from immune checkpoint inhibitors and recommendations for management. *JNCI Cancer Spectrum.* 2018;**2**:pky021.
64. Grande C. Hypothyroidism following radiotherapy for head and neck cancer: multivariate analysis of risk factors. *Radiother Oncol.* 1992;**25**:31–36.
67. Constine LS, Donaldson SS, McDougall IR, et al. Thyroid dysfunction after radiotherapy in children with Hodgkin's disease. *Cancer.* 1984;**53**:878–883.
72. Sklar CA, Kim TH, Ramsay NK. Thyroid dysfunction among long-term survivors of bone marrow transplantation. *Am J Med.* 1982;**73**:688–694.

74. Toubert ME, Socie G, Gluckman E, et al. Short- and long-term follow-up of thyroid dysfunction after allogeneic bone marrow transplantation without the use of preparative total body irradiation. *Br J Haematol.* 1997;**98**:453–457.
79. Morganstein D, Lai Z, Spain L, et al. Thyroid abnormalities following the use of cytotoxic T-lymphocyte antigen-4 and programmed death receptor protein-1 inhibitors in the treatment of melanoma. *Clin Endocrinol.* 2017;**86**:614–620.
82. Iyer PC, Cabanillas ME, Waguespack SG, et al. Immune-related thyroiditis with immune checkpoint inhibitors. *Thyroid.* 2018;**28**:1243–1251.
85. Carroll R, Matfin G. Endocrine and metabolic emergencies: thyroid storm. *Ther Adv Endocrinol Metab.* 2010;**1**:139–145.
87. Haraldsdottir S, Li Q, Villalona-Calero MA, et al. Case of sorafenib-induced thyroid storm. *J Clin Oncol.* 2013;**31**:e262–e264.
96. Constine LS, Woolf PD, Cann D, et al. Hypothalamic-pituitary dysfunction after radiation for brain tumors. *N Engl J Med.* 1993;**328**:87–94.
97. Quigley C, Cowell C, Jimenez M, et al. Normal or early development of puberty despite gonadal damage in children treated for acute lymphoblastic leukemia. *N Engl J Med.* 1989;**321**:143–151.
100. Makari-Judson G, Judson CH, Mertens WC. Longitudinal patterns of weight gain after breast cancer diagnosis: observations beyond the first year. *Breast J.* 2007;**13**:258–265.
101. Saquib N, Flatt SW, Natarajan L, et al. Weight gain and recovery of pre-cancer weight after breast cancer treatments: evidence from the women's healthy eating and living (WHEL) study. *Breast Cancer Res Treat.* 2007;**105**:177–186.
103. Kroenke CH, Chen WY, Rosner B, Holmes MD. Weight, weight gain, and survival after breast cancer diagnosis. *J Clin Oncol.* 2005;**23**:1370–1378.
104. Park SM, Lim MK, Jung KW, et al. Prediagnosis smoking, obesity, insulin resistance, and second primary cancer risk in male cancer survivors: National Health Insurance Corporation Study. *J Clin Oncol.* 2007;**25**:4835–4843.
108. Richardson LC, Pollack LA. Therapy insight: Influence of type 2 diabetes on the development, treatment and outcomes of cancer. *Nat Clin Pract Oncol.* 2005;**2**:48–53.
109. Coughlin SS, Calle EE, Teras LR, et al. Diabetes mellitus as a predictor of cancer mortality in a large cohort of US adults. *Am J Epidemiol.* 2004;**159**:1160–1167.
114. Almawi WY, Tamim H, Azar ST. Clinical review 103: T helper type 1 and 2 cytokines mediate the onset and progression of type I (insulin-dependent) diabetes. *J Clin Endocrinol Metab.* 1999;**84**:1497–1502.
115. Hong AR, Yoon JH, Kim HK, Kang HC. Immune checkpoint inhibitor-induced diabetic ketoacidosis: a report of four cases and literature review. *Front Endocrinol (Lausanne).* 2020;**11**:14.
117. Akturk HK, Kahramangil D, Sarwal A, et al. Immune checkpoint inhibitor-induced Type 1 diabetes: a systematic review and meta-analysis. *Diabet Med.* 2019;**36**:1075–1081.
118. Maamari J, Yeung SJ, Chaftari PS. Diabetic ketoacidosis induced by a single dose of pembrolizumab. *Am J Emerg Med.* 2019;**37**:376 e371–376 e372.
120. Jindal RM, Sidner RA, Milgrom ML. Post-transplant diabetes mellitus. The role of immunosuppression. *Drug Saf.* 1997;**16**:242–257.
123. Anand AJ, Bashey B. Newer insights into cisplatin nephrotoxicity. *Ann Pharmacother.* 1993;**27**:1519–1525.
127. Skinner R, Pearson AD, Price L, et al. Nephrotoxicity after ifosfamide. *Arch Dis Child.* 1990;**65**:732–738.
129. Lupi I, Brancatella A, Cetani F, et al. Activating antibodies to the calcium-sensing receptor in immunotherapy-induced hypoparathyroidism. *J Clin Endocrinol Metab.* 2020;**105**.
130. Piranavan P, Li Y, Brown E, et al. Immune checkpoint inhibitor-induced hypoparathyroidism associated with calcium-sensing receptor-activating autoantibodies. *J Clin Endocrinol Metab.* 2019;**104**:550–556.
132. Win MA, Thein KZ, Qdaisat A, Yeung SJ. Acute symptomatic hypocalcemia from immune checkpoint therapy-induced hypoparathyroidism. *Am J Emerg Med.* 2017;**35**:1039 e1035–1039 e1037.
133. Yeung SC, Chiu AC, Vassilopoulou-Sellin R, Gagel RF. The endocrine effects of nonhormonal antineoplastic therapy. *Endocr Rev.* 1998;**19**:144–172.
135. Cohen J, Gierlowski TC, Schneider AB. A prospective study of hyperparathyroidism in individuals exposed to radiation in childhood. *JAMA.* 1990;**264**:581–584.
137. Liu W, Qdaisat A, Soliman PT, et al. Hypomagnesemia and survival in patients with ovarian cancer who received chemotherapy with carboplatin. *Oncologist.* 2019;**24**:e312–e317.
138. Muallem S, Moe OW. When EGF is offside, magnesium is wasted. *J Clin Invest.* 2007;**117**:2086–2089.
139. Petrelli F, Borgonovo K, Cabiddu M, et al. Risk of anti-EGFR monoclonal antibody-related hypomagnesemia: systematic review and pooled analysis of randomized studies. *Expert Opin Drug Saf.* 2012;**11**(Suppl 1):S9–S19.
142. Vassilopoulou-Sellin R, Brosnan P, Delpassand A, et al. Osteopenia in young adult survivors of childhood cancer. *Med Pediatr Oncol.* 1999;**32**:272–278.

137 Infections in patients with cancer

Harrys A. Torres, MD, FACP, FIDSA ■ Dimitrios P. Kontoyiannis, MD, ScD, FACP, FIDSA ■ Kenneth V.I. Rolston, MD, FACP

Overview

Patients with cancer have increased risk of developing infections, owing both to their underlying disease and its treatment. This risk appears to be greatest in patients with hematologic malignancies and in hematopoietic cell transplant (HCT) recipients. This is due primarily to the development of various immunologic defects such as neutropenia and impaired cellular and/or humoral immunity, each associated with a unique spectrum of infection. Newer therapeutic modalities for the treatment of some cancers are changing the spectrum of infections as are the increasing use of catheters and other medical devices. While bacterial infections are documented most often, opportunistic fungal and viral infections are being encountered with increasing frequency. The morbidity and mortality of infection in cancer patients are generally greater than in the general population. Thus, early diagnosis and the prompt administration of appropriate therapy are of paramount importance. Antimicrobial resistance among these pathogens has become a worldwide problem, which can only be partially tackled by the development of novel agents. Consequently, the importance of conducting frequent epidemiologic surveillance in order to detect local epidemiologic shifts and of infection prevention, infection control, and antimicrobial stewardship cannot be emphasized enough. The number of cancer survivors is steadily increasing. Many of these patients remain immunosuppressed for substantial periods of time. Keeping these survivors healthy and infection free will continue to be a challenge for years to come.

Infection remains a common problem in patients with cancer.[1] Neutropenia, impaired cellular or humoral immunity, the use of catheters and other medical devices, splenectomy, surgery, radiation, nutritional status, and local factors such as obstruction, increase the susceptibility to infection. Each risk factor is associated with a unique set of infections (Table 1). Multiple factors often coexist in the same patient.

Infections primarily associated with neutropenia

A causative pathogen is identified in about 20–25% of febrile episodes in neutropenic patients (microbiologically documented infections). An additional 20–25% have identifiable sites of infection but have negative cultures (clinically documented infections). Approximately 40–45% have neither a clinical focus nor positive cultures (unexplained fever) (Figure 1). Fewer than 5% of febrile episodes are due to noninfectious causes such as transfusion reactions, tumor fever, or drug fever.[2,3] Common sites of infection are the respiratory tract, bloodstream, urinary tract, skin and skin structures, and infections originating from the oropharynx and gastrointestinal tract (Figure 2).

Infections primarily associated with impaired cellular and humoral immunity

Defects in cell-mediated immunity (CMI) are common in patients with lymphoma, in allogeneic HCT recipients, in recipients on high-dose corticosteroid therapy, and in patients treated with nucleoside analogs, monoclonal antibodies, and temozolomide. Infections caused by bacteria such as *Legionella* spp., *Salmonella* spp., *Nocardia* spp., *Listeria monocytogenes*, and *Rhodococcus equi* are common.[4,5] Mycobacterial infections (*Mycobacterium tuberculosis* and nontuberculous mycobacteria) are also common in such patients. *Aspergillus* spp., *Pneumocystis jiroveci*, and fungi (*Cryptococcus neoformans*, *Histoplasma capsulatum*, *Coccidioides immitis*) cause most of the fungal infections.[6,7] Viral infections are predominantly caused by the herpes group of viruses with cytomegalovirus (CMV) being the most frequent. The community respiratory viruses are important causes of morbidity and mortality in allogeneic HCT recipients. Parasitic infections (toxoplasmosis, strongyloidiasis) are also seen more frequently in patients with impaired CMI.[8,9] In patients with impaired humoral immunity, infections caused by encapsulated organisms such as *S. pneumoniae* and *H. influenzae* are common.

Infections in patients with solid tumors

Patients with solid tumors who are not significantly immunosuppressed also develop infections frequently. Risk factors include neutropenia, disruption of normal anatomic barriers (skin, mucosal surfaces), obstruction caused by bulky tumors, radiation damage, surgical procedures, and medical devices.[10] Common sites of infection are summarized in Table 2. Removal of the offending device, and relief of obstruction, are frequently important aspects of the management of these infections.

Spectrum of infection

Bacterial infections
For several decades Gram-positive organisms (GPO) had been the predominant pathogens in neutropenic patients (Table 3).

Holland-Frei Cancer Medicine, Tenth Edition. Edited by Robert C. Bast, John C. Byrd, Carlo M. Croce, Ernest Hawk, Fadlo R. Khuri, Raphael E. Pollock, Apostolia M. Tsimberidou, Christopher G. Willett, and Cheryl L. Willman.
© 2023 John Wiley & Sons, Inc. Published 2023 by John Wiley & Sons, Inc.

Table 1 Defects in host defense mechanisms and common infections associated with malignant diseases.

Disease	Prominent defect	Predominant infections
Acute leukemia, aplastic anemia	Prolonged neutropenia	Gram-positive cocci, Gram-negative bacilli, fungi (Candida, Aspergillus, Zygomycetes, Fusarium, Trichosporon)
Hairy cell leukemia	Neutropenia, impaired lymphocyte function	Gram-negative bacilli, Gram-positive cocci, mycobacteria (including nontuberculous)
Chronic lymphocytic leukemia, multiple myeloma	Hypogammaglobulinemia (impaired humoral immunity)	Encapsulated organisms, Streptococcus pneumoniae; Haemophilus influenzae; Neisseria meningitides
Hodgkin disease	Impaired T-lymphocyte response	Pneumocystis jiroveci, Cryptococcus spp, mycobacteria, Toxoplasma, Listeria monocytogenes, Cryptosporidium, Candida, CMV
Hematopoietic cell transplant recipients	Neutropenia, impaired cellular, and humoral immunity	Gram-positive cocci, Gram-negative bacilli, cytomegalovirus, Candida, Aspergillus, herpes viruses (HSV, VZV, CMV)
Breast cancer	Tissue necrosis, radiation damage, foreign bodies	Gram-positive cocci, Gram-negative bacilli, anaerobes (polymicrobial infections common)
Lung cancer	Local obstruction, tissue necrosis	Gram-positive cocci, Gram-negative bacilli, anaerobes (polymicrobial infections common)
Gynecologic malignancy	Local obstruction, tissue necrosis	Mixed aerobic and anaerobic enteric flora including Enterococcus spp. (polymicrobial infections common)

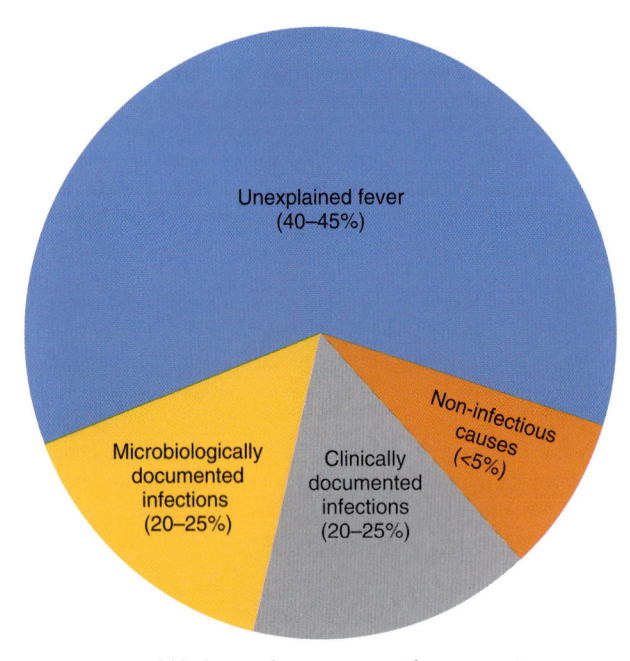

Figure 1 Types of febrile episodes in patients with neutropenia.

Unexplained fever (40–45%)
Microbiologically documented infections (20–25%)
Clinically documented infections (20–25%)
Non-infectious causes (<5%)

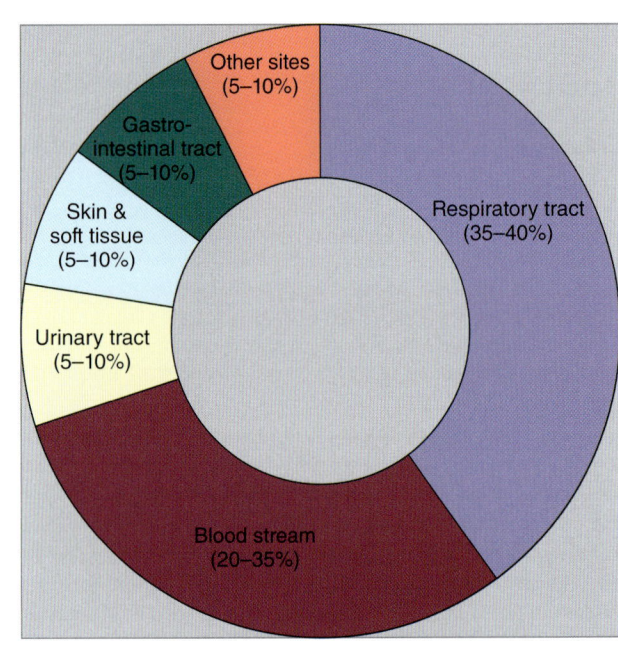

Figure 2 Common sites of infection in patients with neutropenia.

Respiratory tract (35–40%)
Blood stream (20–35%)
Urinary tract (5–10%)
Skin & soft tissue (5–10%)
Gastro-intestinal tract (5–10%)
Other sites (5–10%)

Table 2 Common infections in patients with solid tumors.

Tumor location	Infection site or type
Breast	Wound infection; breast implant infection; cellulitis or lymphangitis related to axillary node dissection; mastitis; breast abscess; bacteremia
Central nervous system (brain; meninges)	Wound infection; epidural/subdural infection; brain abscess; meningitis/ventriculitis; proximal and distal end-shunt-related infections; aspiration pneumonia; urinary tract infection; bacteremia
Genitourinary and prostate	Cystitis; urethritis; acute/chronic pyelonephritis ± bacteremia; catheter-related complicated urinary tract infection (nephrostomy/stents); wound infection; acute/chronic prostatitis; epididymitis, orchitis; pelvic abscess
Hepatobiliary-pancreatic	Wound infection; peritonitis; ascending cholangitis ± bacteremia; hepatic, pancreatic, or subdiaphragmatic abscess
Head and neck	Cellulitis; wound infection; deep facial space infection; mastoiditis/osteomyelitis; sinusitis; aspiration pneumonia; bacteremia; suppurative intracranial phlebitis; meningitis; brain abscess; retropharyngeal; and paravertebral abscesses
Musculoskeletal (muscles, bones, joints)	Wound infections; pyomyositis; lymphangitis; bursitis; synovitis; septic arthritis; osteomyelitis; prosthesis related infections; bacteremia
Upper gastrointestinal	Esophagitis; tracheoesophageal fistula with pneumonitis/lung abscess; gastric perforation and abscess; feeding tube related infections; mediastinitis/osteomyelitis
Lower gastrointestinal	Wound infection; intraabdominal or pelvic abscess; peritonitis (perforation); enterocolitis; urinary tract infection; perianal/perirectal infection; sacral/coccygeal osteomyelitis

Table 3 Bacterial infection in 2223 febrile episodes in neutropenic patients[a].

Infection type[a]	2002–2003		2012–2013	
	No.	%	No.	%
Microbiologically documented	262	26	321	26
Gram-positive	134	51	163	51
Gram-negative	51	20	55	17
Polymicrobial	71	27	92	29
Anaerobic	6	2	11	3
Clinically documented	210	21	298	24
Unexplained fever	521	53	611	50

[a]These data are derived from surveys conducted at the University of Texas MD Anderson Cancer Center, Houston, Texas, USA.

Table 4 Common infectious agents in patients with cancer.

Neutropenia
  Bacteria
    Gram-positive organisms
      Coagulase-negative staphylococci
      Staphylococcus aureus (including MRSA)
      Enterococcus spp. (including VRE)
      Viridans group streptococci
    Gram-negative organisms
      Escherichia coli
      Klebsiella pneumoniae
      Pseudomonas aeruginosa
      Other *Enterobacteriacae*
      Stenotrophomonas maltophilia
  Fungi
    Candida spp.
    Aspergillus spp.
    Zygomycetes
    Fusarium spp.
Cellular immune dysfunction
  Bacteria
    Listeria monocytogenes
    Rhodococcus equi
    Salmonella spp.
    Mycobacteria
    Nocardia spp.
    Legionella spp.
  Fungi
    Aspergillus spp.
    Cryptococcus spp.
    Histoplasma capsulatum
    Coccidioides immitis
    Pneumocystis jiroveci
  Protozoa
    Toxoplasma gondii
  Helminth
    Strongyloides stercoralis
  Viruses
    Cytomegalovirus
    Herpes simplex virus I and II
    Varicella-zoster virus
    Epstein–Barr virus
Humoral immune dysfunction
  Streptococcus pneumoniae
  Haemophilus influenzae

Recently Gram-negative bacilli (GNB) are being isolated with increasing frequency and are now more common than GPO at some centers.[11] A substantial proportion of infections are polymicrobial.[12–15] Common bacterial pathogens are depicted in Table 4. Geographic and institutional variations exist.[16] Clinicians should consider local epidemiology and resistance patterns when initiating empiric antibiotic therapy.

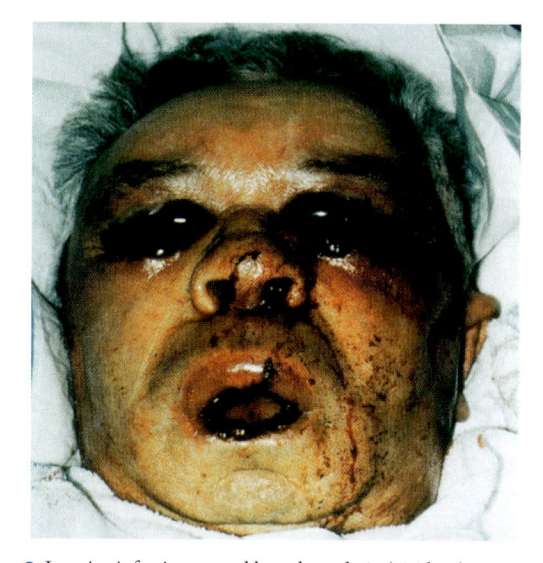

Figure 3 Invasive infection caused by α-hemolytic (viridans) streptococci. Note the hemorrhagic nature of the lesions in this patient with thrombocytopenia.

Gram-positive bacteria

Coagulase-negative staphylococci (CoNS) often cause skin and catheter-related infections.[17] *S. lugdunensis* is a more virulent species of CoNS.[18,19] *Staphylococcus aureus* is often associated with deep-seated infections (deep abscesses, endocarditis) and all patients with *S. aureus* bacteremia should be evaluated for such foci.[20] Methicillin-resistance among *S. aureus* isolates has become common (>50%) at many centers.[21] Many of these isolates have developed tolerance or reduced susceptibility to vancomycin, thereby reducing the efficacy of this agent.[22–26] Alternative therapeutic agents include daptomycin, telavancin, dalbavancin, oritavancin, linezolid, tedizolid, and ceftaroline.[27–29]

Viridans group streptococci (VGS) are mainly encountered in patients with acute leukemia, and in allogeneic HCT recipients.[30] Risk factors include chemotherapy with agents that induce severe oral mucositis, prophylaxis with fluoroquinolones, and treatment of chemotherapy-induced gastritis with antacids or histamine type 2 (H2) antagonists[31,32] Bacteremia is the most common manifestation. Some patients develop a rapidly progressive infection involving the bloodstream, lungs, central nervous system, and skin (Figure 3). This is associated with 25–35% mortality despite aggressive therapy.[33] Of concern are reports that 20–60% of VGS are penicillin-resistant at some institutions.[30,34] Beta-hemolytic streptococci also cause infections in neutropenic patients, but less often than VGS.[35]

The enterococci colonize the lower intestinal tract.[36,37] *Enterococcus faecalis* is the predominant species isolated. Most *E. faecalis* strains are susceptible to penicillin, ampicillin, and vancomycin. Combinations of these agents with aminoglycosides are recommended for serious enterococcal infections. *Enterococcus faecium* often expresses high-level resistance to aminoglycosides, ampicillin, and vancomycin (VRE). Risk factors for infection with VRE include intestinal colonization and the use of antimicrobials such as metronidazole, clindamycin, imipenem, and vancomycin.[38] Established therapeutic options include linezolid, daptomycin, and oritavancin.[39–41] Other Gram-positive pathogens include *Bacillus* spp., *Corynebacterium* spp., *Micrococcus* spp., and *Rothia* spp. (previously, *Stomatococcus mucilaginosus*).[42,43] Nocardiosis is caused by several *Nocardia* species (*Nocardia asteroides* complex, *Nocardia brasiliensis*, and *Nocardia otitidiscaviarum*). The most common sites of infection are the lungs (70%) and soft tissue sites (16%).[44] Establishing a specific diagnosis is of paramount importance as the differential diagnosis is wide. Trimethoprim/sulfamethoxazole (TMP/SMX) remains the backbone of therapy although it is often combined with the carbapenems, tetracyclines, or aminoglycosides. *Listeria monocytogenes* is often acquired by the consumption of raw milk or products (cheese) made from raw milk. Bacteremia (75%) and meningoencephalitis (20%) are the most common manifestations.[45] Mortality is high.

Gram-negative bacteria
The intestinal tract serves as an important source of infection in neutropenic patients. *Escherichia coli*, *Klebsiella* spp., and *Pseudomonas aeruginosa* remain the three primary pathogens.[12,46] Other Enterobacteriaceae (*Citrobacter* spp., *Enterobacter* spp., *Proteus* spp., and *Serratia* spp.) are less common. The proportion of infections caused by nonfermentative GNB (NFGNB) such as *P. aeruginosa*, *Stenotrophomonas maltophilia*, and *Acinetobacter* spp. has increased.[47] *P. aeruginosa* is the most frequently isolated and the most virulent NFGNB and causes between 15% and 20% of these infections. It is also the most common GNB isolated from polymicrobial infections.[15] Infections caused by *S. maltophilia* are being documented more often in patients with hematologic malignancies and in HCT recipients.[48,49] The switch from TMP/SMX, which is active against *S. maltophilia*, to the fluoroquinolones, which generally are not, as preferred agents for prophylaxis, may account for this increase. Other infrequent but important NFGNB include *Achromobacter* spp., *Alcaligenes* spp. Bacteremia is most common, followed by pneumonia, and urinary tract infection. Fever is often the only manifestation of infection. Other manifestations include ecthyma gangrenosum (Figure 4). Polymicrobial infections and infections that are complicated by deep tissue involvement (pneumonia, neutropenic enterocolitis [NEC], perirectal infections) are associated with greater morbidity and mortality.[15,50] The emergence of resistance to β-lactam agents and carbapenems is of great concern.[51–53] Some organisms (*P. aeruginosa* and *Acinetobacter* spp.) have become multidrug resistant (MDR).[54,55] Very few established options to treat such organisms (polymyxins [colistin or polymyxin B], ceftazidime-avibactam, ceftolozane-tazobactam, meropenem-vaborbactam, tigecycline, combination regimens) exist. There is limited experience with newer agents (ceftazidime-avibactam, ceftolozane-tazobactam, and meropenem-vaborbactam) in the setting of infected cancer patients. Ceftolozane/tazobactam and ceftazidime/avibactam have been used successfully in "real-life" experiences for treatment of MDR GNB in patients with hematological malignancies, although data are based mainly on case series and case reports.[56] Many institutions conduct surveillance studies in high-risk patients looking for fecal colonization with VRE, *P. aeruginosa*, extended-spectrum beta-lactamase (ESBL) producers, and carbapenem-resistant Enterobacteriaceae (CRE), since positive surveillance cultures often predict subsequent infection.[57–60]

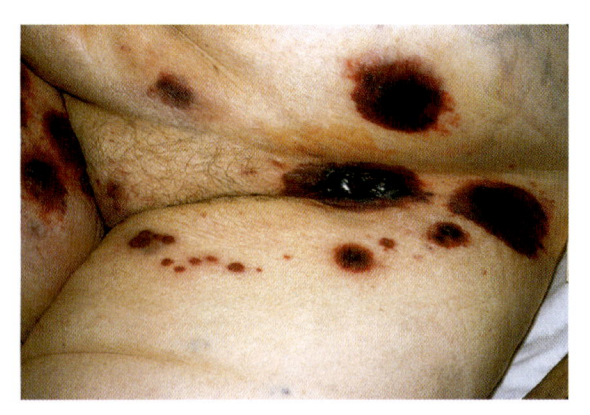

Figure 4 Multiple skin lesions (ecthyma gangrenosum) in a patient with *Pseudomonas aeruginosa* bacteremia.

Impaired CMI is a risk factor for legionellosis. The most common *Legionella* species causing infection is *Legionella pneumophila*. Hospital water systems or human-made building water systems often harbor *Legionella* spp. and many cases of hospital-acquired legionellosis can be traced to such sources.[61] Pneumonia is the most common manifestation. The detection of urinary antigens (to identify the most common cause of legionellosis, *L. pneumophila* serogroup 1) or recovery of the organisms on cultures using special media (to detect all species) is required to make a diagnosis. The fluoroquinolones and macrolides are used most often for treatment and there appears to be no advantage of using them in combination. Nontyphoidal *Salmonella* and *Campylobacter* spp. infections are also seen in patients with impaired CMI.[62]

CMI plays an essential role in the control of mycobacterial infections. Certain cancer groups (e.g., patients from low-income countries, patients with head and neck cancers) are at high risk for these infections. The association of tuberculosis and Hodgkin's disease or hairy cell leukemia has been well established.[63] Pulmonary infection which produces fever cough and weight loss is common. Diffuse pulmonary infiltrates with or without mediastinal enlargement are the most common radiographic findings. Nontuberculous mycobacterial infections are less common.[64,65] They produce pulmonary infections, lymphadenitis, skin and skin structure infections (SSSIs), catheter-related infections, and disseminated disease. The species isolated most often are *M. avium-intracellulare*, *M. abscessus*, *M. chelonae*, *M. fortuitum*, *M. kansasii*, and *M. marinum*. Prolonged, multiple drug therapy is usually administered for progressive infection.[66]

Anaerobes
Anaerobes are frequently involved in deep-seated, polymicrobial infections such as abdominal/pelvic abscesses, NEC, peri-rectal infections, complicated SSSIs, oral infections, and pneumonia.[50,67] The organisms isolated most often include *Peptococcus* spp., *Fusobacterium nucleatum*, *Bacteroides* spp., and *Prevotella* species.[68] *Clostridium difficile* infection (CDI) is a leading infectious cause of diarrhea in cancer patients in whom there is an increased severity of illness, higher mortality, and an increased risk of relapse and complications. Newer diagnostic tests are available including polymerase chain reaction (PCR)-based assays.[69] Metronidazole is now considered inferior to vancomycin for the treatment of CDI.[70] Agents such as rifaximin and nitazoxanide have been used with limited success.[71–73] Fidaxomycin is an oral macrocyclic antibiotic approved for the treatment of CDI,

especially for those individuals at the greatest risk for relapse.[74,75] For patients with cancer, fidaxomicin treatment was superior to vancomycin.[75] Fecal transplants have also been used successfully in this setting and appear to be promising,[76] even in cancer patients[77]; but a strong recommendation to not use fecal microbiota transplantation was made in children and adolescents with cancer.[78] On the other hand, preliminary data reveal the potential of fecal microbiota transplantation in alleviating various cancers linked to intestinal dysbiosis and cancer treatment-associated complications as well as enhancing the efficacy of cancer immunotherapy.[79] Preventive measures for CDI include appropriate infection control practices, antimicrobial stewardship, and improved environment cleaning methods. There is an increased interest in the role of the intestinal microbiome in the outcomes of patients with cancer.[80]

Fungal infections

Prolonged neutropenia (>7 days) is a risk factor for the development of invasive fungal infections (IFIs). The most common causes of IFIs are *Candida* spp. and *Aspergillus* spp.[81] The epidemiology of IFIs has changed substantially over the past 20 years.[82,83] Prior to the availability of agents such as fluconazole, invasive candidiasis was common with *Candida albicans* being the predominant species. The use of azole prophylaxis has led to a decrease in the frequency of candidiasis. Candidemia, often catheter-related, is the most common manifestation, with the alimentary tract being the predominant portal of entry. Recent studies have demonstrated a major shift from *C. albicans* to nonalbicans *Candida* species (*Candida glabrata, Candida tropicalis, Candida krusei,* and *Candida parapsilosis*).[83–85]

There are no characteristic physical signs and symptoms of disseminated candidiasis. Often, the only indication is persistent fever and a gradual worsening of the patient's clinical condition. Some patients have ocular infection. Nearly 10% of patients develop characteristic erythematous macronodular skin lesions. (Figure 5). Treatment should be guided by *in vitro* antifungal susceptibility data.[86] Breakthrough *C. parapsilosis* fungemia may develop during echinocandin therapy, as may *C. glabrata* infection during azole therapy. Echinocandin resistance among *C. glabrata* isolates appears to be increasing.[87] *C. krusei* isolates are resistant to fluconazole. The crude mortality associated with systemic *Candida* infections is ~40%. Guidelines for the management of candidiasis have been published by various societies.[88–91]

Aspergillosis is frequent in patients with hematologic malignancies and persistent neutropenia. Other risk factors include prolonged high-dose corticosteroid therapy, graft-versus-host disease (GVHD), respiratory viral infections, and advanced age.[92] The most common pathogen is *Aspergillus fumigatus*.[93] Infection is usually acquired by inhalation of spores. Outbreaks of aspergillosis associated with construction within or adjacent to the hospital have occurred. More than 70% of infections involve the lungs, and approximately 35% of patients have hematogenous dissemination to other organs.[94] Often, the only evidence of infection is prolonged fever with pulmonary infiltrates that fail to respond to antibacterial therapy. High-resolution CT scanning is helpful in the early diagnosis of aspergillosis.[95,96] Characteristic findings in early-stage disease in neutropenic patients is one or several nodules with a halo of surrounding ground-glass attenuation that represents hemorrhage surrounding a region of pulmonary infarction (Figure 6).[95–97] As neutrophil recovery occurs, the infarcted tissue becomes necrotic and retracts from the viable tissue leaving an air crescent. Aspergillus sino-orbital infection is being diagnosed with increasing frequency in patients with acute leukemia and in HCT recipients, accounting for at least 15% of cases of aspergillosis (Figure 7). Infections may erode through the base of the skull and invade the brain or cause destruction of the paranasal and facial structures and the eye. A localized form of aspergillosis has been

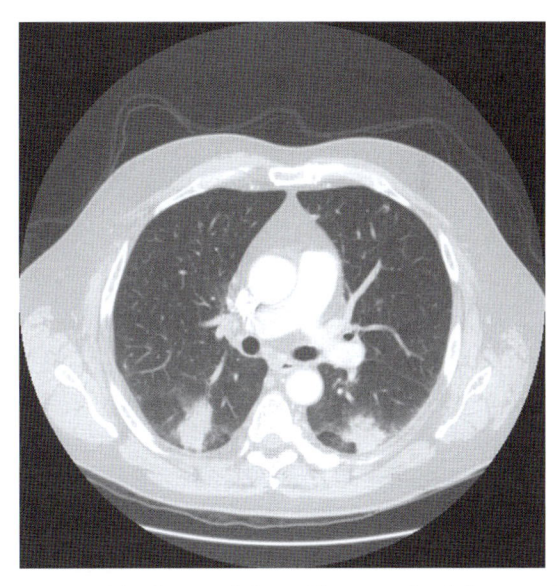

Figure 6 Rounded pulmonary lesions with surrounding halo, compatible with invasive pulmonary aspergillosis.

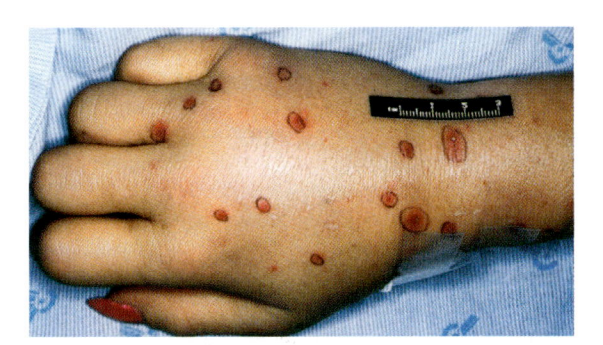

Figure 5 Characteristic macronodular cutaneous lesions in a patient with acute leukemia and disseminated *Candida krusei* infection.

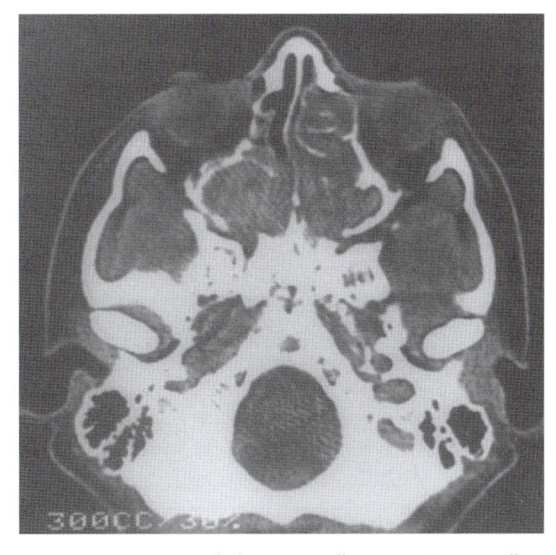

Figure 7 Pansinusitis caused by *Aspergillus* spp. in an allogeneic hematopoietic cell transplant recipient with persistent fever.

described rarely in association with intravascular catheters.[98] These infections are potentially serious because they can disseminate.[98,99] Skin lesions, manifested as sharply defined black eschars, occur in about 5% of patients with disseminated infection. Voriconazole or isavuconazole are the preferred agents for the treatment of invasive or disseminated aspergillosis. Posaconazole and lipid preparations of amphotericin B (AMB) are used more often for salvage therapy or when voriconazole intolerance occurs. Combination therapy with a triazole and an echinocandin may be useful in selected cases of invasive aspergillosis.[86,90,100,101] A randomized trial has shown higher survival in patients with early invasive aspergillosis diagnosed by *Aspergillus* galactomannan treated with voriconazole and anidulafungin than those treated with voriconazole monotherapy.[102]

Cryptococcosis is caused by two species, *C. neoformans,* and *Cryptococcus gatti.* The primary site of infection is the lung. Dissemination usually involves the central nervous system (meningoencephalitis, cryptococcoma). Fever and meningeal symptoms are common. Cerebrospinal fluid (CSF) abnormalities include raised opening pressure, lymphocytosis, elevated proteins, and low glucose levels. Cryptococcal antigen is detected in the CSF and serum in most cases. Induction therapy with AMB or its lipid formulations plus 5-fluorocytosine for 2 weeks followed by maintenance therapy with fluconazole is the standard of care.[103] Histoplasmosis and infections caused by other endemic fungi are less common.[7] They usually cause pulmonary, central nervous system (CNS), or disseminated infection and should be considered in the differential diagnosis in endemic areas although isolated asymptomatic lung nodules (e.g., histoplasmoma) can be seen. *Pneumocystis jiroveci* pneumonia has traditionally been associated with impaired CMI.[104,105] In contrast to patients with HIV/AIDS, the clinical presentation of *Pneumocystis jiroveci* pneumonia is usually sub-acute in cancer patients. Clinical features include fever, a nonproductive cough, and progressive dyspnea. The most common CT findings are diffuse bilateral ground-glass pulmonary infiltrates with apical predominance and peripheral sparing.[106] The diagnosis is often made by demonstrating the organisms on respiratory specimens including biopsy tissue using stains such as methenamine silver or toluidine blue (Figure 8). Staining methods have been supplanted by sensitive serum biomarkers including Beta-D-glucan and semi-quantitative or quantitative PCR.[107,108] TMP/SMX remains the agent of choice for prophylaxis and treatment. Alternative agents include pentamidine, atovaquone, clindamycin plus primaquine, and dapsone plus trimethoprim.[109]

Other opportunistic fungi

Mucormycosis (zygomycosis) is relatively uncommon with the most common pathogens being *Rhizopus* spp., *Mucor* spp., *Lichtheimia* (formerly *Absidia*) *corymbifera*, *Rhizomucor* spp., and *Cunninghamella bertholletiae*. Invasive sinopulmonary infection is the most common form of infection. Some patients develop pansinusitis, rhinocerebral, gastrointestinal, cutaneous, or disseminated infection.[110,111] The clinical presentation of mucormycosis is often indistinguishable from aspergillosis. Mucormycosis should be considered in patients who are immunosuppressed and who develop sinusitis or IFS after prolonged exposure to voriconazole or echinocandins.[112–114] Early diagnosis and administration of antifungal therapy are critical along with debridement of infected tissue. Control of underlying disease and reversal of risk factors, when feasible, is of paramount importance.[86,115] AMB products, posaconazole, and isavuconazole have reliable activity against Mucorales.[116] Lipid preparations of AMB are preferred for initial therapy and the value of combination therapy is unproven.[117]

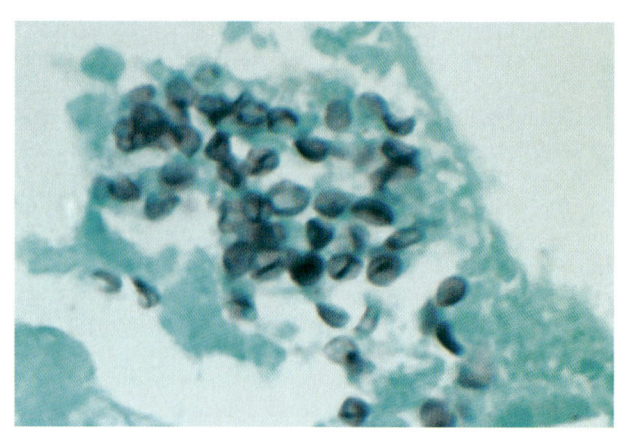

Figure 8 Gomori methenamine silver (GMS) stain from a bronchoalveolar lavage specimen demonstrating multiple organisms in a patient with *Pneumocystis jiroveci* pneumonia.

Therapy is often switched from lipid preparations of AMB to posaconazole or isavuconazole when feasible. *Trichosporon beigelii* can cause disseminated infection, particularly in patients on oral triazoles with severe neutropenia. A variety of skin lesions have been described and occur in approximately 30% of patients. Portals of entry include the gastrointestinal tract, respiratory tract, and intravenous catheter sites. *Fusarium* spp. have emerged as a significant pathogen in leukemia patients.[118] Localized infections of the lung, sinuses, and skin occur, but most patients have disseminated infection. Cutaneous and subcutaneous lesions are frequent.[119] Like *Aspergillus* spp., these organisms invade blood vessels, causing thrombosis and infarction. *Fusarium* spp. can be isolated readily from blood culture or tissue specimens. It may be difficult to distinguish *Fusarium* from some other fungi on histopathologic examination. Recovery from this infection depends on the resolution of neutropenia, and currently available antifungal agents such as voriconazole are marginally effective in the setting of cytopenias.[120,121]

Uncommon mold infections (*Scedosporium* or *Phaecilomycetes* species) or non-*Candida* yeasts (such as *Rhodotorula, Saccharomyces cerevisiae,* or *Geotrichum*) are seen in patients with advanced hematologic cancer and preexposure to other antifungals and are still associated high mortality rates. As is the case of most IFIs, there is a standardized approach in the management that takes into account the multiple factors influencing outcomes, such as the in vitro and pharmacokinetic/pharmacodynamic features of antifungals, the potential of recovery of the host immune system, and possibly surgery. The evolution of the underlying malignant disease is the key determinant of prognosis.[122–124]

Viral infections

Hepatitis viruses

Universal screening of cancer patients for hepatitis C virus (HCV) is recommended given the significant morbidity and mortality associated with chronic infection.[125] A similar screening approach is expected to be approved soon for hepatitis B virus (HBV) given the risk of reactivation. HBV reactivation occurs primarily in patients with chronic HBV (detectable HBV surface antigen or HBV DNA) on cancer treatment. Patients receiving anti-CD20 agents (rituximab, ofatumumab, and obinutuzumab) and HCT recipients are at risk for reactivation in the setting of past HBV (reactive HBV core antibody) without chronic HBV. Reactivation rates dependent on HBV DNA levels, cancer therapy, and type of malignancy, and it can occur among those with chronic HBV (~50% of cases), and among those with past HBV (~20%).[126]

HBV reactivation may vary from asymptomatic elevation of hepatic enzymes (hepatitis flare) to fulminant hepatic failure and death. Early detection of HBV with appropriate screening (HBV surface antigen, HBV core antibody) and quantitative HBV DNA measurements along with administration of antiviral agents (entecavir, tenofovir [Tenofovir disoproxil fumarate, Tenofovir alafenamide]) improves outcome. Lamivudine therapy has fallen out of favor. Unlike HBV reactivation, HCV reactivation seems to have a more indolent course but it can affect the cancer treatment plan.[127]

Viral infections are uncommon in patients with neutropenia unless they are HCT recipients. Herpes viruses are identified most frequently, especially herpes simplex viruses (HSV), varicella-zoster virus (VZV), and CMV. Most adults are HSV seropositive, and reactivation can occur in ~60–80 % of patients undergoing HCT or chemotherapy for hematologic malignancies. Reactivation generally occurs while patients are still severely neutropenic with oral mucositis/ulceration being the most common manifestation. Esophagitis occurs occasionally. Encephalitis and dissemination are uncommon. HSV prophylaxis is recommended in patients undergoing HCT or remission induction therapy for leukemia,[128] as well as those with chimeric antigen receptor-modified T (CAR-T)-cell immunotherapy. Reactivation of latent VZV also occurs and prophylaxis to prevent recurrence of VZV infection in seropositive patients is recommended for the first year following allogeneic HCT.[129,130] Community respiratory viruses, including respiratory syncytial virus (RSV), influenza A and B, and parainfluenza viruses, human metapneumovirus, human coronaviruses, and human rhinoviruses are common among HCT recipients and patients with acute leukemia in whom upper respiratory tract infection can progress to pneumonitis, which is associated with substantial morbidity and mortality,[131] and fungal superinfections.[132] During outbreaks like Middle East respiratory syndrome coronavirus (MERS-CoV), epidemics such as severe acute respiratory syndrome (SARS), or pandemic like coronavirus disease 2019 (COVID-19) cancer patients can be affected. There are sparse cancer-specific data of these diseases not allowing to draw definitive conclusions on clinical features, radiologic presentations, diagnostics methods, treatment recommendations including impact on cancer care, and management of these conditions in patients with malignancies. Close surveillance, major infection-control measure, and global public health responses are required to control the spread of these diseases.[133-138] Testing for respiratory viruses is recommended in high-risk patients. Specimens include nasopharyngeal swabs, washes, or aspirates, tracheal aspirates, and bronchoalveolar lavage specimens. Optimum treatment for most of these viral infections, except for influenza viruses, remains to be determined. Ribavirin therapy for upper respiratory infection with RSV deters progression to pneumonia and may improve overall outcome in HCT recipients.[139]

Reactivation of Epstein–Barr virus (EBV) may occur after HCT or following chemotherapy with purine analogs such as fludarabine. EBV infection may be responsible for Richter transformation or development of Hodgkin disease in patients with chronic lymphocytic leukemia. In recipients of HCT or solid-organ transplants, uncontrolled proliferation of EBV infected B cells may occur, producing posttransplant lymphoproliferative disorders (PTLD). In younger patients, a mononucleosis-like syndrome is a common presentation. Fever, sore throat, and lymphadenopathy are typical findings. Dissemination can occur and can be fulminant and rapidly fatal. It is important to monitor high-risk patients (umbilical cord blood transplants, haploidentical transplants, T-cell depleted transplants) for EBV DNA viral load using PCR assays. Rituximab is recommended for preemptive therapy or the treatment of PTLD.[140,141]

Human Herpesvirus 6 (HHV-6) is being recognized as an important pathogen in HCT recipients.[142,143] Serologic reactivation accompanied by specific manifestations, including fever, rash, pneumonitis, hepatitis, myelosuppression, and neurologic dysfunction, have been described in recipients of HCT, kidney, and liver transplants. HHV-6 viremia is not associated with increased mortality, and routine screening is not necessary.[144,145] Ganciclovir, foscarnet, and cidofovir inhibit viral replication, and therapy with these agents may be useful in patients with severe infections.[146] The investigational agent brincidofovir has also activity against HHV-6.[146] Immunotherapeutic prevention and treatment strategies are being developed.[147,148]

CMV infection occurs frequently in immunocompromised patients, especially those with impaired CMI. It is common in patients undergoing allogeneic HCT and has a negative impact on survival after transplantation.[149] CMV seropositivity in HCT recipients is a major risk factor. Without prophylaxis, 50% to 80% of seropositive patients undergoing HCT reactivate latent infection. CMV seropositivity in the HCT recipient or donor has an impact on the subsequent development of CMV end-organ disease.[150] Other risk factors for CMV infection include total body irradiation, umbilical cord blood transplantation, the use of T-cell depleted stem cells, treatment with purine analogs (fludarabine, cladribine), and monoclonal antibodies against CD20 (rituximab) and CD52 (alemtuzumab), GVHD, and advanced age.[151] CMV pneumonia is the most common presentation (Figure 9). Other manifestations include retinitis, esophagitis, enteritis, hepatitis, myocarditis, and encephalitis. In addition to end-organ disease, CMV infection has been associated with the development of GVHD and secondary bacterial and fungal infections given its immunosuppressive properties. Early detection of CMV infection is important to initiate preventive measures. These measures consist of CMV prophylaxis or preemptive therapy. The prophylactic strategy is mostly with letermovir in HCT recipients. The preemptive strategy consists of the administration of antiviral therapy (ganciclovir, foscarnet) which is initiated upon detection of CMV, using the PCR assay. Viral load-based, risk-adapted, preemptive treatment strategies have successfully prevented CMV disease, with a very low incidence of breakthrough disease.[152] The treatment of end-organ disease, especially pneumonia is unsatisfactory.

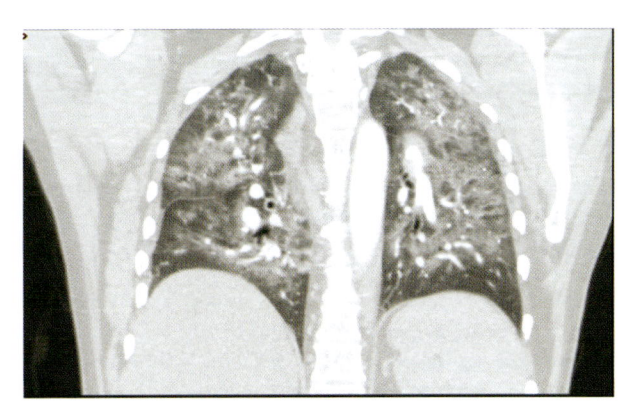

Figure 9 Computerized tomography scan of an allogeneic hematopoietic cell transplant recipient with CMV pneumonitis, showing diffuse bilateral pulmonary infiltrates.

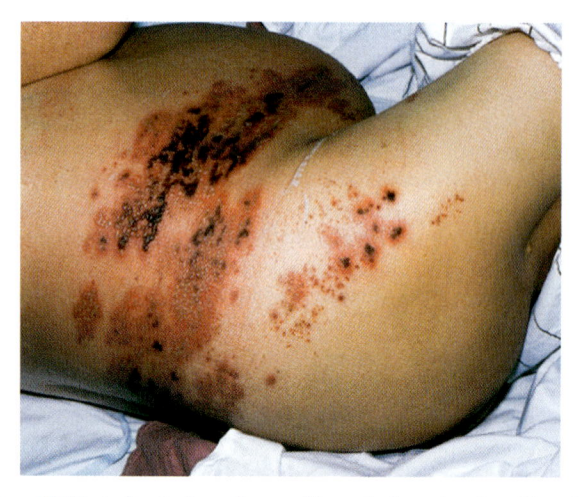

Figure 10 Typical vesicular rash caused by varicella-zoster virus. Note the dermatomal distribution and the hemorrhagic nature of lesions in this patient with thrombocytopenia.

Currently available systemic antiviral agents include ganciclovir, foscarnet, cidofovir, leflunomide, and letermovir. Novel agents such as brincidofovir, maribavir, and cyclopropavir (filociclovir) that are being developed.[146,153,154]

Herpes zoster occurs most often in patients with lymphoproliferative disorders. The infection is characterized by a unilateral vesicular rash in the distribution of one or two adjacent sensory dermatomes (Figure 10). Occasionally, patients develop a generalized varicelliform eruption. The rash is accompanied by pain (zoster-associated pain) that can last for several months. Cutaneous dissemination of herpes zoster occurs in ~35% of patients with cancer, as compared with only 4% of those without cancer. Therapy with corticosteroids, radiation, or antitumor agents facilitates dissemination.

Laboratory confirmation of the diagnosis is generally not required. VZV can be recovered from the vesicular fluid for a few days after the onset of the eruption. Cultures are positive 30–60% of the time. Detection of VZV antigens in skin scrapings using fluorescence microscopy, and detection of VZV DNA, in the CSF or other tissues, using PCR, are more rapid and sensitive diagnostic techniques.

Therapy of VZV infection shortens viral shedding, accelerates the healing of lesions and reduces the frequency of visceral disease. Oral valacyclovir and famciclovir are better absorbed and more effective than acyclovir. Severe infections such as meningoencephalitis, disseminated infection, or pneumonitis require intravenous acyclovir therapy. Therapy with foscarnet or combination therapy with foscarnet and acyclovir should be considered for patients who fail to respond to acyclovir alone.

Other infections
Toxoplasmosis is one of the most common parasitic infestations in man. Disseminated disease generally occurs in immunocompromised individuals with the CNS, heart, and lungs being involved most often.[155] CT or magnetic resonance imaging of the brain reveals multiple hypodense lesions, often with moderate contrast ring enhancement. The diagnosis can be confirmed by serologic testing, PCR, or biopsy. Specific therapy consists of pyrimethamine plus sulfadiazine. Alternative agents such as clindamycin, atovaquone, and TMP/SMX have also been used for treatment and/or prophylaxis.[156] *Strongyloides stercoralis* is a soil-transmitted helminth and lymphoma is the most common malignancy associated with strongyloidiasis. Many infestations are asymptomatic and some produce only eosinophilia.[157] Common clinical features include fever and gastrointestinal symptoms such as diarrhea and abdominal pain/cramping. Immunosuppression often induced by corticosteroids can trigger the development of hyperinfection of dissemination.[9,158] Polymicrobial bacteremia caused by GNB and anaerobes is not uncommon. Diagnostic tests include the demonstration of the organisms in stool and respiratory specimens, and serological (ELISA) methods. Ivermectin is the drug of choice. Screening of high-risk patients (allogeneic HCT recipients, corticosteroid usage) is recommended.[159]

Special situations

Neutropenic enterocolitis
NEC is seen primarily in patients receiving agents that produce severe intestinal mucositis.[50] Clinical features include fever, abdominal pain/cramping, distention, and diarrhea. Complications include bacteremia which is often polymicrobial, hemorrhage, bowel wall perforation, and abscess. The disease usually involves the entire lower intestinal tract. Radiographic examination (preferably CT) reveals evidence of paralytic ileus with lack of bowel gas in the right lower quadrant, distention of the terminal ileum, and >4 mm thickening of the bowel wall, which is considered a hallmark of NEC. Management includes bowel rest, intravenous fluids, and broad-spectrum antibiotics that include coverage for *P. aeruginosa* and anaerobes. Surgical intervention may be necessary to manage complications such as hemorrhage or bowel perforation.

Perianal infections

Perianal infections are estimated to occur in 6% of patients with hematologic neoplasms. More than 90% are neutropenic.[160] The major presenting symptom is pain that is aggravated by defecation. Erythematous, indurated, or ulcerated lesions with tissue necrosis, are common. The infection often occurs at the site of a fissure or hemorrhoid. Digital rectal examination is not recommended. GNB, especially *P. aeruginosa* and *E. coli* are isolated frequently. Therapy includes measures such as sitz baths, warm compresses, stool softeners, analgesics, along with broad-spectrum antibiotics. Empiric antifungal therapy is not recommended. Abscesses, if present, should be drained.[161] Resolution of infection often depends on the recovery of the neutrophil count. Patients with hematologic diseases who recover from perianal infections caused by hemorrhoids or fissures should undergo surgical correction when feasible, to avoid recurrent infections.

Catheter-related infections

Central line-related bloodstream infections have become relatively common.[162] The majority are caused by *Staphylococcus* spp. and other GPO. Other pathogens include *P. aeruginosa*, the Enterobacteriaceae, *S. maltophilia*, and *Candida* spp. Quantitative blood cultures and time to positivity help establish the diagnosis.[163–167] Sequential time to positivity can also predict outcome.[168] Some episodes caused by CoNS can be treated without catheter removal.[169] Catheter removal is usually necessary for infections caused by *S. aureus*, *Acinetobacter*, *Pseudomonas* spp. *S. maltophilia*, *Candida* spp., and nontuberculous mycobacteria. If there are signs of localized infection at the catheter insertion site, or if fever or bacteremia persists despite adequate therapy, catheters must always be removed.[163] Antimicrobial lock therapy may be useful particularly if catheter removal is not feasible.

Antimicrobial impregnated catheters have been shown to reduce the frequency of catheter-associated infections.[162,170]

Therapy of infections in patients with neutropenia

Initial patient evaluation

Febrile neutropenic patients should receive prompt, empiric, broad-spectrum antimicrobial therapy generally via the intravenous route, and at maximal therapeutic doses.[171] Pretreatment evaluation should be performed expeditiously since a delay in instituting empiric therapy can result in diminished response rates.[172] Historical information should be obtained and a thorough physical examination should be performed. Attention should be paid to sites such as the oro-pharynx, lower esophagus, perineum, paranasal sinuses, fingernails, and skin including the armpits, groin, and catheter insertion sites. Cultures from appropriate sites should be obtained. In patients with central venous catheters, cultures from a peripheral site and all lumens of the catheter should be obtained.[173,174] Neutropenic patients with pneumonia may have normal appearing radiographs and CT of the chest should be obtained in these patients when pneumonia is clinically suspected. CT scans of the paranasal sinuses, chest, abdomen, and pelvis should be performed if these sites are potential sources of infection. PET scan is used in patients with persistent fever of unknown origin.[175] Risk assessment should be performed to determine whether the patient requires hospitalization or not.[176] Low-risk febrile neutropenic patients can be treated with out-patient parenteral or oral antibiotic regimens if the infrastructure for out-patient management of such patients is in place.[177–179] All other patients should receive hospital-based therapy. Outpatient therapy can be administered after a short period of hospitalization or for the entire episode.[180–183] It has been shown to be safe and effective in adults and children.[184–186] Outpatient therapy is associated with cost savings, a lower incidence of superinfections with nosocomial pathogens, and improved quality of life for patients and convenience for their caregivers.[177,187] Multiple guidelines for the management of infections in patients with cancer have been published.[171,188–190]

Initial antibiotic therapy

The empiric regimen should be based on local epidemiologic and resistance patterns and should provide coverage against GNB including *P. aeruginosa*, and GPO. This is usually achieved either by administering a single broad-spectrum agent (monotherapy), or antibiotic combinations.[171,189] Tables 5 and 6 list the common therapeutic options in use. No single regimen is optimal. Monotherapy with agents such as carbapenems (meropenem, imipenem, and doripenem but not ertapenem), cefepime, and piperacillin/tazobactam is considered appropriate for ~60% of febrile neutropenic episode especially if no obvious focus of infection can be identified.[171] If resistant GPO infections are likely (e.g., in patients colonized with MRSA or VRE), a combination of these agents with vancomycin, linezolid, or daptomycin is considered appropriate. However, studies have shown that the addition of these agents after a resistant Gram-positive infection has been identified is just as effective as empiric usage. Vancomycin may no longer be adequate at some institutions due to changing susceptibilities, and alternative agents such as daptomycin, dalbavancin, telavancin, and ceftaroline may be considered, although clinical experience with these agents in neutropenic patients is limited.[22,26–28] Combinations of antipseudomonal beta-lactams

Table 5 Common empiric antibiotic regimens for febrile neutropenic patients.

Regimens for low-risk patients
→Oral
  Quinolone + amoxicillin/clavulante
  Quinolone + clindamycin or azithromycin
  Moxifloxacin or levofloxacin (monotherapy)
→Parenteral
  Ceftriaxone or ertapenem ± amikacin
  Aztreonam + clindamycin
  Quinolone ± clindamycin
  Ceftazidime or cefepime

Regimens for moderate to high-risk patients
  Combination regimens
    Aminoglycoside + antipseudomonal penicillin/beta-lactamase inhibitor or cephalosporin or carbapenem, or quinolone (if patient not on quinolone prophylaxis)
    Vancomycin (or linezolid or daptomycin) + antipseudomonal penicillin, or cephalosporin, or carbapenem, or quinolone (if patient not on quinolone prophylaxis)
  Single-agent regimens (monotherapy)
    Extended-spectrum cephalosporin (cefepime)
    Carbapenems (imipenem, meropenem, or dorzipenem, but not ertapenem)
    Antipseudomonal penicillin/beta-lactamse inhibitor (piperacillin/tazobactam)

and aminoglycosides are used to provide synergistic bactericidal activity against GNB. Agents with potent anaerobic activity should be administered when anaerobic infections are likely. The initial regimen may need to be altered depending on the susceptibility of microorganisms isolated, the development of bacterial, fungal, or viral superinfections, or lack of efficacy after administration of the regimen for 3–5 days. All patients need to be carefully monitored for response, toxicity, and the development complications and appropriate changes should be made if the clinical situation or microbiologic data indicate the need.[191] Initial empiric therapy is usually associated with response rates of 65–85% (higher in low-risk patients).[184] Many patients will respond after modification of the initial regimen.[171]

Duration of therapy

Some authorities recommend the continuation of antibiotic therapy in patients with documented infections until recovery of the neutrophil count (i.e., an absolute neutrophil count >500 cells for two consecutive days). This approach is expensive and may not be needed in many patients. It actually represents broad-spectrum prophylaxis after the resolution of infection. Another approach is to continue broad-spectrum antibiotics until all sites of infection have resolved, the causative pathogen, if isolated, has been eradicated, the patient has been treated for a minimum of 7 days and has remained free of symptoms or signs of infection for at least 4 days. This is the case in most patients with unexplained fever. Antibiotic therapy may be discontinued at this point despite the persistence of neutropenia. This approach is less expensive and may be associated with fewer superinfections.[192–194]

Persistent fever

Patients who remain febrile despite antibacterial and antifungal therapy are challenging. They may have resistant bacterial infections, or infections by other pathogens (viruses, parasites). Drug fever or tumor fever may also be present. Extensive, often invasive, diagnostics are necessary in order to make a specific diagnosis and provide appropriate therapy. In patients unable to tolerate

Table 6 Antimicrobial agents commonly used in patients with neutropenia.

Aminoglycosides	
Amikacin	15 mg/kg q24h, IV (monitor levels)
Tobramycin	7 mg/kg q24h, IV (monitor levels)
Antipseudomonal penicillins + β-lactamase inhibitor	
Piperacillin + tazobactam	4.5 g q6h, IV
Cephalosporins	
Cefepime	2 g q8h, IV
Ceftazidime-avibactam	2.5 g q8h, IV
Ceftolozane-tazobactam	1.5–3 g q8h, IV
Carbapenem	
Imipenem/cilastatin	500 mg q6h, IV
Meropenem	1–2 g q8h, IV
Meropenem-vaborbactam	4 g q8h, IV
Monobactam	
Aztreonam	2 g q6h, IV
Quinolones	
Ciprofloxacin	400 mg q8h–q12h, IV or 500–750 mg q12h, PO[a]
Levofloxacin	500 or 750 mg q24 hours[a]
Moxifloxacin	400 mg q24 hours[a]
Others	
Vancomycin	15 mg/kg q12h, IV (monitor levels, target AUC 400–600 if treating MRSA)
Trimethoprim-sulfamethoxazole	10–20 mg/kg/day (invasive infections)[a]
Metronidazole	500 mg IV q8h[a]
Linezolid	600 mg IV q12h[a]
Daptomycin	6–10 mg/kg/d
Tigecycline	Initial loading dose 100 mg, then 50 mg IV q12h
Antifungal agents	
Azoles	
Fluconazole	200–800 mg q24 hours[a]
Itraconazole	200 mg q12 hours[a]
Voriconazole	6 mg/kg loading dose q12 × 2 doses, then 4 mg/kg q12 hours[a]
Posaconazole	Suspension 200 mg q8 hours with food, tablets/IV 300 mg q12 hours × 2, then 300 mg q24 hours[a]
Isavuconazole	Oral 372 mg (isavuconazole 200 mg) q8 hours for six doses, then 372 mg (isavuconazole 200 mg) q24 hours/IV 372 mg (isavuconazole 200 mg) q8 hours for six doses, then 372 mg (isavuconazole 200 mg) q24 hours[a]
Echinocandins	
Caspofungin	70 mg day 1, then 50 mg q24 hours
Micafungin	100 mg q24 hours
Anidulafungin	200 mg day 1, then 100 mg q24 hours
Polyenes	
Amphotericin B deoxycholate	0.3–1 mg/kg/day q24 hours
Amphotericin B liposomal (ambisome)	3–6 mg/kg/day q24 hours
Amphotericin B lipid complex (abelcet)	5 mg/kg/day q24 hours
Antiviral agents	
Acyclovir	5–10 mg/kg q8 hours, IV[a]
Valacyclovir	1 g q8 hours
Ganciclovir	5 mg/kg q12 hours
Valganciclovir	Oral 900 mg q12 hours
Foscarnet	90 mg/kg q12 hours
Cidofovir	5 mg/kg iv once a week, must be given with probenecid 3 g prior to infusion and 1 g 2 and 8 hours postinfusion
Letermovir	Oral, IV 480 mg q24 hours
Ribavirin	10 mg/kg loading dose followed by 20 mg/kg/day divided q8 hours. Available in PO and inhalation, drug is cytotoxic and teratogenic

Abbreviations: AUC, area under the curve; IV, intravenously; MRSA, methicillin-resistant *S. aureus*; PO, orally.
Note: There is limited experience with newer agents such as ceftazidime-avibactam, ceftolozane-tazobactam, and meropenem-vaborbactam in the setting of infected cancer patients with neutropenia.
[a]Preparations are available for both intravenous and oral administration, check dosing for each specific preparation.

invasive procedures, the continuation of the empiric antibacterial and antifungal regimen and the addition of empiric antiviral, or antiparasitic therapy might be necessary.

Other therapeutic modalities

Nearly 15–25% of infections occurring in patients with neutropenia fail to respond to appropriate antimicrobial therapy. In most cases, profound neutropenia persists. The availability of the hematopoietic growth factors has rekindled interest because the administration of granulocyte colony-stimulating factor (G-CSF) to donors increases the number of neutrophils that can be collected.[195–197] Some clinical studies suggest that this approach to white blood cell collection has produced therapeutic benefit in selected recipients.[198,199]

The administration of hematopoietic growth factors to patients receiving cancer chemotherapy reduces the severity and duration of neutropenia and, hence, the frequency of infectious complications.[200] The efficacy of these factors as adjuncts to antibiotic therapy has not been clearly established. It is reasonable to administer these agents to patients with neutrophil counts <500/mm^3 who develop pneumonia, septic shock, sepsis syndrome, or fungal infection because these patients have a poor prognosis without recovery of their neutrophils. These agents should also be considered for patients with documented infections who are failing to respond to appropriate therapy after 24–48 h. The role of G-CSFs appears to be expanding.[201] White blood cell transfusions are cumbersome to administer and may occasionally be beneficial, although data are limited. Similarly, interferon-gamma (IFN-γ) may be beneficial for some bacterial or fungal infections that are not responding to appropriate therapy.[202]

Infection risk of newer oncologic treatments

Based on preliminary data, checkpoint inhibitors (CPIs) per se do not appear to increase the risk of infection.[203] Small, uncontrolled studies suggest that checkpoint molecule blockade may improve patient outcomes in certain infections, but the effect of CPIs on clinical outcomes of infections has not yet been well studied.[203] CPI-mediated enhanced immunity could pose a significant risk of immune reconstitution inflammatory syndrome (IRIS) and autoimmune toxicity, whose treatment with immunosuppressive agents might predispose to opportunistic infections.[203] An increased risk of infections has been reported after CD19-targeted CAR-T cell immunotherapy in patients who had acute lymphoblastic leukemia, more prior antitumor treatment, a higher CAR-T-cell dose, or more severe cytokine release syndrome (CRS).[204] However, the overall incidence and type of infections after CD19 CAR-T-cell immunotherapy was similar to the incidence after other salvage chemo-immunotherapies for relapsed or refractory B-cell malignancies.[204] CAR-T-cell immunotherapy can be complicated by CRS, which can require treatment with corticosteroids and/or tocilizumab, both of which may increase infection risk.[204] In a multivariable analysis of a large study, CRS severity was the only factor associated with infection after CAR-T-cell infusion.[204]

Infection prevention

Suppression of the endogenous microflora, from which most infections arise, is usually achieved by using antimicrobial prophylaxis (bacterial, fungal, viral, and protozoal) during periods of risk. The acquisition of new organisms is reduced by various techniques, including infection control, well-cooked foods, and various isolation techniques or protected environments (PE).

Antibacterial prophylaxis

Prophylactic antimicrobial regimens achieve a major reduction in the patients' microbial burden. The fluoroquinolones are the most commonly used agents for prophylaxis resulting in a significant reduction in the frequency of Gram-negative infections, but with little impact on the frequency of gram-positive infections.[205,206] Although fluoroquinolone prophylaxis is associated with reduced mortality related to gram-negative infections, and in reduced all-cause mortality in some studies, it has also resulted in the emergence of fluoroquinolone resistance among GNB including *E. coli*.[207–209] Its uses remain controversial and it is therefore not recommended routinely, but must be considered only in patients at high risk for bacterial infection, such as those with prolonged neutropenia.[171,188,189] Surveillance for the emergence of resistant organisms is also of utmost importance.[210,211]

Antifungal and antiviral prophylaxis

The increasing frequency of IFIs in high-risk patients with leukemia or HCT recipients has led to the use of antifungal prophylaxis. Historically, fluconazole (and itraconazole) prophylaxis has been shown to decrease both superficial colonization and systemic *Candida* infections. The selection of resistant species (*C. krusei, C. glabratta*) is a potential problem, although these organisms are also seen in "azole naïve" patients. In regards to invasive aspergillosis, the most serious IFI in patients with hematologic cancer and/or HCT, there is high-quality evidence based on randomized controlled studies to recommend posaconazole for prophylaxis in patients with acute myeloid leukemia undergoing induction chemotherapy and those with GVHD following allogeneic HCT.[212–214] There is less strong evidence to guide the selection of antifungal prophylaxis following allogeneic HCT in patients who have no GVHD as well as for patients at intermediate/low risk for aspergillosis such as those with heavily pretreated lymphomas or myelomas. The use of TK inhibitors such as ibrutinib and possibly CAR-T cell therapy in patients with lymphoid malignancies. However, the cost-effectiveness and type of antifungal prophylaxis in these patients remains unclear. Antifungal prophylaxis typically is not indicated in patients with solid tumors.[212–214] TMP/SMX remains the agent of choice for *Pneumocystis jiroveci* prophylaxis.[109] Alternative (but less effective) agents include pentamidine, dapsone, and atovaquone.

Prophylaxis with acyclovir or valacyclovir prevents reactivation of HSV infection in patients undergoing chemotherapy (with or without radiation therapy) before HCT or induction therapy for leukemia or lymphoma. There is no consensus on the most appropriate approach to prevent CMV infection in HCT recipients, but management guidelines are being developed to address whether to give prophylactic or preemptive therapy. Prophylaxis with letermovir is indicated for prevention of CMV reactivation in CMV seropositive adult HCT recipients. Letermovir administered from the time of transplant through day 100 reduced the incidence of CMV infection and all-cause mortality at week 24 in CMV seropositive allogenic HCT recipients.[146,215] Many centers still use a preemptive approach for CMV in HCT recipients rather than a prophylactic approach to minimize toxicity. Preemptive therapy with ganciclovir or foscarnet requires serial testing for CMV (e.g., by PCR of whole blood or plasma) following HCT, treating only those who develop viremia.[152]

Isolation

The reduction of the acquisition of new organisms has been attempted by putting patients at risk into reverse isolation. Patients are also given well-cooked foods and are asked to avoid fresh fruits and vegetables that are frequently contaminated with GNB.

PE provides a combination of the two approaches, i.e., the use of isolation units to protect the patient against nosocomial contamination plus antibiotic regimens to reduce the patient's endogenous flora. The PE generally consists of isolation units, which provide a barrier between the patient and the hospital environment, using aggressive decontamination techniques and filtered air. The patient's food is prepared to minimize contamination. Disinfection of the patient is achieved by using intensive regimens, which include oral nonabsorbable antibiotics. Patients bathe with germicidal soaps and apply topical antibiotic ointments or sprays to areas of heavy microbial contamination.

Because attempts at suppressing the endogenous microflora and those at preventing the acquisition of organisms have not been overwhelmingly successful, other means for infection prevention need to be developed. The hematopoietic growth factors (granulocyte-macrophage [GM]-CSF and G-CSF) have been demonstrated to shorten the duration of neutropenia and to reduce the number of febrile days and of documented infections in some patients. Guidelines suggest that the primary use of these agents is not indicated in patients who were previously untreated and receiving most chemotherapy regimens. The secondary administration of growth factors can decrease the probability of febrile

Table 7 Antimicrobial stewardship strategies.

- Continuing education for all healthcare providers
- Guidelines/pathways for appropriate antimicrobial usage based on local microbiology and susceptibility/resistance
- Formulary interventions restricting specific agents
- Audits of antimicrobial usage with feedback to prescribers
- Introduction of surveillance and decision support programs
- Monitoring outcomes (morbidity, mortality, length of stay) and resistance patterns
- Comprehensive infection control program

neutropenia after a documented occurrence in an earlier cycle. It can also reduce the period of neutropenia and the frequency of infectious complications in patients undergoing high-dose cytotoxic therapy with autologous HCT.

Antimicrobial stewardship

Antimicrobial resistance results in increased morbidity, mortality, and cost of healthcare. Antimicrobial stewardship has become an essential part of the management of patients with cancer. The major goal of antimicrobial stewardship is to optimize antimicrobial usage while reducing unwanted consequences such as toxicity and the selection of resistant organisms.[216,217] Strategies for effective antimicrobial stewardship are listed in Table 7. These strategies are best implemented by an independent, multidisciplinary, antimicrobial stewardship team (MAST).[218]

Perspectives

Infection remains a serious complication for many cancer patients. The spectrum of infection continues to change and the emergence of MDR pathogens has posed serious challenges. Disseminated IFIs have become the leading cause of death in patients with hematologic malignancies, and in HCT recipients. Despite some improvements, the early diagnosis and adequate treatment of many IFIs remain unsatisfactory. Viral infections represent a growing threat particularly in patients with hematologic malignancies and HCT recipients. Parasitic infections remain uncommon except in endemic areas. Although effective therapies are available, toxicity and the need for prolonged maintenance or suppressive therapy can be problematic. The development of risk assessment strategies has led to the recognition of a "low-risk" subset among patients with neutropenia. Treatment strategies such as outpatient, oral therapy have resulted in substantial cost savings, reduction in healthcare-associated infections, and improved quality of life. PE, prophylactic programs, infection control strategies, and the CSFs have reduced the risk of infection in patients with cancer. Antimicrobial stewardship may delay the development of resistant organisms. Newer technological advances should lead to further progress. Nonetheless, the recognition, prevention, diagnosis, and treatment of infections in patients with cancer will continue to challenge us in the foreseeable future, as we work toward the larger goal of eliminating cancer.

Key references

The complete reference list can be found on Vital Source version of this title, see inside front cover.

2   Bow EJ. Neutropenic fever syndromes in patients undergoing cytotoxic therapy for acute leukemia and myelodysplastic syndromes. *Semin Hematol.* 2009;**46**:259–268.

3   Zell JA, Chang JC. Neoplastic fever: a neglected paraneoplastic syndrome. *Support Care Cancer.* 2005;**13**:870–877.

11 Rolston KV, Freifeld AG, Zimmer AJ, et al. Bloodstream infection survey in high-risk oncology patients (BISHOP) with fever and neutropenia in the United States: microbiology data. 28th European Congress of Clinical Microbiology and Infectious Diseases; 2018. April 21–24; Madrid, Spain.

12 Wisplinghoff H, Seifert H, Wenzel RP, Edmond MB. Current trends in the epidemiology of nosocomial bloodstream infections in patients with hematological malignancies and solid neoplasms in hospitals in the United States. *Clin Infect Dis.* 2003;**36**(9):1103–1110.

13 Nesher L, Rolston KV. The current spectrum of infection in cancer patients with chemotherapy related neutropenia. *Infection.* 2014;**42**:5–13.

15 Rolston KV, Bodey GP, Safdar A. Polymicrobial infection in patients with cancer: an underappreciated and underreported entity. *Clin Infect Dis.* 2007;**45**:228–233.

21 Liu C, Bayer A, Cosgrove SE, et al. Clinical practice guidelines by the infectious diseases society of america for the treatment of methicillin-resistant *Staphylococcus aureus* infections in adults and children. *Clin Infect Dis.* 2011;**52**:e18–e55.

32 Bochud PY, Eggiman P, Calandra T, et al. Bacteremia due to viridans streptococci in neutropenic patients with cancer: clinical spectrum and risk factors. *Clin Infect Dis.* 1994;**18**:25–31.

35 Shelburne SA, Tarrand J, Rolston KV. Review of streptococcal bloodstream infections at a comprehensive cancer care center, 2000–2011. *J Infect.* 2013;**66**:136–146.

39 Dubberke ER, Hollands JM, Georgantopoulos P, et al. Vancomycin-resistant enterococcal bloodstream infections on a hematopoietic stem cell transplant unit: are the sick getting sicker? *Bone Marrow Transplant.* 2006;**38**:813–819.

44 Torres HA, Reddy BT, Raad II, et al. Nocardiosis in cancer patients. *Medicine (Baltimore).* 2002;**81**:388–397.

48 Safdar A, Rolston KV. *Stenotrophomonas maltophilia*: changing spectrum of a serious bacterial pathogen in patients with cancer. *Clin Infect Dis.* 2007;**45**:1602–1609.

50 Nesher L, KVI R. Neutropenic enterocolitis, a growing concern in the era of widespread use of aggressive chemotherapy. *Clinical Infectious Diseases.* 2013;**56**:711–717.

51 Boucher HW, Talbot GH, Bradley JS, et al. Bad bugs, no drugs: no ESKAPE! An update from the Infectious Diseases Society of America. *Clin Infect Dis.* 2009;**48**:1–12.

52 Bushnell G, Mitrani-Gold F, Mundy LM. Emergence of New Delhi metallo-β-lactamase type 1-producing enterobacteriaceae and non-enterobacteriaceae: global case detection and bacterial surveillance. *Int J Infect Dis.* 2013;**17**:e325–e333.

64 Chen CY, Sheng WH, Lai CC, et al. Mycobacterial infections in adult patients with hematological malignancy. *Eur J Clin Microbiol Infect Dis.* 2012;**31**:1059–1066.

69 Cohen SH, Gerding DN, Johnson S, et al. Clinical practice guidelines for *Clostridium difficile* infection in adults: 2010 update by the society for healthcare epidemiology of America (SHEA) and the infectious diseases society of America (IDSA). *Infect Control Hosp Epidemiol.* 2010;**31**:431–455.

72 Johnson S, Schriever C, Patel U, et al. Rifaximin redux: treatment of recurrent *Clostridium difficile* infections with rifaximin immediately post-vancomycin treatment. *Anaerobe.* 2009;**15**:290–291.

75 Cornely OA, Miller MA, Fantin B, et al. Resolution of *Clostridium difficile*-associated diarrhea in patients with cancer treated with fidaxomicin or vancomycin. *J Clin Oncol.* 2013;**31**:2493–2499.

78 Diorio C, Robinson PD, Ammann RA, et al. Guideline for the management of *Clostridium difficile* infection in children and adolescents with cancer and pediatric hematopoietic stem-cell transplantation recipients. *J Clin Oncol.* 2018:JCO1800407.

79 Chen D, Wu J, Jin D, et al. Fecal microbiota transplantation in cancer management: current status and perspectives. *Int J Cancer.* 2019;**145**:2021–2031.

80 Galloway-Pena JR, Peterson CB, Malik F, et al. Fecal microbiome, metabolites, and stem cell transplant outcomes: a single-center pilot study. *Open Forum Infect Dis.* 2019;**6**:ofz173.

81 Lewis RE, Cahyame-Zuniga L, Leventakos K, et al. Epidemiology and sites of involvement of invasive fungal infections in patients with haematological malignancies: a 20-year autopsy study. *Mycoses.* 2013;**56**:638–645.

82 Kontoyiannis DP, Marr KA, Park BJ, et al. Prospective surveillance for invasive fungal infections in hematopoietic stem cell transplant recipients, 2001–2006: overview of the Transplant-Associated Infection Surveillance Network (TRANSNET) Database. *Clin Infect Dis.* 2010;**50**:1091–1100.

85 Sipsas NV, Lewis RE, Tarrand J, et al. Candidemia in patients with hematologic malignancies in the era of new antifungal agents (2001–2007): stable incidence but changing epidemiology of a still frequently lethal infection. *Cancer.* 2009;**115**:4745–4752.

89 Groll AH, Castagnola E, Cesaro S, et al. Fourth European Conference on Infections in Leukaemia (ECIL-4): guidelines for diagnosis, prevention, and treatment of invasive fungal diseases in paediatric patients with cancer or allogeneic haemopoietic stem-cell transplantation. *Lancet Oncol.* 2014;**15**:e327–e340.

91 Pappas PG, Kauffman CA, Andes DR, et al. Clinical practice guideline for the management of candidiasis: 2016 update by the Infectious Diseases Society of America. *Clin Infect Dis.* 2016;**62**:e1–e50.

102 Marr KA, Schlamm HT, Herbrecht R, et al. Combination antifungal therapy for invasive aspergillosis: a randomized trial. *Ann Intern Med.* 2015;**162**:81–89.

104 Kamel S, O'Connor S, Lee N, et al. High incidence of *Pneumocystis jirovecii* pneumonia in patients receiving biweekly rituximab and cyclophosphamide, adriamycin, vincristine, and prednisone. *Leuk Lymphoma.* 2010;**51**:797–801.

109 Cooley L, Dendle C, Wolf J, et al. Consensus guidelines for diagnosis, prophylaxis and management of *Pneumocystis jirovecii* pneumonia in patients with haematological and solid malignancies, 2014. *Intern Med J.* 2014;**44**:1350–1363.

117 Kyvernitakis A, Torres HA, Jiang Y, et al. Initial use of combination treatment does not impact survival of 106 patients with haematologic malignancies and mucormycosis: a propensity score analysis. *Clin Microbiol Infect.* 2016;**22**:811 e1–e8.

125 Hwang JP, LoConte NK, Rice JP, et al. Oncologic implications of chronic hepatitis C virus infection. *J Oncol Pract.* 2019;**15**:629–637.

126 Hwang JP, Lok AS. Management of patients with hepatitis B who require immunosuppressive therapy. *Nat Rev Gastroenterol Hepatol.* 2014;**11**:209–219.

127 Torres HA, Hosry J, Mahale P, et al. Hepatitis C virus reactivation in patients receiving cancer treatment: a prospective observational study. *Hepatology.* 2018;**67**:36–47.

131 Hirsch HH, Martino R, Ward KN, et al. Fourth European Conference on Infections in Leukaemia (ECIL-4): guidelines for diagnosis and treatment of human respiratory syncytial virus, parainfluenza virus, metapneumovirus, rhinovirus, and coronavirus. *Clin Infect Dis.* 2013;**56**:258–266.

133 Poutanen SM, Low DE, Henry B, et al. Identification of severe acute respiratory syndrome in Canada. *N Engl J Med.* 2003;**348**:1995–2005.

134 Centers for Disease Control and Prevention. Update: severe respiratory illness associated with a novel coronavirus – worldwide, 2012-2013. *MMWR Morb Mortal Wkly Rep.* 2013;**62**:194–195.

135 Liang W, Guan W, Chen R, et al. Cancer patients in SARS-CoV-2 infection: a nationwide analysis in China. *Lancet Oncol.* 2020;**21**:335–337.

138 Bhimraj A, Morgan RL, Hirsch Shumaker A, et al. Infectious Diseases Society of America Guidelines on the Treatment and Management of Patients with COVID-19 Infection. *Clin Infect Dis.* 2020;**27**:ciaa478.

146 Chemaly RF, Hill JA, Voigt S, Peggs KS. In vitro comparison of currently available and investigational antiviral agents against pathogenic human double-stranded DNA viruses: a systematic literature review. *Antiviral Res.* 2019;**163**:50–58.

147 Zerr DM, Boeckh M, Delaney C, et al. HHV-6 reactivation and associated sequelae after hematopoietic cell transplantation. *Biol Blood Marrow Transplant.* 2012;**18**:1700–1708.

148 Gerdemann U, Keukens L, Keirnan JM, et al. Immunotherapeutic strategies to prevent and treat human herpesvirus 6 reactivation after allogeneic stem cell transplantation. *Blood.* 2013;**121**:207–218.

149 Ljungman P, Griffiths P, Paya C. Definitions of cytomegalovirus infection and disease in transplant recipients. *Clin Infect Dis.* 2002;**34**:1094–1097.

171 Freifeld AG, Bow EJ, Sepkowitz KA, et al. Clinical practice guideline for the use of antimicrobial agents in neutropenic patients with cancer: 2010 update by the infectious diseases society of america. *Clin Infect Dis.* 2011;**52**:e56–e93.

176 Klastersky J, Paesmans M, Rubenstein EB, et al. The multinational association for supportive care in cancer risk index: a multinational scoring system for identifying low-risk febrile neutropenic cancer patients. *J Clin Oncol.* 2000;**18**:3038–3051.

183 Kern WV, Marchetti O, Drgona L, et al. Oral antibiotics for fever in low-risk neutropenic patients with cancer: a double-blind, randomized, multicenter trial comparing single daily moxifloxacin with twice daily ciprofloxacin plus amoxicillin/clavulanic acid combination therapy – EORTC infectious diseases group trial XV. *J Clin Oncol.* 2013;**31**:1149–1156.

188 Flowers CR, Seidenfeld J, Bow EJ, et al. Antimicrobial prophylaxis and outpatient management of fever and neutropenia in adults treated for malignancy: American Society of Clinical Oncology clinical practice guideline. *J Clin Oncol.* 2013;**31**:794–810.

190 Taplitz RA, Kennedy EB, Bow EJ, et al. Outpatient management of fever and neutropenia in adults treated for malignancy: American Society of Clinical Oncology and Infectious Diseases Society of America Clinical Practice Guideline Update. *J Clin Oncol.* 2018;**36**:1443–1453.

205 Bucaneve G, Micozzi A, Menichetti F, et al. Levofloxacin to prevent bacterial infection in patients with cancer and neutropenia. *N Engl J Med.* 2005;**353**:977–987.

206 Cullen M, Steven N, Billingham L, et al. Antibacterial prophylaxis after chemotherapy for solid tumors and lymphomas. *N Engl J Med.* 2005;**353**:988–998.

207 Gafter-Gvili A, Fraser A, Paul M, et al. Antibiotic prophylaxis for bacterial infections in afebrile neutropenic patients following chemotherapy. *Cochrane Database Syst Rev.* 2012;**1**:CD004386.

213 Maertens JA, Girmenia C, Bruggemann RJ, et al. European guidelines for primary antifungal prophylaxis in adult haematology patients: summary of the updated recommendations from the European Conference on Infections in Leukaemia. *J Antimicrob Chemother.* 2018;**73**:3221–3230.

214 Taplitz RA, Kennedy EB, Bow EJ, et al. Antimicrobial prophylaxis for adult patients with cancer-related immunosuppression: ASCO and IDSA Clinical Practice Guideline Update. *J Clin Oncol.* 2018;**36**:3043–3054.

215 Marty FM, Ljungman P, Chemaly RF, et al. Letermovir prophylaxis for cytomegalovirus in hematopoietic-cell transplantation. *N Engl J Med.* 2017;**377**:2433–2444.

218 Tverdek FP, Rolston KV, Chemaly RF. Antimicrobial stewardship in patients with cancer. *Pharmacotherapy.* 2012;**32**:722–734.

138 Oncologic emergencies

Sai-Ching J. Yeung, MD, PhD, FACP ■ Carmen P. Escalante, MD

> **Overview**
>
> Cancer and its treatment can lead to oncologic emergencies. This article discusses the approach to acute emergency problems in cancer patients. A list of emergent problems has been selected for focused discussion. Sudden cardiopulmonary arrest is discussed along with considerations in resuscitation of cancer patients. Arrhythmia, superior vena caval syndrome, pericardial tamponade, and acute hemorrhage are important cardiovascular emergencies. Tumor lysis syndrome can be rapidly fatal, and early recognition and treatment are very important in preventing disastrous outcomes. Pulmonary problems include airway obstruction, pleural effusion, hemoptysis, pneumothorax, and pulmonary embolism. Neurological emergencies include spinal cord compression, brain herniation, and status epilepticus. Neutropenic fever is perhaps the most frequently discussed important topic in oncologic emergency. Other important issues such as immune-related adverse effects of cancer immunotherapy, anaphylaxis, and cytokine release syndrome are also discussed. Oncologists and emergency physicians must be aware of these potentially serious acute complications of cancer patients in order to initiate appropriate treatments in a timely manner.

Introduction

An oncologic emergency is an acute condition that is caused by cancer or its treatment and that requires intervention as soon as possible to avoid mortality or severe morbidity. Cancer patients are more likely to require emergency care than patients without cancer. Physical debilitation, altered hemostasis, and impaired immunity due to malignancy or its treatment also make cancer patients vulnerable to accidents and mishaps in everyday life. Because cancer patients have unique concerns and changes in physiological status, emergency care providers need to adapt to their special needs. Due to page constraints and coverage of some relevant topics in other articles of this encyclopedia, this article will cover only selected topics.[1–3]

Approach to acutely ill cancer patients

Cancer patients often have comorbidities such as coronary heart disease, diabetes mellitus, and chronic obstructive pulmonary disease. Some of these may be attributable to the same risk factors for carcinogenesis (i.e., old age, diet, cigarette smoking, or sedentary lifestyle). Emergency care providers must assess the extent of the malignancy, the response to treatment, the overall prognosis, and the patient's and family's wishes in order to formulate an appropriate treatment plan (Figure 1). The majority of cancer patients who are approaching their ends of life do not want "heroic" measures, and addressing advance directives and do-not-resuscitate (DNR) orders in a timely manner may improve the quality of life in the weeks before death.[1]

First, the patient should be rapidly assessed. This assessment should include the chief complaint, a focused history, vital signs, and a quick overall physical assessment. If the patient is unable to relay the history of present illness, a family member, companion, or caregiver may provide pertinent information. Intervention for unstable vital signs should be initiated immediately. In case of cardiopulmonary arrest, appropriate guidelines are followed (http://www.acls.net/aclsalg.htm).[2] Once the patient is stabilized, thorough history and physical examination should be completed. For the majority of cancer patients with emergencies, a comprehensive evaluation is necessary. The emergency may be due to the cancer, cancer treatments, or comorbid conditions, all of which should be considered in the differential diagnosis.

Circulatory oncologic emergencies

Sudden cardiopulmonary arrest

Most deaths are preceded by cardiopulmonary arrest. Resuscitation is more likely to succeed when cardiopulmonary arrest was caused by an acute reversible insult rather than by a steady irreversible decline in bodily functions. The success rate of resuscitation and the hospital discharge rate of resuscitated patients are similar for cancer patients and noncancer patients.[3] A meta-analysis of inpatient resuscitation (including cancer patients) estimated that the probabilities of successful resuscitation and being discharged alive are about 30% and 12%, respectively.[4] Similarly, for cancer patients with out-of-hospital arrest who received resuscitation at the Emergency Department of a cancer center, the probabilities of successful resuscitation and being discharged alive are 43% and 17%, respectively.[5] The mortality rate of cancer patients in intensive care is about 50%, which is similar to that of severely ill noncancer patients.[6] If a cancer patient has good performance status and is not expected to die soon, reluctance to resuscitate the patient or admit the patient to intensive care is unjustified. A non-end-stage cancer patient in cardiopulmonary arrest should be resuscitated with the same level of intense effort as any patient without cancer. However, when cardiopulmonary arrest occurs as the expected final event, resuscitation is generally futile.

Oncologists should ensure that advance directives (medical power of attorney, living will, and out-of-hospital DNR orders) are discussed with cancer patients and their families. Many informed patients readily sign living wills or appoint health care proxies. Timely recommendation of DNR status may avoid unnecessary trauma to patients, futile efforts, wasted resources, and anguish for family members; this also provides time for open discussion to settle disagreements among the patient and family members.

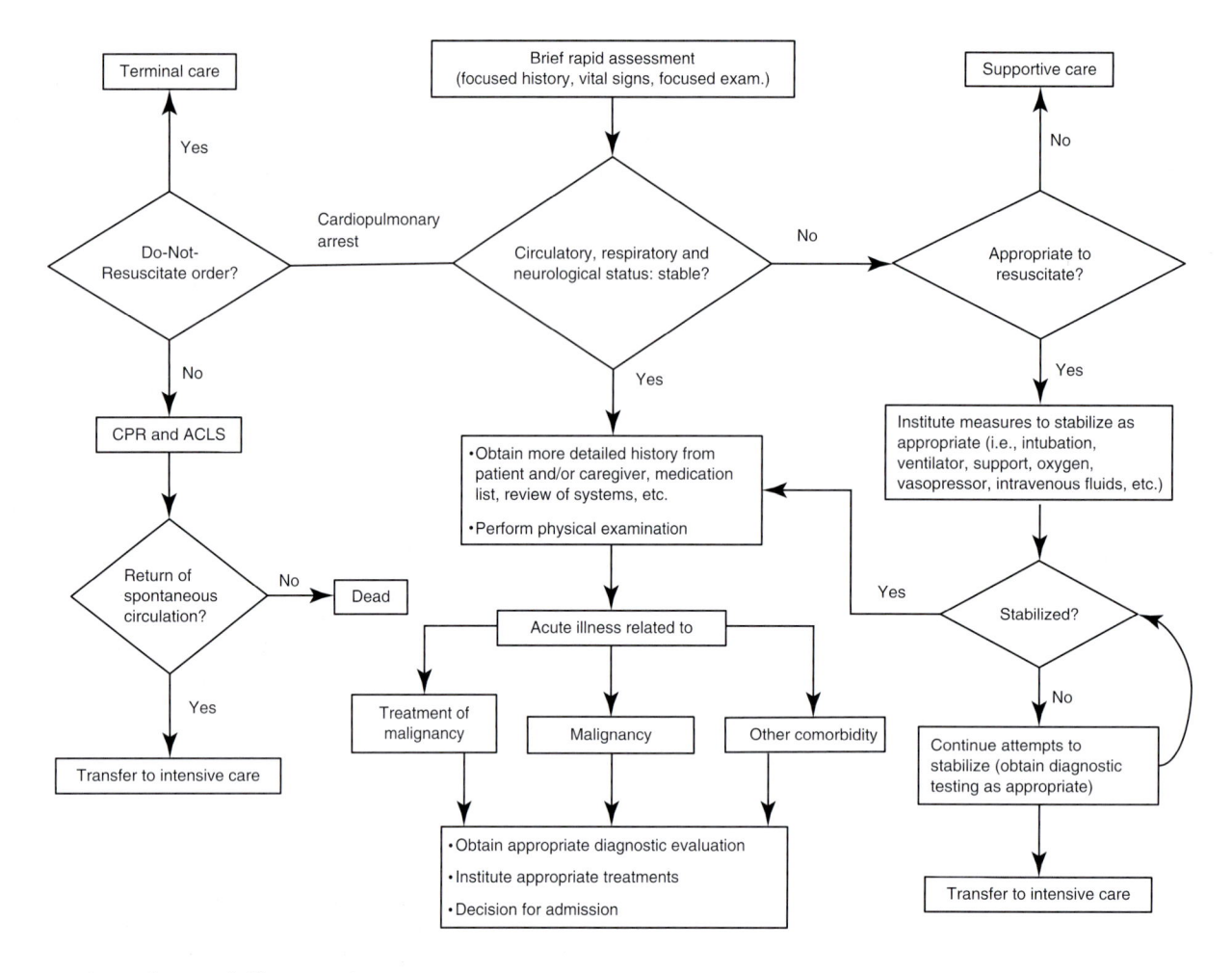

Figure 1 Approach to acutely ill cancer patients.

When a cancer patient presents to a health care facility in impending or full cardiopulmonary arrest, the emergency physician may have never seen the patient before, and assessment of prognosis is difficult and often impossible. The decision to initiate or continue resuscitation should be based on a rapid assessment of the patient's physical condition, a brief history of the events preceding the arrest, and the following factors: (1) duration of arrest, (2) initial cardiac rhythm, (3) rigor mortis or algor mortis, (4) type, stage, and prognosis of cancer, (5) history of cancer treatment and prospects for its success, (6) expressed directives of the patient or family, (7) comorbid conditions, (8) performance and nutritional status, (9) potential quality of life if the patient survives, and (10) advanced age.

The fact that the patient was transported to an emergency center may indicate that death is unexpected, that the family has not yet accepted the patient's grave prognosis, or that the patient or family is seeking relief of symptoms or suffering at the last moments of life. Demands for resuscitation may be motivated by denial of the terminal condition. A questionnaire-based study has found that most cancer patients want to be resuscitated despite poor survival rates and that they want themselves and their next of kin to be involved in the decision-making process.[7] In the absence of clear advance directive, resuscitation may be needed to give the family "closure" by knowing that "everything possible has been done." However, resuscitation of patients with advanced refractory malignancies may be inappropriate when it will only prolong pain and suffering.

Special consideration in resuscitation of cancer patients

Most physicians and health care providers follow the resuscitation algorithms outlined in the advanced cardiac life support protocols (http://www.acls.net/aclsalg.htm).[2] However, identification of specific causes of cardiopulmonary arrest may enable physicians to target efforts to reverse or control the specific causes. Carcinoid crisis is a good example of an uncommon but preventable and treatable cause of cardiopulmonary arrest in cancer patients. The crisis may be precipitated by anesthesia, biopsy, surgery, chemotherapy, or adrenergic drugs (e.g., dopamine and epinephrine). Affected patients may develop refractory hypotension, arrhythmias, and bronchospasm due to massive release of serotonin and other vasoactive peptides from the tumor. Carcinoid crisis can be aborted or treated with octreotide acetate, a somatostatin analogue, 150–500 μg intravenously (IV).[8] Empiric naloxone treatment is recommended for all unresponsive opioid-associated life-threatening emergencies. Resuscitative measures (high-quality chest compressions plus ventilation) should take priority over naloxone. Naloxone may be continued in postarrest care to antagonize long-acting opioids. Cardiac tamponade is another example. If a patient has pulseless electrical activity due to tamponade by a pericardial effusion (e.g., malignant or immune-mediated), resuscitation will not succeed until the pressure on the cardiac chambers is relieved by pericardiocentesis.

Causes of cardiac arrest in cancer patients

In the general population, undiagnosed neoplasm is a rare cause of sudden death. In cancer patients, a review of causes of death found that 4% of patients died of cardiac problems and that 90% of these died from atherosclerosis-related ischemic heart disease.[9] Most causes of cardiopulmonary arrests in cancer patients are related to cancer or antineoplastic therapy, rather than primary cardiac disease.

Tumor-related causes
Tumor-related cardiac problems are usually the result of pericardial involvement (e.g., neoplastic pericarditis, and cardiac tamponade). Tumors can induce arrhythmias by secretion of hormone mediators (e.g., catecholamines by pheochromocytomas, and serotonin by carcinoid tumors) or by direct mechanical irritation of the heart or pericardium. Arrhythmias associated with myocardial tumors, coronary obstruction by tumor, and massive tumor embolization have been reported to cause sudden cardiopulmonary arrest. Cardiac amyloidosis can also lead to intractable congestive heart failure, arrhythmias, conduction disturbances, and sudden death.[10] Other tumor-related causes of arrest include hemorrhage, loss of ventilatory function, and organ failure.

Systemic therapy-related causes
Antineoplastic agents can cause complications (angina, myocardial infarction, congestive heart failure, hypotension, arrhythmia) leading to cardiopulmonary arrest.[11] Doxorubicin may cause electrocardiographic and rhythm changes (mostly benign) in about 30% of patients,[12] and sudden cardiopulmonary arrest in almost 1% of patients.[13] Some drugs (e.g., imatinib, trastuzumab) may interfere with myocardial remodeling after cytotoxic myocardial damage, causing cardiomyopathy and heart failure.[12] High-dose cyclophosphamide may cause ventricular arrhythmia, cardiomyopathy, pericardial effusion, and cardiac arrest.[14] Fluorouracil and capecitabine are associated with acute coronary vasospasm leading to angina and myocardial infarction; they have also been reported to cause acute cardiogenic shock. Hypotension, arrhythmia, and sudden death have been reported with cytokines (interleukin-2 [IL-2], interferons) and monoclonal antibodies. Immune checkpoint inhibitors can cause immune-mediated pericarditis or myocarditis and potentially lead to cardiac arrest.

Radiotherapy-related causes
Radiation can damage the pericardium and heart.[15] Pericarditis may occur shortly or months to years after exposure of the chest to radiation. Radiotherapy can lead to valvular diseases, pericardial effusion, tamponade, pericardial fibrosis, or restrictive cardiomyopathy. The direct toxic effect of radiation can cause electrocardiographic changes, including T-wave abnormalities and atrial arrhythmias. Exposure of the heart to radiation is also associated with coronary artery problems (accelerated atherosclerosis, endarteritis, medial fibrosis, intimal proliferation), leading to myocardial infarction and sudden death.[16]

Arrhythmia

Arrhythmia is a common problem in cancer patients that needs emergency care. Sustained arrhythmia can lead to cardiopulmonary arrest and death; otherwise, the symptoms of intermittent arrhythmia can be subtle. The symptoms are primarily due to the hemodynamic effects. Significant signs and symptoms include isolated or recurrent loss of consciousness (syncope), lightheadedness (dizziness), palpitation, chest pain, dyspnea, and acute neurologic deficits.

Sustained arrhythmia can be diagnosed electrographically readily. However, arrhythmia is often transient or intermittent, causing difficulty in diagnosis. An electrocardiographic rhythm strip or a brief period of continuous monitoring does not exclude latent and potentially serious rhythm disorders. When symptoms suggest arrhythmia, Holter monitoring or event recorders (continuous loop, postevent, or real-time continuous) are indicated to capture the arrhythmia. Analysis of cardiac rhythm may be complicated in cancer patients because they often have exaggerated respiratory variations of the electrical axis and changes in mean QRS voltage that can be confused with heart rhythm irregularity. Such changes may be due to pleural or pericardial effusions, pulmonary surgery (pneumonectomy or lobectomy), or radiation-induced lung damage.

Primary arrhythmia
Primary arrhythmia arises from cardiac and pericardial structures. Common causes of primary arrhythmia in all patients include ischemic disease; increased intracardiac pressure and wall stress; congestive, hypertrophic, and infiltrative cardiomyopathy; and fibrosis. In cancer patients, the causes of primary arrhythmia are primary or metastatic intracardiac tumors, amyloid infiltration, myocarditis (including immune-related adverse effects (irAEs) induced by immune checkpoint inhibitors), pericarditis (including irAEs), pericardial constriction, and cardiomyopathy related to antineoplastic agents (especially anthracyclines and anti-HER2 therapy).[11]

Secondary arrhythmia
Secondary arrhythmia arises from toxic reactions to drugs; increased sympathetic states (severe anxiety, hyperthyroidism, pheochromocytomas, carcinoid tumors, etc.); and abnormal electrolytes (especially hypomagnesemia and hypokalemia in cancer patients). Some cancer drugs are arrhythmogenic (Table 1).[17–21] Acquired QT prolongation due to medications increases the risk for polymorphic ventricular tachycardia (*torsade de pointes*) and sudden death. The US Food and Drug Administration (FDA) warns against a QT interval, corrected using the Fridericia formula, (QTc) >450 ms, and especially concerned if QTc is >500 ms.[22] In addition to chemotherapy, antifungal agents, anti-protozoans, and antibiotics, which are commonly used to treat infectious complications in cancer patients, may prolong the QT interval, potentially leading to arrhythmia. An updated list of QT-prolonging drugs is available at https://crediblemeds.org/pdftemp/pdf/CombinedList.pdf.

Treatment of arrhythmia
Treatment of arrhythmia should be based on both urgency and etiology. For hemodynamically stable arrhythmias of secondary origins, the primary treatment should focus on correcting metabolic derangements (particularly potassium, calcium, and magnesium) and discontinuing culprit drugs. Specific treatment to reverse the causative factor should be administered. When treatment aimed at controlling the cardiac rhythm is necessary, standard guidelines for management of arrhythmia may be followed.[2] Commonly used IV antiarrhythmic drugs are listed in Table 2.

Paroxysmal supraventricular tachycardia (SVT) may be converted back into sinus rhythm in a considerable proportion of cases by vagal maneuvers. Adenosine administered as one or two doses of rapidly injected boluses under electrocardiographic monitoring is frequently effective in restoring sinus heart rhythm. Adenosine is also used to determine the mechanism of the arrhythmia when the diagnosis is unclear on electrocardiograms.

Table 1 Antineoplastic drugs associated with cardiovascular side effects[a].

	Pulmonary HTN	Systemic HTN	Ischemia/ ACS/MI	Reduction in LVEF/CHF	QT prolongation	VT/VF/ Sudden death	Bradycardia/ AVB	AF/ SVT	PE	Myocarditis	Pericarditis/ Pericardial effusion
Immune checkpoint inhibitors											
Atezolizumab										X	X
Avelumab										X	X
Cemiplimab										X	X
Durvalumab										X	X
Ipilimumab										X	X
Nivolumab										X	X
Pembrolizumab										X	X
Kinase inhibitors											
Acalabrutinib								X			
Afatinib		X		X	X			X			
Axitinib		X		X							
Binimetinib				X							
Bosutinib		X			X			X			
Brigatinib		X					X				
Cabozantinib		X			X						
Ceritinib					X		X				
Cobimetinib				X							
Crizotinib					X						
Dabrafenib				X	X						
Dasatinib	X			X	X						
Encorafenib					X						
Entrectinib				X	X						
Erlotinib			X								
Ibrutinib		X				X		X			
Imatinib	X			X							
Lapatinib			X	X	X	X					
Lenvatinib		X		X	X						
Nilotinib	X	X			X	X					
Osimertinib				X	X						
Pazopanib		X		X	X	X					
Ponatinib			X	X		X					
Regorafenib		X									
Ribociclib					X						
Ruxolitinib				X							
Sorafenib		X	X	X	X						
Sunitinib		X		X	X	X					
Trametinib				X	X						
Vandetanib		X		X	X						
Vemurafenib					X						
Zanubrutinib		X						X			
Antibodies											
Bevacizumab		X	X	X							
Elotuzumab		X									
Necitumumab		X		X							
Pertuzumab				X							
Ramucirumab						X					
Trastuzumab									X		
Recombinant fusion protein											
Ziv-aflibercept		X									
Antibody-conjugate											
Ado-trastuzumab emtansine				X							
Fam-trastuzumab deruxtecan-nxki				X							
Inotuzumab ozogamicin					X						
Alkylating agents											
Busulfan				X							
Cisplatin		X	X	X		X		X			
Cyclophosphamide			X	X				X			
Ifosfamide				X				X			
Mitomycin				X							

(continued overleaf)

Table 1 (Continued)

	Pulmonary HTN	Systemic HTN	Ischemia/ ACS/MI	Reduction in LVEF/CHF	QT prolongation	VT/VF/ Sudden death	Bradycardia/ AVB	AF/ SVT	PE	Myocarditis	Pericarditis/ Pericardial effusion
Anthracyclines/anthraquinolones											
Daunorubicin				x							
Doxorubicin				x		x	x	x			
Epirubicin				x							
Idarubicin				x							
Mitoxantrone				x							
Antimetabolites											
5-Fluorouracil			x	x				x			
Capecitabine			x	x		x					
Clofarabine				x							
Cytarabine				x							
Gemcitabine								x			
Topoisomerase I inhibitors											
Irinotecan							x				
Taxanes											
Docetaxel			x	x							
Paclitaxel			x			x	x	x			
Vinca alkaloids											
Vinblastine			x								
Vincristine			x								
Miscellaneous											
Apalutamide			x								
Arsenic trioxide					x						
Belinostat					x					x	
Bortezomib				x							
Carfilzomib				x	x						
Enzalutamide	x	x									
IL-2				x		x		x			
Interferon-alpha			x	x				x			
Panobinostat lactate			x			x					
Pentostatin				x							
Pomalidomide									x		
Thalidomide							x	x			
Trabectedin				x							
Tretinoin (retinoic acid)				x							
Vorinostat					x						

Abbreviations: AF, atrial fibrillation; HTN, hypertension; LVEF, left ventricular ejection fraction; QTcF, QT interval corrected by Fridericia's Formula; VT, ventricular tachycardia; SVT, supraventricular tachycardia.
[a]Source: Adapted from Yeh et al.[17]; Lenihan and Kowey[18]; Guglin et al.[19]; Yeh and Bickford[20]; and Ewer and Ewer[21].

Stable secondary arrhythmia is unlikely to deteriorate into a life-threatening catastrophe. Frequently, secondary arrhythmia presents as ventricular ectopy (sometimes in bigeminy, trigeminy, or other coupled patterns), or supraventricular ectopy (often as intermittent or sustained SVT). Isolated premature ventricular complexes do not require any treatment. Complex forms of ventricular ectopy are often controlled by beta-adrenergic blockers. Amiodarone should be considered for patients with a low left ventricular ejection fraction, but with caution for patients with hepatic insufficiency or underlying thyroid diseases. Rarely, amiodarone can cause hypotension, bradycardia, and QT prolongation that may precipitate torsades de pointes. Except for beta-adrenergic blockers, many antiarrhythmic drugs, especially types 1A, 1C, and 3, are potentially proarrhythmic.[23] Cardiac monitoring during the initiation of antiarrhythmic therapy should be considered because cancer patients may have an increased susceptibility to proarrhythmic effects due to metabolic derangements and concomitant use of other QT-prolonging drugs.

SVT is the most common arrhythmia in cancer patients. While pharmacological agents are used for sustained SVT with stable hemodynamics, elective synchronized cardioversion under conscious sedation should be considered early and planned appropriately. The initial energy level for synchronized cardioversion recommended by the American Heart Association is 100 joules, but an initial shock with an energy level of 200 joules has been recommended by others for the conversion of atrial fibrillation.[24] Higher energy levels for cardioversion are appropriate when cancer patients have concomitant effusions or are significantly overweight. If sinus rhythm can be restored within 48 h of the onset of SVT, anticoagulation therapy may be avoided. However, the time of onset of arrhythmia is not always clear. Intracardiac thrombosis may be excluded by transesophageal echocardiography. In lack of clear evidence for the time of onset, the patient should be anticoagulated prior to cardioversion.

Arrhythmias of structural origin in cancer patients are more difficult to control than arrhythmias of metabolic etiology. In the emergency setting, the therapeutic goals are stabilization of hemodynamics and respiratory status, discovery of correctable pathologic conditions, and control of symptoms. Depending on the etiology of the arrhythmia, emergent consultation with cardiologists and emergent diagnostic or interventional procedures may be required.

Patients with unstable arrhythmia should be treated with aggressive pharmacological or electrical interventions. The interventions should follow established algorithms such as those by the American Heart Association.[25] These interventions include administration of a vasopressor, such as vasopressin or epinephrine (if required); administration of antiarrhythmic drugs such as

Table 2 Commonly used IV antiarrhythmic drugs[a].

Name	Class	Dose	Indication
Adenosine	Nucleoside	6 mg IV over <3 s followed by normal saline 20-mL bolus; second dose and third dose of 12 mg 2 min apart prn	Narrow complex PSVT; PSVT due to atrioventricular node or sinus node reentry
Amiodarone	Class III antiarrhythmic	Cardiac arrest: 300 mg IVP; 150 mg IVP q 3 to 5 min up to 2.2 g/day Stable wide complex tachycardia: 150 mg IV over 10 min; repeat q 10 min prn; maintenance infusion 0.5 mg/min; up to 2.2 g/day	Supraventricular or ventricular tachydysrhythmias; control of rapid atrial tachydysrhythmia in patients with low left ventricular ejection fraction when digoxin is ineffective
Atropine	Anticholinergic	0.5–1 mg IVP q 3–5 min prn up to 0.04 mg/kg	Symptomatic sinus bradycardia; Mobitz type I atrioventricular block; asystole
Digoxin	Digitalis glycoside	Loading dose: 10–15 μg/kg lean body weight in divided doses	To slow ventricular response in atrial fibrillation or atrial flutter; PSVT
Diltiazem	Calcium channel blocker	0.25 mg/kg IV over 2 min; second dose 0.35 mg/kg IV over 2 min, 15 min later prn; maintenance: 5–15 mg/h by titration	To slow ventricular response in atrial fibrillation or atrial flutter; PSVT; to terminate atrioventricular nodal reentrant tachycardia
Esmolol	β-blocker	0.5 mg/kg over 1 min; then infuse at 0.05 mg/kg/min; titrate up to maximum of 0.3 mg/kg/min	PSVT, atrial fibrillation or atrial flutter; reduce incidence of ventricular fibrillation in myocardial infarction or unstable angina
Ibutilide	Class III antiarrhythmic	1 mg IV over 10 min; repeat in 10 min prn	Supraventricular tachycardia including atrial fibrillation or flutter; effective for conversion of atrial fibrillation or flutter of relatively brief duration
Isoproterenol	β-agonist	Infuse 2–10 μg/min; titrate	Symptomatic bradycardia; torsades de pointes refractory to magnesium; β-blocker overdose
Lidocaine	Class IB antiarrhythmic	1–1.5 mg/kg IVP; repeat 0.5–0.75 mg/kg IVP q 5–10 min up to total of 3 mg/kg prn; maintenance: 30–50 μg/kg/min IV	Ventricular tachycardia or ventricular fibrillation; wide-complex tachycardia; significant ventricular ectopy; torsades de pointes
Metoprolol	β-blocker	5 mg slow IVP q 5 min up to a total of 15 mg	PSVT, atrial fibrillation, or atrial flutter; reduce incidence of ventricular fibrillation in myocardial infarction or unstable angina
Propranolol	β-blocker	0.1 mg/kg slow IVP in three divided doses 2–3 min apart	PSVT, atrial fibrillation, or atrial flutter; reduce incidence of ventricular fibrillation in myocardial infarction or unstable angina
Verapamil	Calcium channel blocker	2.5–5 mg IV over 2 min; repeat q 15–30 min prn up to a total of 20 mg	PSVT, atrial fibrillation, or atrial flutter

Abbreviations: A. fib., atrial fibrillation; A. flutter, atrial flutter; AV, atrioventricular; IV, IV; IVP, IV push; LVEF, left ventricular ejection fraction; MI, myocardial infarction; NS, normal saline; prn, as needed; PSVT, paroxysmal supraventricular tachycardia; USA, unstable angina; VF, ventricular fibrillation; VT, ventricular tachycardia.
[a]Source: From ACLS Provider Manual.[2]

amiodarone and lidocaine; electrical cardioversion or defibrillation; airway management; ventilation with oxygen; administration of IV fluid; and chest compression (if required). Emergency treatment of torsades de pointes varies from the standard algorithms for ventricular tachycardia; it entails expedient use of IV magnesium sulfate, electrical overdrive pacing, pharmacological overdrive with isoproterenol, or administration of phenytoin or lidocaine.

Tumor lysis syndrome

Tumor lysis syndrome (TLS) consists of severe hyperphosphatemia, hyperkalemia, hyperuricemia, azotemia, hypocalcemia, and metabolic acidosis (out of proportion to renal insufficiency) due to the massive release of cell contents and degradation products of dead tumor cells into the bloodstream.[26] TLS can occur spontaneously, but it usually occurs within 72 h after chemotherapy in patients with leukemia and lymphoma, but new therapeutic regimens may alter the timing of onset. TLS can also occur in patients with nonhematologic malignancies, including small cell carcinomas, nonsmall cell lung cancer, breast cancer, and ovarian cancer.

The symptoms of TLS are nonspecific. Common symptoms include nausea, vomiting, cloudy urine, weakness, fatigue, and arthralgia. Other signs and symptoms related to metabolic and electrolyte abnormalities include neuromuscular irritability, seizures, muscle weakness, and arrhythmia. Arrhythmia may cause sudden death in patients with TLS.[27] Precipitation of uric acid in the renal tubules may lead to nephropathy and acute renal failure.[28] The acute cause of death in TLS is arrhythmia secondary to severe electrolyte abnormalities (especially hyperkalemia) and renal failure. Early recognition of metabolic abnormalities and prompt treatment can avoid fatal outcomes.

Factors associated with increased risk of TLS include the type of malignancy (e.g., acute lymphocytic leukemia, acute myeloid leukemia with WBC >75,000/μL, Burkitt's lymphoma), responsiveness to therapy, rapid malignant cell turnover, and large tumor burden.[29] Other risk factors are preexisting renal insufficiency, acute renal failure developing shortly after the treatment, and poor response to hydration. Pretreatment serum lactate dehydrogenase levels, which tend to correlate with tumor bulk in lymphoma or lymphocytic leukemia, can predict the development of posttreatment azotemia, but pretreatment hyperuricemia is not predictive. A predictive scoring system for TLS has been proposed based on data from acute myelocytic leukemia patients undergoing induction therapy.[30,31] The score may potentially be used in a risk-based prophylaxis for TLS. Preventive measures should be started early in patients at risk. Aggressive hydration with IV crystalloid fluid up to 3 L/m^2/day may maintain a urine output >100 mL/h with or without diuretics. The xanthine oxidase inhibitor allopurinol (100–300 mg/day orally) may prevent severe hyperuricemia. Febuxostat (40–80 mg/day orally), another xanthine oxidase inhibitor, may be an effective alternative in TLS.[32]

The diagnosis of TLS requires a high level of suspicion because there are few signs or symptoms in the early stage. Routine uric acid and electrolyte screening (including measurement of calcium and phosphorus levels) is indicated in patients with high tumor bulk or hematologic malignancies. The diagnosis of TLS may be based on the Cairo–Bishop definition.[29,33] Once diagnosed, patients with severe TLS should have continuous monitoring of hemodynamic and electrocardiographic parameters in intensive care. The allopurinol dose may be increased up to 900 mg/day. Rasburicase, a recombinant urate oxidase that converts uric acid to allantoin, is highly efficacious in reducing uric acid level. Rasburicase (150–200 µg/kg IV daily, or one-time 3-mg dose[34] with a rescue dose as needed) may be used to prevent or treat urate nephropathy.[35] Increased IV fluid hydration may be coupled with diuresis using loop diuretics (e.g., furosemide) and acetazolamide. Urinary alkalinization by sodium bicarbonate or acetate IV infusion to increase the solubility of urate in urine should only be considered in cases of severe hyperuricemia when rasburicase is not available. Frequent electrolyte measurements (every 4–6 h) may be required. Hyperkalemia should be treated with insulin plus dextrose, calcium, and bicarbonate IV along with oral potassium ion-exchange resins (sodium polystyrene sulfonate). In hyperphosphatemic patients with hypocalcemia, the addition of an oral calcium-based compound (e.g., calcium acetate or calcium carbonate) will reduce phosphate absorption and enhance calcium absorption. IV calcium infusion can potentially cause calcium phosphate precipitation in the presence of severe hyperphosphatemia and should be used cautiously. Dialysis may be required for patients with symptomatic hypocalcemia and a serum phosphorus level >3.3 mmol/L (>10.2 mg/dL). Other indications for dialysis include persistent or refractory azotemia, hyperkalemia, hyperuricemia, oliguria, anuria despite diuretic use, acidemia, and volume overload. Prompt dialysis should be instituted with continued monitoring until biochemical abnormalities resolve. Hemodialysis is the most common mode of dialysis; prolonged hemodialysis sessions, continuous arteriovenous hemodialysis, continuous veno-venous hemofiltration, or continuous renal replacement therapy at a high dialysate or replacement fluid flow rate (>3 L/h) are alternative methods.

Pericardial tamponade

Pericardial tamponade occurs when a pericardial effusion impairs hemodynamics. Accumulation of excess fluid in the pericardial space in cancer patients is due to obstruction of lymphatic drainage and/or excess fluid secretion from tumor nodules on pericardial surfaces. Mesothelioma is the most common malignancy that arises from the pericardium. Carcinoma of the lung and malignant thymoma may involve the pericardium by direct extension. More frequently, malignancies arrive at the pericardium by retrograde lymphangitic spread or hematogenous dissemination. Melanoma is the malignancy most likely to metastasize to the heart. Lymphomas, leukemias, and gastrointestinal neoplasms may also cause pericardial effusions.[36] Cytologic examination of pericardial fluid reveals metastatic disease in 70–80% of cancer patients with pericardial effusion. Nonmalignant causes of pericardial tamponade include pericardial abscess, Candida pericarditis, and complications of central venous catheterization.

Malignant pericardial effusion usually occurs in advanced malignancy and is associated with poor prognosis (median survival time: about 6 months; 1-year survival rate: 28%).[37] More than two-thirds of patients with malignant pericardial effusion are asymptomatic. In symptomatic patients, common complaints are shortness of breath, dyspnea on exertion, chest pain, orthopnea, and general weakness. Findings on physical examination may vary from normal to hemodynamic collapse. Tachycardia, hypotension, jugular venous distention, organomegaly, and edema may indicate compromised cardiac output. The classic findings of cardiac tamponade are determined by both the quantity of pericardial fluid and the rapidity of fluid accumulation. Pulsus paradoxus, an exaggeration of the physiological decrease in systolic blood pressure with inspiration, is a classic but nonspecific finding of cardiac tamponade because it is seen also in patients with lung cancer, significant lung disease, or cor pulmonale.

Diagnosis of pericardial tamponade usually requires additional testing. Low QRS voltage and electrical alternans in electrocardiographs are suggestive findings. Chest radiographs may reveal widening of the mediastinum and cardiac silhouette (Figure 2a,b). Computed tomography (CT) or magnetic resonance (MR) scans frequently detect pericardial effusion as an incidental finding. These studies provide information on the location, loculation, and size of pericardial effusions but do not adequately assess the hemodynamic significance. Two-dimensional echocardiography is the most useful test for diagnosing pericardial effusion and evaluating its hemodynamic significance, that is, the presence of cardiac tamponade. Collapse or compression of the right atrium, diastolic collapse of the right ventricle, and cardiac "rocking" (side-to-side or front-to-back movement) are often observed in cardiac tamponade. Alterations in the respiratory variation of flow across the mitral valve as measured by Doppler shift are also helpful in evaluating the hemodynamics.

Initial management of malignant pericardial effusion depends on the hemodynamic stability. A scoring system may guide the decision for urgent pericardiocentesis.[38] In patients with hemodynamic compromise, ultrasound-guided pericardiocentesis, with placement of a drainage catheter into the pericardial space (Figure 2c), may be performed emergently in the emergency center or intensive care unit (Figure 2d). Complications are rare and may include massive pericardial bleeding and pneumothorax. Pericardial fluid can be drained from the catheter, and the catheter can stay until <50 mL/day of fluid is drained. Fibrinolytic agents may be used to unclog the catheter to facilitate drainage and avoid repeat pericardiocentesis or replacement of the catheter.[39] However, pericardial fluid will usually (>50% of cases) reaccumulate after removal of the catheter. Local application of cytotoxic agents or sclerosing agents to the pericardium can prevent fluid re-accumulation in many patients,[40] but sclerotherapy can be very painful. Creation of a pleuro-pericardial window using a variety of approaches can avoid repeated pericardiocentesis. Percutaneous intrapericardial balloon catheter to create a pleuro-pericardial window[41] laparoscopic transdiaphragmatic creation of a pericardio-peritoneal shunt[42] are alternative approaches. In stable patients, systemic chemotherapy, pericardial radioactive colloid, or thoracic external beam irradiation may be used for tumors that are sensitive to these modalities. Additional radiotherapy should be avoided in patients with significant prior exposure of the heart to radiation.

Acute hemorrhage

Acute gastrointestinal bleeding and genitourinary bleeding are discussed in other articles. Hemoptysis, which can rapidly compromise respiratory function, will be discussed later in this article. This section will cover some less frequent but serious bleeding events: carotid arterial rupture, splenic rupture, and retroperitoneal hemorrhage.

The manifestations of acute hemorrhage depend on the rate and the site of bleeding. In most cases, the site of bleeding is obvious, but sometimes bleeding can be internal and difficult to diagnose. Signs and symptoms of hypovolemia and hypoperfusion include tachycardia, hypotension, oliguria, and depressed mental status. Very often, diagnostic imaging studies or procedures, such as CT scans, ultrasonography, arteriography, or endoscopy, are necessary to diagnose internal bleeding.

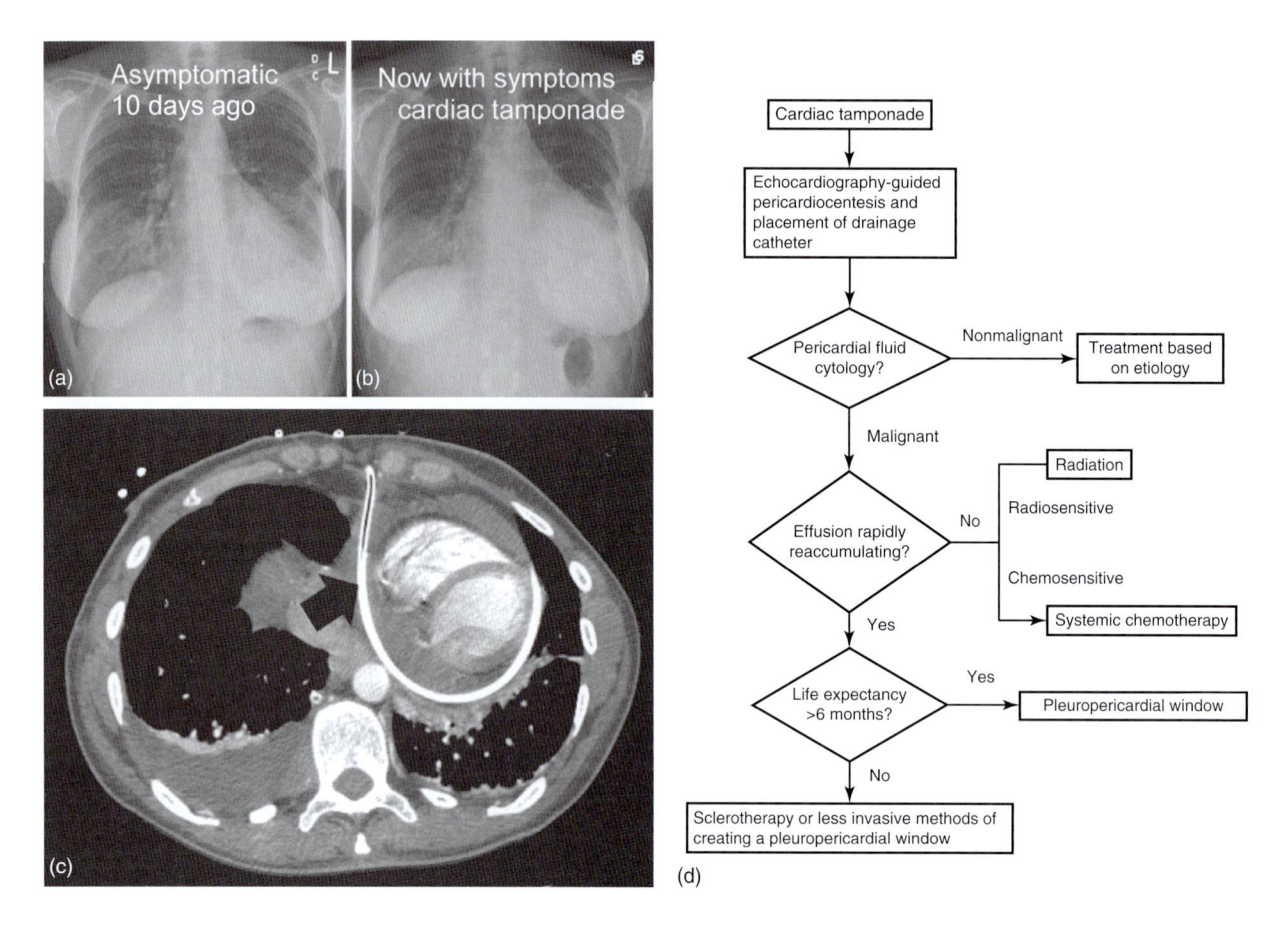

Figure 2 Chest imaging of patients with pericardial tamponade and management algorithm. Widening of mediastinum and cardiac silhouette is evident (b) when compared with a prior chest radiograph (a). Chest CT of a different patient with pericardial tamponade shows the presence of an indwelling drainage catheter (c). An algorithm for management of pericardial effusion is shown (d).

The primary management objectives for acute hemorrhage are to rapidly identify the bleeding source and achieve hemostasis. In the acute setting, direct pressure to compress the bleeding vessel or site should be applied whenever feasible while the cardiopulmonary status is assessed expeditiously. IV fluid resuscitation is vital in maintaining intravascular volume, cardiac output, and adequate vital organ perfusion. Isotonic crystalloid fluids (normal saline, lactated Ringer's solution, Plasmalyte, etc.) should be used as first-line agents because colloids (e.g., gelatins, dextrans, hydroxyethyl starches, albumin) have not been proven to improve survival.[43] Coagulopathy or thrombocytopenia should be corrected immediately by transfusion of blood products. The decision to transfuse red blood cells depends on the hematocrit, hemodynamic stability, persistence of hemorrhage, estimated blood loss, and comorbid diseases (e.g., coronary artery disease and cerebrovascular disease). Typed and cross-matched red blood cells are preferred, but noncross-matched type-specific blood or type-O blood may have to be used in life-threatening cases. Specific therapeutic procedures to control bleeding, such as embolization, balloon tamponade, or surgery, should be performed in a timely manner.

Carotid artery rupture

Most cases of carotid artery "blowout" occur in patients with head and neck cancers. Carotid blowout syndrome may be caused by direct tumor invasion or erosion into the carotid artery or by complications of cancer treatment, for example, postsurgical wound infection, postradiation necrosis, or orocutaneous fistula. It usually occurs as a sudden and massive arterial spurting. Occasionally, ominous minor and transient bleeding (sentinel bleeds) herald the massive blowout. In some cases, bleeding through a fistula into the esophagus or trachea may manifest as massive hematemesis or hemoptysis. Without prompt management, the patient's condition will rapidly deteriorate to hypotension, hypovolemic shock, loss of consciousness, and death.

Hemostasis is of utmost importance. Since neck vessels are accessible to direct manual compression, continuous firm compression should be applied at the site of the carotid artery rupture until the patient arrives at the operating room for surgical treatment. Crystalloid IV fluid resuscitation, prompt transfusion of blood products, and administration of vasopressors should be performed to maintain perfusion of vital organs. Carotid artery rupture has limited surgical options, and surgical ligation of the bleeding carotid artery is associated with high morbidity (25% of patients have neurologic sequelae) and high mortality (40%).[44] Endovascular treatment with vessel sacrifice (embolization or balloon occlusion) or stent placement (covered stent) has become major treatment options.[45,46]

Splenic rupture

The spleen is fragile and vulnerable to rupture from trauma. In cancer patients, spontaneous splenic rupture is relatively rare and is associated with acute leukemia, non-Hodgkin's lymphoma, chronic myelogenous leukemia, hairy cell leukemia, and Hodgkin's lymphoma. Metastases to the spleen in patients with solid tumors such as gastric, prostate, and lung cancer can also cause rupture.

The mechanism of spontaneous splenic rupture is not clear. Minor trauma to the spleen may contribute in some cases. Other contributing factors include splenomegaly, infiltration of the splenic capsule by malignant cells, splenic infarction, thrombocytopenia, coagulopathy, anticoagulation therapy, and disseminated intravascular coagulation.

The typical clinical presentation of splenic rupture involves pain in the left shoulder or abdomen (left upper quadrant), tachycardia, and hypotension. The severity of the signs and symptoms may depend on the extent of bleeding. Diagnostic peritoneal lavage is rarely used in nontraumatic cases; thus, the definitive diagnosis of splenic rupture relies on imaging studies. Contrast-enhanced CT is the diagnostic study of choice; ultrasonography can be performed at bedside for hemodynamically unstable patients to diagnose splenic rupture.[47]

For patients with splenic rupture and hematologic malignancies, prompt splenectomy is necessary because the mortality rate for these patients is extremely high without surgery. In selected patients with contraindications to surgery, selective arterial embolization of the ruptured site may stop the bleeding.[48] Other supportive treatments are IV fluid, supplemental oxygen, pain medications, blood transfusion, and correction of thrombocytopenia and coagulopathy.

Retroperitoneal hemorrhage

Damage to retroperitoneal organs or structures may cause retroperitoneal hemorrhage. Malignancies rarely cause spontaneous retroperitoneal hemorrhage; in such cases, the culprit is usually renal cell carcinoma or adrenal gland neoplasm (primary or metastatic). Anticoagulation, thrombocytopenia, and coagulopathy are predisposing factors. Retroperitoneal or intraperitoneal invasive procedures and placement of a central venous catheter through a femoral vessel can also cause severe retroperitoneal hemorrhage.

Retroperitoneal hemorrhage causes nonspecific signs and symptoms that vary according to the rate of bleeding and the underlying disease. Patients may present with abdominal pain, a tender mass in the flank, tachycardia, and hypotension. Some may have hematuria or hematochezia if the blood somehow finds its way into the ureter or gastrointestinal tract. It is difficult to establish a diagnosis of retroperitoneal hemorrhage on the basis of clinical findings. Maintaining a high level of clinical suspicion and performing early imaging studies are keys to the successful management of retroperitoneal hemorrhage. CT of the abdomen and pelvis is the noninvasive study most commonly used to diagnose retroperitoneal bleeding (Figure 3). Bedside ultrasonography may also rapidly diagnose retroperitoneal bleeding.

The management of retroperitoneal hemorrhage depends on the severity of bleeding and the underlying cause. After the initial stabilizing treatments for acute hemorrhage, the patient should be monitored closely for hemodynamic stability and continued blood loss. In life-threatening situations, most patients require emergent laparotomy to remove the bleeding tumor or organ.[49] Renal cell carcinomas are often hypervascular, and selective arterial embolization may control the bleeding of a renal lesion. External-beam radiation treatment of a bleeding tumor is another option in hemodynamically stable patients with a relatively stable hematocrit.[50]

Superior vena cava syndrome

Superior vena cava (SVC) syndrome refers to a constellation of signs and symptoms resulting from partial or complete obstruction of blood flow through the SVC to the right atrium. The

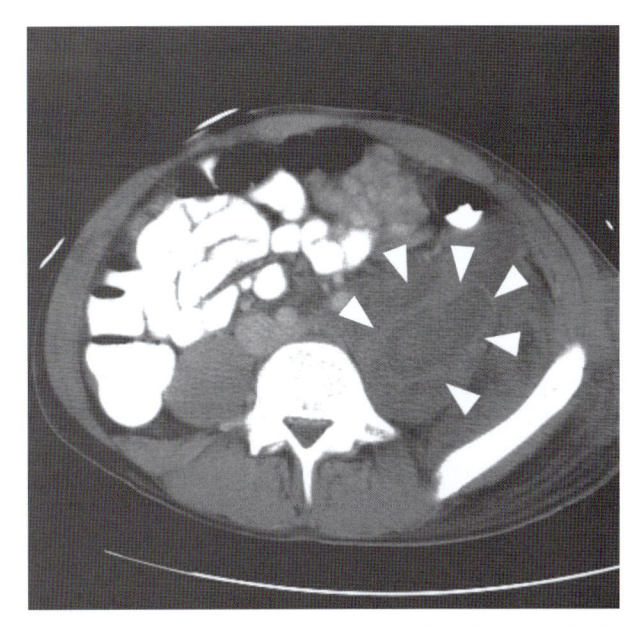

Figure 3 Retroperitoneal bleeding. The CT scan of the abdomen and pelvis of a thrombocytopenic leukemia patient showed a large inhomogeneous retroperitoneal collection (white arrowheads) consistent with a hematoma in the left psoas muscle displacing bowel loops to the right.

obstruction may be caused by compression, invasion, thrombosis, or fibrosis of this vessel. Lung cancer is the leading cause of SVC syndrome; non-Hodgkin lymphoma is the second most common cause.[51,52] Although Hodgkin lymphoma commonly involves the mediastinum, it rarely causes SVC syndrome. Primary mediastinal malignancies like thymoma and germ cell tumors account for <2% of SVC syndrome. Breast cancer is the most common metastatic disease that causes SVC syndrome[53]; other metastatic cancers include gastrointestinal adenocarcinoma, prostate adenocarcinoma, sarcomas, and melanoma. Nonmalignant causes of SVC syndrome include retrosternal goiter, pyogenic infections, sarcoidosis, teratoma, pleural calcification, silicosis, postradiation fibrosis, chemotherapy-induced fibrosis, constrictive pericarditis, and idiopathic mediastinal fibrosis.[52] An increasing cause of SVC syndrome in cancer patients is central venous catheter-induced thrombosis.

Obstruction of the SVC raises the blood pressure in the SVC. Collateral venous circulation often flows through the azygos system. Obstruction below or at the entrance of the azygos veins forces blood to travel in the opposite direction down the azygos and chest wall veins to reach the inferior vena cava. SVC obstruction caused by tumors often develops insidiously over weeks. However, thrombosis may cause a rapid onset of obstruction. Sudden SVC obstruction is a true emergency because the rapid elevation of pressure in the SVC causes increased intracranial pressure, resulting in cerebral edema, intracranial thrombosis or bleeding, and death.

Common symptoms of SVC syndrome are a sensation of fullness and pressure in the head, cough, dyspnea, chest pain, and dysphagia. More significant symptoms include visual disturbances, hoarseness, stupor, seizure, and syncope. Typical signs include venous distention of the neck and chest wall, nonpitting edema of the neck, facial edema, facial plethora, tongue edema, proptosis, retinal vessel dilatation, stridor, and upper-extremity edema. The signs and symptoms are exacerbated by lowering the upper body relative to the heart (i.e., bending forward, stooping, or lying down).

CT, especially contrast-enhanced spiral CT, is the most useful diagnostic study. It not only reveals the site of obstruction and collateral flow but also differentiates extrinsic compression of SVC by tumor from thrombosis. CT also provides anatomical details about the tumor and its surrounding structures, helping to guide biopsy procedures if a histologic diagnosis of the tumor has not been established previously. CT can also detect other emergent complications—such as proximal airway obstruction and pericardial effusion—that frequently coexist with SVC obstruction. If IV iodine contrast is contraindicated, radionuclide venography or MR imaging are alternatives. 3-D contrast-enhanced MR venography may be superior to CT, digital subtraction angiography, and doppler ultrasonography in detecting and determining the extent of thrombo-occlusive disease in chest vessels.[54] Contrast angiography for diagnosis of SVC syndrome is rarely indicated.

The method for establishing the histologic cancer diagnosis may depend on the working diagnosis, location of the tumor, physical status of the patient, comorbid conditions, and available expertise of the health care facility. CT-guided needle biopsy is an alternative to surgical biopsy by thoracotomy or mediastinoscopy.[55] Bronchoscopy may provide the cancer diagnosis in up to 50% of patients with SVC syndrome. If lymph nodes are accessible, excisional biopsy can establish the diagnosis with minimal morbidity. Excisional biopsy is preferred if lymphoma is suspected because the histologic classification of lymphoma is firmly based on lymph node architecture.

In rare emergent situations of impending airway obstruction or increased intracranial pressure, endovascular interventions,[56] including angioplasty, SVC stenting, and pharmaco-mechanical thrombolysis, should be employed immediately. Stenting may be first-line treatment of SVC syndrome[57,58] and can relieve severe symptoms while the histologic diagnosis of the malignancy is being pursued, or when radiation or chemotherapy has failed or not yet taken effect. Stenting provides rapid symptomatic relief in the majority of patients and improves the quality of life. These stents usually remain patent for the rest of the patient's life.[57]

Supplemental oxygen, bed rest with upper body elevation, and sedation may help to lessen the symptoms by lowering venous pressure and cardiac output. The use of diuretics may transiently decrease edema, but the efficacy of diuretics has not been proven, and overdiuresis causes dehydration, which should be avoided to minimize the risk of thrombosis. Corticosteroids (e.g., dexamethasone) may be useful in the presence of airway compromise or increased intracranial pressure. Anticoagulation is controversial despite the presence of superimposed thrombosis in up to 50% of SVC syndrome. Anticoagulation and thrombolysis may be beneficial in situations such as indwelling catheter-induced thrombosis or propagation of the thrombus into the brachiocephalic or subclavian system. However, anticoagulation increases the risk of intracranial bleeding, especially when intracranial pressure is elevated, and may complicate or delay biopsy procedures; therefore, it should be avoided unless a clear indication is identified.

Radiotherapy remains the principal treatment for many patients with malignant SVC syndrome, especially in recurrent disease after chemotherapy or chemo-insensitive tumors such as nonsmall cell lung cancer.[59] In general, radiotherapy is well tolerated, and SVC syndrome symptoms begin to improve in about 1 week. Radiotherapy is also justified if a histologic diagnosis cannot be established in a timely manner. Chemotherapy is the preferred initial treatment of SVC syndrome caused by chemo-sensitive tumors such as small cell lung cancer and lymphoma. Most small cell lung cancer patients experience partial or complete resolution of the signs and symptoms within a couple of weeks. Although SVC obstruction recurs in approximately 25% of cases, salvage chemotherapy and/or radiotherapy can achieve prompt resolution of symptoms in most patients. After chemotherapy for lymphoma, local consolidation with radiotherapy may be beneficial in patients with large cell lymphoma and large mediastinal masses. Cancer invasion of SVC is no longer considered unresectable.[60] Surgical treatment with reconstruction may be indicated for certain tumor types or selected patients.[61]

Respiratory oncologic emergencies

Massive hemoptysis

Approximately 5% of hemoptysis episodes are considered massive. The definition of massive hemoptysis ranges from the expectoration of >100 mL of blood in a single episode to >600 mL in 24 h.[62] Airway bleeding leading to life-threatening airway obstruction, hypotension, aspiration, or anemia is also considered massive hemoptysis. The mortality rate of massive hemoptysis is about 30%, ranging from 5% to 71% depending on the volume of blood expectorated and the rate of bleeding.[63–67] Other factors associated with mortality include low pulmonary reserve, and large amount of blood retained in the lungs.[64] Death attributable to endobronchial and alveolar hemorrhage is usually due to asphyxiation rather than exsanguination.

The primary causes of massive hemoptysis in cancer patients are malignancy, infection, and hemostatic abnormalities. Bronchogenic carcinoma is the most common cause of massive hemoptysis in cancer patients over 40 years old. About 3% of lung cancer patients have fatal hemoptysis,[68] which occurs more commonly in necrotic squamous cell carcinoma than other types of lung cancer. Hemoptysis secondary to lung metastases is most commonly associated with melanoma, breast, kidney, laryngeal, and colon cancers. Other tumors, such as esophageal tumors, may cause massive hemoptysis by direct extension to the tracheobronchial tree. In immunocompromised patients (e.g., patients with hematologic malignancies, bone marrow transplantation, or prolonged neutropenia), necrotizing, angioinvasive fungal infections (aspergillosis, mucormycosis) may cause massive pulmonary hemorrhage.[64] Hemostatic abnormalities such as severe thrombocytopenia and coagulopathy may result from malignancy or its treatments and contribute to hemorrhage. Another factor that can contribute to massive hemoptysis in cancer patients is lung injury by radiation or chemotherapy.

Hemoptysis may be associated with other symptoms such as coughing, dyspnea, hypotension, tachycardia, central cyanosis, and chest pain. Hemodynamic instability may require volume resuscitation. The respiratory status should be initially supported by supplemental oxygen. The American College of Chest Physicians Guidelines recommend securing the airway by endotracheal intubation with a single-lumen tube, and emergent bronchoscopy to identify the bleeding site for endobronchial interventions such as laser or plasma coagulation and electrocautery.[69] Endobronchial interventions may also include administration of topical agents (thrombin), iced saline lavage, injection of epinephrine 1:20,000, and tamponade with a balloon catheter. While rigid bronchoscopes offer improved airway control, ability to suction, and the ability to remove large clots, fiberoptic scopes offer improved access and visualization of the distal airways. Other airway management options include unilateral intubation via the bronchoscope or a double-lumen endotracheal tube to isolate the unaffected lung.

For massive right-sided pulmonary bleeding, the left mainstem bronchus is intubated over the bronchoscope, but unilateral intubation of the right lung in patients with massive left-sided bleeding is not recommended due to the risk of right upper lobe occlusion. For patients bleeding from one lung, lateral decubitus positioning with the affected lung in the dependent position may help to minimize aspiration to the unaffected side. Underlying coagulopathies must be corrected, and cough suppressants may be helpful.

Noe et al.[70] have proposed an algorithm for management of massive hemoptysis, in which CT angiography plays an important role. Together with bronchoscopy and chest X-ray, CT angiography provides information about the tumor, bleeding site, and anatomy of the bronchial and extrabronchial arteries for planning the endovascular intervention. Bronchial artery embolization can be first-line treatment for massive or recurrent hemoptysis as it is safe and effective. Embolization of the bleeding vessel may be performed with Gianturco steel coils, absorbable gelatin pledgets, polyvinyl alcohol foam, or isobutyl-2-cyanoacrylate. Patients in whom embolization fails may benefit from radiotherapy. Emergency lung resection is feasible in selected patients and is generally performed in patients with hemoptysis refractory to the above treatments or bleeding from major pulmonary vessels.[71]

Massive pleural effusion

Approximately 10% of pleural effusions are massive when there is near-complete opacification of the hemithorax on chest X-ray. About two-thirds of massive pleural effusions (Figure 4) have underlying cancer.[72] The malignant causes are lung carcinoma (36%), breast carcinoma (25%), lymphoma (10%), and ovarian carcinoma (5%).[73] Adenocarcinoma accounts for 79% of lung carcinoma cases that metastasize to the pleura.[74] In young adults, lymphoma is the most common cause of malignant pleural effusions.[74] After pneumonia, malignancy is the second leading cause of exudative pleural effusions, and malignancy is the cause of 8–20% of transudative pleural effusions.[75] Other factors causing pleural effusions include local tumor effects (hilar and mediastinal lymphadenopathy causing impaired lymphatic drainage from the pleural space), systemic tumor effects, hypoalbuminemia, complications of cancer treatment [radiotherapy and chemotherapy (e.g., methotrexate, procarbazine, cyclophosphamide, mitomycin, bleomycin, and interleukin-1)], and congestive heart failure.

For some patients, the pleural effusion may be the presenting sign of the malignancy. Common symptoms are cough, dyspnea, and orthopnea, but about one-fourth of malignant pleural effusions are asymptomatic. The presence and severity of these symptoms depend on the volume and the rapidity of fluid accumulation. Fever is occasionally present and may be due to atelectasis or pneumonia. Pleuritic chest pain and pleural friction rubs are not common; when present, they indicate extensive neoplastic involvement of the pleura and chest wall. The pleural effusion caused by lung carcinoma is generally on the same side as the primary lesion.[72] The cause of a pleural effusion is generally diagnosed by thoracentesis. Malignant effusions may appear serous, serosanguinous, or bloody. Fluid analysis discriminates between exudative and transudative effusions.[76] Cytology is more sensitive than percutaneous pleural biopsy to diagnose the cause of the effusion.[74,77] Other more invasive diagnostic options include bronchoscopy, pleuroscopy, video-assisted thoracoscopy, and open pleural biopsy.

Massive pleural effusion causing hemodynamic instability, significant dyspnea, hypoxemia, or mediastinal shift should be treated emergently by thoracentesis. The benefit of a therapeutic thoracentesis without pleurodesis is usually temporary; in approximately 70% of cases, fluid reaccumulates shortly unless effective systemic chemotherapy is administered. If there is no symptomatic improvement after thoracentesis in cancer patients with lung trapping by visceral pleura encasement, placement of an indwelling pleural catheter is not indicated.[78] Otherwise, an indwelling pleural catheter will allow outpatient periodic drainage of pleural fluid to improve symptoms,[79,80] particularly dyspnea, and improve quality-adjusted survival.[81] Some patients may also achieve pleurodesis over time. Chemical pleurodesis should be considered in patients with life expectancy of more than a few months and symptomatic relief after thoracentesis. The effective sclerosing agents, with success rates of 72–90%, are doxycycline, minocycline, bleomycin, and talc.[82,83] Tube thoracostomy may be indicated depending on clinical and radiographic findings and the biochemical characteristics of the effusion:[84] empyema, infected pleural fluid as confirmed by culture or microscopy (e.g., Gram stain), or complicated parapneumonic effusions. Patients in whom thoracoscopic treatment fails and patients with chronic complicated parapneumonic effusions should be considered for open thoracotomy and decortication.

Acute airway obstruction

Acute airway obstruction usually involves the upper airway. Tumors that obstruct by direct extension are primary tumors of the head and neck (base of tongue, larynx, hypopharynx, thyroid, or trachea) and mediastinum (lung cancer, thymoma). Metastatic tumors that may cause upper airway obstruction are cancers of the breast, esophagus, kidney, colon, melanoma, sarcoma, and mediastinal lymphoma. The mechanisms causing the obstruction include extrinsic compression, tumor encroachment, tumor-associated airway edema, and hemorrhage. Nonmalignant causes include food or foreign body aspiration, severe tracheomalacia, tracheal stenosis or stricture, and airway edema (due to hypersensitivity and infections). Severe drug-induced angioedema may occur with angiotensin-converting enzyme inhibitors and paclitaxel. The most common cause of lower airway obstruction

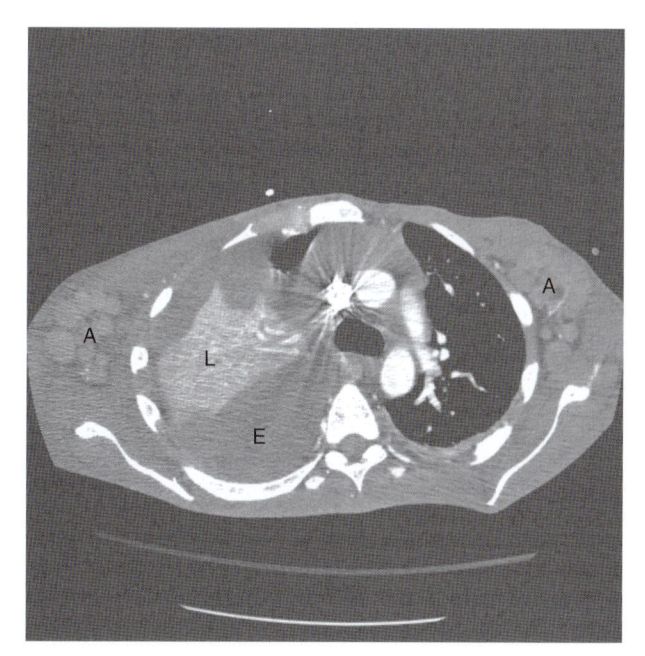

Figure 4 Massive pleural effusion. The CT scan of the chest of a patient with a massive pleural effusion is shown. L, collapsed lung; E, pleural effusion; A, extensive axillary lymphadenopathy.

is primary bronchogenic carcinoma. Other, rare causes of lower airway obstruction are metastases from cancers of the colon, breast, thyroid and kidney, melanoma, lymphoma, and sarcoma. Patients with carcinoid tumors may experience severe bronchospasm due to release of hormone mediators.

Dyspnea may be the only early symptom of airway obstruction. When dyspnea occurs with exertion, the upper airway diameter is usually decreased to 8 mm, whereas when dyspnea occurs at rest, the airway diameter is usually decreased to 5 mm, often coinciding with the development of stridor. As obstruction progresses, orthopnea, tachycardia, diaphoresis, wheezing, stridor, and intercostal muscle retraction may be noted. Stridor is an ominous finding that may be rapidly followed by cyanosis, obtundation, bradycardia, and death.

The oral cavity should be quickly visualized to exclude foreign body aspiration. In most cases of upper airway obstruction, the clinical examination provides the diagnosis. The clinical examination is often corroborated by direct visualization via either laryngoscopy or bronchoscopy depending on the location of the lesion. For lower airway obstruction, chest radiographs identify the obstruction in 75% of cases. CT of the neck and/or chest is very helpful in diagnosing obstruction by tumors. Edema caused by acute infection in a previously narrowed airway should also be considered in the differential diagnosis.

The management of airway obstruction is to reverse or bypass the obstruction. In addition to supplemental oxygen, supportive therapies may include administration of corticosteroids, inhaled racemic epinephrine, bronchodilators, helium–oxygen mixtures, and antibiotics (if infection is suspected). Laryngoscopy or bronchoscopy may be necessary to guide endotracheal intubation in upper airway obstruction.[85] Patients with obstructions involving the upper third of the trachea may require a low tracheotomy. Decisions for surgical interventions depend on extent of the malignancy, responsiveness to antineoplastic treatment, performance status, and comorbid conditions. For central airway obstruction, interventional pulmonary treatments may use rigid or flexible bronchoscopes[86] and may include placement of tracheobronchial stents, balloon bronchoplasty, laser bronchoscopy, endobronchial argon plasma coagulation, photodynamic therapy, cryosurgery, and brachytherapy. Other treatment options include CT-guided radiofrequency ablation, external beam radiotherapy, and surgical debulking or resection.

Pneumothorax

Pneumothoraces in cancer patients are iatrogenic or spontaneous. The majority of pneumothoraces treated in hospitals are iatrogenic.[87] Procedures that may cause a pneumothorax include percutaneous lung biopsy, transbronchial biopsy, insertion of central venous catheters, and insertion of pulmonary artery catheters. Spontaneous pneumothorax is most commonly due to chronic obstructive pulmonary disease. Both primary and metastatic pulmonary neoplasms may also cause pneumothorax. Chemotherapeutic agents associated with pneumothorax include bleomycin, carmustine, and lomustine. Infectious agents associated with pneumothorax include *Staphylococcus*, *Klebsiella*, and *Pseudomonas* species, *Pneumocystis carinii*, and *Mycobacterium* species. Rupture of mycetoma into the pleural space may result in pneumothorax and is associated with *Aspergillus fumigatus* infection, coccidioidomycosis, cryptococcosis, and mucormycosis.

The severity of symptoms at presentation is related to the patient's underlying pulmonary status. Patients may present with respiratory distress, tachypnea, tachycardia, cyanosis, diaphoresis, and agitation. Patients with underlying lung disease often cannot tolerate decreases in vital capacity and have an increased risk for respiratory failure secondary to pneumothorax. Dyspnea is often unrelated to the volume of pneumothorax; however, dyspnea and chest pain are present in almost all cases of significant pneumothorax. The chest pain is frequently acute, pleuritic, and on the affected side. Cough, hemoptysis, and orthopnea are less frequent.

Small pneumothoraces are usually undetectable on physical examination. Examination usually demonstrates tachycardia, absent tactile fremitus, hyperresonance, and absent or decreased breath sounds on the affected side. Patients with large or tension pneumothoraces may have contralateral deviation of the trachea, asymmetrical hyper-expansion, and decreased movement of the affected hemithorax. Patients with a tension pneumothorax may have elevated central venous, pulmonary artery, and right atrial pressures. Hypotension, severe hypoxemia, and respiratory acidosis occur when increased intrapleural pressure impedes venous return. The diagnosis of pneumothorax is confirmed when an upright chest radiograph reveals a visceral pleural line with the absence of lung markings beyond the line. One-third of pneumothoraces are undetected on semi-erect and supine chest radiographs.[88] Pleural ultrasonography may be more accurate than chest radiography to diagnose pneumothorax.[89] However, CT chest is the most accurate.

Patients with small pneumothoraces may be closely observed with supplemental oxygen and serial chest radiographs 3–6 h after the initial radiograph. If there is no expansion of the pneumothorax, the patient may be discharged from observation with appropriate follow-up instructions and repeat radiograph in 12–48 h.[90] For symptomatic, rapidly expanding, and moderate to large (>15% of the ipsilateral pleural space) pneumothoraces, catheter aspiration should be done. Outpatient management with small-caliber intercostal catheters and Heimlich valves has a success rate of 78%.[91] Failure to re-expand or recurrence following catheter aspiration requires tube thoracostomy. Tube thoracostomy is indicated as initial treatment for traumatic pneumothorax, hemothorax, pneumothorax occupying >15% of the ipsilateral pleural space with retained secretions, pneumothorax with lung infections on the affected side, and pneumothorax related to mechanical ventilation/barotrauma. Patients with a persistent air leak due to bronchopleural fistula and patients with only partial lung expansion 5–7 days after a tube thoracostomy should be considered for surgical repair. Chemical pleurodesis may be indicated for recurrent pneumothorax.[92]

Pulmonary embolism

Pulmonary embolism can be difficult to diagnose in cancer patients because the signs and symptoms may be masked by the neoplastic process or complications of cancer treatments. Cancer is an independent risk factor for thromboembolism in addition to other factors such as major trauma/surgery, advanced age, recent myocardial infarction, cerebral vascular accident, immobility, obesity, and history of thrombosis. Compared with patients without malignancies, cancer patients have higher rates of initial thrombosis, thrombosis recurrence, and fatal pulmonary embolism.[93] The risk of thromboembolism in cancer patients without other comorbid conditions is 15–20%. Compared with patients without cancer undergoing similar procedures, cancer patients undergoing surgery have two to three times the risk of developing postoperative deep venous thrombosis.[94]

In most cases, symptoms of pulmonary embolism are vague. Dyspnea, pleuritic chest pain, and tachypnea are present in 97% of patients with confirmed pulmonary embolism.[95,96] The most common presenting symptom is dyspnea. Frequently, patients also have tachycardia. Massive pulmonary embolism may cause syncope. Angina may occur due to right ventricular ischemia. Hemoptysis may rarely occur due to pulmonary infarction 12–36 h after the embolic event. Deep venous thrombosis in the lower extremities is found in <50% of patients with pulmonary embolism. Sometimes, fever and a pleural rub may also be detected.

Pulse oximetry or arterial blood gases may reveal hypoxemia for which supplemental oxygen is needed. Chest radiography is helpful in excluding other causes of the symptoms and occasionally may suggest pulmonary embolism by the presence of a Hampton's hump (dome-shaped and pleura-based lung opacity) or Westermark sign (peripheral radiolucency due to decreased blood flow with or without central pulmonary vessel dilatation). An electrocardiogram commonly shows sinus tachycardia, inverted T waves, or nonspecific ST-T wave abnormalities. Right axis deviation, atrial arrhythmia, right bundle branch block, and P-pulmonale may occur, but the classical S1-Q3-T3 pattern is unusual. The American College of Physicians (ACP) guideline for evaluation of patients with suspected PE has negative predictive value of 99% and sensitivity of 97% in predicting PE in cancer patients;[97] PEs were present in 6% of low-risk 10% of intermediate-risk, and 25% of high-risk patients. In cancer patients, d-dimer has a high negative predictive value and sensitivity for pulmonary embolism, and a normal d-dimer result can exclude pulmonary embolism.[98] However, the predictive performance of D-dimer in cancer patients varies with the type of malignancy, and it performs poorly in excluding venous thromboembolism in lymphoma and leukemia patients.[99]

High-resolution CT pulmonary angiography or spiral CT is the first-line diagnostic test (Figure 5); in case of IV iodine contrast allergy, MR angiography is an alternative. For diagnosis of pulmonary embolism, CT and MR angiography has a sensitivity and a specificity of about 80% and 90%, respectively.[100,101] The negative predictive value of CT angiography is 98%.[102] The radionuclide ventilation-perfusion (V/Q) scan is second line when CT or MR angiography is contraindicated because of renal dysfunction or hypersensitivity. Since emboli in the distal pulmonary vasculature is not reliably detected with CT or MR angiography, patients with strong suspicion of pulmonary embolism but negative findings on either imaging modalities should be considered for contrast pulmonary angiography, the diagnostic gold standard.

Hemodynamically unstable patients should be stabilized by administration of IV fluid and/or inotropic agents as guided by central venous pressure monitoring in intensive care. Oxygen at high concentration via mask or endotracheal tube may be necessary for massive pulmonary embolism. Treatment options for patients with massive pulmonary embolus and hemodynamic instability (i.e., occlusion of >40% of the pulmonary vasculature, right ventricular dysfunction according to echocardiography, and severe hypoxemia) include systemic thrombolysis, catheter-directed thrombolysis, and embolectomy. In pulmonary embolism causing acute right ventricular dysfunction, thrombolytic therapy is associated with decreased all-cause mortality despite increased major bleeding and intracranial hemorrhage.[103] Thrombolysis demands special attention to contraindications related to bleeding risk (especially in the presence of brain metastasis). Due to increased risk for massive bleeding and intracranial hemorrhage but no reduction in mortality, thrombolysis should not be used for normotensive patients with pulmonary embolism.[104] While systemic thrombolysis may be beneficial in massive pulmonary embolism, catheter-directed thrombolysis may cause less major bleeding complications than systemic thrombolysis; the role for catheter-directed thrombolysis remains to be clearly defined.[105] Surgical or catheter embolectomy is reserved for patients in whom other approaches of clot removal have failed.

There are updated guidelines for the management of venous thromboembolism in cancer patients.[106,107] Choices for initial anticoagulation in the ED include low-molecular-weight heparin (LMWH), unfractionated heparin, fondaparinux (a synthetic sulfated pentasaccharide from the antithrombin-binding region of heparin that is an indirect Factor Xa inhibitor), apixaban and rivaroxaban. LMWH is generally preferred over unfractionated heparin. For initial parenteral anticoagulation for cancer patients with newly diagnosed pulmonary embolism and creatinine clearance >30 mL/min. Unfractionated heparin (IV bolus of 80 units/kg followed by continuous infusion at 18 units/kg/h) can be an alternative to LMWH. LMWH has the advantages of not requiring partial thromboplastin time monitoring and IV access. IV unfractionated heparin may be preferred in patients who very probably will need invasive interventions because of its short half-life. IV unfractionated heparin is administered in a bolus injection of 5000–10,000 units, followed by a continuous infusion of 1000–1500 units/h with adjustments to maintain the activated partial thromboplastin time at 1.5–2.0 times the control value. Factor Xa-inhibiting direct oral anticoagulants (DOACs), that is, rivaroxaban,[108] apixaban, and edoxaban, are efficacious for the treatment of cancer-associated venous thromboembolism[107,109–111]; however, DOACs are associated with increased risk of bleeding (especially in the setting of gastrointestinal tract or urinary tract cancers). For initiation of anticoagulation using DOACs, rivaroxaban (15 mg po BID × 21 days, then 20 mg daily) or apixaban (10 mg PO BID × 7 days, then 5 mg BID) are two options. Other DOACs such dabigatran and edoxaban may be used after 5–10 days of initial parenteral anticoagulation. Treatment with vitamin K antagonists (e.g., warfarin) to an international normalized ratio (INR) between 2 and 3 is an inferior alternative for long-term therapy when DOACs and LMWH are not possible. Anticoagulation is contraindicated in the presence of active intracranial bleeding, recent surgery, thrombocytopenia (platelet <50,000/μL), or coagulopathy. Inferior vena cava filters may be considered when anticoagulation is contraindicated or when pulmonary

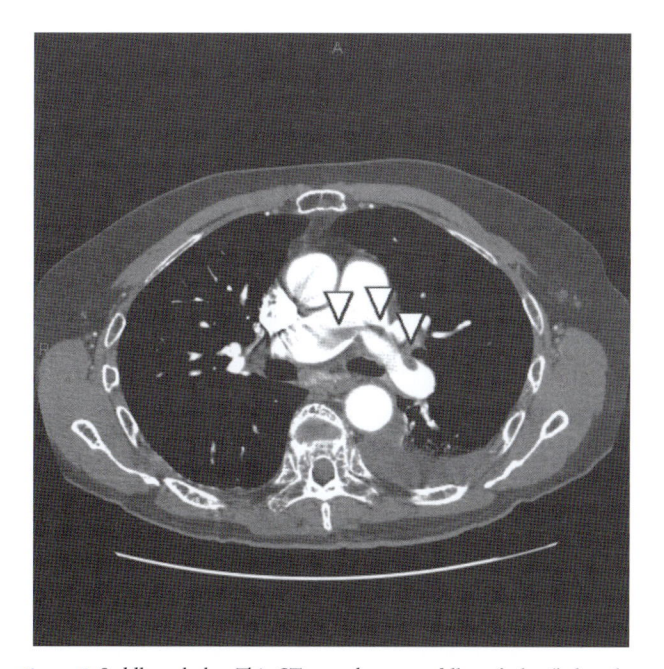

Figure 5 Saddle embolus. This CT scan shows a saddle embolus (below the three arrowheads) at the bifurcation into the pulmonary arteries.

embolism recurs or existing thrombus worsens under optimal therapy, but end-stage cancer patients may gain little benefit and long-term complications can be significant in cancer survivors.[112] Contraindications for anticoagulation should be periodically reassessed so that anticoagulation can resume when it is safe.

For patients with primary brain malignancies, anticoagulation is recommended in the same manner as for patients with other cancers. Many cancer patients with pulmonary embolism may be safely treated as outpatients, especially cases of incidental pulmonary embolism, which are clinically unsuspected and are discovered in CT scans ordered for treatment response evaluation or staging.[107,113] Since the rates of recurrence, morbidity, and mortality in incidental cases are comparable to symptomatic cases, incidental pulmonary embolism should be treated in the same way with initial and long-term anticoagulant therapy as for symptomatic pulmonary embolism except for peripheral subsegmental emboli that are judged to be highly probable imaging artifacts.[114–117]

Neurologic oncologic emergencies

Spinal cord compression

Spinal cord compression occurs in 3–5% of cancer patients and should be considered an emergency because treatment delay may result in irreversible morbidity, including paralysis.[118] In 95% of cases, spinal cord compression is caused by metastases involving the vertebral column (70% in the thoracic spine, 20% in the lumbosacral spine, and 10% in the cervical spine). Metastasis to the thoracic vertebrae is likely to cause problems because of the vulnerable local blood supply and the fact that the spinal canal is narrowest here. Spinal cord compression occurs more frequently in patients with lung, breast, unknown primary, prostate, and renal cell cancer than other malignancies.

Back pain is the most common symptom in spinal cord compression, and patients may present with pain localized to the spine or radicular pain due to neural compression. The pain may worsen with movement, recumbence, coughing, sneezing, or straining. Muscle weakness follows pain and may be accompanied by sensory loss. Once symptoms of autonomic dysfunction, urinary retention, and constipation develop, irreversible paralysis rapidly follows. Paralysis and urinary retention before treatment are predictive of poor outcome. Clinical findings include tenderness elicited by palpation over the involved vertebral segments, muscle weakness, abnormal reflexes, and sensory loss in the distribution of the involved spinal segment and below. Leg ataxia may be present prior to muscle weakness. Patients with autonomic dysfunction may have a palpable bladder, an increased postvoid residual urinary volume, or decreased rectal tone.

Clinical guidelines for diagnosis and management of spinal cord compression are available.[119,120] Patients with spinal cord compression often have abnormalities (e.g., bony erosion and pedicle loss, partial or complete vertebral collapse) on plain radiographs of the spine. However, normal spine radiographs do not exclude epidural metastasis. MR tomography of the spine is the best method for evaluating epidural spinal cord compression (Figure 6). Gadolinium enhancement should be used when there is suspicion of cord compression due to epidural abscess or neurological symptoms due to leptomeningeal metastasis. Gadolinium enhances inflamed tissues and defines anatomic margins. Myelography accompanied by CT may be performed with minimum discomfort. However, when metastatic disease completely blocks the flow of cerebrospinal fluid, myelography does not allow definition of the upper margin of tumor involvement.

Treatment of spinal cord compression aims to improve or prevent loss of neurologic function, provide local tumor control, stabilize the spine, and pain control. Analgesics, especially opioids, should be administered promptly and judiciously because inadequate pain control often delays appropriate physical examination and diagnostic imaging study. When spinal cord compression is suspected, corticosteroid therapy should be administered. Dexamethasone is often used since it has good gastrointestinal absorption and a 36-h half-life. It is controversial whether a high-dose (100 mg) IV bolus followed by maintenance doses (usually 16 mg every 6 h) is necessary.[121] Low doses (4–10 mg every 6 h) may be just as effective with fewer side effects.[120,122] For most patients with spinal cord compression by a radiosensitive malignancy, radiotherapy alone is the standard initial treatment. The outcome of radiotherapy depends on the pretreatment neurologic status and radiosensitivity of the malignancy. Surgical decompression may be appropriate for patients requiring spine stabilization, patients who have had prior radiotherapy in the area of the compression, patients who need tissue for diagnosis, and patients with progression despite appropriate treatment with steroids and radiation but may not be appropriate for patients with advanced malignancy and a limited life expectancy. A meta-analysis has shown that surgical resection followed by radiotherapy may improve ambulation ability and survival better than radiotherapy alone.[123] Chemotherapy may be effective for compression by a chemosensitive malignancy and may also be used in combination with other treatments or sometimes as an alternative when other choices

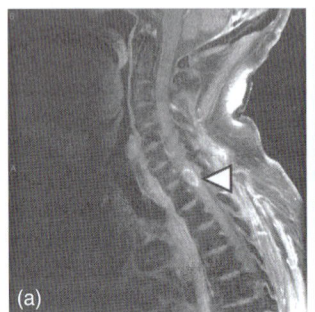

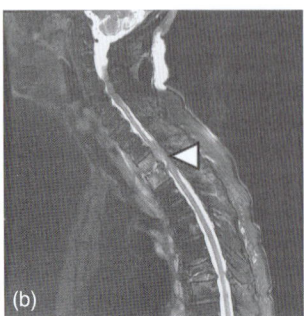

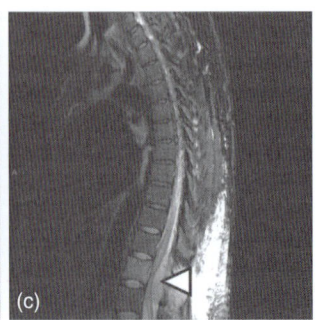

Figure 6 Spinal cord compression. Sagittal MRI images of the spine from three different patients demonstrate an intramedullary lesion (*arrowhead*) in low cervical spine (a), compression of the lower portion of the thoracic spinal cord by metastatic disease in the vertebral body (*arrowhead*) (b), and compression of the upper portion of the lumbar spinal cord by an epidural tumor (*arrowhead*) (c).

are not appropriate (e.g., high operative risks, or near-maximum radiation doses already delivered to the affected area).

Brain herniation

Patients with possible brain herniation should be rapidly assessed, and those with hemodynamic instability should be stabilized with appropriate therapies.[124] Symptoms and physical findings suggestive of brain herniation include changes in the level of consciousness, papilledema, pupillary and eye movement irregularities, nausea, vomiting, meningismus, decorticate or decerebrate posturing, and Cushing reflex (hypertension and bradycardia). If there are findings suggestive of herniation or increased intracranial pressure, an imaging study such as a noncontrast CT of the brain should be performed emergently. MR imaging can provide additional diagnostic information after the patient has been stabilized.

Upon recognition of clinical signs of brain herniation, treatment to decrease intracranial pressure should be instituted immediately, even before brain herniation is documented by imaging studies. Emergency treatments include hyperventilation, administration of mannitol, and steroids. Hyperventilation is the most rapid way to decrease intracranial pressure. Sedate, intubate, and ventilate to achieve a PCO_2 of 25–30 mm Hg, which causes cerebral vasoconstriction, decreases cerebral blood volume, and subsequently decreases intracranial pressure. The benefit of hyperventilation is generally short-lived, and equilibration may occur within a few hours. Mannitol 20–25%, a hyperosmotic agent, is effective within minutes of administration and remains effective for several hours by forming an osmotic gradient between the blood and brain to drive water from the brain to the blood. Mannitol 20–25% is administered IV at 0.5–2.0 g/kg over 20–30 min. Additional doses may be necessary if the patient continues to deteriorate. Corticosteroids should be administered and may be helpful especially when herniation is due to vasogenic edema surrounding intracranial metastases.[125] Dexamethasone is commonly administered at an initial bolus dose of 40–100 mg IV, then 40–100 mg/day in divided doses.

Further treatment in intensive care may include IV infusion of hypertonic saline, propofol, and hypothermia.[124] Neurosurgical intervention such as placement of a ventricular drain or decompressive craniectomy may be necessary if the patient has neurologic deterioration despite appropriate medical management. Treatment should be directed at the underlying cause once intracranial pressure is controlled.

Status epilepticus

Status epilepticus is defined as >5 min of continuous seizure activity or >2 sequential seizures without full recovery between seizures.[126] It can lead to devastating neurologic and systemic consequences, such as neuronal injury and cell death, neurogenic pulmonary edema, and rhabdomyolysis with renal failure. Tumors in the brain cause about 7% of cases of status epilepticus, and these cases have higher short-term mortality than status epilepticus unrelated to tumors.[127]

The etiology of seizures in cancer patients may include structural, metabolic, infectious, and treatment-related causes. In a review of 50 cancer patients presenting to an emergency center with seizures, 16% had seizures due to a new structural lesion, and 52% had previously documented central nervous system lesions.[128] Seizures commonly occur in patients with intracranial tumors. The cancers that commonly metastasize to the brain are lung cancer, breast cancer, melanoma, genitourinary malignancies, and gastrointestinal malignancies.

Neurologic function is often suppressed (confused or unresponsive) postictally. Clinical findings after seizure activity may include bruising or tongue bites, signs of urinary or fecal incontinence, and increases in lactic acid and muscle enzyme levels. It is important to determine whether the patient has previously had seizures and, if so, the type of seizure, medications used for control, and their plasma drug levels. The status, extent, and treatment of the malignancy should also be reviewed. If the event precipitating seizure activity cannot easily be determined, a diagnostic workup should be initiated. Evaluation may include a complete blood cell count, comprehensive metabolic panel, blood cultures, drug screens, and electroencephalography are appropriate. CT brain imaging without IV contrast is necessary.[129] Lumbar puncture may also be indicated depending on the suspected seizure precipitant, the patient's condition, and findings on imaging.

When patients present with status epilepticus, airway, breathing, and circulation should be assessed immediately (Figure 7).[126,129] Cardiopulmonary status should be supported and stabilized according to ACLS algorithms. Hypoglycemia must be first excluded or diagnosed and treated immediately. Anticonvulsant therapy with an IV benzodiazepine (e.g., lorazepam or midazolam) should be administered to halt seizure activity. Generally, lorazepam is used because of its rapid onset of action and longer duration of efficacy. After seizure has stopped, an unconscious patient should be placed on his or her side in the recovery position to prevent aspiration. Airway suctioning and supplemental oxygen may be required. Reversible medical causes of seizures should be corrected. These patients will likely not require long-term anticonvulsant therapy. Patients with status epilepticus due to other causes will require prolonged treatment with an anticonvulsant. Some

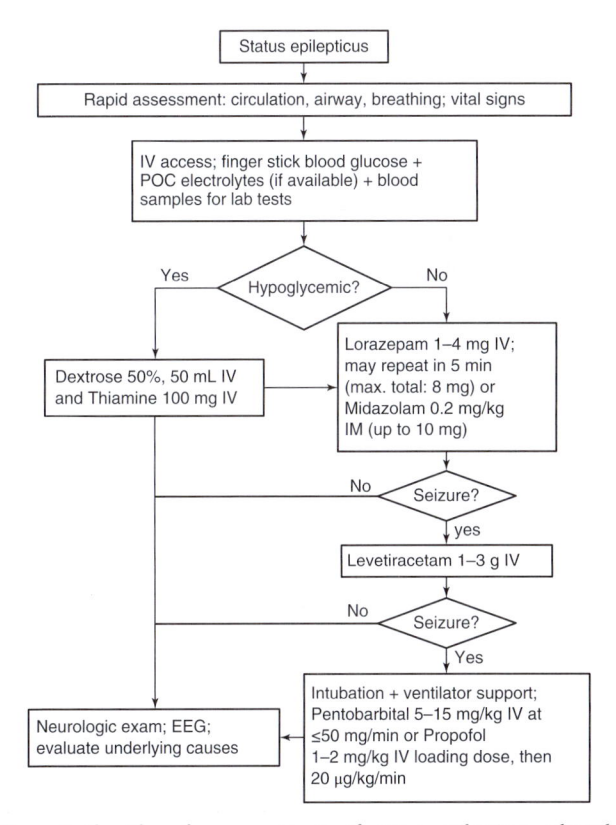

Figure 7 Algorithm for management of status epilepticus adapted for cancer patients. *Abbreviations*: EEG, electroencephalogram; POC, point-of-care bedside testing; IV, IV; IM, intramuscular. Source: Modified from Brophy et al.[126] and Claassen et al.[129]

clinicians prefer levetiracetam in cancer patients because it is not metabolized by the liver and has minimal drug interactions with antineoplastic therapy. For patients with continuing seizure activity despite initial anticonvulsant treatment, escalate to high dose anticonvulsant therapy (e.g., pentobarbital, thiopental, propofol, and midazolam) with complete sedation, intubation/ventilator support, and electroencephalography monitoring in intensive care.

Immune-related oncologic emergencies

Anaphylactic and anaphylactoid reactions to antineoplastic drugs

Anaphylactic reactions to chemotherapy manifest as chest tightness, upper airway obstruction, abdominal pain, bronchospasm, and hypotension; and urticaria and angioedema occur in 90% of cases. Common chemotherapy that may cause anaphylaxis include L-asparaginase, taxanes, anthracyclines, platinum compounds, ifosfamide, cyclophosphamide, procarbazine, teniposide, and etoposide. Important elements in anaphylaxis treatment are early recognition, airway maintenance, and hemodynamic support (Table 3).[130–134]

An infusion-related reaction is an adverse reaction to the infusion of a pharmacologic or biologic substance.[135] and it occurs upon infusion or within a few hours after infusion of a biological.[136] Biological drugs are protein drugs produced using biotechnology, and they include fusion proteins, cytokines, and monoclonal antibodies. Reactions to biological agents may be classified into five types: α-reactions due to massive release of cytokines, β-hypersensitivity because of an immune reaction against the biological agent, χ-immune or cytokine imbalance syndromes manifesting as immunosuppression, autoimmune or inflammatory diseases, δ-symptoms due to cross-reactivity, and ε-symptoms not directly involving the immune system.[137] Cytokines or massive release of cytokines induced by monoclonal antibodies may lead to reactions that vary widely from skin reactions to anaphylaxis (fever, rigor, dyspnea, hypoxia, and hypotension). Infusion-related reactions can manifest hours after the patient has left the outpatient infusion facility, requiring presentation to an ED for acute management.[138]

Acute adverse effects of interferon alfa (IFN-α) occur during the first 2–8 hours. Common symptoms are flu-like, and these side effects may be managed with acetaminophen or nonsteroidal anti-inflammatory drugs and supportive care. High-dose interleukin-2 (IL-2, aldesleukin) is associated with cardiovascular and hemodynamic adverse effects that resemble septic shock.[139] Low-dose IV and subcutaneous IL-2 regimens can be administered in an ambulatory care setting, and delayed reactions may lead to presentation to the ED. Common symptoms include malaise, fatigue, fever, chills, anorexia, nausea, vomiting, arthralgia, myalgia, and pruritus.

Immediate reactions to infusion of antibodies during the first hour after administration are heterogeneous in etiology and presentation (nausea/vomiting, skin reactions, respiratory symptoms, and hemodynamic instability).[140] Some involve release of cytokines (type α); others involve an IgE-mediated hypersensitivity (type β); anaphylaxis with urticaria, and angioedema can occur. Risk factors for having a reaction include the malignancy, concomitant treatments, and current immune status. Drug-related factors include the degree of humanization, method of production, glycosylation pattern, and the allergenic potential of the excipients. Delayed hypersensitivity can appear between 2 h and up to 14 days after infusion,[140] and are often serum sickness-like (e.g., rash, vasculitis, and erythema multiforme). Transient symptoms may be treated and supported similar to anaphylaxis (Table 3). Infusion-related reactions are usually mild to moderate (grade ≤2). Management depends on the severity. In the emergency setting, infusion of the triggering agent should be stopped if not already completed. Respiration and hemodynamics are stabilized according to resuscitation guidelines.[141,142] The supportive symptomatic treatments include antipyretics, histamine type 1 and 2 receptor antagonists, corticosteroids, and meperidine (as needed for rigor and chills).

Table 3 Recommendations for acute management of anaphylaxis in adults.[a]

1. Remove the antigen or delay the absorption of the antigen
2. Assess airway; intubate if there is evidence of laryngeal edema or impending severe airway obstruction; in extreme circumstances when orotracheal intubation or bag/valve/mask ventilation is not effective, cricothyrotomy or catheter jet ventilation may be needed
3. Assess hemodynamics; position the patient supine (or semi-reclining in a position of comfort if dyspneic or vomiting) and elevate the legs
4. Administer epinephrine as first-line treatment
   - In case of a less severe episode: 0.3 mg SQ, 1 mg/mL, repeated at 10- to 20-min intervals
   - In case of a more severe episode: 0.3–0.5 mg IM, 1 mg/mL, repeated at 5- to 10-min intervals
   - In case of shock or airway obstruction: 1 mg/100 mL IV, 0.01–0.02 mg/min, up to a total dose of 0.1 mg
   - In case of persistent shock: May repeat dose or start an IV drip infusing at 2–10 µg/min
   - If patient is over 50 years old or has a history or cardiac problems and life-threatening symptoms exist: Test dose of 0.1–0.15 mg SQ or IM
5. Administer IV crystalloid fluid (normal saline or lactated Ringer's solution)
   - In case of hypotension, administer 1 L over 15 min, then reassess; repeat as needed up to 3 L
6. Administer glucocorticoid:
   - Methylprednisolone 125 mg IV push; may repeat every 4 h if symptoms persist (alternative: hydrocortisone 500 mg, dexamethasone 20 mg, or other potent corticosteroids)
7. Administer antihistamines (both H1 and H2 blockers):
   - Diphenhydramine 25–50 mg IV or IM; repeat every 2–4 h as needed
   - Cimetidine 300 mg IV or famotidine 20 mg IV
8. Inhaled racemic epinephrine via a nebulizer can reduce laryngeal swelling; beta-agonists for bronchospasm and wheezing
9. In case of resistant hypotension:
   - Military antishock trousers or Trendelenburg's position may be helpful
   - Infuse dopamine 5–20 µg/kg/min IV by titration
   - Administer naloxone 0.4–2.0 mg IV every 2 min (maximum 10 mg)
10. In case of beta-blocker-accentuated epinephrine-resistant anaphylaxis:
    - Administer glucagon 1–5 mg IV over 2–5 min
    - Administer terbutaline 0.25 mg SQ
    - Administer isoproterenol 2–10 µg/min IV by titration

Abbreviations: IM, intramuscularly; IV, IV; SQ, subcutaneously.
[a]Source: Adapted from Simons et al.[130]; Lieberman et al.[131]; Boyce et al.[132]; and Muraro et al.[134]

Immune-related adverse events (irAEs)

Monoclonal antibodies that bind and block immune checkpoint proteins (cytotoxic T lymphocyte-associated protein 4 (CTLA4), programmed cell death 1 (PD-1), and programmed cell death ligand 1 (PD-L1)) are used to treat many solid tumors and hematologic malignancies. Harnessing immunity to fight cancer can inadvertently cause autoimmunity, leading to irAEs. The onset of irAE varies widely (from after a single dose[143] to even after treatment discontinuation[144-147]) but is usually around the fourth dose (12–16 weeks after initiation).[148] Cancer patients with moderate or severe irAEs often need emergency care. Existing guidelines from American Society of Clinical Oncology (ASCO),[149] National Comprehensive Cancer Network (NCCN),[150] European Society of Medical Oncology (ESMO),[151] and Society of Immunotherapy for Cancer (SITC) [152] can guide management of irAEs. Severity grading s is based on CTCAE, version 5.0.[135] Immunosuppression with a glucocorticoid is the primary treatment for clinically significant irAEs. Escalation to other immunosuppressants (e.g., infliximab for colitis[153] or mycophenolate mofetil for hepatitis[154]) may be required in steroid-refractory cases or when significant steroid-induced side effects occur. The occurrence of irAEs and subsequent use of immunosuppressive therapy does not seem to affect cancer response rates or antitumor therapeutic activity.[155,156]

Cutaneous irAEs are the most common, occurring in almost half of the patients receiving immune checkpoint inhibitor therapy. The majority are low grade, presenting within the first two cycles of therapy[157-161] with itching, erythema, rash, vesicles, or blisters.[157,160,162,163] Serious cutaneous irAEs occur in about 1–3% of patients, and these include toxic epidermal necrolysis (TEN), drug rash with eosinophilia (DRESS), and Steven-Johnson (SJS), which can be fatal if not recognized and treated with high-dose corticosteroids as inpatient.[150,164-166] GABA agonists (e.g., pregabalin or gabapentin) can be used for severe pruritus.[149,158,162,167]

Cardiac irAEs result from damage by lymphocytic infiltration[168-172]; immune-mediated myocarditis, and pericarditis may present emergently as acute life-threatening events. The onset may be rapid and can lead to cardiac failure, pericardial effusion, or dysrhythmias and are potentially fatal[168,173,174] The incidence of cardiac dysfunction is not clear but is perhaps ≤1%.[168,169]

Endocrine irAEs manifest hormone deficiency or excess. The spectrum of clinical illness ranges from no symptoms to life-threatening endocrine emergencies[175-180] (e.g., adrenal crisis, thyroid storm, myxedema coma, diabetic ketoacidosis). Emergency visits for endocrine irAEs are often related to the thyroid, adrenal, and pituitary glands.[181]

Gastrointestinal irAEs may lead to diarrhea, colitis, pancreatitis, and hepatitis. Corticosteroids are the primary treatment for gastrointestinal toxicities, with escalation to infliximab for severe steroid-refractory colitis.[150,182-184] Vedolizumab can be effective in steroid-refractory and infliximab-resistant enterocolitis.[185,186] Hepatitis and pancreatitis are usually mild, presenting with no or a few nonspecific symptoms but can be severe or even fatal in some cases.[187]

Severe neurologic irAEs is rare (<1%),[146] and usually happens within 1–7 weeks of therapy.[188-190] Seizures, confusion, ataxia, abnormal behavior, or altered consciousness warrant evaluation for encephalitis which occurs in 0.1–0.2% of patients.[191-195] Emergent brain imaging with CT or magnetic resonance imaging (MRI) with and without contrast is indicated. Brain MRI is the imaging modality of choice for evaluation of neurologic irAEs. In neurological irAEs, CSF analyses are consistent with lymphocytic meningitis (with mild to high pleocytosis, negative cultures, elevated protein, and cytopathology negative for malignancy).

Pneumonitis is one of the most serious irAEs and can be fatal.[196-200] New persistent cough or shortness of breath in patients receiving immune checkpoint inhibitors should prompt evaluation for pneumonitis. Patients with grade ≥2 pneumonitis should start glucocorticoids and be closely monitored.[149] Grade ≥3 pneumonitis requires inpatient care, evaluation to exclude infections, and probably consultation with pulmonary and infectious disease experts. Treatment with high-dose glucocorticoids (methylprednisolone, 1–2 mg/kg/day) is indicated, aiming to improve symptoms down to grade ≤1.

Rheumatologic irAEs include primarily arthritis, sicca symptoms (dry eyes, dry mouth, and parotid gland enlargement), and a polymyalgia-like syndrome.[145,201] Among irAEs involving the musculoskeletal system, myositis can be serious. Myositis presents as proximal muscle weakness with an increase in serum muscle enzymes, with or without respiratory complaints.[173,202-214] Myasthenia-like syndromes can present with "dropped heads," bilateral proximal limb muscle weakness, muscle pain, and dyspnea.[202,211] Myositis and myasthenic syndromes can be life-threatening because of CO_2 retention and respiratory failure, and severe rhabdomyolysis may cause renal failure, electrolyte imbalance, and fatal arrhythmia; both would require prompt diagnosis and management. When respiratory compromise is suspected (as prompted by shallow rapid breathing, dyspnea, low oxygen saturation, etc.), ventilatory status should be evaluated with arterial blood gases measurement, peak flows, and/or bedside pulmonary function tests (negative inspiratory force and vital capacity) to determine whether support with positive pressure ventilation or intubate for mechanical ventilation is indicated.

Chimeric antigen receptor (CAR)-T cell therapy

CD19-chimeric antigen receptor (CAR)-T cell therapy is a treatment for certain acute lymphocytic leukemia and large B-cell lymphoma. CAR-T therapy-related toxicities are related to markedly increased circulating cytokines and manifest as two syndromes: cytokine release syndrome (CRS) and immune effector cell-associated neurotoxicity syndrome (ICANS).[215-217] Delayed onset of these side effects may lead to emergency center visits.

Cytokine release syndrome

Symptoms of CRS range from mild "flu-like" to life-threatening inflammatory responses.[218] Symptoms include high-grade fever, hypotension, hypoxia, and/or multi-organ toxicity, which resemble sepsis. Serious CRS is characterized by hypotension and hyperpyrexia that can progress to an uninhibited systemic inflammatory response syndrome with circulatory shock, disseminated intravascular coagulation, vascular leak, and multi-organ system failure. Laboratory abnormalities include cytopenias, elevated creatinine, elevated liver enzymes, impaired coagulation, and elevated C-reactive protein level. Respiratory involvement is common, ranging from tachypnea and cough, hypoxemia with bilateral pulmonary infiltrates on radiography to acute respiratory distress syndrome that require mechanical ventilation.

Management of CRS varies by grade.[216,219] Grade 1: Supportive care should keep the patient well-hydrated using IV fluids with special attention to fluid balance to avoid pulmonary vascular congestion. Grade 2: Hypotension should be treated promptly with IV crystalloid fluid. In patients who are refractory to fluid boluses, management may include therapies that block IL-6 signaling (i.e., anti-IL-6 receptor antibody tocilizumab or anti-IL-6 antibody siltuximab) and glucocorticoids. Grade 3 or 4: Arrhythmias, hemodynamic shock, and respiratory compromise need to be emergently supported. Therapies that block IL-6 signaling and high-dose glucocorticoids are indicated.

Immune effector cell-associated neurotoxicity syndrome (ICANS)

ICANS is a toxic encephalopathy with symptoms of confusion/delirium, headache, word retrieval difficulty, somnolence, hemiparesis, aphasia, hallucinations, cranial nerve palsies, tremors, and occasionally seizures.[216,220–229] ICANS often starts shortly after CAR-T cell infusion while the patients are still hospitalized, but delayed onset may occur after discharge from hospital, leading to emergency department visits. Early signs of ICANS include loss of language coherence, impaired handwriting, and decreased attention span. The diagnosis and evaluation of ICANS may be guided by the Immune Effector Cell-Associated Encephalopathy (ICE) score.[218] Emergent imaging study of the brain using CT or MRI is necessary. Emergent lumbar puncture for cerebrospinal fluid analysis would be indicated in the presence of mental status change and fever (e.g., concurrent CRS) to examine the differential diagnoses of meningitis and encephalitis.

Similar to CRS, the management of ICANS is also grade-based. Grade 1: Supportive care is provided. Increasing the angle of the head of the bed to >30° may minimize the risk of aspiration and improve cerebral venous blood flow. Neurology consultation would facilitate evaluation, including electroencephalogram, evaluation of intracranial pressure, and brain imaging studies. Grade 2: High doses of glucocorticoids (dexamethasone 40 mg/day, or methylprednisolone 1 g/day) is administered until neurologic recovery.[230] Grades 3 and 4: In addition to high-dose glucocorticoids, seizures and status epilepticus need to be treated and controlled. Cerebral edema and increased intracranial pressure may require intensive care,[231] and management with mechanical hyperventilation, acetazolamide, and/or mannitol.[230] In patients with concurrent neurotoxicity and CRS, treatment should include tocilizumab (8 mg/kg) and glucocorticoids until the symptoms resolve.[230]

Other oncologic emergencies

Perforated bowel

Perforation along the gastrointestinal tract is a serious emergency. In cancer patients, common causes are spontaneous perforation secondary to tumor (primary or metastatic) and iatrogenic perforation secondary to endoscopy or cancer treatment. If the wall of the gastrointestinal tract is significantly infiltrated or replaced by tumor, radiotherapy- or chemotherapy-induced tumor necrosis may lead to bowel perforation. Antiangiogenic therapies such as bevacizumab and small molecule inhibitors such as imatinib and sorafenib have been associated with bowel perforation.[232] Bowel perforation can be caused by severe infections like typhlitis and neutropenic enterocolitis.[233] Severe gastroenteritis due to radiotherapy or chemotherapy may lead to severe bowel dilatation/distention and subsequent perforation. Common causes of bowel perforation unrelated to cancer include appendicitis, diverticulitis, and peptic ulcer disease.

Typically, perforation causes acute pain that prompts emergent evaluation. In cases of cervical esophageal perforation, symptoms at presentation may include neck pain, dysphagia, hoarseness, and subcutaneous emphysema. In thoracic esophageal perforation, upper abdominal rigidity, severe retrosternal chest pain, odynophagia, and hematemesis are common. In gastric perforation, acute onset of severe abdominal pain is usually the first symptom. The pain may be associated with nausea and vomiting, and in about 15% of patients, significant bleeding is present. Referred pain to the shoulders may occur because of irritation of the diaphragm. In cases of free perforation into the peritoneal cavity, abdominal distension and signs of peritonitis (severe rebound abdominal tenderness, guarding/rigidity, and absent bowel sounds) may be present.

Fever and leukocytosis with left shift may be present in patients with peritonitis, mediastinitis, or abscess. However, the white blood cell count should be interpreted in the context of recent chemotherapy or use of neutrophil-stimulating cytokines. Amylase levels may be high in intestinal, esophageal, or gastric perforation, and lipase levels may be high in gastric perforation. In cervical esophageal perforation, a plain radiograph of the neck in the lateral view may show air in the deep cervical tissues. Plain radiographs of the chest are also valuable in esophageal perforation as pneumomediastinum may be evident. Free air detected by plain radiographs (upright chest X-ray or abdominal series with upright or decubitus views) (Figure 8) can provide evidence of

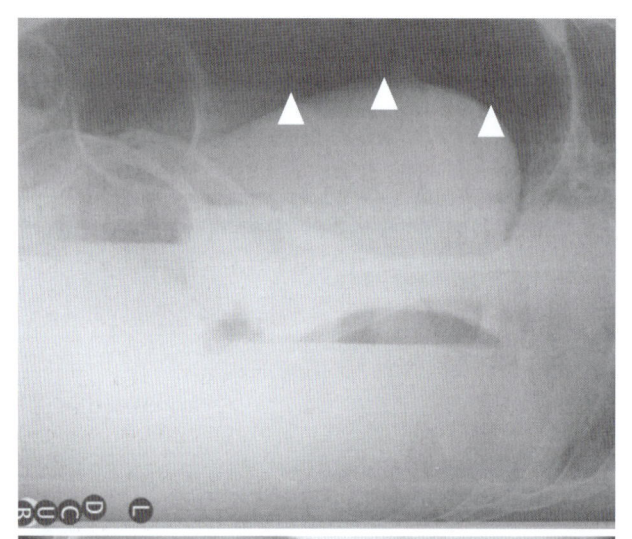

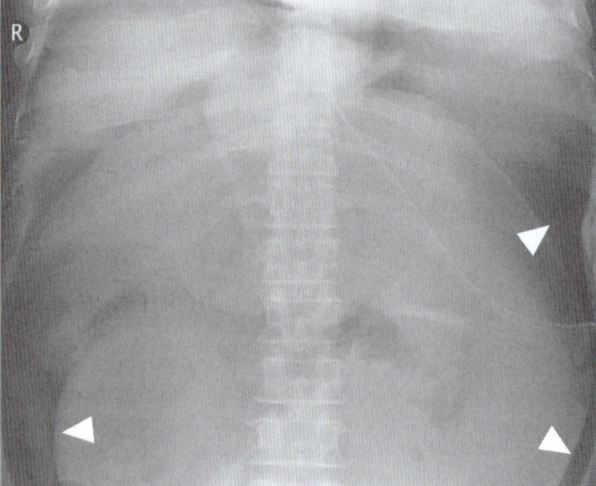

Figure 8 Pneumoperitoneum. A 53-year-old man with multiple myeloma and amyloidosis involving the gastrointestinal tract, undergoing treatment with thalidomide and dexamethasone, presented with acute abdominal pain and abdominal distension. Abdominal radiographs showed intraperitoneal free air (*arrowheads*). Laparotomy revealed bowel perforation secondary to massive colonic distention.

bowel perforation. As for duodenal perforation, plain abdominal radiographs may show air in the retroperitoneal space. Other radiographic signs of perforation include outlining of both sides of the bowel wall by air and visualization of the hepatic ligament. If bowel perforation is highly suspected clinically and the initial studies do not show evidence of perforation, CT scan with oral water-soluble contrast agent (e.g., diatrizoate) is very accurate in diagnosing bowel perforation and can provide detailed information about the location and surrounding anatomy of the perforated structure.

Management of a perforated viscus may be expectant management, expectant management followed by surgery, or immediate surgery. Factors influencing the management are the etiology, size, location and containment of the perforation, the clinical course (development of sepsis), the patient's performance status and quality of life prior to the perforation, the prognosis based on the status of the malignant disease, and comorbid conditions that increase the risk of perioperative mortality. Nonsurgical treatment measures include nasogastric tube suction, administration of broad-spectrum IV antibiotics, IV hydration, parenteral nutrition, and close monitoring.[234] If the patient's condition deteriorates during expectant treatment, then a decision to operate can be made.

Neutropenic fever

Neutrophils are phagocytic white blood cells that defend the human body against infections. Neutropenia is defined as a neutrophil count of ≤1000 cells/μL, absolute neutropenia as neutrophil ≤500 cells/μL, and profound neutropenia as neutrophil ≤100 cells/μL.[235] Neutropenia often occurs in cancer patients as a consequence of intensive chemotherapy or the malignancy. Infection is the leading cause of morbidity and mortality in neutropenic patients. Fever [defined as a single oral temperature >38.3°C (101°F) or >38.0°C (100.4°F) for >1 h] in a neutropenic cancer patient often resolves after empirical systemic broad-spectrum antibiotics (up to about 60% of cases).[236] Neutropenic fever is a true medical emergency, and timely administration of antibiotics may prevent sepsis and death.

Neutropenic patients are immuno-compromised and lack the ability to mount a full inflammatory response to infections. Therefore, any symptom or sign of infection should be investigated fully.[237] Physical examination should include careful inspection of commonly infected sites such as mouth, pharynx, perineum, eyes, vascular access sites, percutaneous catheter sites, and skin. Initial laboratory evaluation should include complete blood cell count, serum creatinine, blood urea nitrogen, transaminases, blood cultures from a peripheral vein and vascular access ports or catheters, urinalysis, urine culture. Chest radiography is indicated for patients with respiratory signs or symptoms.

Further evaluation should be guided by physical findings, signs, and symptoms. Lesions on the mucous membranes and the skin can be viral (e.g., herpes simplex and varicella-zoster), bacterial (e.g., ecthyma gangrenosum), or fungal (e.g., disseminated candidiasis, aspergillosis, or *Fusarium*) infection. Any site of a localized infection should be pursued with aspiration or biopsy for pathogen identification to guide treatment. Sinus symptoms may be due to bacterial or fungal infections, some of which may be invasive and fatal. Abdominal pain, distention, bloody diarrhea, nausea, and vomiting are typical findings in neutropenic enterocolitis.[238] In the presence of diarrhea, stool specimens should be evaluated with for *Clostridium difficile* infection by a toxin assay or polymerase chain reaction. Perianal symptoms may suggest the presence of a perianal abscess. The differential diagnosis of pulmonary disease in febrile neutropenic patients is broad: infection (viral, bacterial, fungal, and protozoan), radiation-induced pathologic conditions, chemotherapy-induced side effects, hemorrhage, and infarction. Correlation of pulmonary symptoms and findings on chest radiographs is a clinical challenge in neutropenic patients. Classic methods of sputum evaluation such as direct examination of stained specimens, culture, and testing of antibiotic sensitivities are now complemented by detecting microbial DNA (polymerase chain reaction) and microbial antigens in bodily fluids or tissues. Serologic tests have also been helpful in identifying infections in neutropenic patients. Nevertheless, findings on chest radiography are abnormal in 17–25% of patients with neutropenic fever despite the absence of pulmonary signs or symptoms,[239] and lung infiltrate on chest X-ray can predict a complicated clinical course.[240] Therefore, if a neutropenic patient is being considered for possible out-patient oral antibiotic therapy, a chest X-ray should be obtained to exclude pulmonary infiltrates even in the absence of pulmonary signs or symptoms.[237]

About 80% of clinicians prescribe antibiotics according to guidelines for neutropenic fever.[241] While guidelines and general statements should be heeded, local epidemiology and clinical practice conditions must also be taken into consideration.[242] The initial management approach of neutropenic fever should be based on risk with subsequent modification based on clinical response.[236,243–245] Both Multinational Association for Supportive Care in Cancer (MASCC) and Clinical Index of Stable Febrile Neutropenia (CISNE) scores can identify low-risk febrile neutropenia.[246,247] For low-risk patients (i.e., MASCC score ≥21 or Talcott group 4) with stable hemodynamics, no comorbidity, and low symptom burden, outpatient treatment with oral fluoroquinolone plus amoxicillin/clavulanate (clindamycin if allergic to penicillin) as initial empiric regimen may be appropriate unless a fluoroquinolone has been used for prophylaxis before fever onset.[248] The patients should receive the initial doses of empirical antibiotics within one hour of triage. Eligibility for outpatient management should be determined by monitoring the patient's condition for at least 4 h. However, successful outpatient management relies on coordination among primary care, oncology, and emergency departments to ensure a rapid response and close follow-up during the outpatient treatment period as well as effective communication between clinicians and patients and their care-takers.[249]

Outside large comprehensive cancer centers, the standard approach for neutropenic fever is inpatient treatment with IV antibiotics.[250] At our institution, high-risk patients with neutropenic fever not eligible for out-patient therapy are admitted for IV antibiotics. Factors associated with prolonged hospital stay in adults with neutropenic fever include hematologic malignancies, high-intensity chemotherapy, long duration of neutropenia, and cultures growing Gram-negative multi-drug-resistant bacteria.[251] Monotherapy with broad-spectrum beta-lactam antibiotics, such as or piperacillin-tazobactam, carbapenems, or the fourth-generation cephalosporin cefepime, is recommended. Adding other antimicrobials (e.g., aminoglycosides, fluoroquinolones, vancomycin, colistin, daptomycin) to the initial regimen in cases with suspected or known antibiotic resistance or serious infections is also indicated. Empirical coverage for Gram-positive organisms with vancomycin is acceptable if a Gram-positive bacterial infection is suspected or known, for example, cellulitis, central venous catheter-related infection, mucositis, or the use of prophylactic antibiotics against Gram-negative bacteria.[236] Vancomycin use in neutropenic fever has more than tripled to 55% in 2010 over 10 years.[241]

If a febrile neutropenic patient does not respond to the initial broad-spectrum antibiotic therapy, additional antibiotics or antifungal therapy is recommended. Fluconazole may be used as initial empirical therapy in patients who have not received prior antifungal prophylaxis. Amphotericin B is beneficial for patients with persistent fever during broad-spectrum antibiotic treatment without antifungal prophylaxis, persistent neutropenia for more than 15 days, or a documented fungal infection. *Candida albicans* and nonalbicans candidal species are important pathogens in leukemia patients and bone marrow transplant recipients, and *Aspergillus* infection causes significant problems in patients with prolonged and profound neutropenia. Other fungi, such as *Fusarium* and *Trichosporon*, are emerging as important pathogens, perhaps owing to increased prevalence of antifungal prophylaxis.

In high-risk patients, especially leukemic patients, a de-escalation approach may be employed instead of the escalation approach discussed above.[244] Patients at risk for infection with resistant pathogens (e.g., methicillin-resistant *Staphylococcus aureus*, vancomycin-resistant *Enterococcus*, extended-spectrum beta-lactamase-producing Gram-negative bacteria, and carbapenemase-producing organisms) and patient with unstable hemodynamics should be treated initially with broad-spectrum antibiotic combinations. Major risk factors for infection with resistant pathogens include prior colonization or infection by resistant organisms and a high local prevalence of resistant pathogens in cultures obtained when fever started in neutropenic patients. De-escalation of antibiotic therapy is based on the culture results and clinical response 72–96 h after initiation of antibiotic therapy.

The adjunct therapy of a myeloid colony-stimulating factor to increase leukocytes in chemotherapy-induced neutropenic fever does not improve overall mortality, although such therapy is associated with shorter durations of fever, neutropenia, and antibiotics use.[252] Although prophylactic colony-stimulating factors should be considered if the risk of chemotherapy-induced neutropenic fever is >20%, starting these factors after fever onset in a neutropenic patient is generally not recommended.[236]

Differentiation syndrome

Differentiation syndrome (DS) was previously called the retinoic acid syndrome because it is a complication of all-*trans* retinoic acid treatment for acute promyelocytic leukemia. DS can also occur in acute promyelocytic leukemia patients treated with arsenic trioxide and patients with relapsed or refractory acute myeloid leukemia who are receiving isocitrate dehydrogenase (IDH) inhibitors.[253] Classic DS has a bimodal distribution with peak incidence in the first and third weeks after initiation of induction therapy for acute promyelocytic leukemia in about 25% of cases.[253–255] IDH inhibitor-induced DS has a median onset time of 48 days (range 10–340 days) for enasidenib (IDH2 inhibitor) and 29 days (range 5–59 days) for ivosidenib (IDH1 inhibitor)[253,256] at lower incidence rates (ivosidenib: 10.6%,[253] and enasidenib: 11.7%[253,257]). IDH inhibitor-induced DS may occur 1 week to 5 months after treatment initiation. Furthermore, IDH inhibitor-induced DS can recur after therapy interruption or dose escalation.[257]

DS involves infiltration of differentiated white blood cells into various organs, causing endothelial activation and release of cytokines and vasoactive factors.[253] DS is a challenging clinical diagnosis because there are no specific laboratory tests or imaging modalities. This life-threatening emergency is characterized by dyspnea, unexplained fever, >5-kg weight gain (from fluid retention), unexplained hypotension, acute renal failure, pulmonary infiltrates, pleural and/or pericardial effusion on imaging.[254,255] White blood cell count $>5 \times 10^9$/L and elevated serum creatinine level are associated with high severity and mortality.[254] Uric acid must be checked, and hyperuricemia management is important.[253,254,257] For patients with renal failure, hemodialysis may be required, and for those without renal failure, fluid overload can be treated with diuretics.[257] Broad-spectrum antibiotics are appropriate because of the overlap with the signs and symptoms of sepsis. Because DS can mimic decompensated heart failure, pneumonia, and sepsis, prompt recognition and diagnosis may be difficult. In the right clinical settings, DS should be treated as soon as suspected because delayed workup and management increase morbidity.[253,258] Early intervention and treatment with corticosteroids (dexamethasone 10 mg/day until symptom resolution) reduce mortality.[254,255]

Sinusoidal occlusion syndrome

Sinusoidal occlusion syndrome (SOS) is a hepatic veno-occlusive disease caused by obliterative terminal hepatic venulitis due to a prothrombotic hypofibrinolytic state. SOS is a serious emergency that happens in 8–14% of patients during the first month after hematopoietic stem cell transplantation. Antibody-drug conjugates, gemtuzumab ozogamicin and inotuzumab ozogamicin are humanized anti-CD33 and anti-CD22 mAb, respectively, conjugated to ozogamicin (a derivative of calicheamicin),[259] and SOS occurs in about 9% of patients with acute myeloid leukemia who receive gemtuzumab ozogamicin,[260–262] around 1% in patients with relapsed or refractory B-cell non-Hodgkin lymphoma who receive inotuzumab ozogamicin, and 13% in patients with relapsed or refractory acute lymphoblastic leukemia who received inotuzumab ozogamicin.[263,264] The triad of hepatomegaly, jaundice, and ascites should raise suspicion of SOS in these clinical settings.

The clinical presentation typically includes hyperbilirubinemia, elevated liver enzyme level, weight gain, ascites, and tender hepatomegaly. The differential diagnosis includes sepsis, graft-versus-host disease, Budd-Chiari syndrome, medication toxicity, congestive heart failure, and viral hepatitis. Grading is based on rate of progression and clinical findings (bilirubin, fluid retention, liver enzyme levels, and increased serum creatinine).[265] With multi-organ failure, the mortality rate is 80%.

Treatment of SOS is mainly supportive. The main challenge for emergency physicians is fluid management because intravascular volume needs to be optimized with crystalloids or colloid solutions without overload to avoid hepatorenal syndrome. Adequate oxygenation and maintenance of oxygen-carrying capacity by transfusion would help to minimize ischemic injury. Potentially toxic drugs should be avoided. The treatment for moderate to severe cases is high-dose glucocorticoids (methylprednisolone 1 mg/kg/day IV).[266]

Conclusion

The above discussion of selected topics in oncologic emergencies would give a glimpse of this developing field. As knowledge accumulates, the textbooks about this field are getting thicker and thicker.[267] The National Institutes of Health sponsored the formation of the Comprehensive Oncologic Emergencies Research Network (CONCERN) in 2015 to accelerate research, synthesis, and translation in the field of oncologic emergency through multi-center collaborations. As the prevalence of cancer survivors grow, oncologists and emergency physicians will increasingly collaborate in patient care.

Key references

The complete reference list can be found on Vital Source version of this title, see inside front cover.

5. Hwang JP, Patlan J, de Achaval S, Escalante CP. Survival in cancer patients after out-of-hospital cardiac arrest. *Support Care Cancer*. 2010;**18**:51–55.
21. Ewer MS, Ewer SM. Cardiotoxicity of anticancer treatments: what the cardiologist needs to know. *Nature Rev Cardiol*. 2010;**7**:564–575.
26. Howard SC, Jones DP, Pui CH. The tumor lysis syndrome. *N Engl J Med*. 2011;**364**:1844–1854.
38. Ristic AD, Imazio M, Adler Y, et al. Triage strategy for urgent management of cardiac tamponade: a position statement of the European Society of Cardiology Working Group on Myocardial and Pericardial Diseases. *Eur Heart J*. 2014;**35**:2279–2284.
43. Annane D, Siami S, Jaber S, et al. Effects of fluid resuscitation with colloids vs crystalloids on mortality in critically ill patients presenting with hypovolemic shock: the CRISTAL randomized trial. *JAMA*. 2013;**310**:1809–1817.
45. Haas RA, Ahn SH. Interventional management of head and neck emergencies: carotid blowout. *Semin Intervent Radiol*. 2013;**30**:245–248.
58. Fagedet D, Thony F, Timsit JF, et al. Endovascular treatment of malignant superior vena cava syndrome: results and predictive factors of clinical efficacy. *Cardiovasc Intervent Radiol*. 2013;**36**:140–149.
63. Jean-Baptiste E. Clinical assessment and management of massive hemoptysis. *Crit Care Med*. 2000;**28**:1642–1647.
69. Simoff MJ, Lally B, Slade MG, et al. Symptom management in patients with lung cancer: diagnosis and management of lung cancer, 3rd ed: American College of Chest Physicians evidence-based clinical practice guidelines. *Chest*. 2013;**143**:e455S–e497S.
79. Putnam JB Jr, Walsh GL, Swisher SG, et al. Outpatient management of malignant pleural effusion by a chronic indwelling pleural catheter. *Ann Thorac Surg*. 2000;**69**:369–375.
81. Ost DE, Jimenez CA, Lei X, et al. Quality-adjusted survival following treatment of malignant pleural effusions with indwelling pleural catheters. *Chest*. 2014;**145**:1347–1356.
85. Patel A, Pearce A. Progress in management of the obstructed airway. *Anaesthesia*. 2011;**66**(Suppl 2):93–100.
92. MacDuff A, Arnold A, Harvey J, Group BTSPDG. Management of spontaneous pneumothorax: British Thoracic Society Pleural Disease Guideline 2010. *Thorax*. 2010;**65**(Suppl 2):ii18–ii31.
97. Qdaisat A, Yeung SJ, Variyam DE, et al. Evaluation of cancer patients with suspected pulmonary embolism: performance of the American College of Physicians Guideline. *J Am Coll Radiol*. 2020;**17**:22–30.
98. King V, Vaze AA, Moskowitz CS, et al. D-dimer assay to exclude pulmonary embolism in high-risk oncologic population: correlation with CT pulmonary angiography in an urgent care setting. *Radiology*. 2008;**247**:854–861.
99. Qdaisat A, Soud RA, Wu CC, et al. Poor performance of D-dimer in excluding venous thromboembolism among patients with lymphoma and leukemia. *Haematologica*. 2019;**104**:e265–e268.
103. Chatterjee S, Chakraborty A, Weinberg I, et al. Thrombolysis for pulmonary embolism and risk of all-cause mortality, major bleeding, and intracranial hemorrhage: a meta-analysis. *JAMA*. 2014;**311**:2414–2421.
107. Key NS, Khorana AA, Kuderer NM, et al. Venous thromboembolism prophylaxis and treatment in patients with cancer: ASCO clinical practice guideline update. *J Clin Oncol*. 2020;**38**:496–520.
117. Qdaisat A, Kamal M, Al-Breiki A, et al. Clinical characteristics, management, and outcome of incidental pulmonary embolism in cancer patients. *Blood Adv*. 2020;**4**:1606–1614.
120. O'Phelan KH, Bunney EB, Weingart SD, Smith WS. Emergency neurological life support: spinal cord compression (SCC). *Neurocrit Care*. 2012;**17**(Suppl 1):S96–S101.
124. Stevens RD, Huff JS, Duckworth J, et al. Emergency neurological life support: intracranial hypertension and herniation. *Neurocrit Care*. 2012;**17**(Suppl 1):S60–S65.
129. Claassen J, Silbergleit R, Weingart SD, Smith WS. Emergency neurological life support: status epilepticus. *Neurocrit Care*. 2012;**17**(Suppl 1):S73–S78.
130. Simons FE, Ardusso LR, Bilo MB, et al. World Allergy Organization anaphylaxis guidelines: summary. *J Allergy Clin Immunol*. 2011;**127**:587–593 e581–522.
133. Campbell RL, Li JT, Nicklas RA, et al. Emergency department diagnosis and treatment of anaphylaxis: a practice parameter. *Ann Allergy, Asthma Immunol*. 2014;**113**:599–608.
140. Corominas M, Gastaminza G, Lobera T. Hypersensitivity reactions to biological drugs. *J Investig Allergol Clin Immunol*. 2014;**24**:212–225; quiz 211p following 225.
141. Rosello S, Blasco I, Garcia Fabregat L, et al. Management of infusion reactions to systemic anticancer therapy: ESMO Clinical Practice Guidelines. *Ann Oncol: Official J Eur Soc Med Oncol*. 2017;**28**:iv100–iv118.
149. Brahmer JR, Lacchetti C, Schneider BJ, et al. Management of immune-related adverse events in patients treated with immune checkpoint inhibitor therapy: American Society of Clinical Oncology Clinical Practice Guideline. *J Clin Oncol*. 2018;**36**:1714–1768.
151. Haanen JBAG, Carbonnel F, Robert C, et al. Management of toxicities from immunotherapy: ESMO clinical practice guidelines for diagnosis, treatment and follow-up. *Ann Oncol*. 2017;**28**:iv119–iv142.
171. Wang DY, Okoye GD, Neilan TG, et al. Cardiovascular toxicities associated with cancer immunotherapies. *Curr Cardiol Rep*. 2017;**19**:21.
174. Fellner A, Makranz C, Lotem M, et al. Neurologic complications of immune checkpoint inhibitors. *J Neurooncol*. 2018;**137**:601–609.
181. El Majzoub I, Qdaisat A, Thein KZ, et al. Adverse effects of immune checkpoint therapy in cancer patients visiting the emergency department of a comprehensive cancer center. *Ann Emerg Med*. 2019;**73**:79–87.
216. Lee DW, Gardner R, Porter DL. Current concepts in the diagnosis and management of cytokine release syndrome (vol 124, pg 188, 2014). *Blood*. 2016;**128**:1533–1533.
218. Lee DW, Santomasso BD, Locke FL, et al. ASBMT consensus grading for cytokine release syndrome and neurological toxicity associated with immune effector cells. *Biol Blood Marrow Transplant*. 2019;**25**(4):625–638.
230. Acharya UH, Dhawale T, Yun S, et al. Management of cytokine release syndrome and neurotoxicity in chimeric antigen receptor (CAR) T cell therapy. *Expert Rev Hematol*. 2019;**12**:195–205.
245. Klastersky J, Paesmans M, Georgala A, et al. Outpatient oral antibiotics for febrile neutropenic cancer patients using a score predictive for complications. *J Clin Oncol*. 2006;**24**:4129–4134.
246. Ahn S, Rice TW, Yeung SJ, Cooksley T. Comparison of the MASCC and CISNE scores for identifying low-risk neutropenic fever patients: analysis of data from three emergency departments of cancer centers in three continents. *Support Care Cancer*. 2018;**26**:1465–1470.
252. Mhaskar R, Clark OA, Lyman G, et al. Colony-stimulating factors for chemotherapy-induced febrile neutropenia. *Cochrane Database Syst Rev*. 2014;**10**:CD003039.
257. Fathi AT, DiNardo CD, Kline I, et al. Differentiation syndrome associated with enasidenib, a selective inhibitor of mutant isocitrate dehydrogenase 2: analysis of a phase 1/2 study. *JAMA Oncol*. 2018;**4**:1106–1110.
258. Luesink M, Pennings JL, Wissink WM, et al. Chemokine induction by all-trans retinoic acid and arsenic trioxide in acute promyelocytic leukemia: triggering the differentiation syndrome. *Blood*. 2009;**114**:5512–5521.
260. Tallman MS, McDonald GB, DeLeve LD, et al. Incidence of sinusoidal obstruction syndrome following Mylotarg (gemtuzumab ozogamicin): a prospective observational study of 482 patients in routine clinical practice. *Int J Hematol*. 2013;**97**:456–464.

PART 13

The Future of Oncology

139 A vision for twenty-first century healthcare

Leroy Hood, MD, PhD ■ Nathan D. Price, PhD ■ James T. Yurkovich

> **Overview**
>
> The convergence of systems science, big data, and patient-activated social networks is leading to the practice of predictive, preventive, personalized, and participatory (P4) Medicine. P4 Medicine has two central thrusts: optimizing wellness and demystifying disease. In this chapter, we will describe current research practices that embody P4 Medicine, providing examples of how these studies have and can continue to integrate with and transform the healthcare system. We will focus on the use of dense longitudinal profiling of an individual's physiological state—so-called "deep phenotyping"—to gain key insights into wellness as well as the onset, progression, treatment, and prevention of disease. Such a systems approach will generate clinically actionable possibilities to enable individuals to optimize wellness and/or avoid disease. We believe that this approach will transform healthcare by decreasing costs, increasing healthcare quality, and promoting innovation in a new paradigm of medical practice.

A vision for healthcare

Healthcare is one of the most significant challenges of our time. Costs are rapidly growing worldwide, but commensurate improvements in health are not being delivered.[1,2] Even though the United States is the biggest healthcare spender per capita in the world, it ranks near the bottom of the top 17 developed nations in survival among those 50-years of age and older[1,3] and has among the highest avoidable mortality rates.[4] Studies on the drivers of health and disease show that approximately 30% of lifetime health is attributable to genetic causes, 60% to environmental and behavioral causes, and only about 10% to healthcare itself, with significant interactions among these factors.[5] Thus, the focus of today's healthcare—which is almost entirely on disease—ignores major aspects of the actual drivers of health. This focus is problematic in the treatment of disease because once biological systems are altered by disease, they often cannot be restored to their fully functional pre-disease state. Major systemic changes are clearly needed to provide the healthcare we need for the twenty-first century. As we will discuss in this chapter, medicine must become predictive and preventive, using longitudinal studies of wellness in individuals to follow and reverse the eventual transitions into disease.

Quantifying wellness and demystifying disease

Understanding wellness is critical to both optimizing human potential and providing fundamental insights into the treatment and prevention of disease. While the healthcare system generally focuses on patients after they become sick, a focus on wellness allows for the identification and examination of the earliest wellness-to-disease transitions so as to study disease at its earliest inception and decipher the underlying initial mechanisms. Over the past several years, the United States healthcare system has invested approximately 97% of its resources to the treatment of disease (i.e., after diagnosis of one or more potentially serious conditions).[6] Further, it has been estimated that over 85% of healthcare costs are spent on the treatment of chronic diseases.[7,8] One of the primary drivers of these trends is the simple fact that we have no gold standard for the quantification of "wellness" and do not know in detail what a healthy physiology looks like.

To transform the current healthcare system, we suggest the adoption of a major thrust: *scientific (or quantitative) wellness*. The key to this transformation lies in a holistic strategy for the longitudinal, high-dimensional study of human health and disease in each individual—a systems biology approach. Such an approach naturally leads to the practice of predictive, preventive, personalized, and participatory (P4) Medicine. This fundamental approach will allow us to apply P4 Medicine to patients and integrate it with the contemporary healthcare system.

In this chapter, we outline this systems biology approach to studying disease and provide examples of deep insights that have been gained through its successful application. We discuss the kinds of data and analytical techniques that can help fuel this approach and discuss how these aspects might be translated from research laboratories to clinical practices. Finally, we describe a massive, real-world project in its nascent stages that promises to integrate systems P4 medicine with healthcare systems and identify challenges facing the widespread adoption of this type of approach. Ultimately, this model will provide the basis for establishing quantitative metrics of wellness and for identifying transitions from wellness to common diseases.

Systems biology as an emerging paradigm

Human biology and disease are complex, much more complex than was widely recognized in the 1970s and 1980s. While great progress was being made in research laboratories around the world, the focus was largely on individual biological components (e.g., proteins, genes, transcripts). This reductionist approach failed to capture the dense, interconnected nature of biological networks and systems. Consider the well-known parable of the elephant and the six blind men. Each man used his sense of touch on a different part of the elephant and characterized the unknown thing by that observation. To one man, the elephant was like a snake (the trunk), while to another it was like a fan (the ear). The ability to identify the unknown object as an elephant requires a holistic approach that integrates all available data. A similar comparison describes how twentieth century biology would attempt to understand how a radio works.[9] The study of biology and medicine suffers from analogous complexities, where we measure one or a few genes or proteins but fail to see the bigger picture. We are constantly faced with a puzzle with missing pieces, and systems biology offers a path forward to decipher these complexities.[10] The emergence of this new integrative discipline,[11] now called "systems science," has led to the transformation of biology and medicine and promises to offer a new, valuable perspective in a variety of topical areas, such as transfusion medicine.[12–15]

In his seminal 1962 book *The Structure of Scientific Revolutions*,[16] Thomas Kuhn highlighted the difficulties in catalyzing paradigm changes in physics due to scientists' conservatism and reluctance to move beyond conventional wisdom to think outside the box. As the field of systems biology began to gain traction in the 1990s and especially in the early 2000s,[11] the paradigm shift from a reductionist to a holistic view of biology was met with broad skepticism[17]—as predicted by Kuhn. Since the 1970s, there have been several paradigm shifts in life science and biomedical research, five of which one of us (Lee Hood) participated in and helped drive:

1. Bringing *engineering to biology* through the development of six instruments that allowed the reading and writing of DNA and proteins. These instruments introduced the concept of high-throughput biological data generation and associated analytic frameworks.[18–20]
2. One of these instruments, the automated DNA sequencer, enabled the *Human Genome Project* and the subsequent production of the complete list of genes. Building on this foundation, lists of encoded proteins, the functional modalities of cells, were generated—resulting in parts lists that together made systems science possible.[21,22] The human genome project also gave us access to all human genetic variability (polymorphisms) and the ability to correlate variants with wellness and disease phenotypes.
3. The emergence of *cross-disciplinary biology*—research teams comprising biologists, chemists, computer scientists, engineers, mathematicians, physicists, and physicians—that spanned many areas of expertise to solve complex biological problems. These collaborative efforts fueled the cycle of biological discovery driving technology that, in turn, drives analytics to understand the mechanisms of biology and ultimately led to key technologies and analytics in genomics, proteomics, cell sorting, single-cell analysis, and large-scale DNA synthesis.[23]
4. In 2000, the founding of the first dedicated systems biology research institute, the Institute for Systems Biology (ISB) (Seattle, WA), to pioneer *systems science* and its necessary technologies and analytics.[24–26] A systems approach to disease led to defining the conceptual framework of twenty-first century medicine, as reviewed herein.
5. The emergence of *systems medicine* and *P4 Medicine* from the application of systems science to disease. The first four paradigm shifts above enabled this revolutionary new approach to study disease, wellness, and medicine.[27–29] The important point was these paradigm changes allowed us for the first time to deal effectively with human complexity through longitudinal, high-dimensional analyses of individual humans. We will discuss several examples of this approach shortly.

In retrospect, these experiences generated useful insights regarding how to catalyze paradigm shifts in modern society.[25]

Multiscale biological systems

The adoption of systems science has provided the conceptual framework and technological tools—both experimental and computational—to gain a deeper understanding of biological information that was previously inaccessible.[30] Human physiology comprises biological networks that operate at distinct, functional phenotypic states spanning multiple physiological scales: molecules, cells, tissues/organs, and the organism (Figure 1). One or more of these biological networks are generally (perhaps always) disease-perturbed well before clinical diagnosis of disease.[28,30,31] Diagnosing and appropriately treating diseases most effectively thus relies on our knowledge of the underlying biological and pathophysiological mechanisms to detect these network perturbations before symptoms arise.

The genome is like a book containing the digital instructions for life.[10,21] This book is composed using the four-letter language of DNA—adenine (A), cytosine (C), guanine (G), and thymine (T), and is packaged into 23 pairs of human chromosomes present in (almost) each of an individual's $\sim 10^{13}$ cells. Approximately 1% of the roughly six billion nucleotide bases code for $\sim 20,000$ units of information ("genes") that are transcribed into RNA copies which are ultimately translated into individual proteins. Genes can be modified chemically or through their interactions with proteins ("epigenetic modifications"), thus modifying their ability to be expressed. The generation of RNA transcripts for individual genes allows for complex regulatory networks that differentially express certain genes according to the needs of individual cell types (up to millions of RNA copies per cell) and chemically alter the expressed transcripts to modify their information content. For example, the neurexin human gene has at least 2000 different RNA transcripts, leading to fascinating questions regarding how many of these unique transcripts represented signal and which are simply noise.[32]

RNA transcripts are translated into proteins, which are the molecular machines of life that determine the functional state of a cell. A 20-letter language corresponding to the 20 amino acids encodes proteins. This language directs the folding of each protein into complex three-dimensional structures that executes the specific functions of life. Proteins may function alone or through interactions with other proteins and other molecules to create complex molecular machines and functional biological networks.

These networks arise from interactions among DNA, RNA, proteins, and small molecules involved in energy metabolism ("metabolites") in the context of various biological networks of life—for example, protein, metabolic, and transcriptional networks. These networks are dynamic in time and are influenced by both the genome and the environment. Networks thus govern how biological systems change over time and mediate critical life processes that include development, physiology, and aging. Perturbations to these networks result in disease.

The study of these networks as a whole—as opposed to analyzing one or a few molecules at a time—allows for the characterization of these dynamic systems that lead directly to observable phenotypic states. Technological developments enable these dynamical networks to be profiled, with tools that allow for the analysis of the complete genome (genomics), all gene modifications (epigenetics), all RNAs (transcriptomics), and many (but not all) metabolites or proteins in a given cell, tissue, or organ (metabolomics and proteomics, respectively). Collectively, these various -omic technologies provide a broad molecular characterization of a physiological state. However, when considering human wellness and disease, it is important to capture higher-level

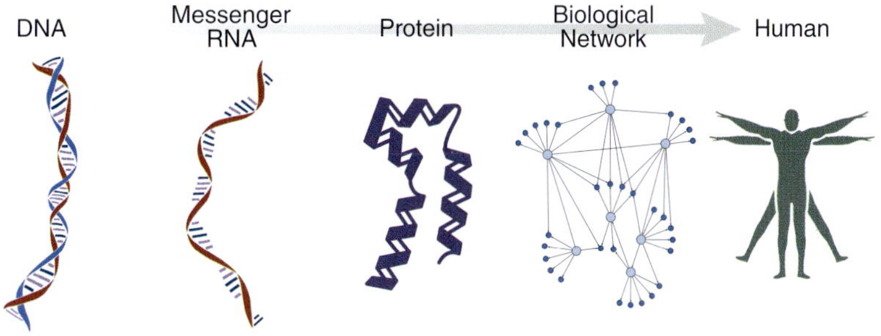

DNA → Messenger RNA → Protein → Biological Network → Human

Figure 1 Individual data clouds capture important physiological data from multiple levels of the informational hierarchy within complex biological organisms.

phenotyping data such as health outcomes (i.e., the consequences of clinical diagnoses), anthropometric measurements (e.g., body mass index, imaging of all organs), environmental factors (e.g., exposures), and meta-information (e.g., age, sex). Thus, a systems approach to medicine focuses on understanding the roles that these molecular mechanisms and environmental exposures play in wellness and disease.

Systems science in biomedicine

The integration of systems science in the practice of healthcare (which we will refer to as "systems medicine") requires the collection of vast amounts of data longitudinally for each individual to characterize wellness and understand individualized physiology to the point where disease transitions can be recognized, understood, and potentially reversed at an early stage. A systems medicine approach must therefore utilize data collected from each individual that will enable the construction of computational models to interpret the data and ultimately suggest personalized treatments. To realize these goals, an enormous amount of data is required—but what should these data look like?

We envision a future in which each person will undergo "deep phenotyping" in order to generate an associated longitudinal data cloud (Figure 2).[33] These data clouds have several important properties. First, the data clouds are *personal*, representing measurements made for an individual. Second, the data clouds are *dense*, comprising billions of data points that come from disparate measurements, including complete genome sequence, transcriptomic, proteomic, metabolomic, quantified self-measurements, clinical chemistries, gut microbiome composition, body and organ imaging, nutrient tracking, environmental measurements, and more. Third, the data clouds are *dynamic*, representing multiple measurements over time. These longitudinal measurements provide snapshots of a person's physiology and environment (defined broadly as all dynamic surroundings that impinge upon the individual, inside and outside the body).[34] Together, these deep-phenotyping data inherently integrate genetic, phenotypic, and environmental information—the three essential components of health assessments.

The analysis of deep-phenotyping data presents enormous challenges in identifying true signal and separating it from the inherent variability (noise) in biological information that is irrelevant to the health questions at hand. Systems approaches, including various machine learning applications, are critical to mining these large datasets for actionable information, identifying potentially small but meaningful signals from large amounts of noise.[35,36] New techniques are constantly being developed that aid in this process,

such as techniques for functional genomics analysis[37] and the application of deep learning and reinforcement learning strategies to deep-phenotyping data.[38]

Deep-phenotyping data can be modeled using a variety of top-down statistical approaches and bottom-up mechanistic approaches. Different data types can be examined in the context of dynamic biological networks—such as those for gene regulation, protein interactions, or metabolism—that mediate processes involved in development, physiology, and aging. These models are then interpreted to understand how perturbations to these networks cause deviations from wellness (manifesting ultimately as disease), revealing fundamental insights into disease mechanisms through experimental validation. This approach allows for the identification of "actionable possibilities" for the optimization of wellness and the avoidance or amelioration of disease,[39] revealing fundamental insights into disease mechanisms and the development of early diagnostics.[40]

Longitudinal deep phenotyping allows for a move away from population averages and toward the practice of using each person as his or her own baseline, referred to as an "N-of-1" study (where the variable N denotes the sample size).[41] Such an approach has been applied in several different areas, including the study of pregnancy,[42] nutrition,[43] and sleep.[44] Further, longitudinal sampling allows for the study of onset and progression of disease. As networks are perturbed by disease, the information that gets processed is altered.[11,45] Assessing the differences between normal and disease-perturbed networks provides deep insights into disease mechanisms, novel diagnostic approaches, and candidate targets for new therapies (Figure 3). While there are many challenges associated with designing such studies on human patients, animal models present one promising and informative research route. We developed an inducible mouse model of prion disease and identified 10 biological networks perturbed over the 22-week progression of the disease.[46] Notably, these networks were perturbed at different points during the course of the disease progression, and their dynamics explained almost all aspects of the disease pathophysiology. Similar inducible models have been developed to study other diseases, like glioblastoma multiforme[47] and acute myeloid leukemia.[48]

The use of deep phenotyping to study human health and disease is growing. Family units present one good opportunity for the identification of disease-related genes through genome sequencing.[49] We have applied whole-genome sequencing to family units in the study of various diseases, resulting in the identification of rare variants in a cluster of genes encoding neural excitability that influence the risk of bipolar disease[50] and dozens of candidate biomarkers for very early preterm birth in growth signaling and inflammation- and immunity-related pathways.[51]

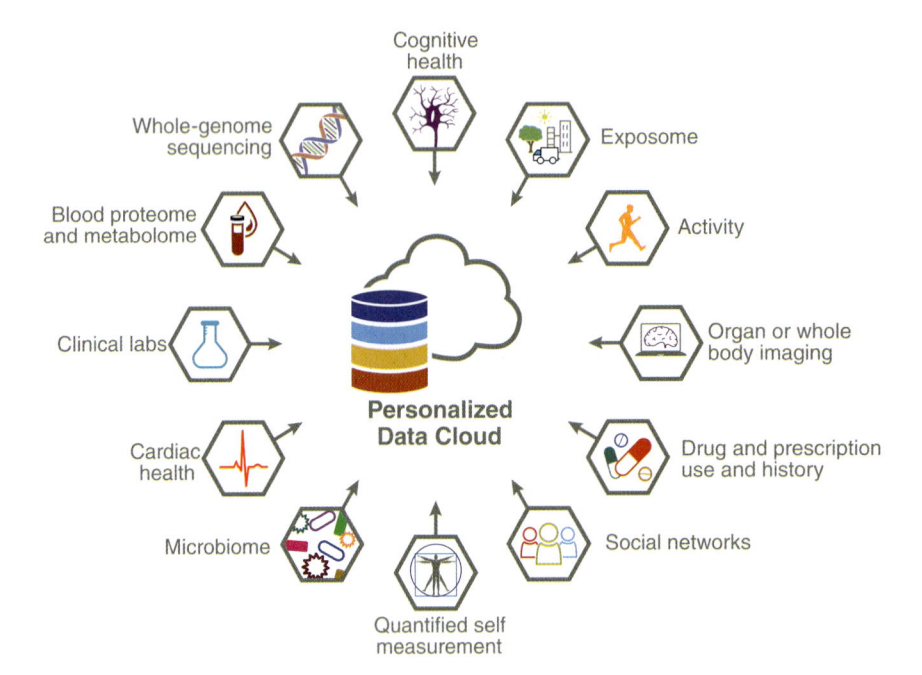

Figure 2 Each human is a "network of networks." These biological networks span from genes and individual molecules (e.g., proteins, metabolites) to cells, tissues, and organs. Together, humans form social networks that encapsulate various levels of interaction. The differences between normal and disease-perturbed networks provides insights into disease mechanisms, early diagnosis, and improved identification of drug target candidates.

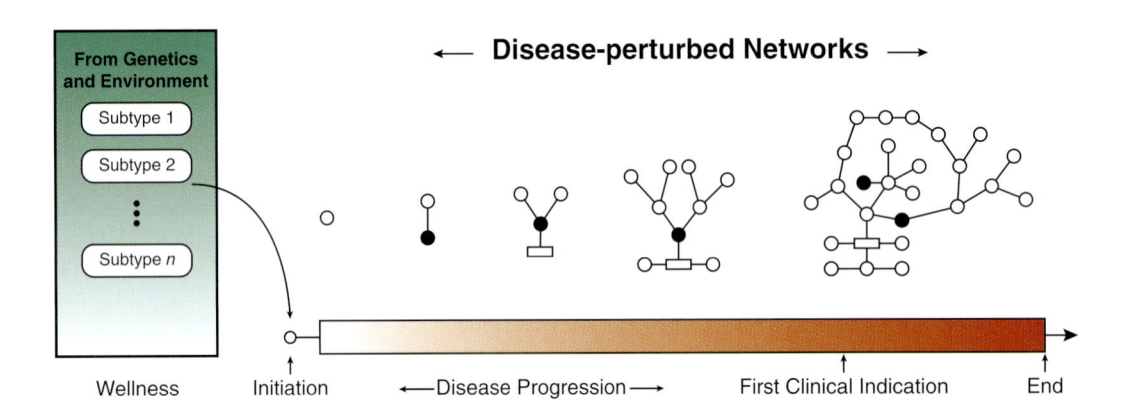

Figure 3 Biological networks are perturbed far in advance of clinical diagnoses. Genetics, lifestyle, and the environment define and influence the networks in the human body, while perturbations to these networks manifest as disease.

Various types of molecular profiling have aided in the study of a variety of diseases, including type 2 diabetes[52] and weight gain/loss.[53]

The first large deep-phenotyping study for scientific wellness was the Pioneer 100 project in which we designed and performed a study of 108 individuals that collected genomes, gut microbiomes, blood metabolomes and proteomes, clinical chemistries, and fitness tracking from wearable devices over a 9-month period.[33] When analyzed, these individual data clouds revealed long lists of "actionable possibilities" derived from the literature that could either improve wellness or avoid or ameliorate disease. The actionable possibilities were delivered to individuals by a coach trained in psychology to facilitate behavior change. Virtually all of the individuals felt their health was strikingly improved at the end of the 9-month experiment. Various computational analyses demonstrated that deep phenotyping can elucidate striking statistical connections among various analytes and genetic risk scores, such as a negative correlation between plasma cystine levels and genetic risk for inflammatory bowel disease. The study required a sophisticated team to manage a host of challenges associated with scientific questions (e.g., which appropriate assays to include, the development of analytical tools to define actionable possibilities), logistics (e.g., sample collection procedures), organization (e.g., formation of a physician advisory panel), and participant engagement. Of the 108 individuals who enrolled in the study, 107 remained in the study throughout its duration and 70% were compliant to coaching recommendations related to the actionable possibilities revealed through analysis of the data.

The high retention and engagement rates were influenced by three elements: (1) coaches were effective in explaining each individual's actionable possibilities and in encouraging individuals to act upon them in accordance with their own health objectives, (2) an understanding how one's own genes interacted with and impacted other types of data encouraged individuals to modify behavior, and (3) observing the positive changes in one's data over time in response to specific lifestyle changes reinforced positive behaviors. The first clinical lab measurements revealed that 91% of the individuals had specific nutritional deficiencies and 68% had inflammatory indicators, both of which are correctable. Three individuals had extremely high levels of mercury; two ate significant amounts of tuna sushi (with high levels of mercury), while the third had mercury from old dental fillings. One of these individuals simply substituted salmon for tuna sushi and within 2-months experienced a halving of the original measured mercury level, while the other two had similar experiences in dealing with the source of this anomaly.

Individual genetic risk for disease can inform about longitudinal measures that should be tracked to see if the disease is manifesting. For example, two individuals were homozygous for the variant that causes hemochromatosis (C282Y). In a subset of such individuals, this disorder can lead to high iron and ferritin levels in the blood. High blood iron levels can attack the skin, joints, pancreas, liver, and/or the heart—potentially leading to arthritis, diabetes, liver cirrhosis/cancer, and/or cardiac decompensation in various combinations. Since this disease often presents with these cardiac complications, individuals may be already chronically ill with diabetes or liver disease. The treatment is simple: send the individuals with the C282Y mutations to their physician to perform the necessary tests for a clinical diagnosis; if positive, the individual can have regular blood draws until normal iron levels are reached. We identified the two individuals with homozygous C282Y genotypes before any serious tissue damage had been done, thus saving the healthcare system significant dollars by avoiding what could have been chronic hemochromatosis. Further, the children of these individuals underwent genetic testing, stopping the trend of an undiagnosed yet treatable disease to future generations.

Using standard cutoff values for fasting serum glucose, we identified 43 individuals (~40%) who had fasting glucose in the prediabetic range at baseline (i.e., were prediabetic). After only 5–6-months of health coaching, seven of these individuals had reverted to normoglycemia, and the overall trend in glucose levels in the population was decreasing.

The integration of two or more different data types (e.g., blood, microbiome, genetics, activity) was also informative. For example, using Genome-wide Association Studies (GWAS), we placed these 107 individuals into five risk categories according to their genetic (GWAS) propensity for Crohn's disease. When the bacterial populations in the gut microbiome were compared against these genetic propensities, two strains of more "pathogenic" bacteria increased as the genetic risk for each group of individuals increased. Thus, we observed an association between the genetics of Crohn's disease susceptibility and changing microbial populations in the gut microbiome; it is not yet clear what the causal association might be or whether there may be a strong actionable possibility here.

One of the clear outcomes of this study was that each of the 107 participants had multiple actionable possibilities. There was a remarkable compliance, with more than 70% of the Pioneers acting upon their actionable possibilities. Two clear conclusions came from this study:

1. Your genes determine your potential, not your destiny. For many conditions, a change in behavior can address genetic limitations.
2. Personalized, comprehensive, and real-time data are empowering. With this knowledge, it is easier and more motivating for one to take responsibility for one's health—one key to beginning to control healthcare costs. This is the fourth P in "P4 Medicine": participatory.

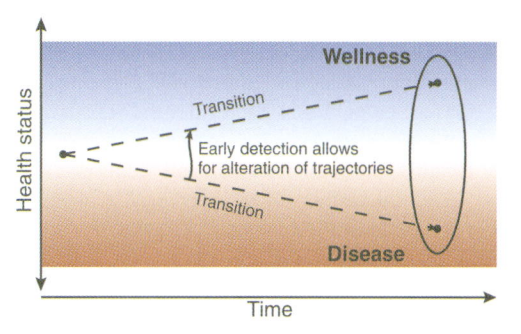

Figure 4 Health status changes over time. An individual's trajectory can maintain or increase wellness, or a trajectory can transition from wellness into a diseased state. Early detection of these transitions—and the identification of actionable possibilities to reverse these transitions—can aid in the optimization of wellness for each individual on a personalized level.

Through a commercial endeavor, we expanded upon this study to generate similar data clouds for almost 5000 individuals, enrolled over a four-and-a-half-year period, to explore targeted aspects of human health. Notably, we have used these vast data to explore gut health,[54] aging,[55] and an individual's genetic predisposition to disease.[56] We also saw more than 100 transitions from wellness to many chronic diseases, especially cancers. By analyzing changes in blood analytes (clinical chemistries, proteins, and metabolites), we were able to identify potential biomarkers for the earliest points of transition from wellness to disease (Figure 4). These candidate early disease transition biomarkers can then be used with systems approaches to understand the nature of the earliest disease-perturbed networks and thus identify therapies that might reverse the disease at it earliest detectable stage. Such an approach becomes exponentially more powerful as the size of the data clouds increase. This approach to prevent chronic diseases from being manifest as a disease phenotype will be an important aspect of disease prevention in the future.

While many human diseases have been connected with the bacterial diversity of the gut microbiome, the molecular effects on the host pathophysiology is largely unknown. Using approximately 1000 blood analytes (clinical labs, metabolites, and proteins), we found that just 40 metabolites (13 of microbial origin) could be used to robustly predict bacterial diversity in the gut.[54] Several of these metabolite biomarkers were previously linked with cardiovascular disease, diabetes, and kidney function. This pilot study suggests that the blood metabolome could serve as a proxy for the measurement of gut microbial health. This metric is important because significant gut microbiome diversity is one component of wellness—and having an easy blood test for this diversity will be useful.

One challenge with human health is defining what exactly "wellness" means. Dr. Dennis Ausiello (Emeritus Chief of Medicine at Harvard Medical School's Massachusetts General Hospital) has previously observed that healthcare is the only industry that does not study its own gold standard—wellness. To this end, we explored deep-phenotyping data for 3558 individuals to compute their "biological age" (the age your body says you are as opposed to the age your birthday says you are). If your biological age is lower than your chronological age, this suggests you are aging in a healthy manner. Thus, biological age represents one general and interpretable metric for wellness we explored within this population of individuals.[55] We found that individuals with most diseases have biological ages that are older than their chronological age (e.g., 300 individuals with type 2 diabetes had biological ages that averaged 6 years greater than their chronological ages).

Importantly, our analysis of longitudinal data points indicated an individual's biological age could be modified beneficially, providing insight into healthy aging. This metric will be extremely important to follow in facilitating "healthy aging" for individuals in the future.

As mentioned previously, it is estimated that approximately 90% of health and disease is attributable to genetic and lifestyle factors.[5] Using calculations of an individual's genetic predisposition to a disease from the genome ("polygenic risk scores"),[57] we examined the link between genetic risk and 55 clinical markers.[56] We were able to demonstrate that individuals with a high genetic risk for LDL cholesterol (a proxy for heart disease) that had high blood levels of LDL cholesterol could not reduce this analyte with lifestyle changes—rather only statins or similar drugs brought their levels down. In contrast, if you were at low genetic risk for LDL cholesterol and had high blood levels, lifestyle, diet, and exercise could bring the level down. The important point is that individuals at high risk for a genetic disease in many cases may have to be treated differently from those with a low risk. Hence, knowing the individual's risks for more than 100 different diseases through existing polygenic risk scores will become essential to adequate patient treatment in the future.

Beyond the Human Genome: integrating genomics and deep phenotyping in clinical practice

For successful integration of this systems approach into modern healthcare, we must make an important distinction between *discovery* and acceptable clinical *application*. The genome sequence is the foundation for both. The research studies described above have focused on the discovery aspect of human health, using vast amounts of data to make connections between various genes, analytes, and lifestyles. As more and more data are collected—made possible by the continued decrease in the prices of the associated technologies[30] and the clinical validation of their results—researchers will be faced with the task of reducing the dimensionality of these data to identify the most informative measurements. It is largely impractical to measure thousands of blood analytes and collect imaging as part of routine medical care, particularly for young, healthy individuals. However, using the genome to identify individuals at greater risk for developing certain diseases allows us to stratify the population and determine those individuals who should perhaps receive deeper phenotyping. For example, an individual with high genetic risk for a particular disease could be a candidate to undergo more regular screening.

To this end, the recently announced Beyond the Human Genome (BHG) project will bring deep phenotyping into routine clinical practice by leveraging cutting-edge technologies to understand how to optimize the health trajectory of each individual. This expansive initiative will bring together academic and industry resources to determine the complete genome sequence and deep phenotyping (analysis of the three classes of blood analytes and the gut microbiome every six months, digital health measurements) on one million patients across the spectrum of human diversity over a period of five years. This effort will require persuading physicians to enroll their patients, creating a biobank for storing blood samples, recruiting vendors to generate the genomic and -omic data, creating the computational platforms to manage the patients and their sample acquisition, sending the blood out to appropriate vendors for the data generation and integrating these data via a computational platform to analyze the genome and phenome data for biological discoveries and health insights.

These data, together with electronic health records (EHRs), will be placed in the cloud where the analytic and integrative analyses will be carried out. BHG will target five primary chronic disease areas: (1) Myelodysplastic syndromes (MDS) and acute myeloid leukemia (AML); (2) cardiovascular disease; (3) type 2 diabetes; (4) Alzheimer's disease; and (5) long COVID-19.

This program will identify currently accepted actionable possibilities and bring them to patients. It will discover thousands of new actionable possibilities from the phenomic data and the integration of genomic, phenomic and EHR data. It will make possible distributed, digital clinical trials matching appropriate patients in an unbelievably powerful manner. It will foster striking new opportunities for innovation, including the formation of both for-profit and non-profit data and analytics companies for the generation and management of thousands of actionable possibilities. Finally, it will hopefully catalyze a movement for other healthcare systems to adopt this new approach to twenty-first century medicine. This program requires extensive strategic partners, from genome sequencing and -omic data generation to one or more technological companies to handle the artificial intelligence (AI) challenges of thousands of actionable possibilities arising -omic data and the integration of all of these data types. It will also require pharma partners to take advantage of the rich opportunities coming from these integrative analyses. We believe this effort—when introduced into the healthcare system—will revolutionize the practice of medicine by bringing to physicians and their patients strikingly new types of actionable possibilities and ultimately it will focus on wellness rather than just disease. We also believe that the generation of this unique set of strategic partners will advance the required technologies, computational tools and even biological understanding of wellness and disease. These data will also result in diverse innovation, such as new intellectual property and new companies.

A systems approach to cancer medicine

Readers of this text may wonder how the systems approach described in this chapter can be applied to the study and treatment of cancers. We recently addressed this question in a review article[30] which outlined several opportunities for the effective utilization of a systems approach. We will discuss several of these areas here in more detail.

The early diagnosis of a cancer is vital to receiving the best treatment. The definition of an individual's normal baseline state is therefore key for the detection of transitions away from this state, as such transition may indicate the early formation of a cancer. For example, cancers shed rare cells into the blood that can be isolated and characterized. New robust technologies are enabling the profiling of single cells, providing new opportunities for early diagnosis from blood samples. Ultimately, the approach we have outlined in this chapter can help by identifying those individuals at high risk for developing cancers, providing insight into a subset of the population who should undergo more regular screening.

Deep phenotyping can be extended beyond whole body physiological to also include tumors, providing insight into potential therapeutic options. Thanks to large-scale pioneering research efforts like The Cancer Genome Atlas (TCGA)[58] and TCGA Pan-Cancer analysis project,[59] and the rise of a related commercial industry, the molecular profiling of tumors is becoming routine practice in many healthcare institutions. A focus on the tumor alone, however, is much too narrow and ultimately fails to capture the complex connections between the tumor and each individual's unique physiology. Thus, an analysis of a patient's germline DNA is important to distinguish newly arising cancer genome variants from variants already present in the individual's germline DNA. It is also possible to identify cell-free DNA (cfDNA) in the blood that reflects changes that have occurred in the tumors—providing insights into the location(s) and disease mechanisms of the cancer.[30] Additionally, as deep phenotyping becomes more prevalent, new insights have been emerging into the role of the microbiome and the immune system in cancer progression and treatment.[60–62]

As research continues to bring new insights into the complexities of cancers, a key aspect of future treatment strategies will likely involve multimodal therapies. Consider the example of HIV/AIDS (human immunodeficiency virus/acquired immunodeficiency syndrome), which exhibits excessive mutation rates in some ways similar to what is seen in cancers. Just as a triple drug therapy helped transform HIV/AIDS from a fatal to a chronic disease,[63] multidrug therapies—potentially combined with lifestyle and other intervention strategies—may have the same opportunity in cancers. The design of such multimodal therapies that work synergistically to combat the disease will require an understanding of the mechanisms underlying the relevant biological networks. The systems approach described in this chapter offers the potential to identify appropriate combinations of therapies on a personalized level.

While these are just a few examples of how systems science and P4 Medicine can be applied to the study and treatment of cancers, we are just at the beginning of exploring these opportunities. There are obvious challenges associated with the cost of these approaches, ultimately providing significant barriers to the large-scale implementation of P4 Medicine. Another important and omnipresent challenge is how to translate research to the clinic. Successful translation requires sparking the interest of clinicians and physicians in emerging research and discoveries. There are many obstacles associated with using new techniques, ranging from infrastructure and implementation to patient care and health. Thus, we need to constantly work to bridge the gap between the laboratory and the clinic to ensure that the progress made through research can be applied to address relevant and important medical questions. How do we catalyze the movement from research to clinic? Researchers must demonstrate success and describe how these successes have the potential to impact patients. Our understanding of complex mechanisms will 1 day provide physicians with a list of assays from which the best diagnostic can be chosen. The ability of researchers to demonstrate success will help ensure the translation of emerging technologies to clinical use.

It is an exciting time for systems science and its expansion into medical practice. We are faced with enormous opportunity to employ cutting-edge science that has driven important discoveries and will continue to impact the way medicine is practiced. The coming years will witness systems medicine transform society and healthcare in profound ways as innovative new technologies are developed that drive scientific discovery toward successful translational applications and personalized patient care. As we move into the twenty-first century, medicine will become increasingly P4, focusing on each individual for the optimization of health according to our unique physiology.

Acknowledgment

J.T.Y.'s effort was supported by the Institute for Systems Biology's Translational Research Fellows Program.

Conflict of interest

The authors declare no competing financial interests.

Key references

The complete reference list can be found on Vital Source version of this title, see inside front cover.

1. de la Maisonneuve C, de la Maisonneuve C, Martins JO. A projection method for public health and long-term care expenditures. *SSRN Electron J*. **1048**:5–40. doi: 10.2139/ssrn.2291541.
2. de la Maisonneuve C, de la Maisonneuve C, Martins JO. The future of health and long-term care spending. *OECD J Econ Stud*. 2015;**2014**:61–96.
3. National Research Council (US) & Institute of Medicine (US). *U.S. Health in International Perspective: Shorter Lives, Poorer Health*. Washington, DC: National Academies Press (US); 2013.
4. Heijink R, Koolman X, Westert GP. Spending more money, saving more lives? The relationship between avoidable mortality and healthcare spending in 14 countries. *Eur J Health Econ*. 2013;**14**:527–538.
5. Schroeder SA. We can do better—improving the health of the American people. *N Engl J Med*. 2007;**357**:1221–1228.
6. Institute of Medicine (US) Roundtable on Evidence-Based Medicine. *The Healthcare Imperative: Lowering Costs and Improving Outcomes: Workshop Series Summary*. Washington, DC: National Academies Press (US); 2011.
7. Van Dyke K. The incredible costs of chronic diseases: why they occur and possible preventions and/or treatments. *J Health Educ Res Dev*. 2016;**4**. doi: 10.4172/2380-5439.1000182.
8. Chapel JM, Ritchey MD, Zhang D, Wang G. Prevalence and medical costs of chronic diseases among adult medicaid beneficiaries. *Am J Prev Med*. 2017;**53**:S143–S154.
9. Lazebnik Y. Can a biologist fix a radio?—Or, what I learned while studying apoptosis. *Cancer Cell*. 2002;**2**:179–182.
10. Yurkovich JT, Palsson BO. Solving puzzles with missing pieces: the power of systems biology. *Proc IEEE*. 2016;**104**:2–7.
11. Ideker T, Galitski T, Hood L. A new approach to decoding life: systems biology. *Annu Rev Genomics Hum Genet*. 2001;**2**:343–372.
12. Yurkovich JT, Palsson BO. Quantitative -omic data empowers bottom-up systems biology. *Curr Opin Biotechnol*. 2018;**51**:130–136.
13. Yurkovich JT, Bordbar A, Sigurjónsson ÓE, et al. Systems biology as an emerging paradigm in transfusion medicine. *BMC Syst Biol*. 2018;**12**:1–9.
14. Yurkovich JT, Yang L, Palsson BO. Systems-level physiology of the human red blood cell is computed from metabolic and macromolecular mechanisms. doi: 10.1101/797258.
15. Paglia G, D'Alessandro A, Rolfsson O, et al. Biomarkers defining the metabolic age of red blood cells during cold storage. *Blood*. 2016;**128**:e43–e50.
16. Kuhn TS. *The Structure of Scientific Revolutions: 50th Anniversary Edition*. Chicago, IL: University of Chicago Press; 2012.
17. Brenner S. Sequences and consequences. *Philos Trans R Soc Lond Ser B Biol Sci*. 2010;**365**:207–212.
18. Hood L. Systems biology: integrating technology, biology, and computation. *Mech Ageing Dev*. 2003;**124**:9–16.
19. Hood L. A personal view of molecular technology and how it has changed biology. *J Proteome Res*. 2002;**1**:399–409.
20. Hood L. Biotechnology and medicine of the future. *JAMA*. 1988;**259**:1837–1844.
21. Hood L, Galas D. The digital code of DNA. *Nature*. 2003;**421**:444–448.
22. Smith LM, Sanders JZ, Kaiser RJ, et al. Fluorescence detection in automated DNA sequence analysis. *Nature*. 1986;**321**:674–679.
23. Hood L. A personal journey of discovery: developing technology and changing biology. *Annu Rev Anal Chem*. 2008;**1**:1–43.
24. Hood L, Rowen L, Galas DJ, Aitchison JD. Systems biology at the Institute for Systems Biology. *Brief Funct Genomics Proteomics*. 2008;**7**:239–248.
25. Hood L, Lessons E. Learned as president of the Institute for Systems Biology (2000–2018). *Genomics Proteomics Bioinformatics*. 2018;**16**:1–9.
26. Kitano H. Systems biology: a brief overview. *Science*. 2002;**295**:1662–1664.
27. Hood L. Systems biology and p4 medicine: past, present, and future. *Rambam Maimonides Med J*. 2013;**4**:e0012.
28. Hood L, Friend SH. Predictive, personalized, preventive, participatory (P4) cancer medicine. *Nat Rev Clin Oncol*. 2011;**8**:184–187.
29. Tian Q, Price ND, Hood L. Systems cancer medicine: towards realization of predictive, preventive, personalized and participatory (P4) medicine. *J Intern Med*. 2012;**271**:111–121.
30. Yurkovich JT, Tian Q, Price ND, Hood L. A systems approach to clinical oncology uses deep phenotyping to deliver personalized care. *Nat Rev Clin Oncol*. 2019;**17**:183–194. doi: 10.1038/s41571-019-0273-6.

31. Kauffman S. Homeostasis and differentiation in random genetic control networks. *Nature*. 1969;**224**:177–178.
32. Rowen L, Young J, Birditt B, et al. Analysis of the human neurexin genes: alternative splicing and the generation of protein diversity. *Genomics*. 2002;**79**: 587–597.
33. Price ND, Magis AT, Earls JC, et al. A wellness study of 108 individuals using personal, dense, dynamic data clouds. *Nat Biotechnol*. 2017;**35**:747–756.
34. Yurkovich JT, Hood L. Blood is a window into health and disease. *Clin Chem*. 2019;**65**:1204–1206.
35. Sung J, Wang Y, Chandrasekaran S, et al. Molecular signatures from omics data: from chaos to consensus. *Biotechnol J*. 2012;**7**:946–957.
36. Ideker T, Dutkowski J, Hood L. Boosting signal-to-noise in complex biology: prior knowledge is power. *Cell*. 2011;**144**:860–863.
37. Baker EJ, Jay JJ, Bubier JA, et al. GeneWeaver: a web-based system for integrative functional genomics. *Nucleic Acids Res*. 2012;**40**:D1067–D1076.
38. Mahmud M, Kaiser MS, Hussain A, Vassanelli S. Applications of deep learning and reinforcement learning to biological data. *IEEE Trans Neural Netw Learn Syst*. 2018;**29**:2063–2079.
39. Hood L, Price ND. Demystifying disease, democratizing health care. *Sci Transl Med*. 2014;**6**:225ed5.
40. Li X-J, Hayward C, Fong P-Y, et al. A blood-based proteomic classifier for the molecular characterization of pulmonary nodules. *Sci Transl Med*. 2013;**5**: 207ra142.
41. Schork NJ. Personalized medicine: time for one-person trials. *Nature*. 2015;**520**: 609–611.
42. Sugawara J, Ochi D, Yamashita R, et al. Maternity log study: a longitudinal lifelog monitoring and multiomics analysis for the early prediction of complicated pregnancy. *BMJ Open*. 2019;**9**:e025939.
43. Schork NJ, Goetz LH. Single-subject studies in translational nutrition research. *Annu Rev Nutr*. 2017;**37**:395–422.
44. Magnuson V, Wang Y, Schork N. Normalizing sleep quality disturbed by psychiatric polypharmacy: a single patient open trial (SPOT). *F1000Res*. 2016;**5**:132.
45. Ideker T, Thorsson V, Ranish JA, et al. Integrated genomic and proteomic analyses of a systematically perturbed metabolic network. *Science*. 2001;**292**:929–934.
46. Hwang D, Lee IY, Yoo H, et al. A systems approach to prion disease. *Mol Syst Biol*. 2009;**5**:252.
47. Song Y, Zhang Q, Kutlu B, et al. Evolutionary etiology of high-grade astrocytomas. *Proc Natl Acad Sci U S A*. 2013;**110**:17933–17938.
48. An J, González-Avalos E, Chawla A, et al. Acute loss of TET function results in aggressive myeloid cancer in mice. *Nat Commun*. 2015;**6**:10071.
49. Roach JC, Glusman G, Smith AFA, et al. Analysis of genetic inheritance in a family quartet by whole-genome sequencing. *Science*. 2010;**328**:636–639.
50. Ament SA, Szelinger S, Glusman G, et al. Rare variants in neuronal excitability genes influence risk for bipolar disorder. *Proc Natl Acad Sci U S A*. 2015;**112**: 3576–3581.
51. Knijnenburg TA, Vockley JG, Chambwe N, et al. Genomic and molecular characterization of preterm birth. *Proc Natl Acad Sci U S A*. 2019;**116**:5819–5827.
52. Schüssler-Fiorenza Rose SM, Contrepois K, Moneghetti KJ, et al. A longitudinal big data approach for precision health. *Nat Med*. 2019;**25**:792–804.
53. Piening BD, Zhou W, Contrepois K, et al. Integrative personal omics profiles during periods of weight gain and loss. *Cell Syst*. 2018;**6**:157–170.e8.
54. Wilmanski T, Rappaport N, Earls JC, et al. Blood metabolome predicts gut microbiome α-diversity in humans. *Nat Biotechnol*. 2019;**37**:1217–1228.
55. Earls JC, Rappaport N, Heath L, et al. Multi-omic biological age estimation and its correlation with wellness and disease phenotypes: a longitudinal study of 3,558 individuals. *J Gerontol A*. 2019;**74**:S52–S60.
56. Zubair N, Conomos MP, Hood L, et al. Genetic predisposition impacts clinical changes in a lifestyle coaching program. *Sci Rep*. 2019;**9**:6805.
57. Torkamani A, Wineinger NE, Topol EJ. The personal and clinical utility of polygenic risk scores. *Nat Rev Genet*. 2018;**19**:581–590.
60. Gopalakrishnan V, Helmink BA, Spencer CN, et al. The influence of the gut microbiome on cancer, immunity, and cancer immunotherapy. *Cancer Cell*. 2018;**33**:570–580.
61. Song M, Chan AT, Sun J. Influence of the gut microbiome, diet, and environment on risk of colorectal cancer. *Gastroenterology*. 2019;**158**(2):322–340. doi: 10.1053/j.gastro.2019.06.048.
62. Barroso-Sousa R, Teles LT. Gut microbiome and breast cancer in the era of cancer immunotherapy. *Curr Breast Cancer Rep*. 2019;**11**:272–276. doi: 10.1007/s12609-019-00346-y.

Index

Page numbers in *italics* indicate figures and/or tables.

A

ABC proteins, 733
abdominoperineal resection (APR), 1172
aberrant signaling pathways, 151–159
Abl inhibitors, 157
Abl kinase inhibitors (AKIs), 512
absolute risk, 396
absorption, 657
    methotrexate, 668
acalabrutinib, 1565
acneiform eruption, of face, *1702*
acquired drug resistance, 734
acral erythema (AE), 1709
    vs. acute GVHD, 1710
    biopsies of, 1709
    incidence, 1709
acral melanoma, 1415
acral reactions
    chemotherapeutic agents associated with, *1703*
    dermatologic complications, 1709–1710
acromegaly, 1860
ACT. *see* adoptive cell therapy (ACT)
actinic keratoses (AKs), 1437, 1704. *see also* solar keratosis
    inflammation of, 1708
activated *ras* genes, 317
acupuncture, 1679
    integrative oncology, 596
acute airway obstruction, 1893–1894
acute emesis, 1674
acute generalized exanthematous pustulosis (AGEP), 1701
acute hemorrhage
    carotid artery rupture, 1890
    management objectives for, 1890
    manifestations of, 1889
    retroperitoneal hemorrhage, 1891
    splenic rupture, 1890–1891
acute leukemia, 873
acute lymphoblastic leukemia (ALL), 132, 840, 1547–1558
    allogeneic stem cell transplantation, 1557
    clinical presentation, 1548
    cytochemistry, 1549
    cytogenetic and molecular abnormalities, 1549
    diagnosis, 1548
    epidemiology and etiology, 1547
    hyperdiploidy, 134
    immunophenotyping, 1549
    methotrexate, 671
    morphology, 1549
    Ph-like ALL, 135
    salvage therapy, 1555
    therapy, 1551
    translocation 1;19, 135
    translocation 8;14, 135
    translocation 9;22, 132
    translocation 12;21, 134
    translocation involving 11q, 134
acute lymphocytic leukemia, 1694
acute myelogenous leukemia, 671
acute myeloid leukemia (AML), 839
    de novo, 131
    and myelodysplastic syndrome (MDS) predisposition syndromes
        familial AML with mutated DDX41, 420
        familial aplastic anemia/MDS with SRP72 mutation, 420
        familial MDS/AML with mutated GATA2 (GATA2 deficiency), 420
        FPD-AML, 419
        thrombocytopenia 5, 420
acute pancreatitis, GI complications, 1824
acute survival phase, 912
acyclovir-resistant HSV, 1812
adamantinoma, 1465
adeno-associated virus vectors, 818
adenocarcinoma, 444, 1084, 1178, 1277, 1649–1650
    of gallbladder, 1109
    lung cancer, 1007
    of unknown primary site, 1648
adenoid cystic carcinoma (ACC), 940
adenomatous atypical hyperplasia (AAH), 1005, 1014
adenomatous polyposis coli (APC)
    APC gene, 80, 81
    characterization, 80
    function of, 81–82
    germline missense mutation, 81
    Wilms tumor, 82–83
adenosine antimetabolites, 688–690
adenosquamous carcinoma, 1236
    of lung, 1008
adenovirus vectors, 819
Adjuvant Chemoradiation Therapy in Stomach Cancer (ARTIST) trial, 1090
adjuvant chemotherapy, 646
    carcinosarcoma, 1356
    leiomyosarcoma, 1356
adjuvant FGFR targeted therapy, 1199
adjuvant immune checkpoint blockade, melanoma, 1421–1422
The Adjuvant Lung Cancer Enrichment Marker Identification and Sequencing Trials (ALCHEMIST), 255
adjuvant mitotane, 966–967
adjuvant radiation, to resected nodal basin, 1422
adjuvant targeted therapy, melanoma, 1422
adjuvant therapy, operable NSCLC, 1018
adoptive cell therapy (ACT), 1694
    chimeric antigen receptor (CAR) T-cell, 625
    NK cytotoxic lymphocytes, 625–626
    tumor-infiltrating lymphocyte therapy, 625
adoptive T-cell therapy, 1178
adrenal cortical carcinoma
    adjuvant mitotane, 966–967
    chemotherapy, 967
    clinical presentation, 964
    diagnosis, evaluation, and pathology, 964–965
    genetics and molecular characterization, 964
    hormonal therapy, 966
    immunotherapy, 968
    mitotane, 966
    neoadjuvant therapy, 967
    radiation therapy, 968
    surgical treatment of localized disease, 965
    targeted radionuclide therapy, 968
    targeted therapy, 968
    treatment of advanced disease, 965–966
adrenal diseases, 1863
adrenal insufficiency, 1863
adrenal metastasis, 1863
adrenocorticotrophic hormone (ACTH), 1855
adrenocorticotropic hormone-secreting adenomas, 946
adult-onset cancer survivors, 911
advance care planning, 568
advanced melanoma, 1424
    cytotoxic agents and combinations with immunotherapy, 1432
    immunotherapy, 1427–1429
    molecularly targeted therapy, 1425–1427
advanced-stage non-small-cell lung cancer, targeted therapy in, *1023*
aerobic glycolysis, 214
Affordable Care Act, 917
aflatoxins
    B1 and G1 activation, 313
    hepatocellular carcinoma, 1096
agonist mAbs, 805
AGS-003, 784
AJCC lung cancer staging system (AJCC8), 1012
AJCC/UICC 8th edition TNM staging system, 1101, *1101*
AK recall reaction, 1708–1709
Akt, 68, 154
Al amyloidosis, 1631

alcohol, 437, 440–441
    hepatocellular carcinoma, 1096
alectinib, 1024
alemtuzumab, 1607, 1844
ALK, 69
ALK inhibitors, 1024
alkylating agents, 646, 1821
    administration schedule effects, 647
    adverse effects, 696–697
    bifunctional, 694–695
    clinical pharmacology, 696
    decomposition and metabolism, 695
    monofunctional, 693–694
    resistance to, 695–696
alkyl sulfonates, 696
allogeneic bone marrow transplantation, 646
allogeneic donor, 834
allogeneic HCT, 833
    graft failure, 836
    graft-*versus*-host-disease (GVHD), 836
    immunodeficiency and infections, 838
    late effects, 839
    miscellaneous noninfectious complications, 839
alopecia, 1705
    chemotherapeutic agents associated with, *1705*
α1-antitrypsin deficiency (AATD), 1097
alpha-fetoprotein (AFP), 513
alternative-end joining (alt-EJ), 547
alternative lengthening of telomeres, 202
alternative splicing, 202
amelanotic melanoma, 1416
American Association for the Study of Liver Disease (AASLD), 1099
American Burkitt lymphoma, 386
American Council of Graduate Medical Education (ACGME) accredited surgical oncology fellowship programs, 542
American Joint Cancer Committee (AJCC) TNM classification, 8th edition, 1110, *1111*
American Society for Clinical Oncology (ASCO), 596
aminopterin (AMT), 667, *668*
amiodarone, 1887
amplicon-based hotspot panels, 495
anaerobes, 1872–1873
anaerobic glycolysis, 214
anal cancer, 905–906
anal margin cancer, 1176
anaphylaxis acute management, recommendations for, *1898*
anaplastic lymphoma kinase (ALK) gene translocations, 510
androgen deprivation therapy (ADT), 1748
aneurysmal bone cyst, 1463
angiogenesis inhibitors *vs.* vascular targeting agents, 231
angiopoietins, 227–228
angiosarcoma (AS), 1445
angiostatin, 229
anorexia/cachexia syndrome (ACS), 572
anterior mediastinal mass, 1049
anthracenediones, 705, 711
anthracyclines, 705, 709–711, 1493
    administration schedule effects, 648
antiangiogenic agents
    in combination with immune checkpoint inhibitors, 233
    in combination with radiotherapy, 233
antiangiogenic effects, of chemotherapy, 231
antiangiogenic therapy
    bowel perforation, 1900
    tumor angiogenesis, 233–243
antiarrhythmic drugs, *1888*
antibacterial prophylaxis, infections, 1879
antibiotic therapy, 1877
antibody-drug conjugates, 1902
anticancer therapies, 667
anti-CD19 CAR T-cell therapy, 625
anti-CD20 monoclonal antibodies, 1564

anticipatory emesis, 1674
antidiabetic medication, 1124
antidotes, 1706
anti-EGFR monoclonal antibodies, 1165
antiemetic agents, for CINV prevention and treatment, 1824
antiemetic therapy, 1673–1681
    classes of antiemetics, 1675
    complementary and alternative medicine (CAM) therapies, 1679
    emetogenic chemotherapy, 1675
    special situations, 1680
    treatment of chemotherapy-induced emesis, 1680
antifungal and antiviral prophylaxis, 1879–1880
antigen-binding site, 834
antimicrobial agents, *1878*
antimicrobial lock therapy, 1876
antimicrobial stewardship strategies, 1880, *1880*
antimitotics, 717
anti-Müllerian hormone (AMH)
    in females, 1840
    in males, 1839
antineoplastic agents, 643
    adjustment based on renal insufficiency, *1754*
antineoplastic drugs, *1886*, *1887*
anti-PD1 antibodies, for advanced melanoma, 1421
antisense oligonucleotides, 205–206
anxiety disorders, 545
APC gene, 80, 81
Apc proteins function, *83*
apoptosis, 56
appendages, tumors arising from, 1446
appendix, 1139–1142
    clinical presentation, 1139
    epithelial neoplasms of, 1139
    neuroendocrine tumors of, 1140
    nonepithelial neoplasms of, 1142
aprepitant, 1678
aprepitant emulsion, 1678
arabinoside (Ara-C), 1821
Arbeitgemeinschaft Internistische Onkologie (AIO), 1091
aromatase-inhibitor-based stimulation protocols, 1844
aromatase inhibitors, 1308
arrhythmia
    primary, 1885
    secondary, 1885
    signs and symptoms, 1885
    treatment of, 1885–1888
arterial chemoembolization, 522
arterial embolization, 521–522
arterial infusion therapy, 521
arterial thromboembolic events, 239
arterial thrombosis, GI complications, 1824
artificial antigen-presenting cells (aAPCs), 830
artificial sweeteners, 449
aryl hydrocarbon receptor repressor (AHRR), 320
AS1411, 205
ASCO Quality Oncology Practice Initiative (QOPI®), 916
asparaginase, 1821
aspartame, 449
Aspergillus fumigatus, 1873
Aspergillus sino-orbital infection, 1873
associated paraneoplastic syndromes, 1050
astrocytic tumors classification, 922
asymptomatic cancers, 3
ataxia telangiectasia, 85
atezolizumab, 1197, 1198, 1429
ATM genes, 1123
atypical mole syndrome/phenotype, 1414
augmented intelligence, 498
auristatin F, 727
autocrine stimulation, 54
autologous HCT, 833
autophagy, 213
avelumab (anti-PD-L1), 1041

axillary lymph node metastases, in women, 1653
axin proteins function, *83*
5-azacytidine (5-AC)
    cellular uptake and metabolism, 684–685
    clinical activity, 685
    clinical pharmacology, 685
    mechanism of action, 685
    toxicities, 685

B

Bacillus Calmette Guerin (BCG), 1194, 1419
bacterial infections, 1869–1871, *1871*
bacterial sepsis, 1735
BAP1, 417, 1032
BAP1 wild-type (BAP1WT) protein, 1033
Bartholin gland carcinoma, 1267–1268
basal cell carcinoma (BCC), 933, 1442
    chemotherapy, 1444
    clinical features, 1443
    definition, 1442
    electrodesiccation and curettage, 1443
    epidemiology, 1442
    Mohs surgery, 1443
    morpheaform, 1443
    radiation therapy, 1444
    surgical excision, 1443
    vulvar area, 1268
basket trials, 620
4-1BB (CD137), 805
B7-CD28 superfamily, 800
B-cell hyperplasia, 386
B-cell maturation antigen (BCMA), 1625–1626
B cell receptor (BCR) inhibitors, 841
BCL-2, 68
BCR-ABL1 fusion gene, 493
Bcr-Abl (T315I) mutant CML, 512
Bcr-Abl oncogene, 157
BCR-ABL tyrosine kinase inhibitors, 1702
    effects on gonadal function, 1843
9-β-D-arabinosyl-2-fluoroadenine monophosphate. *see* fludarabine
Beau's lines, 1705, *1706*
bendamustine, 695
bendamustine-rituximab, 1564
benign bone tumors, 1456
benign teratomas of mediastinum, 1061
benzydamine mouthwash, in oral mucositis prevention, 1824
beta-carotene, 448
bevacizumab, 157, 650, 1165, 1322, 1326, 1694
bexarotene, 1606
BH3 mimetics, 1557
bias and confounders, HSR, 604–605
bifunctional alkylating agents
    alkyl sulfonates, 695
    aziridines, 695
    hexitol epoxides, 695
    nitrogen mustards, 694–695
    nitrosoureas, 695
    structures of, *694*
bifunctional drugs, 693
bile duct cancer
    causative factors, 1114–1115
    clinical presentation, 1115
    diagnostic studies, 1116–1118
    pathology, 1116
    prognostic factors, 1118
    treatment
        liver transplantation, 1119
        locoregional therapy, 1120
        palliation, 1120
        surgery, 1118–1119
        systemic therapy, 1119–1120
bilharzial bladder cancer (BBC)
    benign and paraneoplastic schistosomal bladder lesions, 382–383
    carcinogenic mechanism, 381

diagnosis, 380–381
epidemiology of, 379–380
experimental data for, 383
histopathological type, 379–380
human papilloma virus, 381
late chronic infection, 381
metabolic observations, 381–382
microbiome role, 381
morbidity and mortality rates, 379
binary alignment map (BAM) file, 497
bintrafusp alfa, 788
bioinformatics, 247–258
analog (microarray) to digital (sequencing) transition, 248
analysis and interpretation, 248, 251–252
clustered heat maps, 252
current trends, 258–260
data types and data sources, 252
definition, 247–248
hardware challenges, 248–250
hypothesis-generating and hypothesis-driven research, 252
molecular profiling projects, 254, 255, 256, 259
software challenges, 250
statistical methods, 255, 259
web-based tools, 253
wetware challenges, 250–251
biological hallmarks, of cancer, 7–15
aberrations, 11–13
activating invasion and metastasis, 10
avoiding immune destruction, 11
complex manifestations, 7
deregulating cellular energetics and metabolism, 10–11
enabling replicative immortality, 9
evading growth suppressors, 8
inducing angiogenesis, 9–10
overview, 7
resisting cell death, 8–9
sustaining proliferative signaling, 7–8
therapeutic targeting, 14–15
tumor microenvironments (TMEs), 13–14
biologically therapeutic agents, dose effect for, 641
biologic therapy, gynecologic sarcomas, 1356–1357
biomarker-based cancer tool development, 517
biomarker-based clinical trial designs, 285–290
Basket discovery trial, 287, 288
challenges, 290
master protocol designs, 287
with multiple biomarkers, 290
need, current state, and evolution of, 285
phase I and II trials with companion diagnostics, 285, 286
phase IIa master trials, 286, 287, 288
phase III designs, 288, 289, 290
platform trials, 288
umbrella discovery trial, 286, 288
biomarkers, 505
cancer-specific, 514–515
germline, 514
human papillomavirus and human genital neoplasia, 371
immune biomarkers, in lung cancer, 1010–1011
precision oncology challenges, 626
predictive, 290
serum, 515
testing, endometrial cancer, 1302
urine, 515
biphasic/mixed type, 1032
Birt–Hogg–Dubé syndrome (BHD), 417
bispecific T cell receptor-engaging (BITE), 1694
bisphosphonates, 1721
BKM120, 510
bladder cancer, 446, 511
clinical presentation, 1193
epidemiology, 1191
incidence, 1191

invasive bladder cancer management, 1195–1197
investigation and staging, 1193–1194
metastatic, 1197–1198
molecular determinants, 1191–1193
muscle-invasive, 1192–1193
non-muscle-invasive bladder cancer management, 1194–1195
pathobiology, 1191–1193
prognosis, 1194
uncommon histologic variants, 1198
upper tract tumors, 1198–1199
bladder carcinoma, vaccine trials, 784
bladder outlet and urethral obstruction, 1748
bleeding, GI complications, 1824
bleomycin, cutaneous flagellate hyperpigmentation of, 1707
blinatumomab, 1694
Bloom syndrome, 85
board certification, in surgical oncology, 542
bone lymphoma, 1472
bone marrow
cytokinetics of, 644
transplantation and GvL effect, 789
bone metastases
bisphosphonates, 1721
denosumab, 1722
medical management of, 1721
radiation therapy for, 1724
bone scintigraphy, 1069
bone tumors, 1451–1474
biopsy, 1454
bone lymphoma, 1472
cartilage tumors, 1458–1459
congenital syndromes, 1473–1474
cysts and other tumors, 1463–1464
evaluation, 1451–1453
fibrous tumors, 1459–1461
giant cell tumors, 1461
hemangioma, 1461–1462
limb salvage *versus* amputation, 1455–1456
medical management, 1458
metastatic disease to bone, 1471–1472
myeloma, 1472
operative management, 1456
osteogenic tumors, 1462–1463
overview, 1451
primary bone sarcomas
adamantinoma, 1465
chondrosarcoma, 1465–1467
chordoma, 1467–1468
Ewing sarcoma, 1468
osteosarcoma, 1468–1471
vascular sarcomas, 1471
radiotherapy, 1457–1458
reconstructive alternatives
benign bone tumors, 1456
primary bone sarcomas, 1456–1457
staging, 1453–1454
surgical margins, 1454–1455
borderline tumors, 1315
bortezomib, 1694
bowel and bladder dysfunction, 1685
bowel perforation, 239–240, 1900–1901
brachial plexopathy, 1691
brachytherapy, 543, 544, 1172, 1218
BRAF
colon cancer, 511
melanoma, 511
BRAF inhibitors, 68, 1703–1704
kinase inhibitors effects on gonadal function, 1843
BRAF-mutated melanomas, 1416
B-Raf mutations, 155
BRAF mutations, lung cancer, 510–511
BRAF V600E mutations, 1025
Bragg peak, 544
brain
herniation, 1897

melanoma metastatic to, 1432
toxicity, 1695
brain stem gliomas (BSG), 859
braking radiation, 543
BRCA1, 1123
BRCA2, 1123
BRCA1/2 mutated ovarian cancers, 510
BRCA1 mutations, 84
BRCA2 mutations, 84
BRCA1/2 mutations guide therapy, 508
breakthrough emesis, 1675
breast cancer, 238, 394, 441–442, 869–870, 907
and gynecologic cancer syndromes, 404
methotrexate, 672
and ovarian cancer predispositions, 406–407
and ovarian cancer syndrome, 404–405
vaccine trials, 783–784
5-year relative survival rates, 913
Breast Cancer Prevention Trial (BCPT), 457
breast-conserving surgery, 532
breastfeeding, 437
Bremsstrahlung, 543
brentuximab, 512
brentuximab vedotin, 1607
brigatinib, 1024
bronchiolitis obliterans syndrome (BOS), 839
bronchoscopy, 1069
Burkitt lymphoma, 361, 386
American, 386
Burkitt lymphoma (BL), 903
Buschke–Loewenstein tumor, 1441
busulfan. *see* alkyl sulfonates

C
CA15-3, 513
CA27.29, 513
CA125, 513
cabazitaxel, 721
cabozantinib, 979
calcitriol production, by malignant tumors, 1857
calcium, 447
camptothecin analogs, 707
cancer
biomarkers, 505
causes of, 394
cell immortality, 201–208
chronic inflammation and, 316
family inheritance, 74
medicine, 1912–1913
vs. other abnormal cellular growths, 3
rehabilitation medicine, 585–590
of brain, 585
of breast, 588
head and neck cancer, 587
spinal cord dysfunction, 586
symptoms, 3, 4
vaccines, 820–821
cancer and aging, 877–883
cancer-specific geriatric screening tools, 880–881
comorbidities, 879
comprehensive geriatric assessment, 879–880
geriatric oncology screening tools, 881–882
geriatric syndromes, 878–879
palliative care, 882
physiologic aging and cancer, 877–878
survivorship, 882
cancer and pregnancy, 867–874
acute leukemia, 873
breast cancer, 869–870
cancer treatment, 868
cervical cancer, 871
chronic leukemia, 873
diagnosis and staging, 867–868
epidemiology, 867
Hodgkin disease and non-Hodgkin lymphoma, 871–872
melanoma, 873

cancer and pregnancy (continued)
  ovarian cancer, 872–873
  overview, 867
  radiation, 868
  surgery, 868
  systemic therapy, 868–869
  thyroid cancer, 870–871
  transplacental malignancy and placental metastasis, 873–874
cancer chemoprevention, 453–471
  biology of, 453
  breast, 457–462
  colon and rectum, 455–457
  immune checkpoint inhibitors, 470–471
  lung, 454–455
  prostate, 462–463
  risk modeling, 453
  vaccines, 463–470
cancer epidemiology, 391–400
  case-control studies, 395
  clinical trials, 395
  cohort studies, 395
  cross-sectional and ecological studies, 396
  interpretation, 396
  trends, 400
cancer gene therapy, 817–823
  clinical practice, 823
  gene editing, 819–820
  gene transfer, 817–819
  safety, 823
  targets of, 820–823
cancer genomic data repositories and analysis tools, 108–109
cancer genomics and evolution, 101–122
  cancer evolution, 114–117
  cancer genomic data repositories and analysis tools, 108–109
  cell-free tumor-specific DNA, 114
  clinical implications of cancer genome landscapes, 111–113
  early history of, 102–103
  gene expression microarrays, 105–106
  landmark cancer genomic studies, 106–108
  massively parallel sequencing, 106
  melanoma
    background, 117
    clinical implications, 120–121
    drug resistance and evolution, 121–122
    genetic basis of, 117–118
    genomic landscapes, 118–120
  molecular cytogenetics, 103–105
  molecular genetics, 105
  overview, 101
  vast and varied landscapes of human cancers, 109–111
cancer immunotherapy, 799–814
cancer metabolism, 211–221
  bad table manners of cancer cells, 213
  cancer cells corrupt their neighbors, 219
  clinic, 220–221
  feeding habits in rogue travelers, 219–220
  glutamine and anabolic metabolism, 216–217
  malicious builders, 211
  nucleus, 218
  overview, 211
  traveling electrons, 213–214
  Warburg effect, 214–216
  from yeast to mammals, 212–213
cancer nanotechnology, 825–831
  chemotherapy, 827
  clinical stage, 825
  gene therapy, 829
  hyperthermia therapy, 829
  image-guided surgery, 825
  immunotherapy, 830
  radiotherapy, 829
  recent advances in, 830

cancer of unknown primary site (CUP)
  clinical evaluation, 1647–1649
  comprehensive molecular profiling, 1656
  electron microscopy, 1650
  empiric chemotherapy, 1647, 1655–1656
  histologic examination, 1649–1650
  immunohistochemical staining, 1650
  molecular cancer classifier assays, 1651–1652
  molecular diagnostics, 1656
  pathologic evaluation, 1649–1652
  patient management, 1656–1657
  signs/symptoms, 1647
  site-specific treatment, 1656
  treatment, 1652–1656
  tumor-specific chromosomal abnormalities, 1651
cancerophobia, 5
cancer plasticity
  brachyury, 785
  in tumor progression, 785
cancer predisposition syndromes, 85
cancer progenitor cells (CPCs), 644
cancer registry systems, 294
cancer research, 269–281
  adaptive designs, 275
  adaptive phase II trials, 277
  adaptive phase I trials, 275
  adaptive randomization, 278
  Bayesian approach, 270
  Bayesian updating, 270
  clinical oncology trials, 281
  clinical trial software, 281
  decision analysis, 280
  extraim analyses, 279
  frequentist/Bayesian comparison, 272
  hierarchical modeling, 273, 274
  predictive probabilities, 273
  prior probabilities, 271
  robustness and sensitivity analysis, 272
  seamless phase I/II and phase II/III designs, 277
cancer risk factors, reducing exposure to, 914
cancer-specific biomarkers, 514–515
cancer-specific neo-epitopes, 626
cancer statistics, 391–395
cancer stem cells (CSC), 734
  clinical significance
    dormancy, 184
    metastasis, 183–184
    treatment resistance, 183
  hypothesis
    isolation, identification, and characterization, 177–179
    models of carcinogenesis, 177
    unifying concept in multiple cancers, 177
  plasticity and heterogeneity
    core stemness signaling, 180
    EMT/MET, 180–181
    epigenetic state, 179–180
    microenvironmental control, 183
    signal transduction pathways, 181–183
  therapeutic targeting
    dormancy, 184–185
Candida albicans, 1873
Candida glabrata, 1873
Candida krusei, 1873
Candida parapsilosis, 1873
Candida tropicalis, 1873
cannabidiol (CBD) formulations, 573
capecitabine, 647, 648, 681
  clinical activity, 682
  clinical pharmacology, 682
  mechanism of action, 682
  metabolism, 682
  structure and activation of, *682*
  toxicities, 682
capmatinib, 1025
carbohydrate antigen 19-9 (CA19-9), 513

carboplatin, 698
  clinical pharmacology, 699
  resistance to, 698
  structures of, *697*
carboxylesterase 2 (CES2), 1137
carcinoembryonic antigen (CEA), 513
carcinogen–DNA adduct formation, 307
carcinogenesis, mutations and skin cancer types, 336
carcinogenic N-nitrosamines, 312
carcinogen metabolism, 311, 311, 312
carcinoid crisis, 1884
carcinoid heart disease, 974
carcinoid syndrome, 974
carcinoid tumors, lung, 1008–1009
carcinoma
  pediatric oncology, principles of, 862
  poorly differentiated, 1655
carcinoma *in situ*, 1261
carcinoma-*in-situ* neoplasia, 3
carcinoma of the stomach, 1083–1093
  diagnosis, 1086
  incidence and epidemiology, 1083
  medical oncology, 1089
  molecularly targeted agents and immune therapy, 1091–1092
  multidisciplinary care, 1086–1087
    radiation oncology, 1088–1089
    surgery, 1087–1088
  needs and future directions, 1092–1093
  pathogenesis and natural history
    molecular alterations, 1084–1085
    progression and patterns of metastasis, 1085
  pathology, 1084
  postoperative adjuvant chemotherapy
    integration of multimodal care, 1090
    management of advanced disease, 1090–1091
    monitoring for recurrence, 1090
  risk factors and genetics, 1083–1084
  screening, 1085
  TNM stage classification, 1086
carcinosarcoma, 1301, 1352
  adjuvant chemotherapy, 1356
  chemotherapy, 1355–1356
  ifosfamide-mesna with/without cisplatin combination therapy, 1356
  paclitaxel and carboplatin combination therapy, 1356
  paclitaxel-ifosfamide combination therapy, 1356
  radiation therapy for, 1355
cardiac arrest, in cancer patients, 1885
cardiac irAEs, 1899
cardiac toxicity, 839
cardiac tumors
  clinical presentation of, 1055
  imaging for, 1055
  myxomas, 1057
  papillary fibroelastomas, 1056
  rhabdomyomas, 1057
cardinal manifestations, 3–5
cardio-oncology, 1055
carfilzomib, 1621–1623
CAR-modified immune effector cell strategies, 794–795
CAR-modified T cells, 792–794
Carney triad, 416
carotid artery rupture, 1890
CAR-T cell immunotherapy, 1879
cartilage tumors, 1458–1459
castrate-resistant locally advanced disease, 1224
catheter-related infections, 1876–1877
CD27, 806
CD40, 805
CD56, 972
CD137, 805
CDKN2A (p16), 1123
celecoxib, 1709
cell cycle
  arrest and DNA repair, 547
  control and checkpoints, 546

cell death pathways, 733
cell-free tumor-specific DNA (ctDNA), 114
cell hybridization approach, 74
cell-mediated immunity (CMI), 1869, 1872
central nervous system toxicity, methotrexate, 673–674
central nervous system tumors, methotrexate, 672
cereblon E3 ligase modulators (CELMoDs), 1627
cerebral embolism, 1698
cerebral infarction, 1698
cerebral venous thrombosis, 1698
cerebrovascular complications, 1697
ceritinib, 1024
cervical cancer, 238, 871, 904–905, 1275–1297
   cervical conization, 1285
   clinical symptoms, 1282
   diagnosis, 1282
   evaluation and staging, 1282
   extrafascial hysterectomy, 1286
   incidence and mortality, 1275
   prognostic factors, 1284
   radiation therapy, 1287
   radical hysterectomy, 1286
   radical trachelectomy, 1286
   risk factors for, 1275
   sentinel lymph nodes, 1285
cervical neoplasia, papillomaviruses and, 367–371
   definitions, 367
   HPV and human genital neoplasia
      abnormal pap smear and primary screening, 370–371
      applications to clinical medicine, 370
      clinical management, 371
      prevention, 371
      risk factors, 369–370
      surrogate biomarkers of, 371
   HPV-target cells and mechanism of infection/viral entry, 367–369
   mechanisms of neoplastic transformation, 369
   overview, 367
cetuximab, 157
cfDNA liquid biopsy platforms, 1656
Charcot–Marie–Tooth neuropathy, 1692
checkpoint inhibitor MAbs (CIM), 788
checkpoint inhibitors (CPIs), 1879
chemical carcinogenesis, 305–322
   carcinogen metabolism, 311, 312
   DNA damage and repair, 312–315
   and epigenetics, 308–310
   gene–environment interactions, 310, *311*
   malignant conversion, 308
   microRNAs (miRNAs), 309, 310
   multistage, 305–306
   mutation signatures associated with, 318
   oncogenes and tumor suppressor genes, 317, 318
   precision medicine, molecular epidemiology, and prevention, 319, 321, 322
   racial, gender, and socioeconomic disparities, 315, 316
   tumor initiation, 306, 307
   tumor progression, 308
   tumor promotion, 308
chemical cellulitis, chemotherapeutic agents associated with, *1706*
chemo-induced acral erythema, of palms, *1710*
chemoradiation therapy, 1174
chemoreceptor trigger zone (CTZ), 1673
chemotherapy, 1051, 1174
   cancer nanotechnology, 827
   carcinosarcoma, 1355–1356
   endometrial stromal sarcoma, 1356
   gynecologic sarcomas, 1355–1356
   leiomyosarcoma, 1355–1356
   primary thyroid dysfunction, 1862
   SVC syndrome, 1892
chemotherapy-associated liver injury, 1819
chemotherapy-associated nephrotoxicity, clinical and pathologic features of, *1752–1753*
chemotherapy-induced cystitis, 1748
chemotherapy-induced emesis
   highly emetogenic chemotherapy, 1680
   low-risk chemotherapy, 1680
   minimally emetogenic chemotherapy, 1680
   moderately emetogenic chemotherapy, 1680
chemotherapy-induced hypocalcemia, 1865
chemotherapy-induced nausea and vomiting (CINV), 572, 1673, 1824
chest radiography, lung cancer, 1012–1013
childhood acute lymphoblastic leukemia, agents and curative treatment for, 642, *642*
chimeric antigen receptor modified T (CART), 1566
chimeric antigen receptor (CAR)-T cell therapy, 830, 1557, 1798
   cytokine release syndrome, 1899–1900
   immune effector cell-associated neurotoxicity syndrome, 1900
chlorambucil, 696, 1563
2-chlorodeoxyadenosine, 690
2-chloroethyl-nitrosourea (CENU), 695
chloromas, 850
cholangiocarcinomas. *see* bile duct cancer
chondroblastoma, 1458–1459
chondromas, 1458
chondromyxoid fibroma, 1459
chondrosarcoma, 1465–1467
chordoma, 1467–1468
choriocarcinoma (CCA), 1343
   methotrexate, 671–672
chromatin, 309
chromogranin A (CgA), 972
chromosomal aberrations, in cancer, 125–141
   acute lymphoblastic leukemia (ALL), 132
   acute myeloid leukemia (AML) *de novo*, 131
   chromosome nomenclature, 126
   chronic lymphocytic leukemia (CLL), 135
   chronic myeloid leukemia (CML), 128
   cytogenetic and genetic terminology, *126*
   fluorescence *in situ* hybridization (FISH), 126
   genetic consequences of genomic rearrangements, 125
   multiple myeloma, 136
   myeloproliferative neoplasms (MPNs), 129
   next-generation sequencing (NGS), 128
   non-Hodgkin lymphoma (NHL), 135
   other low-throughput methods, 128
   primary myelodysplastic syndromes (MDS), 130
   single nucleotide polymorphism (SNP) arrays, 128
   solid tumors, 136
   T-cell acute lymphoblastic leukemia, 135
   therapy-related myeloid neoplasms (t-MN), 132
chromosome nomenclature, 126
chromosome 3 translocations, 418
chronic fibrosis, 863
chronic hepatic GVHD, 1823
chronic inflammation and cancer, 316
chronic kidney disease epidemiology (CKD-EPI), 1751
chronic leukemia, 873
chronic lymphocytic leukemia (CLL), 135, 841, 1559–1567
   clinical presentation, 1559
   clinical staging and other prognostic features, 1561
   cytogenetics, 1561
   diagnosis, 1559
   immunobiology and immunophenotype, 1559
   incidence and epidemiology, 1559
   major prognostic markers, 1561
   molecular genetics, 1562
   monoclonal B-cell lymphocytosis, 1559
   natural history, 1561
   treatment, 1562
chronic myelogenous leukemia, 840
   imatinib treatment for, 493
chronic myeloid leukemia (CML), 128, 512, 1537–1545
   cytogenetics, 1539
   definition, 1537
   diagnosis, 1540–1541
   historical perspective, 1537
   incidence and epidemiology, 1537
   molecular biology, 1539–1540
   pathogenesis, 1539
   pathology, 1537
   prognostic classification, 1538
   risk factors, 1537
   staging and prognostic factors, 1541
   treatment
      adverse events, 1544
      algorithm, 1542
      free remission, 1543
      imatinib mesylate, 1541
      options after failure of prior TKI, 1542–1543
      recommendations in CML in 2020, 1544
      second-generation tyrosine kinase inhibitors, 1541
      stem cell transplantation, 1543
chronic pancreatitis, 1125
cigarette smoking and lung cancer, 1005
circulating cell-free DNA (cfDNA), 500
circulating nucleotides, 515–516
circulating tumor cells (CTCs), 500, 515
   detection and isolation of, 501
   technical innovations, 503
circulating tumor DNA (ctDNA), 500, 501, 558
   early cancer detection approach analyses, 501
   liquid biopsy assessment, 502
   resequencing of, 502
   technical innovations, 503
circulatory oncologic emergencies
   acute hemorrhage, 1889–1891
   arrhythmia, 1885–1888
   cardiac arrest, causes of, 1885
   pericardial tamponade, 1889
   resuscitation algorithms, 1884
   sudden cardiopulmonary arrest, 1883–1884
   superior vena cava syndrome, 1891–1892
   tumor lysis syndrome, 1888–1889
cirrhosis, 374, 1095
cisplatin, *535*, 697–698, 1421
   clinical pharmacology, 698–699
   nephrotoxicity, 1749
   resistance to, 698
   structures of, *697*
cisplatin plus gemcitabin, 1114
cisplatin-prodrug BTP-114, 698
c-Jun, 384
cladribine, 690
clearance, drug, 658
clear cell adenocarcinoma, of vagina, 1271–1272
clear cell carcinoma, 1300
clear cell chondrosarcoma, 1467
clinical cancer genomic testing, 493
clinical dosage schedules, methotrexate, 670, *670*
clinical germline genetic testing, 493
Clinical Index of Stable Febrile Neutropenia (CISNE) score, 1901
Clinical Laboratory Improvement Amendments (CLIA) certification, 620
clinically atypical nevi (CAN), 1414
clinical stage, cancer nanotechnology, 825
clinical target volume (CTV), 1019
clinical trials
   biomarker-based designs
      challenges, 290
      master protocol designs, *287*
      with multiple biomarkers, 290
      need, current state, and evolution of, 285
      phase I and II trials with companion diagnostics, 285, 286
      phase IIa master trials, 286–288
      phase III designs, 288–290
clinical trials management systems (CTMS), 294–295
clofarabine, 690
clonal hematopoiesis, 1579–1585
   chemotherapy, 1583

clonal hematopoiesis (continued)
  clinical consequences of, 1581
  current management approaches, 1584
  definitions, 1579
  determinants of transformation, 1582
  hematopoietic cell transplantation, 1584
  risk factors for, 1581
Clonorchis sinensis, 385
Clostridium difficile-associated diarrhea, 1814–1815
Clostridium difficile infection (CDI), 1872
cloud computing, 249
cluster A personality traits, 546
cluster B personality traits, 546
cluster C personality traits, 547
clustered heat maps (CHMs), 252
CML. *see* chronic myeloid leukemia (CML)
CMV infection, 1875–1876
coagulase-negative staphylococci (CoNS), 1871
Cockayne syndrome (CS), 335–336
Cockcroft–Gault formula, 1751, *1753*
coffee, 449
coinhibitory ligand–receptor interactions, *801*
Coley's toxins, 799
colitis
  neutropenic enterocolitis, 1816
  radiation-induced proctitis and, 1817–1818
  secondary to immune-modulatory, antineoplastic agents, 1816–1817
Cologuard® test, 508
colony-stimulating factor production, 1859
colorectal cancer (CRC), 235–236, 437–440, 1147–1165
  adjuvant therapy for
    biologic agents, 1160
    5-fluorouracil-based regimens, 1159
    irinotecan-based regimens, 1160
    oxaliplatin-based regimens, 1159–1160
  epidemiology, 1147
  genetics
    APC gene, 1148
    BRAF gene, 1149
    DCC gene, 1148
    inherited syndromes, 1149–1150
    K-*ras* proto-oncogene, 1148
    p53 gene, 1148
    polymorphisms, 1150
  metastatic
    anti-EGFR monoclonal antibodies, 1165
    bevacizumab, 1165
    capecitabine/XELOX, 1164
    FOLFIRI, 1164
    FOLFOX, 1163–1164
    FOLFOXIRI, 1164–1165
  preoperative work-up and staging
    colonoscopy, 1151
    laboratory work, 1151
    staging, 1151–1152
    staging system, 1152
  presentation, 1150
  profile, CUP patients, 1653
  risk factors
    age and racial background, 1147
    alcohol and tobacco, 1148
    diabetes mellitus and hyperinsulinemia, 1148
    diet and lifestyle, 1148
    inflammatory bowel disease, 1148
    personal or family history, 1147–1148
    protective effect of NSAID and aspirin, 1148
  screening
    colonoscopy, 1151
    CT colonography, 1151
    flexible sigmoidoscopy, 1151
    stool-based screening methods, 1150
  surgical management of
    abdominal perineal resection with total mesorectal excision, 1156
    antibiotic administration, 1154
    bowel preparation, 1152

laparoscopic colectomy, 1156–1157
left-sided colon cancers, 1154
local excision, 1155
local recurrence, 1159
low anterior resection with total mesorectal excision, 1156
lymphadenectomy, 1156
management of carcinoma in a polyp, 1154
obstructing colon cancers, 1158
perforated colon cancers, 1158
rectal cancers, 1155
right-sided colon cancers, 1154
robotic colectomy, 1157–1158
sigmoid colon cancers, 1154
subtotal colectomy, 1154
surveillance following resection, 1158
synchronous and metachronous lesions, 1156
synchronous distant metastases, 1158
total proctocolectomy, 1155
transverse colon cancers, 1154
5-year relative survival rates, *913*
colorectal cancer syndromes, 407
colorectal metastases, 525–526
combination chemotherapy, 642
  in clinic, 649
  drug resistance
    implications of, 650–651
    reversal of, 651
    tumor cell heterogeneity and, 649–650
  experimental models of, 651–652
  vs. holotherapy, *651*
  rationales for, 649
combined modality therapy, 1078
comparative effectiveness research (CER), 606
complementary and alternative medicine (CAM), 593, 594, 1679
complementary and integrative medicine (CIM), 593
complementary DNA, 28–30
complete hydatidiform mole (CHM), 1343
complete pathological response (CPR), 1010
completion lymphadenectomy (CLND), 1419
comprehensive molecular profiling, CUP, 1656
computed tomography (CT), 519
  scan, lung cancer, 1013–1016
cone-beam CT, 544
congenital melanocytic nevi, 1414
congenital syndromes, 1473–1474
conjunctival melanoma (CM), 935
constipation, 570
  GI complications, 1823
contiguous gene syndrome, 82
contrast-enhanced spiral CT, SVC syndrome, 1892
contrast radiography, 1068
conventional osteosarcoma, 1469–1470
COPD-like small airway epithelium transcriptome signature, 320
copy number high (serous-like) tumors, 1302
copy number low/microsatellite stable group, 1302
copy number variants (CNVs), 102
core biopsy, 1016
core stemness signaling, 180
corticosteroid-induced osteopenia, 1724
corticosteroids, 1566, 1677, 1709
costimulatory ligand–receptor interactions, *801*
COVID-19 pandemic, 400, 1195, 1875
Cowden syndrome, 409–410, 418
CPI-associated colitis, 1816
CPI-mediated hepatitis, 1822
CPI-mediated hepatotoxicity, 1821
  management of, 1822
CRAM file, 497
cranial neuropathies, 1690
cranial/peripheral nerve metastases
  pathogenesis, 1690
  symptoms and signs, 1690
Creutzfeldt–Jakob disease, 1736
CRISPR/Cas9 gene therapy, 39–42

crizotinib, 494, 510, 1024
cross-sectional study, 396
cross-validation, 499
CRS. *see* cytokine release syndrome (CRS)
CRS-207, 784
CRS-207 vaccines, 784
cryoablation, 1717
  for painful metastatic lesions, 528
cryopreservation, 1844
  of embryos and unfertilized oocytes, 1844
  of ovarian tissue, 1844
cryosurgery, 1441
Cryptococcosis, 1874
Cryptococcus gatti, 1874
Cryptococcus neoformans, 1874
Cryptosporidium parvum, 387
CSA and CSB proteins, 336
CSC marker expression, 178
CT-based structural rigidity analysis (CTRA), 1721
ctDNA analysis, 619
CTLA-4. *see* cytotoxic lymphocyte antigen-4 (CTLA-4)
CTLA-4 blocking antibodies, 1421
CTNNB1, 82
CT urography, 1194
CUP. *see* cancer of unknown primary site (CUP)
cutaneous AS (cAS), 1446
cutaneous eruption of lymphocyte recovery, 1710
cutaneous flagellate hyperpigmentation, of bleomycin, *1707*
cutaneous irAEs, 1899
cutaneous reactions, 1701
  associated with chemotherapy, *1702*
  diagnosis and management of, *1711*
cutaneous squamous cell carcinoma (cSCC), 1442
CX-3543, 205
cyclin-dependent kinase inhibitor 2A (CDKN2A), 1030
cyclin-dependent kinase inhibitor 2A (*CDKN2A*) locus, 79–80
cyclin-dependent kinase 4 (INK4) protein inhibitor, 79
cyclobutane pyrimidine dimer (CPD), 333
cyclophosphamide, 696, 1842
CYP2D6 variants, 664
cytarabine, 1689
  administration schedule effects, 647
cytochrome P450 (CYP), 310
cytochrome P450 3A4, 645
cytokine release syndrome (CRS), 1792, 1899–1900
cytokines, 1704–1705
cytokine therapy, of melanoma, 1431
cytokinetics, 646
  of tumor, chemotherapy dose effects, 644
cytology
  NSCLC, 1009
  sputum, lung cancer, 1016
cytomegalovirus, 1734
cytopathology, 1033
cytosine antimetabolites, 683–685
cytosine arabinoside (ara-C), 1694
  clinical activity, 684
  clinical pharmacology, 684
  mechanism of action, 684
  metabolism, 683–684
  toxicities, 684
cytotoxic chemotherapeutic agents, 641
cytotoxic chemotherapy, 977
  effect, on gonadal function
    in boys, 1840–1841
    in men, 1841
    in prepubertal girls, 1841
    in women, 1841–1843
  melanoma, 1421
  recurrent endometrial cancer treatment, 1306
cytotoxicity, general mechanisms of, 693
cytotoxic lymphocyte antigen-4 (CTLA-4), 800–803
cytotoxics, 999
cytotoxic T-lymphocyte-associated antigen 4 (CTLA-4) blockade, 1427, *1428*

D

dabrafenib, 1025
dacarbazine, 694, 1432
damage-associated molecular patterns (DAMP), 1030
daratumumab, 1619, 1624–1625
"data integration," 251
daunorubicin, 714
DCVax-L, 785
ddTRAP (droplet digital telomeric repeat amplification protocol), 202
decitabine
　cellular uptake and metabolism, 684–685
　clinical activity, 685
　clinical pharmacology, 685
　mechanism of action, 685
　toxicities, 685
dedifferentiated chondrosarcoma, 1467
deep phenotyping, 1907
defibrotide, 1823
delayed emesis, 1674
delirium, 547
delirium management, 574
denosumab, 1722, 1858
2′-Deoxy-5-(trifluoromethyl) uridine, 682–683
depressive disorders, treatment of
　anxiety disorders, 545
　personality clusters and potential impact, 546
　suicide risk, 544
　trauma and stressor-related disorders, 545
dermatofibrosarcoma protuberans (DFSP), 1445
dermatologic complications, of cancer chemotherapy, 1701–1712
　acral reactions, 1709–1710
　alopecia, 1705
　cutaneous eruption of lymphocyte recovery, 1710
　extravasation reactions, 1706–1707
　nail reactions, 1705–1706
　pigmentary changes, 1707
　radiation-associated reactions, 1707–1709
　stomatitis, 1705
dermis, tumors arising from, 1445
desmoplastic melanoma, 1416
desquamation phase of hand-and-foot syndrome, *1709*
diabetes mellitus, 1124, 1864
　hepatocellular carcinoma, 1096
diarrhea
　C. difficile-associated, 1814–1815
　chemotherapy and radiation, 1813–1814
　CMV, 1816
　differential diagnosis of, *1814*
　GI complications, 1813–1818
diet and nutrition, 433–451
　current research, 446–449
　methodologic issues in, 433–435
　overview, 433
　prevention of cancer recurrence long-term complication of therapy, 451
　public health guidelines, 435–446
　survivorship, 449–451
dietary patterns, 446–447
dietary supplements, 437
differentiation syndrome (DS), 1902
diffuse alveolar hemorrhage (DAH), 839, 1793
diffuse astrocytic tumors, 927
diffuse large B-cell lymphoma (DLBCL), 841, 902–903
diffuse neuroendocrine system (DES), 971–979
　clinical features of, 973
　cytotoxic chemotherapy, 977
　epidemiology, 971
　gastrointestinal neuroendocrine tumors (GI-NETS), 974
　histology and staging of, 973
　imaging, 974
　inherited syndromes with associated neuroendocrine tumors, 978
　liver-directed therapies, 976
　MEN-2 and MEN-3 syndromes, 978
　molecular alterations, 973
　neuroendocrine markers, 972
　neurofibromatosis-1 (NF-1), 979
　pancreatic NET (PNET) (ISLET-cell tumors), 974
　peptide receptor radiotherapy (PRRT), 977
　pheochromocytomas, 979
　somatostatin analogs, 976
　somatostatin and somatostatin receptors, 973
　targeted therapies, 977
　tuberous sclerosis (TS), 979
　von Hippel–Lindau (VHL), 979
diffusing capacity of the lung for carbon monoxide (DLCO), 1017
difluoromethylornithine (DFMO), 455
digital pathology and artificial intelligence, 498–499
dihydrofolate reductase (DHFR) inhibitor, 667
dihydropyrimidine dehydrogenase (DPD), 664
dimethyl sulfoxide (DMSO), 1707
diphencyprone (DPCP), 1420
direct intra-tumoral percutaneous ethanol injection, 523–524
direct oral anticoagulants (DOACs), 1895
displacement loop (D-loop), 201
distribution
　drug, 658
　methotrexate, 668–669
DNA
　alkylating and platinum-based drugs, 693
　alterations, 28
　damage
　　chemical carcinogenesis, 312, 313, 314, 315
　　response, 545
　microarray analysis, 30
　repair, diseases of, 335–336
　sunlight induced photoproducts in, 333–334
　UV photoproducts in, 334
DNA methyltransferase inhibitors (DNMTi), 787
DNA mismatch repair (MMR), 84, *85*
DNA mismatch repair gene defects, 84
DNA-repair
　chemical carcinogenesis, 312, 313, 314, 315
　genes, 313, *314*
　mechanisms, 546
　in normal tissues, 547
DNA topoisomerase targeting drugs, 701–714
　mechanisms of action, 701–705
　overview, 701
　perspectives, 714
　pharmacogenomics, 712–714
　TOP2 inhibitors, 709–712
　topoisomerase biology, 701
　topoisomerase I inhibitors, 705–709
docetaxel, 721, 1693
dopamine D2, 1673
dopamine receptor antagonists, 1677
dose-dense chemotherapy, 646
dose effect
　adjuvant chemotherapy, 646
　and clinical trials, 645
　factors influencing, 643
　real-time pharmacokinetics and patient safety, 645
　in sensitive tumors, 645–646
dose fractionation, 1725
dose proportionality, 659
dose selection, 645
double-minute chromosomes (DMs), 59
double-strand DNA breaks, 315
doxorubicin, 522, 713–714, 1821
　administration, 648
　recurrent endometrial cancer treatment, 1306
driver alterations, 615
drug availability and access
　precision oncology challenges, 626
drug–drug interactions, *1753*, 1754
drug-eluting beads (DEBs), 522
drug hypersensitivity reactions, 1701
drug-induced nephrotoxicity, monitoring for, 1751–1754
drug interactions, methotrexate, 670
drug reaction with eosinophilia and systemic syndrome (DRESS), 1701
drug resistance
　chemotherapy dose effects, 644
　and clinical circumvention, 731–735
　　acquired drug resistance and tumor heterogeneity, 734
　　avert or overcome, 735
　　cancer stem cells and lineage plasticity, 734
　　genetic mechanisms, 732
　　metabolic mechanisms, 732
　　to multiple agents, 733
　　to single agents, 731
　implications of, 650–651
　reversal of, 651
　tumor cell heterogeneity and, 649–650
　　cytokinetics, 650
　　modulation, 650
　　synchronization, 650
Dubois BSA formula, 645
duvelisib, 1565
dye exclusion assays, 178
dynamic instability, 717
dysplastic nodules, hepatocellular carcinoma, 1097
dyspnea, 573
　airway obstruction, 1894

E

E1A oncoprotein, 76
early-stage epithelial cancer treatment
　early-stage borderline tumors management, 1318
　early-stage mucinous carcinoma management, 1318
　invasive early-stage low-risk disease management, 1317–1318
　staging surgery, 1317
Eastern Cooperative Oncology Group (ECOG), 1118
EBRT, 543
echinocandins, 1812
ecological fallacy, 396
ecological study, 396
ectopic ACTH production, 1855–1857
ectopic endocrine paraneoplastic syndromes
　ectopic ACTH production, 1855–1857
　growth hormone and prolactin, 1860
　human chorionic gonadotropin, 1858
　hypercalcemia, 1857–1858
　hypoglycemia, 1858
　renin production, 1859
　syndrome of inappropriate antidiuretic hormone, 1858–1859
　tumor-induced osteomalacia, 1859
educational resources, integrative oncology, 596
effusion, cancer presentation, 5
EGFR family, 230–231
EGFR T790M resistance mutations, 516
EGFR tyrosine kinase inhibitor (TKI)
　afatinib, 1023
　dacomitinib, 1023
　erlotinib, 1023
　gefitinib, 1023
　osimertinib, 1023
elastic nets, 499
electrolyte/mineral metabolism, disorders of
　hypercalcemia, 1865
　hypernatremia, 1865
　hypocalcemia, 1865
　hypomagnesemia, 1865
　hyponatremia, 1864–1865
electronic health records (EHRs), 293–294
electron microscopy, CUP evaluation, 1650
elimination, drug, 658
elimination phase, of immune evasion, 799
elotuzumab, 1624
embryonal rhabdomyosarcomas, 1272, 1357

embryonal tumors, classification, 924
emergency surgery, 541
emetogenic chemotherapy, 1675
EML4-ALK fusion oncogene, 494
empiric chemotherapy, cancer of unknown primary site, 1655–1656
empiric naloxone treatment, 1884
emtansine, 727
enchondromatosis, 1473
The Encyclopedia of DNA Elements (ENCODE), 255
endemic Burkitt lymphoma (eBL)
 sickle-cell trait in, 385
endobronchial US-guided transbronchial needle aspiration (EBUS-TBNA), 1017
endocrine functions
 oncologic complications of
  adrenal diseases, 1863
  electrolyte/mineral metabolism, disorders of, 1864–1865
  energy balance and glucose metabolism, 1864
  hypothalamic–pituitary dysfunction, 1860–1861
  lipid metabolism, disorders of, 1864
  metabolic bone diseases, 1865–1866
  primary thyroid dysfunction, 1861–1863
  sexual dysfunction, 1864
endocrine hyperactivity syndromes, 5
endocrine irAEs, 1899
endocrine syndromes, 412
endodermal sinus tumor, 1272
endogenous inhibitors of angiogenesis, 228–230
endogenous retroviruses, 356
endometrial cancer, 445, 1299–1309
 biomarker testing, 1302
 diagnosis, 1302
 epidemiology, 1299
 genomic alterations, 1301
 histologic types, 1302
 histopathology, 1303
 hormone receptor status, 1303
 imaging, 1302
 laboratory evaluation, 1302
 lymphovascular space invasion, 1303
 molecular subtypes of, 1301–1302
 myometrial invasion, 1303
 pathology, 1300–1302
 PI3K pathway, 1301
 positive peritoneal cytology, 1303
 primary disease treatment, 1303–1306
 prognostic factors, 1302–1303
 race, 1303
 Ras/Raf/MEK/ERK pathway, 1301
 recurrent disease treatment, 1306–1309
 risk factors, 1299–1300
 staging, 1302, 1303
 tumor grade, 1302–1303
endometrial hyperplasia, 1300
endometrial stromal sarcoma (ESS), 1351, 1354
endometrioid adenocarcinoma, 1300
endoscopic mucosal resection, 1068
endoscopic ultrasonography, 1069
endostatin, 229–230
energy balance and glucose metabolism, 1864
energy-dense "fast" foods, 436
enfortumab vedotin, 1197
engineered protein expression, 37–38
engraftment, 836
enhanced permeability and retention (EPR) effect, 827, 831
enostosis, 1462
ensemble methods, 499
Enterococcus faecalis, 1871–1872
entrectinib, 615
environmental carcinogenesis, 306
eosinophilic pneumonia (EP), 1793
ependymal tumors, classification, 924
ependymoma, 859, 929

epidemic-type gastric cancer, 1084
epidemiology, lung cancer, 1005
epidermal growth factor receptor (EGFR), 126, 211, 1694, 1701–1702
 lung cancer, 510
epidermal growth factor receptor TKIs
 effects on gonadal function, 1843
epidermis, tumors arising from, 1437
epidural spinal cord compression (ESCC), 1725
epigenetics and chemical carcinogenesis, 308–310
epigenetic therapies
 clinical trials, 787–788
 vaccine plus epigenetic modulators, 786–787
 vaccine plus other immunomodulators, 788
epigenomics, 321
epipodophyllotoxins, 711
Epi proColon™, 507
epirubicin, 714
 cisplatin, and 5-FU (ECF) chemotherapy, 1089
epithelial-mesenchymal transition (EMT), 10, 180–181, 785, 786, 1032
epithelial ovarian, fallopian tube, and peritoneal cancer, 1311–1326
 advanced-stage epithelial cancer treatment
  adjuvant chemotherapy with platinum compounds and taxanes, 1320
  advanced-stage low-grade serous cancer ovarian cancer management, 1323
  advanced stage mucinous ovarian cancers, 1323
  bevacizumab, 1322
  cytoreductive surgery, 1319–1320
  dose-dense chemotherapy, 1320–1321
  follow-up examinations, 1323–1324
  intraperitoneal chemotherapy, 1321
  maintenance with chemotherapy and targeted therapies, 1322
  neoadjuvant chemotherapy, 1321–1322
  PARP-inhibitors, 1322–1323
  treatment assessment, 1323
 BRCA1 to BRCA2 mutations or multigene panel testing, 1313
 diagnosis, 1316
 early-stage epithelial cancer treatment
  early-stage borderline tumors management, 1318
  early-stage mucinous carcinoma management, 1318
  invasive early-stage low-risk disease management, 1317–1318
  staging surgery, 1317
 epidemiology and etiology
  etiology, 1311–1312
  incidence, prevalence and mortality, 1311
 genetic predisposition
  BRCA1 and BRCA2, 1312
  hereditary ovarian cancer, 1312
  Lynch syndrome, 1312
  management of, 1312–1313
 molecular, cellular, and clinical biology
  borderline tumors, 1315
  classification and pathology, 1314
  clinical symptoms, 1316
  invasive histotypes, 1314–1315
  low-grade serous carcinomas (LGSC), 1315
  patterns of spread, 1315–1316
 prevention, 1312
 prognosis, 1318–1319
 recurrent epithelial cancer treatment
  chemotherapy, 1324
  hormonal therapy, 1326
  immunotherapy, 1326
  palliative radiotherapy, 1326
  PARP-inhibitors, 1326
  platinum-resistant disease, 1325–1326
  platinum-sensitive disease, 1324
  targeted therapies, 1324–1325, 1326

 screening
  CA125, 1317
  women at high risk, 1317
epithelial to mesenchymal transition (EMT), 733
epithelial tumors, histologic classification of, 1276
epithelioid hemangioendothelioma (EHE), 1106
epithelioid trophoblastic tumor (ETT), 1343, 1347
epothilones, 724
Epstein–Barr virus (EBV)
 clinical aspects, 360–362
 expressed during productive infection, 360
 gene expression in transformed lymphocytes, 359–360
 infection, 1875
equilibrium phase, of immune evasion, 799
ERB B1 gene, 66
ERB B2 gene, 65
ErbB2 gene, 153
eribulin, 727
erythema multiforme (EM), 1701
erythropoietin, 1859
escape phase, of immune evasion, 799
esophageal candidiasis, 1811
esophageal disorders, GI complications, 1811–1813
esophagitis
 bacterial, 1813
 causes of, 1812
 fungal infections, 1811–1812
 malignant dysphagia, 1813
 pill-induced, 1813
 radiation-induced, 1811
 viral infections, 1812–1813
esophagus, 1065–1080
 anatomy and histology, 1065
 biologic staging, 1070
 bone scintigraphy, 1069
 bronchoscopy, 1069
 combined modality therapy, 1078
 contrast radiography, 1068
 CT, 1069
 diagnosis, 1067
 endoscopic mucosal resection, 1068
 endoscopic ultrasonography, 1069
 endoscopy, 1068
 epidemiology, 1066
 etiology, 1065
 immunomodulatory therapy, 1077
 magnetic resonance imaging, 1069
 minimally invasive surgical staging, 1070
 neck ultrasonography, 1069
 palliative therapy, 1080
 positron emission tomography, 1069
 pretreatment assessment, 1067
 radiation therapy, 1074
 single-agent chemotherapy, 1076
 staging evaluation, 1068
 surgery, 1071
 systemic therapy, 1075
 therapy, 1071
 TNM staging system, 1070
 treatment, 1067
ESR1 gene, 70
essential thrombocytosis, 1633
estramustine, 1866
estrogen receptor positive (ER+), 734
ethanol, 523
etoposide, 711–712, 714
 administration schedule effects, 648
European leukemiaNET risk stratification, 840
euthyroid sick syndrome, 1861
everolimus, 977
ewing sarcoma (EWS), 1468
 pediatric bone tumors, 856
ewing sarcoma family of tumors (EWSFT), 856
The Exceptional Responders Initiative, 255
excretion
 methotrexate, 670

exogenous glucocorticoid therapy, 1860
exome sequencing, 128
exposome, 320, 322, 398, *399*
expressive art therapies, 595
extended pleurectomy decortication (EPD), 1037
extended survival phase, 912
external beam, 543
external beam radiation therapy (EBRT), 528, 956
external validity, HSR, 605
extracellular signal-regulated kinase (ERK), 155
extracorporeal photopheresis, 1607
extragonadal germ cell tumor syndrome, 1654
extramammary Paget disease (EMPD), 1446
extrapleural pneumonectomy (EPP), 1036
extravasated cytotoxic agents, 1706
extravasation reactions, 1706–1707
eye cancers, 933–941

F

fallopian tube sarcomas, 1357
familial adenomatous polyposis (FAP), 408–409, 508, 1084, 1473. *see* adenomatous polyposis coli (APC)
familial AML with mutated DDX41, 420
familial aplastic anemia/MDS with SRP72 mutation, 420
familial atypical multiple-mole/melanoma syndrome (FAMMM), 411
familial breast cancer, 84
familial hypocalciuric-hypercalcemia (FHH), 414
familial isolated primary hyperparathyroidism (FIHP), 414
familial lymphoproliferative disorders, 421
familial MDS/AML with mutated GATA2 (GATA2 deficiency), 420
familial melanoma, 1414
familial pancreatic cancer (FPC), 410–411
familial platelet disorder with propensity to myeloid malignancy (FPD-AML), 419
fam-trastuzumab deruxtecan-nxki, 708
Fanconi anemia, 85
FASTQ, 497
FDA approved checkpoint immunotherapy, *802, 803*
FDA biomarker-based therapeutic approvals, 493, *494*
febrile episodes, types of, *1870*
febrile neutropenic patients, 1877
fecal immunochemical test (FIT), 507
feedback-controlled dosing, 665
female urethral carcinoma, 1242
fever of unknown origin, cancer presentation, 5
FGFR, 69
fiberoptic bronchoscopy (FOB), 1016
fibroblast growth factor (FGF), 153, 226
fibroblast growth factor receptor (FGFR) signaling, 511
fibrous cortical defects, 1460–1461
fibrous dysplasia, 1459–1460
fibrous tumors, 1459–1461
fidaxomicin, 1815, 1872
financial challenges, in precision oncology, 626
financial toxicity, 917
first-pass effect, 657
FISH, 515
fish oil, 448
fistula formation, GI complications, 1824
"flash" radiation therapy, 548
floor of mouth (FOM), 986
fluconazole, 1812
fludarabine, 688, *689*
fludarabine–cyclophosphamide–rituximab (FCR), 1563
fluorescence-guided surgery (FGS), 825
fluorescence *in situ* hybridization (FISH), 126, 129, 493
fluorodeoxyglucose (FDG)-avidity, 1716
fluorodeoxyglucose (FDG)-PET/CT, 1034
fluorodeoxyuridine (FUDR), 647, 681
fluorodeoxyuridine monophosphate (FdUMP), 650
5-fluoro-2′-deoxyuridine (5-FdU) triphosphate, 207
fluoropyrimidines, 664
fluoropyrimidines, administration schedule effects, 647

5-fluorouracil (5-FU), 1694
 antineoplastic agent, 679
 clinical pharmacology, 681
 clinical use and indications, 681
 mechanism of action, 680–681
 metabolism, 680
 toxicities, 681
5-fluorouracil-based chemotherapy, 511
5-fluorouracil-based regimens, 1159
fluticasone, azithromycin, and montelukast (FAM), 839
folate, 447
folate antagonists, 667–677
 adverse effects, 672–674
 aminopterin, 667, *668*, 675
 clinical dosage schedules, 670
 function, 667
 historical overview, 667
 methotrexate (*see* methotrexate (MTX))
 pemetrexed, 676
 pralatrexate, 676
 resistance to antifolates, 674–675
FOLFOX-based chemotherapy regimens, 522
folic acid structure, *668*
follicular lymphoma (FL), 841
follow-up care guidelines, for cancer survivors, *916*
folylpolyglutamate synthetase (FPGS), 667
food preservation, processing, and preparation, 437
forced expiratory volume after 1 second (FEV1), 1017
fosaprepitant, 1678
FoundationOne Liquid CDx, 516
frailty in older adults with cancer, 878–879
French Action Clinique Coordonnées en Cancérologie Digestive (ACCORD-07) study, 1089
5-FU, 1821
 effect on AK, 1709
 severity of diarrhea with, 1813
fumarate hydratase (FH), 218
fungal infections, 1873–1874
Fusarium spp., 1874

G

gain-of-function approaches, 42
gallbladder cancer, 1109–1114
 causative factors, 1109–1110
 clinical presentation, 1110–1111
 diagnostic studies, 1111–1112
 pathology, 1110
 treatment
  chemotherapy, 1113
  palliation, 1114
  radiation therapy, 1113–1114
  resection, 1112–1113
gallbladder, schistosomiasis, 384
Gardner syndrome, 80, 1473
gastric and gastroesophageal junction cancer, 236
gastric cancer, 1083
 hereditary, 410
gastric outlet obstruction, 1114
gastrinoma syndrome, 975. *see also* Zollinger–Ellison syndrome (ZES)
 MEN-1 syndrome and, 978
gastroenteropancreatic neuroendocrine tumors (GEP-NET), 971
 classification of, *973*
gastroesophageal junction (GEJ) tumors, 1086
gastrointestinal adverse events, 727
gastrointestinal cancer, methotrexate, 672
gastrointestinal (GI) complications, 1811–1824
 acute pancreatitis, 1824
 arterial thrombosis, 1824
 bleeding, 1824
 constipation, 1823
 diarrhea, 1813–1818
 esophageal disorders, 1811–1813
 fistula formation, 1824
 GI perforation, 1824
 graft-*versus*-host disease, 1818–1819

 nausea and vomiting, 1824
 oral and gastrointestinal mucositis, 1824
gastrointestinal irAEs, 1899
gastrointestinal mucositis (GIM), 1824
gastrointestinal neuroendocrine tumors (GI-NETS), 974
gastrointestinal toxicity, methotrexate, 673
GATA6, 1137
gatekeeper genes, 305
gatekeeper mutations, 732
gateway cloning, 23
gemcitabine, *535*, 685
gemcitabine, administration schedule effects, 647
gemtuzumab ozogamicin, 1902
gene activation, 60
gene amplification, 59
gene analysis
 DNA alterations, 28
 nucleotide sequencing, 24–28
 polymerase chain reaction, 24
 Southern blotting, 23–24
gene cloning, 21–23
gene-directed enzyme prodrug therapy, 205
gene editing, 819–820
gene–environment interactions, 310, *311*
gene expression, 398
gene expression microarrays, 105–106
gene fusion, 60
gene therapy, 205
 cancer nanotechnology, 829
genetic epidemiology, 397
genetic mechanisms
 activation of alternative signaling pathways, 732
 altered gene and protein expression, 732
 mutation of drug targets, 732
genetic predisposition, 863
gene transfer, 53, 817–819
genitourinary cancer, methotrexate, 672
Genome Data Analysis Centers (GDACs), 255
genome-wide association studies (GWAS), 397, 848
genome-wide mutational signatures
 historical significance, 498
 supervised mutational signatures, 498
 unsupervised mutational signatures, 498
genomic and sequencing informatics, 296
genomics, 261–268
The Genotype-Tissue Expression Project (GTEx), *255*
geriatric oncology screening tools, 881–882
geriatric syndromes, 878–879
germ cell tumors (GCTs), 1048
 malignant, *861*
 pediatric oncology, principles of, 860
germline biomarkers, 514
germline oncogene mutations, 73
gestational trophoblastic neoplasia (GTN), 1343–1348
 clinical presentation and diagnosis, 1344
 EMACO regimen, *1346*
 hCG follow-up and relapse, 1348
 high-risk GTN management, 1346
 histopathologic classification of, 1343
 incidence of, 1343
 low-risk GTN
  primary therapy of, 1345–1346
  salvage therapy of, 1346
 management of, 1345
 pretreatment evaluation and staging of, 1345
 quiescent, 1348
 risk factors for, 1343
 scoring system for, *1344*
 stage IV GTN management, 1346–1347
 staging and risk assessment, 1344–1345
 therapy results, 1348
giant aggressive keratoacanthomas, 1440
giant cell tumors, 1461
Giardia lamblia, 386
Gibson cloning, 23
Gilbert's syndrome, 1820

gingival and buccal mucosa, 986
GI perforation, 1824
GITR. see glucocorticoid-induced TNFR (GITR)
glial neoplasms, 859
glioblastoma, 238, 927
   vaccine trials, 785
gliomas, 139, 238
gliosarcoma, 927
glove-and-stocking distribution, 724
glucagonoma, 975
glucarpidase, 1750
Glucksberg grading system, *838*
glucocorticoids-induced TNFR (GITR), 805
glucocorticoids, 1857
glutaminolysis, 216
GNAQ/11 gene mutations, 1423
gonadal complications, 1839–1846
gonadal function
   assessment of
      in females, 1839–1840
      in males, 1839
   associated with antineoplastic agents, *1840*
   cytotoxic chemotherapy effects, 1840–1843
   protective measures (fertility preservation)
      for children, 1845
      for men, 1844
      for women, 1844–1845
   radiation impact on, 1839
   radiation therapy effects, 1843
   targeted therapy effects, 1843–1844
gonadotropin deficiency, 1864
gonadotropin-releasing hormone
   recurrent endometrial cancer treatment, 1308
G-protein coupled receptors (GPCRs), 156
G-quadruplex formation, 201
G-quadruplex stabilizers, 204–205
gradient boosting, 499
graft failure, 836
   significant risk factors for, *838*
graft-*versus*-host disease (GVHD), 836, 1837
   acute, 1818–1819
   chronic, 1819
   GI complications, 1818–1819
   of liver, 1823
gram-negative bacteria, 1872
gram-positive bacteria, 1871–1872
gram-positive organisms (GPO), 1869
granulocyte colony-stimulating factor (G-CSF)
   administration, 1878, 1879
granulocyte monocyte colony-stimulating factor (GMCSF), 855
granulocyte transfusion, 1731
Granulomatous disease, 1795
Graves' disease, 1863
great vessels tumors, 1059
γ-retroviral vectors, 817–818
grief and bereavement, 574
GRN163L (Imetelstat), 206, 208
GRNVAC1, 205
gross tumor volume, in lung cancer patient, 1019
growth factors, 54
   receptors, 54
growth factor signaling
   and cancer therapy, 157–159
   inhibition of downstream signaling, 159
   with Tyr kinase activity, 151–153
growth fraction (GF) of tumor
   chemotherapy dose effects, 644
growth hormone and prolactin, 1860
growth hormone-secreting pituitary adenomas, 945
Gsk3p proteins function, 83
GTPase-activating proteins (GAPs), 155
guanine antimetabolites, 686–688
guanine nucleotide exchange factor (GEF), 155
GVAX vaccines, 784
gynecologic sarcomas, 1351–1357
   amplifications, 1352

chemotherapy, 1355–1356
clinical profile, 1352
deletions, 1352
diagnosis, 1353
endometrial stromal lesions, 1351
epidemiology, 1351
hormone and biologic therapy, 1356–1357
imaging studies, 1353
incidence, 1351
molecular and genetic alterations, 1352
morcellation, 1354
mutations, 1352
nonuterine, 1357
pathology, 1351
patterns of spread, 1352
postsurgical therapy for, 1354
prognosis, 1353–1354
prognostic factors, 1353–1354
radiation oncology, 1354–1355
risk factors, 1351
surgical treatment, 1354
TNM and FIGO staging classification, 1353, *1353*
translocations, 1352
tumor biomarkers, 1352

H

hallmarks of cancer. *see* biological hallmarks, of cancer
hamartomatous polyposis syndromes, 409
hand-and-foot syndrome, *1709*
hand-foot skin reaction (HFSR), 1702, 1703, 1710, *1710*
haploidentical HCT, 834
head and neck cancers (HNCs), 587, 981–1002
   anatomy, 982
   diagnosis and staging, 982–984
   general principles of treatment, 984
   hypopharynx, 988–989
   incidence, 981
   larynx, 989–991
   methotrexate, 672
   mortality, 981
   nasopharynx
      presentation and staging, 991
      treatment, 991–992
   nose and paranasal sinuses, 992–993
   oral cavity
      floor of mouth (FOM), 986
      gingival and buccal mucosa, 986
      lips, 985
      retromolar trigone, 986
      tongue, 985–986
   oral premalignancy, 984–985
   oropharynx, 986–988
   pathologic assessment and biology, 982
   radiation therapy
      combined surgery and radiotherapy, 998
      hypofractionation, 996
      intensity-modulated radiotherapy (IMRT), 997
      particle therapy, 997
      photon radiation, 996
      technologic advances, 996
   salivary glands
      anatomy, 993
      histopathology, 993–994
      systemic therapy, 995
      treatment, 994–995
   systemic therapy, 1002
      angiogenesis, 1000
      concurrent chemotherapy and radiation, 999
      cytotoxics, 999
      epidermal growth factor receptor, 1000
      gene therapy, 1001
      immunotherapy, 1001–1002
      induction chemotherapy, 998–999
      novel therapeutics, 999–1000
      phosphatidylinositol-3 kinase (PI3K), 1001
   tobacco, 982
head, and neck squamous cell carcinoma (HNSCC), 981

healthcare
   twenty-first century (*see* twenty-first century healthcare)
   vision for, 1907
health care quality, for cancer survivors, 916–917
health information technology (HIT) systems
   cancer registry systems, 294
   clinical trials management systems (CTMS), 294–295
   electronic health records, 293–294
   genomic and sequencing informatics, 296
   picture archiving and communications systems (PACS), 295
   tissue banking informatics, 296–297
health-related quality of life (HRQOL), 1084
health services research (HSR), 599–609
   bundled episodes of care, 608
   comparative effectiveness research, 606
   cost-effectiveness analysis, 608
   costs, 607
   disciplines, 600
   implementation science, 609
   meta-analyses and systematic reviews, 605
   mixed methods, 608–609
   modeling, 605
   observational studies, 601–602
   overview, 599
   patient-reported outcomes, 607
   qualitative methods, 608
   quality of care, 606
   quality of life, 607
   randomized controlled trials, 600–601
   secondary data sources, 602–603
   significance, 599
   statistical analyses, 603–605
   study designs, 600
healthy weight, 435–436
heart tumors, 1055–1060
Hedgehog signaling, 181
hemangioma of bone, 1461–1462
hematologic complications and blood bank support, 1729–1736
   abnormalities in platelet function, 1731
   alloimmunization, 1732, 1733
   blood component support posttransplantation, 1736
   causes of pancytopenia
      associated processes, 1730
      chemotherapy related, 1729
      disease related, 1729
      gamma radiation related, 1729–1730
   granulocyte transfusion, 1731
   leukopenia, 1731
   platelet transfusion
      clinical and laboratory assessment, 1732
      indications for therapeutic and prophylactic, 1732
   platelet transfusion support, 1731–1732
   red cells and red cell suppor
      anemia, 1730
      red cell transfusion, 1730
      therapeutic antibody treatments interfering with pretransfusion red cell testing, 1730–1731
   single-and multiple-donor platelets, 1732
   thrombocytopenia, 1731
   transfusion-associated GVHD
      definition, 1733–1734
      historic perspective, 1733
      strategies for prevention, 1734
   transfusion of fresh frozen plasma, 1733
   transfusion-related infectious diseases
      bacterial sepsis, 1735
      Creutzfeldt–Jakob disease, 1736
      cytomegalovirus, 1734
      hepatitis B, 1734
      hepatitis C, 1734
      human immunodeficiency virus, 1735
      human T-cell lymphotropic virus type 1, 1735
      parasitic diseases, 1735
      pathogen inactivation in blood products, 1735

West Nile virus (WNV), 1735
Zika virus (ZIKV), 1735
hematologic malignancies, 418
hematologic toxicity, methotrexate, 672–673
hematopoietic cell transplantation (HCT), 833–842
  acute lymphoblastic leukemia, 840
  acute myeloid leukemia, 839
  allogeneic donor, 834
  allogeneic transplantation, 833
  autologous transplantation, 833
  chronic lymphocytic leukemia, 841
  chronic myelogenous leukemia, 840
  complications after, *837*
  conditioning, 834, *835*
  diffuse large B-cell lymphoma (DLBCL), 841
  diseases treated with, *834*
  follicular lymphoma (FL), 841
  histocompatibility complex (MHC), 833
  HLA matching and donor selection, 834
  Hodgkin lymphoma, 841
  mantle cell lymphoma (MCL), 841
  multiple myeloma, 841
  myelodysplastic syndromes, 840
  risk assessment, 835
  solid tumors, 842
  T-cell and NK/T-cell lymphoma, 841
hematopoietic growth factors, 1878
hematopoietic stem cell transplant (HSCT), 850, 1566, 1608
hemibody irradiation (HBI), 1727
hemochromatosis, hepatocellular carcinoma, 1096–1097
hemodialysis, 1889
hemolytic-uremic syndrome (HUS), 1749, 1751
hemostasis, 1890
hepatic abnormalities
  biochemical tests, differential diagnosis of, *1820*
  causes of, *1820*
hepatic angiosarcoma, 1106
hepatic artery immunoembolization, 526
hepatic artery vasoocclusive therapy, 976
hepatic complications, 1811–1824
  of cancer treatment, 1819–1823
hepatic metastases, interventional radiology, 525–526
hepatic metastasis chemotherapy
  adjuvant therapy after, 1163
  conversion therapy, 1162
  neoadjuvant therapy, 1163
hepatic radioembolization, 522
hepatic steatosis, 1820
hepatic transplantation, 976
hepatic vascular interventions
  arterial chemoembolization, 522
  arterial embolization, 521–522
  arterial infusion therapy, 521
  hepatic radioembolization, 522
  interventional radiology, 521–524
  local tissue ablation, 523–524
  portal vein embolization, 524
hepatic venous gradient (HVPG) measurement, 1822
hepatitis A virus cellular receptor 2 (HAVCR2), 804
hepatitis B virus (HBV), 373, 1734, 1820, 1874–1875
hepatitis C virus (HCV), 376, 1734, 1874
hepatitis viruses, 373–377, 1874–1876
hepatocellular carcinoma (HCC), 377, 906
  chemoembolization, 524–525
  incidence and epidemiology, 1095
  interventional radiology, 524–525
  kinase inhibitors for, 524
  nodular, 524
  pathogenesis and natural history, 1099
  pathology
    combined HCC and cholangiocarcinoma, 1099
    dysplastic nodules, 1097
    early HCC, 1097–1098
    fibrolamellar, 1099
    macroscopic presentation of HCC, 1098
    microscopic presentation, 1098–1099
  prevention, 1097
  risk factors
    aflatoxins, 1096
    alcohol, 1096
    α1-antitrypsin deficiency (AATD), 1097
    diabetes mellitus, 1096
    hemochromatosis, 1096–1097
    hypothyroidism, 1097
    obesity, 1096
    viral hepatitis (HBV and HCV), 1095–1096
  screening and diagnosis, 1099
  staging, 1099–1101
  treatment
    locoregional ablation therapies, 1102–1103
    orthotopic liver transplantation (OLT), 1102
    surgical resection, 1101–1102
    systemic treatment, 1103–1104
    transarterial chemoembolization (TACE), 1103
hepatocyte growth factor (HGF), 732
hepatoma, 238, 373–377
hepatotoxicity, 1821–1822
  methotrexate, 673
HER2-derived peptide vaccines, 783
hereditary breast and ovarian cancer syndrome (HBOC), 411
hereditary cancer syndromes, 403–422
  BAP1, 417
  Birt–Hogg–Dubé syndrome (BHD), 417
  breast and ovarian cancer syndrome, 404–405
  breast cancer and gynecologic cancer syndromes, 404
  Carney triad, 416
  chromosome 3 translocations, 418
  colorectal cancer syndromes, 407
  Cowden syndrome, 409–410, 418
  endocrine syndromes, 412
  familial adenomatous polyposis, 408–409
  familial lymphoproliferative disorders, 421
  familial pancreatic cancer (FPC), 410–411
  FAMMM, 411
  gastric cancer, 410
  genitourinary syndromes
    breast and ovarian cancer syndrome, 412
    HOXB13, 412
    prostate cancer, 412
  hamartomatous polyposis syndromes, 409
  HBOC and moderate penetrance genes, 411
  HDGC, 410
  hematologic malignancies, 418
  hereditary pancreatitis, 411
  hereditary predispositions to acute lymphoblastic leukemia (ALL), 421
  high-risk breast cancer syndromes (CDH1, PTEN, STK11)
    Cowden syndrome, 405
    hereditary diffuse gastric cancer, 406
    Peutz–Jeghers syndrome, 406
  HLRCC, 417
  HPRC, 417
  inherited bone marrow failure syndromes
    dyskeratosis congenita/telomeropathies, 421
    fanconi anemia, 420
  Li–Fraumeni syndrome, 405
  Lynch syndrome, 406
  Lynch syndrome (hereditary nonpolyposis colorectal cancer), 407–408
  MAX, TMEM127, 415
  MDS and AML
    familial AML with mutated DDX41, 420
    familial aplastic anemia/MDS with SRP72 mutation, 420
    familial MDS/AML with mutated GATA2 (GATA2 deficiency), 420
    FPD-AML, 419
    thrombocytopenia 2, 419–420
    thrombocytopenia 5, 420
  MiTF, 417
  moderate risk breast and ovarian cancer predispositions, 406–407
  multiple endocrine neoplasia type 1, 412–413
  multiple endocrine neoplasia type 2 (MEN2), 413–414
  Von Hippel–Lindau, and neurofibromatosis type 1, 415–416
  oligopolyposis syndromes, 409
  pancreatic adenocarcinomas, 410
  pancreatic cancer risk in FPC families, 411
  paraganglioma/ pheochromocytoma syndromes, 414
  parathyroid diseases
    familial hypocalciuric-hypercalcemia (FHH), 414
    familial isolated primary hyperparathyroidism (FIHP), 414
    hyperparathyroidism-jaw tumor syndrome (HPT-JT), 414
    multiple endocrine neoplasia type 4 (MEN4), 414
  PCC/PGL, 416
  Peutz–Jeghers syndrome, 409, 411
  potential genetic risks, 412
  renal cell carcinoma syndromes, 416
  risk assessment and risk models, 403–404
  SDH-RCC, 417
  SDHx, 415
  special considerations for genetic counseling and testing, 421–422
  testicular cancer, 418
  TSC, 417–418
  upper urinary tract cancer, 418
  Von Hippel–Lindau syndrome, 416
hereditary diffuse gastric cancer (HDGC), 410, 1083
hereditary leiomyomatosis and renal cell cancer (HLRCC), 417
hereditary nonpolyposis colorectal cancer (HNPCC), 84, 508, 1084, 1123, 1312
hereditary pancreatitis, 411, 1124
hereditary papillary renal cancer (HPRC), 417
hereditary syndromes, 455
herpesviruses, 359–364
  clinical aspects
    Kaposi sarcoma, 363
    multicentric castleman disease, 364
    primary effusion lymphomas, 364
  Epstein–Barr virus
    clinical aspects, 360–362
    expressed during productive infection, 360
    gene expression in transformed lymphocytes, 359–360
  KSHV and malignancies, 362
  properties of, 359
  viral proteins, 362–363
HIF-1a transcription factor, 84
high-dose chemotherapy, 641
high dose per fraction/ablative radiation therapy, 548
highly emetogenic chemotherapy (HEC), 1680
high mobility group box 1 protein (HMGB1), 1030
high-throughput reverse-phase protein lysate array (RPPA) proteomic technology, 514
histamine H1 receptors, 1673
histone deacetylase (HDAC) inhibitors, 1607, 1624
HLA complex, 833. *see also* major histocompatibility complex (MHC) region
HNPCC. *see* hereditary nonpolyposis colorectal cancer (HNPCC)
Hodgkin disease and non-Hodgkin lymphoma, 871–872
hodgkin lymphoma, 361, 841, 904, 1569–1578
  epidemiology and etiology, 1569–1570
  history, 1569
  immunologic abnormalities in patients, 1570
  immunophenotype and biology, 1572
  principles of treatment in
    chemotherapy, 1574
    early-stage cHL, 1574–1575
    favorable risk, 1575

hodgkin lymphoma (continued)
    new agents in, 1577
    radiotherapy, 1573
    of relapsed/refractory Hodgkin lymphoma
        management, 1576–1577
    risk-adapted interim PET, 1574
    treatment, 1576
    unfavorable risk, 1575–1576
    special populations
        elderly, 1577
        HIV, 1578
        NLPHL, 1577
        pregnancy, 1577
    staging, 1573
    subtypes, 1570–1572
homo-vanillic acid (HVA), 854
hormone receptors (HR)
    breast cancer, 508–509
    endometrial cancer, 1303
hormone replacement therapy (HRT), 457
hormone therapy
    gynecologic sarcomas, 1356–1357
    recurrent endometrial cancer treatment, 1307–1308
hospice, 574
host defense mechanisms, defects in, 1870
host somatic mutations, 375
host–tumor interactions, 733
HPV-associated malignancies
    vaccine trials, 782
HPV infection, 1169
HSR. see health services research (HSR)
HSV esophagitis, 1812, 1812
hTERTα splice variant, 203
The Human Cell Atlas (HCA), 255
human chemical carcinogenesis, 305, 306
human chorionic gonadotropin (hCG), 513, 1858
human diet assessment, 434
The Human Genome Project, 255
human hepatitis viruses, 373
human herpesvirus 6 (HHV-6), 1875
human immunodeficiency virus (HIV), 354–356, 1170, 1735
human papilloma virus (HPV)
    based screening, 507
    and human genital neoplasia
        abnormal pap smear and primary
            screening, 370–371
        applications to clinical medicine, 370
        clinical management, 371
        prevention, 371
        risk factors, 369–370
        surrogate biomarkers of, 371
    infection, 1169
    related OPCs, 512
    vaccines, 782
human T-cell lymphotropic virus type 1, 1735
The Human Tumor Atlas Network (HTAN), 255
human whole-genome sequencing, 250
hybridization-based enrichment, 495
4-hydroxy-cyclophosphamide, 695
5-hydroxytryptophan (5-HTP), 972
hypercalcemia, 1857–1858
    calcitriol production by malignant tumors, 1857
    localized osteolytic bone resorption, 1857
    of malignancy, 1724
    malignancy-related, 1857
    parathyroid hormone-related protein, 1857
    therapy of, 1857
hyperdiploidy, 134
hyperlipidemia, 1864
hyperparathyroidism-jaw tumor syndrome
    (HPT-JT), 414
hyperpigmentation, 1705, 1706, 1707
    chemotherapeutic agents associated with, 1707
hyperprolactinemia, 1864
hypersensitivity pneumonitis, 1792
hypertension, 239

hyperthermia therapy
    cancer nanotechnology, 829
hyperthermic intraperitoneal chemotherapy
    (HIPEC), 1490
hyperthermic isolated limb perfusion (HILP), 1491
    in melanoma, 1419
hyperthyroidism, 1863
hypnosis, in cancer patients, 595
hypogammaglobulinemia, 1051
hypoglycemia, 1858
hypopharynx, 988–989
hypothalamic/pituitary axes, dynamic testing of, 1856
hypothalamic–pituitary dysfunction, 1860–1861
hypothyroidism, 1861
    hepatocellular carcinoma, 1097
hypoxia chemotherapy dose effects, 644
hypoxia-inducible factor 1 (HIF1), 230, 644
hypoxia-inducible transcription factors (HIF), 9

I

ibrutinib, 1564
ICANS. see immune effector cell-associated
    neurotoxicity syndrome (ICANS)
[131]I-containing compounds, 1862–1863
ICOS. see inducible T cell costimulator (ICOS)
idelalisib, 1565
idiopathic pneumonia syndrome (IPS), 839
ifosfamide, 645, 695, 696, 1355, 1864, 1865
    toxic effects of, 1866
image-guided radiation therapy (IGRT), 1218
image-guided surgery, cancer nanotechnology, 825
imaging, 519
imatinib, 157, 493, 643, 1843
    targeted therapy, 512
imiquimod, 1263, 1420
immune biomarkers, in lung cancer, 1010–1011
immune checkpoint inhibitor-related diarrhea and
    enterocolitis, management of, 1817
immune checkpoint inhibitors (ICIs), 470–471,
    648–649, 1010, 1694, 1704, 1844
immune checkpoint molecules
    combination strategies, 804–805
    cytotoxic lymphocyte antigen-4 (CTLA-4), 800–803
    lymphocyte activation gene-3 (LAG-3), 804
    programmed cell death-1 (PD-1), 803–804
    T-cell Ig and mucin-domain-containing-3, 804
    T cell immunoreceptor with Ig and ITIM
        domains, 804
    V-domain Ig suppressor of T cell activation, 804
immune checkpoint therapy, 800
    clinical challenges with, 806–807
immune CPI, for cancer treatment, 1820–1821
immune editing, 799
Immune Effector Cell-Associated Encephalopathy
    (ICE) score, 1900
immune effector cell-associated neurotoxicity
    syndrome (ICANS), 1900
immune evasion
    mechanisms, 1010
    phases of, 799
immune-mediated colitis, 1817
immune modulatory agents, 1816
immune-related adverse events (irAEs), 1899
immune-related biomarkers, for checkpoint blockade
    agents, 621
immune-related oncologic emergencies
    anaphylactic and anaphylactoid reactions, 1898
    chimeric antigen receptor-T cell therapy, 1899–1900
    immune-related adverse events, 1899
immune surveillance, 799
immune thyroiditis, 1862
immune tolerance, 799
immunoglobulin superfamily (IgSF), 800
immunohistochemical staining, CUP, 1650
immunohistochemistry (IHC), 1033
immunologic agents, nephrotoxicity, 1751

immunologically—mediated drug hypersensitivity
    reactions, 1703
immunomodulators
    cytokines, 1704–1705
    immune checkpoint inhibitors, 1704
immunomodulatory therapy, 1077
immunotherapeutic vaccines, 1178
immunotherapy, 205, 1053, 1421, 1432
    adoptive cell therapies (ACTs), 1694
    for advanced melanoma, 1427–1429
    cancer nanotechnology, 830
    clinically effective strategies, 799, 800
    effects on gonadal function, 1844
    immune checkpoint inhibitors (ICIs), 1694
    immune checkpoint therapy, 800
    immune editing, 799
    immune surveillance, 799
    immune tolerance, 799
    primary thyroid dysfunction, 1862
    recurrent endometrial cancer treatment, 1308–1309
    stimulatory immune receptors, 805–806
    targetable immune checkpoint molecules, 800–805
IMP321 (eftilagimod alpha), 804
indocyanine green (ICG), 825
indoor tanning, 1413
inducible T cell costimulator (ICOS), 805
infections, 1869–1880
    antifungal and antiviral prophylaxis, 1879–1880
    associated with impaired cellular and humoral
        immunity, 1869–1880
    associated with neutropenia, 1869
    catheter-related, 1876–1877
    common sites of, 1870
    duration of therapy, 1877–1879
    fungal, 1873–1874
    in patients with solid tumors, 1869, 1870
    perianal, 1876
    persistent fever, 1877–1878
    prevention, 1879
    risk of oncologic treatments, 1879
    spectrum of, 1869–1873
    therapy in neutropenia patients, 1877
    viral, 1874–1876
infectious diseases, 1125
infertility protective measures
    for children, 1845
    for men, 1844
    for women, 1844–1845
inflammation, 12
Initiative for Molecular Profiling and Advanced Cancer
    Therapy (IMPACT), 556
INK4A, 79
INK4B, 79
innovative trial designs, precision oncology, 620, 622
inoperable locally advanced NSCLC
    combined modality therapy for stage III, 1020
    radiation therapy, 1019
    stage IV NSCLC, treatment of, 1021
        without driver alterations, 1021–1022
inotuzumab ozogamicin, 1902
insertional mutagenesis, 50, 350–351
insulinomas, 975
    robotic enucleation of, 533
integrated PET/CT, lung cancer, 1016
integrative oncology, 593–598
    bio-psychosocial model of health care, 597
    in clinical practice, 596–598
    communication, 594
    definitions, 593
    educational resources, 596
    evidence, 594–595
    guidelines, 596
    mind-body practices, 594–595
    Tai Chi/Qigong effects, 595–596
    utilization, 593–594
    yoga, 595

intensity modulated radiation therapy (IMRT), 997, 1019, 1037, 1175, 1217
  advanced vulvar tumor, 1267
intercellular communication, in multicellular organisms, 151
interferon, 1606
interferon-alpha (IFN-α), 1705
interindividual variation
  and gene–environment interactions, 310, *311*
interleukin-2 (IL-2), 1431, 1705
  erythematous rash associated with, *1710*
intermittent dosing, use of, 648
internal gross tumor volume (IGTV), 1019
internal target volume (ITV), 1019
internal validity, HSR, 605
International Breast Cancer Intervention Study (IBIS-I), 457
The International Cancer Genome Consortium (ICGC), *255*
international cancer survivorship care models, 914
The International HapMap Project, *255*
interventional radiology, 521–529
  genitourinary interventions, 526–527
  hepatic metastases, 525–526
  hepatic vascular interventions, 521–524
  hepatocellular carcinoma, 524–525
  palliative therapy, 528
  partial splenic embolization, 529
  percutaneous biopsy, 529
  stent placement for venous stenosis, 529
  thoracic interventions, 527–528
  vena cava filter placement, 528–529
intra-arterial regional perfusion therapies, 1419
intracavitary radiation therapy (ICRT), 1288
intracranial germ-cell tumors (IGCTs), 859
intraepithelial neoplasia, 3
intrahepatic cholangiocarcinoma, *535*
  diagnosis, 1104–1105
  incidence and epidemiology, 1104
  pathology, 1104
  risk factors, 1104
  staging, 1105
  treatment, 1105–1106
intralesional (IL) therapy, 1439
intralesional therapy in melanoma, 1419
intramedullary nailing, 1718
in-transit recurrent melanoma, management of, 1419–1420
intrathecal MTX administration, side effect of, 673–674
intrinsic resistance, methotrexate, 674–675
intrinsic tumor cell sensitivity, chemotherapy dose effects, 643
invasive bladder cancer
  adjuvant chemotherapy, 1196–1197
  definitive surgery, 1195
  laparoscopic radical cystectomy, 1195
  neoadjuvant (preemptive) cytotoxic chemotherapy, 1196
  neoadjuvant (preemptive) targeted therapies, 1196
  radiotherapy, 1195–1196
invasive carcinomas
  of vagina, 1270–1271
  of vulvar area, 1265–1267
invasive infection, by α-hemolytic streptococci, *1871*
invasive mediastinal staging, 1012
invasive tumors, lung cancers, 1007–1010
Investigation of Serial Studies to Predict Your Therapeutic Response With Imaging And moLecular Analysis 2 (I-SPY2) trial, 625
in vivo serial dilution CSC assays, 179
iodized oil, 522
ionizing radiation, 325–331
  adaptive responses, 327
  bystander effects, 327
  cell killing, 325
  chromosomal aberrations, 326
  development, 325
  DNA damage, 327
  general characteristics of, 328
  genetic susceptibility to, 329
  human epidemiologic studies, 329
  mutagenesis, 325
  radiation-induced genomic instability, 326
ipilimumab, 1421
ipilimumab monotherapy, 801–803
ipsilateral/bilateral tonsillectomy, 1648
irAEs. *see* immune-related adverse events (irAEs)
irinotecan, 664, 706–707, 712–713
  based regimens, 1160
irreversible electroporation (IRE), 523, 524, 1135
irritants, 1706
isatuximab, 1625
isocitrate dehydrogenase (IDH), 70
  inhibitor-induced DS, 1902
isolated limb infusion, 1419, 1491
I-SPY2 trial, 625
itraconazole, 1812
ixazomib, 1623–1624

J

JNK, 155
joint arthroplasty, 1719
juvenile polyposis syndrome (JPS), 409, 1084

K

Kaposi sarcoma, 363, 898–902
Kaposi sarcoma-associated herpesvirus (KSHV) and malignancies, 362
karzinoide, 973
keratoacanthoma (KA), 1439
keratoderma, 1704
Ki67, 1352
kinases, 63. *see also* kinome
kinome, 63
Ki-ras gene mutations, 317
KIT, 66, 511
  melanoma, 511
KRAS
  colon cancer, 511
  G12C mutations, 1025
Kryder's law, 249

L

label retention, 178
laboratory evaluation, endometrial cancer, 1302
lactate dehydrogenase (LDH), 513
LAG-3. *see* lymphocyte activation gene-3 (LAG-3)
LAG525, 804
Lambert–Eaton myasthenic syndrome (LEMS), 1698
lamivudine, 1820
landmark cancer genomic studies, 106–108
Langerhans cell histiocytosis, 1464
laparoscopic radical cystectomy, invasive bladder cancer, 1195
laparoscopic radical nephroureterectomy, 1199
lapatinib, 1821
large-cell carcinoma, lung, 1008
large-cell neuroendocrine carcinoma (LCNEC), 1009
large core dense vesicles (LCDV), 972
large intestine, *S. japonicum* infestation, 383
larotrectinib, 615, 1025, 1137
larynx
  advanced laryngeal cancer, 990–991
  glottic cancers, 989–990
  subglottic cancers, 990
  supraglottic cancers, 989
laxatives, 1823
Legionella pneumophila, 1872
leiomyosarcoma
  adjuvant chemotherapy, 1356
  adriamycin-ifosfamide combination therapy, 1356
  chemotherapy, 1355–1356
  gemcitabine-docetaxel combination therapy, 1356

lenalidomide, 1607
lentigo maligna melanoma (LMM), 1415
lentiviral vectors, 818
lepidic-predominant adenocarcinoma (LPA), 1014
leptomeningeal metastasis (LM)
  diagnosis, 1687
  frequency of, *1687*
  pathophysiology of, 1686, *1688*
  symptoms and signs, 1687
  treatment, 1687
less common GEP-NETS, 975
leukemia, vaccine trials, 785
leukopenia, 1731
leukopoietin, 1859
leydig cell function, 1841
Li–Fraumeni syndrome, 405
limited-stage SCLC, radiation therapy, 1025
lineage plasticity, 734
lineage tracing studies, 179
lipid metabolism, disorders of, 1864
liposomal irinotecan, 708
lips, 985
liquid biopsy, 128, 515
  advantages, 500
  challenges, 500–501
  circulating cell-free DNA, 500
  circulating tumor cells, 500
  circulating tumor DNA, 500
  comprehensive cancer genomic analyses, 499, *500*
  early detection and diagnosis, 501
  innovations and emerging technologies, 503
  minimal residual disease, 502
  NGS multigene panel assay, 502
  therapeutic decision making, 501–502
  therapeutic response, 502
liver cancer, 445
  schistosomiasis and, 384
liver-directed therapies, 976
liver fluke, 385
liver function tests, 1820
liver tumors pediatric oncology, principles of, 862
LMS, 1352
  radiation therapy for, 1354
lobectomy, lung cancer, 1018
localized osteolytic bone resorption, 1857
localized primary disease
  combined preoperative chemotherapy and RT, 1490
  "pediatric" sarcomas and adjuvant therapy, 1490–1491
  radiotherapy
    brachytherapy, 1488
    dose fractionation issues, 1485–1486
    EBRT, 1488
    essential elements in the treatment planning of external beam radiotherapy, 1485
    intensity-modulated radiotherapy, 1487–1488
    methods of radiotherapy delivery, 1487
    radiation dose and target volumes, 1486–1487
    rationale for combining radiotherapy with surgery, 1485
    sequencing of radiotherapy and surgery, 1487
  surgery
    amputation, 1483
    combined-modality limb-sparing treatment, 1484
    general issues, 1483
    management of regional lymph nodes, 1484–1485
    satisfactory surgical margins to omit radiotherapy, 1484
  systemic therapy
    adjuvant systemic therapy following primary surgical resection, 1488–1489
    preoperative (neoadjuvant) chemotherapy, 1489–1490
    regional administration of chemotherapy, 1490
locally advanced pancreatic cancer, 1134
local tissue ablation, 523–524

locoregional recurrent melanoma
  management of, 1419–1420
long-read sequencing (cDNA and direct RNA
  sequencing), 32–33
loperamide, 1814
lorlatinib, 510, 1024
loss-of-function approaches, 38–39
loss of heterozygosity (LOH), 852
low fidelity DNA polymerases, 334–335
low-grade serous carcinomas (LGSC), 1315
low-molecular-weight heparin (LMWH), 1895
low-risk chemotherapy, 1680
low-risk GTN
  primary therapy of, 1345–1346
  salvage therapy of, 1346
lubiprostone, 1823
lumbosacral plexopathy, 1691
lung ablation, 527–528
lung adjuvant cisplatin evaluation (LACE), 1018
lung cancer, 443, 906, 1005–1027
  clinical manifestations of, 1011
  epidemiology, 1005
  imaging of, 1012–1016
  immune biomarkers, 1010–1011
  intrathoracic spread of, 1011
  invasive studies of, 1016–1017
  methotrexate, 672
  molecular pathogenesis, 1005–1006
  noninvasive studies of, 1012–1016
  NSCLC (see non-small-cell lung cancer (NSCLC))
  pathology of, 1006–1010
  risk factors, 1005
  SCLC (see small-cell lung carcinoma (SCLC))
  signs and symptoms, 1011
  targeted therapy, 1023–1025
  vaccine trials, 784
  work-up and staging of, 1012
  5-year relative survival rates, *913*
lung-MAP study, 290
lutenizing hormone releasing hormone (LHRH), 1723
lycopene, 448
lymphadenectomy for node-positive disease, 1419
lymphatic drainage, of vagina, *1270*
lymph node metastasis, 1352
lymph node sampling, 1012
lymphocyte activation gene-3 (LAG-3), 804
lymphoma, 902–904
  CD20 and other biomarkers, 512
  methotrexate, 671
  schistosomiasis and, 384
lymphomas, 1059
lymphoproliferative disease, 360–361
lymphovascular space invasion, endometrial cancer, 1303
Lynch syndrome, 406, 498, 1084, 1300, 1312. *see* hereditary nonpolyposis colorectal cancer (HNPCC)
  hereditary nonpolyposis colorectal cancer, 407–408

M

machine learning, 498
macronodular cutaneous lesions, *1873*
macroscopic complete resection (MCR), 1036
Maffucci syndrome, 1473
magnetic resonance imaging, 1069
magnetothermal therapy, 829
major histocompatibility complex (MHC) region, 833
major pathological response (MPR), 1010
malaria
  Burkitt lymphoma incidences, 385
  chromosomal aberrations, 386
  and EBV, 386
  lymphomagenesis, 386
male urethral carcinoma, 1242
malignancy-related hypercalcemia, 1857
malignant airway obstruction, 1779–1808
  clinical presentation, 1779

diagnostic evaluation, 1779
differential diagnosis, 1779
management, 1780
malignant cells, 1687
malignant conversion, 308
malignant diseases, infections associated with, *1870*
malignant dysphagia, 1813
malignant GCT
  clinical characteristics, 1062
  epidemiology, 1061
  etiology, 1061
  histopathology, 1061
  nonseminomatous GCT, 1062
  seminomas, 1062
malignant germ cell tumors, *861*
malignant melanoma, 1413–1433
malignant mixed Müllerian tumors (MMMTs), 1301
malignant pleural effusions (MPEs), 1780
malignant pleural mesothelioma (MPM), 1029–1041
  etiology, 1029
  genetic predisposition to, 1032
  genomic abnormalities, 1030
  histologic subtypes, 1032
  imaging, 1034
  invasive staging, 1034
  laboratory evaluation, 1032
  molecular biology of, 1030
  NGS and other metatranscriptomic studies, 1030
  radiation therapy for, 1038
  salvage combination checkpoint inhibitor therapies, 1041
  staging and prognosis, 1035
  surgery, 1036
  symptoms and signs, 1032
  systemic chemotherapy for, 1039
  tumor markers, 1033
malignant primary cardiac tumors
  lymphomas, 1059
  mesothelioma, 1059
  sarcomas, 1058
malignant tumors of the adrenal gland, 961–968
  adrenal cortical carcinoma, 964–968
  benign adrenal tumors, 961
  pheochromocytoma and paraganglioma, 961–962
mammalian Raf isoforms, 155
mammalian target of rapamycin (mTOR) inhibitors, 1751
mantle cell lymphoma (MCL), 841
mass, 4
massage, integrative oncology, 595–596
massive hemoptysis, 1892–1893
massively parallel sequencing, cancer genomics and evolution, 106
massive pleural effusion, 1893
mass spectrometry-based unbiased approaches, 515
Master Registry of Oncology Outcomes Associated with Testing and Treatment (ROOT) study, 625
matched-unrelated donors (MUDs), 834
maximum tolerated dose (MTD), 655
MAX, TMEM127, 415
MD Anderson Cancer Center IMPACT study, 621–622
MD Anderson IMPACT2 randomized trial, 624
MDS. *see* myelodysplastic syndromes (MDS)
mechanism of action
  5-Azacytidine (5-AC), 685
  capecitabine, 682
  2-Chlorodeoxyadenosine, 690
  clofarabine, 690
  cytosine arabinoside (ara-C), 684
  decitabine, 685
  5-Fluorodeoxyuridine, 681
  5-Fluorouracil (5-FU), 680–681
  gemcitabine, 685
  6-mercaptopurine, 686
  methotrexate, 667–668
  nelarabine, 688

6-thioguanine, 686
trifluridine, 682
mechanisms of oncogenesis, 349
mediastinoscopy, 1017
medical oncology, 553–564
  economic aspects of diagnosis and treatment, 562
  ethnic diversity, genetic differences, health disparities, and impact, 562
  evolution of systemic cancer therapy, 555–556
  goals of care and advanced care planning, 561
  opportunities and challenges, 562–564
  overview, 553
  patient enrollment on clinical trials, 560
  personalized medicine
    choice of therapy based on circulating tumor DNA (ctDNA), 558
    choice of therapy based on tumor tissue analysis, 556–558
  primary, adjuvant, and neoadjuvant chemotherapy, 555
  principles of care
    evidence-based medicine and standards of practice, 559
    first do no harm, 558
    laws of therapeutics, 558
    monitoring and treatment of comorbidities, 559–560
    monitoring response to therapy, 559
    prioritization of the patient's therapeutic goals, 558
  role of, 553–555
  role of supportive care, 560–561
Medical Research Council Adjuvant Gastric Infusional Chemotherapy (MAGIC) trial, 1089
medullary thyroid carcinoma (MTC), 971, 978
  treatment of, 978–979
medulloblastoma, 858
mees lines, 1705
megaprostheses
  skeletal complications, 1719
MEK inhibitors, 1704
  effects on gonadal function, 1843
melanocortin receptor 1 (MC1R), 1416
melanomas, 336, *337*, 873, 1178
  adjuvant immune checkpoint blockade, 1421–1422
  adjuvant therapy for resected, high-risk melanoma, 1421–1423
  advanced (see advanced melanoma)
  amelanotic, 1416
  atypical mole syndrome/phenotype, 1414
  background, 117
  clinical features, *1415*
  clinical implications, 120–121
  clinical presentation, 1414–1415
  clinicopathologic subtypes, 1415
  congenital melanocytic nevi, 1414
  cytokine therapy, 1431
  dermatologic principles, 1413–1414
  desmoplastic, 1416
  drug resistance and evolution, 121–122
  environmental factors, 1413
  epidemiology and etiology, 1413
  genetic basis of, 117–118
  genetic predisposition and familial melanoma, 1414
  genetics and molecular pathology, 1416–1417
  genomic landscapes, 118–120
  host factors, 1413–1414
  intratumoral immunomodulatory therapy, 1420
  metastatic to the brain, 1432
  neoadjuvant therapy, 1432
  pathologic features, 1415
  pediatric oncology, principles of, 862
  prognostic factors, 1414
  risk assessment, 1414
  risk factors, 1413–1414
  stage IV, 1420–1421
  surgical management, 1417–1421
  surveillance for high-risk patients, 1422–1423

tumor-infiltrating lymphocyte therapy, 1433
uveal, 1423–1424
vaccine trials, 782–783
vaginal area, 1272
vulvar area, 1268–1269
melflufen, 1627
melphalan, 695, 696, 1419
men
  gonadal function
    assessment, 1839
    cytotoxic chemotherapy effect, 1841
    radiation therapy effect, 1841
  infertility protective measures, 1844
  with skeletal metastases, treatment, 1653–1655
mendelian randomization, 400
meningioma, 930
MEN-1 syndromes, 978
  and gastrinoma, 978
  medical and surgical management, 978
  and parathyroid lesions, 978
MEN-2 syndromes, 978
  and pheochromocytoma, 979
MEN-3 syndromes, 978
6-mercaptopurine (6-MP), 686, *687*, 1821
Merkel cell carcinoma (MCC), 1444
mesenchymal chondrosarcoma, 1467
mesothelioma, 1059
  vaccine trials, 784
mesothelioma and radical surgery (MARS), 1037
messenger RNA (mRNA), 398
metabolic bone diseases, 1865–1866
metabolic mechanisms, drug resistance
  altered drug metabolism, 732
  decreased drug accumulation, 731
metabolismm methotrexate, 669–670
metabolomics, 398
meta-iodo-benzyl-guanidine (MIBG), 545, 854
metastatic bladder cancer
  cytotoxic chemotherapy, 1197
  targeted agents and innovative approaches, 1197–1198
metastatic cardiac tumors, 1059
metastatic castrate-resistant disease (mCRPC), 1228
metastatic colorectal cancer
  anti-EGFR monoclonal antibodies, 1165
  bevacizumab, 1165
  capecitabine/XELOX, 1164
  FOLFIRI, 1164
  FOLFOX, 1163–1164
  FOLFOXIRI, 1164–1165
metastatic disease, 1177
  immunotherapy, 1187
  prognostic factors, 1184
  surgery, 1184
  targeted therapy, 1185
  VEGF ligand-directed therapy, 1185
  VEGF receptor tyrosine kinase inhibitors, 1185
metastatic disease, soft tissue sarcomas
  chemotherapy for
    anthracyclines and ifosfamide, 1492
    beyond anthracyclines and ifosfamide, 1493–1494
    dose–response relationships, 1493
    doxorubicin, 1493
    encapsulated anthracyclines, 1493
    eribulin, 1494
    natural history of, 1492
    newer agents, 1494
    single-agent *versus* combination chemotherapy, 1493
    trabectidin (ET-743, ecteinascidin), 1494
  clinical problem, 1491
  individualized therapy, 1492
  resection of, 1492
metastatic disease to bone, 1471–1472
metastatic GTN, 1344
metastatic prostate cancer, 1225
metastatic tumors, 1448

metastatic UM, 1424
MET gene, 68
methemoglobinemia, 1795
methotrexate (MTX), 1688, 1692
  absorption, 668
  acquired resistance, 675
  acute myelogenous leukemia, 671
  administration schedule effects, 647
  adverse effects, 672–674
  clinical dosage schedules, 670, *670*
  combination chemotherapy with, *671*
  distribution, 668–669
  drug interactions, 670
  excretion, 670
  intrinsic resistance, 674–675
  mechanisms of action, 667–668
  metabolism, 669–670
  neoplastic disease treatment, 671–672
  nephrotoxicity, 1749–1750
  pharmacogenomics, 670
  pharmacokinetics, 668–670
  polyglutamates, 667
  primary site of action, *668*
methylations sensitive sequencing, 37
methylnaltrexone, 1823
methylxanthines, 673
metronidazole, 1872
MIA. *see* minimally invasive adenocarcinoma (MIA)
microbiome, 399, 1125
microbiota, 1125
microenvironmental control of cancer stem cell plasticity, 183
micronite filters, 1029
microphthalmia-associated transcription factor (MiTF), 417
microRNAs (miRNAs), 63
  chemical carcinogenesis, 309, 310
microsatellite instability, 498
  colon cancer, 511
  digital pathology and machine learning to predict, *499*
microsatellite instability (MSI), 1301
microsatellite instability-high (MSI-H) phenotype, of colorectal cancer, 498
microtubule depolymerizing drugs
  auristatin F, 727
  emtansine, 727
  monomethyl auristatin E, 727
microtubule destabilizing drugs
  eribulin, 727
  microtubule depolymerizing drugs, 727
  vinca alkaloids, 724
microtubule inhibitors (MTIs), 717–729
  in clinical development, *722*
  in clinical oncology, *719–721*
  described, 717
  mechanisms of resistance, 728
  microtubule destabilizing drugs, 724
  microtubule stabilizing drugs, 718
  tubulin and microtubules, 717
  tubulin dynamic equilibrium, *718*
microtubule stabilizing drugs
  epothilones, 724
  taxanes, 718
microwave ablation, of lung metastases, 528
mind-body practices, integrative oncology, 594–595
mind–body therapies, 1679
mindfulness-based cancer recovery (MBCR), 595
mindfulness-based stress reduction (MBSR), 595
minimally emetogenic chemotherapy, 1680
minimally invasive adenocarcinoma (MIA), 1007
minimally invasive pancreatectomy, 1130
minimal residual disease (MRD), 849
mismatch repair (MMR), 732
mismatch repair proficient (MMRp) tumors, 1308
mitogen activated protein kinase kinase (MAPKK), 155

mitomycin-C
  versus cisplatin, 1174
  nephrotoxicity, 1751
mitosis-activated kinase (MAPK) pathway, 1446
mitosis-karyorrhexis index (MKI), 854
mitotane, 966–967
MMR-deficient cancers, 84
moagmulizumab, 1607
moderately emetogenic chemotherapy, 1680
Mohs surgery, 1441
molar pregnancy, 1343–1348. *see also* gestational trophoblastic neoplasia
  incidence of, 1343
  risk factors for, 1343
molecular biology, 652
  targeted therapy, 651
molecular biology, genetics, and translational models, 19–47
  epigenetic regulation, 36–37
  gain-of-function approaches, 42
  gene analysis
    DNA alterations, 28
    nucleotide sequencing, 24–28
    polymerase chain reaction, 24
    Southern blotting, 23–24
  gene cloning, 21–23
  gene editing with CRISPR/Cas9, 39–42
  gene probes and hybridization, 23
  gene structure
    functional components of the gene, 19–20
    genes and gene expression, 19
    structural considerations, 20
  loss-of-function approaches, 38–39
  mouse models of, 45–47
  mRNA transcript analysis
    complementary DNA, 28–30
    DNA microarray analysis, 30
    Northern blotting, 28
    reverse-transcriptase polymerase chain reaction (RT-PCR), 30–31
    sequence-based gene expression profiling, 30
    structural considerations, 28
    transcriptomic sequencing, 31–35
  organoids
    background, 42
    cancer research applications, 42–43
    natural habitat, 43–44
    new therapeutic strategies, 44–45
  overview, 19
  protein analysis
    engineered protein expression, 37–38
    sodium dodecyl sulfate–polyacrylamide gel electrophoresis (SDS–PAGE), 37
  restriction endonucleases and recombinant DNA, 21
molecular biomarkers
  in breast and ovarian cancer screening, prevention and detection, 508
  for cancer monitoring, 512–514
  in cervical cancer screening, prevention and detection, 507
  in colon cancer screening, prevention and detection, 508
  in colorectal cancer screening, prevention and detection, 507
  for elevated risk individuals, 507
  in esophageal cancer screening, prevention and detection, 507
  in hepatocellular cancer screening, prevention and detection, 507
  in lung cancer screening, prevention and detection, 506
  in ovarian cancer screening, prevention and detection, 507
  for predicting outcomes and therapy responsiveness, 508–512
  in prostate cancer screening, prevention and detection, 506–507

molecular biomarkers (continued)
  recommendations, 516–517
  screening and early cancer detection, 505–506
  validation challenges, 516
molecular cancer classifier assays, in CUP evaluation
  accuracy, 1651
  vs. immunohistochemical staining, 1652
molecular cancer epidemiology, 319
molecular cytogenetics, 103–105
molecular diagnostics, 505–517
molecular epidemiology, 397–400
  exposome, 398, 399
  gene expression, 398
  genetic epidemiology, 397
  and genetics, 397
  Mendelian randomization, 400
  metabolomics, 398
  microbiome, 399
molecular genetics, 105
molecularly targeted agents
  phase I and II trials of, 285, 286
  sequential/simultaneous administration of, 1429–1431
molecularly targeted therapy
  for advanced melanoma, 1425–1427
molecular medicine, 285
molecular profiling, 254, 255, 256, 259, 493
molecular targets, for cancer treatment, 641, 642
monoclonal antibodies, 157
  effects on gonadal function, 1844
monofunctional alkylating agents, 693–694, 694
monomethyl auristatin E (MMAE), 727
mononuclear phagocyte system (MPS), 830
morpheaform BCCs, 1443
mouse double minute 2 (MDM2), 77
MRI, lung cancer, 1016
mRNA transcript analysis
  complementary DNA, 28–30
  DNA microarray analysis, 30
  Northern blotting, 28
  reverse-transcriptase polymerase chain reaction (RT-PCR), 30–31
  sequence-based gene expression profiling, 30
  structural considerations, 28
  transcriptomic sequencing, 31–35
MSI "hypermutated" tumors, 1302
mTOR inhibitors, 1703
mTOR kinase inhibitors
  effects on gonadal function, 1844
MT-stabilizing drugs, 717
MTX therapy, 1821
mucinous adenocarcinomas, 1236
mucocutaneous reactions, cytotoxic chemotherapeutic drugs, 1702
mucormycosis, 1874
mucositis, 1828, 1837
MUC-1 tumor-associated antigen, 781
Muir–Torre syndrome (MTS), 1439, 1448
Müllerian adenosarcomas, 1357
multi-cancer early detection (MCED) approach, 508
multicentric castleman disease (MCD), 364, 904
multidrug resistance protein (MRP), 733
multifocal extraovarian serous carcinoma, 1652
multigene prognostic test, 495
multikinase inhibitors, 1702–1703
multi-leaf collimator, 544
Multinational Association for Supportive Care in Cancer (MASCC) score, 1901
multinucleated giant cells, 851
multiomics approach, 495
multiparameter gene expression profiles, breast cancer, 509
multiple biomarkers, clinical trial design with, 290
multiple endocrine neoplasia 3 (MEN3), 1448
multiple endocrine neoplasia (MEN) syndromes, 971
multiple endocrine neoplasia type 1 (MEN1), 412–413

multiple endocrine neoplasia type 2 (MEN2), 413–414, 415–416
multiple endocrine neoplasia type 4 (MEN4), 414
multiple fraction radiation therapy (MFRT), 1725
multiple hypothesis-testing trap, 252–253
multiple mucosal neuromas, 1448
multiple myeloma, 136
  hematopoietic cell transplantation (HCT), 841
multiple osteochondromatosis, 1473
multiple skin lesions (ecthyma gangrenosum), 1872
multiple tumor suppressor 1 (MTS1), 79
multiplex ligation-dependent probe amplification (MLPA), 1030
multistage carcinogenesis, 305–306
multivariable analyses, HSR, 604
multivariable versus univariate analyses, HSR, 603–604
muscarinic, 1673
muscle-invasive bladder cancer, classes of, 1192–1193
musculoskeletal ablation, 528
mutagenic effects, methotrexate, 674
mutant-template human telomerase RNA (MT-hTERC), 207
mutations
  oncogenes, 57
  skin cancer types, 336
  to-resistance theory, 646
mutator phenotype, 305
MUTYH-associated polyposis (MAP), 408–409
MUTYH gene, germline mutations in, 81
MVAC regimen, 1197
myasthenia gravis, 1050
mycophenolate mofetil (MMF), 837
mycosis fungoides (MF), 1603–1608
  diagnosis, 1603
  hematopoietic stem cell transplant, 1608
  incidence and epidemiology, 1603
  pathogenesis and natural history, 1603
  prognostic factors and biomarkers, 1604
  skin-directed therapies, 1605
  staging, 1604
  systemic biologic therapies, 1606
  systemic cytotoxic chemotherapy, 1607
  systemic therapy, 1606
  treatment, 1604
myeloablative conditioning (MAC), 834–835
myelodysplastic syndromes (MDS), 130, 840, 1501–1515
  classification, 1501–1502
  diagnosis, 1508–1509
  diagnostic dilemmas
    anti-tumor necrosis factor (anti-TNF) and the immunomodulatory imide drugs (IMiDs), 1510
    bone marrow transplantation, 1514
    chemotherapy, 1513
    clinical management, 1514–1515
    epigenetic combinations, 1512
    erythropoietin, 1510
    hypomethylating agents, 1511
    iron chelation, 1511
    myeloid growth factors, 1510
    novel agents in combination with HMA agents, 1513
    novel immunotherapy combinations, 1513–1514
    pathogenesis and relation to leukemic transformation, 1509–1510
    signal inhibitors—multikinase inhibitors, 1513
    use of HMAs as MDS therapy in the community, 1512
  etiology, 1503
  future directions, 1515
  pathobiology
    bone marrow microenvironment, 1505
    clinical and laboratory features, 1507–1508
    clonal origin, 1503–1505
    cytogenetics, 1505–1507
    signal transduction, 1505
myelofibrosis, 1637

myeloma, 1472
myeloproliferative neoplasms (MPNs), 129, 1633–1642
  biology, 1633
  presentation, 1633
myelosuppression, 727
myometrial invasion, endometrial cancer, 1303
myxomas, 1057

N

nab-paclitaxel, 721
nail abnormalities and associated chemoagents, 1706
naloxegol, 1823
nasopharyngeal carcinoma, 361
nasopharynx
  presentation and staging, 991
  treatment, 991–992
National Comprehensive Cancer Network (NCCN), 596
National Surgical Adjuvant Breast and Bowel Project (NSABP), 1300
nausea and vomiting
  anticipatory, 1680
  breakthrough, 1680
  multiple day chemotherapy-induced, 1680
  palliative care, 571
  pathophysiology of, 1673
  radiation-induced nausea and vomiting (RINV), 1681
  types of, 1674
nausea, GI complications, 1824
NCI-MATCH, 624
NCI-MPACT (Molecular Profiling-Based Assignment of Cancer Therapy) trial, 624–625
near-infrared light (NIR), 829
necrolytic migratory erythema (NME), 975
nectin-4, 511
nelarabine, 688
neoadjuvant (preemptive) cytotoxic chemotherapy, 1196
neoadjuvant (preemptive) targeted therapies, 1196
neoadjuvant therapy
  of melanoma, 1432
  operable NSCLC, 1018
neoantigen vaccines, 783
neoplasms of unknown primary site, 1647–1657
neoplastic disease treatment, methotrexate, 671–672
neoplastic meningitis, methotrexate, 672
nephroblastoma. see Wilms tumor
nephron-sparing surgery, 852, 1199
nephrotoxicity, 239
  cisplatin, 1749
  drug-induced, monitoring for, 1751–1754
  immunologic agents, 1751
  methotrexate, 1749–1750
  mitomycin C, 1751
  nitrosoureas, 1751
  targeted therapies, 1751
  therapeutic agents associated with, 1749
netupitant, 1678
neuroblastoma (NB) pediatric oncology, principles of, 853
neurocysticercosis, 387
neuroendocrine carcinoma, 1650
  unknown primary site, 1648–1649
neuroendocrine markers, 972
neuroendocrine metastases, 526
neuroendocrine tumor (NET), 1047, 1235
  high-grade, 1655
  low-grade, 1654
  lung, 1008, 1009
  relative incidence of, 972
neurofibromatosis 1 (NF1), 83
  diffuse neuroendocrine system (DES), 979
neurofibromatosis 2 (NF2), 83, 1030
neurofibromin, 83
neurokinin 1 (NK-1), 1673
neurologic complications, cancer of, 1683–1699
  cranial and peripheral nerve metastases, 1689

leptomeningeal metastasis (LM), 1686
  nonmetastatic, 1691
  spinal metastases, 1683
neurologic irAEs, 1899
neurologic oncologic emergencies
  brain herniation, 1897
  spinal cord compression, 1896–1897
  status epilepticus, 1897–1898
neuron-specific enolase (NSE), 972
neuro-oncological ventra antigen 1 (NOVA1), 203
neutropenia, definition, 1901
neutropenic enterocolitis, 1816
neutropenic fever, 1901–1902
neutrophilic dermatoses, 1703
next-generation sequencing (NGS), 26–27, 128, 397
  technology, 493, 494, 1030
    applications in clinical practice, 494–495
    paired tumor-normal samples for somatic testing, 496–497
    RNA sequencing, 497
    somatic alterations, annotation and curation of, 497
    targeted gene panels, 495
    whole exome sequencing, 496
    whole-genome sequencing, 496
  of tumor and ctDNA, 615–619
next-generation tumor-targeted T cells, 795–796
NGS-based ctDNA testing, 619
NGS liquid biopsy assays, 502
NHS-IL12, 788
nitrosoureas, nephrotoxicity, 1751
nivolumab, 1422, 1656
nivolumab (anti-PD-1), 1041
nivolumab and ipilimumab combination therapy, 615
NK-1 receptor antagonists, 1678
NK/T cell lymphomas, HCT, 841
nodular lymphocyte-predominant Hodgkin lymphoma (NLPHL), 851
nodular melanoma, 1414, 1415
nodular regenerative hyperplasia (NRH), 1821
"N-of-1" trials, 620
non-AIDS-defining cancers
  anal cancer, 905–906
  breast cancer, 907
  hepatocellular carcinoma (HCC), 906
  lung cancer, 906
  prostate cancer, 906–907
nonalcoholic fatty liver disease (NAFLD), 1096
nonangiogenic tumors, 223–224
nonbacterial thrombotic endocarditis (NBTE), 1698
noncamptothecin TOP1 inhibitors, 707
nonfunctioning PNET, 975
nongenotoxic carcinogens, 312
non-Hodgkin lymphoma (NHL), 135, 238, 841, 871–872, 902–903
  pediatric oncology, principles of, 850
nonintegrating virus vectors, 819
noninvasive papillary carcinoma, 1191
noninvasive radiographic imaging techniques endometrial cancer, 1302
nonmelanoma skin cancer (NMSC), 336, 1437, 1438
nonmetastatic complications, cancer of
  cerebrovascular complications of, 1697
  chemotherapy, 1688
  cytosine arabinoside, 1694
  5-fluorouracil, 1694
  immunotherapy, 1694
  methotrexate, 1692
  paraneoplastic neurologic syndromes, 1698
  platins, 1693
  radiation therapy, 1687, 1695
  seizures and tumor-related epilepsy, 1696
  small molecule and antibody targeted therapies, 1694
  taxanes, 1693
  vinca alkaloids, 1691
nonmetastatic GTN, 1344

non-muscle-invasive bladder cancer management, 1194–1195
nonmyeloablative conditioning (NMA), 835
nonnegative matrix factorization, 498
nonossifying fibromas and fibrous cortical defects, 1460–1461
nonrhabdomyosarcoma soft tissue sarcomas (NRSTS), 858
nonseminomatous GCT
  chemotherapy, 1063
  recurrent/progressive disease, 1063
  residual mass, 1063
non-small-cell lung cancer (NSCLC), 139, 236–238
  adenocarcinomas, molecular abnormalities associated with, *1006*
  CUP patients, 1653
  forms, histopathologic characteristics of, *1008*
  gefitinib and erlotinib treatment, 494
  high tumor mutational burden, 619
  histological classification, 1009
  inoperable locally advanced, treatment of (*see* inoperable locally advanced NSCLC)
  neoadjuvant therapies, pathological assessment of, *1010*
  operable, treatment of (*see* operable NSCLC)
nonuterine gynecologic sarcomas
  fallopian tube, 1357
  ovary, 1357
  vagina, 1357
  vulva, 1357
nonviral vectors including transposons, 819
Northern blotting, 28
nose and paranasal sinusesm treatment, 992–993
Notch pathway, 156
Notch signaling, 181–182
NRAS
  colon cancer, 511
  melanoma, 511
NSCLC not otherwise specified (NOS), 1009
NTRK, 69
  fusion-positive cancers, 141
  inhibitors, 615
nuclear factor kappa B (NF-*k*B), 1030
nucleotide excision repair mechanism, 334
nucleotide sequencing, 24–28
Nutritional Prevention Cancer Trial (NCP), 455
nutrition improvement, 914

O

obesity, 1124
  hepatocellular carcinoma, 1096
  and metabolic syndrome, 1864
obstructive jaundice, 1114
octopus studies, 620
octreotide, 1814
ocular surface squamous neoplasia (OSSN), 934
oligodendroglial tumors, classification, 922
oligodendrogliomas, 928
oligopolyposis syndromes, 409
olive oil, 448
Ollier disease, 1473
omega-3 fatty acids, 448
"omics" technologies, 321, 516
oncofetal antigens, 781
oncogene addiction-growth factor signaling, 644
oncogene and suppressor gene products, 781
oncogenes, 49–70, 73, 74
  Akt expression, 68
  ALK, 69
  BCL-2, 68
  BRAF, 68
  chromosomal rearrangements, 59
  discovery and identification of, 50
  ERB B1 gene, 66
  ERB B2 gene, 65
  ESR1 gene, 70
  FGFR, 69

gene activation, 60
gene amplification, 59
gene fusion, 60
growth factor receptors, 54
growth factors, 54
initiation and progression of neoplasia, 64
isocitrate dehydrogenases (IDH), 70
kinases, 63
KIT and PDGFRA, 66
MET gene, 68
micrornas (miRNAs), 63
mutations, 57
NTRK, 69
phosphatases, 63
phosphatidylinositol 3-kinases (PI3K), 63
PIK3CA, 68
programed cell death regulation, 56
protein overexpression and constitutive phosphorylation, 63
proto-oncogenes, and their functions, 53
RAS, 67
RET, 67
ROS1, 69
signal transducers, 56
target of new drugs, 65
transcription factors, 56
and tumor suppressor genes, 317, 318
oncologic complications, of endocrine functions
  adrenal diseases, 1863
  electrolyte/mineral metabolism, disorders of, 1864–1865
  energy balance and glucose metabolism, 1864
  hypothalamic–pituitary dysfunction, 1860–1861
  lipid metabolism, disorders of, 1864
  metabolic bone diseases, 1865–1866
  primary thyroid dysfunction, 1861–1863
  sexual dysfunction, 1864
oncologic emergencies, 1883–1902
  acutely ill cancer patients, 1883, *1884*
  circulatory, 1883–1892
  description, 1883
  differentiation syndrome, 1902
  immune-related, 1898–1900
  neurologic, 1896–1898
  neutropenic fever, 1901–1902
  perforated bowel, 1900–1901
  respiratory, 1892–1896
  sinusoidal occlusion syndrome, 1902
oncometabolites, 218
Oncotype DX, 495, 509, *509*
operable NSCLC
  adjuvant and neoadjuvant therapy, 1018
  radiation therapy, 1018
  surgery, 1017–1018
opioid analgesics, *570*
opioid-induced constipation (OIC), 1823
Opisthorchis felineus, 385
Opisthorchis viverrini-associated CCA, 385
opsoclonus/myoclonus syndrome (OMS), 854
optic nerve glioma, 940
oral cavity
  floor of mouth (FOM), 986
  gingival and buccal mucosa, 986
  larynx, and oropharynx cancers, 443–444
  lips, 985
  retromolar trigone, 986
  tongue, 985–986
oral complications, 1827–1838
  of chemotherapy, 1832
  graft-*versus*-host disease, 1837
  mucositis, 1837
  osteonecrosis, 1834
  pretreatment assessment, 1827
oral cryotherapy, oral mucositis pevention, 1824
oral mucositis, 1824
orbit cancers, 933–941
organic foods, 448–449

organoids
	background, 42
	cancer research applications, 42–43
	natural habitat, 43–44
	new therapeutic strategies, 44–45
oropharyngeal cancer (OPC), 512
oropharyngeal candidiasis (OPC), 1812
oropharynx
	soft palate and pharyngeal wall, 988
	tongue base, 988
	tonsil, 987–988
orthotopic liver transplantation (OLT), 1823
osimertinib, 510
osteoblastoma, 1462–1463
osteochondroma, 1459
osteofibrous dysplasia, 1461
osteogenic sarcoma, methotrexate, 672
osteogenic tumors, 1462–1463
osteoid osteoma, 1462
osteomalacia, 1866
	tumor-induced, 1859
osteopoikilosis, 1473
osteoporosis, 674, 1865–1866
osteoradionecrosis, 1831
osteosarcoma (OS), 1468–1471
	pediatric bone tumors, 855
osteosarcomas, 75
ototoxicity, 1693
outpatient therapy, 1877
ovarian cancer, 238, 445–446, 872–873
ovarian sarcomas, 1357
OX-40, 805
oxaliplatin, 698
	clinical pharmacology, 699
	resistance to, 698
	structures of, 697
oxaliplatin-based regimens, 1159–1160
oxaliTEX, 698

P

p38, 155
p53, 230
paclitaxel, 1693
	in recurrent endometrial cancer, 1307
Paget disease, 1263
pain cancer presentation, 4
pain management, palliative care, 569
paired tumor-normal samples
	genomic profiling by NGS, 496
	for somatic testing, 496–497
PALB2, 1123
palifermin, oral mucositis pevention, 1824
palliative care, 567–575, 882
	advance care planning, 568
	anorexia/cachexia syndrome (ACS), 572
	communication, 568
	constipation, 570
	dyspnea, 573
	grief and bereavement, 574
	hospice, 574
	nausea and vomiting, 571
	pain management, 569
	physician aid in dying, 574
	symptom management, 568
	terminal phase, 573
	whole patient assessment, 567
palliative surgery, 541
palliative therapy, 528, 1080, 1083
palmoplantar hyperkeratosis, 1704
p14 Alternative Reading Frame (p14^ARF), 79, 81
Pan Cancer Analysis of Whole Genomes (PCAWG), 255
The PanCancer Analysis of Whole Genomes (PCAWG), 255
The PanCancer Atlas, 255
pancreatic cancer, 238, 445, 1123–1137
	adjuvant (postoperative) therapy, 1131
	clinical management of, 1137
	emergence of precision medicine, 1136
	epidemiology, 1123
	etiologic factors, 1123
	hereditary, 410
	locally advanced pancreatic cancer, 1134
	molecular events in, 1125
	pathology, 1127
	potential biomarker-driven precision therapy, 1137
	presentation, diagnosis, and staging, 1127
	systemic therapy, 1135
	treatment modalities in, 1129
	vaccine trials, 784
pancreatic neuroendocrine tumors (PNET), 971
pancreaticoduodenectomy, 1130
pancytopenia, causes of
	associated processes, 1730
	chemotherapy related, 1729
	disease related, 1729
	gamma radiation related, 1729–1730
papillary fibroelastomas, 1056
papillomaviruses and cervical neoplasia, 367–371
	definitions, 367
	HPV and human genital neoplasia
		abnormal pap smear and primary screening, 370–371
		applications to clinical medicine, 370
		clinical management, 371
		prevention, 371
		risk factors, 369–370
		surrogate biomarkers of, 371
	HPV-target cells and mechanism of infection/viral entry, 367–369
	mechanisms of neoplastic transformation, 369
	overview, 367
para-aortic metastasis, 1294
paraneoplastic neurologic syndromes, 1698, 1698
paraneoplastic syndromes, 5
	lung cancer, 1011
parasites, 379–387
	Giardia lamblia, 386
	liver fluke, 385
	malaria, 385–386
	schistosomiasis
		and bladder cancer, 379–383
		and cancer of other sites, 383–385
parasitic diseases, 1735
parathyroid diseases
	familial hypocalciuric-hypercalcemia (FHH), 414
	familial isolated primary hyperparathyroidism (FIHP), 414
	hyperparathyroidism-jaw tumor syndrome (HPT-JT), 414
	multiple endocrine neoplasia type 4 (MEN4), 414
parathyroid hormone-related protein (PTHrP), 1857
parathyroid lesions, MEN-1 syndrome, 978
parathyroid tumors, pheochromocytoma, 971
PARP enzymes, 510
PARP-inhibitors, 1326
partial splenic embolization, 529
passenger/hitchhiker alterations, 615
pathology, lung cancer, 1006–1010
pazopanib, 1357, 1821
PDGFRA, 66
PD1-PDL1 targeted immune-oncology agents, 1197
pediatric bone tumors
	ewing sarcoma (EWS), 856
	nonrhabdomyosarcoma soft tissue sarcomas (NRSTS), 858
	osteosarcoma (OS), 855
	pediatric oncology, principles of, 855
	rhabdomyosarcoma (RMS), 857
	soft tissue sarcomas, 857
pediatric oncology, principles of, 847–864
	acute lymphoblastic leukemia (ALL), 847
	acute myeloid leukemia (AML), 850
	central nervous system tumors, 858
	epidemiology, 847
	Hodgkin lymphoma (HL), 851
	late effects and quality of survivorship, 862
	less-frequently encountered tumors, 860
	neuroblastoma (NB), 853
	non-Hodgkin lymphoma (NHL), 850
	pediatric bone tumors, 855
	renal tumors, 852
pediatric tumors, 1059
pelvic exenteration, 540
pembrolizumab, 512, 615, 803, 1021–1022, 1136, 1197, 1607, 1656
	anti-PD-1, 1041
	recurrent endometrial cancer treatment, 1308
pemetrexed, 676
penile squamous cell carcinoma (PSCC), 1239
penis cancer, 1239–1243
	chemotherapy, 1241
	diagnosis, 1239
	epidemiology and etiology, 1239
	prognosis, 1241
	radiotherapy, 1241
	surgical treatment, 1240
	tumor staging, 1240
pentose phosphate pathway (PPP), 214
pentostatin, 688
people living with human immunodeficiency viruses (PLWH), 895–908
	cervical cancer, 904–905
	epidemiology, 895–898
	general management issues, 907–908
	Kaposi sarcoma, 898–902
	lymphoma, 902–904
	non-AIDS-defining cancers, 905–907
	overview, 895
peptide-based MAGE-A3 vaccine, 784
peptide receptor radiotherapy (PRRT), 977
percutaneous biliary drainage, 528
percutaneous biliary stenting, 528
percutaneous biopsy, 529
percutaneous hepatic perfusion (PHP) of chemotherapy, 1424
perforated bowel, 1900–1901
perforation, cancer presentation, 5
periacetabular lesions, treatment of, 1720
perianal infections, 1876
pericardial tamponade, 1889
peri-engraftment respiratory distress syndrome (PERDS), 839
peripheral blood stem cell and marrow transplantation, 646
peripheral bronchoscopy, 1017
peripheral intrahepatic cholangiocarcinoma, 1116
peripherally active μ-opioid receptor antagonists (PAMORA), 1823
peripheral neuropathy, 699, 1691, 1693
peripheral primitive neuroectodermal tumors (PPNET), 856
peritoneal carcinomatosis, 1144
	treatment for women with, 1652–1653
peritoneal papillary serous carcinoma, 1652
peritoneum, 1142–1144
	peritoneal carcinomatosis, 1144
	primary peritoneal mesothelioma, 1142
	primary peritoneal serous carcinoma, 1143
	pseudomyxoma peritonei, 1143
permanent survival phase, 912
persistence, drug resistance, 733
persistent chemotherapy-induced alopecia (PCIA), 1705
personality traits
	cluster A, 546
	cluster B, 546
	cluster C, 547
personalized medicine, 321
	choice of therapy based on circulating tumor DNA (ctDNA), 558
	choice of therapy based on tumor tissue analysis, 556–558

Peutz–Jeghers syndrome (PJS), 406, 409, 411, 1084
p53 function, 77–78, *79*
p-glycoprotein, 731
pharmacogenomics, methotrexate, 670
pharmacokinetics
  dose effects, 645
  linearity, 659
  methotrexate, 668–670
  real-time pharmacokinetics and patient safety, 645
pharmacology of small-molecule anticancer agents, 655–665
  anticancer therapies and their mechanisms of action, 655, *656*
  approaches to reduce variability
    feedback-controlled dosing, 665
    population pharmacokinetic strategies, 665
    therapeutic drug monitoring, 664–665
  overview, 655
  pharmacodynamic concepts, 659–660
  pharmacokinetic concepts, 656–659
  sources of variability
    age, 660
    body size and body composition, 660
    drug interactions, 661–663
    inherited genetic factors, 663–664
    pathophysiologic changes, 661
phase 1b trial of avelumab (anti-PD-L1), 968
phase I and II trials, of molecularly targeted agents, 285, 286
pheochromocytoma
  diffuse neuroendocrine system (DES), 979
  MEN-2 and, 979
  and parathyroid tumors, 971
pheochromocytoma/paraganglioma
  chemotherapy, 963
  clinical presentation, 962
  diagnosis and evaluation, 962–963
  genetics and molecular characterization, 962
  surgical treatment of localized disease, 963
  targeted and immunotherapy, 964
  targeted radionuclide therapy, 963
  treatment of advanced disease, 963
philadelphia chromosome translocation, 493
Ph-like ALL, 135, 847
phosphaplatin (PT-112), 698
phosphatase and tensin homolog (PTEN), 1447
phosphatases, 63
phosphatidylinositol 3-kinases (PI3K), 63
photodynamic therapy (PDT), 829, 1439
photosensitivity, 1709
photothermal therapy (PTT), 829
phototoxicity, chemotherapeutic agents, *1708*
physical activity, 436
  improving, 914
physician aid in dying, 574. *see also* physician-assisted death (PAD)
physician-assisted death (PAD), 574
physiologic aging and cancer
  biological age, 878
  cardiopulmonary, 877
  gastrointestinal tract, 878
  hematopoietic/immune system, 878
  renal, 877
picture archiving and communications systems (PACS), 295
PI3K/AKT pathway, 1703
PI-3-K and survival signaling, 153–154
PIK3CA, 68, 154
PIK-related protein kinases (PIKKs), 545
PI-3-K signaling, 154–155
pill-induced esophagitis, 1813
p16^{INK4A} protein, 79, 80
pituitary neoplasms, 943–946
  adrenocorticotropic hormone-secreting adenomas, 946
  classification, 943
  growth hormone-secreting pituitary adenomas, 945

prolactin-secreting pituitary adenomas, 944
TSH-secreting pituitary adenomas, 946
placental site trophoblastic tumor (PSTT), 1343, 1347
planning target volume (PTV), 1019
plant-based diet, 436
plasma cell disorders, 1611–1631
  Al amyloidosis, 1631
  allogeneic stem cell transplantation, 1620
  biology
    cell surface phenotype, 1612–1613
    cellular origin of MM, 1613
    immune microenvironment in MM, 1614–1615
    molecular pathogenesis of MM, 1615–1616
    role of adhesion molecules, cytokines, and BM stromal cells, 1613–1614
    somatic mutations and interclonal diversity, 1616
  clinical features, 1611–1612
  combination therapy, 1618–1619
  complications
    bone disease, 1628–1629
    hyperviscosity, 1629
    infections, 1629
    renal failure, 1629
  daratumumab, 1619
  diagnostic criteria, 1611
  epidemiology, 1611
  high-dose melphalan and autologous stem cell transplant, 1619
  immunomodulatory drugs, 1616–1618
  under investigation
    cereblon E3 ligase modulators (CELMoDs), 1627
    checkpoint inhibition, 1627
    melflufen, 1627
    targeting specific mutations, 1627
    venetoclax, 1627
  maintenance therapy, 1620–1621
  minimal residual disease (MRD), 1621
  monoclonal gammopathy
    of renal significance, 1630
    of undetermined significance, 1629
  multiple myeloma, 1611
  plasmacytomas, 1630
  prognostic factors, 1616
  proteasome inhibitors, 1618
  relapsed disease
    B-cell maturation antigen (BCMA), 1625–1626
    carfilzomib, 1621–1623
    choosing therapy in, 1626–1627
    daratumumab, 1624–1625
    elotuzumab, 1624
    histone deacetylase (HDAC) inhibitors, 1624
    isatuximab, 1625
    ixazomib, 1623–1624
    pomalidomide, 1623
    selinexor, 1625
  smoldering multiple myeloma, 1630
plate and screw fixation, 1718
platelet-derived growth factor receptor A (PDGFRA), 511
platform studies, 620
platins, 1693
platinum antitumor compounds
  adverse effects, 699
  carboplatin, 698
  cisplatin, 697–698
  clinical pharmacology, 698–699
  oxaliplatin, 698
platinum-containing regimens, 1137
platinum-resistant disease, 1325–1326
platinum-sensitive disease, 1324
PLWH. *see* people living with human immunodeficiency viruses (PLWH)
PML-RAR fusion protein, 156
Pneumocystis jiroveci pneumonia, 1874
pneumonectomy, lung cancer, 1018
pneumonitis, 1899
pneumothorax, 1894

POLE, 498
  "ultramutated" tumors, 1302
Pol H, 334
Pol I, 334
Pol K, 334
polycythemia, 1859
Polycythemia vera, 1635
polyethylene glycol-conjugated (pegylated) IFN-α, 1421
polyglutamates, methotrexate, 667
polymerase chain reaction (PCR), 24, 1439
polymerase proofreading-associated polyposis syndrome (PPAP), 498
Pol Z, 334
pomalidomide, 1623
popcorn cells, 851
population pharmacokinetics, 665
portal vein embolization (PVE), 524
positive peritoneal cytology
  endometrial cancer, 1303
positron emission tomography (PET), 1069
  bile duct cancer, 1117
  imaging, 519
  lung cancer, 1016
posterior reversible encephalopathy syndrome (PRES), 1694
postmolar GTN, 1344
postreplication repair, 315
postsurgical respiratory insufficiency, 1784
posttranscriptional and epigenetic alterations, 203
poxvirus-based brachyury vaccines, 786
pralatrexate, 676
p105-Rb function, 76–77
precision immunotherapy trials
  adoptive cell therapy, 625–626
  personalized vaccines (vaccinomics), 626
precision medicine, 319
  in oncology drug development, 613–626 (*see* precision oncology)
precision oncology, 494
  advanced bioinformatics analysis, 297–298
  challenges, 626
  future perspectives, 626
  immunotherapy in, 615
  innovative trial designs, 620, *622*
  new drug approval, 615
  overview, 613–615, *614*
  quantitative imaging informatics, radiomics, and computational pathology, 298
  real-world data, 620–621
  research workspace architecture, 297
  trials of targeted therapy
    I-SPY2, 625
    MD Anderson Cancer Center IMPACT study, 621–622
    MD Anderson IMPACT2 randomized trial, 624
    NCI-MATCH, 624
    NCI-MPACT, 624–625
    PREDICT family trials, 622
    ROOT, 625
    SHIVA randomized trial, 622
    TAPUR, 624
    WINTHER genomic/transcriptomic trial, 622–624
precursor lesions, lung cancers, 1007
PREDICT family trials, 622
predictive biomarkers, 290
predisposition to cancer, 5
preexisting liver disease, effect of, 1820–1821
pregnancy-associated breast cancers (PABCs), 867
pregnancy, cancer and, 867–874
  acute leukemia, 873
  breast cancer, 869–870
  cancer treatment, 868
  cervical cancer, 871
  chronic leukemia, 873
  diagnosis and staging, 867–868
  epidemiology, 867

pregnancy, cancer and (continued)
    Hodgkin disease and non-Hodgkin lymphoma, 871–872
    melanoma, 873
    ovarian cancer, 872–873
    overview, 867
    radiation, 868
    surgery, 868
    systemic therapy, 868–869
    thyroid cancer, 870–871
    transplacental malignancy and placental metastasis, 873–874
pregnancy, outcomes of, 1845–1846
premalignant vaginal disease, 1269–1270
preneoplasia, 224–225
prepubertal girls
    cytotoxic chemotherapy effect, on gonadal function, 1841
primary, adjuvant, and neoadjuvant chemotherapy, 555
primary arrhythmia, 1885
primary bone sarcomas, 1456–1457
    adamantinoma, 1465
    chondrosarcoma, 1465–1467
    chordoma, 1467–1468
    Ewing sarcoma, 1468
    osteosarcoma, 1468–1471
    vascular sarcomas, 1471
primary central nervous system lymphoma (PCNSL), 903, 929
    high-dose MTX regimen, 671
primary cutaneous melanoma
    management of, 1417
    width of excision for, 1434
primary effusion lymphomas, 364
primary germ cell tumors (GCT), 1061–1063
    benign teratomas of mediastinum, 1061
    chemotherapy, 1062
    malignant GCT, 1061
    pretreatment evaluation and staging, 1062
    radiation therapy, 1063
    residual mass, 1063
    treatment of nonseminomatous GCT, 1063
primary liver cancer, 1095–1106
    definition, 1095
    epithelioid hemangioendothelioma, 1106
    hepatic angiosarcoma, 1106
    hepatocellular carcinoma
        pathogenesis and natural history, 1099
        pathology, 1097–1099
        prevention, 1097
        risk factors, 1095–1097
        screening and diagnosis, 1099
        staging, 1099–1101
        treatment, 1101–1104
    intrahepatic cholangiocarcinoma
        diagnosis, 1104–1105
        incidence and epidemiology, 1104
        pathology, 1104
        risk factors, 1104
        staging, 1105
        treatment, 1105–1106
primary myelodysplastic syndromes (MDS), 130
primary neoplasms, 921–931
    chemotherapy, 927
    classification, 921
    clinical presentation, 924
    diagnostic neuroimaging, 924
    epidemiology, 921
    radiation therapy, 927
    risk factors, 921
    supportive therapy, 926
    surgery, 926
primary thyroid dysfunction, 1861–1863
    chemotherapy, 1862
    euthyroid sick syndrome, 1861
    hypothyroidism, 1861
    immunotherapy, 1862

    radiation, 1861–1862
    serum thyroid hormone-binding protein abnormalities, 1861
    targeted therapy, 1862
    thyroidectomy, 1862–1863
ProBE method, 517
procedure-tract metastases (PTMs), 1039
processed foods, 436
prochlorperazine, 1677
prodrug-metabolizing enzymes, 820
professional education, on survivorship, 916
progestins recurrent endometrial cancer treatment, 1307–1308
programed cell death regulation, 56
programmed cell death-1 (PD-1), 803–804
programmed cell death-ligand 1 (PD-L1), 800, 1010
programmed cell death-ligand 2 (PD-L2), 803
programmed cell death protein 1 (PD-1), 1010. see programmed cell death-1 (PD-1)
    blocking antibodies, 1429
progressive multifocal leukoencephalopathy (PML), 1694
prolactin-secreting pituitary adenomas, 944
proopiomelanocortin (POMC), 1855
prophylactic antiviral therapy, 1820
prophylactic cranial irradiation, SCLC, 1026
prophylaxis, antifungal and antiviral, 1879–1880
prospective cohort study, 395
prostate cancer, 140, 442–443, 906–907, 1201–1237
    active surveillance, 1214
    biochemical recurrence, 1212
    curative therapy for, 1215
    early detection of, 1206
    genetic risk factors and molecular pathogenesis, 1204
    histologic features of, 1203
    hormone and growth factor signaling, 1205
    imaging, 1210
    mCRPC, 1212
    neurovascular bundle dissection, 1217
    normal anatomic and histologic features, 1201
    premalignant prostatic lesions, 1203
    prevention, 1213
    staging of, 1208
    vaccine trials, 783
    5-year relative survival rates, 913
Prostate Health Index (PHI), 507
prostate-specific antigen (PSA), 506–507, 513–514
prostate-specific membrane antigen (PSMA), 827
PROSTVAC, 783
protein analysis
    engineered protein expression, 37–38
    sodium dodecyl sulfate–polyacrylamide gel electrophoresis (SDS–PAGE), 37
protein overexpression, 63
proton therapy, 1218
proto-oncogenes, 53
prucalopride, 1823
pruritic diffuse erythroderma, 1704
pseudoencapsulation approach, 540
Pseudomonas aeruginosa, 1872
pseudomyxoma peritonei, 1143
pseudo-sarcoma botryoides, 1272
psycho-oncology, 543–548
    clinical management, 543
    cluster A personality traits, 546
    cluster B personality traits, 546
    cluster C personality traits, 547
    delirium, 547
    depressive disorders, 544
psychosocial conditions, identification and management of, 914
psychosocial issues, 1846
pulmonary embolism, 1894–1896
    diagnosis of, 1895
    symptoms of, 1894
pulmonary fibrosis, 863
pulmonary function testing (PFT), 1017

pulmonary hemorrhage, 239
Pulmonary hypertension, 1793
pulmonary toxicity, methotrexate, 674
pulmonary veno-occlusive disease, 1793
pulsus paradoxus, 1889
purine and pyrimidine-targeted antimetabolites, 643
purine antimetabolites, 685
pylorus preservation, 1130
pyrimidine antimetabolites
    adenosine antimetabolites, 688–690
    cytosine antimetabolites, 683–685
    guanine antimetabolites, 686–688
    purine antimetabolites, 685
    thymidine antimetabolites, 682–683
    uracil antimetabolites, 679–682
[6-4] pyrimidine dimer ([6-4]PD), 333

Q

quality of care, HSR, 606
quantitative reverse-transcription polymerase chain reaction (qRT-PCR), 129
quiescent gestational trophoblastic neoplasia, 1348

R

radiation
    enhancement, 1707
    on gonadal function, impact, 1839
    interactions
        with biological molecules, 545
        with immune system, 548
    nephritis, 1749
    primary thyroid dysfunction, 1861–1862
    recall, 1708
radiation-associated cAS (RAAS), 1446
radiation-associated reactions
    chemotherapeutic agents implicated in, 1708
    photosensitivity, 1709
    radiation enhancement, 1707
    radiation recall, 1708
radiation-induced cystitis, 1748–1749
radiation-induced DNA damage, 545
radiation-induced genomic instability, 326
radiation-induced nausea and vomiting (RINV), 1681
radiation-induced painless thyroiditis, 1863
radiation-induced proctitis and colitis, 1817–1818
radiation-induced secondary tumors, 331
radiation oncology
    gynecologic sarcomas, 1354–1355
    principles of, 543–550
        beam production for external beam radiotherapy, 543
        brachytherapy, 544
        cell cycle arrest and DNA repair in normal tissues, 547
        cell cycle control and checkpoints, 546
        DNA damage response, 545
        DNA repair mechanisms, 546
        "flash" radiation therapy, 548
        fundamental principles, 543
        high dose per fraction/ablative radiation therapy, 548
        modern beam modulation and treatment planning, 544
        radiation-induced DNA damage, 545
        radiation interactions with biological molecules, 545
        radiation interactions with immune system, 548
        radiation therapy imaging and target localization, 544
        radiosensitization, 547
radiation technique, 1726
radiation therapy, 1074
    bone metastases for, 1724
    for carcinosarcoma, 1355
    on gonadal function, 1843
    imaging and target localization, 544

inoperable locally advanced NSCLC, 1019
in-transit and locoregional recurrent melanoma, 1420
for LMS, 1354
mesothelioma for
  after extrapleural pneumonectomy, 1038
  after pleurectomy/decortication (P/D) or unresectable disease, 1039
  alternative radiation therapy approaches, 1039
  summary recommendations on, 1039
operable NSCLC, 1018
pregnancy outcomes, 1846
small-cell lung carcinoma (SCLC), 1025
radical cystectomy, invasive bladder cancer, 1195
radical prostatectomy, 1224
radioembolization, 1424
  with yttrium-90, 524–525
radiofrequency ablation (RFA), 976, 1717
radioisotopes, 1727
radiosensitization, 547
radiotherapy
  cancer nanotechnology, 829
  invasive bladder cancer, 1195–1196
  recurrent endometrial cancer treatment, 1306
  related cardiac problems, 1885
  SVC syndrome, 1892
Raf and cancer, 155
RAI therapy, 955
random forests, 499
randomized phase II design analysis strategy, *286*
randomized trial, 395
RAS, 67, 230
  and cancer, 155
  proteins, 154–155
  signaling downstream, 155
rasburicase, 1889
RAS-MAPK signal transduction pathway, 1192
ras mutations, 781
Ras-Raf-mitogen activated protein kinase (MAPK) pathway, 155
RB1 gene analysis, 75–77
real-time pharmacokinetics and patient safety, 645
receptor occupancy (RO), of surface glycoprotein target, 645
receptor Tyr kinases (RTKs)
  families of, 151, *152*
  intracellular effectors of, 154, *154*
recessive cancer predisposition syndromes, 85
recombinant DNA, 21
recombinant *S. cerevisiae*–brachyury vaccine, 786
rectal cancer. *see also* colorectal cancer (CRC)
  adjuvant chemotherapy and radiation, 1162
  indication, 1161
  neoadjuvant chemotherapy and radiation, 1161
  short-course radiation, 1161
  total neoadjuvant therapy, 1161
  watch and wait nonoperative management, 1162
recurrent epithelial cancer treatment
  chemotherapy, 1324
  hormonal therapy, 1326
  immunotherapy, 1326
  palliative radiotherapy, 1326
  PARP-inhibitors, 1326
  platinum-resistant disease, 1325–1326
  platinum-sensitive disease, 1324
  targeted therapies, 1324–1325, 1326
red cell hypoplasia, 1050
red meats, 436–437
Reduction by Dutasteride of Prostate Cancer Events (REDUCE) study, 462
Reed–Sternberg (RS) cells, 851
refractory emesis, 1675
regional lymph nodes, management of, 1417–1419
regularized regression methods, 499
regulated cell death (RCD) pathways, 733
regulatory challenges, in precision oncology, 626
reirradiation, 1726
renal ablation, 526–527

renal artery embolization, for renal cell carcinoma, 526
renal cancer profile, CUP patients, 1653–1654
renal cell carcinoma (RCC), 139, 234–235, 1181–1188
  clinical presentation, 1181
  CUP patients, 1653–1654
  epidemiology, 1181
  pathophysiology, 1181
  syndromes, 416
  treatment, 1182
  vaccine trials, 784
renal toxicity methotrexate, 673
renal tumors, 852, 853
renin production, 1859
replication by-pass mechanism, 334
replication cycle, 348
replicative senescence, 201
resectability, defined, 540
respiratory oncologic emergencies
  acute airway obstruction, 1893–1894
  massive hemoptysis, 1892–1893
  massive pleural effusion, 1893
  pneumothorax, 1894
  pulmonary embolism, 1894–1896
restriction endonucleases and recombinant DNA, 21
resuscitation of cancer patients, 1884
RET, 67
ret gene, 153
retinoblastoma (RB), 74
  autosomal dominant inheritance mode, 75
  deoxyribonucleic acid probes, 75
  pediatric oncology, principles of, 860
  RB1 gene analysis, 75–77
  syndrome, 1474
  TP53 gene analysis, 77–78
  "two-hit" hypothesis, 75
retinoblastoma protein (pRB), function of, 77, *78*
retinoic acid syndrome. *see* differentiation syndrome (DS)
retrievable IVC filters, prophylactic placement of, 529
retromolar trigone, 986
retroperitoneal hemorrhage, 1891
retroperitoneal sarcomas (RPS)
  chemoradiation approaches, 1497
  radiotherapy for, 1496
retrospective cohort study, 395
retroviral vectors, 817
  and gene therapy, 356–357
reverse S sign of golden, 1013
reverse transcription-polymerase chain reaction (RT-PCR), 30–31, 856
reversible posterior leukoencephalopathy syndrome (RPLS), 239
RF ablation, painful metastatic lesions, 528
rhabdomyomas, 1057
rhabdomyosarcoma (RMS), 939
  pediatric bone tumors, 857
rheumatologic irAEs, 1899
RHPS4, 204
ribonucleoprotein cellular reverse transcriptase, 201
Richter's syndrome, 1566
rituximab, 1566
RNA interference (RNAi), 38–39, 829
RNA sequencing (RNA-Seq), 497
RNA tumor viruses, 347–357
  classification, 347
  endogenous retroviruses, 356
  genomic structure, 348
  growth stimulation and two-step oncogenesis, 351–352
  HIV, 354–356
  insertional mutagenesis, 350–351
  mechanisms of oncogenesis, 349
  oncogene capture, 349–350
  overview, 347
  replication cycle, 348
  retroviral vectors and gene therapy, 356–357

structure, 347–348
transactivation, 352–354
viral genome and gene products, 348
robotic-assisted thoracic surgery (RATS) lung cancer, 1018
rolapitant, 1679
ROOT trial, 625
ROS-1, 69
  gene translocations, 510
Rothmund–Thomson syndrome, 1474
rucaparib, 501, 648

S

saccharin, 449
sacituzumab govitecan-hziy, 709
s-adenosyl-homocysteine (SAH), 668
sanger sequencing, 24–26, 1030
sarcomas, 136, 1058, 1179
  botryoides, 1272
  historical perspective, 1351
  vulvar area, 1269
sarcomatoid carcinomas, 1236
  of lung, 1008
sarcomatoid type, 1032
SBRT, 1020
Schistosoma mansoni-associated colorectal cancer, 384
Schistosomiasis japonica and CRC, 383
screening
  second primary cancers, 913
  strategies, 505
  test criteria, 506
screening programs, cancer diagnosis, 5
SDHx, 415
sebaceous adenoma, 1448
sebaceous carcinoma, 1446
secondary arrhythmia, 1885
secondary cytoreduction, 1324
secondary surgical cytoreduction, 1306
second-generation DHFR inhibitor. *see* pralatrexate
seizures and tumor-related epilepsy, 1696
selective internal radiation therapy (SIRT), 1424
selenium, 448
Selenium and Vitamin E Cancer Prevention Trial (SELECT), 455
self-expanding esophageal stent, *1814*
self-expanding metal stents (SEMS), 1813
self-fusion, 60
selinexor, 1625
selpercatinib (LOXO-292), 1024
seminomas
  chemotherapy, 1062
  malignant GCT, 1062
  radiation therapy, 1063
  residual mass, 1063
sentinel lymphadenectomy, 540
sentinel lymph node biopsy
  ASCO-SSO recommendations for, *1417*
  role of, 1417–1419
sentinel lymph node biopsy (SLNB), 1264–1265
SEPT9, 501
sequence-based gene expression profiling, 30
serotonin (5-HT3), 1673
  and metabolites, 972
  receptor antagonists, 1676
serum biomarkers, 515
serum CA125, 507
serum thyroid hormone-binding protein abnormalities, 1861
SETDB1, 1030
SETD2 tumor suppressor gene, 1030
sexual dysfunction, 1864
Sézary syndrome (SS), 1603–1608
  diagnosis, 1603
  hematopoietic stem cell transplant, 1608
  incidence and epidemiology, 1603
  pathogenesis and natural history, 1603
  prognostic factors and biomarkers, 1604

Sézary syndrome (SS) (continued)
  skin-directed therapies, 1605
  staging, 1604
  systemic biologic therapies, 1606
  systemic cytotoxic chemotherapy, 1607
  systemic therapy, 1606
  treatment, 1604
shelterin complex, 201
SHERLOCK, 40–41
SHIVA randomized trial, 622
short-read sequencing, 32
signaling pathways
  aberrantly deregulated in cancer, 156
  of receptor Tyr kinases (RTKs), 153–155
signal transducers, 56
signal transducers and activators of transcription (STATs), 156
signet ring cell, 1236
simple bone cyst, 1463–1464
single-agent activity, in uterine sarcomas, *1355*
single-agent chemotherapy, 1076
  stage I GTN treatment, 1346, *1346*
single-agent cytotoxic chemotherapy, for endometrial cancer, *1307*
single binary biomarker, phase III designs with
  prospective–retrospective designs, 289
  run-in designs, 290
  stratification designs, 288
  targeted (enrichment) designs, 288, *289*
single-cell sequencing (scRNA seq), 35
single metastatic lesion treatment, 1654
single nucleotide polymorphism (SNP)
  arrays, 128
  microarrays, 397
sinonasal undifferentiated carcinoma (SNUC), 993
sinusoidal obstruction syndrome (SOS), 839, 1822–1823
sinusoidal occlusion syndrome (SOS), 1902
sipuleucel-T vaccine, 783
sirolimus, 837
SIR-Spheres, 522
skeletal complications, 1715–1727
  corticosteroid-induced osteopenia, 1724
  evaluation of, 1715
  hypercalcemia of malignancy, 1724
  intramedullary nailing, 1718
  joint arthroplasty, 1719
  medical management of, 1721
  megaprostheses, 1719
  options for treatment, 1717
  periacetabular lesions, treatment of, 1720
  plate and screw fixation, 1718
  principles of pathologic fracture, 1717
  radiation therapy for, 1724
  resection without reconstruction, 1720
  solitary lesions of bone, 1715
  spine lesions, 1720
  treatment of painful metastases and impending fractures, 1720
  tumor-induced osteomalacia (TIO), 1724
skeletal-related events (SREs), *1716*
skin cancers, 1437–1448
  epidemiology of, 333–334
  frequency and age of onset, 333
  metastatic tumors, 1448
  sunlight spectrum and wavelengths responsible for, 333
  tumors arising from appendages, 1446
  tumors arising from dermis, 1445
  tumors arising from epidermis, 1437
  ultraviolet radiation, 1437
skin carcinogenesis, genetic factors, 334–335
skin toxicity, methotrexate, 674
SLC43A3, 207
small-cell lung carcinoma (SCLC), 1009
  prophylactic cranial irradiation, 1026
  radiation therapy, 1025
  surgery, 1025
  systemic therapy, 1026–1027
small cell undifferentiated bladder cancer, 1198
small interfering RNA (siRNA), 829
small intestinal NETS (Si-NETS), 971
small-molecule inhibitors, 205–206
small molecule oral kinase inhibitors (SMOKIs), 1488
smoking, 1124
smoldering multiple myeloma, 1630
Society for Integrative Oncology (SIO), 596
sodium dodecyl sulfate–polyacrylamide gel electrophoresis (SDS–PAGE), 37
soft palate and pharyngeal wall, 988
soft tissue sarcomas, 238, 1477–1498
  biopsy, 1480–1481
  clinical presentation, 1479
  conventional prognostic factors, 1482–1483
  etiology, 1477–1478
  functional outcome and morbidity of treatment, 1497
  gastrointestinal stromal tumors, 1495–1496
  histopathologic classification
    histologic grade, 1479–1480
    methods of classification, 1479
  imaging, 1480
  immunotherapy for, 1498
  localized primary disease of the extremities, treatment of
    radiotherapy, 1485–1488
    surgery, 1483–1485
    systemic therapy, 1488–1490
  locally advanced disease, treatment of, 1491
  management of local recurrence, 1494–1495
  metastatic disease, treatment of
    chemotherapy for, 1492–1494
    clinical problem, 1491
    resection of, 1492
  molecularly and pathologically based sarcoma management, 1498
  pediatric bone tumors, 857
  potential molecular prognostic factors, 1483
  retroperitoneal sarcomas
    chemoradiation approaches, 1497
    radiotherapy for, 1496
  screening, 1478
  sites of origin, 1478
  staging, 1481–1482
solar keratosis, 1437
solid tumors
  FDA approved targeted therapies, *616–617*
  gliomas, 139
  hematopoietic cell transplantation (HCT), 842
  indications for checkpoint inhibitors of, *618–619*
  non-small-cell lung cancer (NSCLC), 139
  NTRK-fusion-positive cancers, 141
  prostate cancer, 140
  renal cell carcinoma (RCC), 139
  sarcomas, 136
  testicular cancer, 139
soluble mesothelin-related peptides (SMRP), 1033
somatic alterations, annotation and curation of, 497
somatic cell genetic studies, tumorigenesis, 74
somatic mutations, 74
  in cancer genomes, 318
somatic single-nucleotide variants (SNVs), 102
somatic testing, paired tumor-normal samples, 496–497
somatostatin analogs, 976
somatostatinomas, 975
somatostatin receptors, 973
somatostatin receptor scintigraphy (SRS), 974
sorafenib, 1702, 1703, 1843
sotorasib, 1025
southern blotting, 23–24
soy products, 448
special populations, cancer survivors in, 917
spectral karyotyping (SKY), 103
sperm cryopreservation, 1844
sphere formation assay, 178–179
spinal cord compression, 1896–1897
spinal cord dysfunction (SCD), 586
spinal cord toxicity, 1696
spinal metastases
  clinical findings and diagnosis, 1684
  pathophysiology of, 1684
  treatment, 1685
spine lesions, 1720
spleen tyrosine kinase (SYK), 728
splenic rupture, 1890–1891
sporadic colorectal cancer, 456
sputum cytology, lung cancer, 1016
squamous carcinoma, 1650
  involving cervical/supraclavicular lymph nodes, 1654
  involving inguinal lymph nodes, 1654
  of unknown primary site, 1648
squamous cell carcinoma (SCC), 1239, 1277, 1440
  chest wall invasion and cavitation in, 1014, *1014*
  histopathologic and molecular changes, 1005, *1006*
  incidence, 1704
  lung, 1007
  with vemurafenib therapy, *1704*
squamous cell carcinoma of the anal canal (SCCA), 1169–1179
  brachytherapy, 1175
  diagnosis of, 1171
  epidemiology, 1169
  gross anatomy, 1169
  HIV infection, 1170
  HPV infection, 1169
  intensity-modulated radiation therapy, 1175
  molecular characterization of, 1170
  natural history of, 1171
  pathology of, 1170
  prognostic factors, 1171
  response evaluation, 1175
  staging of, 1171
  treatment, 1172–1175
squamous cell carcinomas, 1263
  vulvar area, treatment of, *1267*
squamous cell esophageal cancer, 444
S sign of Golden, 1013
stage IV GTN management
  EMAEP regimen, 1346–*1347*
  radiation therapy, 1347
  surgery, 1347
stage IV melanoma, surgical metastasectomy for, 1420–1421
staging, endometrial cancer, 1302, *1303*
STAT3, 384
status epilepticus, 1897–1898
stent placement, for venous stenosis, 529
Stevens–Johnson Syndrome (SJS), 1701
Stewart–Treves syndrome, 1446
stimulant laxatives, 1823
stimulatory immune receptors
  4-1BB (CD137), 805
  CD27, 806
  CD40, 805
  glucocorticoid-induced TNFR (GITR), 805
  inducible T cell costimulator (ICOS), 805
  OX-40, 805
stomach cancer (noncardia), 445
streptozocin, 1865
stress management, 595
stromal-derived factor-1 (SDF-1), 833
Strongyloides stercoralis, 387, 1876
structural variants (SVs), 102
Study of Tamoxifen and Raloxifene (STAR), 459
succinate dehydrogenase (SDH), 218
succinate dehydrogenase-deficient renal cancer, 417
sudden cardiopulmonary arrest, 1883–1884
sugar, 449
suicide gene therapy (Ad-hTR-NTR), 205
suicide risk, 544
sunitinib, 977, 1702, 1703
sunlight induced photoproducts, in DNA, 333–334

superficial spreading melanoma, 1415
superior vena cava (SVC) syndrome, 1011
  cause of, 1891
  chemotherapy, 1892
  contrast-enhanced spiral CT, 1892
  obstruction of, 1891
  radiotherapy, 1892
  symptoms, 529, 1891
SuperSigs, 498
supervised mutational signatures, 498
supportive care, for high-dose methotrexate treatment, 673
supportive expressive group therapy, 595
suppressor of mothers against decapentaplegic (SMAD) transcription factors, 156
supraventricular tachycardia (SVT), 1885, 1887
surgery
  invasive bladder cancer, 1195
  operable NSCLC, 1017–1018
  recurrent endometrial cancer treatment, 1306
  small-cell lung carcinoma (SCLC), 1025
surgical extirpation, 535
surgical oncologists, role of, 533–534
surgical oncology
  advances in, 532, 533
  emergency surgery, 541
  future of, 541–542
  history of, 532–533
  innovations, 532
  in modern era, 533–535
  multidisciplinary management, 534–535
  palliative surgery, 541
  principles of, 531–542
  pseudoencapsulation approach, 540
  surgical management components, cancer patients
    biopsy and diagnosis, 535
    cancer operations, types of, 539–541
    operative considerations, 539
    preoperative preparation, 538–539
    prevention, 535
    quality control, 541
    tumor spread patterns, 537–538
surgical resection, 531
  principles of, 531
surveillance
  for high-risk melanoma patients, 1422–1423
  for recurrence, survivorship, 913
survivorship, 449–451, 911–917
  awareness of, 911
  care
    clinical practice guidelines for, 916, 916
    components of, 913
    coordination of, 915–916
    delivery models, 914–915
    implementation of, 914–915
    plan and treatment, 915
    self-management approach, 914
  definition, 912
  evolution of concept, 912
  financial impact, 917
  health care quality evaluation, 916–917
  management guidelines, 914
  professional education, resources for, 916
  screening for second primary cancers, 913–914
  significance, 912–913
  in special populations, 917
  surveillance for recurrence, 913
SV40, 77
Sweet's syndrome, 1703
symptom management, 568
synaptic-like microvesicles (SLMV), 972
synaptophysin (p38), 972
syndrome of inappropriate antidiuretic hormone (SIADH), 1858–1859
synthetic lethality, 735
systemic chemotherapy, mesothelioma for
  first-line immunotherapy for, 1040

intrapleural strategies, 1040
  maintenance therapy for, 1040
  newer neoadjuvant or adjuvant systemic therapy, 1039
  nivolumab (anti-PD-1), 1041
  salvage chemotherapy for, 1040
  salvage immunotherapies, 1041
  for unresectable, 1040
systemic therapy
  in-transit and locoregional recurrent melanoma, 1420
  pregnancy outcomes, 1845–1846
  related cardiac problems, 1885
  small-cell lung carcinoma (SCLC), 1026–1027
systems biology, 261–268
  extrinsic, 261
  intrinsic, 261
systems science, 1908

T

tacrolimus, 1864
Tai Chi/Qigong effects, 595–596
talimogene laherparepvec (TVEC), 1420
  for melanoma treatment, 783
tamoxifen, 493, 664, 1299–1300, 1842, 1845
  recurrent endometrial cancer treatment, 1308
Targeted Agent and Profiling Utilization Registry (TAPUR) study, 624
targeted cancer therapeutics
  BCR-ABL tyrosine kinase inhibitors, 1702
  BRAF inhibitors, 1703–1704
  epidermal growth factor receptor inhibitors, 1701–1702
  MEK inhibitors, 1704
  mTOR inhibitors, 1703
  multikinase inhibitors, 1702–1703
targeted delivery of TOP1 inhibitors, 708
targeted gene panels, 128, 495
targeted therapy, 1052
  on gonadal function
    BCR-ABL tyrosine kinase inhibitors, 1843
    BRAF kinase inhibitors, 1843
    epidermal growth factor receptor TKIs, 1843
    immunotherapy, effects of, 1844
    MEK inhibitors, 1843
    monoclonal antibodies, effects of, 1844
    mTOR kinase inhibitors, 1844
    vascular endothelial growth factor TKIs, 1843
  nephrotoxicity, 1751
  primary thyroid dysfunction, 1862
  recurrent endometrial cancer treatment, 1308
taxanes, 1693
  adverse events, 723
  clinical pharmacology and indications, 721
  drug interactions, 723
  mechanism of action, 718
TBNA biopsy, 1017
T cell activation, 799
T-cell acute lymphoblastic leukemia, 135
T-cell Ig and mucin-domain-containing-3 (TIM-3), 804
T cell immunoreceptor with Ig and ITIM domains (TIGIT), 804
T cell immunotherapy of cancer, 789–797
  bone marrow transplantation and the GvL effect, 789
  CAR-modified immune effector cell strategies, 794–795
  CAR-modified T cells, 792–794
  next-generation tumor-targeted T cells, 795–796
  TCR-modified T cells, 791–792
  tumor-infiltrating lymphocytes, 791
  virus-specific T cells, 789–791
T-cell lymphomas, HCT, 841
T cell-mediated anti-tumor response, 799
TCR-modified T cells, 791–792
tea, 449
tegaserod, 1823
telehealth, 563
telemedicine, 563

teletherapy, 543
telomelysin (OBP-301), 205
telomerase
  for cancer therapy
    antisense oligonucleotides, 205–206
    gene therapy, 205
    G-quadruplex stabilizers, 204–205
    immunotherapy, 205
    small-molecule inhibitors, 205–206
  inhibitors, challenges for, 206–207
  mutant hTERC and wild type hTERC-targeted siRNA overexpression, 207
  telomere uncapping approach, 207–208
telomerase reverse transcriptase (TERT), 201, 202, 1030
telomere dysfunction induced foci (TIF) assay, 201
telomere looping, 201
telomere position effect over long distances (TPE-OLD), 201
telomeres (TTAGGG)$_n$
  length, 201
  senescence and crisis, 201
  techniques used, 202
telomere uncapping approach, 207
telomeric repeat-containing RNA (TERRA), 201
temozolomide, 694, 696, 1821
teniposide, 712
teratogenic effects, methotrexate, 674
terminal phase, 573
testicular cancer, 139, 418
testicular sperm extraction, 1844
tetrahydrocannabinol (THC), 573
The Cancer Genome Atlas (TCGA), 255
  endometrial cancer, 1301
The Therapeutically Applicable Research to Generate Effective Treatments (TARGET), 255
therapeutic cancer vaccines, 781
therapeutic drug monitoring (TDM), 664
therapy-related myeloid neoplasms (t MN), 132
therapy-related secondary AML (t-AML), 712
TheraSphere microspheres, 522
theta-mediated end joining (TMEJ), 547
6-thio-2' deoxyguanosine (6-thio-dG), 207, 208
6-thioguanine (6-TG), 686, 687
thiopurine S-methyltransferase (TPMT), 664
thipurines, 664
thoracic spine, 1683
thoracoscopy, 1017
three-dimensional conformal radiotherapy (3D-CRT), 1019
thrombocytopenia 5, 420
thromboembolic disease, 1793
thrombopoietin, 1859
thrombospondin-1, 229
thymic carcinomas, 1046
thymic lymphomas, 1048
thymic tumors, 1043–1054
  anatomy, 1044
  embryology, 1044
  epidemiology, 1043
  gene signatures, 1048
  incidence, 1043
  radiotherapy, 1051
  surgery, 1051
  systemic therapy, 1051
thymidine antimetabolites, 682–683
thymidylate synthase variants, 664
thymomas
  clinical features of, 1050
  pathology, 1044
  vs. thymic carcinomas, 1048
  World Health Organization classification, 1045
thyroid cancer, 870–871
thyroid carcinoma profile, CUP patients, 1654
thyroidectomy, primary thyroid dysfunction, 1862–1863
thyroid neoplasms, 949–959
  diagnostic evaluation, 952

thyroid neoplasms (*continued*)
  epidemiology, 949
  external beam radiation therapy, 956
  genomics of, 951
  history, 949
  imaging, 952
  incidence, 949
  isolated or limited recurrence locations, 957
  long-term remission, 957
  monitoring, 956
  pathology, 950
  postsurgical assessment of, 954
  progressive multi-location/distant disease, 958
  RAI therapy, 955
  reoperation, 956
  residual and recurrent, 957
  risk factors for, 950
  surgery and active surveillance, 953
  TSH suppression therapy, 955
thyrotoxicosis, 1863
TIGIT. *see* T cell immunoreceptor with Ig and ITIM domains (TIGIT)
TIM-3. *see* T-cell Ig and mucin-domain-containing-3 (TIM-3)
tipiracil
  clinical activity, 683
  clinical pharmacology, 683
  mechanism of action, 682
  metabolism, 682
  toxicities, 683
tissue acquisition, 1129
tissue banking informatics, 296–297
tissue homeostasis, 73
tissue-lineage antigens, 781
tissue-specific biomarkers, 514
TLS. *see* tumor lysis syndrome (TLS)
TMB, 498
T1 melanomas, 1417, *1418*
TMPyP4, 204
TNFRSF7, 806
toll-like receptor 7 (TLR7), 1439
tongue, 985–986
  base, 988
tonsil, 987–988
TOP2 inhibitors, 709–712
topoisomerase biology, 701
topoisomerase I inhibitors, 705–709
topotecan, 705–706
total body irradiation (TBI), 834
total body radiotherapy-based regimens, 646
toxic epidermal necrolysis (TEN), 1701
toxic erythema of chemotherapy, 1701
toxicities
  capecitabine, 682
  2-Chlorodeoxyadenosine, 690
  clofarabine, 690
  cytosine arabinoside (ara-C), 684
  decitabine, 685
  5-Fluorodeoxyuridine, 681
  5-Fluorouracil (5-FU), 681
  gemcitabine, 685
  6-mercaptopurine, 686
  nelarabine, 688
  6-thioguanine, 686
  trifluridine, 683
Toxoplasma gondii, 387
toxoplasmosis, 1876
TP53 gene analysis, 77–78
TP53 tumor suppressor gene, molecular analysis of, 318
trabectedin, 694, 696
traditional Chinese medicine (TCM), 596
transarterial chemoembolization (TACE), 1103, 1424
transcatheter arterial hepatic chemoembolization, 522
transcervical mediastinoscopy, 1017
transcription-coupled repair (TCR), 334
transcription factor E3 (TFE3) gene, 853
transcription factors, 56

transcriptomic sequencing, 31–35
transfection assay, 53
transforming growth factor-α (TGFα) signaling, 156
transfusion-related infectious diseases
  bacterial sepsis, 1735
  Creutzfeldt–Jakob disease, 1736
  cytomegalovirus, 1734
  hepatitis B, 1734
  hepatitis C, 1734
  human immunodeficiency virus, 1735
  human T-cell lymphotropic virus type 1, 1735
  parasitic diseases, 1735
  pathogen inactivation in blood products, 1735
  West Nile virus (WNV), 1735
  Zika virus (ZIKV), 1735
trans-jugular intrahepatic portosystemic stent-shunt (TIPS), 1823
translesion synthesis (TLS), 732
  DNA polymerases, 315
transport-mediated multiple drug resistance (MDR), 733
transthoracic percutaneous needle aspiration biopsy (TPNAB), 1016
transvaginal sonography (TVS), 507
trastuzumab, 157, 509
trastuzumab emtansine (T-DM1), 1821
trastuzumab therapy
  stage IV HER2/neu+ breast cancer, 784
traveling electrons, 213–214
treatment-related mortality (TRM), 834
tremelimumab, 803
tremelimumab (anti-CTLA-4), 1041
trichilemmoma, 1447
trichothiodystrophy (TTD), 336
Trichomonas vaginalis, 387
Trichuris suis, 387
trifluridine
  clinical activity, 683
  clinical pharmacology, 683
  mechanism of action, 682
  metabolism, 682
  toxicities, 683
Trypanosoma cruzi, 387
TSH-secreting pituitary adenomas, 946
TSH suppression therapy, 955
tuberous sclerosis (TS), 979
tuberous sclerosis complex (TSC), 417–418
tubulin binders, 648
tumor agnostic approach, 613
tumor agnostic therapies, 512
tumor angiogenesis, 223–243
  antiangiogenic therapy, 233–240
  biology, 224–225
  historic background, 224
  nonangiogenic tumors, 223–224
  overview, 223
  preclinical and clinical studies of antiangiogenic therapy, 240–243
  regulators of, 225–231
  therapeutic approaches to targeting tumor vasculature, 231–233
tumor-associated antigens (TAAs), 781
  specific immunotherapy, 205
tumor burden, chemotherapy dose effects, 643–644
tumor cells, aberrations affecting growth factor receptors, 153
tumor development, genetic basis for, 73–74
tumor heterogeneity, 734
tumor hypoxia, chemotherapy dose effects, 644
tumorigenesis, somatic cell genetic studies of, 74
tumorigenicity, 74
tumor-induced hypoglycemia, 1858
tumor-induced osteomalacia (TIO), 1724, 1859
tumor-infiltrating lymphocyte (TIL), 791
  in melanoma, 1433
tumor initiation, 305
tumor lysis syndrome (TLS), 1888–1889

tumor markers, 1687
tumor microenvironments (TMEs), 13–14, 265, 733
tumor mutational burden (TMB), 512
tumor necrosis factor-alpha (TNF-α), 1030
tumor necrosis factor receptor superfamily (TNFRSF), 800
tumor occlusion of essential conduit, 4
tumor progression, cancer plasticity in, 785
tumor-promoting immune cell infiltration, 12
tumor-related cardiac problems, 1885
tumor-specific antigens, 781
tumor-specific chromosomal abnormalities, CUP diagnosis, 1651
tumor-specific replication-competent adenoviral (hTERTp-TRAD) gene therapy approach, 205
tumor suppressor genes (TSGs), 8, 73–86, 1126
  adenomatous polyposis coli (*see* adenomatous polyposis coli (APC))
  CDKN2A locus, 79–80
  and hereditary cancers, 85, *86*
  NF1 and 2 genes, 83–84
  required for genetic stability maintenance, 84
  retinoblastoma (*see* retinoblastoma)
tumor suppressor miRNAs, 310
tumstatin, 230
twenty-first century healthcare, 1907–1913
  cancer medicine, 1912–1913
  integrating genomics and deep phenotyping in clinical practic, 1912
  multiscale biological systems, 1908–1909
  quantifying wellness and demystifying disease, 1907
  systems biology as an emerging paradigm, 1907–1908
  systems science in biomedicine, 1909–1912
"two-hit" hypothesis, 75
Tyr kinase inhibitors, 157–159
tyrosine kinase inhibitors (TKIs), 126, 732, 840, 1862

U
UGT1A1 variants, 664
UK Familial Ovarian Cancer Study (UKFOCCS), 1317
ulceration
  cancer presentation, 4
ultraviolet B (UVB) radiation, 1437
ultraviolet radiation carcinogenesis, 333–337
umbrella studies, 620
undifferentiated endometrial sarcoma (UES), 1351
unsupervised mutational signatures, 498
upper aerodigestive tract (UADT), 982
upper tract tumors
  chemotherapy, 1199
  radiotherapy, 1199
  surgical treatment, 1198–1199
upper urinary tract cancer, 418
uracil antimetabolites, 679–682
ureteral obstruction, 1747–1748
urethra cancer, 1239–1243
  diagnosis and staging, 1242
  epidemiology and risk factors, 1242
  female urethral carcinoma, 1242
  male urethral carcinoma, 1242
  neoadjuvant and adjuvant therapy, 1243
  surgical management, 1242
urinary bladder cancer, 446
urinary tract obstruction, 1747–1748
urine biomarkers, 515
urologic complications, 1747–1754
  cystitis, 1748–1749
  nephritis, 1749
  nephrotoxicity, 1749–1754
  urinary tract obstruction, 1747–1748
urothelial carcinoma (UC), 1191–1199. *see also* bladder cancer
  gene expression profiling, 1192
  molecular pathway alterations, *1193*
  noninvasive/invasive disease, 1191
urothelial tumorigenesis and progression model, *1192*
US cancer statistics, 392

uterine endometrial stromal tumors, 1352
uterine sarcomas, classification of, *1352*
uterine serous carcinoma (USC), 1300, *1301*
UVA, 333
    importance of, 337
UVB, 333
    importance of, 337
UVC, 333
uveal melanoma (UM), 935, 1423–1424
UV photoproducts
    mutagenicity of, 334–335
    recognition in DNA, 334
UV recall reaction, 1708

V

vaccines
    clinical trials, 782–785
    therapy, targets for, 781, *782*
    types of, 782
vagina
    clear cell adenocarcinoma of, 1271–1272
    invasive carcinomas of, 1270–1271
    melanomas, 1272
    premalignant vaginal disease, 1269–1270
vaginal carcinoma
    defined, 1269
    FIGO staging classification for, *1270*
    symptom of, 1269
    treatment scheme for, *1271*
    tumors in young females, 1272
vaginal sarcomas, 1357
valganciclovir, 1812
vancomycin, 1815
    in neutropenic fever, 1901
vandetanib, 979
vanillylmandelic acid (VMA), 854
variant annotation, 497
variant call format (VCF) file, 497
variant calling, 497
variant of uncertain significance (VUS), 497
varlilumab (CDX-1127), 806
vascular endothelial growth factor (VEGF)
    family, 226
    pathway inhibitors
        mechanisms of resistance to, 240–241
        potential biomarkers for, 241–243
    receptor, 1446
    signal transduction, 226–227
    therapy, 1751
    TKIs
        effects on gonadal function, 1843
vascular endothelial growth factor receptor (VEGFR) inhibitors, 1702
vascular sarcomas, 1471
vasoactive intestinal polypeptide (VIP)oma, 975
V-domain Ig suppressor of T cell activation (VISTA), 804, 1032

vemurafenib, 159
vena cava filter placement, 528–529
vena caval syndrome, 529
venetoclax, 1565, 1627
veno-occlusive disease (VOD), 839. *see* sinusoidal obstruction syndrome (SOS)
venous stenosis, stent placement for, 529
verrucous carcinoma, vulvar area, 1268
vertebral metastases, 1683
vesicants, 1706
Veterans Affairs Larynx, 991
VHL gene, 84
video-assisted thoracic surgery (VATS), lung cancer, 1018
video-assisted thoracoscopy (VATS), 1017
vinblastine, 726
vinca alkaloids, 1691
    adverse events, 726
    clinical pharmacology and indications, 726
    drug interactions, 726
    mechanism of action, 725
vincristine, 726
vindesine, 726
vinflunine, 726
vinorelbine, 726
viral genome and gene products, 348
viral hepatitis (HBV and HCV), 1095–1096
viral infections, 1874–1876
viral proteins, 362–363
Viridans group streptococci (VGS), 1871
virotherapy or viral oncolysis, 820
virus-specific T cells, 789–791
VISTA. *see* V-domain Ig suppressor of T cell activation (VISTA)
Vitamin A, 447
Vitamin C, 447
Vitamin D, 447
Vitamin E, 447
vitiligo, 1707
    chemotherapeutic agents associated with, *1707*
volumetric-modulated arc therapy (VMAT), 1019
vomiting, GI complications, 1824
von Hippel–Lindau (VHL)
    diffuse neuroendocrine system (DES), 979
    and neurofibromatosis type 1, 415–416
    syndrome, 83–84, 416
Von Recklinghausen's disease, 83
v-sis oncogene of simian sarcoma virus, 151
vulvar cancer
    advanced tumor, 1267
    clinical stage IA treatment, 1265
    clinical stage I/II treatment, 1265–1269
    incidence and epidemiology, 1261
    intraepithelial neoplasias, 1261–1263
    invasive vulvar carcinomas, 1263
    Paget disease, 1263

    recurrences, 1267
    risk factors, 1261
    survival rate, *1268*
    TNM classification and staging of, *1264*
vulvar dysplasias, classifications of, *1262*
vulvar intraepithelial neoplasias (VIN), 1261–1263
vulvar sarcomas, 1357
VZV infection, 1876

W

Warburg effect, 214–216, 1032
wedge resection, lung cancer, 1018
weight loss, cancer presentation, 4
Werner syndrome, 978, 1474
West Nile virus (WNV), 1735
whole exome sequencing (WES), 496
    limitations of, 497
whole-genome sequencing (WGS), 128, 496
whole patient assessment, 567
wild-type human telomerase RNA (WT-hTERC), 207
Wilms tumor (WT), 852
    gene, 82–83
Wilms tumor 1 (*WT1*) gene, 83
WINTHER genomic/transcriptomic trial, 622–624
WNT/APC pathway, 81
Wnt signaling, 182–183
    aberrant activation of, 156
women
    with axillary lymph node metastases, treatment, 1653
    cytotoxic chemotherapy effect, on gonadal function, 1841–1843
    gonadal function
        cytotoxic chemotherapy effect on, 1841–1843
        radiation therapy effect on, 1843
    gonadal function assessment, 1839–1840
    infertility protective measures, 1844–1845
    peritoneal carcinomatosis treatment, 1652–1653

X

xanthine oxidase inhibitor, 1888
xeroderma pigmentosum, 85
xeroderma pigmentosum (XP), 335, 337
xerostomia, 1830

Y

yellow nail syndrome (YNS), 1705
yoga, 595
yttrium-90 (^{90}Y) microspheres, 522

Z

zika virus (ZIKV), 1735
zinc supplement, soral mucositis pevention, 1824
Zollinger–Ellison syndrome (ZES), 975